KAPLAN & SADOCK'S
SYNOPSIS OF PSYCHIATRY

TWELFTH EDITION

Editorial Assistant

Arya Shah, M.D.

Resident in Psychiatry
Brigham and Women's Hospital/Harvard Medical School Program
Boston, Massachusetts

Contributing Editors

Caroly S. Pataki, M.D.

Clinical Professor of Psychiatry and the Biobehavioral Sciences, Keck School
of Medicine at the University of Southern California;
Director, Child and Adolescent Psychiatry Residency Training Program,
University of Southern California, Los Angeles, California

Norman Sussman, M.D.

Professor of Psychiatry, New York University School of Medicine;
Director, Treatment Resistant Depression Program and Co-director, Continuing Education
in Psychiatry, Department of Psychiatry;
Attending Psychiatrist, Tisch Hospital, New York, New York

KAPLAN & SADOCK'S
SYNOPSIS OF PSYCHIATRY

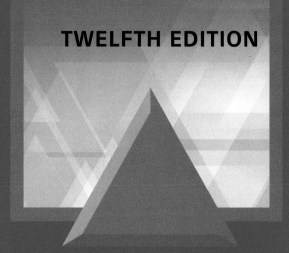

TWELFTH EDITION

EDITORS

Robert Joseph Boland, M.D.

Vice-Chair for Education
Department of Psychiatry
Brigham and Women's Hospital
Associate Professor
Harvard Medical School
Boston, Massachusetts

Marcia L. Verduin, M.D.

Associate Dean for Students
Professor of Psychiatry
Department of Medical Education
Department of Clinical Sciences
University of Central Florida College of Medicine
Orlando, Florida

CONSULTING EDITOR

Pedro Ruiz, M.D.

Clinical Professor
Menninger Department of Psychiatry and
Behavioral Sciences
Baylor College of Medicine

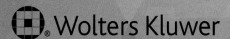

Philadelphia • Baltimore • New York • London
Buenos Aires • Hong Kong • Sydney • Tokyo

Not authorized for sale in United States, Canada, Australia, New Zealand, Puerto Rico, and U.S. Virgin Islands

Acquisitions Editor: Chris Teja
Development Editor: Ariel S. Winter
Editorial Coordinator: Ashley Pfeiffer
Editorial Assistant: Maribeth Wood
Marketing Manager: Kirsten Watrud
Production Project Manager: Bridgett Dougherty
Design Coordinator: Stephen Druding
Manufacturing Coordinator: Beth Welsh
Prepress Vendor: Aptara, Inc.

12th edition

9 8 7 6 5 4 3 2 1

Printed in China

Library of Congress Cataloging-in-Publication Data

Names: Boland, Robert Joseph, editor. | Verduin, Marcia L., editor. | Ruiz,
    Pedro, 1936- editor. | Shah, Arya, editor. | Sadock, Benjamin J., 1933-
    Kaplan & Sadock's synopsis of psychiatry.
Title: Kaplan & Sadock's synopsis of psychiatry / editors, Robert Joseph
    Boland, Marcia L. Verduin; consulting editor, Pedro Ruiz; editorial
    assistant, Arya Shah.
Other titles: Kaplan and Sadock's synopsis of psychiatry
Description: Twelfth edition. | Philadelphia : Wolters Kluwer, 2022. |
    Preceded by Kaplan & Sadock's synopsis of psychiatry / Benjamin James
    Sadock, Virginia Alcott Sadock, Pedro Ruiz. Eleventh edition. 2015. |
    Includes bibliographical references and index.
Identifiers: LCCN 2020056686 | ISBN 9781975145569 (paperback)
Subjects: MESH: Mental Disorders
Classification: LCC RC454 | NLM WM 140 | DDC 616.89–dc23
LC record available at https://lccn.loc.gov/2020056686

Preface

"No one can replace him, Sir; I am only his successor."

Thomas Jefferson would routinely say this when asked if he was replacing Benjamin Franklin as Minister to France. Although not quite the same historical scale, this aptly describes our feelings about taking over as editors for *Kaplan & Sadock's Synopsis of Psychiatry*.

The Synopsis was one of the first psychiatry books we encountered and was our "Bible" during our respective training years. As we became educators, it was the book that we recommended to our students and residents. In our roles as editors of the Psychiatry Resident-In-Training Examination®, administered by the American College of Psychiatrists to virtually all trainees in the United States, the *Synopsis* was the book we would most often turn to when deciding whether a given question on the test was within the accepted body of knowledge for all psychiatrists.

As we approach the book again from this new perspective, the time we have spent editing and revising the book has only given renewed respect for this fantastic work. The previous authors have done an incredible job of creating a book that is comprehensive, approachable, and frankly enjoyable to read.

Much of our approach to this new edition has been careful, and we have preserved much of the previous editions, often verbatim. Our edits have been either to incorporate discoveries in our rapidly growing field or to reorganize the book in a way we think practical for a new generation of psychiatrists. We have emphasized the clinical material upfront. The underlying science and theory of the field have been moved later in the book. This reorganization does not reflect any value or order of importance; it is meant to be practical: one can imagine a busy trainee grabbing the book during the day to answer a crucial question about the diagnosis or management of a patient, and later that day, with, hopefully, more time for reflection, sitting down and reading further to understand their patient more deeply.

Whenever we could, we grouped disorders syndromally. Thus, we first discuss the various depressive disorders' phenomenology as a group before discussing diagnosis and, eventually, treatment. This approach was a strategic choice as much modern research no longer groups patients by clinical diagnoses, and many incorporate larger groupings: depressed patients or psychotic patients, for example. That said, in deference to Emerson, we did not let our desire for organization and consistency become so rigid as to be foolish, and in cases where the disorders within a chapter are fundamentally different, we did create separate sections for each.

We realize that some may worry that our "practical" approach might take away some of the artistry of this book. Indeed, we no longer include many paintings, creative photos, and other artistic touches that were a defining part of previous volumes. These are personal choices reflecting on our personal approaches. We certainly do not wish to wring out all of the personality from the book, and we hope that our preservation of much of the prose, case histories, and historical references keep some of what made the previous volumes special.

The other philosophy we bring to this work is that mental health is part of physical health, and one cannot discuss psychiatric disease except within the context of all medicines. Even the term "mind—body" seems obsolete and implying a divide that does not exist. We were frequently reminded of this as we edited during the COVID-19 pandemic and witnessed in our patients, faculty, and trainees how a simple virus can wreak such havoc on the psyche.

HISTORY

This textbook evolved as a condensation of the *Comprehensive Textbook of Psychiatry*. That book is an extensive, two-volume work with many contributions by experts in the field. It helps those who require an exhaustive, detailed, and encyclopedic survey of the entire field. That work aims at all levels of expertise in the field who desire an up-to-date work that is as comprehensive as possible. This textbook is aimed more at the trainee, who needs a brief and more condensed statement of the field of psychiatry. Although, in essence, this book derives from the *Comprehensive Textbook of Psychiatry*, different purposes for each work result in a divergence. However, although we have reworked some sections of this book and written new content, we still owe an outstanding debt of gratitude to the more than 2,000 contributors to the current and previous editions of the *Comprehensive Textbook of Psychiatry*, all of whom have allowed us to synopsize their work. At the same time, we must accept responsibility for the modifications and changes in the new work.

COMPREHENSIVE TEACHING SYSTEM

This textbook forms one part of a comprehensive system developed to facilitate the teaching of psychiatry and the behavioral sciences. At the head of the system is the *Comprehensive Textbook of Psychiatry*, which is global in depth and scope; it is designed for and used by psychiatrists, behavioral scientists, and all workers in the mental health field. *Synopsis of Psychiatry* is a briefer, highly modified, and current version useful for medical students, psychiatric residents, practicing psychiatrists, and mental health professionals. Two special editions derived from the *Synopsis*, *Concise Textbook of Clinical Psychiatry* and *Concise Textbook of Child and Adolescent Psychiatry*, contain descriptions of all psychiatric disorders, including their diagnosis and treatment in adults and children, respectively. They will be useful for clinical clerks and psychiatric residents who need a succinct overview of the management of clinical problems. Another part of the system, *Study Guide and Self-Examination Review of Psychiatry*, consists of multiple-choice questions and answers; it is designed for students of psychiatry and for clinical psychiatrists who require a review of the behavioral sciences and general psychiatry in preparation for a variety of examinations. The questions are consistent with the format used by most standardized examinations. Other parts of the system are the various editions of the pocket handbooks: *Pocket Handbook of Clinical Psychiatry, Pocket Handbook of Psychiatric Drug Treatment, Pocket Handbook of Emergency Psychiatric Medicine,* and *Pocket Handbook of Primary Care Psychiatry.* Those books cover the diagnosis and treatment of psychiatric disorders, psychopharmacology, psychiatric emergencies, and primary care psychiatry, respectively, and are designed and written to be carried by clinical clerks and practicing physicians, whatever their specialty, for a quick reference. Finally, *Comprehensive Glossary of Psychiatry and Psychology* provides written definitions for psychiatrists and other physicians, psychologists, students, other mental health professionals, and the public. Together, these books create multiple approaches to the teaching, study, and learning of psychiatry.

CLASSIFICATION OF DISORDERS

DSM-5

The American Psychiatric Association published the fifth edition of the *American Psychiatric Association's Diagnostic and Statistical Manual of Mental Disorders* in 2013; it is commonly called the DSM-5. It contains the official nomenclature used by psychiatrists and other mental health professionals in the United States, and many other countries also use the manual. The psychiatric disorders discussed in the textbook are consistent with and follow that nosology. We have chosen not to directly reproduce the DSM-5 criteria in either prose or table form. We expect that most psychiatrists and trainees already have access to the DSM-5; if not, we do highly recommend it. We include some tables outlining the primary symptoms, time courses, and other criteria associated with the major diagnoses to aid the reader with diagnostic reasoning.

ICD-10

Readers also should be aware of a parallel classification system developed by the World Health Organization (WHO) called the *International Statistical Classification of Diseases and Related Health Problems* (ICD-10). There are textual differences between DSM and ICD, but according to treaties between the United States and the WHO, the diagnostic code numbers are identical to ensure uniform national and international psychiatric statistics. ICD diagnoses and numerical codes are accepted by Medicare, Medicaid, and private insurance companies for reimbursement purposes. ICD-10 is a comprehensive list of all medical diagnoses, not just psychiatric. It tends to be descriptive and allows more judgment than the DSM-5, which contains fixed numbers of criteria. ICD-10 is also older than DSM-5 and contains diagnoses no longer included in the newer manual. ICD-11 is currently available in draft form and is online at the WHO's website. The ICD-11 is more aligned with DSM-5. The WHO plans for this new edition of the ICD to go into effect in 2022. As much of the world still uses ICD-10 (including the United States, especially for billing purposes), we include it in our tables devoted to diagnostic reading. The reader will note the many similarities between DSM-5 and ICD-10 in those tables, as well as some interesting differences.

CASE HISTORIES

Case histories are an integral part of *Synopsis.* They are used extensively throughout the text to add clarity and bring life to the clinical disorders described. Cases come from various sources. Many are from the Sadocks' hospital colleagues or the Sadocks' own experience at Bellevue Hospital in New York. We have preserved most of these case studies as we believe that they expertly illustrate the sometimes abstract concepts described, and we thank the many contributors of those cases for allowing the Synopsis to use these cases in past and future editions.

REFERENCES

Each section in *Synopsis* ends with several citations that include reviews of the literature and references in addition to relevant chapters in our more extensive textbook, *Comprehensive Textbook of Psychiatry.* References are limited in number; in part, this was to conserve space, but more importantly, we are mindful that modern-day readers consult Internet databases such as *PubMed* and *Google Scholar* to stay abreast of the most current literature, and we encourage that trend.

ACKNOWLEDGMENTS

We sincerely appreciate the work of our distinguished Editorial Assistant, Arya Shah, M.D., who helped us to update much of the work, including epidemiology and much other research. Dr. Shah also took on the challenge of reviewing DSM-5 and ICD-10 to create the diagnostic comparative tables, which are new to this edition.

We also wish to thank our colleagues and friends at our respective departments. This impressive group includes the members of the Department of Psychiatry at the Brigham and Women's Hospital. A special thanks to David Silbersweig, M.D., the Chair of Psychiatry at the Brigham and Women's, who offered invaluable advice and mentorship throughout the creation of this work, and to Deborah German, M.D., the Vice President for Health Affairs and Dean of the College of Medicine at the University of Central Florida, for her support, encouragement, and mentorship.

We would also thank our many friends in psychiatry and medicine who live throughout the country. One of them, Josepha Cheong, M.D., at the University of Florida, has dubbed us an "Invisible College," and this is an apt description of the loose network of dear friends, many of them leaders in their fields, who are available at any time to offer advice, counsel, critique, and perspective, all delivered with an infectious sense of humor.

We want to take this opportunity to acknowledge those who have translated this and other *Kaplan & Sadock* books into foreign languages, including Chinese, Croatian, French, German, Greek, Indonesian, Italian, Japanese, Polish, Portuguese, Romanian, Russian, Spanish, and Turkish, in addition to a special Asian and international student edition.

A special thanks to the editorial team at Wolters Kluwer, who were patient with us as we took on this work. We put their patience to the test during the pandemic, and the editorial team was both supportive and encouraging as we helped manage the ramifications of the disease on our respective home fronts while we worked on this edition. Particular thanks go to Chris Teja, our Acquisitions Editor; Anne Malcolm, the Associate Director for Content Development; Ariel Winter, our Development Editor; Ashley Pfeiffer, our Editorial Coordinator; Karan Rana, our Project Manager and Bridgett Dougherty, the Vendor Manager.

Our most tremendous thanks go to Benjamin and Virginia Sadock. Sadly, the pandemic has required that we only know them through their reputations and electronic communication. We do thank them for trusting us with their brainchild. We cannot replace them, but we hope we can still do them proud.

INTERVIEW

Our Meeting with the Sadocks

In planning for this book, we were hoping to visit Benjamin and Virginia Sadock. However, like so many things, the pandemic made that impossible. We settled for a Zoom meeting. We wished to hear some of the book's history and get some advice from the experts. We also wanted to understand the goals and values that motivated them to take on this monumental task. Most of all, we just wanted to meet the people who were responsible for this fantastic work. So we joined the video call with great anticipation, not knowing what to expect.

Meeting people you have only known by reputation can play out in various ways. In this case, the experience was a lovely one. Ben and Virginia turned out to be a warm and friendly couple who were very gracious. They were a smart and energetic pair who played well off each other, at times reflective, other times witty, and always surprisingly humble. They were also happy to tell us about their life's work. They explained that the history of the *Synopsis* began with the *Comprehensive Textbook*, first published in 1967. It was initially about 1,000 pages, with about 200 contributors, edited by Harold Kaplan and Benjamin. Now, of course, it is closer to 5,000 pages with thousands of contributors. Still, even then, it was a massive book, so eventually, they had the idea to try to condense it into something that could be used by medical students and residents. They explained that they did a "cut and paste" of the more extensive book for the first edition of the *Synopsis*. We asked them to clarify and found that they meant a *literal* cutting up of portions of the *Comprehensive Textbook* with an X-ACTO knife, which they then pasted together to form the first edition, calling it the *Modern Synopsis of the Comprehensive Textbook of Psychiatry*. Several editions later, they shortened the title. They explained that as they continued to write new editions of the *Synopsis*, the authors felt that simply extracting bits from the *Comprehensive Textbook* read poorly. They gradually translated the grander work into their words while keeping some of the original book's prose until it became the hybrid between a multiple-contributor and consistently authored work that exists today.

They recalled that, sadly, Harold Kaplan died in 1998 while working on the seventh edition of the *Synopsis*, which is when Virginia became an official author. Benjamin clarified "official," as she had long been unofficially contributing to the book. Virginia noted that, among other things, she helped to add a female perspective to the book—a critical perspective: she was, she noted, only one of eight women in her class at New York Medical College.

They felt that an important goal for them in writing the *Synopsis* was to address their growing concern with the rise of technology and corporate medicine and their dehumanizing effect on medical education. Medical students, they felt, were trained to be "robotic physicians." This dilemma is a problem all academic physicians still worry about as we heap more checklists, protocols, and electronic record-keeping on physicians. They hoped that their book could help to restore some humanism in psychiatric education.

Thus, although there has always been much science and groundbreaking research in the book, they have always kept the practicing physician in mind, which was easy for them as they continued to treat patients as they wrote the book. Indeed, the book is enormously popular among practicing psychiatrists. However, they related their surprise when they found that many nonpsychiatrists were also buying the book, including psychologists, various therapists, and many other professionals involved in treating patients with mental illnesses.

The Sadocks noted that there had been specific challenges, such as keeping up to date with the many revisions of the American Psychiatric Association's *Diagnostic and Statistical Manual of Mental Disorders* (DSM). Although they acknowledge the occasional competition between these two popular books, they see the DSM and the *Synopsis* as complementary, with the DSM defining and their book explaining.

Much of their advice involved the aesthetics of the work. We were impressed with Virginia and Ben's careful thought to details such as the layout, the color scheme, and even the quality of paper used. Their advice helped us appreciate the importance of the work as a whole, including the book's look and feel.

In discussing the book's more than 50-year history, it was clear that the Sadocks rightly took a great deal of pride from their masterpiece. They described being somewhat critical about their first edition, and each time working to make the book better. They felt that their most recent 11th edition was as near to perfect as they could make it. Clearly, the book has grown from the "cut-and-paste" work of the first edition into a thoughtful work with an engaging style and a humanistic approach that incorporates art, history, philosophy, and many case studies. It also grew from a work that, as they related, was initially difficult to interest a publisher in, to become one of the most popular books in psychiatry. Most importantly, they rightfully took great pride in achieving their original goals of creating a work that moves beyond the checklist and outline style that defines many references, to a work that reflects both the art and science of medicine, emphasizing the whole patient.

The meeting ended with their blessing and good wishes. For us, it was a revelation and a great chance to gain some insight into the passion that goes into creating great work. We can only hope that we can learn from their advice and work and try our best to continue the book in the rich tradition that they have built. We also hope that they remain in the excellent health and spirits we encountered when we virtually met and that we can meet in person sometime soon.

Bob Boland and Marcy Verduin. 10/16/2020.

Contents

1 ▲

Examination and Diagnosis
of the Psychiatric Patient

PSYCHIATRIC INTERVIEW, HISTORY, AND MENTAL STATUS EXAMINATION

The psychiatric interview is the most crucial element in the evaluation and care of persons with mental illness. A significant purpose of the initial psychiatric interview is to obtain information that will establish a criteria-based diagnosis. This process, helpful in the prediction of the course of the illness and the prognosis, leads to treatment decisions. A well-conducted psychiatric interview provides a multidimensional understanding of the disorder's biopsychosocial elements. It provides the information necessary for the psychiatrist, in collaboration with the patient, to develop a person-centered treatment plan.

Equally important, the interview itself is often an essential part of the treatment process. From the very first moments of the encounter, the interview shapes the nature of the patient–physician relationship, which can have a profound influence on the outcome of treatment. The settings in which the psychiatric interview takes place include psychiatric inpatient units, medical nonpsychiatric inpatient units, emergency rooms, outpatient offices, nursing homes, other residential programs, and correctional facilities. The length of time for the interview, and its focus, will vary depending on the setting, the specific purpose of the interview, and other factors (including concurrent competing demands for professional services).

Nevertheless, some basic principles and techniques are essential for all psychiatric interviews, and these will be the focus of this section. There are particular issues in the evaluation of children that will not be addressed. This section focuses on the psychiatric interview of adult patients.

General Principles

Agreement as to Process. At the beginning of the interview, the psychiatrist should introduce themself and, depending on the circumstances, may need to identify why he or she is speaking with the patient. Unless implicit (the patient coming to the office), consent to proceed with the interview should be obtained, and the nature of the interaction and the approximate (or specific) amount of time for the interview should be stated. The patient should be encouraged to identify any elements of the process that he or she wishes to alter or add.

A crucial issue is whether the patient is, directly or indirectly, seeking the evaluation voluntarily or has been brought involuntarily for the assessment. This issue should be established before the interview begins, and this information will guide the interviewer, especially in the early stages of the process.

Privacy and Confidentiality. Issues concerning confidentiality are crucial in the evaluation/treatment process and may need to be discussed on multiple occasions. Health Insurance Portability and Accountability Act (HIPAA) regulations must be carefully followed, and the appropriate paperwork must be presented to the patient.

Confidentiality is an essential component of the patient–doctor relationship. The interviewer should make every attempt to ensure that others cannot overhear the content of the interview. Sometimes, in a hospital unit or other institutional setting, this may be difficult. If the patient is sharing a room with others, an attempt should be made to use a different place for the interview. If this is not feasible, the interviewer may need to avoid specific topics or indicate that these issues can be discussed later when privacy can be ensured. Generally, in the beginning, the interviewer should suggest that the content of the session(s) will remain confidential except for what needs to be shared with the referring physician or treatment team. Some evaluations, including forensic and disability evaluations, are less confidential, and what is discussed may be shared with others. In those cases, the interviewer should be explicit in stating that the session is not confidential and identify who will receive a report of the evaluation. This information should be carefully and thoroughly documented in the patient's record.

A special issue concerning confidentiality is when the patient indicates that he or she intends to harm another person. When the psychiatrist's evaluation suggests that this might indeed happen, the psychiatrist may have a legal obligation to warn the potential victim. (The law concerning notification of a potential victim varies by state.) Psychiatrists should also consider their ethical obligations. Part of this obligation may be met by appropriate clinical measures such as increasing the dose of antipsychotic medication or hospitalizing the patient.

Often members of the patient's family, including spouse, adult children, or parents, come with the patient to the first session or are present in the hospital or other institutional setting when the psychiatrist first sees the patient. If a family member wishes to talk to the psychiatrist, it is generally preferable to meet with the family member(s) and the patient together after the session and after the patient's consent has been obtained. The psychiatrist should not bring up material the patient has shared but listen to the input from family members and discuss items that the patient introduces during the joint session. Occasionally, when family members have not asked to be seen, the psychiatrist may feel that including a family member or caregiver might be helpful and raise this subject with the patient. This may be the case when the patient is not able to communicate effectively. As always, the patient must give consent except if the psychiatrist determines that the patient is a danger to himself or herself or others. Sometimes family members might telephone the psychiatrist. Except in an emergency, consent should be obtained from the patient before the psychiatrist speaks to the relative. As indicated above, the psychiatrist should not bring up material that the patient has shared but listen to the input from the family member. The patient should be told when a family member has contacted the psychiatrist even if the patient has given consent for this to occur.

In educational and, occasionally, forensic settings, there may be occasions when the session is recorded. The patient must be fully informed about the recording and how the recording will be used. The length of time the recording will be kept and how access to it will be restricted must be discussed. Occasionally in educational settings, one-way mirrors may be used as a tool to allow trainees to benefit from the observation of an interview. The patient should be informed of the use of the one-way mirror and the category of the observers and be reassured that the rules of confidentiality also bound the observers. The patient's consent for proceeding with the recording or use of the one-way mirror must be obtained, and it should be made clear that the patient's receiving care will not be determined by whether he or she agrees to its use. These devices will have an impact on the interview that the psychiatrist should be open to discussing as the session unfolds.

Respect and Consideration.   As should happen in all clinical settings, the patient must be treated with respect, and the interviewer should be considerate of the circumstances of the patient's condition. The patient is often experiencing considerable pain or other distress and frequently is feeling vulnerable and uncertain of what may happen. Because of the stigma of mental illness and misconceptions about psychiatry, the patient may be especially concerned, or even frightened, about seeing a psychiatrist. The skilled psychiatrist is aware of these potential issues and interacts in a manner to decrease, or at least not increase the distress. The success of the initial interview will often depend on the physician's ability to alleviate excessive anxiety.

Rapport/Empathy.   Respect for and consideration of the patient will contribute to the development of rapport. In the clinical setting, rapport can be defined as the harmonious responsiveness of the physician to the patient and the patient to the physician. It is crucial that patients increasingly feel that the evaluation is a joint effort and that the psychiatrist is genuinely interested in their story. Empathic interventions ("*That must have been very difficult for you*" or "*I'm beginning to understand how awful that felt*") further increase the rapport. Frequently a nonverbal response (raised eyebrows or leaning toward the patient) or a very brief response ("*Wow*") will be similarly effective. Empathy is understanding what the patient is thinking and feeling. It occurs when the psychiatrist can put himself or herself in the patient's place while at the same time maintaining objectivity. For the psychiatrist to truly understand what the patient is thinking and feeling requires an appreciation of many issues in the patient's life. As the interview progresses, the patient's story unfolds, and patterns of behaviors become evident, and it becomes clearer what the patient may have experienced. Early in the interview, the psychiatrist may not be as fully confident of where the patient is or was (although the patient's nonverbal cues can be very beneficial). If the psychiatrist is uncertain about the patient's

experience, it is often best not to guess but to encourage the patient to continue. Head nodding, putting down one's pen, leaning toward the patient, or a brief comment, "*I see,*" can accomplish this objective and simultaneously indicate that this is important material. The large majority of empathic responses in an interview are nonverbal.

An essential ingredient in empathy is retaining objectivity. Maintaining objectivity is crucial in a therapeutic relationship, and it differentiates empathy from identification. With identification, psychiatrists not only understand the emotion but also experience it to the extent that they lose the ability to be objective. This blurring of boundaries between the patient and psychiatrist can be confusing and distressing to many patients, especially to those who, as part of their illness, already have significant boundary problems (e.g., individuals with borderline personality disorder). Identification can also be draining to the psychiatrist and lead to disengagement and, ultimately, burnout.

Patient–Physician Relationship.   The patient–physician relationship is the core of the practice of medicine. (For many years, the term used was "physician–patient" or "doctor–patient," but the order is sometimes reversed to reinforce that the treatment should always be patient-centered.) Although the relationship between any single patient and physician will vary depending on each of their personalities and past experiences as well as the setting and purpose of the encounter, there are general principles that, when followed, help to ensure that the relationship established is helpful.

The patient comes to the interview seeking help. Even in those instances when the patient arrives on the insistence of others (i.e., spouse, family, courts), assistance may be sought by the patient in dealing with the person requesting or requiring the evaluation or treatment. This desire for help motivates the patient to share with a stranger information and feelings that are distressing, personal, and often private. The patient is willing, to various degrees, to do so because of a belief that the doctor has the expertise, by training and experience, to be of help. Right from the very first encounter (sometimes the initial phone call), the patient's willingness to share is increased or decreased depending on the verbal and often the nonverbal interventions of the physician and other staff. As the physician's behaviors demonstrate respect and consideration, rapport begins to develop. This rapport is increased as the patient feels safe and comfortable. If the patient feels secure that what is said in the interview remains confidential, he or she will be more open to sharing.

The sharing is reinforced by the nonjudgmental attitude and behavior of the physician. The patient may have been exposed to considerable negative responses, actual or feared, to their symptoms or behaviors, including criticism, disdain, belittlement, anger, or violence. Being able to share thoughts and feelings with a nonjudgmental listener is generally a positive experience.

There are two additional essential ingredients in a helpful patient–physician relationship. One is the demonstration by physicians that they understand what the patient is stating and emoting. It is not enough that the physician understands what the patient is relating, thinking, and feeling; this understanding must be conveyed to the patient if it is to nurture the therapeutic relationship. The interview is not just an intellectual exercise to arrive at a supportable diagnosis. The other essential ingredient in a helpful patient–physician relationship is the recognition by the patient that the physician cares. As the patient becomes aware that the physician not only understands but also cares, trust increases, and the therapeutic alliance becomes stronger.

The genuineness of the physician reinforces the patient–physician relationship. Being able to laugh in response to a humorous comment, admit a mistake, or apologize for an error that inconvenienced the patient (e.g., being late for or missing an appointment) strengthens the therapeutic alliance. It is also essential to be flexible in the interview and responsive to patient initiatives. If the patient brings in an item, for example, a photo that he or she wants to show the psychiatrist, it is good to look at it, ask questions, and thank the patient for sharing it. Much can be learned about the family history and dynamics from such a seemingly sidebar moment. Also, the therapeutic alliance is strengthened. The psychiatrist should be mindful of the reality that there are no irrelevant moments in the interview room.

At times patients will ask questions about the psychiatrist. A good rule of thumb is that questions about the physician's qualifications and position should generally be answered directly (e.g., board certification, hospital privileges). On occasion, such a question might be a sarcastic comment ("Did you really go to medical school?"). In this case, it would be better to address the issue that provoked the comment rather than respond concretely. There is no easy answer to the question of how the psychiatrist should respond to personal questions ("Are you married?" "Do you have children?" "Do you watch football?"). Advice on how to respond will vary depending on several issues, including the type of psychotherapy being used or considered, the context in which the question is asked, and the wishes of the psychiatrist. Often, especially if the patient is being, or might be, seen for insight-oriented psychotherapy, it is useful to explore why the question is being asked. The question about children may be precipitated by the patient wondering if the psychiatrist has had personal experience in raising children, or more generally does the psychiatrist have the skills and expertise necessary to meet the patient's needs. In this instance, part of the psychiatrist's response may be that he or she has had considerable experiences in helping people deal with issues of parenting. For patients being seen for supportive psychotherapy or medication management, answering the question, especially if it is not very personal, such as "Do you watch football?" is entirely appropriate. A significant reason for not directly answering personal questions is that the interview may become psychiatrist-centered rather than patient-centered.

Occasionally, again depending on the nature of the treatment, it can be helpful for the psychiatrist to share some personal information even if it is not asked directly by the patient. The purpose of the self-revelation should always be to strengthen the therapeutic alliance to be helpful to the patient. Personal information should not be shared to meet the psychiatrist's needs.

Conscious/Unconscious. Unconscious processes must be considered to understand more fully the patient–physician relationship. The reality is that the majority of mental activity remains outside of conscious awareness. In the interview, unconscious processes may be suggested by tangential references to an issue, slips of the tongue or mannerisms of speech, what is not said or avoided, and other defense mechanisms. For example, phrases such as "to tell you the truth" or "to speak frankly" suggest that the speaker does not usually tell the truth or speak frankly. In the initial interview, it is best to note such mannerisms or slips but not to explore them. It may or may not be helpful to pursue them in subsequent sessions. In the interview, transference and countertransference are very significant expressions of unconscious processes. *Transference* is the process of the patient unconsciously and inappropriately displacing onto individuals in his or her current life those patterns of behavior and emotional reactions that originated with significant figures from earlier in life, often childhood. In the clinical situation, the displacement is onto the psychiatrist, who is usually an authority figure or a parent surrogate. The psychiatrist must recognize that the transference may be driving the behaviors of the patient, and the interactions with the psychiatrist may be based on distortions that have their origins much earlier in life. The patient may be angry, hostile, demanding, or obsequious not because of the reality of the relationship with the psychiatrist but because of former relationships and patterns of behaviors. Failure to recognize this process can lead to the psychiatrist inappropriately reacting to the patient's behavior as if it were a personal attack on the psychiatrist.

Similarly, *countertransference* is the process where the physician unconsciously displaces onto the patient patterns of behaviors or emotional reactions as if he or she were a significant figure from earlier in the physician's life. Psychiatrists should be alert to signs of countertransference issues (missed appointments by the psychiatrist, boredom, or sleepiness in a session). Supervision or consultations can be helpful as can personal therapy in helping the psychiatrist recognize and deal with these issues.

Although the patient comes for help, there may be forces that impede the movement to health. Resistances are the processes, conscious or unconscious, that interfere with the therapeutic objectives of treatment. The patient is generally unaware of the impact of these feelings, thinking, or behaviors, which take many different forms, including exaggerated emotional responses, intellectualization, generalization, missed appointments or acting out behaviors. Resistance may be fueled by repression, which is an unconscious process that keeps issues or feelings out of awareness. Because of repression, patients may not be aware of the conflicts that may be central to their illness. In insight-oriented psychotherapy, interpretations are interventions that undo the process of repression and allow the unconscious thoughts and feelings to come to awareness so that they can be handled. As a result of these interventions, the primary gain of the symptom, the unconscious purpose that it serves, may become apparent. In the initial session, interpretations are generally avoided. The psychiatrist should make a note of potential areas for exploration in subsequent sessions.

Person-Centered and Disorder-Based Interviews. A psychiatric interview should be person- (patient-) centered. That is, the focus should be on understanding the patient and enabling the patient to tell his or her story. The individuality of the patient's experience is a central theme, and the patient's life history is elicited, subject to the constraints of time, the patient's willingness to share some of this material, and the skill of the interviewer. Adolf Meyer's "life-charts" were graphic representations of the material collected in this endeavor and were a core component of the "psychobiological" understanding of the illness. The patient's early life experiences, family, education, occupation(s), religious beliefs and practices, hobbies, talents, relationships, and losses are some of the areas that, in concert with genetic and biologic variables, contribute to the development of the personality. An appreciation of these experiences and their impact on the person is necessary for forming an understanding of the patient. It is not only the history that should be person-centered. The resulting treatment plan must be based on the patient's goals, not the psychiatrist's. Numerous studies have demonstrated that often the patient's goals for treatment (e.g., safe housing) are not the same as the psychiatrist's (e.g., decrease in hallucinations). This dichotomy can often be traced to the interview where the focus was not sufficiently person-centered but instead was exclusively or mostly symptom-based. Even when the interviewer asks explicitly about the patient's goals and aspirations, the patient, having been exposed on numerous occasions to what a professional is interested in hearing about, may attempt to focus on "acceptable" or "expected" goals rather than his or her own goals. The patient should be explicitly encouraged to identify his or her goals and aspirations in his or her own words.

Traditionally, medicine has focused on illness and deficits rather than strengths and assets. A person-centered approach focuses on strengths and assets as well as deficits. During the assessment, it is often helpful to ask the patient, "*Tell me about some of the things you do best,*" or, "*What do you consider your greatest asset?*" A more open-ended question, such as "*Tell me about yourself,*" may elicit information that focuses more on either strengths or deficits depending on several factors, including the patient's mood and self-image.

Safety and Comfort.   Both the patient and the interviewer must feel safe. This includes physical safety. On occasion, especially in hospital or emergency room settings, this may require that other staff be present or that the door to the room where the interview is conducted be left ajar. In emergency room settings, it is generally advisable for the interviewer to have a clear, unencumbered exit path. Patients, especially if psychotic or confused, may feel threatened and need to be reassured that they are safe, and the staff will do everything possible to ensure their safety. Sometimes it is useful to explicitly state and sometimes demonstrate that there is sufficient staff to prevent a situation from spiraling out of control. For some, often psychotic patients who are fearful of losing control, this can be reassuring. The interview may need to be shortened or quickly terminated if the patient becomes more agitated and threatening. Once issues of safety have been assessed (and for many outpatients, this may be accomplished within a few seconds), the interviewer should inquire about the patient's comfort and continue to be alert to the patient's comfort throughout the interview. A direct question may be helpful in not only making the patient feel more comfortable but also in enhancing the patient–doctor relationship. This might include, "Are you warm enough?" or "Is that chair comfortable for you?" As the interview progresses, if the patient desires tissues or water, it should be provided.

Time and Number of Sessions.   For an initial interview, 45 to 90 minutes are generally allotted. For inpatients on a medical unit or at times for confused patients, in considerable distress, or psychotic, the length of time that can be tolerated in one sitting may be 20 to 30 minutes or less. In those instances, several brief sessions may be necessary. Even for patients who can tolerate longer sessions, more than one session may be required to complete an evaluation. The clinician must accept the reality that the history obtained is never complete or entirely accurate. An interview is dynamic, and some aspects of the assessment are ongoing, such as how a patient responds to exploration and consideration of new material that emerges. If the patient is coming for treatment, as the initial interview progresses, the psychiatrist makes decisions about what can be continued in subsequent sessions.

Process of the Interview

Before the Interview.   For outpatients, the first contact with the psychiatrist's office is often a telephone call. Whoever is receiving the call must understand how to respond if the patient is acutely distressed, confused, or expresses suicidal or homicidal intent. If the receiver of the call is not a mental health professional, the call should be transferred to the psychiatrist or other mental health professional, if available. If not available, the caller should be directed to a psychiatric emergency center or an emergency hotline. The receiver of the call should obtain the name and phone number of the caller and offer to initiate the call to the hotline if the caller prefers that.

Most calls are not of such an urgent nature. The receptionist (or whoever receives the call) should obtain the information that the setting has deemed relevant for the first contact. Although the requested information varies considerably, it generally includes the name, age, address, and telephone number(s) of the patient, who referred the patient, the reason for the referral, and insurance information. The patient is given relevant information about the office, including the length of time for the initial session, fees, and whom to call if there are additional questions. In many practices, the psychiatrist will contact the patient to discuss the reason for the appointment and to determine if indeed an appointment appears warranted. The timing of the appointment should reflect the apparent urgency of the problem. Asking the patient to bring information about past psychiatric and medical treatments as well as a list of medications (or preferably the medications themselves) can be very helpful. Frequently a patient is referred to the psychiatrist or a psychiatric facility. If possible, reviewing records that precede the patient can be quite beneficial. Some psychiatrists prefer not to read records before the initial interview so that prior evaluations will not unduly influence their initial view of the patient's problems. Whether or not records are reviewed, the reason for the referral must be understood as clearly as possible. This is especially important for forensic evaluations where the reason for the referral and the question(s) posed will help to shape the assessment. Often, especially in the outpatient setting, a patient is referred to the psychiatrist by a primary care physician or other health care provider. Although not always feasible, communicating with the referring professional before the evaluation can be very helpful. It is critical to determine whether the patient is referred for only an evaluation with the ongoing treatment to be provided by the primary care physician or mental health provider (e.g., social worker) or if the patient is being referred for evaluation and treatment by the psychiatrist.

If the court refers the patient or a lawyer or some other non–treatment-oriented agency such as an insurance company, the goals of the interview may be different from diagnosis and treatment recommendations. These goals can include determination of disability, questions of competence or capacity, or determining, if possible, the cause or contributors of the psychiatric illness. In these particular circumstances, the patient and clinician are not entering a treatment relationship, and often the usual rules of confidentiality do not apply. This limited confidentiality must be explicitly established with the patient and must include a discussion of who will be receiving the information gathered during the interview.

The Waiting Room.   When the patient arrives for the initial appointment, he or she is often given forms to complete. These generally include demographic and insurance information. Also, the patient receives information about the practice (including contact information for evenings and weekends) and HIPAA-mandated information that must be read and signed. Many practices also ask for a list of medications, the name and address of the primary care physician, and the identification of major medical problems and allergies. Sometimes the patient is asked what his or her primary reason is for coming to the office. Increasingly, some psychiatrists ask the patient to fill out a questionnaire or a rating scale that identifies significant symptoms. Such scales include the Patient

Health Questionnaire 9 (PHQ-9) or the Quick Inventory of Depression Symptomatology Self Report (QIDS-SR), which are scales of depressive symptoms based on the *Diagnostic and Statistical Manual of Mental Diseases* (DSM).

The Interview Room. The interview room itself should be relatively soundproof. The decor should be pleasant and not distracting. If feasible, it is a good idea to give the patient the choice of a soft chair or a hard-back chair. Sometimes the selection of the chair or how the chair is chosen can reveal characteristics of the patient. Many psychiatrists suggest that the interviewer's chair and the patient's chair be of relatively equal height so that the interviewer does not tower over the patient (or vice versa). It is generally agreed that the patient and the psychiatrist should be seated approximately 4 to 6 ft apart. The psychiatrist should not be sitting behind a desk. The psychiatrist should dress professionally and be well-groomed. Distractions should be kept to a minimum. Unless there is an urgent matter, there should be no telephone or beeper interruptions during the interview. The patient should feel that the time has been set aside just for him or her and that for this designated time, he or she is the exclusive focus of the psychiatrist's attention.

Initiation of the Interview. The patient is greeted in the waiting room by the psychiatrist who, with a friendly face, introduces themself, extends a hand, and, if the patient reciprocates, gives a firm handshake. If the patient does not extend their hand, it is probably best not to comment at that point but warmly indicate the way to the interview room. The refusal to shake hands is probably an important issue, and the psychiatrist can keep this in mind for a potential inquiry if it is not brought up subsequently by the patient. Upon entering the interview room, if the patient has a coat, the psychiatrist can offer to take the coat and hang it up. The psychiatrist then indicates where the patient can sit. A brief pause can be helpful as there may be something the patient wants to say immediately. If not, the psychiatrist can inquire if the patient prefers to be called Mr. Smith, Thomas, or Tom. If this question is not asked, it is best to use the last name as some patients will find it presumptive to be called by their first name, especially if the interviewer is many years younger. These first few minutes of the encounter, even before the formal interview begins, can be crucial to the success of the interview and the development of a helpful patient–doctor relationship. The patient, who is often anxious, forms an initial impression of the psychiatrist and begins to make decisions as to how much can be shared with this doctor. Psychiatrists can convey interest and support by exhibiting a warm, friendly face and other nonverbal communications such as leaning forward in their chair. It is generally useful for the psychiatrist to indicate how much time is available for the interview. The patient may have some questions about what will happen during this time, confidentiality, and other issues, and these questions should be answered directly by the psychiatrist. The psychiatrist can then continue with an open-ended inquiry, "*Why don't we start by you telling me what has led to your being here,*" or simply, "*What has led to your being here?*" Often the response to this question will establish whether or not the patient has been referred. When a referral has been made, it is important to elicit from the patient his or her understanding of why he or she has been referred. Not uncommonly, the patient may be uncertain as to why he or she has been referred or may even feel angry at the referrer, often a primary care physician.

Open-Ended Questions. As the patient responds to these initial questions, the psychiatrist must interact in a manner that allows the patient to tell his or her story. This is the primary goal of the data collection part of the interview to elicit the patient's story of his or her health and illness. Open-ended questions are a necessity to accomplish this objective. Open-ended questions identify an area but provide minimal structure as to how to respond. A typical open-ended question is, "*Tell me about your pain.*" This is in contrast to closed-ended questions that provide much structure and narrow the field from which a response may be chosen. "*Is your pain sharp?*" The ultimate closed-ended question leads to a "yes" or "no" answer. In the initial portion of the interview, questions should be primarily open-ended. As the patient responds, the psychiatrist reinforces the patient continuing by nodding or other supportive interventions. As the patient continues to share his or her story about an aspect of his or her health or illness, the psychiatrist may ask some increasingly closed-ended questions to understand some of the specifics of the history. Then, when that area is understood, the psychiatrist may make a transition to another area again using open-ended questions and eventually closed-ended questions until that area is well described. Hence, the interview should not be a single funnel of open-ended questions in the beginning and closed-ended questions at the end of the interview but rather a series of funnels, each of which begins with open-ended questions.

Elements of the Initial Psychiatric Interview

The interview is now well launched into the present illness. Table 1-1 lists the sections or parts of the initial psychiatric interview. Although not necessarily obtained during the interview in precisely this order, these are the categories that conventionally have been used to organize and record the elements of the evaluation.

The two overarching elements of the psychiatric interview are patient history and the mental status examination. The patient history is based on the subjective report of the patient and, in some cases, the account of collaterals, including other health care providers, family, and other caregivers. The mental status examination, on the other hand, is the interviewer's objective tool similar to the physical examination in other areas of medicine. The physical examination, although not part of the interview itself, is included because of its potential relevance in the psychiatric diagnosis and also because it usually is included as part of the psychiatric evaluation, especially in the inpatient setting. (Also, much relevant information can be verbally obtained by the physician as parts of the physical examination are performed.) Similarly, the formulation, diagnosis, and treatment plan are included because they are products of the interview and also influence the course of the interview

Table 1-1
Parts of the Initial Psychiatric Interview

   I. Identifying data
  II. Source and reliability
 III. Chief complaint
  IV. Present illness
   V. Past psychiatric history
  VI. Substance use/abuse
 VII. Past medical history
VIII. Family history
  IX. Developmental and social history
   X. Review of systems
  XI. Mental status examination
 XII. Physical examination
XIII. Formulation
 XIV. DSM-5 diagnoses
  XV. Treatment plan

dynamically as the interview moves back and forth pursuing, for example, whether specific diagnostic criteria are met or whether potential elements of the treatment plan are realistic. Details of the psychiatric interview are discussed below.

I. Identifying Data.
This section is brief, one or two sentences, and typically includes the patient's name, age, sex, marital status (or significant other relationship), race or ethnicity, and occupation. Often the referral source is also included.

II. Source and Reliability.
It is important to clarify where the information has come from, primarily if others have provided information or records reviewed, and the interviewer's assessment of how reliable the data are.

III. Chief Complaint.
This should be the patient's presenting complaint, ideally in his or her own words. Examples include, "I'm depressed" or "I have a lot of anxiety."

A 64-year-old man presented in a psychiatric emergency room with a chief complaint, "I'm melting away like a snowball." He had become increasingly depressed over 3 months. Four weeks before the emergency room visit, he had seen his primary care physician who had increased his antidepressant medication (imipramine) from 25 to 75 mg and also added hydrochlorothiazide (50 mg) because of mild hypertension and slight pedal edema. Over the ensuing 4 weeks, the patient's condition deteriorated. In the emergency department, he was noted to have a depressed mood, hopelessness, weakness, significant weight loss, and psychomotor retardation and was described as appearing "depleted." He also seemed to be dehydrated, and blood work indicated he was hypokalemic. Examination of his medication revealed that the medication bottles had been mislabeled; he was taking 25 mg of imipramine (generally a nontherapeutic dose) and 150 mg of hydrochlorothiazide. He was indeed, "melting away like a snowball." Fluid and potassium replacement and a therapeutic dose of an antidepressant resulted in significant improvement.

IV. History of Present Illness.
The present illness is a chronologic description of the evolution of the symptoms of the current episode. Also, the account should include any other changes that have occurred during this same period in the patient's interests, interpersonal relationships, behaviors, personal habits, and physical health. As noted above, the patient may provide much of the essential information for this section in response to an open-ended question such as, *"Can you tell me in your own words what brings you here today?"* Other times the clinician may have to lead the patient through parts of the presenting problem. Details that should be gathered include the length of time that the current symptoms have been present and whether there have been fluctuations in the nature or severity of those symptoms over time. ("I have been depressed for the past 2 weeks" vs. "I've had depression all my life"). The presence or absence of stressors should be established, and these may include situations at home, work, school, legal issues, medical comorbidities, and interpersonal difficulties. Also important are factors that alleviate or exacerbate symptoms such as medications, support, coping skills, or time of day. The essential questions to be answered in the history of the present illness include what (symptoms), how much (severity), how long, and associated factors. It is also essential to identify why the patient is seeking help now and what are the "triggering" factors ("I'm here now because my girlfriend told me if I don't get help with this nervousness she is going to leave me."). Identifying the setting in which the illness

Table 1-2
Psychiatric Review of Systems

1. Mood
   A. Depression: Sadness, tearfulness, sleep, appetite, energy, concentration, sexual function, guilt, psychomotor agitation or slowing, interest. A common pneumonic used to remember the symptoms of major depression is SIGECAPS (**S**leep, **I**nterest, **G**uilt, **E**nergy, **C**oncentration, **A**ppetite, **P**sychomotor agitation or slowing, **S**uicidality).
   B. Mania: Impulsivity, grandiosity, recklessness, excessive energy, decreased need for sleep, increased spending beyond means, talkativeness, racing thoughts, hypersexuality.
   C. Mixed/Other: Irritability, liability.
2. Anxiety
   A. Generalized anxiety symptoms: Where, when, who, how long, how frequent.
   B. Panic disorder symptoms: How long until peak, somatic symptoms including racing heart, sweating, shortness of breath, trouble swallowing, sense of doom, fear of recurrence, agoraphobia.
   C. Obsessive-compulsive symptoms: Checking, cleaning, organizing, rituals, hang-ups, obsessive thinking, counting, rational vs. irrational beliefs.
   D. Posttraumatic stress disorder: Nightmares, flashbacks, startle response, avoidance.
   E. Social anxiety symptoms.
   F. Simple phobias, for example, heights, planes, spiders, etc.
3. Psychosis
   A. Hallucinations: Auditory, visual, olfactory, tactile.
   B. Paranoia.
   C. Delusions: TV, radio, thought broadcasting, mind control, referential thinking.
   D. Patient's perception: Spiritual or cultural context of symptoms, reality testing.
4. Other
   A. Attention-deficit/hyperactivity disorder symptoms.
   B. Eating disorder symptoms: Binging, purging, excessive exercising.

began can be revealing and helpful in understanding the etiology of or significant contributors to the condition. If any treatment has been received for the current episode, it should be defined in terms of who saw the patient and how often, what was done (e.g., psychotherapy or medication), and the specifics of the modality used. Also, is that treatment continuing and, if not, why not? The psychiatrist should be alert for any hints of abuse by former therapists as this experience, unless addressed, can be a significant impediment to a healthy and helpful therapeutic alliance.

Often it can be helpful to include a psychiatric review of systems in conjunction with the history of the present illness to help rule in or out psychiatric diagnoses with pertinent positives and negatives. This may help to identify whether some comorbid disorders or disorders are actually more bothersome to the patient but are not initially identified for a variety of reasons. This review can be split into four major categories of mood, anxiety, psychosis, and other (Table 1-2). The clinician will want to ensure that these areas are covered in the comprehensive psychiatric interview.

V. Past Psychiatric History.
In the past psychiatric history, the clinician should obtain information about all psychiatric illnesses and their course over the patient's lifetime, including symptoms and treatment. Because comorbidity is the rule rather than the exception, also to prior episodes of the same illness (e.g., past episodes of depression in an individual who has a major depressive disorder), the psychiatrist should also be alert for the signs and symptoms of other psychiatric disorders. Description of past symptoms should

include when they occurred, how long they lasted, and the frequency and severity of episodes.

Past treatment episodes should be reviewed in detail. These include outpatient treatment such as psychotherapy (individual, group, couple, or family), day treatment or partial hospitalization, inpatient treatment, including voluntary or involuntary, and what precipitated the need for the higher level of care, support groups, or other forms of treatment such as vocational training. Medications and other modalities such as electroconvulsive therapy (ECT), light therapy, or alternative treatments should be carefully reviewed. One should explore what was tried (may have to offer lists of names to patients), how long and at what doses they were used (to establish the adequacy of the trials), and why they were stopped. Essential questions include what the response to the medication or modality and whether there were side effects was. It is also helpful to establish whether there was reasonable compliance with the recommended treatment. The psychiatrist should also inquire whether a diagnosis was made, what it was, and who made the diagnosis. Although a diagnosis made by another clinician should not be automatically accepted as valid, it is essential information that can be used by the psychiatrist in forming his or her opinion.

Special consideration should be given to establishing a lethality history that is important in the assessment of current risk. Past suicidal ideation, intent, plan, and attempts should be reviewed, including the nature of attempts, perceived lethality of the attempts, save potential, suicide notes, giving away things, or other death preparations. Violence and homicidality history will include any violent actions or intent. Specific questions about domestic violence, legal complications, and the outcome of the victim may help define this history more clearly. History of nonsuicidal self-injurious behavior should also be covered, including any history of cutting, burning, banging head, and biting oneself. The feelings, including relief of distress that accompany or follow the behavior, should also be explored as well as the degree to which the patient has gone to hide the evidence of these behaviors.

VI. Substance Use, Abuse, and Addictions.

A careful review of substance use, abuse, and addictions are essential to the psychiatric interview. The clinician should keep in mind that this information may be difficult for the patient to discuss, and a nonjudgmental style will elicit more accurate information. If the patient seems reluctant to share such information, specific questions may be helpful (e.g., *"Have you ever used marijuana?"* or *"Do you typically drink alcohol every day?"*). History of use should include which substances have been used, including alcohol, drugs, medications (prescribed or not prescribed to the patient), and routes of use (oral, snorting, or intravenous). The frequency and amount of use should be determined, keeping in mind the tendency for patients to minimize or deny use that may be perceived as socially unacceptable. Also, there are many misconceptions about alcohol that can lead to erroneous data. The definition of alcohol may be misunderstood, for example, "No, I don't use alcohol," yet later in the same interview, "I drink a fair amount of beer." Also, the amount of alcohol can be confused with the volume of the drink: "I'm not worried about my alcohol use. I mix my drinks, and I add a lot of water." in response to a follow-up question, *"How much bourbon? Probably three or four shots?"* Tolerance, the need for increasing amounts of use, and any withdrawal symptoms should be established to help determine abuse versus dependence. The impact of use on social interactions, work, school, legal consequences, and driving while intoxicated (DWI) should be covered. Some

psychiatrists use a brief standardized questionnaire, the CAGE or RAPS4, to identify alcohol abuse or dependence.

CAGE includes four questions: Have you ever **C**ut down on your drinking? Have people **A**nnoyed you by criticizing your drinking? Have you ever felt bad or **G**uilty about your drinking? Have you ever had a drink the first thing in the morning, as an **E**ye-opener, to steady your nerves or get rid of a hangover? The Rapid Alcohol Problem Screen 4 (RAPS4) also consists of four questions: Have you ever felt guilty after drinking (**R**emorse), could not remember things said or did after drinking (**A**mnesia), failed to do what was normally expected after drinking (**P**erform), or had a morning drink (**S**tarter)?

Any periods of sobriety should be noted, including the length of time and setting such as in jail, legally mandated, and so forth. A history of treatment episodes should be explored, including inpatient detoxification or rehabilitation, outpatient treatment, group therapy, or other settings including self-help groups, Alcoholics Anonymous (AA) or Narcotics Anonymous (NA), halfway houses, or group homes.

Current substance abuse or dependence can have a significant impact on psychiatric symptoms and treatment course. The patient's readiness for change should be determined, including whether they are in the precontemplative, contemplative, or action phase. Referral to the appropriate treatment setting should be considered.

Other vital substances and addictions that should be covered in this section include tobacco and caffeine use, gambling, eating behaviors, and Internet use. Exploration of tobacco use is especially crucial because persons abusing substances are more likely to die as a result of tobacco use than because of the identified abused substance. Gambling history should include casino visits, horse racing, lottery, and scratch cards, and sports betting. Addictive type eating may include binge eating disorder. Overeaters Anonymous (OA) and Gamblers Anonymous (GA) are 12-step programs, similar to AA, for patients with addictive eating behaviors and gambling addictions.

VII. Past Medical History.

The past medical history includes an account of major medical illnesses and conditions as well as treatments, both past, and present. Any past surgeries should also be reviewed. It is essential to understand the patient's reaction to these illnesses and the coping skills employed. The past medical history is an important consideration when determining potential causes of mental illness as well as comorbid or confounding factors and may dictate possible treatment options or limitations. Medical illnesses can precipitate a psychiatric disorder (e.g., anxiety disorder in an individual recently diagnosed with cancer), mimic a psychiatric disorder (hyperthyroidism resembling an anxiety disorder), be precipitated by a psychiatric disorder or its treatment (a metabolic syndrome in a patient on a second-generation antipsychotic medication), or influence the choice of treatment of a psychiatric disorder (renal disorder and the use of lithium carbonate). It is vital to pay special attention to neurologic issues, including seizures, head injury, and pain disorder. Any known history of prenatal or birthing problems or issues with developmental milestones should be noted. In women, a reproductive and menstrual history is essential as well as a careful assessment of the potential for current or future pregnancy. (*"How do you know you are not pregnant?"* may be answered with "Because I have had my tubes tied" or "I just hope I'm not.")

A careful review of all current medications is critical. This should include all current psychiatric medications with attention to how long they have been used, compliance with schedules, the effect of the medications, and any side effects. It is often helpful to be very specific in determining compliance and side effects, including asking questions such as, *"How many days of the week are you able to actually take this medication?"* or *"Have you noticed any change in your sexual function since starting this medication?"* as the patient may not spontaneously offer this information, which may be embarrassing or perceived to be treatment interfering.

Nonpsychiatric medications, over-the-counter medications, sleep aids, herbal, and alternative medications should also be reviewed. These can all potentially have psychiatric implications, including side effects or produce symptoms, as well as potential medication interactions dictating treatment options. Optimally the patient should be asked to bring all medications currently being taken, prescribed or not, over-the-counter preparations, vitamins, and herbs to the interview.

Allergies to medications must be covered, including which medication and the nature of the extent of, and the treatment of the allergic response. Psychiatric patients should be encouraged to have adequate and regular medical care. The sharing of appropriate information among the primary care physicians, other medical specialists, and the psychiatrist can be beneficial for optimal patient care. The initial interview is an opportunity to reinforce that concept with the patient. At times a patient may not want the information to be shared with his or her primary care physician. This wish should be respected, although it may be useful to explore if there is some information that can be shared. Often patients want to restrict certain social or family information (e.g., an extramarital affair) but are comfortable with other details (medication prescribed) being shared.

VIII. Family History.
Because many psychiatric illnesses are familial and a significant number of those have a genetic predisposition, if not cause, a careful review of family history is an essential part of the psychiatric assessment. Furthermore, an accurate family history helps not only in defining a patient's potential risk factors for specific illnesses but also the formative psychosocial background of the patient. Psychiatric diagnoses, medications, hospitalizations, substance use disorders, and lethality history should all be covered. The importance of these issues is highlighted, for example, by the evidence that, at times, there appears to be a familial response to medications, and a family history of suicide is a significant risk factor for suicidal behaviors in the patient. The interviewer must keep in mind that the diagnosis ascribed to a family member may or may not be accurate, and some data about the presentation and treatment of that illness may be helpful. Medical illnesses present in family histories may also be significant in both the diagnosis and the treatment of the patient.

An example is a family history of diabetes or hyperlipidemia affecting the choice of antipsychotic medication that may carry a risk for the development of these illnesses in the patient. Family traditions, beliefs, and expectations may also play a significant role in the development, expression, or course of the illness. Also, the family history is essential in identifying potential support as well as stresses for the patient and, depending on the degree of disability of the patient, the availability and adequacy of likely caregivers.

IX. Developmental and Social History.
The developmental and social history reviews the stages of the patient's life. It is an essential tool in determining the context of psychiatric symptoms and illnesses and may identify some of the significant factors in the evolution of the disorder. Frequently, current psychosocial stressors will be revealed in the course of obtaining a social history. It can often be helpful to review the social history chronologically to ensure all information is covered.

Any available information concerning prenatal or birthing history and developmental milestones should be noted. For the large majority of adult patients, such information is not readily available, and when it is, it may not be entirely accurate. Childhood history will include childhood home environments, including members of the family and social environment, including the number and quality of friendships. A detailed school history including how far the patient went in school and how old he or she was at that level, any special education circumstances or learning disorders, behavioral problems at school, academic performance, and extracurricular activities should be obtained. Childhood physical and sexual abuse should be carefully queried.

Work history will include types of jobs, performance at jobs, reasons for changing jobs, and current work status. The nature of the patient's relationships with supervisors and coworkers should be reviewed. The patient's income, financial issues, and insurance coverage, including pharmacy benefits, are often significant issues.

Military history, where applicable, should be noted, including rank achieved, combat exposure, disciplinary actions, and discharge status. Marriage and relationship history, including sexual preferences and current family structure, should be explored. This should include the patient's capacity to develop and maintain stable and mutually satisfying relationships as well as issues of intimacy and sexual behaviors. Current relationships with parents, grandparents, children, and grandchildren are an essential part of social history. Legal history is also relevant, especially any pending charges or lawsuits. The social history also includes hobbies, interests, pets, and leisure time activities and how this has fluctuated over time. It is important to identify cultural and religious influences on the patient's life and current religious beliefs and practices. A brief overview of the sexual history is given in Table 1-3.

Table 1-3
Sexual History

1. Screening questions
   a. Are you sexually active?
   b. Have you noticed any changes or problems with sex recently?
2. Developmental
   a. Acquisition of sexual knowledge
   b. Onset of puberty/menarche
   c. Development of sexual identity and orientation
   d. First sexual experiences
   e. Sex in romantic relationship
   f. Changing experiences or preferences over time
   g. Sex and advancing age
3. Clarification of sexual problems
   a. Desire phase
      Presence of sexual thoughts or fantasies:
         When do they occur and what is their object?
         Who initiates sex and how?
   b. Excitement phase
      Difficulty in sexual arousal (achieving or maintaining erections, lubrication), during foreplay and preceding orgasm
   c. Orgasm phase
      Does orgasm occur?
      Does it occur too soon or too late?
      How often and under what circumstances does orgasm occur?
      If orgasm does not occur, is it because of not being excited or lack of orgasm despite being aroused?
   d. Resolution phase
      What happens after sex is over (e.g., contentment, frustration, continued arousal)?

X. Review of Systems.   The review of systems attempts to capture any current physical or psychological signs and symptoms not already identified in the present illness. Particular attention is paid to neurologic and systemic symptoms (e.g., fatigue or weakness). Illnesses that might contribute to the presenting complaints or influence the choice of therapeutic agents should be carefully considered (e.g., endocrine, hepatic, or renal disorders). Generally, the review of systems is organized by the major systems of the body.

XI. Mental Status Examination.
The mental status examination (MSE) is the psychiatric equivalent of the physical examination in the rest of medicine. The MSE explores all the areas of mental functioning and denotes evidence of signs and symptoms of mental illnesses. Data are gathered for the mental status examination throughout the interview from the initial moments of the interaction, including what the patient is wearing and their general presentation. Most of the information does not require direct questioning, and the information gathered from observation may give the clinician a different dataset than patient responses. Direct questioning augments and rounds out the MSE. The MSE provides the clinician with a snapshot of the patient's mental status at the time of the interview and is useful for subsequent visits to compare and monitor changes over time. The psychiatric MSE includes cognitive screening most often in the form of the Mini-Mental Status Examination (MMSE), but the MMSE is not to be confused with the MSE overall. The components of the MSE are presented in this section in the order one might include them in the written note for organizational purposes. Still, as noted above, the data are gathered throughout the interview.

APPEARANCE AND BEHAVIOR.   This section consists of a general description of how the patient looks and acts during the interview. Does the patient appear to be his or her stated age, younger or older? Is this related to the patient's style of dress, physical features, or style of interaction? Items to be noted include what the patient is wearing, including body jewelry, and whether it is appropriate for the context. For example, a patient in a hospital gown would be appropriate in the emergency room or inpatient unit but not in an outpatient clinic. Distinguishing features, including disfigurations, scars, and tattoos, are noted. Grooming and hygiene also are included in the overall appearance and can be clues to the patient's level of functioning.

The description of a patient's behavior includes a general statement about whether he or she is exhibiting acute distress and then a more specific statement about the patient's approach to the interview. The patient may be described as cooperative, agitated, disinhibited, disinterested, and so forth. Once again, appropriateness is an essential factor to consider in the interpretation of the observation. If a patient is brought involuntarily for examination, it may be appropriate, certainly understandable, that he or she is somewhat uncooperative, especially at the beginning of the interview.

MOTOR ACTIVITY.   Motor activity may be described as normal, slowed (bradykinesia), or agitated (hyperkinesia). This can give clues to diagnoses (e.g., depression vs. mania) as well as confounding neurologic or medical issues. Gait, freedom of movement, any unusual or sustained postures, pacing, and hand wringing are described. The presence or absence of any tics should be noted, as should be jitteriness, tremor, apparent restlessness, lip-smacking, and tongue protrusions. These can be clues to adverse reactions or side effects of medications such as tardive dyskinesia, akathisia, or parkinsonian features from antipsychotic medications or suggestion

of symptoms of illnesses such as attention-deficit/hyperactivity disorder (ADHD).

SPEECH.   Evaluation of speech is an integral part of the MSE. Elements considered include fluency, amount, rate, tone, and volume. Fluency can refer to whether the patient has full command of the English language as well as potentially more subtle fluency issues such as stuttering, word-finding difficulties, or paraphasic errors. (A Spanish-speaking patient with an interpreter would be considered not fluent in English, but an attempt should be made to establish whether he or she is fluent in Spanish.) The evaluation of the amount of speech refers to whether it is normal, increased, or decreased. Decreased amounts of speech may suggest several different things ranging from anxiety or disinterest to thought blocking or psychosis. Increased amounts of speech often (but not always) are suggestive of mania or hypomania. A related element is the speed or rate of speech. Is it slowed or rapid (pressured)? Finally, speech can be evaluated for its tone and volume. Descriptive terms for these elements include irritable, anxious, dysphoric, loud, quiet, timid, angry, or childlike.

MOOD.   The terms *mood* and *affect* vary in their definition, and several authors have recommended combining the two elements into a new label, "emotional expression." Traditionally, *mood* is defined as the patient's internal and sustained emotional state. Its experience is subjective, and hence it is best to use the patient's own words in describing his or her mood. Terms such as "sad," "angry," "guilty," or "anxious" are common descriptions of mood.

AFFECT.   *Affect* differs from mood in that it is the expression of mood or what the patient's mood appears to be to the clinician. Affect is often described with the following elements: quality, quantity, range, appropriateness, and congruence. Terms used to describe the quality (or tone) of a patient's affect include dysphoric, happy, euthymic, irritable, angry, agitated, tearful, sobbing, and flat. Speech is often an essential clue to the assessment of affect, but it is not exclusive. Quantity of affect is a measure of its intensity. Two patients, both described as having depressed affect can be very different if one is described as mildly depressed and the other as severely depressed. The range can be restricted, normal, or labile. *Flat* is a term that has been used for a severely restricted range of affect that is described in some patients with schizophrenia. Appropriateness of affect refers to how the affect correlates to the setting. A patient who is laughing at a solemn moment of a funeral service is described as having an inappropriate affect. Affect can also be congruent or incongruent with the patient's described mood or thought content. A patient may report feeling depressed or describe a depressive theme but do so with laughter, smiling, and no suggestion of sadness.

THOUGHT CONTENT.   Essentially, thought content is what thoughts are occurring to the patient. This is inferred by what the patient spontaneously expresses, as well as responses to specific questions aimed at eliciting particular pathology. Some patients may perseverate or ruminate on specific content or thoughts. They may focus on material that is considered obsessive or compulsive. *Obsessional thoughts* are unwelcome and repetitive thoughts that intrude into the patient's consciousness. They are generally ego alien and resisted by the patient. *Compulsions* are repetitive, ritualized behaviors that patients feel compelled to perform to avoid an increase in anxiety or some dreaded outcome. Another broad category of thought content pathology is delusions. *Delusions* are false, fixed ideas that are not shared by others and can be divided into bizarre and nonbizarre (nonbizarre delusions refer to thought content that is not true but is not out of the realm of possibility). Common delusions include grandiose, erotomanic, jealous, somatic, and persecutory. It is often helpful to suggest delusional content to patients who may have learned not to spontaneously discuss them. Questions that can be helpful include, "*Do you ever feel like someone is following you or out to get you?*" and "*Do you feel like the TV or radio has a special message for you?*" An affirmative answer to the latter question indicates an "idea of reference." Paranoia can be closely related to delusional material and can range from "soft" paranoia, such as general suspiciousness, to more severe forms that impact daily functioning. Questions that elicit paranoia can include asking about the patient worrying about cameras, microphones, or the government.

Suicidality and homicidality fall under the category of thought content, but here are discussed separately because of their particular importance in being addressed in every initial psychiatric interview. Simply asking if someone is suicidal or homicidal is not adequate. One must get a sense of ideation, intent, plan, and preparation. Although completed suicide is hugely challenging to predict accurately, there are identified risk factors, and these can be used in conjunction with an evaluation of the patient's intent and plan for acting on thoughts of suicide.

THOUGHT PROCESS. Thought process differs from thought content in that it does not describe what the person is thinking but rather how the thoughts are formulated, organized, and expressed. A patient can have normal thought process with significantly delusional thought content. Conversely, there may be generally normal thought content but significantly impaired thought process. Normal thought process is typically described as linear, organized, and goal-directed. With flight of ideas, the patient rapidly moves from one thought to another, at a pace that is difficult for the listener to keep up with, but all of the ideas are logically connected. The circumstantial patient overincludes details and material that is not directly relevant to the subject or an answer to the question but does eventually return to address the subject or answer the question. Typically the examiner can follow a circumstantial train of thought, seeing connections between the sequential statements. Tangential thought process may at first appear similar, but the patient never returns to the original point or question. The tangential thoughts are seen as irrelevant and related in a minor, insignificant manner. Loose thoughts or associations differ from circumstantial and tangential thoughts in that with loose thoughts it is difficult or impossible to see the connections between the sequential content. Perseveration is the tendency to focus on a specific idea or content without the ability to move on to other topics. The perseverative patient will repeatedly come back to the same topic despite the interviewer's attempts to change the subject. Thought blocking refers to a disordered thought process in which the patient appears to be unable to complete a thought. The patient may stop midsentence or midthought and leave the interviewer waiting for the completion. When asked about this, patients will often remark that they don't know what happened and may not remember what was being discussed. Neologisms refer to a new word or condensed combination of several words that is not a true word and is not readily understandable. However, sometimes the intended meaning or partial meaning may be apparent. Word salad is speech characterized by confused, and often repetitious, language with no apparent meaning or relationship attached to it. A description of formal thought disorders is given in Table 1-4.

PERCEPTUAL DISTURBANCES. Perceptual disturbances include hallucinations, illusions, depersonalization, and derealization. Hallucinations are perceptions in the absence of stimuli to account

Table 1-4
Formal Thought Disorders

Circumstantiality. Overinclusion of trivial or irrelevant details that impede the sense of getting to the point.

Clang associations. Thoughts are associated by the sound of words rather than by their meaning (e.g., through rhyming or assonance).

Derailment. (Synonymous with loose associations.) A breakdown in both the logical connection between ideas and the overall sense of goal directedness. The words make sentences, but the sentences do not make sense.

Flight of ideas. A succession of multiple associations so that thoughts seem to move abruptly from idea to idea; often (but not invariably) expressed through rapid, pressured speech.

Neologism. The invention of new words or phrases or the use of conventional words in idiosyncratic ways.

Perseveration. Repetition of out of context words, phrases, or ideas.

Tangentiality. In response to a question, the patient gives a reply that is appropriate to the general topic without actually answering the question. Example:
Doctor: "Have you had any trouble sleeping lately?"
Patient: "I usually sleep in my bed, but now I'm sleeping on the sofa."

Thought blocking. A sudden disruption of thought or a break in the flow of ideas.

for them. Auditory hallucinations are the hallucinations most frequently encountered in the psychiatric setting. Other hallucinations can include visual, tactile, olfactory, and gustatory (taste). In the North American culture, nonauditory hallucinations are often clues that there is a neurologic, medical, or substance withdrawal issue rather than a primary psychiatric issue. In other cultures, visual hallucinations have been reported to be the most common form of hallucinations in schizophrenia. The interviewer should make a distinction between a real hallucination and a misperception of stimuli (illusion). Hearing the wind rustle through the trees outside one's bedroom and thinking a name is being called is an illusion. Hypnagogic hallucinations (at the interface of wakefulness and sleep) may be normal phenomena. At times patients without psychosis may hear their name called or see flashes or shadows out of the corners of their eyes. In describing hallucinations, the interviewer should include what the patient is experiencing, when it occurs, how often it occurs, and whether or not it is uncomfortable (ego-dystonic). In the case of auditory hallucinations, it can be useful to learn if the patient hears words, commands, or conversations and whether the voice is recognizable to the patient.

Depersonalization is a feeling that one is not oneself or that something has changed. Derealization is a feeling that one's environment has changed in some strange way that is difficult to describe.

COGNITION. The elements of cognitive functioning that should be assessed are alertness, orientation, concentration, memory (both short and long term), calculation, fund of knowledge, abstract reasoning, insight, and judgment.

Note should be made of the patient's level of alertness. The amount of detail in assessing cognitive function will depend on the purpose of the examination and also what has already been learned in the interview about the patient's level of functioning, performance at work, handling daily chores, balancing one's checkbook, among others. Also, the psychiatrist will have already elicited data concerning the patient's memory for both remote and recent past. A general sense of intellectual level and how much schooling the patient has had can help distinguish intelligence and educational

Table 1-5
Questions Used to Test Cognitive Functions in the Sensorium Section of the Mental Status Examination

1. Alertness	(Observation)
2. Orientation	What is your name? Who am I? What place is this? Where is it located? What city are we in?
3. Concentration	Starting at 100, count backward by 7 (or 3). Say the letters of the alphabet backward starting with Z. Name the months of the year backward starting with December.
4. Memory: Immediate	Repeat these numbers after me: 1, 4, 9, 2, 5.
Recent	What did you have for breakfast? What were you doing before we started talking this morning? I want you to remember these three things: a yellow pencil, a cocker spaniel, and Cincinnati. After a few minutes I'll ask you to repeat them.
Long term	What was your address when you were in the third grade? Who was your teacher? What did you do during the summer between high school and college?
5. Calculations	If you buy something that costs $3.75 and you pay with a $5 bill, how much change should you get? What is the cost of three oranges if a dozen oranges cost $4.00?
6. Fund of knowledge	What is the distance between New York and Los Angeles? What body of water lies between South America and Africa?
7. Abstract reasoning	Which one does not belong in this group: a pair of scissors, a canary, and a spider? Why? How are an apple and an orange alike?

issues versus cognitive impairment that might be seen in delirium or dementia. Table 1-5 presents an overview of the questions used to test cognitive function in the mental status examination.

ABSTRACT REASONING. Abstract reasoning is the ability to shift back and forth between general concepts and specific examples. Having the patient identify similarities between like objects or concepts (apple and pear, bus and airplane, or a poem and a painting) as well as interpreting proverbs can be useful in assessing one's ability to abstract. Cultural and educational factors and limitations should be kept in mind when assessing the ability to abstract. Occasionally, the inability to abstract or the idiosyncratic manner of grouping items can be dramatic.

INSIGHT. Insight, in the psychiatric evaluation, refers to the patient's understanding of how he or she is feeling, presenting, and functioning as well as the potential causes of his or her psychiatric presentation. The patient may have no insight, partial insight, or full insight. A component of insight often is reality testing in the case of a patient with psychosis. An example of intact reality testing would be, "I know that there are not really little men talking to me when I am alone, but I feel like I can see them and hear their voices." As indicated by this example, the amount of insight is not an indicator

of the severity of the illness. A person with psychosis may have good insight, while a person with a mild anxiety disorder may have little or no insight.

JUDGMENT. Judgment refers to the person's capacity to make good decisions and act on them. The level of judgment may or may not correlate to the level of insight. A patient may have no insight into his or her illness but have good judgment. It has been traditional to use hypothetical examples to test judgment, for example, *"What would you do if you found a stamped envelope on the sidewalk?"* It is better to use real situations from the patient's own experience to test judgment. The important issues in assessing judgment include whether a patient is doing things that are dangerous or going to get him or her into trouble and whether the patient can effectively participate in his or her own care. Significantly impaired judgment can be cause for considering a higher level of care or more restrictive setting such as inpatient hospitalization. Table 1-6 lists some common questions for the psychiatric history and mental status.

XII. Physical Examination. The inclusion and extent of physical examination will depend on the nature and setting of the psychiatric interview. In the outpatient setting, little or no physical examination may be routinely performed, while in the emergency room or inpatient setting, a more complete physical examination is warranted. Vital signs, weight, waist circumference, body mass index, and height may be important measurements to follow particularly given the potential effects of psychiatric medications or illnesses on these parameters. The Abnormal Involuntary Movement Scale (AIMS) is an important screening test to be followed when using antipsychotic medication to monitor for potential side effects such as tardive dyskinesia. A focused neurologic evaluation is an important part of the psychiatric assessment.

In those instances where a physical examination is not performed the psychiatrist should ask the patient when the last physical examination was performed and by whom. As part of the communication with that physician, the psychiatrist should inquire about any abnormal findings.

XIII. Formulation. The culmination of the data-gathering aspect of the psychiatric interview is developing a formulation and diagnosis (diagnoses) as well as recommendations and treatment planning. In this part of the evaluation process, the data gathering is supplanted by data processing where the various themes contribute to a biopsychosocial understanding of the patient's illness. Although the formulation is placed near the end of the reported or written evaluation, it is developed as part of a dynamic process throughout the interview as new hypotheses are created and tested by further data that are elicited. The formulation should include a brief summary of the patient's history, presentation, and current status. It should include discussion of biologic factors (medical, family, and medication history) as well as psychological factors such as childhood circumstances, upbringing, and past interpersonal interactions and social factors including stressors, and contextual circumstances such as finances, school, work, home, and interpersonal relationships. These elements should lead to a differential diagnosis of the patient's illness (if any) as well as a provisional diagnosis. Finally, the formulation should include a summary of the safety assessment, which contributes to the determination of the level of care recommended or required.

XIV. Treatment Planning. The assessment and formulation will appear in the written note correlating to the psychiatric interview. Still, the discussion with the patient may only be a summary

Table 1-6
Common Questions for Psychiatric History and Mental Status

Topic	Questions	Comments and Clinical Hints
Identifying data	Be direct in obtaining identifying data. Request specific answers.	If patient cannot cooperate, get information from family member or friend; if referred by a physician, obtain medical record.
Chief complaint (CC)	Why are you going to see a psychiatrist? What brought you to the hospital? What seems to be the problem?	Records answers verbatim; a bizarre complaint points to psychotic process.
History of present illness (HPI)	When did you first notice something happening to you? Were you upset about anything when symptoms began? Did they begin suddenly or gradually?	Record in patient's own words as much as possible. Get history of previous hospitalizations and treatment. Sudden onset of symptoms may indicate drug-induced disorder.
Previous psychiatric and medical disorders	Did you ever lose consciousness? Have a seizure?	Ascertain extent of illness, treatment, medications, outcomes, hospitals, doctors. Determine whether illness serves some additional purpose (secondary gain).
Personal history	Do you know anything about your birth? If so, from whom? How old was your mother when you were born? Your father?	Older mothers (>35) have high risk for Down syndrome babies; older fathers (>45) may contribute damaged sperm, producing deficits including schizophrenia.
Childhood	Toilet training? Bed-wetting? Sex play with peers? What is your first childhood memory?	Separation anxiety and school phobia are associated with adult depression; enuresis is associated with fire setting. Childhood memories before the age of 3 are usually imagined, not real.
Adolescence	Adolescents may refuse to answer questions, but they should be asked. Adults may distort memories of emotionally charged experiences. Sexual molestation?	Poor school performance is a sensitive indicator of emotional disorder. Schizophrenia begins in late adolescence.
Adulthood	Open-ended questions are preferable. Tell me about your marriage. Be nonjudgmental; What role does religion play in your life, if any? What is your sexual preference in a partner?	Depending on the chief complaint, some areas require more detailed inquiry. Manic patients frequently go into debt or are promiscuous. Overvalued religious ideas are associated with paranoid personality disorder.
Sexual history	Are there or have there been any problems or concerns about your sex life? How did you learn about sex? Has there been any change in your sex drive?	Be nonjudgmental. Asking *when* masturbation began is a better approach than asking *do you* or *did you ever* masturbate.
Family history	Have any members in your family been depressed? Alcoholic? In a mental hospital? Describe your living conditions. Did you have your own room?	Genetic loading in anxiety, depression, schizophrenia. Get medication history of family (medications effective in family members for similar disorders may be effective in patient).
Mental Status		
General appearance	Introduce yourself and direct patient to take a seat. In the hospital, bring your chair to bedside; do not sit on the bed.	Unkempt and disheveled in cognitive disorder, pinpoint pupils in narcotic addiction, withdrawal and stooped posture in depression.
Motoric behavior	Have you been more active than usual? Less active? You may ask about obvious mannerisms, such as, "I notice that your hand still shakes, can you tell me about that?" Stay aware of smells, such as alcoholism/ketoacidosis.	Fixed posturing, odd behavior in schizophrenia. Hyperactive with stimulant (cocaine) abuse and in mania. Psychomotor retardation in depression; tremors with anxiety or medication side effect (lithium). Eye contact is normally made during the interview. Minimal eye contact in schizophrenia. Scanning of environment in paranoid states.
Attitude during interview	You may comment about attitude: "You seem irritated about something; is that an accurate observation?"	Suspiciousness in paranoia; seductive in hysteria; apathetic in conversion disorder (*la belle indifference*); punning (*witzelsucht*) in frontal lobe syndromes.
Mood	How do you feel? How are your spirits? Do you have thoughts that life is not worth living or that you want to harm yourself? Do you have plans to take your own life? Do you want to die? Has there been a change in your sleep habits?	Suicidal ideas in 25% of depressives; elation in mania. Early morning awakening in depression; decreased need for sleep in mania.
Affect	Observe nonverbal signs of emotion, body movements, facies, rhythm of voice (prosody). Laughing when talking about sad subjects, such as death, is inappropriate.	Changes in affect usual with schizophrenia: loss of prosody in cognitive disorder, catatonia. Do not confuse medication adverse effect with flat affect.
Speech	Ask patient to say "Methodist Episcopalian" to test for dysarthria.	Manic patients show pressured speech; paucity of speech in depression; uneven or slurred speech in cognitive disorders.

Table 1-6
Common Questions for Psychiatric History and Mental Status (*Continued*)

Topic	Questions	Comments and Clinical Hints
Perceptual disorders	Do you ever see things or hear voices? Do you have strange experiences as you fall asleep or upon awakening? Has the world changed in any way? Do you have strange smells?	Visual hallucinations suggest schizophrenia. Tactile hallucinations suggest cocainism, delirium tremens (DTs). Olfactory hallucinations common in temporal lobe epilepsy.
Thought content	Do you feel people want to harm you? Do you have special powers? Is anyone trying to influence you? Do you have strange body sensations? Are there thoughts that you can't get out of your mind? Do you think about the end of the world? Can people read your mind? Do you ever feel the TV is talking to you? Ask about fantasies and dreams.	Are delusions congruent with mood (grandiose delusions with elated mood) or incongruent? Mood-incongruent delusions point to schizophrenia. Illusions are common in delirium. Thought insertion is characteristic of schizophrenia.
Thought process	Ask meaning of proverbs to test abstraction, such as, "People in glass houses should not throw stones." Concrete answer is, "Glass breaks." Abstract answers deal with universal themes or moral issues. Ask similarity between bird and butterfly (both alive), bread and cake (both food).	Loose associations point to schizophrenia; flight of ideas to mania; inability to abstract to schizophrenia, brain damage.
Sensorium	What place is this? What is today's date? Do you know who I am?	Delirium or dementia shows clouded or wandering sensorium. Orientation to person remains intact longer than orientation to time or place.
Remote memory (long-term memory)	Where were you born? Where did you go to school? Date of marriage? Birthdays of children? What were last week's newspaper headlines?	Patients with dementia of the Alzheimer type retain remote memory longer than recent memory. Gaps in memory may be localized or filled in with confabulatory details. Hypermnesia is seen in paranoid personality.
Immediate memory (very short-term memory)	Ask patient to repeat six digits forward, then backward (normal responses). Ask patient to try to remember three nonrelated items; test patient after 5 min.	Loss of memory occurs with cognitive, dissociative, or conversion disorder. Anxiety can impair immediate retention and recent memory. Anterograde memory loss (amnesia) occurs after taking certain drugs, such as benzodiazepines. Retrograde memory loss occurs after head trauma.
Concentration and calculation	Ask patient to count from 1 to 20 rapidly; do simple calculations (2×4, 4×9); do serial 7 test (i.e., subtract 7 from 100 and keep subtracting 7). How many nickels in $1.35?	Rule out medical cause for any defects vs. anxiety or depression (pseudodementia). Make tests congruent with educational level of patient.
Information and intelligence	Distance from New York City to Los Angeles. Name some vegetables. What is the largest river in the United States?	Check educational level to results. Rule out mental retardation, borderline intellectual functioning.
Judgment	What is the thing to do if you find an envelope in the street that is sealed, stamped, and addressed?	Impaired in brain disease, schizophrenia, borderline intellectual functioning, intoxication.
Insight level	Do you think you have a problem? Do you need treatment? What are your plans for the future?	Impaired in delirium, dementia, frontal lobe syndrome, psychosis, borderline intellectual functioning.

From Sadock BJ, Sadock V. *Kaplan and Sadock's Pocket Handbook of Clinical Psychiatry*. Philadelphia, PA: Lippincott Williams & Wilkins, 2010, with permission.

of this assessment geared toward the patient's ability to understand and interpret the information. Treatment planning and recommendations, in contrast, are integral parts of the psychiatric interview and should be explicitly discussed with the patient in detail.

The first part of treatment planning involves determining whether a treatment relationship is to be established between the interviewer and patient. Cases, where this may not be the case, include if the interview was done in consultation, for a legal matter or as a third-party review, or in the emergency room or other acute setting. If a treatment relationship is not being started, then the patient should be informed as to what the recommended treatment is (if any). In some instances, this may not be voluntary (as in the case of an involuntary hospitalization). In most cases, there should be a discussion of the options available so that the patient can participate in the decisions about the next steps. If a treatment

relationship is being initiated, then the structure of that treatment should be discussed. Will the primary focus be on medication management, psychotherapy, or both? What will the frequency of visits be? How will the clinician be paid for service, and what are the expectations for the patient to be considered engaged in treatment?

Medication recommendations should include a discussion of possible therapeutic medications, the risks and benefits of no medication treatment, and alternative treatment options. The prescriber must obtain informed consent from the patient for any medications (or other treatments) initiated.

Other clinical treatment recommendations may include referral for psychotherapy, group therapy, chemical dependency evaluation or treatment, or medical assessment. There also may be recommended psychosocial interventions, including case management, group home or assisted living, social clubs, support groups such as a mental health alliance, the National Alliance for the Mentally Ill, and AA.

Collaboration with primary care doctors, specialists, or other clinicians should always be a goal, and proper patient consent must be obtained for this. Similarly, family involvement in a patient's care can often be a useful and integral part of treatment and requires proper patient consent.

A thorough discussion of safety planning and contact information should occur during the psychiatric interview. The clinician's contact information, as well as after-hours coverage scheme, should be reviewed. The patient needs to be informed of what he or she should do in the case of an emergency, including using the emergency room or calling 911 or available crisis hotlines.

Techniques

General principles of the psychiatric interview, such as the patient–doctor relationship, open-ended interviewing, and confidentiality, are described above. Also, to the general principles, several specific techniques can be useful in obtaining information in a manner consistent with the general principles. These helpful techniques can be described as facilitating interventions and expanding interventions. Some interventions are generally counterproductive and interfere with the goals of helping the patient tell his or her story and reinforcing the therapeutic alliance.

Facilitating Interventions.   These are some of the interventions that are effective in enabling the patient to continue sharing his or her story and also help promote a positive patient–doctor relationship. At times some of these techniques may be combined in a single intervention.

REINFORCEMENT.   Reinforcement interventions, although seemingly simplistic, are very important in the patient sharing material about himself or herself and other influential individuals and events in the patient's life. Without these reinforcements, often, the interview will become less productive. A brief phrase such as "I see," "Go on," "Yes," "Tell me more," "Hmm," or "Uh-huh" all convey the interviewer's interest in the patient continuing. These phrases must fit naturally into the dialogue.

REFLECTION.   By using the patient's words, the psychiatrist indicates that he or she has heard what the patient is saying and conveys an interest in hearing more.

This response is not a question. A question, with a slight inflection at the end, calls for some clarification. It should also not be said with a tone that is challenging or disbelieving but rather as a statement of fact. The fact is that this is the patient's experience that the psychiatrist hears. Sometimes it is helpful to paraphrase the patient's statement, so it doesn't sound like it is coming from anautomation.

SUMMARIZING.   Periodically during the interview, it is helpful to summarize what has been identified about a certain topic. This provides the opportunity for the patient to clarify or modify the psychiatrist's understanding and possibly add new material. When new material is introduced, the psychiatrist may decide to continue with a further exploration of the previous discussion and return to the new information at a later point.

EDUCATION.   At times in the interview, it is helpful for the psychiatrist to educate the patient about the interview process.

REASSURANCE.   It is often appropriate and helpful to provide reassurance to the patient. For example, accurate information about the usual course of an illness can decrease anxiety, encourage the patient to continue to discuss his or her illness, and strengthen his or her resolve to continue in treatment. It is generally inappropriate for psychiatrists to reassure patients when the psychiatrist does not know what the outcome will be. In these cases, psychiatrists can assure patients they will continue to be available and will help in whatever way they can.

ENCOURAGEMENT.   It is difficult for many patients to come for a psychiatric evaluation. Often they are uncertain as to what will happen, and receiving encouragement can facilitate their engagement. Psychiatrists should be careful not to overstate the patient's progress in the interview. The psychiatrist may provide the patient with feedback about his or her efforts, but the secondary message should be that there is more work to be done.

ACKNOWLEDGMENT OF EMOTION.   The interviewer needs to acknowledge the expression of emotion by the patient. This frequently leads to the patient sharing more feelings and being relieved that he or she can do so. Sometimes a nonverbal action, such as moving a tissue box closer, can suffice or be used adjunctly. If the display of the emotion is clear (e.g., patient openly crying), then it is not helpful to comment directly on the expression of the emotion. It is better to comment on the associated feelings.

HUMOR.   At times the patient may make a humorous comment or tell a brief joke. It can be beneficial if the psychiatrist smiles, laughs, or even, when appropriate, add another punch line. This sharing of humor can decrease tension and anxiety and reinforce the interviewer's genuineness. It is crucial to be certain that the patient's comment was indeed meant to be humorous and that the psychiatrist clearly conveys that he or she is laughing with the patient, not at the patient.

SILENCE.   Careful use of silence can facilitate the progression of the interview. The patient may need time to think about what has been said or to experience a feeling that has arisen in the interview. The psychiatrist, whose own anxiety results in any silence quickly being terminated, can retard the development of insight or the expression of feeling by the patient. On the other hand, extended or repeated silences can deaden an interview and become a struggle as to who can outwait the other. If the patient is looking at his or her watch or looking about the room, then it might be helpful to comment, "*It looks like there are other things on your mind.*" If the patient has become silent and looks like he or she is thinking about the subject, then the psychiatrist might ask, "*What thoughts do you have about that?*"

NONVERBAL COMMUNICATION.   In many good interviews, the most common facilitating interventions are nonverbal. Nodding of the head, body posture including leaning toward the patient, body positioning becoming more open, moving the chair closer to the patient, putting down the pen and folder, and facial expressions including arching of eyebrows all indicate that the psychiatrist is concerned, listening attentively, and engaged in the interview. Although these interventions can be constructive, they can also be overdone, especially if the same action is repeated too frequently or done exaggeratedly. The interviewer does not want to reinforce the popular caricature of a psychiatrist nodding his or her head repeatedly regardless of the content of what is being said or the emotion being expressed.

EXPANDING INTERVENTIONS.   Several interventions can be used to expand the focus of the interview. These techniques are helpful when the line of discussion has been sufficiently mined, at least for the time being, and the interviewer wants to encourage the patient to talk about other issues. These interventions are most successful when a degree of trust has been established in the interview, and the patient feels that the psychiatrist is nonjudgmental about what is being shared.

CLARIFYING.   At times carefully clarifying what the patient has said can lead to unrecognized issues or psychopathology.

A 62-year-old widow describes how it feels since her husband died 14 months ago. She repeatedly comments that "everything is empty inside." The resident interprets this as meaning her world feels empty without her spouse and makes this interpretation on a few occasions. The patient's nonverbal cues suggest that she is not on the same wavelength. The supervisor asks the patient to clarify what she means by "empty inside." After some avoidance, the patient states that she is indeed empty inside; all her organs are missing—they have "disappeared."

The resident's interpretation may have been psychodynamically accurate, but a somatic delusion was not identified. The correct identification of what the patient was saying led to an exploration of other thoughts and other delusions were uncovered. This vignette of "missing" the delusion is an example of the interviewer "normalizing" what the patient is saying. The interviewer was using secondary process thinking in understanding the words of the patient, while the patient was using primary process thinking.

ASSOCIATIONS.   As the patient describes his or her symptoms, other areas are related to a symptom that should be explored. For example, the symptom of nausea leads to questions about appetite, bowel habits, weight loss, and eating habits. Also, experiences that are temporally related may be investigated. When a patient is talking about his or her sleeping pattern, it can be a good opportunity to ask about dreams.

LEADING.   Often, continuing the story can be facilitated by asking a "what," "when," "where," or "who" question. Sometimes the psychiatrist may suggest or ask about something that has not been introduced by the patient but that the psychiatrist surmises may be relevant.

PROBING.   The interview may point toward an area of conflict, but the patient may minimize or deny any difficulties. Gently encouraging the patient to talk more about this issue may be quite productive.

TRANSITIONS.   Sometimes transitions occur very smoothly. The patient is talking about her primary education major in college and the psychiatrist asks, "*Did that lead to your work after college?*" On other occasions, the transition means moving to a different area of the interview, and a bridge statement is useful.

REDIRECTING.   A difficult technique for unseasoned interviewers is redirecting the focus of the patient. If the interviewer is concentrating on reinforcing the patient's telling of his or her story, it can be especially difficult to move the interview in a different direction. However, this is often crucial to a successful interview because of the time constraints and the necessity to obtain a broad overview of the patient's life as well as the current problems. Also, the patient may, for conscious or often unconscious reasons, avoid certain important areas, and need guidance in approaching these subjects. Redirection can be used when the patient changes the topic or when the patient continues to focus on a nonproductive or well-covered area.

Obstructive Interventions.   Although supportive and expanding techniques facilitate the gathering of information and the development of a positive patient–doctor relationship, several other interventions are not helpful for either task. Some of these activities are in the same categories as the more useful interventions but are unclear, unconnected, poorly timed, and not responsive to the patient's issues or concerns.

CLOSED-ENDED QUESTIONS.   A series of closed-ended questions early in the interview can retard the natural flow of the patient's story and reinforces the patient giving one word or brief answers with little or no elaboration.

A patient can be a partner in the interview unless the psychiatrist blocks them. Many patients, some of whom have previous experiences in therapy, come prepared to talk about even painful matters. Over time, psychiatrists, especially if they have had the benefit of supervision, learn from patients, and refine their interviewing skills.

COMPOUND QUESTIONS.   Some questions are difficult for patients to respond to because more than one answer is being sought.

WHY QUESTIONS.   Especially early in the psychiatric interview, "why" questions are often nonproductive. Very often, the answer to that question is one of the reasons that the patient has sought help.

JUDGMENTAL QUESTIONS OR STATEMENTS.   Judgmental interventions are generally nonproductive for the issue at hand and also inhibit the patient from sharing even more private or sensitive material. Instead of telling a patient that particular behavior was right or wrong, it would be better for the psychiatrist to help the patient reflect on how successful that behavior was.

MINIMIZING PATIENT'S CONCERNS.   In an attempt to reassure patients, psychiatrists sometimes make the error of minimizing a concern. This can be counterproductive in that rather than being reassured, and the patient may feel that the psychiatrist does not understand what he or she is trying to express. It is much more productive to explore the concern; there is likely much more material that has not yet been shared.

PREMATURE ADVICE.   Advice given too early is often bad advice because the interviewer does not yet know all of the variables. Also, it can preempt the patient from arriving at a plan for himself or herself.

PREMATURE INTERPRETATION.   Even if it is accurate, a premature interpretation can be counterproductive as the patient may respond defensively and feel misunderstood.

TRANSITIONS.   Some transitions are too abrupt and may interrupt essential issues that the patient is discussing.

NONVERBAL COMMUNICATION.   The psychiatrist that repeatedly looks at a watch turns away from the patient, yawns, or refreshes the computer screen conveys boredom, disinterest, or annoyance. Just as reinforcing nonverbal communications can be powerful facilitators of a good interview, these obstructive actions can quickly shatter an interview and undermine the patient–doctor relationship.

Closing of Interview.   The last 5 to 10 minutes of the interview are crucial and are often not given sufficient attention by inexperienced interviewers. It is essential to alert the patient to the remaining time: "*We have to stop in about 10 minutes.*" Not infrequently, a patient will have kept an important issue or question until the end of the interview, and having at least a brief time to identify the issue is helpful. If there is to be another session, then the psychiatrist can indicate that this issue will be addressed at the beginning of the next session or ask the patient to bring it up at that time. If the patient repeatedly brings up important information at the end of sessions, then this should be explored as to its meaning. If the patient spontaneously brings up no such item, then it can be useful to ask the patient if any other issues have not been covered that the patient wanted to share. If such an issue can be dealt with in short order, then it should be; if not, then it can be put on the agenda for the next session. It can also be useful to allow the patient to ask a question: "*I've asked you a lot of questions today. Are there any other questions you'd like to ask me at this point?*"

If this interview was to be a single evaluative session, then a summary of the diagnosis and options for treatment should generally be shared with the patient (exceptions may be a disability or forensic evaluation for which it was established at the outset that a report would be made to the referring entity). If a primary care physician referred the patient, then the psychiatrist also indicates that he or she will communicate with the primary care physician and share the findings and recommendations. If this was not to be a single session and the patient will be seen again, then the psychiatrist may indicate that he or she and the patient can work further on the treatment plan in the next session. A mutually agreed upon time is arrived at, and the patient is escorted to the door.

Motivational Interviewing.   Motivational interviewing is a technique used to motivate the patient to change his or her maladaptive behavior. The therapist relies on empathy to convey understanding, provides support by noting the patient's strengths, and explores the ambivalence and conflicting thoughts or feelings the patient may have about change. Guidance is provided in the interview by imparting information about issues (e.g., alcoholism, diabetes) while at the same time getting the patient to talk about resistances to altering behavior. It has been used effectively in persons with substance use disorders to get them to join AA, to help change lifestyles, or to enter psychotherapy. It has the potential to combine diagnosis and therapy in a single interview with the patient and can be applied to a wide range of mental disorders.

Medical Record

Most psychiatrists take notes throughout the interview. Generally, these are not verbatim recordings, except for the chief complaint or other key statements. Many psychiatrists use a form that covers the basic elements in the psychiatric evaluation. Occasionally, patients may have questions or concerns about note-taking. These concerns, which often have to do with confidentiality, should be discussed (and during this discussion, notes should not be taken). After the discussion, it is rare for a patient to insist that notes not be taken. It is much more common for patients to feel comfortable about the note-taking, feeling reassured that their experiences and feelings are important enough to be written. However, too much attention to the record can be distracting. Eye contact must be maintained as much as possible during the note-taking. Otherwise, patients will feel that the record is more important than what they are saying. Also, the interviewer may miss nonverbal communications that can be more important than the words being recorded.

Increasingly, the electronic health record (EHR) is now being used throughout medicine. There are great advantages of computerized records, including rapid retrieval of information, appropriately sharing data among various members of the health care team, access to important data in an emergency, decreasing errors, and as a tool for research and quality improvement activities. Evidence-based practice guidelines can also be integrated with EHRs so that information or recommendations can be provided at the point of service. However, the use of computers can also present significant challenges to the developing patient–physician relationship. Frequently, physicians using computers during an interview will turn away from the patient to enter data. Especially in a psychiatric interview, this can be very disruptive to a smooth and dynamic interaction. As improved technology becomes more widespread (e.g., the use of notepads held in the lap) and psychiatrists become more accustomed to using the equipment, some of these disruptions can be minimized.

Cultural Issues

Culture can be defined as a common heritage, a set of beliefs, and values that set expectations for behaviors, thoughts, and even feelings. Several culture-bound syndromes that are unique to a particular population have been described (see Chapter 34). Culture can influence the presentation of illness, the decision when and where to seek care, the decision as to what to share with the physician, and the acceptance of and participation in treatment planning. Often, individuals from a minority population may be reluctant to seek help from a physician who is from the majority group, especially for emotional difficulties. Some minority groups have strong beliefs in faith healers, and in some areas of the US "root doctors" carry significant influence. These beliefs may not be apparent in the interview as the patient may have learned to be quite guarded about such matters. A patient may only report that he or she is "frightened" and not discuss the reality that this fear began when he or she realized someone was working "roots" on him or her. The psychiatrist needs to be alert to the possibility that the patient's thoughts about what has happened may be unusual from a traditional Western medical perspective and at the same time recognize that these culturally shared beliefs are not indications of psychosis. By being humble, open, and respectful the psychiatrist increases the possibility of developing a trusting working relationship with the patient and learning more about the patient's actual experiences.

The psychiatrist clearly understanding what the patient is saying, and the patient clearly understanding what the psychiatrist is saying are crucial for an effective interview. It is not just both being fluent in the language of the interview, but the psychiatrist should also be aware of common slang words and phrases that the patient, depending on their cultural background, may use. If the psychiatrist does not understand a particular phrase or comment, then he or she should ask for clarification. If the patient and psychiatrist are not both fluent in the same language, then an interpreter is necessary.

Interviewing with an Interpreter.   When translation is needed, it should be provided by a non–family-member professional interpreter. Translation by family members is to be avoided because (1) a patient, with a family member as an interpreter, may justifiably be very reluctant to discuss sensitive issues, including suicidal ideation or drug use, and (2) family members may be hesitant to portray a patient's deficits accurately. Both of these issues make accurate assessment very difficult.

It is helpful to speak with the interpreter before the interview to clarify the goals of the exam. If the interpreter does not primarily work with psychiatric patients, then it is important to highlight the need for verbatim translation even if the responses are disorganized or tangential. If the translator is not aware of this issue, then the psychiatrist may have difficulty diagnosing thought disorders or cognitive deficits. Occasionally, the patient will say several sentences in response to a question, and the interpreter will remark, "He said it's okay." The interpreter should again be reminded that the psychiatrist wants to hear everything that the patient is saying.

It is helpful to place the chairs in a triangle so that the psychiatrist and patient can maintain eye contact. The psychiatrist should continue to refer to the patient directly to maintain the therapeutic connection rather than speaking to the interpreter. The examiner may need to take a more directive approach and interrupt the patient's responses more frequently to allow for accurate and timely translation.

Once the interview is concluded, it may be helpful to again meet briefly with the interpreter. If the interpreter is especially knowledgeable about the patient's cultural background, they may be able to provide helpful insights regarding cultural norms.

Interviewing the Difficult Patient

Patients with Psychosis. Patients with psychotic illnesses are often frightened and guarded. They may have difficulty with reasoning and thinking clearly. Also, they may be actively hallucinating during the interview, causing them to be inattentive and distracted. They may have suspicions regarding the purpose of the interview. All of these possibilities are reasons that the interviewer may need to alter the usual format and adapt the interview to match the capacity and tolerance of the patient.

Auditory hallucinations are the most common hallucinations in psychiatric illnesses in North America. Many patients will not interpret their experiences as hallucinations, and it is useful to begin with a more general question: "*Do you ever hear someone talking to you when no one else is there?*" The patient should be asked about the content of the hallucinations, the clarity, and the situations in which they occur. Often it is helpful to ask the patient about a specific instance and if he or she can repeat verbatim the content of the hallucination. It is important to specifically ask if the patient has ever experienced command hallucinations, hallucinations in which a patient is ordered to perform a specific act. If so, the nature of the commands should be clarified, specifically if the commands have ever included orders to harm himself or herself or others, and if the patient has ever felt compelled to follow the commands.

The validity of the patient's perception should not be dismissed, but it is helpful to test the strength of the belief in the hallucinations: "*Does it seem that the voices are coming from inside your head? Who do you think is speaking to you?*"

Other perceptual disturbances should be explored, including visual, olfactory, and tactile hallucinations. These disturbances are less common in psychiatric illness and may suggest a primary medical etiology to the psychosis.

The psychiatrist should be alert for cues that psychotic processes may be part of the patient's experience during the interview. It is usually best to ask directly about such behaviors or comments.

By definition, patients with delusions have fixed false beliefs. With delusions, as with hallucinations, it is important to explore the specific details. Patients are often very reluctant to discuss their beliefs, as many have had their beliefs dismissed or ridiculed. They may ask the interviewer directly if the interviewer believes the delusion. Although an interviewer should not directly endorse the false belief, it is rarely helpful to challenge the delusion, particularly in the initial examination directly. It can be useful to shift the attention back to the patient's rather than the examiner's beliefs and

acknowledge the need for more information: "*I believe that what you are experiencing is frightening and I would like to know more about your experiences.*"

For patients with paranoid thoughts and behaviors, it is important to maintain a respectful distance. Their suspiciousness may be increased by an overly warm interview. It may be helpful to avoid sustained direct eye contact, as this may be perceived as threatening. Harry Stack Sullivan recommended that rather than sitting face to face with the patient who is paranoid, the psychiatrist might sit more side by side, "looking out" with the patient. Interviewers should keep in mind that they themselves may become incorporated into the paranoid delusions, and it is helpful to ask directly about such fears: "*Are you concerned that I am involved?*" The psychiatrist should also ask whether there is a specific target related to paranoid thinking. When asked regarding thoughts about hurting others, the patient may not disclose plans for violence. Exploration of the patient's plan on how to manage his or her fears may elicit information regarding violence risk: "*Do you feel you need to protect yourself in any way? How do you plan to do so?*" If there is some expression of possible violence toward others, the psychiatrist then needs to do further risk assessment. This is further discussed in the section below on hostile, agitated, and violent patients.

Depressed and Potentially Suicidal Patients. The depressed patient may have particular difficulty during the interview as he or she may have cognitive deficits as a result of the depressive symptoms. The patients may have impaired motivation and may not spontaneously report their symptoms. Feelings of hopelessness may contribute to a lack of engagement. Depending on the severity of symptoms, patients may need more direct questioning rather than an open-ended format.

A suicide assessment should be performed for all patients, including prior history, family history of suicide attempts and completed suicides, and current ideation, plan, and intent. An open-ended approach is often helpful: "*Have you ever had thoughts that life wasn't worth living?*" It is important to detail prior attempts. The lethality risk of prior attempts and any potential triggers for the attempt should be clarified. This can help with assessing the current risk.

The patient should be asked about any current thoughts of suicide, and if thoughts are present, what is the patient's intent. Some patients will describe having thoughts of suicide but do not intend to act on these thoughts or wish to be dead. They report that although the thoughts are present, they have no intent to act on the thoughts. This is typically referred to as passive suicidal ideation. Other patients will express their determination to end their life and are at higher risk. The presence of psychotic symptoms should be assessed. Some patients may have hallucinations compelling them to hurt themselves even though they do not have a desire to die.

If the patient reports suicidal ideation, they should be asked if they have a plan to end his or her life. The specificity of the plan should be determined and whether the patient has access to the means to complete the plan. The interviewer should pursue this line of questioning in detail if the patient has taken any preparatory steps to move forward with the plan. (A patient who has purchased a gun and has given away important items would be at high risk.)

If the patient has not acted upon these urges, then it is helpful to ask what has prevented him or her from acting on these thoughts: "*What do you think has kept you from hurting yourself?*" The patient may disclose information that may decrease their acute risk, such as religious beliefs that prohibit suicide or awareness of the impact of suicide on family members. This information is essential to keep in mind during treatment especially if these preventative factors change. (A patient who states he or she could never abandon a beloved pet may be at increased risk if the pet dies.)

Although the psychiatric interview intends to build rapport and gather information for treatment and diagnosis, the patient's safety must be the priority. If the patient is viewed to be at imminent risk, then an interview may need to be terminated, and the interviewer must take action to secure the safety of the patient.

Hostile, Agitated, and Potentially Violent Patients.   Safety for the patient and the psychiatrist is the priority when interviewing agitated patients. Hostile patients are often interviewed in emergency settings, but angry and agitated patients can present in any setting. If interviewing in an unfamiliar setting, then the psychiatrist should familiarize himself or herself with the office setup, paying particular attention to the chair placement. The chairs should ideally be placed in a way in which both the interviewer and patient could exit if necessary and not be obstructed. The psychiatrist should be aware of any available safety features (emergency buttons or number for security) and should be familiar with the facility's security plan. If the psychiatrist is aware in advance that the patient is agitated, then he or she can take additional preparatory steps such as having security closely available if necessary.

As increased stimulation can be agitating for a hostile patient, care should be taken to decrease excess stimulation as much as feasible. The psychiatrist should be aware of their own body position and avoid postures that could be seen as threatening, including clenched hands or hands behind the back.

The psychiatrist should approach the interview in a calm, direct manner and take care not to bargain or promise to elicit cooperation in the interview: "*Once we finish here, you will be able to go home.*" These tactics may only escalate agitation.

As stated above, the priority must be safety. An intimidated psychiatrist who is fearful regarding his or her physical safety will be unable to perform an adequate assessment. Similarly, a patient who feels threatened will be unable to focus on the interview and may begin to escalate thinking that he or she needs to defend himself or herself. An interview may need to be terminated early if the patient's agitation escalates. Generally, unpremeditated violence is preceded by a period of gradually escalating psychomotor agitation such as pacing, loud speech, and threatening comments. At this point, the psychiatrist should consider whether other measures are necessary, including assistance from security personnel or need for medication or restraint.

If the patient makes threats or gives some indication that he or she may become violent outside the interview setting, then further assessment is necessary. Because a past history of violence is the best predictor of future violence, past episodes of violence should be explored as to setting, what precipitated the episode, and what was the outcome or potential outcome (if the act was interrupted). Also, what has helped in the past in preventing violent episodes (medication, timeout, physical activity, or talking to a particular person) should be explored. Is there an identified victim and is there a plan for the violent behavior? Has the patient taken steps to fulfill the plan? Depending on the answers to these questions the psychiatrist may decide to prescribe or increase antipsychotic medication, recommend hospitalization, and perhaps, depending on the jurisdiction, notify the threatened victim.

Deceptive Patients.   Psychiatrists are trained to diagnose and treat psychiatric illness. Although psychiatrists are well trained in eliciting information and maintaining awareness for deception, these abilities are not foolproof. Patients lie or deceive their psychiatrists for many different reasons. Some are motivated by secondary gain (e.g., for financial resources, absence from work, or for a supply of medication). Some patients may deceive, not for an external advantage, but for the psychological benefits of assuming a sick role. As noted above, unconscious processes may result in events or feelings being outside the patient's awareness.

There are no current biologic markers to validate a patient's symptoms definitively. Psychiatrists are dependent on the patient's self-report. Given these limitations, it may be useful, especially when there is a question about the patient's reliability (possibly related to inconsistencies in the patient's report), to gather collateral information regarding the patient. This allows the psychiatrist to have a more broad understanding of the patient outside the interview setting, and discrepancies in symptom severity between self-report and collateral information may suggest deception. Some psychological tests can help in further evaluating the reliability of the patient.

PHYSICAL EXAMINATION OF THE PSYCHIATRIC PATIENT

Confronted with a patient who has a mental disorder, the psychiatrist must decide whether a medical, surgical, or neurologic condition may be the cause. Once satisfied that no disease process can be held accountable, then the diagnosis of mental disorder not attributable to a medical illness can be made. Although psychiatrists do not perform routine physical examinations of their patients, knowledge, and understanding of physical signs and symptoms is part of their training, which enables them to recognize signs and symptoms that may indicate possible medical or surgical illness. For example, palpitations can be associated with mitral valve prolapse, which is diagnosed by cardiac auscultation. Psychiatrists are also able to recognize and treat the adverse effects of psychotropic medications, which are used by an increasing number of patients seen by psychiatrists and nonpsychiatric physicians.

Some psychiatrists insist that every patient has a complete medical workup; others may not. Whatever their policy, psychiatrists should consider patients' medical status at the outset of a psychiatric evaluation. Psychiatrists must often decide whether a patient needs a medical examination and, if so, what it should include—most commonly, a thorough medical history, including a review of systems, a physical examination, and relevant diagnostic laboratory studies. A recent study of 1,000 medical patients found that in 75 percent of cases, no cause of symptoms (i.e., subjective complaints) could be found, and a psychological basis was assumed in 10 percent of those cases.

History of Medical Illness

In the course of conducting a psychiatric evaluation, the information should be gathered about known bodily diseases or dysfunctions, hospitalizations and operative procedures, medications are taken recently or at present, personal habits and occupational history, family history of illnesses, and specific physical complaints. Information about medical illnesses should be gathered from the patient, the referring physician, and the family, if necessary.

Information about previous episodes of illness may provide valuable clues about the nature of the present disorder. For example, a distinctly delusional disorder in a patient with a history of several similar episodes that responded promptly to diverse forms of treatment strongly suggests the possibility of substance-induced psychotic disorder. To pursue this lead, the psychiatrist should order a drug screen. The history of a surgical procedure may also be useful; for instance, a thyroidectomy suggests hypothyroidism as the cause of depression.

Depression is an adverse effect of several medications prescribed for hypertension. Medication taken in a therapeutic dosage occasionally reaches high concentrations in the blood. Digitalis intoxication, for example, can occur under such circumstances and result in impaired mental functioning. Proprietary drugs can cause or contribute to an anticholinergic delirium. The psychiatrist, therefore, must inquire about over-the-counter remedies as well as prescribed medications. A history of herbal intake and alternative therapy is essential, given their increased use.

An occupational history may also provide essential information. Exposure to mercury can result in complaints suggesting a psychosis, and exposure to lead, as in smelting, can produce a cognitive disorder. The latter clinical picture can also result from imbibing moonshine whiskey with high lead content.

In eliciting information about specific symptoms, the psychiatrist brings medical and psychological knowledge into full play. For example, the psychiatrist should elicit sufficient information from the patient complaining of headaches to predict whether the pain results from an intracranial disease that requires neurologic testing. Also, the psychiatrist should be able to recognize that the pain in the right shoulder of a hypochondriacal patient with abdominal discomfort may be the classic referred pain of gallbladder disease.

Review of Systems

An inventory by systems should follow the open-ended inquiry. The review can be organized according to organ systems (e.g., liver, pancreas), functional systems (e.g., gastrointestinal), or a combination of the two, as in the outline presented in the following subsections. In all cases, the review should be comprehensive and thorough. Even if a psychiatric component is suspected, a complete workup is still indicated.

Head.   Many patients give a history of headache; its duration, frequency, character, location, and severity should be ascertained. Headaches often result from substance abuse, including alcohol, nicotine, and caffeine. Vascular (migraine) headaches are precipitated by stress. Temporal arteritis causes unilateral throbbing headaches and can lead to blindness. Brain tumors are associated with headaches as a result of increased intracranial pressure, but some may be silent, the first signs being a change in personality or cognition.

> A 63-year-old woman in treatment for depression began to complain of difficulties in concentration. The psychiatrist attributed the complaint to the depressive disorder; however, when the patient began to complain of balance difficulties, magnetic resonance imaging was obtained, which revealed the presence of meningioma.

A head injury can result in subdural hematoma and, in boxers, can cause progressive dementia with extrapyramidal symptoms. The headache of subarachnoid hemorrhage is sudden, severe, and associated with changes in the sensorium. Normal-pressure hydrocephalus can follow a head injury or encephalitis and be associated with dementia, shuffling gait, and urinary incontinence. Dizziness occurs in up to 30 percent of persons, and determining its cause is challenging and often complicated. A change in the size or shape of the head may be indicative of Paget disease.

Eye, Ear, Nose, and Throat.   Visual acuity, diplopia, hearing problems, tinnitus, glossitis, and bad taste are covered in this area. A patient taking antipsychotics who gives a history of twitching about the mouth or disturbing movements of the tongue may be in the early and potentially reversible stage of tardive dyskinesia. Impaired vision can occur with thioridazine (Mellaril) in high doses (over 800 mg a day). A history of glaucoma contraindicates drugs with anticholinergic effects. Complaints of bad odors may be a symptom of temporal lobe epilepsy rather than schizophrenia. Aphonia may be hysterical. The late stage of cocaine abuse can result in perforations of the nasal septum and difficulty breathing. A transitory episode of diplopia may herald multiple sclerosis. Delusional disorder is more common in hard of hearing persons than in those with normal hearing. Transient blue-tinged vision can occur when using sildenafil (Viagra) or similar drugs.

Respiratory System.   Cough, asthma, pleurisy, hemoptysis, dyspnea, and orthopnea are considered in this subsection. Hyperventilation is suggested if the patient's symptoms include all or a few of the following: onset at rest, sighing respirations, apprehension, anxiety, depersonalization, palpitations, inability to swallow, numbness of the feet and hands, and carpopedal spasm. Dyspnea and breathlessness can occur in depression. In pulmonary or obstructive airway disease, the onset of symptoms is usually insidious, whereas, in depression, it is sudden. In depression, breathlessness is experienced at rest, shows little change with exertion, and can fluctuate within a matter of minutes; the onset of breathlessness coincides with the onset of a mood disorder and is often accompanied by attacks of dizziness, sweating, palpitations, and paresthesias.

In obstructive airway disease, patients with the most advanced respiratory incapacity experience breathlessness at rest. Most striking and of greatest assistance in making a differential diagnosis is an emphasis placed on the difficulty in inspiration experienced by patients with depression and on the difficulty in expiration experienced by patients with pulmonary disease. Bronchial asthma has sometimes been associated with a childhood history of extreme dependence on the mother. Patients with bronchospasm should not receive propranolol (Inderal) because it can block catecholamine-induced bronchodilation; propranolol is specifically contraindicated for patients with bronchial asthma because epinephrine given to such patients in an emergency will not be effective. Patients taking angiotensin-converting enzyme (ACE) inhibitors can develop a dry cough as an adverse effect of the drug.

Cardiovascular System.   Tachycardia, palpitations, and cardiac arrhythmia are among the most common signs of anxiety about which the patient may complain. Pheochromocytoma usually produces symptoms that mimic anxiety disorders, such as rapid heartbeat, tremors, and pallor. Increased urinary catecholamines are diagnostic of pheochromocytoma. Patients taking guanethidine (Ismelin) for hypertension should not receive tricyclic drugs, which reduce or eliminate the antihypertensive effect of guanethidine. A history of hypertension can preclude the use of MAOIs because of the risk of a hypertensive crisis if such patients with hypertension inadvertently ingest foods high in tyramine. Patients with suspected cardiac disease should have an electrocardiogram before tricyclics or lithium (Eskalith) is prescribed. A history of substernal pain should be evaluated, and the clinician should keep in mind that psychological stress can precipitate angina-type chest pain in the presence of normal coronary arteries. Patients taking opioids should never receive MAOIs; the combination can cause cardiovascular collapse.

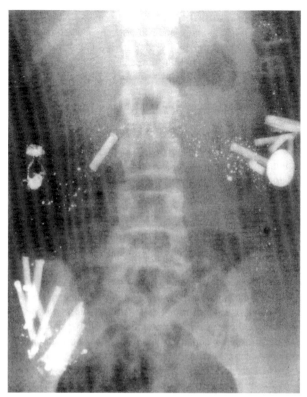

FIGURE 1-1

A mentally ill patient who is a habitual swallower of foreign objects. Included in his colonic lumen are 13 thermometers and 8 pennies. The dense, round, almost punctate densities are globules of liberated liquid mercury. (Courtesy of Stephen R. Baker, M.D. and Kyunghee C. Cho, M.D.)

Gastrointestinal System. Such topics as appetite, distress before or after meals, food preferences, diarrhea, vomiting, constipation, laxative use, and abdominal pain relate to the gastrointestinal system. A history of weight loss is common in depressive disorders, but depression can accompany the weight loss caused by ulcerative colitis, regional enteritis, and cancer. Atypical depression is accompanied by hyperphagia and weight gain. Anorexia nervosa is accompanied by severe weight loss in the presence of normal appetite. Avoidance of certain foods may be a phobic phenomenon or part of an obsessive ritual. Laxative abuse and induced vomiting are common in bulimia nervosa. Constipation can be caused by opioid dependence and psychotropic drugs with anticholinergic side effects. Cocaine or amphetamine abuse causes a loss of appetite and weight loss. Weight gain can occur under stress or in association with atypical depression. Polyphagia, polyuria, and polydipsia are the triad of diabetes mellitus. Polyuria, polydipsia, and diarrhea are signs of lithium toxicity. Some patients take enemas routinely as part of paraphilic behavior, and anal fissures or recurrent hemorrhoids may indicate anal penetration by foreign objects. Some patients may ingest foreign objects that produce symptoms that can be diagnosed only by x-ray (Fig. 1-1).

Genitourinary System. Urinary frequency, nocturia, pain or burning on urination, and changes in the size and the force of the stream are some of the signs and symptoms emanating from the genitourinary system. Anticholinergic adverse effects associated with antipsychotics and tricyclic drugs can cause urinary retention in men with prostate hypertrophy. Erectile difficulty and retarded ejaculation are also common adverse effects of these drugs, and

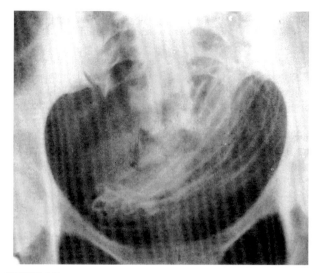

FIGURE 1-2

A patient brought to the emergency room with lower abdominal pain. X-ray shows a nasogastric tube folded into the bladder. The patient would insert the tube into his urethra as part of a masturbatory ritual (urethral eroticism). (Courtesy of Stephen R. Baker, M.D. and Kyunghee C. Cho, M.D.)

retrograde ejaculation occurs with thioridazine. A baseline level of sexual responsiveness before using pharmacologic agents should be obtained. A history of STDs—for example, gonorrheal discharge, chancre, herpes, and pubic lice—may indicate sexual promiscuity or unsafe sexual practices.

In some cases, the first symptom of acquired immune deficiency syndrome (AIDS) is the gradual onset of mental confusion leading to dementia. Incontinence should be evaluated carefully, and if it persists, further investigation for more extensive disease should include a workup for HIV infection. Drugs with anticholinergic adverse effects should be avoided in men with prostatism. Urethral eroticism, in which catheters or other objects are inserted into the urethra, can cause infection or laceration (Fig. 1-2).

Orgasm causes prostatic contractions, which may artificially raise prostate-specific antigen (PSA) and give a false-positive result for prostatic cancer. Men scheduled to have a PSA test should avoid masturbation or coitus for 7 to 10 days before the test.

Menstrual History. A menstrual history should include the age of the onset of menarche (and menopause, if applicable); the interval, regularity, duration, and amount of flow of periods; irregular bleeding; dysmenorrhea; and abortions. Amenorrhea is characteristic of anorexia nervosa and also occurs in women who are psychologically stressed. Women who are afraid of becoming pregnant or who have a wish to be pregnant may have delayed periods. *Pseudocyesis* is false pregnancy with complete cessation of the menses. Perimenstrual mood changes (e.g., irritability, depression, and dysphoria) should be noted. Painful menstruation can result from uterine disease (e.g., myomata), from psychological conflicts about the menses, or from a combination of the two. Some women report a perimenstrual increase in sexual desire. The emotional reaction associated with abortion should be explored because it can be mild or severe.

General Observation

An important part of the medical examination is subsumed under the broad heading of general observation—visual, auditory, and olfactory. Such nonverbal clues as posture, facial expression, and mannerisms should also be noted.

Visual Inspection.   Scrutiny of the patient begins at the first encounter. When the patient goes from the waiting room to the interview room, the psychiatrist should observe the patient's gait. Is the patient unsteady? Ataxia suggests diffuse brain disease, alcohol or other substance intoxication, chorea, spinocerebellar degeneration, weakness based on a debilitating process, and an underlying disorder, such as myotonic dystrophy. Does the patient walk without the usual associated arm movements and turn in a rigid fashion, such as a toy soldier, as is seen in early Parkinson disease? Does the patient have asymmetry of gait, such as turning one foot outward, dragging a leg, or not swinging one arm, suggesting a focal brain lesion?

As soon as the patient is seated, the psychiatrist should direct attention to grooming. Is the patient's hair combed, are the nails clean, and are the teeth brushed? Has clothing been chosen with care and is it appropriate? Although inattention to dress and hygiene is common in mental disorders—in particular, depressive disorders—it is also a hallmark of cognitive disorders. Lapses, such as mismatching socks, stockings, or shoes, may suggest a cognitive disorder.

The patient's posture and automatic movements or the lack of them should be noted. A stooped, flexed posture with a paucity of automatic movements may be caused by Parkinson disease or diffuse cerebral hemispheric disease or be an adverse effect of antipsychotics. An unusual tilt of the head may be adopted to avoid eye contact, but it can also result from diplopia, a visual field defect, or focal cerebellar dysfunction. Frequent quick, purposeless movements are characteristic of anxiety disorders, but they are equally characteristic of chorea and hyperthyroidism. Tremors, although commonly seen in anxiety disorders, may point to Parkinson disease, essential tremor, or adverse effects of psychotropic medication. Patients with essential tremor sometimes seek psychiatric treatment because they believe the tremor must be caused by unrecognized fear or anxiety, as others often suggest. Unilateral paucity or excess of movement suggests focal brain disease.

The patient's appearance is then scrutinized to assess general health. Does the patient appear to be robust or is there a sense of ill health? Does looseness of clothing indicate recent weight loss? Is the patient short of breath or coughing? Does the patient's general physiognomy suggest a specific disease? Men with Klinefelter syndrome have a feminine fat distribution and lack the development of secondary male sex characteristics. Acromegaly is usually immediately recognizable by the large head and jaw.

What is the patient's nutritional status? Recent weight loss, although often seen in depressive disorders and schizophrenia, may be caused by gastrointestinal disease, diffuse carcinomatosis, Addison disease, hyperthyroidism, and many other somatic disorders. Obesity can result from either emotional distress or organic disease. Moon facies, truncal obesity, and buffalo hump are striking findings in Cushing syndrome. The puffy, bloated appearance seen in hypothyroidism and the massive obesity and periodic respiration seen in Pickwickian syndrome are easily recognized in patients referred for psychiatric help. Hyperthyroidism is indicated by exophthalmos.

The skin frequently provides valuable information. The yellow discoloration of hepatic dysfunction and the pallor of anemia are reasonably distinctive. Intense reddening may be caused by carbon monoxide poisoning or by photosensitivity resulting from porphyria or phenothiazines. Eruptions can be manifestations of such disorders as SLE (e.g., the butterfly on the face), tuberous sclerosis with adenoma sebaceum, and sensitivity to drugs. A dusky purplish cast to the face, plus telangiectasia, is almost pathognomonic of alcohol abuse.

Careful observation may reveal clues that lead to the correct diagnosis in patients who create their skin lesions. For example, the location and shape of the lesions and the time of their appearance may be characteristic of dermatitis factitia.

The patient's face and head should be scanned for evidence of disease. Premature whitening of the hair occurs in pernicious anemia, and thinning and coarseness of the hair occur in myxedema. In alopecia areata, patches of hair are lost, leaving bald spots; hair-pulling disorder (trichotillomania) presents a similar picture. Pupillary changes are produced by various drugs—constriction by opioids and dilation by anticholinergic agents and hallucinogens. The combination of dilated and fixed pupils and dry skin and mucous membranes should immediately suggest the likelihood of atropine use or atropine-like toxicity. The diffusion of the conjunctiva suggests alcohol abuse, cannabis abuse, or obstruction of the superior vena cava. Flattening of the nasolabial fold on one side or weakness of one side of the face—as manifested in speaking, smiling, and grimacing—may be the result of focal dysfunction of the contralateral cerebral hemisphere or Bell palsy. A drooping eyelid may be an early sign of myasthenia gravis.

The patient's state of alertness and responsiveness should be evaluated carefully. A psychological problem may cause drowsiness and inattentiveness, but they are more likely to result from organic brain dysfunction, whether secondary to an intrinsic brain disease or an exogenous factor, such as substance intoxication.

Listening.   Listening intently is just as important as looking intently for evidence of somatic disorders. Slowed speech is characteristic not only of depression but also of diffuse brain dysfunction and subcortical dysfunction; unusually rapid speech is characteristic of manic episodes and anxiety disorders and also of hyperthyroidism. A weak voice with a monotonous tone may be a clue to Parkinson disease in patients who complain mainly of depression. A slow, low-pitched, hoarse voice should suggest the possibility of hypothyroidism; this voice quality has been described as sounding like a drowsy, slightly intoxicated person with a bad cold and a plum in the mouth. A soft or tremulous voice accompanies anxiety.

Difficulty initiating speech may be owing to anxiety or stuttering or may indicate Parkinson disease or aphasia. Easy fatigability of speech is sometimes a manifestation of an emotional problem, but it is also characteristic of myasthenia gravis. Patients with these complaints are likely to be seen by a psychiatrist before the correct diagnosis is made.

Word production, as well as the quality of speech, is important. Mispronounced or incorrectly used words suggest a possibility of aphasia caused by a lesion of the dominant hemisphere. The same possibility exists when the patient perseverates, has trouble finding a name or a word, or describes an object or an event in an indirect fashion (paraphasia). When not consonant with patients' socioeconomic and educational levels, coarseness, profanity, or inappropriate disclosures may indicate loss of inhibition caused by dementia.

Smell.   Smell may also provide useful information. The unpleasant odor of a patient who fails to bathe suggests a cognitive or a depressive disorder. The odor of alcohol or substances used to hide it is revealing in a patient who attempts to conceal a drinking problem. Occasionally, a uriniferous odor calls attention to bladder dysfunction secondary to a nervous system disease. Characteristic odors are also noted in patients with diabetic acidosis, flatulence, uremia, and hepatic coma. Precocious puberty can be associated with the smell of adult sweat produced by mature apocrine glands.

A 23-year-old woman was referred to a psychiatrist for a second opinion. She had been diagnosed 6 months earlier with schizophrenia after complaining of smelling foul odors that were considered to be hallucinatory. She had been placed on antipsychotic medication (perphenazine) and was compliant despite the side effects of tremor and lethargy. Although there was some improvement in her symptoms, they did not remit entirely. The consulting psychiatrist obtained an electroencephalogram, which showed abnormal waveforms consistent with a diagnosis of temporal lobe epilepsy. The antipsychotic medication was replaced with an anticonvulsant (phenytoin), after which she no longer experienced an olfactory hallucination, nor did she have to endure the unpleasant side effects of the previous medication.

Physical Examination

Patient Selection. The nature of the patient's complaints is critical in determining whether a complete physical examination is required. Complaints fall into the three categories of body, mind, and social interactions. Bodily symptoms (e.g., headaches and palpitations) call for a thorough medical examination to determine what part if any, somatic processes play in causing the distress. The same can be said for mental symptoms such as depression, anxiety, hallucinations, and persecutory delusions, which can be expressions of somatic processes. If the problem is limited to the social sphere (e.g., long-standing difficulties in interactions with teachers, employers, parents, or a spouse), there may be no particular indication for a physical examination. Personality changes, however, can result from a medical disorder (e.g., early Alzheimer disease) and cause interpersonal conflicts.

Psychological Factors. Even a routine physical examination may evoke adverse reactions; instruments, procedures, and the examining room may be frightening. A simple running account of what is being done can prevent much needless anxiety. Moreover, if the patient is consistently forewarned of what will be done, the dread of being suddenly and painfully surprised recedes. Comments such as "There's nothing to this" and "You don't have to be afraid because this won't hurt" leave the patient in the dark and are much less reassuring than a few words about what actually will be done.

Although the physical examination is likely to engender or intensify a reaction of anxiety, it can also stir up sexual feelings. Some women with fears or fantasies of being seduced may misinterpret an ordinary movement in the physical examination as a sexual advance. Similarly, a delusional man with homophobic fears may perceive a rectal examination as a sexual attack. Lingering over the examination of a particular organ because an unusual but normal variation has aroused the physician's scientific curiosity is likely to raise concern in the patient that a severe pathologic process has been discovered. Such a reaction may be profound in an anxious or hypochondriacal patient.

The physical examination occasionally serves a psychotherapeutic function. Anxious patients may be relieved to learn that, despite troublesome symptoms, no evidence is found of the serious illness that they fear. The young person who complains of chest pain and is confident that the pain heralds a heart attack can usually be reassured by the report of normal findings after a physical examination and electrocardiogram. The reassurance relieves only the worry occasioned by the immediate episode, however. Unless psychiatric treatment succeeds in dealing with the determinants of the reaction, recurrent episodes are likely.

Sending a patient who has a deeply rooted fear of malignancy for still another test that is intended to be reassuring is usually unrewarding. Some patients may have a false fixed belief that a disorder is present.

During the performance of the physical examination, an observant physician may note indications of emotional distress. For instance, during genital examinations, a patient's behavior may reveal information about sexual attitudes and problems, and these reactions can be used later to open this area for exploration.

Timing of the Physical Examination. Circumstances occasionally make it desirable or necessary to defer a complete medical assessment. For example, a delusional or manic patient may be combative, resistive, or both. In this instance, a medical history should be elicited from a family member, if possible, but unless a pressing reason exists to proceed with the examination, it should be deferred until the patient is tractable.

For psychological reasons, it may be ill-advised to recommend a medical assessment at the time of an initial office visit. Because of today's increased sensitivity and openness about sexual matters and a tendency to turn quickly to psychiatric help, young men may complain about their failure to consummate their first coital attempt. After taking a detailed history, the psychiatrist may conclude that the failure was because of situational anxiety. If so, neither a physical examination nor psychotherapy should be recommended; they would have the undesirable effect of reinforcing the notion of pathology. Should the problem be recurrent, further evaluation would be warranted.

Neurologic Examination. If the psychiatrist suspects that the patient has an underlying somatic disorder, such as diabetes mellitus or Cushing syndrome, a referral is usually made for diagnosis and treatment. The situation is different when a cognitive disorder is suspected. The psychiatrist often chooses to assume responsibility in these cases. At some point, however, a thorough neurologic evaluation may be indicated.

During the history-taking process in such cases, the patient's level of awareness, attentiveness to the details of the examination, understanding, facial expression, speech, posture, and gait are noted. It is also assumed that a thorough mental status examination will be performed. The neurologic examination is carried out with two objectives in mind: to elicit (1) signs pointing to focal, circumscribed cerebral dysfunction, and (2) signs suggesting diffuse, bilateral cerebral disease. The first objective is met by the routine neurologic examination, which is designed primarily to reveal asymmetries in the motor, perceptual, and reflex functions of the two sides of the body, caused by focal hemispheric disease. The second objective is met by seeking to elicit signs that have been attributed to diffuse brain dysfunction and to frontal lobe disease. These signs include the sucking, snout, palmomental, and grasp reflexes and the persistence of the glabella tap response. Regrettably, except for the grasp reflex, such signs do not correlate strongly with the presence of underlying brain pathology.

Other Findings. Psychiatrists should be able to evaluate the significance of findings uncovered by consultants. With a patient who complains of a lump in the throat (globus hystericus) and who is found on examination to have hypertrophied lymphoid tissue, it is tempting to wonder about a causal relation. How can a clinician be sure that the finding is not incidental? Has the patient been known to have hypertrophied lymphoid tissue at a time when no complaint was made? Do many persons with hypertrophied lymphoid tissue never experience the sensation of a lump in the throat?

With a patient with multiple sclerosis who complains of an inability to walk but, on neurologic examination, has only mild spasticity and a unilateral Babinski sign, it is tempting to ascribe the symptom to the neurologic disorder. However, the complaint may be aggravated by emotional distress. The same holds for a patient with profound dementia in whom a small frontal meningioma is seen on CT scan. Dementia is not always correlated with the findings. Significant brain atrophy could cause very mild dementia, and minimal brain atrophy could cause significant dementia.

A lesion is often found that can account for a symptom, but the psychiatrist should make every effort to separate an incidental finding from a causative one and to distinguish a lesion merely found in the area of the symptom from a lesion producing the symptom.

Patients Undergoing Psychiatric Treatment

While patients are being treated for psychiatric disorders, psychiatrists should be alert to the possibility of intercurrent illnesses that call for diagnostic studies. Patients in psychotherapy, particularly those in psychoanalysis, may be all too willing to ascribe their new symptoms to emotional causes. Attention should be given to the possible use of denial, especially if the symptoms seem to be unrelated to the conflicts currently in focus.

Not only may patients in psychotherapy be likely to attribute new symptoms to emotional causes, but sometimes their therapists do so as well. The danger of providing psychodynamic explanations for physical symptoms is ever-present.

Symptoms such as drowsiness and dizziness and signs such as a skin eruption and a gait disturbance, common adverse effects of psychotropic medication, call for a medical reevaluation if the patient fails to respond in a reasonable time to changes in the dose or the kind of medication prescribed. If patients who are receiving tricyclic or antipsychotic drugs complain of blurred vision (usually an anticholinergic adverse effect) and the condition does not recede with a reduction in dose or a change in medication, they should be evaluated to rule out other causes. In one case, the diagnosis proved to be toxoplasma chorioretinitis. The absence of other anticholinergic adverse effects, such as a dry mouth and constipation, is an additional clue alerting the psychiatrist to the possibility of a concomitant medical illness.

Early in the illness, there may be few, if any, positive physical or laboratory results. In such instances, especially if the evidence of psychic trauma or emotional conflicts is glaring, all symptoms are likely to be regarded as psychosocial in origin, and new symptoms are also seen in this light. Indications for repeating portions of the medical workup may be missed unless the psychiatrist is alert to clues suggesting that some symptoms do not fit the original diagnosis and, instead, point to a medical illness. Occasionally, a patient with an acute illness, such as encephalitis, is hospitalized with the diagnosis of schizophrenia, or a patient with a subacute illness, such as carcinoma of the pancreas, is treated in a private office or clinic with the diagnosis of a depressive disorder. Although it may not be possible to make the correct diagnosis at the time of the initial psychiatric evaluation, continued surveillance, and attention to clinical details usually provide clues leading to the recognition of the cause.

The likelihood of intercurrent illness is higher with some psychiatric disorders than with others. Substance abusers, for example, because of their life patterns, are susceptible to infection and are likely to suffer from the adverse effects of trauma, dietary deficiencies, and poor hygiene. Depression decreases the immune response.

When somatic and psychological dysfunctions are known to coexist, the psychiatrist should be thoroughly conversant with the patient's medical status. In cases of cardiac decompensation, peripheral neuropathy, and other disabling disorders, the nature and degree of impairment that can be attributed to the physical disorder should be assessed. It is important to answer the question: Does the patient exploit a disability, or is it ignored or denied with resultant overexertion? To answer this question, the psychiatrist must assess the patient's capabilities and limitations, rather than make sweeping judgments based on a diagnostic label.

Special vigilance about medical status is required for some patients in treatment for somatoform and eating disorders. Such is the case for patients with ulcerative colitis who are bleeding profusely and for patients with anorexia nervosa who are losing appreciable weight. These disorders can become life-threatening.

Importance of Medical Screening.   Numerous articles have called attention to the need for thorough medical screening of patients seen in psychiatric inpatient services and clinics. (A similar need has been demonstrated for the psychiatric evaluation of patients seen in medical inpatient services and clinics.) The concept of *medical clearance* remains ambiguous and has meaning in the context of psychiatric admission or clearance for transfers from different settings or institutions. It implies that no medical condition exists to account for the patient's condition.

Among identified psychiatric patients, from 24 to 60 percent have been shown to suffer from associated physical disorders. In a survey of 2,090 psychiatric clinic patients, 43 percent were found to have associated physical disorders; of these, almost half the physical disorders had not been diagnosed by the referring sources. (In this study, 69 patients were found to have diabetes mellitus, but only 12 of these cases had been diagnosed before referral.)

Expecting psychiatrists to be experts in internal medicine is unrealistic, but they should be able to recognize or have a high suspicion of physical disorders when they are present. Moreover, they should make appropriate referrals and collaborate in treating patients who have both physical and mental disorders.

Psychiatric symptoms are nonspecific; they can herald medical as well as psychiatric illness. They often precede the appearance of definitive medical symptoms. Some psychiatric symptoms (e.g., visual hallucinations, distortions, and illusions) should evoke a high level of suspicion of medication toxicity.

The medical literature abounds with case reports of patients whose disorders were initially considered emotional but ultimately proved to be secondary to medical conditions. The data in most of the reports revealed features pointing toward organicity. Diagnostic errors arose because such features were accorded too little weight.

THE PSYCHIATRIC REPORT AND MEDICAL RECORD

Psychiatric Report

This section complements the previous section, "Psychiatric Interview, History, and Mental Status Examination," in that it provides a comprehensive outline on how to write the psychiatric report (see Table 1-7). The need to follow some sort of outline in gathering data about a person to make a psychiatric diagnosis is universally

Table 1-7
Psychiatric Report

I. Psychiatric History
  A. Identification: Name, age, marital status, sex, occupation, language if other than English, race, nationality, and religion if pertinent; previous admissions to a hospital for the same or a different condition; with whom the patient lives
  B. Chief complaint: Exactly why the patient came to the psychiatrist, preferably in the patient's own words; if that information does not come from the patient, note who supplied it
  C. History of present illness: Chronologic background and development of the symptoms or behavioral changes that culminated in the patient's seeking assistance; patient's life circumstances at the time of onset; personality when well; how illness has affected life activities and personal relations—changes in personality, interests, mood, attitudes toward others, dress, habits, level of tenseness, irritability, activity, attention, concentration, memory, speech; psychophysiological symptoms—nature and details of dysfunction; pain—location, intensity, fluctuation; level of anxiety—generalized and nonspecific (free floating) or specifically related to particular situations, activities, or objects; how anxieties are handled—avoidance, repetition of feared situation, use of drugs or other activities for alleviation
  D. Past psychiatric and medical history: (1) Emotional or mental disturbances—extent of incapacity, type of treatment, names of hospitals, length of illness, effect of treatment; (2) psychosomatic disorders: hay fever, arthritis, colitis, rheumatoid arthritis, recurrent colds, skin conditions; (3) medical conditions: follow customary review of systems—sexually transmitted diseases, alcohol or other substance abuse, at risk for acquired immunodeficiency syndrome (AIDS); (4) neurologic disorders: headache, craniocerebral trauma, loss of consciousness, seizures, or tumors
  E. Family history: Elicited from patient and from someone else, because quite different descriptions may be given of the same persons and events; ethnic, national, and religious traditions; other persons in the home, descriptions of them—personality and intelligence—and what has become of them since patient's childhood; descriptions of different households lived in; present relationships between patient and those who were in family; role of illness in the family; family history of mental illness; where does patient live—neighborhood and particular residence of the patient; is home crowded; privacy of family members from each other and from other families; sources of family income and difficulties in obtaining it; public assistance (if any) and attitude about it; will patient lose job or apartment by remaining in the hospital; who is caring for children
  F. Personal history (anamnesis): History of the patient's life from infancy to the present to the extent it can be recalled; gaps in history as spontaneously related by the patient; emotions associated with different life periods (painful, stressful, conflictual) or with phases of life cycle
    1. Early childhood (Birth through age 3)
      a. Prenatal history and mother's pregnancy and delivery: Length of pregnancy, spontaneity and normality of delivery, birth trauma, whether patient was planned and wanted, birth defects
      b. Feeding habits: Breast-fed or bottle-fed, eating problems
      c. Early development: Maternal deprivation, language development, motor development, signs of unmet needs, sleep pattern, object constancy, stranger anxiety, separation anxiety
      d. Toilet training: Age, attitude of parents, feelings about it
      e. Symptoms of behavior problems: Thumb sucking, temper tantrums, tics, head bumping, rocking, night terrors, fears, bed-wetting or bed soiling, nail biting, masturbation
      f. Personality and temperament as a child: Shy, restless, overactive, withdrawn, studious, outgoing, timid, athletic, friendly patterns of play, reactions to siblings
    2. Middle childhood (ages 3–11): Early school history—feelings about going to school, early adjustment, sex identification, conscience development, punishment; social relationships, attitudes toward siblings and playmates
    3. Later childhood (prepuberty through adolescence)
      a. Peer relationships: Number and closeness of friends, leader or follower, social popularity, participation in group or gang activities, idealized figures; patterns of aggression, passivity, anxiety, antisocial behavior
      b. School history: How far the patient went, adjustment to school, relationships with teachers—teacher's pet or rebellious—favorite studies or interests, particular abilities or assets, extracurricular activities, sports, hobbies, relationships of problems or symptoms to any school period
      c. Cognitive and motor development: Learning to read and other intellectual and motor skills, minimal cerebral dysfunction, learning disabilities—their management and effects on the child
      d. Particular adolescent emotional or physical problems: Nightmares, phobias, masturbation, bed-wetting, running away, delinquency, smoking, drug or alcohol use, weight problems, feeling of inferiority
      e. Psychosexual history
        i. Early curiosity, infantile masturbation, sex play
        ii. Acquiring of sexual knowledge, attitude of parents toward sex, sexual abuse
        iii. Onset of puberty, feelings about it, kind of preparation, feelings about menstruation, development of secondary sexual characteristics
        iv. Adolescent sexual activity: Crushes, parties, dating, petting, masturbation, wet dreams and attitudes toward them
        v. Attitudes toward same and opposite sex: Timid, shy, aggressive, need to impress, seductive, sexual conquests, anxiety
        vi. Sexual practices: Sexual problems, homosexual and heterosexual experiences, paraphilias, promiscuity
      f. Religious background: Strict, liberal, mixed (possible conflicts), relation of background to current religious practices
    4. Adulthood
      a. Occupational history: Choice of occupation, training, ambitions, conflicts; relations with authority, peers, and subordinates; number of jobs and duration; changes in job status; current job and feelings about it
      b. Social activity: Whether patient has friends or not; is patient withdrawn or socializing well; social, intellectual, and physical interests; relationships with same sex and opposite sex; depth, duration, and quality of human relations

Table 1-7
Psychiatric Report (*Continued*)

      c. Adult sexuality
          i. Premarital sexual relationships, age of first coitus, sexual orientation
          ii. Marital history: Common-law marriages, legal marriages, description of courtship and role played by each partner, age at marriage, family planning and contraception, names and ages of children, attitudes toward raising children, problems of any family members, housing difficulties if important to the marriage, sexual adjustment, extramarital affairs, areas of agreement and disagreement, management of money, role of in-laws
          iii. Sexual symptoms: Anorgasmia, impotence, premature ejaculation, lack of desire
          iv. Attitudes toward pregnancy and having children; contraceptive practices and feelings about them
          v. Sexual practices: Paraphilias such as sadism, fetishes, voyeurism; attitude toward fellation, cunnilingus; coital techniques, frequency
      d. Military history: General adjustment, combat, injuries, referral to psychiatrists, type of discharge, veteran status
      e. Value systems: Whether children are seen as a burden or a joy; whether work is seen as a necessary evil, an avoidable chore, or an opportunity; current attitude about religion; belief in heaven and hell
   G. Summation of the examiner's observations and impressions derived from the initial interview
II. Mental Status
  A. Appearance
    1. Personal identification: May include a brief nontechnical description of the patient's appearance and behavior as a novelist might write it; attitude toward examiner can be described here—cooperative, attentive, interested, frank, seductive, defensive, hostile, playful, ingratiating, evasive, guarded
    2. Behavior and psychomotor activity: Gait, mannerisms, tics, gestures, twitches, stereotypes, picking, touching examiner, echopraxia, clumsy, agile, limp, rigid, retarded, hyperactive, agitated, combative, waxy
    3. General description: Posture, bearing, clothes, grooming, hair, nails; healthy, sickly, angry, frightened, apathetic, perplexed, contemptuous, ill at ease, poised, old looking, young looking, effeminate, masculine; signs of anxiety—moist hands, perspiring forehead, restlessness, tense posture, strained voice, wide eyes; shifts in level of anxiety during interview or with particular topic
  B. Speech: Rapid, slow, pressured, hesitant, emotional, monotonous, loud, whispered, slurred, mumbled, stuttering, echolalia, intensity, pitch, ease, spontaneity, productivity, manner, reaction time, vocabulary, prosody
  C. Mood and affect
    1. Mood (a pervasive and sustained emotion that colors the person's perception of the world): How does patient say he or she feels; depth, intensity, duration, and fluctuations of mood—depressed, despairing, irritable, anxious, terrified, angry, expansive, euphoric, empty, guilty, awed, futile, self-contemptuous, anhedonic, alexithymic
    2. Affect (the outward expression of the patient's inner experiences): How examiner evaluates patient's affects—broad, restricted, blunted or flat, shallow, amount and range of expression; difficulty in initiating, sustaining, or terminating an emotional response; is the emotional expression appropriate to the thought content, culture, and setting of the examination; give examples if emotional expression is not appropriate
  D. Thinking and perception
    1. Form of thinking
      a. Productivity: Overabundance of ideas, paucity of ideas, flight of ideas, rapid thinking, slow thinking, hesitant thinking; does patient speak spontaneously or only when questions are asked, stream of thought, quotations from patient
      b. Continuity of thought: Whether patient's replies really answer questions and are goal directed, relevant, or irrelevant; loose associations; lack of causal relations in patient's explanations; illogic, tangential, circumstantial, rambling, evasive, perseverative statements, blocking or distractibility
      c. Language impairments: Impairments that reflect disordered mentation, such as incoherent or incomprehensible speech (word salad), clang associations, neologisms
    2. Content of thinking
      a. Preoccupations: About the illness, environmental problems; obsessions, compulsions, phobias; obsessions or plans about suicide, homicide; hypochondriacal symptoms, specific antisocial urges or impulses
    3. Thought disturbances
      a. Delusions: Content of any delusional system, its organization, the patient's convictions as to its validity, how it affects his or her life: persecutory delusions—isolated or associated with pervasive suspiciousness; mood congruent or mood incongruent
      b. Ideas of reference and ideas of influence: How ideas began, their content, and the meaning the patient attributes to them
    4. Perceptual disturbances
      a. Hallucinations and illusions: Whether patient hears voices or sees visions; content, sensory system involvement, circumstances of the occurrence; hypnagogic or hypnopompic hallucinations; thought broadcasting
      b. Depersonalization and derealization: Extreme feelings of detachment from self or from the environment
    5. Dreams and fantasies
      a. Dreams: Prominent ones, if patient will tell them; nightmares
      b. Fantasies: Recurrent, favorite, or unshakable daydreams
  E. Sensorium
    1. Alertness: Awareness of environment, attention span, clouding of consciousness, fluctuations in levels of awareness, somnolence, stupor, lethargy, fugue state, coma
    2. Orientation
      a. Time: Whether patient identifies the day correctly; or approximate date, time of day; if in a hospital, knows how long he or she has been there; behaves as though oriented to the present
      b. Place: Whether patient knows where he or she is
      c. Person: Whether patient knows who the examiner is and the roles or names of the persons with whom in contact
    3. Concentration and calculation: Subtracting 7 from 100 and keep subtracting 7s; if patient cannot subtract 7s, can easier tasks be accomplished—4×9; 5×4; how many nickels are in $1.35; whether anxiety or some disturbance of mood or concentration seems to be responsible for difficulty

(continued)

Table 1-7
Psychiatric Report (*Continued*)

    4. Memory: Impairment, efforts made to cope with impairment—denial, confabulation, catastrophic reaction, circumstantiality used to conceal deficit: whether the process of registration, retention, or recollection of material is involved
      a. Remote memory: Childhood data, important events known to have occurred when the patient was younger or free of illness, personal matters, neutral material
      b. Recent past memory: Past few months
      c. Recent memory: Past few days, what did patient do yesterday, the day before, have for breakfast, lunch, dinner
      d. Immediate retention and recall: Ability to repeat six figures after examiner dictates them—first forward, then backward, then after a few minutes' interruption; other test questions; did same questions, if repeated, call forth different answers at different times
      e. Effect of defect on patient: Mechanisms patient has developed to cope with defect
    5. Fund of knowledge: Level of formal education and self-education; estimate of the patient's intellectual capability and whether capable of functioning at the level of his or her basic endowment; counting, calculation, general knowledge; questions should have relevance to the patient's educational and cultural background
    6. Abstract thinking: Disturbances in concept formation; manner in which the patient conceptualizes or handles his or her ideas; similarities (e.g., between apples and pears), differences, absurdities; meanings of simple proverbs (e.g., "A rolling stone gathers no moss") answers may be concrete (giving specific examples to illustrate the meaning) or overly abstract (giving generalized explanation); appropriateness of answers
  F. Insight: Degree of personal awareness and understanding of illness
    1. Complete denial of illness
    2. Slight awareness of being sick and needing help but denying it at the same time
    3. Awareness of being sick but blaming it on others, on external factors, on medical or unknown organic factors
    4. Intellectual insight: Admission of illness and recognition that symptoms or failures in social adjustment are due to irrational feelings or disturbances, without applying that knowledge to future experiences
    5. True emotional insight: Emotional awareness of the motives and feelings within, of the underlying meaning of symptoms; does the awareness lead to changes in personality and future behavior; openness to new ideas and concepts about self and the important persons in his or her life
  G. Judgment
    1. Social judgment: Subtle manifestations of behavior that are harmful to the patient and contrary to acceptable behavior in the culture; does the patient understand the likely outcome of personal behavior and is patient influenced by that understanding; examples of impairment
    2. Test judgment: Patient's prediction of what he or she would do in imaginary situations (e.g., what patient would do with a stamped addressed letter found in the street)
III. Further Diagnostic Studies
  A. Physical examination
  B. Neurologic examination
  C. Additional psychiatric diagnostic studies
  D. Interviews with family members, friends, or neighbors by a social worker
  E. Psychological, neurologic, or laboratory tests as indicated: Electroencephalogram, computed tomography scan, magnetic resonance imaging, tests of other medical conditions, reading comprehension and writing tests, test for aphasia, projective or objective psychological tests, dexamethasone-suppression test, 24-hour urine test for heavy metal intoxication, urine screen for drugs of abuse
IV. Summary of Findings
  Summarize mental symptoms, medical and laboratory findings, and psychological and neurologic test results, if available; include medications patient has been taking, dosage, duration. Clarity of thinking is reflected in clarity of writing. When summarizing the mental status (e.g., the phrase "Patient denies hallucinations and delusions" is not as precise as "Patient denies hearing voices or thinking that he is being followed."). The latter indicates the specific question asked and the specific response given. Similarly, in the conclusion of the report one would write "Hallucinations and delusions were not elicited."
V. Diagnosis
  Diagnostic classification is made according to DSM-5. The diagnostic numerical code should be used from DSM-5 or ICD-10. It might be prudent to use both codes to cover current and future regulatory guidelines.
VI. Prognosis
  Opinion about the probable future course, extent, and outcome of the disorder; good and bad prognostic factors; specific goals of therapy
VII. Psychodynamic Formulation
  Causes of the patient's psychodynamic breakdown—influences in the patient's life that contributed to present disorder; environmental, genetic, and personality factors relevant to determining patient's symptoms; primary and secondary gains; outline of the major defense mechanism used by the patient
VIII. Comprehensive Treatment Plan
  Modalities of treatment recommended, role of medication, inpatient or outpatient treatment, frequency of sessions, probable duration of therapy; type of psychotherapy; individual, group, or family therapy; symptoms or problems to be treated. Initially, treatment must be directed toward any life-threatening situations such as suicidal risk or risk of danger to others that require psychiatric hospitalization. Danger to self or others is an acceptable reason (both legally and medically) for involuntary hospitalization. In the absence of the need for confinement, a variety of outpatient treatment alternatives are available: day hospitals, supervised residences, outpatient psychotherapy or pharmacotherapy, among others. In some cases, treatment planning must attend to vocational and psychosocial skills training and even legal or forensic issues.
  Comprehensive treatment planning requires a therapeutic team approach using the skills of psychologists, social workers, nurses, activity and occupational therapists, and a variety of other mental health professionals, with referral to self-help groups (e.g., Alcoholics Anonymous [AA]) if needed. If either the patient or family members are unwilling to accept the recommendations of treatment and the clinician thinks that the refusal of the recommendations may have serious consequences, the patient, parent, or guardian should sign a statement to the effect that the recommended treatment was refused.

recognized. The one that follows calls for including a tremendous amount of potential information about the patient, not all of which need be obtained, depending on the circumstances in the case. Beginning clinicians are advised to get as much information as possible; more experienced clinicians can pick and choose among the series of questions they might ask. In all cases, however, the person is best understood within the context of his or her life events.

The psychiatric report covers both the psychiatric history and the mental status. The history, or *anamnesis* (from the Greek meaning "to remember"), describes life events within the framework of the life cycle, from infancy to old age, and the clinician should attempt to elicit the emotional reaction to each event as remembered by the patient. The mental status examination covers what the patient is thinking and feeling at the moment and how he or she responds to specific questions from the examiner. Sometimes it may be necessary to report, in detail, the questions asked and the answers received; but this should be kept to a minimum, so that the report does not read like a verbatim transcript. Nevertheless, the clinician should try to use the patient's own words as much as possible, especially when describing certain symptoms such as hallucinations or delusions.

Finally, the psychiatric report includes more than the psychiatric history and mental status. It also includes a summary of positive and negative findings and an interpretation of the data. It has more than descriptive value; it has meaning that helps provide an understanding of the case. The examiner addresses critical questions in the report: Are future diagnostic studies needed, and, if so, which ones? Is a consultant needed? Is a comprehensive neurologic workup, including an electroencephalogram (EEG) or computed tomography (CT) scan, needed? Are psychological tests indicated? Are psychodynamic factors relevant? Has the cultural context of the patient's illness been considered? The report includes a diagnosis made according to the 5th edition of the *Diagnostic and Statistical Manual of Mental Disorders* (DSM-5). Prognosis is also discussed in the report, with good and bad prognostic factors listed. The report concludes with a discussion of a treatment plan and makes firm recommendations about the management of the case.

Medical Record

The psychiatric report is a part of the medical record; however, the medical record is more than the psychiatric report. It is a narrative that documents all events that occur during treatment, most often referring to the patient's stay in the hospital. Progress notes record every interaction between doctor and patient; reports of all special studies, including laboratory tests; and prescriptions and orders for all medications. Nurses' notes help describe the patient's course: Is the patient beginning to respond to treatment? Are there times during the day or night when symptoms get worse or remit? Are there adverse effects or complaints by the patient about prescribed medication? Are there signs of agitation, violence, or mention of suicide? If the patient requires restraints or seclusion, are the proper supervisory procedures being followed? The medical record tells what happened to the patient since first making contact with the health care system. It concludes with a discharge summary that provides a concise overview of the patient's course with recommendations for future treatment, if necessary. Evidence of contact with a referral agency should be documented in the medical record to establish continuity of care if further intervention is necessary.

Use of the Record.   The medical record is not only used by physicians. It is also used by regulatory agencies and managed

Table 1-8
Medical Record

There shall be an individual record for each person admitted to the psychiatric inpatient unit. Patient records shall be safeguarded for confidentiality and should be accessible only to authorized persons. Each case record shall include:
Legal admission documents
Identifying information on the individual and family
Source of referral, date of commencement of service, and name of staff member carrying overall responsibility for treatment and care
Initial, intercurrent, and final diagnoses, including psychiatric or mental retardation diagnoses in official terminology
Reports of all diagnostic examinations and evaluations, including findings and conclusions
Reports of all special studies performed, including x-rays, clinical laboratory tests, clinical psychological testing, electroencephalograms, and psychometric tests
The individual written plan of care, treatment, and rehabilitation
Progress notes written and signed by all staff members having significant participation in the program of treatment and care
Summaries of case conferences and special consultations
Dated and signed prescriptions or orders for all medications, with notation of termination dates
Closing summary of the course of treatment and care
Documentation of any referrals to another agency

Adapted from the 1995 guidelines of the New York State Office of Mental Health.

care companies to determine the length of stay, quality of care, and reimbursement to doctors and hospitals. In theory, the inpatient medical record is accessible to authorized persons only and is safeguarded for confidentiality. In practice, however, absolute confidentiality cannot be guaranteed. Guidelines for what material needs to be incorporated into the medical record are provided in Table 1-8.

The medical record is also crucial in malpractice litigation. Robert I. Simon summarized the liability issues as follows:

Properly kept medical records can be the psychiatrist's best ally in malpractice litigation. If no record is kept, numerous questions will be raised regarding the psychiatrist's competence and credibility. This failure to keep medical records may also violate state statutes or licensing provisions. Failure to keep medical records may arise out of the psychiatrist's concern that patient treatment information be totally protected. Although this is an admirable ideal, in real life, the psychiatrist may be legally compelled under certain circumstances to testify directly about confidential treatment matters.

Outpatient records are also subject to scrutiny by third parties under certain circumstances, and psychiatrists in private practice are under the same obligation to maintain a record of the patient in treatment as the hospital psychiatrist. Table 1-9 lists documentation issues of concern to third-party payers.

Personal Notes and Observations.   According to laws relating to access to medical records, some jurisdictions (such as in the Public Health Law of New York State) have a provision that applies to a physician's personal notes and observations. *Personal notes* are defined as "a practitioner's speculations, impressions (other than tentative or actual diagnosis) and reminders." The data are maintained only by the clinician and cannot be disclosed to any other person, including the patient. Psychiatrists concerned about material that may prove damaging or otherwise hurtful to the patient if released to a third party may consider using this provision to maintain doctor–patient confidentiality.

Psychotherapy Notes.   Psychotherapy notes include details of transference, fantasies, dreams, personal information about persons

Table 1-9
Documentation Issues

Are patient's areas of dysfunction described? From the biologic, psychological, and social points of view?

Is alcohol or substance abuse addressed?

Do clinical activities happen at the expected time? If too late or never, why?

Are issues identified in the treatment plan and followed in progress notes?

When there is a variance in the patient's outcome, is there a note in the progress notes to that effect? Is there also a note in the progress notes reflecting the clinical strategies recommended to overcome the impediments to the patient's improvement?

If new clinical strategies are implemented, how is their impact evaluated? When?

Is there a sense of multidisciplinary input and coordination of treatment in the progress notes?

Do progress notes indicate the patient's functioning in the therapeutic community and its relationship to their discharge criteria?

Can one extrapolate from the patient's behavior in the therapeutic community how he or she will function in the community at large?

Are there notes depicting the patient's understanding of his or her discharge planning? Family participation in discharge planning must be entered in the progress notes with their reaction to the plan.

Do attending progress notes bridge the differences in thinking of other disciplines?

Are the patient's needs addressed in the treatment plan?

Are the patient's family's needs evaluated and implemented?

Is patient and family satisfaction evaluated in any way?

Is alcohol and substance abuse addressed as a possible contributor to readmission?

If the patient was readmitted, are there indications that previous records were reviewed, and, if the patient is on medication other than that prescribed on discharge, is there a rationale for this change?

Do the progress notes identify the type of medication used and the rationale for increase, decrease, discontinuation, or augmentation of medication?

Are medication effects documented, including dosages, response, and adverse or other side effects?

Note: Documentation issues are of concern to third-party payers, such as insurance companies and health maintenance organizations who examine patients' charts to see if the areas listed above are covered. In many cases, however, the review is conducted by persons with little or no background in psychiatry or psychology who do not recognize the complexities of psychiatric diagnosis and treatment. Payments to hospitals, doctors, and patients are often denied because of what such reviewers consider to be the so-called inadequate documentation.

with whom the patient interacts, and other intimate details of the patient's life. They may also include the psychiatrist's comments on his or her countertransference and feelings toward the patient. Psychotherapy notes should be kept separate from the rest of the medical records.

Patient Access to Records. Patients have a legal right to access their medical records. This right represents society's belief that the responsibility for medical care has become a collaborative process between doctor and patient. Patients see many different physicians, and they can be more effective historians and coordinators of their care with such information.

Psychiatrists must be careful in releasing their records to the patient if, in their judgment, the patient can be harmed emotionally as a result. Under these circumstances, the psychiatrist may choose to prepare a summary of the patient's course of treatment, holding back material that might be hurtful—especially if it were to get into

the hands of third parties. In malpractice cases, however, it may not be possible to do so. When litigation occurs, the entire medical record is subject to discovery. Psychotherapy notes are usually protected, but not always. If psychotherapy notes are ordered to be produced, the judge would probably review them privately and select what is relevant to the case in question.

Blogs. Blogs or weblogs are used by persons who wish to record their day-to-day experiences or to express their thoughts and feelings about events. Physicians should be especially cautious about such activities because they are subject to discovery in lawsuits. Pseudonyms and aliases offer no protection because they can be traced. Writing about patients on blogs is a breach of confidentiality. In one case, a doctor detailed his thoughts about a lawsuit that included hostile comments about the plaintiff and his attorney. His blog was discovered inadvertently and was used against him in court. Physicians are advised not to use blogs to vent emotions and to write nothing that they would not write for attribution even if their identity were discovered.

E-Mail. Physicians are increasingly using e-mail as a quick and efficient way to communicate not only with patients but also with other doctors about their patients; however, it is a public document and should be treated as such. The dictum of not diagnosing or prescribing medication over the telephone to a patient one has not examined should also apply to e-mail. It is not only dangerous but also unethical. All e-mail messages should be printed to include with the paper chart unless electronic archives are regularly backed up and secure.

Ethical Issues and the Medical Record. Psychiatrists continually make judgments about what is appropriate material to include in the psychiatric report, the medical record, the case report, and other written communications about a patient. Such judgments often involve ethical issues. In a case report, for example, the patient should not be identifiable, a position made clear in the American Psychiatric Association's (APA's) *Principles of Medical Ethics with Annotations Especially Applicable to Psychiatry,* which states that published case reports must be suitably disguised to safeguard patient confidentiality without altering material to provide a less-than-complete portrayal of the patient's actual condition. In some instances, obtaining a written release from the patient that allows the psychiatrist to publish the case may also be advisable, even if the patient is appropriately disguised.

Psychiatrists sometimes include material in the medical record that is specifically directed toward warding off future culpability if liability issues are ever raised. This may include having advised the patient about specific adverse effects of medication to be prescribed.

Health Insurance Portability and Accountability Act (HIPAA). The HIPAA was passed in 1996 to address the medical delivery system's mounting complexity and its rising dependence on electronic communication. The act orders that the federal Department of Health and Human Services (HHS) develop rules protecting the transmission and confidentiality of patient information, and all units under HIPAA must comply with such rules.

Two rules were finalized in February 2003: the Transaction Rule and the Privacy Rule (see Tables 1-10 and 1-11). The Transaction Rule facilitates transferring health information effectively and efficiently using regulations created by the HHS that established a uniform set of formats, code sets, and data requirements. The Privacy Rule, administered by the Office of Civil Rights (OCR) at HHS,

Table 1-10
Transaction Rule Code Sets

Health care information: The Transactions Rule defines standards and establishes code sets and forms to be used for electronic transaction that involve the following health care information:
Claims or equivalent encounter information
Eligibility inquiries
Referral certification and authorization
Claims status inquiries
Enrollment and disenrollment information
Payment and remittance advice
Health plan premium payments
Coordination of benefits

Code sets: Under the Transaction Rule, the following code sets are required for filing claims with Medicare:
Procedure codes
American Medical Association Current Procedural Terminology codes
Healthcare Common Procedure Coding System codes
Diagnosis codes
International Classification of Disease, 10th edition, clinical modification, codes
Drugs and biologicals
National Drug Codes
Dental codes
Code on dental procedures
Nomenclature for dental services

Adapted from Jaffe E. HIPAA basics for psychiatrists. *Psych Pract Manage Care.* 2002;8:15.

Table 1-11
Patient's Rights under the Privacy Rule

Physician must give the patient a written notice of his or her privacy rights, the privacy policies of the practice, and how patient information is used, kept, and disclosed. A written acknowledgment should be taken from the patient verifying that he or she seen such notice.
Patients should be able to obtain copies of their medical records and to request revisions to those records within a stated amount of time (usually 30 days). Patients do not have the right to see psychotherapy notes.
Physicians must provide the patient with a history of most disclosures of his or her medical history on request. There are some exceptions. The APA Committee on Confidentiality has developed a model document for this requirement.
Physicians must obtain authorization from the patient for disclosure of information other than for treatment, payment, and health care operations (these three are considered to be routine uses, for which consent is not required). The APA Committee on Confidentiality has developed a model document for this requirement.
Patients may request another means of communication of their protected information (i.e., request that the physician contact them at a specific phone number or address).
Physicians cannot generally limit treatment to obtaining patient authorization for disclosure of the patient's information for nonroutine uses.
Patients have the right to complain about Privacy Rule violations to the physician, their health plan, or to the secretary of HHS.

APA, American Psychiatric Association; HHS, Department of Health and Human Services.
Adapted from Jaffe E. HIPAA basics for psychiatrists. *Psych Pract Manage Care.* 2002;8:15.

protects the confidentiality of patient information. This means that a patient's medical information belongs to the patient and that the patient has the right to access it, except for psychotherapy notes, which are deemed as property of the psychotherapist who wrote them.

In 2003, the Privacy Rule was executed. Under the Privacy Rule, there are certain guidelines by which every practice must abide:

1. Every practice must establish written privacy procedures. These include administrative, physical, and technical safeguards that establish who has access to the patient's information, how this information is used within the facility, and when the information will and will not be disclosed to others.
2. Every practice must take steps to make sure that its business associates protect the privacy of medical records and other health information.
3. Every practice must train employees to comply with the rule.
4. Every practice must have a designated person to serve as a privacy officer. If it is an individual practice or private practice, this person can be the physician.
5. Every practice must establish complaint procedures for patients who wish to ask or to complain about the privacy of their records.

The OCR at HHS is responsible for making sure that Privacy Rule is enforced; however, it is not clear as to how it will be done. One method expressed by the government is a complaint-driven system in which the OCR will respond to complaints made by patients concerning confidentiality violations or denied access to records, all of which are covered under HIPAA. In such cases, OCR may follow up and audit compliance.

The APA's Committee on Confidentiality, along with legal experts, has developed a set of sample forms. They are part of the APA's HIPAA educational packet, which can be obtained on the APA website (www.psych.org/). On the website, there are

also recommendations for enabling physicians to comply with HIPAA.

PSYCHIATRIC RATING SCALES

The term *psychiatric rating scales* encompasses a variety of questionnaires, interviews, checklists, outcome assessments, and other instruments that are available to inform psychiatric practice, research, and administration. Psychiatrists must keep up with significant developments in rating scales for several reasons. Most critically, many such scales are useful in psychiatric practice for monitoring patients over time or for providing information that is more comprehensive than what is generally obtained in a routine clinical interview. Also, health care administrators and payors are increasingly requiring standardized assessments to justify the need for services or to assess the quality of care. Lastly, but equally important, rating scales are used in research that informs the practice of psychiatry, so familiarity with them provides a deeper understanding of the results of that research and the degree to which it applies to psychiatric practice.

Potential Benefits and Limitations of Rating Scales in Psychiatry

The key role of rating scales in psychiatry and elsewhere is to standardize the information collected across time and by various observers. This standardization ensures a consistent, comprehensive evaluation that may aid treatment planning by establishing a diagnosis, ensuring a thorough description of symptoms, identifying comorbid conditions, and characterizing other factors affecting treatment response. Also, the use of a rating scale can establish a baseline for follow-up of the progression of an illness over time or in response to specific interventions. This is particularly useful when more than one clinician is involved—for instance, in a group practice or in the conduct of psychiatric research.

Also to standardization, most rating scales also offer the user the advantages of a formal evaluation of the measure's performance characteristics. This allows the clinician to know to what extent a given scale produces reproducible results (reliability) and how it compares to more definitive or established ways of measuring the same thing (validity).

Types of Scales and What They Measure

Scales are used in psychiatric research and practice to achieve a variety of goals. They also cover a broad range of areas and use a broad range of procedures and formats.

Measurement Goals. Most psychiatric rating scales in common use fall into one or more of the following categories: making a diagnosis; measuring severity and tracking change in specific symptoms, in general functioning, or overall outcome; and screening for conditions that may or may not be present.

Constructs Assessed. Psychiatric practitioners and investigators assess a broad range of areas, referred to as *constructs,* to underscore the fact that they are not simple, direct observations of nature. These include diagnoses, signs and symptoms, severity, functional impairment, quality of life, and many others. Some of these constructs are relatively complex and are divided into two or more domains (e.g., positive and negative symptoms in schizophrenia or mood and neurovegetative symptoms in major depression).

CATEGORICAL VERSUS CONTINUOUS CLASSIFICATION. Some constructs are viewed as *categorical* or classifying, whereas others are seen as *continuous* or measuring. Categorical constructs describe the presence or absence of a given attribute (e.g., competency to stand trial) or the category best suited to a given individual among a finite set of options (e.g., assigning a diagnosis). Continuous measures provide a quantitative assessment along a continuum of intensity, frequency, or severity. Also, to symptom severity and functional status, multidimensional personality traits, cognitive status, social support, and many other attributes are generally measured continuously.

The distinction between categorical and continuous measures is by no means absolute. *Ordinal* classification, which uses a finite, ordered set of categories (e.g., unaffected, mild, moderate, or severe) stands between the two.

Measurement Procedures. Rating scales differ in measurement methods. Issues to be considered include format, raters, and sources of information.

FORMAT. Rating scales are available in a variety of formats. Some are simply checklists or guides to observation that help the clinician achieve a standardized rating. Others are self-administered questionnaires or tests. Still, others are formal interviews that may be *fully structured* (i.e., specifying the exact wording of questions to be asked) or *partly structured* (i.e., providing only some specific wording, along with suggestions for additional questions or probes).

RATERS. Some instruments are designed to be administered by doctoral-level clinicians only, whereas others may be administered by psychiatric nurses or social workers with more limited clinical experience. Other instruments are designed primarily for use by lay raters with little or no experience with psychopathology.

SOURCE OF INFORMATION. Instruments also vary in the source of information used to make the ratings. Information may be obtained solely from the patient, who generally knows the most about his or her condition. In some instruments, some or all of the information may be obtained from a knowledgeable informant. When the construct involves limited insight (e.g., cognitive disorders or mania) or significant social undesirability (e.g., antisocial personality or substance abuse), other informants may be preferable. Informants may also be helpful when the subject has limited ability to recall or report symptoms (e.g., delirium, dementia, or any disorder in young children). Some rating scales also allow or require information to be included from medical records or patient observation.

Assessment of Rating Scales

In clinical research, rating scales are mandatory to ensure interpretable and potentially generalizable results. They are selected based on coverage of the relevant constructs, expense (based on the nature of the raters, purchase price if any, and necessary training), length and administration time, comprehensibility to the intended audience, and quality of the ratings provided. In clinical practice, one considers these factors and, also, whether a scale would provide more or better information than what would be obtained in ordinary clinical practice or would contribute to the efficiency of obtaining that information. In either case, the assessment of quality is based on *psychometric,* or mind-measuring, properties.

Psychometric Properties. The two principal psychometric properties of a measure are *reliability* and *validity.* Although these words are used almost interchangeably in everyday speech, they are distinct in the context of evaluating rating scales. Scales should be *reliable,* or consistent and repeatable even if performed by different raters at different times or under different conditions, and they should be *valid* or accurate in representing the actual state of nature.

RELIABILITY. *Reliability* refers to the consistency or repeatability of ratings and is mainly empirical. An instrument is more likely to be reliable if the instructions and questions are clearly and simply worded, and the format is easy to understand and score. There are three standard ways to assess reliability: *internal consistency, interrater,* and *test–retest.*

INTERNAL CONSISTENCY. Internal consistency assesses agreement among the individual items in a measure. This provides information about reliability because each item is viewed as a single measurement of the underlying construct. Thus, the coherence of the items suggests that each is measuring the same thing.

INTERRATER AND TEST–RETEST RELIABILITY. Interrater (also called *interjudge* or *joint*) reliability is a measure of agreement between two or more observers evaluating the same subjects using the same information. Estimates may vary with assessment conditions—for instance, estimates of interrater reliability based on video-taped interviews tend to be higher than those based on interviews conducted by one of the raters. Test–retest evaluations measure reliability only to the extent that the subject's true condition remains stable in the time interval.

ISSUES IN INTERPRETING RELIABILITY DATA.   When interpreting reliability data, it is important to bear in mind that reliability estimates published in the literature may not generalize to other settings. Factors to consider are the nature of the sample, the training and experience of the raters, and the test conditions. Issues regarding the sample are especially critical. In particular, reliability tends to be higher in samples with high variability in which it is easier to discriminate among individuals.

VALIDITY.   *Validity* refers to conformity with truth, or a gold standard that can stand for truth. In the categorical context, it refers to whether an instrument can make correct classifications. In the continuous context, it refers to accuracy, or whether the score assigned can be said to represent the true state of nature. Although reliability is an empirical question, validity is partly theoretical—for many constructs measured in psychiatry, there is no absolute underlying truth. Even so, some measures yield more useful and meaningful data than others do. Validity assessment is generally divided into face and content validity, criterion validity, and construct validity.

Face and Content Validity.   *Face validity* refers to whether the items appear to assess the construct in question. Although a rating scale may purport to measure a construct of interest, a review of the items may reveal that it embodies a very different conceptualization of the construct. For instance, an insight scale may define *insight* in either psychoanalytic or neurologic terms. However, items with a transparent relationship to the construct may be a disadvantage when measuring socially undesirable traits, such as substance abuse or malingering. *Content validity* is similar to face validity but describes whether the measure provides good balanced coverage of the construct and is less focused on whether the items give the appearance of validity. Content validity is often assessed with formal procedures such as expert consensus or factor analysis.

Criterion Validity.   *Criterion validity* (sometimes called *predictive* or *concurrent validity*) refers to whether or not the measure agrees with a gold standard or criterion of accuracy. Suitable gold standards include the long form of an established instrument for a new, shorter version, a clinician-rated measure for a self-report form, and blood or urine tests for measures of drug use. For diagnostic interviews, the generally accepted gold standard is the **L**ongitudinal, **E**xpert, **A**ll **D**ata (LEAD) standard, which incorporates expert clinical evaluation, longitudinal data, medical records, family history, and any other sources of information.

Construct Validity.   When an adequate gold standard is not available—a frequent state of affairs in psychiatry—or when additional validity data are desired, construct validity must be assessed. To accomplish this, one can compare the measure to *external validators. These attributes* bear a well-characterized relationship to the construct under study but are not measured directly by the instrument. External validators used to validate psychiatric diagnostic criteria and the diagnostic instruments that aim to operationalize them include the course of illness, family history, and treatment response. For example, when compared with schizophrenia measures, mania measures are expected to identify more individuals with a remitting course, a family history of major mood disorders, and a good response to lithium.

Selection of Psychiatric Rating Scales

The scales discussed below cover various areas such as diagnosis, functioning, and symptom severity, among others. Selections were made based on coverage of major areas and common use in clinical research or current (or potential) use in clinical practice. Only a few of the many scales available in each category are discussed here.

Disability Assessment.   One of the most widely used scales to measure disability was developed by the World Health Association (WHO), known as the WHO Disability Assessment Schedule, now in its second iteration (WHODAS 2.0). It is self-administered and measures disability along several parameters such as cognition, interpersonal relations, work and social impairment, among many others. It can be taken at intervals along the course of a person's illness and is reliable in tracking changes that indicate a positive or negative response to therapeutic interventions or course of illness (Table 1-12).

Several assessment scales were developed for inclusion in the 5th edition of the *Diagnostic and Statistical Manual of Mental Disorders* of the American Psychiatric Association, (DSM-5); however, they were developed by and intended for use by research psychiatrists and are not as well tested as the WHO scales. It is expected that, in time, they will eventually be better adapted for clinical use. Some clinicians may wish to use the scales known as *Cross-Cutting Symptom Measure Scales,* but at this time, the WHO scale is recommended for general use.

Psychiatric Diagnosis.   Instruments assessing psychiatric diagnoses are central to psychiatric research and may be useful in clinical practice as well. However, they tend to be rather long, especially with individuals reporting many symptoms, potentially requiring many follow-up questions. When such instruments are evaluated, it is essential to ensure they implement the current diagnostic criteria and cover the diagnostic areas of interest.

STRUCTURED CLINICAL INTERVIEW FOR DSM (SCID).   The SCID begins with a section on demographic information and clinical background. Then there are seven diagnostic modules focused on different diagnostic groups: mood, psychotic, substance abuse, anxiety, somatic, eating, and adjustment disorders; the modules can be administered separately. Both required and optional probes are provided and skip outs are suggested where no further questioning is warranted. All available information, including that from hospital records, informants, and patient observation, should be used to rate the SCID. The SCID is designed to be administered by experienced clinicians and is generally not recommended for use by lay interviewers. Also, formal training in the SCID is required, and training books and videos are available to facilitate this. Although the primary focus is research with psychiatric patients, a nonpatient version (with no reference to a chief complaint) and a more clinical version (without as much detailed subtyping) are also available. Reliability data on the SCID suggest that it performs better on more severe disorders (e.g., bipolar disorder or alcohol dependence) than on milder ones (e.g., dysthymia). Validity data are limited, as the SCID is more often used as the gold standard to evaluate other instruments. It is considered the standard interview to verify the diagnosis in clinical trials and is extensively used in other forms of psychiatric research. Although its length precludes its use in routine clinical practice, the SCID can sometimes be useful to ensure a systematic evaluation in psychiatric patients—for instance, on admission to an inpatient unit or at intake into an outpatient clinic. It is also used in forensic practice to ensure a formal and reproducible examination.

Psychotic Disorders.   A variety of instruments are used for patients with psychotic disorders. Those discussed here are

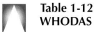

Table 1-12
WHODAS 2.0

World Health Organization Disability Assessment Schedule 2.0
36-item version, self-administered

Patient Name:_____   Age:_____   Sex: Male   Female   Date: _____

This questionnaire asks about <u>difficulties due to health/mental health conditions</u>. Health conditions include **diseases or illnesses, other health problems that may be short or long lasting, injuries, mental or emotional problems, and problems with alcohol or drugs.** Think back over the **past 30 days** and answer these questions thinking about how much difficulty you had doing the following activities. For each question, please circle only **one** response.

Numeric Scores Assigned to Each of the Items:	1	2	3	4	5	Clinician Use Only		
						Raw Item Score	Raw Domain Score	Average Domain Score

In the <u>last 30 days</u>, how much difficulty did you have in:

Understanding and Communicating

		1	2	3	4	5	Raw Item Score	Raw Domain Score	Average Domain Score
D1.1	<u>Concentrating</u> on doing something for <u>ten minutes</u>?	None	Mild	Moderate	Severe	Extreme or cannot do			
D1.2	<u>Remembering</u> to do <u>important things</u>?	None	Mild	Moderate	Severe	Extreme or cannot do			
D1.3	<u>Analyzing and finding solutions to problems</u> in day-to-day life?	None	Mild	Moderate	Severe	Extreme or cannot do		30	5
D1.4	<u>Learning</u> a <u>new task</u> for example, learning how to get to a new place?	None	Mild	Moderate	Severe	Extreme or cannot do			
D1.5	<u>Generally understanding</u> what people say?	None	Mild	Moderate	Severe	Extreme or cannot do			
D1.6	<u>Starting and maintaining</u> a <u>conversation</u>?	None	Mild	Moderate	Severe	Extreme or cannot do			

Getting Around

		1	2	3	4	5	Raw Item Score	Raw Domain Score	Average Domain Score
D2.1	<u>Standing</u> for <u>long periods</u>, such as 30 minutes?	None	Mild	Moderate	Severe	Extreme or cannot do			
D2.2	<u>Standing up</u> from sitting down?	None	Mild	Moderate	Severe	Extreme or cannot do			
D2.3	<u>Moving</u> around <u>inside your home</u>?	None	Mild	Moderate	Severe	Extreme or cannot do		25	5
D2.4	<u>Getting out</u> of your <u>home</u>?	None	Mild	Moderate	Severe	Extreme or cannot do			
D2.5	<u>Walking a long distance</u>, such as a kilometer (or equivalent)?	None	Mild	Moderate	Severe	Extreme or cannot do			

Self-care

		1	2	3	4	5	Raw Item Score	Raw Domain Score	Average Domain Score
D3.1	<u>Washing</u> your <u>whole body</u>?	None	Mild	Moderate	Severe	Extreme or cannot do			
D3.2	Getting <u>dressed</u>?	None	Mild	Moderate	Severe	Extreme or cannot do			
D3.3	<u>Eating</u>?	None	Mild	Moderate	Severe	Extreme or cannot do		20	5
<u>D3.4</u>	Staying <u>by yourself</u> for a <u>few days</u>?	None	Mild	Moderate	Severe	Extreme or cannot do			

Getting Along with People

		1	2	3	4	5	Raw Item Score	Raw Domain Score	Average Domain Score
D4.1	<u>Dealing</u> with people <u>you do not know</u>?	None	Mild	Moderate	Severe	Extreme or cannot do			
D4.2	<u>Maintaining a friendship</u>?	None	Mild	Moderate	Severe	Extreme or cannot do			
D4.3	<u>Getting along</u> with people who are <u>close</u> to you?	None	Mild	Moderate	Severe	Extreme or cannot do		25	5
D4.4	<u>Making new friends</u>?	None	Mild	Moderate	Severe	Extreme or cannot do			
D4.5	<u>Sexual</u> activities?	None	Mild	Moderate	Severe	Extreme or cannot do			

Table 1-12
WHODAS 2.0 (*Continued*)

Numeric Scores Assigned to Each of the Items:	1	2	3	4	5	Clinician Use Only		
						Raw Item Score	Raw Domain Score	Average Domain Score
Life Activities–Household								
D5.1 Taking care of your <u>household responsibilities</u>?	None	Mild	Moderate	Severe	Extreme or cannot do			
D5.2 Doing most important household tasks <u>well</u>?	None	Mild	Moderate	Severe	Extreme or cannot do		__20__	__5__
D5.3 Getting all of the household work <u>done</u> that you needed to do?	None	Mild	Moderate	Severe	Extreme or cannot do			
D5.4 Getting your household work done as <u>quickly</u> as needed?	None	Mild	Moderate	Severe	Extreme or cannot do			
Life Activities–School/Work								
D5.5 Your day-to-day <u>work/school</u>?	None	Mild	Moderate	Severe	Extreme or cannot do			
D5.6 Doing your most important work/school tasks <u>well</u>?	None	Mild	Moderate	Severe	Extreme or cannot do		__20__	__5__
D5.7 Getting all of the work <u>done</u> that you need to do?	None	Mild	Moderate	Severe	Extreme or cannot do			
D5.8 Getting your work done as <u>quickly</u> as needed?	None	Mild	Moderate	Severe	Extreme or cannot do			
Participation in Society								
In the past <u>30 days:</u>								
D6.1 How much of a problem did you have in <u>joining in community activities</u> (for example, festivities, religious, or other activities) in the same way as anyone else can?	None	Mild	Moderate	Severe	Extreme or cannot do			
D6.2 How much of a problem did you have because of <u>barriers or hindrances</u> around you?	None	Mild	Moderate	Severe	Extreme or cannot do			
D6.3 How much of a problem did you have <u>living with dignity</u> because of the attitudes and actions of others?	None	Mild	Moderate	Severe	Extreme or cannot do			
D6.4 How much <u>time</u> did <u>you</u> spend on your health condition or its consequences?	None	Mild	Moderate	Severe	Extreme or cannot do		__40__	__5__
D6.5 How much have <u>you</u> been <u>emotionally affected</u> by your health condition?	None	Mild	Moderate	Severe	Extreme or cannot do			
D6.6 How much has your health been a <u>drain on the financial resources</u> of you or your family?	None	Mild	Moderate	Severe	Extreme or cannot do			
D6.7 How much of a problem did your <u>family</u> have because of your health problems?	None	Mild	Moderate	Severe	Extreme or cannot do			
D6.8 How much of a problem did you have in doing things <u>by yourself</u> for <u>relaxation or pleasure</u>?	None	Mild	Moderate	Severe	Extreme or cannot do			
General Disability Score (Total):							__180__	__5__

Table 1-13
Brief Psychiatric Rating Scale

DEPARTMENT OF HEALTH AND HUMAN SERVICES PUBLIC HEALTH SERVICE	PATIENT NUMBER – – – –	DATA GROUP bprs	EVALUATION DATE $\overline{M}\,\overline{D}\,\overline{Y}$
Alcohol, Drug Abuse, and Mental Health Administration NIMH Treatment Strategies in Schizophrenia Society	PATIENT NAME		
Brief Psychiatric Rating Scale – Anchored Overall and Gorham	RATER NUMBER		

RATER NUMBER – – –	EVALUATION TYPE (Circle)
	1. Baseline 4. Major evaluation 7. During open meds 10. Study completion 2. 4-wk minor 5. Other 8. Stop open minds 3. Start double-blind 6. Start open meds 9. Early termination

Introduce all questions with "During the past week have you…"

[a]1. **Somatic Concern:** Degree of concern over present bodily health. Rate the degree to which physical health is perceived as a problem by the patient, whether complaints have a realistic basis or not. Do not rate mere reporting of somatic symptoms. Rate only concern for (or worrying about) physical problems (real or imagined). **Rate on the basis of reported (i.e., subjective) information pertaining to the past week.**
   1 = Not reported
   2 = Very Mild: occasionally is somewhat concerned about body, symptoms, or physical illness
   3 = Mild: occasionally is moderately concerned, or often is somewhat concerned
   4 = Moderate: occasionally is very concerned, or often is moderately concerned
   5 = Moderately Severe: often is very concerned
   6 = Severe: is very concerned most of the time
   7 = Very Severe: is very concerned nearly all of the time
   8 = Cannot be assessed adequately because of severe formal thought disorder, uncooperativeness, or marked evasiveness/guardedness; or Not assessed

2. **Anxiety:** Worry, fear, or overconcern for present or future: Rate solely on the basis of verbal report of patient's own subjective experiences pertaining to the past week.
   Do not infer anxiety from physical signs or from neurotic defense mechanisms. Do not rate if restricted to somatic concern.
   1 = Not reported
   2 = Very Mild: occasionally feels somewhat anxious
   3 = Mild: occasionally feels moderately anxious, or often feels somewhat anxious
   4 = Moderate: occasionally feels very anxious, or often feels moderately anxious
   5 = Moderately Severe: often feels very anxious
   6 = Severe: feels very anxious most of the time
   7 = Very Severe: feels very anxious nearly all of the time
   8 = Cannot be assessed adequately because of severe formal thought disorder, uncooperativeness, or marked evasiveness/guardedness; or Not assessed

3. **Emotional Withdrawal:** Deficiency in relating to the interviewer and to the interview situation. Overt manifestations of this deficiency include poor/absence of eye contact, failure to orient oneself physically toward the interviewer, and a general lack of involvement or engagement in the interview. Distinguish from BLUNTED AFFECT, in which deficits in facial expression, body gesture, and voice pattern are scored.
   1 = Not observed
   2 = Very Mild: e.g., occasionally exhibits poor eye contact
   3 = Mild: e.g., as above, but more frequent
   4 = Moderate: e.g., exhibits little eye contact, but still seems engaged in the interview and is appropriately responsive to all questions
   5 = Moderately Severe: e.g., stares at floor or orients self away from interviewer but still seems moderately engaged
   6 = Severe: e.g., as above, but more persistent or pervasive
   7 = Very Severe: e.g., appears "spacey" or "out of it" (total absence of emotional relatedness) and is disproportionately uninvolved or unengaged in the interview (DO NOT SCORE IF EXPLAINED BY DISORIENTATION)
   8 = Cannot be assessed adequately because of severe formal thought disorder, uncooperativeness, or marked evasiveness/guardedness; or Not assessed

4. **Conceptual Disorganization:** Degree of speech incomprehensibility. Include any type of formal thought disorder (e.g., loose associations, incoherence, flight of ideas, neologisms). DO NOT include mere circumstantiality or pressured speech, even if marked. DO NOT rate on the basis of the patient's subjective impressions (e.g., "my thoughts are racing. I can't hold a thought," "My thinking gets all mixed up"). Rate ONLY on the basis of observations made during the interview.
   1 = Not observed
   2 = Very Mild: e.g., somewhat vague, but of doubtful clinical significance
   3 = Mild: e.g., frequently vague, but the interview is able to progress smoothly; occasional loosening of associations
   4 = Moderate: e.g., occasional irrelevant statements, infrequent use of neologisms, or moderate loosening of associations
   5 = Moderately Severe: as above, but more frequent
   6 = Severe: formal thought disorder is present for most of the interview, and the interview is severely strained
   7 = Very Severe: e.g., appears "spacey" or "out of it" (total absence of emotional relatedness) and is disproportionately uninvolved or unengaged in the interview (DO NOT SCORE IF EXPLAINED BY DISORIENTATION)

Table 1-13
Brief Psychiatric Rating Scale (*Continued*)

DEPARTMENT OF HEALTH AND HUMAN SERVICES PUBLIC HEALTH SERVICE	PATIENT NUMBER – – – –	DATA GROUP bprs	EVALUATION DATE $\overline{M}\,\overline{D}\,\overline{Y}$
Alcohol, Drug Abuse, and Mental Health Administration NIMH Treatment Strategies in Schizophrenia Society	PATIENT NAME		
Brief Psychiatric Rating Scale – Anchored Overall and Gorham	RATER NUMBER		

RATER NUMBER – – –	EVALUATION TYPE (*Circle*)
	1. Baseline 4. Major evaluation 7. During open meds 10. Study completion 2. 4-wk minor 5. Other 8. Stop open minds 3. Start double-blind 6. Start open meds 9. Early termination

5. **Guilt Feelings:** Overconcern or remorse for past behavior. Rate on the basis of the patient's subjective experiences of guilt as evidenced by verbal report pertaining to the past week. Do not infer guilt feelings from depression, anxiety, or neurotic defenses.
   1 = Not reported
   2 = Very Mild: occasionally feels somewhat guilty
   3 = Mild: occasionally feels moderately guilty, or often feels somewhat guilty
   4 = Moderate: occasionally feels very guilty, or often feels moderately guilty
   5 = Moderately Severe: often feels very guilty
   6 = Severe: feels very guilty most of the time, or encapsulated delusion of guilt
   7 = Very Severe: agonizing constant feelings of guilt, or pervasive delusion(s) of guilt
   8 = Cannot be assessed adequately because of severe formal thought disorder, uncooperativeness, or marked evasiveness/guardedness; or Not assessed

6. **Tension:** Rate motor restlessness (agitation) observed during the interview.
   DO NOT rate on the basis of subjective experiences reported by the patient. Disregard suspected pathogenesis (e.g., tardive dyskinesia).
   1 = Not reported
   2 = Very Mild: e.g., occasionally fidgets
   3 = Mild: e.g., frequently fidgets
   4 = Moderate: e.g., constantly fidgets, or frequently fidgets, wrings hands and pulls clothing
   5 = Moderately Severe: e.g., constantly fidgets, wrings hands and pulls clothing
   6 = Severe: e.g., cannot remain seated (i.e., must pace)
   7 = Very Severe: e.g., paces in a frantic manner

7. **Mannerisms and Posturing:** Unusual and unnatural motor behavior.
   Rate only abnormality of movements. Do not rate simple heightened motor activity here. Consider frequency, duration, and degree of bizarreness. Disregard suspected pathogenesis.
   1 = Not observed
   2 = Very Mild: odd behavior but of doubtful clinical significance, e.g., occasional unprompted smiling, infrequent lip movements
   3 = Mild: strange behavior but not obviously bizarre, e.g., infrequent head-tilting (side to side) in a rhythmic fashion, intermittent abnormal finger movements
   4 = Moderate: e.g., assumes unnatural position for a brief period of time, infrequent tongue protrusions, rocking, facial grimacing
   5 = Moderately Severe: e.g., assumes and maintains unnatural position throughout interview, unusual movements in several body areas
   6 = Severe: as above, but more frequent, intense, or pervasive
   7 = Very Severe: e.g., bizarre posturing throughout most of the interview, continuous abnormal movements in several body areas

[a]8. **Grandiosity:** Inflated self-esteem (self-confidence), or inflated appraisal of one's talents, powers, abilities, accomplishments, knowledge, importance, or identity. Do not score mere grandiose quality of claims (e.g., "I'm the worst sinner in the world," "The entire country is trying to kill me") unless the guilt/persecution is related to some special, exaggerated attributes of the individual. Also, the patient must claim exaggerated attributes: e.g., if patient denies talents, powers, etc., even if he or she states that others indicate that he or she has these attributes, this item should not be scored. Rate on the basis of reported (i.e., subjective) information pertaining to the past week.
   1 = Not reported
   2 = Very Mild: e.g., is more confident than most people, but of only possible clinical significance
   3 = Mild: e.g., definitely inflated self-esteem or exaggerates talents somewhat out of proportion to the circumstances
   4 = Moderate: e.g., inflated self-esteem clearly out of proportion to the circumstances or suspected grandiose delusion(s)
   5 = Moderately Severe: e.g., a single (definite) encapsulated grandiose delusion, or multiple (definite) encapsulated grandiose delusion, or multiple (definite) fragmentary grandiose delusions
   6 = Severe: e.g., a single (definite) grandiose delusion/delusional system, or multiple (definite) grandiose delusions that the patient seems preoccupied with
   7 = Very Severe: e.g., as above, but nearly all conversation is directed toward the patient's grandiose delusion(s)
   8 = Cannot be assessed adequately because of severe formal thought disorder, uncooperativeness, or marked evasiveness/guardedness; or Not assessed

(continued)

Table 1-13
Brief Psychiatric Rating Scale (*Continued*)

DEPARTMENT OF HEALTH AND HUMAN SERVICES PUBLIC HEALTH SERVICE	PATIENT NUMBER – – – –	DATA GROUP bprs	EVALUATION DATE $\overline{}\,\overline{}\,\overline{}$ M D Y
Alcohol, Drug Abuse, and Mental Health Administration NIMH Treatment Strategies in Schizophrenia Society	PATIENT NAME		
Brief Psychiatric Rating Scale – Anchored Overall and Gorham	RATER NUMBER		

RATER NUMBER – – –	EVALUATION TYPE (*Circle*)			
	1. Baseline	4. Major evaluation	7. During open meds	10. Study completion
	2. 4-wk minor	5. Other	8. Stop open minds	
	3. Start double-blind	6. Start open meds	9. Early termination	

[a]9. **Depressive Mood:** Subjective report of feeling depressed, blue, "down in the dumps," etc. Rate only degree of reported depression. Do not rate on the basis of inferences concerning depression based upon general retardation and somatic complaints. Rate on the basis of report (i.e., subjective) information pertaining to the past week.
   1 = Not reported
   2 = Very Mild: occasionally feels somewhat depressed
   3 = Mild: occasionally feels moderately depressed, or often feels somewhat depressed
   4 = Moderate: occasionally feels very depressed, or often feels moderately depressed
   5 = Moderately Severe: often feels very depressed
   6 = Severe: feels very depressed most of the time
   7 = Very Severe: feels very depressed nearly all of the time
   8 = Cannot be assessed adequately because of severe formal thought disorder, uncooperativeness, or marked evasiveness/guardedness; or Not assessed

[a]10. **Hostility:** Animosity, contempt, belligerence, disdain for other people outside the interview situation. Rate solely on the basis of the verbal report of feelings and actions of the patient toward others during the past week. Do not infer hostility from neurotic defenses, anxiety, somatic complaints.
   1 = Not reported
   2 = Very Mild: occasionally feels somewhat angry
   3 = Mild: often feels somewhat angry, or occasionally feels moderately angry
   4 = Moderate: occasionally feels very angry, or often feels moderately angry
   5 = Moderately Severe: often feels very angry
   6 = Severe: has acted on his anger by becoming verbally or physically abusive on one or two occasions
   7 = Very Severe: has acted on his anger on several occasions
   8 = Cannot be assessed adequately because of severe formal thought disorder, uncooperativeness, or marked evasiveness/guardedness; or Not Assessed

[a]11. **Suspiciousness:** Belief (delusional or otherwise) that others have now, or have had in the past, malicious or discriminatory intent toward the patient. On the basis of verbal report, rate only those suspicions which are currently held whether they concern past or present circumstances. Rate on the basis of reported (i.e., subjective) information pertaining to the past week.
   1 = Not reported
   2 = Very Mild: rare instances of distrustfulness which may or may not be warranted by the situation
   3 = Mild: occasional instances of suspiciousness that are definitely not warranted by the situation
   4 = Moderate: more frequent suspiciousness, or transient ideas of reference
   5 = Moderately Severe: pervasive suspiciousness, frequent ideas of reference, or an encapsulated delusion
   6 = Severe: definite, delusion(s) of reference or persecution that is (are) not wholly pervasive (e.g., an encapsulated delusion)
   7 = Very Severe: as above, but more widespread, frequent, or intense
   8 = Cannot be assessed adequately because of severe formal thought disorder, uncooperativeness, or marked evasiveness/guardedness; or Not assessed

[a]12. **Hallucinatory Behavior:** Perceptions (in any sensory modality) in the absence of an identifiable external stimulus. Rate only those experiences that have occurred during the last week. DO NOT rate "voices in my head," or "visions in my mind" unless the patient can differentiate between these experiences and his or her thoughts.
   1 = Not reported
   2 = Very Mild: suspected hallucinations only
   3 = Mild: definite hallucinations, but insignificant, infrequent, or transient (e.g., occasional formless visual hallucinations, a voice calling the patient's name)
   4 = Moderate: as above, but more frequent or extensive (e.g., frequently sees the devil's face, two voices carry on lengthy conversations)
   5 = Moderately Severe: hallucinations are experienced nearly every day, or are a source of extreme distress
   6 = Severe: as above, and has had a moderate impact on the patient's behavior (e.g., concentration difficulties leading to impaired work functioning)
   7 = Very Severe: as above, and has had a severe impact (e.g., attempts suicide in response to command hallucinations)
   8 = Cannot be assessed adequately because of severe formal thought disorder, uncooperativeness, or marked evasiveness/guardedness; or Not assessed

Table 1-13
Brief Psychiatric Rating Scale (*Continued*)

DEPARTMENT OF HEALTH AND HUMAN SERVICES PUBLIC HEALTH SERVICE	PATIENT NUMBER _ _ _ _	DATA GROUP bprs	EVALUATION DATE M D Y
Alcohol, Drug Abuse, and Mental Health Administration NIMH Treatment Strategies in Schizophrenia Society	PATIENT NAME		
Brief Psychiatric Rating Scale – Anchored Overall and Gorham	RATER NUMBER		

RATER NUMBER _ _ _	EVALUATION TYPE (*Circle*)		
	1. Baseline	4. Major evaluation	7. During open meds 10. Study completion
	2. 4-wk minor	5. Other	8. Stop open minds
	3. Start double-blind	6. Start open meds	9. Early termination

13. **Motor Retardation:** Reduction in energy level evidenced in slowed movements. Rate on the basis of observed behavior of the patient only. Do not rate on the basis of the patient's subjective impression of his or her own energy level.
   1 = Not observed
   2 = Very Mild: Very Mild and of doubtful clinical significance
   3 = Mild: e.g., conversation is somewhat retarded, movements somewhat slowed
   4 = Moderate: e.g., conversation is noticeably retarded but not strained
   5 = Moderately Severe: e.g., conversation is strained, moves very slowly
   6 = Severe: e.g., conversation is difficult to maintain, hardly moves at all
   7 = Very Severe: e.g., conversation is almost impossible, does not move at all throughout interview

14. **Uncooperativeness:** Evidence of resistance, unfriendliness, resentment, and lack of readiness to cooperate with the interviewer. Rate only on the basis of the patient's attitude and responses to the interviewer and the interview situation. Do not rate on the basis of reported resentment or uncooperativeness outside the interview situation.
   1 = Not observed
   2 = Very Mild: e.g., does not seem motivated
   3 = Mild: e.g., seems evasive in certain areas
   4 = Moderate: e.g., monosyllabic, fails to elaborate spontaneously, somewhat unfriendly
   5 = Moderately Severe: e.g., expresses resentment and is unfriendly throughout the interview
   6 = Severe: e.g., refuses to answer a number of questions
   7 = Very Severe: e.g., refuses to answer most questions

15. **Unusual Thought Content:** Severity of delusions of any type—consider conviction, and effect on actions. Assume full conviction if patient has acted on his or her beliefs. Rate on the basis of reported (i.e., subjective) information pertaining to past week.
   1 = Not reported
   2 = Very Mild: delusion(s) suspected or likely
   3 = Mild: at times, patient questions his or her belief(s) (partial delusion)
   4 = Moderate: full delusional conviction, but delusion(s) has little or no influence on behavior
   5 = Moderately Severe: full delusional conviction, but delusion(s) has only occasional impact on behavior
   6 = Severe: delusion(s) has significant effect, e.g., neglects responsibilities because of preoccupation with belief that he/she is God
   7 = Very Severe: delusion(s) has major impact, e.g., stops eating because believes food is poisoned

16. **Blunted Affect:** Diminished affective responsivity, as characterized by deficits in facial expression, body gesture, and voice pattern. Distinguish from EMOTIONAL WITHDRAWAL, in which the focus is on interpersonal impairment rather than affect. Consider degree and consistency of impairment. Rate based on observations made during interview.
   1 = Not reported
   2 = Very Mild: e.g., occasionally seems indifferent to material that is usually accompanied by some show of emotion
   3 = Mild: e.g., somewhat diminished facial expression, or somewhat monotonous voice or somewhat restricted gestures
   4 = Moderate: e.g., as above, but more intense, prolonged, or frequent
   5 = Moderately Severe: e.g., flattening of affect, including at least two of the three features: severe lack of facial expression, monotonous voice or restricted body gestures
   6 = Severe: e.g., profound flattening of affect
   7 = Very Severe: e.g., totally monotonous voice, and total lack of expressive gestures throughout the evaluation

17. **Excitement:** Heightened emotional tone, including irritability and expansiveness (hypomanic affect). Do not infer affect from statements of grandiose delusions. Rate based on observations made during interview.
   1 = Not reported
   2 = Very Mild and of doubtful clinical significance
   3 = Mild: e.g., irritable or expansive at times
   4 = Moderate: e.g., frequently irritable or expansive
   5 = Moderately Severe: e.g., constantly irritable or expansive; or, at times, enraged or euphoric
   6 = Severe: e.g., enraged or euphoric throughout most of the interview
   7 = Very Severe: e.g., as above, but to such a degree that the interview must be terminated prematurely

(*continued*)

Table 1-13
Brief Psychiatric Rating Scale (*Continued*)

DEPARTMENT OF HEALTH AND HUMAN SERVICES PUBLIC HEALTH SERVICE	PATIENT NUMBER — — — —	DATA GROUP bprs	EVALUATION DATE M̄ D̄ Ȳ
Alcohol, Drug Abuse, and Mental Health Administration NIMH Treatment Strategies in Schizophrenia Society	PATIENT NAME		
Brief Psychiatric Rating Scale – Anchored Overall and Gorham	RATER NUMBER		

RATER NUMBER — — —	EVALUATION TYPE (*Circle*)
	1. Baseline 4. Major evaluation 7. During open meds 10. Study completion
	2. 4-wk minor 5. Other 8. Stop open minds
	3. Start double-blind 6. Start open meds 9. Early termination

18. **Disorientation:** Confusion or lack of proper association for person, place or time.
Rate based on observations made during interview.
1 = Not reported
2 = Very Mild: e.g., seems somewhat confused
3 = Mild: e.g., indicated 1982 when, in fact, it is 1983
4 = Moderate: e.g., indicates 1978
5 = Moderately Severe: e.g., is unsure where he/she is
6 = Severe: e.g., has no idea where he/she is
7 = Very Severe: e.g., does not know who he/she is
8 = Cannot be assessed adequately because of severe formal thought disorder, uncooperativeness, or marked evasiveness/guardedness; or Not assessed

19. **Severity of Illness:** Considering your total clinical experience with this patient population, how mentally ill is the patient at this time?
1 = Normal, not at all ill
2 = Borderline mentally ill
3 = Mildly ill
4 = Moderately ill
5 = Markedly ill
6 = Severely ill
7 = Among the most severely ill patients

20. **Global Improvement:** Rate total improvement whether or not, in your judgment, it is due to treatment. At baseline assessment, mark "Not assessed" for item 20. For assessments up to the start of double-blind medication, rate Global Improvement compared to baseline. For assessments following the start of double-blind medication, rate Global Improvement compared to the start of double-blind.
1 = Very much improved
2 = Much improved
3 = Minimally improved
4 = No change
5 = Minimally worse
6 = Much worse
7 = Very much worse
8 = Not assessed

ᵃRatings based primarily on verbal report.
From Sadock BJ, Sadock VA, Ruiz P. *Kaplan & Sadock's Comprehensive Textbook of Psychiatry*. 9th ed. Philadelphia, PA: Lippincott Williams & Wilkins; 2009:1043, with permission.

symptom severity measures. A developing consensus suggests that the distinction between positive and negative symptoms in schizophrenia is worthwhile, and more recently developed instruments implement this distinction.

BRIEF PSYCHIATRIC RATING SCALE (BPRS). The BPRS (Table 1-13) was developed in the late 1960s as a short scale for measuring the severity of psychiatric symptomatology. It was designed primarily to assess change in psychotic inpatients and covers a broad range of areas, including thought disturbance, emotional withdrawal and retardation, anxiety and depression, and hostility and suspiciousness. The reliability of the BPRS is good to excellent when raters are experienced, but this is difficult to achieve without substantial training; a semistructured interview has been developed to increase reliability. Validity is also good as measured by correlations with other measures of symptom severity, especially those assessing schizophrenia symptomatology. The BPRS has been used extensively for decades as an outcome measure in treatment studies

of schizophrenia; it functions well as a measure of the change in this context and offers the advantage of comparability with earlier trials. However, it has been largely supplanted in more recent clinical trials by the newer measures described below. Also, given its focus on psychosis and associated symptoms, it is only suitable for patients with fairly significant impairment. Its use in clinical practice is less well supported, in part because considerable training is required to achieve the necessary reliability.

POSITIVE AND NEGATIVE SYNDROME SCALE (PANSS). The PANSS was developed in the late 1980s to remedy perceived deficits in the BPRS in the assessment of positive and negative symptoms of schizophrenia and other psychotic disorders by adding additional items and providing careful anchors for each. The PANSS requires a clinician rater because it requires considerable probing and clinical judgment. A semistructured interview guide is available. Reliability for each scale is reasonably high, with excellent internal consistency and interrater reliability. Validity also appears good based on correlation with other symptom severity measures and factor analytic validation of the subscales. The PANSS has become the standard tool for assessing clinical outcome in treatment studies of schizophrenia and other psychotic disorders and is easy to administer reliably and sensitive to change with treatment. Its high reliability and good coverage of both positive and negative symptoms make it excellent for this purpose. It may also be useful for tracking severity in clinical practice, and its clear anchors make it easy to use in this setting.

SCALE FOR THE ASSESSMENT OF POSITIVE SYMPTOMS (SAPS) AND SCALE FOR THE ASSESSMENT OF NEGATIVE SYMPTOMS (SANS). The SAPS and SANS (Tables 1-14 and 1-15) were designed to provide a detailed assessment of positive and negative symptoms of schizophrenia and may be used separately or in tandem. SAPS assesses hallucinations, delusions, bizarre behavior, and thought disorder, and SANS assesses affective flattening, poverty of speech, apathy, anhedonia, and inattentiveness. The SAPS and SANS are mainly used to monitor treatment effects in clinical research.

Mood Disorders.

The domain of mood disorders includes both unipolar and bipolar disorder, and the instruments described here assess depression and mania. For mania, the issues are similar to those for psychotic disorders in that limited insight and agitation may hinder accurate symptom reporting, so clinician ratings, including observational data, are generally required. Rating depression, on the other hand, depends, to a substantial extent, on subjective assessment of mood states, so interviews and self-report instruments are both common. Because depression is common in the general population and involves significant morbidity and even mortality, screening instruments—especially those using a self-report format—are potentially quite useful in primary care and community settings.

HAMILTON RATING SCALE FOR DEPRESSION (HAM-D). The HAM-D was developed in the early 1960s to monitor the severity of major depression, with a focus on somatic symptomatology. The 17-item version is the most commonly used version, although versions with different numbers of items, including the 24-item version in Table 1-16, have been used in many studies as well. The 17-item version does not include some of the symptoms for depression in DSM-III and its successors, most notably the so-called reverse neurovegetative signs (increased sleep, increased appetite, and psychomotor retardation). The HAM-D was designed for clinician raters but has been used by trained lay administrators as well. Ratings are completed by the examiner based on the patient interview and observations. A structured interview guide has been developed to improve reliability. The ratings can be completed in 15 to 20 minutes. Reliability is good to excellent, particularly when the structured interview version is used. Validity appears good based on correlation with other depression symptom measures. The HAM-D has been used extensively to evaluate a change in response to pharmacologic and other interventions and, thus, offers the advantage of comparability across a broad range of treatment trials. It is more problematic in the elderly and the medically ill, in whom the presence of somatic symptoms may not be indicative of major depression.

BECK DEPRESSION INVENTORY (BDI). The BDI was developed in the early 1960s to rate depression severity, with a focus on behavioral and cognitive dimensions of depression. The current version, the Beck-II, has added more coverage of somatic symptoms and covers the most recent 2 weeks. Earlier versions are focused on the past week or even shorter intervals, which may be preferable for monitoring treatment response. The scale can be completed in 5 to 10 minutes. Internal consistency has been high in numerous studies. Test–retest reliability is not consistently high, but this may reflect changes in underlying symptoms. Validity is supported by correlation with other depression measures. The principal use of the BDI is as an outcome measure in clinical trials of interventions for major depression, including psychotherapeutic interventions. Because it is a self-report instrument, it is sometimes used to screen for major depression.

Anxiety Disorders.

The anxiety disorders addressed by the measures below include panic disorder, generalized anxiety disorder, posttraumatic stress disorder (PTSD), and obsessive-compulsive disorder (OCD). When anxiety measures are examined, it is important to be aware that there have been significant changes over time in how anxiety disorders are defined. Both panic and OCD are relatively recently recognized, and the conceptualization of generalized anxiety disorder has shifted over time. Thus, older measures have somewhat less relevance for diagnostic purposes, although they may identify symptoms causing considerable distress. Whether reported during an interview or on a self-report rating scale, virtually all measures in this domain, like the measures of depression discussed above, depend on subjective descriptions of inner states.

HAMILTON ANXIETY RATING SCALE (HAM-A). The HAM-A (Table 1-17) was developed in the late 1950s to assess anxiety symptoms, both somatic and cognitive. Because the conceptualization of anxiety has changed considerably, the HAM-A provides limited coverage of the "worry" required for a diagnosis of generalized anxiety disorder and does not include the episodic anxiety found in panic disorder. A score of 14 has been suggested as the threshold for clinically significant anxiety, but scores of 5 or less are typical in individuals in the community. The scale is designed to be administered by a clinician, and formal training or the use of a structured interview guide is required to achieve high reliability. A computer-administered version is also available. Reliability is fairly good based on internal consistency, interrater, and test–retest studies. However, given the lack of specific anchors, reliability should not be assumed to be high across different users in the absence of formal training. Validity appears good based on correlation with other anxiety scales but is limited by the relative lack of coverage of domains critical to the modern understanding of anxiety disorders. Even so, the HAM-A has been used extensively to monitor treatment response in clinical trials of generalized anxiety disorder and may also be useful for this purpose in clinical settings.

PANIC DISORDER SEVERITY SCALE (PDSS). The PDSS was developed in the 1990s as a brief rating scale for the severity of panic disorder. It was based on the Yale-Brown Obsessive-Compulsive Scale and has seven items, each of which is rated on an item-specific, 5-point Likert scale. The seven items address frequency of attacks, distress associated with attacks, anticipatory anxiety, phobic avoidance, and impairment. Reliability is excellent based on interrater studies, but, in keeping with the small number of items and multiple dimensions, internal consistency is limited. Validity is supported by correlations with other anxiety measures, both at the total and item levels; lack of correlation with the HAM-D; and, more recently, by brain imaging studies. Growing experience with the PDSS suggests that it is sensitive to change

Table 1-14
Scale for the Assessment of Positive Symptoms (SAPS)

0 = None	1 = Questionable	2 = Mild	3 = Moderate	4 = Marked	5 = Severe

Hallucinations

1 *Auditory hallucinations* The patient reports voices, noises, or other sounds that no one else hears.   0 1 2 3 4 5

2 *Voices commenting* The patient reports a voice which makes a running commentary on his [her] behavior or thoughts.   0 1 2 3 4 5

3 *Voices conversing* The patient reports hearing two or more voices conversing.   0 1 2 3 4 5

4 *Somatic or tactile hallucinations* The patient reports experiencing peculiar physical sensations in the body.   0 1 2 3 4 5

5 *Olfactory hallucinations* The patient reports experiencing unusual smells which no one else notices.   0 1 2 3 4 5

6 *Visual hallucinations* The patient sees shapes or people that are not actually present.   0 1 2 3 4 5

7 *Global rating of hallucinations* This rating should be based on the duration and severity of the hallucinations and their effects on the patient's life.   0 1 2 3 4 5

Delusions

8 *Persecutory delusions* The patient believes he [she] is being conspired against or persecuted in some way.   0 1 2 3 4 5

9 *Delusions of jealousy* The patient believes his [her] spouse is having an affair with someone.   0 1 2 3 4 5

10 *Delusions of guilt or sin* The patient believes that he [she] has committed some terrible sin or done something unforgivable.   0 1 2 3 4 5

11 *Grandiose delusions* The patient believes he [she] has special powers or abilities.   0 1 2 3 4 5

12 *Religious delusions* The patient is preoccupied with false beliefs of a religious nature.   0 1 2 3 4 5

13 *Somatic delusions* The patient believes that somehow his [her] body is diseased, abnormal, or changed.   0 1 2 3 4 5

14 *Delusions of reference* The patient believes that insignificant remarks or events refer to him [her] or have some special meaning.   0 1 2 3 4 5

15 *Delusions of being controlled* The patient feels that his [her] feelings or actions are controlled by some outside force.   0 1 2 3 4 5

16 *Delusions of mind reading* The patient feels that people can read his [her] mind or know his [her] thoughts.   0 1 2 3 4 5

17 *Thought broadcasting* The patient believes that his [her] thoughts are broadcast so that he himself [she herself] or others can hear them.   0 1 2 3 4 5

18 *Thought insertion* The patient believes that thoughts that are not his [her] own have been inserted into his [her] mind.   0 1 2 3 4 5

19 *Thought withdrawal* The patient believes that thoughts have been taken away from his [her] mind.   0 1 2 3 4 5

20 *Global rating of delusions* This rating should be based on the duration and persistence of the delusions and their effect on the patient's life.   0 1 2 3 4 5

Bizarre Behavior

21 *Clothing and appearance* The patient dresses in an unusual manner or does other strange things to alter his [her] appearance.   0 1 2 3 4 5

22 *Social and sexual behavior* The patient may do things considered inappropriate according to usual social norms (e.g., masturbating in public).   0 1 2 3 4 5

23 *Aggressive and agitated behavior* The patient may behave in an aggressive, agitated manner, often unpredictably.   0 1 2 3 4 5

24 *Repetitive or stereotyped behavior* The patient develops a set of repetitive actions or rituals that he [she] must perform over and over.   0 1 2 3 4 5

25 *Global rating of bizarre behavior* This rating should reflect the type of behavior and the extent to which it deviates from social norms.   0 1 2 3 4 5

Positive Formal Thought Disorder

26 *Derailment* A pattern of speech in which ideas slip off track onto ideas obliquely related or unrelated.   0 1 2 3 4 5

27 *Tangentiality* Replying to a question in an oblique or irrelevant manner.   0 1 2 3 4 5

28 *Incoherence* A pattern of speech which is essentially incomprehensible at times.   0 1 2 3 4 5

29 *Illogicality* A pattern of speech in which conclusions are reached which do not follow logically.   0 1 2 3 4 5

30 *Circumstantiality* A pattern of speech which is very indirect and delayed in reaching its goal idea.   0 1 2 3 4 5

31 *Pressure of speech* The patient's speech is rapid and difficult to interrupt; the amount of speech produced is greater than that considered normal.   0 1 2 3 4 5

32 *Distractible speech* The patient is distracted by nearby stimuli which interrupt his [her] flow of speech.   0 1 2 3 4 5

33 *Clanging* A pattern of speech in which sounds rather than meaningful relationships govern word choice.   0 1 2 3 4 5

34 *Global rating of positive formal thought disorder* This rating should reflect the frequency of abnormality and degree to which it affects the patient's ability to communicate.   0 1 2 3 4 5

Inappropriate Affect

35 *Inappropriate affect* The patient's affect is inappropriate or incongruous, not simply flat or blunted.   0 1 2 3 4 5

Table 1-15
Scale for the Assessment of Negative Symptoms (SANS)

0 = None	1 = Questionable	2 = Mild	3 = Moderate	4 = Marked	5 = Severe

Affective Flattening or Blunting

1 *Unchanging facial expression* The patient's face appears wooden, changes less than expected as emotional content of discourse changes. — 0 1 2 3 4 5

2 *Decreased spontaneous movements* The patient shows few or no spontaneous movements, does not shift position, move extremities, etc. — 0 1 2 3 4 5

3 *Paucity of expressive gestures* The patient does not use hand gestures, body position, etc., as an aid to expressing his ideas. — 0 1 2 3 4 5

4 *Poor eye contact* The patient avoids eye contact or "stares through" interviewer even when speaking. — 0 1 2 3 4 5

5 *Affective nonresponsivity* The patient fails to smile or laugh when prompted. — 0 1 2 3 4 5

6 *Lack of vocal inflections* The patient fails to show normal vocal emphasis patterns, is often monotonic. — 0 1 2 3 4 5

7 *Global rating of affective flattening* This rating should focus on overall severity of symptoms, especially unresponsiveness, eye contact, facial expression, and vocal inflections. — 0 1 2 3 4 5

Alogia

8 *Poverty of speech* The patient's replies to questions are restricted in *amount* tend to be brief, concrete, and unelaborated. — 0 1 2 3 4 5

9 *Poverty of content of speech* The patient's replies are adequate in amount but tend to be vague, overconcrete, or overgeneralized, and convey little information. — 0 1 2 3 4 5

10 *Blocking* The patient indicates, either spontaneously or with prompting, that his [her] train of thought was interrupted. — 0 1 2 3 4 5

11 *Increased latency of response* The patient takes a long time to reply to questions; prompting indicates the patient is aware of the question. — 0 1 2 3 4 5

12 *Global rating of alogia* The core features of alogia are poverty of speech and poverty of content. — 0 1 2 3 4 5

Avolition-apathy

13 *Grooming and hygiene* The patient's clothes may be sloppy or soiled, and he [she] may have greasy hair, body odor, etc. — 0 1 2 3 4 5

14 *Impersistence at work or school* The patient has difficulty seeking or maintaining employment, completing school work, keeping house, etc. If an inpatient, cannot persist at ward activities, such as occupational therapy, playing cards, etc. — 0 1 2 3 4 5

15 *Physical anergia* The patient tends to be physically inert. He [she] may sit for hours and does not initiate spontaneous activity. — 0 1 2 3 4 5

16 *Global rating of avolition-apathy* Strong weight may be given to one or two prominent symptoms if particularly striking. — 0 1 2 3 4 5

Anhedonia-asociality

17 *Recreational interests and activities* The patient may have few or no interests. Both the quality and quantity of interests should be taken into account. — 0 1 2 3 4 5

18 *Sexual activity* The patient may show a decrease in sexual interest and activity, or enjoyment when active. — 0 1 2 3 4 5

19 *Ability to feel intimacy and closeness* The patient may display an inability to form close or intimate relationships, especially with the opposite sex and family. — 0 1 2 3 4 5

20 *Relationships with friends and peers* The patient may have few or no friends and may prefer to spend all of his [her] time isolated. — 0 1 2 3 4 5

21 *Global rating of anhedonia-asociality* This rating should reflect overall severity, taking into account the patient's age, family status, etc. — 0 1 2 3 4 5

Attention

22 *Social inattentiveness* The patient appears uninvolved or unengaged. He [she] may seem spacey. — 0 1 2 3 4 5

23 *Inattentiveness during mental status testing* Tests of "serial 7s" (at least five subtractions) and spelling *world* backward: Score: 2 = 1 error; 3 = 2 errors; 4 = 3 errors. — 0 1 2 3 4 5

24 *Global rating of attention* This rating should assess the patient's overall concentration, clinically and on tests. — 0 1 2 3 4 5

From Nancy C. Andreasen, M.D., Ph.D., Department of Psychiatry, College of Medicine, The University of Iowa, Iowa City, IA 52242, with permission.

with treatment and is useful as a change measure in clinical trials or other outcome studies for panic disorder, as well as for monitoring panic disorder in clinical practice.

CLINICIAN-ADMINISTERED PTSD SCALE (CAPS). The CAPS includes 17 items required to make the diagnosis, covering all four criteria: (1) the event itself, (2) reexperiencing of the event, (3) avoidance, and (4) increased arousal. The diagnosis requires evidence of a traumatic event, one symptom of reexperiencing, three of

avoidance, and two of arousal (typically, an item is counted if the frequency is rated at least 1 and intensity is at least 2). The items can also be used to generate a total PTSD severity score obtained by summing the frequency and intensity scales for each item. The CAPS also includes several global rating scales for the impact of PTSD symptomatology on social and occupational functioning, for general severity, for recent changes, and the validity of the patient's report. The CAPS must be administered by a trained clinician and requires 45 to 60 minutes to complete, with follow-up examinations

Table 1-16
Hamilton Rating Scale for Depression

For each item select the "cue" which best characterizes the patient.

1: Depressed mood (Sadness, hopeless, helpless, worthless)
 0 Absent
 1 These feeling states indicated only on questioning
 2 These feeling states spontaneously reported verbally
 3 Communicates feeling states nonverbally—i.e., through facial expression, posture, voice, and tendency to weep
 4 Patient reports VIRTUALLY ONLY these feeling states in his spontaneous verbal and nonverbal communication

2: Feelings of guilt
 0 Absent
 1 Self-reproach, feels he has let people down
 2 Ideas of guilt or rumination over past errors or sinful deeds
 3 Present illness is a punishment. Delusions of guilt.
 4 Hears accusatory or denunciatory voices and/or experiences threatening visual hallucinations

3: Suicide
 0 Absent
 1 Feels life is not worth living
 2 Wishes he were dead or any thoughts of possible death to self
 3 Suicide ideas or gesture
 4 Attempts at suicide (any serious attempt rates 4)

4: Insomnia early
 0 No difficulty falling asleep
 1 Complains of occasional difficulty falling asleep—i.e., more than ¼ hour
 2 Complains of nightly difficulty falling asleep

5: Insomnia middle
 0 No difficulty
 1 Patient complains of being restless and disturbed during the night
 2 Waking during the night—any getting out of bed rates 2 (except for purpose of voiding)

6: Insomnia late
 0 No difficulty
 1 Waking in early hours of the morning but goes back to sleep
 2 Unable to fall asleep again if gets out of bed

7: Work and activities
 0 No difficulty
 1 Thoughts and feelings of incapacity, fatigue, or weakness related to activities, work, or hobbies
 2 Loss of interest in activity, hobbies, or work—either directly reported by patient, or indirect in listlessness, indecision, and vacillation (feels he has to push self to work or activities)
 3 Decrease in actual time spent in activities or decrease in productivity. In hospital, rate 3 if patient does not spend at least 3 hours a day in activities (hospital job or hobbies) exclusive of ward chores
 4 Stopped working because of present illness. In hospital, rate 4 if patient engages in no activities except ward chores, or if patient fails to perform ward chores unassisted

8: Retardation (Slowness of thought and speech; impaired ability to concentrate; decreased motor activity)
 0 Normal speech and thought
 1 Slight retardation at interview
 2 Obvious retardation at interview
 3 Interview difficult
 4 Complete stupor

9: Agitation
 0 None
 1 "Playing with" hands, hair, etc.
 2 Hand-wringing, nail biting, hair pulling, biting of lips

10: Anxiety psychic
 0 No difficulty
 1 Subjective tension and irritability
 2 Worrying about minor matters
 3 Apprehensive attitude apparent in face or speech
 4 Fears expressed without questioning

11: Anxiety somatic

0 Absent	Physiologic concomitants of anxiety, such as:
1 Mild	
2 Moderate	Gastrointestinal—dry mouth, wind, indigestion, diarrhea, cramps, belching
3 Severe	Cardiovascular—palpitations, headaches
4 Incapacitating	Respiratory—hyperventilation, sighing Urinary frequency Sweating

12: Somatic symptoms gastrointestinal
 0 None
 1 Loss of appetite but eating without staff encouragement Heavy feelings in abdomen
 2 Difficulty eating without staff urging; requests or requires laxatives or medication for bowels or medication for GI symptoms

13: Somatic symptoms general
 0 None
 1 Heaviness in limbs, back, or head. Backaches, headache, muscle aches. Loss of energy and fatigability
 2 Any clear-cut symptom rates 2

14: Genital symptoms

0 Absent	Symptoms such as:
1 Mild	Loss of libido
2 Severe	Menstrual disturbances

15: Hypochondriasis
 0 Not present
 1 Self-absorption (bodily)
 2 Preoccupation with health
 3 Frequent complaints, requests for help, etc.
 4 Hypochondriacal delusions

16: Loss of weight
 When rating by history
 0 No weight loss
 1 Probable weight loss associated with present illness
 2 Definite (according to patient) weight loss
 On weekly ratings by ward psychiatrist, when actual weight changes are measured
 0 Less than 1 lb weight loss in week
 1 Greater than 1 lb weight loss in week
 2 Greater than 2 lb weight loss in week

17: Insight
 0 Acknowledges being depressed and ill
 1 Acknowledges illness but attributes cause to bad food, climate, overwork, virus, need for rest, etc.
 2 Denies being ill at all

18: Diurnal variation

AM	PM		
0	0	Absent	If symptoms are worse in the morning or
1	1	Mild	evening, note which it is and rate
2	2	Severe	severity of variation

Table 1-16
Hamilton Rating Scale for Depression (*Continued*)

19: Depersonalization and derealization
   0 Absent
   1 Mild   Such as:
   2 Moderate   Feeling of unreality
   3 Severe   Nihilistic ideas
   4 Incapacitating

20: Paranoid symptoms
   0 None
   1
   Suspiciousness
   2
   3 Ideas of reference
   4 Delusions of reference and persecution

21: Obsessional and compulsive symptoms
   0 Absent
   1 Mild
   2 Severe

22: Helplessness
   0 Not present
   1 Subjective feelings which are elicited only by inquiry
   2 Patient volunteers his helpless feelings
   3 Requires urging, guidance, and reassurance to accomplish ward chores or personal hygiene
   4 Requires physical assistance for dress, grooming, eating, bedside tasks, or personal hygiene

23: Hopelessness
   0 Not present
   1 Intermittently doubts that "things will improve" but can be reassured
   2 Consistently feels "hopeless" but accepts reassurances
   3 Expresses feelings of discouragement, despair, pessimism about future, which cannot be dispelled
   4 Spontaneously and inappropriately perseverates: "I'll never get well" or its equivalent

24: Worthlessness (Ranges from mild loss of esteem, feelings of inferiority, self-deprecation to delusional notions of worthlessness)
   0 Not present
   1 Indicates feelings of worthlessness (loss of self-esteem) only on questioning
   2 Spontaneously indicates feelings of worthlessness (loss of self-esteem)
   3 Different from 2 by degree. Patient volunteers that he is "no good," "inferior," etc.
   4 Delusional notions of worthlessness—i.e., "I am a heap of garbage" or its equivalent

From Hamilton M. A rating scale for depression. *J Neurol Neurosurg Psychiatry*. 1960;23:56, with permission.

Table 1-17
Hamilton Anxiety Rating Scale

Instructions: This checklist is to assist the physician or psychiatrist in evaluating each patient as to his degree of anxiety and pathologic condition. Please fill in the appropriate rating:

NONE = 0	MILD = 1	MODERATE = 2	SEVERE = 3	SEVERE, GROSSLY DISABLING = 4

Item		Rating
Anxious	Worries, anticipation of the worst, fearful anticipation, irritability	_____
Tension	Feelings of tension, fatigability, startle response, moved to tears easily, trembling, feelings of restlessness, inability to relax	_____
Fears	Of dark, of strangers, of being left alone, of animals, of traffic, of crowds	_____
Insomnia	Difficulty in falling asleep, broken sleep, unsatisfying sleep and fatigue on waking, dreams, nightmares, night-terrors	_____
Intellectual (cognitive)	Difficulty in concentration, poor memory	_____
Depressed mood	Loss of interest, lack of pleasure in hobbies, depression, early waking, diurnal swing	_____
Somatic (muscular)	Pains and aches, twitching, stiffness, myoclonic jerks, grinding of teeth, unsteady voice, increased muscular tone	_____
Somatic (sensory)	Tinnitus, blurring of vision, hot and cold flushes, feelings of weakness, picking sensation	_____
Cardiovascular symptoms	Tachycardia, palpitations, pain in chest, throbbing of vessels, fainting feelings, missing beat	_____
Respiratory symptoms	Pressure or constriction in chest, choking feelings, sighing, dyspnea	_____
Gastrointestinal symptoms	Difficulty in swallowing, wind, abdominal pain, burning sensations, abdominal fullness, nausea, vomiting, borborygmi, looseness of bowels, loss of weight, constipation	_____
Genitourinary symptoms	Frequency of micturition, urgency of micturition, amenorrhea, menorrhagia, development of frigidity, premature ejaculation, loss of libido, impotence	_____
Autonomic symptoms	Dry mouth, flushing, pallor, tendency to sweat, giddiness, tension headache, raising of hair	_____
Behavior at interview	Fidgeting, restlessness or pacing, tremor of hands, furrowed brow, strained face, sighing or rapid respiration, facial pallor, swallowing, belching, brisk tendon jerks, dilated pupils, exophthalmos	_____

ADDITIONAL COMMENTS
Investigator's signature:

From Hamilton M. The assessment of anxiety states by rating. *Br J Psychiatry*. 1959;32:50, with permission.

somewhat briefer. It has demonstrated reliability and validity in multiple settings and multiple languages, although it has had more limited testing in the setting of sexual and criminal assault. It performs well in the research setting for diagnosis and severity assessment but is generally too long for use in clinical practice.

YALE–BROWN OBSESSIVE-COMPULSIVE SCALE (YBOCS). The YBOCS was developed in the late 1980s to measure the severity of symptoms in OCD. It has 10 items rated based on a semistructured interview. The first five items concern obsessions: the amount of time that they consume, the degree to which they interfere with normal functioning, the distress that they cause, the patient's attempts to resist them, and the patient's ability to control them. The remaining five items ask parallel questions about compulsions. The semistructured interview and ratings can be completed in 15 minutes or less. A self-administered version has recently been developed and can be completed in 10 to 15 minutes. Computerized and telephone use have also been found to provide acceptable ratings. Reliability studies of the YBOCS show good internal consistency, interrater reliability, and test–retest reliability over a 1-week interval. Validity appears good, although data are fairly limited in this developing field. The YBOCS has become the standard instrument for assessing OCD severity and is used in virtually every drug trial. It may also be used clinically to monitor treatment response.

Substance Use Disorders.

Substance use disorders include abuse and dependence on both alcohol and drugs. These disorders, particularly those involving alcohol, are common and debilitating in the general population, so screening instruments are particularly helpful. Because these behaviors are socially undesirable, underreporting of symptoms is a significant problem; thus, the validity of all substance use measures is limited by the honesty of the patient. Validation against drug tests or other measures is of great value, particularly when working with patients who have known substance abuse.

CAGE. The CAGE was developed in the mid-1970s to serve as a very brief screen for significant alcohol problems in a variety of settings, which could then be followed up by clinical inquiry. CAGE is an acronym for the four questions that comprise the instrument: (1) Have you ever felt you should Cut down on your drinking? (2) Have people Annoyed you by criticizing your drinking? (3) Have you ever felt bad or Guilty about your drinking? (4) Have you ever had a drink first thing in the morning to steady your nerves or to get rid of a hangover (Eye-opener)? Each "yes" answer is scored as 1, and these are summed to generate a total score. Scores of 1 or more warrant follow-up, and scores of 2 or more strongly suggest significant alcohol problems. The instrument can be administered in a minute or less, either orally or on paper. Reliability has not been formally assessed. Validity has been assessed against a clinical diagnosis of alcohol abuse or dependence, and these four questions perform surprisingly well. Using a threshold score of 1, the CAGE achieves excellent sensitivity and fair to good specificity. A threshold of 2 provides still greater specificity but at the cost of a drop in sensitivity. The CAGE performs well as an extremely brief screening instrument for use in primary care or in psychiatric practice focused on problems unrelated to alcohol. However, it has limited ability to pick up early indicators of problem drinking that might be the focus of preventive efforts.

ADDICTION SEVERITY INDEX (ASI). The ASI was developed in the early 1980s to serve as a quantitative measure of symptoms and functional impairment due to alcohol or drug disorders. It covers demographics, alcohol use, drug use, psychiatric status, medical status, employment, legal status, and family and social issues. Frequency, duration, and severity are assessed. It includes both subjective and objective items reported by the patient and observations made by the interviewer.

Eating Disorders.

Eating disorders include anorexia nervosa, bulimia, and binge-eating disorder. A wide variety of instruments, particularly self-report scales, are available. Because of the secrecy that may surround dieting, bingeing, purging, and other symptoms, validation against other indicators (e.g., body weight for anorexia or dental examination for bulimia) may be very helpful. Such validation is particularly critical for patients with anorexia, who may lack insight into their difficulties.

EATING DISORDERS EXAMINATION (EDE). The EDE was developed in 1987 as the first interviewer-based comprehensive assessment of eating disorders, including diagnosis, severity, and an assessment of subthreshold symptoms. A self-report version (the EDE-Q), as well as an interview for children, have since been developed. The EDE focuses on symptoms during the preceding 4 weeks, although longer-term questions are included to assess diagnostic criteria for eating disorders. Each item on the EDE has a required probe with suggested follow-up questions to judge severity, frequency, or both, which are then rated on a 7-point Likert scale. For the self-report version, subjects are asked to make similar ratings of frequency or severity. The instrument provides both global severity ratings and ratings on four subscales: restraint, eating concern, weight concern, and shape concern. The interview, which must be administered by a trained clinician, requires 30 to 60 minutes to complete, whereas the self-report version can be completed more quickly. Reliability and validity data for both the EDE and EDE-Q are excellent, although the EDE-Q may have greater sensitivity for binge-eating disorder. The EDE performs well in both the diagnosis and the detailed assessment of eating disorders in the research context. It also has the sensitivity to change as is required for use in clinical trials or monitoring of individual therapy. Even in the research setting, however, the EDE is relatively lengthy for repeated use, and the EDE-Q may be preferable for some purposes. Although the EDE is too lengthy for routine clinical practice, the EDE or EDE-Q might help provide a comprehensive assessment of a patient with a suspected eating disorder, particularly during an evaluation visit or on entry into an inpatient facility.

BULIMIA TEST-REVISED (BULIT-R). The BULIT-R was developed in the mid-1980s to provide both a categorical and a continuous assessment of bulimia. Patients with bulimia typically score above 110, whereas patients without disordered eating typically score below 60. The instrument can be completed in approximately 10 minutes. The BULIT-R shows high reliability based on studies of internal consistency and test–retest reliability in multiple studies. High correlations support validity with other bulimia assessments. The recommended cutoff of 104 suggested to identify probable cases of bulimia shows high sensitivity and specificity for a clinical diagnosis of bulimia nervosa. With cutoffs between 98 and 104, the BULIT-R has been used successfully to screen for cases of bulimia nervosa. As with any screening procedure, follow-up by clinical examination is indicated for individuals scoring positive; clinical follow-up is particularly critical because the BULIT-R does not distinguish clearly between different types of eating disorders. The BULIT-R may also be useful in clinical and research practice to track symptoms over time or in response to treatment. However, more detailed measures of the frequency and severity of bingeing and purging may be preferable in research settings.

Cognitive Disorders.   A wide variety of measures of dementia are available. Most involve cognitive testing and provide objective, quantifiable data. However, scores vary by educational level in subjects without dementia, so these instruments tend to be most useful when the patient's baseline scores are known. Other measures focus on functional status, which can be assessed based on a comparison with a description of the subject's baseline function; these types of measures generally require a knowledgeable informant and, thus, may be more cumbersome to administer but tend to be less subject to educational biases. A third type of measure focuses on the associated behavioral symptoms that are frequently seen in demented patients.

MINI-MENTAL STATE EXAMINATION (MMSE).   The MMSE is a 30-point cognitive test developed in the mid-1970s to provide a bedside assessment of a broad array of cognitive functions, including orientation, attention, memory, construction, and language. It can be administered in less than 10 minutes by a busy doctor or a technician and scored rapidly by hand. The MMSE has been extensively studied and shows excellent reliability when raters refer to consistent scoring rules. Validity appears good based on correlations with a wide variety of more comprehensive measures of mental functioning and clinicopathologic correlations.

Since its development in 1975, the MMSE was widely distributed in textbooks, pocket guides, and on websites and has been used at the bedside. In 2001 the authors granted a worldwide exclusive license to Psychological Assessment Resources (PAR) to publish, distribute, and manage all intellectual property rights to the test. A licensed version of the MMSE, officially called the MMSE-2, must now be purchased from PAR per test. The MMSE form is gradually disappearing from textbooks, websites, and clinical tool kits.

In an article in the *New England Journal of Medicine* (2011;365:2447–2449) John C. Newman and Robin Feldman concluded: "The restrictions on the MMSE's use present clinicians with difficult choices: increase practice costs and complexity, risk copyright infringement, or sacrifice 30 years of practical experience and validation to adopt new cognitive assessment tools."

NEUROPSYCHIATRIC INVENTORY (NPI).   The NPI was developed in the mid-1990s to assess a wide range of behavioral symptoms that are often seen in Alzheimer disease and other dementing disorders. The current version rates 12 areas: delusions, hallucinations, dysphoria, anxiety, agitation/aggression, euphoria, disinhibition, irritability/lability, apathy, aberrant motor behavior, nocturnal disturbances, appetite, and eating. The standard NPI is an interview with a caregiver or other informant that can be performed by a clinician or trained lay interviewer and requires 15 to 20 minutes to complete. There is also a nursing home interview version, the NPI-NH, and a self-report questionnaire, the NPI-Q. For each area, the NPI asks whether a symptom is present and, if so, assesses the frequency, severity, and associated caregiver distress. The instrument has demonstrated reliability and validity and is useful to screen for problem behaviors in both clinical and research settings. Because of the detailed frequency and severity ratings, it is also helpful to monitor change with treatment.

SCORED GENERAL INTELLIGENCE TEST (SGIT).   This test was developed and validated by N. D. C. Lewis at the New York State Psychiatric Institute in the 1930s. It is one of the few tests that attempts to measure general intelligence that can be administered by the clinician during the psychiatric interview. A decline in general intelligence will be seen in cognitive disorders, and the SGIT can alert the clinician to begin a workup for disease states that interfere with cognition. This test deserves more widespread use (Table 1-18).

Personality Disorders and Personality Traits.   Personality may be conceptualized categorically as personality disorders or dimensionally as personality traits, which may be viewed as normal or pathologic. The focus here is on personality disorders and the maladaptive traits generally viewed as their milder forms. Ten personality disorders are divided into three clusters. Patients tend not to fall neatly into DSM personality categories; instead, most patients who meet the criteria for one personality disorder also meet the criteria for at least one other, particularly within the same cluster. This and other limitations in the validity of the constructs themselves make it difficult to achieve validity in personality measures. Personality measures include both interviews and self-report instruments. Self-report measures are appealing in that they require less time and may appear less threatening to the patient. However, they tend to overdiagnose personality disorders. Because many of the symptoms suggesting personality problems are socially undesirable and because patients' insight tends to be limited, clinician-administered instruments, which allow for probing and patient observation, may provide more accurate data.

PERSONALITY DISORDER QUESTIONNAIRE (PDQ).   The PDQ was developed in the late 1980s as a simple self-report questionnaire designed to provide a categorical and dimensional assessment of personality disorders. The PDQ includes 85 yes–no items intended primarily to assess the diagnostic criteria for personality disorders. Within the 85 items, two validity scales are embedded to identify underreporting, lying, and inattention. There is also a brief clinician-administered Clinical Significance Scale to address the impact of any personality disorder identified by the self-report PDQ. The PDQ can provide categorical diagnoses, a scaled score for each, or an overall index of personality disturbance based on the sum of all of the diagnostic criteria. Overall scores range from 0 to 79; normal controls tend to score below 20, personality disordered patients generally score above 30, and psychotherapy outpatients without such disorders tend to score in the 20 to 30 range.

Childhood Disorders.   A wide variety of instruments are available to assess mental disorders in children. Despite this rich array of instruments, however, the evaluation of children remains difficult for several reasons. First, the child psychiatric nosology is at an earlier stage of development, and construct validity is often problematic. Second, because children change markedly with age, it is virtually impossible to design a measure that covers children of all ages. Lastly, because children, particularly young children, have limited ability to report their symptoms, other informants are necessary. This often creates problems because there are frequent disagreements among child, parent, and teacher reports of symptoms, and the optimal way to combine information is unclear.

CHILD BEHAVIOR CHECKLIST (CBCL).   The CBCL is a family of self-rated instruments that survey a broad range of difficulties encountered in children from preschool through adolescence. One version of the CBCL is designed for completion by parents of children between 4 and 18 years of age. Another version is available for parents of children between 2 and 3 years of age. Children between 11 and 18 years of age complete the Youth Self-Report and the Teacher Report Form is completed by teachers of school-age children. The scale includes not only problem behaviors but

Table 1-18
Scored General Intelligence Test (SGIT)

<u>Indications</u>: When a cognitive disorder is suspected because of apparent intellectual defects, impairment in the ability to make generalizations, the ability to maintain a trend of thought, or to show good judgment, a scored test can be of value.

<u>Directions</u>: Ask the following questions as part of the mental status examination. A conversational manner should be used and the questions may be adapted to cultural differences.

<u>Scoring</u>: If the patient obtains a score of 25 or under (out of a maximum of 40), it is indicative of a cognitive problem and further examination should follow.

<u>Questions</u>: There are 13 questions that follow.

1. What are houses made of? (Any material you can think of) 1–4
   One point for each item, up to four.
2. What is sand used for? .... 1, 2, or 4
   Four points for manufacture of glass. Two points for mixing with concrete, road building, or other constructive use. One point for play or sandboxes. Credit not cumulative.
3. If the flag floats to the south, from what direction is the wind? 3
   Three points for north, no partial credits. It is permissible to say: "Which way is the wind coming from?"
4. Tell me the names of some fish. 1–4
   One point for each, up to four. If the subject stops with one, encourage him or her to go on.
5. At what time of day is your shadow shortest? 3
   Noon, three points. If correct response is suspected of being a guess, inquire why.
6. Give the names of some large cities. 1–4
   One point for each, up to four. When any state is named as a city, no credit, that is, New York unless specified as New York City. No credit for hometown, except when it is an outstanding city.
7. Why does the moon look larger than the stars? .... 2, 3, or 4
   Make it clear that the question refers to any particular star, and give assurance that the moon is actually smaller than any star. Encourage the subject to guess. Two points for "Moon is lower down." Three points for nearer or closer. Four points for generalized statement that nearer objects look larger than more distant objects.
8. What metal is attracted by a magnet? .... 2 or 4
   Four points for iron, two for steel.
9. If your shadow points to the northeast, where is the sun? 4
   Four points for southwest, no partial credits.
10. How many stripes are in the American flag? 2
    Thirteen, two points. A subject who responds 50 may be permitted to correct the mistake. Explain, if necessary, that the white stripes are included as well as the red ones.
11. What does ice become when it melts? 1
    Water, one point.
12. How many minutes in an hour? 1
    60, one point.
13. Why is it colder at night than in the daytime? 1–2
    Two points for "sun goes down," or any recognition of direct rays of sun as source of heat. Question may be reversed: "What makes it warmer in the daytime than at night?" Only one point for answer to reverse question.

This test was developed and validated by N. D. C. Lewis, M.D.
From Sadock BJ, Sadock VA. *Pocket Handbook of Clinical Psychiatry*. 5th ed. Philadelphia, PA: Lippincott Williams & Wilkins, 2010, with permission.

also academic and social strengths. Each version includes approximately 100 items scored on a 3-point Likert scale. Scoring can be done by hand or computer, and normative data are available for each of the three subscales: problem behaviors, academic functioning, and adaptive behaviors. A computerized version is also available. The CBCL does not generate diagnoses but, instead, suggests cutoff scores for problems in the "clinical range." Parent, teacher, and child versions all show high reliability on the problem subscale, but the three informants frequently do not agree with one another. The CBCL may be useful in clinical settings as an adjunct to clinical evaluation, as it provides a good overall view of symptomatology and may also be used to track change over time. It is used frequently for similar purposes in research involving children and, thus, can be compared with clinical experience. The instrument does not, however, provide diagnostic information, and its length limits its efficiency for tracking purposes.

DIAGNOSTIC INTERVIEW SCHEDULE FOR CHILDREN (DISC). The current DISC, the DISC-IV, covers a broad range of DSM diagnoses, both current and lifetime. It has nearly 3,000 questions but is structured with a series of stem questions that serve as gateways to each diagnostic area, with the remainder of each section skipped if the subject answers no. Subjects who enter each section have very few skips, so complete diagnostic and symptom scale information can be obtained. Child, parent, and teacher versions are available. Computer programs are available to implement diagnostic criteria and generate severity scales based on each version or to combine parent and child information. A typical DISC interview may take more than 1 hour for a child, plus an additional hour for a parent. However, because of the stem question structure, the actual time varies widely with the number of symptoms endorsed. The DISC was designed for lay interviewers. It is relatively complicated to administer, and formal training programs are highly recommended. The reliability of the DISC is only fair to good and generally better for the combined child and parent interview. Validity judged against a clinical interview by a child psychiatrist is also fair to good—better for some diagnoses and better for the combined interview. The DISC is well tolerated by parents and children and can be used to supplement a clinical interview to ensure comprehensive diagnostic coverage. Because of its inflexibility, some clinicians find it uncomfortable to use, and its length makes it less than optimal for use in clinical practice. However, it is frequently used in a variety of research settings.

CONNERS RATING SCALES.   The Conners Rating Scales are a family of instruments designed to measure a range of childhood and adolescent psychopathology. They are most commonly used in the assessment of ADHD. The main uses of the Conners Rating Scales are in screening for ADHD in school or clinic populations and following changes in symptom severity over time; sensitivity to change in response to specific therapies has been demonstrated for most versions of the Conners Rating Scales. There are teacher, parent, and self-report (for adolescents) versions and both short (as few as 10 items) and long (as many as 80 items, with multiple subscales) forms. Reliability data are excellent for the Conners Rating Scales. However, the teacher and parent versions tend to show poor agreement. Validity data suggest that the Conners Rating Scales are excellent at discriminating between ADHD patients and normal controls.

AUTISM DIAGNOSTIC INTERVIEW-REVISED (ADI-R).   The Autism Diagnostic Interview (ADI) was developed in 1989 as a clinical assessment of autism and related disorders. The ADI-R was developed in 2003 to provide a shorter instrument with a better ability to discriminate autism from other developmental disorders. The instrument has 93 items, is designed for individuals with a mental age greater than 18 months, and covers three broad areas, consistent with the diagnostic criteria for autism: language and communication; reciprocal social interactions; and restricted, repetitive, and stereotyped behaviors and interests. There are three versions: one for lifetime diagnosis, one for current diagnosis, and one for patients under age 4 focused on an initial diagnosis. It must be administered by a clinician trained in its use and takes about 90 minutes to complete. When clinicians are properly trained, it has good to excellent reliability and validity but performs poorly in the setting of severe developmental disabilities. It is generally intended for the research setting when a thorough assessment of autism is required but may have use in clinical practice as well.

CLINICAL NEUROPSYCHOLOGY AND INTELLECTUAL ASSESSMENT OF ADULTS

Clinical neuropsychology is a specialty in psychology that examines the relationship between behavior and brain functioning in the realms of cognitive, motor, sensory, and emotional functioning. The clinical neuropsychologist integrates the medical and psychosocial history with the reported complaints and the pattern of performance on neuropsychological procedures to determine whether results are consistent with a particular area of brain damage or a specific diagnosis.

Neuroanatomical Correlates

The early history of neuropsychology was driven in large part by the goal of linking behavioral deficits to specific neuroanatomical areas of dysfunction or damage. Although this historic assessment method helped to validate neuropsychological tests that are commonly used today, the localizing function of neuropsychological assessment is now considered less important in light of recent advances in neuroimaging techniques. Increasing knowledge in the neurosciences has also led to a more sophisticated view of brain–behavior relationships, in which complex cognitive, perceptual, and motor

Table 1-19
Selected Neuropsychological Deficits Associated with Left or Right Hemisphere Damage

Left Hemisphere	Right Hemisphere
Aphasia	Visuospatial deficits
Right–left disorientation	Impaired visual perception
Finger agnosia	Neglect
Dysgraphia (aphasic)	Dysgraphia (spatial, neglect)
Dyscalculia (number alexia)	Dyscalculia (spatial)
Constructional apraxia (details)	Constructional apraxia (Gestalt)
Limb apraxia	Dressing apraxia Anosognosia

From Sadock BJ, Sadock VA, Ruiz P. *Kaplan & Sadock's Comprehensive Textbook of Psychiatry*. 9th ed. Philadelphia, PA: Lippincott Williams & Wilkins; 2009, with permission.

activities are controlled by neural circuits rather than single structures within the brain. An understanding of these brain–behavior relationships is particularly helpful when evaluating patients with focal damage. It is crucial to ensure that the neuropsychological evaluation adequately assesses relevant behavior that is likely to be associated with that area and its interconnecting pathways.

Hemispheric Dominance and Intrahemispheric Localization.   Many functions are mediated by both the right and left hemispheres. However, critical qualitative differences between the two hemispheres can be demonstrated in the presence of lateralized brain injury. Various cognitive skills that have been linked to the left or right hemisphere in right-handed individuals are listed in Table 1-19. Although language is the most apparent function that is mostly controlled by the left hemisphere, especially among right-handed individuals, the left hemisphere is also generally considered to be dominant for limb praxis (i.e., performing complex movements, such as brushing teeth, to command, or imitation). It has been associated with the cluster of deficits identified as Gerstmann syndrome (i.e., finger agnosia, dyscalculia, dysgraphia, and right–left disorientation). In contrast, the right hemisphere is thought to play a more critical role in controlling visuospatial abilities and hemispatial attention, which are associated with the clinical presentations of constructional apraxia and neglect, respectively.

Although lateralized deficits such as these are typically characterized in terms of *damage* to the right or left hemisphere, it is essential to keep in mind that the patient's performance can also be described in terms of *preserved* brain functions. In other words, it is the remaining intact brain tissue that drives many behavioral responses following an injury to the brain and not only the absence of critical brain tissue.

LANGUAGE DISORDERS.   Appreciation for the special role of the left hemisphere in the control of language functions in most right-handed individuals has been validated in many studies. These include the results of sodium amytal testing in epilepsy surgery patients, as well as the incidence of aphasia following unilateral stroke to the left versus right hemisphere. Although it is rare for right-handed individuals to be right hemisphere dominant for language, it does occur in about 1 percent of the cases. Hemispheric dominance for language in left-handed individuals varies. About two-thirds of left-handed individuals are left-hemisphere dominant for language, while about 20 percent each are right hemisphere dominant or bilaterally dominant.

Several classification systems have been developed over the years for describing various patterns of language breakdown. A standard method takes into account the presence or absence of three key features: (1) fluency, (2) comprehension, and (3) repetition (i.e., intact ability to repeat verbally presented words or phrases).

Broca Aphasia. *Broca Aphasia* (also called *nonfluent* or *expressive aphasia*) has traditionally been characterized by nonfluent speech but intact auditory comprehension and somewhat impaired repetition. It has long been thought to be associated with damage to Broca area (i.e., left inferior frontal convolution) or Brodmann area 44 (Fig. 1-3). However, more recent neuroimaging data in stroke patients have shown that the full syndrome of Broca aphasia, including *agrammatism* (telegraphic speech), is found only in the presence of more extensive damage, which encompasses the suprasylvian area from Broca area to the posterior extent of the Sylvian fissure.

Wernicke Aphasia. *Wernicke aphasia* (also called *fluent* or *receptive aphasia*) is characterized by fluent speech, impaired comprehension, and somewhat impaired repetition. It has been associated with damage to Wernicke area in the region of the superior temporal gyrus. The impaired ability to comprehend language directly affects the individual's ability to self-monitor language output and may be related to a breakdown of the syntactic structure of language. Unlike patients with Broca aphasia, who are usually painfully aware of their communication difficulty, patients with Wernicke

aphasia are typically not aware of their communication problems because Wernicke area is critical for comprehending their speech as well as the language of others. This lack of insight is similar to the condition of *anosognosia,* in which patients fail to appreciate their deficits, and presents an incredibly frustrating condition for many family members and caregivers.

Conduction Aphasia. Patients with *conduction aphasia* demonstrate relatively intact auditory comprehension and spontaneous speech, due to the preservation of Wernicke and Broca areas. However, the ability to repeat words and phrases is specifically impaired and has traditionally been attributed to damage to the arcuate fasciculus, which interconnects Wernicke and Broca areas. This type of aphasia is much more subtle and tends to have a less negative impact on daily functioning.

Global Aphasia. Another common classification, *global aphasia,* is characterized by impairment in all three dimensions of fluency, comprehension, and repetition due to damage to the core language areas on the lateral surface of the left hemisphere. In reality, many aphasic patients cannot be neatly classified within a specific system because the pattern of deficits does not precisely fit clear, descriptive categories. Detailed language assessment of most aphasic patients typically demonstrates deficits in all three areas, although the degree of deficit among the three areas varies.

LIMB APRAXIA. Limb apraxia and other cognitive-motor skills deficits are more commonly seen with left than with right hemisphere damage. However, Kathleen Haaland and Deborah Harrington reviewed data showing that the difference in the incidence of limb apraxia after left or right hemisphere damage is not as great as with language, suggesting that left hemisphere dominance for disorders of complex movement is not as strong as that for language. Although limb apraxia has not traditionally been considered to be of substantial functional importance, more recently, new information suggests it may significantly affect rehabilitation outcome. *Conceptual apraxia* might result in using the wrong object to perform a movement, such as attempting to use a toothbrush to eat. Finally, sequencing errors and ideational errors can lead to disrupted activities, such as trying to light a candle before striking the match.

ARITHMETIC. Arithmetic skills can be impaired after either left or right hemisphere damage. Left hemisphere damage, especially of the parietal lobe, produces difficulty in reading and appreciating the symbolic meaning of numbers (*number dyslexia*). Left hemisphere damage also can be associated with an impaired conceptual understanding of the arithmetic problem (*anarithmetria*). In contrast, the deficits in arithmetic computation that can accompany right hemisphere damage are more likely to be observed in written problems. These emerge as problems with the spatial aspects of arithmetic, such as errors resulting from hemispatial visual neglect, poor alignment of columns, or visual misperceptions and rotations that can confuse signs for addition and multiplication.

SPATIAL DISORDERS. Right hemisphere damage in right-handed individuals is frequently associated with deficits in visuospatial skills. Common assessment techniques include drawings and constructional or spatial assembly tasks.

Visuospatial Impairment. Distinctive qualitative errors in constructing block designs and in drawing a complex geometric configuration (e.g., Rey–Osterrieth Complex Figure test) can be seen with either right or left hemisphere damage. In the presence of lateralized damage to the right hemisphere, impaired performance often

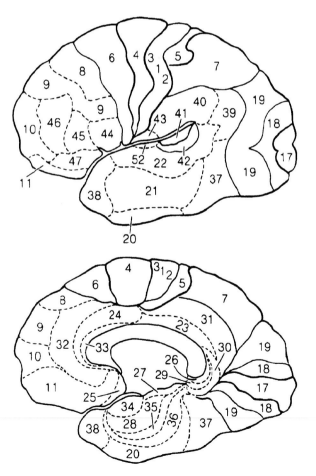

FIGURE 1-3
Brodmann areas of the human cortex, showing convex surface (*top*) and medial surface (*bottom*). (From Elliott HC. *Textbook of Neuroanatomy*. Philadelphia, PA: Lippincott; 1969, with permission.)

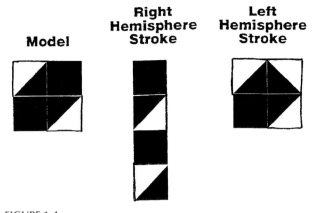

FIGURE 1-4
Examples of block design construction seen in a right hemisphere stroke patient and a left hemisphere stroke patient. (From Sadock BJ, Sadock VA, Ruiz P. *Kaplan & Sadock's Comprehensive Textbook of Psychiatry*. 9th ed. Philadelphia, PA: Lippincott Williams & Wilkins; 2009, with permission.)

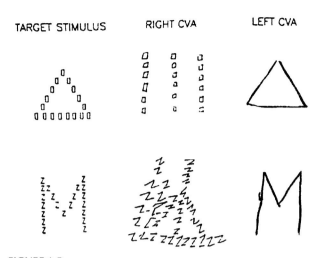

FIGURE 1-5
Global local target stimuli with drawings from memory by a patient with right hemisphere cerebrovascular accident (CVA) and by a patient with left hemisphere CVA. (From Robertson LC, Lamb MR. Neuropsychological contributions to theories of part/whole organization. *Cogn Psychol*. 1991;23:325, with permission from Elsevier Science.)

reflects the patient's inability to appreciate the "Gestalt" or global features of a design. In the example shown in Figure 1-4, this is seen in the patient's failure to maintain the 2 × 2 matrix of blocks and instead of converting this matrix into a column of four blocks. In contrast, damage to the left hemisphere commonly results in inaccurate reproduction of internal details of the design, including improper orientation of individual blocks. However, the 2 × 2 matrix (i.e., the Gestalt) is more likely to be preserved. Many neuropsychologists emphasize that a neuropsychological understanding of the impairment depends not just on a set of test scores but also on a qualitative description of the type of error. This often allows the impairment to be linked to a specific neuroanatomical region as well as enabling a better understanding of the mechanisms of the deficit for rehabilitation purposes. This qualitative focus on the type of error is similar to the *pathognomonic* approach that is often used by behavioral neurologists.

In another example, damage to the right hemisphere tends to be associated with a decreased appreciation of global features of visual stimuli. In contrast, left hemisphere damage tends to be associated with the decreased analysis of local features and detail. This notion is illustrated in Figure 1-5, where a patient with left hemisphere damage focuses on the larger Gestalt of the triangle or letter M with no regard for the internal characters that make up the designs. In contrast, the "local" approach of a patient with right hemisphere damage emphasizes the internal details (small rectangles or letter Z) without an appreciation of the Gestalt that is formed by the internal details. This example also illustrates the important point that behavioral responses (including errors) are driven as much by preserved regions of intact brain functioning as by the loss of other regions of brain functioning.

Neglect. *Neglect syndromes* are characterized by failure to detect visual or tactile stimuli or to move the limb in the contralateral hemispace. They are most commonly associated with right hemisphere damage in the parietal region, but damage to other areas within the cerebral cortex and subcortical areas can also produce this problem. Although neglect syndromes have a similar incidence and may co-occur with visual field cuts or somatosensory deficits, the neglect syndrome is distinct and not explained by any motor or sensory problems that may be present. Visual neglect can be assessed with line cancellation and line bisection tasks, in which the paper is placed at the patient's midline, and the patient is asked to

either cross out all of the lines on the page or to bisect the single line presented. The method of double simultaneous stimulation or visual extinction is another standard procedure for demonstrating the deficit. Neglect syndromes can have devastating functional effects on safety and the ability to live independently and should be taken into account as a standard consideration in the evaluation process.

Dressing Apraxia. The syndrome of *dressing apraxia* tends to arise in association with spatial deficits following right hemisphere damage. The resulting difficulty in coordinating the spatial and tactual demands of dressing can be seen in the patient's difficulty in identifying the top or bottom of a garment, as well as right–left confusion in inserting his or her limbs into the garment. As a result, dressing time can be painfully protracted, and the patient may present with a greater level of functional dependence than might otherwise be expected from the assessment of simple motor or spatial skills alone.

MEMORY DISORDERS. Memory complaints constitute the most common referral to neuropsychology. A thorough neuropsychological examination of memory considers the modality (e.g., verbal vs. spatial) in which the material is presented, as well as presentation formats that systematically assess different aspects of the information-processing and storage system that forms the basis for memory. Accumulated research indicates that specialized processing of verbal and spatial memory material tends to be differentially mediated by the left and right hemispheres, respectively. Also, to interhemispheric differences in functional localization, specific memory problems can be associated with a breakdown at any stage in the information-processing model of memory. These stages include (1) registration of the material through *attention*, (2) initial processing and encoding of the material within *short-term memory*, also known as *working memory*, (3) consolidation and storage of material in *long-term memory*, and (4) *retrieval* processes, in which material moves from long-term memory storage back into consciousness. A great advantage of neuropsychological assessment is that these various types of memory problems can be readily isolated and described in the course of the examination procedures. Once identified, the specific nature of the deficit can then have important implications for diagnosis, treatment, and prognosis.

Encoding. The initial encoding of new material can be influenced by a variety of factors, including deficits in attention, language, and spatial processing abilities. It is usually measured by the immediate recall of newly learned information (e.g., narrative stories or designs) or by demonstrating the ability to learn new material that has been presented across multiple "learning trials" (e.g., word lists). Attention itself is a relatively fragile cognitive function that can be affected by many factors, including neurologically based disorders (e.g., head injury or acute confusional state) and psychiatric disorders (e.g., depression or anxiety), so it is a crucial aspect of a proper assessment of memory.

Storage and Retrieval. Deficits in recall can be associated with impaired storage of information, or it can be due to impaired retrieval, in which case the material is still present but not readily accessible. The best way of differentiating these problems is to examine *recognition memory,* in which a patient is typically asked to choose from a set of multiple-choice alternatives or to discriminate target words from *false-positive* foils. If the patient demonstrates accurate recognition but poor recall, then the problem most likely lies in poor retrieval. However, if recognition is impaired, then the problem is more likely to be related to impaired storage of new information. This distinction is important because different neuroanatomical structures subserve the functions of retrieval and storage. Impaired storage is more often associated with dysfunction of the medial temporal lobe (MTL)-diencephalic systems, whereas impaired retrieval can be associated with a variety of structures, including the frontal lobes.

EXECUTIVE FUNCTION. The prefrontal lobes and their interconnections to the rest of the brain are known to play an important role in *executive functions,* which are essential in planning and organizing, self-monitoring, and controlling complex problem-solving responses. Damage to the frontal lobes also has been associated with significant personality changes. This was historically exemplified by the famous 19th-century case of Phineas Gage, who became irresponsible, socially inappropriate, and unable to carry out plans after a tamping iron was blown through his frontal lobes. As conceptualized by Muriel Lezak, the executive functions include volition (i.e., formulation of a goal, motivation to achieve the goal, and awareness of one's own ability to achieve the goal), planning, purposive action (response selection and initiation, maintenance, switching, and stopping), and execution, which involves self-monitoring and self-correction as well as control of the spatiotemporal aspects of the response. Hemispheric differences in the control of executive functions by the frontal lobes have not been as well documented as in the parietal and temporal lobes.

MOTOR SKILLS. The neuropsychological evaluation commonly includes formal tests of motor skills, such as measures of finger tapping speed, grip strength, and fine motor dexterity. These tests, which have demonstrated validity and reliability, are useful for assessing lateralized motor impairment and have implications for functioning in daily life as well as vocational planning.

General Referral Issues

Referents turn to neuropsychology for many reasons that include differential diagnosis, baseline measurement, and treatment planning, as well as opinions regarding causality and decisional capacity. Because many referents have limited experience and knowledge of the scope of neuropsychology, it is both reasonable and essential for the neuropsychologist to take an active role in

refining the specific questions that are asked and providing realistic information about the limitations of the consultation.

Level of Functioning. A common referral issue involves documentation of the level of functioning for a variety of purposes, including assessment of change or capacity to make decisions, especially in the presence of diagnoses such as dementia, stroke, and head injury.

Differential Diagnosis. Like any other diagnostic procedure, the results of a neuropsychological examination must be interpreted in light of all available information, including the history and any associated medical factors that are documented or reported for the individual. Many neurologic and psychiatric disorders have similar clusters of symptoms in common, with complaints of concentration or memory problems being among the most frequently reported problems.

AGE- OR STRESS-RELATED COGNITIVE CHANGE. Many middle-aged and older adults have concerns about everyday concentration and memory failures. With heightened public awareness about conditions such as Alzheimer disease, an increasing number of these individuals seek evaluations for these concerns. Neuropsychological testing provides a detailed, objective picture of different aspects of memory and attention, which can be helpful in reassuring healthy persons about their abilities. It also offers an opportunity for assessing undetected mood or anxiety disorders that may be reflected in cognitive concerns and for offering suggestions about mnemonic strategies that can sharpen everyday function.

A 77-year-old, left-handed man with a high school education was referred for neuropsychological assessment by his primary care physician after the patient mentioned a recent episode of getting turned around while driving. Results of the neuropsychological assessment indicated variable performance on tests of attention and concentration. His performance was excellent on tests of memory, language, and executive problem-solving abilities, but visual-spatial and constructional abilities were moderately impaired.

MILD TRAUMATIC BRAIN INJURY. Traumatic brain injury (TBI) is usually classified as mild, moderate, or severe. However, the vast majority of TBI cases referred for neuropsychological consultation involve mild TBI. A significant proportion of persons who have suffered a mild TBI complain of problems with attention and inefficient information processing, memory, and mood, also to headache or other forms of pain, for many months after the injury. Neuropsychological testing plays a crucial role in determining the extent of objective cognitive deficit and examining the possible role of psychological factors in perpetuating cognitive problems.

The neuropsychologist should bear in mind that many patients with mild TBI are involved in litigation, which can complicate the neuropsychologist's ability to identify the causes for impairment. Although outright malingering is probably relatively infrequent, subtle presentations of chronic illness behavior should be a prominent consideration when potential legal settlements or disability benefits are in question. This is a particularly important factor in the case of mild head injury, when subjective complaints may be disproportionate to the objectively reported circumstances of the injury, especially because most follow-up studies of mild head injury indicate a return to neuropsychological baseline with no objective evidence of significant cognitive sequelae after 3 to 12 months following injury.

POSTSTROKE SYNDROMES.   After the acute phase of recovery from stroke, patients may be left with residual deficits, which can affect memory, language, sensory/motor skills, reasoning, or mood. Neuropsychological testing can help to identify areas of strength, which can be used in planning additional rehabilitation and can provide feedback on the functional implications of residual deficits for work or complex activities of daily living. Assessment of functional skills can also be helpful to a psychiatrist who is managing mood and behavioral symptoms or dealing with family caregivers.

DETECTING EARLY DEMENTIA.   Conditions that particularly warrant neuropsychological assessment for early detection and potential treatment include HIV-related cognitive deficits and normal pressure hydrocephalus. When concerns about a person's memory functioning are expressed by relatives instead of the patient, there is a higher probability of a neurologic basis for the functional problems. Neuropsychological testing, combined with a good clinical history and other medical screening tests, can be highly effective in distinguishing early dementia from the mild changes in memory and executive functioning that can be seen with normal aging. Neuropsychological evaluation is particularly helpful in documenting cognitive deterioration and differentiating among different forms of dementia. An additional incentive for early diagnosis of dementia now lies in the fact that a portion of patients with early dementia may be candidates for memory-enhancing therapies (e.g., acetylcholinesterase inhibitors), and testing can provide an objective means of monitoring treatment efficacy.

DISTINGUISHING DEMENTIA AND DEPRESSION.   A substantial minority of patients with severe depression exhibit serious generalized impairment of cognitive functioning. Also, to problems with attention and slowing of thought and action, there may be significant forgetfulness and problems with reasoning. By examining the pattern of cognitive impairment, neuropsychological testing can help to identify a dementia syndrome that is associated with depression, usually known as *depression-related cognitive dysfunction.* Mixed presentations are also common, in which symptoms of depression coexist with various forms of cognitive decline and exacerbate the effects of cognitive dysfunction beyond what would be expected from the neurologic impairment alone. Neuropsychological testing, in this case, can be beneficial by providing a baseline for measuring the effect of antidepressants or other therapy in alleviating cognitive and mood symptoms.

A 75-year-old man with a Ph.D. in the social sciences sought neuropsychological reexamination for ongoing memory complaints, stating that "several of my friends have Alzheimer's." In an initial examination 1 year prior, he had performed in the expected range (above average) for most procedures, despite variable performance on measures of attention and concentration. Results of the follow-up examination again clustered in the expected above-average range with uneven performance on measures of attention. On list learning tests of memory, his initial learning of a word list was lower than expected. Still, delayed retention of the material was above average, with excellent discrimination of target items on a recognition subtest. He also endorsed a large number of symptoms of depression on a self-report inventory.

Change in Functioning Over Time.   Because many neurologic diagnoses carry clear expectations regarding normal rates

of recovery and decline over time, it is frequently important to reexamine a given patient with follow-up neuropsychological assessment after 6 months to a year. For example, it might be essential to monitor declines in independent functioning that could be associated with progressive dementia or to identify improvement following a stroke or tumor resection. Follow-up examinations also provide an opportunity to objectively examine complaints of long-standing or worsening cognitive sequelae following mild head trauma, even though the current literature indicates that the most significant proportion of recovery of function is likely to occur over the initial 6 months to 1-year postinjury. Although continuing subtle signs of recovery can continue after that period, failure to improve following the injury—or a worsening of complaints—would suggest the possibility of contributing psychological factors or the existence of a preexisting or coexisting condition, such as substance abuse, dementia, or outright malingering.

Assessment of Decision-Making Capacity.   Neuropsychologists are often asked to assist in determining an individual's capacity to make decisions or to manage personal affairs. Neuropsychological testing can be useful in these cases by documenting areas of significant impairment and by identifying areas of strength and well-preserved skills. Opinions about decision-making capacity are seldom based on test findings alone. Usually, they rely heavily on information gleaned from the clinical interview, collateral interviews with family or caregivers, and direct observations (e.g., in-home assessment) of everyday function. Appraisal of an individual's level of insight and capacity to appreciate his or her limitations is typically the most critical aspect of the assessment. State statutes generally define standards for decision-making capacity, and, of course, the ultimate determination of competence rests in the authority of the presiding judge. However, the neuropsychologist or other health care professional can play a significant role in shaping the judge's ruling by providing a professional opinion that is supported by compelling behavioral data that have strong face validity. As a general rule of thumb, consideration of decision-making capacity is usually best approached in the narrowest possible sense to infringe as little as possible on the individual's freedom to represent his or her interests. Therefore, consultation requests for assessment of decision-making capacity should identify specific areas of decision making and behavior that are of concern. Frequent concerns having to do with decision-making capacity involve the areas of (1) financial and legal matters, (2) health care and medical treatment, and (3) ability to live independently. Some capacity issues involve higher standards, such as the ability to drive, the ability to work, or practice in a given profession (e.g., air traffic controller, surgeon, or financial advisor). In such cases, the neuropsychologist needs to rely on normative expectations that are appropriate for the type of activity, as well as the patient's demographics.

Forensic Evaluation.   Neuropsychological evaluation of individuals in matters of criminal or civil law usually requires specialized knowledge beyond expertise in neuropsychology. Neuropsychologists are frequently called upon as experts in matters involving head injury, especially in the case of mild head injury associated with a motor vehicle accident. As a distinct subspecialty, this area of practice requires the integration of knowledge of statutes, laws, precedents, and legal procedures as well as expertise in identifying and describing the impact of an injury or event on cognitive, emotional, and behavioral functioning.

Approaches to Neuropsychological Assessment

The neuropsychological examination systematically assesses functioning in the realms of attention and concentration, memory, language, spatial skills, sensory and motor abilities, as well as executive functioning and emotional status. Because deficits in cognitive performance can only be interpreted in comparison to a person's long-standing or *premorbid level of functioning,* overall intellectual abilities are typically examined to measure the current level of overall functioning and to identify any changes in intellectual functioning. Psychological contributions to performance are also considered concerning personality and coping style, emotional lability, presence of thought disorder, developmental history, and significant past or current stressors. The expertise of the neuropsychologist lies in integrating findings that are obtained from many diverse sources, including the history, clinical presentation, and several dozen discrete performance scores that make up the neuropsychological data.

Battery Approach.   The battery approach, exemplified by the Halstead–Reitan Neuropsychological Test Battery (HRNTB) or the Neuropsychological Assessment Battery (NAB), grew directly out of the psychometric tradition in psychology. This approach typically includes a large variety of tests that measure most cognitive domains as well as sensory and motor skills. Traditionally, all parts of the test battery are administered regardless of the patient's presenting problem, although the NAB has a screening examination that covers all appropriate domains. The battery approach has the advantage of identifying issues that the patient might not have mentioned and that the medical history may not necessarily predict. However, it has the disadvantage of being very time-consuming (i.e., 6- to 8-hour examination for the HRNTB).

Hypothesis Testing Approach.   The qualitative hypothesis testing approach is historically best exemplified by the work of Alexander Luria and more recently developed as the Boston Process Approach by Edith Kaplan and her colleagues. It is characterized by a detailed evaluation of areas of functioning that are related to the patient's complaints and predicted areas of impairment, with relatively less emphasis on aspects of functioning that are less likely to be impaired. The hypothesis testing approach has been particularly helpful in illuminating the differential roles of the two hemispheres, as discussed above. This approach has the advantage of efficiently honing in on areas of impairment and producing a detailed description of the deficits from a cognitive processing standpoint. Still, it has the shortcoming of potentially overlooking unexpected areas of deficits.

Screening Approaches.   Many practitioners have moved away from strict battery or hypothesis testing approaches since the 1990s and developed more flexible and efficient screening approaches. In this model, the neuropsychologist utilizes a core set of screening procedures as a first step in determining whether a diagnosis can be made with less information or whether additional testing is necessary to identify more subtle problems. Therefore, a screening protocol that efficiently assesses the major areas of neuropsychological functioning may or may not be followed by more detailed testing in selected areas that might provide a better understanding of the reasons for the deficits demonstrated on the screening evaluation.

Mental Status Examinations.   In some cases, usually involving very acute or severe cognitive impairment, it is simply not feasible to administer extensive cognitive examination procedures, so the neuropsychologist might appropriately rely on bedside mental status examination or very brief cognitive screening procedures to address the referral issues. However, research has shown that, even with brief screening procedures, the systematic use of a structured examination format can significantly increase the accuracy of detecting cognitive impairment.

One of the most widely used screening instruments for documenting gross changes in mental status is the Mini-Mental State Examination (MMSE). However, it is essential to note that the MMSE does have distinct limitations. Other than serial seven countings, the MMSE does not assess executive functions, which are often impaired in dementing patients. Also, the MMSE is likely to underestimate the prevalence of cognitive deficits in well-educated older persons with early Alzheimer disease or in younger adults with focal brain injury. Still, it is more likely to overestimate the presence of cognitive deficits in persons with little education. Therefore, cutoff scores should be adjusted for age and education before concluding that impairment is present. Although mental status examinations can be beneficial in screening for gross signs of cognitive impairment, they do not provide a sufficient foundation for diagnosing specific etiologies of cognitive impairment, and they are not interchangeable with neuropsychological testing.

Domains of Formal Neuropsychological Assessment

The past decade has seen a virtual explosion in the growth of more sophisticated and better-standardized tests and procedures for neuropsychological evaluation. A list of examples of standard neuropsychological tests and techniques is provided in Table 1-20.

Interview.   The clinical interview provides the single best opportunity for identifying the patient's concerns and questions, eliciting a direct description of current complaints from the patient, and understanding the context of the patient's history and current circumstances. Although the patient typically serves as the primary interview source, it is crucial to seek corroborating information for the patient's account from interviews with caregivers or family members as well as a thorough review of relevant records, such as medical and mental health treatment, educational, and employment experiences.

Intellectual Functioning.   Assessment of intellectual functioning serves as the cornerstone of the neuropsychological examination. The Wechsler Intelligence Scales have represented the traditional gold standard in intellectual assessment for many years, based on carefully developed normative standards. The scope and variety of subtests on which the summary IQ values are based also provide useful benchmarks against which to compare performance on other tests of specific abilities. The latest revision of this instrument, the Wechsler Adult Intelligence Scale III (WAIS-III), offers the additional advantage of greatly extended age norms (ages 16 to 89) that are directly related to normative performances on the Wechsler Memory Scale III (WMS-III). The Wechsler Intelligence Scales utilize a broad set of complex verbal and visuospatial tasks that have traditionally been summarized as a verbal IQ, a performance IQ, and full-scale IQ. In the context of a neuropsychological examination, the patient's performance across the procedures provides useful information regarding long-standing abilities as well as current functioning. Most neuropsychologists recognize that the summary IQ values provide only a ballpark range for

Table 1-20
Selected Tests of Neuropsychological Functioning

Area of Function	Comment
Intellectual Functioning	
Wechsler Intelligence Scales	Age-stratified normative references; appropriate for adults up to age 89, adolescents, and young children
Shipley Scale	Scale Brief (20-min) paper-and-pencil measure of multiple-choice vocabulary and open-ended verbal abstraction
Attention and Concentration	
Digit Span	Auditory–verbal measure of simple span of attention (*digits forward*) and cognitive manipulation of increasingly longer strings of digits (*digits backward*)
Visual Memory Span	Visual–spatial measure of ability to reproduce a spatial sequence in forward and reverse order
Paced Auditory Serial Addition Test (PASAT)	Requires double tracking to add pairs of digits at increasing rates; particularly sensitive to subtle simultaneous processing deficits, especially in head injury
Digit Vigilance Test	Timed measure of speed and accuracy in cancelling a specific digit on a page of random digits; directly examines an individual's tendency to sacrifice either speed or accuracy in favor of the other
Memory	
Wechsler Memory Scale III	Comprehensive set of subtests measuring attention and encoding, retrieval, and recognition of various types of verbal and visual material with both immediate recall and delayed retention; excellent age-stratified normative comparisons for adults up to age 89 with intellectual data for direct comparison
California Verbal Learning Test II	Documents encoding, recognition, and both immediate and 30-min recall; affords examination of possible learning strategies as well as susceptibility to semantic interference with alternate and short forms available
Fuld Object Memory Evaluation	Selective reminding format requires patient to identify objects tactually, then assesses consistency of retrieval and storage as well as ability to benefit from cues; normative reference group is designed for use with older individuals
Benton Visual Retention Test	Assesses memory for 10 geometric designs after 10-s exposures; requires graphomotor response
Brief Visuospatial Memory Test—Revised	Serial learning approach used to assess recall and recognition memory for an array of six geometric figures; six alternate forms
Language	
Boston Diagnostic Aphasia Examination	Comprehensive assessment of expressive and receptive language functions
Boston Naming Test—Revised	Documents word finding difficulty in a visual confrontation format
Verbal Fluency	Measures ability to fluently generate words within semantic categories (e.g., animals) or phonetic categories (e.g., words beginning with "S")
Token Test	Systematically assesses comprehension of complex commands using standard token stimuli that vary in size, shape, and color
Visuospatial-Constructional	
Judgment of Line Orientation	Ability to judge angles of lines on a page presented in a match-to-sample format
Facial Recognition	Assesses matching and discrimination of unfamiliar faces
Clock Drawing	Useful screening technique is sensitive to organization and planning as well as constructional ability
Rey–Osterrieth Complex Figure test	Ability to draw and later recall a complex geometric configuration; sensitive visual memory as well as executive deficits in development of strategies and planning
Motor	
Finger Tapping	Standard measure of simple motor speed; particularly useful for documenting lateralized motor impairment
Grooved Pegboard	Ability to rapidly place notched pegs in slotted holes; measures fine finger dexterity as well as eye–hand coordination
Grip Strength	Standard measure of lateralizing differences in strength
Executive Functions	
Wisconsin Card Sorting Test	Measure of problem-solving efficiency is particularly sensitive to executive deficits of perseveration and impaired ability to flexibly generate alternative strategies in response to feedback
Category Test	This measure of problem-solving ability also examines ability to benefit from feedback while flexibly generating alternative response strategies; regarded as one of the most sensitive measures of general brain dysfunction in the Halstead–Reitan Battery
Trail-Making Test	Requires rapid and efficient integration of attention, visual scanning, and cognitive sequencing
Delis–Kaplan Executive Function System (D-KEFS)	Battery of measures that are sensitive to executive functions

(continued)

Table 1-20
Selected Tests of Neuropsychological Functioning (*Continued*)

Area of Function	Comment
Psychological Factors	
Beck Depression Inventory	Brief (5–10 min) self-report measure that is sensitive to symptoms of depression; best for screening depression in adults up to late middle age, who can be expected to frankly report symptoms; available in standard (21 four-choice items) or short (13-item) form
Geriatric Depression Scale	30-item self-report screen for symptoms of depression; the yes–no format is less cognitively demanding than other scales
Minnesota Multiphasic Personality Inventory 2	This psychometrically developed self-report instrument remains highly useful for documenting quantitative levels of self-reported symptoms that can be objectively compared with known populations; drawbacks include administration time (567 true–false questions, requires about 1–1.5 hr or more) for frail individuals, and the emphasis on pathologic features for persons who are generally psychologically healthy; advantages include well-developed validity scales and availability of many symptom-specific subscales that have been identified over the years

characterizing an individual's general level of functioning. Therefore, it is usually more appropriate and meaningful to characterize an individual's intellectual functioning in terms of the range of functioning (e.g., borderline, low average, average, high average, or superior) that is represented by the IQ value rather than the specific value itself.

Careful examination of the individual's performance across the various verbal and performance subtests can provide information regarding the patient's pattern of strengths and weaknesses as well as the degree to which these performance characteristics are consistent with the history and performance on other aspects of the neuropsychological examination. Tests of long-standing knowledge, such as for vocabulary or general information, provide a basis for estimating an individual's long-standing (or premorbid) level of intellectual abilities, which in turn can help to gauge the degree to which an individual may have deteriorated.

The verbal IQ and performance IQ (VIQ and PIQ) have historically been reported to be associated with left and right hemisphere functioning, respectively. However, more recent research indicates that, also to language and spatial skills, the subtests of the Wechsler Intelligence Scales reflect other contributions such as speed, sustained concentration, and novel experience. Therefore, experienced neuropsychologists do not merely assume that a discrepancy between VIQ and PIQ is due to unilateral hemispheric damage. Important clues to the nature of the contributing problem can often be gleaned by considering the pattern of performance across other aspects of the examination and by carefully analyzing the types of errors that are observed.

Attention. Attention underlies performance in virtually all other areas of functioning. It should always be considered a potential contributor to impairment on any tests that require sustained concentration and vigilance or rapid integration of new information. Measures of attention and concentration have traditionally been included in the Wechsler Intelligence and Wechsler Memory Scales to assess orientation and "freedom from distractibility." These procedures also provide a useful basis for "previewing" the individual's ability to comprehend, process information, and otherwise engage in the assessment process. *Digit span* requires patients to repeat longer strings of digits increasingly as a way of assessing the ability to process relatively simple information. In contrast, *digit span backward* reflects more complex simultaneous processing and cognitive manipulation demands or working memory.

Memory. Complaints of memory problems constitute one of the most common reasons for referral to neuropsychology. As described above, the neuropsychologist utilizes an information-processing approach to assess memory problems that might involve difficulty with encoding, retrieval, or storage of new information. The WMS-III is the latest revision of a widely used battery of subtests that utilizes several measures of attention, memory, and new learning ability.

Language. The assessment of language examines both expressive abilities and comprehension. However, most neuropsychologists screen for language impairment rather than administer an extensive formal language assessment battery, such as the Boston Diagnostic Aphasia Examination. Expressive language is commonly assessed by measures of *verbal fluency,* which require the patient to rapidly generate words within semantic (e.g., names of animals) and phonetic categories (e.g., words beginning with specified letters of the alphabet).

Visuospatial Functions. Complex visuospatial abilities can be assessed through procedures that were developed in Arthur Benton's laboratory, such as *facial recognition* and *judgment of line orientation*. Measures of visual constructional ability examine the person's ability to draw spatial designs or assemble two- or three-dimensional figures (see Fig. 1-5). Also, to the significant visuospatial component, these tasks reflect the contributions of executive planning and organizational abilities. More impaired individuals can be asked to copy simple geometric forms, such as a Greek cross or intersecting pentagons, to examine visuospatial abilities that are less influenced by planning and organization.

The widely used technique of *clock drawing* provides a surprisingly sensitive measure of planning and organization, especially for older individuals who are at risk for dementia. Although problems involving poor organization, perseveration, and possible neglect are apparent in the drawing that is illustrated in Figure 1-6, more subtle difficulties can also be detected, especially when a patient's performance is evaluated in light of premorbid expectations.

Sensory and Motor Functions. *Double simultaneous stimulation* in the visual, tactile, and auditory modalities is a standard component of the HRNTB. It can be useful for assessing the integrity of basic sensory functions as well as neglect if deficits are

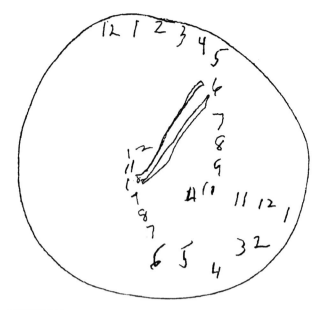

FIGURE 1-6

Clock drawing by a patient with vascular dementia, showing poor planning and organization, perseveration, and possible neglect. (From Sadock BJ, Sadock VA, Ruiz P. *Kaplan & Sadock's Comprehensive Textbook of Psychiatry*. 9th ed. Philadelphia, PA: Lippincott Williams & Wilkins; 2009, with permission.)

present on one side only on the bilateral simultaneous trials and not when stimulation is unilateral. *Grip strength* and rapid *finger tapping* are commonly used measures of motor strength and speed that are sensitive to lateralized brain dysfunction.

Executive Functions.   One of the most critical aspects of the neuropsychological examination lies in the assessment of higher *executive* functions, which play an essential role in the planning and initiation of independent activities, self-monitoring of performance, inhibition of inappropriate responses, switching between tasks, and planning and control of complex motor and problem-solving responses. Although the prefrontal lobes have long been regarded as a vital component in mediating these functions, more recent developments in the neurosciences have also led to an increased appreciation for the essential role that is played by extensive cerebral interconnections between subcortical and cortical regions of the brain.

Psychological Factors.   A key component of any neuropsychological examination involves consideration of the degree to which long-standing personality or other psychological factors (including current stressors) might contribute to the patient's presentation. Common techniques for assessing personality and psychological factors include the Minnesota Multiphasic Personality Inventory 2 (MMPI-2) and paper and pencil techniques, such as the Beck Depression Inventory II.

Assessment of Effort and Motivation.   Because the results of neuropsychological examinations may eventually be introduced as evidence in litigation or other forensic proceedings or be used for determining disability compensation, the neuropsychologist must address any possible concerns about effort and motivation as a routine matter. Several instruments have been developed recently that directly assess a patient's level of effort and motivation to perform at his or her best. Normative research indicates that patients with

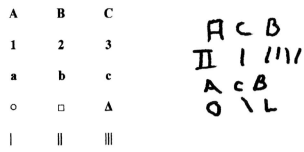

FIGURE 1-7

Rey's Memory Test with example of a response that is typical of exaggerated "memory" problems. (From Sadock BJ, Sadock VA, Ruiz P. *Kaplan & Sadock's Comprehensive Textbook of Psychiatry*. 9th ed. Philadelphia, PA: Lippincott Williams & Wilkins; 2009, with permission.)

histories of bona fide brain injury or even dementia perform close to perfect levels on many such instruments, so poor performance suggests poor effort or tendencies to exaggerate symptoms. Many other indicators of effort are based on the pattern of an individual's performance on standard procedures in a neuropsychological examination.

> A 32-year-old woman with 13 years' education was seen for disability evaluation, claiming current "trouble remembering things." Her account of personal history was vague, and she "forgot" information, such as her birth date and mother's maiden name. Response latencies were extremely long, even for highly familiar information (e.g., count from 1 to 20), she could not repeat more than three digits forward consistently, and on a word list learning procedure, she was not able to correctly recognize more items (only five) than she could freely recall (also five). Despite otherwise fluent language, she was only able to generate five examples of animals in 1 minute. When asked to recall 15 items on a procedure (Rey's Memory Test) that is presented as a challenging task, but in reality is fairly simple, her performance demonstrated exaggerated errors of commission (Fig. 1-7). The evaluation concluded that current levels of cognitive functioning could not be conclusively established due to overt symptoms exaggeration.

Therapeutic Discussion of Results

A critical component of the neuropsychological examination process is found in the opportunity to discuss the results of the examination with the patient and family or other caregivers. This meeting can represent a potential therapeutic opportunity to educate and clarify individual and relationship issues, which can impact the identified patient's functioning. If the patient's active cooperation in the initial examination has been appropriately enlisted, then the patient will be prepared to invest value and confidence in the findings of the examination. At the time of the discussion of the results, it is useful to review the goals of the examination with the patient and supportive family or caregivers and to clarify the expectations of those who are present. Typically, these sessions will include information about the patient's diagnosis, with emphasis on the natural course and prognosis as well as compensation and coping strategies for the patient and family. Given the impact of chronic neurologic disease on the family system as well as the patient, explicit discussion of these issues is critical in maximizing adjustment to brain injury. It is equally important to relate the impact of the results on the patient's current living circumstances, future goals, and course of adjustment. It is not unusual for strong emotions and underlying tensions within family relationships to come to light in the context of honest discussion, so the results discussion can represent a significant therapeutic opportunity to model effective communication and problem-solving techniques.

PERSONALITY ASSESSMENT: ADULTS AND CHILDREN

Personality is defined as an individual's enduring and pervasive motivations, emotions, interpersonal styles, attitudes, and traits. Personality assessment is the systematic measurement of these personality characteristics. Personality tests measure such difficult-to-define concepts as depression, anger, and anxiety. Even more challenging personality concepts such as somatization, ability to delay gratification or suicide potential can be quantified using personality assessment. Personality assessment can be of utmost importance in the scientific study of psychology and psychiatry.

Purposes of Psychological Testing

Personality testing can be an expensive undertaking. A considerable amount of time is required to administer, score, and interpret psychological test results. Personality testing should not be routinely obtained from all psychiatric patients. Personality testing can be helpful with selective patients from both a clinical and a cost–benefit analysis perspective.

Assisting in Differential Diagnosis.   Psychiatric diagnosis can be difficult and, at times, confusing exercise. However, knowing a patient's diagnosis is essential to treatment, as a proper diagnosis can assist in understanding the etiology of the presenting psychiatric problem and the prognosis of the disorder.

A 49-year-old man had abruptly resigned his position as an accountant and decided he was going to start an oil exploration business. He had never worked in the oil business and knew nothing about the profession. The patient had received a revelation from an unknown entity through an auditory hallucination. This voice told him he would become quite wealthy in the business if he would simply follow the directions given to him. Around this time, the patient had a marked change in personality. Although his grooming was formally very neat and appropriate, he became disheveled. He began sleeping about 3 hours a night. He became somewhat agitated and talked loudly to those around him.

The differential diagnosis, in this case, includes schizophrenia and bipolar disorder. Psychological testing might help assist in this differential diagnosis, as well as in the formulation of a treatment plan.

Aiding in Psychotherapy.   Psychological tests can be useful in psychotherapy. The usefulness of these tests can be even more important for short-term, problem-centered therapy, where understanding the patient and his or her problem must be accomplished quickly. Psychological assessment can be used in pretreatment planning, assessing progress once therapy begins, and in evaluating the effectiveness of therapy. Patients need to have objective information about themselves at the time of therapy if they are to go about changing themselves productively. Personality tests, particularly objective tests, allow patients to compare themselves to objective norms and evaluate the extent and magnitude of their problem. Testing also can reveal areas of the patient's life that may be problematic but for which the patient may not have a full appreciation. Information about patients' willingness to disclose information about themselves can also be helpful. Psychological tests may reveal considerable information concerning the patient's inner life, feelings, and images, which may make therapy progress faster. Psychological testing can provide baseline information at the beginning of therapy, and repeat testing can then be used to assess the change that occurred during therapy.

Providing Narrow-Band Assessment.   *Narrow-band personality tests* measure a single personality characteristic or a few related characteristics. *Broad-bank personality tests,* on the other hand, are designed to measure a wide spectrum of personality characteristics. A psychiatrist may need answers to specific questions, such as those that arise when assessing the degree of clinical depression, measuring the intensity of the state or trait anxiety, or, possibly, quantifying the amount of a patient's anger. Such quantification can help measure severity or in providing a baseline for future assessment.

Psychometric Properties of Personality Assessment Instruments

The quality of personality tests varies widely. On the one hand, there are well-constructed, empirically validated instruments, and, on the other hand, there are "psychological tests" that one can find in the Sunday supplement of the newspaper or on the Internet. Evaluating the usefulness of particular psychological instruments can be challenging, even to the well informed.

Normative Sample.   To construct a personality test, a representative sample of subjects (normative sample) should be administered the test to establish expected performance. Fundamental issues, such as the size and representativeness of the sample used to construct the test, must be evaluated. To illustrate this point, the Minnesota Multiphasic Personality Inventory 2 (MMPI-2), a well-constructed instrument, initially tested approximately 2,900 subjects. However, about 300 subjects were eliminated because of test invalidity or incompleteness of needed information.

Test Characteristics.   Any psychological test must be completed, in its entirety, by the intended test taker to be useful. If the questions are offensive or are difficult to understand, then the individual taking the test may not complete all items. These omissions can create problems, especially when normative tables are used to interpret results.

Validity Issues.   Perhaps the most crucial characteristic in evaluating the scientific merit of a given personality test is the validity of the instrument. Does the test measure what it purports to measure? If a test is designed to measure depression, does it indeed measure depression? Although validity may seem like a simple issue to address, it can become complex, especially when attempting to measure such characteristics as self-esteem, assertiveness, hostility, or self-control.

FACE VALIDITY.   *Face validity* refers to the content of the test items themselves. In other words, do the items appear to measure what they purport to measure? One problem with face validity is that professionals differ in their subjective appraisal of individual items.

CRITERIA AND CONSTRUCT VALIDITY.   Although face validity refers to the degree that test items appear on the surface to measure what the instrument, as a whole, purports to measure, *criterion validity* uses data outside the test itself to measure validity. For example, if a test were designed to measure hypochondria, one would expect that a patient with high scores would have more visits to the physician's office, complain of more physical symptoms, and use prescribed and over-the-counter medications more extensively.

CONCURRENT AND PREDICTIVE VALIDITY.   To determine test *concurrent validity,* external measures are obtained at the same time that the test is given to the sample of subjects. Thus, the concurrent validity of the test reveals that, at a given point of time, high scorers on a test may be more likely than low scorers on a test to manifest the behavior reflected in the criteria (e.g., more physician visits or more medication for a hypochondriac patient). Occasionally, however, a test developer is interested in predicting future events. The *discriminant validity* of a test tells whether the test can discriminate between known groups of patients at a given time. Is a measure of depression able to statistically differentiate among mild, moderate, and severe major depressive disorder?

FACTOR VALIDITY.   Factor validity utilizes a multivariate statistical technique known as *factor analysis* to determine if certain significant groups of items on a given test empirically cluster together. For example, on a personality test measuring depression, do items concerning vegetative symptoms tend to covary together?

Reliability.   *Reliability* refers to the degree that a test measures what it purports to measure, consistently. The key word here is *consistently.* There are several means of checking reliability, including test–retest reliability, internal consistency reliability, and parallel form reliability.

TEST–RETEST RELIABILITY.   *Test–retest reliability* is obtained by simply administering the same test on two occasions to a group of subjects and statistically correlating the results. The correlation coefficient should be at least 0.80 if the two tests were administered within 2 weeks of each other, and if the trait in question is stable.

INTERNAL CONSISTENCY RELIABILITY.   Another approach to determining *internal consistency reliability* is to divide a given test into two equal parts and statistically correlate the two halves for the test with each other. This technique determines the *split-half reliability* of a test. The first half of the test should be highly correlated with the second half of the test if the test is consistently measuring what it purportedly measures. Alternatively, the odd-numbered items could be correlated with the even-numbered items (*odd–even consistent reliability*). A reliability coefficient of 0.80 to 0.85 is needed to demonstrate usefulness in most circumstances. However, the higher the reliability as measured by the correlation coefficient, the better the test instrument.

PARALLEL FORM RELIABILITY.   Sometimes, two separate forms of the same test are needed. For example, if the process of taking a test at one point in time would by itself influence a patient's score the second time he or she took the same test, then parallel forms of the tests are needed. *Parallel forms* of a test measure the same construct but use different items to do so. To ensure that the test does measure the same construct, the correlation coefficient between the two parallel forms of the same test is computed. Such parallel form reliability should be at least 0.90 or higher.

USE OF STANDARD ERROR OF MEASUREMENT TO ASSESS RELIABILITY. Another way to assess the usefulness of a given test is to examine the test's standard error of measurement (SEM), which should be included in the test's manual. The SEM is a single statistic that is used to estimate what the score of a given patient would be on the test if the patient retook the same test within a short time.

Adult Psychological Tests

Objective Personality Tests.   *Objective personality tests* are rather straightforward in approach. Patients are usually asked specific and standard questions in a structured written or oral format. Each patient is typically asked the same question. The data obtained from a given patient are compared to similar data obtained from the normative group. The degree to which the patient deviates from the norm is noted and is used in the interpretive process. The patient's responses are scored according to certain agreed-upon criteria. The obtained scores are then compared with normative tables and often converted to standardized scores or percentiles, or both. The MMPI-2 is an example of an objective personality test. Table 1-21 lists a sample of objective personality test along with a brief description and brief list of strengths and weaknesses.

MINNESOTA MULTIPHASIC PERSONALITY INVENTORY.   The MMPI-2 is relatively easy to administer and score and takes approximately 1.5 hours for most patients to complete. It consists of 567 true or false questions concerning a wide variety of issues and requires only eighth-grade reading comprehension. Scoring of the MMPI-2 involves adding up the number of responses on numerous scales and comparing the results to certain normative information. Interpretation of the MMPI-2 is more straightforward than with many other tests.

When a patient takes the MMPI-2, questions are not grouped in any particular order to aid in interpretation. Various items in the MMPI-2 can be selected, sorted, and analyzed according to various criteria.

A new version of the MMPI-2 was developed in 2008, the MMPI-2 Restructured Form (MMPI-2 RF). It contains 338 questions and allows less time to administer. The MMPI-2 RF is meant to be an alternative to the MMPI-2, not a replacement.

PERSONALITY ASSESSMENT INVENTORY (PAI).   Another increasingly popular objective personality test is the Personality Assessment Inventory (PAI). This test consists of 344 items that are written at a fourth-grade reading level. This reading level ensures that most patients can complete it without experiencing any reading problems. The PAI takes about 45 to 50 minutes to complete for most patients. The PAI was normed on 1,000 community-dwelling individuals stratified according to sex, race, and age. There are no separate norms for male and female as there are in the MMPI. Also, data were gathered on 1,246 clinical subjects and 1,051 college students in the normative process. The clinical subjects were drawn from a variety of different clinical settings, including inpatient psychiatric facilities (25 percent), outpatient psychiatric facilities (35 percent), correctional institutions (12 percent), medical settings (2 percent), and substance abuse treatment programs (15 percent).

The PAI has 11 clinical scales. These main clinical scales are similar to the MMPI-2 clinical scales and measure such personality issues as somatic concerns, depression, paranoia, borderline features, or alcohol or drug problems. The PAI also has five treatment-related scales that are designed to address such issues as treatment rejection, suicide ideation, or aggression.

Projective Personality Test.   Projective personality tests, in contrast to objective personality instruments, are more indirect and unstructured. Unlike objective tests in which the patient

Table 1-21
Objective Measures of Personality

Name	Description	Strengths	Weaknesses
Minnesota Multiphasic Personality Inventory-2 (MMPI-2)	567 Items; true–false; self-report format; 20 primary scales	Current revision of MMPI that has updated the response booklet; revised scaling methods and new validity scores; new normative data	Preliminary data indicate that the MMPI-2 and the MMPI can provide discrepant results; normative sample biased toward upper socioeconomic status; no normative data for adolescents
Million Clinical Multiaxial Inventory (MCMI)	175 Items; true–false; self-report format; 20 primary scales	Brief administration time; corresponds well with diagnostic classifications	In need of more validation research; no information on disorder severity; needs revision for DSM-5
Million Clinical Multiaxial Inventory-II (MCMI-II)	175 Items; true–false; self-report format; 25 primary scales	Brief administration time	High degree of item overlap in various scales; no information on disorder or trait severity
16 Personality Factor Questionnaire (16 PF)	True–false; self-report format; 16 personality dimensions	Sophisticated psychometric instrument with considerable research conducted on nonclinical populations	Limited usefulness with clinical populations
Personality Assessment Inventory (PAI)	344 Items; Likert-type format; self-report; 22 scales	Includes measures of psychopathology, personality dimensions, validity scales, and specific concerns to psychotherapeutic treatment	The inventory is new and has not yet generated a supportive research base
California Personality Inventory (CPI)	True–false; self-report format; 17 scales	Well-accepted method of assessing patients who do not present with major psychopathology	Limited usefulness with clinical populations
Jackson Personality Inventory (JPI)	True–false; self-report format; 15 personality scales	Constructed in accord with sophisticated psychometric techniques; controls for response sets	Unproved usefulness in clinical settings
Edwards Personal Preference Schedule (EPPS)	Forced choice; self-report format	Follows Murray's theory of personology; accounts for social desirability	Not widely used clinically because of restricted nature of information obtained
Psychological Screening Inventory (PSI)	103 Items; true–false; self-report format	Yields four scores, which can be used as screening measures on the possibility of a need for psychological help	The scales are short and have correspondingly low reliability
Eysenck Personality Questionnaire (EPQ)	True–false; self-report format	Useful as a screening device; test has a theoretical basis with research support	Scales are short, and items are transparent as to purpose; not recommended for other than a screening device
Adjective Checklist (ACL)	True–false; self-report or informant report	Can be used for self-rating or other rating	Scores rarely correlate highly with conventional personality inventories
Comrey Personality Scales (CPS)	True–false; self-report format; eight scales	Factor analytic techniques used with a high degree of sophistication in test constructed	Not widely used; factor analytic interpretation problems
Tennessee Self-Concept Scale (TSCS)	100 Items; true–false; self-report format; 14 scales	Brief administration time yields considerable information	Brevity is also a disadvantage, lowering reliability and validity; useful as a screening device only

Courtesy of Robert W. Butler, Ph.D. and Paul Satz, Ph.D.

may simply mark true or false to given questions, the variety of responses to projective personality tests are almost unlimited. Instructions are usually very general, allowing the patient's fantasies to be expressed. The patient generally does not know how his or her responses will be scored or analyzed. Consequently, trying to fake the test becomes difficult. Projective tests typically do not measure one particular personality characteristic, such as "type A personality" (e.g., narrow-band measurement). Instead, they are designed to assess one's personality as a whole (e.g., broad-band measurement).

Projective tests often focus on "latent" or unconscious aspects of personality. Psychologists and others differ in the degree to which they rely on "unconscious" information. In many projective techniques, the patient is simply shown a picture of something and asked to tell what the picture reminds him or her of. An underlying assumption of projective techniques (projective hypothesis) is that, when presented with an ambiguous stimulus, such as an inkblot, for which there are an almost unlimited number of responses, the patient's responses will reflect fundamental aspects of his or her personality. The ambiguous stimulus is a sort of screen on which the individual projects his or her own needs, thoughts, or conflicts. Different persons have different thoughts, needs, and conflicts and, hence, have widely different responses. A schizophrenic's responses often reflect a rather bizarre, idiosyncratic view of the world.

Table 1-22 lists the common projective tests together with a description and strengths and weaknesses for each test.

RORSCHACH TEST. Herman Rorschach, a Swiss psychiatrist, developed the first significant use of projective techniques around

Table 1-22
Projective Measures of Personality

Name	Description	Strengths	Weaknesses
Rorschach test	10 Stimulus cards of inkblots, some colored, others achromatic	Most widely used projective device and certainly the best researched; considerable interpretative data available	Some Rorschach interpretive systems have unimproved validity
Thematic Apperception Test (TAT)	20 Stimulus cards depicting a number of scenes of varying ambiguity	A widely used method that, in the hands of a well-trained person, provides valuable information	No generally accepted scoring system results in poor consistence in interpretation; time-consuming administration
Sentence completion test	A number of different devices available, all sharing the same format with more similarities than differences	Brief administration time; can be a useful adjunct to clinical interviews if supplied beforehand	Stimuli are obvious as to intent and subject to easy falsification
Holtzman Inkblot Technique (HIT)	Two parallel forms of inkblot cards with 45 cards per form	Only one response is allowed per card, making research less troublesome	Not widely accepted and rarely used; not directly comparable to Rorschach interpretive strategies
Figure drawing	Typically human forms but can involve houses or other forms	Quick administration	Interpretive strategies have typically been unsupported by research
Make-a-Picture Story (MAPS)	Similar to TAT; however, stimuli can be manipulated by the patient	Provides idiographic personality information through thematic analysis	Minimal research support; not widely used

Courtesy of Robert W. Butler, Ph.D. and Paul Satz, Ph.D.

1910. The Rorschach test is the most frequently used projective personality instrument (Fig. 1-8). The test consists of 10 ambiguous symmetrical inkblots. The inkblot card appears as if a blot of ink were poured onto a piece of paper and folded over—hence, the symmetrical appearance.

Minimal interaction between the examiner and the patient occurs while the Rorschach is administered, which ensures standardization procedures are upheld. The examiner writes down verbatim what the patient says during the above-described "free association" or "response proper" phase. If the patient rotates the card during his or her response, then the examiner makes the appropriate notation on the test protocol. After the patient has given answers to all 10 cards, an inquiry phase of administration begins. The examiner asks the patient to go through the cards again and help the examiner see the responses he or she gave. The examiner reads the patient's initial response and asks the patient to point out what he or she saw and explain what made it look like that to him or her. An almost unlimited range of responses is possible with the Rorschach test and most projective tests.

THEMATIC APPERCEPTION TEST. Although the Rorschach test is the most frequently used projective personality test, the Thematic Apperception Test (TAT) is probably in second place. Many clinicians will include both the TAT and the Rorschach test in a battery of tests for personality assessment. The TAT consists of a series of 10 black-and-white pictures that depict individuals of both sexes and of different age groups, who are involved in a variety of different activities. An example of a TAT card is presented in Figure 1-9.

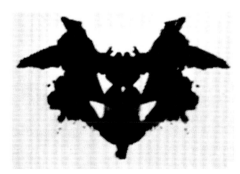

FIGURE 1-8
Card I of the Rorschach test. (From Hermann Rorschach, Rorschach®-Test. Copyright © Verlag Hans Hubar AG, Bern, Switzerland, 1921, 1948, 1994, with permission.)

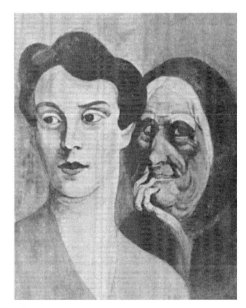

FIGURE 1-9
Card 12F of the Thematic Apperception Test. (Reprinted from Henry A. Murray, Thematic Apperception Test, Harvard University Press, Cambridge, MA. Copyright © 1943 President and Fellows of Harvard College, © 1971 Henry A. Murray, with permission.)

Henry Murray developed the TAT in 1943 at the Harvard Psychological Clinic. The stories that the patient makes up concerning the pictures, according to the projective hypothesis, reflect the patient's own needs, thoughts, feelings, stresses, wishes, desires, and views of the future. According to the theory underlying the test, a patient identifies with a particular individual in the picture. This individual is called the *hero*. The hero is usually close to the age of the patient and frequently of the same sex, although not necessarily so. Theoretically, the patient would attribute his or her own needs, thoughts, and feelings to this hero. The forces present in the hero's environment represent the *press* of the story, and the *outcome* is the resolution of the interaction between the hero's needs and desires and the press of the environment.

SENTENCE COMPLETION TEST.   Although a projective instrument, the sentence completion test is much more direct in soliciting responses from the patient. He or she is simply presented with a series of incomplete sentences and is asked to complete the sentence with the first response that comes to mind. The following are examples of possible incomplete sentences:

My father seldom…
Most people don't know that I'm afraid of…
When I was a child, I…
When encountering frustration, I usually…

The purpose of the test is to elicit, in a somewhat indirect manner, information about the patient that cannot be elicited from other measures. Because the patient responds in writing, the examiner's time is limited. The length of time it takes to complete the sentence completion varies greatly depending on the number of incomplete sentences. Tests can range from less than 10 sentences to greater than 75.

Behavioral Assessment.   Behavioral assessment involves the direct measurement of a given behavior. Rather than focus primarily on human characteristics, such as repression, ego strength, or self-esteem (vague terms to a behaviorist), strict behavioral measurement concentrates on the direct measurement that can be observed, such as several temper tantrums per unit of time, duration, and intensity and number of hyperventilation episodes, or the number of cigarettes smoked per 24-hour period.

Although early strict behaviorists would count only observable behaviors, a broader definition of behavior has emerged, under which just about anything people do—whether it is overt such as crying, swearing, or hand-washing or covert such as feeling and thinking—is considered behavior.

DIRECT COUNTING OF BEHAVIOR.   Measuring overt behavior is direct and can be done by the patient himself or herself, a family member, or an impartial observer.

Cognitive behavior therapists use these measurements to establish baselines of a given undesirable behavior (i.e., violent thoughts that the patient may wish to reduce). Similarly, therapists can measure behavior that the patient wants to increase (time studying, time out of bed, or distance walked on a treadmill). Follow-up measures of the same behavior monitor progress and quantify improvement.

MEDICAL ASSESSMENT AND LABORATORY TESTING IN PSYCHIATRY

Two recent issues have pushed medical assessment and laboratory testing in psychiatric patients to the forefront of attention for most clinicians: the widespread recognition of the pervasive problem of metabolic syndrome in clinical psychiatry and the shorter life expectancy of psychiatric patients compared with that of the general population. Factors that may contribute to medical comorbidity include abuse of tobacco, alcohol, and drugs, poor dietary habits, and obesity. Further, many psychotropic medications are associated with health risks that include obesity, metabolic syndrome, and hyperprolactinemia. Consequently, monitoring the physical health of psychiatric patients has become a more prominent issue.

A logical and systematic approach to the use of medical assessment and laboratory testing by the psychiatrist is vital to achieving the goals of arriving at accurate diagnoses, identifying medical comorbidities, implementing appropriate treatment, and delivering cost-effective care. Concerning the diagnosis or management of medical disease, it is crucial to consult with colleagues in other specialties. Good clinicians recognize the limits of their expertise and the need for consultation with their nonpsychiatric colleagues.

Physical Health Monitoring

Monitoring the physical health of psychiatric patients has two goals: to provide appropriate care for existing illnesses and to protect the patient's current health from possible future impairment. Disease prevention should begin with a clear concept of the condition to be avoided. Ideally, in psychiatry, this would be a focus on commonly found conditions that could be a significant source of morbidity or mortality. It is clear that in psychiatry, a small number of clinical problems underlie a significant number of impairments and premature deaths.

Role of History and Physical Examination

A thorough history, including a review of systems, is the basis for a comprehensive patient assessment. The history guides the clinician in the selection of laboratory studies that are relevant for a specific patient. Many psychiatric patients, owing to their illnesses, are not capable of providing sufficiently detailed information. Collateral sources of information, including family members and prior clinicians and their medical records, may be particularly helpful in the assessment of such patients.

The patient's medical history is an important component of the history. It should include notation of prior injuries and, in particular, head injuries that resulted in loss of consciousness and other causes of unconsciousness. The patient's medical history also should note pain conditions, ongoing medical problems, prior hospitalizations, prior surgeries, and a list of the patient's current medications. Toxic exposures are another important component of the medical history. Such exposures are often workplace-related.

The social history contains many of the details relevant to the assessment of character pathology, including risk factors for personality disorders as well as information relevant to the assessment of major disorders. Commonly, the social history includes a legal history, information about family and other significant relationships, and an occupational history.

In evaluating patients who appear demented, the role of the physical examination is to elucidate possible causative factors such as the cogwheel rigidity and tremor associated with Parkinson disease or neurologic deficits suggestive of prior strokes. Standard laboratory studies commonly assessed in dementia patients include a complete blood count (CBC), serum electrolytes, liver function tests (LFTs), blood urea nitrogen (BUN), creatinine

(Cr), thyroid function tests, serum B_{12}, and folate levels, Venereal Disease Research Laboratory (VDRL) test, and a urinalysis. Currently, there is no clear clinical indication for testing for the apolipoprotein E epsilon 4 allele. Often, a CT scan is performed if there are focal neurologic findings, and an electroencephalogram (EEG) may be performed if there is delirium. When patients are delirious, the neurologic examination may be complicated by inattention due to altered levels of consciousness. Delirium workup often includes the same laboratory workup described above for dementia. Urine or blood cultures, chest radiograph, neuroimaging studies, or EEG also may be appropriate.

Imaging of the Central Nervous System

Imaging of the central nervous system (CNS) can be broadly divided into two domains: structural and functional. Structural imaging provides detailed, noninvasive visualization of the morphology of the brain. Functional imaging provides a visualization of the spatial distribution of specific biochemical processes. Structural imaging includes x-ray, CT, and magnetic resonance imaging (MRI). Functional imaging includes PET, single-photon emission computed tomography (SPECT), fMRI, and magnetic resonance spectroscopy (MRS). With the limited exception of PET scanning, functional imaging techniques are still considered research tools that are not yet ready for routine clinical use.

Magnetic Resonance Imaging. MRI scans are used to distinguish structural brain abnormalities that may be associated with a patient's behavioral changes. These studies provide the clinician with images of anatomical structures viewed from cross-sectional, coronal, or oblique perspectives. MRI scans can detect a large variety of structural abnormalities. The MRI is particularly useful in examining the temporal lobes, the cerebellum, and the deep subcortical structures. It is unique in its ability to identify periventricular white matter hyperintensities. MRI scans are useful in examining the patient for particular diseases, such as nonmeningeal neoplasms, vascular malformations, seizure foci, demyelinating disorders, neurodegenerative disorders, and infarctions. The advantages of MRI include the absence of ionizing radiation and the absence of iodine-based contrast agents. MRI scans are contraindicated when the patient has a pacemaker, aneurysm clips, or ferromagnetic foreign bodies.

Computed Tomography. CT scans are used to identify structural brain abnormalities that may contribute to a patient's behavioral abnormalities. These studies provide the clinician with cross-sectional x-ray images of the brain. CT scans can detect a large variety of structural abnormalities in the cortical and subcortical regions of the brain. CT scans are useful when a clinician is looking for evidence of a stroke, subdural hematoma, tumor, or abscess. These studies also permit visualization of skull fractures. CT scans are the preferred modality when there is suspicion of a meningeal tumor, calcified lesions, acute subarachnoid or parenchymal hemorrhage, or acute parenchymal infarction.

CT scans may be performed with or without contrast. The purpose of contrast is to enhance the visualization of diseases that alter the blood–brain barrier, such as tumors, strokes, abscesses, and other infections.

Positron Emission Tomography. PET scans are performed predominantly at university medical centers. PET scans require a positron emission tomograph (the scanner) and a cyclotron to create the relevant isotopes. This type of scan involves the detection and measurement of emitted positron radiation after the injection of a compound that has been tagged with a positron-emitting isotope. Typically, PET scans use fluorodeoxyglucose (FDG) to measure regional brain glucose metabolism. Glucose is the principal energy source for the brain. These scans can provide information about the relative activation of brain regions because regional glucose metabolism is directly proportionate to neuronal activity. Brain FDG scans are useful in the differential diagnosis of dementing disease. The most consistent finding in the PET literature is the pattern of temporal-parietal glucose hypometabolism in patients with Alzheimer type dementia.

PET scanning using FDDNP (2-(1-{6-[(2-[fluorine-18]fluoroethyl)(methyl)amino]-2-naphthyl}-ethylidene) malononitrile) can differentiate between normal aging, mild cognitive impairment, and Alzheimer disease by determining regional cerebral patterns of plaques and tangles associated with Alzheimer disease. FDDNP binds to the amyloid senile plaques and tau neurofibrillary tangles. FDDNP appears to be superior to FDG PET in differentiating Alzheimer's patients from those with mild cognitive impairment and subjects with normal aging and no cognitive impairment.

Single-Photon Emission Computed Tomography. SPECT is available in most hospitals but is rarely used to study the brain. SPECT is more commonly used to study other organs, such as the heart, liver, and spleen. Some recent work, however, attempts to correlate SPECT brain imaging with mental disorders.

Functional Magnetic Resonance Imaging. fMRI is a research scan used to measure regional cerebral blood flow. Often, fMRI data are superimposed on conventional MRI images, resulting in detailed brain maps of brain structure and function. The measurement of blood flow involves the use of the heme molecule as an endogenous contrast agent. The rate of flow of heme molecules can be measured, resulting in an assessment of regional cerebral metabolism.

Magnetic Resonance Spectroscopy. MRS is another research method to measure regional brain metabolism. MRS scans are performed on conventional MRI devices that have had specific upgrades to their hardware and software. The upgrades permit the signal from protons to be suppressed and other compounds to be measured. (Conventional MRI images are, in reality, a map of the spatial distribution of protons found in water and fat.)

Magnetic Resonance Angiography. Magnetic resonance angiography (MRA) is a method for creating three-dimensional maps of cerebral blood flow. Neurologists and neurosurgeons more commonly use this test. Psychiatrists rarely use it.

Toxicology Studies

Urine drugs of abuse screens are immunoassays that detect barbiturates, benzodiazepines, cocaine metabolites, opiates, phencyclidine, tetrahydrocannabinol, and tricyclic antidepressants. These rapid tests provide results within an hour. However, they are screening tests; additional testing is required to confirm the results of this screening.

Testing to determine blood concentrations of certain psychotropic medications enables the clinician to ascertain whether blood levels of medications are at therapeutic, subtherapeutic, or toxic levels. Psychiatric symptoms are not uncommon when prescribed medications are at toxic levels. In the debilitated and the elderly, pathologic symptoms may occur at therapeutic concentrations. The normal reference range varies between laboratories. It is essential to check with the laboratory performing the test to obtain the normal reference range for that laboratory.

Testing for drugs of abuse is usually performed on urine specimens. It also may be performed on specimens of blood, breath (alcohol), hair, saliva, and sweat. Urine screens provide information about the recent use of frequently abused drugs such as alcohol, amphetamines, cocaine, marijuana, opioids, and phencyclidine along with 3,4-methylenedioxymethamphetamine (MDMA) (ecstasy). Many substances may produce false positives with urine drug screening tests. When a false positive is suspected, a confirmatory test may be requested.

Comprehensive qualitative toxicology screening is usually performed by liquid and gas chromatography. This may require many hours to perform and is rarely done in routine clinical situations. It is usually performed in patients with unexplained toxicity and an atypical clinical picture.

Qualitative toxicology assessments may be useful in managing patients who have overdosed when combined with clinical assessment and knowledge of when the ingestion occurred.

Drug Abuse. Patients are frequently unreliable when reporting their drug abuse history. Drug-induced mental disorders often resemble primary psychiatric disorders. Furthermore, substance abuse can exacerbate preexisting mental illness. Indications for ordering a drug abuse screen include unexplained behavioral symptoms, a history of illicit drug use or dependence in a new patient evaluation, or a high-risk background (e.g., criminal record, adolescents, and prostitutes). A drug abuse screen is also frequently used to monitor patient abstinence during treatment of substance abuse. Such tests can be ordered on a scheduled or random basis. Many clinicians believe random testing may be more accurate in the assessment of abstinence. The tests also may help to motivate the patient.

Other laboratory data may suggest a problem with a substance use disorder. An increase in the mean corpuscular volume is associated with alcohol use disorder. Liver enzymes may be increased with alcohol use disorder or from hepatitis B or C acquired from intravenous (IV) drug abuse. Serologic testing for hepatitis B or C can confirm that diagnosis. IV drug abusers are at risk for bacterial endocarditis. If bacterial endocarditis is suspected, a further medical workup is indicated.

TESTED SUBSTANCES. Routine tests are available for phencyclidine (PCP), cocaine, tetrahydrocannabinol (THC; also known as *marijuana*), benzodiazepines, methamphetamine, and its metabolite amphetamine, morphine (Duramorph), codeine, methadone (Dolophine), propoxyphene (Darvon), barbiturates, lysergic acid diethylamide (LSD), and MDMA.

Drug screening tests may have high false-positive rates. This is often due to the interaction of prescribed medication with the test, resulting in false-positive results and a lack of confirmatory testing. False-negative tests are common as well. False-negative results may be due to problems with specimen collection and storage.

Testing is most commonly performed on urine, although serum testing is also possible for most agents. Hair and saliva testing are also available in some laboratories. Alcohol can also be detected in the breath (breathalyzer). Except for alcohol, drug levels are not usually determined. Instead, only the presence or absence of the drug is determined. There is usually not a meaningful or useful correlation between the level of the drug and clinical behavior. The

Table 1-23
Drugs of Abuse that Can Be Detected in Urine

Drug	Length of Time Detected in Urine
Alcohol	7–12 hr
Amphetamine	48–72 hr
Barbiturate	24 hr (short acting); 3 wk (long acting)
Benzodiazepine	3 days
Cocaine	6–8 hr (metabolites 2–4 days)
Codeine	48 hr
Heroin	36–72 hr
Marijuana	2–7 days
Methadone	3 days
Methaqualone	7 days
Morphine	48–72 hr

length of time that a substance can be detected in the urine is listed in Table 1-23.

Alcohol. There is no single test or finding on physical examination that is diagnostic for alcohol use disorder. The history of the pattern of alcohol ingestion is most important in making the diagnosis. Laboratory test results and findings on physical examination may help to confirm the diagnosis. In patients with acute alcohol intoxication, a blood alcohol level (BAL) may be useful. A high BAL in a patient who clinically does not show significant intoxication is consistent with tolerance. Significant clinical evidence of intoxication with a low BAL should suggest intoxication with additional agents. Intoxication is commonly found with levels between 100 and 300 mg/dL. The degree of alcohol intoxication can also be assessed using the concentration of alcohol in expired respirations (breathalyzer). Chronic alcohol use is commonly associated with other laboratory abnormalities, including elevation in liver enzymes, such as aspartate aminotransferase (AST), which is usually greater than serum alanine aminotransferase (ALT). Bilirubin also is often elevated. Total protein and albumin may be low, and prothrombin time (PT) may be increased. A macrocytic anemia may be present.

Alcohol use disorder may be associated with rhinophyma, telangiectasias, hepatomegaly, and evidence of trauma on physical examination. In withdrawal, patients may have hypertension, tremulousness, and tachycardia.

Laboratory studies in patients who abuse alcohol may reveal macrocytosis. This occurs in most patients who consume four or more drinks per day. Elevations in AST and ALT characterize alcoholic liver disease, typically in a ratio of AST to ALT of 2:1 or greater. The γ-glutamyl transpeptidase (GGT) level may be elevated. Carbohydrate-deficient transferrin (CDT) may be helpful in the identification of chronic heavy alcohol use. It has a sensitivity of 60 to 70 percent and a specificity of 80 to 90 percent.

BAL is used to legally define intoxication in the determination of whether an individual is driving under the influence. The legal limit in many states is 80 mg/dL. However, clinical manifestations of intoxication vary with an individual's degree of alcohol tolerance. At the same BAL, an individual who chronically abuses alcohol may exhibit less impairment than an alcohol-naive individual. Generally, a BAL in the range of 50 to 100 mg/dL is associated with impaired judgment and coordination and levels greater than 100 mg/dL produce ataxia.

Environmental Toxins.

Specific toxins are associated with a variety of behavioral abnormalities. Exposure to toxins commonly occurs through occupation or hobbies.

Aluminum intoxication can cause a dementia-like condition. Aluminum can be detected in the urine or blood.

Arsenic intoxication may cause fatigue, loss of consciousness, anemia, and hair loss. Arsenic can be detected in urine, blood, and hair.

Manganese intoxication may present with delirium, confusion, and a parkinsonian syndrome. Manganese may be detected in urine, blood, and hair.

Symptoms of mercury intoxication include apathy, poor memory, lability, headache, and fatigue. Mercury can be detected in urine, blood, and hair.

Manifestations of lead intoxication include encephalopathy, irritability, apathy, and anorexia. Lead can be detected in blood or urine. Lead levels typically are assessed by collecting a 24-hour urine sample. The free erythrocyte protoporphyrin test is a screening test for chronic lead intoxication. This test is commonly coupled with a blood lead level. The Centers for Disease Control and Prevention specify that a lead level greater than 5 μg/dL requires further evaluation, and above 20 μg/dL requires a thorough investigation of the home and other possible sources of lead exposure. The incidence of lead toxicity in children has been falling recently.

Significant exposure to organic compounds, such as insecticides, may produce behavioral abnormalities. Many insecticides have strong anticholinergic effects. There are no readily available laboratory tests to detect these compounds. Poison control centers may assist in the identification of appropriate testing facilities.

Volatile Solvent Inhalation.

Volatile substances produce vapors that are inhaled for their psychoactive effect. The most commonly abused volatile solvents include gasoline, glue, paint thinner, and correction fluid (white-out). The aerosol propellants from cleaning sprays, deodorant sprays, and whipped cream containers may be abused. Nitrites, such as amyl nitrite ("poppers") and butyl nitrite vials ("rush"), and anesthetic gases, such as chloroform, ether, and nitrous oxide, are also abused.

Chronic abuse of volatile solvents is associated with damage to the brain, liver, kidneys, lung, heart, bone marrow, and blood. Abuse may produce hypoxia or anoxia. Signs of abuse include short-term memory loss, cognitive impairment, slurred and "scanning" speech, and tremor. Cardiac arrhythmias may occur. Exposure to toluene, which is present in many cleaning solutions, paints, and glues, has been associated with loss of clear gray–white matter differentiation and with brain atrophy on MRI scans. Methemoglobinemia has occurred with butyl nitrite abuse. Chronic use of volatile solvents is associated with the production of panic attacks and an organic personality disorder. Chronic use may also produce impairment in working memory and executive cognitive function.

Serum Medication Concentrations

Serum concentrations of psychotropic medications are assessed to minimize the risk of toxicity to patients receiving these medications and to ensure the administration of amounts sufficient to produce a therapeutic response. This is particularly true for medications with therapeutic blood levels. Medication levels are often influenced by hepatic metabolism. This metabolism occurs via the action of enzymes in the liver.

Acetaminophen.

Acetaminophen may produce hepatic necrosis, which in some cases may be fatal. Acetaminophen is one of the most frequently used agents in intentional drug overdoses and is a common cause of overdose-related deaths. Toxicity is associated with levels greater than 140 mcg/mL at 4 hours from ingestion in patients without preexisting liver disease. Chronic abusers of alcohol are particularly vulnerable to the effects of an overdose. Acetylcysteine (Mucomyst) treatment must occur promptly after an overdose to prevent hepatotoxicity.

Salicylate Toxicity.

Aspirin is frequently ingested in overdose. Consequently, serum salicylate levels often are obtained in overdose cases. Some rheumatic patients may chronically ingest large amounts of salicylate for therapeutic reasons. Ingestion of 500 mg/kg of aspirin may be fatal. Most patients will develop symptoms of toxicity when salicylate levels are greater than 40 mg/dL. Common symptoms of toxicity include acid–base abnormalities, tachypnea, tinnitus, nausea, and vomiting. In cases of severe toxicity, symptoms may include hyperthermia, altered mental status, pulmonary edema, and death.

Antipsychotic Agents

CLOZAPINE. Clozapine (Clozaril) levels are trough levels determined in the morning before administration of the morning dose of medication. A therapeutic range for clozapine has not been established; however, a level of 100 mg/mL is widely considered to be the minimum therapeutic threshold. At least 350 mg/mL of clozapine is considered to be necessary to achieve therapeutic response in patients with refractory schizophrenia. The likelihood of seizures and other side effects increase with clozapine levels greater than 1,200 mg/mL or doses greater than 600 mg per day or both. Clozapine is a common cause of leukopenia in psychiatry. When moderate to severe leucopenia develops, clozapine treatment must be interrupted, but patients may be retreated with clozapine in the future.

Mood Stabilizers

CARBAMAZEPINE. Carbamazepine (Tegretol) may produce changes in the levels of white blood cells, platelets, and, under rare circumstances, red blood cells. Anemia, aplastic anemia, leucopenia, and thrombocytopenia may all occur but are rare. Pretreatment evaluations typically include CBC.

Carbamazepine may produce hyponatremia. This hyponatremia is usually mild and does not produce clinical symptoms. However, carbamazepine may cause the syndrome of inappropriate secretion of antidiuretic hormone (SIADH). Carbamazepine may produce a variety of congenital abnormalities, including spina bifida and anomalies of the fingers. Manifestations of toxicity may include nausea, vomiting, urinary retention, ataxia, confusion, drowsiness, agitation, or nystagmus. At very high levels, symptoms may also include cardiac dysrhythmias, seizures, and respiratory depression.

LITHIUM. Lithium (Eskalith) has a narrow therapeutic index. Consequently, blood levels of lithium must be monitored to achieve therapeutic dosing and avoid toxicity. Side effects are dose-dependent. Symptoms of toxicity include tremors, sedation, and confusion. At higher levels, delirium, seizures, and coma may occur. Symptoms of toxicity may begin to manifest with serum levels of greater than 1.2 mEq/L and are common with levels greater than 1.4 mEq/L. Elderly or debilitated patients may show signs of toxicity with levels of less than 1.2 mEq/L.

VALPROATE.   Because of the risk of hepatotoxicity, ranging from mild dysfunction to hepatic necrosis, pretreatment LFTs are usually obtained. More commonly valproate (valproic acid [Depakene] and divalproex [Depakote]) may cause a sustained elevation in liver transaminase levels of as much as three times the upper limit of normal.

Valproate may increase the risk of congenital disabilities. A pretreatment urine pregnancy test is usually obtained in women of childbearing years. Women should be cautioned to use adequate contraception.

Hematologic abnormalities are also possible and include leucopenia and thrombocytopenia. Treatment with valproate may increase serum ammonia levels. It is prudent to obtain an ammonia level in a patient undergoing valproate treatment who presents with altered mental status or lethargy. Acute pancreatitis may also occur.

Antidepressants

MONOAMINE OXIDASE INHIBITORS.   Treatment with monoamine oxidase inhibitors (MAOIs) can cause orthostasis and, rarely, hypertensive crisis. Baseline blood pressure measurement should be obtained before the initiation of treatment, and blood pressure should be monitored during treatment.

There are no meaningful blood levels for MAOIs, and direct monitoring of MAOI blood levels is not clinically indicated. Treatment with MAOIs is occasionally associated with hepatotoxicity. For this reason, LFTs usually are obtained at the initiation of treatment and periodically after.

TRICYCLIC AND TETRACYCLIC ANTIDEPRESSANTS.   Routine laboratory studies obtained before initiation of tricyclic or tetracyclic antidepressants (TCAs) typically include CBC, serum electrolytes, and LFTs. Because TCAs affect cardiac conduction, clinicians also may obtain an electrocardiogram (ECG) to assess for the presence of abnormal cardiac rhythms and prolonged PR, QRS, and QTc complexes before initiation of these medications.

Neuroleptic Malignant Syndrome

Neuroleptic malignant syndrome (NMS) is a rare, potentially fatal consequence of neuroleptic administration. The syndrome consists of autonomic instability, hyperpyrexia, severe extrapyramidal symptoms (i.e., rigidity), and delirium. Sustained muscle contraction results in peripheral heat generation and muscle breakdown. Muscle breakdown contributes to elevated levels of creatine kinase (CK). Peripheral heat generation with impaired central mechanisms of thermoregulation results in hyperpyrexia. Myoglobinuria and leukocytosis are common. Hepatic and renal failure may occur. Liver enzymes become elevated with liver failure. Patients may die from hyperpyrexia, aspiration pneumonia, renal failure, hepatic failure, respiratory arrest, or cardiovascular collapse. Treatment includes discontinuation of the neuroleptic, hydration, administration of muscle relaxants, and general supportive nursing care.

A typical laboratory workup for NMS includes a CBC, serum electrolytes, BUN, Cr, and CK. A urinalysis, including an assessment of urine myoglobin, is also usually performed. As part of the differential diagnosis, blood and urine cultures are performed as part of a fever workup. Pronounced elevations in the white blood cell (WBC) count may occur in NMS. White blood cell counts are typically in the range from 10,000 to 40,000 per mm³.

Muscle Injury.   Serum CK levels may rise in response to repeated intramuscular (IM) injections, prolonged or agitated periods in restraint, or NMS. Dystonic reactions from neuroleptic administration may also result in elevated levels of CK.

Electroconvulsive Therapy

ECT is usually reserved for patients with the most treatment-resistant depression. Typical laboratory tests obtained before the administration of ECT include a CBC, serum electrolytes, urinalysis, and LFTs. However, no specific laboratory tests are required in the pre-ECT evaluation. Usually, an ECG is also obtained. A spinal x-ray series is no longer considered routinely indicated because of the low risk of spinal injury associated with modern administration techniques that use paralyzing agents. A comprehensive medical history and physical examination are useful screening tools to identify possible conditions that could complicate treatment.

Endocrine Evaluations

Endocrine disease is of great relevance to psychiatry. Management of psychiatric illness is complicated by comorbid endocrine disease. Endocrine illness frequently has psychiatric manifestations. For these reasons, screening for endocrine disease is often of relevance to the psychiatrist.

Adrenal Disease.   Adrenal disease may have psychiatric manifestations, including depression, anxiety, mania, dementia, psychosis, and delirium. However, patients with adrenal disease rarely come to the attention of psychiatrists. Assessment and management of these patients are best done in conjunction with specialists.

Low plasma levels of cortisol are found in Addison disease. These patients may have symptoms that are also common in psychiatric conditions, including fatigue, anorexia, weight loss, and malaise. Patients may also have memory impairment, confusion, or delirium. Depression or psychosis with hallucinations and delusions may occur.

Elevated levels of cortisol are seen in Cushing syndrome. About half of all patients with Cushing syndrome develop psychiatric symptoms. These symptoms may include lability, irritability, anxiety, panic attacks, depressed mood, euphoria, mania, or paranoia. Cognitive dysfunctions may include cognitive slowing and poor short-term memory. Symptoms usually improve when cortisol normalizes. If not, or if symptoms are severe, psychiatric treatment may be necessary.

Cortisol levels are not useful in the assessment or management of primary psychiatric disease. In particular, the dexamethasone-suppression test (DST) remains a research tool in psychiatry that is not used in routine clinical care.

Anabolic Steroid Use.   The use of anabolic steroids has been associated with irritability, aggression, depression, and psychosis. Athletes and bodybuilders are common abusers of anabolic steroids. Urine specimens can be used to screen for these agents. Because so many compounds have been synthesized, a variety of tests may be required to confirm the diagnosis, depending on the compound that has been used. Consultation with a specialist is advised. Generally, androgens other than testosterone can be detected by gas chromatography and mass spectroscopy.

Antidiuretic Hormone.   Arginine vasopressin (AVP), also called antidiuretic hormone (ADH), is decreased in central diabetes insipidus (DI). DI may be central (due to the pituitary or hypothalamus) or nephrogenic. Nephrogenic DI may be acquired or due to an inherited X-linked condition. Lithium-induced DI is an example of an acquired form of DI. Lithium has been shown to decrease the sensitivity of renal tubules to AVP. Patients with central DI respond to the administration of vasopressin with a decrease in urine output. Secondary central DI may develop in response to head trauma that produces damage in the pituitary or hypothalamus.

About one-fifth of patients taking lithium develop polyuria, and a more considerable amount may have some degree of impairment in concentrating urine. Chronic treatment with lithium is a common cause of nephrogenic DI. However, there are other causes of polyuria in lithium-treated patients also to nephrogenic DI. Primary polydipsia is common and is often associated with the dry mouth associated with many psychiatric medications. Central diabetes has also been associated with lithium treatment.

Excessive secretion of AVP results in increased retention of fluid in the body. This condition is called SIADH. Water retention in SIADH causes hyponatremia. SIADH may develop in response to injury to the brain or from medication administration (including phenothiazines, butyrophenones, carbamazepine, and oxcarbazepine). The hyponatremia associated with this condition may produce delirium.

Human Chorionic Gonadotropin.

Human chorionic gonadotropin (hCG) can be assessed in the urine and blood. The urine test for hCG is the basis for the commonly used urine pregnancy test. This immunometric test can detect pregnancy approximately 2 weeks after an expected menstrual period has passed. Routine tests are most accurate when performed 1 to 2 weeks after a missed period and are not reliably accurate until the 2-week period has passed. However, there are ultrasensitive urine hCG tests that can accurately detect pregnancy 7 days after fertilization. Pregnancy tests often are obtained before initiating certain psychotropic medications, such as lithium, carbamazepine, and valproate, which are associated with congenital anomalies.

Parathormone.

Parathormone (parathyroid hormone) modulates serum concentrations of calcium and phosphorus. Dysregulation in this hormone and the resulting production of abnormalities in calcium and phosphorus may produce depression or delirium.

Prolactin.

Prolactin levels may become elevated in response to the administration of antipsychotic agents. Elevations in serum prolactin result from the blockade of dopamine receptors in the pituitary. This blockade produces an increase in prolactin synthesis and release.

Cerebral MRI is not usually performed if the patient is taking an antipsychotic drug known to cause hyperprolactinemia, and the magnitude of the prolactin elevation is consistent with drug-induced causes.

Prolactin levels may briefly rise after a seizure. For this reason, prompt measurement of a prolactin level after possible seizure activity may assist in differentiating a seizure from a pseudoseizure.

Thyroid Hormone.

The disease of the thyroid is associated with many psychiatric manifestations. Thyroid disease is most commonly associated with depression and anxiety but may also give rise to symptoms of panic, dementia, and psychosis. Thyroid disease may mimic depression. It is challenging to achieve euthymia if a patient is not euthyroid.

Systemic Lupus Erythematosus.

Systemic lupus erythematosus (SLE) is an autoimmune disorder. Tests for SLE are based on the detection of antibodies formed as part of the disease.

Antinuclear antibodies are found in virtually all patients with SLE. Antibody levels also are used to monitor the severity of the illness. A fluorescent test is used to detect antinuclear antibodies. This test can be positive in a variety of rheumatic diseases.

For this reason, a positive result usually is followed by additional tests, including a test to detect anti-deoxyribonucleic acid (DNA) antibodies. Anti-DNA antibodies, when associated with antinuclear antibodies, are strongly suggestive of a diagnosis of lupus. Anti-DNA antibodies are followed to monitor the response to treatment.

Psychiatric manifestations of lupus include depression, dementia, delirium, mania, and psychosis. About 5 percent of patients with lupus present with symptoms of psychosis, including hallucinations and delusions.

Pancreatic Function.

Measurement of serum amylase is used to monitor pancreatic function. Elevations in amylase levels may occur in alcohol-abusing patients who develop pancreatitis. Serum amylase levels also may be fractionated into salivary and pancreatic components.

Clinical Chemistry

Serum Electrolytes.

Serum electrolyte levels may be useful in the initial evaluation of a psychiatric patient. Levels of serum electrolytes often are abnormal in patients with delirium. Abnormalities also may occur in response to the administration of psychotropic medications. Low serum chloride levels may occur in eating disorder patients who purge by self-induced vomiting. Serum bicarbonate levels may be elevated in patients who purge or who abuse laxatives. Bicarbonate levels are commonly low in patients who hyperventilate in response to anxiety.

Hypokalemia may be present in eating disorder patients who purge or abuse laxatives and in psychogenic vomiting. Diuretic abuse by eating disorder patients also may produce hypokalemia. Low levels of potassium are associated with weakness and fatigue. Characteristic ECG changes occur with hypokalemia and consist of cardiac arrhythmias, U waves, flattened T waves, and ST-segment depression.

Eating disorder patients with anorexia nervosa or bulimia nervosa usually receive a relatively standard set of laboratory studies, including serum electrolytes (particularly potassium and phosphorus), blood glucose, thyroid function tests, liver enzymes, total protein, serum albumin, BUN, Cr, CBC, and ECG. Serum amylase is often assessed in bulimic patients.

Magnesium levels may be low in alcohol-abusing patients. Low magnesium levels are associated with agitation, confusion, and delirium. If untreated, convulsions and coma may follow.

Low levels of serum phosphorus may be present in eating disorder patients with purging behavior. Phosphorus levels may also be low in anxiety patients who hyperventilate. Hyperparathyroidism may produce low serum phosphorus levels. Elevated serum phosphorus levels are seen in hypoparathyroidism.

Hyponatremia is seen in psychogenic polydipsia and SIADH and in response to certain medications, such as carbamazepine. Low sodium levels are associated with delirium.

Serum calcium abnormalities are associated with a variety of behavioral abnormalities. Low serum calcium levels are associated with depression, delirium, and irritability. Elevated levels are associated with depression, psychosis, and weakness. Laxative abuse, common in eating disorder patients, can be associated with hypocalcemia. Hypocalcemia secondary to hypoparathyroidism may occur in patients who have undergone surgery for thyroid disease.

Serum copper levels are low in Wilson disease, a rare abnormality in copper metabolism. Copper is deposited in the brain and liver, resulting in decreased intellectual functioning, personality changes, psychosis, and a movement disorder. Symptoms are usually present in the second and third decades of life. Laboratory assessment for Wilson disease includes the measurement of serum ceruloplasmin, the transport protein for copper, which is low, and urine copper, measured in a 24-hour specimen, which is elevated.

Renal Function. Tests of renal function include BUN and Cr. Other relevant laboratory studies include routine urinalysis and Cr clearance. An elevated BUN often results in lethargy or delirium. BUN is commonly elevated with dehydration. Elevations in BUN often are associated with impaired clearance of lithium. A less sensitive index of renal function is Cr. Elevations in Cr may indicate extensive renal impairment. Elevated levels occur when approximately 50 percent of the nephrons are damaged.

Cr clearance is often assessed in patients taking lithium. It is a sensitive measurement of renal function. The test is performed in a well-hydrated patient by collecting all of the patient's urine for 24 hours. During the midpoint of the 24-hour collection period, a serum Cr level also is obtained. The resulting data are used to calculate the patient's Cr clearance. Usually, the laboratory performs the calculation.

Elevated levels of porphobilinogen are found in the urine of symptomatic patients with acute intermittent porphyria. Symptoms of this disease include psychosis, apathy, or depression, along with intermittent abdominal pain, neuropathy, and autonomic dysfunction. If urine porphobilinogen levels are elevated when the patient is symptomatic, collection of a 24-hour urine specimen for quantitative assessment of porphobilinogen and aminolevulinic acid is indicated.

Liver Function. LFTs commonly include the serum aminotransferases, alkaline phosphatase, γ-glutamyl transpeptidase, and tests of synthetic function, usually the serum albumin concentration and prothrombin time, and the serum bilirubin, which reflects hepatic transport capability.

Elevations in AST may occur with diseases of the liver, heart, lungs, kidneys, and skeletal muscle. In patients with alcohol-induced liver disease, AST typically is more elevated than ALT. In viral- and drug-induced liver disease, ALT is often elevated. Serum GGT is elevated in hepatobiliary disease, including alcohol-induced liver disease and cirrhosis.

Alkaline phosphatase elevations occur in many diseases, including diseases of the liver, bone, kidney, and thyroid. Levels of alkaline phosphatase may be elevated in response to some psychiatric medications, most notably the phenothiazines.

Serum ammonia levels are often elevated in patients with hepatic encephalopathy. High levels are associated with the delirium of hepatic encephalopathy. Serum ammonia levels also may be elevated in patients undergoing treatment with valproate.

Serum bilirubin is an index of hepatic and bile duct function. Prehepatic, unconjugated, or indirect bilirubin and posthepatic, conjugated, or direct bilirubin are often assessed to help elucidate the origin of the elevation in bilirubin.

Lactate dehydrogenase (LDH) may be elevated in diseases of the liver, skeletal muscle, heart, and kidney. It is also elevated in pernicious anemia.

Vitamins

FOLATE AND B$_{12}$. Folate and B$_{12}$ deficiencies are common in patients who abuse alcohol. Folate and B$_{12}$ deficiencies are associated with dementia; delirium; psychosis, including paranoia;

fatigue; and personality change. Folate and B$_{12}$ can be directly measured. Low folate levels may be found in patients who use contraceptive pills or other forms of estrogen, who drink alcohol, or who take phenytoin.

Infectious Disease Testing

Testing for sexually transmitted diseases (STDs) has become common, given the current frequency of these diseases. Some psychiatric illnesses, such as mania and substance abuse, are associated with a higher risk of contracting STDs. STDs include herpes simplex virus types 1 and 2, chlamydia, hepatitis viruses, gonorrhea, syphilis, and human immunodeficiency virus (HIV). Risk factors for STD include contact with sex workers, drug abuse, prior history of STDs, meeting partners on the Internet, multiple sex partners, a new sex partner, and being young or unmarried. Other diseases to think about are Epstein–Barr virus and gonorrhea.

Intravenous Drug Use. The IV route is used for many substances of abuse. Most commonly, heroin, amphetamines, and cocaine are used alone or in combination via the IV route. Because needles often are contaminated, IV drug users are at risk for bacterial endocarditis, hepatitis B and C, HIV infection, and acquired immunodeficiency syndrome (AIDS) from HIV infection. It has been estimated that over 60 percent of new cases of hepatitis C occur in individuals with a history of injecting illicit drugs.

CBC AND SERUM BLOOD CULTURES. The use of contaminated needles or nonsterile injection sites places IV drug users at risk for bacterial infections, including abscesses, bacteremia, and bacterial endocarditis. Findings on physical examination suggestive of endocarditis, possible bacteremia, or abscess necessitate obtaining a CBC to rule out an elevated WBC count. Blood cultures should be obtained from at least two different sites if the patient is febrile or if findings are suggestive of bacteremia or endocarditis, and internal medicine consultation should be obtained.

Syphilis. The fluorescent treponemal antibody absorption (FTA-ABS) test detects antibodies against *Treponema pallidum* spirochetes and is more sensitive and specific than nontreponemal tests for syphilis. The test is used to confirm positive screening tests for syphilis, such as the rapid plasma reagin (RPR) test and the VDRL test. The FTA-ABS test is also used when neurosyphilis is suspected. Once positive, a patient usually remains so for life. False-positive results may occur in patients with SLE.

Viral Hepatitis. Several types of viruses can cause viral hepatitis. Viral hepatitis produces abnormalities in LFTs, including elevation of liver enzymes, especially ALT. Symptoms range from mild flu-like manifestations to rapidly progressive and fatal liver failure. Psychiatric manifestations include depression, anxiety, weakness, and psychosis. Viral hepatitis can also impair the metabolism of psychotropic medications that are metabolized by the liver. Impaired liver metabolism requires an adjustment of the dose of medications metabolized by the liver or consideration of agents that are less affected by alterations in liver metabolism. Viruses causing hepatitis include hepatitis A virus (HAV), hepatitis B virus (HBV), hepatitis C virus (HCV), and hepatitis D virus (HDV) (delta agent).

The WBC is normal to low in patients with hepatitis, especially in the preicteric phase. Large atypical lymphocytes occasionally are present. Rarely, aplastic anemia follows an episode of acute hepatitis not caused by any of the known hepatitis viruses. Mild proteinuria is common, and bilirubinuria often precedes the appearance of jaundice. Acholic stools frequently are present during the icteric phase. Strikingly elevated AST or ALT occurs early, followed by elevations of bilirubin and alkaline phosphatase. In a minority of patients, elevations of bilirubin and alkaline phosphatase persist after aminotransferase levels have normalized. Cholestasis may be substantial in acute hepatitis A. Marked prolongation of the PT in severe hepatitis correlates with increased mortality.

Chronic hepatitis, characterized by elevated aminotransferase levels for more than 6 months, develops in 1 to 2 percent of immunocompetent adults with acute hepatitis B. More than 80 percent of all persons with acute hepatitis C develop chronic hepatitis, which, in many cases, progresses slowly. Ultimately, cirrhosis develops in as many as 30 percent of those with chronic hepatitis C and 40 percent of those with chronic hepatitis B; the risk of cirrhosis is even higher in patients coinfected with both viruses or with HIV. Patients with cirrhosis are at risk, with a rate of 3 to 5 percent per year, of hepatocellular carcinoma. Even in the absence of cirrhosis, patients with chronic hepatitis B—particularly those with active viral replication—are at an increased risk.

Electroencephalogram

The EEG assesses regional cerebral cortical electrical activity. Clinical neuroscience has a long history of using EEG. The EEG can be used in different ways to study specific brain states or activities by modifications to the technique of data collection or the data themselves. EEG data can be displayed on paper tracings in the manner of conventional EEG recordings. Alternatively, the data can be digitized, and the digitized data can be transformed, often using a Fourier transformation, to yield color-coded topographic brain maps of regional activity. The collection periods can be prolonged, and the data can be electronically displayed along with video monitoring of the patient to provide telemetry assessments of patients with epilepsy. Telemetry assessments are typically performed to correlate behavioral abnormalities with brain electrical activity as part of the workup of seizure disorders. Prolonged periods of EEG recording during sleep, when coupled with a recording of a limited lead ECG and facial muscle activity, result in the sleep EEG or polysomnography. Many clinicians also use the EEG to monitor ECT administration.

Clinicians use the EEG to localize seizure foci and to evaluate delirium. The EEG and its topographical descendants have not found an exact role in the diagnostic assessment of psychiatric patients. The EEG is usually used in psychiatry to rule out nonpsychiatric diseases, such as seizure disorders or delirium, as a cause of psychiatric symptoms. When the differential diagnosis includes strokes, tumors, subdural hematomas, or dementia, the yield is usually higher with imaging tests. Not surprisingly, the yield is the highest in patients with a history of a seizure disorder or a clinical history that is strongly suggestive of a recent seizure or other organic illness. Such clinical features would include a history of altered consciousness, atypical hallucinations (e.g., olfactory), head injury, and automatism. Also, the EEG is commonly obtained when there is an abnormal CT or MRI. It is important to remember that seizures are a clinical diagnosis; a normal EEG does not rule out the possibility of a seizure disorder.

Evoked Potential. Evoked potential (EP) testing is the measurement of the EEG response to specific sensory stimulation. The stimulation may be visual, auditory, or somatosensory. During visual EPs, the patient is exposed to flashing lights or a checkerboard pattern. With auditory EP, the patient hears a specific tone. In somatosensory EP, the patient experiences an electrical stimulation to an extremity. These stimuli repeatedly occur while the patient undergoes a routine EEG. Using a computer, the responses to these stimuli are recorded and averaged. The time frame is measured in milliseconds. These tests are useful in neurology and neurosurgery. For example, they assist in the assessment of demyelinating disorders such as multiple sclerosis (MS). In psychiatry, EP testing may help in the differentiation of organic from functional impairments. A classical example is the use of EP testing to evaluate possible hysterical blindness. The usefulness of these tests in psychiatry is still under investigation.

Polysomnography. Polysomnography is used to assess disorders of sleep by concurrently assessing the EEG, ECG, blood oxygen saturation, respiration, body temperature, electromyogram, and electrooculogram. Polysomnography has demonstrated an increase in the overall amount of rapid eye movement (REM) sleep and a shortened period before the onset of REM sleep (decreased REM latency) in patients with major depression. These studies may assist in differentiating depression from other conditions that mimic depression. For example, patients who appear depressed from dementia do not have decreased REM latency or an increase in the amount of REM sleep.

Electrocardiogram

The ECG is a graphical representation of the electrical activity of the heart. Abnormalities in this activity correlate with cardiac pathology. The ECG is most commonly used in psychiatry to assess the side effects of psychotropic medications.

Ziprasidone has been associated with a dose-related prolongation of the QTc interval. There is a known association of fatal arrhythmias (e.g., torsades de pointes) with QTc prolongation from some other medications. For this reason, clinicians usually obtain an ECG before initiation of treatment with ziprasidone. Ziprasidone is contraindicated in patients with a known history of QTc prolongation (including congenital long QT syndrome), with recent acute myocardial infarction, or with uncompensated heart failure. Bradycardia, hypokalemia or hypomagnesemia, or the concurrent use of other drugs that prolong the QTc interval all increase the risk of severe arrhythmias. Ziprasidone should be discontinued in patients who have persistent QTc measurements greater than 500 milliseconds.

Like ziprasidone, thioridazine has been associated with prolongation of the QTc interval in a dose-related manner. Prolongation of the QTc interval has been associated with torsades de pointes arrhythmias and sudden death. An ECG should be obtained before initiating treatment with thioridazine to rule out QTc prolongation. Many other antipsychotics can along prolong the QTc interval particularly in patients with preexisting arrhythmia.

TCAs are, at times, associated with ECG changes. Anticholinergic effects may increase heart rate. Prolongation of the PR, QT, and QRS intervals, along with ST-segment and T-wave abnormalities, may occur. The TCAs can cause or increase preexisting atrioventricular or bundle branch block. When the QTc exceeds 0.440 seconds, a patient is at an increased risk for sudden death due to cardiac arrhythmias. Many clinicians obtain an ECG before beginning a TCA in a patient older than 40 years of age and any patient with known cardiovascular disease.

Lithium therapy can cause benign reversible T-wave changes, which can impair sinoatrial (SA) node function and can cause heart block. ECGs are often obtained before initiation of treatment with lithium and in cases of lithium toxicity or overdose.

Psychiatrists, when treating patients with specific psychiatric diagnoses, also use the ECG. Eating disorder patients commonly have low potassium levels that may result in abnormal ECG recordings. As the serum potassium drops below normal, T waves become flat (or inverted), and U waves may appear.

Holter Monitoring. Holter monitoring is the continuous recording of a patient's ECG activity for a sustained period (e.g., 24 hours). Patients are ambulatory during this time. It is useful for the evaluation of dizziness, palpitations, and syncope. It is commonly used in the evaluation of patients with panic disorder who manifest cardiac symptoms.

Cardiac Ultrasound. Cardiac ultrasound is the visualization of cardiac anatomy by the use of computer-transformed echoes of ultrasound. It is commonly used in the evaluation of mitral valve prolapse. There is an unclear association between mitral valve prolapse and panic attacks and anxiety disorders.

NEUROIMAGING

The primary observation of structural and functional brain imaging in neuropsychiatric disorders such as dementia, movement disorders, demyelinating disorders, and epilepsy has contributed to a greater understanding of the pathophysiology of neurologic and psychiatric illnesses and helps practicing clinicians in difficult diagnostic situations.

Neuroimaging methodologies allow measurement of the structure, function, and chemistry of the living human brain. Over the past decade, studies using these methods have provided new information about the pathophysiology of psychiatric disorders that may prove to be useful for diagnosing illness and for developing new treatments. Computed tomographic (CT) scanners, the first widely used neuroimaging devices, allowed assessment of structural brain lesions such as tumors or strokes. MRI scans, developed next, distinguish gray and white matter better than CT scans do and allow visualizations of smaller brain lesions as well as white matter abnormalities. Also, to structural neuroimaging with CT and MRI, a revolution in functional neuroimaging has enabled clinical scientists to obtain unprecedented insight into the diseased human brain. The foremost techniques for functional neuroimaging include PET and SPECT.

Uses of Neuroimaging

Indications for Ordering Neuroimaging in Clinical Practice

NEUROLOGIC DEFICITS. In a neurologic examination, any change that can be localized to the brain or spinal cord requires neuroimaging. Neurologic examination includes mental status, cranial nerves, motor system, coordination, sensory system, and reflex components. The mental status examination assesses arousal, attention, and motivation; memory; language; visuospatial function; complex cognition; and mood and affect. Consultant psychiatrists should consider a workup, including neuroimaging for patients with new-onset psychosis and acute changes in mental status. The clinical examination always assumes priority, and neuroimaging is ordered based on clinical suspicion of a CNS disorder.

DEMENTIA. Loss of memory and cognitive abilities affects more than 10 million persons in the United States and will affect an

increasing number as the population ages. Reduced mortality from cancer and heart disease has increased life expectancy and has allowed persons to survive to the age of onset of degenerative brain disorders, which have proved more challenging to treat. Depression, anxiety, and psychosis are common in patients with dementia. The most common cause of dementia is Alzheimer disease, which does not have a characteristic appearance on routine neuroimaging but, instead, is associated with diffuse loss of brain volume.

One treatable cause of dementia that requires neuroimaging for diagnosis is *normal pressure hydrocephalus,* a disorder of the drainage of cerebrospinal fluid (CSF). This condition does not progress to the point of acutely increased intracranial pressure but stabilizes at a pressure at the upper end of the normal range. The dilated ventricles, which may be readily visualized with CT or MRI, exert pressure on the frontal lobes. A gait disorder is almost uniformly present; dementia, which may be indistinguishable from Alzheimer disease, appears less consistently. Relief of the increased CSF pressure may completely restore gait and mental function.

Infarction of the cortical or subcortical areas, or stroke, can produce focal neurologic deficits, including cognitive and emotional changes. Strokes are easily seen on MRI scans. Depression is common among stroke patients, either because of direct damage to the emotional centers of the brain or because of the patient's reaction to the disability. Depression, in turn, can cause pseudodementia. Also, to major strokes, extensive atherosclerosis in brain capillaries can cause countless tiny infarctions of brain tissue; patients with this phenomenon may develop dementia as fewer and fewer neural pathways participate in cognition. This state, called *vascular dementia* (or Vascular Neurocognitive Disorder in DSM-5), is characterized on MRI scans by patches of increased signal in the white matter.

Certain degenerative disorders of basal ganglia structures, associated with dementia, may have a characteristic appearance on MRI scans. Huntington disease typically produces atrophy of the caudate nucleus; thalamic degeneration can interrupt the neural links to the cortex (Fig. 1-10).

Space-occupying lesions can cause dementia. Chronic subdural hematomas and cerebral contusions, caused by head trauma, can produce focal neurologic deficits or may only produce dementia. Brain tumors can affect cognition in several ways. Skull-based meningiomas can compress the underlying cortex and impair its processing. Infiltrative glial cell tumors, such as astrocytoma or glioblastoma multiforme, can cut off communication between brain centers by interrupting white matter tracts. Tumors located near the ventricular system can obstruct the flow of CSF and gradually increase the intracranial pressure.

Chronic infections, including neurosyphilis, cryptococcosis, tuberculosis, and Lyme disease, can cause symptoms of dementia and may produce a characteristic enhancement of the meninges, especially at the base of the brain. Serologic studies are needed to complete the diagnosis. HIV infection can cause dementia directly, in which case is seen as a diffuse loss of brain volume, or it can allow a proliferation of Creutzfeldt–Jakob virus to yield progressive multifocal leukoencephalopathy, which affects white matter tracts and appears as increased white matter signal on MRI scans.

Chronic demyelinating diseases, such as multiple sclerosis, can affect cognition because of white matter disruption. Multiple sclerosis plaques are easily seen on MRI scans as periventricular patches of increased signal intensity.

Any evaluation of dementia should consider medication effects, metabolic derangements, infections, and nutritional causes that may not produce abnormalities on neuroimaging.

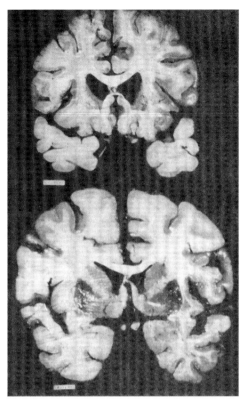

FIGURE 1-10
Brain slices. **Top:** Huntington disease. Atrophy of caudate nucleus and lentiform nuclei with dilatation of lateral ventricle. **Bottom:** Normal brain. (From Fahn S. Huntington disease. In: Rowland LP, ed. *Merritt's Textbook of Neurology*. 10th ed. Philadelphia, PA: Lippincott Williams & Wilkins; 2000:659, with permission.)

Indications for Neuroimaging in Clinical Research

ANALYSIS OF CLINICALLY DEFINED GROUPS OF PATIENTS. Psychiatric research aims to categorize patients with psychiatric disorders to facilitate the discovery of neuroanatomical and neurochemical bases of mental illness. Researchers have used functional neuroimaging to study groups of patients with such psychiatric conditions as schizophrenia, affective disorders, and anxiety disorders, among others. In schizophrenia, for example, neuropathologic volumetric analyses have suggested a loss of brain weight, specifically of gray matter. A paucity of axons and dendrites appears present in the cortex, and CT and MRI may show compensatory enlargement of the lateral and third ventricles. Specifically, the temporal lobes of persons with schizophrenia appear to lose the most volume relative to healthy persons. Recent studies have found that the left temporal lobe is generally more affected than the right. The frontal lobe may also have abnormalities, not in the volume of the lobe, but in the level of activity detected by functional neuroimaging. Persons with schizophrenia consistently exhibit decreased metabolic activity in the frontal lobes, especially during tasks that require the prefrontal cortex. As a group, patients with schizophrenia are also more likely to have an increase in ventricular size than are healthy controls.

Disorders of mood and affect can also be associated with loss of brain volume and decreased metabolic activity in the frontal lobes. Inactivation of the left prefrontal cortex appears to depress mood; inactivation of the right prefrontal cortex elevates it. Among anxiety disorders, studies of OCD with conventional CT and MRI have shown either no specific abnormalities or a smaller caudate nucleus. Functional PET and SPECT studies suggest abnormalities in the corticolimbic, basal ganglia, and thalamic structures in the disorder. When patients are experiencing OCD symptoms, the orbital prefrontal cortex shows abnormal activity. A partial normalization of caudate glucose metabolism appears in patients taking medications such as fluoxetine or clomipramine or undergoing behavior modification.

Functional neuroimaging studies of persons with ADHD either have shown no abnormalities or have shown a decreased volume of the right prefrontal cortex and the right globus pallidus. Also, whereas usually the right caudate nucleus is larger than the left caudate nucleus, persons with ADHD may have caudate nuclei of equal size. These findings suggest dysfunction of the right prefrontal-striatal pathway for control of attention.

ANALYSIS OF BRAIN ACTIVITY DURING PERFORMANCE OF SPECIFIC TASKS. Many original conceptions of different brain region functions emerged from observing deficits caused by local injuries, tumors, or strokes. Functional neuroimaging allows researchers to review and reassess classic teachings in the intact brain. Most work, to date, has been aimed at language and vision. Although many technical peculiarities and limitations of SPECT, PET, and fMRI have been overcome, none of these techniques has demonstrated clear superiority. Studies require carefully controlled conditions, which subjects may find arduous. Nonetheless, functional neuroimaging has contributed major conceptual advances, and the methods are now limited mainly by the creativity of the investigative protocols.

Studies have been designed to reveal the functional neuroanatomy of all sensory modalities, gross and fine motor skills, language, memory, calculations, learning, and disorders of thought, mood, and anxiety. Unconscious sensations transmitted by the autonomic nervous system have been localized to specific brain regions. These analyses provide a basis for comparison with results of studies of clinically defined patient groups and may lead to improved therapies for mental illnesses.

Specific Techniques

CT Scans. In 1972, CT scanning revolutionized diagnostic neuroradiology by allowing imaging of the brain tissue in live patients. CT scanners are currently the most widely available and convenient imaging tools available in clinical practice; practically, every hospital emergency room has immediate access to a CT scanner at all times. CT scanners effectively take a series of head x-ray pictures from all vantage points, 360 degrees around a patient's head. The amount of radiation that passes through, or is not absorbed from, each angle is digitized and entered into a computer. The computer uses matrix algebra calculations to assign a specific density to each point within the head and displays these data as a set of two-dimensional images. When viewed in sequence, the images allow mental reconstruction of the shape of the brain.

The CT image is determined only by the degree to which tissues absorb x-irradiation. The bony structures absorb high amounts of irradiation and tend to obscure details of neighboring structures, an especially troublesome problem in the brainstem, which is surrounded by a thick skull base. Within the brain itself, there is relatively little difference in the attenuation between gray matter and white matter in x-ray images. Although the gray–white border is usually distinguishable, details of the gyral pattern may be difficult to appreciate in CT scans. Certain tumors may be invisible on CT because they absorb as much irradiation as the surrounding normal brain.

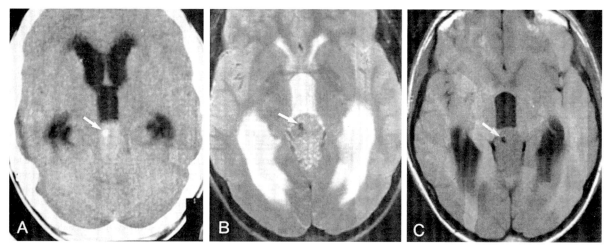

FIGURE 1-11

Comparison of computed tomography (CT) and magnetic resonance imaging (MRI). **A:** CT scan in the axial plane at the level of the third ventricle. The cerebrospinal fluid (CSF) within the ventricles appears black, the brain tissue appears gray, and the skull appears white. There is very poor discrimination between the gray and white matter of the brain. The *arrow* indicates a small calcified lesion in a tumor of the pineal gland. Detection of calcification is one role in which CT is superior to MRI. **B:** T2-weighted image of the same patient at roughly the same level. With T2, the CSF appears white, the gray matter appears gray, the white matter is clearly distinguished from the gray matter; the skull and indicated calcification appear black. Much more detail of the brain is visible than with CT. **C:** T1-weighted image of the same patient at roughly the same level. With T1, the CSF appears dark, the brain appears more uniformly gray, and the skull and indicated calcification appear black. T1 MRI images are the most similar to CT images. (Reprinted from Grossman CB. *Magnetic Resonance Imaging and Computed Tomography of the Head and Spine*. 2nd ed. Baltimore, MD: Williams & Wilkins; 1996:101, with permission.)

Appreciation of tumors and areas of inflammation, which can cause changes in behavior, can be increased by intravenous infusion of iodine-containing contrast agents. Iodinated compounds, which absorb much more irradiation than the brain, appear white. The intact brain is separated from the bloodstream by the blood–brain barrier, which normally prevents the passage of the highly charged contrast agents. The blood–brain barrier, however, breaks down in the presence of inflammation or fails to form within tumors and thus allows accumulation of contrast agents. These sites appear whiter than the surrounding brain. Iodinated contrast agents must be used with caution in patients who are allergic to these agents or shellfish.

With the introduction of MRI scanning, CT scans have been supplanted as the nonemergency neuroimaging study of choice (Fig. 1-11). The increased resolution and delineation of detail afforded by MRI scanning is often required for diagnosis in psychiatry. Also, performing the most detailed study available inspires the most confidence in the analysis. The only component of the brain better seen on CT scanning is calcification, which may be invisible on MRI.

MRI Scans. MRI scanning entered clinical practice in 1982 and soon became the test of choice for clinical psychiatrists and neurologists. The technique does not rely on the absorption of x-rays but is based on nuclear magnetic resonance (NMR). The principle of NMR is that the nuclei of all atoms are thought to spin about an axis, which is randomly oriented in space. When atoms are placed in a magnetic field, the axes of all odd-numbered nuclei align with the magnetic field. The axis of a nucleus deviates away from the magnetic field when exposed to a pulse of radiofrequency electromagnetic radiation oriented at 90 or 180 degrees to the magnetic field. When the pulse terminates, the axis of the spinning nucleus realigns itself with the magnetic field, and during this realignment, it emits its own radiofrequency signal. MRI scanners collect the emissions of individuals, realigning nuclei, and use computer analysis to generate a series of two-dimensional images that represent the brain. The images can be in the axial, coronal, or sagittal planes.

By far, the most abundant odd-numbered nucleus in the brain belongs to hydrogen. The rate of realignment of the hydrogen axis is determined by its immediate environment, a combination of both the nature of the molecule of which it is a part and the degree to which it is surrounded by water. Hydrogen nuclei within fat realign rapidly, and hydrogen nuclei within water realign slowly. Hydrogen nuclei in proteins and carbohydrates realign at intermediate rates.

Routine MRI studies use three different radiofrequency pulse sequences. The two varied parameters are the duration of the radiofrequency excitation pulse and the length of the time that data are collected from the realigning nuclei. Because T1 pulses are brief and data collection is brief, hydrogen nuclei in hydrophobic environments are emphasized. Thus, fat is bright on T1, and CSF is dark. The T1 image most closely resembles that of CT scans and is most useful for assessing overall brain structure. T1 is also the only sequence that allows contrast enhancement with the contrast agent gadolinium-diethylenetriamine pentaacetic acid (gadolinium-DTPA). As with the iodinated contrast agents used in CT scanning, gadolinium remains excluded from the brain by the blood–brain barrier, except in areas where this barrier breaks down, such as inflammation or tumor. On T1 images, gadolinium-enhanced structures appear white.

T2 pulses last four times as long as T1 pulses, and the collection times are also extended to emphasize the signal from hydrogen nuclei surrounded by water. Thus, brain tissue is dark, and CSF is white on T2 images. Areas within the brain tissue that have abnormally high water content, such as tumors, inflammation, or strokes, appear brighter on T2 images. T2 images reveal brain pathology most clearly. The third routine pulse sequence is the proton density or balanced sequence. In this sequence, a short radio pulse is followed by a prolonged period of data collection, which equalizes the density of the CSF and the brain and allows the distinction of tissue changes immediately adjacent to the ventricles.

An additional technique, sometimes used in clinical practice for specific indications, is fluid-attenuated inversion recovery (FLAIR). In this method, the T1 image is inverted and added to the T2 image

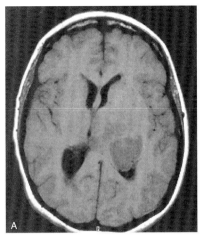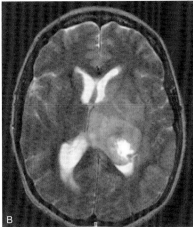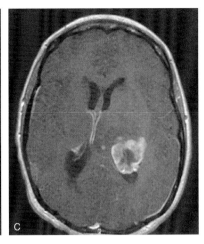

FIGURE 1-12

Three axial images from a 46-year-old woman who was hospitalized for the first time for depression and suicidality following the end of a long-standing relationship. A malignant neoplasm extending into the posterior aspect of the left lateral ventricle is clearly seen in all three images. Images **A** and **B** are T1 and T2 weighted, respectively. Image **C** demonstrates the effects of postcontrast enhancement. (Courtesy of Craig N. Carson, M.D. and Perry F. Renshaw, M.D.)

to double the contrast between gray matter and white matter. Inversion recovery imaging is useful for detecting sclerosis of the hippocampus caused by temporal lobe epilepsy and for localizing areas of abnormal metabolism in degenerative neurologic disorders.

MRI magnets are rated in teslas (T), units of magnetic field strength. MRI scanners in clinical use range from 1.5 to 3.0 T. Higher field–strength scanners produce images of markedly higher resolution. In research settings for humans, magnets as powerful as 7.0 T are used (and a few centers have used magnetic fields greater than 10 T in humans); for animals, magnets greater than 20 T are used. Unlike the well-known hazards of x-irradiation, exposure to electromagnetic fields of the strength used in MRI machines has not been shown to damage biologic tissues.

MRI scans cannot be used for patients with pacemakers or implants of ferromagnetic metals. MRI involves enclosing a patient in a narrow tube, in which the patient must remain motionless for up to 20 minutes. The radiofrequency pulses create a loud banging noise that may be obscured by music played in headphones. A significant number of patients cannot tolerate the claustrophobic conditions of routine MRI scanners and may need an open MRI scanner, which has less power and thus produces images of lower resolution. The resolution of brain tissue of even the lowest power MRI scan, however, exceeds that of CT scanning. Figure 1-12 reveals that a brain tumor is the cause of a patient's depression.

MRI APPLICATIONS TO DEMENTIA. Several MRI changes, including an increased number of subcortical hyperintensities, generalized atrophy, and ventricular enlargement, are associated with normal aging. However, it is well established that some changes seem more specific to the diagnosis of Alzheimer disease and may be clinically useful in formulating the diagnosis and prognosis of the disorder. MRI evidence of MTL atrophy appears to be most closely associated with the disorder. One approach that may help to improve the clinical utility of MRI in the diagnosis and prognosis of Alzheimer disease and other forms of dementia is to follow the rate of change in brain structure over time. Longitudinal follow-up studies have shown the rates of volume loss to be significantly greater in subjects with prodromal Alzheimer disease (up to 5 percent brain volume per year) compared with those experiencing normal age-related reductions (0.1 percent brain volume per year).

MRI APPLICATIONS TO ALCOHOL DEPENDENCE. MRI studies have been the principal tool to describe in vivo the many sources of neurotoxicity associated with alcoholism, including (1) the direct neurotoxic and gliotoxic effect of ethanol, (2) the neurotoxic effects of poor nutrition that often accompany the abuse of alcohol, (3) the excitotoxicity associated with the ethanol withdrawal state, and (4) the possible disruption in adult-neurogenesis-associated ethanol intoxication and withdrawal. These studies documented a striking age dependence of the overall neurotoxicity associated with alcoholism.

Magnetic Resonance Spectroscopy. Whereas routine MRI detects hydrogen nuclei to determine brain structure, MRS can detect several odd-numbered nuclei (Table 1-24). The ability of MRS to detect a wide range of biologically important nuclei allows the use of the technique to study many metabolic processes. Although the resolution and sensitivity of MRS machines are poor compared with those of currently available PET and SPECT devices, the use of stronger magnetic fields will improve this feature to some extent in the future. MRS can image nuclei with an odd number of protons and neutrons. The unpaired protons and neutrons (nucleons) appear naturally and are nonradioactive. As in MRI, the nuclei align themselves in the strong magnetic field produced by an MRS device. A radiofrequency pulse causes the nuclei of interest to absorb and then emit energy. The readout of an MRS device is usually in the form of a spectrum, such as those for phosphorus-31 and hydrogen-1 nuclei, although the spectrum can also be converted into a pictorial image of the brain. The multiple peaks for each nucleus reflect that the same nucleus is exposed to different electron environments (electron clouds) in different molecules. The hydrogen-1 nuclei in a molecule of creatine, therefore, have a different chemical shift (position in the spectrum) than the hydrogen-1 nuclei in a choline molecule, for example. Thus, the position in the spectrum (the chemical shift) indicates the identity of the molecule in which the nuclei are present. The height of the peak for a reference standard of the molecule indicates the amount of the molecule present.

The MRS of the hydrogen-1 nuclei is best at measuring *N*-acetylaspartate (NAA), creatine, and choline-containing molecules, but MRS can also detect glutamate, glutamine, lactate, and

Table 1-24
Nuclei Available for In Vivo Magnetic Resonance Spectroscopy[a]

Nucleus	Natural Abundance	Sensitivity	Relative Potential Clinical Uses
^{1}H	99.99	1.00	Magnetic resonance imaging (MRI) Analysis of metabolism Identification of unusual metabolites Characterization of hypoxia
^{19}F	100.00	0.83	Measurement of pO_2 Analysis of glucose metabolism Measurement of pH Noninvasive pharmacokinetics
^{7}Li	92.58	0.27	Pharmacokinetics
^{23}Na	100.00	0.09	MRI
^{31}P	100.00	0.07	Analysis of bioenergetics Identification of unusual metabolites Characterization of hypoxia Measurement of pH
^{14}N	93.08	0.001	Measurement of glutamate, urea, ammonia
^{39}K	93.08	0.0005	Similar to sodium (^{23}Na) but less specific, hence rarely used
^{13}C	1.11	0.0002	Analysis of metabolite turnover rate Pharmacokinetics of labeled drugs
^{17}O	0.04	0.00001	Measurement of metabolic rate
^{2}H	0.02	0.000002	Measurement of perfusion

[a]Natural abundance is given as percentage abundance of the isotope of interest. Nuclei are tabulated in order of decreasing relative sensitivity; relative sensitivity is calculated by multiplying the relative sensitivity for equal numbers of nuclei (at a given field strength) by the natural abundance of that nucleus. A considerable gain in relative sensitivity can be obtained by isotopic enrichment of the nucleus of choice or by the use of novel pulse sequences.
Reprinted from Dager SR, Steen RG with minor adaptations. Applications of magnetic resonance spectroscopy to the investigation of neuropsychiatric disorders. *Neuropsychopharmacology.* 1992;6:249, with permission.

myoinositol. Although glutamate and γ-aminobutyric acid (GABA), the major amino acid neurotransmitters, can be detected by MRS, the biogenic amine neurotransmitters (e.g., dopamine) are present in concentrations too low to be detected with the technique. MRS of phosphorus-31 can be used to determine the pH of brain regions and the concentrations of phosphorus-containing compounds (e.g., adenosine triphosphate [ATP] and guanosine triphosphate [GTP]), which are important in the energy metabolism of the brain.

MRS has revealed decreased concentrations of NAA in the temporal lobes and increased concentrations of inositol in the occipital lobes of persons with dementia of the Alzheimer type. In a series of subjects with schizophrenia, decreased NAA concentrations were found in the temporal and frontal lobes. MRS has been used to trace the levels of ethanol in various brain regions. In panic disorder, MRS has been used to record the levels of lactate, whose intravenous infusion can precipitate panic episodes in about three-fourths of patients with either panic disorder or major depression. Brain lactate concentrations were found to be elevated during panic attacks, even without provocative infusion.

Additional indications include the use of MRS to measure concentrations of psychotherapeutic drugs in the brain. One study used MRS to measure lithium (Eskalith) concentrations in the brains of patients with bipolar disorder and found that lithium concentrations in the brain were half those in the plasma during depressed and euthymic periods but exceeded those in the plasma during manic episodes. Some compounds, such as fluoxetine and trifluoperazine (Stelazine), contain fluorine-19, which can also be detected in the brain and measured by MRS. For example, MRS has demonstrated that it takes 6 months of steady use for fluoxetine to reach maximal

concentrations in the brain, which equilibrate at about 20 times the serum concentrations.

MRS IN DEMENTIA. MRS presents the opportunity to noninvasively obtain measures of several neurochemicals related to neurotransmission, energy metabolism, and cellular function. Studies using MRS have shown a trend for a general reduction in NAA measures with increasing age in MTL and frontal cortical brain regions. The studies in MCI and Alzheimer disease report patients with these disorders have decreased levels of NAA and increased levels of myoinositol (a form of inositol normally found in the brain that contributes to osmotic regulation) compared with those of age-matched comparison subjects.

MRS IN SCHIZOPHRENIA. MRS has been applied widely in studies of cortical chemistry in schizophrenia. These studies documented reductions in NAA levels in many cortical and limbic brain regions in schizophrenic individuals and smaller reductions in family members of people diagnosed with schizophrenia. Other metabolites have been measured in MRS studies of schizophrenic patients. The most interesting finding may be the description of normal or low levels of glutamate and increased levels of glutamine in medication-free patients with schizophrenia. One preliminary study suggested that glutamine elevations were not present in medication-free patients who were receiving benzodiazepines, drugs that would be predicted to suppress excitatory neurotransmission.

MRS IN ALCOHOL DEPENDENCE. MRS studies evaluating NAA and choline have provided neurochemical evidence that complements the MRI findings related to the emergence and recovery from alcohol-related neurotoxicity. MRS studies of GABA have provided insights into alterations in cortical inhibitory neurotransmissions associated with the recovery from alcohol dependence. During acute withdrawal, cortical GABA levels appear to be normal. With recovery from alcohol dependence, cortical GABA levels appear to decline and may be significantly below the level seen in healthy subjects with extended sobriety.

Functional MRI.   Recent advances in data collection and computer data processing have reduced the acquisition time for an MRI image to less than 1 second. A new sequence of particular interest to psychiatrists is the T2 or blood oxygen level-dependent (BOLD) sequence, which detects levels of oxygenated hemoglobin in the blood. Neuronal activity within the brain causes a local increase in blood flow, which in turn increases the local hemoglobin concentration. Although neuronal metabolism extracts more oxygen in active areas of the brain, the net effect of neuronal activity is to increase the local amount of oxygenated hemoglobin. This change can be detected nearly in real-time with the T2 sequence, which thus detects the functionally active brain regions. This process is the basis for the technique of fMRI.

What fMRI detects is not brain activity per se, but blood flow. The volume of the brain in which blood flow increases exceeds the volume of activated neurons by about 1 to 2 cm and limits the resolution of the technique. Sensitivity and resolution can be improved with the use of nontoxic, ultrasmall iron oxide particles. Thus, two tasks that activate clusters of neurons 5 mm apart, such as recognizing two different faces, yield overlapping signals on fMRI and so are usually indistinguishable by this technique. fMRI is useful to localize neuronal activity to a particular lobe or subcortical nucleus and has even been able to localize activity to a single gyrus. The method detects tissue perfusion, not neuronal metabolism. In contrast, PET scanning may give information specifically about neuronal metabolism.

No radioactive isotopes are administered in fMRI, a great advantage over PET and SPECT. A subject can perform a variety of tasks, both experimental and control, in the same imaging session. First, a routine T1 MRI image is obtained; then, the T2 images are superimposed to allow more precise localization. Acquisition of sufficient images for study can require 20 minutes to 3 hours, during which time the subject's head must remain in exactly the same position. Several methods, including a frame around the head and a special mouthpiece, have been used. Although realignments of images can correct for some head movement, small changes in head position may lead to erroneous interpretations of brain activation.

fMRI has recently revealed unexpected details about the organization of language within the brain. Using a series of language tasks requiring semantic, phonemic, and rhyming discrimination, one study found that rhyming (but not other types of language processing) produced a different pattern of activation in men and women. Rhyming activated the inferior frontal gyrus bilaterally in women, but only on the left in men. In another study, fMRI revealed a previously suspected, but unproved, neural circuit for lexical categories, interpolated between the representations for concepts and those for phonemes. This novel circuit was located in the left anterior temporal lobe. Data from patients with dyslexia (reading disorder) doing simple rhyming tasks demonstrated a failure to activate Wernicke area and the insula, which were active in normal subjects doing the same task.

Sensory functions have also been mapped in detail with fMRI. The activation of the visual and auditory cortices has been visualized in real-time. In a recent intriguing study, the areas that were activated while a subject with schizophrenia listened to speech were also activated during auditory hallucinations. These areas included the primary auditory cortex as well as higher-order auditory processing regions. fMRI is the imaging technique most widely used to study brain abnormality related to cognitive dysfunction.

fMRI OF DEMENTIA.   fMRI methods provide information that can potentially be used in the study, diagnosis, and prognosis of Alzheimer disease and other forms of dementia as well as proving insights into normal age-related changes in cognitive processing. Evidence that aging is associated with weaker and more diffused activations as well as decreased hemispheric lateralization, suggests either compensation for lost regional intensity or dedifferentiation of processing. The weaker activation, especially prefrontal, suggests potential encoding-stage dysfunctions associated with aging. fMRI studies have consistently demonstrated that patients with Alzheimer disease have decreased fMRI activation in the hippocampus and related structures within the MTL during the encoding of new memories compared with cognitively intact older subjects. More recently, fMRI studies of subjects at risk for Alzheimer disease, by their genetics or evidence of minimal cognitive impairment, have yielded variable results with some studies suggesting there may be a phase of paradoxically increased activation early in the course of prodromal Alzheimer disease.

fMRI OF ALCOHOL DEPENDENCE.   fMRI studies have provided insights into the functional consequences of alcoholism-related neurotoxicity. Studies suggest that recovering alcohol-dependent patients show abnormal activation patterns in the frontal cortex, thalamus, striatum, cerebellum, and hippocampus related to impairments in attention, learning and memory, motor coordination, and inhibitory control of behavior. Studies have begun to explore pharmacologic modulation of resting circuit activity to probe mechanisms underlying circuit dysfunction in alcoholism, illustrated by blunted responses to benzodiazepines.

SPECT Scanning.   Manufactured radioactive compounds are used in SPECT to study regional differences in cerebral blood flow within the brain. This high-resolution imaging technique records the pattern of photon emission from the bloodstream according to the level of perfusion in different regions of the brain. As with fMRI, it provides information on the cerebral blood flow, which is highly correlated with the rate of glucose metabolism, but does not measure neuronal metabolism directly.

SPECT uses compounds labeled with single photon-emitting isotopes: iodine-123, technetium-99m, and xenon-133. Xenon-133 is a noble gas that is inhaled directly. The xenon quickly enters the blood and is distributed to areas of the brain as a function of regional blood flow. Xenon-SPECT is thus referred to as the *regional cerebral blood flow* (rCBF) *technique*. For technical reasons, xenon-SPECT can measure blood flow only on the surface of the brain, which is an important limitation. Many mental tasks require communication between the cortex and subcortical structures, and this activity is poorly measured by xenon-SPECT.

Assessment of blood flow over the whole brain with SPECT requires the injectable tracers, technetium-99m-D,L-hexamethyl-propyleneamine oxime (HMPAO [Ceretec]) or iodoamphetamine (Spectamine). These isotopes are attached to molecules that are highly lipophilic and rapidly cross the blood–brain barrier and enter cells. Once inside the cell, the ligands are enzymatically converted to charged ions, which remain trapped in the cell. Thus, over time, the tracers are concentrated in areas of relatively higher blood flow. Although blood flow is usually assumed to be the major variable tested in HMPAO SPECT, local variations in the permeability of the blood–brain barrier and in the enzymatic conversion of the ligands within cells also contribute to regional differences in signal levels.

Also, to these compounds used for measuring blood flow, iodine-123–labeled ligands for the muscarinic, dopaminergic, and serotonergic receptors, for example, can be used to study these receptors by SPECT technology. Once photon-emitting compounds reach the brain, detectors surrounding the patient's head pick up their light emissions. This information is relayed to a computer, which constructs a two-dimensional image of the isotope's distribution within a slice of the brain. A critical difference between SPECT and PET is that in SPECT a single particle is emitted, whereas in PET two particles are emitted; the latter reaction gives a more precise location for the event and better resolution of the image. Increasingly, for both SPECT and PET studies, investigators are performing prestudy MRI or CT studies, then superimposing the SPECT or PET image on the MRI or CT image to obtain a more accurate anatomical location for the functional information. SPECT is useful in diagnosing decreased or blocked cerebral blood flow in stroke victims. Some have described abnormal flow patterns in the early stages of Alzheimer disease that may aid in early diagnosis.

PET Scanning. The isotopes used in PET decay by emitting positrons, antimatter particles that bind with and annihilate electrons, thereby giving off photons that travel in 180-degree opposite directions. Because detectors have twice as much signal from which to generate an image as SPECT scanners have, the resolution of the PET image is higher than with SPECT. A wide range of compounds can be used in PET studies, and the resolution of PET continues to be refined closer to its theoretical minimum of 3 mm, which is the distance positrons move before colliding with an electron. Relatively few PET scanners are available because they require an onsite cyclotron to make the isotopes.

The most commonly used isotopes in PET are fluorine-18 (^{18}F), nitrogen-13, and oxygen-15. These isotopes are usually linked to another molecule, except in the case of oxygen-15 (^{15}O). The most commonly reported ligand has been [^{18}F]fluorodeoxyglucose (FDG), an analog of glucose that the brain cannot metabolize. Thus, the brain regions with the highest metabolic rate and the highest blood flow take up the most FDG but cannot metabolize and excrete the usual metabolic products. The concentration of ^{18}F builds up in these neurons and is detected by the PET camera. Water-15 ($H_2^{15}O$) and nitrogen-13 are used to measure blood flow, and ^{15}O can be used to determine the metabolic rate. Glucose is by far the predominant energy source available to brain cells, and its use is thus a highly sensitive indicator of the rate of brain metabolism. ^{18}F-labeled 3,4-dihydroxyphenylalanine (DOPA), the fluorinated precursor to dopamine, has been used to localize dopaminergic neurons.

PET has been used increasingly to study normal brain development and function as well as to study neuropsychiatric disorders. Concerning brain development, PET studies have found that glucose use is greatest in the sensorimotor cortex, thalamus, brainstem, and cerebellar vermis when an infant is 5 weeks of age or younger. By 3 months of age, most areas of the cortex show increased use, except for the frontal and association cortices, which do not begin to exhibit an increase until the infant is 8 months of age. An adult pattern of glucose metabolism is achieved by the age of 1 year, but use in the cortex continues to rise above adult levels until the child is about 9 years of age when use in the cortex begins to decrease and reaches its final adult level in the late teen years.

In another study, subjects listened to a rapidly presented list of thematically related words. When asked to recall words in the thematic category that may or may not have been on the list, some subjects falsely recalled that they had heard words that were not on the list. By PET scanning, the hippocampus was active during both true and false recollections, whereas the auditory cortex was only active during recollection of words that were heard. When pressed to determine whether memories were true or false, subjects activated the frontal lobes. FDG studies have also investigated pathology in neurologic disorders and psychiatric disorders. Two other types of studies used precursor molecules and receptor ligands. The dopamine precursor dopa has been used to visualize pathology in patients with Parkinson disease, and radiolabeled ligands for receptors have been useful in determining the occupancy of receptors by specific psychotherapeutic drugs. Neurochemical findings from PET radiotracer scan are listed in Table 1-25.

For example, dopamine receptor antagonists such as haloperidol block almost 100 percent of D_2 receptors. The atypical antipsychotic drugs block serotonin 5-HT_2 receptors also to D_2 receptors; hence, they are referred to as *serotonin-dopamine receptor antagonists*. The case study presented illustrates the potential diagnostic value of three-dimensional PET imaging.

> Patient A is a 70-year-old man who had gotten more forgetful, to the point that his family was worried about him. The patient's family was interested in getting a diagnostic workup to evaluate the possible causes of his memory disorder. His PET scan showed that he had functional parietotemporal decrease, which corroborated other neurologic evaluations, suggesting that he had Alzheimer disease. The patient was treated with tacrine (Cognex) and benefited from some stabilization of his symptoms. (Courtesy of Joseph C. Wu, M.D., Daniel G. Amen, M.D., and H. Stefan Bracha, M.D.)

Pharmacologic and Neuropsychological Probes. With both PET and SPECT and eventually, with MRS, more studies and possibly more diagnostic procedures will use pharmacologic and neuropsychological probes. The purpose of such probes is to stimulate particular regions of brain activity, so that, when compared with a baseline, workers can reach conclusions about the functional correspondence to particular brain regions. One example of the approach is the use of PET to detect regions of the brain involved in the processing of shape, color, and velocity in the visual system. Another example is the use of cognitive activation tasks (e.g., the Wisconsin Card Sorting Test) to study frontal blood flow in patients with schizophrenia. A key consideration in the evaluation of reports that measure blood flow is the establishment of actual baseline value in the study design. Typically, the reports use an awake, resting state, but there is variability in whether the patients have their eyes closed or their ears blocked; both conditions can affect brain function. There is also variability in such baseline brain function factors as sex, age, anxiety about the test, nonpsychiatric drug treatment, vasoactive medications, and time of day.

▲ 1.2 Children and Adolescents

A comprehensive evaluation of a child is composed of interviews with the parents, the child, and other family members, gathering information regarding the child's current school functioning; and often, a standardized assessment of the child's intellectual level and academic achievement. In some cases, standardized measures of developmental level and neuropsychological assessments

Table 1-25
Neurochemical Findings from Positron Emission Tomography Radiotracer Scans

Dopamine	Decreased uptake of dopamine in striatum in parkinsonian patients
	Dopamine release higher in patients with schizophrenia than in controls
	High dopamine release associated with positive symptoms in schizophrenia
Receptors	
• D_1 receptor	Lower D_1 receptor binding in prefrontal cortex of patients with schizophrenia compared with controls; correlates with negative symptoms
• D_2 receptor	Schizophrenia associated with small elevations of binding at D_2 receptor
• Serotonin type 1A (5-HT_{1A})	Reduction in receptor binding in patients with unipolar major depression
Transporters	
• Dopamine	Amphetamine and cocaine cause an increase in dopamine
	Tourette disorder shows increase in dopamine transporter system (may account for success of dopamine blocking therapies)
• Serotonin	Serotonin binding is low in depression, alcoholism, cocainism, binge eating, and impulse control
Metabolism	
• Nicotine	Cigarette smoking inhibits monamine oxidase activity in brain
• Amyloid-β Deposits	Can be visualized in vivo with positron emission tomography
Pharmacology	Plasma levels of cocaine peak at 2 min
	D_2 receptor occupancy lasts for several weeks after discontinuation of antipsychotic medication
	D_2 receptor occupancy is lower for atypical antipsychotics than typical antipsychotics (may account for decrease in extrapyramidal side effects)
	Low doses (10–20 mg) of selective serotonin reuptake inhibitors cause occupancy of up to 90% of serotonin receptors

are useful. The child rarely initiates psychiatric evaluations, so we must obtain information from the family and the school to understand the reasons for the evaluation. In some cases, the court or a child protective service agency may initiate a psychiatric evaluation. Children can be excellent informants about symptoms related to mood and inner experiences, such as psychotic phenomena, sadness, fears, and anxiety. However, they often have difficulty with the chronology of symptoms and are sometimes reticent about reporting behaviors that have gotten them into trouble. Very young children often cannot articulate their experiences verbally and do better, showing their feelings and preoccupations in a play situation. Assessment of a child or adolescent includes identifying the reasons for referral; assessing the nature and extent of the child's psychological and behavioral difficulties; and determining family, school, social, and developmental factors that may be influencing the child's emotional well-being.

The first step in the comprehensive evaluation of a child or adolescent is to obtain a full description of the current concerns and a history of the child's previous psychiatric and medical problems. This evaluation is often done with the parents for school-age children, whereas we may choose to see adolescents first, to get their perception of the situation. A direct interview and observation of the child are usually next, followed by psychological testing when indicated.

Clinical interviews offer the most flexibility in understanding the evolution of problems and in establishing the role of environmental factors and life events, but they may not systematically cover all psychiatric diagnostic categories. To increase the breadth of information generated, we may use semistructured interviews such as the *Kiddie Schedule for Affective Disorders and Schizophrenia for School-Age Children* (K-SADS); structured interviews such as the *National Institute for Mental Health Diagnostic Interview Schedule for Children Version IV* (NIMH DISC-IV); and rating scales, such as the *Child Behavior Checklist* and *Connors Parent or Teacher Rating Scale for ADHD.*

It is not uncommon for interviews from different sources, such as parents, teachers, and school counselors, to reflect different or even contradictory information about a given child. When faced with conflicting information, we must determine whether apparent contradictions reflect an accurate picture of the child in different settings. Once obtaining a complete history from the parents, we should examine the child and assess the child's current functioning at home and school. Once we complete the evaluation and psychological testing, we can use all the available information to make a best-estimate diagnosis and can then make recommendations.

Once we obtain clinical information about a given child or adolescent, it is our task to determine whether that child meets the criteria for one or more psychiatric disorders according to the Fifth Edition of the *Diagnostic and Statistical Manual of Mental Disorders* (DSM-5). Whereas clinical situations requiring intervention do not always fall within the context of a given psychiatric disorder, the importance of identifying psychiatric disorders when they arise is to facilitate meaningful investigation of childhood psychopathology.

CLINICAL INTERVIEWS

To conduct a useful child interview, we must be familiar with typical development to place the child's responses in the proper perspective. For example, a young child's discomfort on separation from a parent and a school-age child's lack of clarity about the purpose of the interview is perfectly normal. Furthermore, behavior that is normal in a child at one age, such as temper tantrums in a 2-year-old, takes on a different meaning, for example, in a teenager. Chapter 32 presents a detailed discussion of healthy childhood development.

The interviewer's first task is to engage the child and develop a rapport so that the child is comfortable. The interviewer should inquire about the child's concept of the purpose of the interview and should ask what the parents have told the child. If the child appears to be confused about the reason for the interview, the examiner may opt to summarize the parents' concerns in a developmentally appropriate and supportive manner. During the interview with the child, we seek to learn about the child's relationships with family members and peers, academic achievement, and peer relationships in school, and the child's pleasurable activities. An estimate of the child's cognitive functioning is a part of the mental status examination.

The extent of confidentiality in child assessment correlates with the age of the child. In most cases, almost all specific information can appropriately be shared with the parents of a very young child, whereas the privacy and permission of an older child or adolescent are necessary before we can share any information with parents. We should inform school-age and older children that if we become concerned that any child is dangerous to himself or herself or others, we must share this information with parents and, at times, additional adults. As part of our assessment, we must determine whether that child is safe in his or her environment and must develop an index of suspicion about whether the child is a victim of abuse or neglect. Whenever there is a suspicion of child maltreatment, we are required to inform the local child protective service agency.

Toward the end of the interview, the child may be asked in an open-ended manner whether he or she would like to bring up anything else. We should complement each child for his or her cooperation and thank them for participating in the interview, and the interview should end on a positive note.

Infants and Young Children

Assessments of infants usually begin with the parents present, because very young children may be frightened by the interview situation; the interview with the parents present also allows us to assess the parent–infant interaction. Infants may be referred for a variety of reasons, including high levels of irritability, difficulty being consoled, eating disturbances, poor weight gain, sleep disturbances, withdrawn behavior, lack of engagement in play, and developmental delay. We should assess areas of functioning that include motor development, activity level, verbal communication, ability to engage in play, problem-solving skills, adaptation to daily routines, relationships, and social responsiveness.

We should use our observations during the interview and well as standardized developmental measures to determine a child's developmental level of functioning. Observations of play reveal a child's developmental level and reflect the child's emotional state and preoccupations. The examiner can interact with an infant age 18 months or younger in a playful manner by using such games as peek-a-boo. We may observe children between the ages of 18 months and 3 years in a playroom. Children ages 2 years or older may exhibit symbolic play with toys, revealing more in this mode than through conversation. The use of puppets and dolls with children younger than 6 years of age is often an effective way to elicit information, particularly if questions are directed to the dolls, rather than to the child.

School-Age Children

Some school-age children are at ease when conversing with an adult; others may show fear, anxiety, poor verbal skills, or oppositional behavior. School-age children can usually tolerate a 45-minute session. The room should be sufficiently spacious for the child to move around, but not so large as to reduce intimate contact between the examiner and the child. We may reserve part of the interview for unstructured play, and various toys can be made available to capture the child's interest and to elicit themes and feelings. Children in lower grades may be more interested in the toys in the room, whereas by the sixth grade, children may be more comfortable with the interview process and less likely to show spontaneous play.

The first part of the interview explores the child's understanding of the reasons for the meeting. We should reassure the child that they are not here because they are "in trouble." Techniques that can facilitate disclosure of feelings include asking the child to draw peers, family members, a house, or anything else that comes to mind. We can then question the child about the drawings. We may ask children to reveal three wishes, to describe the best and worst events of their lives, and to name a favorite person to be stranded with on a desert island. Games such as Donald W. Winnicott's "squiggle," in which the examiner draws a curved line and then the child and the examiner take turns continuing the drawing, may facilitate conversation.

Questions that are partially open-ended with some multiple choices may elicit the best answers from school-age children. Simple, closed (yes or no) questions may not elicit sufficient information, and entirely open-ended questions can overwhelm a school-age child who cannot construct a chronologic narrative. These techniques often result in a shoulder shrug from the child. The use of indirect commentaries—such as, "I once knew a child who felt very sad when he moved away from all his friends"—is helpful, although we must be careful not to lead the child into confirming what the child thinks we want to hear. School-age children respond well to clinicians who help them compare moods or feelings by asking them to rate feelings on a scale of 1 to 10.

Adolescents

Adolescents usually have distinct ideas about why the evaluation was initiated, and can usually give a chronologic account of the recent events leading to the evaluation, although some may disagree with the need for the evaluation. We should communicate the value of hearing the story from an adolescent's point of view and must be careful to reserve judgment and not assign blame. Adolescents may be concerned about confidentiality, and clinicians can assure them that permission will be requested from them before we share any specific information with parents, except in situations involving danger to the adolescent or others, in which case we must sacrifice confidentiality. We can approach adolescents in an open-ended manner; however, when silences occur during the interview, we should attempt to reengage the patient. We can explore what the adolescent believes the outcome of the evaluation will be (change of school, hospitalization, removal from the home, removal of privileges).

Some adolescents approach the interview with apprehension or hostility but open up when it becomes evident that we are neither punitive nor judgmental. We must be aware of our responses to adolescents' behavior (countertransference) and stay focused on the therapeutic process even in the face of defiant, angry, or difficult teenagers. We should set appropriate limits and should postpone or discontinue an interview if they feel threatened or if they become destructive or self-injurious. Every interview should include an exploration of suicidal thoughts, assaultive behavior, psychotic symptoms, substance use, and knowledge of safe sexual practices along with a sexual history. Once we establish rapport, many adolescents appreciate the opportunity to tell their side of the story and may reveal things that they have not disclosed to anyone else.

Family Interview

An interview with parents and the patient may take place first or may occur later in the evaluation. Sometimes, an interview with the entire family, including siblings, can be enlightening. During it, we can observe the interactions between the parents and children. Our job is to maintain a nonthreatening atmosphere in which each member of the family can speak freely without feeling that we are taking sides with any particular member. Although child psychiatrists generally function as advocates for the child, we must validate each family member's feelings in this setting, because lack of communication often contributes to the patient's problems.

Parents

The interview with the patient's parents or caretakers is necessary to get a chronologic picture of the child's growth and development. We should obtain a thorough developmental history and details of any stressors or significant events that have influenced the child's development. We should also elicit the parents' view of the family dynamics, their marital history, and their emotional adjustment. The family's psychiatric history and the upbringing of the parents are pertinent. Parents are usually the best informants about the child's early development and previous psychiatric and medical illnesses. They may be better able to provide an accurate chronology of past evaluations and treatment. In some cases, especially with older children and adolescents, the parents may be unaware of significant current symptoms or social difficulties of the child. Clinicians elicit the parents' formulation of the causes and nature of their child's problems and ask about their expectations for the current assessment.

DIAGNOSTIC INSTRUMENTS

The two main types of diagnostic instruments used by clinicians are diagnostic interviews and questionnaires. We administer diagnostic interviews to either children or their parents, which should elicit sufficient information on various aspects of functioning in order to determine whether the child meets DSM-5 criteria.

Semistructured interviews, or "interviewer-based" interviews, such as K-SADS and the *Child and Adolescent Psychiatric Assessment* (CAPA), serve as guides. They help us clarify answers to questions about symptoms. Structured interviews, or "respondent-based" interviews, such as NIMH DISC-IV, the *Children's Interview for Psychiatric Syndromes* (ChIPS), and the *Diagnostic Interview for Children and Adolescents* (DICA), provide a script for the interviewer without interpretation of the patient responses during the interview process. Two other diagnostic instruments, the *Dominic-R* and the *Pictorial Instrument for Children and Adolescents* (PICA-III-R), use pictures as cues along with an accompanying question to elicit information about symptoms, which can be especially useful for young children as well as for adolescents.

Diagnostic instruments systematically aid the collection of information. Diagnostic instruments, even the most comprehensive, however, cannot replace clinical interviews because clinical interviews are superior in understanding the chronology of symptoms, the interplay between environmental stressors and emotional responses, and developmental issues. Clinicians often find it helpful to combine data from diagnostic instruments with clinical material gathered in a comprehensive evaluation.

Questionnaires can cover a broad range of symptom areas, such as the *Achenbach Child Behavior Checklist,* or they can focus on a particular type of symptomatology, such as the *Connors Parent Rating Scale for ADHD.*

Semistructured Diagnostic Interviews

Kiddie Schedule for Affective Disorders and Schizophrenia for School-Age Children (K-SADS). The K-SADS is intended for children and adolescents from 6 to 18 years of age. It contains multiple items with some space for further clarification of symptoms. It elicits information on current diagnosis and symptoms present in the previous year. Another version can also ascertain lifetime diagnoses. This instrument has been used extensively, especially in the evaluation of mood disorders, and includes measures of impairment caused by symptoms. There is also a form for parents as well as the child. The schedule takes about 1 to 1.5 hours to administer. The interviewer should have some training in the field of child psychiatry, but need not be a psychiatrist.

Child and Adolescent Psychiatric Assessment (CAPA). The CAPA is an "interviewer-based" instrument that can be used for children from 9 to 17 years of age. It comes in modular form so that we can focus on particular diagnostic entities without having to give the entire interview. It covers disruptive behavior disorders, mood disorders, anxiety disorders, eating disorders, sleep disorders, elimination disorders, substance use disorders, tic disorders, schizophrenia, PTSD, and somatization symptoms. It focuses on the 3 months before the interview, called the "primary period." In general, it takes about 1 hour to administer. It has a glossary to help clarify symptoms, and it provides separate ratings for the presence and severity of symptoms. The CAPA can be used to obtain information that applies to DSM-5 diagnoses. Training is necessary to administer this interview, and the interviewer must be prepared to use some clinical judgment in interpreting elicited symptoms.

Structured Diagnostic Interviews

National Institute of Mental Health Interview Schedule for Children Version IV (NIMH DISC-IV). The NIMH DISC-IV is a highly structured interview designed to assess more than 30 DSM-IV diagnostic entities administered by trained "laypersons." Although developed for DSM-IV, it can still be helpful diagnoses in DSM-5. It is available in parallel child and parent forms. The parent form can be used for children from 6 to 17 years of age, and the direct child form of the instrument was designed for children from 9 to 17 years of age. A computer scoring algorithm is available. This instrument assesses for diagnoses present within the last 4 weeks, and also within the last year. Because it is a fully structured interview, the instructions serve as a complete guide for the questions, and the examiner need not have any knowledge of child psychiatry to administer the interview correctly.

Children's Interview for Psychiatric Syndromes (ChIPS). The ChIPS is a highly structured interview designed for use by trained interviewers with children from 6 to 18 years of age. It is composed of 15 sections, and it elicits information on psychiatric symptoms as well as psychosocial stressors targeting 20 psychiatric disorders, according to DSM-IV criteria; however, it also applies to diagnoses in DSM-5. There are parent and child forms. It takes approximately 40 minutes to administer the ChIPS. Diagnoses covered include depression, mania, ADHD, separation disorder, OCD, conduct disorder, substance use disorder, anorexia, and bulimia.

The ChIPS is a screening instrument for clinicians and a diagnostic instrument for clinical and epidemiologic research.

Diagnostic Interview for Children and Adolescents (DICA).

The current version of the DICA was developed in 1997 to assess information resulting in diagnoses according to either DSM-IV or DSM-III-R. This instrument is relevant to DSM-5 as well. Although designed as a highly structured interview, it can be used in a semistructured format. This means that, although interviewers are allowed to use additional questions and probes to clarify elicited information, the method of probing is standardized so that all interviewers will follow a specific pattern. When using the interview with younger children, more flexibility is built-in, allowing interviewers to deviate from written questions to ensure that the child understands the question. Parent and child interviews are expected to be used. The DICA is designed for use with children 6 to 17 years of age and generally takes 1 to 2 hours to administer. It covers externalizing behavior disorders, anxiety disorders, depressive disorders, and substance abuse disorders, among others.

Pictorial Diagnostic Instruments

Dominic-R.

The Dominic-R is a pictorial, fully structured interview designed to elicit psychiatric symptoms from children 6 to 11 years of age. The pictures illustrate abstract emotional and behavioral content of diagnostic entities according to the DSM-III-R; however, information gleaned from this instrument also applies in conjunction with clinical information to the DSM-5. The instrument uses a picture of a child called "Dominic," who is experiencing the symptom in question. Some symptoms have more than one picture, with a brief story. Each picture includes a question about the situation depicted and whether the child has experienced something similar. Diagnostic entities covered by the Dominic-R include separation anxiety, generalized anxiety, depression and dysthymia, ADHD, oppositional defiant disorder, conduct disorder, and specific phobia. The symptom list is comprehensive; however, the interview does not explicitly ask about the frequency, duration, or age of onset of the symptom. The paper version of this interview takes about 20 minutes, and the computerized version of this instrument takes about 15 minutes. Trained lay-interviewers can administer this interview. Computerized versions of this interview are available with pictures of a child who is white, black, Latino, or Asian.

Pictorial Instrument for Children and Adolescents (PICA-III-R).

PICA-III-R is composed of 137 pictures organized in modules and designed to cover five diagnostic categories, including disorders of anxiety, mood, psychosis, disruptive disorders, and substance use disorder. It is designed to be administered by clinicians and can be used for children and adolescents ranging from 6 to 16 years of age. The PICA-III_R provides a categorical (diagnosis present or absent) and a dimensional (range of severity) assessment. This instrument presents pictures of a child experiencing emotional, behavioral, and cognitive symptoms. The clinician asks the child, "How much are you like him/her?" and a five-point rating scale with pictures of a person with open arms in increasing degrees is shown to the child to help the child identify the severity of the symptoms. It takes about 40 minutes to 1 hour to administer the interview. This instrument was designed for DSM-III-R but is useful for DSM-5 diagnoses. This assessment can be used to aid in clinical interviews and research diagnostic protocols.

QUESTIONNAIRES AND RATING SCALES

Achenbach Child Behavior Checklist

The parent and teacher versions of the *Achenbach Child Behavior Checklist* cover a broad range of symptoms and several positive attributes related to academic and social competence. The checklist presents items related to mood, frustration tolerance, hyperactivity, oppositional behavior, anxiety, and various other behaviors. The parent version consists of 118 items to be rated 0 (not true), 1 (sometimes true), or 2 (very true). The teacher version is similar, but without the items that apply only to home life. Profiles were developed based on normal children of three different age groups (4 to 5, 6 to 11, and 12 to 16).

Such a checklist identifies specific problem areas that we might otherwise overlook, and it may point out areas in which the child's behavior deviates from that of normal children of the same age group. The checklist does not make diagnoses.

Revised Achenbach Behavior Problem Checklist

Consisting of 150 items that cover a variety of childhood behavioral and emotional symptoms, the *Revised Achenbach Behavior Problem Checklist* discriminates between clinic-referred and nonreferred children. Separate subscales correlate in the appropriate direction with other measures of intelligence, academic achievement, clinical observations, and peer popularity. As with the other broad rating scales, this instrument can help elicit a comprehensive view of a multitude of behavioral areas, but it does not make psychiatric diagnoses.

Connors Abbreviated Parent–Teacher Rating Scale for ADHD

In its original form, the *Connors Abbreviated Parent–Teacher Rating Scale for ADHD* consisted of 93 items rated on a 0 to 3 scale, subgrouped into 25 clusters, including problems with restlessness, temper, school, stealing, eating, and sleeping. Over the years, multiple versions of this scale were developed and used to aid in the systematic identification of children with ADHD. A highly abbreviated form of this rating scale, the *Connors Abbreviated Parent–Teacher Questionnaire,* was developed in 1973. It consists of 10 items that assess both hyperactivity and inattention.

Brief Impairment Scale

A newly validated 23-item instrument suitable to obtain information on children ranging from 4 to 17 years, the *Brief Impairment Scale* (BIS) evaluates three domains of functioning: interpersonal relations, school/work functioning, and care/self-fulfillment. This scale is administered to an adult informant about his or her child, does not take long to administer, and provides a global measure of impairment along the above three dimensions. This scale does not make clinical decisions on individual patients, but it can provide information on the degree of impairment that a given child is experiencing in a particular area.

COMPONENTS OF THE CHILD PSYCHIATRIC EVALUATION

Psychiatric evaluation of a child includes a description of the reason for the referral, the child's past and present functioning, and any test results. Table 1-26 gives an outline of the evaluation.

Table 1-26
Child Psychiatric Evaluation

Identifying data
Identified patient and family members
Source of referral
Informants
History
Chief complaint
History of present illness
Developmental history and milestones
Psychiatric history
Medical history, including immunizations
Family social history and parents' marital status
Educational history and current school functioning
Peer relationship history
Current family functioning
Family psychiatric and medical histories
Current physical examination
Mental status examination
Neuropsychiatric examination (when applicable)
Developmental, psychological, and educational testing
Formulation and summary
DSM-5 diagnosis
Recommendations and treatment plan

Identifying Data

Identifying data for a child includes the child's gender, age, as well as the family constellation surrounding the child.

History

A comprehensive history contains information about the child's current and past functioning from the child's report, from clinical and structured interviews with the parents, and information from teachers and previous treating clinicians. We usually obtain the chief complaint and the history of the present illness from both the child and the parents. Naturally, the child will articulate the situation according to his or her developmental level. The parents are usually the best source for determining the child's developmental history. Past clinicians can help augment the psychiatric and medical histories. The child's report is critical for understanding the current situation regarding peer relationships and adjustment to school. Adolescents are the best informants regarding knowledge of safe sexual practices, drug or alcohol use, and suicidal ideation. The parents are usually the best source to understand the family's psychiatric and social histories and family functioning.

Mental Status Examination

We should obtain a detailed description of the child's current mental functioning through observation and specific questioning. Table 1-27 presents an outline of the mental status examination, and Table 1-28 lists components of a comprehensive neuropsychiatry mental status.

Physical Appearance. The examiner should document the child's size, grooming, nutritional state, bruising, head circumference, physical signs of anxiety, facial expressions, and mannerisms.

Table 1-27
Mental Status Examination for Children

1. Physical appearance
2. Parent–child interaction
3. Separation and reunion
4. Orientation to time, place, and person
5. Speech and language
6. Mood
7. Affect
8. Thought process and content
9. Social relatedness
10. Motor behavior
11. Cognition
12. Memory
13. Judgment and insight

Parent–Child Interaction. Before the interview, the examiner can observe the interactions between parents and the child in the waiting area. How the parents and child interact, both verbally and emotionally, are pertinent.

Separation and Reunion. The examiner should note how the child responds to separation from a parent, and how they react to the reunion. Either lack of affect at separation and reunion or severe distress on separation or reunion can indicate problems in the parent–child relationship or other psychiatric disturbances.

Orientation to Time, Place, and Person. Impairments in orientation can reflect neurologic damage, low intelligence, or a thought disorder. The age of the child must be kept in mind, however, because very young children may not know the date, other chronologic information, or the name of the interview site.

Speech and Language. The examiner should evaluate the child's speech and language acquisition. Is it appropriate for the child's age? A disparity between expressive language usage and receptive language is notable. The examiner should also note the child's rate of speech, rhythm, latency to answer, the spontaneity of speech, intonation, articulation of words, and prosody. Echolalia, repetitive stereotypical phrases and unusual syntax are significant psychiatric findings. Children who do not use words by age 18 months or who do not use phrases by ages 2.5 to 3 years, but who have a history of typical babbling and responding appropriately to nonverbal cues, are probably developing typically. The examiner should consider the possibility that a hearing loss is contributing to a speech and language deficit.

Mood. A child's sad expression, lack of appropriate smiling, tearfulness, anxiety, euphoria, and anger are valid indicators of mood, as are verbal admissions of feelings. Persistent themes in play and fantasy also reflect the child's mood.

Affect. The examiner should note the child's range of emotional expressivity, appropriateness of affect to thought content, ability to move smoothly from one affect to another, and sudden labile emotional shifts.

Thought Process and Content. In evaluating a thought disorder in a child, we must always consider what is typical for the child's age and what is deviant for any age group. The evaluation of thought-form considers loosening of associations, excessive magical thinking, perseveration, echolalia, the ability to distinguish fantasy from reality, sentence coherence, and the ability to reason

Table 1-28
Neuropsychiatric Mental Status Examination[a]

A. General Description
  1. General appearance and dress
  2. Level of consciousness and arousal
  3. Attention to environment
  4. Posture (standing and seated)
  5. Gait
  6. Movements of limbs, trunk, and face (spontaneous, resting, and after instruction)
  7. General demeanor (including evidence of responses to internal stimuli)
  8. Response to examiner (eye contact, cooperation, ability to focus on interview process)
  9. Native or primary language
 	
B. Language and Speech
  1. Comprehension (words, sentences, simple and complex commands, and concepts)
  2. Output (spontaneity, rate, fluency, melody or prosody, volume, coherence, vocabulary, paraphasic errors, complexity of usage)
  3. Repetition
  4. Other aspects
    a. Object naming
    b. Color naming
    c. Body part identification
    d. Ideomotor praxis to command
 	
C. Thought
  1. Form (coherence and connectedness)
  2. Content
    a. Ideational (preoccupations, overvalued ideas, delusions)
    b. Perceptual (hallucinations)
	D. Mood and Affect
	  1. Internal mood state (spontaneous and elicited; sense of humor)
	  2. Future outlook
	  3. Suicidal ideas and plans
	  4. Demonstrated emotional status (congruence with mood)
	
	E. Insight and Judgment
	  1. Insight
	    a. Self-appraisal and self-esteem
	    b. Understanding of current circumstances
	    c. Ability to describe personal psychological and physical status
	  2. Judgment
	    a. Appraisal of major social relationships
	    b. Understanding of personal roles and responsibilities
	
	F. Cognition
	  1. Memory
	    a. Spontaneous (as evidenced during interview)
	    b. Tested (incidental, immediate repetition, delayed recall, cued recall, recognition; verbal, nonverbal; explicit, implicit)
	  2. Visuospatial skills
	  3. Constructional ability
	  4. Mathematics
	  5. Reading
	  6. Writing
	  7. Fine sensory function (stereognosis, graphesthesia, two-point discrimination)
	  8. Finger gnosis
	  9. Right–left orientation
	  10. "Executive functions"
	  11. Abstraction

[a]Questions should be adapted to the age of the child.
Courtesy of Eric D. Caine, M.D. and Jeffrey M. Lyness, M.D.

logically. The evaluation of thought content considers delusions, obsessions, themes, fears, wishes, preoccupations, and interests.

Suicidal ideation is always a part of the mental status examination for children who are sufficiently verbal to understand the questions and old enough to understand the concept. Generally, children of average intelligence who are older than 4 years of age have some understanding of what is real and what is make-believe and may be asked about suicidal ideation, although a firm concept of the permanence of death may not be present until several years later.

We should also assess for aggressive thoughts and homicidal ideation. Perceptual disturbances, such as hallucinations, are also assessed. Very young children are expected to have short attention spans and may change the topic and conversation abruptly without exhibiting a symptomatic flight of ideas. Transient visual and auditory hallucinations in very young children do not necessarily represent major psychotic illnesses, but they do deserve further investigation.

Social Relatedness. We should assess the appropriateness of the child's response to the interviewer, general level of social skills, eye contact, and degree of familiarity or withdrawal in the interview process. Overly friendly or familiar behavior may be as troublesome as extremely retiring and withdrawn responses. The examiner assesses the child's self-esteem, general and specific areas of confidence, and success with family and peer relationships.

Motor Behavior. The motor behavior part of the mental status examination includes observations of the child's coordination and activity level and ability to pay attention and carry out developmentally appropriate tasks. It also involves involuntary movements,

tremors, motor hyperactivity, and any unusual focal asymmetries of muscle movement.

Cognition. We also should assess the child's intellectual functioning and problem-solving abilities. We can estimate the relative level of intelligence from a child's general information, vocabulary, and comprehension. For a specific assessment of the child's cognitive abilities, we can use a standardized test.

Memory. School-age children should be able to remember three objects after 5 minutes and to repeat five digits forward and three digits backward. Anxiety can interfere with the child's performance, but an apparent inability to repeat digits or to add simple numbers may reflect brain damage, mental retardation, or learning disabilities.

Judgment and Insight. The child's view of the problems, reactions to them, and suggested solutions may give us a good idea of the child's judgment and insight. Also, the child's understanding of what he or she can realistically do to help and what we can do adds to the assessment of the child's judgment.

Neuropsychiatric Assessment

A neuropsychiatric assessment is appropriate for children suspected of having a psychiatric disorder that coexists with neuropsychiatric impairment, or psychiatric symptoms that may be caused by neuropsychiatric dysfunction, or a neurologic disorder. Although a neuropsychiatric assessment is not sufficient in most cases to make a psychiatric diagnosis, neuropsychological profiles have been, in some cases, correlated with particular psychiatric symptoms and syndromes. For example, neuropsychological differences in executive function, language, and memory functions, as well as measures of mood and anxiety, have been found between youth with histories of childhood maltreatment and those without it. The neuropsychiatric evaluation combines information from neurologic, neuropsychological testing, and mental status examinations. The neurologic examination can identify asymmetrical abnormal signs (hard signs) that may indicate lesions in the brain. A physical examination can evaluate the presence of physical stigmata of particular syndromes in which neuropsychiatric symptoms or developmental aberrations play a role (e.g., fetal alcohol syndrome, Down syndrome).

A neuropsychiatric examination also includes neurologic soft signs and minor physical anomalies. Loretta Bender coined the term *neurological soft signs* in the 1940s to describe the nondiagnostic abnormalities in the neurologic examinations of children with schizophrenia. Soft signs do not indicate focal neurologic disorders, but they are associated with a wide variety of developmental disabilities and frequently occur in children with low intelligence, learning disabilities, and behavioral disturbances. Soft signs may refer to both behavioral symptoms (which are sometimes associated with brain damage, such as severe impulsivity and hyperactivity), physical findings (including contralateral overflow movements), and a variety of nonfocal signs (e.g., mild choreiform movements, poor balance, mild incoordination, asymmetry of gait, nystagmus, and the persistence of infantile reflexes). Soft signs include those that are normal in a young child, but become abnormal when they persist in an older child and those that are abnormal at any age. The *Physical and Neurological Examination for Soft Signs* (PANESS) is an instrument used with children up to the age of 15 years. It consists of 15 questions about the general physical status and medical history and 43 physical tasks (e.g., touch your finger to your nose, hop on one foot to the end of the line, tap quickly with your finger). Neurologic soft signs are useful to note, but they are not useful in making a specific psychiatric diagnosis.

Minor physical anomalies or dysmorphic features occur with a higher than usual frequency in children with developmental disabilities, learning disabilities, speech and language disorders, and hyperactivity. As with soft signs, the documentation of minor physical anomalies is part of the neuropsychiatric assessment, but it is rarely helpful in the diagnostic process and does not imply a good or bad prognosis. Minor physical anomalies include a high-arched palate, epicanthal folds, hypertelorism, low-set ears, transverse palmar creases, multiple hair whorls, a large head, a furrowed tongue, and partial syndactyl of several toes.

When considering a seizure disorder in the differential diagnosis or a structural abnormality in the brain, electroencephalography (EEG), CT, or MRI may be indicated.

Developmental, Psychological, and Educational Testing

Psychological testing, structured developmental assessments, and achievement testing are valuable in evaluating a child's developmental level, intellectual functioning, and academic difficulties. A measure of adaptive functioning (including the child's competence in communication, daily living skills, socialization, and motor skills) is the most definitive way to determine the level of intellectual disability in a child. Table 1-29 outlines the general categories of psychological tests.

Development Tests for Infants and Preschoolers.   The *Gesell Infant Scale,* the *Cattell Infant Intelligence Scale, Bayley Scales of Infant Development,* and the *Denver Developmental Screening Test* include developmental assessments of infants as young as 2 months of age. When used with very young infants, the tests focus on sensorimotor and social responses to a variety of objects and interactions. When using these instruments with older infants and preschoolers, the emphasis is on language acquisition. The *Gesell Infant Scale* measures development in four areas: motor, adaptive functioning, language, and social.

An infant's score on one of these developmental assessments is not a reliable way to predict a child's future IQ in most cases. Infant assessments are valuable, however, in detecting developmental deviation and mental retardation and in raising suspicions of a developmental disorder. Whereas infant assessments rely heavily on sensorimotor functions, intelligence testing in older children and adolescents includes later-developing functions, including verbal, social, and abstract cognitive abilities.

Intelligence Tests for School-Age Children and Adolescents.   The most widely used test of intelligence for school-age children and adolescents is the third edition of the *Wechsler Intelligence Scale for Children* (WISC-III-R). It can be given to children from 6 to 17 years of age and yields a verbal IQ, a performance IQ, and a combined full-scale IQ. The verbal subtests consist of vocabulary, information, arithmetic, similarities, comprehension, and digit span (supplemental) categories. The performance subtests include block design, picture completion, picture arrangement, object assembly, coding, mazes (supplemental), and symbol search (supplemental). The IQ computation does not include the scores of the supplemental subtests.

Each subcategory is scored from 1 to 19, with 10 being the average score. An average full-scale IQ is 100; 70 to 80 represents borderline intellectual function; 80 to 90 is in the low average range; 90 to 109 is average; 110 to 119 is a high average, and above 120 is in the superior or very superior range. The multiple breakdowns of the performance and verbal subscales allow great flexibility in identifying specific areas of deficit and scatter in intellectual abilities. Because a large part of intelligence testing measures abilities used in academic settings, the breakdown of the WISC-III-R can also point out skills in which a child is weak and may benefit from remedial education.

The *Stanford-Binet Intelligence Scale* covers an age range from 2 to 24 years. It relies on pictures, drawings, and objects for very young children and verbal performance for older children and adolescents. This intelligence scale, the earliest version of an intelligence test of its kind, leads to a mental age score as well as an IQ.

The *McCarthy Scales of Children's Abilities* and the *Kaufman Assessment Battery for Children* are two other intelligence tests that are available for preschool and school-age children. They do not cover adolescents.

LONG-TERM STABILITY OF INTELLIGENCE.   Although a child's intelligence is relatively stable throughout the school-age years and adolescence, some factors can influence intelligence and a child's score on an intelligence test. The intellectual functions of children with severe mental illnesses and of those from deprived and neglectful environments may decrease over time, whereas the IQs of children with intensively enriched environments may increase over time. Factors that influence a child's score on a given test of intellectual functioning and, thus, affect the accuracy of the test are motivation, emotional state, anxiety, and cultural milieu. The interactions between cognitive ability and anxiety and depression and psychosis are complex. One study of 4,405 youth from the Canadian National

Table 1-29
Commonly Used Child and Adolescent Psychological Assessment Instruments

Test	Age/Grades	Data Generated and Comments
Intellectual Ability		
Wechsler Intelligence Scale for Children—Third Edition (WISC-III-R)	6–16	Standard scores: verbal, performance and full-scale IQ; scaled subtest scores permitting specific skill assessment.
Wechsler Adult Intelligence Scale—(WAIS-III)	16–adult	Same as WISC-III-R.
Wechsler Preschool and Primary Scale of Intelligence—Revised (WPPSI-R)	3–7	Same as WISC-III-R.
Kaufman Assessment Battery for Children (K-ABC)	2.6–12.6	Well-grounded in theories of cognitive psychology and neuropsychology. Allows immediate comparison of intellectual capacity with acquired knowledge. Scores: Mental Processing Composite (IQ equivalent); sequential and simultaneous processing and achievement standard scores; scaled mental processing and achievement subtest scores; age equivalents; percentiles.
Kaufman Adolescent and Adult Intelligence Test (KAIT)	11–85+	Composed of separate Crystallized and Fluid scales. Scores: Composite Intelligence Scale; Crystallized and Fluid IQ; scaled subtest scores; percentiles.
Stanford-Binet, 4th Edition (SB:FE)	2–23	Scores: IQ; verbal, abstract/visual, and quantitative reasoning; short-term memory; standard age.
Peabody Picture Vocabulary Test—III (PPVT-III)	4–adult	Measures receptive vocabulary acquisition; standard scores, percentiles, age equivalents.
Achievement		
Woodcock–Johnson Psycho-Educational Battery—Revised (W-J)	K–12	Scores: reading and mathematics (mechanics and comprehension), written language, other academic achievement; grade and age scores, standard scores, percentiles.
Wide Range Achievement Test—3, Levels 1 and 2 (WRAT-3)	Level 1: 1–5 Level 2: 12–75	Permits screening for deficits in reading, spelling, and arithmetic; grade levels, percentiles, stanines, standard scores.
Kaufman Test of Educational Achievement, Brief and Comprehensive Forms (K-TEA)	1–12	Standard scores: reading, mathematics, and spelling; grade and age equivalents, percentiles, stanines. Brief Form is sufficient for most clinical applications; Comprehensive Form allows error analysis and more detailed curriculum planning.
Wechsler Individual Achievement Test (WIAT)	K–12	Standard scores: basic reading, mathematics reasoning, spelling, reading comprehension, numerical operations, listening comprehension, oral expression, written expression. Co-normal with WISC-III-R.
Adaptive Behavior		
Vineland Adaptive Behavior Scales	Normal: 0–19 Retarded: All ages	Standard scores: adaptive behavior composite and communication, daily living skills, socialization, and motor domains; percentiles, age equivalents, developmental age scores. Separate standardization groups for normal, visually handicapped, hearing impaired, emotionally disturbed, and retarded.
Scales of Independent Behavior—Revised	Newborn–adult	Standard scores: four adaptive (motor, social interaction, communication, personal living, community living) and three maladaptive (internalized, asocial, and externalized) areas; General Maladaptive Index and Broad Independence cluster.
Attentional Capacity		
Trail Making Test	8–adult	Standard scores, standard deviations, ranges; corrections for age and education.
Wisconsin Card Sorting Test	6.6–adult	Standard scores, standard deviations, T-scores, percentiles, developmental norms for number of categories achieved, perseverative errors, and failures to maintain set; computer measures.
Behavior Assessment System for Children (BASC)	4–18	Teacher and parent rating scales and child self-report of personality permitting multireporter assessment across a variety of domains in home, school, and community. Provides validity, clinical, and adaptive scales. ADHD component avails.
Home Situations Questionnaire—Revised (HSQ-R)	6–12	Permits parents to rate child's specific problems with attention or concentration. Scores for number of problem settings, mean severity, and factor scores for compliance and leisure situations.
ADHD Rating Scale	6–12	Score for number of symptoms keyed to DSM cutoff for diagnosis of ADHD; standard scores permit derivation of clinical significance for total score and two factors (Inattentive-Hyperactive and Impulsive-Hyperactive).

Table 1-29
Commonly Used Child and Adolescent Psychological Assessment Instruments (*Continued*)

Test	Age/Grades	Data Generated and Comments
School Situations Questionnaire (SSQ-R)	6–12	Permits teachers to rate a child's specific problems with attention or concentration. Scores for number of problem settings and mean severity.
Child Attention Profile (CAP)	6–12	Brief measure allowing teachers' weekly ratings of presence and degree of child's inattention and overactivity. Normative scores for inattention, overactivity, and total score.
Projective Tests		
Rorschach Inkblots	3–adult	Special scoring systems. Most recently developed and increasingly universally accepted is John Exner's Comprehensive System (1974). Assesses perceptual accuracy, integration of affective and intellectual functioning, reality testing, and other psychological processes.
Thematic Apperception Test (TAT)	6–adult	Generates stories that are analyzed qualitatively. Assumed to provide especially rich data regarding interpersonal functioning.
Machover Draw-A-Person Test (DAP)	3–adult	Qualitative analysis and hypothesis generation, especially regarding subject's feelings about self and significant others.
Kinetic Family Drawing (KFD)	3–adult	Qualitative analysis and hypothesis generation regarding an individual's perception of family structure and sentient environment. Some objective scoring systems in existence.
Rotter Incomplete Sentences Blank	Child, adolescent, and adult forms	Primarily qualitative analysis, although some objective scoring systems have been developed.
Personality Tests		
Minnesota Multiphasic Personality Inventory-Adolescent (MMPI-A)	14–18	1992 version of widely used personality measure, developed specifically for use with adolescents. Standard scores: 3 validity scales, 14 clinical scales, additional content and supplementary scales.
Millon Adolescent Personality Inventory (MAPI)	13–18	Standard scores for 20 scales grouped into three categories: Personality styles; expressed concerns; behavioral correlates. Normed on adolescent population. Focuses on broad functional spectrum, not just problem areas. Measures 14 primary personality traits, including emotional stability, self-concept level, excitability, and self-assurance.
Children's Personality Questionnaire	8–12	Generates combined broad trait patterns including extraversion and anxiety.
Neuropsychological Screening Tests and Test Batteries		
Developmental Test of Visual-Motor Integration (VMI)	2–16	Screening instrument for visual motor deficits. Standard scores, age equivalents, percentiles.
Benton Visual Retention Test	6–adult	Assesses presence of deficits in visual-figure memory. Mean scores by age.
Benton Visual Motor Gestalt Test	5–adult	Assesses visual-motor deficits and visual-figural retention. Age equivalents.
Reitan-Indiana Neuropsychological Test Battery for Children	5–8	Cognitive and perceptual-motor tests for children with suspected brain damage.
Halstead–Reitan Neuropsychological Test Battery for Older Children	9–14	Same as Reitan-Indiana.
Luria-Nebraska Neuropsychological Battery: Children's Revision LNNB:C	8–12	Sensory-motor, perceptual, cognitive tests measuring 11 clinical and 2 additional domains of neuropsychological functioning. Provides standard scores.
Developmental Status		
Bayley Scales of Infant Development-Second Edition	16 days–42 mo	Mental, motor, and behavior scales measuring infant, development. Provides standard scores.
Mullen Scales of Early Learning	Newborn–5 yr	Language and visual scales for receptive and expressive ability. Yields age scores and T scores.

Adapted from Racusin G, Moss N. Psychological assessment of children and adolescents. In: Lewis M, ed. *Child and Adolescent Psychiatry: A Comprehensive Textbook.* Philadelphia, PA: Williams Wilkins; 1991, with permission.

Longitudinal Study of Children and Youth (NLSCY), by Weeks and colleagues (2013) found that more exceptional cognitive ability was associated with less risk for anxiety and depressive symptoms in youth from 12 to 13 years of age, however, by ages 14 to 15 years, cognitive ability did not affect the odds of anxiety or depression.

Perceptual and Perceptual Motor Tests. The *Bender Visual-Motor Gestalt Test* can be given to children between the ages of 4 and 12 years. The test consists of a set of spatially related figures that the child copies. The number of errors determines the score. Although not a diagnostic test, it is useful in identifying developmentally age-inappropriate perceptual performances.

Personality Tests. Personality tests are not of much use in making diagnoses, and they are less satisfactory than intelligence tests concerning norms, reliability, and validity, but they can help elicit themes and fantasies.

The Rorschach test is a projective technique in which ambiguous stimuli—a set of bilaterally symmetrical inkblots—are shown to a child, who then describes what he or she sees in each. The hypothesis is that the child's interpretation of the vague stimuli reflects the basic characteristics of their personality. The examiner notes the themes and patterns.

A more structured projective test is the *Children's Apperception Test* (CAT), which is an adaptation of the *Thematic Apperception Test* (TAT). The CAT consists of cards with pictures of animals in scenes that are somewhat ambiguous but are related to parent–child and sibling issues, caretaking, and other relationships. The child describes what is happening and tells a story about the scene. The choice to use animals for the pictures is because some believe that children might respond more readily to animal images than to human figures.

Drawings, toys, and play are also applications of projective techniques used to evaluate children. Dollhouses, dolls, and puppets have been especially helpful in allowing a child a nonconversational mode in which to express a variety of attitudes and feelings. Play materials that reflect household situations are likely to elicit a child's fears, hopes, and conflicts about the family.

Projective techniques have not fared well as standardized instruments. Rather than being considered tests, projective techniques are better used as additional clinical modalities.

Educational Tests. Achievement tests measure the attainment of knowledge and skills in a particular academic curriculum. The *Wide-Range Achievement Test-Revised* (WRAT-R) consists of tests of knowledge and skills and timed performances of reading, spelling, and mathematics. It is used with children from 5 years of age to adulthood. The test yields a score that we can compare to the average expected score for the child's chronologic age and grade level.

The *Peabody Individual Achievement Test* (PIAT) includes word identification, spelling, mathematics, and reading comprehension.

The *Kaufman Test of Educational Achievement,* the *Gray Oral Reading Test-Revised* (GORT-R), and the *Sequential Tests of Educational Progress* (STEP) are achievement tests that determine whether a child has achieved the educational level expected for his or her grade level. Often, children whose achievement is significantly lower than expected for their grade level in one or more subjects exhibit a specific learning disorder.

Biopsychosocial Formulation. Our task is to integrate all of the information obtained into a formulation that takes into account the biologic predisposition, psychodynamic factors, environmental stressors, and life events that have led to the child's current level of functioning. We must consider psychiatric disorders and any specific physical, neuromotor, or developmental abnormalities in the formulation of etiologic factors for current impairment. Our conclusions are an integration of clinical information along with data from standardized psychological and developmental assessments. The psychiatric formulation includes an assessment of family function as well as the appropriateness of the child's educational setting. We should then determine the child's overall safety in his or her current situation, and report any suspected maltreatment to the local child protective service agency. We then consider the child's overall well-being regarding growth, development, and academic and play activities.

Diagnosis

Structured and semistructured (evidence-based) assessment tools often enhance a clinician's ability to make the most accurate diagnoses. These instruments described earlier include the K-SADS, the CAPA, and the NIMH DISC-IV interviews. The advantages of including an evidence-based instrument in the diagnostic process include decreasing potential clinician bias to make a diagnosis without all of the necessary symptoms information and serving as guides for us to consider each symptom that could contribute to a given diagnosis. These data can enable us to optimize his expertise to make challenging judgments regarding child and adolescent disorders, which may possess overlapping symptoms. Our ultimate task includes making all appropriate diagnoses according to the DSM-5. Some clinical situations do not fulfill the criteria for DSM-5 diagnoses, but cause impairment and require psychiatric attention and intervention. Clinicians who evaluate children are frequently in the position of determining the impact of the behavior of family members on the child's well-being. In many cases, a child's level of impairment is related to factors extending beyond a psychiatric diagnosis, such as the child's adjustment to his or her family life, peer relationships, and educational placement.

RECOMMENDATIONS AND TREATMENT PLAN

To recommend treatment, we should use our formulation, integrating all of the data gained during our assessments. Optimal treatment often flows from this formulation. That is, identification of a biologic predisposition to a particular psychiatric disorder may be clinically relevant to inform a psychopharmacologic recommendation. An understanding of the psychodynamic interactions between family members may lead a clinician to recommend treatment that includes a family component. Educational and academic problems addressed in the formulation may lead to a recommendation to seek a more effective academic placement. We should also take into account the overall social situation of the child or adolescent when recommending treatment. Of utmost important—and at the top of our recommendation list—is the physical and emotional safety of a child or adolescent.

The child or adolescent's family, school life, peer interactions, and social activities often have a direct impact on the child's success in overcoming his or her difficulties. The psychological education and cooperation of a child or adolescent's family are essential ingredients in the successful application of treatment recommendations. Patients and families often see communications that balance the observed positive qualities of the child and family with the weak areas as more helpful than a focus only on the problem areas. Finally, the most successful treatment plans are those developed cooperatively between us, the child, and the family.

INTELLECTUAL DISABILITY PSYCHIATRIC INTERVIEW AND TESTS

Psychiatric Interview

A psychiatric interview of a child or adolescent with intellectual disability requires a high level of sensitivity in order to elicit information at the appropriate intellectual level while remaining respectful of the patient's age and emotional development. The patient's verbal abilities, including receptive and expressive language, can be initially screened by observing the communication between the caretakers and the patient. If the patient communicates mostly through gestures or sign language, the parents may serve as interpreters. Patients with milder forms of intellectual disability are often well aware of their differences from others and their failures and may be anxious and ashamed during the interview. Approaching patients with a clear, supportive, concrete explanation of the diagnostic process, particularly patients with sufficiently receptive language ability, may allay anxiety and fears. Providing support and praise in language appropriate to the patient's age and understanding is beneficial. Subtle direction, structure, and reinforcement may be necessary to keep patients focused on the task or topic.

In general, the psychiatric examination of an intellectually disabled child or adolescent should reveal how the patient has coped with stages of development. Frustration tolerance, impulse control, and over-aggressive motor and sexual behavior are essential areas of attention in the interview. It is equally crucial to elicit the patient's self-image, areas of self-confidence, and an assessment of tenacity, persistence, curiosity, and willingness to explore the environment.

Structured Instruments, Rating Scales, and Psychological Assessment

In children and adolescents who have acquired language, we usually use one of several standardized instruments that include numerous domains of cognitive function. For children ages 6 to 16 years, the Wechsler Intelligence Test for Children is most common, and for children ages 3 to 6 years, the most commonly used is the Wechsler Preschool and Primary Scale of Intelligence-Revised. The Stanford-Binet Intelligence Scale, Fourth Edition, has the advantage that it can be administered to children even younger, starting at the age of 2 years. The Kaufman Assessment Battery for Children is appropriate for children ages 2½ to 12½ years, whereas the Kaufman Adolescent and Adult Intelligence Test apply to a wide range of ages, from 11 to 85 years. All of these standardized instruments evaluate cognitive abilities across multiple domains, including verbal, performance, memory, and problem-solving. Standardized instruments measuring adaptive function (functions of "everyday" life) assume that adaptive skills increase with age, and that adaptation may vary across different settings such as school, peer relationships, and family life. The Vineland Adaptive Behavior Scales can be used in infants through youth 18 years of age and includes four basic domains including *Communication* (Receptive, Expressive, and Written); *Daily Living Skills (*Personal, Domestic, and Community); *Socialization (*Interpersonal Relations, Play and Leisure, and Coping Skills); *Motor Skills* (Fine and Gross).

Several behavioral rating scales exist for the population with intellectual disabilities. General behavioral rating scales include the Aberrant Behavior Checklist (ABC) and the Developmental Behavior Checklist (DBC). The Behavior Problem Inventory (BPI) is a useful screening instrument for self-injurious, aggressive, and stereotyped behaviors. The Psychopathology Inventory for Mentally Retarded Adults (PIMRA) helps identify the presence of comorbid psychiatric symptoms and disorders.

Examining clinicians can use several screening instruments for developmental and intellectual delay or disability in infants and toddlers. However, the controversy over the predictive value of infant psychological tests is heated. Some report the correlation of abnormalities during infancy with later abnormal functioning as very low, and others report it to be very high. The correlation rises in direct proportion to the age of the child at the time of the developmental examination. Some exercises such as copying geometric figures, the *Goodenough Draw-a-Person Test,* the *Kohs Block Test,* and geometric puzzles all are useful quick screening tests of visual-motor coordination. For infants, the *Gesell* and *Bayley scales* and the *Cattell Infant Intelligence Scale* are useful.

The *Peabody Vocabulary Test* is the most widely used picture-based vocabulary test. Other tests often found useful in detecting intellectual disability are the *Bender Gestalt Test* and the *Benton Visual Retention Test.* The psychological evaluation should assess perceptual, motor, linguistic, and cognitive abilities.

Physical Examination

Various parts of the body may demonstrate identifying characteristics of specific perinatal and prenatal events or conditions associated with intellectual disabilities. For example, the configuration and the size of the head may offer clues to a variety of conditions, such as microcephaly, hydrocephalus, or Down syndrome. A patient's facial characteristics, for example, hypertelorism, a flat nasal bridge, prominent eyebrows, epicanthal folds, may provide clues to a recognizable syndrome such as FAS. Additional facial characteristics including corneal opacities, retinal changes, low-set, and small or misshapen ears, a protruding tongue, and disturbance in dentition may be stigmata of a variety of known syndromes. The facial expression, color, and texture of the skin and hair, a high-arched palate, the size of the thyroid gland, and the proportions of a child's trunk and extremities may offer clues for particular syndromes. We should measure the circumference of the head as part of the clinical investigation. Dermatoglyphics (studying skin markings) may offer another diagnostic tool because unique ridge patterns and flexion creases on the hand occur in persons who are intellectually disabled, including chromosomal disorders and rubella. Table 1-30 lists syndromes with intellectual disability and their behavioral phenotypes.

Neurologic Examination

Sensory impairments frequently occur among persons with intellectual disabilities. For example, hearing impairment occurs in 10 percent of persons with intellectual disability, a rate that is four times that of the general population. Visual disturbances can range from blindness to disturbances of spatial concepts, design recognition, and concepts of body image. Seizure disorders occur in about 10 percent of intellectually disabled populations and one-third of those with severe intellectual disabilities. Neurologic abnormalities increase in incidence and severity in direct proportion to the degree of intellectual disability. Disturbances in motor areas cause abnormalities of muscle tone (spasticity or hypotonia), reflexes (hyperreflexia), and involuntary movements (choreoathetosis). Less disability may also be associated with clumsiness and poor coordination.

Table 1-30
Syndromes with Intellectual Disability and Behavioral Phenotypes

Disorder	Pathophysiology	Clinical Features and Behavioral Phenotype
Down syndrome	Trisomy 21, 95% nondisjunction, approx. 4% translocation; 1/1,000 live births: 1:2,500 in women less than 30 yr old, 1:80 over 40 yr old, 1:32 at 45 yr old; possible overproduction of β-amyloid due to defect at 21q21.1	Hypotonia, upward-slanted palpebral fissures, midface depression, flat wide nasal bridge, simian crease, short stature, increased incidence of thyroid abnormalities and congenital heart disease Passive, affable, hyperactivity in childhood, stubborn; verbal > auditory processing, increased risk of depression, and dementia of the Alzheimer type in adulthood
Fragile X syndrome	Inactivation of *FMR-1* gene at X q27.3 due to CGG base repeats, methylation; recessive; 1:1,000 male births, 1:3,000 female; accounts for 10–12% of intellectual disability in males	Long face, large ears, midface hypoplasia, high arched palate, short stature, macroorchidism, mitral valve prolapse, joint laxity, strabismus Hyperactivity, inattention, anxiety, stereotypies, speech and language delays, IQ decline, gaze aversion, social avoidance, shyness, irritability, learning disorder in some females; mild intellectual disability in affected females, moderate to severe in males; verbal IQ > performance IQ
Prader–Willi syndrome	Deletion in 15q12 (15q11–15q13) of paternal origin; some cases of maternal uniparental disomy; dominant 1/10,000 live births; 90% sporadic; candidate gene: small nuclear ribonucleoprotein polypeptide (SNRPN)	Hypotonia, failure to thrive in infancy, obesity, small hands and feet microorchidism, cryptorchidism, short stature, almond-shaped eyes, fair hair and light skin, flat face, scoliosis, orthopedic problems, prominent forehead and bitemporal narrowing Compulsive behavior, hyperphagia, hoarding, impulsivity, borderline to moderate intellectual disability, emotional lability, tantrums, excess daytime sleepiness, skin picking, anxiety, aggression
Angelman syndrome	Deletion in 15q12 (15q11–15q13) of maternal origin; dominant; frequent deletion of γ-aminobutyric acid (GABA) B-3 receptor subunit, prevalence unknown but rare, estimated 1/20,000–1/30,000	Fair hair and blue eyes (66%); dysmorphic faces including wide smiling mouth, thin upper lip, and pointed chin; epilepsy (90%) with characteristic EEG; ataxia; small head circumference, 25% microcephalic Happy disposition, paroxysmal laughter, hand flapping, clapping; profound intellectual disability; sleep disturbance with nighttime waking; possible increased incidence of autistic features; anecdotal love of water and music
Cornelia de Lange syndrome	Lack of pregnancy-associated plasma protein A (PAPPA) linked to chromosome 9q33; similar phenotype associated with trisomy 5p, ring chromosome 3; rare (1/40,000–1/100,000 live births); possible association with 3q26.3	Continuous eyebrows, thin downturning upper lip, microcephaly, short stature, small hands and feet, small upturned nose, anteverted nostrils, malformed upper limbs, failure to thrive Self-injury, limited speech in severe cases, language delays, avoidance of being held, stereotypic movements, twirling, severe to profound intellectual disability
Williams syndrome	1/20,000 births; hemizygous deletion that includes elastin locus chromosome 7q11–23; autosomal dominant	Short stature, unusual facial features including broad forehead, depressed nasal bridge, stellate pattern of the iris, widely spaced teeth, and full lips; elfinlike facies; renal and cardiovascular abnormalities; thyroid abnormalities; hypercalcemia Anxiety, hyperactivity, fears, outgoing, sociable, verbal skills > visual spatial skills
Cri-du-chat syndrome	Partial deletion 5p; 1/50,000; region may be 5p15.2	Round face with hypertelorism, epicanthal folds, slanting palpebral fissures, broad flat nose, low-set ears, micrognathia; prenatal growth retardation; respiratory and ear infections; congenital heart disease; gastrointestinal abnormalities Severe intellectual disability, infantile catlike cry, hyperactivity, stereotypies, self-injury
Smith–Magenis syndrome	Incidence unknown, estimated 1/25,000 live births; complete or partial deletion of 17p11.2	Broad face; flat midface; short, broad hands; small toes; hoarse, deep voice Severe intellectual disability; hyperactivity; severe self-injury including hand biting, head banging, and pulling out finger- and toenails; stereotyped self-hugging; attention seeking; aggression; sleep disturbance (decreased REM)
Rubinstein–Taybi syndrome	1/250,000, approx. male = female; sporadic; likely autosomal dominant; documented microdeletions in some cases at 16p13.3	Short stature and microcephaly, broad thumb and big toes, prominent nose, broad nasal bridge, hypertelorism, ptosis, frequent fractures, feeding difficulties in infancy, congenital heart disease, EEG abnormalities, seizures Poor concentration, distractible, expressive language difficulties, performance IQ > verbal IQ; anecdotally happy, loving, sociable, responsive to music, self-stimulating behavior; older patients have mood lability and temper tantrums
Tuberous sclerosis complex 1 and 2	Benign tumors (hamartomas) and malformations (hamartias) of central nervous system (CNS), skin, kidney, heart; dominant; 1/10,000 births; 50% TSC 1, 9q34; 50% TSC 2, 16p13	Epilepsy, autism, hyperactivity, impulsivity, aggression; spectrum of intellectual disability from none (30%) to profound; self-injurious behaviors, sleep disturbances

Table 1-30
Syndromes with Intellectual Disability and Behavioral Phenotypes (*Continued*)

Disorder	Pathophysiology	Clinical Features and Behavioral Phenotype
Neurofibromatosis type 1 (NF1)	1/2,500–1/4,000; male = female; autosomal dominant; 50% new mutations; more than 90% paternal NF1 allele mutated; *NFI* gene 17q11.2; gene product is neurofibromin thought to be tumor suppressor gene	Variable manifestations; café-au-lait spots, cutaneous neurofibromas, Lisch nodules; short stature and macrocephaly in 30–45 Half with speech and language difficulties; 10% with moderate to profound intellectual disability; verbal IQ > performance IQ; distractible, impulsive, hyperactive, anxious; possibly associated with increased incidence of mood and anxiety disorders
Lesch–Nyhan syndrome	Defect in hypoxanthine guanine phosphoribosyl-transferase with accumulation of uric acid; Xq26–27; recessive; rare (1/10,000–1/38,000)	Ataxia, chorea, kidney failure, gout Often severe self-biting behavior; aggression; anxiety; mild to moderate intellectual disability
Galactosemia	Defect in galactose-1-phosphate uridyltransferase or galactokinase or empiramase; autosomal recessive; 1/62,000 births in the United States	Vomiting in early infancy, jaundice, hepatosplenomegaly; later cataracts, weight loss, food refusal, increased intracranial pressure and increased risk for sepsis, ovarian failure, failure to thrive, renal tubular damage Possible intellectual disability even with treatment, visuospatial deficits, language disorders, reports of increased behavioral problems, anxiety, social withdrawal, and shyness
Phenylketonuria	Defect in phenylalanine hydroxylase (PAH) or cofactor (biopterin) with accumulation of phenylalanine; approximately 1/11,500 births; varies with geographical location; gene for PAH, 12q22–24.1; autosomal recessive	Symptoms absent neonatally, later development of seizures (25% generalized), fair skin, blue eyes, blond hair, rash Untreated: mild to profound intellectual disability, language delay, destructiveness, self-injury, hyperactivity
Hurler syndrome	1/100,000; deficiency in α-L-iduronidase activity; autosomal recessive	Early onset; short stature, hepatosplenomegaly; hirsutism, corneal clouding, death before age 10 yr, dwarfism, coarse facial features, recurrent respiratory infections Moderate to severe intellectual disability, anxious, fearful, rarely aggressive
Hunter syndrome	1/100,000, X-linked recessive; iduronate sulfatase deficiency; X q28	Normal infancy; symptom onset at age 2–4 yr; typical coarse faces with flat nasal bridge, flaring nostrils; hearing loss, ataxia, hernia common; enlarged liver and spleen, joint stiffness, recurrent infections, growth retardation, cardiovascular abnormality Hyperactivity, intellectual disability by 2 yr; speech delay; loss of speech at 8–10 yr; restless, aggressive, inattentive, sleep abnormalities; apathetic, sedentary with disease progression
Fetal alcohol syndrome	Maternal alcohol consumption (trimester III > II > I); 1/3,000 live births in Western countries; 1/300 with fetal alcohol effects	Microcephaly, short stature, midface hypoplasia, short palpebral fissure, thin upper lip, retrognathia in infancy, micrognathia in adolescence, hypoplastic long or smooth philtrum Mild to moderate intellectual disability, irritability, inattention, memory impairment

Table by B. H. King, M.D., R. M. Hodapp, Ph.D., and E. M. Dykens, Ph.D.

▲ 1.3 Geriatric Patients

PSYCHIATRIC EXAMINATION OF THE OLDER PATIENT

Psychiatric history taking and the mental status examination of older adults follow the same format as for younger adults; however, because of the high prevalence of cognitive disorders in older persons, psychiatrists must determine whether a patient understands the nature and purpose of the examination. When a patient is cognitively impaired, an independent history should be obtained from a family member or caretaker. The patient still should be seen alone—even in cases of clear evidence of impairment—to preserve the privacy of the doctor–patient relationship and to elicit any suicidal thoughts or paranoid ideation, which may not be voiced in the presence of a relative or nurse.

When approaching the examination of the older patient, it is essential to remember that older adults differ markedly from one another. The approach to examining the older patient must take into account whether the person is a healthy 75-year-old who recently retired from a second career or a frail 96-year-old who just lost the only surviving relative with the death of the 75-year-old care-giving daughter.

Psychiatric History

A complete psychiatric history includes preliminary identification (name, age, sex, marital status), chief complaint, history of the present illness, history of previous illnesses, personal history, and family history. A review of medications (including over-the-counter medications), both current and recent, is also essential.

Patients older than age 65 often have subjective complaints of minor memory impairments, such as forgetting persons' names and misplacing objects. Minor cognitive problems also can occur because of anxiety in the interview situation. These age-associated memory impairments are of no significance; the term *benign senescent forgetfulness* has been used to describe them.

A patient's childhood and adolescent history can provide information about personality organization and give important clues about coping strategies and defense mechanisms used under stress. A history of learning disability or minimal cerebral dysfunction is significant. The psychiatrist should inquire about friends, sports, hobbies, social activity, and work. The occupational history should include the patient's feelings about work, relationships with peers, problems with authority, and attitudes toward retirement. The patient also should be questioned about plans for the future. What are the patient's hopes and fears?

The family history should include a patient's description of parents' attitudes and adaptation to their old age and, if applicable, information about the causes of their deaths. Alzheimer disease is transmitted as an autosomal-dominant trait in 10 to 30 percent of the offspring of parents with Alzheimer disease; depression and alcohol dependence also run in families. The patient's current social situation should be evaluated. Who cares for the patient? Does the patient have children? What are the characteristics of the patient's parent–child relationships? A financial history helps the psychiatrist evaluate the role of economic hardship in the patient's illness and to make realistic treatment recommendations.

The marital history includes a description of the spouse and the characteristics of the relationship. If the patient is a widow or a widower, the psychiatrist should explore how grieving was handled. If the loss of the spouse occurred within the past year, the patient is at high risk for an adverse physical or psychological event.

The patient's sexual history includes sexual activity, orientation, libido, masturbation, extramarital affairs, and sexual symptoms (e.g., impotence and anorgasmia). Young clinicians may have to overcome their own biases about taking a sexual history: Sexuality is an area of concern for many geriatric patients, who welcome the chance to talk about their sexual feelings and attitudes.

Mental Status Examination

The mental status examination offers a cross-sectional view of how a patient thinks, feels, and behaves during the examination. With older adults, a psychiatrist may not be able to rely on a single examination to answer all of the diagnostic questions. Repeat mental status examinations may be needed because of fluctuating changes in the patient's family.

General Description. A general description of the patient includes appearance, psychomotor activity, attitude toward the examiner, and speech activity.

Motor disturbances (e.g., shuffling gait, stooped posture, "pill-rolling" movements of the fingers, tremors, and body asymmetry) should be noted. Involuntary movements of the mouth or tongue may be adverse effects of phenothiazine medication. Many depressed patients seem to be slow in speech and movement. Mask-like facies occurs in Parkinson disease.

The patient's speech may be pressured in agitated, manic, and anxious states. Tearfulness and overt crying occur in depressive and cognitive disorders, especially if the patient feels frustrated about being unable to answer one of the examiner's questions. The presence of a hearing aid or another indication that the patient has a hearing problem (e.g., requesting repetition of questions) should be noted.

The patient's attitude toward the examiner—cooperative, suspicious, guarded, ingratiating—can give clues about possible transference reactions. Because of transference, older adults can react to younger physicians as if the physicians were parent figures, despite the age difference.

Functional Assessment. Patients older than 65 years of age should be evaluated for their capacity to maintain independence and to perform the activities of daily life, which include toileting, preparing meals, dressing, grooming, and eating. The degree of functional competence in their everyday behaviors is an essential consideration in formulating a treatment plan for these patients.

Mood, Feelings, and Affect. Suicide is a leading cause of death of older persons, and an evaluation of a patient's suicidal ideation is essential. Loneliness is the most common reason cited by older adults who consider suicide. Feelings of loneliness, worthlessness, helplessness, and hopelessness are symptoms of depression, which carries a high risk of suicide. Nearly 75 percent of all suicide victims suffer from depression, alcohol abuse, or both. The examiner should specifically ask the patient about any thoughts of suicide: Does the patient feel life is no longer worth living? Does the patient think he or she would be better off dead or, when dead, would no longer be a burden to others? Such thoughts—significantly when associated with alcohol abuse, living alone, the recent death of a spouse, physical illness, and somatic pain—indicate a high suicidal risk.

Disturbances in mood states, most notably depression and anxiety, can interfere with memory functioning. An expansive or euphoric mood may indicate a manic episode or may signal a dementing disorder. Frontal lobe dysfunction often produces *witzelsucht,* which is the tendency to make puns and jokes and then laugh aloud at them.

The patient's affect may be flat, blunted, constricted, shallow, or inappropriate, all of which can indicate a depressive disorder, schizophrenia, or brain dysfunction. Such affects are significant abnormal findings, although they are not pathognomonic of a specific disorder. Dominant lobe dysfunction causes *dysprosody,* an inability to express emotional feelings through speech intonation.

Perceptual Disturbances. Hallucinations and illusions by older adults can be transitory phenomena resulting from decreased sensory acuity. The examiner should note whether the patient is confused about time or place during the hallucinatory episode; confusion points to an organic condition. It is particularly important to ask the patient about distorted body perceptions. Because brain tumors and other focal pathology can cause hallucinations, a diagnostic workup may be indicated. Brain diseases cause perceptive impairments; agnosia, the inability to recognize and interpret the significance of sensory impressions, is associated with organic brain diseases. The examiner should note the type of agnosia. Types of agnosia include denial of illness (anosognosia), denial of a body part (atopognosia), and inability to recognize objects (visual agnosia) or faces (prosopagnosia).

Language Output. The language output category of the geriatric mental status examination covers the aphasias, which are disorders of language output related to organic lesions of the brain. The best described are nonfluent or Broca aphasia, fluent or Wernicke aphasia, and global aphasia, a combination of fluent and nonfluent aphasias. In nonfluent or Broca aphasia, the patient's understanding remains intact, but the ability to speak is impaired. The patient cannot pronounce "Methodist Episcopalian." Words are generally mispronounced, and speech may be telegraphic. A simple test for Wernicke aphasia is to point to some everyday objects—such as a pen or a pencil, a doorknob, and a light switch—and ask the patient to name them. The patient also may be unable to demonstrate the use of simple objects, such as a key and a match (ideomotor apraxia).

Visuospatial Functioning.　Some decline in visuospatial capability is expected with aging. Asking a patient to copy figures or a drawing may help assess the function. A neuropsychological assessment should be performed when visuospatial functioning is impaired.

Thought.　Disturbances in thinking include neologisms, word salad, circumstantiality, tangentiality, loosening of associations, flight of ideas, clang associations, and blocking. The loss of the ability to appreciate nuances of meaning (abstract thinking) may be an early sign of dementia. Thinking is then described as concrete or literal.

Thought content should be examined for phobias, obsessions, somatic preoccupations, and compulsions. Ideas about suicide or homicide should be discussed. The examiner should determine whether delusions are present and how such delusions affect the patient's life. Delusions may be present in nursing home patients and may have been a reason for admission. Ideas of reference or influence should be described. Patients who are hard of hearing can be classified mistakenly as paranoid or suspicious.

Sensorium and Cognition.　*Sensorium* concerns the functioning of the special senses; *cognition* concerns information processing and intellect. The survey of both areas, known as the neuropsychiatric examination, consists of the clinician's assessment and a comprehensive battery of psychological tests.

CONSCIOUSNESS.　A sensitive indicator of brain dysfunction is an altered state of consciousness in which the patient does not seem to be alert, shows fluctuations in levels of awareness, or seems to be lethargic. In severe cases, the patient is somnolescent or stuporous.

ORIENTATION.　Impairment in orientation to time, place, and person is associated with cognitive disorders. Cognitive impairment often is observed in mood disorders, anxiety disorders, factitious disorders, conversion disorder, and personality disorders, especially during periods of severe physical or environmental stress. The examiner should test for orientation to place by asking the patient to describe his or her present location. Orientation to a person may be approached in two ways: Does the patient know their name, and are nurses and doctors identified as such? Time is tested by asking the patient the date, the year, the month, and the day of the week. The patient also should be asked about the length of time spent in a hospital, during what season of the year, and how the patient knows these facts. Greater significance is given to difficulties concerning person than to difficulties of time and place, and more significance is given to orientation to place than to orientation to time.

MEMORY.　Memory usually is evaluated in terms of immediate, recent, and remote memory. Immediate retention and recall are tested by giving the patient six digits to repeat forward and backward. The examiner should record the result of the patient's capacity to remember. Persons with unimpaired memory usually can recall six digits forward and five or six digits backward. The clinician should be aware that the ability to do well on digit-span

tests is impaired in very anxious patients. Remote memory can be tested by asking for the patient's place and date of birth, the patient's mother's name before she was married, and the names and birthdays of the patient's children.

In cognitive disorders, recent memory deteriorates first. Recent memory assessment can be approached in several ways. Some examiners give the patient the names of three items early in the interview and ask for recall later. Others prefer to tell a brief story and ask the patient to repeat it verbatim. We can test for recent memory by asking for the patient's place of residence, including the street number, the method of transportation to the hospital, and some current events. If the patient has a memory deficit, such as amnesia, careful testing should be performed to determine whether it is retrograde amnesia (loss of memory before an event) or anterograde amnesia (loss of memory after the event). Retention and recall also can be tested by having the patient retell a simple story. Patients who confabulate make up new material in retelling the story.

INTELLECTUAL TASKS, INFORMATION, AND INTELLIGENCE.　Various intellectual tasks can be presented to estimate the patient's fund of general knowledge and intellectual functioning. Counting and calculation can be tested by asking the patient to subtract 7 from 100 and to continue subtracting 7 from the result until the number 2 is reached. The examiner records the responses as a baseline for future testing. The examiner can also ask the patient to count backward from 20 to 1 and can record the time necessary to complete the exercise.

The patient's fund of general knowledge is related to intelligence. The patient can be asked to name the president of the United States, to name the three largest cities in the United States, to give the population of the United States, and to give the distance from New York to Paris. The examiner must take into account the patient's educational level, socioeconomic status, and general life experience in assessing the results of some of these tests.

READING AND WRITING.　It may be necessary for the clinician to examine the patient's reading and writing and to determine whether the patient has a specific speech deficit. The examiner may have the patient read a simple story aloud or write a short sentence to test for a reading or writing disorder. Whether the patient is right-handed or left-handed should be noted.

JUDGMENT.　*Judgment* is the capacity to act appropriately in various situations. Does the patient show impaired judgment? What would the patient do on finding a stamped, sealed, addressed envelope in the street? What would the patient do if he or she smelled smoke in a theater? Can the patient discriminate? What is the difference between a dwarf and a boy? Why are couples required to get a marriage license?

Neuropsychological Evaluation

A thorough neuropsychological examination includes a comprehensive battery of tests that can be replicated by various examiners and can be repeated over time to assess the course of a specific illness. The most widely used test of current cognitive functioning is the Mini-Mental State Examination (MMSE), which assesses orientation, attention, calculation, immediate and short-term recall, language, and the ability to follow simple commands. The MMSE is used to detect impairments, follow the course of an illness, and monitor the patient's treatment responses. It is not used to make a formal diagnosis. The maximal MMSE score is 30. Age and educational level influence cognitive performance.

The assessment of intellectual abilities is performed with the Wechsler Adult Intelligence Scale-Revised (WAIS-R), which gives verbal, performance, and full-scale IQ scores. Some test results, such as those of vocabulary tests, hold up as aging progresses; results of other tests, such as tests of similarities and digit-symbol substitution, do not. The performance part of the WAIS-R is a more sensitive indicator of brain damage than the verbal part.

Visuospatial functions are sensitive to the normal aging process. The Bender Gestalt Test is one of a large number of instruments used to test visuospatial functions; another is the Halstead–Reitan Battery, which is the most complex battery of tests covering the entire spectrum of information processing and cognition. Depression, even in the absence of dementia, often impairs psychomotor performance, especially visuospatial functioning and timed motor performance. The Geriatric Depression Scale is a useful screening instrument that excludes somatic complaints from its list of items. The presence of somatic complaints on a rating scale tends to confound the diagnosis of a depressive disorder.

Medical History. Elderly patients have more concomitant, chronic, and multiple medical problems and take more medications than younger adults; many of these medications can influence their mental status. The medical history includes all significant illnesses, trauma, hospitalizations, and treatment interventions. The psychiatrist should also be alert to underlying medical illness. Psychiatric symptoms may first manifest infections, metabolic and electrolyte disturbances, and myocardial infarction and stroke. Depressed mood, delusions, and hallucinations may precede other symptoms of Parkinson disease by many months. On the other hand, a psychiatric disorder can also cause such somatic symptoms as weight loss, malnutrition, and inanition of severe depression.

A careful review of medications (including over-the-counter medications, laxatives, vitamins, tonics, and lotions) and even substances recently discontinued is critical. Drug effects can be long-lasting and may induce depression (e.g., antihypertensives), cognitive impairment (e.g., sedatives), delirium (e.g., anticholinergics), and seizures (e.g., neuroleptics). The review of medications must include sufficient detail to identify misuse (overdose, underuse) and relate medication use to special diets. A dietary history is also essential; deficiencies and excesses (e.g., protein, vitamins) can influence physiologic function and mental status.

EARLY DETECTION AND PREVENTION STRATEGIES

Many age-related illnesses develop insidiously and gradually progress over the years. The most common cause of late-life cognitive impairment, Alzheimer disease, is characterized neuropathologically by a gradual accumulation of neuritic plaques and neurofibrillary tangles in the brain. Clinically, a progression of cognitive decline is seen, which begins with mild memory loss and ends with severe cognitive and behavioral deterioration.

Because it will likely be simpler to prevent neural damage than to repair it once it occurs, investigators are developing strategies for early detection and prevention of age-related illnesses, such as Alzheimer disease. Considerable progress has been made in the detection component of this strategy, using brain imaging technologies, such as PET and fMRI, in combination with genetic risk measures. With these approaches, subtle brain changes can now be detected that progress and can be followed over time. Such surrogate markers allow clinical scientists to track disease progression and to test novel treatments designed to decelerate brain aging. Clinical trials of cholinesterase inhibitor drugs, anticholesterol drugs, anti-inflammatory drugs, and others (e.g., vitamin E) are in progress to determine if such treatments delay the onset of Alzheimer disease or the progression of brain metabolic or cognitive decline.

Novel approaches to measuring the physical evidence of Alzheimer disease, the plaques, and tangles in the cerebral cortex, have been successful in initial studies and will likely facilitate the testing of innovative treatments designed to rid the brain of these pathognomonic lesions. Scientists may not be able to cure Alzheimer disease in its advanced stages, but they may be able to delay its onset effectively, thus helping patients live longer without the debilitating manifestations of the disease, including cognitive decline.

References

Achenbach TM, Dumenci L, Rescorla LA. *Ratings of Relations between DSM-IV Diagnostic Categories and Items of the CBCL/6–18, TRF, and YSR.* Burlington, VT: University of Vermont, Research Center for Children, Youth, & Families; 2001.

Adams RL, Culbertson JL. Personality assessment: adults and children. In: Sadock BJ, Sadock VA, Ruiz P, eds. *Kaplan & Sadock's Comprehensive Textbook of Psychiatry.* 9th ed. Philadelphia, PA: Lippincott Williams & Wilkins; 2009:951.

Aggarwal NK, Zhang XY, Stefanovics E, Chen da C, Xiu MH, Xu K, Rosenheck RA. Rater evaluations for psychiatric instruments and cultural differences: the positive and negative syndrome scale in China and the United States. *J Nerv Ment Dis.* 2012;200(9):814–820.

Allott K, Proffitt TM, McGorry PD, Pantelis C, Wood SJ, Cumner M, Brewer WJ. Clinical neuropsychology within adolescent and young-adult psychiatry: conceptualizing theory and practice. *Appl Neuropsychol Child.* 2013;2(1):47–63.

American Psychiatric Association. *Diagnostic and Statistical Manual of Mental Disorders.* 5th ed. Arlington, VA: American Psychiatric Association; 2013.

Arnone D, McKie S, Elliott R, Thomas EJ, Downey D, Juhasz G, Williams SR, Deakin JF, Anderson IM. Increased amygdala responses to sad but not fearful faces in major depression: relation to mood state and pharmacological treatment. *Am J Psychiatry.* 2012;169(8):841–850.

Aronne LJ, Segal KR. Weight gain in the treatment of mood disorders. *J Clin Psychiatry.* 2003;64(Suppl 8):22–29.

Balzer DG, Steffens DC. *Essentials of Geriatric Psychiatry.* 2nd ed. Arlington, VA: American Psychiatric Association; 2012.

Baron DA, Baron DA, Baron DH. Laboratory testing for substances of abuse. In: Frances RJ, Miller SI, Mack AH, eds. *Clinical Textbook of Addictive Disorders.* 3rd ed. New York: Guilford; 2011:63.

Beck A, Wüstenberg T, Genauck A, Wrase J, Schlagenhauf F, Smolka MN, Mann K, Heinz A. Effect of brain structure, brain function, and brain connectivity on relapse in alcohol-dependent patients. *Arch Gen Psychiatry.* 2012;69(8):842.

Bird HR, Canino GJ, Davies M, Ramirez R, Chavez L, Duarte C, Shen S. The Brief Impairment Scale (BIS): a multidimensional scale of functional impairment for children and adolescents. *J Am Acad Child Adolesc Psychiatry.* 2005;44(7):699–707.

Björklund A, Dunnett SB. Dopamine neuron systems in the brain: an update. *Trends Neurosci.* 2007;30(5):194–202.

Blacker D. Psychiatric rating scales. In: Sadock BJ, Sadock VA, Ruiz P, eds. *Kaplan & Sadock's Comprehensive Textbook of Psychiatry.* 9th ed. Philadelphia, PA: Lippincott Williams & Wilkins; 2009:1032.

Blumenthal JA, Sherwood A, Babyak MA, Watkins LL, Smith PJ, Hoffman BM, O'Hayer CV, Mabe S, Johnson J, Doraiswamy PM, Jiang W, Schocken DD, Hinderliter AL. Exercise and pharmacological treatment of depressive symptoms in patients with coronary heart disease: results from the UPBEAT (Understanding the Prognostic Benefits of Exercise and Antidepressant Therapy) study. *J Am Coll Cardiol.* 2012;60(12):1053.

Boosman H, Visser-Meily JM, Winken I, van Heugten CM. Clinicians' views on learning in brain injury rehabilitation. *Brain Inj.* 2013;27(6):685–688.

Borairi S, Dougherty DD. The use of neuroimaging to predict treatment response for neurosurgical interventions for treatment-refractory major depression and obsessive-compulsive disorder. *Harvard Rev Psychiatry.* 2011;19(3):155.

Bram AD. The relevance of the Rorschach and patient-examiner relationship in treatment planning and outcome assessment. *J Pers Assess.* 2010;92(2):91.

Cahn B, Polich J. Meditation states and traits: EEG, ERP, and neuroimaging studies. *Psychol Consciousness Theory Res Pract.* 2013;1(S):48–96.

Calamia M, Markon K, Tranel D. Scoring higher the second time around: meta-Analyses of practice effects in neuropsychological assessment. *Clin Neuropsychologist.* 2012;26(4):543–570.

Cernich AN, Chandler L, Scherdell T, Kurtz S. Assessment of co-occurring disorders in veterans diagnosed with traumatic brain injury. *J Head Trauma Rehabil.* 2012;27(4):253–260.

Chan RCK, Stone WS, Hsi X. Neurological and neuropsychological endophenotypes in schizophrenia spectrum disorders. In: Ritsner MS, ed. *Handbook of Schizophrenia Spectrum Disorders*. New York: Springer; 2011:325.

Chue P, Kovacs CS. Safety and tolerability of atypical antipsychotics in patients with bipolar disorder: prevalence, monitoring, and management. *Bipolar Disord.* 2003;5(Suppl 2):62–79.

Cleary MJ, Scott AJ. Developments in clinical neuropsychology: implications for school psychological services. *J School Health*. 2011;81(1):1–7.

Cormac I, Ferriter M, Benning R, Saul C. Physical health and health risk factors in a population of long-stay psychiatric patients. *Psychol Bull*. 2005;29:18–20.

Daniel M, Gurczynski J. Mental status examination. In: Segal DL, Hersen M, eds. *Diagnostic Interviewing*. 4th ed. New York: Springer; 2010:61.

Dawson P, Guare R. *Executive Skills in Children and Adolescents: A Practical Guide to Assessment and Intervention*. 2nd ed. New York: Gilford; 2010.

De Bellis MD, Wooley DP, Hooper SR. Neuropsychological findings in pediatric maltreatment: relationship of PTSD, dissociative symptoms and abuse/neglect indices to neurocognitive outcomes. *Child Maltreat*. 2013;18(3):171–183.

DeShong HL, Kurtz JE. Four factors of impulsivity differentiate antisocial and borderline personality disorders. *J Pers Disord*. 2013;27(2):144–156.

de Waal MWM, van der Weele GM, van der Mast RC, Assendelft WJJ, Gussekloo J. The influence of the administration method on scores of the 15-item Geriatric Depression Scale in old age. *Psychiatry Res*. 2012;197(3):280–284.

Doss AJ. Evidence-based diagnosis: incorporating diagnostic instruments into clinical practice. *J Am Acad Child Adolesc Psychiatry*. 2005;44(9):947–952.

Dougall N, Lambert P, Maxwell M, Dawson A, Sinnott R, McCafferty S, Springbett A. Deaths by suicide and their relationship with general and psychiatric hospital discharge: 30-year record linkage study. *Br J Psychiatry*. 2014;204(4):267–273.

Flanagan DP, Harrison PL, eds. *Contemporary Intellectual Assessment*. 3rd ed. Theories, Tests, and Issues. New York: Guilford; 2012.

Fletcher JM, Lyon RG, Fuchs LS, Barnes MA. *Learning Disabilities: From Identification to Intervention*. New York: Guilford; 2007.

Fornito A, Bullmore ET. Does fMRI have a role in personalized health care for psychiatric patients? In: Gordon E, Koslow SH, eds. *Integrative Neuroscience and Personalized Medicine*. New York: Oxford University Press; 2011:55.

Foster NL. Validating FDG-PET as a biomarker for frontotemporal dementia. *Exp Neurol*. 2003;184(Suppl 1):S2–S8.

Frazier JA, Giuliano AJ, Johnson JL, Yakuris L, Youngstrom EA, Breiger D, Sikich L, Findling RL, McClellan J, Hamer RM, Vitiello B, Lieberman JA, Hooper SA. Neurocognitive outcomes in the treatment of early-onset schizophrenia Spectrum Disorders Study. *J Am Acad Child Adolesc Psychiatry*. 2012;51:496–505.

Garden G. Physical examination in psychiatric practice. *Adv Psychiatr Treat*. 2005; 11:142–149.

Gearing RE, Townsend L, Elkins J, El-Bassel N, Osterberg L. Strategies to predict, measure, and improve psychosocial treatment adherence. *Harv Rev Psychiatry*. 2014;22(1):31–45.

Gibbons RD, Weiss DJ, Pilkonis PA, Frank E, Moore T, Kim JB, Kupfer DJ. Development of a computerized adaptive test for depression. *Arch Gen Psychiatry*. 2012;69(11):1104–1112.

Guze BH, James M. Medical assessment and laboratory testing in psychiatry. In: Sadock BJ, Sadock VA, Ruiz P, eds. *Kaplan & Sadock's Comprehensive Textbook of Psychiatry*. 9th ed. Philadelphia, PA: Lippincott Williams & Wilkins; 2009:995.

Guze BH, Love MJ. Medical assessment and laboratory testing in psychiatry. In: Sadock BJ, Sadock VA, eds. *Kaplan & Sadock's Comprehensive Textbook of Psychiatry*. 8th ed. Vol. 1. Philadelphia, PA: Lippincott Williams & Wilkins; 2005:916.

Hamilton J. Clinician's guide to evidence-based practice. *J Am Acad Child Adolesc Psychiatry*. 2005;44(5):494–498.

Hamilton J. The answerable question and a hierarchy of evidence. *J Am Acad Child Adolesc Psychiatry*. 2005;44(6):596–600.

Hentschel AG, Livesley W. Differentiating normal and disordered personality using the General Assessment of Personality Disorder (GAPD). *Pers Mental Health*. 2013;7(2):133–142.

Hodgson R, Adeyamo O. Physical examination performed by psychiatrists. *Int J Psychiatr Clin Pract*. 2004;8(1):57–60.

Hoff HA, Rypdal K, Mykletun A, Cooke DJ. A prototypicality validation of the Comprehensive Assessment of Psychopathic Personality model (CAPP). *J Pers Disord*. 2012;26(3):414–427.

Holt DJ, Coombs G, Zeidan MA, Goff DC, Milad MR. Failure of neural responses to safety cues in schizophrenia. *Arch Gen Psychiatry*. 2012;69(9):893–903.

Holtz JL. *Applied Clinical Neuropsychology: An Introduction*. New York: Springer; 2011.

Hooper SR, Giulano AJ, Youngstrom EA, Breiger D, Sikich L, Frazier JA, Findling RL McClellan J, Hamer RM, Vitiello B, Lieberman JA. Neurocognition in early-onset schizophrenia and schizoaffective disorders. *J Am Acad Child Adolesc Psychiatry*. 2010;49(1):52–60.

Hopwood CJ, Moser JS. Personality assessment inventory internalizing and externalizing structure in college students: invariance across sex and ethnicity. *Pers Individ Dif*. 2011;50:116.

Howieson DB, Lezak MD. The neuropsychological evaluation. In: Yudosfky SC, Hales RE, eds. *Essentials of Neuropsychiatry and Behavioral Neurosciences*. 2nd ed. Arlington, VA: American Psychiatric Publishing; 2010:29.

Israel S, Moffitt TE, Belsky DW, Hancox RJ, Poulton R, Roberts B, Thomson WM, Caspi A. (2014). Translating personality psychology to help personalize preventive medicine for young adult patients. *J Pers Soc Psychol*. 2014;106(3):484–498.

Jeste D. Geriatric psychiatry: introduction. In: Sadock BJ, Sadock VA, Ruiz P, eds. *Kaplan & Sadock's Comprehensive Textbook of Psychiatry*. 9th ed. Philadelphia, PA: Lippincott Williams & Wilkins; 2009:3932.

Jura MB, Humphrey LA. Neuropsychological and cognitive assessment of children. In: Sadock BJ, Sadock VA, Ruiz P, eds. *Kaplan & Sadock's Comprehensive Textbook of Psychiatry*. 9th ed. Philadelphia, PA: Lippincott Williams & Wilkins; 2009:973.

Kavanaugh B, Holler KI, Selke G. A neuropsychological profile of childhood maltreatment within an adolescent inpatient sample. *Appl Neuropsychol Child*. 2015;4(1):9–19.

Keedwell PA, Linden DE. Integrative neuroimaging in mood disorders. *Curr Opin Psychiatry*. 2013;26(1):27–32.

Kestenbaum CJ. The clinical interview of the child. In: Wiener JM, Dulcan MK, eds. *The American Psychiatric Publishing Textbook of Child and Adolescent Psychiatry*. 3rd ed. Washington, DC: American Psychiatric Publishing, Inc.; 2004:103–111.

Kim HF, Schulz PE, Wilde EA, Yudosfky SC. Laboratory testing and imaging studies in psychiatry. In: Hales RE, Yudosfky SC, Gabbard GO, eds. *Essentials of Psychiatry*. 3rd ed. Arlington, VA: American Psychiatric Publishing; 2011:15.

King RA, Schwab-Stone ME, Thies AP, Peterson BS, Fisher PW. Psychiatric examination of the infant, child, and adolescent. In: Sadock BJ, Sadock VA, eds. *Kaplan & Sadock's Comprehensive Textbook of Psychiatry*. 9th ed. Vol. II. Philadelphia, PA: Lippincott Williams & Wilkins; 2009:3366.

Kolanowski AM, Fick DM, Yevchak AM, Hill NL, Mulhall PM, McDowell JA. Pay attention! The critical importance of assessing attention in older adults with dementia. *J Gerontol Nurs*. 2012;38(11):23–27.

Korja M, Ylijoki M, Japinleimu H, Pohjola P, Matomäki J, Kuśmierek H, Mahlman M, Rikalainen H, Parkkola R, Kaukola T, Lehtonen L, Hallman M, Haataja L. Apolipoprotein E, brain injury and neurodevelopmental outcome of children. *Genes Brain Beh*. 2013;28(4):435–445.

Lambert TJ, Velakoulis D, Pantelis C. Medical comorbidity in schizophrenia. *Med J Aust*. 2003;178(Suppl):S67–S70.

Leentjens AFG, Dujardin K, Marsh L, Richard IH, Starkstein SE, Martinez-Martin P. Anxiety rating scales in Parkinson's disease: a validation study of the Hamilton anxiety rating scale, the Beck anxiety inventory, and the hospital anxiety and depression scale. *Mov Disord*. 2011;26(3):407–415.

Lewis DA, Gonzalez-Burgos G. Pathophysiologically based treatment interventions in schizophrenia. *Nat Med*. 2006;12(9):1016–1022.

Lim HK, Aizenstein HJ. Recent findings and newer paradigms of neuroimaging research in geriatric psychiatry. *J Geriatr Psychiatry Neurol*. 2014;27(1):3–4.

Lyndenmayer JP, Czobor P, Volavka J, Sheitman B, McEvoy JP, Cooper TB, Chakos M, Lieberman JA. Changes in glucose and cholesterol levels in patients with schizophrenia treated with typical or atypical antipsychotics. *Am J Psychiatry*. 2003;160:290–296.

Lyneham HJ, Rapee RM. Evaluation and treatment of anxiety disorders in the general pediatric population: a clinician's guide. *Child Adolesc Psychiatr Clin N Am*. 2005;14(4):845–861.

Marder SR, Essock SM, Miller AL, Buchanan RW, Casey DE, Davis JM, Kane JM, Lieberman J, Schooler NR, Covell N, Stroup S, Weissman EM, Wirshing DA, Hall CS, Pogach L, Xavier P, Bigger JT, Friedman A, Kleinber D, Yevich S, Davis B, Shon S. Health monitoring of patients with schizophrenia. *Am J Psychiatry*. 2004;161(9):1334–1349.

Mason GF, Krystal JH, Sanacora G. Nuclear magnetic resonance imaging and spectroscopy: basic principles and recent findings in neuropsychiatric disorders. In: Sadock BJ, Sadock VA, Ruiz P, eds. *Kaplan & Sadock's Comprehensive Textbook of Psychiatry*. 9th ed. Philadelphia, PA: Lippincott Williams & Wilkins; 2009:248.

Matson JL, Hess JA, Mahan S, Fodstad JC, Neal D. Assessment of the relationship between diagnoses of ASD and caregiver symptom endorsement in adults diagnosed with intellectual disability. *Res Dev Disabil*. 2013;34(1):168–173.

Mattis S, Papolos D, Luck D, Cockerham M, Thode HC Jr. Neuropsychological factors differentiating treated children with pediatric bipolar disorder from those with attention-deficit/hyperactivity disorder. *J Clin Experi Neuropsychology*. 2011;33(1):74–84.

McDowell I, Newell C. *Measuring Health: A Guide to Rating Scales and Questionnaires*. New York: Oxford University Press; 2006.

McIntyre KM, Norton JR, McIntyre JS. Psychiatric interview, history, and mental status examination. In: Sadock BJ, Sadock VA, Ruiz P, eds. *Kaplan & Sadock's Comprehensive Textbook of Psychiatry*. 9th ed. Philadelphia, PA: Lippincott Williams & Wilkins; 2009:886.

Meszaros ZS, Perl A, Faraone SV. Psychiatric symptoms in systemic lupus erythematosus: a systematic review. *J Clin Psychiatry*. 2012;73(7):993–1001.

Migo EM, Williams SCR, Crum WR, Kempton MJ, Ettinger U. The role of neuroimaging biomarkers in personalized medicine for neurodegenerative and psychiatric disorders. In: Gordon E, Koslow SH, eds. *Integrative Neuroscience and Personalized Medicine*. New York: Oxford University Press; 2011:141.

Minden SL, Feinstein A, Kalb RC, Miller D, Mohr DC, Patten SB, Bever C, Schiffer RB, Gronseth GS, Narayanaswami P. Evidence-based guideline: assessment and management of psychiatric disorders in individuals with MS Report of the Guideline Development Subcommittee of the American Academy of Neurology. *Neurology*. 2014;82(2):174–181.

Mordal J, Holm B, Mørland J, Bramness JG. Recent substance intake among patients admitted to acute psychiatric wards: physician's assessment and on-site urine testing compared with comprehensive laboratory analyses. *J Clin Psychopharm*. 2010;30(4):455–459.

Morgan JE, Ricker JH. *Textbook of Clinical Neuropsychology*. New York: Psychology Press; 2008.

Morgenstern J, Naqvi NH, Debellis R, Breiter HC. The contributions of cognitive neuroscience and neuroimaging to understanding mechanisms of behavior change in addiction. *Psychol Addict Behav*. 2013;27(2):336–350.

Ng B, Atkins M. Home assessment in old age psychiatry: a practical guide. *Adv Psychiatry Treat*. 2012;18:400.

Oberheim NA, Wang X, Goldman S, Nedergaard M. Astrocytic complexity distinguishes the human brain. *Trends Neurosci*. 2006;29(10):547–553.

Pachet A, Astner K, Brown L. Clinical utility of the mini-mental status examination when assessing decision-making capacity. *J Geriatr Psychiatry Neurol*. 2010;23(1):3–8.

Pataki CS. Child psychiatry: introduction and overview. In: Sadock BJ, Sadock VA, eds. *Kaplan & Sadock's Comprehensive Textbook of Psychiatry*. 9th ed. Philadelphia, PA: Lippincott Williams & Wilkins; 2009:3335.

Pavletic AJ, Pao M, Pine DS, Luckenbaugh DA, Rosing DR. Screening electrocardiograms in psychiatric research: implications for physicians and healthy volunteers. *Int J Clin Pract*. 2014;68(1):117–121.

Pennington B. *Diagnosing Learning Disorders: A Neuropsychological Framework*. 2nd ed. New York: Guilford; 2008.

Perez VB, Swerdlow NR, Braff DL, Näätänen R, Light GA. Using biomarkers to inform diagnosis, guide treatments and track response to interventions in psychotic illnesses. *Biomark Med*. 2014;8(1):9–14.

Philips ML, Vieta E. Identifying functional neuroimaging biomarkers of bipolar disorder. In: Tamminga CA, Sirovatka PJ, Regier DA, van Os J, eds. *Deconstructing Psychosis: Refining the Research Agenda for DSM-V*. Arlington, VA: American Psychiatric Association; 2010:131.

Posner K, Brown GK, Stanley B, Brent DA, Yershova KV, Oquendo MA, Currier GW, Melvin GA, Greenhill L, Shen S, Mann JJ. The Columbia–Suicide Severity Rating Scale: initial validity and internal consistency findings from three multisite studies with adolescents and adults. *Am J Psychiatry*. 2011;168(12):1266–1277.

Puig-Antich J, Orraschel H, Tabrizi MA, Chambers W. *Schedule for Affective Disorders and Schizophrenia for School-Age Children-Epidemiologic Version*. New York: New York State Psychiatric Institute and Yale School of Medicine; 1980.

Purgato M, Barbui C. Dichotomizing rating scale scores in psychiatry: a bad idea? *Epidemiol Psychiatric Sci*. 2013;22(1):17–19.

Recupero PR. The mental status examination in the age of the internet. *J Am Acad Psychiatry Law*. 2010;38(1):15–26.

Robert G, Le Jeune F, Lozachmeur C, Drapier S, Dondaine T, Péron J, Travers D, Sauleau P, Millet B, Vérin M, Drapier D. Apathy in patients with Parkinson disease without dementia or depression: a PET study. *Neurology*. 2012;79(11):1155.

Roffman JL, Silverman BC, Stern TA. Diagnostic rating scales and laboratory testing. In: Stern TA, Fricchione GL, Cassem NH, Jellinek M, Rosenbaum JF, eds. *Massachusetts General Hospital Handbook of General Hospital Psychiatry*. 6th ed. Philadelphia, PA: Saunders; 2010:61.

Rosse RB, Deutsch LH, Deutsch SI. Medical assessment and laboratory testing in psychiatry. In: Sadock BJ, Sadock VA, eds. *Kaplan & Sadock's Comprehensive Textbook of Psychiatry*. 7th ed. Vol. 1. Philadelphia, PA: Lippincott Williams & Wilkins; 2000:732.

Rush J, First MB, Blacker D, eds. *Handbook of Psychiatric Measures*. 2nd ed. Washington, DC: American Psychiatric Press; 2007.

Ryan JJ, Gontkovsky ST, Kreiner DS, Tree HA. Wechsler adult intelligence scale–fourth edition performance in relapsing–remitting multiple sclerosis. *J Clin Exp Neuropsychol*. 2012;34(6):571–579.

Saczynski JS, Marcantonio ER, Quach L, Fong TG, Gross A, Inouye SK, Jones RN. Cognitive trajectories after postoperative delirium. *N Engl J Med*. 2012;367(1):30–39.

Samuel DB, Hopwood CJ, Krueger RF, Patrick CJ. Comparing methods for scoring personality disorder types using maladaptive traits in DSM-5. *Assessment*. 2013; 20(3):353–361.

Saunders RD, Keshavan MS. Physical and neurologic examinations in neuropsychiatry. *Semin Clin Neuropsychiatry*. 2002;7(1):18–29.

Scholle SH, Vuong O, Ding L, Fry S, Gallagher P, Brown JA, Hays RD, Cleary PD. Development of and field test results for the CAHPS PCMH survey. *Med Care*. 2012;50(Suppl):S2–S10.

Schulte P. What is an adequate trial with clozapine? Therapeutic drug monitoring and time to response in treatment refractory schizophrenia. *Clin Pharmacokinet*. 2003;42(7):607–618.

Schuppert HM, Bloo J, Minderaa RB, Emmelkamp PM, Nauta MH. Psychometric evaluation of the Borderline Personality Disorder Severity Index-IV—adolescent version and parent version. *J Pers Disord*. 2012;26(4):628–640.

Simon RI. *Clinical Psychiatry and the Law*. American Psychiatric Pub; 2003.

Staley JK, Krystal JH. Radiotracer imaging with positron emission tomography and single photon emission computed tomography. In: Sadock BJ, Sadock VA, Ruiz P, eds. *Kaplan & Sadock's Comprehensive Textbook of Psychiatry*. 9th ed. Philadelphia, PA: Lippincott Williams & Wilkins; 2009:273.

Staller JA. Diagnostic profiles in outpatient child psychiatry. *Am J Orthopsychiatry*. 2006;76(1):98–102.

Stark D, Thomas S, Dawson D, Talbot E, Bennett E, Starza-Smith A. Paediatric neuropsychological assessment: an analysis of parents' perspectives. *Soc Care Neurodisabil*. 2014;5:41–50.

Stowell KR, Florence P, Harman HJ, Glick RL. Psychiatric evaluation of the agitated patient: consensus statement of the American Association for Emergency Psychiatry project BETA psychiatric evaluation workgroup. *West J Emerg Med*. 2012;13:11.

Strickland CM, Drislane LE, Lucy M, Krueger RF, Patrick CJ. Characterizing psychopathy using DSM-5 personality traits. *Assessment*. 2013;20(3):327–338.

Suchy Y. *Clinical Neuropsychology of Emotions*. New York: Guilford; 2011.

Swanda RM, Haaland KY. Clinical neuropsychology and intellectual assessment of adults. In: Sadock BJ, Sadock VA, Ruiz P, eds. *Kaplan & Sadock's Comprehensive Textbook of Psychiatry*. 9th ed. Philadelphia, PA: Lippincott Williams & Wilkins; 2009:935.

Thakur ME, Blazer DG, Steffens DC, eds. *Clinical Manual of Geriatric Psychiatry*. Arlington, VA: American Psychiatric Publishing; 2014.

Thapar A, Hammerton G, Collishaw S, Potter R, Rice F, Harold G, Craddock N, Thapar A, Smith DJ. Detecting recurrent major depressive disorder within primary care rapidly and reliably using short questionnaire measures. *Br J Gen Pract*. 2014; 64(618):e31–e37.

Tolin DF, Frost RO, Steketee G. A brief interview for assessing compulsive hoarding: the hoarding rating scale-interview. *Psychiatry Rev*. 2010;178(1):147–152.

Vannest J, Szaflarski JP, Eaton KP, Henkel DM, Morita D, Glauser TA, Byars AW, Patel K, Holland SK. Functional magnetic resonance imaging reveals changes in language localization in children with benign childhood epilepsy with centrotemporal spikes. *J Child Neurol*. 2013;28(4):435–445.

Weeks M, Wild TC, Poubidis GB, Naiker K, Cairney J, North CR, Colman I. Childhood cognitive ability and its relationship with anxiety and depression in adolescence. *J Affect Disord*. 2013 http://dx.doi.org/10.1016/j.jad.2013.08.019.

Williams L, Hermens D, Thein T, Clark C, Cooper N, Clarke S, Lamb C, Gordon E, Kohn M. Using brain-based cognitive measures to support clinical decisions in ADHD. *Pediatr Neurol*. 2010;42(2):118–126.

Wilson KCM, Green B, Mottram P. Overview of rating scales in old age psychiatry. In: Abou-Saleh MT, Katona C, Kumar A, eds. *Principles and Practice of Geriatric Psychiatry*. 3rd ed. Hoboken, NJ: Wiley; 2011.

Winters NC, Collett BR, Myers KM. Ten-year review of rating scales, VII: scales assessing functional impairment. *J Am Acad Child Adolesc Psychiatry*. 2005;44(4):309–338.

Youngstrom EA, Duax J. Evidence-based assessment of pediatric bipolar disorder. Part 1: base rate and family history. *J Am Acad Child Adolesc Psychiatry*. 2005;44(7):712–717.

2 ▲

Neurodevelopmental Disorders and Other Childhood Disorders

This section contains disorders typically found in children. Some disorders are disorders of development and invariably present during childhood or adolescence. Others are more common disorders, such as depression or anxiety, that may have unique presentations or treatment issues in children.

▲ 2.1 Intellectual Disability

Intellectual disability (ID), formerly known as *mental retardation,* can be caused by a range of environmental and genetic factors that lead to a combination of cognitive and social impairments. The American Association on Intellectual and Developmental Disability (AAIDD) defines intellectual disability as a disability characterized by significant limitations in both intellectual functioning (reasoning, learning, and problem-solving) and in adaptive behavior (conceptual, social, and practical skills) that emerges before the age of 18 years.

The widespread acceptance of this definition has led to the international consensus that an assessment of both social adaptation and intelligence quotient (IQ) is necessary to determine the level of intellectual disability. Measures of adaptive function assess competency in social functioning, understanding of societal norms, and performance of everyday tasks, whereas measures of intellectual function focus on cognitive abilities. Although individuals with a given intellectual level do not all have identical levels of adaptive function, epidemiologic data suggest that a person's intellectual level and level of adaptive function largely determine the prevalence of intellectual disability and typically correspond closely with cognitive ability.

In the *Diagnostic and Statistical Manual of Mental Disorders,* Fifth Edition (DSM-5), various levels of severity of intellectual disability are determined based on adaptive functioning, not on IQ scores. DSM-5 has adopted this change in emphasis from prior diagnostic manuals because adaptive functioning determines the level of support that is required. Furthermore, IQ scores are less valid in the lower portions of the IQ range. Deciding the severity level of intellectual disability, according to DSM-5, includes an assessment of functioning in a conceptual domain (e.g., academic skills), a social domain (e.g., relationships), and a practical domain (e.g., personal hygiene).

As it is older, the International Classification of Diseases, 10th Edition (ICD-10) continues to rely on IQ as the main determiner of severity; this is being revised for the next edition.

Societal approaches to children with intellectual disabilities have shifted significantly over time. Historically, in the mid-1800s, many children with intellectual disabilities were placed in residential, educational facilities based on the belief that with sufficient intensive training, these children would be able to return to their families and function in society at a higher level. However, many residential programs increased in size, and eventually, the focus began to shift from intensive education to custodial care. Residential settings for children with an intellectual disability received their maximal use in the mid-1900s until public awareness of the crowded, unsanitary, and, in some cases, abusive conditions sparked the movement toward "deinstitutionalization." A vital force in the deinstitutionalization of children with intellectual disability was the philosophy of "normalization" in living situations, and "inclusion" in educational settings. Since the late 1960s, placing children with intellectual disabilities into institutions is rare, and the concepts of normalization and inclusion remain prominent among advocacy groups and parents.

The passage of Public Law 94–142 (the Education for all Handicapped Children Act) in 1975 mandates that the public school system provides appropriate educational services to all children with disabilities. The Individuals with Disabilities Act in 1990 extended and modified the above legislation. Currently, the provision of public education for all children, including those with disabilities, "within the least restrictive environment" is mandated by law.

In addition to the educational system, advocacy groups, including the Council for Exceptional Children (CEC) and the Arc of the United States (The Arc), are well-known parental lobbying organizations for children with intellectual disability and were instrumental in advocating for Public Law 94–142. The American Association on Intellectual and Developmental Disabilities (AAIDD) is the most prominent advocacy organization in this field. It has been very influential in educating the public about and supporting research and legislation relating to intellectual disability.

The AAIDD promotes a view of intellectual disability as a functional interaction between an individual and the environment, rather than a static designation of a person's limitations. Within this conceptual framework, a child or adolescent with an intellectual disability is determined to need intermittent, limited, extensive, or pervasive "environmental support" concerning a specific set of adaptive function domains. These include communication, self-care, home living, social or interpersonal skills, use of community resources, self-direction, functional academic skills, work, leisure, health, and safety.

The United Nations Convention on the Rights of Persons with Disabilities (2006) has created a forum to promote the full social inclusion of people with intellectual disabilities. Through its recognition and focus on social barriers, this international forum aims

Table 2-1
Intellectual Disability

	DSM-5	ICD-10
Diagnostic name	Intellectual Disability (Intellectual Developmental Disorder)	Mental Retardation
Duration	The symptoms arise during development	Occurs during the developmental period
Symptoms	Deficits in: • Reasoning • Abstraction • Judgment • Learning • Adaptive functioning	Incomplete mental development Affects skills related to intelligence: • Cognitive • Language • Motor • Social abilities
Psychosocial consequences of symptoms	Symptoms delay developmental milestones, achieving independence and social functioning	
Severity specifiers	Profound Severe Moderate Mild	Estimated by IQ: Mild: 50–69 Moderate: 35–49 Severe: 20–34 Profound: <20

to provide protections for individuals with intellectual disabilities and to seek more inclusion of those with intellectual disabilities in social, civic, and educational activities.

NOMENCLATURE

The accurate definition of intellectual disability has been a challenge for clinicians over the centuries. All current classification systems underscore that intellectual disability is more than a cognitive deficit. That is, it also includes impaired social adaptive function. According to DSM-5, we should only make a diagnosis of intellectual disability when there are deficits in intellectual functioning and deficits in adaptive functioning (Table 2-1). Once intellectual

disability is recognized, we determine the level of severity by the level of adaptive functional impairment.

CLASSIFICATION

DSM-5 criteria for intellectual disability include significantly subaverage general intellectual functioning associated with concurrent impairment in adaptive behavior manifested before the age of 18. The diagnosis is made independent of coexisting physical or mental disorders. Table 2-2 presents an overview of developmental levels in communication, academic functioning, and vocational skills expected of persons with various degrees of intellectual disability.

Table 2-2
Developmental Characteristics of Intellectual Disability

Level of Intellectual Disability	Preschool Age (0–5 yr) Maturation and Development	School Age (6–20 yr) Training and Education	Adult (21 yr and Above) Social and Vocational Adequacy
Profound	Gross disability; minimal capacity for functioning in sensorimotor areas; needs nursing care; constant aid and supervision required	Some motor development present; may respond to minimal or limited training in self-help	Some motor and speech development; may achieve very limited self-care; needs nursing care
Severe	Poor motor development; speech minimal; generally unable to profit from training in self-help; little or no communication skills	Can talk or learn to communicate; can be trained in elemental health habits; profits from systematic habit training; unable to profit from vocational training	May contribute partially to self-maintenance under complete supervision; can develop self-protection skills to a minimal useful level in controlled environment
Moderate	Can talk or learn to communicate; poor social awareness; fair motor development; profits from training in self-help; can be managed with moderate supervision	Can profit from training in social and occupational skills; unlikely to progress beyond second-grade level in academic subjects; may learn to travel alone in familiar places	May achieve self-maintenance in unskilled or semiskilled work under sheltered conditions; needs supervision and guidance when under mild social or economic stress
Mild	Can develop social and communication skills; minimal retardation in sensorimotor areas; often not distinguished from normal until later age	Can learn academic skills up to approximately sixth-grade level by late teens; can be guided toward social conformity	Can usually achieve social and vocational skills adequate for minimal self-support, but may need guidance and assistance when under unusual social or economic stress

Adapted from *Mental Retarded Activities of the US Department of Health, Education and Welfare*. Washington, DC: US Government Printing Office; 1989:2, with permission.

If we choose to use a standardized test of intelligence—which is still a common practice—the term *significantly subaverage* is defined as an IQ of approximately 70 or below or two standard deviations below the mean for the particular test. We can measure adaptive functioning by using a standardized scale, such as the *Vineland Adaptive Behavior Scale.* This scale scores communications, daily living skills, socialization, and motor skills (up to 4 years, 11 months) and generates an adaptive behavior composite that correlates with the expected skills at a given age.

Approximately 85 percent of individuals who have an intellectual disability fall within the DSM-5 mild intellectual disability category. This category requires an IQ between 50 and 70 and an adaptive function severity in the mild range. Adaptive function includes skills such as communication, self-care, social skills, work, leisure, and understanding of safety. Genetic, environmental, and psychosocial factors all influence intellectual disability. A host of subtle environmental and developmental factors, including subclinical lead intoxication and prenatal exposure to drugs, alcohol, and other toxins, can contribute to intellectual disability. Specific genetic syndromes associated with intellectual disability such as fragile X syndrome, Down syndrome, and Prader–Willi syndrome have characteristic patterns of social, linguistic, and cognitive development and typical behavioral manifestations.

DEGREES OF SEVERITY OF INTELLECTUAL DISABILITY

DSM-5 classifies the severity levels of intellectual disability as mild, moderate, severe, and profound. "Borderline intellectual functioning," a term previously used to describe individuals with an IQ in the range of 70 to 80, is no longer described as a diagnosis in DSM-5, and is instead listed as a condition that may be the focus of clinical attention; although DSM-5 does not offer any criteria.

Mild intellectual disability represents approximately 85 percent of persons with intellectual disabilities. Children with mild intellectual disabilities often are not identified until the first or second grade, when academic demands increase. By late adolescence, they often acquire academic skills at approximately a sixth-grade level. Specific causes for intellectual disability are often unidentified in this group. Many adults with mild intellectual disabilities can live independently with appropriate support and raise their own families. IQ for this level of adaptive function may typically range from 50 to 70.

Moderate intellectual disability represents about 10 percent of persons with intellectual disabilities. Most children with a moderate intellectual disability acquire language and can communicate adequately during early childhood. They are challenged academically and often are not able to achieve above a second- to third-grade level. During adolescence, socialization difficulties often set these persons apart, and a great deal of social and vocational support is beneficial. As adults, individuals with moderate intellectual disability may be able to perform semiskilled work under appropriate supervision. IQ for this level of adaptive function may typically range from 35 to 50.

Severe intellectual disability represents about 4 percent of individuals with intellectual disabilities. They may be able to develop communication skills in childhood and often can learn to count as well as recognize words that are critical to functioning. In this group, the cause for the intellectual disability is more likely to be identified than in milder forms of intellectual disability. In adulthood,

persons with severe intellectual disability may adapt well to supervised living situations, such as group homes, and may be able to perform work-related tasks under supervision. IQ in individuals with this level of adaptive function may typically range from 20 to 35.

Profound intellectual disability constitutes approximately 1 to 2 percent of individuals with intellectual disabilities. Most individuals with profound intellectual disabilities have identifiable causes for their condition. Children with profound intellectual disabilities may be taught some self-care skills and learn to communicate their needs, given the appropriate training. IQ in individuals with this level of adaptive function may typically be less than 20.

The DSM-5 also includes a disorder called "Unspecified Intellectual Disability" (Intellectual Developmental Disorder), reserved for individuals over the age of 5 years who are difficult to evaluate but likely have an intellectual disability. Individuals with this diagnosis may have sensory or physical impairments such as blindness or deafness, or concurrent mental disorders, making it challenging to administer standard assessment tools.

CLINICAL FEATURES

Mild intellectual disability may not be recognized or diagnosed in a child until school challenges the child's social and communication skills. Cognitive deficits include reduced ability to abstract and egocentric thinking, both of which become more readily evident as a child reaches middle childhood. Children with milder intellectual disabilities may function academically at the high elementary level and may acquire vocational skills sufficient to support themselves in some cases; however, social assimilation may be problematic. Communication deficits, poor self-esteem, and dependence may further contribute to a relative lack of social spontaneity.

Moderate levels of intellectual disability are significantly more likely to be observed at a younger age since communication skills develop more slowly, and social isolation may ensue in the elementary school years. Academic achievement is usually limited to the middle-elementary level. Children with moderate intellectual deficits benefit from individual attention focused on the development of self-help skills. However, these children are aware of their deficits and often feel alienated from their peers and frustrated by their limitations. They continue to require a relatively high level of supervision but can become competent at occupational tasks in supportive settings.

Severe intellectual disability is typically evident in the preschool years; affected children have minimal speech and impaired motor development. Some language development may occur in the school-age years. By adolescence, if the language has not improved significantly, nonverbal forms of communication may have evolved. Behavioral approaches are useful means to promote some self-care, although those with severe intellectual disabilities generally need extensive supervision.

Children with profound intellectual disabilities require constant supervision and are severely limited in both communication and motor skills. By adulthood, some speech development may be present, and simple self-help skills may be acquired. Clinical features frequently observed in populations with intellectual disability, either in isolation or as part of a mental disorder, include hyperactivity, low frustration tolerance, aggression, affective instability, repetitive and stereotypic motor behaviors, and self-injurious behaviors. Self-injurious behaviors occur more frequently and with higher intensity in more severe intellectual disability.

Dylan was a full-term infant, the second child born to his 42-year-old mother, a medical technician, and a 48-year-old father, a high school basketball coach. The pregnancy was unremarkable, and Dylan's sister, who was 2 years older, was healthy and developing typically. The family lived in a rural town in the Midwest.

Dylan was an extremely fussy, active newborn with extended periods of crying that the pediatrician labeled classic colic. As a newborn, Dylan seemed to have large ears and strabismus, which the pediatrician said would probably resolve spontaneously. At 2 months of age, at a regular pediatric visit, a systolic heart murmur was heard, and electrocardiography (ECG) revealed a mitral valve prolapse. Because Dylan was not cyanotic and had no other cardiac symptoms, his pediatrician monitored him without specific treatment. Although Dylan became less fussy over time, he remained very active, did not sleep through the night, and was a picky eater, refusing solid foods.

Milestones were slightly delayed, with Dylan sitting unassisted at 10 months and walking at 18 months. He had delayed language, and, although his first words appeared at 20 months, Dylan had always made his wants and needs known. Dylan's parents were concerned about his activity level and his developmental delays compared with his sister; however, the pediatrician reassured them that boys often develop more slowly than girls in the first 2 years.

When Dylan was 3 years of age, his preschool teacher noted that he was unable to pay attention, and he was hyperactive compared to his classmates, prompting his parents to obtain a developmental evaluation. Results showed modest delays in cognitive, linguistic, and motor functioning, with a developmental quotient (DQ) of 74. Dylan was inattentive, shy, and anxious, and he had poor eye contact. Enrolled in a special kindergarten, Dylan remained in a combination of special education and mainstreamed classes throughout his academic life.

At 7 years of age, the school psychologist evaluated Dylan, and results indicated that he met the criteria for a "learning disability" profile. Dylan had an overall IQ of 66, with close to normal functioning in short-term memory and pronounced deficits in long-term memory, expressive language, and visual–spatial functioning. Dylan struggled with writing tasks and arithmetic but loved science. Due to his significant problems with inattention and hyperactivity, Dylan was placed on Concerta, which was beneficial, and titrated up to 54 mg/day. He displayed transient, intense interests in unusual items, such as vacuum cleaners. When Dylan reached the older elementary grades, he began to have more difficulty socially, and some peers bullied him about being in special education and teased for his long head and big ears.

As he entered adolescence, Dylan became increasingly anxious, so much so that he occasionally rubbed his hands or rocked, and he "fretted" about day-to-day issues and what would happen next. His long-term sensitivities to loud sounds seemed to wane slightly, but he developed fears of storm clouds and dogs and refused to ride on elevators. Dylan became tearful and upset after his older sister left for a party, and worried that she might have a car accident. Dylan was very shy and would occasionally pace with worry and complain of stomachaches, but he attended school and had a small group of acquaintances in the Special Olympics bowling league. He enjoyed activities that did not involve much talking or sustained attention.

When Dylan was 17 years of age, his parents happened to watch a television documentary on genetic causes of intellectual disability. They were overwhelmed by the similarities between Dylan and some of the people described in the program. They later described the experience as a "jolt." They had always accepted Dylan, quirks and all, and had stopped pushing their doctors for reasons "why" when Dylan was a preschooler. Nevertheless, they immediately called the informational number offered in the show, and within 2 months, genetic tests confirmed a diagnosis of fragile X syndrome.

Although Dylan's day-to-day life did not change dramatically after the diagnosis, his parents reported a big difference in their approach to his shyness, restricted interests, and inattention. Dylan later received a selective serotonin reuptake inhibitor (SSRI) for anxiety, which decreased his social anxiety and facilitated activities with a few peers. Dylan's parents reported a mixture of feelings at having such a late diagnosis—disappointment in their doctors, relief in finally knowing, and twinges of guilt. They were energized by Dylan's positive responses to treatments for his attentional and anxiety symptoms and were pleased with Dylan's recent increased interest in sharing activities with classmates and peers.

A negative self-image and poor self-esteem are standard features of mildly and moderately intellectually disabled persons who are aware of their social and academic differences from others. Given their experience of repeated failure and disappointment in being unable to meet their parents' and society's expectations, they may also fall progressively behind younger siblings. Communication difficulties further increase their vulnerability to feelings of ineptness and frustration. Inappropriate behaviors, such as withdrawal, are common. The perpetual sense of isolation and inadequacy is related to feelings of anxiety, anger, dysphoria, and depression.

DIAGNOSIS

The diagnosis of intellectual disability occurs after obtaining the history, using information from a standardized intellectual assessment, and a standardized measure of adaptive function indicating that a child is significantly below the expected level in both areas. The severity of the intellectual disability is determined based on the level of adaptive function. A history and psychiatric interview are useful in obtaining a longitudinal picture of the child's development and functioning. Examination of physical signs, neurologic abnormalities, and in some cases, laboratory tests can help ascertain the cause and prognosis.

History

When we take the history, which may elucidate pathways to intellectual disability, we should pay particular attention to the mother's pregnancy, labor, and delivery; the presence of a family history of intellectual disability; consanguinity of the parents; and known familial hereditary disorders.

Chapter 1 details some approaches to interviewing and examining children with intellectual disabilities.

Laboratory Examination

Laboratory tests that may elucidate the causes of intellectual disability include chromosomal analysis, urine and blood testing for metabolic disorders, and neuroimaging. Chromosomal abnormalities are the most common known cause of intellectual disability.

Chromosome Studies.   When multiple physical anomalies, developmental delays, and intellectual disability present together, we should order chromosome analysis. Current techniques can identify chromosomal regions with specific fluorescent in situ hybridization (FISH) markers, enabling the identification of microscopic deletions in up to 7 percent of persons with moderate to severe intellectual disability. A history of growth retardation, the presence of microcephaly, a family history of intellectual disability, short stature, hypertelorism, and other facial abnormalities increase the risk of finding subtelomeric defects.

Amniocentesis, in which clinicians remove a small amount of amniotic fluid from the amniotic cavity transabdominally at about 15 weeks of gestation, has been useful for diagnosing prenatal chromosomal abnormalities. Its use is considered when an increased fetal risk exists, such as with increased maternal age. Amniotic fluid cells, mostly fetal in origin, are cultured for cytogenetic and biochemical studies.

Chorionic villi sampling (CVS) is a screening technique to determine fetal chromosomal abnormalities. It is done at 8 to 10 weeks of gestation, 6 weeks earlier than amniocentesis. The results are available in a short time (hours or days) and, if the result is abnormal, it is possible to decide to terminate the pregnancy within the first trimester. The procedure has a miscarriage risk between 2 and 5 percent; the risk in amniocentesis is lower (1 in 200). A noninvasive blood test called MaterniT21 is a proprietary prenatal test that detects abnormalities of chromosomes 21, 18, 13, X, and Y. It is highly specific for Down syndrome. There is a slight risk of miscarriage.

Urine and Blood Analysis.   Lesch–Nyhan syndrome, galactosemia, PKU, Hurler syndrome (Fig. 2-1), and Hunter syndrome (Fig. 2-2) are examples of disorders characterized by an intellectual disability that we can identify through assays of the appropriate enzyme or organic or amino acids. Enzymatic abnormalities in chromosomal disorders, such as Down syndrome, promise to become useful diagnostic tools.

Electroencephalography.   Whenever considering a seizure disorder, we should request electroencephalography (EEG). "Nonspecific" EEG changes, characterized by slow frequencies with bursts of spikes and sharp or blunt wave complexes, are found with higher frequency among populations with intellectual disability than in the general population; however, these findings do not elucidate specific diagnoses.

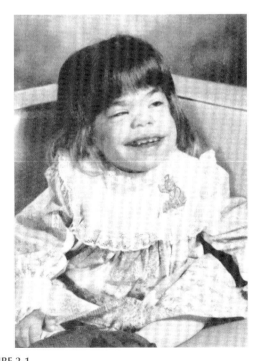

FIGURE 2-1

A 6-year-old girl with Hurler syndrome. Her care has involved a class for seriously multihandicapped children, attention to cardiac problems, and special counseling for patients. (Courtesy of L.S. Syzmanski, M.D. and A.C. Crocker, M.D.)

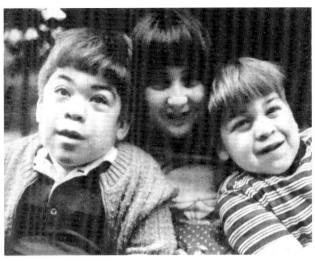

FIGURE 2-2

Two brothers, age 6 and 8 years, with Hunter syndrome, shown with their developmentally normal older sister. They have had significant developmental delay, trouble with recurrent respiratory infection, and behavioral abnormalities. (Courtesy of L.S. Syzmanski, M.D. and A.C. Crocker, M.D.)

Neuroimaging.   Neuroimaging studies with populations of intellectually disabled patients using either computerized tomography (CT) or magnetic resonance imaging (MRI) have found high rates of abnormalities in those patients with microcephaly, significant delay, cerebral palsy, and profound disability. Among patients with intellectual disability, seizures, microcephaly or macrocephaly, loss of previously acquired skills, or neurologic signs such as dystonia, spasticity, or altered reflexes all are indications for neuroimaging.

Although clinically not diagnostic, neuroimaging studies are currently also utilized to gather data that may eventually uncover biologic mechanisms contributing to intellectual disability. Structural MRI, functional MRI (fMRI), and diffusion tensor imaging (DTI) are useful in current research. For example, current data suggest that individuals with fragile X syndrome and concurrent attentional deficits are also more likely to show aberrant frontal–striatal pathways on MRI than those patients without attentional problems. MRI is also useful to elucidate myelination patterns. MRI studies can also provide a baseline for comparison of a later, potentially degenerative process in the brain.

Hearing and Speech Evaluations.   We should evaluate a patient's hearing and speech routinely. Speech development may be the most reliable criterion in investigating intellectual disability. Various hearing impairments often occur in persons who are intellectually disabled, but in some instances, hearing impairments can simulate intellectual disability. The commonly used methods of hearing and speech evaluation, however, require the patient's cooperation and, thus, are often unreliable in severely disabled persons.

DIFFERENTIAL DIAGNOSIS

By definition, an intellectual disability must begin before the age of 18. In some cases, severe child maltreatment in the form of neglect or abuse may contribute to delays in development, which can appear to be an intellectual disability. However, these damages are partially reversible when a child grows up in a corrective, enriched, and stimulating environment. Sensory disabilities, especially deafness and blindness, can be mistaken for intellectual disability when a lack of awareness of the sensory deficit leads to inappropriate testing. Expressive and receptive speech disorders may give the impression of intellectual disability in a child of average intelligence, and cerebral palsy may be mistaken for intellectual disability. Chronic, debilitating medical diseases may depress and delay a child's functioning and achievement despite average intelligence. Seizure disorders, especially uncontrolled, may contribute to persisting intellectual disability. Specific syndromes leading to isolated handicaps such as failure to read (alexia), failure to write (agraphia), or failure to communicate (aphasia), may occur in a child of average and even superior intelligence. Children with learning disorders (which can coexist with intellectual disability) experience a delay or failure of development in a specific area, such as reading or mathematics, but they usually develop in other areas. In contrast, children with intellectual disabilities show delays in most areas of development.

Intellectual disability and autism spectrum disorder (ASD) often coexist; 70 to 75 percent of those with ASD have an IQ below 70. Also, epidemiologic data indicate that ASD occurs in approximately 19.8 percent of persons with intellectual disabilities. Children with ASD have relatively more severe impairment in social relatedness and language than other children with the same level of intellectual disability.

A child younger than the age of 18 years with significant adaptive functional impairment, with an IQ less than 70, who also meets diagnostic criteria for dementia, will receive both a diagnosis of dementia and intellectual disability. However, a child whose IQ drops below 70 after the age of 18 years with newly acquired cognitive impairment will receive only the diagnosis of dementia.

COMORBIDITY

Many psychiatric disorders are common with intellectual disabilities, including depressive disorders, attention-deficit disorders, anxiety and neurologic disorders.

Attention-Deficit/Hyperactivity Disorder

Estimates of attention-deficit/hyperactivity disorder (ADHD) and ADHD-like symptoms among children with subaverage intelligence, genetic disorders, and developmental delay are estimated to be significantly higher than rates in the community.

Neurologic Disorders

Seizure disorders occur more frequently in individuals with intellectual disabilities than in the general population, and prevalence rates for seizures increase proportionally to the severity level of intellectual disability. A review of psychiatric disorders in children and adolescents with intellectual disability and epilepsy found that approximately one-third had comorbid autism spectrum disorder. The combination of intellectual disability, epilepsy, and autism spectrum disorder may occur in 0.07 percent of the general population.

COURSE AND PROGNOSIS

Although the underlying intellectual impairment does not improve, in most cases of intellectual disability, the level of adaptation increases with age and can be influenced positively by an enriched and supportive environment. In general, persons with mild and moderate intellectual disabilities have the most flexibility in adapting to various environmental conditions. Comorbid psychiatric disorders negatively impact overall prognosis. When psychiatric disorders co-occur with intellectual disabilities, standard treatments for comorbid mental disorders are often beneficial; however, less robust responses and increased vulnerability to side effects of psychopharmacologic agents are common.

TREATMENT

Interventions for children and adolescents with intellectual disabilities incorporate an assessment of social, educational, psychiatric, and environmental needs. Intellectual disability is associated with a variety of comorbid psychiatric disorders that often require specific treatment, in addition to psychosocial support. Of course, when preventive measures are available, the optimal approach includes primary, secondary, and tertiary interventions.

Prevention

Primary Prevention.   Primary prevention comprises actions taken to eliminate or reduce the conditions that lead to the development of intellectual disability, as well as associated disorders. For example, screening babies for PKU, and administrating a low phenylalanine diet when PKU is present, significantly alters the emergence of intellectual disability in those affected children. Additional primary prevention steps include education of the general public about strategies to prevent intellectual disability, such as abstinence from alcohol during pregnancy, continuing efforts of health professionals to ensure and upgrade public health policies, and legislation to provide optimal maternal and child health care. Family and genetic counseling help reduce the incidence of intellectual disability in a family with a history of a genetic disorder.

Secondary and Tertiary Prevention.   Prompt attention to medical and psychiatric complications of intellectual disability can diminish their course (secondary prevention) and minimize the sequelae or consequent disabilities (tertiary prevention). Hereditary metabolic and endocrine disorders, such as PKU and hypothyroidism, can be treated effectively in an early stage by dietary control or hormone replacement therapy.

Psychosocial Interventions

Educational Interventions.   Educational settings for children with intellectual disability should include a comprehensive program that addresses academics and training in adaptive skills, social skills, and vocational skills. Particular attention should focus on communication and efforts to improve the quality of life.

Behavioral and Cognitive-Behavioral Interventions.   The difficulties in adaptation among the intellectual disability populations are widespread and so varied that several interventions alone or in combination may be beneficial. Behavior therapy has been used for many years to shape and enhance social behaviors and to control and minimize aggressive and destructive behaviors. Positive reinforcement for desired behaviors and benign punishment (e.g., loss of privileges) for objectionable behaviors has been helpful. Cognitive therapy, such as dispelling false beliefs and relaxation exercises with self-instruction, has also been recommended for intellectually disabled persons who can follow the instructions. Psychodynamic therapy has been used with patients and their families to decrease conflicts about expectations that result in persistent anxiety, rage, and depression. Psychiatric treatment modalities require modifications that take into consideration the patient's level of intelligence.

Family Education.   One of the most critical areas that we can address is educating the family of a child or adolescent with intellectual disability about ways to enhance competence and self-esteem while maintaining realistic expectations for the patient. The family often finds it challenging to balance the fostering of independence and the providing of a nurturing and supportive environment for an intellectually disabled child, who is likely to experience some rejection and failure outside the family context. The parents may benefit from continuous counseling or family therapy and should be allowed opportunities to express their feelings of guilt, despair, anguish, recurring denial, and anger about their child's disorder and future. We should give the parents all the necessary and current medical information regarding causes, treatment, and other pertinent areas (e.g., specialized training and the correction of sensory defects).

Social Intervention.   One of the most prevalent problems among persons with an intellectual disability is a sense of social isolation and social skills deficits. Thus, improving the quantity and quality of social competence is a critical part of their care. Special Olympics International is the most extensive recreational sports program geared for this population. In addition to providing a forum to develop physical fitness, Special Olympics also enhances social interactions, friendships, and (hopefully) general self-esteem.

Psychopharmacologic Interventions

Pharmacologic approaches to the treatment of behavioral and psychological symptoms in children with an intellectual disability follow the paradigms of the evidence-based literature on treatment for all children with psychiatric disorders. However, given the paucity of randomized trials in the childhood intellectual disability population, an empirical approach must also be taken.

Treating Comorbid Disorders and Symptoms

AGGRESSION, IRRITABILITY, AND SELF-INJURIOUS BEHAVIOR.   Antipsychotic medicine may be useful for reducing challenging behaviors. Among the antipsychotics, both aripiprazole and risperidone had reasonable effect sizes in multiple studies. However, we should view these findings cautiously as many of the studies had significant methodologic limitations. Overall, the consensus seems to be that antipsychotics are helpful in the short term. Among them, aripiprazole and risperidone have the majority of studies and show effect sizes in the moderate to large range. There is little evidence on the long-term use of these medications. Given the significant side effects (weight gain, sedation, cardiovascular risks, extrapyramidal side effects, and increased prolactin levels, which are of particular concern in children), we should be very cautious when choosing to use these medications beyond an acute crisis.

Other medications, such as anticonvulsants and antioxidants, may be helpful; however, the data are not conclusive. GABA analogs, such as piracetam, may have promise, but the supportive data are limited.

ATTENTION-DEFICIT/HYPERACTIVITY DISORDER.   The existing data for the treatment of ADHD and ADHD-like symptoms in youth with sub-average intelligence and developmental disorders suggest that agents, particularly stimulants used to treat ADHD in typically developing children, provide some degree of benefit to children with intellectual disability and ADHD. However, these children experience more side effects than ADHD children without an intellectual disability. Thus, recommendations regarding the treatment of ADHD in children and adolescents with comorbid intellectual disability include close monitoring for side effects. Studies of methylphenidate treatment in those mildly intellectually disabled with ADHD show significant improvement in the ability to maintain attention and to stay focused on tasks. Methylphenidate treatment studies have not shown evidence of long-term improvement in social skills or learning. Risperidone may be beneficial in reducing symptoms of ADHD in this population; however, as with all antipsychotics, it has substantial side effects. Thus stimulant medications are the preferred choice.

In addition to stimulants and antipsychotics, clonidine has been used clinically in this population, especially to ameliorate hyperactivity and impulsivity. Although there are scant data, clinical ratings by parents and clinicians suggest its efficacy. Atomoxetine may also help for this population.

DEPRESSIVE DISORDERS.   The identification of depressive disorders among individuals with intellectual disabilities requires careful evaluation since they are easy to miss when behavioral problems are prominent. There have been anecdotal reports of disinhibition in response to SSRIs in intellectually disabled individuals with ASD. Given the relative safety of SSRI antidepressants, it is reasonable to try them when a child with an intellectual disability is depressed.

STEREOTYPICAL MOTOR MOVEMENTS.   Antipsychotic medications are used in the treatment of repetitive self-stimulatory behaviors in children with intellectual disability when these behaviors are either harmful to the child or disruptive. Anecdotal reports indicate that these agents may diminish self-stimulatory behaviors; however, there is no improvement seen in adaptive behavior. Obsessive-compulsive symptoms often overlap with the repetitive stereotypical behaviors seen in children and adolescents with intellectual disability, particularly in those with comorbid ASD. SSRIs such as fluoxetine, fluvoxamine, paroxetine, and sertraline have efficacy for treating obsessive-compulsive symptoms in children and adolescents and may have some efficacy for stereotyped motor movements.

EXPLOSIVE RAGE BEHAVIOR.   Antipsychotic medications, particularly risperidone, are typically used for the treatment of explosive rage. As with the treatment of aggression, there is a need for more data investigating this use. β-Adrenergic receptor antagonists (β-blockers), such as propranolol, have been anecdotally reported to result in fewer explosive rages in some children with intellectual disability and ASD.

Services and Support for Children with Intellectual Disability

Early Intervention.   Early intervention programs serve individuals for the first 3 years of life. Such services are generally provided by the state and begin with a specialist visiting the home for several hours per week. Since the passage of Public Law 99–457, the Education of the Handicapped Amendments of 1986, the emphasis is on early intervention services for the entire family. Agencies are required to develop an Individualized Family Service Plan (IFSP) for each family, which identifies specific interventions to best help the family and child.

School. From ages 3 to 21 years, school is responsible by law to provide appropriate educational services to children and adolescents with intellectual disability in the United States. Two laws codified these mandates, Public Law 94–142, the Education for all Handicapped Children Act of 1975, and the Individuals with Disabilities Act (IDEA) of 1990. Through these laws, public schools must develop and provide an individualized educational program for each student with intellectual disability, determined at a meeting designated as the Individualized Education Plan (IEP) with school personnel and the family. Schools should educate the children in the "least restrictive environment" that will allow the child to learn.

Supports. A wide variety of organized groups and services are available for children with intellectual disability and their families. These include short-term respite care, which allows families a break and is generally set up by state agencies. Other programs include the Special Olympics, which allows children with intellectual disabilities to participate in team sports and sports competitions. Many organizations also exist for families who wish to connect with others who have children with intellectual disabilities.

EPIDEMIOLOGY

The majority of population-based prevalence estimates for intellectual disability in developing countries range from 10 to 15 per 1,000 children. The prevalence of intellectual disability at any one time is estimated to range from 1 to 3 percent of the population in Western societies. The incidence of intellectual disability is difficult to calculate because mild disabilities may be unrecognized until middle childhood. In some cases, even when the intellectual function is limited, adaptive social skills may not be challenged until late childhood or early adolescence. The highest incidence of intellectual disability is reported in school-age children, with a peak at ages 10 to 14 years. Intellectual disability is about 1.5 times more common among males than females.

Prevalence

Epidemiologic surveys indicate that up to two-thirds of children and adults with intellectual disabilities have comorbid psychiatric disorders, and this rate is several times higher than that in community samples without intellectual disability. The prevalence of psychopathology appears to correlate with the severity of the intellectual disability; the more severe the intellectual disability, the higher the risk for coexisting psychiatric disorders. An epidemiologic study found that 40.7 percent of intellectually disabled children between 4 and 18 years of age met the criteria for at least one additional psychiatric disorder.

The severity of intellectual disability influences the risk of particular comorbid psychiatric disorders. Disruptive and conduct-disorder behaviors occur more frequently in those diagnosed with mild intellectual disability. In contrast, those with more severe intellectual disabilities are more likely to meet criteria for autism spectrum disorder and exhibit symptoms such as self-stimulation and self-mutilation. Comorbidity of psychiatric disorders with intellectual disability in children do not appear to correlate with age or gender. Children diagnosed with profound intellectual disabilities are less likely to exhibit comorbid psychiatric disorders.

Psychiatric disorders among persons with intellectual disabilities vary and include mood disorders, schizophrenia, ADHD, and conduct disorder. Children diagnosed with severe intellectual disabilities have an unusually high rate of comorbid autism spectrum disorder. Approximately 2 to 3 percent of those with an intellectual disability meet diagnostic criteria for schizophrenia, which is several times higher than the rate for the general population. Up to 50 percent of children and adults with intellectual disabilities meet the criteria for a mood disorder as measured on an appropriate depression scale. However, a limitation of these studies is that these instruments are not standardized within intellectual disability populations. Frequent psychiatric symptoms that occur in children with intellectual disability, outside the context of a full psychiatric disorder, include hyperactivity and short attention span, self-injurious behaviors (e.g., head-banging and self-biting), and repetitive stereotypical behaviors (hand-flapping and toe-walking). In children and adults with milder forms of intellectual disability, negative self-image, low self-esteem, poor frustration tolerance, interpersonal dependence, and a rigid problem-solving style are frequent.

ETIOLOGY

Etiologic factors in intellectual disability can be genetic, developmental, environmental, or a combination. Genetic causes include chromosomal and inherited conditions; developmental and environmental factors include prenatal exposure to infections and toxins; and environmental or acquired factors include prenatal trauma (e.g., prematurity) and sociocultural factors. The severity of intellectual disability may relate to the timing and duration of a given trauma as well as to the degree of exposure to the central nervous system (CNS). In about three-fourths of persons diagnosed with severe intellectual disability, there is an identifiable cause, whereas the etiology is apparent in only about half of those diagnosed with mild intellectual disability. No cause is known for three-fourths of persons with IQ ranging from 70 to 80 and variable adaptive functioning. Among chromosomal disorders, Down syndrome and fragile X syndrome are the most common disorders that usually produce at least moderate intellectual disability. A prototype of a metabolic disorder associated with an intellectual disability is phenylketonuria (PKU). Deprivation of nutrition, nurturance, and social stimulation can potentially contribute to the development of at least mild forms of intellectual disability. Current knowledge suggests that genetic, environmental, biologic, and psychosocial factors work additively to the emergence of intellectual disability.

Genetic Etiologic Factors in Intellectual Disability

Single-Gene Causes. One of the most well-known single-gene causes of intellectual disability is fragile X syndrome, a mutation of the *FMR1* gene. It is the most common and first X-linked gene to be identified as a direct cause of intellectual disability. Abnormalities in autosomal chromosomes are frequently associated with intellectual disability. In contrast, aberrations in sex chromosomes can result in characteristic physical syndromes that do not include intellectual disability (e.g., Turner syndrome with XO and Klinefelter syndrome with XXY, XXXY, and XXYY variations). Some children with Turner syndrome have average to superior intelligence. An agreement exists on a few predisposing factors for chromosomal disorders—among them, advanced maternal age, increased age of the father, and x-ray radiation.

Visible and Submicroscopic Chromosomal Causes of Intellectual Disability. Trisomy 21 (Down syndrome) is a prototype of a cytogenetically visible abnormality that accounts for about two-thirds of the 15 percent of intellectual disability attributable to visible abnormal cytogenetics. Other microscopically visible chromosomal abnormalities associated with intellectual disability include deletions, translocations, and supernumerary marker chromosomes. Typically, microscopic chromosome analysis can identify abnormalities of 5 to 10 million base pairs or higher.

Submicroscopic identification requires the use of microarrays that can identify losses of chromosomal segments too small to be picked up by light microscopy. The altered copy number variants (CNVs) in submicroscopic segments of the chromosome are associated with up to 13 to 20 percent of cases of intellectual disability. That is, the genes associated with a particular developmental abnormality are in the critical regions of the pathogenic CNVs.

Genetic Intellectual Disability and Behavioral Phenotype

Specific and predictable behaviors are associated with certain genetically based cases of intellectual disability. These behavioral phenotypes are a syndrome of observable behaviors that occur with a significantly higher probability than expected among those individuals with a specific genetic abnormality.

Examples of behavioral phenotypes occur in genetically determined syndromes such as fragile X syndrome, Prader–Willi syndrome, and Down syndrome in which we can expect specific behavioral manifestations. Persons with fragile X syndrome have incredibly high rates (up to three-fourths of those studied) of ADHD. High rates of aberrant interpersonal behavior and language function often meet the criteria for autistic disorder and avoidant personality disorder. Prader–Willi syndrome is almost always associated with compulsive eating disturbances, hyperphagia, and obesity. Socialization is an area of weakness, especially in coping skills. Externalizing behavior problems—such as temper tantrums, irritability, and arguing—seem to be heightened in adolescence.

Down Syndrome.   The etiology of Down syndrome, known to be caused by an extra copy of the entire chromosome 21, makes it one of the more complicated disorders. The original description

of Down syndrome, first made by the English physician Langdon Down in 1866, was based on physical characteristics associated with subnormal mental functioning. Since then, Down syndrome has been the most investigated, and most discussed, syndrome in intellectual disability. Recent data have suggested that Down syndrome may be more amenable to postnatal interventions to address the cognitive deficits that it produces than was previously thought. Although still in the early stages of animal research, data from experiments with one mouse model, the Ts65Dn, indicate that pharmacologic interventions may influence learning and memory deficits known to occur in Down syndrome.

Phenotypically, children with Down syndrome have characteristic physical attributes, including slanted eyes, epicanthal folds, and a flat nose. Figure 2-3 illustrates the typical features.

There are three types of chromosomal aberrations in Down syndrome, which complicate the diagnosis. They are:

1. Patients with trisomy 21 (three chromosomes 21, instead of the usual two) represent the overwhelming majority; they have 47 chromosomes, with an extra chromosome 21. The mothers' karyotypes are normal. A nondisjunction during meiosis, occurring for unknown reasons, is held responsible for the disorder.
2. Nondisjunction occurring after fertilization in any cell division results in mosaicism, a condition in which there are both normal and trisomic cells in various tissues.
3. In translocation, a fusion occurs of two chromosomes, usually 21 and 15, resulting in a total of 46 chromosomes, despite the presence of an extra chromosome 21. The disorder, unlike trisomy 21, is usually inherited, and the translocated chromosome may occur in unaffected parents and siblings. The asymptomatic carriers have only 45 chromosomes.

Approximately 6,000 babies are affected with Down syndrome in the United States annually, which makes the incidence of Down syndrome 1 in every 700 births, or 15 per 10,000 live births. For women older than 32 years of age, the risk of having a child with Down syndrome (trisomy 21) is about 1 in 100 births, but when translocation is present, the risk is about 1 in 3. Most children

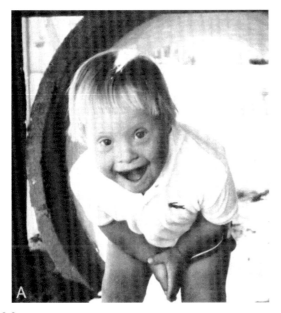 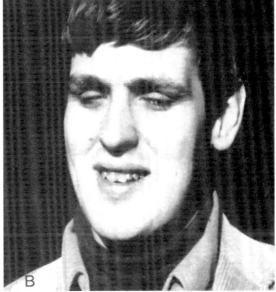

FIGURE 2-3
Down Syndrome and Fragile X Syndrome. **A.** An young child with Down syndrome. **B.** A young adult with fragile X syndrome. (Courtesy of L.S. Syzmanski, M.D. and A.C. Crocker, M.D.)

with Down syndrome are mildly to moderately intellectually disabled, with a minority having an IQ above 50. Cognitive development appears to progress normally from birth to 6 months of age; IQ scores gradually decrease from near normal at 1 year of age to about 30 to 50 as development proceeds. The decline in intellectual function may not be readily apparent. Infant tests may not reveal the full extent of the deficits. According to anecdotal clinical reports, children with Down syndrome are typically placid, cheerful, and cooperative and adapt quickly at home. With adolescence, the picture changes: youth with Down syndrome may experience more social and emotional difficulties and behavior disorders, and there is an increased risk for psychotic disorders.

In Down syndrome, language function is a relative weakness, whereas sociability and social skills, such as interpersonal cooperation and conformity with social conventions, are relative strengths. Children with Down syndrome typically manifest deficits in scanning the environment; they are more likely to focus on a single stimulus, leading to difficulty noticing environmental changes. A variety of comorbid psychiatric disorders emerge in persons with Down syndrome; however, the rates appear to be lower than in children with intellectual disability and an autism spectrum disorder.

The diagnosis of Down syndrome is relatively simple in an older child, but it is often tricky in newborn infants. The most important signs in a newborn include general hypotonia; oblique palpebral fissures; abundant neck skin; a small, flattened skull; high cheekbones; and a protruding tongue. The hands are broad and thick, with a single palmar transversal crease, and the little fingers are short and curved inward. Moro reflex is weak or absent. More than 100 signs or stigmata may occur in Down syndrome, but rarely all in one person. Commonly occurring physical problems in Down syndrome include cardiac defects, thyroid abnormalities, and gastrointestinal problems. Life expectancy was once drastically limited to about the age of 40. However, it is now significantly increased, although still shorter than those without intellectual disability.

Down syndrome includes deterioration in language, memory, self-care skills, and problem-solving by the third decade of life. Postmortem studies of individuals with Down syndrome older than age 40 have shown a high incidence of senile plaques and neurofibrillary tangles, similar to those seen in Alzheimer disease. Neurofibrillary tangles are known to occur in a variety of degenerative diseases, whereas senile plaques seem to be found most often in Alzheimer disease and Down syndrome.

Fragile X Syndrome.   Fragile X syndrome is the second most common single cause of intellectual disability. The syndrome results from a mutation on the X chromosome at what is known as the fragile site (Xq27.3). The fragile site occurs in only some cells, and it may be absent in asymptomatic males and female carriers. Much variability is present in both genetic and phenotypic expression. Fragile X syndrome occurs in about 1 of every 1,000 males and 1 of every 2,000 females. The typical phenotype includes a large, long head and ears, short stature, hyperextensible joints, and postpubertal macroorchidism (see Figure 2-3). Associated intellectual disability ranges from mild to severe. The behavioral profile of persons with the syndrome includes a high rate of ADHD, learning disorders, and autism spectrum disorder. Deficits in language function include rapid perseverative speech with abnormalities in combining words into phrases and sentences. Persons with fragile X syndrome seem to have relatively strong skills in communication and socialization; their intellectual functions seem to decline in the pubertal period. Often, female carriers are less impaired than males

with fragile X syndrome, but females can also manifest the typical physical characteristics and may have a mild intellectual disability.

Prader–Willi Syndrome.   Prader–Willi syndrome likely results from a small deletion involving chromosome 15, occurring sporadically. Its prevalence is less than 1 in 10,000. Persons with the syndrome exhibit compulsive eating behavior and often obesity, intellectual disability, hypogonadism, small stature, hypotonia, and small hands and feet.

Cat's Cry (Cri-du-Chat) Syndrome.   Children with cat's cry syndrome have a deletion in chromosome 5. They are typically severely intellectually disabled and show many signs often associated with chromosomal aberrations, such as microcephaly, low-set ears, oblique palpebral fissures, hypertelorism, and micrognathia. The characteristic cat-like cry that gave the syndrome its name is caused by laryngeal abnormalities that gradually change and disappear with increasing age.

Phenylketonuria (PKU).   Ivar Asbjörn Fölling first described PKU in 1934 as an inborn error of metabolism. PKU is transmitted as a recessive autosomal Mendelian trait and occurs in about 1 of every 10,000 to 15,000 live births. For parents who have already had a child with PKU, the chance of having another child with PKU is 20 to 25 percent of successive pregnancies. PKU is reported predominantly in persons of North European origin; a few cases may occur in African Americans, Yemenite Jews, and Asians. The underlying metabolic defect in PKU is an inability to convert phenylalanine, an essential amino acid, to paratyrosine because of the absence or inactivity of the liver enzyme phenylalanine hydroxylase, which catalyzes the conversion. Therefore, PKU is mostly preventable with a screening for it, which, if positive, should be followed with a low phenylalanine diet. Other types of hyperphenylalaninemia exist, but are rare and often fatal.

Most patients with PKU are severely intellectually disabled, but some have borderline or average intelligence. Eczema, vomiting, and convulsions occur in about one-third of all patients. Although the clinical picture varies, typically, children with PKU are reported to be hyperactive and irritable. They frequently exhibit temper tantrums and often display bizarre movements of their bodies and upper extremities, including twisting hand mannerisms. Verbal and nonverbal communication is commonly severely impaired or nonexistent. The child has reduced coordination, and they have many perceptual difficulties.

Currently, the Guthrie inhibition assay is a widely applied screening test using a bacteriologic procedure to detect phenylalanine in the blood. In the United States, screening newborn infants for PKU is routine. Early diagnosis is essential, because a low-phenylalanine diet, in use since 1955, significantly improves both behavior and developmental progress. The best results seem to be obtained with early diagnosis and the start of dietary treatment before the child is 6 months of age. Dietary treatment, however, is not without risk. Phenylalanine is an essential amino acid, and its omission from the diet can lead to severe complications such as anemia, hypoglycemia, or edema. The dietary treatment of PKU continues indefinitely. Children who receive a diagnosis before the age of 3 months and have an optimal dietary regimen may have average intelligence. A low-phenylalanine diet does not reverse intellectual disability in untreated older children and adolescents with PKU, but the diet does decrease irritability and abnormal EEG changes and does increase social responsiveness and attention span. The parents of children with PKU and some of the children's unaffected siblings are heterozygous carriers.

Rett Syndrome.

Rett syndrome, now diagnosed in the DSM-5 as a form of autism spectrum disorder, is believed to be caused by a dominant X-linked gene. It is degenerative and affects only females. In 1966, Andreas Rett reported on 22 girls with a severe progressive neurologic disability. Deterioration in communications skills, motor behavior, and social functioning starts at about 1 year of age. Symptoms include ataxia, facial grimacing, teeth-grinding, and loss of speech. Intermittent hyperventilation and a disorganized breathing pattern are characteristic while the child is awake. Stereotypical hand movements, including hand-wringing, are typical. Progressive gait disturbance, scoliosis, and seizures occur. Severe spasticity is usually present in middle childhood. Cerebral atrophy occurs with decreased pigmentation of the substantia nigra, which suggests abnormalities of the dopaminergic nigrostriatal system.

Associated features include seizures in up to 75 percent of affected children and disorganized EEG findings with some epileptiform discharges in almost all young children with Rett syndrome, even in the absence of clinical seizures. An additional associated feature is irregular respiration, with episodes of hyperventilation, apnea, and breath-holding. The disorganized breathing occurs in most patients while they are awake; during sleep, the breathing usually normalizes. Many patients with Rett syndrome also have scoliosis. As the disorder progresses, muscle tone seems to change from an initial hypotonic condition to spasticity to rigidity.

Although children with Rett syndrome may live for well over a decade after the onset of the disorder, after 10 years, many patients are wheelchair-bound, with muscle wasting, rigidity, and virtually no language ability. Long-term receptive and expressive communication and socialization abilities remain at a developmental level of less than 1 year.

Dana was born as a full-term and healthy baby after an uncomplicated pregnancy. An amniocentesis had been obtained because of advanced maternal age of 40 years, and findings were normal. At birth, Dana received good Apgar scores and her weight, height, and head circumference were all near the 50th percentile. Her development during the first months of life was unremarkable. At approximately 8 months of age, her development seemed to wane, and her interest in the environment, including the social environment, declined. Dana's developmental milestones failed to progress, and she became markedly delayed; she was just starting to walk at her second birthday and had no spoken language. Evaluation at that time revealed that head growth had decelerated. Self-stimulatory behaviors emerged, and in addition, marked cognitive and communicative delays were noted on formal testing. Dana began to lose purposeful hand movements and developed unusual stereotypical hand-washing behaviors. By age 6, her EEG was abnormal and abnormal hand movements were prominent. Subsequently, Dana developed truncal ataxia and breath-holding spells, and motor skills further deteriorated. (Adapted from Fred Volkmar, M.D.)

Neurofibromatosis.

Also called *von Recklinghausen's* disease, neurofibromatosis is the most common of the neurocutaneous syndromes caused by a single dominant gene, which may be inherited or occur as a new mutation. The disorder occurs in about 1 of 5,000 births and is characterized by café-au-lait spots on the skin and by neurofibromas, including optic gliomas and acoustic neuromas, caused by abnormal cell migration. Mild intellectual disability occurs in up to one-third of those with the disease.

Tuberous Sclerosis.

Tuberous sclerosis is the second most common of the neurocutaneous syndromes; a progressive intellectual disability occurs in up to two-thirds of all affected persons. It occurs in about 1 of 15,000 persons who inherit it through autosomal dominant transmission. Seizures are present in all those with intellectual disability, and in two-thirds of those without. Infantile spasms may occur as early as 6 months of age. The phenotypic presentation includes adenoma sebaceum and ash-leaf spots, identifiable with a slit lamp.

Childhood Disintegrative Disorder.

The previous diagnosis of childhood disintegrative disorder, now included in autism spectrum disorder, is characterized by marked regression in several areas of functioning after at least 2 years of apparently normal development. Childhood disintegrative disorder, also called *Heller syndrome* and *disintegrative psychosis,* was described in 1908 as a deterioration over several months of intellectual, social, and language function occurring in 3- and 4-year-olds with previously normal function. After the deterioration, the children closely resembled children with autistic disorder.

Ron's early history was within normal limits. By age 2, he was speaking in sentences, and his development appeared to be proceeding appropriately. At 3½ years of age, he abruptly exhibited a period of marked behavioral regression shortly after the birth of a sibling. Ron lost previously acquired skills in communication and was no longer toilet trained. Ron became more withdrawn and less interested in social interaction, exhibiting various self-stimulatory behaviors repeatedly. Comprehensive medical examination failed to reveal any conditions that might account for this developmental regression. Behaviorally, Ron exhibited features of autism spectrum disorder. At follow-up at age 12, he spoke only an occasional single word and had severe mental retardation. (Adapted from Fred Volkmar, M.D.)

Lesch–Nyhan Syndrome.

Lesch–Nyhan syndrome is a rare disorder caused by a deficiency of an enzyme involved in purine metabolism. The disorder is X-linked; patients have intellectual disability, microcephaly, seizures, choreoathetosis, and spasticity. The syndrome is also associated with severe compulsive self-mutilation by biting the mouth and fingers. Lesch–Nyhan syndrome is another example of a genetically determined syndrome with a specific, predictable behavioral pattern.

Adrenoleukodystrophy.

The most common of several disorders of sudanophilic cerebral sclerosis, adrenoleukodystrophy is characterized by diffuse demyelination of the cerebral white matter resulting in visual and intellectual impairment, seizures, spasticity, and progression to death. Adrenocortical insufficiency accompanies the cerebral degeneration. A sex-linked gene located on the distal end of the long arm of the X chromosome transmits the disorder. The clinical onset is generally between 5 and 8 years of age, with early seizures, disturbances in gait, and mild intellectual impairment. Abnormal pigmentation reflecting adrenal insufficiency sometimes precedes the neurologic symptoms, and attacks of crying are frequent. Spastic contractures, ataxia, and swallowing disturbances are also frequent. Although the course is often rapidly progressive, some patients may have a relapsing and remitting course.

Maple Syrup Urine Disease.

The clinical symptoms of maple syrup urine disease appear during the first week of life. The infant deteriorates rapidly and has decerebrate rigidity, seizures, respiratory irregularity, and hypoglycemia. If untreated, maple syrup urine disease is usually fatal in the first months of life, and the survivors have a severe intellectual disability. Some variants have transient ataxia and only mild intellectual disability. Treatment follows the general principles established for PKU and consists of a diet deficient in the three involved amino acids—leucine, isoleucine, and valine.

Other Enzyme Deficiency Disorders.   We have identified several enzyme deficiency disorders associated with intellectual disability, and are adding more as discoveries are made, including Hartnup disease, galactosemia, and glycogen-storage disease. Table 2-3 lists 30 significant disorders with inborn errors of metabolism, hereditary transmission patterns, defective enzymes, clinical signs, and relation to intellectual disability.

Acquired and Developmental Factors

Prenatal Period.   Essential prerequisites for the overall development of the fetus include the mother's physical, psychological, and nutritional health during pregnancy. Many illnesses and conditions can affect fetal brain development, including uncontrolled diabetes, anemia, emphysema, hypertension, and long-term use of alcohol and narcotic substances. Maternal infections during pregnancy, especially viral infections, have been known to cause fetal damage and intellectual disability. The extent of fetal damage depends on several factors. These factors include the type and severity of the viral infection and the gestational age of the fetus.

Rubella (German Measles).   Rubella has replaced syphilis as the primary cause of congenital malformations and intellectual disability caused by maternal infection. The children of affected mothers may show several abnormalities, including congenital heart disease, intellectual disability, cataracts, deafness, microcephaly, and microphthalmia. Timing is crucial because the extent and frequency of the complications are inversely related to the duration of the pregnancy at the time of maternal infection. When mothers become infected in the first trimester of pregnancy, 10 to 15 percent of the children are affected. This incidence rises to almost 50 percent when the infection occurs in the first month of pregnancy. Undetected subclinical forms of maternal infection can complicate the situation. Immunization can prevent maternal rubella.

Cytomegalic Inclusion Disease.   In many cases, cytomegalic inclusion disease remains dormant in the mother. Some children are stillborn, and others have jaundice, microcephaly, hepatosplenomegaly, and radiographic findings of intracerebral calcification. Children with intellectual disability from the disease frequently have cerebral calcification, microcephaly, or hydrocephalus. Positive findings of the virus in throat and urine cultures and the recovery of inclusion-bearing cells in the urine all can confirm the diagnosis.

Syphilis.   Syphilis in pregnant women was once the leading cause of various neuropathologic changes in their offspring, including intellectual disability. Today, the incidence of syphilitic complications of pregnancy fluctuates with the incidence of syphilis in the general population. Some recent alarming statistics from several major cities in the United States indicate that there is still no room for complacency.

Toxoplasmosis.   The mother can transmit toxoplasmosis to the fetus. It causes mild or severe intellectual disability and, in severe cases, hydrocephalus, seizures, microcephaly, and chorioretinitis.

Herpes Simplex.   The herpes simplex virus can be transmitted transplacentally, although the most common mode of infection is during birth. Microcephaly, intellectual disability, intracranial calcification, and ocular abnormalities may result.

Human Immunodeficiency Virus (HIV).   Cognitive impairments are well known to be associated with the transmission of HIV from mothers to their babies. HIV may have both direct and indirect influences on the developing brain. A subset of infants born infected with HIV may develop progressive encephalopathy, intellectual disabilities, and seizures within the first year of life. Fortunately, over the last two decades, there has been a dramatic decrease in perinatal HIV transmission due to a combination of antiviral agents provided to mothers during pregnancy and delivery, obstetric interventions that reduce risk, and administration of zidovudine (ZDV) as prophylaxis for 6 weeks to newborns exposed to HIV. In the United States, the annual number of HIV infections through perinatal transmission had declined about 40 percent over the last 5 years and is dramatically less than the 1990s when the transmission was at its peak. In 2015 the rates were less than 1 percent in white and Hispanic/Latino HIV-infected mothers. However, that rate is about five times greater in African American mothers with HIV. Vertical transmission of HIV from mother to child around the world, especially in Africa, is also considerable.

Fetal Alcohol Syndrome.   Fetal alcohol syndrome (FAS) results from prenatal alcohol exposure and can lead to a wide range of problems in the newborn. According to the Centers for Disease Control and Prevention, FAS in the United States occurs at a rate ranging from 0.2 to 1.5 per 1,000 live births. FAS is one of the leading preventable causes of intellectual disability and physical disabilities. Table 2-4 lists the typical characteristics of FAS, and Figure 2-4 demonstrates examples of the typical defects.

The entire syndrome occurs in up to 15 percent of babies born to women who regularly ingest large amounts of alcohol. Babies born to women who consume alcohol regularly during pregnancy have a high incidence of ADHD, learning disorders, and intellectual disability without facial dysmorphism.

Prenatal Drug Exposure.   Prenatal exposure to opioids, such as heroin, often results in infants who are small for their gestational age, with head circumference below the tenth percentile and withdrawal symptoms that appear within the first 2 days of life. The withdrawal symptoms of infants include irritability, hypertonia, tremor, vomiting, a high-pitched cry, and an abnormal sleep pattern. Seizures are unusual, but the withdrawal syndrome can be life-threatening to infants if it is untreated. Diazepam, phenobarbital, chlorpromazine, and paregoric have been used to treat neonatal opioid withdrawal. The long-term sequelae of prenatal opioid exposure are not fully known; the children's developmental milestones and intellectual functions may be within the normal range, but they have an increased risk for impulsivity and behavioral problems. Infants prenatally exposed to cocaine are at high risk for low birth weight and premature delivery. In the early neonatal period, they may have transient neurologic and behavioral abnormalities, including abnormal results on EEG studies, tachycardia, poor feeding patterns, irritability, and excessive drowsiness. The

Table 2-3
Impairment in Disorders with Inborn Errors of Metabolism

Disorder	Hereditary Transmission[a]	Enzyme Defect	Prenatal Diagnosis	Intellectual Disability	Clinical Signs
I. LIPID METABOLISM					
Niemann-Pick disease					
Group A, infantile		Unknown			Hepatomegaly
Group B, adult	A.R.	Sphingomyelinase	+	±	Hepatosplenomegaly
Groups C and D, intermediate		Unknown	−	+	Pulmonary infiltration
Infantile Gaucher disease	A.R.	β-Glucosidase	+	±	Hepatosplenomegaly, pseudobulbar palsy
Tay–Sachs disease	A.R.	Hexosaminidase A	+	+	Macular changes, seizures, spasticity
Generalized gangliosidosis	A.R.	β-Galactosidase	+	+	Hepatosplenomegaly, bone changes
Krabbe disease	A.R.	Galactocerebroside β-Galactosidase	+	+	Stiffness, seizures
Metachromatic leukodystrophy	A.R.	Cerebroside sulfatase	+	+	Stiffness, developmental failure
Wolman disease	A.R.	Acid lipase	+	−	Hepatosplenomegaly, adrenal calcification, vomiting, diarrhea
Farber lipogranulomatosis	A.R.	Acid ceramidase	+	+	Hoarseness, arthropathy, subcutaneous nodules
Fabry disease	X.R.	β-Galactosidase	+	−	Angiokeratomas, renal failure
II. MUCOPOLYSACCHARIDE METABOLISM					
Hurler syndrome MPS I	A.R.	Iduronidase	+	+	?
Hurler disease II	X.R.	Iduronate sulfatase	+	+	?
Sanfilippo syndrome III	A.R.	Various sulfatases (types A–D)	+	+	Varying degrees of bone changes, hepatosplenomegaly, joint restriction, etc.
Morquio disease IV	A.R.	N-Acetylgalactosamine-6-sulfate sulfatase	+	−	?
Maroteaux–Lamy syndrome VI	A.R.	Arylsulfatase B	+	±	?
III. OLIGOSACCHARIDE AND GLYCOPROTEIN METABOLISM					
I-cell disease	A.R.	Glycoprotein N-acetylglucos-aminyl-phospho transferase	+	+	Hepatomegaly, bone changes, swollen gingivae
Mannosidosis	A.R.	Mannosidase	+	+	Hepatomegaly, bone changes, facial coarsening
Fucosidosis	A.R.	Fucosidase	+	+	Same as above
IV. AMINO ACID METABOLISM					
Phenylketonuria	A.R.	Phenylalanine hydroxylase	−	+	Eczema, blonde hair, musty odor
Hemocystinuria	A.R.	Cystathionine β-synthetase	+	+	Ectopia lentis, Marfan-like phenotype, cardiovascular anomalies
Tyrosinosis	A.R.	Tyrosine amine transaminase	−	+	Hyperkeratotic skin lesions, conjunctivitis
Maple syrup urine disease	A.R.	Branched-chain ketoacid decarboxylase	+	+	Recurrent ketoacidosis
Methylmalonic acidemia	A.R.	Methylmalonyl-CoA mutase	+	+	Recurrent ketoacidosis, hepatomegaly, growth retardation
Propionic acidemia	A.R.	Propionyl-CoA carboxylase	+	+	Same as above
Nonketotic hyperglycinemia	A.R.	Glycine cleavage enzyme	+	+	Seizures
Urea cycle disorders	Mostly A.R.	Urea cycle enzymes	+	+	Recurrent acute encephalopathy, vomiting
Hartnup disease	A.R.	Renal transport disorder	−	−	None consistent
V. OTHERS					
Galactosemia	A.R.	Galactose-1-phosphate uridyltransferase	+	+	Hepatomegaly, cataracts, ovarian failure
Wilson's hepatolenticular degeneration	A.R.	Unknown factor in copper metabolism	−	±	Liver disease, Kayser-Fleischer ring, neurologic problems
Menkes kinky-hair disease	X.R.	Same as above	+	−	Abnormal hair, cerebral degeneration
Lesch–Nyhan syndrome	X.R.	Hypoxanthine guanine phosphoribosyltransferase	+	+	Behavioral abnormalities

[a]A.R., autosomal recessive transmission; X.R., X-linked recessive transmission.
Adapted from Leroy JC. Hereditary, development, and behavior. In: Levine MD, Carey WB, Crocker AC, eds. *Developmental-Behavioral Pediatrics.* Philadelphia, PA: WB Saunders; 1983:315, with permission.

Table 2-4
Characteristics of Fetal Alcohol Syndrome

Growth retardation of prenatal origin (height, weight)
Facial dysmorphism
   Microcephaly (head circumference below the third percentile)
   Hypertelorism (large distance between eyes)
   Microphthalmia (small eyeballs)
   Short palpebral fissures
   Inner epicanthal folds
   Midface hypoplasia (underdevelopment)
   Smooth or short philtrum
   Thin upper lip
   Short, turned up nose
Cardiac Defects
Central nervous system (CNS) manifestations
   Delayed development
   Hyperactivity
   Attention deficits
   Learning disabilities
   Intellectual deficits
   Seizures

physiologic and behavioral abnormalities are from cocaine intoxication, not withdrawal, as cocaine excretion may take up to a week after.

Complications of Pregnancy.   Toxemia of pregnancy and uncontrolled maternal diabetes present hazards to the fetus and can potentially result in intellectual disability. Maternal malnutrition during pregnancy often results in prematurity and other obstetrical complications. Vaginal hemorrhage, placenta previa, premature separation of the placenta, and prolapse of the cord can damage the fetal brain by causing anoxia.

Perinatal Period.   Some evidence indicates that premature infants and infants with low birth weight are at high risk for neurologic and subtle intellectual impairments that may not be apparent until their school years. Infants who sustain intracranial hemorrhages or show evidence of cerebral ischemia are especially vulnerable to cognitive abnormalities. The degree of neurodevelopmental impairment generally correlates with the severity of the intracranial

hemorrhage. Recent studies have documented that, among children with low birth weight (less than 1 kg), 20 percent had significant disabilities, including cerebral palsy, intellectual disability, autism, and low intelligence with severe learning problems. Very premature children and those who had intrauterine growth retardation were at high risk for developing both social problems and academic difficulties. Socioeconomic deprivation can also affect the adaptive function of these vulnerable infants. Early intervention may improve their cognitive, language, and perceptual abilities.

Acquired Childhood Disorders

Infection.   The most severe infections affecting cerebral integrity are encephalitis and meningitis. The universal use of the measles vaccine had virtually eliminated measles encephalitis. However, a recent refusal by some individuals and communities to vaccinate their children has increased the risk of this as well as subacute sclerosing panencephalitis, a rare and usually fatal degenerative disease that can occur years after the infection. Antibacterial agents have reduced the incidence of other bacterial infections, at least in the developed world. Viruses now cause most episodes of encephalitis. Sometimes a clinician must retrospectively consider a probable encephalitic component in a previously unknown illness with a high fever. A delayed diagnosis of meningitis, even when followed by antibiotic treatment, can seriously affect a child's cognitive development. Thrombotic and purulent intracranial phenomena secondary to septicemia are rarely seen today except in small infants.

Head Trauma.   The best-known causes of head injury in children that produce developmental handicaps, including seizures, are motor vehicle accidents (household accidents are the most common cause of head injuries, such as falls from tables, open windows, and on stairways). Child maltreatment is a frequent cause of head traumas or intracranial trauma such as bleeding due to "shaken baby" syndrome.

Asphyxia.   Brain damage due to asphyxia associated with near-drowning is not an uncommon cause of intellectual disability.

Long-Term Exposures.   Long-term exposure to lead is a well-established cause of compromised intelligence and learning skills.

FIGURE 2-4

Fetal alcohol syndrome. Photographs of children with "fetal-alcohol syndrome." **A.** Severe case. **B.** Slightly affected child. Note in both children the short palpebral fissures and hypoplasia of the maxilla. Usually, the defect includes other craniofacial abnormalities. Cardiovascular defects and limb deformities are also common symptoms of the fetal alcohol syndrome. (From Langman J. *Medical Embryology*. 7th ed. Philadelphia, PA: Williams & Wilkins; 1995:108, with permission.)

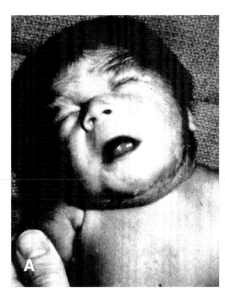
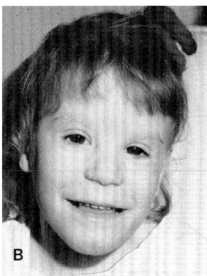

Intracranial tumors of various types and origins, surgery, and chemotherapy can also adversely affect brain function.

Environmental and Sociocultural Factors

Mild intellectual disability is associated with significant deprivation of nutrition and nurturance. Children who have endured these conditions are at risk for a host of psychiatric disorders, including mood disorders, posttraumatic stress disorder (PTSD), and attentional and anxiety disorders. A prenatal environment compromised by poor medical care and poor maternal nutrition may be contributing factors in the development of mild intellectual disability. Teenage pregnancies are at risk for mild intellectual disability in the baby due to the increased risk of obstetrical complications, prematurity, and low birth weight. Poor postnatal medical care, malnutrition, exposure to toxic substances such as lead, and potential physical trauma are additional risk factors for mild intellectual disabilities. Child neglect and inadequate caretaking may deprive an infant of both physical and emotional nurturances, leading to failure to thrive syndromes.

▲ 2.2 Communication Disorders

Communication disorders range from mild delays in acquiring language to expressive or mixed receptive–expressive disorders, phonologic disorders, and stuttering, which may remit spontaneously or persist into adolescence or even adulthood. Language delay is one of the most common very early childhood developmental delays, affecting up to approximately 7 percent of 5-year-olds. The rates of language disorders are understandably higher in preschoolers than in school-age children; rates were close to 20 percent of 4-year-olds in the Early Language in Victoria Study (ELVS). To communicate effectively, children must have a mastery of multiple aspects of language—that is, the ability to understand and express ideas—using words and speech to express themselves in vernacular language. In DSM-5, Language Disorder includes both expressive and mixed receptive–expressive problems. DSM-5 speech disorders include Speech Sound Disorder (formerly known as Phonologic Disorder) and Childhood-Onset Fluency Disorder (Stuttering). Children with expressive language deficits have difficulties expressing their thoughts with words and sentences at a level of sophistication expected for their age and developmental level in other areas. These children may struggle with a limited vocabulary, speak in sentences that are short or ungrammatical, and often present descriptions of situations that are disorganized, confusing, and infantile. They may be slow to develop an understanding and a memory of words compared with others their age. Children with language disorders are at higher risk for developing reading difficulties. Current expert consensus considers reading comprehension impairment a form of language impairment, distinct from other reading deficits such as dyslexia.

Language and speech are pragmatically intertwined, despite the distinct categories of language disorders and speech disorders in DSM-5. Language competence spans four domains: phonology, grammar, semantics, and pragmatics. *Phonology* refers to the ability to produce sounds that constitute words in a given language and the skills to discriminate the various phonemes (sounds that

are made by a letter or group of letters in a language). A child must be able to produce the sounds of a word to imitate them. *Grammar* designates the organization of words and the rules for placing words in an order that makes sense in that language. *Semantics* refers to the organization of concepts and the acquisition of words themselves. A child draws from a mental list of words to produce sentences. Children with language impairments exhibit a wide range of difficulties with semantics that includes acquiring new words, storage and organization of known words, and word retrieval. Speech and language evaluations that are sufficiently broad to test all of the other skill levels will be more accurate in evaluating a child's remedial needs. *Pragmatics* is a branch of linguistics concentrating on the skill of using language. It involves the ability to understand the context of one's speech and how to interact and converse. It requires not only understanding the literal meaning of a sentence but also the speaker's intention. By age 2 years, toddlers without speech or language delay may know a few words or up to 200 words, and by age 3 years, most children understand the basic rules of language and can converse effectively. Table 2-5 provides an overview of typical milestones in language and nonverbal development.

Over the last decade, there have been an increasing number of investigative studies of speech and language interventions with positive outcomes identified in numerous areas of language. These include improvements in expressive vocabulary, syntax usage, and overall phonologic development. Most interventions are targeted strategies for the child's particular deficit and delivered by speech and language therapists.

LANGUAGE DISORDER

Language disorder consists of difficulties in the acquisition and use of language across many modalities, including spoken and written, due to deficits in comprehension or production based on both expressive and receptive skills. These deficits include reduced vocabulary, limited abilities in forming sentences using the rules of grammar, and impairments in conversing based on difficulties using vocabulary to connect sentences in descriptive ways. Table 2-6 lists the approaches to diagnosing language disorders.

Expressive Language Deficits

Expressive language deficits are present when a child demonstrates a selective deficit in expressive language development relative to receptive language skills and nonverbal intellectual function. Infants and young children with typically developing expressive language will laugh and coo by about 6 months of age, babble and verbalize syllables such as *mama* or *dada* by about 9 months, and by 1 year, babies imitate vocalizations and can often speak at least one word. Expressive speech and language generally continue to develop in a stepwise fashion, so that at a year and a half, children typically can say a handful of words, and by 2 years, children generally are combining words into simple sentences. By the age of 2½ years, children can name actions in a picture and can make themselves understood through their verbalizations about half of the time. By 3 years, most children can speak understandably and can name a color and describe what they see with several adjectives. At 4 years, children typically can name at least four colors and can converse understandably. In the early years, before entering preschool, the development of proficiency in vocabulary and language usage is highly variable and influenced by the

Table 2-5
Language Development

Age and Stage of Development	Mastery of Comprehension	Mastery of Expression
0–6 mo	Shows startle response to loud or sudden sounds; Attempts to localize sounds, turning eyes or head; Appears to listen to speakers, may respond with smile; Recognizes warning, angry, and friendly voices; Responds to hearing own name	Has vocalizations other than crying; Has differential cries for hunger, pain; Makes vocalizations to show pleasure; Plays at making sounds; Babbles (a repeated series of sounds)
7–11 mo Attending-to-Language	Shows listening selectivity (voluntary control over responses to sounds); Listens to music or singing with interest; Recognizes "no," "hot," own name; Looks at pictures being named for up to 1 min; Listens to speech without being distracted by other sounds	Responds to own name with vocalizations; Imitates the melody of utterances; Uses jargon (own language); Has gestures (shakes head for no); Has exclamation ("oh-oh"); Plays language games (pat-a-cake, peekaboo)
12–18 mo Single-Word	Shows gross discriminations between dissimilar sounds (bells vs. dog vs. horn vs. mother's or father's voice); Understands basic body parts, names of common objects; Acquires understanding of some new words each week; Can identify simple objects (baby, ball, etc.) from a group of objects or pictures; Understands up to 150 words by age 18 mo	Uses single words (mean age of first word is 11 mo; by age 18 mo, child is using up to 20 words); "Talks" to toys, self, or others using long patterns of jargon and occasional words; Approximately 25% of utterances are intelligible; All vowels articulated correctly; Initial and final consonants often omitted
12–24 mo Two-Word Messages	Responds to simple directions ("Give me the ball") Responds to action commands ("Come here," "Sit down") Understands pronouns (me, him, her, you) Begins to understand complex sentences ("When we go to the store, I'll buy you some candy")	Uses two-word utterances ("Mommy sock," "all gone," "ball here"); Imitates environmental sounds in play ("moo," "mmm, mmm," etc.); Refers to self by name, begins to use pronouns; Echoes two or more last words of sentences; Begins to use three-word telegraphic utterances ("all gone ball," "me go now"); Utterances 26–50% intelligible; Uses language to ask for needs
24–36 mo Grammar Formation	Understands small body parts (elbow, chin, eyebrow); Understands family name categories (grandma, baby) Understands size (little one, big one) Understands most adjectives Understands functions (why do we eat, why do we sleep)	Uses real sentences with grammatical function words (can, will, the, a); Usually announces intentions before acting; "Conversations" with other children, usually just monologues; Jargon and echolalia gradually drop from speech; Increased vocabulary (up to 270 words at 2 yr, 895 words at 3 yr); Speech 50–80% intelligible; P, b, m articulated correctly; Speech may show rhythmic disturbances
36–54 mo Grammar Development	Understands prepositions (under, behind, between) Understands many words (up to 3,500 at 3 yr, 5,500 at 4 yr) Understands cause and effect (What do you do when you're hungry? cold?) Understands analogies (Food is to eat, milk is to ____)	Correct articulation of n, w, ng, h, t, d, k, g; Uses language to relate incidents from the past; Uses wide range of grammatical forms: plurals, past tense, negatives, questions; Plays with language: rhymes, exaggerates; Speech 90% intelligible, occasional errors in the ordering of sounds within words; Able to define words; Egocentric use of language rare; Can repeat a 12-syllable sentence correctly; Some grammatical errors still occur
55 mo on True Communication	Understands concepts of number, speed, time, space; Understands left and right; Understands abstract terms; Is able to categorize items into semantic classes	Uses language to tell stories, share ideas, and discuss alternatives; Increasing use of varied grammar; Spontaneous self-correction of grammatical errors; Stabilizing of articulation f, v, s, z, l, r, th, and consonant clusters; Speech 100% intelligible

Reprinted from Rutter M, Hersov L, eds. *Child and Adolescent Psychiatry*. London: Blackwell; 1985, with permission.

amount and quality of verbal interactions with family members. After beginning school, the level of verbal engagement in school can significantly influence a child's language skills. A child with expressive language deficits may demonstrate a verbal intellectual level that appears to be depressed compared with the child's overall IQ. A child with expressive language problems is likely to function below the expected levels of acquired vocabulary, correct tense usage, complex sentence constructions, and word recall. Children with expressive language deficits often present verbally as younger than their age. Language disability can be acquired during childhood (e.g., secondary to a trauma or a neurologic disorder), although less frequently, or it can be developmental; it is usually congenital, without an apparent cause. Most childhood language disorders fall into the developmental category. In either case, deficits in receptive skills (language comprehension) or expressive skills (ability to use language) can occur. Expressive language disturbance often appears in the absence of comprehension difficulties, whereas receptive dysfunction generally diminishes proficiency in the expression of language. Children with expressive language disturbance alone have better prognoses, and less interference with learning, than children with mixed receptive–expressive language disturbances.

Table 2-6
Language Disorders

	DSM-5	ICD-10
Diagnostic name	Language Disorder	Specific Developmental Disorders of Speech and Language
Duration	Onset during early development	Onset during early development
Symptoms	Difficulties with acquiring language skills, symptoms include decreased/limited: • Vocabulary • Sentence structure • Discourse Symptoms beginning during school-age years (but may become obvious during later part of academic career)	**Specific speech articulation disorder:** speech sounds **Expressive language disorder:** spoken language **Receptive language disorder:** understanding of language **Acquired aphasia with epilepsy (Landau–Kleffner):** sudden loss of expressive and receptive skills after onset of paroxysmal EEG abnormalities **Other development disorders of speech and language:** e.g., lisping
Exclusions (not result of):	Age appropriate language development Sensory impairment Motor dysfunction Intellectual disability A neurologic disorder Another medical disorder	Mechanical speech abnormality Sensory impairment Mental retardation Neurologic disorder (aphasias, etc.) Environmental factors

Although language use depends on both expressive and receptive skills, the degree of deficits in a given individual may be severe in one area, and hardly impaired at all in the other. Thus, language disorders can exist in children with expressive language disturbance in the absence of receptive language problems, or both receptive and expressive language syndromes can be present. In general, when receptive skills are sufficiently impaired to warrant a diagnosis, expressive skills are also impaired. In DSM-5, a language disorder is not limited to developmental language disabilities; it also includes acquired forms of language disturbances. To meet the DSM-5 criteria for language disorder, patients must have scores on standardized measures of expressive or receptive language markedly below those of standardized nonverbal IQ subtests and standardized tests.

Clinical Features.   Children with expressive language deficits are vague when telling a story and use many filler words such as "stuff" and "things" instead of naming specific objects.

The essential feature of expressive deficits in language disorder is marked impairment in the development of age-appropriate expressive language, which results in the use of verbal or sign language markedly below the expected level given a child's nonverbal intellectual capacity. Language understanding (decoding) skills remain relatively intact. When severe, the disorder becomes recognizable by about the age of 18 months, when a child fails to utter spontaneously or even echo single words or sounds. Even simple words, such as "Mama" and "Dada," are absent from the child's active vocabulary, and the child points or uses gestures to indicate desires. The child seems to want to communicate, maintains eye contact, relates well to the mother, and enjoys games such as pat-a-cake and peek-a-boo. The child's vocabulary is severely limited. At 18 months, the child may only point at common objects when they are named.

When a child with expressive language deficits begins to speak, language impairment gradually becomes apparent. Articulation is often immature; numerous articulation errors occur but are inconsistent, particularly with such sounds as *th, r, s, z, y,* and *l,* which the child either omits or substitutes with other sounds.

By the age of 4 years, most children with expressive language disturbance can speak in short phrases but may have difficulty retaining new words. After beginning to speak, they acquire language more slowly than do most children. Their use of various grammatical structures is also markedly below the age-expected level, and they may have delayed milestones. Emotional problems involving poor self-image, frustration, and depression may develop in school-age children.

Diagnosis.   We should diagnose a language disorder of the expressive disturbance type when a child has a selective deficit in language skills and is functioning well in nonverbal areas. Markedly below-age-level verbal or sign language, accompanied by a low score on standardized expressive verbal tests, is diagnostic of expressive deficits in language disorder. Although expressive language deficits often occur in children with autism spectrum disorders, these disturbances also frequently occur in the absence of autism spectrum disorder and are characterized by the following features: limited vocabulary, simple grammar, and variable articulation. "Inner language" or the appropriate use of toys and household objects is present. One assessment tool, the *Carter Neurocognitive Assessment,* itemizes and quantifies skills in areas of social awareness, visual attention, auditory comprehension, and vocal communication even when there are compromised expressive language and motor skills in very young children—up to 2 years of age. Also, we should administer standardized expressive language and nonverbal intelligence tests. Observations of children's verbal and sign language patterns in various settings (e.g., schoolyard, classroom, home, and playroom) and during interactions with other children help ascertain the severity and specific areas of a child's impairment and aid in early detection of behavioral and emotional complications. Family history should include the presence or absence of expressive language disorder among relatives.

Damien was a friendly, alert, and hyperactive 2-year-old, whose expressive vocabulary was limited to only two words (*mama, daddy*). He used these words one at a time in inappropriate situations. He supplemented his infrequent verbal communications with pointing and other simple gestures to request desired objects or actions. He was unable to communicate for other purposes (e.g., commenting or protesting). Damien appeared to be developing typically in other areas, especially in gross motor skills, although his fine motor skills were also poor. Damien sat, stood, and walked, and played happily with other children, enjoying activities and toys that were appropriate for 2-year-olds. Although he had a history of frequent ear infections, a recent hearing test revealed normal hearing. Despite his expressive limitations, Damien exhibited age-appropriate comprehension for the names of familiar objects and actions and simple verbal instructions (e.g., "Put that down." "Get your shirt." "Clap your hands."). However, due to his hyperactivity and impulsivity, he often required multiple directions to complete a simple task.

Despite Damien's slow start in language development, his pediatrician had reassured his parents that most of the time, toddlers like Damien spontaneously overcome their initial slow start in language development. Fortunately, Damien's language delay spontaneously remitted by the time he entered preschool at 3½ years of age, although he showed symptoms of an attention-deficit/hyperactivity disorder.

Jessica was a sociable, active 5-year-old, who presented with a language disorder. She was well-liked in kindergarten despite her language deficits and played with many of her classmates. During an activity in which each student recounted the story of Little Red Riding Hood to her doll, Jessica's classmate's story began: "Little Red Riding Hood was taking a basket of food to her grandmother who was sick. A bad wolf stopped Red Riding Hood in the forest. He tried to get the basket away from her, but she would not give it to him."

Jessica tried to avoid participating, but when called on, her version sounded quite different. Jessica struggled and came up with: "Riding Hood going to grandma house. Her taking food. Bad wolf in a bed. Riding Hood say, what big ears, and grandma? Hear you, dear. What big eyes, grandma? See you, dear. What big mouth, grandma? Eat you all up!"

Jessica's story was characteristic of expressive language deficits at her age: including short, incomplete sentences; simple sentence structures; omission of grammatical function words (e.g., *is* and *the*) and inflectional endings (e.g., possessives and present tense verbs); problems in question formation; and incorrect use of pronouns (e.g., *her* for *she*). Jessica, however, understood the story as well as her classmates. Jessica also demonstrated adequate comprehension skills in her kindergarten classroom, where she readily followed the teacher's complex, multistep verbal instructions (e.g., "After you write your name in the top left corner of your paper, get your crayons and scissors, put your library books under your chair, and line up at the back of the room.").

Ramon was a quiet, sullen 8-year-old boy whose expressive language problems had improved over time and were no longer evident in play with peers. His speech now rarely contained the incomplete sentences and grammatical errors that were so evident when he was younger. Ramon's expressive problems, however, were still impairing him in tasks involving abstract use of language, and he was struggling in his third-grade academic work. An example was Ramon's explanation of a recent science experiment: "The teacher had stuff in some jars. He poured it, and it got pink. The other thing made it white." Although each sentence was grammatical, his explanation was difficult to follow, because he vaguely explained critical ideas and details. Ramon also showed problems in word-finding, and he relied on vague and nonspecific terms, such as *thing, stuff,* and *got.*

In the first and second grades, Ramon had struggled to keep up with his classmates in reading, writing, and other academic skills. By third grade, however, the increasing demands for written work were beyond his abilities. Ramon's written work was disorganized and lacked specificity. Also, classmates began to tease him about his difficulties, and he was ashamed of his disability and reacted quite aggressively, often leading to physical fighting. Nonetheless, Ramon continued to show

relatively good comprehension of spoken language, including classroom teaching concerning abstract concepts. He also comprehended sentences that were grammatically and conceptually complex (e.g., "The car the truck hit had hubcaps that were stolen. Had it been possible, she would have notified us by mail or by phone.")

PATHOLOGY AND LABORATORY EXAMINATION. Children with speech and language disorders should have an audiogram to rule out hearing loss.

Course and Prognosis.

The prognosis for expressive language disturbance worsens the longer it persists in a child; prognosis is also dependent on the severity of the disorder. Studies of infants and toddlers who are "late talkers" concur that 50 to 80 percent of these children master language skills that are within the expected level during the preschool years. Most children with language delays later catch up in their preschool years. Other comorbid disorders may influence the outcome of expressive language deficits. If children do not develop mood disorders or disruptive behavior problems, the prognosis is better. The rapidity and extent of recovery depend on the severity of the disorder, the child's motivation to participate in speech and language therapy, and the timely initiation of therapeutic interventions. The presence or absence of hearing loss, or intellectual disability, impedes remediation and leads to a worse prognosis. Up to 50 percent of children with mild expressive language disorder recover spontaneously without any sign of language impairment, but those children with a severe expressive speech disorder may persist in exhibiting some symptoms into middle childhood or later.

Current literature shows that children who demonstrate poor comprehension, poor articulation, or poor academic performance tend to continue to have problems in these areas at follow-up 7 years later. There is also an association between particular language impairment profiles and persistent mood and behavior problems. Children with poor comprehension associated with expressive difficulties seem to be more socially isolated and impaired concerning peer relationships.

Differential Diagnosis.

Language disorders are associated with various psychiatric disorders, including other learning disorders and ADHD, and in some cases, the language disorder is challenging to separate from another dysfunction. In mixed receptive–expressive language disorder, language comprehension (decoding) is markedly below the expected age-appropriate level, whereas in expressive language disorder, language comprehension remains within normal limits.

In autism spectrum disorders, children often have impaired language, symbolic and imagery play, appropriate use of gesture, or capacity to form typical social relationships. In contrast, children with expressive language disorder become very frustrated with their disorder and are usually highly motivated to make friends despite their disability.

Children with acquired aphasia or dysphasia have a history of early normal language development; the disordered language had its onset after head trauma or other neurologic disorder (e.g., a seizure disorder). Children with selective mutism have normal language development. Often these children will speak only in front of family members (e.g., mother, father, and siblings). Children affected by selective mutism are socially anxious and withdrawn outside the family. Table 2-7 lists the differential diagnosis for language disorders.

Table 2-7
Differential Diagnosis of Language Disorder

	Hearing Impairment	Intellectual Disability	Autism Spectrum Disorder	Expressive Language Deficits Disturbance	Receptive–Expressive Language Deficits Disturbance	Selective Mutism	Speech Sound Disorder
Language comprehension	–	–	–	+	–	+	+
Expressive language	–	–	–	–	–	Variable	+
Audiogram	–	+	+	+	Variable	+	+
Articulation	–	–	– (Variable)	– (Variable)	– (Variable)	+	–
Inner language	+	+ (Limited)	–	+	+ (Slightly limited)	+	+
Uses gestures	+	+ (Limited)	–	+	+	+ (Variable)	+
Echoes	–	+	+ (Inappropriate)	+	+	+	+
Attends to sounds	Loud or low frequency only	+	–	+	Variable	+	+
Watches faces	+	+	–	+	+	+	+
Performance	+	–	+	+	+	+	+

+, normal; –, abnormal.
Adapted from Dennis Cantwell, M.D. and Lorian Baker, Ph.D, 1991.

Comorbidity. Children with language disorders have above-average rates of comorbid psychiatric disorders. In one large study of children with speech and language disorders, the most common comorbid disorders were ADHD (19 percent), anxiety disorders (10 percent), oppositional defiant disorder, and conduct disorder (7 percent combined). Children with expressive language disorder are also at higher risk for a speech disorder, receptive difficulties, and other learning disorders. Many disorders—such as reading disorder, developmental coordination disorder, and other communication disorders—are associated with expressive language disturbance. Children with expressive language disturbance often have some receptive impairment, although not always sufficiently significant for the diagnosis of language disorder on this basis. Speech sound disorder, formerly known as phonologic disorder, is commonly found in young children with a language disorder, and neurologic abnormalities exist in some children, including soft neurologic signs, depressed vestibular responses, and EEG abnormalities.

Treatment. The primary goals for early childhood speech and language treatment are to guide children and their parents toward greater production of meaningful language. There are more data to support improvements through speech and language interventions for expressive language deficit in young school-age children with primary deficits than in preschool children. A study investigating Parent–Child Interaction Therapy (PCIT) for school-age children with expressive language impairment found that PCIT was particularly efficacious in improving a child's verbal initiation, mean length of utterances, and the proportion of child-to-parent utterances. A large-scale randomized trial of a yearlong intervention targeting preschoolers with language delay in Australia found that a community-based program did not affect language acquisition in 2- and 3-year-olds. Given the high rate of spontaneous remission of language deficits in preschoolers, and less than robust effects of interventions for children that are young, treatment for expressive language disorder is generally not initiated unless it persists after the preschool years. Various techniques may help a child improve their use of such parts of speech as pronouns, correct tenses, and question forms. Direct interventions use a speech and language pathologist who works directly with the child. Mediated interventions, in which a speech and language professional teaches a child's teacher or parent how to promote therapeutic language techniques, have also been efficacious. Language therapy works on using words to improve communication strategies and social interactions, as well. Such therapy consists of behaviorally reinforced exercises and training with phonemes (sound units), vocabulary, and sentence construction. The goal is to increase the number of phrases by using block-building methods and conventional speech therapies.

Etiology. The specific causes of the expressive components of language disorder are likely to be multifactorial. Scant data are available on the specific brain structure of children with a language disorder. However, limited MRI studies suggest that language disorders are associated with diminished left-right brain asymmetry in the perisylvian and planum temporale regions. Results of one small MRI study suggested possible inversion of brain asymmetry (right > left). Left-handedness or ambilaterality appears to be associated with expressive language problems with more frequency than righthandedness. Evidence shows that language disorders occur more frequently within some families, and several studies of twins show significant concordance for monozygotic twins for language disorders. Environmental and educational factors also likely contribute to developmental language disorders.

Mixed Receptive and Expressive Deficits

Children with both receptive and expressive language impairment may have impaired ability in sound discrimination, deficits in auditory processing, or poor memory for sound sequences. Children with mixed receptive–expressive disturbance have impaired skills in the expression and reception (understanding and comprehension) of spoken language. The expressive difficulties in these children may be similar to those of children with only expressive language disturbance, which is characterized by limited vocabulary, use of simple sentences, and short sentence usage. Children with receptive language difficulties may be experiencing additional deficits in basic auditory processing skills, such as discriminating between sounds, rapid sound changes, the association of sounds and symbols, and the memory of sound sequences. These deficits may lead to a whole host of communication barriers for a child, including a lack of understanding of questions or directives from others, or inability to follow the conversations of peers or family members. Teachers or parents may initially misattribute communication difficulties as behavioral problems, delaying the recognition of the actual diagnosis.

We can measure the essential features of mixed receptive–expressive language disturbance on standardized tests; both receptive (comprehension) and expressive language development scores fall substantially below those obtained from standardized measures of nonverbal intellectual capacity. Language difficulties must be sufficiently severe to impair academic achievement or daily social communication.

Clinical Features. The essential clinical feature of this language disturbance is a significant impairment in both language comprehension and language expression. In the mixed type, expressive impairments are similar to those of expressive language disturbance but can be more severe. The clinical features of the receptive component of the disorder typically appear before the age of 4 years. Severe forms are apparent by the age of 2 years; mild forms may not become evident until age 7 (second grade) or older when language becomes complex. Children with language disorder characterized by mixed receptive–expressive disturbance show markedly delayed and below-normal ability to comprehend (decode) verbal or sign language, although they have age-appropriate nonverbal intellectual capacity. Patients with receptive dysfunction also are impaired in verbal or sign expression (encoding) of language. The clinical features of mixed receptive–expressive language disturbance in children between the ages of 18 and 24 months result from a child's failure to utter a single phoneme spontaneously or to mimic another person's words.

Many children with mixed receptive–expressive language deficits have auditory sensory difficulties and compromised ability to process visual symbols, such as explaining the meaning of a picture. They have deficits in integrating both auditory and visual symbols—for example, recognizing the common attributes of a toy truck and a toy passenger car. Whereas at 18 months, a child with expressive language deficits only comprehends simple commands and can point to familiar household objects when told to do so, a child of the same age with mixed receptive–expressive language disturbance typically cannot either point to everyday objects or obey simple commands. A child with mixed receptive–expressive language deficits may appear to be deaf. He or she responds appropriately to sounds from the environment, but not to spoken language. If the child later starts to speak, the speech contains numerous articulation errors, such as omissions, distortions, and substitutions of phonemes. Language acquisition is much slower for children with mixed receptive–expressive language disturbance than for other children of the same age.

Children with mixed receptive–expressive language disturbance have difficulty recalling early visual and auditory memories and recognizing and reproducing symbols in a proper sequence. Some children with mixed receptive–expressive language deficits have a partial hearing defect for true tones, an increased threshold of auditory arousal, and an inability to localize sound sources. Seizure disorders and reading disorders are more common among the relatives of children with mixed receptive–expressive problems than in the general population.

Diagnosis. Children with mixed receptive–expressive language deficits develop language more slowly than their peers and have trouble understanding conversations that peers can follow. In mixed receptive–expressive language disorder, receptive dysfunction coexists with expressive dysfunction. Therefore, we should give standardized tests for both receptive and expressive language abilities to anyone suspected of having a language disorder with mixed receptive–expressive disturbance.

A markedly below-expected level of comprehension of verbal or sign language with intact age-appropriate nonverbal intellectual capacity, confirmation of language difficulties by standardized receptive language tests, and the absence of autism spectrum disorder, confirm the diagnosis of mixed receptive–expressive language deficits; however, in DSM-5, these deficits are included in the diagnosis of language disorder.

PATHOLOGY AND LABORATORY EXAMINATION. All children thought to have mixed receptive–expressive language disturbance should have an audiogram to rule out or confirm the presence of deafness or auditory deficits. A history of the child and family and observation of the child in various settings help to clarify the diagnosis.

Jenna was a pleasant 2-year-old who did not yet use any spoken words and did not respond to simple commands without gestures. She made her needs known with vocalizations and simple gestures (e.g., showing or pointing) such as those typically used by younger children. She seemed to understand the names for only a few familiar people and objects (e.g., *mommy, daddy, cat, bottle,* and *cookie*). Compared with other children her age, she had a small comprehension vocabulary and showed limited understanding of simple verbal directions (e.g., "Get your doll." "Close your eyes."). Nonetheless, her hearing was reasonable, and her motor and play skills were developing as expected for her age. She showed interest in her environment and the activities of the other children at her daycare.

Lena was a shy, reserved 5-year-old who grew up in a bilingual home. Lena's parents and older siblings spoke English and Cantonese proficiently. Her grandparents, who lived in the same home, spoke only Cantonese. Lena began to understand and speak both languages much later than her older siblings had. Throughout her preschool years, Lena continued to develop slowly in comprehension and production. At the start of kindergarten, Lena understood fewer English words for objects, actions, and relations than her classmates did. Lena was unable to follow complicated classroom instructions, particularly those that involved words for concepts of time (e.g., *tomorrow, before,* or *day*) and space (e.g., *behind, next to,* or *under*). It was also hard for Lena to match one of several pictures to a syntactically complex sentence that she had heard (e.g., "It was not the train she was waiting for." "Because he had already completed his work, he was not kept after school."). Lena played with other children but only rarely tried to speak with them, which led to her classmates ostracizing her. Lena's attempts at conversations usually broke down because she misinterpreted what others said or could not express her thoughts clearly.

Consequently, her classmates generally ignored her, preferring instead to play with more verbally competent peers. Lena's infrequent interactions further limited her opportunities to learn and to practice her already weak language skills. Lena also showed limited receptive and expressive skills in Cantonese, as revealed by an assessment conducted with the assistance of a Cantonese interpreter. Nonetheless, her nonverbal cognitive and motor skills were within the normal range for her age. Lena was quite proficient in solving spatial and numerical problems, provided they were presented on paper and were not word problems.

Mark received a diagnosis of Language Disorder, based on mixed receptive–expressive deficits when he was a preschooler. By 7 years of age, he had also received the comorbid diagnoses of reading disorder and ADHD. This combination of language, reading, and attention problems made it virtually impossible for Mark to succeed in school, although he was able to engage his peers during free play. His comprehension and attention difficulties limited his ability to understand and to learn valuable information or to follow classroom instructions or discussions. Mark fell further and further behind his classmates. He was also disadvantaged because he could read only a few familiar words. This disadvantage meant that Mark was neither motivated nor able to learn academic information outside of the classroom by reading. Mark received tutoring and speech and language interventions, and despite some improvements, he continued to lag behind his classmates academically. Despite his academic problems, however, Mark made friends during sports activities in which he excelled, and continued to show nonverbal intellectual skills within the average range.

Differential Diagnosis.   Children with language disorder characterized by mixed receptive–expressive deficits have a deficit in language comprehension as well as in language production. The receptive deficit may be overlooked at first, because the expressive language deficit may be more prominent. In expressive language disturbance alone, comprehension of spoken language (decoding) remains within age norms. Children with speech sound disorder and child-onset fluency disorder (stuttering) have normal expressive and receptive language competence, despite the speech impairments.

Most children with mixed receptive–expressive language disturbance have a history of variable and inconsistent responses to sounds; they respond more often to environmental sounds than to speech sounds (Table 2-7). We should also rule out intellectual disability, selective mutism, acquired aphasia, and autism spectrum disorder.

Comorbidity.   Children with mixed receptive–expressive deficits are at high risk for additional speech and language disorders, learning disorders, and additional psychiatric disorders. About half of children with these deficits also have pronunciation difficulties leading to speech sound disorder, and about half also have a reading disorder. These rates are significantly higher than the comorbidity found in children with only expressive language problems. ADHD is present in at least one-third of children with mixed receptive–expressive language disturbances.

Course and Prognosis.   The overall prognosis for language disorder with mixed receptive–expressive disturbance is less favorable than that for expressive language disturbance alone. When the mixed disorder is identified in a young child, it is usually severe, and the short-term prognosis is poor. Language develops at a rapid rate in early childhood, and young children with the disorder may appear to be falling behind. Given the likelihood of comorbid learning disorders and other mental disorders, there is a guarded prognosis. Young children with severe mixed receptive–expressive language deficits are likely to have learning disorders in the future. In children with mild versions, it may take several years to identify the mixed disorder, and the disruption in everyday life may be less overwhelming than that in severe forms of the disorder. Over the long run, some children with mixed receptive–expressive language disturbance achieve close to normal language functions. The prognosis for children who have mixed receptive–expressive language disturbances varies widely and depends on the nature and severity of the damage.

Treatment.   Children with mixed receptive–expressive language disturbance should have a comprehensive speech and language evaluation, given the complexities of having both deficits. Some controversy exists as to whether remediation of receptive deficits before expressive deficits improves the overall efficacy of treatment. A review of the literature indicates that it is not more beneficial to address receptive deficits before expressive, and, in some cases, remediation of expressive language may reduce or eliminate the need for receptive language remediation. Thus, current recommendations are either to address both simultaneously, or to provide interventions for the expressive component first, and then address the receptive language. Preschoolers with mixed receptive–expressive language problems optimally receive interventions designed to promote social communication and literacy as well as oral language. For children at the kindergarten level, the optimal intervention includes direct teaching of key pre-reading skills as well as social skills training. An important early goal of interventions for young children with mixed receptive–expressive language disturbance is the achievement of rudimentary reading skills, in that these skills are protective against the academic and psychosocial ramifications of falling behind early on in reading. Some language therapists favor a low-stimuli setting, in which they give children individual linguistic instruction. Others recommend integrating speech and language instruction into a varied setting with several children whom they teach several language structures simultaneously. Often, a child with receptive and expressive language deficits will benefit from a small, special-educational setting that allows more individualized learning.

Psychotherapy may be helpful for children with mixed language disorder who have associated emotional and behavioral problems. We should pay particular attention to evaluating the child's self-image and social skills. Family counseling in which parents and children can develop more effective, less frustrating means of communicating may be beneficial.

Epidemiology.   Mixed receptive–expressive language deficits occur less frequently than expressive deficits; however, epidemiologic data are scant regarding specific prevalence rates. The language disturbance is believed to occur in about 5 percent of preschoolers and persists in about 3 percent of school-age children. It is less common than expressive language disturbance. Mixed receptive–expressive language disorder is likely twice as prevalent in boys as in girls.

Etiology.   Language disorders most likely have multiple determinants, including genetic factors, developmental brain abnormalities, environmental influences, neurodevelopmental immaturity, and auditory processing features in the brain. As with expressive language disturbance alone, there is evidence of familial aggregation of mixed receptive–expressive language deficits. Twin studies implicate a genetic contribution to this disorder, but there is no proven mode of genetic transmission. Some studies of children with various speech and language disorders have also shown cognitive deficits, notably slower processing of tasks involving naming objects, as well as fine motor tasks. Slower myelinization of neural pathways may account for the slow processing found in children with developmental language disorders. Several studies suggest an underlying impairment of auditory discrimination because most children with the disorder are more responsive to environmental sounds than to speech sounds.

SPEECH SOUND DISORDER

Children with speech sound disorder have difficulty pronouncing speech sounds correctly due to omissions of sounds, distortions of sounds, or atypical pronunciation. Formerly called phonologic disorder, typical speech disturbances in speech sound disorder include omitting the last sounds of the word (e.g., saying *mou* for *mouse* or *drin* for *drink*), or substituting one sound for another (saying *bwu* instead of *blue* or *tup* for *cup*). Distortions in sounds can occur when children allow too much air to escape from the side of their mouths while saying sounds like *sh* or producing sounds like *s* or *z* with their tongue protruded. Speech sound errors can also occur in patterns because a child has an interrupted airflow instead of a steady airflow preventing their pronouncing words (e.g., *pat* for *pass* or *bacuum* for *vacuum*). Children with a speech sound disorder can be mistaken for younger children because of their difficulties in producing speech sounds correctly. We make a diagnosis of a speech sound disorder by comparing the skills of a given child with the expected skill level of others of the same age. The disorder results in errors in whole words because of incorrect pronunciation of consonants, substitution of one sound for another, omission of entire phonemes, and, in some cases, dysarthria (slurred speech because of incoordination of speech muscles) or dyspraxia (difficulty planning and executing speech). Speech sound development likely depends on both linguistic and motor development that we must integrate to produce sounds.

Speech sound disturbances such as dysarthria and dyspraxia are not diagnosed as speech sound disorder if they are known to have a neurologic basis, according to DSM-5. Thus, speech sound abnormalities accounted for by cerebral palsy, cleft palate, deafness or hearing loss, traumatic brain injury, or neurologic conditions are not diagnosed as speech sound disorder. Articulation difficulties not associated with a neurologic condition are the most common components of speech sound disorder in children. Articulation deficits include poor articulation, sound substitution, and speech sound omission, and give the impression of "baby talk." Typically, these deficits are not caused by anatomical, structural, physiologic, auditory, or neurologic abnormalities. They vary from mild to severe and result in speech that ranges from entirely intelligible to unintelligible.

Clinical Features

Children with speech sound disorder have a delay in, or are incapable of, producing accurate speech sounds typical for their age, intelligence, and dialect. The sounds are often substitutions—for example, the use of *t* instead of *k*—and omissions, such as leaving off the final consonants of words. We can usually recognize speech sound disorder in early childhood. In severe cases, we can recognize it between 2 and 3 years of age. In less severe cases, the disorder may not be apparent until the age of 6 years. A child's articulation is disordered when it is significantly behind that of most children at the same age level, intellectual level, and educational level.

In very mild cases, a single speech sound (i.e., phoneme) may be affected. When a single phoneme is affected, it is usually one that is acquired late in normal language acquisition. The speech sounds most frequently misarticulated are also those acquired late in the developmental sequence, including *r, sh, th, f, z, l,* and *ch.* In severe cases and young children, sounds such as *b, m, t, d, n,* and *h* may be mispronounced. One or many speech sounds may be affected, but vowel sounds are not among them.

Children with speech sound disorder cannot articulate specific phonemes correctly and may distort, substitute, or even omit the affected phonemes. With omissions, the phonemes are absent entirely—for example, bu for blue, ca for car, or whaa? For what's that? With substitutions, children may replace difficult phonemes with incorrect ones—for example, wabbit for rabbit, fum for thumb, or whath dat? For what's that? With distortions, the child may approximate the correct phoneme but articulate it incorrectly. Rarely, additions (usually of the vowel uh) occur—for example, puhretty for pretty, what's uh that uh? For what's that?

Omissions are the most severe type of misarticulating, with substitutions the next most serious, and distortions the least severe type. Omissions, which are most frequent in the speech of young children, usually occur at the ends of words or in clusters of consonants (ka for car, scisso for scissors). Distortions, which are found mainly in the speech of older children, result in a sound that is not part of the speaker's dialect. Distortions may be the last type of misarticulating remaining in the speech of children whose articulation problems have mostly remitted. The most common types of distortions are the lateral slip—in which a child pronounces s sounds with the airstream going across the tongue, producing a whistling effect—and the palatal or lisp—in which the s sound, formed with the tongue too close to the palate, produces a ssh sound effect.

The misarticulating of children with speech sound disorder is often inconsistent and random. A child may pronounce a phoneme correctly one time and incorrectly another time. Misarticulating is most common at the ends of words, in long and syntactically complex sentences, and during rapid speech.

Omissions, distortions, and substitutions also usually occur in the speech of young children learning to talk. However, whereas young, typically speaking children soon replace their misarticulating, children with speech sound disorder do not. Even as children with articulation problems grow and finally acquire the correct phoneme, they may use it only in newly acquired words and may not correct the words learned earlier that they have been mispronouncing for some time.

Most children eventually outgrow speech sound disorder, usually by the third grade. After the fourth grade, however, spontaneous recovery is unlikely, and so it is essential to try to remediate the disorder before the development of complications. Often, beginning kindergarten or school precipitates the improvement when recovery from speech sound disorder is spontaneous. Children who have not shown spontaneous improvement by the third or fourth grade should have speech therapy. Speech therapy should be initiated at an early age for children whose articulation is significantly unintelligible and who are troubled by their inability to speak clearly.

Children with speech sound disorder may have various concomitant social, emotional, and behavioral problems, mainly when comorbid expressive language problems are present. Children with chronic expressive language deficits and severe articulation impairment are the ones most likely to suffer from psychiatric problems.

Martin was a talkative, likable 3-year-old with virtually unintelligible speech, despite excellent receptive language skills and normal hearing. Martin's level of expressive language development was difficult to quantify due to his very poor pronunciation. The rhythm and melody of his speech, however, suggested that he was trying to produce multiword utterances, as would be expected at his age. Martin produced only a few vowels (/ee/, /ah/, and /oo/), some early developing consonants (/m/, /n/, /d/, /t/, /p/, /b/, /h/, and /w/), and limited syllables. This reduced sound repertoire made many of his spoken words indistinguishable from one another (e.g., he said *bahbah* for *bottle, baby,* and *bubble,* and he used *nee* for *knee, need,* and *Anita* [his sister]). Moreover, he consistently omitted consonant sounds at the end of words and in consonant cluster sequences (e.g., /tr-/, /st-/, /-nt/, and /-mp/). Understandably, on occasion, Martin reacted with frustration and tantrums to his difficulties in making his needs understood.

Brad was a pleasant, cooperative 5-year-old, who was recognized as early as preschool to have articulation problems, and these persisted into kindergarten. His language comprehension skills and hearing were within normal limits. He showed some mild expressive language problems, however, in the use of certain grammatical features (e.g., pronouns, auxiliary verbs, and past-tense word endings) and in the formulation of complex sentences. He correctly produced all vowel sounds and most of the early developing consonants, but he was inconsistent in his attempts to produce later-developing consonants (e.g., /r/, /l/, /s/, /z/, /sh/, /th/ ,and /ch/). Sometimes, he omitted them; sometimes, he substituted other sounds for them (e.g., /w/ for /r/ or /f/ for /th/); occasionally, he even produced them correctly. Brad had particular problems in correctly producing consonant cluster sequences and multisyllabic words. Cluster sequences had omitted or incorrect sounds (e.g., *blue* might be produced as *bue* or *bwue,* and *hearts* as

hots or *hars*). Multisyllabic words had syllables omitted (e.g., *efant* for *elephant* and *getti* for *spaghetti*) and sounds mispronounced or even transposed (e.g., *aminal* for *animal* and *lemon* for *melon*). Strangers were unable to understand approximately 80 percent of Brad's speech. Brad often spoke more slowly and clearly than usual, however, when asked to repeat something, as he often was.

Jane was a hyperactive 8-year-old, with a history of significant speech delay. During her preschool and early school years, she had overcome many of her earlier speech errors. A few late-developing sounds (/r/,/l/, and/th/), however, continued to pose a challenge for her. Jane often substituted /f/ or /d/ for/th/and produced /w/ for /r/ and /l/. Overall, her speech was easily understood, despite these minor errors. Nonetheless, she became somewhat aggressive with her peers because of the teasing she received from her classmates about her speech.

Diagnosis

The essential feature of speech sound disorder is a child's delay or failure to produce developmentally expected speech sounds, especially consonants, resulting in sound omissions, substitutions, and distortions of phonemes. A rough guideline for clinical assessment of children's articulation is that normal 3-year-olds correctly articulate *m, n, ng, b, p, h, t, k, q,* and *d;* ordinary 4-year-olds correctly articulate *f, y, ch, sh,* and *z;* and typical 5-year-olds correctly articulate *th, s,* and *r.*

Speech sound disorder cannot be accounted for by structural or neurologic abnormalities, and typically, normal language development accompanies it. Table 2-8 lists the diagnostic approaches to speech sound disorder.

Differential Diagnosis

The differential diagnosis of speech sound disorder includes a careful determination of symptoms, severity, and possible medical conditions that might be producing the symptoms. First, we must

Table 2-8
Speech Sound Disorder

	DSM-5	ICD-10
Diagnostic name	Speech Sound Disorder	Specific Speech Articulation Disorder
Duration	Onset during early development	Onset during early development

Symptoms	Difficulty producing spoken sounds
	Difficult to understand
	Limits social/academic/occupational achievement
		Disorder of speech sounds. Examples:
		• Developmental disorder:
		  • phonologic disorder
		  • speech articulation disorder
		• Dyslalia
		• Functional speech articulation disorder
		• Lalling

Exclusions (not result of):	Mechanical disorders of speech or hearing (e.g., deafness, cleft palate) A neurologic disorder Another medical disorder	Aphasia NOS Apraxia Hearing loss Mental retardation With language developmental disorder: • Expressive • Receptive
Comments		ICD groups this with the language disorder as per Table 2-6

Table 2-9
Differential Diagnosis of Speech Sound Disorder

Criteria	Speech Sound Dysfunction due to Structural or Neurologic Abnormalities (Dysarthria)	Speech Sound Dysfunction due to Hearing Impairment	Speech Sound Disorder	Speech Sound Dysfunction Associated with Intellectual Disability, Autism Spectrum Disorder, Developmental Dysphasia, Acquired Aphasia, or Deafness
Language development	Within normal limits	Within normal limits unless hearing impairment is serious	Within normal limits	Not within normal limits
Examination	Possible abnormalities of lips, tongue, or palate; muscular weakness, incoordination, or disturbance of vegetative functions, such as sucking or chewing	Hearing impairment shown on audiometric testing	Normal	
Rate of speech	Slow; marked deterioration of articulation with increased rate	Normal	Normal; possible deterioration of articulation with increased rate	
Phonemes affected	Any phonemes, even vowels	*f, th, sh,* and *s*	*r, sh, th, ch, dg, j, f, v, s,* and *z* are most commonly affected	

Adapted from Dennis Cantwell, M.D. and Lorian Baker, Ph.D., 1991.

determine that the misarticulating is sufficiently severe to impair the child, rather than a normative developmental process of learning to speak. Second, we must determine that no physical abnormalities account for the articulation errors and must rule out neurologic disorders that may cause dysarthria, hearing impairment, mental retardation, and pervasive developmental disorders. Third, we must obtain an evaluation of receptive and expressive language to determine that the speech difficulty is not solely attributable to the disorders, as mentioned earlier.

Neurologic, oral structural, and audiometric examinations may be necessary to rule out physical factors that cause certain types of articulation abnormalities. Children with dysarthria, a disorder caused by structural or neurologic abnormalities, differ from children with speech sound disorder in that dysarthria is less likely to remit spontaneously and may be more difficult to remediate. Drooling, slow, or uncoordinated motor behavior, abnormal chewing or swallowing, and awkward or slow protrusion and retraction of the tongue indicate dysarthria. A slow rate of speech also indicates dysarthria (Table 2-9).

Comorbidity

More than half of children with speech sound disorder have some difficulty with language. Disorders most commonly present with speech sound disorders are language disorder, reading disorder, and developmental coordination disorder. Enuresis may also accompany the disorder. A delay in reaching speech milestones (e.g., first word and first sentence) occurs in some children with speech sound disorder, but most children with the disorder begin speaking at the appropriate age. Children with both speech sound and language disorders are at the highest risk for attentional problems and specific learning disorders. Children with speech sound disorder in the absence of language disorder have a lower risk of comorbid psychiatric disorders and behavioral problems.

Course and Prognosis

Spontaneous remission of symptoms is common in children whose misarticulating involves only a few phonemes. Children who persist in exhibiting articulation problems after the age of 5 years may be experiencing a myriad of other speech and language impairments so that it is appropriate to perform a comprehensive evaluation at that time. Children older than age 5 with articulation problems are at higher risk for auditory perceptual problems. Spontaneous recovery is rare after the age of 8 years. Some debate exists regarding the relationship between articulation problems and reading disorder or dyslexia. A recent study comparing children with phonologic problems only, with children who had dyslexia only, and those with both phonologic difficulties and dyslexia concluded that children with both disorders have somewhat distinct profiles and are comorbid disorders rather than one mixed disorder.

Treatment

Two main approaches can successfully improve speech sound difficulties. The first one, the *phonologic approach,* is usually chosen for children with extensive patterns of multiple speech sound errors that may include final consonant deletion or consonant cluster reduction. Exercises in this approach to treatment focus on the guided practice of specific sounds, such as final consonants, and when mastering that skill, extending the practice to use it in meaningful words and sentences. The other approach, the *traditional approach,* is used for children who produce substitution or distortion errors in just a few sounds. In this approach, the child practices the production of the problem sound while we provide immediate feedback and cues concerning the correct placement of the tongue and mouth for improved articulation. Children who have errors in articulation because of abnormal swallowing resulting in tongue thrust and lisps should receive exercises to improve their swallowing patterns and, in turn, improve their speech. A speech-language pathologist typically provides speech therapy, yet parents can learn to provide adjunctive help by practicing techniques used in the treatment. Early intervention can be helpful, because, for many children with mild articulation difficulties, even several months of intervention may be helpful in early elementary school. In general, when a child's articulation and intelligibility is noticeably different from peers by 8 years of age, speech deficits often lead to problems with peers, learning, and self-image, especially when the disorder is so severe that many consonants are misarticulated, and when errors involve omissions and substitutions of phonemes, rather than distortions.

Children with persistent articulation problems are likely to be teased or ostracized by peers and may become isolated and demoralized. Therefore, it is crucial to give support to children with phonologic disorders and, whenever possible, to support prosocial activities and social interactions with peers. Parental counseling and monitoring of child–peer relationships and school behavior can help minimize social impairment in children with speech sound and language disorder.

Epidemiology

Epidemiologic studies suggest that the prevalence of speech sound disorder is at least 3 percent in preschoolers, 2 percent in children 6 to 7 years of age, and 0.5 percent in 17-year-old adolescents. Approximately 7 to 8 percent of 5-year-old children in one large community sample had speech sound production problems of developmental, structural, or neurologic origins. Another study found that up to 7.5 percent of children between the ages of 7 and 11 years had speech sound disorders. Of those, 2.5 percent had speech delay (deletion and substitution errors past the age of 4 years), and 5 percent had residual articulation errors beyond the age of 8 years. Speech sound disorders occur much more frequently than disorders with a known structural or neurologic origin. Speech sound disorder is approximately two to three times more common in boys than in girls. It is also more common among first-degree relatives of patients with the disorder than in the general population. Although speech sound mistakes are quite common in children younger than 3 years of age, these mistakes are usually self-corrected by age 7 years. Misarticulating after the age of 7 years is likely to represent a speech sound disorder. The prevalence of speech sound disorders reportedly falls to 0.5 percent by mid to late adolescence.

Etiology

Contributing factors leading to speech disturbance may include perinatal problems, genetic factors, and auditory processing problems. Given the high rates of spontaneous remission in very young children, there may be a maturational delay in the developmental brain process underlying speech in some cases. The likelihood of neuronal cause is supported by the observation that children with speech sound disorder are also more likely to manifest "soft neurologic signs" as well as language disorder and a higher-than-expected rate of reading disorder. Data from twin studies implicate genetic factors, as they show concordance rates for monozygotic twins that are higher than chance.

Articulation disorders caused by structural or mechanical problems are rare. Articulation problems not caused by speech sound disorder could represent a neurologic impairment, such as dysarthria and apraxia or dyspraxia. Dysarthria results from an impairment in the neural mechanisms regulating the muscular control of speech. This impairment can occur in congenital conditions, such as cerebral palsy, muscular dystrophy, or head injury, or because of infectious processes. Apraxia or dyspraxia is characterized by difficulty in the execution of speech, even when no apparent paralysis or weakness of the muscles used in speech exists.

Environmental factors may play a role in speech sound disorder, but constitutional factors seem to make the most significant contribution. The high proportion of speech sound disorder in individual families implies a genetic component in the development of this disorder. Developmental coordination disorder and coordination in the mouth, such as in chewing and blowing the nose, may be associated.

CHILD-ONSET FLUENCY DISORDER (STUTTERING)

Child-onset fluency disorder (stuttering) usually begins during the first years of life and is characterized by disruptions in the normal flow of speech by involuntary speech motor events. Stuttering can include a variety of specific disruptions of fluency, including sound or syllable repetitions, sound prolongations, dysrhythmic phonations, and complete blocking or unusual pauses between sounds and syllables of words. In severe cases, the stuttering may include accessory or secondary attempts to compensate, such as respiratory, abnormal voice phonations, or tongue clicks. Associated behaviors, such as eye blinks, facial grimacing, head jerks, and abnormal body movements, may be observed before or during the disrupted speech.

Early intervention is necessary because children who receive early intervention can be more than seven times more likely to have full resolution of their stuttering. In severe and some untreated cases, stuttering can become an entrenched pattern that is more challenging to remediate later in life and is associated with significant psychological and social distress. When stuttering becomes chronic, persisting into adulthood, the rate of concurrent social anxiety disorder is between 40 and 60 percent.

Diagnosis

The diagnosis of childhood-onset fluency disorder (stuttering) is not difficult when the clinical features are apparent and well developed, and each of the following four phases (described in the next section) are readily recognized. Diagnostic difficulties can arise when evaluating for stuttering in young children because some preschool children experience transient dysfluency. It may not be clear whether the nonfluent pattern is part of normal speech and language development or whether it represents the initial stage in the development of stuttering. The child should be referred to a speech therapist if incipient stuttering is suspected. Table 2-10 compares the approaches to diagnosing stuttering.

Clinical Features

Stuttering usually appears between the ages of 18 months and 9 years, with two sharp peaks of onset between the ages of 2 to 3.5 years and 5 to 7 years. Some, but not all, stutterers have other speech and language problems, such as phonologic disorder and expressive language disorder. Stuttering does not begin suddenly; it typically develops over weeks or months with a repetition of initial consonants, whole words that are usually the first words of a phrase, or long words. As the disorder progresses, the repetitions become more frequent, with consistent stuttering on the most

Table 2-10
Child Onset Fluency Disorder (Stuttering)

	DSM-5	ICD-10
Diagnostic name	Childhood-Onset Fluency Disorder (Stuttering)	Stuttering (stammering)
Duration	Onset of symptoms during the developmental period	
Symptoms	Fluency/speech abnormalities: • Repetition of sounds/ syllables • Prolonging sounds or consonants • Using broken words • Blocking/pausing • Frequent word substitution (circumlocution) • Excess physical tension during word production • Repeating monosyllabic words	Speech characterized by: • Repetition or prolongation of sounds or words • Frequent pauses
Psychosocial consequences of symptoms	Causing severe anxiety and/or impairment in areas of functioning	Resulting in disruption of normal flow or rhythm of speech
Exclusions (not result of):	Speech-motor or sensory issues Neurologic injury Another medical condition Another mental disorder Note: later-onset cases after the developmental period are coded as "adult-onset fluency disorder"	Tic disorders

important words or phrases. Even after it develops, stuttering may be absent during oral readings, singing, and talking to pets or inanimate objects.

There are four gradually evolving phases in the development of stuttering:

▶ **Phase 1** occurs during the preschool period. Initially, the difficulty tends to be episodic and appears for weeks or months between long interludes of normal speech. A high percentage of recovery from these periods of stuttering occurs. During this phase, children stutter most often when excited or upset, when they seem to have a great deal to say, and under other conditions of communicative pressure.

▶ **Phase 2** usually occurs in the elementary school years. The disorder is chronic, with few, if any, intervals of normal speech. Affected children become aware of their speech difficulties and regard themselves as stutterers. In phase 2, the stuttering occurs mainly with the significant parts of speech—nouns, verbs, adjectives, and adverbs.

▶ **Phase 3** usually appears after the age of 8 years and up to adulthood, most often in late childhood and early adolescence. During phase 3, stuttering comes and goes mainly in response to specific situations, such as reciting in class, speaking to strangers, making purchases in stores, and using the telephone. Some words and sounds are more difficult than others.

▶ **Phase 4** typically appears in late adolescence and adulthood.

Stutterers show vivid, fearful anticipation of stuttering. Words, sounds, and situations can all be intimidating. Word substitutions and circumlocutions are common. Stutterers avoid situations requiring speech and show other evidence of fear and embarrassment.

Stutterers may have associated clinical features: vivid, fearful anticipation of stuttering, with avoidance of particular words, sounds, or situations in which stuttering is anticipated; and eye blinks, tics, and tremors of the lips or jaw. Frustration, anxiety, and depression are common among those with chronic stuttering.

Differential Diagnosis

Normal speech dysfluency in preschool years is challenging to differentiate from incipient stuttering. In stuttering occurs more nonfluencies, part-word repetitions, sound prolongations, and disruptions in voice airflow through the vocal tract. Children who stutter appear to be tense and uncomfortable with their speech pattern, in contrast to young children who are nonfluent in their speech but seem to be at ease. Spastic dysphonia is a stuttering-like speech disorder distinguished from stuttering by the presence of an abnormal breathing pattern.

Cluttering is a speech disorder characterized by erratic and dysrhythmic speech patterns of rapid and jerky spurts of words and phrases. In cluttering, those affected are usually unaware of the disturbance, whereas after the initial phase of the disorder, stutterers are aware of their speech difficulties. Cluttering is often an associated feature of expressive language disturbance.

Comorbidity

Very young children who stutter typically show some delay in the development of language and articulation without additional disorders of speech and language. Preschoolers and school-age children who stutter exhibit an increased incidence of social anxiety, school refusal, and other anxiety symptoms. Older children who stutter also do not necessarily have comorbid speech and language disorders, but often manifest anxiety symptoms and disorders. When stuttering persists into adolescence, social isolation occurs at higher rates than in the general adolescent population. Stuttering is also associated with a variety of abnormal motor movements, upper body tics, and facial grimaces. Other disorders that coexist with stuttering include phonologic disorder, expressive language disorder, mixed receptive–expressive language disorder, and ADHD.

Course and Prognosis

The course of stuttering is often long term, with periods of partial remission lasting for weeks or months and exacerbations occurring most frequently when a child is under pressure to communicate. In children with mild cases, 50 to 80 percent recover spontaneously. School-age children who stutter chronically may have impaired peer relationships as a result of teasing and social rejection. These children may face academic difficulties, especially if they persistently avoid speaking in class. Stuttering is associated with anxiety disorders in chronic cases, and approximately half of individuals with persistent stuttering have social anxiety disorder.

Treatment

There are several evidence-based treatments for stuttering. One such treatment is the Lidcombe Program, which uses an operant conditioning model in which parents use praise for periods in which the child does not stutter, and intervene when the child does stutter to request the child to self-correct the stuttered word. This treatment program is primarily administered at home by parents, under the supervision of a speech and language therapist. A second treatment program in clinical trials is a family-based, PCIT that identifies stressors possibly associated with increased stuttering and aims to diminish these stressors. A third treatment under investigation in clinical trials relies on the knowledge that speaking each syllable in time to a particular rhythm has led to diminished stuttering in adults. This treatment program appears to be promising when administered early on, to preschoolers.

Distinct forms of interventions have historically helped stuttering. The first approach, direct speech therapy, targets modification of the stuttering response to fluent-sounding speech by systematic steps and rules of speech mechanics that the person can practice. The other form of therapy for stuttering targets diminishing tension and anxiety during speech. These treatments may utilize breathing exercises and relaxation techniques to help children slow the rate of speaking and modulate speech volume. Relaxation techniques use the premise that it is nearly impossible to be relaxed and stutter in the usual manner at the same time—current interventions for stuttering use individualized combinations of behavioral distraction, relaxation techniques, and directed speech modification.

Stutterers who have a poor self-image, comorbid anxiety disorders, or depressive disorders are likely to require additional treatments with cognitive-behavioral therapy (CBT) or pharmacologic agents such as one of the selective serotonin reuptake inhibitor (SSRI) antidepressants.

An approach to stuttering proposed by the Speech Foundation of America is labeled self-therapy, based on the premise that stuttering is not a symptom, but a behavior that can be modified. Stutterers can learn to control their difficulty partly by modifying their feelings about stuttering and attitudes toward it and partly by modifying the deviant behaviors associated with their stuttering blocks. The approach includes desensitizing, reducing the emotional reaction to and fears of, stuttering, and substituting positive action to control the moment of stuttering.

Epidemiology

An epidemiologic survey of 3- to 17-year-olds derived from the United States National Health Interview Surveys reports that the prevalence of stuttering is approximately 1.6 percent. Stuttering tends to be most common in young children and has often resolved spontaneously as the child ages. The typical age of onset is 2 to 7 years of age, with 90 percent of children exhibiting symptoms by age 7 years. Approximately 65 to 80 percent of young children who stutter are likely to have a spontaneous remission over time. According to the DSM-5, the rate dips to 0.8 percent by adolescence. Stuttering affects about three to four males for every one female. The disorder is significantly more common among family members of affected children than in the general population. Reports suggest that for male persons who stutter, 20 percent of their male children and 10 percent of their female children will also stutter.

Etiology

Converging evidence indicates that the cause of stuttering is multifactorial, including genetic, neurophysiologic, and psychological factors that predispose a child to have poor speech fluency. Although research evidence does not indicate that anxiety or conflicts cause stuttering or that persons who stutter have more psychiatric disturbances than those with other forms of speech and language disorders, stressful situations can exacerbate stuttering.

Other theories about the cause of stuttering include organic models and learning models. Organic models include those that focus on incomplete lateralization or abnormal cerebral dominance. Several studies using EEG found that stuttering males had right hemispheric α-suppression across stimulus words and tasks; nonstutterers had left hemispheric suppression. Some studies of stutterers have noted an overrepresentation of lefthandedness and ambidexterity. Twin studies and striking gender differences in stuttering indicate that stuttering has some genetic basis.

Learning theories about the cause of stuttering include the semantogenic theory, in which stuttering is a learned response to normative early childhood disfluencies. Another learning model focuses on classical conditioning, in which the stuttering becomes conditioned to environmental factors. In the cybernetic model, speech is a process that depends on appropriate feedback for regulation; stuttering is hypothesized to occur because of a breakdown in the feedback loop. The observations that white noise reduces stuttering and delayed auditory feedback produces stuttering in regular speakers lend support to the feedback theory.

The motor functioning of some children who stutter appears to be delayed or slightly abnormal. The observation of difficulties in speech planning exhibited by some children who stutter suggests that higher-level cognitive dysfunction may contribute to stuttering. Although children who stutter do not routinely exhibit other speech and language disorders, family members of these children often exhibit an increased incidence of a variety of speech and language disorders. Stuttering is most likely to be caused by a set of interacting variables that include both genetic and environmental factors.

SOCIAL (PRAGMATIC) COMMUNICATION DISORDER

Social (pragmatic) communication disorder is a newly added diagnosis to DSM-5 characterized by persistent deficits in using verbal and nonverbal communication for social purposes in the absence of restricted and repetitive interests and behaviors. Examples of observable deficits include difficulty in understanding and following social rules of language, gesture, and social context. This deficit may limit a child's ability to communicate effectively with peers, in academic settings, and family activities. For successful

Table 2-11
Social (Pragmatic) Communication Disorder

	DSM-5	ICD-10
Diagnostic name	Social (Pragmatic) Communication Disorder	Developmental disorder of speech and language, unspecified
Duration	Begins in the early developmental period	
Symptoms	Difficulties with verbal/nonverbal communication in social situations. Examples include difficulties with: • Greetings • Sharing information • Matching conversational tone • Matching conversation context • Following normal rules for social conversations • Understanding implied meanings	(No criteria listed)
Psychosocial consequences of symptoms	Causing functional limitation	
Exclusions (not result of):	• Another medical condition • Another neurologic condition • Another mental disorder • Autism spectrum disorder • Intellectual disability • Global developmental delay	

social and pragmatic communication, a child or adolescent must integrate gestures, language, and social context of a given interaction to correctly infer its meaning. Thus, the child or adolescent must understand another speaker's "intention" of the communication with verbal and nonverbal cues. This understanding requires that they understand the environmental and social context of the interaction. One of the reasons DSM-5 introduced the diagnosis of social (pragmatic) communication disorder was to include those children with social communication impairment who do not exhibit restrictive and repetitive interests and behaviors and therefore do not fulfill the criteria for autism spectrum disorders. Pragmatic communication encompasses the ability to infer meaning in a given communication by not only understanding the words used but also integrating the phrases into their prior understanding of the social environment. Social (pragmatic) communication disorder is a new disorder; however, the concept of children with social communication deficits without repetitive and restrictive interests and behaviors has been identified for many years and is often associated with delayed language acquisition and language disorder.

Clinical Features

Social (pragmatic) communication disorder is an impaired ability to use verbal and nonverbal communication for social purposes effectively and occurs in the absence of restricted and repetitive interests and behaviors. Although the preceding deficits begin in the early developmental period, we would rarely make the diagnosis in a child younger than 4 years of age. In milder cases, the difficulties may not become apparent until adolescence, with its associated increased demands for language and social understanding. The deficits in social communication lead to impairment in function in social situations, in developing relationships, and in family and academic settings.

Diagnosis

According to the DSM-5, all of the following features must be present in order to meet diagnostic criteria: (1) Deficits in using

appropriate communication such as greeting or sharing information in a social situation or context. (2) Impaired ability to modulate the tone, level, or vocabulary used in social communication to match the listener and the situation, such as inability to simplify communication when speaking to a young child. (3) Impaired ability in following the rules for conversations such as taking turns or rephrasing a statement for clarification and failure to recognize and respond socially appropriately to verbal and nonverbal feedback. (4) Difficulty understanding things that are not explicitly stated, impaired ability to make inferences, understand humor, or interpret socially ambiguous stimuli.

The diagnosis of social (pragmatic) communication disorder can be difficult to distinguish from mild variants of autism spectrum disorder in which repetitive and restricted interests and behaviors are minimal. There are discrepant data regarding how many children previously diagnosed with autism would be excluded from the DSM-5 criteria, which now focus on only two symptom domains: social communication deficits and restricted, repetitive interests and behaviors. In one study, only 60.6 percent of children who had previously met the criteria for autistic spectrum disorder in the previous edition of the DSM met DSM-5 criteria for autistic spectrum disorder. However, in another study, up to 91 percent of patients with autism continued to meet the same DSM-5 criteria.

The essential features of social (pragmatic) communication disorder are persistently impaired social pragmatic communication resulting in limited effective communication, compromised social relationships, and difficulties with academic or occupational achievement.

Table 2-11 lists the diagnostic approach to social (pragmatic) communication disorder.

Differential Diagnosis

The primary diagnostic consideration in social (pragmatic) communication disorder is autism spectrum disorder. The two disorders are most easily distinguished when the prominence of restricted and repetitive interests and behaviors characteristic of autistic spectrum disorder is present. However, in many cases of autism, restrictive interests and repetitive behaviors manifest more prominently in the early developmental period and are not apparent in older childhood. However, even when these features are not observable, if we can obtain them in the patient's history, we would diagnose autism rather than social (pragmatic) communication disorder. We should consider social (pragmatic) communication disorder only when the restricted interests and repetitive behaviors have never been present. ADHD may overlap with a social (pragmatic) communication disorder in social communication disturbance; however, the core features of ADHD are not likely to be confused with autism spectrum disorder.

In some cases, however, the two disorders may coexist. Another childhood disorder with socially impairing symptoms that may overlap with social (pragmatic) communication disorder is social anxiety disorder. In social anxiety disorder, however, social communication skills are present, but not manifested in feared social situations. In social (pragmatic) communication disorder, appropriate social communication skills are not present in any setting. Both social anxiety disorder and social (pragmatic) communication disorder may occur comorbidly, however, and children with social (pragmatic) communication disorder may be at higher risk for social anxiety disorder. Finally, intellectual disability may be confused with social (pragmatic) communication disorder, in that social communication skills may be deficits in children with intellectual disability. We should only make a diagnosis of social (pragmatic) communication disorder when social communication skills are more severe than intellectual disability.

Comorbidity

Social (pragmatic) communication disorder is commonly associated with language disorder, consisting of diminished vocabulary for expected age, deficits in receptive skills, as well as impaired ability to use expressive language. ADHD is often concurrent with social (pragmatic) communication disorder. Specific learning disorders with impairments in reading and writing are also commonly comorbid disorders with social (pragmatic) communication disorder. Although some symptoms of social anxiety disorder may overlap with social (pragmatic) communication disorder, the full disorder of social anxiety disorder may emerge comorbidly with social (pragmatic) communication disorder.

Course and Prognosis

The course and outcome of social (pragmatic) communication disorder are highly variable and dependent on both the severity of the disorder and potential interventions administered. By age 5 years, most children demonstrate enough speech and language to be able to discern the presence of deficits in social communication. However, in the milder forms of the disorder, social communication deficits may not be identified until adolescence, when language and social interactions are sufficiently complex that deficits stand out. Many children have significant improvement over time; however, even so, some early pragmatic deficits may cause lasting impairment in social relationships and academic progress. There is a newly growing body of investigations on therapeutic interventions that may affect future outcomes of social (pragmatic) communication disorder.

Treatment

There are few data to date to inform an evidence-based treatment for social (pragmatic) communication disorder or to sufficiently distinguish it from other disorders with overlapping symptoms such as autism spectrum disorder, ADHD, and social anxiety disorder. A randomized controlled trial (RCT) of a social communication intervention explicitly directed at children with social (pragmatic) communication disorder aimed at three areas of communication: (1) social understanding and social interaction; (2) verbal and nonverbal pragmatic skills, including conversation; and (3) language processing, involving making inferences, and learning new words. Although the primary outcome measure in this study did not show significant differences for the intervention group versus the "treatment as usual" group, there were several ratings by parents and teachers that demonstrate potential improvements in social communication skills after a 20-session intensive intervention for social (pragmatic) communication disorder. Continued investigation is necessary to both validate the preceding results and to promote evidence-based treatments for children with social (pragmatic) communication disorder.

Epidemiology

It is difficult to estimate the prevalence of social (pragmatic) communication disorder. Nevertheless, a body of literature has documented a profile of children who present with these persistent difficulties in pragmatic language, who do not meet the criteria for autism spectrum disorder.

Etiology

A family history of communication disorders, autism spectrum disorder, or specific learning disorder all appear to increase the risk for social (pragmatic) communication disorder. This increased risk suggests that genetic influences are contributing factors in the development of this disorder. The etiology of social (pragmatic) communication disorder, however, is likely to be multifactorial, and given its frequent comorbidity with both language disorder and ADHD, developmental and environmental influences are also likely to play a role.

UNSPECIFIED COMMUNICATION DISORDER

Disorders that do not meet the diagnostic criteria for any specific communication disorder fall into the category of unspecified communication disorder. An example is voice disorder, in which the patient has an abnormality in pitch, loudness, quality, tone, or resonance. To be coded as a disorder, the voice abnormality must be sufficiently severe to impair academic achievement or social communication. Operationally, speech production includes five interacting subsystems, including respiration (airflow from the lungs), phonation (sound generation in the larynx), resonance (shaping of the sound quality in the pharynx and nasal cavity), articulation (modulation of the sound stream into consonant and vowel sounds with the tongue, jaw, and lips), and suprasegmentalia (speech rhythm, loudness, and intonation). These systems work together to convey information, and voice quality conveys information about the speaker's emotional, psychological, and physical status. Thus, voice abnormalities can cover a broad area of communication as well as indicate many different types of abnormalities.

Cluttering is not a disorder in the DSM-5, but it is an associated speech abnormality in which a disturbed rate and rhythm of speech impair intelligibility. ICD-10 does include it as a behavioral disorder usually occurring in childhood or adolescence. Speech is erratic and dysrhythmic and consists of rapid, jerky spurts that are inconsistent with standard phrasing patterns. The disorder usually occurs in children between 2 and 8 years of age; in two-thirds of cases, the patient recovers spontaneously by early adolescence. Cluttering is associated with learning disorders and other communication disorders.

▲ 2.3 Autism Spectrum Disorder

Autism spectrum disorder (previously known as pervasive developmental disorders), describes a wide range of impairments in social communication and restricted and repetitive behaviors. It is a phenotypically heterogeneous group of neurodevelopmental syndromes, with polygenic heritability. Before DSM-5, five overlapping disorders captured the spectrum: *autistic disorder, Asperger disorder, childhood disintegrative disorder, Rett syndrome,* and *pervasive developmental disorder not otherwise specified.* These differed by the level of severity, specific syndrome, and in some cases underlying pathology. ICD-10 continues to follow this approach to a degree. However, the recent clinical consensus has shifted the conceptualization of autism spectrum disorder toward a continuum model in which heterogeneity of symptoms is inherent in the disorder. DSM-5 collapses the core diagnostic impairments into two domains: deficits in social communication, and restricted and repetitive behaviors. Aberrant language development and usage are no longer considered a core feature of autism spectrum disorder. This diagnostic change, is based, in part, on recent studies in siblings with diagnoses of autistic disorder, suggesting that symptom domains may be transmitted separately and that aberrant language development and usage is not a defining feature, but an associated feature in some individuals with autism spectrum disorder. Autism spectrum disorder is typically evident during the second year of life, and in severe cases, a lack of developmentally appropriate interest in social interactions may be noted even in the first year. Some studies suggest that a decline in social interaction may ensue between the first and second years of life. However, in milder cases, core impairments in autism spectrum disorder may not be identified for several more years. Although language impairment is not a core diagnostic criterion in autism spectrum disorder, clinicians and parents share concerns about a child who, by 12 to 18 months, has not developed any language, and delayed language accompanied by diminished social behavior are frequently the heralding symptoms in autism spectrum disorder. In up to 25 percent of cases of autism spectrum disorder, some language develops and is subsequently lost. Autism spectrum disorder in children with normal intellectual function and mild impairment in language function may not be identified until middle childhood when both academic and social demands increase. Children with autism spectrum disorder often exhibit intense, idiosyncratic interest in a narrow range of activities, resist change, and typically do not respond to their social environment per their peers.

According to the DSM-5, the diagnostic criteria for autism spectrum disorder include deficits in social communication and restricted interests, which present in the early developmental period. However, when subtle, the child's caregivers may not identify the symptoms until several years later. Approximately one-third of children who meet the DSM-5 criteria for autism spectrum disorder show intellectual disability.

Rett syndrome was in DSM-IV and remains in ICD-10. This disorder appeared to occur exclusively in females and is characterized by normal development for at least 6 months, followed by stereotyped hand movements, a loss of purposeful motions, diminishing social engagement, poor coordination, and decreasing language use. In the formerly labeled *childhood disintegrative disorder,* development progresses normally for approximately 2 years, after which the child shows a loss of previously acquired skills in two or more of the following areas: language use, social responsiveness, play, motor skills, and bladder or bowel control. The former *Asperger disorder* is an impairment in social relatedness and repetitive and stereotyped patterns of behavior without delay or marked aberrant language development and usage. In Asperger disorder, cognitive abilities and significant adaptive skills are age-appropriate, although social communication is impaired. A survey of children undertaken with the former autism spectrum disorders revealed that the average age of diagnosis was 3.1 years for children with autistic disorder, 3.9 years for children diagnosed with pervasive developmental disorder not otherwise specified, and 7.2 years for those youth with Asperger disorder. Children with autism spectrum disorder who exhibited severe language deficits received an autism spectrum disorder diagnosis, on average, a year earlier than children without impairment in language. Children with autism spectrum disorder who exhibited repetitive behaviors such as hand-flapping, toe-walking, and odd play were diagnosed with autism spectrum disorders at a younger age than those who did not exhibit such behaviors. The current DSM-5 autism spectrum disorder criteria provide specifiers for the severity of the main domains of impairment and also specifiers for the presence or absence of language impairment and intellectual impairment.

DIAGNOSIS AND CLINICAL FEATURES

Table 2-12 describes the diagnostic approaches to autism spectrum disorder.

Core Symptoms of Autism Spectrum Disorder

Persistent Deficits in Social Communication and Interaction. Children with autism spectrum disorder characteristically do not conform to the expected level of reciprocal social skills and spontaneous nonverbal social interactions. Infants with autism spectrum disorder may not develop a social smile, and as older babies may lack the anticipatory posture for being picked up by a caretaker. Less frequent and poor eye contact is common during childhood and adolescence compared to other children. The social development of children with autism spectrum disorder is characterized by atypical, but not absent, attachment behavior. Children with autism spectrum disorder may not explicitly acknowledge or differentiate the most influential persons in their lives—parents, siblings, and teachers—and on the other hand, may not react as strongly to being left with a stranger compared to others their age. Children with autism spectrum disorder often feel and display extreme anxiety when someone disrupts their usual routine. By the time children with this disorder reach school age, their social skills may have increased, and social withdrawal may be less obvious, particularly in higher-functioning children. An observable deficit, however, often remains in spontaneous play with peers and in subtle social abilities that promote developing friendships. The social behavior of children with autism spectrum disorder is often awkward and may be inappropriate. In older school-age children, social impairments may be manifested in a lack of conventional back and forth conversation, fewer shared interests, and less body and facial gestures during conversations. Cognitively, children with

Table 2-12
Autism Spectrum Disorder

	DSM-5	ICD-10
Diagnostic name	Autism Spectrum Disorder	Childhood Autism
Duration	Begins in the early developmental period	Occurs during development, begins before age 3
Symptoms	Deficits in social interaction. Example deficits: • Emotional reciprocity/appropriate response to social interactions • Nonverbal communication/eye contact/ body language/gesturing and/or facial expression • Forming/developing/maintaining relationships and friendships Restricted/repetitive behaviors or interests. Examples: • Stereotyped motor movements • Rigid about daily routines/rituals • Restricted/fixed interests • Hyper- or hyporeactivity to sensations	Abnormal: • Social functioning • Communication • Behavior (repetitive/restricted)
Required number of symptoms	Symptoms from each category above	
Psychosocial consequences of symptoms	Functional impairment	
Exclusions (not result of):	Intellectual disability Global developmental delay	Atypical autism—symptoms do not meet all diagnostic criteria for childhood autism Asperger Syndrome—difficulties in social interaction similar to that found in autism, in addition to restricted interests; however, no deficits in language or cognition are seen
Symptom Specifiers	*With or without accompanying intellectual impairment* *With or without accompanying language impairment* *Associated with another neurodevelopmental, mental or behavioral disorder* *With catatonia*	
Severity specifiers	For social impairment: **mild, moderate, severe** For behavioral patterns: **mild, moderate, severe**	

autism spectrum disorder are frequently more skilled in visual–spatial tasks than in tasks requiring skill in verbal reasoning.

One observation of the cognitive style of children with autism spectrum disorder is an impaired ability to infer the feelings or emotional state of others around them. That is, individuals with autism spectrum disorder have difficulty with making attributions about the motivation or intentions of others (also termed "theory of mind") and thus have difficulty developing empathy. The lack of a "theory of mind" produces difficulties interpreting the social behavior of others and leads to a lack of social reciprocation.

Individuals with autism spectrum disorder generally desire friendships, and higher functioning children may be aware that their lack of spontaneity and poor skills in responding to the emotions and feelings of their peers are significant obstacles in developing friendships. Children with autism spectrum disorder are often avoided or shunned by peers who expect them to conform to their mainstream activities and experience their behavior as awkward and alienating. Adolescents and adults with autism spectrum disorder often desire romantic relationships, and for some, their increase in social competence and skills over time enables them to develop long-term relationships.

Restricted, Repetitive Patterns of Behavior, Interests, and Activities. From the first years of life, in a child with autism spectrum disorder, developmentally expected exploratory play is restricted and muted. They may not use toys and objects in a typical manner. Instead, they often manipulate the toys in a ritualistic manner, with fewer symbolic features. Children with autism spectrum disorder generally do not show the level of imitative play or abstract pantomime that other children of their age exhibit spontaneously. The activities and play of children with autism spectrum disorder may appear more rigid, repetitive, and monotonous than their peers. Ritualistic and compulsive behaviors are common in early and middle childhood. Children with autism spectrum disorder often seem to enjoy spinning, banging, and watching water flow. Frank compulsive behaviors are not uncommon among children with autism spectrum disorder, such as lining up objects, and not infrequently a child with autism spectrum disorder may exhibit a strong attachment to a particular inanimate object. Children with autism spectrum disorder who are severely intellectually disabled have increased rates of self-stimulatory and self-injurious behaviors. Stereotypies, mannerisms, and grimacing emerge most frequently when a child with autism spectrum disorder is in a less-structured situation. Children with autism spectrum disorder often find transitions and change intimidating. Moving to a new house, rearranging furniture in a room, or even a change such as eating a meal before a bath when the reverse was the routine, may evoke panic, fear, or temper tantrums in a child with autism spectrum disorder.

Associated Physical Characteristics. At first glance, children with autism spectrum disorder do not show any physical signs indicating the disorder. Children with autism spectrum disorder, overall, do exhibit higher rates of minor physical anomalies, such as ear malformations, and others that may reflect abnormalities in fetal development of those organs along with parts of the brain.

A higher-than-expected number of children with autism spectrum disorder do not show early handedness and lateralization and remain ambidextrous at an age when most children establish cerebral dominance. Children with autism spectrum disorder may have a higher incidence of abnormal dermatoglyphics (e.g., fingerprints) than those in the general population. This finding may suggest a disturbance in neuroectodermal development.

Associated Behavioral Symptoms that May Occur in Autism Spectrum Disorder

Disturbances in Language Development and Usage. Deficits in language development and difficulty using language to communicate ideas are not among the core criteria for diagnosing autism spectrum disorder; however, they occur in a subset of those individuals with autism spectrum disorder. Some children with autism spectrum disorder are not merely reluctant to speak, and their speech abnormalities do not result from a lack of motivation. Language deviance, as much as language delay, is characteristic of more severe subtypes of autism spectrum disorder. Children with severe autism spectrum disorder have significant difficulty putting meaningful sentences together, even when they have extensive vocabularies. When children with autism spectrum disorder with delayed language learn to converse fluently, their conversations may impart information without typical prosody or inflection.

In the first year of life, a typical pattern of babbling may be minimal or absent. Some children with autism spectrum disorder vocalize noises—clicks, screeches, or nonsense syllables—in a stereotyped fashion, without a seeming intent of communication. Unlike most young children who generally have better receptive language skills than expressive ones, children with autism spectrum disorder may express more than they understand. Words and even entire sentences may drop in and out of a child's vocabulary. It is not atypical for a child with autism spectrum disorder to use a word once and then not use it again for a week, a month, or years. Children with autism spectrum disorder may exhibit speech that contains echolalia, both immediate and delayed, or stereotyped phrases that seem out of context. These language patterns are frequently associated with pronoun reversals. A child with autistic disorder might say, "You want the toy" when she means that she wants it. Difficulties in articulation are also common. Many children with autistic disorder use peculiar voice quality and rhythm. About 50 percent of autistic children never develop useful speech. Some of the brightest children show a particular fascination with letters and numbers. Children with autism spectrum disorder sometimes excel in specific tasks or have special abilities; for example, a child may learn to read fluently at preschool age (hyperlexia), often astonishingly well. Very young children with autism spectrum disorder who can read many words, however, have little comprehension of the words read.

Intellectual Disability. About 30 percent of children with autism spectrum disorder are intellectually disabled. Of those, about 30 percent of children function in the mild to moderate range, and about 45 to 50 percent are severe to profoundly intellectually disabled. The IQ scores of autism spectrum disorder children with intellectual impairments tend to reflect the most severe problems with verbal sequencing and abstraction skills, with relative strengths in visuospatial or rote memory skills. This finding suggests the importance of defects in language-related functions.

Irritability. Broadly defined, irritability includes aggression, self-injurious behaviors, and severe temper tantrums. These phenomena are common in children and adolescents with autism spectrum disorder. Severe temper tantrums may be difficult to subdue, and self-injurious behaviors are often problematic to control. Everyday situations can cause these symptoms in which one would expect a youth to transition from one activity to another, sit in a classroom setting, or remain still when they desire to run around. In children with autism spectrum disorder who are lower functioning and have intellectual deficits, aggression may emerge unexpectedly without an obvious trigger or purpose, and self-injurious behaviors such as head banging, skin picking, and biting oneself may also occur.

Instability of Mood and Affect. Some children with autism spectrum disorder exhibit sudden mood changes, with bursts of laughing or crying without an apparent reason. It is difficult to learn more about these episodes if the child cannot express the thoughts related to the affect.

Response to Sensory Stimuli. Children with autism spectrum disorder may overrespond to some stimuli and underrespond to other sensory stimuli (e.g., to sound and pain). It is not uncommon for a child with autism spectrum disorder to appear deaf, at times showing little response to a normal speaking voice; on the other hand, the same child may show intent interest in the sound of a wristwatch. Some children have a heightened pain threshold or an altered response to pain. Indeed, some children with autism spectrum disorder do not respond to an injury by crying or seeking comfort. Some youth with autism spectrum disorder perseverate on a sensory experience; for example, they frequently hum a tune or sing a song or commercial jingle before saying words or using speech. Some particularly enjoy vestibular stimulation—spinning, swinging, and up-and-down movements.

Hyperactivity and Inattention. Hyperactivity and inattention are both common behaviors in young children with autism spectrum disorder. Lower than average activity level is less frequent; when present, it often alternates with hyperactivity. Short attention span, poor ability to focus on a task, may also interfere with daily functioning.

Precocious Skills. Some individuals with autism spectrum disorder have precocious or splinter skills of high proficiency, such as prodigious rote memories or calculating abilities, usually beyond the capabilities of their conventional peers. Other potential precocious abilities in some children with autism spectrum disorder include hyperlexia, an early ability to read well (even though they cannot understand what they read), memorizing and reciting, and musical abilities (singing or playing tunes or recognizing musical pieces).

Insomnia. Insomnia is a frequent sleep problem among children and adolescents with autism spectrum disorder, estimated to occur in 44 to 83 percent of school-age children.

Minor Infections and Gastrointestinal Symptoms. Young children with autism spectrum disorder can have a higher-than-expected incidence of upper respiratory infections and other minor infections. They may also have febrile seizures. Some do not become febrile when they have a minor infection, and they may not have the typical malaise. The children can also have a great many gastrointestinal symptoms. These include such symptoms as excessive burping, constipation, and loose bowel movements. In other children, behavior problems and relatedness seem to improve noticeably during a minor illness, and in some, such changes are a clue to physical illness.

Assessment Tools

A standardized instrument that can be very helpful in eliciting comprehensive information regarding autism spectrum disorder is the *Autism Diagnostic Observation Schedule-Generic* (ADOS-G).

Brett was the first of two children born to middle-class parents both in their early 40s after a difficult pregnancy, with induced labor at 36 weeks due to fetal distress. As an infant, Brett was undemanding and relatively placid; he did not have colic, and motor development proceeded appropriately, but he had delayed language development. Brett's parents first became concerned about his development when he was 18 months of age and still not speaking; however, upon questioning, they noted that, in comparison to other toddlers in his playgroup, Brett had seemed less interested in social interaction and the social games with toddlers and adults. Stranger anxiety became marked at 18 months, much later compared to the other toddlers in his daycare program. Brett would become extremely upset if his usual daycare worker was not present and would tantrum until his mother took him home. Brett's pediatrician initially reassured his parents that he was a "late talker"; however, when Brett was 24 months old, he was referred for a developmental evaluation. At 24 months, motor skills were age-appropriate. His language and social development, however, were severely delayed, and he was resistant to changes in routine and unusually sensitive to aspects of the inanimate environment. Brett's play skills were quite limited, and he played with toys in repetitive and idiosyncratic ways. His younger sister, now 12 months, was beginning to say a few words, and the family history was negative for language and developmental disorders. A comprehensive medical evaluation revealed a normal EEG and CT scan; genetic screening and chromosome analysis were routine as well.

Brett was diagnosed with autism spectrum disorder, and he started a special education program where he gradually began to speak. His speech was extremely literal and characterized by monotonic voice quality and an occasional pronoun reversal. Brett often spoke and was able to make his needs known; however, his language was odd, and the other toddlers did not play with him. Brett pursued mainly solo activities and remained quite isolated. By age 5 years, Brett was quite attached to his mother and often became separation anxious and upset when she went out, exhibiting severe tantrums. Brett also had developed several self-stimulatory behaviors, such as waving his fingers in front of his eyes. His extreme sensitivity to change continued over the next few years. Intelligence testing revealed a full-scale IQ in the average range with relative weakness in the verbal subtests compared to the performance subtests. In the fourth grade, Brett began to have severe behavioral problems at school and at home. Brett was unable to complete his classwork, would wander around the classroom, and would begin to tantrum when the teacher insisted that he sit in his seat. Brett would sometimes begin screaming so loudly that he had to leave the classroom. He would then become upset and throw all of his books off his desk in a rage, sometimes inadvertently hitting other students. It took him up to 2 hours to calm down. At home, Brett would fly into a tantrum if anyone touched his things, and he would become stubborn and belligerent when asked to do anything that he was not expecting. Brett's tantrum behavior continued into middle school, and by the eighth grade, when he was 13 years old, these behaviors became so severe that the school warned his parents that he was becoming unmanageable.

Brett was evaluated by a child and adolescent psychiatrist who recommended a social skills group for him and prescribed risperidone. Brett's tantrums became less frequent and less severe. Brett seemed calmer and did not become physically out of control during tantrums. Brett continued in middle school in a combination of special education classes and regular classes. Brett's social skills group was helpful in terms of teaching him how to approach peers in ways that would lead to less rejection. Brett had made some acquaintances, and by the time he started high school, he had acquired two friends who would come to his home and play video games with him. Brett knew that he was different from the other students, but he had trouble articulating what was different about him. Brett continued in high school with a combination of special and regular education and had plans to attend a community college and live at home for the first year. (Adapted from a case by Fred Volkmar, M.D.)

DIFFERENTIAL DIAGNOSIS

Disorders to consider in the differential diagnosis of autism spectrum disorder include social (pragmatic) communication disorder, the newly described DSM-5 communication disorder; schizophrenia with childhood-onset; congenital deafness or severe hearing disorder; and psychosocial deprivation. It is also challenging to make the diagnosis of autism spectrum disorder because of its potentially overlapping symptoms with childhood schizophrenia, intellectual disability syndromes with behavioral symptoms, and language disorders. Given the many concurrent problems often encountered in autism spectrum disorder, Michael Rutter and Lionel Hersov suggested a stepwise approach to the differential diagnosis.

Social (Pragmatic) Communication Disorder

Patients with this disorder have difficulty with conforming to typical storytelling, understanding the rules of social communication through language, exemplified by a lack of conventional greeting of others, taking turns in a conversation, and responding to verbal and nonverbal cues of a listener. Other forms of language impairment may accompany social communication disorder such as delay in learning language or expressive and receptive difficulties. Social communication disorder occurs with higher frequency in relatives of individuals with autism spectrum disorder, which increases the difficulty in discriminating this disorder from autism spectrum disorder. Although relationships may be negatively affected by social communication disorder, this disorder does not include restricted or repetitive behaviors and interests, as autism spectrum disorder does.

Childhood-Onset Schizophrenia

Schizophrenia is rare in children younger than 12 years and almost nonexistent before the age of 5 years. Characterized by hallucinations or delusions, childhood-onset schizophrenia has a lower incidence of seizures and intellectual disability and poor social skills. Table 2-13 compares autism spectrum disorder and schizophrenia with childhood-onset.

Intellectual Disability with Behavioral Symptoms

Children with intellectual disability may exhibit behavioral symptoms that overlap with some autism spectrum disorder features. The main differentiating features between autism spectrum disorder and intellectual disability are that children with intellectual disability

Table 2-13
Autism Spectrum Disorder versus Childhood-Onset Schizophrenia

Criteria	Autism Spectrum Disorder	Schizophrenia (with Onset before Puberty)
Age of onset	Early developmental period	Rarely under the age of 5
Incidence	1%	<1 in 10,000
Sex ratio (M:F)	4:1	1.67:1 (slight preponderance of males)
Family history of schizophrenia	Not increased	Likely Increased
Prenatal and perinatal complications	Increased	Not increased
Behavioral characteristics	Poor social relatedness; may have aberrant language, speech or echolalia; stereotyped phrases; may have stereotypies, repetitive behaviors	Hallucinations and delusions; thought disorder
Adaptive functioning	Impaired	Deterioration in functioning
Level of intelligence	Wide range, may be intellectually disabled (30%)	Usually within normal range, may be low average normal
Pattern of IQ	Typical higher performance than verbal	More even
Grand mal seizures	4–32%	Low incidence

Adapted from Magda Campbell, M.D. and Wayne Green, M.D.

syndromes generally display global impairments in both verbal and nonverbal areas. In contrast, children with autism spectrum disorder are relatively weak in social interactions compared to other areas of performance. Children with intellectual disability generally relate verbally and socially to adults and peers per their mental age, and they exhibit a relatively even profile of limitations.

Language Disorder

Some children with language disorders also have autism spectrum disorder features, which may present a diagnostic challenge. Table 2-14 summarizes the significant differences between autism spectrum disorder and language disorders.

Congenital Deafness or Hearing Impairment

Because children with autism spectrum disorder may appear mute or lack language development, we should rule out hearing impairment or congenital deafness. Differentiating factors include the following: infants with autism spectrum disorder may babble only infrequently, whereas deaf infants often have a history of relatively normal babbling that then gradually tapers off and may stop at 6 months to 1 year of age. Deaf children generally respond only to loud sounds, whereas children with autism spectrum disorder may ignore loud or normal sounds and respond to soft or low sounds. Most importantly, an audiogram or auditory-evoked potentials indicate a significant hearing loss in deaf children. Deaf children

Table 2-14
Autism Spectrum Disorder versus Language Disorder

Criteria	Autism Spectrum Disorder	Language Disorder
Incidence	1%	5 of 10,000
Sex ratio (M:F)	4:1	Equal or almost equal sex ratio
Family history of speech delay or language problems	<25% cases	<25% cases
Associated deafness	Very infrequent	Not infrequent
Nonverbal communication (e.g., gestures)	Impaired	Actively utilized
Language abnormalities (e.g., echolalia, stereotyped phrases out of context)	Present in a subset	Uncommon
Articulation problems	Infrequent	Frequent
Intellectual level	Impaired in a subset (about 30%)	Uncommon, less frequently severe
Patterns of intelligence quotient (IQ) tests	Typically lower on verbal scores than performance scores	Often verbal scores lower than performance scores
Impaired social communication, restricted and repetitive behaviors	Present	Absent or, if present, mild
Imaginative play	Often impaired	Usually intact

Adapted from Magda Campbell, M.D. and Wayne Green, M.D.

usually seek out nonverbal social communication with regularity and seek social interactions with peers and family members more consistently than children with autism spectrum disorder.

Psychosocial Deprivation

Severe neglect, maltreatment, and lack of parental care can lead children to appear apathetic, withdrawn, and alienated. They may have delayed language and motor skills. Children with these signs generally improve when placed in a favorable and enriched psychosocial environment, but such improvement is not the case with children with autism spectrum disorder.

COURSE AND PROGNOSIS

Autism spectrum disorder is typically a lifelong, albeit heterogeneous disorder with highly variable severity and prognosis. Children with autism spectrum disorder and IQs above 70 with average adaptive skills, who develop communicative language by ages 5 to 7 years, have the best prognoses. A longitudinal study comparing symptoms in children with high-IQ autism spectrum disorder at the age of 5 years, with their symptoms at age 13 through young adulthood, found that a small proportion no longer met criteria for autism spectrum disorder. Most of these youth demonstrated positive changes in communication and social domains over time. Early intensive behavioral interventions can provide a profound positive impact on many children with the disorder, and in some cases, lead to recovery and function in the average range.

The symptoms that do not seem to improve substantively over time with early behavioral interventions are related to ritualistic and repetitive behaviors. However, currently, evidence-based behavioral interventions specifically targeting repetitive behaviors may ameliorate them. The prognosis of a given child with autism spectrum disorder is generally improved if the home environment is supportive.

TREATMENT

The goals of treatment for children with autism spectrum disorder are to target core behaviors to improve social interactions, communication, broaden strategies to integrate into schools, develop meaningful peer relationships, and increase long-term skills in independent living. Psychosocial treatment interventions aim to help children with autism spectrum disorder to develop skills in social conventions, increase socially acceptable and prosocial behavior with peers, and to decrease odd behavioral symptoms. In many cases, a child may require language and academic remediation. Also, treatment goals generally include the reduction of irritable and disruptive behaviors that may emerge in school and at home and may exacerbate during transitions. Children with intellectual disability require developmentally appropriate behavioral interventions to reinforce socially acceptable behaviors and encourage self-care skills. Also, parents of children with autism spectrum disorder often benefit from psychoeducation, support, and counseling in order to optimize their relationships and effectiveness with their children. Comprehensive treatment for autism spectrum disorder, including intensive behavioral programs, parent training and participation, and academic/educational interventions, have provided the most promising results. Components of these comprehensive treatments include expanding social skills, communication, and language, often through practicing imitation, joint attention, social reciprocity, and play in a directed but child-centered

manner. Five RCTs of early intensive, comprehensive behavioral interventions targeting core features of autism spectrum disorder in children ranging in age from 2 to 5 years of age have shown increases in language acquisition, social interactions, and educational achievement at the end of the study period compared to control groups. The study periods ranged from 12 weeks to several years, and the settings were at home, in a clinic, or at school. The next section describes some comprehensive treatment models or adapted versions based on these studies.

Psychosocial Interventions

Early Intensive Behavioral and Developmental Interventions

UCLA/LOVAAS-BASED MODEL. This intensive and manualized intervention primarily utilizes techniques derived from applied behavior analysis, given on a one-to-one basis for many hours per week. A therapist and a child will work on practicing specific social skills, language usage, and other target play skills, with reinforcement and rewards provided for accomplishments and mastery of skills.

EARLY START DENVER MODEL (ESDM). Interventions occur in naturalistic settings such as in daycare, at home, and during play with other children. Parents learn to be co-therapists and provide the training at home while educational settings also provide the interventions. The focus of the interventions is on developing basic play skills and relationship skills and integrating applied behavior analysis into the interventions. This approach is focused on training for very young children and occurs within the context of the child's daily routine.

PARENT TRAINING APPROACHES. This includes Pivotal Response Training, in which parents learn to facilitate social and communication development within the home and during activities by targeting gateway or pivotal social behaviors for mastery by the child, with the expectation that once they master these central social skills, a natural generalizing of social behaviors would follow. The approach integrates extensive parent and family components into this type of intervention. Once parents learn the interventions, they gradually increase the frequency until they occur throughout the day with the child. Another example of a parent training approach is the Hanen More Than Words Program.

Social Skills Approaches

SOCIAL SKILLS TRAINING. Typically provided by therapeutic leaders to children of various ages in a group setting with peers, children are given guided practice in initiating social conversation, greetings, initiating games, and joint attention. The approach includes emotion identification and regulation in practice with recognizing and learning how to label emotions in given social situations, learning to attribute appropriate emotional reactions in others, and social problem-solving techniques. The goals are that with practice in the group setting, the child will be able to use the techniques in less-structured settings and internalize strategies to interact positively with peers.

Behavioral Interventions (BIs) and Cognitive-Behavioral Therapy (CBT) for Repetitive Behaviors and Associated Symptoms

BEHAVIORAL THERAPY. Applied behavioral analysis is somewhat effective in reducing some repetitive behaviors in children and adolescents with autism spectrum disorder. Early intervention helps for repetitive self-injurious behaviors; behavioral interventions may need to be combined with pharmacologic treatments to manage the symptoms adequately.

COGNITIVE-BEHAVIORAL THERAPY. There is a significant evidence base from RCTs for the efficacy of CBT for symptoms of anxiety, depression, and obsessive-compulsive disorders (OCDs) in children. There are fewer controlled trials of this treatment in children with autism spectrum disorder, although there are at least two published studies in which CBT was used to treat repetitive behavior in individuals with autism spectrum disorder.

Interventions for Comorbid Symptoms in Autism Spectrum Disorder

NEUROFEEDBACK. This modality can influence symptoms of ADHD, anxiety, and increased social interaction by providing computer games or other games which reinforce the desired behavior. At the same time, the child wears electrodes that monitor electrical activity in the brain. The aim is to influence brainwave activity to prolong or produce electrical activity present during the desired behaviors. This modality is still under investigation in the treatment of symptoms in autism spectrum disorder.

INSOMNIA. Insomnia is a prevalent concern among children and adolescents with autism spectrum disorder, and both behavioral and pharmacologic interventions may improve this condition. The most common behavioral intervention for insomnia in autism spectrum disorder is based on changing the parents' behavior first toward the child at bedtime and throughout the night, such that there is a removal of reinforcement and attention for being awake, leading to gradual extinction of the "staying awake" behavior. Several studies using massage therapy before bedtime in children with autism spectrum disorder between the ages of 2 years and 13 years provided an improvement in falling asleep and a sense of relaxation.

Educational Interventions for Children with Autism Spectrum Disorder

TREATMENT AND EDUCATION OF AUTISTIC AND COMMUNICATION-RELATED HANDICAPPED CHILDREN (TEACCH). Originally developed at the University of North Carolina at Chapel Hill in the 1970s, TEACCH involves structured teaching based on the notion that children with autism spectrum disorder have difficulty with perception. This teaching method incorporates many visual supports and a picture schedule to aid in teaching academic subjects as well as socially appropriate responses. Caregivers arrange the physical environment to support visual learning, and the day is structured to promote autonomy and social relatedness.

BROAD-BASED APPROACHES. These educational plans include a blend of teaching strategies that use behavioral analysis and also focus on language remediation. Behavioral reinforcement is provided for socially acceptable behaviors while teaching academic subjects. TEACCH can be part of a broader special educational program for autism spectrum disorder.

COMPUTER-BASED APPROACHES AND VIRTUAL REALITY. Computer-based and virtual reality approaches use computer programs to teach language acquisition and reading skills. This approach provides the child with a sense of mastery. It also delivers a behaviorally based instruction in a modality that is appealing for the child. The Let's Face It! program is a computerized game that helps to teach children with autism spectrum disorder to recognize faces. It consists of seven interactive computer games that target changes in facial expression, attention to the eye region of the face, holistic face recognition, and identifying emotional expression. An RCT of this program with children with autism spectrum disorder provided evidence that after 20 hours of face training with Let's Face It!, compared to the control group, the trained children demonstrated improvement in their ability to focus on the eye region of a face and improved their analytic and holistic face-processing skills. Several studies using virtual reality environments to teach children with autism spectrum disorder social skills and interaction have provided evidence of their value. In one study, a virtual café for children with autism spectrum disorder allowed the children to practice ordering and paying for drinks and food by navigation with the use of a computer mouse.

Psychopharmacological Interventions

Psychopharmacological interventions in autism spectrum disorder help ameliorate behavioral symptoms rather than core features of autism spectrum disorder. Target symptoms include irritability, broadly including aggression, temper tantrums, and self-injurious behaviors, hyperactivity, impulsivity, and inattention.

Irritability. Two second-generation antipsychotics, risperidone, and aripiprazole, have been approved by the Food and Drug Administration (FDA) in the United States for treatment of irritability in individuals with autism spectrum disorder. Risperidone, a high-potency antipsychotic with combined dopamine (D_2) and serotonin ($5-HT_2$) receptor antagonist properties, has been shown to subdue aggressive or self-injurious behaviors in children with and without autism spectrum disorder. There have been seven RCTs, three reanalysis studies, and two add-on studies, which have converged to confirm risperidone as an efficacious pharmacologic treatment for irritability in children and adolescents with autism spectrum disorder. Typical doses range from 0.5 to 1.5 mg. Some of the preschoolers in this study were also receiving intensive behavioral treatments. Risperidone is considered the first-line of medication treatment for children and adolescents with autism spectrum disorder who exhibit severe irritability. Despite its efficacy, risperidone's main side effects of weight gain and increased appetite, metabolic side effects such as hyperglycemia, prolactin elevation, and dyslipidemia, along with other common adverse effects such as fatigue, drowsiness, dizziness, and drooling, have limited its use in some individuals. Risperidone should be used with caution in individuals with underlying cardiac abnormalities or hypotension, since risperidone may contribute to orthostatic hypotension. In further continuation studies of risperidone in the treatment of irritability in autism spectrum disorder, persistent efficacy and tolerability were found over 6 months, with a rapid return of symptoms in good responders when discontinuing the risperidone. Other drugs studied in the treatment of irritability in autism spectrum disorder include aripiprazole and olanzapine.

Two extensive studies utilizing aripiprazole in the treatment of tantrums, aggression, and self-injury in children and adolescents with autism spectrum disorder found that aripiprazole was both efficacious and safe. Doses ranged from 5 to 15 mg/day. The main side effects included sedation, dizziness, insomnia, akathisia, nausea, and vomiting. Although weight gain was not as pronounced as with risperidone, it was still considered a moderate adverse event, with approximately 1.3 to 1.5 kg gained during an 8-week study period. The weight gain was similar at the lower and higher doses. Olanzapine, which blocks $5-HT_{2A}$ and D_2 receptors and also blocks muscarinic receptors, has been studied in children and adolescents with autism spectrum disorder for the treatment of irritability with a trend toward a positive response; however, significant weight gain of approximately 3.5 kg occurred. The main side effect was sedation.

Hyperactivity, Impulsivity, and Inattention. There have been several randomized placebo-controlled trials of methylphenidate for the treatment of hyperactivity, impulsivity, and inattention in children and adolescents with autism spectrum disorder. The Research Units of Pediatric Psychopharmacology found methylphenidate to be at least moderately efficacious at doses of 0.25 to 0.5 mg/kg for youth with autism spectrum disorder and ADHD symptoms. The efficacy of methylphenidate in this population was less effective than in children with ADHD without autism spectrum disorder, and children with autism spectrum disorder developed more frequent side effects, including increased irritability, compared to ADHD children. A study of methylphenidate in the treatment of hyperactivity and inattention in preschoolers with autism spectrum disorder found the stimulant safe and relatively efficacious; half of the preschoolers developed side effects including increased stereotypies, gastrointestinal upset, sleep problems, and emotional lability. Among nonstimulants, one double-blind placebo-controlled study of hyperactivity, impulsivity, and inattention using atomoxetine in children with autism spectrum disorder found that it was significantly more effective than placebo. Side effects included sedation, irritability, constipation, and nausea. Clonidine, an α-agonist, has also been studied in children with autism spectrum disorder for the treatment of hyperactivity with mixed results. Guanfacine may also help in some cases.

Repetitive and Stereotypic Behavior. Antidepressants and mood stabilizers have been studied for the treatment of these core symptoms of autism spectrum disorder. One study with fluoxetine found the medication group only slightly better and not significantly better than the placebo group regarding the target symptoms, and another trial with escitalopram found no difference between groups. Risperidone, however, was found to be effective in targeting irritability, and restrictive and repetitive behaviors were improved. One study using valproate in a 12-week trial with 55 children with a mean age of 9½ years with autism spectrum disorder found that those who were considered responders to irritability also spent less time engaging in repetitive behaviors.

Agents Administered for Behavioral Impairment in Autism Spectrum Disorder Based On Open Trials. Quetiapine is an antipsychotic with more potent $5-HT_{2A}$ than D_2 receptor blocking properties. Although there are only open-label trials with this agent, some experts use this when risperidone and olanzapine fail or are intolerable. Doses range from 50 to 200 mg/day. Adverse effects include drowsiness, tachycardia, agitation, and weight gain.

Clozapine has a heterocyclic chemical structure that is related to certain first-generation antipsychotics, such as loxapine, although clozapine carries a lower risk of extrapyramidal symptoms. It is not generally used in the treatment of aggression and self-injurious behavior unless those behaviors coexist with psychotic symptoms. The most severe adverse effect is agranulocytosis, which necessitates monitoring white blood cell count weekly during clozapine use. Its use is generally limited to treatment-resistant psychotic patients.

Ziprasidone has receptor-blocking properties at the $5-HT_{2A}$ and D_2 receptor sites and carries little risk of extrapyramidal and antihistaminic effects. No guidelines exist for its use in autistic children with aggressive and self-injurious behaviors; clinicians sometimes use it to treat these behaviors in treatment-resistant children. In studies of its use in adults with schizophrenia, dose ranges of 40 to 160 mg were effective. Adverse effects include sedation, dizziness, and lightheadedness. Before using this medication, the clinician should check an electrocardiogram.

Lithium is efficacious in children with aggression without autism spectrum disorder, and it is used clinically in the treatment of aggressive or self-injurious behaviors when antipsychotic medications are not helpful.

Agents Used for Behavioral Impairment in Autism Spectrum Disorder without Evidence of Efficacy. A double-blind study investigated the efficacy of amantadine, which blocks *N*-methyl-D-aspartate (NMDA) receptors, in the treatment of behavioral disturbance, such as irritability, aggression, and hyperactivity, in children with autism. Some researchers have suggested that abnormalities of the glutamatergic system may contribute to the emergence of autism spectrum disorders. High glutamate levels occur in children with the formerly labeled Rett syndrome. In the amantadine study, 47 percent of children on amantadine were "improved" per their parents, and 37 percent of children on placebo were rated "improved" by parents in irritability and hyperactivity, although this difference was not statistically significant. Investigators rated the children on amantadine "significantly improved" for hyperactivity. A double-blind, placebo-controlled study of the efficacy of the anticonvulsant lamotrigine on hyperactivity in children with autism showed high rates of placebo improvement in ratings of hyperactivity, which were similar to response on the medication.

Clomipramine is sometimes used but lacks RCTs to provide evidence of positive results. Fenfluramine, which reduces blood serotonin levels, has also been used but appears to be ineffective. Improvement does not seem to be associated with a reduction in blood serotonin levels. Naltrexone, an opioid receptor antagonist, has been investigated without much success, based on the notion that blocking endogenous opioids would reduce autistic symptoms.

Tetrahydrobiopterin, a coenzyme that enhances the action of enzymes, was studied. However, the results were not significant. Post hoc analysis of the three core symptoms of autism—social interaction, communication, and stereotyped behaviors—revealed a significant improvement in social interaction score after 6 months of active treatment. There was a positive correlation between social response and IQ. These results suggest that there is a possible effect of tetrahydrobiopterin on the social functioning of children with autism.

A case report suggested that low-dose venlafaxine was efficacious in three adolescents and young adults with autistic disorder with self-injurious behavior and hyperactivity. The dose of venlafaxine used was 18.75 mg/day, and the efficacy continued over 6 months.

Complementary and Alternative Medicine (CAM) Approaches to Autism Spectrum Disorder

Complementary and alternative medicine (CAM) is a group of nontraditional treatments used in conjunction with conventional treatments. Safe interventions that target both core and associated behavioral features of autism spectrum disorder with unknown efficacy include the following: music therapy, to promote communication and expression, and yoga, to promote attention and decrease activity level. A biologically based practice that appears to be safe and efficacious is melatonin, which reduces sleep-onset latency in children. Other biologic practices that appear to be safe but with unknown efficacy include vitamin C, multivitamins, essential fatty acids, and the amino acids carnosine and carnitine. Secretin is ineffective in RCTs in the treatment of autism spectrum disorder.

EPIDEMIOLOGY

Prevalence

The diagnostic rate for autism spectrum disorders has increased over the last two decades, and currently 1 in 54 children is diagnosed with autism spectrum disorder in the United States. Autistic disorder, based on DSM-IV-TR criteria, is believed to occur at a rate of about 8 cases per 10,000 children (0.08 percent). By definition, the onset of autism spectrum disorder is in the early developmental period; however, some children go undetected until they are much older. Because of this delay between onset and diagnosis, the prevalence rates increase with age in young children.

Sex Distribution

Autism spectrum disorder is diagnosed four times more often in boys than in girls. In clinical samples, girls with autism spectrum disorder more often exhibit intellectual disability than boys. One potential explanation for this is that girls with autism spectrum disorder without an intellectual disability may be less likely to be identified, referred clinically, and diagnosed.

ETIOLOGY AND PATHOGENESIS

Genetic Factors

Family and twin studies suggest that autism spectrum disorder has a significant heritable contribution; however, it does not appear to be fully penetrant. Although up to 15 percent of cases of autism spectrum disorder appear to be associated with a known genetic mutation, in most cases, its expression is dependent on multiple genes. Family studies have demonstrated increased rates of autism spectrum disorder in siblings of an index child, as high as 50 percent in some families with two or more children with autism spectrum disorder. Siblings of a child with autism spectrum disorder are also at increased risk for a variety of developmental impairments in communication and social skills, even when they do not meet the criteria for autism spectrum disorder.

The concordance rate of autistic disorder in two extensive twin studies was 36 percent in monozygotic pairs versus 0 percent in dizygotic pairs in one study and about 96 percent in monozygotic pairs versus about 27 percent in dizygotic pairs in the second study. High rates of cognitive impairments, in the nonautistic twin in monozygotic twins with perinatal complications, suggest that contributions of perinatal environmental factors interact with genetic vulnerability differentially in autism spectrum disorder.

The heterogeneity in the expression of symptoms in families with autism spectrum disorder suggests that there are multiple patterns of genetic transmission. Studies indicate that both an increase and decrease in specific genetic patterns may be risk factors for autism spectrum disorder. In addition to specific genetic factors, gender plays a substantial role in the expression of autism spectrum disorder. Genetic studies have identified two biologic systems involved in autism spectrum disorder: the consistent finding of elevated platelet serotonin (5-HT) and the mTOR, that is, mammalian target of rapamycin–linked synaptic plasticity mechanisms, which is disrupted in autism spectrum disorder. These will be discussed further in the next section.

Several genetic disorders cause autism spectrum disorder symptoms as part of a broader phenotype. The most common of these inherited disorders is fragile X syndrome, an X-linked recessive disorder that is present in 2 to 3 percent of individuals with autism spectrum disorder. Fragile X syndrome exhibits a nucleotide repeat in the 5' untranslated region of the *FMNR1* gene, resulting in symptoms of autism spectrum disorder. Children with fragile X syndrome characteristically exhibit intellectual disability, gross and fine motor impairments, an unusual facies, macroorchidism, and significantly diminished expressive language ability. Tuberous sclerosis, another genetic disorder characterized by multiple benign tumors, inherited by autosomal dominant transmission, is found with higher frequency among children with autism spectrum disorder. Up to 2 percent of children with autism spectrum disorder also have tuberous sclerosis.

Researchers who screened the DNA of more than 150 pairs of siblings with autism spectrum disorder found evidence of two regions on chromosomes 2 and 7 containing genes that may contribute to autism spectrum disorder. Additional genes hypothesized to be involved in autism spectrum disorder are on chromosomes 16 and 17.

Biomarkers in Autism Spectrum Disorder

Autism spectrum disorder is associated with several biomarkers, potentially resulting from interactions of genes and environmental factors, which then influence neuronal function, dendrite development, and contribute to altered neuronal information processing. Researchers have identified several biomarkers of abnormal signaling in the 5-HT system, the mTOR-linked synaptic plasticity mechanisms, and alterations of the γ-aminobutyric acid (GABA) inhibitory system.

The first biomarker identified in autism spectrum disorder was elevated serotonin in whole blood, almost exclusively in the platelets. Platelets acquire 5-HT through the process of SERT (serotonin transporter), known to be hereditary, as they pass through the intestinal circulation. The genes that mediate SERT (*SLC64A*), and the 5-HT receptor 5-HT$_{2A}$ gene (*HTR2A*) are known to be more heritable than autism spectrum disorder, and encode the same protein in the platelets and the brain. Because 5-HT is known to be involved in brain development, the changes in 5-HT regulation may lead to alterations in neuronal migration and growth in the brain.

Both structural and functional neuroimaging studies have suggested specific biomarkers associated with autism spectrum disorder. Several studies found increased total brain volume in children younger than 4 years of age with autism spectrum disorder, whose neonatal head circumferences were within normal limits or slightly below. By about age 5 years, however, 15 to 20 percent of children with autism spectrum disorder developed macrocephaly. Additional studies found confirmatory data in samples of infants who later had autism spectrum disorder, who exhibited normal head circumferences at birth; by 4 years, 90 percent had larger brain volumes than controls, with 37 percent of the disordered group meeting criteria for macrocephaly. In contrast, structural magnetic resonance imaging (sMRI) studies of children with autism spectrum disorder ranging from 5 to 16 years did not find mean values of total brain volume increased. One study followed the size of the amygdala in youth with autism spectrum disorder in the first few years of life, and similarly, found an increased size in the first few years of life, followed by a decrease in size over time. Several studies have found enlarged striatum in young children with autism spectrum disorder, with a positive correlation of striatal size with the frequency of repetitive behaviors. The dynamic process of the atypical and changing total brain volume observed in children with autism spectrum disorder lends support for the overarching hypothesis that there are sensitive periods or "critical periods" within the brain's plasticity, which when disrupted, may contribute to the emergence of autism spectrum disorder.

Functional MRI (fMRI) studies have focused on identifying biomarkers; that is, the functional brain correlates of various observed core symptoms in autism spectrum disorder. fMRI studies of children, adolescents, and adults with autism spectrum disorder have employed tasks including face perception, neutral face tasks, "theory of mind" deficits, language and communication impairments, working memory, and repetitive behaviors. fMRI studies have provided evidence that individuals with autism spectrum disorder tend to scan faces differently than controls, in that they focus more on the mouth region of the face rather than on the eye region and rather than scanning the entire face multiple times, individuals with autism spectrum disorder focus more on individual features of the face. In response to socially relevant stimuli, researchers have concluded that individuals with autism spectrum disorder have greater amygdala hyperarousal. In terms of "theory of mind," that is, the ability to attribute emotional states to others, and to oneself, fMRI studies find differences in activation in brain regions such as the right temporal lobe and other areas of the brain known to become activated in controls during tasks involving the theory of mind. This difference has been hypothesized by some researchers to represent dysfunction of the mirror neuron system (MNS). Atypical patterns of frontal lobe activation have been found in multiple studies of autism spectrum disorder during face processing tasks, suggesting that this area of the brain may be critical in social perception and emotional reasoning. Decreased activation in individuals with autism spectrum disorder in the left frontal regions of the brain during memory and language-based tasks led researchers to hypothesize that individuals with autism spectrum disorder utilized more visual strategies during language processing than controls did.

Both sMRI and fMRI research have contributed to demonstrating brain correlates of core impairments observed in individuals with autism spectrum disorder.

Immunologic Factors

Several reports have suggested that immunologic incompatibility (i.e., maternal antibodies directed at the fetus) may contribute to autistic disorder. The lymphocytes of some autistic children react with maternal antibodies, which raise the possibility that embryonic neural tissues damage during gestation. These reports usually reflect single cases rather than controlled studies, and this hypothesis is still under investigation.

Prenatal and Perinatal Factors

A higher-than-expected incidence of prenatal and perinatal complications seems to occur in infants who later have autism spectrum disorder. The most significant prenatal factors associated with autism spectrum disorder in the offspring are advanced maternal and paternal age at birth, maternal gestational bleeding, gestational diabetes, and first-born baby. Perinatal risk factors for autism spectrum disorder include umbilical cord complications, birth trauma, fetal distress, small for gestational age, low birth weight, low 5-minute Apgar score, congenital malformation, ABO blood group system or Rh factor incompatibility and hyperbilirubinemia. Many of the obstetrical complications that are associated with risk for autism spectrum disorder are also risk factors for hypoxia, which may be an underlying risk factor itself. There is no sufficient evidence to implicate any one single perinatal or prenatal factor in autism spectrum disorder etiology, and a genetic predisposition to autism spectrum disorder may be interacting with perinatal factors.

Comorbid Neurologic Disorders

EEG abnormalities and seizure disorders occur with higher-than-expected frequency in individuals with autism spectrum disorder. Four percent to 32 percent of individuals with autism spectrum disorder have grand mal seizures at some time, and about 20 to 25 percent show ventricular enlargement on computed tomography (CT) scans. Various EEG abnormalities occur in 10 to 83 percent of children with the previously defined autistic disorder, and although no EEG finding is specific to autistic disorder, there is some indication of failed cerebral lateralization. The current consensus is that autism spectrum disorder is a set of behavioral syndromes caused by a multitude of factors acting on the CNS.

Psychosocial Theories

Studies comparing parents of children with autism spectrum disorder with parents of typical children have shown no significant differences in child-rearing skills. Researchers have disproved earlier speculations that parental emotional factors contribute to the development of autism spectrum disorder.

▲ 2.4 Attention-Deficit/ Hyperactivity Disorder

ADHD is a neuropsychiatric condition affecting preschoolers, children, adolescents, and adults around the world, characterized by a pattern of diminished sustained attention, and increased impulsivity or hyperactivity. Based on family history, genotyping, and neuroimaging studies, there is clear evidence to support a biologic basis for ADHD. Although multiple regions of the brain and several neurotransmitters contribute to the emergence of symptoms, dopamine continues to be a focus of investigation regarding ADHD symptoms. The prefrontal cortex of the brain is a focus of interest because of its high utilization of dopamine and its reciprocal connections with other brain regions involved in attention, inhibition, decision-making, response inhibition, working memory, and vigilance. ADHD affects up to 5 to 8 percent of school-age children, with 60 to 85 percent of those diagnosed as children continuing to meet criteria for the disorder in adolescence, and up to 60 percent continuing to be symptomatic into adulthood. Children, adolescents, and adults with ADHD often have significant impairment in academic functioning as well as in social and interpersonal situations. ADHD is frequently associated with comorbid disorders, including learning disorders, anxiety disorders, mood disorders, and disruptive behavior disorders.

The DSM-5 has made several changes to the diagnostic criteria of ADHD in youth and adults. Whereas in the past, ADHD symptoms had to be present by age 7 years, in DSM-5, "several inattentive or hyperactive-impulsive symptoms" must be present by age 12 years. Previously, there were two subtypes: Inattentive and Hyperactive/Impulsive type. In DSM-5, however, subtypes have been replaced by the following three specifiers, which largely denote the same groups: (1) combined presentation, (2) predominantly inattentive presentation, and (3) predominantly hyperactive/impulsive presentation. Additional changes in DSM-5 include permitting a comorbid ADHD and autism spectrum diagnosis. Finally, in DSM-5, for adolescents 17 years and older and adults, only five symptoms, rather than six symptoms of either inattention or hyperactivity and impulsivity, are required. Also, DSM-5 added symptoms to its list to reflect different presentations across the life span. To confirm a diagnosis of ADHD, impairment from inattention or hyperactivity and impulsivity must be present in at least two settings and interfere with developmentally appropriate social or academic functioning.

ADHD has historically been described in the literature using different terminology. In the early 1900s, impulsive, disinhibited, and hyperactive children—many of whom also had neurologic damage due to encephalitis—were grouped under the label *hyperactive syndrome.* In the 1960s, a heterogeneous group of children with poor coordination, learning disabilities, and emotional lability, but without specific neurologic disorders, were described as having "minimal brain damage"; however, over time, it became clear that this was an inappropriate term. There are many explanations for ADHD symptoms, including theories of abnormal arousal and reduced ability to modulate emotions. This theory was initially supported by the observation that stimulant medications increased sustained attention and improved focus. ADHD is one of the most well-researched childhood psychiatric disorders with several evidence-based treatments.

CLINICAL FEATURES

ADHD can have its onset in infancy, although it is rarely recognized until a child is at least toddler age. More commonly, infants with ADHD are active in the crib, sleep little, and cry a great deal.

In school, children with ADHD may attack a test rapidly but may answer only the first two questions. They may be unable to wait to be called on in school and may respond before everyone else. At home, caregivers cannot put them off for even a minute. Impulsiveness and an inability to delay gratification are characteristic. Children with ADHD are often susceptible to accidents.

The most cited characteristics of children with ADHD, in order of frequency, are hyperactivity, attention deficit (short attention span, distractibility, perseveration, failure to finish tasks, inattention, poor concentration), impulsivity (action before thought, abrupt shifts in activity, lack of organization, jumping up in class), memory and thinking deficits, specific learning disabilities, and speech and hearing deficits. Associated features often include perceptual-motor impairment, emotional lability, and developmental coordination disorder. A significant percentage of children with ADHD show behavioral symptoms of aggression and defiance. School difficulties, both learning and behavioral, commonly exist with ADHD. Comorbid communication disorders or learning disorders that hamper the acquisition, retention, and display of knowledge complicate the course of ADHD.

A psychiatrist evaluated Justin, a 9-year-old boy, after his teacher informed his adoptive parents that she was unable to manage Justin's impulsive and aggressive behaviors in the classroom. Justin was attending public school and was in a regular classroom with two resource room periods per day to help him with reading and math. Justin also received speech therapy once a week. Justin's adoptive parents knew very little about his biologic family other than that his biologic mother was known to be a polydrug abuser. Currently, she was incarcerated. His parents adopted Justin as an infant, and the pediatrician had told his adoptive parents that Justin was entirely healthy at birth. However, ever since kindergarten, Justin's teachers had complained that Justin did "not seem to listen," had "poor concentration," and was unable to stay in his

seat. Because Justin was an engaging and cute child, his teachers in kindergarten and first grade made accommodations for him in their classrooms despite their complaints. When Justin entered the second grade, however, it became clear that he was struggling with reading and writing, and the school initiated an individualized educational program (IEP). Justin was provided with resource room periods for remediation during the school day but continued to have additional problems getting along with his peers during lunch, and even at recess. Justin was often arguing or fighting with other children, who said that he did not know the rules of their games. Justin became angry when his peers criticized him, and he would often push his classmates. At home, Justin's adoptive parents were becoming more and more frustrated with Justin because he seemed to take hours to do a few math problems and was unable to write a paragraph without much help. Justin would become easily annoyed when frustrated with himself and then run around the house in a silly and disruptive manner. Justin was a good-hearted child who seemed to get along best with children who were younger than he was. Justin did not seem to make any close friends among his classmates, and the teachers indicated that Justin's peers sometimes avoided him because he was too rough during play, and he did not follow the rules of their games. Justin had a difficult time waiting for his turn, and when reprimanded, he became easily provoked. Consequently, Justin became alienated and often bullied by his classmates. Justin was aware that he was not able to keep up with the classwork, and he told his adoptive parents that he was just "stupid." Although Justin acted in a rambunctious and impulsive manner, he also appeared sad, and one day after a fight with several peers, he told his adoptive parents that he was going to "kill" himself. At this point, Justin's parents became worried and decided that Justin's teacher was right, and they would seek a psychiatric evaluation for Justin. During the initial evaluation with a child and adolescent psychiatrist, Justin was a well-developed, cute, and active child, who appeared distracted and fidgety and somewhat sad. When asked about it, Justin said that he wanted to do "better" in school but that nobody liked him, he was failing his classes, and that he did not like doing homework. He denied suicidal thoughts and reported that he had only said that to his parents because he was angry at his peers. Justin admitted that it was tough for him to understand his school work and impossible to complete his assignments. The evaluation included several parent and teacher rating scales. These included The Child Behavior Checklist and the SNAP Rating Scale. Justin's teacher and parents endorsed similar symptoms, including poor organization, inability to follow directions, being forgetful in daily activities, impulsivity, with several episodes of running into the street without looking, blurting things out in the classroom without raising his hand, and recurrent fights with peers. Justin looked dejected in school when he was excluded from play activities by peers, and sullen or angry at home when his parents asked him to read or do homework. Based on the clinical history, the rating scales, and the teacher's report, a diagnosis of attention-deficit/hyperactivity disorder, with the DSM-5 specifier of combined presentation, was made. Also, Justin had a mood disorder with depressed mood, which did not qualify for major depression. The suggested treatment plan included a behavioral plan allowing Justin to receive rewards for effort on his homework along with a trial of stimulant medication. An extensive medical history and recent physical examination did not reveal any systemic illnesses. After obtaining a normal ECG, the psychiatrist started Justin on a trial dose of a short-acting stimulant, methylphenidate at 10 mg, to determine if he could tolerate a stimulant without any unexpected sensitivities. Justin had no adverse effects, and soon the doctor switched him to a long-acting formulation (Concerta), 36 mg, which would last between 10 and 12 hours. Justin became more vigilant in class and seemed to be less restless and more focused, and his teacher reported that he was not getting out of his seat as often, although he continued to blurt out in class inappropriately, and he continued to have difficulty following directions and forgetting things. Because Justin was not experiencing any adverse effects and was still displaying some ADHD symptoms, his psychiatrist increased his Concerta to 54 mg/day. At this dose, Justin was better at sitting and finishing his classwork and homework. However, he began to have significant problems with insomnia and was becoming fatigued from not being able to fall asleep until about 2 AM on a nightly basis. The child and adolescent psychiatrist and Justin's parents discussed two options to address insomnia. One was to add a dose of short-acting clonidine in the evenings to cause a calming effect along with some sedative properties. The other was to initiate a methylphenidate transdermal patch, which could be applied to deliver a similar dose of methylphenidate throughout the day, and the patch could be removed at approximately 4 PM or 5 PM to determine which produced the desired effect for the target symptoms for the most optimal amount of time. Because the patch may deliver medication for an hour or so after its removal, Justin would need to try several different removal times to find the optimal treatment time. Justin's family and his child psychiatrist determined that it would be the best next step for Justin to try the transdermal patch rather than add medication to treat his insomnia. Justin was tried on the transdermal 20-mg patch and found that if it was removed by 5 PM, he was able to fall asleep within 30 to 45 minutes after getting into bed. Despite some mild erythema around the site of the patch, Justin experienced no other side effects and was glad that he did not have to take pills each morning. It was determined by Justin's parents, teachers, and child and adolescent psychiatrist that Justin's ADHD symptoms were now under much-improved control. Justin began to receive better grades, and his self-esteem improved. However, Justin still had difficulties with peers and felt that he was not making as many friends as he wanted. Justin's child psychiatrist suggested that Justin receive weekly social skills group therapy that was led by a psychologist who had experience with group interventions for children with ADHD. At first, Justin did not want to attend these sessions, but after a few sessions, during which the group praised Justin for his appropriate interactions, he decided he liked the group. Over time, he even invited a few of his peers from the group to his home to play. The combination of the medication and the social skills group resulted in a significant improvement in Justin's ADHD symptoms. It also improved the quality of his relationships with peers and even his family. (Adapted from Greenhill LL, Hechtman LI. Attention-deficit/hyperactivity disorder. In: Sadock BJ, Sadock VA, Ruiz P, eds. *Kaplan & Sadock's Comprehensive Textbook of Psychiatry*. 9th ed. Vol. 2. Philadelphia, PA: Lippincott Williams & Wilkins; 2009:3571.)

DIAGNOSIS

We can elicit the principal signs of inattention, impulsivity, and hyperactivity from a detailed history of a child's early developmental patterns along with direct observation of the child, especially in situations that require sustained attention. Hyperactivity may be more severe in some situations (e.g., school) and less marked in others (e.g., one-on-one interviews), and may be less evident in pleasant structured activities (sports). The diagnosis of ADHD requires persistent, impairing symptoms of either hyperactivity/impulsivity or inattention in at least two different settings. For example, most children with ADHD have symptoms in school and at home. Table 2-15 outlines the diagnostic criteria for ADHD.

Distinguishing features of ADHD are short attention span and high levels of distractibility for chronologic age and developmental level. In school, children with ADHD often exhibit difficulties following instructions and require increased individualized attention from teachers. At home, children with ADHD frequently have difficulty complying with their parents' directions and may need to be asked multiple times to complete relatively simple tasks. Children with ADHD typically act impulsively, are emotionally labile, explosive, lack focus, and are irritable.

Children for whom hyperactivity is a predominant feature are more likely to be referred for treatment earlier than are children whose primary symptoms are attention deficit. Children with the combined inattentive and hyperactive-impulsive symptoms of ADHD, or predominantly hyperactive-impulsive symptoms of ADHD, are more apt to have a stable diagnosis over time and to exhibit comorbid conduct disorder than those children with inattentive ADHD. Specific learning disorders in the areas of reading, arithmetic, language, and writing frequently occur in association with ADHD. We should assess global development to rule out other sources of inattention.

School history and teachers' reports are critical in evaluating whether a child's difficulties in learning and school behavior are caused primarily by inattention or compromised understanding of the academic material. In addition to intellectual limitations, poor performance in school may result from maturational problems, social rejection, mood disorders, anxiety, or poor self-esteem due to learning disorders. Assessment of social relationships with siblings, peers, and adults, and engagement in free and structured activities may yield valuable diagnostic clues to the presence of ADHD.

The mental status examination in a given child with ADHD who is aware of his or her impairment may reflect a demoralized or depressed mood; however, we would not expect to see a thought disorder or impaired reality testing. A child with ADHD may exhibit distractibility and perseveration and signs of visual-perceptual, auditory-perceptual, or language-based learning disorders. A neurologic examination may reveal visual, motor, perceptual, or auditory discriminatory immaturity or impairments without overt signs of visual or auditory disorders. Children with ADHD often have problems with motor coordination and difficulty copying age-appropriate figures, rapid alternating movements, right-left discrimination, ambidexterity, reflex asymmetries, and a variety of subtle nonfocal neurologic signs (soft signs).

If there are indications of possible absence spells, clinicians should obtain a neurologic consultation and an EEG to rule out seizure disorders. A child with an unrecognized temporal lobe seizure focus may have behavior disturbances which can resemble those of ADHD.

Pathology and Laboratory Examination

Evaluation for ADHD includes a comprehensive psychiatric and medical history. This history includes prenatal, perinatal, and toddler information. Complications during the mother's pregnancy are also informative. Medical problems that may produce symptoms overlapping with ADHD include petit mal epilepsy, hearing and visual impairments, thyroid abnormalities, and hypoglycemia. A thorough cardiac history should be taken, including an investigation of the life history of syncope, family history of sudden death, and a cardiac examination of the child. Although it is reasonable to obtain electrocardiography (ECG) study before treatment, if any cardiac risk factors are present, a cardiology consultation and examination are warranted. No specific laboratory measures are pathognomonic of ADHD.

A continuous performance task, a computerized task in which a child presses a button each time a particular sequence of letters or numbers flashes on a screen, is not specifically a useful diagnostic tool for ADHD; however, it may be useful in comparing a child's performance before and after medication treatment, particularly at different doses. Children with poor attention tend to make errors of omission—that is, they fail to press the button when the sequence has flashed. Impulsivity causes errors of commission, in which an

Table 2-15
Attention-Deficit/Hyperactivity Disorder

	DSM-5	ICD-10
Diagnostic name	Attention-Deficit/Hyperactivity Disorder	Hyperkinetic Disorders Disturbance of activity and attention
Duration	≥6 mo Symptoms present before the age of 12	Usually occurs before the age of 5
Symptoms	Inattention: • Poor attention to detail/frequent mistakes • Hard to maintain attention/focus • When spoken to, appears not to listen • Poor follow through on tasks • Poor organizational skills • Procrastinates from tasks requiring attention • Loses things • Distractible • Forgetfulness Hyperactivity/impulsivity: • Fidgety/restless • Cannot stay seated • Runs/climbs inappropriately • Cannot do things quietly (e.g., play) • Cannot keep still • Inappropriately talkative • Inappropriately blurts out answers • Cannot wait his turn • Interrupts others	Cannot engage in activities requiring prolonged attention Disorganized about completing tasks Excess activity May have: • Impulsivity • Recklessness • Social disinhibition
Required number of symptoms	≥6 of each category (≥5 for age ≥17) Symptoms occur in >1 setting	
Psychosocial consequences of symptoms	Functional impairment	
Exclusions (not result of):	Another mental illness	Hyperkinetic conduct disorder—referring to symptoms present in the context of conduct disorder
Symptom Specifiers	**Combined presentation** **Predominantly inattentive presentation** **Predominantly hyperactive/impulsive presentation**	
Course specifiers	**In partial remission:** last 6 mo, symptoms continue but less than required for diagnosis	
Severity specifiers	**Mild:** minimal symptoms required for diagnosis; Minor functional impairment **Moderate:** Intermediate symptoms and impairment **Severe:** Severe symptoms, marked impairment	

impulsive child cannot resist pushing the button, even when the desired sequence has not yet appeared on the screen.

DIFFERENTIAL DIAGNOSIS

A temperamental constellation of high activity level and short attention span, in the normal range for the child's age, and without impairment, should be ruled out. Differentiating these temperamental characteristics from the cardinal symptoms of ADHD before the age of 3 years is difficult, mainly because of the overlapping features of an ordinarily immature nervous system and the emerging signs of visual-motor-perceptual impairments frequently seen in ADHD. It is critical to evaluate for anxiety. Anxiety can accompany ADHD as a symptom or comorbid disorder, and anxiety can manifest with overactivity and easy distractibility.

It is not uncommon for a child with ADHD to become demoralized or, in some cases, to develop depressive symptoms in reaction to persistent frustration with academic difficulties and resulting in

low self-esteem. Mania and ADHD share many core features, such as excessive verbalization, motoric hyperactivity, and high levels of distractibility. Also, in children with mania, irritability seems to be more common than euphoria. Although mania and ADHD can coexist, children with bipolar I disorder exhibit more waxing and waning of symptoms than those with ADHD. Recent follow-up data for children who met the criteria for ADHD and subsequently developed bipolar disorder suggest that certain clinical features occurring during ADHD predict future mania. Children with ADHD who had developed bipolar I disorder at 4-year follow-up had a higher co-occurrence of additional disorders and a higher family history of bipolar disorders and other mood disorders than children without bipolar disorder.

Frequently, oppositional defiant disorder, or conduct disorder and ADHD, may coexist, and when that occurs, we should diagnose both disorders. We must also distinguish specific learning disorders from ADHD; a child may be unable to read or do mathematics because of a learning disorder, rather than because of inattention. ADHD often coexists with one or more learning problems, including deficits in reading, mathematics, or written expression.

The DSM-5 includes Unspecified ADHD as a category for disturbances of inattention or hyperactivity that cause impairment, but do not meet the full criteria for ADHD.

COURSE AND PROGNOSIS

The course of ADHD is variable. Symptoms persist into adolescence in 60 to 85 percent of cases, and into adult life in approximately 60 percent of cases. The remaining 40 percent of cases may remit at puberty or in early adulthood. In some cases, the hyperactivity may disappear, but the decreased attention span and impulse-control problems persist. Overactivity is usually the first symptom to remit, and distractibility is the last. ADHD does not usually remit during middle childhood. A family history of the disorder predicts persistence, as do adverse life events, and comorbidity with conduct symptoms, depression, and anxiety disorders. When remission occurs, it is usually between the ages of 12 and 20. After remission, the child can go on to have a productive adolescence and adult life, satisfying interpersonal relationships, and few significant sequelae. Most patients with the disorder, however, undergo partial remission and are vulnerable to antisocial behavior, substance use disorders, and mood disorders. Learning problems often continue throughout life.

In about 60 percent of cases, some symptoms persist into adulthood. Those who persist with the disorder may show diminished hyperactivity but remain impulsive and accident-prone. Although the educational attainments of people with ADHD as a group are lower than those of people without ADHD, early employment histories do not differ from those of people with similar educations.

Children with ADHD whose symptoms persist into adolescence are at higher risk for developing conduct disorder. Children with both ADHD and conduct disorder are also at risk for developing substance use disorders. The development of substance use disorders among ADHD youth in adolescence appears to be more related to the presence of conduct disorder rather than to ADHD.

Most children with ADHD have some social difficulties. Socially dysfunctional children with ADHD have significantly higher rates of comorbid psychiatric disorders and experience more problems with behavior in school as well as with peers and family members. Overall, the outcome of ADHD in childhood seems to be related to the degree of persistent comorbid psychopathology, primarily conduct disorder, social disability, and chaotic family factors. For optimal outcomes, it is essential to ameliorate children's social functioning, diminish aggression, and improve family situations as early as possible.

TREATMENT

Pharmacotherapy

Pharmacologic treatment is considered the first line of treatment for ADHD. CNS stimulants are the first choice of agents in that they have the highest efficacy with generally mild tolerable side effects. Children, adolescents, and adults with known cardiac risks and abnormalities should not use stimulants. In healthy youths, both short- and sustained-release preparations have excellent safety records. The newer preparations aim to maximize the target effects and minimize the adverse effects in individuals with ADHD who obtain a partial response from methylphenidate or whose dose was limited by side effects.

Current strategies favor once a day sustained-release stimulant preparations for their convenience and diminished rebound side effects. Advantages of the sustained-release preparations are that a single dose will sustain the effects all day, and the medication is sustained at an approximately even level in the body throughout the day. In general the immediate-release preparations are expected to last 1 to 4 hours and extended-release preparations are expected to last up to 8 hours, with exceptions for the transdermal patch, which lasts an hour after it is removed.

Nonstimulant medications approved by the FDA in the treatment of ADHD include atomoxetine, a norepinephrine uptake inhibitor. Unlike the stimulants, atomoxetine carries with it a black-box warning for potential increases in suicidal thoughts or behaviors and requires children with ADHD to be monitored for these symptoms, similarly to children taking antidepressants. α-agonists, including clonidine and guanfacine, are also useful in treating ADHD. The FDA has approved the extended-release form of clonidine and the extended-release form of guanfacine for the treatment of ADHD in children 6 years and older. Antidepressants, such as bupropion, have been used with variable success in the treatment of ADHD. Table 2-16 indicates FDA-approved ages for ADHD medications.)

Stimulant Medications.   Methylphenidate and amphetamine preparations are dopamine agonists; however, the precise mechanism of the stimulant's central action remains unknown. Methylphenidate preparations are highly effective in up to three-fourths of children with ADHD, with relatively few adverse effects. Concerta, the 10- to 12-hour extended-release OROS (osmotic controlled-release extended delivery system) form of methylphenidate, is administered once daily in the morning and is useful during school hours as well as after school during the afternoon and early evening. Both shorter forms of methylphenidate and Concerta have similar common adverse effects, including headaches, stomachaches, nausea, and insomnia. Some children experience a rebound effect, in which they become mildly irritable and appear to be slightly hyperactive for a brief period when the medication wears off. In children with a history of motor tics, we should observe them as, in some cases, methylphenidate can exacerbate the tics, whereas, in other children, the tics are unaffected or even improved. Because tics wax and wane, it is essential to observe their patterns over some time. Another common concern about the use of methylphenidate preparations over long periods is potential growth suppression. During periods of use, methylphenidate may cause slightly decreased rates of growth, and if used over many years continuously without any drug holidays, experts have noted a growth suppression of about several centimeters. When given "drug holidays" on weekends or summers, children tend to eat more and also make up the growth. The methylphenidate products can improve ADHD children's scores on tasks of vigilance, such as on math calculation tests, the continuous performance task, and paired associations. Transdermal methylphenidate is available for children and adolescents. Advantages of this preparation include an alternative for children who have difficulties swallowing pills, and that the patch can individualize how many hours per day a given child with ADHD receives the medication. This option is useful because a child with ADHD who needs the medication in the late afternoons to do homework but develops insomnia if the medication is still present after dinner can remove the patch at the desired time. Thus, individualized delivery time may be provided for each child by how many hours they wear the patch.

In contrast, oral sustained-release forms of methylphenidate are those in which the release time continues for 12 hours after

Table 2-16
FDA Approval for ADHD Medications

Medication	Generic Name	FDA Approval Age (yr)
Methylphenidate		
Concerta	Methylphenidate (OROS long acting)	6 and older
Ritalin	Methylphenidate	6 and older
Ritalin LA	Methylphenidate (long acting)	6 and older
Metadate ER	Methylphenidate (extended release)	6 and older
Metadate CD	Methylphenidate (extended release)	6 and older
Methylin	Methylphenidate (oral solution and chewable tablet)	6 and older
Daytrana	Methylphenidate (patch)	6 and older
Adhansia XR	Methylphenidate (extended release)	6 and older
Aptensio XR	Methylphenidate (extended release)	6 and older
Cotempla XR-ODT	Methylphenidate (extended-release orally disintegrating tablet)	6–17
Jornay PM	Methylphenidate (extended release)	6 and older
Quillichew	Methylphenidate (extended-release chewable)	6 and older
Quillivant ER	Methylphenidate (extended-release suspension)	6 and older
Dexmethylphenidate		
Focalin	Dexmethylphenidate	6 and older
Focalin XR	Dexmethylphenidate (extended release)	6 and older
Dextroamphetamine		
Dexedrine	Dextroamphetamine	3 and older
Amphetamine		
Adzenys ER	Amphetamine (extended-release suspension)	6–12
Adzenys XR-ODT	Amphetamine (extended-release orally disintegrating tablet)	6–17
Dynavel XR	Amphetamine (extended-release suspension)	6 and older
Evekeo	Amphetamine	3 and older
Evekeo ODT	Amphetamine (orally disintegrating tablet)	6–17
Dextroamphetamine/amphetamine		
Adderall	Dextroamphetamine/amphetamine	3 and older
Adderall XR	Dextroamphetamine/amphetamine (extended release)	6 and older
Mydayis	Dextroamphetamine/amphetamine (extended release)	13 and older
Lisdexamfetamine		
Vyvanse	Lisdexamfetamine	6 and older
Nonstimulants		
Strattera	Atomoxetine	6 and older
Alpha Agonists		
Kapvay	Clonidine (extended release)	6–17
Intuniv	Guanfacine (extended release)	6–17

swallowing the pill. A double-blind, randomized study in children with ADHD who wore the methylphenidate patch for 12 hours at a time, showed the efficacy of the patch preparation doses ranging from patches delivering 0.45 to 1.8 mg/hr of methylphenidate. A delay in the onset of the transdermal medication effect was approximately an hour. Side effects were similar to oral preparations of methylphenidate. Approximately half of the children exhibited at least minor erythematous reactions to the patch; however, these side effects are usually well tolerated by children on the patch. Dextroamphetamine and dextroamphetamine/amphetamine salt combinations are usually the second drugs of choice when methylphenidate fails.

CNS STIMULANT SIDE EFFECTS. CNS stimulants are generally well tolerated, and the current consensus is that once a day dosing is preferable for convenience and to minimize rebound side effects. Long-term tolerability of once-daily mixed amphetamine salts

has shown mild side effects, most commonly decreased appetite, insomnia, and headache. There are a variety of strategies for children or adolescents with ADHD who respond favorably to methylphenidate, but for whom insomnia has become a significant problem. Clinical strategies to manage insomnia include the use of diphenhydramine (25 to 75 mg), a low dose of trazodone (25 to 50 mg), or the addition of an α-adrenergic agent, such as guanfacine. In some cases, insomnia may attenuate on its own after several months of treatment.

Nonstimulant Medications. Atomoxetine HCl is a norepinephrine uptake inhibitor approved by the FDA for the treatment of ADHD in children age 6 years and older. The mechanism of action is not well understood, but likely involves selective inhibition of the presynaptic norepinephrine transporter. Atomoxetine absorbs well in the gastrointestinal tract, and it reaches maximal plasma levels in 1 to 2 hours after ingestion. It is useful for inattention as well as impulsivity in children and adults with ADHD. Its half-life is approximately 5 hours and is given twice daily in most cases. The most common side effects include diminished appetite, abdominal discomfort, dizziness, and irritability. In some cases, there were increases in blood pressure and heart rate. Atomoxetine is metabolized by the cytochrome P450 (CYP) 2D6 hepatic enzyme system. A small fraction of the population are poor metabolizers of CYP 2D6–metabolized drugs, and, for those individuals, plasma concentrations of the drug may increase as much as fivefold for a given dose of medication. Drugs that inhibit CYP 2D6, including fluoxetine, paroxetine, and quinidine, may lead to increased plasma levels of this medication. Despite its short half-life, research suggests that atomoxetine can reduce symptoms of ADHD in children during the school day when administered once daily. Another recent study of a combination of atomoxetine alone and combined with fluoxetine in the treatment of 127 children with ADHD and symptoms of anxiety or depression suggested that atomoxetine alone can lead to improvements in mood and anxiety. Children who received combined atomoxetine and fluoxetine experienced more significant increases in blood pressure and pulse than those taking atomoxetine only.

α-Agonists, both short-acting and the extended-release forms of clonidine hydrochloride and guanfacine, are FDA approved for the treatment of ADHD in children and adolescents from 6 to 7 years of age. Clonidine, a centrally acting α_2-adrenergic receptor agonist, likely exerts its effect on the prefrontal cortex, although the mechanism of action is unknown. It is available in 0.1-mg and 0.2-mg tablets, and is generally used twice daily, once in the morning and once at night, to provide an around-the-clock effect. Clonidine is initiated at 0.1 mg at bedtime, with incremental weekly increases of 0.1 mg. The maximum dose recommended is 0.2 mg twice daily. The extended-release formulation is not interchangeable with the short-acting clonidine. Because it is also an antihypertensive agent, it causes a decrease in blood pressure and heart rate. We should monitor vital signs in patients, especially during initiation and titration of the dose. Common side effects include somnolence, headache, upper abdominal pain, and fatigue. When tapering the drug, the rate should be no more than 0.1 mg every 3 to 7 days.

Extended-release guanfacine is a once-a-day medication for children between 6 and 17 years of age, available in 1-mg, 2-mg, 3-mg, and 4-mg tabs. It is swallowed whole with liquids, and the patient should not take it with a high-fat meal. It is initiated as a 1-mg tab daily and titrated by 1 mg/day at 1-week intervals. The maximum dose approved is 4 mg/day. As a monotherapy, improvement in ADHD symptoms occurs at 0.05 to 0.08 mg/kg once daily. As an adjunctive treatment, optimal doses are reported to range from 0.05 to 0.12 mg/kg/day. Common side effects include somnolence, sedation, fatigue, nausea, hypotension, insomnia, and dizziness. We should monitor the heart rate and blood pressure. When discontinuing the drug, one should use a gradual taper, decreasing by 1 mg every 3 to 7 days.

α-Adrenergic agents, including the short- and extended-release preparations of guanfacine and clonidine, are sometimes preferred treatments in children with ADHD and comorbid tic disorders when stimulants exacerbated the tics. Bupropion is somewhat useful for some children and adolescents in the treatment of ADHD. One multisite, double-blind, placebo-controlled study found a positive result regarding the efficacy of bupropion. No further studies have compared bupropion with other stimulants. There is a higher risk of seizures at doses of 400 mg/day or more.

Few data confirm the efficacy of SSRIs in the treatment of ADHD, but due to the frequency of comorbid depression and anxiety with ADHD, in cases of comorbidity, the SSRIs are likely to be considered at least in conjunction with a stimulant.

We should not use tricyclic drugs for ADHD due to potential cardiac arrhythmia effects. The reports of sudden death in at least four children with ADHD using desipramine have made the tricyclic antidepressants an unlikely choice. Antipsychotics may treat refractory severely hyperactive children and adolescents who are significantly dysfunctional. Antipsychotics are generally not chosen in the treatment of ADHD due to the risks of tardive dyskinesia, withdrawal dyskinesia, neuroleptic malignant syndrome, and weight gain.

Modafinil, another type of CNS stimulant, a narcolepsy treatment, may help treat adults with ADHD. Only one randomized, double-blind, placebo-controlled study of the efficacy and safety of modafinil film-coated tablets in approximately 250 adolescents with ADHD showed that 48 percent of those on active treatment were rated as "much" or "very much" improved compared with 17 percent of patients receiving placebo. The dosage range was from 170 to 425 mg administered once daily, titrated to optimal doses based on efficacy and tolerability. Modafinil failed to receive FDA approval based on a Stevens–Johnson skin rash that occurred in a patient during the trial. The most common side effects included insomnia, headache, and decreased appetite.

Some clinicians use venlafaxine, especially for children and adolescents, with combinations of ADHD and depression or anxiety features. No clear empirical evidence supports the use of venlafaxine in the treatment of ADHD.

One open-label report of reboxetine, a selective norepinephrine reuptake inhibitor that is not available in the US, in 31 children and adolescents with ADHD who were resistant to methylphenidate treatment, suggested that this agent may have efficacy. In this open trial, reboxetine was initiated and maintained at 4 mg/day. The most common side effects included drowsiness, sedation, and gastrointestinal symptoms. Reboxetine and other new agents in this class await controlled studies.

Monitoring Pharmacologic Treatment

STIMULANTS. Stimulant medications have adrenergic effects and cause moderate increases in blood pressure and pulse rate. At baseline, the most recent American Academy of Child and Adolescent Psychiatry (AACAP) practice parameters recommend the following workup before starting the use of stimulant medications: physical examination, blood pressure, pulse, weight, and height. Screening electrocardiograms are recommended prior to initiating stimulant medications, particularly if there is a family history or risk factors for cardiac disease.

Children and adolescents using stimulants should have their height, weight, blood pressure, and pulse checked quarterly and have a physical examination annually. Monitoring starts with the initiation of medication. Because school performance is most markedly affected, we should give individual attention and effort to establishing and maintaining a close collaborative working relationship with a child's school personnel. In most patients, stimulants reduce overactivity, distractibility, impulsiveness, explosiveness, and irritability. No evidence indicates that medications directly improve any existing impairments in learning, although when the attention deficits diminish, children can learn more effectively. Also, medication can improve self-esteem when children are no longer constantly reprimanded for their behavior. Children treated with medications should be taught the purpose of the medication and encouraged to describe any side effects that they may be experiencing.

Psychosocial Interventions

Psychosocial interventions for children with ADHD include psychoeducation, academic organization skills remediation, parent training, behavior modification in the classroom and at home, CBT, and social skills training. There are various studies of social skills groups, behavioral training for parents of children with ADHD, and behavioral interventions at school and home, alone and in combination with medication management for ADHD. Evaluation and treatment of coexisting learning disorders or additional psychiatric disorders are essential.

When we help children structure their environment, their anxiety diminishes. Parents and teachers should work together to develop concrete expectations for the child, and a system of rewards when the child meets these expectations.

A common goal of therapy is to help parents of children with ADHD recognize and promote the notion that, although the child may not "voluntarily" exhibit symptoms of ADHD, he or she is still capable of being responsible for meeting reasonable expectations. We should also help parents recognize that, despite their child's difficulties, every child faces the usual tasks of maturation, including the significant building of self-esteem when they develop a sense of mastery. Therefore, children with ADHD do not benefit from being exempted from the requirements, expectations, and planning applicable to other children. Parental training is an integral part of the psychotherapeutic interventions for ADHD. Most parental training helps parents develop usable behavioral interventions with positive reinforcement that target both social and academic behaviors.

Group therapy aimed at both refining social skills and increasing self-esteem and a sense of success may be beneficial for children with ADHD who have great difficulty functioning in group settings, especially in school. A recent year-long group therapy intervention in a clinical setting for boys with the disorder described the goals as helping the boys improve skills in game-playing and feeling a sense of mastery with peers. The researchers asked the boys to do a fun task, in pairs, and then they were gradually asked to do projects in a group. The researchers directed them on how to follow instructions, wait, and pay attention, and praised them for successful cooperation.

Multimodal Treatment Study of Children with ADHD (MTA Study)

The National Institute of Mental Health (NIMH)–supported Multimodal Treatment Study of Children with ADHD (The MTA Cooperative Group, 1999) was a 14-month–long randomized clinical trial involving six clinical sites comparing four treatment strategies. More than 500 children diagnosed with DSM-IV ADHD, combined type, were randomly assigned to (1) systematic medication management utilizing an initial placebo-controlled titration and t.i.d. dosing 7 days per week and monthly 30-minute clinic visits, (2) behavior therapy consisting of 27 sessions of group parent training, eight individual parent sessions, an 8-week summer treatment program, 12 weeks of classroom administered behavior therapy with a half-time aide, and 10 teacher consultation sessions, (3) a combination of medication and behavior therapy, or (4) usual community care. All groups showed improvement over baseline; however, a combination of medication management and behavior therapy led to a greater reduction in symptoms in children with ADHD alone or ADHD and oppositional defiant disorder than behavior therapy alone or community care. The combination treatment had significantly better outcomes for those children with ADHD and anxiety or mood disorders compared to behavioral treatment and community care. Combined treatment but not medication management was superior for improvement in oppositional and aggressive symptoms, anxiety and mood symptoms, teacher-rated social skills, parent–child relationships, and reading achievement. Furthermore, the mean dose of medication per day was less in the combination group than in the medication-only management group.

A follow-up of the MTA sample at 6 and 8 years revealed that the clinical presentation of the disorder, including the severity of ADHD, comorbid conduct disturbance, and intellect, were more reliable predictors of later functioning than the type of treatment received in childhood during the 14-month study period. The children maintained the improvements as long as they continued treatment, but 3 years after treatment, there was no difference between groups.

Overall, the evidence suggests that medication and psychosocial interventions for the combined type of ADHD in childhood provide the broadest benefit in functioning for this population. This recommendation is especially pertinent given the comorbidity of learning disorders, anxiety, mood disorders, and other disruptive behavior disorders that occur in children with ADHD.

EPIDEMIOLOGY

Rates of ADHD are 7 to 8 percent in prepubertal elementary school children. Epidemiologic studies suggest that ADHD occurs in about 5 percent of youth, including children and adolescents, and about 2.5 percent of adults. The rate of ADHD in parents and siblings of children with ADHD is two to eight times greater than in the general population. ADHD is more prevalent in boys than in girls, with the ratio ranging from 2:1 to as high as 9:1. First-degree biologic relatives (e.g., siblings of probands with ADHD) are at high risk for developing ADHD as well as other psychiatric disorders, including disruptive behavior disorders, anxiety disorders, and depressive disorders. Siblings of children with ADHD are also at higher risk than the general population for learning disorders and academic difficulties. The parents of children with ADHD show an increased incidence of substance use disorders. Symptoms of ADHD are often present by age 3 years, but unless they are very severe, the diagnosis is frequently not made until the child is in kindergarten or elementary school when teacher information is available comparing the index child peers of the same age.

ETIOLOGY

Data suggest that the etiology of ADHD is mainly genetic, with a heritability of approximately 75 percent. ADHD symptoms are the product of complex interactions of neuroanatomical and neurochemical systems evidenced by data from twin and adoption family genetic studies, dopamine transport gene studies, neuroimaging studies, and neurotransmitter data. Most children with ADHD have no evidence of gross structural damage in the CNS. In some cases, contributory factors for ADHD may include prenatal toxic exposures, prematurity, and prenatal mechanical insult to the fetal nervous system. Some have suggested that food additives, colorings, preservatives, and sugar are possible contributing causes of hyperactive behavior; however, studies have not confirmed these theories. No research has established artificial food coloring nor sugar as causes of ADHD. There is no clear evidence that omega-3 fatty acids are beneficial in the treatment of ADHD.

Genetic Factors

Evidence for a significant genetic contribution to ADHD has emerged from family studies, which reveal an increased concordance in monozygotic compared to dizygotic twins, as well as a marked increased risk of two to eight times for siblings as well as parents of an ADHD child, compared to the general population. Clinically, one sibling may have impulsivity/hyperactivity symptoms predominantly, and others may have predominantly inattention symptoms. Up to 70 percent of children with ADHD meet criteria for a comorbid psychiatric disorder, including learning disorders, anxiety disorders, mood disorder, conduct disorders, and substance use disorders. Several hypotheses of the mode of transmission of ADHD have been proposed, including a sex-linked hypothesis, which would explain the significantly increased rates of ADHD in males. Other theories have focused on a model of interaction of multiple genes that produces the various symptoms of ADHD. Numerous investigations continue to identify specific genes involved in ADHD. Cook and colleagues have found an association of the dopamine transporter gene (DAT1) with ADHD, although data from other research groups have not confirmed that result. Family studies and population-based studies have found an association between the dopamine four receptor seven-repeat allele (DRD4) gene and ADHD. Most molecular research on ADHD has focused on genes that influence the metabolism or action of dopamine. Continued investigation is necessary to clarify the complex relationships between multiple interactive genes and the emergence of ADHD.

Neurochemical Factors

Many neurotransmitters are likely associated with ADHD symptoms; however, dopamine is a primary focus of clinical investigation, and the prefrontal cortex has been implicated based on its role in attention and regulation of impulse control. Animal studies have shown that other brain regions such as locus ceruleus, which consists predominantly of noradrenergic neurons, also play a significant role in attention. The noradrenergic system includes the central system (originating in the locus ceruleus) and the peripheral sympathetic system. Dysfunction in peripheral epinephrine, which causes the hormone to accumulate peripherally, may potentially feedback to the central system and "reset" the locus ceruleus to a lower level. In part, hypotheses regarding the neurochemistry of ADHD have arisen from the predictable effect of medications. Stimulants, known to be the most effective medications in the treatment of ADHD, affect both dopamine and norepinephrine, leading to neurotransmitter hypotheses that may include dysfunction in both the adrenergic and dopaminergic systems. Stimulants increase catecholamine concentrations by promoting their release and blocking their uptake.

Neurophysiologic Factors

EEG studies in ADHD children and adolescents over the last several decades have found evidence of increased theta activity, especially in the frontal regions. Further studies of youth with ADHD have provided data showing elevated beta activity in their EEG studies. Clarke and colleagues, studying EEG findings in children and adolescents over the last two decades, found that those ADHD children with the combined type of ADHD were the ones who showed significantly elevated beta activity on EEG, and further studies indicate that these youth also tend to show increased mood lability and temper tantrums. The current investigation of EEG in youth with ADHD has identified behavioral symptom clusters among children with similar EEG profiles.

Neuroanatomical Aspects

Researchers have hypothesized networks within the brain for promoting components of attention, including focusing, sustaining attention, and shifting attention. They describe neuroanatomical correlations for the superior and temporal cortices with focusing attention; external parietal and corpus striatal regions with motor executive functions; the hippocampus with encoding of memory traces; and the prefrontal cortex with shifting from one stimulus to another. Further hypotheses suggest that the brainstem, which contains the reticular thalamic nuclei function, is involved in sustained attention. A review of MRI, positron emission tomography (PET), and single-photon emission computerized tomography (SPECT) suggests that populations of children with ADHD show evidence of both decreased volume and decreased activity in prefrontal regions, anterior cingulate, globus pallidus, caudate, thalamus, and cerebellum. PET scans have also shown that female adolescents with ADHD have globally lower glucose metabolism than both control female and male adolescents without ADHD. One theory postulates that the frontal lobes in children with ADHD do not adequately inhibit lower brain structures, an effect leading to disinhibition.

Developmental Factors

Higher rates of ADHD are present in children who were born prematurely and whose mothers had infections during pregnancy. Perinatal insult to the brain during early infancy caused by infection, inflammation, and trauma may, in some cases, be contributing factors in the emergence of ADHD symptoms. Children with ADHD exhibit nonfocal (soft) neurologic signs at higher rates than those in the general population. Reports in the literature indicate that September is a peak month for births of children with ADHD with and without comorbid learning disorders. The implication is that prenatal exposure to winter infections during the first trimester may contribute to the emergence of ADHD symptoms in some susceptible children.

Psychosocial Factors

Severe chronic abuse, maltreatment, and neglect are associated with specific behavioral symptoms that overlap with ADHD, including poor attention and poor impulse control. Predisposing factors may include the child's temperament and genetic–familial factors.

ADULT MANIFESTATIONS OF ADHD

We usually think of ADHD as a childhood condition resulting in delayed development of impulse control. Historically, many experts thought that, by adolescence, patients would grow out of the disorder. However, in the last few decades, many more adults with ADHD have been identified, diagnosed, and successfully treated. Longitudinal follow-up has shown that up to 60 percent of children with ADHD have persistent impairment from symptoms into adulthood. Genetic studies, brain imaging, and neurocognitive and pharmacologic studies in adults with ADHD have replicated findings demonstrated in children with ADHD. Increased public awareness and treatment studies within the last decade have led to widespread acceptance of the need for diagnosis and treatment of adults with ADHD.

Diagnosis and Clinical Features

The clinical phenomenology of ADHD features inattention and manifestations of impulsivity prevailing as the core of this disorder. A leading figure in the development of criteria for adult manifestations of ADHD is Paul Wender, from the University of Utah, who began his work on adult ADHD in the 1970s. Wender developed criteria for adults (Table 2-17). They included a retrospective diagnosis of ADHD in childhood and evidence of current impairment from ADHD symptoms in adulthood. Furthermore, evidence exists of several additional symptoms that are typical of adult behavior as opposed to childhood behaviors.

In adults, residual signs of the disorder include impulsivity and attention deficit (e.g., difficulty in organizing and completing work, inability to concentrate, increased distractibility, and sudden decision-making without thought of the consequences). Many people with the disorder have a secondary depressive disorder associated with low self-esteem related to their impaired performance and which affects both occupational and social functioning.

Brett was a 26-year-old man convinced by his new wife to seek an evaluation for his distractibility, forgetfulness, and "not listening" after a minor traffic accident. After consulting his mother, Brett reported that in grade school, he was often "in trouble" for talking out of turn, and his mother recalled teachers' reports that Brett often made careless mistakes on tests, forgot his assignments, and had great difficulty sitting still. Although as a young child people considered him to be intellectually gifted, when Brett got to the third grade, his grades were only average, and he seemed more interested in getting his work done quickly than correctly. Brett was talkative and loud and enjoyed sports, although he was not particularly talented at them. Nevertheless, Brett had acquaintances and superficial friends because he was likable, funny, and even entertaining. Brett had no idea what he wanted to do when he grew up, and during his senior year in high school, he neglected to finish any of his college applications on time and ended up attending a community college part-time. During the 2 years after high school, Brett held down a series of jobs only briefly, including a construction job, a waiter position in a restaurant, and a Fed-Ex driver, and then decided that he wanted to become an actor. Brett went on a series of auditions but found that he would become distracted and did poorly remembering his lines and even spaced out during readings. Despite that, he acted in one commercial.

Brett reported that he had never had problems with the abuse of drugs or alcohol, and he occasionally drank beer socially. During his evaluation with a child and adolescent psychiatrist, Brett disclosed that his most significant difficulties were with tasks that seemed boring to him. He had difficulty maintaining his attention, was easily distracted, felt restless most of the time, and became frustrated when he had to sit still for long periods. Brett endorsed six inattentive and five hyperactive/impulsive symptoms on a DSM ADHD Checklist of current symptoms. Brett met the diagnostic criteria for adult ADHD, combined presentation, with a probable onset in childhood. Brett's medical history was negative for all major illnesses, and neither he nor his parents had a history of cardiac abnormalities. He took no prescribed medications. After discussing the situation with his psychiatrist and his wife, Brett decided that he would like to try a stimulant medication. A trial of a once-a-day extended-release formulation of stimulant medication was selected: Adderall XR 10 mg.

At his first follow-up visit, a week later, Brett reported that he felt a slight effect from this medication, but it was not enough to improve his functioning, so Brett and his psychiatrist agreed that he would increase his dose to 20 mg/day. At his next follow-up appointment, Brett reported that he had noticed a significant improvement in his ability to focus, concentrate, and remember his lines in auditions. He had just received a small part in an upcoming movie. Brett and his wife were both thrilled with the results, and Brett continued to return for monthly follow-up visits. (Adapted from McGough J. Adult manifestations of attention-deficit/hyperactivity disorder. In: Sadock BJ, Sadock VA, Ruiz P, eds. *Kaplan & Sadock's Comprehensive Textbook of Psychiatry.* 9th ed. Philadelphia, PA: Lippincott Williams & Wilkins; 2009:3577.)

Differential Diagnosis

A diagnosis of ADHD is likely when adults describe symptoms of inattention and impulsivity as a life-long problem, not as episodic events. The overlap of ADHD and hypomania, bipolar II disorder, and cyclothymia is controversial and challenging to sort out retrospectively. Clear-cut histories of discrete episodes of hypomania and mania, with or without periods of depression, are suggestive of a mood disorder rather than a clinical picture of ADHD; however, ADHD may have predated the emergence of a mood disorder in some individuals. In such a case, ADHD and bipolar disorder may be comorbid. Adults with an early history of chronic school difficulties related to paying attention, activity level, and impulsive behavior are generally diagnosed with ADHD, even when a mood disorder occurs later in life. Anxiety disorders can coexist with ADHD and are less complicated than hypomania to distinguish from it.

Course and Prognosis

The prevalence of ADHD diminishes over time, although at least half of children and adolescents may have the disorder into adulthood. Many children, initially diagnosed with ADHD, combined presentation, exhibit fewer impulsive-hyperactive symptoms as

---

Table 2-17
Utah Criteria for Adult Attention-Deficit/ Hyperactivity Disorder (ADHD)

I. Retrospective childhood ADHD diagnosis
  A. Narrow criterion: met DSM-IV criteria in childhood by parent interview[a]
  B. Broad criterion: both (1) and (2) are met as reported by patient[b]
    1. Childhood hyperactivity
    2. Childhood attention deficits
II. Adult characteristics: five additional symptoms, including ongoing difficulties with inattentiveness and hyperactivity and at least three other symptoms:
  A. Inattentiveness
  B. Hyperactivity
  C. Mood lability
  D. Irritability and hot temper
  E. Impaired stress tolerance
  F. Disorganization
  G. Impulsivity
III. Exclusions: not diagnosed in presence of severe depression, psychosis, or severe personality disorder

[a]Parent report aided with 10-item *Parent Rating Scale of Childhood Behavior.*
[b]Patient self-report of retrospective childhood symptoms aided by *Wender Utah Rating Scale.*

they get older and, by the time they are adults, will meet criteria for ADHD, predominantly inattentive presentation. As with children, adults with ADHD demonstrate higher rates of learning disorders, anxiety disorders, mood disorders, and substance use disorders compared with the general population.

Treatment

The treatment of ADHD in adults targets pharmacotherapy, mainly long-acting stimulants, similar to that used with children and adolescents with ADHD. In adults, only the long-acting stimulants are FDA approved in the treatment of ADHD. Signs of a positive response are an increased attention span, decreased impulsiveness, and improved mood. Psychopharmacological therapy may be needed indefinitely. Clinicians should use standard ways to monitor drug response and patient compliance.

Epidemiology

Among adults, evidence suggests an approximate 4 percent prevalence of ADHD in the population. ADHD in adulthood is generally diagnosed by self-report, given the lack of school information and observer information available; therefore, it is more challenging to make an accurate diagnosis.

▲ 2.5 Specific Learning Disorder

Specific learning disorder in youth is a neurodevelopmental disorder produced by the interactions of heritable and environmental factors that influence the brain's ability to perceive or process verbal and nonverbal information efficiently. Children with the disorder have persistent difficulty learning academic skills in reading, written expression, or mathematics, beginning in early childhood, which is inconsistent with the overall intellectual ability of a child. Children with specific learning disorder often find it challenging to keep up with their peers in certain academic subjects, whereas they may excel in others. Several academic skills may be compromised in specific learning disorder include reading single words and sentences fluently, written expression and spelling, and calculation and solving mathematical problems. Specific learning disorder results in underachievement that is unexpected based on the child's potential as well as the opportunity to have learned more. Specific learning disorder in reading, spelling, and mathematics appears to aggregate in families. There is an increased risk of four to eight times in first-degree relatives for reading deficits, and about five to ten times for mathematics deficits, compared to the general population. Specific learning disorder occurs two to three times more often in males than in females. Learning problems in a child or adolescent identified in this manner can establish eligibility for academic services through the public school system.

The American Psychiatric Association's DSM-5, combines the DSM-IV diagnoses of reading disorder, mathematics disorder, and disorder of written expression and learning disorder not otherwise specified into a single diagnosis: Specific learning disorder. Learning deficits in reading, written expression, and mathematics in the DSM-5 are designated using specifiers. ICD-10 continues to separate the disorders. DSM-5 notes that the term *dyslexia* is an equivalent term describing a pattern of learning difficulties, including deficits in accurate or fluent word recognition, poor decoding, and poor spelling skills. *Dyscalculia* is an alternative term referring to a pattern of deficits related to learning arithmetic facts, processing numerical information, and performing accurate calculations. Table 2-18 lists the approaches to diagnosis of specific learning disorder.

Specific learning disorder of all types affects approximately 10 percent of youth. This disorder represents approximately half of all public school children who receive special education services in the United States. In 1975, Public Law 94–142 (the Education for All Handicapped Children Act, now known as the Individual with Disabilities Education Act [IDEA]) mandated all states to provide free and appropriate educational services to all children. Since that time, the number of children identified with learning disorders has increased, and a variety of definitions of learning disabilities have arisen. For this diagnosis, a child's achievement must be significantly lower than expected in one or more of the following: reading skills, comprehension, spelling, written expression, calculation, mathematical reasoning, or the learning problems interfere with academic achievement or activities of daily living. It is common for specific learning disorder to include more than one area of skill deficits.

Children with specific learning disorder in the area of reading can be identified by poor word recognition, slow reading rate, and impaired comprehension compared with most children of the same age. Current data suggest that most children with reading difficulties have deficits in speech sound processing skills, regardless of their IQ. In DSM-5, there is no longer a diagnostic criterion for specific learning disorder comparing the specific deficit to overall IQ. The current consensus is that children with reading impairment have trouble with word recognition and "sounding out" words because they cannot efficiently process and use phonemes (the smaller bits of words that are associated with particular sounds). An epidemiologic study found four profiles, including (1) weak reading, (2) weak language, (3) weak math, or (4) combined weak math and reading, accounting for 70 percent of children with specific learning impairments. Low scores in short-term memory for speech sounds characterized the profile with weak language, whereas, low speech sound awareness was associated with the weak reading group, but not the weak language group. Finally, in another study, it was found that the weak math group did not show speech sound deficits.

Severe specific learning disorder may make it agonizing for a child to succeed in school, often leading to demoralization, low self-esteem, chronic frustration, and compromised peer relationships. Specific learning disorder is associated with an increased risk of comorbid disorders, including ADHD, communication disorders, conduct disorders, and depressive disorders. Adolescents with specific learning disorder are at least 1.5 times more likely to drop out of school, approximating rates of 40 percent. Adults with specific learning disorder are at increased risk for difficulties in employment and social adjustment. Specific learning disorder often extends to skills deficits in multiple areas such as reading, writing, and mathematics.

Moderate to high heritability contributes to specific learning disorder, and it appears that many cognitive traits are polygenic. Also, there is pleiotropy; that is, the same genes may affect the skills necessary for diverse learning tasks. Factors such as perinatal injury and specific neurologic conditions may contribute to the development of specific learning disorder. Conditions such as lead poisoning, FAS, and in utero drug exposure are also associated with increased rates of specific learning disorder.

Table 2-18
Specific Learning Disorder

	DSM-5	ICD-10
Diagnostic name	Specific Learning Disorder	Specific Developmental Disorders of Scholastic Skills • Specific reading disorder • Specific spelling disorder • Specific disorder of arithmetical skills • Mixed disorder of scholastic skills
Duration	≥6 mo Symptoms beginning during school-age years, may not be apparent until later	
Symptoms	Difficulties with learning or academics. Example difficulties: • Reading (slow/inaccurate) • Reading comprehension • Spelling • Written expression • Numbers/calculation • Math reasoning	Deficits in the specific domain (reading, spelling, arithmetic) relevant to the above listed disorder
Exclusions (not result of):	Intellectual disability Visual or auditory impairment Another mental disorder Another medical disorder Psychosocial adversity Inadequate education	Intellectual disability Mental age Visual impairment Inadequate education
Symptom specifiers	**With impairment in reading** **With impairment in written expression** **With impairment in mathematics**	
Severity specifiers	**Mild:** minimal accommodations or support needed in school **Moderate:** some accommodations needed **Severe:** intensive individualized and specialized teaching most of the time in school	

SPECIFIC LEARNING DISORDER WITH IMPAIRMENT IN READING

Reading impairment is present in up to 75 percent of children and adolescents with a specific learning disorder. Students who have learning problems in other academic areas most commonly experience difficulties with reading as well.

Reading impairment is characterized by difficulty in recognizing words, slow and inaccurate reading, poor comprehension, and difficulties with spelling. Reading impairment is often comorbid with other disorders in children, particularly ADHD. The historical term *developmental alexia* defines a developmental deficit in recognizing printed symbols. The term was simplified to *dyslexia* in the 1960s. Dyslexia was used extensively for many years to describe a reading disability syndrome that often included speech and language deficits and right-left confusion. Reading impairment is frequently accompanied by disabilities in other academic skills, and the term dyslexia remains as an alternate term for a pattern of reading and spelling difficulties.

Clinical Features

We can usually identify children with reading disabilities by the age of 7 years (second grade). Reading difficulty may be apparent among students in classrooms that expect reading skills earlier. Children can sometimes compensate for reading disorders in the early elementary grades by the use of memory and inference, particularly in children with high intelligence. In such instances, the disorder may not be apparent until age 9 (fourth grade) or later.

Children with reading impairment make many errors in their oral reading. The errors include omissions, additions, and distortions of words. Such children have difficulty in distinguishing between printed letter characters and sizes, especially those that differ only in spatial orientation and length of a line. The problems in managing printed or written language can pertain to individual letters, sentences, and even a page. The child's reading speed is slow, often with minimal comprehension. Most children with reading disability have an age-appropriate ability to copy from a written or printed text, but nearly all spell poorly.

Associated problems include language difficulties: discrimination, and difficulty in sequencing words properly. A patient might start with a word that occurs midway or at the end of a written sentence. Most children with reading disorder dislike and avoid reading and writing. They become anxious when confronted with demands that involve printed language. Many children with specific learning disorders who do not receive remedial education have a sense of shame and humiliation because of their continuing failure and subsequent frustration. The intensity of these feelings grows over time. Older children tend to be angry and depressed and exhibit poor self-esteem.

Jackson, a 10-year-old boy, was referred for evaluation of failing to complete in-class assignments and homework and failing tests in reading, spelling, and arithmetic. For the past 2 years (grades 5 and 6), he had been attending a particular education class every morning in the local community school, based on an assessment from the second grade. A subsequent psychoeducational assessment by a clinical psychologist confirmed reading problems. Jackson was eligible for a full-day special education class, after which he started attending a program with eight other students ranging from 6 to 12 years of age.

Clinical interview with his parents revealed a healthy pregnancy and neonatal period, and a history of language delay. In preschool and kindergarten, Jackson had difficulty with rhyming games and showed a lack of interest in books and preferred to play with construction toys. In the first grade, Jackson had more difficulty learning to read than other boys in his class and continued to have problems pronouncing multisyllabic words (e.g., he said "aminals" for "animals" and "sblanation" for "explanation"). Family history was positive for reading deficits and ADHD. Jackson's father disclosed a history of personal reading problems, and Jackson's older brother, 15 years of age, had ADHD, for which he took stimulant medication. Jackson's parents were concerned about his poor focus in school and wondered whether he had ADHD. In the clinical interview with Jackson, he rarely made eye contact, mumbled a lot, and struggled to find the right words (e.g., manifested many false starts, hesitations, and nonspecific terms, such as "the thing that you draw … um … pencil—no … um … lines with"). He admitted to disliking school, adding, "Reading is boring and stupid—I'd rather be skateboarding." Jackson complained about how much reading he was given—even in math—and commented, "Reading takes so much time. By the time I figure out a word, I can't remember what I just read, and so have to read the stuff again."

Psychoeducational assessment included the Wechsler Intelligence Scale for Children-IV, Clinical Evaluation of Language Fundamentals-IV (CELF-IV), the Wechsler Individual Achievement Test-II, and self-ratings of anxiety, depression, and self-esteem. Results indicated low-average verbal and above-average performance IQ, poor word attack and word identification skills (below 12th percentile), poor comprehension (below ninth percentile), poor spelling (below sixth percentile), weak comprehension of oral language (below 16th percentile), elevated but subthreshold scores on the Children's Depression Inventory, and low self-esteem. Although Jackson manifested symptoms of inattention, restlessness, and oppositional behavior (mainly at school), he did not meet the criteria for ADHD. Jackson met DSM-5 criteria for a specific learning disorder, with deficits in reading and written expression. Recommendations included continuation in special education plus attendance at a summer camp specializing in children with reading disorder, as well as ongoing monitoring of self-esteem and depressive traits.

At 1-year follow-up, Jackson and his parents reported striking improvements in his reading, overall school performance, mood, and self-esteem. Both Jackson and his family felt that the specialized instruction provided during the summer camp was beneficial. The program had provided one-on-one focused and explicit instruction for 1 hour a day for a total of 70 hours. Jackson explained that he had been taught "like a game plan" to read, and challenged the clinician to give him a "really tough long word to read." He demonstrated strategies that he had learned to read the word "unconditionally" and also explained what it meant. To boost his fluency in reading and comprehension, he was provided with assignments to read along with audio-taped versions of books, use of graphic organizers to facilitate reading comprehension, and continued participation in the summer camp reading program. (Adapted from Rosemary Tannock, Ph.D.)

Diagnosis

Reading impairment is diagnosed when a child's reading achievement is significantly below that expected of a child of the same age. Characteristic diagnostic features include difficulty recalling, evoking, and sequencing printed letters and words, processing sophisticated grammatical constructions, and making inferences. School failure and ensuing poor self-esteem can exacerbate the problems as a child becomes more consumed with a sense of failure and spends less time focusing on academic work. Students with reading impairment are entitled to an educational evaluation through the school district to determine eligibility for special education services. Special education classification, however, is not uniform across states or regions, and students with identical reading difficulties may be eligible for services in one region, but ineligible in another.

Pathology and Laboratory Examination.   No specific physical signs or laboratory measures are helpful in the diagnosis of reading deficits. Psychoeducational testing, however, is critical in determining these deficits. The diagnostic battery generally includes a standardized spelling test, written composition, processing, and using oral language, design copying, and judgment of the adequacy of pencil use. The reading subtests of the *Woodcock-Johnson Psycho-Educational Battery-Revised* and the *Peabody Individual Achievement Test-Revised* are useful in identifying reading disability. A screening projective battery may include human-figure drawings, picture-story tests, and sentence completion. The evaluation should also include systematic observation of behavioral variables.

Differential Diagnosis

Reading deficits are often accompanied by comorbid disorders, such as language disorder, disability in written expression, and ADHD. Data indicate that children with reading disability consistently present difficulties with linguistic skills, whereas children with ADHD only do not. Children with reading disability without ADHD, however, may have some overlapping deficits in cognitive inhibition. For example, they perform impulsively on continuous performance tasks. Deficits in expressive language and speech discrimination, along with reading disorder, may lead to a comorbid diagnosis of language disorder. We should differentiate reading impairment from intellectual disability syndromes in which reading, along with most other skills, are below the achievement expected for a child's chronologic age. Intellectual testing helps to differentiate global deficits from more specific reading difficulties.

We can detect poor reading skills resulting from inadequate schooling by comparing a given child's achievement with classmates on reading performance on standardized reading tests. We should rule out hearing and visual impairments with screening tests.

Comorbidity

Children with reading difficulties are at high risk for additional learning deficits, including mathematics and written expression. The DSM-5 Language disorder, also known as specific language impairment, has traditionally been viewed as distinct from dyslexia and dyscalculia. Children with language disorder have poor word knowledge, limited abilities to form accurate sentence structure, and impairments in the ability to put words together to produce clear explanations. Children with language disorder may have delayed development of language acquisition, and difficulties with grammar and syntactical knowledge. Specific learning disorder in the areas of reading and mathematics frequently occur comorbidly with language disorder. In one study, 19 percent to 63 percent of reading disorder patients also had language impairment.

Conversely, reading impairment occurs in 12.5 to 85 percent of individuals with language disorder. In twin studies, reading impairments are significantly higher in those children with specific learning impairment and family members of children with the disorder. There are also high rates of comorbidity between reading impairment and mathematics impairment; in some studies, the comorbidity is as high as 60 percent. It appears that children with both reading and math impairment may perform more poorly in mathematics; however, the reading skills of the comorbid children were no different from children who had only reading disorder and not math disorder.

Comorbid psychiatric disorders are also frequent, such as ADHD, oppositional defiant disorder, conduct disorders, and depressive disorders, especially in adolescents. Data suggest that up to 25 percent of children with reading impairment may have comorbid ADHD. Alternately, between 15 and 30 percent of children diagnosed with ADHD have specific learning disorder. Family studies suggest that ADHD and reading impairment may share some degree of heritability. That is, some genetic factors contribute to both reading impairment and attentional syndromes. Youth with reading impairments have higher than average rates of depression on self-report measures and experience higher levels of anxiety symptoms than children without specific learning disorder. Furthermore, children with reading impairment are at increased risk for poor peer relationships and exhibit less skill in responding to subtle social cues.

Course and Prognosis

Children with a reading disability may gain knowledge of printed language during their first 2 years in grade school without remedial assistance. By the end of the first grade, many children with reading problems have learned how to read a few words; however, by the third grade, keeping up with classmates is exceedingly hard without remedial educational intervention. When remediation is instituted early, in milder cases, it may not be necessary after the first or second grade. In severe cases and depending on the pattern of deficits and strengths, remediation may continue into the middle and high school years.

Treatment

Remediation strategies for children with reading impairments focus on direct instruction that leads a child's attention to the connections between speech sounds and spelling. Effective remediation programs begin by teaching the child to make accurate associations between letters and sounds. This approach relies on the theory that the core deficits in reading impairments are related to difficulty recognizing and remembering the associations between letters and sounds. After mastering individual letter-sound associations, remediation can target more significant components of reading, such as syllables and words. We can determine the exact focus of any reading program only after an accurate assessment of a child's specific deficits and weaknesses. Positive strategies include small, structured reading groups that offer individual attention and make it easier for a child to ask for help.

Children and adolescents with reading difficulties are entitled to an individual education program (IEP) provided by the public school system. However, for high school students with persistent reading disorders and ongoing difficulties with decoding and word identification, IEP services may not be sufficient to remediate their problems. A study of students with reading disorders in 54 schools indicated that, at the high school level, specific goals are not adequately met solely through school remediation. High schoolers with persisting reading difficulties may likely have more benefit from individualized reading remediation.

Reading instruction programs such as the Orton Gillingham and Direct Instructional System for Teaching and Remediation (DISTAR) approaches begin by concentrating on individual letters and sounds, advance to the mastery of simple phonetic units, and then blend these units into words and sentences. Thus, if children learn to cope with graphemes, they will learn to read. Other reading remediation programs, such as the Merrill program, and the *Science Research Associates, Inc. (SRA) Basic Reading Program,* begin by introducing whole words first and then teach children how to break them down and recognize the sounds of the syllables and the individual letters in the word. Another approach teaches children with reading disorders to recognize whole words through the use of visual aids and bypasses the sounding-out process. One such program is called the *Bridge Reading Program.* The Fernald method uses a multisensory approach that combines teaching whole words with a tracing technique so that the child has kinesthetic stimulation while learning to read the words.

Epidemiology

An estimated 4 to 8 percent of youth in the United States have been identified with dyslexia, encompassing a variety of reading, spelling, and comprehension deficits. Three to four times as many boys as girls have reading impairments in clinically referred samples. In epidemiologic samples, however, rates of reading impairments are much closer among boys and girls. Boys with reading impairment are referred for psychiatric evaluation more often than girls due to comorbid ADHD and disruptive behavior problems. There is no apparent gender differential among adults who report reading difficulties.

Etiology

Data from cognitive, neuroimaging and genetic studies suggest that reading impairment is a neurobiologic disorder with a significant genetic contribution. It reflects a deficiency in processing sounds of speech sounds, and thus, spoken language. Children who struggle with reading most likely also have a deficit in speech sound processing skills. Children with this deficit cannot adequately identify the parts of words that denote specific sounds, leading to difficulty in recognizing and "sounding out" words. Youths with reading impairment are slower than peers in naming letters and numbers. The core deficits for children with reading impairment include poor processing of speech sounds and deficits in comprehension, spelling, and sounding out words.

Because reading impairment typically includes a language deficit, we believe that the left brain is the anatomical site of this dysfunction. Several studies using MRI have suggested that the planum temporale in the left brain shows less asymmetry than the same site in the right brain in children with both language disorders and specific learning disorder. PET studies have led some researchers to conclude that left temporal blood flow patterns during language tasks differ between children with and without learning disorders. Cell analysis studies suggest that, in reading impaired individuals, the visual magnocellular system (which typically contains large cells) contains more disorganized and smaller cell bodies than expected. Studies indicate that 35 to 40 percent of first-degree relatives of children with reading deficits also have reading disability. Several studies have suggested that chromosome 6 maps to phonologic awareness (i.e., the ability to decode sounds and sound out words).

Furthermore, the ability to identify single words maps to chromosome 15. Impairment in reading and spelling likely links to susceptibility loci on multiple chromosomes. Although a recent research study identified a locus on chromosome 18 as a strong influence on single-word reading and phoneme awareness, generalist genes are likely responsible for learning disorders. Many genes believed to be associated with specific learning disorder may also influence normal variation in learning abilities. Also, genes that affect abilities in reading, for example, are also hypothesized to affect written expression and potentially mathematics skills.

Several historical hypotheses about the origin of reading deficits are now known to be untrue. The first myth is that visual-motor problems cause reading impairments, sometimes called *scotopic sensitivity syndrome.* There is no evidence that children with reading impairment have visual problems or difficulties with their visual-motor system. The second false theory is that allergies can cause, or contribute to, reading disability. Finally, unsubstantiated theories have implicated the cerebellar–vestibular system as the source of reading disabilities.

Research in cognitive neuroscience and neuropsychology supports the hypothesis that encoding processes and working memory, rather than attention or long-term memory, are areas of weakness for children with reading impairment. One study found an association between dyslexia and birth in May, June, and July, suggesting that prenatal exposure to maternal infectious illness, such as influenza, in the winter months may contribute to reading disabilities. Complications during pregnancy and prenatal and perinatal difficulties are common in the histories of children with reading disabilities. Meager birth weight and severely premature children are at higher risk for specific learning disorder. Children born very preterm are at increased risk for minor motor, behavioral, and specific learning disorder.

An increased incidence of reading impairment occurs in intellectually average children with cerebral palsy and epilepsy. Children with postnatal brain lesions in the left occipital lobe, resulting in right visual-field blindness, experience reading impairments. Similarly, youths with lesions in the splenium of the corpus callosum that blocks the transmission of visual information from the intact right hemisphere to the language areas of the left hemisphere experience reading impairments.

Children malnourished for long periods during early childhood are at increased risk of compromised performance cognition, including reading.

SPECIFIC LEARNING DISORDER WITH IMPAIRMENT IN MATHEMATICS

Children with mathematics difficulties have difficulty learning and remembering numerals, cannot remember basic facts about numbers, and are slow and inaccurate in computation. There are four groups of skills for which children with this disorder have poor achievement: linguistic skills (those related to understanding mathematical terms and converting written problems into mathematical symbols), perceptual skills (the ability to recognize and understand symbols and order clusters of numbers), mathematical skills (basic addition, subtraction, multiplication, division, and following the sequencing of basic operations), and attentional skills (copying figures correctly and observing operational symbols correctly). There are a variety of terms used over the years to denote various difficulties with math skills, including *dyscalculia, congenital arithmetic disorder, acalculia, Gerstmann syndrome,* and *developmental arithmetic disorder;* these terms have been used to denote the difficulties present in mathematics disorder. Core deficits in dyscalculia are in processing numbers, and good language abilities are needed for accurate counting, calculating, and understanding mathematical principles.

Mathematics deficits can, however, occur in isolation or conjunction with language and reading impairments. According to the DSM-5, the diagnosis of specific learning disorder with impairment in mathematics consists of deficits in arithmetic counting and calculations, difficulty remembering mathematics facts, and potentially counting on fingers instead. Additional deficits include difficulty with mathematical concepts and reasoning, leading to difficulties in applying procedures to solve quantitative problems. These deficits lead to skills that are substantially below what is typical for the child's age and cause significant interference in academic success, as documented by standardized academic achievement testing.

Clinical Features

Common features of mathematics deficit include difficulty learning number names, remembering the signs for addition and subtraction, learning multiplication tables, translating word problems into computations, and performing calculations at the expected pace. We can detect most children with mathematics deficits during the second and third grades in elementary school. A child with poor mathematics abilities typically has problems with concepts, such as counting and adding even one-digit numbers, compared with classmates of the same age. During the first 2 or 3 years of elementary school, a child with poor mathematics skill may just get by in mathematics by relying on rote memory. However, soon, as mathematics problems require discrimination and manipulation of spatial and numerical relations, a child with mathematics difficulties is overwhelmed.

Some investigators have classified mathematics deficiencies into the following categories: difficulty learning to count meaningfully, difficulty mastering cardinal and ordinal systems, difficulty performing arithmetic operations, and difficulty envisioning clusters of objects as groups. Children with mathematics difficulty have trouble associating auditory and visual symbols, understanding the conservation of quantity, remembering sequences of arithmetic steps, and choosing principles for problem-solving activities. Children with these problems are presumed to have good auditory and verbal abilities; however, in many cases, the mathematics deficits may occur in conjunction with reading, writing, and language problems. In these cases, the other deficiencies may compound the impairment of poor mathematics skill.

Mathematics difficulty, in fact, often coexists with other disorders affecting reading, expressive writing, coordination, and language. Spelling problems, deficits in memory or attention, and emotional or behavioral problems may be present. Young grade-school children may exhibit specific learning problems in reading and writing, and we should evaluate these children for mathematics deficits. The exact relationship between mathematics deficits and the deficits in language and dyslexia is not clear. Although children with language disorder do not necessarily experience mathematics deficiencies, these conditions often coexist, and both are associated with impairments in decoding and encoding processes.

Lena, an 8-year-old girl, was referred for evaluation of impairing problems in attention and academic achievement, which were first noted in kindergarten but were now causing difficulty at home and school. Lena attended a regular third-grade class in a local public school, which she had been attending since midway through kindergarten.

Lena's history included a mild delay in speech acquisition (e.g., first words at approximately 18 months of age and short sentences at approximately 3 years of age). However, otherwise, she had no major developmental problems until kindergarten, when her teacher had raised concerns about inattentiveness, difficulty following instructions, and her difficulty in mastering basic number concepts (e.g., inaccurate counting of sets of objects). A speech, language, and hearing assessment completed at the end of kindergarten revealed mild language problems that did not warrant specific intervention. School reports from grades 1 and 2 noted ongoing concerns about inattention, poor reading skills, and difficulty mastering simple arithmetic facts, and "making careless mistakes in copying numbers from the board and in doing addition and subtraction." These problems continued through grade 2, despite some in-school accommodations (e.g., moving Lena's seat closer to the teacher) and modifications (e.g., providing her with printed sheets of arithmetic problems, so she did not need to copy them herself). Lena's parents reported a 3-year history of losing things, fidgeting at the dinner table, and difficulty concentrating on games and homework and forgetting to bring notes to and from school. The psychological assessment included the Wechsler Intelligence Scale for Children-III, Clinical Evaluation of Language Fundamentals-IV, Comprehensive Test of Phonological Processing, and the Woodcock-Johnson Psycho-Educational Battery–III. Results indicated average intelligence, with relatively weaker performance on tests of perceptual organization, weak phonologic (speech sound) awareness, mild deficits in receptive and expressive language, and reading and arithmetic abilities that were well below grade level. Parent and teacher ratings on a standardized behavior questionnaire (Conners' Rating Scales-Long Form) were above the clinical threshold for ADHD.

Lena was given a diagnosis of ADHD, predominantly inattentive type, and specific learning disorder with impairment in reading, based on the history, school achievement, and standardized assessment. She did not meet the criteria for communication disorder, and her doctors thought that her mathematics problems did not cause impairment like her reading disorder and ADHD did. Recommendations included the following: family psychoeducation clarifying the ADHD and specific learning disorder, remedial interventions for reading, and treatment of her ADHD with a long-acting stimulant agent.

At 1-year follow-up, Lena and her parents reported noticeable improvement with inattention, but ongoing problems with reading and more significant deficits in mathematics. Her clinicians added mathematics remediation to her weekly schedule. Two years later, when Lena was 11 years of age, her parents called for an "urgent reevaluation" due to a sudden worsening of her difficulties at home and school. Clinical evaluation revealed adequate stimulant treatment response of her ADHD, more marked deficits in reading speed accuracy compared to others her age, and significant deficits in mathematics. Lena's parents reported that she had started lying about having mathematics homework or refused to do it, was suspended from mathematics class twice in the past 3 months because of oppositional behavior, and had failed sixth-grade mathematics. Lena acknowledged disliking and worrying about math: "whenever the teacher starts asking questions and looks in my direction, my mind just goes blank, and I feel sort of shaky—it's so bad in tests that I have to leave class to get myself together." At this point, her team noted an additional component of anxiety to be contributing to her school impairments. Added recommendations included increased specific educational remediation for mathematics. At follow-up, Lena reported that the resource teacher had taught her some helpful strategies to address her mathematics anxiety, as well as ways of classifying word problems and differentiating critical information from irrelevant information. She continued to be a robust responder to long-acting stimulants for her ADHD and had only minimal difficulties concentrating on homework after school. (Adapted from case material by Rosemary Tannock, Ph.D.)

Diagnosis

We make a diagnosis of specific learning disorder in mathematics when a child's skill in mathematical reasoning, or calculation, remains significantly below that expected for that child's age, for at least 6 months, even when administering remedial interventions. Many different skills contribute to mathematics proficiency. These include linguistic skills, conceptual skills, and computational skills. Linguistic skills involve being able to understand mathematical terms, understand word problems, and translate them into the proper mathematical process. Conceptual skills involve the recognition of mathematical symbols and being able to use mathematical signs correctly. Computational skills include the ability to line up numbers correctly and to follow the "rules" of the mathematical operation.

Pathology and Laboratory Examination. No physical signs or symptoms indicate mathematics disorder, but educational testing and standardized measurement of intellectual function are necessary to make this diagnosis. The *Keymath Diagnostic Arithmetic Test* measures several areas of mathematics, including knowledge of mathematical content, function, and computation. It assesses ability in mathematics of children in grades 1 to 6.

Course and Prognosis

A child with a specific learning disorder in mathematics is usually identifiable by the age of 8 years (third grade). In some children, the disorder is apparent as early as 6 years (first grade); in others, it may not be apparent until age 10 (fifth grade) or later. Too few data are currently available from longitudinal studies to predict patterns of developmental and academic progress of children classified as having mathematics disorder in early school grades. On the other hand, children with a moderate mathematics disorder who do not receive intervention may have complications, including continuing academic difficulties, shame, poor self-concept, frustration, and depression. These complications can lead to reluctance to attend school and demoralization about academic success.

Differential Diagnosis

We should differentiate mathematics deficits from global causes of impaired functioning such as intellectual disability. Inadequate schooling can affect a child's arithmetic performance. Conduct disorder or ADHD can occur comorbidly with specific learning disorder in mathematics, and, in these cases, we would make both diagnoses.

Comorbidity

Mathematics deficits are comorbid with deficits in both reading and written expression. Children with mathematics difficulties may also be at higher risk for expressive language problems and developmental coordination disorder.

Treatment

It is best to treat mathematics difficulties for children with early interventions that lead to improved skills in basic computation. The presence of specific learning disorder in reading, along with mathematics difficulties, can impede progress; however, children are quite responsive to remediation in early grade school. Children with indications of mathematics disorder as early as in kindergarten require help in understanding which digit in a pair is larger, counting abilities, identification of numbers, and remembering sequences of numbers. Flashcards, workbooks, and computer games can be a viable part of this treatment. One study indicated that mathematics instruction is most helpful when the focus is on problem-solving activities, including word problems, rather than only computation. *Project MATH,* a multimedia self-instructional or group-instructional in-service training program, has been successful for some children with mathematics disorder. Computer programs can be helpful and can increase compliance with remediation efforts.

Social skills deficits can contribute to a child's hesitation in asking for help, so a child identified with a mathematics disorder may benefit from gaining positive problem-solving skills in the social arena as well as in mathematics.

Epidemiology

Mathematics disability alone is estimated to occur in about 1 percent of school-age children, that is about one of every five children with specific learning disorder. Epidemiologic studies have indicated that up to 6 percent of school-age children have some difficulty with mathematics, with a prevalence of 3.5 to 6.5 for impairing forms of dyscalculia. Although specific learning disorder overall occurs two to three times more often in males, mathematics deficits may be relatively more frequent in girls than reading deficits. Many studies of learning disorders in children have grouped reading, writing, and mathematics disability, which makes it more difficult to ascertain the precise prevalence of mathematics disability.

Etiology

Mathematics deficiency, as with other areas of specific learning disorder, has a significant genetic contribution. Comorbidity with reading deficits is common and in the range of 17 percent up to 60 percent. One theory proposed a neurologic deficit in the right cerebral hemisphere, particularly in the occipital lobe areas. These regions are responsible for processing visual–spatial stimuli that, in turn, are responsible for mathematical skills. This theory, however, has received little support in subsequent neuropsychiatric studies.

The causes of deficits in mathematics are multifactorial, including genetic, maturational, cognitive, emotional, educational, and socioeconomic factors. Prematurity and very low birth weight are also risk factors for specific learning disorder, including mathematics. Compared with reading abilities, arithmetic abilities seem to depend more on the amount and quality of instruction.

SPECIFIC LEARNING DISORDER WITH IMPAIRMENT IN WRITTEN EXPRESSION

Written expression is the most complex skill acquired to convey an understanding of language and to express thoughts and ideas. Writing skills are highly correlated with reading for most children; however, for some youth, reading comprehension may far surpass their ability to express complex thoughts. Written expression, in some cases, is a sensitive index of more subtle deficits in language usage that typically are not detected by standardized reading and language tests.

Deficits in written expression include writing skills that are significantly below the expected level for a child's age and education. Such deficits impair the child's academic performance and writing in everyday life. Components of writing disorder include poor spelling, errors in grammar and punctuation, and poor handwriting. Spelling errors are among the most common difficulties for a child with a writing disorder. Spelling mistakes are most often phonetic errors; that is, an erroneous spelling that sounds like the correct spelling. Examples of common spelling errors are: fone for phone or beleeve for believe.

Historically, experts considered dysgraphia (i.e., poor writing skills) a reading disorder; however, it is now clear that impairment in written expression can occur on its own. Terms once used to describe writing disability include *spelling disorder* and *spelling dyslexia.* Writing disabilities are often associated with other forms of specific learning disorders; however, impaired writing ability may be identified later than other forms because it is generally acquired later than verbal language and reading.

In contrast with the DSM-5, which includes specific learning disorder in written expression, ICD-10 includes a separate specific spelling disorder.

Clinical Features

Youth with impairments in written expression struggle early in grade school with spelling words and expressing their thoughts according to age-appropriate grammatical norms. Their spoken and written sentences contain an unusually large number of grammatical errors and poor paragraph organization. Affected children commonly make simple grammatical errors, even when writing a short sentence. For example, despite constant reminders, affected youth frequently fail to capitalize the first letter of the first word in a sentence, and fail to end the sentence with a period. Typical features of impaired written expression include spelling errors, grammatical errors, punctuation errors, poor paragraph organization, and poor handwriting.

In higher grades in school, affected youth's written sentences become more conspicuously primitive, odd, and inaccurate compared to what is typical for students at their grade level. For youth with impaired written expression, word choices are often erroneous and inappropriate, paragraphs are disorganized and not in proper sequence, and spelling accuracy becomes increasingly difficult as their vocabulary becomes more extensive and more abstract. Associated features of writing impairments may include reluctance to go to school, refusal to do assigned written homework, and concurrent academic difficulties in other areas.

Many children with impaired written expression understandably become frustrated and angry, and harbor feelings of shame and inadequacy regarding poor academic achievement. In some cases, depressive disorders can result from a growing sense of isolation, estrangement, and despair. Young adults with impaired written expression who do not receive remedial intervention continue to have writing skills deficits and a persistent sense of incompetence and inferiority.

Brett, an 11-year-old boy, was referred for evaluation of increasing problems in school over 2 years, including failure to complete assigned schoolwork and homework, inattention and oppositional behavior, and deteriorating grades and test scores. At the time of assessment, he was in a regular fifth-grade class in a public school, which he had been attending since grade 1.

Clinical interview with parents revealed that Brett had a twin brother (monozygotic) with a history of language problems for which he had received speech-language therapy in the preschool years and remedial reading in the primary grades. Brett, however, had not exhibited difficulty in speech or language development, according to parental reports and scores on standardized tests of oral language administered in the preschool years. His current and previous school reports indicate that Brett participated well in class discussions and had no difficulty in reading or mathematics; however, his written work was far below grade level. In each of the last 2 years, his teachers had expressed increasing concerns about Brett's refusal to complete written work, failure to hand in homework, daydreaming and fidgeting in class, and withdrawal from class activities. Brett admitted to an increasing dislike of school and especially writing assignments. He explained, "It's writing, writing all day long—even in math and science. I know how to do the problems and the experiments, but I hate having to write it all down—my mind just goes blank." Brett complained, "My teacher is always on me, telling me that I'm lazy and haven't done enough and that my writing is atrocious. He tells me I've got a bad attitude—so why would I want to go to school?" Brett and his parents reported that, over the past year, he has been down, increasingly frustrated with school, and has refused to do homework. They all agree that Brett has had a few brief episodes of depressed mood.

Testing by a clinical psychologist revealed average to high-average scores on the verbal and performance scales of the Wechsler Intelligence Scale for Children-III and average scores on the reading and arithmetic subtests of the Wide Range Achievement Test-3 (WRAT-3). However, scores on the WRAT-3 spelling subtest were below the 9th percentile, which was significantly below expectations for age and ability. Examination of his spelling errors revealed that his spelling was typically phonologically accurate (i.e., could plausibly be pronounced to sound like the target word). However, he used letter sequences that did not resemble English, regardless of pronunciation (e.g., "houses" was written as "howssis," "phones" was written as "fones," and "exact" was "egzakt"). Moreover, his performance was well below age and grade on standardized tests of written expression (TOWL-3), as well as on a brief (5-minute) informal assessment of expository text generation on a favorite topic (e.g., newspaper article on recent sports event). During the 5-minute writing activity, he frequently stared out the window, shifted positions, and chewed on his pencil. He would often get up to sharpen his pencil and sigh when he put pencil to paper, writing slowly and laboriously. At the end of 5 minutes, he had produced three short sentences without any punctuation or capitalization that were barely legible, containing several misspellings and grammatical errors, and that were not linked semantically. By contrast, later in the assessment, he described the sporting event with detail and enthusiasm. A speech-language evaluation revealed average scores on standard tests of oral language (Clinical Evaluation of Language Fundamentals-IV). However, he omitted sounds or syllables in a multisyllabic word in a nonword repetition test, which was sensitive to mild residual language impairments and written language impairments.

The clinical team formulated a diagnosis of specific learning disorder with impairment in written expression, based on Brett's inability to compose written text, poor spelling, and grammatical errors, without problems in reading or mathematics or a history of language impairments. He did not meet full diagnostic criteria for any other DSM-5 disorder, including oppositional defiant disorder, ADHD, or mood disorder. Recommendations included the following: psychoeducation, the need for educational accommodations (e.g., provision of additional time for test-taking and written assignments, specific educational intervention to facilitate written expression and to teach note-taking, and use of specific computer software to support written composition and spelling), and counseling should his depressed mood continue or worsen. (Adapted from case material from Rosemary Tannock, Ph.D.)

Diagnosis

The DSM-5 diagnosis of specific learning disorder with impairment in written expression depends on a child's poor ability to use punctuation and grammar accurately in sentences, inability to organize paragraphs or to articulate ideas in writing. Poor performance on composing written text may also include poor handwriting and impaired ability to spell and to place words sequentially in coherent sentences, compared to others of the same age. In addition to spelling mistakes, youth with impaired written expression make grammatical mistakes, such as using incorrect tenses,

forgetting words in sentences, and placing words in the wrong order. Punctuation may be incorrect, and the child may have a reduced ability to remember which words begin with capital letters. Additional symptoms of impaired written expression include the formation of letters that are not legible, inverted letters, and mixtures of capital and lowercase letters in a given word. Other features of writing disorders include poor organization of written stories, which lack critical elements such as "where," "when," and "who" or clear expression of the plot.

Pathology and Laboratory Examination.   Whereas no physical signs of a writing disorder exist, educational testing helps to make a diagnosis of writing disorder. Diagnosis depends on a child's writing performance being markedly below expected production for his age, as confirmed by an individually administered standardized expressive writing test. Currently available tests of written language include the Test of Written Language (TOWL), the Diagnostic Evaluation of Writing Skills (DEWS), and the Test of Early Written Language (TEWL). We should also evaluate for impaired vision and hearing.

When there are impairments in written expression, we should administer a standardized intelligence test, such as WISC-R to determine the child's overall intellectual capacity.

Course and Prognosis

Specific learning disorder with impairment in writing, reading, and mathematics often coexist, and additional language disorder may be present as well. A child with all of the above disabilities will likely be diagnosed with language disorder first and impaired written expression last. In severe cases, an impaired written expression is apparent by age 7 (second grade); in less severe cases, the disorder may not be apparent until age 10 (fifth grade) or later. Youth with mild and moderate impairment in written expression fare well if they receive timely remedial education early in grade school. Severely impaired written expression requires continual, extensive remedial treatment through the late part of high school and even into college.

The prognosis depends on the severity of the disorder, the age or grade when starting the remedial intervention, the length and continuity of treatment, and the presence or absence of associated or secondary emotional or behavioral problems.

Differential Diagnosis

It is crucial to determine whether disorders such as ADHD or major depression are interfering with a child's focus and thereby preventing the production of adequate writing in the absence of a specific writing impairment. If true, treatment for the other disorder should improve a child's writing performance. Commonly comorbid disorders with writing disability are language disorder, mathematics disorder, developmental coordination disorder, disruptive behavior disorders, and ADHD.

Comorbidity

Children with impaired writing ability are significantly more likely to have language disorder and impairments in reading and mathematics compared to the general population of youth. ADHD occurs with higher frequency in children with writing disability than in the general population. Youth with specific learning disorder, including writing disability, are at higher risk for social skills difficulties, and some develop poor self-esteem and depressive symptoms.

Treatment

Remedial treatment for writing disability includes direct practice in spelling and sentence writing as well as a review of grammatical rules. Intensive and continuous administration of individually tailored, one-on-one expressive and creative writing therapy appears to influence a favorable outcome. Teachers in some special schools devote as much as 2 hours a day to such writing instruction. This intervention largely depends on the relationship between the child and the writing specialist. Success or failure in sustaining the patient's motivation affects the treatment's long-term efficacy. Associated secondary emotional and behavioral problems should be given prompt attention, with appropriate psychiatric treatment and parental counseling.

Epidemiology

The prevalence of specific learning disorder with impairment in written expression occurs in the range of 5 to 15 percent of school-age children. Over time, specific learning disorder remits in many youths, leading to a persistent rate of specific learning disorder of 4 percent in adults. The gender ratio in writing deficits is two to three to one in boys compared with girls. Impaired written expression often occurs along with deficits in reading, but not always.

Etiology

Causes of writing disability are likely similar to those of reading disorder, that is, underlying deficits in using the components of language related to letter sounds. Genetic factors are a significant factor in the development of writing disability. Writing difficulties often accompany language disorder, leading an affected child to have trouble with understanding grammatical rules, finding words, and expressing ideas clearly. According to one hypothesis, impairment in written expression may result from combined effects of language disorder and reading disorder. Most youths with impaired written expression have first-degree relatives with similar difficulties. Children with limited attention spans and high levels of distractibility may find writing an arduous task.

▲ 2.6 Motor Disorders

DEVELOPMENTAL COORDINATION DISORDER

Developmental coordination disorder is a neurodevelopmental disorder in which a child's fine or gross motor coordination is slower, less accurate, and more variable than in peers of the same age. Affecting about 5 to 6 percent of school-age children, 50 percent of children with developmental coordination disorder also have comorbid ADHD or dyslexia. A meta-analysis of recent research on developmental coordination disorder concluded that three general areas of deficits contribute to the disorder: (1) Poor predictive control of motor movements; (2) deficits in rhythmic coordination and timing; and (3) deficits in executive functions, including working memory, inhibition, and attention.

Children with developmental coordination disorder struggle to perform the motor activities of daily life, such as jumping, hopping, running, or catching a ball. Children with coordination problems may also agonize over using utensils, tying their shoelaces,

or writing. A child with developmental coordination disorder may exhibit delays in achieving motor milestones, such as sitting, crawling, and walking, because of clumsiness, and yet excel at verbal skills.

Developmental coordination disorder, thus, may be characterized by either clumsy gross or fine motor skills, resulting in poor performance in sports and even in academic achievement because of poor writing skills. A child with developmental coordination disorder may bump into things more often than siblings or drop things. In the 1930s, the term *clumsy child syndrome* began to be used in the literature to denote a condition of awkward motor behaviors not due to any specific neurologic disorder or damage. This term continues to be used to identify imprecise or delayed gross and fine motor behavior in children, resulting in subtle motor inabilities but often significant social rejection. Gross and fine motor impairment in developmental coordination disorder is not from a medical condition, such as cerebral palsy, muscular dystrophy, or a neuromuscular disorder. Currently, specific indications are that perinatal problems, such as prematurity, low birth weight, and hypoxia may contribute to the emergence of developmental coordination disorders. Children with developmental coordination disorder are at higher risk for language and learning disorders. A strong association exists between speech and language problems and coordination problems, as well as an association of coordination difficulties with hyperactivity, impulsivity, and reduced attention span.

Children with developmental coordination disorder may resemble younger children because of their inability to master motor activities typical for their age group. For example, children with developmental coordination disorder in elementary school may not be adept at bicycle riding, skateboarding, running, skipping, or hopping. In the middle school years, children with this disorder may have trouble in team sports, such as soccer, baseball, or basketball. Fine motor skill manifestations of developmental coordination disorder typically include clumsiness using utensils and difficulty with buttons and zippers in the preschool-age group. In older children, using scissors and more complex grooming skills, such as styling hair or putting on makeup, is difficult. Peers often ostracize children with developmental coordination disorder because of their poor skills in many sports, and they often have longstanding difficulties with peer relationships. DSM-5 categorizes developmental coordination disorder as a Motor Disorder, along with stereotypic movement disorder and tic disorders.

Clinical Features

The clinical signs suggesting the existence of developmental coordination disorder are evident as early as infancy in some cases, when a child begins to attempt tasks requiring motor coordination. The essential clinical feature is significantly impaired performance in motor coordination. The difficulties in motor coordination may vary with a child's age and developmental stage (Table 2-19).

In infancy and early childhood, the disorder may manifest in delays in developmental motor milestones, such as turning over, crawling, sitting, standing, walking, buttoning shirts, and zipping up pants. Between the ages of 2 and 4 years, clumsiness appears in almost all activities requiring motor coordination. Affected children cannot hold objects and drop them easily, their gait may be unsteady, they often trip over their own feet, and they may bump into other children while attempting to go around them. Older children may display impaired motor coordination in table games, such as putting together puzzles or building blocks, and in any type of ball game. Although no specific features are pathognomonic of developmental

Table 2-19
Manifestations of Developmental Coordination Disorder

Gross Motor Manifestations

Preschool age

Delays in reaching motor milestones, such as sitting, crawling, and walking

Balance problems: falling, getting bruised frequently, and poor toddling

Abnormal gait

Knocking over objects, bumping into things, and destructiveness

Primary-school age

Difficulty with riding bikes, skipping, hopping, running, jumping, and doing somersaults

Awkward or abnormal gait

Older

Poor at sports, throwing, catching, kicking, and hitting a ball

Fine Motor Manifestations

Preschool age

Difficulty learning dressing skills (tying, fastening, zipping, and buttoning)

Difficulty learning feeding skills (handling knife, fork, or spoon)

Primary-school age

Difficulty assembling jigsaw pieces, using scissors, building with blocks, drawing, or tracing

Older

Difficulty with grooming (putting on makeup, blow-drying hair, and doing nails)

Messy or illegible writing

Difficulty using hand tools, sewing, and playing piano

---

coordination disorder, there is a delay in developmental milestones. Many children with the disorder also have speech and language difficulties. Older children may have secondary problems, including academic difficulties, as well as poor peer relationships based on social rejection. Children with motor coordination problems are more likely to have problems understanding subtle social cues, and their peers often reject them. A recent study indicated that children with motor difficulties perform more poorly on scales that measure the recognition of static and changing facial expressions of emotion. This finding is likely to be correlated to the clinical observations that children with motor coordination have difficulties in social behavior and peer relationships.

Billy was brought for evaluation of suicidal ideation at 8 years of age, after complaining to his parents that peers were bullying him for being "bad" in sports and that nobody liked him. He only had one friend who also laughed at him sometimes, because he always dropped the ball and he looked "funny" while running. He was so upset about being rejected by peers when he tried to play sports that he refused to go to physical education class. Instead, he voluntarily went to the school counselor's office and stayed there until the period was over. Billy was already irritated with a diagnosis of ADHD for which he took medication.

On top of that, he had difficulty with reading. Billy became so distraught that one day he told his school counselor that he wanted to kill himself. A developmental history revealed that he was delayed for sitting, which he finally did at 10 months of age, and he could not walk without falling over until 30 months of age. Billy's parents were aware that he was very clumsy, but they believed that he would outgrow that. Even at 8 years of age, Billy's parents reported that, during meals, Billy often spilled his drinks and was quite awkward when he used a fork. Some of his food typically fell off of his fork or spoon before it reached his mouth, and he had great difficulty using a knife and a fork.

A comprehensive assessment of fine and gross motor skills demonstrated the following: Billy was able to hop, but he could not skip without briefly stopping after each step. Billy could stand with both feet together but was unable to stand on tiptoe. Although Billy could catch a ball, he held a ball bounced to himself at chest level, and was unable to catch a ball bounced to him on the ground from a distance of 15 ft. The Bruininks–Oseretsky Test of Motor Development, a test of agility and coordination, revealed functioning levels commensurate with those of an average 6-year-old child.

Billy was referred to a neurologist for a comprehensive evaluation because he appeared to be generally weak, and his muscles seemed floppy. Neurologic evaluation was negative for diagnosable neurologic disorders, and his muscle strength was normal, despite his appearance. Based on the negative neurologic examination and the finding of the Bruininks-Oseretsky Test of Motor Development, Billy had a diagnosis of developmental coordination disorder. Billy's symptoms included mild hypotonia and fine motor clumsiness.

After the diagnosis of developmental coordination disorder was made, in addition to his already diagnosed ADHD and reading disorder, his treatment plan included private sessions with an occupational therapist who used perceptual-motor exercises to improve Billy's fine motor skills, targeting writing and use of utensils. His clinician requested an Individualized Educational Plan (IEP) evaluation from the school to obtain an adaptive physical education program. Also, the clinical team requested that he have a reading tutor and that he sit close to the front of the classroom. Billy was enrolled in a treatment program using motor imagery training to reduce his clumsiness and improve coordination.

Billy was relieved to be receiving help, especially for his reading and for sports activities, and no longer felt suicidal. Over 3 months of treatment, Billy showed a noticeable improvement in his reading. His mood improved further, mainly because he was receiving praise from his teachers and parents. Billy's classmates were not picking on him the way they used to. As Billy began to feel better about himself, he began to play sports informally with his peers, although not competitively. Billy was granted an adaptive physical education program in school, and he was not required to play on teams. Instead, he practiced throwing and catching a ball and playing basketball with a staff member.

Billy continued to show some degree of clumsiness, especially in his fine motor skills over the next few years, yet he was cooperative, with the occupational therapy interventions, his mood was bright, and he demonstrated continual improvement. (Courtesy of Caroly Pataki, M.D. and Sarah Spence, M.D.)

Diagnosis

The diagnosis of developmental coordination disorder depends on poor performance in activities requiring coordination for a child's age and intellectual level. Diagnosis is based on a history of the child's delay in achieving early motor milestones, as well as on direct observation of current deficits in coordination. An informal screen for developmental coordination disorder involves asking the child to perform tasks involving gross motor coordination (e.g., hopping, jumping, and standing on one foot); fine motor coordination (e.g., finger-tapping and shoelace tying); and hand–eye coordination (e.g., catching a ball and copying letters). We should consider what is expected for a child's age to judge possible poor performance. A mildly clumsy child, but whose functioning is not impaired, does not qualify for a diagnosis of developmental coordination disorder. Table 2-20 compares the diagnostic approaches to developmental coordination disorder.

The diagnosis may be associated with below-normal scores on performance subtests of standardized intelligence tests and

Table 2-20
Developmental Coordination Disorder

	DSM-5	ICD-10
Diagnostic name	Developmental Coordination Disorder	Specific Developmental Disorder of Motor Function
Duration	Occurs during early developmental period	
Symptoms	Delayed development of motor coordination	Significant impairment in motor coordination
Psychosocial consequences of symptoms	Functional impairment (self-care, play, other functions)	
Exclusions (not result of):	Another neurologic condition Intellectual disability Visual impairment	General intellectual retardation A specific congenital or neurologic disorder

by normal or above-normal scores on verbal subtests. Specialized tests of motor coordination can be useful, such as the *Bender Visual Motor Gestalt Test,* the *Frostig Movement Skills Test Battery,* and the *Bruininks-Oseretsky Test of Motor Development.* We should take into account the child's age, and ensure that there is not a better explanation, such as a neurologic or neuromuscular condition. Examination, however, may occasionally reveal slight reflex abnormalities and other soft neurologic signs.

Differential Diagnosis

The differential diagnosis includes medical conditions that produce coordination difficulties (e.g., cerebral palsy and muscular dystrophy). In autism spectrum disorder and intellectual disability, coordination usually does not stand out as a significant deficit compared with other skills. Children with neuromuscular disorders may exhibit more global muscle impairment rather than clumsiness and delayed motor milestones. Neurologic examination and workup usually reveal more extensive deficits in neurologic conditions than in developmental coordination disorder. Extremely hyperactive and impulsive children may be physically careless because of their high levels of motor activity. Clumsy gross and fine motor behavior and ADHD, as well as reading difficulties, are highly associated.

Comorbidity

Developmental coordination disorder is strongly associated with ADHD, specific learning disorder, particularly in reading, as well as language disorder. Children with coordination difficulties have higher-than-expected rates of language disorder, and studies of children with language disorder report very high rates of "clumsiness." Developmental coordination disorder is also associated, but less strongly, with specific learning disorder with impairment in mathematics, and in written expression. A study of children with developmental coordination disorder reported that, although motor coordination is critical for accuracy in tasks that require speed, poor

motor coordination does not correlate with the degree of inattention. Thus, in children comorbid for ADHD and developmental coordination disorder, children with the most severe ADHD do not necessarily have the worst developmental coordination disorder. Functional neuroimaging, pharmacologic, and neuroanatomical studies suggest that motor coordination depends on the integration of sensory input and an action response, not purely through sensorimotor function and higher-level thinking. Investigations of comorbid developmental coordination disorder and ADHD are trying to ascertain whether this comorbidity is due to overlapping genetic factors.

Peer relationship problems are common among children with developmental coordination disorders because of rejection that often occurs along with their poor performance in sports and games that require good motor skill. Adolescents with coordination problems often exhibit poor self-esteem and academic difficulties. Recent studies underscore the importance of attention to both victimization of children and adolescents with developmental motor coordination by peers and the potential resulting damage to self-worth. Children and adolescents with developmental coordination disorder often are victims of bullying and have higher rates of poor self-esteem that often deserves clinical attention.

Course and Prognosis

Historically, experts believed that developmental coordination spontaneously improved over time. However, longitudinal studies have shown that motor coordination problems can persist into adolescence and adulthood. When mild to moderate clumsiness is persistent, some children can compensate by developing interests in other skills. Some studies suggest a more favorable outcome for children who have average or above-average intellectual capacity, in that they come up with strategies to develop friendships that do not depend on physical activities. Clumsiness typically persists into adolescence and adult life. One study following a group of children with developmental coordination problems over a decade found that the clumsy children remained less dexterous, showed poor balance and continued to be physically awkward. The affected children were also more likely to have both academic problems and poor self-esteem. Children with developmental coordination disorder have also been shown to be at higher risk for obesity, have difficulties with running, and are at greater risk of future cardiovascular diseases.

Treatment

Interventions for children with developmental coordination disorder utilize multiple modalities, including visual, auditory, and tactile materials targeting perceptual-motor training for specific motor tasks. Two broad categories of interventions are the following: (1) deficit-oriented approaches, including sensory integration therapy, sensorimotor-oriented treatment, and process-oriented treatment; and (2) task-specific interventions, including neuromotor task training and cognitive orientation to daily occupational performance (CO-OP). More recently, therapists incorporate motor imagery into treatment. These approaches involve visual imagery exercises using a computer; they have a broad range of foci, including predictive timing for motor tasks, relaxation and mental preparation, visual modeling of fundamental motor skills, and mental rehearsal of various tasks. This type of intervention derives from the notion that improved internal representation of a movement task will improve a child's actual motor behavior.

The treatment of developmental coordination disorder generally includes versions of sensory integration programs and modified physical education. Sensory integration programs, usually administered by occupational therapists, consist of physical activities that increase awareness of motor and sensory function. For example, a child who bumps into objects often might be given the task of trying to balance on a scooter, under supervision, to improve balance and body awareness. Therapists often give children with difficulty writing letters tasks to increase awareness of hand movements. School-based occupational therapies for motor coordination problems in writing include utilizing mechanisms that provide resistance or vibration during writing exercises, to improve grip, and practicing vertical writing on a chalkboard to increase arm strength and stability while writing. These programs have been shown to improve the legibility of student's writing, but not necessarily speed, because students learn to write with greater accuracy and deliberate letter formation. Currently, many schools also allow and may even encourage children with coordination difficulties that affect writing to use computers to aid in writing reports and long papers.

Adaptive physical education programs help children enjoy exercise and physical activities without the pressures of team sports. These programs generally incorporate certain sports actions, such as kicking a soccer ball or throwing a basketball. Children with coordination disorder may also benefit from social skills groups and other prosocial interventions. The Montessori technique may promote motor skill development, especially with preschool children, because this educational program emphasizes the development of motor skills. Small studies have suggested that exercise in rhythmic coordination, practicing motor movements, and learning to use word processing keyboards may be beneficial. Parental counseling may help reduce parents' anxiety and guilt about their child's impairment, increase their awareness, and facilitate their confidence to cope with the child.

An investigation of children with developmental coordination disorder showed positive results using a computer game designed to improve the ability to catch a ball. These children were able to improve their game scores by practicing virtual catching without specific instructions on how to utilize the visual cues. This has implications for treatment, in that certain types of motor task coordination can be positively influenced through the practice of specific motor tasks, even without overt instructions.

Epidemiology

The prevalence of developmental coordination disorder is about 5 to 6 percent of school-age children. The male-to-female ratio in referred populations tends to show increased rates of the disorder in males, but schools refer boys more often for testing and special education evaluations. About two males for every one female are affected.

Etiology

The causes of developmental coordination disorder are multifactorial and likely include both genetic and developmental factors. Risk factors postulated to contribute to this disorder include prematurity, hypoxia, perinatal malnutrition, and low birth weight. Prenatal exposure to alcohol, cocaine, and nicotine likely contribute to both low birth weight and cognitive and behavioral abnormalities. Children born prematurely have developmental coordination disorder rates of up to 50 percent. Researchers have proposed that the

cerebellum may be the neurologic substrate for comorbid cases of developmental coordination disorder and ADHD. Neurochemical abnormalities and parietal lobe lesions may contribute to coordination deficits. Studies of postural control, that is, the ability to regain balance after being in motion, indicate that children with developmental coordination disorder who have adequate balance when standing still are unable to accurately correct for movement, resulting in impaired balance, compared with other children. A study concluded that, in children with developmental coordination disorder, neural signals from the brain to particular muscles involved in balance are neither being optimally sent or received. These findings have also implicated the cerebellum as a potential anatomical site for the dysfunction of developmental coordination disorder. There are several theories regarding the mechanisms of developmental coordination disorder. One example, called the automatization deficit hypothesis, suggests that similar to dyslexia, children with developmental coordination disorder have difficulty developing automatic motor skills. Another popular suggestion is called the internal modeling deficit hypothesis, which suggests that children with developmental coordination disorder are unable to perform the typical internal cognitive models that predict the sensory consequences of motor commands. In both scenarios, the cerebellum plays a vital role in motor coordination and developmental coordination disorder.

STEREOTYPIC MOVEMENT DISORDER

Stereotypic movements include a diverse range of repetitive behaviors that usually emerge in the early developmental period, appear to lack a clear function, and sometimes cause an interruption in daily life. These movements are typically rhythmic, such as hand flapping, body rocking, hand waving, hair-twirling, lip-licking, skin picking, or self-hitting. Stereotypic movements often appear to be self-soothing or self-stimulating; however, they can result in self-injury in some cases. Stereotypic movements appear to be involuntary; however, they frequently can be suppressed with a concentrated effort. Stereotypic movement disorder occurs with increased frequency in children with autism spectrum disorder and intellectual disability, but they also exist in typically developing children. Stereotypic movements, such as head-banging, face slapping, eye-poking, or hand-biting, can cause significant self-harm. Nail-biting, thumb-sucking, and nose-picking are often not included as symptoms of stereotypic movement disorder because they rarely cause impairment. When impairment occurs, however, they can be included in stereotypic movement disorder. Stereotypic movements share several features with tics, including the repetitive, seemingly involuntary, and characteristically identical nature of the movements each time they are displayed. However, distinguishing features of stereotypical movements compared to tics include a younger age of onset, lack of changing anatomical locations, lack of premonitory "urge," and decreased response to medication management.

According to DSM-5, stereotypic movement disorder includes repetitive, seemingly driven, and purposeless motor behavior that interferes with social, academic, or other activities and may result in self-harm.

Diagnosis and Clinical Features

The presence of multiple repetitive stereotyped symptoms tends to occur frequently among children with autism spectrum disorder and intellectually disability, particularly when the

Table 2-21
Stereotypic Movement Disorder

	DSM-5	ICD-10
Diagnostic name	Stereotypic Movement Disorder	Stereotyped Movement Disorders
Duration	Onset during the developmental period	
Symptoms	Repetitive/seemingly purposeless movements	Movements that are: Voluntary Repetitive Stereotyped Seemingly purposeless Movements outside of any other psychiatric or neurologic condition; may include such things as repeatedly rocking, hand-flapping, or biting
Psychosocial consequences of symptoms	Marked interference in activities and functioning	
Exclusions (not result of):	Substance use Another medical condition Another mental disorder Another neurodevelopmental disorder	Tic disorder Trichotillomania Nail biting Nose-picking Another neurologic disorder (i.e., movement disorders) Another mental disorder
Symptom specifiers	With self-injurious behavior Without self-injurious behavior Associated with known medical or genetic condition, neurodevelopmental disorder or environmental factor	
Severity specifiers	**Mild:** symptoms easily suppressed by sensory stimulus or distraction **Moderate:** significant behavioral modification needed to control symptoms **Severe:** continuous measures taken to prevent harm or injury	

intellectual disability is severe. Patients with multiple stereotyped movements frequently have other significant mental disorders, including disruptive behavior disorders or neurologic conditions. In extreme cases, severe mutilation and life-threatening injuries can result from self-inflicted trauma. Table 2-21 compares the diagnostic approaches to diagnosing stereotypic movement disorder.

Head-Banging. Head-banging exemplifies a stereotypic movement disorder that can result in functional impairment. Typically, head-banging begins during infancy, between 6 and 12 months of age. Infants strike their heads with a definite rhythmic and monotonous continuity against the crib or another hard surface. They seem to be absorbed in the activity, which can persist until they become exhausted and fall asleep. The head-banging is often transitory but sometimes persists into middle childhood. Head-banging that is a component of temper tantrums differs from stereotypic head-banging and ceases after the tantrums, and controlling their secondary gains.

Nail-Biting. Nail-biting begins as early as 1 year of age and increases in incidence until age 12. Most cases are not sufficiently severe to meet the DSM-5 diagnostic criteria for stereotypic movement disorder. In rare cases, children cause physical damage to the fingers themselves, usually by associated biting of the cuticles, which leads to secondary infections of the fingers and nail beds. Nail-biting seems to occur or increase in intensity when a child is either anxious or stressed. Some of the most severe nail-biting occurs in children with severe or profound intellectual disability. However, many nail-biters have no obvious emotional disturbance.

Tim, a 14-year-old with autism spectrum disorder (ASD) and severe intellectual disability, was evaluated when he transferred to a new private school for children with ASD. Observed in his classroom, he was a small boy who appeared younger than his age. He held his hands in his pockets and spun around in place. When offered a toy, he took it and manipulated it for a while. When prompting him to engage in various tasks that required that he take his hands out of his pockets, he began hitting his head with his hands. If the teacher held his hands, he hit his head with his knees. He was adept in contorting himself so that he could hit or kick himself in almost any position, even while walking. Soon, his face and forehead were covered with bruises.

He had delayed development in all spheres, and he never developed language. He lived at home and attended a special educational program. His self-injurious behaviors developed early in life, and, when his parents tried to stop him, he became aggressive. Gradually, he became too difficult to manage in public school, and, at 5 years of age, his parents placed him in a special school. The self-abusive and self-restraining (i.e., holding his hands in his pockets) behavior was present throughout his stay there, and, virtually all of the time, he tried several second-generation antipsychotics with only minimal improvement. Although the psychiatrist's notes mentioned some improvement in his self-injurious behavior, it was continuing and fluctuating. The school system transferred him to a new school because of lack of progress and difficulties in managing him as he became bigger and stronger. His intellectual functioning was within the 34 to 40 intelligence quotient (IQ) range. His adaptive skills were poor. He required full assistance in self-care, could not provide even for his own simple needs and required constant supervision for his safety.

In a few months, Tim settled into the routine in his new school. His self-injurious behavior fluctuated. He could reduce or stop the behavior by restraining himself. For example, he learned to hold his hands in his pockets or inside his shirt. He also might manipulate an object with his hands. If left to himself, he could contort himself, while holding his hands inside his shirt. Because the stereotypic self-injurious and self-restraining behavior interfered with his daily activities and education, it became a primary focus of a behavior modification program. For a few months, he did well, especially when he developed a good relationship with a new teacher, who was firm, consistent, and nurturing. With him, Tim could successfully engage in some school tasks. When the teacher left, Tim regressed. To prevent injuries, the staff started blocking his self-hitting with a pillow. They offered him activities that he liked and in which he could engage without resorting to self-injury. After several months, his antipsychotic medication was slowly discontinued, over 11 months, without any behavioral deterioration. (Adapted from case material from Bhavik Shah, M.D.)

Pathology and Laboratory Examination.   No specific laboratory measures are helpful in the diagnosis of stereotypic movement disorder.

Differential Diagnosis

The differential diagnosis of stereotypic movement disorder includes OCD and tic disorders, both of which are exclusionary criteria in DSM-5. Although stereotypic movements can often be voluntarily suppressed, and are not spasmodic, it is difficult to differentiate these features from tics in all cases. A study of stereotyped movements compared with tics found that stereotyped movements tended to be longer in duration, and displayed more rhythmic qualities than tics. Tics seemed to occur more when a child was in an "alone" condition, rather than when the child was in a play condition, whereas stereotypic movements occurred with the same frequency in these two different conditions. Stereotypic movements seem to be self-soothing, whereas tics are often associated with distress.

Differentiating dyskinetic movements from stereotypic movements can be difficult. Because antipsychotic medications can sometimes suppress stereotypic movements, clinicians should note any stereotypic movements before initiating treatment with an antipsychotic agent. Stereotypic movement disorder may be diagnosed concurrently with substance-related disorders (e.g., amphetamine use disorders), severe sensory impairments, CNS and degenerative disorders (e.g., Lesch–Nyhan syndrome), and severe schizophrenia.

Course and Prognosis

The duration and course of stereotypic movement disorder vary, and the symptoms may wax and wane. Up to 60 to 80 percent of normal toddlers show transient rhythmic activities that seem purposeful and comforting and tend to disappear by 4 years of age. When stereotypic movements emerge more severely later in childhood, they typically range from brief episodes occurring under stress to an ongoing pattern in the context of a chronic condition,

such as ASD or intellectual disability. Even in chronic conditions, stereotypic behaviors may come and go. In many cases, stereotypic movements are prominent in early childhood and diminish as the child ages.

The severity of the dysfunction caused by stereotypic movements varies with the frequency, amount, and degree of associated self-injury. Children who exhibit frequent, severe, self-injurious stereotypic behaviors have the poorest prognosis. Repetitive episodes of head-banging, self-biting, and eye-poking can be difficult to control without physical restraints. Most nail-biting is benign and often does not meet the diagnostic criteria for stereotypic movement disorder. In severe cases in which the child repetitively damages his nail beds, bacterial and fungal infections can occur. Although chronic stereotypic movement disorders can severely impair daily functioning, several treatments help control the symptoms.

Treatment

When stereotypic movements occur in the absence of any other symptoms or disorders, they may not warrant pharmacologic treatment. Treatment modalities yielding the most promising effects include behavioral techniques, such as habit reversal and differential reinforcement of other behavior, as well as pharmacologic interventions. A recent report on utilizing both habit reversal (in which the therapist trains the child to replace the undesired repetitive behavior with a more acceptable behavior) and reinforcement for reducing the unwanted behavior, indicated that these treatments had efficacy among 12 typically developing children between 6 and 14 years. One case report detailed a successful habit reversal treatment of a 3-year-old with severe stereotypic movements, which was largely implemented at home by her parents.

Pharmacologic interventions have been used in clinical practice to minimize self-injury in children whose stereotyped movements caused significant harm to their bodies. Small open-label studies have reported some benefit from atypical antipsychotics, and case reports have indicated the use of SSRIs in the management of self-injurious stereotypies. The dopamine receptor antagonists have been tried most often for treating stereotypic movements and self-injurious behavior. The SSRI agents may be influential in diminishing stereotypies; however, this is still under investigation. Open trials suggest that both clomipramine and fluoxetine may decrease self-injurious behaviors and other stereotypic movements in some patients.

Epidemiology

Repetitive movements are common in infants and young children, with greater than 60 percent of parents of children between the ages of 2 and 4 years reporting transient emergence of these behaviors. The most frequent age of onset is in the second year of life. Epidemiologic surveys estimate that up to 7 percent of otherwise typically developing children exhibit stereotypic behaviors. A prevalence of about 15 to 20 percent in children younger than the age of 6 years has been reported for displaying stereotypic behavior, with diminishing rates over time. The prevalence of self-injurious behaviors, however, is in the range of 2 to 3 percent among children and adolescents with intellectual disability. Stereotypic movements appear to occur in about twice as many boys as girls. Determining which cases are sufficiently severe to confirm a diagnosis of stereotypic movement disorder may be difficult. Stereotypic behaviors occur in 10 to 20 percent of children with intellectual disability, with increased rates being proportional to the level of severity.

Self-injurious behaviors frequently occur in genetic syndromes, such as Lesch–Nyhan syndrome and children with sensory impairments, such as blindness and deafness.

Etiology

The etiology of stereotypic movement disorder includes environmental, genetic, and neurobiologic factors. Although the neurobiologic mechanisms of stereotypic movement disorder have yet to be proven, given their similarity to other involuntary movements, stereotypic movement disorder is hypothesized to originate from the basal ganglia. Dopamine and serotonin are likely to be involved in their emergence. Dopamine agonists tend to induce or increase stereotypic behaviors, whereas dopamine antagonists sometimes decrease them. One study found that 17 percent of typically developing children with stereotypic movement disorder had a first-degree relative with the disorder, and 25 percent had a first- or second-degree relative with stereotypic movement disorder. Transient stereotypic behaviors in very young children can be considered a normal developmental phenomenon. Genetic factors likely play a role in some stereotypic movements, such as the X-linked recessive deficiency of enzymes leading to Lesch–Nyhan syndrome, which has predictable features including intellectual disability, hyperuricemia, spasticity, and self-injurious behaviors. Other minimal stereotypic movements that do not usually cause impairment (e.g., nail-biting) appear to run in families as well. Some stereotypic behaviors seem to emerge or become exaggerated in situations of neglect or deprivation; such behaviors as head-banging correlate with psychosocial deprivation.

TOURETTES DISORDER

Tics are neuropsychiatric events characterized by brief, rapid motor movements or vocalizations in response to irresistible premonitory urges. Although frequently rapid, tics may include more complex patterns of movements and longer vocalizations. Converging evidence from many lines of research suggests that the production of tics involves dysfunction in the basal ganglia region of the brain, particularly of dopaminergic transmission in the cortico-striato-thalamic circuits. Because tic disorders are significantly more common in children than in adults, the postulated alterations in dopamine circuitry in many affected children appear to improve over time. Tics may be transient or chronic, with a waxing and waning course. Tics typically emerge at age 5 to 6 years of age and tend to reach their highest severity between 10 and 12 years. About one half to two-thirds of children with tic disorders will be much improved or in remission by adolescence or early adulthood. We distinguish tic disorder by the type of tics, their frequency, and the pattern in which they emerge over time. Motor tics most commonly affect the muscles of the face and neck, such as eye-blinking, head-jerking, mouth-grimacing, or head-shaking. Typical vocal tics include throat-clearing, grunting, snorting, and coughing. Tics are repetitive muscle contractions resulting in movements or vocalizations that are involuntary. However, patients can sometimes voluntarily suppress them. Children and adolescents may exhibit tic behaviors that occur after a stimulus or in response to a premonitory internal urge.

The most widely studied and most severe tic disorder is Gilles de la Tourette syndrome, also known as Tourette disorder. Georges Gilles de la Tourette (1857–1904) first described a patient with a syndrome, which became known as Tourette disorder in 1885, while he was studying with Jean-Martin Charcot in France. De la

Tourette noted a syndrome in several patients that included multiple motor tics, coprolalia, and echolalia. Tics often consist of motions we might use in volitional movements. One half to two-thirds of children with Tourette disorder exhibit a reduction in or complete remission of tic symptoms during adolescence. There are many common comorbid psychiatric disorders and behavioral problems likely to emerge along with Tourette disorder. For example, the relationship between Tourette disorder, ADHD, and OCD is not clear. Epidemiologic surveys indicate that more than half of children with Tourette disorder also meet criteria for ADHD. There appears to be a bidirectional relationship between Tourette disorder and OCD, with 20 to 40 percent of Tourette disorder patients meeting full criteria for OCD. First-degree relatives of patients with OCD have higher rates of tic disorders compared to the general population.

There are a few small reports suggesting that the obsessive-compulsive symptoms most likely to occur in Tourette disorder are characteristically related to ordering and symmetry, counting, and repetitive touching. In contrast, OCD symptoms in the absence of tic disorders usually stem from fears of contamination and fear of harming. Motor and vocal tics can be simple or complex. *Simple motor tics* are those composed of repetitive, rapid contractions of functionally similar muscle groups—for example, eye-blinking, neck-jerking, shoulder-shrugging, and facial-grimacing. Common *simple vocal tics* include coughing, throat-clearing, grunting, sniffing, snorting, and barking. *Complex motor tics* appear to be more purposeful and ritualistic than simple tics. Common *complex motor tics* include grooming behaviors, the smelling of objects, jumping, touching behaviors, echopraxia (imitation of observed behavior), and copropraxia (display of obscene gestures). *Complex vocal tics* include repeating words or phrases out of context, coprolalia (use of obscene words or phrases), palilalia (a person repeating their own words), and echolalia (repetition of the last-heard words of others).

Although older children and adolescents with tic disorders may be able to suppress their tics for minutes or hours, young children are often not cognizant of their tics or experience their urges to perform their tics as irresistible. Sleep, relaxation, or absorption in activity can all attenuate tics. Tics often disappear during sleep.

Diagnosis and Clinical Features

A diagnosis of Tourette disorder depends on a history of multiple motor tics that generally emerge over months or years and the emergence of at least one vocal tic at some point. According to the DSM-5, tics may wax and wane in frequency but must have persisted for more than a year since the first tic emerged to meet the diagnosis. The average age of onset of tics is between 4 and 6 years of age, although in some cases, tics may occur as early as 2 years of age. The peak age for the severity of tics is between 10 and 12 years of age. For a diagnosis of Tourette disorder, the onset must occur before the age of 18 years. Table 2-22 compares the diagnostic approaches to Tourette disorder.

In Tourette disorder, typically, the initial tics are in the face and neck. Over time, the tics tend to occur in a downward progression. The most commonly described tics are those affecting the face and head, the arms and hands, the body and lower extremities, and the respiratory and alimentary systems. In these areas, the tics take the form of grimacing; forehead puckering; eyebrow-raising; eyelid-blinking; winking; nose-wrinkling; nostril-trembling; mouth-twitching; displaying the teeth; biting the lips and other parts;

Table 2-22
Tourette Disorder

	DSM-5	ICD-10
Diagnostic name	Tourette Disorder	Combined Vocal and Multiple Motor Tic Disorder (de la Tourette)
Duration	>1 yr duration (may include waxing or waning) Onset before the age of 18	Presents in childhood/adolescence Usually persists into adulthood
Symptoms	Motor/vocal tics	Motor tics ≥1 Vocal tic
Exclusions (not result of):	Substance use Another medical illness If symptoms of ONLY motor OR vocal tics, diagnosis would be of "Persistent (Chronic) Motor or Vocal Tic Disorder"	NOTE: for tics that don't meet above criteria, consider: Tic Disorder—Presence of a tic, defined as an involuntary, fast, repeated and nonrhythmic motor movement or vocal production that is sudden and seemingly purposeless. Such tics are experienced as urges that are strong, but that can be suppressed variably. Transient tic disorder (lasting <12 mo) Chronic motor or vocal tic disorder (lasting longer than a year)

tongue-extruding; protracting the lower jaw; nodding, jerking, or shaking the head; twisting the neck; looking sideways; head-rolling; hand-jerking; arm-jerking; plucking fingers; writhing fingers; fist-clenching; shoulder-shrugging; foot, knee, or toe shaking; walking peculiarly; body writhing; jumping; hiccupping; sighing; yawning; snuffing; blowing through the nostrils; whistling; belching; sucking or smacking sounds; and clearing the throat. Several assessment instruments are currently available that are useful in making diagnoses of tic disorders, including comprehensive self-report assessment tools, such as the *Tic Symptom Self Report* and the *Yale Global Tic Severity Scale,* administered by a clinician (Table 2-23).

Because Tourette disorder is frequently comorbid with attentional, obsessional, and oppositional behaviors, these symptoms often emerge before the tics. In some studies, more than 25 percent of children with Tourette disorder received stimulants for a diagnosis of ADHD before receiving a diagnosis of Tourette disorder. The most frequent initial symptom is an eye-blink tic, followed by a head tic or a facial grimace. Most complex motor and vocal symptoms emerge several years after the initial symptoms. Coprolalia, a very unusual symptom involving shouting or speaking socially unacceptable or obscene words, occurs in less than 10 percent of patients and rarely in the absence of comorbid psychiatric disturbance. Mental coprolalia—in which a patient experiences a sudden, intrusive, socially unacceptable thought or obscene word—occurs more often than coprolalia. In severe cases, physical self-injury has occurred due to tic behaviors.

Jake, age 10 years, came to the Tourette Disorder Clinic for an evaluation of motor tics in the head and neck, occasional coughing and grunting, and a new symptom of throat-clearing many times per day. Jake had a history of ADHD, which included significant hyperactivity and impulsive and oppositional behavior. He is a fifth-grade student in a regular class at the local public school. Before the consultation, parent and teacher ratings, including the *Child Behavior Checklist* (CBCL), *Swanson, Nolan, and Pelham-IV* (SNAP-IV), *Conners' Parent and Teacher Questionnaires, Tic Symptom Self-Report* (TSSR), and medical history survey, were sent to his family. His mother and the classroom teacher rated him well above the norm for hyperactivity, inattention, and impulsiveness. He was failing several subjects in school, often argued with adults, was occasionally aggressive, and had few friends. His tics were moderate.

Jake's mother recalled difficulties with overactivity, oppositional and defiant behaviors, and behavior since preschool. At age 5, due to his activity level and argumentative and aggressive behavior, his kindergarten teacher encouraged the family to obtain a psychiatric consultation. Jake's pediatrician made a diagnosis of ADHD and recommended a trial of Concerta (methylphenidate extended-release tablets) at 36 mg/day, which Jake began in the first grade. Within a week of starting medication, Jake's overly active and impulsive

Table 2-23
Clinical Assessment Tools in Tic Disorders

Domain	Type	Reliability and Validity	Sensitive to Change
Tics			
Tic Symptom Self-Report	Parent/self	Good	Yes
Yale Global Tic Severity Scale	Clinician	Excellent	Yes
Attention-Deficit/Hyperactivity Disorder			
Swanson, Nolan, and Pelham-IV	Parent/teacher	Excellent	Yes
Abbreviated Conners' Questionnaire	Parent/teacher	Excellent	Yes
Obsessive-Compulsive Disorder			
Yale-Brown Obsessive Compulsive Scale and Children's Yale-Brown Obsessive Compulsive Scale	Clinician	Excellent	Yes
National Institute of Mental Health Global Obsessive Compulsive Rating Scale	Clinician	Excellent	Yes
General			
Child Behavior Checklist	Parent/teacher	Excellent	No

behavior showed a dramatic improvement; however, he remained argumentative and oppositional. However, when on his Concerta, Jake was able to stay in his seat and complete his work and was better able to wait his turn on the playground. The next few months went well; however, by early spring, Jake seemed to be returning to some of his old ways. He disrupted the class, talking out of turn and getting out of his seat. After an increase in Concerta to 54 mg/day, in the spring of his first-grade year, however, he began showing motor and phonic tics consisting of head-jerking, facial movements, coughing, and grunting. He discontinued the Concerta to see if this made a difference and, although the tics transiently decreased, they came back in full force within a month. In hindsight, Jake's mother recalled that Jake had exhibited eye blinking and grunting before starting the Concerta, but she had dismissed these events as unimportant, and they did not seem to disrupt Jake's daily life.

While Jake was off Concerta during a period when he began middle school in the sixth grade, he was disruptive to his classes, and he began to be severely teased by several classmates for his impulsivity, frequent motor tics, and loud grunting and throat clearing. Jake became despondent and began to refuse to go to school. At this point, his parents and clinicians decided to place Jake in a special education class. However, after several months of this placement, Jake felt worse about himself, despised school, and begged to be returned to regular classes. At this point, Jake's pediatrician made the referral to a child and adolescent psychiatrist at a local university Tourette Disorder Clinic.

During his evaluation at the Tourette Disorder Clinic, Jake was a healthy child who was the product of an uncomplicated pregnancy, labor, and delivery, and whose developmental milestones were appropriate. Intellectual testing completed by the school psychologist revealed a full-scale IQ of 105. Jake's mother noted that Jake has had longstanding trouble falling asleep but sleeps through the night. Jake has always been described as argumentative and easily frustrated with frequent outbursts of temper; however, when he is not having a tantrum, his mood is generally upbeat.

Jake was noted by the child and adolescent psychiatrist to be of average height and weight with no dysmorphic features. His speech was rapid in tempo but normal in tone and volume. His speech is coherent and developmentally appropriate, without evidence of thought disorder; however, he had vocal tics, including grunting, coughing, and noticeable throat clearing. Jake denied depressed mood or suicidal ideation, although he reported distress about everyday issues such as being teased by peers, not having enough friends, and his poor school performance. Jake also denied recurring worries about contamination or harm coming to him or family members, or fears of acting on unwanted impulses. Other than mild touching habits involving the need to touch objects with each hand three times or in combinations of three, Jake denies repetitive rituals. Several motor tics occurred during the evaluation session, including blinking, head-jerking, and shoulder tics. Jake was restless and easily distracted throughout the session and often needed assistance with entertaining himself when not directly involved in the conversation.

Given the history of enduring motor and phonic tics, confirmed by direct observation, the diagnosis of Tourette disorder and ADHD, as well as oppositional defiant disorder, were confirmed.

Jake and his family attended several sessions with the child and adolescent psychiatrist to learn about the waxing and waning nature of tic symptoms and the natural history of Tourette disorder, as well as ADHD. Jake and his family were heartened to hear that, in general, tics tend to be at their maximum around his age, and it was somewhat likely that Jake's tics would lessen over time or possibly fully remit. Jake began seeing a behavioral psychologist specializing in habit reversal training. In this treatment, Jake learned to engage in a behavior physically incompatible with his tic (a competing response) each time he experienced the urge to perform this tic. The competing response for Jake's shoulder tic, which consisted of raising his shoulders as far as he could, was to gently press his shoulders down and extend his neck each time he felt the urge to engage in this tic. With repeated practice of his competing response, Jake's urge to engage in this tic greatly diminished to the point where he was able to manage the urge without performing the tic. The treatment team referred Jake to a child and adolescent psychiatrist who decided to re-start the Concerta at 36 mg/day and titrated it back up to 54 mg/day without worsening of the tics. Jake responded well to his behavioral therapy, and over 8 weeks, he had learned how to become aware of the urges that occurred before his tics and to replace his usual tics with less-distressing and less-disruptive behaviors.

However, when Jake entered the seventh grade, he had an exacerbation of his motor and vocal tics and was also touching objects repeatedly throughout the day. Jake again became despondent, not wanting to go to school. It was decided by his psychologist to add relaxation training to his behavioral treatment, and his child and adolescent psychiatrist added another medication to his pharmacologic regimen. His psychiatrist prescribed risperidone, 0.5 mg/day, which was titrated up to 1 mg twice daily. Jake became stabilized within a month and was able to continue in his school and even went to some parties. Jake and his parents understood the waxing and waning nature of his tics and were hopeful that they would begin to see some decrease in his tic symptoms within the next few years. At follow-up, when Jake was 15 years of age, Jake had minimal tic symptoms; an occasional eye blink and rare throat clearing was all that was observable. Jake was not currently in behavioral treatment. However, over the years, he had, on a few occasions, received some booster therapy sessions to brush up on his habit reversal training when he had a minor exacerbation of tics. Jake had been taken off his risperidone 2 years before without exacerbation of tics. Jake continued well controlled on Concerta, did well in school, and became more popular after joining the soccer team. (Adapted from L. Scahill M.S.N., Ph.D. and J.F. Leckman, M.D.)

Pathology and Laboratory Examination. No specific laboratory diagnostic test exists for Tourette disorder, but many patients with Tourette disorder have nonspecific abnormal EEG findings. CT and MRI scans have revealed no specific structural lesions, although about 10 percent of all patients with Tourette disorder show some nonspecific abnormality on CT scans.

Differential Diagnosis

We should differentiate tics from other movements and movement disorders (e.g., dystonic, choreiform, athetoid, myoclonic, and hemiballismic movements) and the neurologic diseases that they may characterize (e.g., Huntington disease, parkinsonism, Sydenham chorea, and Wilson disease), as listed in Table 2-24. We should also distinguish tremors, mannerisms, and stereotypic movement disorder (e.g., head-banging or body-rocking) from tic disorders. Stereotypic movement disorders, including movements such as rocking, hand-gazing, and other self-stimulatory behaviors, seem to be voluntary and often produce a sense of comfort, in contrast to tic disorders. Although tics in children and adolescents may or may not feel controllable, they rarely produce a sense of well-being. Compulsions are sometimes difficult to distinguish from complex tics and may be on the same continuum biologically. Tic disorders may also occur comorbidly with mood disturbances. In a recent survey, the greater the severity of tics, the higher the probability of both aggressive and depressive symptoms in children. When a child experiences an exacerbation of tic symptoms, behavior and mood also seem to deteriorate.

Course and Prognosis

Tourette disorder is a childhood-onset neuropsychiatric disorder characterized by both motor and vocal tics, which usually emerge

Table 2-24
Differential Diagnosis of Tic Disorders

Disease or Syndrome	Age at Onset	Associated Features	Course	Predominant Type of Movement
Hallervorden-Spatz	Childhood–adolescence	May be associated with optic atrophy, club feet, retinitis pigmentosa, dysarthria, dementia, ataxia, emotional lability, spasticity, autosomal recessive inheritance	Progressive to death in 5–20 yr	Choreic, athetoid, myoclonic
Dystonia musculorum deformans	Childhood–adolescence	Autosomal recessive inheritance commonly, primarily among Ashkenazi Jews; a more benign autosomal dominant form also occurs	Variable course, often progressive but with rare remissions	Dystonia
Sydenham chorea	Childhood, usually 5–15 yr	More common in females, usually associated with rheumatic fever (carditis elevated ASO titers)	Usually self-limited	Choreiform
Huntington disease	Usually 30–50 yr, but childhood forms are known	Autosomal dominant inheritance, dementia, caudate atrophy on CT scan	Progressive to death in 10–15 yr after onset	Choreiform
Wilson disease (hepatolenticular degeneration)	Usually 10–25 yr	Kayser–Fleischer rings, liver dysfunction, inborn error of copper metabolism; autosomal recessive inheritance	Progressive to death without chelating therapy	Wing-beating tremor, dystonia
Hyperreflexias (including latah, myriachit, Jumping Frenchman of Maine)	Generally in childhood (dominant inheritance)	Familial; may have generalized rigidity and autosomal inheritance	Nonprogressive	Excessive startle response; may have echolalia, coprolalia, and forced obedience
Myoclonic disorders	Any age	Numerous causes, some familial, usually no vocalizations	Variable, depending on cause	Myoclonus
Myoclonic dystonia	5–47 yr	Nonfamilial, no vocalizations	Nonprogressive	Torsion dystonia with myoclonic jerks
Paroxysmal myoclonic dystonia with vocalization	Childhood	Attention, hyperactive, and learning disorders; movements interfere with ongoing activity	Nonprogressive	Bursts of regular, repetitive clonic (less tonic) movements and vocalizations
Tardive Tourette syndrome	Variable (after antipsychotic medication use)	Reported to be precipitated by discontinuation or reduction of medication	May terminate after increase or decrease of dosage	Orofacial dyskinesias, choreoathetosis, tics, vocalization
Neuroacanthocytosis	Third or fourth decade	Acanthocytosis, muscle wasting, parkinsonism, autosomal recessive inheritance	Variable	Orofacial dyskinesia and limb chorea, tics, vocalization
Encephalitis lethargica	Variable	Shouting fits, bizarre behavior, psychosis, Parkinson disease	Variable	Simple and complex motor and vocal tics, coprolalia, echolalia, echopraxia, palilalia
Gasoline inhalation	Variable	Abnormal EEG; symmetrical theta and theta bursts frontocentrally	Variable	Simple motor and vocal tics
Postangiographic complications	Variable	Emotional lability, amnestic syndrome	Variable	Simple motor and complex vocal tics, palilalia
Postinfectious	Variable	EEG: occasional asymmetrical theta bursts before movements, elevated ASO titers	Variable	Simple motor and vocal tics, echopraxia
Posttraumatic	Variable	Asymmetrical tic distribution	Variable	Complex motor tics
Carbon monoxide poisoning	Variable	Inappropriate sexual behavior	Variable	Simple and complex motor and vocal tics, coprolalia, echolalia, palilalia
XYY genetic disorder	Infancy	Aggressive behavior	Static	Simple motor and vocal tics

Table 2-24
Differential Diagnosis of Tic Disorders (*Continued*)

Disease or Syndrome	Age at Onset	Associated Features	Course	Predominant Type of Movement
XXY and 9p mosaicism	Infancy	Multiple physical anomalies, mental retardation	Static	Simple motor and vocal tics
Duchenne muscular dystrophy (X-linked recessive)	Childhood	Mild intellectual disability	Progressive	Motor and vocal tics
Fragile X syndrome	Childhood	Intellectual disability, facial dysmorphism, seizures, autistic features	Static	Simple motor and vocal tics, coprolalia
Developmental and perinatal disorders	Infancy, childhood	Seizures, EEG and CT abnormalities, psychosis, aggressivity, hyperactivity, Ganser syndrome, compulsivity, torticollis	Variable	Motor and vocal tics, echolalia

ASLO, Antistreptolysin O; CT, computed tomography; EEG, electroencephalogram.

in early childhood, with a natural history leading to reduction or complete resolution of tics symptoms in most cases by adolescence or early adulthood. During childhood, individual tic symptoms may decrease, persist, or increase, and new symptoms may replace old ones. Severely afflicted persons may have serious emotional problems, including major depressive disorder. Impairment may also be associated with the motor and vocal tic symptoms of Tourette disorder; however, in many cases, interference in function is exacerbated by comorbid ADHD and OCD, both of which frequently coexist with the disorder. When the above three disorders are comorbid, severe social, academic, and occupational problems may ensue. Although most children with Tourette disorder will experience a decline in the frequency and severity of tic symptoms during adolescence, at present, no clinical measures exist to predict which children may have persistent symptoms into adulthood. Children with mild forms of Tourette disorder often have satisfactory peer relationships, function well in school, and develop adequate self-esteem, and may not require treatment.

Treatment

Psychoeducation is a useful intervention in order for families to gain an understanding of the variability of tics, the natural history of the disorder, and ways to support stress reduction. Families need to be well-informed advocates for their children since it is easy to misinterpret tics as a child's purposeful misbehavior, rather than a response to an irresistible urge. The subjective distress of the child and the functional disruptions caused by the disorder argue for active treatment. In mild cases, children with tic disorders who are functioning well socially and academically may not seek, nor require treatment. In more severe cases, peers may ostracize children with tic disorders, and the tics can disrupt academic work. We should consider a variety of interventions, including psychosocial, pharmacologic, and school-based. A scale to measure tic severity, the *Premonitory Urge for Tics Scale* (PUTS), is internally consistent and correlates with overall tic severity in youths over 10 years of age.

The European clinical guidelines for Tourette syndrome and other tic disorders summarized and reviewed the evidence-based treatments for Tourette disorder and developed a consensus for psychosocial and pharmacologic treatments. This guideline recommends that both behavioral and pharmacologic interventions be considered in more severe cases, with behavioral interventions

typically the first line of treatment. Indications for treatment include, but are not limited to, the following clinical presentations. Tics require treatment when they cause social and emotional problems, depression, or isolation. Children who are prone to severe persistent complex motor tics or loud vocal tics may be the objects of bullying and social rejection. In these cases, depressive symptoms commonly result. Tic reduction and psychoeducation to the school may help preserve healthy social relationships, and to diminish depressive and anxiety symptoms. Tics may also lead to impairment in academic achievement. School difficulties in children with Tourette disorder are not uncommon, and reduction in tics may support increased academic success. Tics may also lead to physical discomfort, based on the repetitive musculoskeletal exertion, especially concerning head and neck tics. In some children with Tourette disorder, tics can worsen headaches and migraines. Behavioral and pharmacologic interventions can both target tic reductions, which can lead to improved quality of life.

Evidence-Based Behavioral and Psychosocial Treatment.
The Canadian guidelines for the evidence-based treatment of tic disorders: behavioral therapy, deep brain stimulation and transcranial magnetic stimulation, and a large multi-site RCT of "Comprehensive Behavioral Intervention for Tics," (CBIT) both found converging evidence supporting *habit-reversal training* and *exposure and response prevention* as efficacious treatments for tic reduction. In an RCT of CBIT, 61 children received habit reversal training as their main component of treatment, and they also received relaxation treatment and a functional intervention to identify situations that worsened or sustained tics and strategies to decrease exposure to these situations. The control group of 65 children received supportive psychotherapy and psychoeducation. After 10 weeks of treatment, the intervention group had a significantly reduced Yale Global Tic Severity Scale Total Tic score compared with the control group.

HABIT REVERSAL. The primary components of habit reversal are awareness training, in which the child uses self-monitoring to enhance awareness of tic behaviors and the premonitory urges or sensations, indicating that a tic is about to occur. In competing-response training, the patient learns to voluntarily perform a behavior that is physically incompatible with the tic, contingent on the onset of the premonitory urge or the tic itself, blocking expression of the tic. The competing-response strategy relies on the self-reported observations of patients that tics occur in response to irresistible premonitory urges in order to diminish the urge. Performing the tic satisfies or reduces the premonitory urges, thus reinforcing the tics, and over time they become repeated entrenched behaviors. Competing-response training is different from voluntary tic suppression in that the patient initiates a voluntary behavior to manage the premonitory urge and thus disrupts the reinforcement of the tic, rather than merely trying to suppress the tic. Successful competing-response training significantly reduces the premonitory urge and can decrease or eliminate the urge. For motor tics, the patient may choose a less noticeable behavior, whereas for vocal tics, slow rhythmic breathing is the most common voluntary competing response. Patients can perform competing responses without disrupting usual activities.

EXPOSURE AND RESPONSE PREVENTION.   The rationale for this treatment relies on the notion that tics occur as a conditioned response to unpleasant premonitory urges, and since the tics reduce the urge, they become associated with the premonitory urge. Each time the tic reduces the urge, this strengthens the association. Rather than using competing responses, as in habit-reversal training, exposure and response prevention asks the patient to suppress tics for increasingly prolonged periods in order to break the association between the urges and the tics. Theoretically, if a patient learns to resist performing the tic in response to the urge for long enough periods, the urge may become more tolerable, or attenuate, and the need to perform the tic may diminish.

Many other behavioral interventions, such as relaxation training, self-monitoring, bio (neuro) feedback, and cognitive-behavioral treatment (CBT), are not useful for reducing tics on their own. However, it may help to include some of these strategies in comprehensive treatment programs for children with tic disorders who are receiving habit-reversal training. Habit reversal has been the most extensively researched behavioral treatment for tic disorders; it is highly effective and is currently the first-line behavioral treatment for tic disorders.

Evidence-Based Pharmacotherapy.

Several reviews of pharmacologic treatments for tics suggest that the following classes of pharmacologic agents have an evidence base for treating tics: typical and atypical antipsychotics; noradrenergic agents; and alternative treatments such as tetrabenazine, topiramate, and tetrahydrocannabinol.

ATYPICAL AND TYPICAL ANTIPSYCHOTIC AGENTS.   Risperidone, with its high affinity for dopamine D_2 and serotonin 5-HT_2 receptors, is the most well-studied atypical antipsychotic in the treatment of tics. There is considerable evidence for its efficacy. Multiple randomized, controlled studies in children and adolescents have shown favorable results compared to placebo as well as in head-to-head studies with the typical antipsychotics haloperidol and pimozide. Risperidone was associated with fewer adverse events compared to typical antipsychotics; however, it can cause weight gain, metabolic side effects, and hyperprolactinemia. In a randomized, double-blind, parallel-group study of Tourette disorder comparing risperidone to pimozide, risperidone showed superiority in reducing comorbid obsessive-compulsive symptoms as well as reducing tics. In other randomized clinical trials, risperidone reduced tics in children, adolescents, and adults with mean daily doses of 2.5 mg with a range of 1 to 6 mg.

Haloperidol and pimozide are the two most well-investigated and FDA-approved antipsychotic agents in the treatment of Tourette disorder. However, atypical antipsychotics such as risperidone are often first-line agents due to their safer side-effect profiles. Both haloperidol and pimozide are efficacious in multiple randomized clinical trials in the treatment of Tourette disorder. Both haloperidol and pimozide present significant risks for extrapyramidal side effects; in a long-term naturalistic follow-up study, haloperidol produces more significant acute dyskinesia and dystonia compared to pimozide.

A third typical antipsychotic, fluphenazine, has been used in the United States for many years in the treatment of tic disorders in the absence of robust data supporting its efficacy. A small controlled study of fluphenazine, trifluphenazine, and haloperidol found similar reductions in tics; however, haloperidol has more extrapyramidal side effects and more sedation. The frequency of sedation, dystonia, and akathisia of typical antipsychotics, probably due to their predominant dopaminergic blockade in the nigrostriatal pathways, limits their use and increases the appeal of the atypical antipsychotics. Risperidone and pimozide had equal efficacy in one study of children, adolescents, and adults with Tourette disorder.

Aripiprazole has become a pharmacologic agent of interest in the treatment of tic disorders due to its mode of action; in addition to its D_2 receptor antagonistic actions, aripiprazole is also a partial D_2 and 5-HT_{1A} receptor agonist and a 5-HT_{2A} antagonist. A multisite double-blind controlled study of aripiprazole in children with Tourette disorder in China found a reduction in tic behaviors in about 60 percent of the aripiprazole group compared to about 64 percent reduction in a group treated with tiapride, a benzamide with selective D_2 receptor antagonism. There was no significant difference between the two groups. Although sedation and sleep disturbance are common side effects with aripiprazole, weight gain is less pronounced than with risperidone.

Olanzapine and ziprasidone are also efficacious in the treatment of tic disorders in at least one RCT. Sedation and weight gain were prominent side effects with olanzapine, and potential QT prolongation was an issue with ziprasidone. Quetiapine is a potentially useful agent in the treatment of tics, with its higher affinity for 5-HT_2 receptors than for D_2 receptors. However, randomized clinical trials are needed. Clozapine, contrary to many other atypical antipsychotics, is not useful in the treatment of tics.

NORADRENERGIC AGENTS.   Noradrenergic agents, including clonidine and guanfacine, as well as atomoxetine, are frequently used in children as primary treatments or adjunctive treatments for comorbid ADHD and tics. Several studies have provided some evidence for the efficacy of clonidine, an α_2-adrenergic agent, in the treatment of tics in children, adolescents, and adults with tic disorders. The largest randomized trial with oral clonidine compared to placebo found a modest reduction in tics with clonidine. A multisite randomized, double-blind placebo-controlled trial using the clonidine patch in the treatment of tic disorders in children found a significant improvement in tic symptoms (about 69 percent) compared to about 47 percent of the children in the control group. The usual dose range for clonidine is from 0.05 mg orally three times daily to 0.1 mg four times daily, and for guanfacine, it is from 1 to 4 mg/day. When used in these dosage ranges, adverse effects of the α-adrenergic agents may include drowsiness, headache, irritability, and occasional hypotension.

Guanfacine can treat children with ADHD successfully, although its efficacy regarding reducing tics is controversial. In one randomized clinical trial treating 34 children with ADHD and tics, guanfacine was superior to placebo in the reduction of tics. In another double-blind placebo-controlled trial of 24 children with Tourette disorder, guanfacine was not superior to placebo.

Atomoxetine, a selective norepinephrine reuptake inhibitor, was found to reduce both tics and ADHD symptoms in a multicenter industry trial of 148 children. Atomoxetine also reduced both tics and ADHD in a subgroup of patients in this study who had Tourette disorder. Additional studies are needed to confirm the safety and efficacy of atomoxetine in the treatment of children with Tourette disorder.

Given the frequent comorbidity of tic behaviors and obsessive-compulsive symptoms or disorders, the SSRIs have been used alone or in combination with antipsychotics in the treatment of Tourette disorder. They seem to be useful, however, there have not been controlled trials yet to determine the effect of SSRIs on tic reduction.

Although clinicians must weigh the risks and benefits of using stimulants in cases of severe hyperactivity and comorbid tics, data suggest that methylphenidate does not increase the rate or intensity of motor or vocal tics in most children with hyperactivity and tic disorders.

ALTERNATIVE AGENTS: TETRABENAZINE, TOPIRAMATE, AND TETRAHYDROCANNABINOL

Tetrabenazine. A vesicular monoamine transporter type 2 inhibitor, tetrabenazine depletes presynaptic dopamine and serotonin and blocks postsynaptic dopamine receptors. There are no randomized clinical trials of this agent in the treatment of Tourette disorder in children; however, clinical experience suggests that this agent may have benefit in tic reduction. In a follow-up of 2 years of treatment in 77 children and adolescents, one study reports tic reduction improvement in 80 percent of subjects. Side effects of this agent include sedation, parkinsonism, depression, insomnia, anxiety, and akathisia.

Topiramate. A GABAergic drug, used primarily as an anticonvulsant, topiramate, was effective for reducing tics in a small randomized clinical trial of children and adults with Tourette disorder. Side effects were minimal. Although this does not confirm its efficacy, GABA-modulating agents deserve further study in the treatment of tic disorders.

Tetrahydrocannabinol. A small randomized trial suggested that tetrahydrocannabinol (THC) may be safe and efficacious in the treatment of tics without neuropsychological impairment. In this trial, reported adverse effects included dizziness, fatigue, and dry mouth. Potential additional side-effects include anxiety, depressive symptoms, tremor, and insomnia. This small trial does not confirm efficacy for this agent in the treatment of tics. Instead, it raises questions about the potential improvements in treatment-resistant tic disorders using this agent.

In summary, the most significant evidence for the safe and efficacious pharmacologic treatment of Tourette disorder seems to be associated with the atypical antipsychotics, in particular, risperidone. Pharmacologic treatment may be combined with and enhanced by a variety of behavioral interventions such as habit reversal and school interventions that may diminish stressful situations in the school environment.

Epidemiology

The estimated prevalence of Tourette disorder ranges from 3 to 8 per 1,000 school-age children. Males are affected between two and four times more often than females. The unique features of Tourette disorder, in which tics wax and wane and may change in character, frequency, and severity over relatively short periods, have made ascertainment of its prevalence challenging. Furthermore, remission of tics is particularly age-dependent in that tics tend to emerge and increase from ages 5 to 10 years of age, and in many cases, decrease in frequency and severity after the age of 10 to 12 years. At age 13 years, however, using stringent criteria, the prevalence rate for Tourette disorder drops to 0.3 percent. The lifetime prevalence of Tourette disorder is estimated to be approximately 1 percent.

Etiology

Genetic Factors. Twin studies, adoption studies, and segregation analysis studies all support a genetic basis, albeit a complex one, for Tourette disorder. Twin studies indicate that concordance for the disorder in monozygotic twins is significantly higher than that in dizygotic twins. Tourette disorder and chronic motor or vocal tic disorder are likely to occur in the same families; this lends support to the view that the disorders are part of a genetically determined spectrum. The sons of mothers with Tourette disorder seem to be at the highest risk for the disorder. Evidence in some families suggests an autosomal dominant transmission for Tourette disorder. Studies of an extended family pedigree suggest that transmission of Tourette disorder is bilinear; that is, Tourette disorder appears to be inherited through an autosomal pattern in some families, intermediate between dominant and recessive. A study of 174 unrelated probands with Tourette disorder identified a higher than chance occurrence of a rare sequence variant in SLITRK1, believed to be a candidate gene on chromosome 13q31.

Up to half of all patients with Tourette disorder also have ADHD, and up to 40 percent of those with Tourette disorder also have OCD. These frequent comorbidities with Tourette disorder can lead to a plethora of overlapping symptoms. Family studies have provided compelling evidence for the association between tic disorders and OCD. First-degree relatives of persons with Tourette disorder are at high risk for the development of Tourette disorder, chronic motor or vocal tic disorder, and OCD. The current understanding of the genetic bases of Tourette disorder implicates multiple vulnerability genes that may serve to mediate the type and severity of tics. Candidate genes associated with Tourette disorder include dopamine receptor genes, dopamine transporter genes, several noradrenergic genes, and serotonergic genes.

Neuroimaging Studies. A functional magnetic resonance imaging (fMRI) study of brain activity 2 seconds before and after a tic found that paralimbic and sensory association areas were involved. Furthermore, evidence suggests that voluntary tic suppression involves deactivation of the putamen and globus pallidus, along with partial activation of regions of the prefrontal cortex and caudate nucleus. Compelling, but indirect, evidence of dopamine system involvement in tic disorders includes the observations that pharmacologic agents that antagonize dopamine (haloperidol, pimozide, and fluphenazine) suppress tics and that agents that increase central dopaminergic activity (methylphenidate, amphetamines, and cocaine) tend to exacerbate tics. The relation of tics to neurotransmitter systems is complex and not yet well understood; for example, in some cases, antipsychotic medications, such as haloperidol, are not effective in reducing tics, and the effect of stimulants on tic disorders reportedly varies. In some cases, Tourette disorder has emerged during treatment with antipsychotic medications.

More direct analyses of the neurochemistry of Tourette disorder have been possible utilizing brain proton magnetic resonance spectroscopy (MRS). Neuroimaging studies using cerebral blood flow in PET and SPECT suggest that alterations of activity may occur in various brain regions in patients with Tourette disorder compared to controls, including the frontal and orbital cortex, striatum, and putamen. An investigation examining the cellular neurochemistry of patients with Tourette disorder utilizing MRS of the frontal cortex, caudate nucleus, putamen, and thalamus demonstrated that these patients had a reduced amount of choline and *N*-acetylaspartate in the left putamen along with reduced levels bilaterally in the putamen. In the frontal cortex, patients with Tourette disorder were found to have lower concentrations of *N*-acetylaspartate bilaterally, lower levels of creatine on the right side, and reduced myoinositol on the left side. These results suggest that deficits in the density of neuronal and nonneuronal cells are present in patients with the disorder. Abnormalities in the noradrenergic system have been implicated in some cases by the reduction of tics with clonidine. This adrenergic agonist reduces the release of norepinephrine in the CNS and, thus, may reduce activity in the dopaminergic system. Abnormalities in the basal ganglia are known to result in various movement disorders, such as Huntington disease, and are likely sites of disturbance in Tourette disorder.

Immunologic Factors and Postinfection.   An autoimmune process and, in particular, one that is secondary to group A β-hemolytic streptococcal infection, is a potential mechanism for the development of tics and obsessive-compulsive symptoms in some cases. Data have been conflicting and controversial, and this mechanism appears to be unlikely as an etiology of Tourette disorder in most cases. One case-control study found little evidence of the development or exacerbation of tics, or obsessions or compulsions, in children with well-documented and treated group A β-hemolytic streptococcal infections.

PERSISTENT (CHRONIC) MOTOR OR VOCAL TIC DISORDER

Chronic motor or vocal tic disorder is defined as the presence of either motor tics or vocal tics, but not both. Tics may wax and wane but must have persisted for more than 1 year since the first tic onset to meet the diagnosis for persistent (chronic) motor or vocal tic disorder. According to DSM-5, this disorder must have its onset before the age of 18 years. We would not diagnose chronic motor or vocal tic disorder if the patient already has Tourette disorder.

Diagnosis and Clinical Features

The onset of chronic motor or vocal tic disorder typically occurs in early childhood. Chronic vocal tics are considerably rarer than chronic motor tics. Chronic vocal tics, in the absence of motor tics, are typically less conspicuous than the vocal tics in Tourette disorder. The vocal tics are usually not loud or intense and are not mainly from the vocal cords; they consist of grunts or other noises caused by thoracic, abdominal, or diaphragmatic contractions.

Differential Diagnosis

We should differentiate chronic motor tics from a variety of other motor movements, including choreiform movements, myoclonus, restless legs syndrome, akathisia, and dystonias. Involuntary vocal utterances can occur in certain neurologic disorders, such as Huntington disease and Parkinson disease.

Course and Prognosis

Children whose tics emerge between the ages of 6 and 8 years seem to have the best outcomes. Symptoms often last for 4 to 6 years and remit in early adolescence. Children whose tics involve the limbs or trunk may have less prompt remission than those with only facial tics.

Treatment

The treatment of chronic motor or vocal tic disorder depends on several factors, including the severity and frequency of the tics; the patient's subjective distress; the effects of the tics on school or work, job performance, and socialization; and the presence of any other concomitant mental disorder. Psychotherapy may help minimize the secondary social difficulties caused by severe tics. Behavioral techniques, particularly habit reversal treatments, are effective in treating chronic motor or vocal tic disorder. When severe, atypical antipsychotics such as risperidone may reduce the tics. If not effective, typical antipsychotics such as pimozide or haloperidol may be helpful. Behavioral interventions are the first line of treatment.

Epidemiology

The rate of chronic motor or vocal tic disorder is 100 to 1,000 times greater than that of Tourette disorder in school-age children. School-age boys are at the highest risk. The estimated prevalence of chronic motor or vocal tic disorder is from 1 to 2 percent.

Etiology

Chronic motor or vocal tic disorder, as well as Tourette disorder, tend to aggregate in the same families. Twin studies have found a high concordance for either Tourette disorder or chronic motor tics in monozygotic twins. This finding supports the importance of hereditary factors in the transmission of tic disorders.

▲ 2.7 Feeding and Eating Disorders of Infancy or Early Childhood

Feeding and eating disorders of infancy and childhood are persistent disturbances in eating or eating-related behaviors that can lead to significant impairments in physical health and psychosocial functioning. The DSM-5 category *Feeding and Eating Disorders* includes three disorders that are often, but not always, associated with infancy and early childhood: pica, rumination disorder, and avoidant/restrictive food intake disorder (formerly known as feeding disorder of infancy or early childhood). As these are specialized diagnoses that are usually made in collaboration between a pediatrician, a child psychiatrist, and often a pediatric gastroenterologist, we discuss them only briefly. Anorexia nervosa, bulimia nervosa, and binge-eating disorder are also part of that DSM category, however they are more often associated with young adulthood and we discuss them in Chapter 13.

PICA

Pica is persistent eating of nonnutritive substances. Typically, no specific biologic abnormalities account for pica. In many cases, we only discover the disorder when medical problems such as intestinal obstruction, intestinal infections, or poisonings arise, such as lead poisoning due to the ingestion of lead-containing paint chips.

Pica is more frequent in the context of autism spectrum disorder or intellectual disability; we only diagnose pica when it is of sufficient severity and persistence to warrant clinical attention. Pica can emerge in young children, adolescents, or adults; however, a minimum of 2 years of age is suggested by DSM-5 in the diagnosis of pica, in order to exclude developmentally appropriate mouthing of objects by infants that may accidentally result in ingestion. Pica occurs in both males and females, and in rare cases, a cultural belief in the spiritual or medicinal benefit of ingesting nonfood substances may be the cause. In this context, we would not diagnose pica. Among adults, certain forms of pica, including geophagia (clay eating) and amylophagia (starch eating), have been reported in pregnant women.

Diagnosis and Clinical Features

Eating nonedible substances repeatedly after 18 months of age is not typical; however, DSM-5 suggests a minimum age of 2 years when making a diagnosis of pica. Pica behaviors, however, may begin in infants 12 to 24 months of age. Specific substances ingested vary with their accessibility, and they increase with a child's mastery of locomotion, and the resultant increased independence and decreased parental supervision. Typically, infants may ingest paint, plaster, string, hair, and cloth, whereas older toddlers and young children with pica may ingest dirt, animal feces, small stones, and paper. The clinical implications can be benign or life-threatening, depending on the objects ingested. Among the most severe complications are lead poisoning (usually from lead-based paint), intestinal parasites after ingestion of soil or feces, anemia and zinc deficiency after ingestion of clay, severe iron deficiency after ingestion of large quantities of starch, and intestinal obstruction from the ingestion of hairballs, stones, or gravel. Except in autism spectrum disorder and intellectual disability, pica often remits by adolescence. Pica associated with pregnancy is usually limited to the pregnancy itself.

Chantal was 2½ years of age when her mother urgently brought her to her pediatrician due to severe abdominal pain and lack of appetite. Chantal's mother complained that she still put everything in her mouth but refused to eat regular food. The pediatrician observed Chantal to be pale, thin, and withdrawn. She sucked her thumb and quietly looked down while her mother reported that Chantal often chewed on newspapers and put plaster in her mouth.

The medical examination revealed that Chantal was anemic and suffered from lead poisoning. She was hospitalized, and a child psychiatric evaluation revealed that Chantal's mother was overwhelmed, caring for five young children, and had little affection for Chantal. Chantal's mother was a single mother, living with her five children and four other family members in a three-bedroom apartment in an old housing project. Her 7-year-old daughter had behavior problems, and her 6- and 4-year-old sons were impulsive and hyperactive and required constant supervision. Chantal's 18-month-old sister was an engaging and active little girl, whereas Chantal was withdrawn, and would sit quietly, rocking herself, sucking her thumb, or chewing on newspaper.

The treatment plan included the involvement of social services and protective services to remove any lead paint from the walls in their current apartment, seek better living arrangements for the family, and provide a safe environment for the children. Chantal's mother received guidance in enrolling Chantal in a preschool program, and her older sister and two brothers in an after-school program that provided structure and stimulation, and some respite time for her mother. Chantal, her mother, and her younger sister started family therapy to help

---

their mother's understanding of her children's needs and to increase her positive interactions with Chantal. Once Chantal's mother felt more supported and less overwhelmed, she was able to become more empathic and warm toward Chantal. When Chantal began chewing on paper, her mother learned to instead engage her in a play activity rather than screaming at her and grabbing her mouth. Chantal and her mother continued in therapy for a year, during which their relationship gradually became more interactive and warm, while Chantal's chewing behaviors decreased, and even her thumb sucking abated.

Pathology and Laboratory Examination. No single laboratory test confirms or rules out a diagnosis of pica, but several laboratory tests are useful because abnormal levels of lead are sometimes associated. Levels of iron and zinc in serum should be determined and corrected if low. In rare cases, when this is the etiology, giving the patient oral iron and zinc may ameliorate the pica. A hemoglobin level should be determined to rule out anemia.

Differential Diagnosis

The differential diagnosis of pica includes avoidance of food, anorexia, or rarely iron and zinc deficiencies. Pica may occur in conjunction with failure to thrive and be comorbid with schizophrenia, autism spectrum disorder, and Kleine–Levin syndrome. In psychosocial dwarfism, a dramatic but reversible endocrinologic and behavioral form of failure to thrive, children often show bizarre behaviors, including ingesting toilet water, garbage, and other nonnutritive substances. Lead intoxication may be associated with pica. In children who exhibit pica that warrants clinical intervention, along with a known medical disorder, we should diagnose both disorders.

In some areas of the world and among certain cultures, such as the Australian aborigines, rates of pica in pregnant women are reportedly high. According to DSM-5, however, if such practices are culturally accepted, the diagnostic criteria for pica are not met.

Course and Prognosis

The prognosis for pica is usually good, and typically in children with normal intellectual function, pica generally remits spontaneously within several months. In childhood, pica usually resolves with increasing age; in pregnant women, pica resolves after delivery. In some adults with pica, particularly those who also have autism spectrum disorder and intellectual disability, pica can continue for years. Follow-up data on these populations are too limited to permit conclusions.

Treatment

The first step in determining the appropriate treatment of pica is to investigate the specific situation whenever possible. When pica occurs in the context of child neglect or maltreatment, those circumstances must be immediately corrected. Exposure to toxic substances, such as lead, must also be eliminated. No definitive treatment exists for pica per se beyond education and behavior modification. Treatments emphasize psychosocial, environmental, behavioral, and family guidance approaches. It is essential to address significant psychosocial stressors. When lead is present in the surroundings, it must be eliminated or rendered inaccessible, or the child and their family should move.

When pica persists in the absence of any toxic manifestations, we should use behavioral techniques. Techniques include positive reinforcement, modeling, behavioral shaping, and overcorrection treatment. Increasing parental attention, stimulation, and emotional nurturance may yield positive results. A study found that pica occurred most frequently in impoverished environments, and in some patients, correcting an iron or zinc deficiency has eliminated pica. Medical complications (e.g., lead poisoning) that develop secondarily to the pica also require treatment.

Epidemiology

The prevalence of pica is unclear. A survey of a large clinic population reported that 75 percent of 12-month-old infants and 15 percent of 2- to 3-year-old toddlers placed nonnutritive substances in their mouth; however, this behavior is developmentally appropriate and typically does not result in ingestion. Pica is common among children and adolescents with autism spectrum disorder and intellectual disability. Up to 15 percent of persons with severe intellectual disability have engaged in pica. Pica appears to affect both sexes equally.

Etiology

Pica is most often a transient disorder that typically lasts for several months and then remits. In younger children, those with developmental speech and social developmental delays are more likely to have it. Among adolescents with pica, a substantial number of them exhibited depressive symptoms and using substances. Nutritional deficiencies in minerals such as zinc or iron (found in, e.g., dirt or ice) may rarely be a cause. In some cases of pica, we also find severe child maltreatment in the form of parental neglect and deprivation. Lack of supervision, as well as in adequate feeding of infants and toddlers, may increase the risk of pica.

RUMINATION DISORDER

Rumination is an effortless and painless regurgitation of partially digested food into the mouth soon after a meal, which is either swallowed or spit out. We can observe rumination in developmentally normal infants who put their thumb or hand in the mouth, suck their tongue rhythmically, and arch their back to initiate regurgitation. We may observe this pattern in infants who receive inadequate emotional interaction and have learned to soothe and may stimulate themselves through rumination. However, rumination syndromes also occur in children and adolescents, in which case rumination is a functional gastrointestinal disorder. The pathophysiology of rumination is not well understood; however, it often involves a rise in intragastric pressure generated by either voluntary or unintentional contraction of the abdominal wall muscles causing movement of gastric contents back up into the esophagus. The onset of the disorder can occur in infancy, childhood, or adolescence. In infants, it typically occurs between 3 and 12 months of age, and once the regurgitation occurs, the food may be swallowed or spit out. Infants who ruminate strain with their backs arched and head back to bring the food back into their mouths and appear to find the experience pleasurable. Infants who are "experienced" ruminators can bring up the food through tongue movements and may not spit out the food at all, but hold it in their mouths and re-swallow it. The disorder is not common in older children, adolescents, and adults. It varies in severity and is sometimes associated with medical conditions, such as hiatal hernia, leading to esophageal reflux. In its most severe form, the disorder can cause malnutrition and be fatal.

We can diagnose rumination disorder even if an infant is a healthy weight. Failure to thrive, therefore, is not a necessary criterion of this disorder, but it is sometimes a sequela. According to DSM-5, the disorder must be present for at least 1 month after a period of normal functioning, and not better accounted for by gastrointestinal illness, or psychiatric or medical conditions.

Doctors have recognized rumination for hundreds of years. An awareness of the disorder is essential to avoid misdiagnosis and unwarranted tests and treatment. *Rumination* comes from the Latin *ruminare,* which means, "to chew the cud." The Greek equivalent is *merycism,* the act of regurgitating food from the stomach into the mouth, re-chewing the food, and re-swallowing it.

Diagnosis and Clinical Features

The DSM-5 notes that the essential feature of the disorder is repeated regurgitation and re-chewing of food for at least 1 month after a period of normal functioning. Patients bring partially digested food into their mouth without nausea, retching, or disgust; on the contrary, it may appear to be pleasurable. This activity may be distinguished from vomiting by painless and purposeful movements observable in some infants who induce it. The food is then ejected from the mouth or swallowed. A characteristic position of straining and arching of the back, with the head held back, is observed. The infant makes sucking movements with the tongue and gives the impression of gaining considerable satisfaction from the activity. Usually, the infant is irritable and hungry between episodes of rumination.

Initially, rumination may be challenging to distinguish from the regurgitation that frequently occurs in healthy infants. In infants with persistent and frequent rumination behaviors, however, the differences are apparent. Although spontaneous remissions are common, secondary complications can develop, such as progressive malnutrition, dehydration, and lowered resistance to disease. Failure to thrive, with the absence of growth and developmental delays in all areas, can occur in the most severe cases. Additional complications may occur if the mother of a given infant with rumination becomes discouraged by the persistent symptoms, viewing it as her feeding failure, as this may lead to more tension and more rumination after feedings.

Luca was 9 months old when his pediatrician referred him to a gastroenterologist, and by his gastroenterologist for psychiatric evaluation due to persistent and frequent rumination. Luca was born full-term and had developed typically until 6 weeks of age when he began to regurgitate large amounts of milk just after feedings. He was evaluated and diagnosed with gastroesophageal reflux, and the gastroenterologist had his mother thicken his feedings. Luca responded well to the treatment; his regurgitation diminished, and he gained weight adequately. Luca continued to do well, and his mother decided to go back to work when Luca was 8 months old. Luca's mother transitioned his care to a young nanny who cared for Luca while she worked. Luca and the nanny seemed to have a warm relationship; however, he started again to regurgitate his meals soon after his mother left the house. The regurgitation seemed to increase in frequency and intensity within 2 weeks of the mother's return to work. At this point, Luca regurgitated after almost every meal, and he was losing weight. A gastroenterologist evaluated Luca, and during the barium swallow, his doctor noted that Luca put his hand in his mouth, which seemed to induce the regurgitation. Luca was administered some medication for gastroesophageal reflux; however, he continued to induce regurgitation after meals with increasing frequency, prompting the psychiatric consultation.

Observation of mother and infant during feeding at home revealed that as soon as Luca finished feeding, he purposefully placed his hand in his mouth and induced the regurgitation. When his mother restricted his hand, Luca moved his tongue back and forth in a rhythmic manner until he regurgitated again. Luca engaged in this rhythmic tongue movement repeatedly, even when he could not bring up any more milk, and appeared to be enjoying this behavior.

Due to Luca's poor nutritional state and moderate dehydration, the doctor hospitalized him and inserted a nasojejunal tube for feedings. When Luca was awake during feedings, a special duty nurse or his parents played with him and distracted him during attempts to put his hand in his mouth or thrust his tongue rhythmically. Luca became increasingly engaged in this playful activity, and his ruminative activity decreased accordingly. After 1 week in the hospital, they started small feedings; however, Luca again successfully was able to bring up his food by his rumination activity, and the treatment team had to stop oral feedings. At this point, Luca's mother decided to stop working and take Luca home to continue an intensive behavioral "distracting" intervention in order to interrupt his rumination during meals. Luca's mother started small feedings while playing with him during and after feedings, and was able to interest him in other activities so that he would not ruminate. After 4 weeks of slow increments in his feedings, Luca was able to take all his feedings by mouth without ruminating, and they removed his nasojejunal tube. Luca and his mother continued to use stimulating and distracting activities during and just after meals, which over time, became more attractive to Luca than his previous ruminating behavior.

Pathology and Laboratory Examination. No specific laboratory examination is pathognomonic of rumination disorder; however, rumination disorder is not uncommonly associated with gastrointestinal abnormalities. Clinicians should evaluate other physical causes of vomiting, such as pyloric stenosis and hiatal hernia, before making the diagnosis of rumination disorder. Rumination disorder can lead to states of malnutrition and dehydration. In very severe cases, laboratory measures of endocrinologic function, serum electrolytes, and a hematologic workup may determine the need for medical intervention.

Differential Diagnosis

To make the diagnosis of rumination disorder, clinicians must rule out primary gastrointestinal congenital anomalies, infections, and other medical illnesses that could account for frequent regurgitation. Pyloric stenosis is usually associated with projectile vomiting and is generally evident before 3 months of age when rumination has its onset. Rumination occurs with both autism spectrum disorder and intellectual disability in which stereotypic behaviors and eating disturbances are not uncommon. Rumination behavior may occur comorbidly in youth with severe anxiety disorders as well. Rumination disorder may also occur in patients with other eating disorders, such as anorexia nervosa and bulimia nervosa.

Course and Prognosis

Rumination disorder has a high rate of spontaneous remission. Indeed, many cases of rumination disorder may develop and remit without ever being diagnosed. Limited data are available about the prognosis of rumination disorder in adolescents and adults. Behavioral interventions using habit-reversal techniques may significantly lead to improved prognosis.

Treatment

The treatment of rumination disorder is often a combination of education and behavioral techniques. Sometimes, an evaluation of the mother–child relationship reveals deficits that can be influenced by offering guidance to the mother. Behavioral interventions, such as habit-reversal, can reinforce an alternate behavior that becomes more compelling than the behaviors leading to regurgitation. Aversive behavioral interventions, such as squirting lemon juice into the infant's mouth whenever rumination occurs, have been used in the past to diminish rumination behavior. Although aversive behavioral interventions have anecdotal support, current recommendations support the use of habit-reversal techniques.

When features of child maltreatment or neglect may have contributed to rumination behaviors in an infant, treatments include improvement of the child's psychosocial environment, increased tender loving care from the mother or caretakers, and psychotherapy for the mother or both parents. Anatomical abnormalities, such as hiatal hernia, are not uncommon and must be evaluated, in some cases leading to surgical repair. In severe cases in which malnutrition and weight loss have occurred, treatment may include jejunal tube placement before implementing other treatments.

Medication is not a standard part of the treatment of rumination. Case reports, however, cite a variety of medications, including metoclopramide, cimetidine, and even antipsychotics such as haloperidol, as helpful. The treatment of adolescents with rumination disorder is often complicated and includes a multidisciplinary approach consisting of individual psychotherapy, nutritional intervention, and pharmacologic treatment for frequent comorbid anxiety and depressive symptoms.

Epidemiology

Rumination is a rare disorder. It seems to be more common among male infants and emerges between 3 months and 1 year of age. It persists more frequently among children, adolescents, and adults with intellectual disability. Adults with rumination usually are normal weight.

Etiology

Rumination is associated with high intragastric pressure and the ability to contract the abdominal wall to cause retrograde movement of the gastric contents into the esophagus. Several studies have elucidated other gastrointestinal symptoms such as gastroesophageal reflux that may accompany rumination.

In a study of 2,163 children in Sri Lanka between the ages of 10 and 16 years, it was found that rumination behaviors were present in 5.1 percent of boys and 5.0 percent of girls. In 94.5 percent of youth who ruminated, the regurgitation occurred in the first hour after the meal, and 73.6 percent reported re-swallowing of the regurgitated food, whereas the rest spit it out. Only 8.2 percent of this sample reported daily episodes of regurgitation, whereas 62.7 percent experienced weekly symptoms. Associated gastrointestinal symptoms reported in this sample included abdominal pain, bloating, and weight loss. Approximately 20 percent of youth with rumination in this sample also experienced other gastrointestinal symptoms. Another survey of 147 patients from 5 to 20 years of age found the mean age of onset of rumination was 15 years, and these patients were symptomatic after each meal; 16 percent of this sample met criteria for a psychiatric disorder, 3.4 percent had anorexia or bulimia nervosa, and 11 percent had a surgical procedure.

Additional gastrointestinal symptoms in this sample included abdominal pain in 38 percent, constipation in 21 percent, nausea in 17 percent, and diarrhea in 8 percent. In some cases, vomiting secondary to gastroesophageal reflux or an acute illness precedes a pattern of rumination that lasts for several months. In many cases, children classified as ruminators have gastroesophageal reflux or hiatal hernia.

It appears, for some infants, that the rumination behavior is self-soothing or produces a sense of relief, leading to a continuation of behaviors to bring it about. In youth with autism spectrum disorder or intellectual disability, rumination may serve as a self-stimulatory behavior. Overstimulation and tension is likely a contributing factor in rumination. Behaviorists attribute persistent rumination to the positive reinforcement of pleasurable self-stimulation and to the attention a baby receives from others as a consequence of the disorder.

AVOIDANT/RESTRICTIVE FOOD INTAKE DISORDER

Avoidant/restrictive food intake disorder, formerly known as feeding disorder of infancy or early childhood, is characterized by a lack of interest in food, or its avoidance based on the sensory features of the food or the perceived consequences of eating. This newly included DSM-5 disorder adds more detail about the nature of the eating problems and includes adolescents and adults. The disorder is manifested by a persistent failure to meet nutritional or energy needs, as evidenced by one or more of the following: significant weight loss or failure to achieve expected weight, nutritional deficiency, dependence on enteral feedings or nutritional supplements, or marked interference with psychosocial functioning. It may take the form of outright food refusal, food selectivity, eating too little, food avoidance, and delayed self-feeding. We should not make the diagnosis in the context of anorexia nervosa or bulimia nervosa, or if caused by a medical condition, by another mental disorder, or by a genuine lack of available food.

Infants and children with the disorder may be withdrawn, irritable, apathetic, or anxious. Because of the avoidant behavior during feeding, there is less touching and holding between mothers and infants during the feeding process compared with other children. Some reports suggest that food avoidance or restriction may be relatively longstanding; however, in many cases, normal adult functioning is eventually achieved.

Differential Diagnosis

We should differentiate the disorder from structural problems with the infants' gastrointestinal tract that may be contributing to discomfort during the feeding process. Because feeding disorders and organic causes of swallowing difficulties often coexist, it is essential to rule out medical reasons for feeding difficulties. A study of videofluoroscopic evaluation of children with feeding and swallowing problems revealed that clinical evaluation was 92 percent accurate in identifying those children at increased risk of aspiration. This type of evaluation is necessary before psychotherapeutic interventions in cases where a medical contribution to feeding problems is suspected.

Course and Prognosis

Most infants identified with feeding disorder within the first year of life and who receive treatment do not go on to develop malnutrition,

growth delay, or failure to thrive. When feeding disorders have their onset later, in children 2 to 3 years of age, growth and development can be affected when the disorder lasts for several months. In older children or adolescents, the feeding disorder typically interferes with social functioning until treated. About 70 percent of infants who persistently refuse food in the first year of life continue to have some eating problems during childhood.

> Jennifer was 6 months old when she saw a child psychiatrist for feeding difficulties, irritability, and poor weight gain since birth. She was small and slight, but she did not appear to be lethargic or malnourished. Her parents were college-educated, and both had pursued their professional careers until Jennifer was born. Although Jennifer was full-term and weighed 7 pounds at birth, she had been unable to breastfeed due to turning away and not ingesting enough milk. When she was 4 weeks old, Jennifer's mother had reluctantly switched her to bottle feedings because Jennifer was losing weight. Although her intake improved somewhat on bottle feedings, she gained weight very slowly and was still less than 8 lb at 3 months of age. Since then, she had gained a minimal amount each month to maintain a low but adequate weight. Jennifer's mother appeared tired and described that Jennifer would drink only up to about 6 oz at a time, or two bites of baby food, and then wiggle and cry; and refuse to continue with the feeding. However, after a few hours, she might cry again as if she were hungry. However, she could not settle her into a good rhythm of feeding and continued attempts to feed her would lead her to cry inconsolably. Jennifer's mother described approximately 10 to 15 attempts at feeding her both liquids and solids in 24 hours. Jennifer was reported to be an irritable and fussy infant, who cried multiple times during the day and at night, and woke her family often during the night with her crying. Jennifer's developmental milestones, such as sitting up, tracking, and making sounds, were normal.
>
> The observation of mother–infant interactions during feeding and play revealed that Jennifer was a very alert and wiggly baby who had difficulty sitting still. While drinking from the bottle, she would kick her feet and move around, and if the bottle slipped out of her mouth, she did not try to recapture it. When eating baby foods, she was not interested, and her mother had to coax her to open her mouth. This upset Jennifer, and she would start crying. Jennifer's mother reported that she was always anxious during meals, and would try to convince Jennifer to take spoonfuls of baby food while sitting in her high chair. After repeated unsuccessful attempts of adequate feeding, Jennifer and her mother both appeared exhausted and took a break.
>
> The history and examination revealed that Jennifer was a very active and excitable baby who had difficulty keeping calm during feedings. After reviewing the videotape with the mother, the therapist explored ways in which the mother could better facilitate calming Jennifer before and during meals. Using a quiet corner in the house and singing to Jennifer before meals resulted in Jennifer remaining calmer during meals, and she was able to drink more substantial amounts of milk, eat more solid foods, and waited longer between meals. This improvement, in turn, relieved her mother's anxiety and helped both to have calmer interactions. (Adapted by Caroly Pataki, M.D.)

Treatment

Most interventions for feeding disorders aim to optimize the interaction between the mother and infant during feedings and identifying any factors that can be changed to promote better ingestion. The psychiatrist helps the mother to become more aware of the infant's stamina for the length of individual feedings, the infant's biologic regulation patterns, and the infant's fatigue level to increase the level of engagement between mother and infant during feeding.

Some experts have proposed a transactional model of intervention for infants who exhibit the "difficult" temperamental traits of emotional intensity, stubbornness, lack of hunger cues, and irregular eating and sleeping patterns. The treatment includes education for the parents regarding the temperamental traits of the infant, exploration of the parents' anxieties about the infant's nutrition, and training for the parents regarding changing their behaviors to promote internal regulation of eating in the infant. Parents are encouraged to feed the infant regularly at 3- to 4-hour intervals and offer only water between meals. The parents learn to deliver praise to the infant for any self-feeding efforts, regardless of the amount of food ingested. Furthermore, parents learn to limit any distracting stimulation during meals and give attention and praise to positive eating behaviors rather than intense negative attention to inappropriate behavior during meals. This training process for parents is intense and is brief. Many parents can facilitate improved eating patterns in the infant as a result. If the mother or caregiver is unable to participate in the intervention, it may be necessary to include additional caregivers to contribute to feeding the infant. In rare cases, an infant may require hospitalization until they receive adequate nutrition. If an infant tires before ingesting an adequate amount of nutrition, it may be necessary to begin treatment with the placement of a nasogastric tube for supplemental oral feedings.

For older children with failure-to-thrive syndromes, hospitalization and nutritional supplementation may be necessary. Medication is not a standard component of treatment for feeding disorders; however, there are anecdotal reports of preadolescents with failure-to-thrive and feeding disorders who were comorbid for anxiety and mood symptoms and who received enteral nutritional interventions in addition to risperidone, and who were observed to have an increase in oral intake and accelerated weight gain.

Epidemiology

Between 15 and 35 percent of infants and young children have transient feeding difficulties. A study of restrictive eating difficulties in Swedish 9- and 12-year-olds found that restrictive eating problems were present in 0.6 percent of their sample. However, another study of avoidant eating patterns in young children in Germany found that some degree of avoidance was present in up to 53 percent of children. Thus, we should separate avoidant eating behaviors without impairment of nutritional state or psychosocial functioning from restricted eating disturbances leading to significant functional impairment. A survey of feeding problems in nursery school children revealed a prevalence of 4.8 percent with equal gender distribution. In that study, children with feeding problems exhibited more somatic complaints, and mothers of affected infants exhibited an increased risk of anxiety symptoms. Data from community samples estimate a prevalence of failure to thrive syndromes in approximately 3 percent of infants, with approximately half of those infants exhibiting feeding disorders.

▲ 2.8 Trauma- and Stressor-Related Disorders in Children

This section includes disorders in which a traumatic or significantly stressful event is a necessary diagnostic criterion, according to the DSM-5. Included here are reactive attachment disorder, disinhibited social engagement disorder, and PTSD. ICD-10 also includes a category of disorders of social functioning with onset specific to childhood and adolescence. Although we cover PTSD in Chapter 10, it can present differently in children and has important implications for child development. Hence we discuss that in this chapter.

DSM-IV divided reactive attachment disorder into two subtypes: emotionally withdrawn/inhibited and indiscriminately social/disinhibited. In DSM-5, however, the preceding two subtypes have been defined as two distinct disorders, with the DSM-5 reactive attachment disorder equivalent to the previous emotionally withdrawn/inhibited subtype, and disinhibited social engagement disorder representing the previous social disinhibited subtype.

REACTIVE ATTACHMENT DISORDER AND DISINHIBITED SOCIAL ENGAGEMENT DISORDER

Reactive attachment disorder and disinhibited social engagement disorder are clinical disorders characterized by aberrant social behaviors in a young child that reflect grossly negligent parenting and maltreatment that disrupted the development of normal attachment behavior. A diagnosis of either reactive attachment disorder or disinhibited social engagement disorder rests on the presumption that the cause is caregiving deprivation. DSM-III was the first to define the disorder in 1980. It derives from attachment theory, which describes the quality of a child's affective relationship with primary caregivers, usually parents. This fundamental relationship is the product of a young child's need for protection, nurturance, and comfort, and the interaction of the parents and child in fulfilling these needs.

Based on observations of a young child and parents during a brief separation and reunion, designated the "strange situation procedure," pioneered by Mary Ainsworth and colleagues, researchers have designated a child's basic pattern of attachment to be characterized as secure, insecure, or disorganized. Children who exhibit secure attachment behavior experience their caregivers as emotionally available and appear to be more exploratory and well adjusted than children who exhibit insecure or disorganized attachment behavior. Insecure attachment results from a young child's perception that the caregiver is not consistently available. In contrast, disorganized attachment behavior in a child results from experiencing both the need for proximity to the caregiver and apprehension in approaching the caregiver. These early patterns of attachment influence a child's future capacities for affect regulation, self-soothing, and relationship building. According to the DSM-5, reactive attachment disorder is a consistent pattern of emotionally withdrawn responses toward adult caregivers, limited positive affect, sadness, and minimal social responsiveness to others, and concomitant neglect, deprivation, and lack of appropriate nurturance from caregivers. Reactive attachment disorder is, presumably, due to grossly pathologic caregiving received by the child. The pattern of care may exhibit a disregard for a child's emotional or physical needs or repeated changes of caregivers, as when a child is frequently relocated during foster care. The symptoms are not due to autism spectrum disorder, and the child must have a developmental age of at least 9 months.

Pathologic caretaking can result in two distinct disorders: reactive attachment disorder, in which the disturbance takes the form of the child's constantly failing to initiate and respond to most social interactions in a developmentally normal way; and disinhibited social engagement disorder, in which the disturbance takes the form of undifferentiated, unselective, and inappropriate social relatedness, with familiar and unfamiliar adults.

In disinhibited social engagement disorder, according to DSM-5, a child actively approaches and interacts with unfamiliar adults in an overly familiar way, either verbally or physically. They check for or seek out their caregiver less often and are willing to go with unfamiliar adults without hesitation. These behaviors in disinhibited social engagement disorder are not accounted for by impulsivity, although socially disinhibited behavior is predominant. These patterns of disinhibited, developmentally inappropriate behaviors are presumed to be caused by pathogenic caregiving. Thus, for both reactive attachment disorder and disinhibited social engagement disorder, aberrant caretaking is presumed to be the predominant cause of the child's inappropriate behaviors. However, there have been cases of less severe disturbances in parenting that may also be associated with young children who exhibit some characteristics of reactive attachment disorder or disinhibited social engagement disorder.

These disorders may also result in a picture of failure to thrive, in which an infant shows physical signs of malnourishment and does not exhibit the expected developmental motor and verbal milestones.

Diagnosis and Clinical Features

Children with reactive attachment disorder and disinhibited social engagement disorder may initially be identified by a preschool teacher or by a pediatrician based on direct observation of the child's inappropriate social responses. These diagnoses rely at least partially on documented evidence of pervasive disturbance of attachment leading to inappropriate social behaviors present before the age of 5 years. The clinical picture varies greatly, depending on a child's chronologic and mental ages, but expected social interaction and liveliness are not present. Often, the child is not progressing developmentally or is frankly malnourished. Perhaps the most common clinical picture of an infant with reactive attachment disorder is the nonorganic failure to thrive. Such infants usually exhibit hypokinesis, dullness, listlessness, and apathy, with poverty of spontaneous activity. Infants look sad, joyless, and miserable. Some infants also appear frightened and watchful, with a radar-like gaze.

Table 2-25 compares the diagnostic approaches to reactive attachment disorder, and Table 2-26 compares them for disinhibited social engagement disorder.

Infants may exhibit delayed responsiveness to a stimulus that would elicit fright or withdrawal from a healthy infant. Infants with failure to thrive and reactive attachment disorder appear significantly malnourished, and many have protruding abdomens. Occasionally, they have foul-smelling, celiac-like stools. In unusually severe cases, a clinical picture of marasmus appears.

The infant's weight is often below the third percentile and markedly below the appropriate weight for his or her height. If serial weights are available, the weight percentiles may have decreased progressively because of an actual weight loss or a failure to gain weight as height increases. Head circumference is usually average for the infant's age. Muscle tone may be weak. The skin may be colder and paler or more mottled than the skin of a healthy child. Laboratory findings may indicate coincident malnutrition, dehydration, or concurrent illness. Bone age is usually retarded. Growth hormone levels are usually normal or elevated, a finding suggesting that growth failure in these children is secondary to caloric deprivation and malnutrition. Cortisol secretion in children with reactive attachment disorder or disinhibited social engagement disorder is lower than in typically developing children. For children with failure to thrive, improvement physically and weight gain generally rapidly occurs after hospitalization.

Socially, the infants with reactive attachment disorder usually show little spontaneous activity and a marked diminution of both initiative toward others and reciprocity in response to the caregiving adult or examiner. Both mother and infant may be indifferent to

Table 2-25
Reactive Attachment Disorder

	DSM-5	ICD-10
Diagnostic name	Reactive Attachment Disorder	Reactive Attachment Disorder of Childhood
Duration	Begins < age 5	Begins < age 5
Symptoms	Emotional inhibition, rarely seeking or responding to comfort when distressed Social and emotional disturbance: • ↓ emotional/social responsiveness • ↓ affect • Fear, sadness or irritability in non-threatening interactions with adults History of insufficient care: • Neglect • Deprivation • Repeated changes in caregivers • Institutional care Child has developmental age of ≥9 mo	Abnormal social relationships Emotional disturbances that are reactive to environmental change *May be present:* Fear Aggression Hypervigilance Failure to thrive History of neglect or abuse
Required number of symptoms	Symptoms in each category ≥2 of the social/emotional disturbance symptoms	
Exclusions (not result of):	Autism spectrum disorder	Asperger syndrome Disinhibited attachment disorder of childhood
Course specifiers	**Persistent:** >12 mo	
Severity specifiers	**Severe:** all symptoms, high severity	

Table 2-26
Disinhibited Social Engagement Disorder

	DSM-5	ICD-10
Diagnostic name	Disinhibited Social Engagement Disorder	Disinhibited Attachment Disorder of Childhood
Duration		Begins during the first 5 yr of age
Symptoms	Disinhibited social behavior: • ↓ hesitation around adult strangers • ↑ familiarity with adult strangers • ↓ checking back with caregivers in unfamiliar situations • Willing/less hesitant to go off with an adult stranger History of insufficient care: • Neglect • Deprivation • Repeated changes in caregivers • Institutional care	Abnormal pattern of social functioning • Nonselective attachment behavior • Attention seeking • Overly friendly behaviors
Required number of symptoms	Each category ≥2 symptoms of disinhibited social behavior All of the above, with child having developmental age of ≥9 mo	
Exclusions (not result of):	ADHD	Asperger syndrome Hyperkinetic disorder Reactive attachment disorder of childhood
Course specifiers	***Persistent:*** >12 mo	
Severity specifiers	***Severe:*** if all symptom criteria met at relatively high level	

separation on hospitalization or to termination of subsequent hospital visits. The infants frequently show none of the normal upset, fretting, or protest about hospitalization. Older infants usually show little interest in their environment. They may not play with toys, even if encouraged; however, they rapidly or gradually take an interest in and relate to their caregivers in the hospital.

Children with disinhibited social engagement disorder appear to be overly friendly and familiar with little fear.

His adoptive parents brought a 7-year-old boy for evaluation because of hyperactivity and inappropriate social behavior at school. They adopted him at 4 years of age, after living most of his life in a Chinese orphanage in which he received care from a rotating shift of caregivers. Although he had been below the 5th percentile for height and weight on arrival, he quickly approached the 15th percentile in his new home. However, his adoptive parents were frustrated by his inability to bond with them. They had initially worried about an intellectual problem, although testing and his capacity to engage almost any adult and many children verbally suggested otherwise. He appeared to be too friendly, talking to anyone and often following strangers willingly. He showed little empathy when others were hurt, and yet he would sit on the laps of teachers and students without asking. He was frequently injured because of seemingly reckless behavior, although he had an extremely high pain tolerance. His parents focused on problem behaviors at home to decrease his impulsive behavior, which improved with much prompting; however, he remained oddly overfriendly at home and in school. The psychiatrist diagnosed the child with disinhibited social engagement disorder. (Adapted from Neil W. Boris, M.D. and Charles H. Zeanah, Jr., M.D.)

Pathology and Laboratory Examination. Although no single specific laboratory test can make a diagnosis, many

children with reactive attachment disorder have disturbances of growth and development. Thus, establishing a growth curve and examining the progression of developmental milestones may help determine whether associated phenomena, such as failure to thrive, are present.

Differential Diagnosis

The differential diagnosis of reactive attachment disorder and disinhibited social engagement disorder must take into account that many other psychiatric disorders may arise in conjunction with maltreatment, including depressive disorders, anxiety disorders, and PTSD. Psychiatric disorders to consider in the differential diagnosis include language disorders, autism spectrum disorder, intellectual disability, and metabolic syndromes. Children with autism spectrum disorder are typically well nourished and of age-appropriate size and weight, and are generally alert and active, despite their impairments in reciprocal social interactions. Significant intellectual disability is often present in children with an autism spectrum disorder, whereas when intellectual disability occurs with reactive attachment disorder or disinhibited social engagement disorder, it is generally relatively mild. Children with disinhibited social engagement disorder often show comorbid ADHD, PTSD, and language disorder or delay. Furthermore, children with disinhibited social engagement disorder symptoms may have complex neuropsychiatric problems.

Course and Prognosis

Most of the data available on the natural course of children with reactive attachment disorder and disinhibited social engagement disorder come from follow-up studies of children in residential facilities with histories of severe neglect. Findings from these studies suggest that children with reactive attachment disorder, who are later adopted into caring environments, improve in their attachment behaviors and may normalize over time. Children with disinhibited social engagement disorder, however, appear to have more difficulty developing attachments to new caregivers. Children with disinhibited social engagement disorder who exhibit indiscriminate social behavior also tend to have poor peer relationships. The duration and severity of the neglect influence the prognosis for both disorders. The degree of resulting impairment does as well. Constitutional and nutritional factors interact in children, who may either respond resiliently to treatment or continue to fail to thrive. The amount of treatment and rehabilitation that the family receives affects the child. Children who have multiple problems stemming from pathogenic caregiving may recover physically faster and more completely than they do emotionally.

Treatment

The first consideration in treating reactive attachment disorder or disinhibited social engagement disorder is a child's safety. Thus, the management of these disorders must begin with a comprehensive assessment of the current level of safety and adequate caregiving. When there is suspicion of maltreatment persisting in the home, usually, the first decision is whether to hospitalize the child or to attempt treatment while the child remains in the home. If we suspect neglect or emotional, physical, or sexual abuse, we must report it to the appropriate law enforcement and child protective services in the area. The therapeutic strategy depends on the child's physical and emotional state and the level of pathologic caregiving. We should determine the nutritional status of the child and the presence of ongoing physical abuse or threat. Hospitalization is necessary for children with malnourishment.

Along with an assessment of the child's physical well-being, an evaluation of the child's emotional condition is essential. Immediate intervention must address the parents' awareness and capacity to participate in altering the injurious patterns that have heretofore ensued. The treatment team must begin to improve the unsatisfactory relationship between caregiver and child. This intervention usually requires extensive and intensive therapy and education with the mother or with both parents when possible.

In one study, parents of 120 children between 11.7 and 31.9 months, identified as being at risk for neglect, were randomly assigned to an intervention for at-risk parents called Attachment and Biobehavioral Catch-up (ABC) or to a control intervention. The purpose of the ABC intervention was to decrease frightening behavior toward the infant by parents and to increase sensitive and nurturing interactions between parents and infants. The investigators manualized the intervention to guide the parents in how to provide those interactions with their infants. They evaluated the children after 10 sessions, and the 60 children who received the ABC intervention showed significantly lower rates of disorganized attachment (32 percent), and higher rates of secure attachment (52 percent) compared to those who received the control intervention (disorganized attachment 57 percent; secure attachment 33 percent). The authors concluded that we could enhance parental nurturance and sensitivity through a comprehensive and explicit intervention such as the ABC intervention, and can measure significant improvements in attachment behaviors in young children after 10 sessions.

The caregiver–child relationship is the basis of the assessment of reactive attachment disorder and disinhibited social engagement

disorder symptoms and the substrate from which to modify attachment behaviors. Structured observations allow a clinician to determine the range of attachment behaviors established with various family members. We may work closely with the caregiver and the child to facilitate higher sensitivity in their interactions. Three primary psychotherapeutic modalities help promote bonds between children and caregivers. First, a clinician can target the caregiver to promote positive interaction with a child who does not yet have the repertoire to respond positively. Second, a clinician can work with the child and the caregiver together as a dyad to advocate for practicing appropriate positive reinforcement for each other. Through the use of videotapes, therapists can view parent–child interactions and suggest modifications to increase positive engagement. The third modality for clinical intervention is through individual work with the child. Working with the child and caregiver together is often more effective in producing more emotionally meaningful exchanges than working with the parent or child individually.

Psychosocial interventions for families in which a child has reactive attachment disorder or disinhibited social engagement disorder include (1) psychosocial support services, including hiring a homemaker, improving the physical condition of the apartment, or obtaining adequate housing, improving the family's financial status, and decreasing the family's isolation; (2) psychotherapeutic interventions, including individual psychotherapy, psychotropic medications, and family or marital therapy; (3) educational counseling services, including mother–infant or mother–toddler groups, and counseling to increase awareness and understanding of the child's needs and to develop parenting skills; and (4) provisions for close monitoring of the progression of the patient's emotional and physical well-being. Sometimes, separating a child from the stressful home environment temporarily, as in hospitalization, allows the child to break out of the accustomed pattern. A neutral setting, such as the hospital, is the best place to start with families who are genuinely available emotionally and physically for intervention. If interventions are not feasible or inadequate or if they fail, we must consider placing the child with relatives or in foster care, adoption, or in a group home or residential treatment facility.

Epidemiology

Few data exist on the prevalence, sex ratio, or familial pattern of reactive attachment disorder and disinhibited social engagement disorder. Both disorders probably occur in less than 1 percent of the population. A study of 1,646 children aged 6 to 8 years old, living in a deprived sector of urban United Kingdom, found that the prevalence of reactive attachment disorder in this population was 1.4 percent. However, other studies of selected high-risk populations have estimated that about 10 percent of young children with documented neglectful and grossly pathologic caregiving exhibit reactive attachment disorder, and up to 20 percent of children in this situation exhibit disinhibited social engagement disorder. In a retrospective report of children in one county of the United States who were removed from their homes because of neglect or abuse before the age of 4 years, 38 percent exhibited signs of either reactive attachment disorder or disinhibited social engagement disorder. Another study established the reliability of the diagnosis by reviewing videotaped assessments of at-risk children interacting with caregivers, along with a structured interview with the caregivers. Given that pathogenic care, including maltreatment, occurs more frequently in the presence of general psychosocial risk factors, such as poverty, disrupted families, and mental illness among caregivers, these circumstances are likely to increase the risk of reactive attachment disorder and disinhibited social engagement disorder.

Etiology

The core features of reactive attachment disorder and disinhibited social engagement disorder are disturbances of normal attachment behaviors. The inability of a young child to develop normative social interactions that culminate in aberrant attachment behaviors in reactive attachment disorder is inherent in the disorder's definition. Reactive attachment disorder and disinhibited social engagement disorder are presumably due to maltreatment of the child, including emotional neglect, physical abuse, or both. Grossly pathogenic care of an infant or young child by the caregiver presumably causes the markedly disturbed social relatedness that is evident. The emphasis is on the unidirectional cause; that is, the caregiver does something inimical or neglects to do something essential for the infant or child. In evaluating a patient for whom such a diagnosis is appropriate, however, clinicians should consider the contributions of each member of the caregiver–child dyad and their interactions. Clinicians should weigh such things as infant or child temperament, deficient or defective bonding, a developmentally disabled child, and a particular caregiver–child mismatch. The likelihood of neglect increases with a parental psychiatric disorder, substance abuse, intellectual disability, the parent's harsh upbringing, social isolation, deprivation, and premature parenthood (i.e., adolescent). These factors compromise parental ability to attend to the needs of the child, as the parents focus primarily on their existence. Frequent changes of the primary caregivers, for example, from multiple foster care placements or repeated lengthy hospitalizations, may also lead to impaired attachment. In the general population, a study of 1,600 children found that those children with reactive attachment disorder/disinhibited social engagement disorder showed a constellation of symptoms characterized by early symptomatic syndromes eliciting neurodevelopmental clinical examinations (ESSENCE). Some of the associated symptoms in children with reactive attachment disorder/disinhibited social engagement disorder include a higher risk of failure to gain weight as neonates, feeding difficulty, and poor impulse control. These traits are likely to emerge because of both genetic and environmental factors. The authors found that children with reactive attachment disorder/disinhibited social engagement disorder were more likely to have multiple psychiatric comorbidities, lower IQs compared to the general population, and more behavioral problems. Thus, a broad assessment may be necessary to identify symptoms and disorders associated with reactive attachment disorder/disinhibited social engagement disorder.

POSTTRAUMATIC STRESS DISORDER OF INFANCY, CHILDHOOD, AND ADOLESCENCE

Posttraumatic stress disorder (PTSD), formerly grouped with anxiety disorders, now has its own chapter in DSM-5 along with other disorders caused by trauma or stress. Chapter 10 describes this disorder in detail. The purpose here is to focus on how the disorder presents in children.

In the United States, the rates of children and adolescents exposed to violence and traumatic events are incredibly high. In a nationally representative sample of children and adolescents, exposure to a traumatic event was 60 percent, with a lifetime rate ranging from 80 to 90 percent. Traumatic events can include physical or sexual abuse, domestic violence, motor vehicle accidents, severe medical illnesses, or natural or human-created disasters. A significant number of children and adolescents who experience traumatic events will develop PTSD. In children younger than the age of 6 years, spontaneous and intrusive memories may be expressed in their play, or occur in frightening dreams; it may be challenging to connect these intrusive thoughts to a traumatic event. The child may also display inexplicable agitation, fear, or disorganization.

Diagnosis and Clinical Features

For PTSD to ensue, exposure to a traumatic event consisting of either direct personal experience or witnessing an event involving the threat of death, serious injury, or severe harm must occur. The most common traumatic exposures for children and adolescents include physical or sexual abuse; domestic, school, or community violence; being kidnapped; terrorist attacks; motor vehicle or household accidents; or disasters, such as floods, hurricanes, tornadoes, fires, explosions, or airline crashes. A child with PTSD experiences either intrusive memories of the event, recurrent frightening dreams, dissociative reactions including flashbacks in which the child feels as if the traumatic event is recurring, or intense psychological distress when exposed to reminders of the trauma.

Symptoms of PTSD include *reexperiencing* the traumatic event in at least one of the following ways. Children may have intrusive thoughts, memories, or images that spontaneously recur, or body sensations that remind them of the event. In very young children, it is common to observe play that includes elements of the traumatic event, or behaviors, such as inappropriate sexual behaviors. Children may experience periods during which they either act or feel as though the event is taking place presently; this is a dissociative event usually described by adults as "flashbacks."

Another critical symptom cluster of PTSD is *avoidance,* in which children may make active physical efforts to avoid the places, people, or situations that would present traumatic reminders of the event. The third cluster of diagnostic criteria for PTSD is negative alterations in cognition and mood following the trauma. In children 6 years or younger, according to DSM-5, negative alterations in cognition may take the form of socially withdrawn behavior, reduction of expressing positive emotions, diminished interest in play, and feelings of shame, fear, and confusion. In children older than 6 years of age, these may take the form of an inability to remember parts of a traumatic event, that is, *psychological amnesia* or persistent negative feelings about oneself, including horror, anger, guilt, or shame. After a traumatic event, children may experience a sense of detachment from their usual play activities ("psychological numbing") or a diminished capacity to feel emotions. Older adolescents may express a fear that they expect to die young (sense of foreshortened future).

Other typical responses to traumatic events include symptoms of hyperarousal that were not present before the traumatic exposure, such as difficulty falling asleep or staying asleep, hypervigilance regarding safety, and increased checking that doors are locked or exaggerated startle reaction. In some children, hyperarousal can present as a generalized inability to relax with increased irritability, outbursts, and impaired ability to concentrate.

To meet the diagnostic criteria for PTSD, according to the DSM-5, the symptoms must be present for at least 1 month and cause distress and impairment in critical functional areas of life. When all of the diagnostic symptoms of PTSD are met following the traumatic event, persist for at least 3 days, but resolve within 1 month, we diagnose it as acute stress disorder. When the full syndrome of PTSD persists beyond 3 months, it is chronic PTSD. In some cases, the PTSD symptoms increase over time, and it is not until more than 6 months have elapsed after the exposure to the trauma that the whole syndrome emerges; in that case, the diagnosis is PTSD, delayed onset.

It is not uncommon for children and adolescents with PTSD to experience feelings of guilt, mainly if they have survived the trauma and others in the situation did not. They may blame themselves for the demise of the others and may go on to develop a comorbid depressive episode. Childhood PTSD is also associated with increased rates of other anxiety disorders, depressive episodes, substance use disorders, and attentional difficulties. DSM-5 includes a specifier *With dissociative symptoms,* which can present as either *Depersonalization,* in which there are recurrent experiences of feeling detached, as if outside of one's own body, or *Derealization,* in which the world feels unreal, dreamlike, and distant. A final specifier, *With delayed expression,* indicates that the full diagnostic criteria were not met until 6 months after the traumatic event, although some symptoms may present earlier.

Pathology and Laboratory Examination.   Although reports indicate some alterations in both neurophysiologic and neuroimaging studies of children and adolescents with PTSD, no current laboratory tests can help in making this diagnosis.

Differential Diagnosis

Several overlapping symptoms exist between childhood PTSD and presentations of childhood anxiety disorders, such as separation anxiety disorder, OCD, or social anxiety disorder, in which recurrent intrusive thoughts or avoidant behaviors occur. Children with depressive disorders often exhibit withdrawal and a sense of isolation from peers as well as guilt about life events over which they have no control. Irritability, poor concentration, sleep disturbance, and decreased interest in usual activities occur in both PTSD and major depressive disorder.

Children who have lost a loved one in a traumatic event may go on to experience both PTSD and a major depressive disorder when bereavement persists beyond its expected course. Children with PTSD may also be confused with children who have disruptive behavior disorders because they often show poor concentration, inattention, and irritability. It is critical to elicit a history of traumatic exposure and evaluate the chronology of the trauma and the onset of the symptoms to make an accurate diagnosis of PTSD.

Course and Prognosis

For some children and adolescents with milder forms of PTSD, symptoms may persist for 1 to 2 years, after which they diminish and attenuate. In more severe circumstances, however, PTSD syndromes persist for many years or decades in children and adolescents, with spontaneous remission in only a portion of them.

The prognosis of untreated PTSD has become an issue of growing concern for researchers and clinicians who have documented a variety of severe comorbidities and psychobiological abnormalities associated with PTSD. In one study, children and adolescents with severe PTSD were at risk for decreased intracranial volume, diminished corpus callosum area, and lower IQs compared to children without PTSD. Children and adolescents with histories of physical and sexual abuse have higher rates of depression and suicidality themselves and in their offspring as well. This risk highlights the importance of early recognition and treatment

of PTSD that may significantly improve the long-term outcome among youth.

Treatment

Trauma-Focused Cognitive-Behavioral Therapy.   Randomized clinical trials have provided evidence for the efficacy of trauma-focused CBT in the treatment of PTSD in children and adolescents. We would administer this treatment over 10 to 16 treatment sessions. The treatment includes nine components itemized in the acronym PRACTICE. Trauma-focused CBT entails the inclusion of gradual exposure to feared stimuli as a critical element. Such stimuli encompass places, people, sounds, and situations. The first component of trauma-focused CBT is *Psychoeducation* regarding the nature of typical emotional and physiologic reactions to traumatic events and PTSD. Next, *Parenting Skills* involve sessions focused on guiding parents on providing praise, administering a time out, contingency reinforcement programs, and troubleshooting for specific symptoms in a given child. Component 3 is *Relaxation,* in which children learn to utilize muscle relaxation, focused breathing, affective modulation, thought-stopping, and other cognitive techniques to diminish feelings of helplessness and distress. Component 4 is *Affective Expression and Modulation,* geared to help children and their parents to identify their feelings, interrupt disturbing thoughts with positive imagery, and teach positive self-talk and social skills building. Component 5 is *Cognitive coping and processing,* which deals specifically with reviewing the Cognitive Triangle, in which the therapist and child explore the relationship between thoughts, feelings, and behaviors. The child would learn to challenge unhelpful thoughts with practice. In Component 6, *Trauma narrative,* the story of the traumatic event and its sequelae are developed over time by the child, with the therapist's support, using a depiction of words, art, or another creative form. Eventually, they share this with the parent. Component 7, *In Vivo Exposure and Mastery of Trauma Reminders,* is a session that reviews with the child how to deal with situations that are a reminder of the trauma and how to maintain control over distressing feelings associated with it. Component 8 is *Conjoint Child-Parent Sessions*; this component may involve several sessions in which the child and parent share their understanding of the process of the therapy and the gains that they have made. Finally, Component 10, *Enhancing future safety,* involves sessions that focus on the changes made in the family to ensure the safety of the child. These final sessions also promote healthy communication between the child and the parents.

A variant of trauma-focused CBT for PTSD is called *eye movement desensitization and reprocessing* (EMDR), in which the therapist combines exposure and cognitive reprocessing interventions with directed eye movements. This technique is not as well accepted as the more extensive trauma-focused CBT detailed above.

Cognitive-Behavioral Intervention for Trauma in Schools (CBITS).   CBITS is an intervention that administers treatment in the school setting for children who screen positive for PTSD and whose parents agree to treatment in school. It consists of ten weekly group sessions, one to three individual imaginal exposure sessions, two to four optional sessions with parents, and one parent education session. Similar to trauma-focused CBT (TF-CBT), CBITS incorporates psychoeducation, relaxation training, cognitive coping skills, gradual exposure to traumatic memories through a narrative, in vivo exposure, and affect modulation, cognitive restructuring, and social problem-solving. In one RCT, 86 percent of students in the CBITS group reported significantly decreased PTSD symptoms compared to the waitlist controls. Students who received CBITS also reported lower depression scores. Among parents whose children received CBITS treatment, 78 percent reported decreased psychosocial problems in their children. After CBITS treatment, the children sustained improvements in both the PTSD and depression symptoms at 6 months.

Structured Psychotherapy for Adolescents Responding to Chronic Stress (SPARCS).

SPARCS consists of a group intervention, generally administered in 16 sessions, with a focus on the needs of adolescents between the ages of 12 and 19 years who have lived with chronic trauma and may also carry a diagnosis of PTSD. Investigators have tested SPARCS in a trial of multicultural teens and young adults with moderate or severe trauma exposure. Most of the participants were female and comprised multiple ethnic groups: 67 percent African American; 12 percent Latino; 21 percent Caucasian. SPARCS demonstrated efficacy in reducing traumatic stress symptoms, mainly in the largest group, the African American group. SPARCS utilizes cognitive-behavioral techniques and also incorporates many of the components of TF-CBT. Also, SPARCS includes mindfulness techniques and relaxation.

Trauma Affect Regulation: Guide for Education and Therapy (TARGET).

TARGET, an affect regulation therapy, combines CBT components, such as cognitive processing, with affect modulation. We would usually consider this for adolescents between the ages of 13 and 19 who experience maltreatment or chronic traumatic exposure to such things as community violence or domestic violence. It usually requires 12 sessions, which focus on past or current situations. As with SPARCS treatment, gradual exposure may occur in the context of recounting past trauma but is not a core component of the treatment. A randomized trial with 59 delinquent girls aged 13 to 17 years who met full or partial criteria for PTSD found that TARGET reduced anxiety, anger, depression, and PTSD cognitions. TARGET is a promising treatment for girls with histories of delinquency, especially to reduce anger and to enhance optimism and self-efficacy.

Psychopharmacological Treatment.

Clinicians have used several pharmacologic agents to treat children and adolescents with PTSD, often focused on diminishing intrusive thoughts, hyperarousal, and avoidance, with some success and mixed results. Given the frequent comorbidity of depressive disorder, anxiety disorders, and behavioral problems associated with PTSD, we might use a multitude of psychopharmacological agents.

Psychiatrists often use antidepressant agents as adjuncts to psychosocial treatments in youth with PTSD. Although sertraline and paroxetine are approved by the FDA in the treatment of PTSD in adults, there is scant evidence to support their use for the core symptoms of PTSD in youth. An RCT of TF-CBT plus sertraline compared to TF-CBT plus placebo in 24 children with PTSD found that both groups had a significant reduction in PTSD symptoms, with no significant difference between the groups. One multicenter placebo-controlled study of 131 children aged 6 to 17 years with PTSD tested sertraline over 10 weeks. Results showed sertraline to be a safe treatment; however, it was not effective when compared to placebo. An RCT using citalopram did not show the superiority of citalopram over placebo in the treatment of core PTSD symptoms. There is, however, evidence suggesting that the use of SSRIs in traumatized children with burns may be preventive regarding the

development of PTSD. Published literature demonstrates that up to 50 percent of children with moderate to severe burns develop PTSD. Thus preventive strategies are essential. A randomized controlled study of sertraline to prevent PTSD found that children who received sertraline, flexibly dosed between 25 and 150 mg/day, had a decrease in parent-reported symptoms of PTSD over 8 weeks compared to a placebo group. Among the child-reported symptoms, however, there was no significant difference between the two groups.

Psychiatrists sometimes use antiadrenergic agents to treat dysregulation of the noradrenergic system in adults and youth with PTSD. α_2-Agonists such as clonidine and guanfacine, for example, have been used to decrease norepinephrine release, whereas centrally acting β-antagonists such as propranolol, and α_1-antagonists such as prazosin, are hypothesized to improve hyperarousal and intrusive thoughts through attenuation of norepinephrine postsynaptically. Although there are some data in adults with PTSD to support the use of these agents, there are mainly case reports for youths. There is a suggestion that guanfacine may reduce nightmares in children with PTSD and that clonidine may diminish symptoms of reenactment of traumatic events in children. One report of propranolol treatment in 11 pediatric patients with PTSD from sexual or physical abuse with a mean age of 8.5 years, who exhibited agitation and hyperarousal, indicated some decrease in symptoms in 8 of the 11 children studied. Another open study of transdermal clonidine treatment of preschoolers with PTSD suggests that clonidine may be efficacious in this population in decreasing activation and hyperarousal. An additional open trial of oral clonidine with dosage ranges of 0.05 to 0.1 mg twice daily similarly suggests that this medication may provide some relief for the symptoms of hyperarousal, impulsivity, and agitation in young children with PTSD.

Second-generation antipsychotics such as risperidone, olanzapine, quetiapine, ziprasidone, and aripiprazole have been studied in adults with PTSD with mixed results. Risperidone and aripiprazole both have FDA approval for use in children and adolescents with aggression, severe behavioral dyscontrol, and severe psychiatric disorders; however, there are no controlled trials with children with PTSD. For example, there is one case series of three preschool-age children who exhibited symptoms of acute stress disorder and who had severe thermal burns improved after being treated with risperidone.

In children and adolescents with PTSD, there is one open-label trial of carbamazepine and one trial of sodium valproate. In the carbamazepine trial, all 28 improved at blood levels of 10 to 11.5 micrograms/mL. In the sodium valproate trial, there was some improvement at higher doses of the drug.

Clinicians also use benzodiazepines to treat anxiety symptoms in patients with PTSD, although there are no controlled trials to support their use in youth with PTSD.

Given that many children and adolescents with PTSD have comorbid depressive and anxiety disorders, we would recommend SSRIs as a first-line pharmacologic option.

Epidemiology

Epidemiologic studies of children 9 to 17 years of age have found 3-month prevalence rates of PTSD ranging from 0.5 to 4 percent. An epidemiologic survey of preschoolers aged 4 to 5 years found a rate of 1.3 percent of PTSD.

Children exposed chronically to trauma, such as child abuse, or traumas resulting in a broader disruption of entire communities, such as war, have the highest risk of developing PTSD. In addition to the staggering rate of the full-blown disorder of PTSD among youth, several studies indicate that most children exposed to severe or chronic trauma develop PTSD symptoms sufficiently severe to disrupt functioning, even in the absence of the full diagnosis.

Etiology

Biologic Factors. Risk factors in children for developing PTSD include preexisting anxiety disorders and depressive disorders. A prospective study found that among children exposed to traumatic events, those with anxiety disorders and teacher ratings of externalizing behavior problems by the age of 6 years were at increased risk for PTSD. Furthermore, children with an IQ higher than 115 at age 6 years were at lower risk for developing PTSD. Also, among children exposed to trauma, those who developed PTSD were at higher risk of developing comorbid disorders such as depression. This comorbidity suggests that a genetic predisposition for anxiety disorders, as well as a family history indicating an increased risk of depressive disorders, may predispose a trauma-exposed child to develop PTSD. Children with PTSD exhibit increased excretion of adrenergic and dopaminergic metabolites, smaller intracranial volume and corpus callosum, memory deficits, and lower IQs compared with age-matched controls. Adults with PTSD have been found to have an overactive amygdala and decreased hippocampal volume. Whether the above findings are sequelae of PTSD or markers of vulnerability to the disorder remains a focus of investigation.

Psychological Factors.   Although the exposure to trauma is the initial etiologic factor in the development of PTSD, the enduring symptoms typical of PTSD, such as avoidance of the place where the trauma occurred, can be conceptualized, in part, as the result of both classical and operant conditioning. Extreme physiologic responses may accompany the fear of a given traumatic event, such as an adolescent who was terrorized by an attack by a group of students near a school, who then develops an extreme adverse physiologic reaction each time he or she is near the school. This reaction is an example of classical conditioning in that a neutral cue (the school) has become paired with an intensely fearful past event. Operant conditioning occurs when a child learns to avoid traumatic reminders to prevent distressing feelings from arising. For example, if a child was in a motor vehicle accident, the child may then refuse to ride in cars altogether to prevent adverse physiologic reactions and fear from occurring.

Another mechanism in developing and maintaining symptoms of PTSD is through modeling, which is a form of learning. For example, when parents and children experience traumatic events, such as natural disasters, children may emulate parental responses, such as avoidance, withdrawal, or extreme expressions of fear, and "learn" to respond to their memories of the traumatic event in the same manner.

Social Factors. Family support and reactions to traumatic events in children may play a significant role in the development of PTSD in that adverse parental emotional reactions to a child's abuse may increase that child's risk of developing PTSD. Lack of parental support and psychopathology among parents—especially maternal depression—have been identified as risk factors in the development of PTSD after a child experiences a traumatic event.

▲ 2.9 Depressive Disorders and Suicide in Children and Adolescents

Chapter 7 discusses depressive disorders in detail. This section focuses on the presentation of this disorder in youths.

Depressive disorders in youth represent a significant public health concern, in that they are prevalent and result in long-term adverse effects on the individual's cognitive, social, and psychological development. These disorders affect approximately 2 to 3 percent of children and up to 8 percent of adolescents, so the need for early identification and access to evidence-based interventions such as CBTs and antidepressant agents, is essential. Although significant depression runs in families, with the highest risk in children whose parents experienced early-onset depression, twin studies have demonstrated that major depression is only moderately heritable, approximately 40 to 50 percent, highlighting environmental stressors and adverse events as significant contributors to major depressive disorder in youth. The core features of major depression in children, adolescents, and adults bear a striking resemblance; however, the developmental level of the child or adolescent influences the clinical presentation. The DSM-5 uses the same criteria for major depressive disorder in youth as in adults, except that for children and adolescents, *irritable mood* may replace a *depressed mood* in the diagnostic criteria.

Most children and adolescents with depressive disorders neither attempt nor complete suicide; however, severely depressed youth often have suicidal ideation, and suicide remains the most severe risk of major depression. Nevertheless, many depressed youths do not ever have suicidal ideation, and many children and adolescents who engage in suicidal behavior do not have a depressive disorder. There is epidemiologic evidence to suggest that depressed youth with recurrent active suicidal ideation, including a plan, and who have made prior attempts, are at higher risk to complete suicide, compared to youth who express only passive suicidal ideation.

Mood disorders in children and adolescents have been studied increasingly over the last two decades, culminating in large sample multisite RCTs such as the Treatment of Adolescent Depression Study (TADS), which provides evidence of the efficacy of both CBT as well as SSRIs. Furthermore, when the preceding modalities are combined, the highest efficacy is achieved. Increased recognition of depressive disorders in preschool populations has sparked clinicians and researchers to develop psychosocial interventions such as the Parent–Child Interaction Therapy Emotion Development (PCIT-ED), which target treatment specifically for this age group. The expression of disturbed and depressed mood appears to vary with the developmental stage. Very young children with major depression are sad, listless, or apathetic, even though they may not articulate these feelings verbally. Perhaps surprisingly, mood-congruent auditory hallucinations occur in young children with major depression. Somatic complaints such as headaches and stomachaches, withdrawn and sad appearance, and poor self-esteem are more universal symptoms. Patients in late adolescence with more severe forms of depression often display pervasive anhedonia, severe psychomotor retardation, delusions, and a sense of hopelessness. Symptoms that appear with the same frequency, regardless of age and developmental status, include suicidal ideation, depressed or irritable mood, insomnia, and diminished ability to concentrate.

Developmental issues, however, influence the expression of depressive symptoms. For example, unhappy young children who exhibit recurrent suicidal ideation are rarely able to propose a realistic suicide plan or to carry out such a plan. Children's moods are especially vulnerable to the influences of severe social stressors, such as chronic family discord, abuse and neglect, and academic failure. Many young children with major depressive disorder have histories of abuse, neglect, and families with significant psychosocial burdens such as parental mental illness, substance abuse, or poverty. Children who develop depressive disorders amid acute toxic family stressors may have remission of depressive symptoms when the stressors diminish or when in a more nurturing family environment. Depressive disorders are generally episodic, albeit typically lasting close to a year; however, their onset may be insidious and remain unidentified until significant impairment in peer relationships, deterioration in academic function, or withdrawal from activities emerges. ADHD, oppositional defiant disorder, and conduct disorder are not infrequently comorbid with a major depressive episode. In some cases, conduct disturbances or disorders occur in the context of a major depressive episode and resolve with the resolution of the depressive episode. Clinicians must clarify the chronology of the symptoms to determine whether a given behavior (e.g., poor concentration, defiance, or temper tantrums) was present before the depressive episode and is unrelated to it or whether the behavior is occurring for the first time and is related to the depressive episode.

DIAGNOSIS AND CLINICAL FEATURES

Major Depressive Disorder

It is easiest to diagnose major depressive disorder in children when the disorder is acute and occurs in a child without previous psychiatric symptoms. Often, however, the onset is insidious, and the disorder occurs in a child who has had several years of difficulties with hyperactivity, separation anxiety disorder, or intermittent depressive symptoms.

A major depressive episode in a prepubertal child is likely to be manifest by somatic complaints, psychomotor agitation, and mood-congruent hallucinations. Anhedonia is also frequent, but anhedonia, as well as hopelessness, psychomotor retardation, and delusions, are more common in adolescent and adult major depressive episodes than in those of young children. Adults have more problems than depressed children and adolescents with sleep and appetite. In adolescence, negativistic or frankly antisocial behavior and the use of alcohol or illicit substances can occur and may justify the additional diagnoses of oppositional defiant disorder, conduct disorder, and substance use disorder. Feelings of restlessness, irritability, aggression, reluctance to cooperate in family ventures, withdrawal from social activities, and isolation from peers often occur in adolescents. School difficulties are likely. Depressed adolescents may become less attentive to personal appearance and show increased sensitivity to rejection by peers and in romantic relationships.

Children can be reliable reporters about their emotions, relationships, and difficulties in psychosocial functions. They may, however, refer to depressive feelings in terms of anger, or feeling "mad" rather than sad. Clinicians should assess the duration and periodicity of the depressive mood to differentiate relatively universal, short-lived, and sometimes frequent periods of sadness, usually after a frustrating event, from a valid, persistent depressive mood. The younger the child, the more imprecise his or her time estimates are likely to be.

Mood disorders tend to be chronic if they begin early. Childhood-onset may be the most severe form of mood disorder and tends to

appear in families with a high incidence of mood disorders and alcohol use disorder. The children are likely to have such secondary complications as conduct disorder, alcohol and other substance use disorders, and antisocial behavior. Functional impairment associated with a depressive disorder in childhood extends to practically all areas of a child's psychosocial world; school performance and behavior, peer relationships, and family relationships all suffer. Only highly intelligent and academically oriented children with no more than a moderate depression can compensate for their difficulties in learning by substantially increasing their time and effort. Otherwise, school performance is invariably affected by a combination of difficulty concentrating, slowed thinking, lack of interest and motivation, fatigue, sleepiness, depressive ruminations, and preoccupations. Sometimes a clinician may misdiagnose a learning disorder as major depression. Learning problems secondary to depression, even when longstanding, are corrected rapidly after a child's recovery from the depressive episode.

Children and adolescents with severe forms of major depressive disorder may have hallucinations or delusions. Usually, these psychotic symptoms are thematically consistent with the depressed mood, occur with the depressive episode (usually at its worst), and do not include certain types of hallucinations (such as conversing voices and a commenting voice, which are specific to schizophrenia). Depressive hallucinations usually consist of a single voice speaking to the person from outside his or her head, with derogatory or suicidal content. Depressive delusions center on themes of guilt, physical disease, death, nihilism, deserved punishment, personal inadequacy, and (sometimes) persecution. These delusions are rare in prepuberty, probably because of cognitive immaturity, but are present in about half of psychotically depressed adolescents.

Alcohol or drug use can complicate adolescent depression. One study found that up to 17 percent of adolescents with depressive disorder received an initial evaluation due to substance abuse.

Persistent Depressive Disorder (Dysthymia)

In children and adolescents, persistent depressive disorder consists of a depressed or irritable mood for most of the day, for more days than not, for at least 1 year. DSM-5 notes that in children and adolescents, irritable mood can replace the depressed mood criterion for adults and that the duration criterion is not 2 years but 1 year for children and adolescents. According to the DSM-5 diagnostic criteria, two or more of the following symptoms must accompany the depressed or irritable mood: low self-esteem, hopelessness, poor appetite or overeating, insomnia or hypersomnia, low energy or fatigue, or poor concentration or difficulty making decisions. During the year of the disturbance, these symptoms do not resolve for more than 2 months at a time. Also, the diagnostic criteria for dysthymic disorder specify that during the first year, no major depressive episode emerges. To meet the DSM-5 diagnostic criteria for persistent depressive disorder, a child must not have a history of a manic or hypomanic episode. Persistent depressive disorder is also not diagnosed if the symptoms occur exclusively during a chronic psychotic disorder or if they are the direct effects of a substance or a general medical condition. DSM-5 provides specifiers for early-onset (before 21 years of age) or late-onset (after 21 years of age).

A child or adolescent with persistent depressive disorder may have had a major depressive episode before developing persistent depressive disorder; however, it is much more common for a child with persistent depressive disorder for more than 1 year to develop a concurrent episode of major depressive disorder. In this case, both depressive diagnoses apply (double depression). Persistent depressive disorder in youth is known to have an average age of onset that is several years earlier than the typical onset of major depressive disorder. Occasionally, youth fulfill the criteria for persistent depressive disorder, except that their episode does not last for a whole year, or they experience remission from symptoms for more than 2 months. These mood presentations in youth may predict additional mood disorder episodes in the future. Current knowledge suggests that the longer, more recurrent, and less directly related to social stress these episodes are, the higher the likelihood of future severe mood disorder. When minor depressive episodes follow a significant stressful life event by less than 3 months, it is more likely to be an adjustment disorder.

Bereavement

Bereavement is a state of grief related to the death of a loved one, which presents with an overlap of symptoms characteristic of a major depressive episode. Typical depressive symptoms associated with bereavement include feelings of sadness, insomnia, diminished appetite, and, in some cases, weight loss. Grieving children may become withdrawn and appear sad and avoid even their favorite activities.

In DSM-5, bereavement is not a mental disorder; however, uncomplicated bereavement is a condition that may be a focus of clinical attention. Children during a typical bereavement period may also meet the criteria for major depressive disorder. Symptoms indicating major depressive disorder exceeding typical bereavement include intense guilt related to issues beyond those surrounding the death of the loved one, preoccupation with death other than thoughts about being dead to be with the deceased person, morbid preoccupation with worthlessness, marked psychomotor retardation, prolonged severe functional impairment, and hallucinations other than transient perceptions of the voice of the deceased person.

The duration of bereavement varies; in children, the duration may depend partly on the support system in place. For example, a child may feel devastated and abandoned if they have to leave their home after the death of an only parent. Children who lose loved ones may feel a sense of guilt that death may have occurred because they were "bad" or did not perform as expected.

Ryan was a 12-year-old seventh grader in middle school who was brought to the emergency room in handcuffs by police after walking into oncoming traffic right after school. Ryan walked in front of a city bus; the driver began honking at the boy who kept ambling into the traffic. Two police stationed in their car across the street from the school heard the bus honking and noticed Ryan and confronted him. The police were about to issue the boy a citation for crossing against the red light; however, when they inquired as to why he had crossed against the traffic light, he informed them that he was trying to kill himself. The police handcuffed Ryan, placed him in the police car without a struggle, and brought him to the local hospital's emergency room. Ryan's mother was contacted and met her son in the emergency room. Ryan was physically intact, without injury, and a team of child psychiatrists evaluated him. When asked what had happened, Ryan became tearful. He said he walked in front of the bus in the hope of being hit and killed. Ryan reported that numerous peers had bullied him over the last 2 years because he is short and overweight. Ryan reported that on this day, a girl in his class had pushed him down and

started hitting him and laughing at him. Ryan reported that peer teased and assaulted him and called him stupid and fat. Ryan has some friends who usually defend him, but on this day, his friends were not close by, and he became desperate. Ryan disclosed, however, that even before this day, he has been sad for the last 2 years and thought about suicide recurrently over the last year.

Ryan was a relatively good student, earning good grades, especially in math, although he was failing history. Upon a separate interview with Ryan's mother, she did not know of any of Ryan's problems. She felt the team was mistaken and that she should take Ryan home.

Ryan had previously seen a counselor in school a few times last year, but the issues of depression or suicide did not come up. Ryan has an older brother and a younger brother who are well adjusted. When interviewing Ryan and his mother together, Ryan was able with some encouragement to let his mother know how depressed, hopeless, and suicidal he felt, and why. Ryan's mother burst into tears, and Ryan tried to comfort his mother.

Ryan was placed on a 72-hour hold and referred to a children's psychiatric inpatient unit for further evaluation and treatment. There the team treated him with an SSRI antidepressant as well as psychoeducation and family sessions. He and his family continued treatment after his hospitalization.

Pathology and Laboratory Examination

No laboratory test is useful for diagnosis. If a child or adolescent also complains of symptoms of hypothyroidism, that is, dry skin, coldness, lethargy, for example, then a screening test for thyroid function may be indicated.

Rating scales for depressive symptoms administered by us to the child and parent may be helpful in the evaluation. The Children's Depression Rating Scale-Revised (CDRS-R) is a 17-item instrument administered by the clinician separately to the parent and child or adolescent. The clinician scores a rating for each item using the information from both the parent and the child. The scale assesses affective, somatic, cognitive, and psychomotor symptoms. A cumulative score of 40 is a marker for moderate depression and a score of 45 or higher for significant depression.

DIFFERENTIAL DIAGNOSIS

A substance-induced mood disorder may be challenging to differentiate from other mood disorders until detoxification occurs. Anxiety symptoms and disorders often coexist with depressive disorders. Of particular importance in the differential diagnosis is the distinction between agitated depressive or manic episodes and ADHD, in which the persistent excessive activity and restlessness are confusing. Prepubertal children generally do not show classic forms of agitated depression, such as hand-wringing and pacing. Instead, an inability to sit still, irritability, and frequent temper tantrums are the most common symptoms. Sometimes, the correct diagnosis becomes evident only after remission of the depressive episode.

COURSE AND PROGNOSIS

The course and prognosis of major depression in youths depend on the severity of illness. Also important is the rapidity of interventions, and the degree of response to the interventions. In general, 90 percent of youth recover from a first episode of moderate to severe major depressive disorder within 1 to 2 years. The age of onset, episode severity, and the presence of comorbid disorders also influence course and prognosis. In general, the younger the age of onset, the higher the recurrence of multiple episodes, and the presence of comorbid disorders predict a poorer prognosis. The mean length of an untreated episode of major depression in children and adolescents is about 8 to 12 months; the cumulative probability of recurrence is 20 to 60 percent within 2 years and 70 percent by 5 years. The most significant risk for relapse is in the 6 months to 1 year after discontinuing treatment. Depressed children who live in families with high levels of chronic conflict are more likely to have relapses. The relapse rate for childhood depression into adulthood is also high. In a community sample, 45 percent of adolescents with a history of major depression developed another episode of major depression in early adulthood.

Youth with major depression are at higher risk for the development of a future bipolar disorder, compared to adults. Overall estimates of children with an episode of major depression developing bipolar disorder are about 20 to 40 percent. Clinical characteristics of a depressive episode in youth suggesting the highest risk of developing bipolar I disorder include hallucinations and delusions, psychomotor retardation, and a family history of bipolar illness. In a longitudinal study of prepubertal children with major depression, 33 percent developed bipolar I disorder, whereas 48 percent went on to develop bipolar II or bipolar disorder not otherwise specified by early adulthood.

Depressive disorders are associated with short- and long-term peer relationship difficulties and complications, compromised academic achievement, and persistently low self-esteem. Persistent depressive disorder has an even more protracted recovery than major depressive disorder; the mean episode length is about 4 years. Early-onset persistent depressive disorder is associated with significant risks of comorbidity with major depressive disorder (70 percent), bipolar disorder (13 percent), and future substance abuse (15 percent). The risk of suicide, which accounts for about 12 percent of adolescent mortalities, is significant among adolescents with depressive disorders.

TREATMENT

The AACAP practice parameters, as well as a consensus of experts who developed the Texas Children's Medication Algorithm Project (TMAP), made evidence-based recommendations for the treatment of children and adolescents with depressive disorders. These include psychoeducation and supportive interventions for youth with mild forms of depression. For youth with moderate to severe depression or recurrent episodes of major depression with significant impairment and with active suicidal thoughts or behaviors or psychosis, the optimal intervention includes both pharmacotherapy and CBT. CBT or interpersonal therapy (IPT) alone may be sufficient for moderate depression, especially when continuing treatment for 6 months or longer.

Psychiatric Hospitalization

We should assess for suicidal thoughts, behaviors, and a history of suicidal behavior in every child or adolescent with major depression. Safety is the most immediate consideration in assessing depression in youth, that is, a determination as to whether immediate psychiatric hospitalization is necessary. Depressed children and adolescents who express suicidal thoughts or behaviors most often require some extended evaluation in the safety of the psychiatric hospital to provide maximal protection from self-destructive impulses and behaviors.

Evidence-Based Treatment Studies

The Treatment for Adolescents with Depression Study (TADS) divided 439 adolescents between 12 and 17 years of age into three treatment groups of 12 weeks, composed of either fluoxetine alone (10 to 40 mg/day), fluoxetine with the same dose range in combination with CBT, or CBT alone. Based on ratings of the *Children's Depression Rating Scale-Revised* (CDRS-R), combination treatment had significantly superior response rates compared with either treatment alone. Based on CGI scores at 12 weeks, rates of much or very much improved were 71 percent for the combined treatment group, 60.6 percent for the fluoxetine group, 43.2 percent for the CBT alone group, and 34.4 percent for the placebo group. At 12 weeks, combination treatment was the optimal strategy in the treatment of adolescent depression. By the end of 9 months of treatment, however, response rates for each group had converged, so that response for the combination group was 86 percent, fluoxetine group response was about 81 percent, and CBT-alone group response rate was 81 percent. The long-term effectiveness of treatments for adolescent depression demonstrates that for moderately ill adolescents, fluoxetine, CBT, or the combination is efficacious. However, the addition of CBT to fluoxetine decreased persistent suicidal ideation and potential treatment-related emergence of suicidal ideation.

A second large multicenter randomized placebo-controlled trial, Treatment of SSRI-Resistant Depression in Adolescents (TORDIA), included adolescents with major depression who had not responded to a 2-month trial with an SSRI antidepressant. The investigators in this study randomly assigned 334 adolescents between 12 and 18 years of age to a different SSRI agent (either citalopram, paroxetine, citalopram, or another antidepressant class, venlafaxine) with or without concurrent CBT. The SSRI plus CBT group and the venlafaxine plus CBT group had higher response rates of improvement (54.8 percent) than the group on medications alone (40.5 percent). There were no differences found in the response rates between antidepressant agents.

Psychosocial Interventions

CBT is an efficacious intervention for the treatment of moderately severe depression in children and adolescents. CBT aims to challenge maladaptive beliefs and enhance problem-solving abilities and social competence. A review of controlled cognitive-behavioral studies in children and adolescents revealed that, as with adults, both children and adolescents showed consistent improvement with these methods. Other "active" treatments, including relaxation techniques, were also shown to be helpful as an adjunctive treatment for mild to moderate depression. Findings from one large controlled study comparing cognitive-behavioral interventions with nondirective supportive psychotherapy and systemic behavioral family therapy showed that 70 percent of adolescents had some improvement with each of the interventions; cognitive-behavioral intervention had the most rapid effect. Another controlled study comparing a brief course of CBT with relaxation therapy favored the cognitive-behavioral intervention. At a 3- to 6-month follow-up, however, no significant differences existed between the two treatment groups. This effect resulted from relapse in the cognitive-behavioral group, along with continued recovery in some patients in the relaxation group. Factors that seem to interfere with treatment responsiveness include the presence of comorbid anxiety disorder that probably was present before the depressive episode. Longer-term CBT is efficacious in the treatment of depression and has the advantage of mitigating suicidal ideation.

Interpersonal psychotherapy (IPT) focuses on improving depression through a focus on ways in which depression interferes with interpersonal relationships and overcoming these challenges. The four main areas of focus with interpersonal psychotherapy include loss, interpersonal disputes, role transition, and interpersonal deficits. A modification of interpersonal therapy to more specifically address depression for adolescents (IPT-A) includes a focus on separation from parents, authority figures, peer pressures, and dyadic relationships. IPT-A has been studied on an outpatient basis as well as in a school-based clinic setting. A 12-week study of 48 adolescents with major depression randomly assigned to IPT-A or clinical monitoring found that the group receiving IPT-A showed decreased depressive symptoms, increased social functioning, and improved problem solving compared to the other group. In the school-based health clinic, depressed adolescents were randomly assigned to IPT-A or treatment as usual for 16 weeks. Trained clinic staff administered the treatment. At the end of 16 weeks, those adolescents receiving IPT-A had more significant symptom reduction and improved overall functioning, especially older and more severely depressed adolescents seemed to benefit most significantly.

PCIT-ED for preschool depression, a modification of PCIT historically used in the treatment of disruptive disorders for children, was piloted in an RCT for 54 depressed preschoolers. Fifty-four depressed young children from ages 3 to 7 years received either PCIT-ED or psychoeducation with their caregivers. PCIT-ED was manualized and consisted of three modules conducted over 14 sessions in 12 weeks. The core modules of PCIT—Child-Directed Interaction (CDI) and Parent-Directed Interaction (PDI)—were utilized and limited to four sessions each. The focus of these modules is to strengthen the parent–child relationship by coaching parents in positive play techniques, giving effective directives to the child, and responding to disruptive behavior in firm but not punitive ways. The novel portion of the treatment targeting the preschool depression consisted of a 6-week Emotion Development (ED) module, which focused on helping the parent to be a more effective emotion guide and affect regulator for the child. As part of the ED module, the parent learns to accurately recognize their emotions as well as the child's and serves to help regulate the child's emotions. The team developed a psychoeducation control condition, Developmental Education and Parenting Intervention (DEPI), for parents using small group sessions. The DEPI condition was designed to educate parents about child development and emphasized emotional and social development without individual coaching or practice with behavioral techniques as provided in the PCIT-ED group. Primary outcome measures included parent's report of the child's symptoms of depression using a structured instrument, the Preschool Age Psychiatric Assessment (PAPA), and the investigators measured depression severity pretreatment and posttreatment using parent ratings on the Preschool Reelings Checklist-Scale Version (PFC-S), a 20-item checklist. Results revealed that both groups showed significant improvement, with particular improvement in the PCIT-ED group concerning emotion recognition, child executive functioning, and parenting stress. This pilot study indicates that PCIT-ED is a promising novel intervention for preschool depression that deserves further investigation.

Pharmacotherapy

Fluoxetine and escitalopram have FDA approval in the treatment of major depression in adolescents. Three RCTs of fluoxetine in depressed children and adolescents demonstrate its efficacy. The common side effects are similar as for adults: headache, gastrointestinal symptoms, sedation, and insomnia.

Short-term randomized clinical trials have demonstrated the efficacy of citalopram and sertraline compared with placebo in the treatment of major depression in children and adolescents. Sertraline was efficacious in two multicenter, double-blind, placebo-controlled trials of 376 children and adolescents. The doses of sertraline ranged from 50 to 200 mg a day or placebo. Nearly 70 percent of the subjects had a greater than 40 percent decrease in depression rating scale scores (compared with 56 percent in the placebo group). The most common side effects are anorexia, vomiting, diarrhea, and agitation.

Citalopram has been demonstrated in one RCT in the United States to be efficacious in 174 children and adolescents treated with citalopram at doses of 20 to 40 mg a day or placebo for 8 weeks. Significantly more of the group on citalopram showed improvement compared with placebo on the depression rating scale (CDRS-R). A significantly increased response rate (response defined as less than 28 on CDRS-R) of 35 percent occurred in the citalopram group, compared with 24 percent of the placebo group. Common side effects that emerged included headache, nausea, insomnia, rhinitis, abdominal pain, dizziness, fatigue, and flu-like symptoms.

RCTs to date that have not shown efficacy on primary outcome measures include those using mirtazapine and tricyclic antidepressants. A meta-analysis of SSRI trials in depressed children and adolescents found the efficacy of SSRIs compared to placebo with an average response rate of 60 percent for the SSRI compared to 49 percent for placebo.

Starting doses of SSRIs for prepubertal children are lower than doses recommended for adults, but adolescents usually use the same doses as adults.

A potential side effect of SSRIs in depressed children is behavioral activation or induction of hypomanic symptoms. We should discontinue the medication in those cases to see if the symptoms resolve. Activation due to SSRIs, however, does not necessarily predict a diagnosis of bipolar disorder.

Venlafaxine was effective in the TORDIA study; however, adverse effects, including increased blood pressure, have made this agent a second-line choice compared to the SSRIs.

Tricyclic antidepressants lack good data and have significant cardiac risks, including arrhythmias, and we do not recommend them.

FDA Warning and Suicidality. In September 2004, the FDA received information from their Psychopharmacologic Drug and Pediatric Advisory Committee indicating, based on their review of reported suicidal thoughts and behavior among depressed children and adolescents who participated in randomized clinical trials with nine different antidepressants, an increased risk of suicidality in those children who were on active antidepressant medications. Although there were no suicides, the rates of suicidal thinking and behaviors were 2 percent for patients on placebo, versus 4 percent among patients on antidepressant medications. The FDA, following the recommendation of their advisory committees, instituted a "black-box" warning to the health professional label of all antidepressant medication indicating the increased risk of suicidal thoughts and behaviors in children and adolescents, and the need for close monitoring for these symptoms. Several reviews since 2004, however, concluded that the data do not indicate a significant increase in the risk of suicide or serious suicide attempts after starting treatment with antidepressant drugs.

Duration of Treatment. Based on available longitudinal data and the natural history of major depression in children and adolescents, current recommendations include maintaining antidepressant treatment for 1 year in a depressed child who has achieved a good response, and to then discontinue the medication at a time of relatively low stress for a medication-free period.

Pharmacologic Treatment Strategies for Resistant Depression.
Pharmacologic recommendations, per an expert consensus panel that developed the TMAP, as well as the Treatment of SSRI-resistant Adolescents with Depression Study (TORDIA), in the treatment of children or adolescents who have not responded to treatment with an SSRI agent, is to change to another SSRI medication. If a child is not responsive to the second SSRI medication, then either a combination of antidepressants or augmentation strategies may be reasonable choices as well as an antidepressant from another class of medications.

Electroconvulsive Therapy

ECT is rarely used for adolescents, although published case reports indicate its efficacy in adolescents with depression and mania. Currently, case reports suggest that ECT may be a relatively safe and useful treatment for adolescents who have persistent severe affective disorders, particularly with psychotic features, catatonic symptoms, or persistent suicidality.

EPIDEMIOLOGY

Depressive disorders increase in frequency with increasing age in the general population. Mood disorders among preschool-age children are estimated to occur in about 0.3 percent of community samples, and 0.9 percent in clinic settings. The prevalence of major depression in school-age children is 2 to 3 percent. Depression in referred samples of school-age children occurs at the same frequency in boys as in girls, with some surveys indicating a slightly increased rate among boys. In adolescents, the prevalence rate of major depression is from 4 to 8 percent and two to three times more likely in females than males. By age 18 years, the cumulative incidence of major depression is 20 percent. Children with a family history of major depression in a first-degree relative are about three times more likely to develop the disorder than in those without family histories of affective disorders. The prevalence of persistent depressive disorder in children ranges from 0.6 to 4.6 percent and in adolescence increases to 1.6 to 8 percent. Children and adolescents with persistent depressive disorder have a high likelihood of developing major depressive disorder at some point after 1 year of persistent depressive disorder. The rate of developing a major depression on top of persistent depressive disorder (double depression) within 6 months of persistent depressive disorder is estimated to be about 9.9 percent.

Among psychiatrically hospitalized children and adolescents, the rates of major depressive disorder are close to 20 percent for children and 40 percent for adolescents.

ETIOLOGY

Considerable evidence indicates that major depression in youth is the same fundamental disorder experienced by adults and that its neurobiology is likely to be an interaction of genetic vulnerability and environmental stressors. The etiology of the depressive disorders is discussed in Chapter 7.

SUICIDE

In the United States, suicide is the third leading cause of death among adolescents, after accidental death and homicide. Throughout the world, suicide rarely occurs in children who have not reached puberty. In the last 15 years, the rates of both completed suicide and suicidal ideation have decreased among adolescents. This decrease appears to coincide with the increase in SSRI medications prescribed to adolescents with mood and behavioral disturbance.

Suicidal Ideation and Behavior

Suicidal ideation, gestures, and attempts are frequently, but not always, associated with depressive disorders. Reports indicate that as many as half of suicidal individuals express suicidal intentions to a friend or a relative within 24 hours before enacting suicidal behavior.

Suicidal ideation occurs in all age groups and with the highest frequency in children and adolescents with severe mood disorders. More than 12,000 children and adolescents are hospitalized in the United States each year because of suicidal threats or behavior, but completed suicide is rare in children younger than 12 years of age. A young child is hardly capable of designing and carrying out a realistic suicide plan. Cognitive immaturity seems to play a protective role in preventing even children who wish they were dead from committing suicide. Completed suicide occurs about five times more often in adolescent boys than in girls, although the rate of suicide attempts is at least three times higher among adolescent girls than among boys. Suicidal ideation is not a static phenomenon; it can wax and wane with time. The decision to engage in suicidal behavior may be made impulsively without much forethought, or the decision may be the culmination of prolonged rumination.

The method of the suicide attempt influences the morbidity and completion rates, independent of the severity of the intent to die at the time of the suicidal behavior. The most common method of completed suicide in children and adolescents is the use of firearms, which accounts for about two-thirds of all suicides in boys and almost one-half of suicides in girls. The second most common method of suicide in boys, occurring in about one-fourth of all cases, is hanging; in girls, about one-fourth commit suicide through the ingestion of toxic substances. Carbon monoxide poisoning is the next most common method of suicide in boys, but it occurs in less than 10 percent; suicide by hanging and carbon monoxide poisoning are equally frequent among girls and account for about 10 percent each. Additional risk factors in suicide include a family history of suicidal behavior, exposure to family violence, impulsivity, substance abuse, and availability of lethal methods. Gender differences in nonfatal suicidal behavior among ninth-grade adolescents in a survey of students in 100 high schools found that 19.8 percent of female students had serious suicidal thoughts, and 10.8 percent of females attempted suicide. In male students, 9.3 percent had a history of suicidal thoughts, and 4.9 percent attempted suicide. In this study, female students showed evidence of higher levels of mood and anxiety problems, whereas males had a slightly higher level of disruptive behavior problems. Female students reported higher levels of depression, anxiety, somatic complaints, and increased levels of emotional and behavioral problems than males. In young adolescents, even without meeting full criteria for psychiatric disorders, females report more psychopathology along with a higher likelihood of nonfatal suicidal behavior.

Diagnosis and Clinical Features

The characteristics of adolescents who attempt suicide and those who complete suicide are similar, and up to 40 percent of suicidal persons have made a previous attempt. Direct questioning of children and adolescents about suicidal thoughts is necessary because studies have consistently shown that caregivers are frequently unaware of these ideas in their children. Suicidal thoughts (i.e., children talking about wanting to harm themselves) and suicidal threats (e.g., children stating that they want to jump in front of a car) are more common than suicide completion.

Most older adolescents with suicidal behavior meet the criteria for one or more psychiatric disorders, often including major depressive disorder, bipolar disorder, and psychotic disorders. Youth with mood disorders in combination with substance abuse and a history of aggressive behavior are at particularly high risk for suicide. The most common precipitating factors in younger adolescent suicide completers appear to be impending disciplinary actions, impulsive behavioral histories, and access to loaded guns, particularly in the home. Adolescents without mood disorders with histories of disruptive and violent, aggressive, and impulsive behavior may be susceptible to suicide during family or peer conflicts. High levels of hopelessness, poor problem-solving skills, and a history of aggressive behavior are risk factors for suicide. A less common profile of an adolescent who completes suicide is one of high achievement and perfectionistic character traits facing a perceived failure, such an academically proficient adolescent humiliated by a poor grade on an examination.

Findings from a World Health Organization mental health survey reveals that a range of psychiatric disorders increases the risk of suicidal ideation across the lifespan. Youth with psychiatric disorders characterized by severe anxiety and poor impulse control are at higher risk to act on suicidal ideation. In psychiatrically disturbed and vulnerable adolescents, suicide behavior may represent impulsive responses to recent stressors. Typical precipitants of suicidal behavior include conflicts and arguments with family members and boyfriends or girlfriends. Alcohol and other substance use can further predispose an already vulnerable adolescent to suicidal behavior. In other cases, an adolescent attempts suicide in anticipation of punishment after being caught by the police or other authority figures for a forbidden behavior.

About 40 percent of youth who complete suicide had previous psychiatric treatment, and about 40 percent had made a previous suicide attempt. A child who has lost a parent by any means before age 13 is at higher risk for mood disorders and suicide. The precipitating factors include loss of face with peers, a broken romance, school difficulties, unemployment, bereavement, separation, and rejection. There are reports of clusters of suicides that occur among adolescents who know one another and go to the same school. Suicidal behavior can precipitate other such attempts within a peer group through identification—so-called copycat suicides. Some studies have found a transient increase in adolescent suicides after television programs in which the central theme was the suicide of a teenager.

The tendency of disturbed young persons to imitate highly publicized suicides has been referred to as *Werther syndrome,* after the protagonist in Johann Wolfgang von Goethe's novel, *The Sorrows of Young Werther.* The novel, in which the hero kills himself, was banned in some European countries after its publication more than 200 years ago because of a rash of suicides by young men who read it; some dressed like Werther before killing themselves or left the book open at the passage describing his death. In general, although imitation may play a role in the timing of suicide attempts by vulnerable adolescents, the overall suicide rate does not seem to increase when media exposure increases. In contrast, direct exposure to peer suicide increases the risk of depression and PTSD rather than suicide.

Treatment

The prognostic significance of suicidal ideation and behaviors in adolescents ranges from relatively low lethality to high risk for completion. One of the challenges in addressing suicide is to identify children and adolescents with suicidal ideation, and particularly to treat those who have untreated psychiatric disorders, as the risk of completed suicide increases with age, as does the onset of an untreated psychiatric disorder. We should always evaluate adolescents who come to medical attention because of suicidal attempts to determine whether hospitalization is necessary. Pediatric patients who present to the emergency room with suicidal ideation benefit from an intervention that occurs in the emergency room to ensure that the patient is transitioned to outpatient care when hospitalization is not necessary. We should hospitalize youths who fall into high-risk groups until the acute suicidality is no longer present. Adolescents at higher risk include those who have made previous suicide attempts, especially with a lethal method, males older than 12 years of age with histories of aggressive behavior or substance abuse, use of a lethal method, and severe major depressive disorder with social withdrawal, hopelessness, and persistent suicidal ideation.

Relatively few adolescents evaluated for suicidal behavior in a hospital emergency room subsequently receive ongoing psychiatric treatment. Factors that may increase the probability of psychiatric treatment include psychoeducation for the family in the emergency room, diffusing acute family conflict, and setting up an outpatient follow-up during the emergency room visit. Emergency room discharge plans often include providing an alternative if suicidal ideation reoccurs, and a telephone hotline number provided to the adolescent and the family in case suicidal ideation reappears.

Scant data exist to evaluate the efficacy of various interventions in reducing suicidal behavior among adolescents. CBT alone and in combination with SSRIs decreased suicidal ideation in depressed adolescents over time in the TADS, a large multisite study; however, these interventions do not work immediately, so we should take safety precautions for high-risk situations. Dialectical behavior therapy (DBT), a long-term behavioral intervention useful for individuals or groups of patients, can reduce suicidal behavior in adults, but there are no significant studies in adolescents. Components of DBT include mindfulness training to improve self-acceptance, assertiveness training, instruction on avoiding situations that may trigger self-destructive behavior, and increasing the ability to tolerate psychological distress. This approach warrants investigation among adolescents.

Given the reduction in completed suicide among adolescents over the last decade, during the same period in which SSRI treatment in the adolescent population has markedly risen, SSRIs may have been instrumental in this effect. Given the risk of the increased rate of suicidal thoughts and behaviors among depressed children and adolescents (indicated in randomized clinical trials with antidepressant medications and leading to the "black-box" warning for all antidepressants for depressed youth), we must closely monitor youths for increased suicidality while taking antidepressants.

Epidemiology

In a study of 9- to 16-year-olds in 3 months, passive suicidal thoughts were approximately 1 percent, suicidal ideation with a plan was 0.3 percent, and suicide attempt was 0.25 percent. In adolescents 14 to 18 years, the current rate of suicidal ideation was 2.7 percent, and the annual incidence was 4.3 percent. Among this population of adolescents, the lifetime prevalence of suicide attempts was 7.1 percent, with a much higher rate of suicidal behavior for girls than for boys: 10.1 percent compared to 3.8 percent. Completed suicide rates in youth are much less common in children and younger teens 10 to 14 years, with a slighter lower rate of 0.95 per 100,000 for females compared to 1.71 per 100,000 for males. In older adolescents 15 to 19 years of age, completed suicide is considerably lower for females, 3.52 per 100,000 compared to males, 12.65 per 100,000 in the United States in 2004.

Etiology

Universal features in adolescents who resort to suicidal behaviors are the inability to synthesize viable solutions to ongoing problems and the lack of coping strategies to deal with immediate crises. Therefore, a narrow view of the options available to deal with recurrent family discord, rejection, or failure contributes to a decision to commit suicide.

Genetic Factors.   Completed suicide and suicidal behavior are two to four times more likely to occur in individuals with a first-degree family member with similar behavior. Family suicide risk studies support a genetic contribution to suicidal behavior. There is also a higher concordance for suicide among monozygotic twins compared to dizygotic twins. Recent studies have investigated the possible contributions of the short allele of the serotonin transporter promoter polymorphism (5-HTTLPR) to suicidal behaviors, although, to date, the evidence has not been consistent. Current studies are seeking to investigate correlations between genetic vulnerability and environment and timing interactions as multiple variables that may interact to increase the risk of suicidal behavior.

Biologic Factors.   Investigators have found a relationship between altered central serotonin with suicide as well as impulsive aggression. This relationship is also true in adults. Studies document a reduction in the density of serotonin transporter receptors in the prefrontal cortex and serotonin receptors among individuals with suicidal behaviors. Postmortem studies in adolescents who have completed suicide show the most significant alterations in the prefrontal cortex and hippocampus, brain regions that are also associated with emotion regulation and problem-solving. These studies have found altered serotonin metabolites, alteration in $5-HT_{2A}$ binding, and decreased activity of protein kinase A and C. Decreased levels of the serotonin metabolite 5-hydroxyindoleacetic acid (5-HIAA) are found in the cerebrospinal fluid (CSF) of depressed adults who attempted suicide by violent methods. Meta-analyses suggest an association between the short S-allele of the serotonin transporter promoter gene and depression as well as suicidal behavior, particularly when combined with adverse life events.

Psychosocial Factors.   Although severe major depressive illness is the most significant risk factor for suicide, increasing its risk by 20 percent, many severely depressed individuals are not suicidal. A sense of hopelessness, impulsivity, recurrent substance use, and a history of aggressive behavior have been associated with an increased risk of suicide. Exposure to violent and abusive homes results in a wide range of psychopathological symptoms. Aggressive, self-destructive, and suicidal behaviors seem to occur with the greatest frequency among youth who have endured chronically stressful family lives. The most significant family risk factor for suicidal behavior is maltreatment, including physical and sexual abuse and neglect. The single largest association is between sexual abuse

and suicidal behavior. Large community studies have provided data suggesting that youth at risk for suicidal behavior include those who feel disconnected, isolated, or alienated from peers. Sexual orientation is a risk factor, with increased rates of suicidal behavior of two to six times among youth who identify themselves as gay, lesbian, or bisexual. Protective factors mitigating the risk of suicidal behavior are youth who have a secure connection to school and peers, even in the face of other risk factors.

▲ 2.10 Early-Onset Bipolar Disorder

Early-onset bipolar disorder has been recognized in children as a rare disorder with greater continuity with its adult counterpart when it occurs in adolescents than in prepubertal children. Over the last decade, there has been a significant increase in the diagnosis of bipolar I disorder made in youth referred to psychiatric outpatient clinics and inpatient units. Questions have arisen regarding the phenotype of bipolar disorder in youth, mainly because of the continuous irritability and mood dysregulation and lack of discrete mood episodes in most prepubertal children who have received the diagnosis. The "atypical" bipolar symptoms among prepubertal children often include extreme mood dysregulation, severe temper tantrums, intermittent aggressive or explosive behavior, and high levels of distractibility and inattention. This constellation of mood and behavior disturbance in the majority of prepubertal children with a current diagnosis of bipolar disorder is nonepisodic, although some fluctuation in mood may occur. The high frequency of the above symptoms in combination with chronic irritability has led to the inclusion of a new mood disorder in youth in DSM-5 called *Disruptive Mood Dysregulation Disorder,* and we discuss that in the next section. Many children with nonepisodic mood disorders often have past histories of severe ADHD, making the diagnosis of bipolar disorder even more complicated. Family studies of children with ADHD have not revealed an increased rate of bipolar I disorder. Children with "atypical" bipolar disorders, however, are frequently severely impaired, are challenging to manage in school and at home, and often require psychiatric hospitalization. Longitudinal follow-up studies are underway with groups of children diagnosed with subthreshold bipolar disorders and nonepisodic mood disorders, to determine how many will develop classic bipolar disorder. In one recent study of 140 children with bipolar disorder not otherwise specified (i.e., the presence of distinct manic symptoms but subthreshold for manic episodes), 45 percent developed bipolar I or bipolar II illness over a follow-up period of 5 years. In another study, investigators followed 84 children with "severe mood dysregulation" who also had at least three manic symptoms plus distractibility for approximately 2 years. The investigators found that only one child experienced a hypomanic or mixed episode. Although childhood severe mood dysregulation is common in community samples—one study reported a lifetime prevalence of 3.3 percent in youth 9 to 19 years of age—its relationship to future bipolar disorder remains questionable. A longitudinal community-based study that followed children and adolescents with nonepisodic irritability over 20 years found that these children were at higher risk for depressive disorders and generalized anxiety disorder than bipolar disorders.

Among adults and older adolescents with bipolar disorder who present with classic manic episodes, a major depressive episode typically precedes a manic episode. A classic manic episode in an adolescent, similar to in a young adult, may emerge as a distinct departure from a preexisting state often characterized by grandiose and paranoid delusions and hallucinatory phenomena. According to DSM-5, the criteria for a manic episode in children or adults are the same. We discuss these in Chapter 6.

When mania appears in an adolescent, there is a high incidence of psychotic features, including delusions and hallucinations, which most typically involve grandiose notions about their power, worth, and relationships. Persecutory delusions and flight of ideas are also common. Overall, gross impairment of reality testing is common in adolescent manic episodes. In adolescents with major depressive disorder destined for bipolar I disorder, those at highest risk have family histories of bipolar I disorder and exhibit acute, severe depressive episodes with psychosis, hypersomnia, and psychomotor retardation.

DIAGNOSIS AND CLINICAL FEATURES

Early-onset bipolar disorder often includes extreme irritability that is severe and persistent and may include aggressive outbursts and violent behavior. In between outbursts, children with the broad diagnosis may continue to be angry or dysphoric. It is rare for a prepubertal child to exhibit grandiose thoughts or euphoric mood; for the most part, children diagnosed with early-onset bipolar disorder are intensely emotional with a fluctuating but overriding negative mood. Current diagnostic criteria for bipolar disorders in children and adolescents in DSM-5 are the same as those used in adults (see Chapter 6, Tables 6-2 and 6-3). The clinical picture of early-onset bipolar disorder, however, is complicated by the prevalence of comorbid psychiatric disorders.

Pathology and Laboratory Examination

No specific laboratory indices are currently helpful in making the diagnosis of bipolar disorders among children and adolescents.

DIFFERENTIAL DIAGNOSIS

The most critical clinical entities to distinguish from early-onset bipolar disorder are also the disorders with which it is most frequently comorbid. Included are ADHD, oppositional defiant disorder, conduct disorder, anxiety disorders, and depressive disorders.

Although childhood ADHD tends to have its onset earlier than pediatric mania, current evidence from family studies supports the presence of ADHD and bipolar disorders as highly comorbid in children, and the concurrence is not because of the overlapping symptoms that the two disorders share. In a recent study of more than 300 children and adolescents who attended a psychopharmacology clinic and received a diagnosis of ADHD, bipolar disorder was also evident in almost one-third of those children with ADHD who had combined–type and hyperactive-types. It was less frequent (i.e., in less than 10 percent) in children with ADHD, inattentive-type.

COMORBIDITY

ADHD is the most common comorbid condition among youth with early-onset bipolar disorder and occurs in up to 90 percent of prepubertal children and up to 50 percent of adolescents diagnosed with bipolar disorder. Comorbid ADHD creates a significant source of diagnostic confusion in children with early-onset bipolar disorder

since the two disorders share many diagnostic criteria, including distractibility, hyperactivity, and talkativeness. Even when removing the overlapping symptoms from the diagnostic count, a significant percentage of children with bipolar disorder continued to meet the full criteria for ADHD. This implies that both disorders, with their distinct features, are present in many cases.

Children and adolescents with bipolar disorder have higher-than-expected rates of panic and other anxiety disorders. In youth with the narrow phenotype of bipolar disorders, up to 77 percent have an anxiety disorder. The lifetime prevalence of panic disorder was 21 percent among subjects with the broader phenotype of bipolar disorder compared with 0.8 percent in those without mood disorders. Patients diagnosed with bipolar disorder who have comorbid high levels of anxiety symptoms are reported as adults to have higher risks of alcohol abuse and suicidal behavior. On the other hand, children who exhibit the broader phenotype of bipolar disorder are at higher risk of going on to have anxiety disorders as well as depressive disorders.

Jeanie is a 13-year-old adopted teen who was hospitalized after assaulting her adoptive mother, causing bruises on her arms and legs from Jeanie's kicks and punches. Jeanie had a long history of excessively severe tantrums, which include assaultive and self-injurious behavior, since before her parents adopted her when she was three. Jeanie had always been a child who was irritable and explosive, with a short fuse, who could blow up with minimal provocation, even when things were going her way. Jeanie had become increasingly hard to manage at home, refused to go to school, yelled and screamed for hours on a daily basis, and often hit and kicked her adoptive parents by the time she was 10 years old. Jeannie was in residential treatment from age 11 to almost 13, where the clinicians diagnosed her with bipolar disorder and started lithium and citalopram. She was doing so well there that Jeanie's adoptive mother decided to take her home. After a few weeks at home, however, Jeanie began to decompensate, having daily explosive tantrums, becoming aggressive and out of control. On multiple occasions, she had hurt herself and her adoptive mother and father. Upon arriving at the hospital, Jeanie was calm; however, her adoptive mother refused to consider taking her home until undergoing a full psychiatric evaluation and treatment for unsafe behaviors. The child psychiatrist initially evaluated Jeanie, after which she went to a pediatric inpatient unit to await a psychiatric bed. The psychiatrist learned that Jeanie had been born prematurely to a teenage mother and placed in multiple foster homes until she was adopted. Jeanie was a small girl who appeared younger than her stated age, although her demeanor was bossy and pedantic. Jeanie's biologic family history was unknown, and although she had at least one stigmata of fetal alcohol syndrome, her IQ was in the average range, and there was no other evidence to corroborate this possibility. On mental status examination in the hospital, Jeanie reported that things were fine, that she was not depressed, and that she did not get along with kids her age but that she had a few friends. Jeanie admitted that she had a bad temper and that she did not remember what she did after she was in a rage. Jeanie's affect was odd, and she seemed to enjoy having the psychiatrist as her audience. Jeanie denied suicidal ideation or past attempts and denied having been a danger to herself or her adoptive parents. Jeanie seemed annoyed when she was asked about the reasons for her placement in a residential facility, and she became irritable when questioned about the reasons for her current admission. The team then transferred Jeanie to an adolescent psychiatric inpatient unit to start a trial of an atypical antipsychotic. The team recommended that her psychiatrist reconsider a more structured school program, either a day program or residential facility. The diagnosis of bipolar disorder remained in question, as she did not meet the narrow phenotype for this disorder.

COURSE AND PROGNOSIS

There are several pathways regarding the course and prognosis of children diagnosed with early-onset bipolar disorder. Those who present with severe mood dysregulation at an early age, without discrete mood cycles, are most likely to develop anxiety and depressive disorders as they mature. Youths who present in adolescence with a recognizable manic episode are most likely to continue to meet the criteria for bipolar I disorder in adulthood. In both cases, long-term impairment is considerable.

A longitudinal study of 263 child and adolescent inpatients and outpatients with bipolar disorder followed for an average of 2 years found that approximately 70 percent recovered from their index episode within that period. Half of these patients had at least one recurrence of a mood disorder during this time, more frequently a depressive episode than a mania. There were no differences in the rates of recovery for children and adolescents whose diagnosis was bipolar I disorder, bipolar II disorder, or bipolar disorder not otherwise specified. However, those whose diagnosis was bipolar disorder not otherwise specified had a significantly longer duration of illness before recovery, with less frequent recurrences once they recovered. About 19 percent of patients changed polarity once per year or less, 61 percent shifted five or more times per year, about half cycled more than ten times per year, and about one-third cycled more than 20 times per year. Predictors of more rapid cycling included lower socioeconomic status (SES), presence of lifetime psychosis, and bipolar disorder not otherwise specified diagnosis. Over the follow-up period, about 20 percent of subjects with bipolar II disorder converted to bipolar I disorder, and 25 percent of the bipolar disorder not otherwise specified subjects developed bipolar I disorder or bipolar II disorder during the follow-up period.

Similar to the natural history of bipolar disorders in adults, children have a wide range of symptom severity in manic and depressed episodes. The more frequent diagnostic conversions from bipolar II disorder to bipolar I disorder among children and adolescents, compared with adults, highlight the lack of stability of the bipolar II disorder diagnosis in youth. This is also the case concerning conversion from bipolar disorder not otherwise specified to other bipolar disorders. When bipolar disorder occurs in young children, recovery rates are lower. Also, there is a higher likelihood mixed states and rapid cycling, and higher rates of polarity changes compared with those who develop bipolar disorders in late adolescence or early adulthood.

TREATMENT

Treatment of early-onset bipolar disorder incorporates multimodal interventions including pharmacotherapy, psychoeducation, psychosocial intervention with the family and the child, and school interventions to optimize a child's school adjustment and achievement.

Pharmacotherapy

Two classes of medications—atypical antipsychotics and mood-stabilizing agents—are the most well-studied agents that provide efficacy in the treatment of early-onset bipolar disorders. Eight RCTs have shown the efficacy of atypical antipsychotic agents in the treatment of bipolar disorder in youth between the ages of 10 and 17 years. These studies compared an atypical antipsychotic to placebo, or compared an atypical antipsychotic to a mood stabilizer, or added an antipsychotic to a mood-stabilizing agent. The atypical antipsychotics included olanzapine, quetiapine, risperidone, aripiprazole, and ziprasidone. All five of the atypical antipsychotic studies demonstrated significant efficacy in the treatment of early-onset bipolar manic or mixed states. A recent trial comparing quetiapine and valproate found that both were efficacious, but the quetiapine was superior in the speed of its effect. In another trial comparing risperidone and sodium valproate treatment for bipolar disorder in youth, risperidone had more rapid improvement and a higher final reduction in manic symptoms compared to sodium valproate.

Mood-stabilizing agents have been used in open trials and anecdotally with early-onset bipolar illness with little evidence of efficacy at this time. In trials using lithium or sodium valproate for the treatment of early-onset bipolar disorder, responses were less robust compared to results with atypical antipsychotics. Controlled trials have provided some evidence suggesting that lithium is efficacious in the management of aggression behavior disorders. Although lithium is approved for adolescent mania, more research is needed to know if lithium is useful for more classic forms of mania in adolescents. The Collaborative Lithium Trials (CoLT) established a set of protocols to establish the safety and potential efficacy of lithium in youth, and to develop studies to provide evidence-based dosing of lithium for youth. A group of researchers studied the first-dose pharmacokinetics of lithium carbonate in youth and found that clearance and volume correlate with total body weight in youth, and particularly with fat-free mass. The difference in body size was consistent with the pharmacokinetics of lithium metabolism in children and adults. An open-label trial of lamotrigine in the treatment of bipolar depression among youth provides possible support for its use in children and adolescents.

Current evidence suggests a faster response and a more robust effect with atypical antipsychotics compared to mood-stabilizing agents in the treatment of early-onset bipolar disorder. However, given the severity and impairment of bipolar disorder in youth, when there is only partial recovery, we should consider adding another agent.

Psychosocial Treatment

Psychosocial treatment interventions for early-onset bipolar illness have included a family-focused treatment. This treatment consists of several sessions of psychoeducation, then sessions focusing on current stressors and a mood management plan, and then several sessions of communication enhancement training and problem-solving skills training. The use of this type of intervention for youths diagnosed with bipolar disorder or at risk (by family history or subthreshold symptoms) is of value. Adjunctive family-focused psychoeducational treatment modified for children and adolescents reduces the relapse rate. Children and adolescents treated with mood-stabilizing agents in addition to a psychosocial intervention showed improvement in depressive symptoms, manic symptoms, and behavioral disturbance over 1 year.

A year-long trial of a modified Family Focused Treatment-High Risk in youth with bipolar disorder showed significant improvement in mood disturbance, especially depressive mood and hypomania, and improved psychosocial functioning. Family-focused treatment for high-risk youth is a promising intervention that deserves further investigation as a longitudinal follow-up to determine the course of youth at risk to develop bipolar disorder.

EPIDEMIOLOGY

The prevalence rates of bipolar disorder among youth vary depending on the age group studied, and on whether the diagnostic criteria are applied narrowly, restricting it to discrete mood episodes or more broadly, to include nonepisodic mood and behavioral states. In younger children, bipolar disorder is infrequent, with no cases of bipolar I disorder identified in children between the ages of 9 and 13 years by the Great Smokey Mountain Study. However, severe mood dysregulation, often a prominent feature in prepubertal children receiving a diagnosis of bipolar disorder, was found in 3.3 percent of an epidemiologic sample. In adolescents, bipolar disorder is more frequent, found to range from 0.06 to 0.1 percent of the general population of 16-year-olds in studies using a narrow definition of bipolar I disorder. The prevalence of subthreshold symptoms of bipolar illness was 5.7 percent in one study to at least 10 percent in another. Follow-up studies into adulthood revealed that the subthreshold manic symptoms predicted high levels of impairment with progression to depression and anxiety disorders, not bipolar I or II disorders.

Community use of the diagnosis of bipolar disorder in youth has increased markedly over the last 15 years in both outpatient and inpatient psychiatric settings. One survey suggested there was a 40-fold increase in the diagnosis of early-onset bipolar disorder at outpatient clinics from the 1990s to the 2000s. Furthermore, from 2000 through 2006, the rate of youth hospitalized with a primary diagnosis of bipolar disorder nearly doubled.

ETIOLOGY

Genetic Factors

High rates of bipolar disorder occur in the relatives of the narrow phenotype of early-onset bipolar disorder compared to young adult-onset of bipolar disorder. The high rates of comorbid ADHD among children with early-onset bipolar disorder have led to questions regarding the co-transmission of these disorders in family members. However, children with the broader phenotype of bipolar disorder, that is, severe mood dysregulation without episodes of mania, have not been found to have higher rates of bipolar disorder in family members, which suggests that the narrow and broad phenotypes of bipolar disorder may be distinct and separate entities. Nearly 25 percent of adolescent offspring of families with probands with bipolar disorder experienced a mood disorder by the age of 17 years old, compared to 4 percent of controls, with approximately 8 percent representing bipolar I, bipolar II, or bipolar disorder not otherwise specified. Most of the risk in the offspring, therefore, is for unipolar major depressive disorder. Disruptive behavior disorders did not increase, in a longitudinal study, in the offspring of families with a bipolar proband, compared to controls. The combination of ADHD and bipolar disorder is not found as frequently in relatives of children with ADHD alone compared with first-degree relatives of children with the combination.

Although bipolar disorder appears to have a significant heritable component, its mode of inheritance remains unknown. Several research groups have concluded that early-onset bipolar disorder is a more severe form of the illness, characterized by more mixed episodes, greater psychiatric comorbidity, more lifetime psychotic symptoms, poorer response to prophylactic lithium treatment, and a greater heritability. The European collaborative study of early-onset bipolar disorder (France, Germany, Ireland, Scotland, Switzerland, England, and Slovenia) carried out a genome-wide linkage analysis of both the narrow and the broad phenotype of early-onset bipolar disorder. This group concluded that a genetic factor located in the 2q14 region is either specifically involved in the etiology of early-onset bipolar disorder, or that a gene in this region exerts influence as a modifier of other genes in the development of bipolar disorder in this age group. Other linkage regions that were found by this collaborative did not pertain only to the early-onset group of bipolar disorder, suggesting that there may be some genetic factors common to early-onset and adult-onset bipolar disorder. This conclusion is consistent with the increased incidence of adult-onset bipolar disorder among siblings of early-onset disease. Further genome-wide studies are needed to elucidate the genetic etiology of early-onset bipolar disorder.

Neurobiologic Factors

Converging data suggest that early-onset bipolar disorder is associated with both structural and functional brain alterations in prefrontal cortical and subcortical regions associated with the processing and regulation of emotional stimuli. MRI studies suggest that altered development of white matter and a decreased amygdalar volume are found more frequently in this population than in the general population.

Functional MRI (fMRI) studies are essential in that they can identify altered brain function in vulnerable populations such as youth with early-onset bipolar disorder at baseline. They can also elucidate functional changes toward normalization in brain functioning after various treatments, and potentially identify pretreatment neural predictors of good response to various treatments. An fMRI study of pediatric bipolar patients documented pretreatment brain activity and posttreatment effects of a trial of risperidone versus sodium valproate. This double-blind study included 24 unmedicated manic patients with a mean age of 13 years, randomized to either risperidone or sodium valproate treatment, and 14 healthy controls examined over 6 weeks. Before treatment, the patient group showed increased amygdala activity compared to healthy controls, which was poorly controlled by the higher ventrolateral prefrontal cortex (VLPFC) and the dorsolateral prefrontal cortex (DLPFC), which exert influence on the amygdala to control emotional regulation and processing. Increased amygdala activity at baseline predicted poorer treatment response to both risperidone and sodium valproate in the patient group. Patients were given an affective color-matching word task involving matching positive words (i.e., happiness, achievement, success), negative words (i.e., disappointment, depression, or rejection), or neutral words, with one of two colored circles displayed on a screen while administering the fMRI. Higher pretreatment right amygdala activity during a word task with positive and negative words in the risperidone group and higher pretreatment left amygdala activity with a positive word task in the sodium valproate group, predicted a poor response on the Young Mania Rating Scale. Increased amygdala activity in early-onset bipolar patients might be a potential biomarker predicting resistance and poor treatment response to both risperidone and sodium valproate.

Neuropsychological Studies

Impairments in verbal memory, processing speed, executive function, working memory, and attention are common in early-onset bipolar disorder. Data suggest that on tasks of working memory, processing speed, and attention, children and adolescents with comorbid bipolar disorder and ADHD demonstrate more pronounced impairments compared with those without ADHD. Other studies found that children with bipolar disorder make a higher number of emotion recognition errors compared with controls. The children more frequently identified faces as "angry" when presented with adult faces; however, these errors did not occur when they looked at children's faces. Impaired perception of facial expression also occurs in studies of adults with bipolar disorder.

▲ 2.11 Disruptive Mood Dysregulation Disorder

Disruptive mood dysregulation disorder, a new inclusion in the DSM-5, describes severe, developmentally inappropriate, and recurrent temper outbursts at least three times per week, along with a persistently irritable or angry mood between temper outbursts. To meet diagnostic criteria, the symptoms must be present for at least a year, and the onset of symptoms must be present by the age of 10 years old. Clinicians usually diagnose these children with bipolar disorder or a combination of oppositional defiant disorder, ADHD, and intermittent explosive disorder. Recent longitudinal data suggest, however, that these children do not typically develop classic bipolar disorder in late adolescence or early adulthood. Instead, studies suggest that youth with chronic irritability and severe mood dysregulation are at higher risk for future unipolar depressive disorders and anxiety disorders. Some experts include hyperarousal as a symptom, but DSM-5 does not.

DIAGNOSIS AND CLINICAL FEATURES

The DSM-5 diagnostic criteria for disruptive mood dysregulation disorder require outbursts that are grossly out of proportion to the situation. These temper outbursts present with verbal rages or physical aggression toward people or property and are inappropriate for the child's developmental level. Temper outbursts occur, on average, three or more times per week, with variations in mood between outbursts. Symptoms must exhibit before age 10 years, be present for at least 12 months, and be present within at least two settings (i.e., home and school). We would not diagnose this in children younger than 6 years or older than 18 years. In between temper outbursts, the child's mood is persistently irritable and angry, and this mood is observable by others, such as parents, teachers, or peers. A diagnosis of bipolar disorder would take precedence over this one, and the symptoms cannot occur only during a major depressive episode. Table 2-27 compares the diagnostic approaches.

Daniel, a 12-year-old seventh-grade boy, was brought to his pediatrician by his mother. His rages and inappropriate tantrums were exasperating her. Daniel was on the floor in the waiting room, pounding his hands on the floor, yelling at his mother, "Get me out of here!" and crying. His mother had bruises on both legs from Dylan's kicks, and she appeared distressed. Daniel's mother walked into the office, leaving Daniel on the floor in the waiting room and burst into tears. "I cannot deal with him anymore." She recounted the problems that Daniel had been having for the last 2 years: Severe recurrent tantrums four to five times/week. "He tantrums like a 6-year-old, and even when he is not having a tantrum, he is perpetually angry and irritable." She reported that Daniel had lost all of his friends due to his short fuse and frequent verbal and physical outbursts. He was almost always irritable, even on his birthday. Daniel's mother wonders whether there is anything physically wrong with him, but physical examination and routine blood tests reveal no abnormalities. Daniel's tantrums had lessened somewhat last summer during the 2-month summer vacation; however, as soon as school resumed, he was back to consistent irritability. After an interview with Daniel, his pediatrician determined that he was not acutely

Table 2-27
Disruptive Mood Dysregulation Disorder

	DSM-5	ICD-10
Diagnostic name	Disruptive Mood Dysregulation Disorder	Unspecified Behavioral and Emotional Disorders with onset usually occurring in childhood and adolescence
Duration	Outbursts occurring ≥3/wk Occurs for ≥12 mo No more than 3 mo during that time when criteria not met Onset between ages 6 and 10 yr	
Symptoms	• Recurrent inappropriate outbursts (verbal/physical) • Developmentally inappropriate • Irritable/angry most days between outbursts • Irritable/mad most days	
Required number of symptoms	All the above	
Exclusions (not result of):	• Another mental disorder • Substance use • Another neurologic disorder Cannot co-occur with: 　• Oppositional defiant disorder 　• Intermittent explosive disorder 　• Bipolar disorder	

suicidal; however, he required urgent psychotherapeutic intervention. Daniel started cognitive-behavioral therapy with a clinical psychologist and also saw a child and adolescent psychiatrist for possible medication. Daniel resisted psychotherapy; however, after several sessions, Daniel's parents felt more hopeful than they had in a long time, and learned that Daniel's problems were not "all their fault." Daniel agreed to begin a trial of fluoxetine, titrated to 30 mg over several weeks, and after about a month, it became clear that his irritability had diminished noticeably. Daniel still had many problems with peers, and he still had one or two tantrums per week; however, the tantrums were becoming less prolonged and less intense. Daniel seemed genuinely happy when a classmate invited him to a birthday party, and he was able to interact successfully with his peers during the party without any conflicts. Daniel continues to benefit from CBT, and he remains on fluoxetine 40 mg a day. Daniel is still a "temperamental" boy, but he is doing well in school, has rekindled several friendships, and can participate in family gatherings without a major tantrum.

DIFFERENTIAL DIAGNOSIS

Bipolar Disorder

Disruptive mood dysregulation disorder closely resembles the broad phenotype of bipolar disorder. Although not episodic, it has been theorized by some clinicians and researchers that the chronic and persistent symptoms of mood disturbance and irritability may be an early developmental presentation of bipolar disorder. Disruptive mood dysregulation, however, does not meet formal diagnostic criteria for mania in bipolar disorder, because irritability in disruptive mood dysregulation disorder is chronic and nonepisodic.

Oppositional Defiant Disorder

Disruptive mood dysregulation disorder is similar to oppositional defiant disorder in that they both include irritability, temper outbursts, and anger. Oppositional defiant disorder includes symptoms of annoyance and defiance, which disruptive mood dysregulation disorder does not have. Disruptive mood dysregulation disorder requires that irritable outbursts be present in at least two settings, whereas oppositional defiant disorder requires that they be present in only one setting.

COMORBIDITY

Disruptive mood dysregulation disorder often co-occurs with other psychiatric disorders. The most common comorbidities are ADHD (94 percent), oppositional defiant disorder (84 percent), anxiety disorders (47 percent), and major depressive disorder (20 percent). The relationship of severe mood dysregulation and disruptive mood dysregulation disorder to bipolar disorder has been a topic of clinical investigation. Some experts consider youths with severe mood dysregulation and hyperarousal symptoms to be part of the broad phenotype of pediatric bipolar disorder. However, the term "severe mood dysregulation" was utilized by researchers for these youth because it remains unclear whether these youth go on to meet the criteria for a bipolar disorder. Disruptive mood dysregulation disorder is not considered episodic and may coexist with ADHD. Current evidence does not support its continuity with an emerging bipolar disorder.

COURSE AND PROGNOSIS

Disruptive mood dysregulation disorder is a chronic disorder. Longitudinal studies thus far have shown that patients with disruptive mood dysregulation disorder in childhood have a high risk of progressing to major depressive disorder, dysthymic disorder, and anxiety disorders over time.

TREATMENT

The current treatment of disruptive mood dysregulation focuses on symptomatic interventions because we do not understand its etiology. If disruptive mood dysregulation disorder is confirmed to resemble unipolar depression and anxiety disorders in its pathophysiology, and it is often comorbid with ADHD, then SSRIs and stimulants would likely be the pharmacologic agents of first choice. However, if the pathophysiology of disruptive mood dysregulation disorder is like that of bipolar disorder, then first-line treatments for youth would include atypical antipsychotic agents and mood stabilizers. There are scant treatment studies of disruptive mood dysregulation disorder in the literature. One controlled trial of youths with symptoms of severe mood dysregulation and ADHD symptoms who did not respond to stimulants responded to sodium valproate combined with behavioral psychotherapy compared to placebo and behavioral psychotherapy. There are treatment studies underway of youth who exhibit symptoms of severe mood dysregulation utilizing an SSRI plus a stimulant compared to a stimulant and placebo.

Psychosocial interventions such as cognitive-behavioral psychotherapy are likely to be an essential component of treatment for youth with disruptive dysregulation disorder, and psychosocial interventions targeting children diagnosed with bipolar disorder may be beneficial.

EPIDEMIOLOGY

Most of the epidemiologic data applied to disruptive mood dysregulation disorder come from children and adolescents with severe mood dysregulation, which includes hyperarousal symptoms. Because disruptive mood dysregulation disorder differs from severe mood dysregulation disorder only in the absence of hyperarousal symptoms, the epidemiologic data from the severe mood dysregulation disorder studies is a useful proxy for disruptive mood dysregulation disorder. Severe mood dysregulation has a lifetime prevalence of 3 percent in children aged 9 to 19 years. Within that percentage, males (78 percent) are more prevalent than females (22 percent). The mean age of onset is 5 to 11 years of age.

▲ 2.12 Disruptive Behaviors of Childhood

Disruptive behaviors, especially oppositional patterns and aggressive behaviors, are among the most frequent reasons for child and adolescent psychiatric evaluation. Demonstration of impulsive and oppositional behaviors are developmentally normative in young children; many youths who continue to display excessive patterns in middle childhood will find other forms of expression as they mature and will no longer demonstrate these behaviors in adolescence or adulthood. The origin of stable patterns of oppositional defiant behavior is widely accepted as a convergence of multiple contributing factors, including biologic, temperamental, learned, and psychological conditions. Risk factors for the development of aggressive behavior in youth include childhood maltreatment such as physical or sexual abuse, neglect, emotional abuse, and overly harsh and punitive parenting.

OPPOSITIONAL DEFIANT DISORDER

Oppositional defiant disorder describes enduring patterns of negativistic, disobedient, and hostile behavior toward authority figures, as well as an inability to take responsibility for mistakes, leading to placing blame on others. Children with oppositional defiant disorder frequently argue with adults and become easily annoyed by others, leading to a state of anger and resentment. Children with oppositional defiant disorder may have difficulty in the classroom and with peer relationships, but generally do not resort to physical aggression or significantly destructive behavior.

In contrast, children with conduct disorder engage in severe, repeated acts of aggression that can cause physical harm to themselves and others and frequently violate the rights of others.

In oppositional defiant disorder, a child's temper outbursts, active refusal to comply with rules, and annoying behaviors exceed expectations for these behaviors for children of the same age. The disorder is an enduring pattern of negativistic, hostile, and defiant behaviors in the absence of significant violations of the rights of others.

Diagnosis and Clinical Features

Children with oppositional defiant disorder often argue with adults, lose their temper, and are angry, resentful, and easily annoyed by others at a level and frequency that is outside of the expected range for their age and developmental level. Frequently, youth with oppositional defiant disorder actively defy adults' requests or rules and deliberately annoy other persons. They tend to blame others for their own mistakes and misbehavior, more often than is appropriate for their developmental age. Manifestations of the disorder are almost invariably present in the home, but they may not be present at school or with other adults or peers. In some cases, the child has symptoms outside the home from the start; in others, it starts at home and later moves beyond that. Typically, symptoms of the disorder are most evident in interactions with adults or peers whom the child knows well. Thus, a child with oppositional defiant

disorder may not show signs of the disorder when examined clinically. Although children with oppositional defiant disorder may be aware that others disapprove of their behavior, they may still justify it as a response to unfair or unreasonable circumstances. The disorder appears to cause more distress to those around the child than to the child. Table 2-28 compares the diagnostic approaches to oppositional defiant disorder.

The DSM-5 has divided oppositional defiant disorder into three types: angry/irritable mood, argumentative/defiant behavior, and vindictiveness. A child may meet diagnostic criteria for oppositional defiant disorder with a 6-month pattern of at least four symptoms from the three types above. Angry/Irritable children with oppositional defiant disorder often lose their tempers, are easily annoyed, and feel irritable much of the time. Argumentative/Defiant children display a pattern of arguing with authority figures and adults such as parents, teachers, and relatives. Children with this type of oppositional defiant disorder actively refuse to comply with requests, deliberately break the rules, and purposely annoy others. These children often do not take responsibility for their actions, and often blame others for their misbehavior. Children with the Vindictive type of oppositional defiant disorder are spiteful and have shown vindictive or spiteful actions at least twice in 6 months to meet the diagnostic criteria.

Chronic oppositional defiant disorder or irritability almost always interferes with interpersonal relationships and school performance. Peers often reject these children, and they may become isolated and lonely. Despite adequate intelligence, they may do poorly or fail in school due to their lack of cooperation, reduced participation, and inability to accept help. Secondary to these difficulties are low self-esteem, poor frustration tolerance, depressed mood, and temper outbursts. Adolescents who are ostracized may turn to alcohol and illegal substances as a modality to fit in with peers. Chronically irritable children often develop mood disorders in adolescence or adulthood.

Pathology and Laboratory Examination.   No specific laboratory tests or pathologic findings help diagnose oppositional

Table 2-28
Oppositional Defiant Disorder

	DSM-5	ICD-10
Diagnostic name	Oppositional Defiant Disorder	Oppositional Defiant Disorder
Duration	≥6 mo For age <5: occurs more days than not For age ≥5: occurs at least 1/wk	
Symptoms	• Losing temper • Sensitive/easily annoyed • Angry/resentful • Arguing with authority figures • Refusing request from authorities or rules • Deliberately annoys others • Blames others for mistakes/behaviors • Spiteful/Vindictiveness (at least 2× in 6 mo)	Defined as a conduct disorder in younger children Predominant symptoms: • Disobedience • Defiance • Disruptive behavior
Required number of symptoms	≥4 symptoms	
Psychosocial consequences of symptoms	Marked distress and/or impairment	
Exclusions (not result of):	Substance use Another mental illness	No delinquent, severely aggressive or dissocial behaviors
Severity specifiers	**Mild:** symptoms in 1 setting **Moderate:** symptoms in 2 settings **Severe:** symptoms in ≥3 settings	

defiant disorder. Because some children with oppositional defiant disorder become physically aggressive and violate the rights of others as they age, they may share some characteristics with people with high levels of aggression, such as low CNS serotonin.

Differential Diagnosis

Oppositional behaviors are both healthy and adaptive within an expected range at specific developmental stages. We should distinguish periods of normative negativism from oppositional defiant disorder. Developmentally appropriate oppositional behavior is neither considerably more frequent nor more intense than that seen in other children of the same mental age. According to the DSM-5, we should not diagnose oppositional defiant disorder in the presence of disruptive mood dysregulation disorder. (See Section 2.11 for a further discussion of disruptive mood dysregulation disorder.)

Oppositional defiant behavior occurring temporarily in reaction to a stressor should be diagnosed as an adjustment disorder. When features of oppositional defiant disorder appear during conduct disorder, schizophrenia, or a mood disorder, we should not diagnose oppositional defiant disorder. Oppositional and negativistic behaviors can also be present in ADHD, cognitive disorders, and mental retardation. Whether we diagnose oppositional defiant disorder along with ADHD depends on the severity, pervasiveness, and duration of such behavior. Some young children who receive a diagnosis of oppositional defiant disorder go on in several years to meet the criteria for conduct disorder. Some investigators believe that the two disorders may be developmental variants of each other, with conduct disorder being the natural progression of oppositional defiant behavior when a child matures. Most children with oppositional defiant disorder, however, do not later meet the criteria for conduct disorder, and up to one-fourth of children with oppositional defiant disorder may not meet the diagnosis several years later.

The subtype of oppositional defiant disorder that tends to progress to conduct disorder is one in which aggression is prominent, for example, the Angry/Irritable type and the Vindictive type. Many children who have ADHD and oppositional defiant disorder develop conduct disorder before the age of 12 years. Many children who develop conduct disorder have a history of oppositional defiant disorder. Overall, the current consensus is that two subtypes of oppositional defiant disorder may exist. One type, which is likely to progress to conduct disorder, includes some symptoms of conduct disorder (e.g., fighting, bullying). The other type, which is characterized by less aggression and fewer antisocial traits, does not progress to conduct disorder. However, in either case, when both oppositional defiant disorder and conduct disorder are present, according to DSM-5, they may be diagnosed concurrently.

Jackson, age 8 years, was brought to the clinic for evaluation of irritability, negativity, and defiant behavior by his mother. She complained that he had frequent, prolonged tantrums, triggered by not "getting his way." Jackson's mother described the tantrums as consisting of shouting, cursing, crying, slamming doors, and sometimes throwing books or objects on the floor. Jackson had been having troubles in school as well, and his teacher had reported to the family that he seemed to have a habit of provoking other students as well as the teacher by making noises, rocking in his seat, and whistling in class. Recently, at home, Jackson was kicking his foot against his mother's chair, and she asked him to stop. He looked at her and continued to kick her chair until she became angry and sent him to his room. He then started yelling and stated that he wasn't doing anything and that his mother was just picking on him. Jackson's mother reported that she has given up on asking him to help with chores because it inevitably results in an argument. Jackson appeared sullen and irritable during the interview. He insisted that his problems are all his mother's fault, and she is always nagging him unfairly. During the interview with his mother, Jackson interrupted her several times to say that she was lying, and contradicted her story. Despite Jackson's behavioral problem, he has been able to succeed academically and scores highly on standardized tests. His mother reports that Jackson used to have some friends in kindergarten, but as he aged, he has lost almost all of his friends because he has difficulty sharing his things and tends to be bossy. Jackson's mother reports that ever since his sister was born when he was 2 years old, he has been aggressive and rivalrous toward her. Jackson's parents separated and divorced when he was 3. He has had no contact with his father since then. Jackson's mother was depressed for a year after the divorce until she sought treatment. She has always felt guilty that his father is not in his life, and Jackson blames her for not having his father around. She believes his behaviors have become worse since she recently started dating again.

Course and Prognosis

The course of oppositional defiant disorder depends on the severity of the symptoms and the ability of the child to develop more adaptive responses to authority. The stability of oppositional defiant disorder varies over time, with approximately 25 percent of children with the disorder no longer meeting diagnostic criteria. Persistence of oppositional defiant symptoms poses an increased risk of additional disorders, such as mood disorders, conduct disorder, and substance use disorders. Positive outcomes are more likely for intact families who can modify their expression of demands and give less attention to the child's argumentative behaviors.

An association exists between oppositional defiant disorder and ADHD, as well as with mood disorders. In children who have a long history of aggression and oppositional defiant disorder, there is a higher risk of the development of conduct disorder and later substance use disorders. Parental psychopathology, such as antisocial personality disorder and substance abuse, appears to be more common in families with children who have oppositional defiant disorder than in the general population, which creates additional risks for chaotic and troubled home environments. The prognosis for oppositional defiant disorder in a child depends somewhat on family functioning and the development of comorbid psychopathology.

Treatment

The primary treatment of oppositional defiant disorder is family intervention using both direct training of the parents in child management skills and careful assessment of family interactions. The goals of this intervention are to reinforce more prosocial behaviors and to diminish undesired behaviors at the same time. Cognitive-behavioral therapists emphasize teaching parents how to alter their behavior to discourage the child's oppositional behavior by diminishing attention to it, and Parent Child Interaction therapy focuses on selectively reinforcing and praising appropriate behavior and ignoring or not reinforcing undesired behavior.

Children with oppositional defiant behavior may also benefit from individual psychotherapy in which they role-play and "practice" more adaptive responses. In the therapeutic relationship, the child can learn new strategies to develop a sense of mastery and success in social situations with peers and families. In the safety of a more "neutral" relationship, children may discover that they are capable of less provocative behavior. Often, we must help restore the child's self-esteem must before they can make more positive responses to external control. Parent–child conflict strongly predicts conduct problems; patterns of harsh physical and verbal punishment, particularly evoke the emergence of aggression in children. Replacing harsh, punitive parenting and increasing positive parent–child interactions may positively influence the course of oppositional and defiant behaviors.

Epidemiology

Oppositional and negativistic behavior, in moderation, is developmentally normal in early childhood and adolescence. Epidemiologic studies of negativistic traits in nonclinical populations found such behavior in 16 to 22 percent of school-age children. Although oppositional defiant disorder can begin as early as 3 years of age, it typically is noted by 8 years of age and usually not later than early adolescence. Oppositional defiant disorder occurs at rates ranging from 2 to 16 percent with increased rates reported in boys before puberty, and an equal sex ratio reported after puberty. The prevalence of oppositional defiant behavior in males and females diminishes in youth older than 12 years of age.

Etiology

The most dramatic example of typical oppositional behavior peaks between 18 and 24 months, the "terrible twos," when toddlers are dramatically expressing their growing autonomy. Pathology begins when this developmental phase persists abnormally, authority figures overreact, or oppositional behavior recurs considerably more frequently than in most children of the same mental age. Among the criteria included in oppositional defiant disorder, irritability appears to be the one most predictive of later psychiatric disorders, whereas the other elements may be considered components of temperament.

Children exhibit a range of temperamental predispositions to strong will, stable preferences, or high assertiveness. Parents who model more extreme ways of expressing and enforcing their own will may contribute to the development of chronic struggles with their children, which the children then reenact with other authority figures. What begins for an infant as an effort to establish self-determination may become transformed into an exaggerated behavioral pattern. In late childhood, environmental trauma, illness, or chronic incapacity, such as mental retardation, can trigger oppositionality as a defense against helplessness, anxiety, and loss of self-esteem. Another normative oppositional stage occurs in adolescence as an expression of the need to separate from the parents and to establish an autonomous identity.

Classic psychoanalytic theory implicates unresolved conflicts as fueling defiant behaviors targeting authority figures. Behaviorists have observed that in children, oppositionality may be a reinforced, learned behavior through which a child exerts control over authority figures; for example, if having a temper tantrum when making a request of the child coerces the parents to withdraw their request, then tantrum behavior becomes strongly reinforced. Also, increased parental attention during a tantrum can reinforce the behavior.

CONDUCT DISORDER

Aggressive patterns of behavior are among the most frequent reasons psychiatrists see children and adolescents. Although the demonstration of impulsive behaviors is developmentally normative in children, many youths who continue to display excessive patterns of aggression in middle childhood generally require intervention. Children who develop enduring patterns of aggressive behaviors that begin in early childhood and violate the fundamental rights of peers and family members, however, may be destined for an entrenched pattern of conduct disordered behaviors over time. Controversy remains as to whether a set of "voluntary" behaviors can constitute a valid psychiatric disorder or whether it is more accurate to see them as maladaptive responses to adverse events, harsh or punitive parenting, or a threatening environment. Longitudinal studies have demonstrated that, for some youth, early patterns of disruptive behavior may become a lifelong pervasive repertoire culminating in adult antisocial personality disorder. The etiology of enduring patterns of aggressive behavior is widely accepted as a convergence of multiple contributing factors, including biologic, temperamental, learned, and psychological conditions. Risk factors for the development of aggressive behavior in youth include childhood maltreatment such as physical or sexual abuse, neglect, emotional abuse, and overly harsh and punitive parenting. Chronic exposure to violence in the media, including television, video games, and music videos, may promote lower levels of empathy in children, which may add a risk factor for the development of aggressive behavior.

Conduct disorder is an enduring set of behaviors in a child or adolescent that evolves, usually characterized by aggression and violation of the rights of others. Youth with conduct disorder often demonstrate behaviors in the following four categories: physical aggression or threats of harm to people, destruction of their property or that of others, theft or acts of deceit, and frequent violation of age-appropriate rules. Conduct disorder is associated with many other psychiatric disorders, including ADHD, depression, and learning disorders. It is also associated with certain psychosocial factors, including childhood maltreatment, harsh or punitive parenting, family discord, lack of appropriate parental supervision, lack of social competence, and low socioeconomic level. The DSM-5 criteria require three persistent specific behaviors of 15 conduct disorder symptoms listed, over the past 12 months, with at least one of them present in the past 6 months. Conduct disorder symptoms include bullying, threatening, or intimidating others, and staying out at night despite parental prohibition. DSM-5 also specifies that when truancy from school is a symptom, it begins before 13 years of age. The disorder may be diagnosed in a person older than 18 years only if the person does not meet the criteria for antisocial personality disorder.

DSM-5 includes specifiers denoting the severity of the disorder, including "mild" in which there are few conduct problems above those needed to make the diagnosis and behaviors cause only minor harm to others. In "moderate" cases, symptoms exceed the minimum; however, there is less confrontation that may cause harm to individuals than in "severe" cases. According to DSM-5, the "severe" level shows many conduct problems over the minimal diagnostic criteria or conduct problems that cause considerable harm to others. DSM-5 has also added the following specifier: "With limited prosocial emotions." For this, the individual must show a persistent interpersonal and emotional pattern that can be characterized by at least two of the following: (1) Lack of remorse or guilt, (2) callous lack of empathy, (3) unconcerned about performance, (4) shallow or deficient affect. Individuals with conduct disorder who qualify for this specifier are more likely to have a childhood-onset type and meet the criteria for a "severe" disorder. Children with conduct disorder engage in severe, repeated acts of aggression that can cause physical harm to themselves and others and frequently violate the rights of others. Children with conduct disorder usually have behaviors characterized by aggression to persons or animals, destruction of property, deceitfulness or theft, and multiple violations of rules, such as truancy from school. These behavioral patterns cause distinct difficulties in school life as well as in peer relationships. Conduct disorder has three subtypes based on the age of onset of the disorder. Childhood-onset subtype, in which at least one symptom has emerged repeatedly before age 10 years; adolescent-onset type, in which no characteristic persistent symptoms occur until after age 10 years; and unspecified-onset, in which age of onset is unknown. Although some young children show persistent patterns of behavior consistent with violating the rights of others or destroying property, the diagnosis of conduct disorder in children appears to increase with age. Epidemiologic surveys indicate that geographic locations representing a broad range of different cultures are not associated with significant variability in prevalence rates of either oppositional defiant disorder or conduct disorder. A longitudinal study of population density and antisocial behaviors in youth found no relationship in children 4 to 13 years of age between conduct problems and density of the living area. However, higher rates of conduct problems were self-reported by youths 10 to 17 years who lived in higher-density communities.

Diagnosis and Clinical Features

Conduct disorder does not develop overnight. Instead, many symptoms evolve until a consistent pattern develops that involves violating the rights of others. Very young children are unlikely to meet the criteria for the disorder because they are not developmentally able to exhibit the symptoms typical of older children with conduct disorder. A 3-year-old does not break into someone's home, steal with confrontation, force someone into sexual activity, or deliberately use a weapon that can cause serious harm. School-age children, however, can become bullies, initiate physical fights, destroy property, or set fires. Table 2-29 compares the diagnostic approaches to conduct disorder.

The average age of onset of conduct disorder is younger in boys than in girls. Boys most commonly meet the diagnostic criteria by 10 to 12 years of age, whereas girls met them closer to 14 to 16 years of age.

Children who meet the criteria for conduct disorder express their overt aggressive behavior in various forms. Aggressive antisocial

Table 2-29
Conduct Disorder

	DSM-5	ICD-10
Diagnostic name	Conduct Disorder	Conduct Disorder
Duration	≥1 criteria for ≥6 mo Other symptoms occur over ≥12 mo	≥6 mo
Symptoms	• Bullying others • Initiating physical fights • Using weapon to inflict serious harm • Physical cruelty to others • Physical cruelty to animals • Confronting and robbing someone • Forcing sex • Fire setting • Property damage • Breaking into properties • Lying for personal gain • Stealing valuable items • Staying out late against parent's will < age 13 • Running away from home ≥2 times (or once with prolonged absence) • Frequent truancy <age 13	Repeated and pervasive pattern of antisocial behavior • Aggression • Defiance May be • Angry • Cruel • Bullying • Destructive • Lying • Truant/running away from home
Required number of symptoms	≥3	
Exclusions (not result of):		Age appropriate behavior
Symptom specifiers	**With limited prosocial emotions:** demonstrating at least two of the following over 12 mo in multiple contexts: • *Lack of remorse or guilt* • *Callous—lack of empathy* • *Unconcerned about performance* • *Shallow or deficient affect*	Conduct disorder confined to the family context (within nuclear family) Unsocialized conduct disorder (predominant aggression, often toward other children) Socialized conduct disorder (despite aggression, there is good integration into their peer group)
Course specifiers	**Childhood onset type:** < age 10 **Adolescent onset type:** ≥ age 10 **Unspecified onset**	
Severity specifiers	**Mild:** minimal symptoms, minor harm/consequences **Moderate:** intermediate symptoms and consequences **Severe:** many symptoms, considerable harm caused	

behavior can take the form of bullying, physical aggression, and cruel behavior toward peers. Children may be hostile, verbally abusive, impudent, defiant, and negativistic toward adults. Persistent lying, frequent truancy, and vandalism are common. In severe cases, destructiveness, stealing, and physical violence often occur. Some adolescents make little effort to conceal their antisocial behavior. Sexual behavior and regular use of tobacco, liquor, or illicit psychoactive substances begin unusually early for such children and adolescents. Suicidal thoughts, gestures, and acts are frequent in children and adolescents with conduct disorder who are in conflict with peers, family members, or the law and are unable to problem-solve their difficulties.

Some children with aggressive behavioral patterns have impaired social attachments, as evidenced by their difficulties with peer relationships. Some may befriend a much older or younger person or have superficial relationships with other antisocial youngsters. Many children with conduct problems have poor self-esteem, although they may project an image of toughness. They may lack the skills to communicate in socially acceptable ways and appear to have little regard for the feelings, wishes, and welfare of others. Children and adolescents with conduct disorders often feel guilt or remorse for some of their behaviors, but try to blame others to avoid punishment.

Many children and adolescents with conduct disorder suffer from the deprivation of having few of their dependency needs met and may have had either overly harsh parenting or a lack of appropriate supervision. The deficient socialization of many children and adolescents with conduct disorder can be expressed in physical violation of others and, for some, in sexual violation of others. Severe punishments for behavior in children with conduct disorder almost invariably increase their maladaptive expression of rage and frustration rather than ameliorating the problem.

In evaluation interviews, children with aggressive conduct disorders are typically uncooperative, hostile, and provocative. Some have a superficial charm and compliance until they discuss their problem behaviors. Then, they often deny any problems. If the interviewer persists, the child may attempt to justify misbehavior or become suspicious and angry about the source of the examiner's information and perhaps bolt from the room. Most often, the child becomes angry with the examiner and expresses resentment of the examination with open belligerence or sullen withdrawal. Their hostility is not limited to adult authority figures, but they also direct it to their peers and younger children. They often bully those who are smaller and weaker. By boasting, lying, and expressing little interest in a listener's responses, such children reveal their lack of trust in adults to understand their position.

Evaluation of the family situation often reveals severe marital disharmony, which initially may center on disagreements about the management of the child. Because of a tendency toward family instability, parent surrogates are often in the picture. Children with conduct disorder are more likely to be unplanned or unwanted babies. The parents of children with conduct disorder, especially the father, have higher rates of antisocial personality disorder or alcohol use disorder. Aggressive children and their families show a stereotyped pattern of impulsive and unpredictable verbal and physical hostility. A child's aggressive behavior rarely seems directed toward any definable goal and offers little pleasure, success, or even sustained advantages with peers or authority figures.

In other cases, conduct disorder includes repeated truancy, vandalism, and physical severe aggression or assault against others by a gang, such as mugging, gang fighting, and beating. Usually, children who become part of a gang have the skills for age-appropriate friendships. They are likely to show concern for the welfare of their friends or their gang members and are unlikely to blame them or inform on them. In most cases, gang members have a history of adequate or even excessive conformity during early childhood that ended when the youngster became a member of the delinquent peer group, usually in preadolescence or during adolescence. Also present in history is some evidence of early problems, such as marginal or poor school performance, mild behavior problems, anxiety, and depressive symptoms. Some family social or psychological pathology is usually evident. Patterns of paternal discipline are rarely ideal and can vary from harshness and excessive strictness to inconsistency or relative absence of supervision and control. The mother has often protected the child from the consequences of early mild misbehavior but does not seem to encourage delinquency actively. Delinquency, also called juvenile delinquency, is most often associated with conduct disorder but can also result from other psychological or neurologic disorders.

Pathology and Laboratory Examination. No specific laboratory test or neurologic pathology helps make the diagnosis of conduct disorder. Some evidence indicates that amounts of certain neurotransmitters, such as serotonin in the CNS, are low in some persons with a history of violent or aggressive behavior toward others or themselves. Whether this association is related to the cause or is the effect of violence or is unrelated to the violence is not clear.

Differential Diagnosis

Disturbances of conduct, including impulsivity and aggression, may occur in many childhood psychiatric disorders, ranging from ADHD to oppositional defiant disorder, to disruptive mood dysregulation disorder, to major depression, to bipolar disorder, specific learning disorders, and psychotic disorders. Therefore, clinicians must obtain a comprehensive history of the chronology of the symptoms to determine whether the conduct disturbance is a transient or an enduring pattern. Isolated acts of aggressive behavior do not justify a diagnosis of conduct disorder; an entrenched pattern must be present. The relationship of conduct disorder to oppositional defiant disorder is still under debate. Typically, we think of oppositional defiant disorder as a mild precursor of conduct disorder, without the violation of rights, likely to be diagnosed in younger children who may be at risk for conduct disorder. Children who progress from oppositional defiant disorder to conduct disorder over time maintain their oppositional characteristics, and some evidence indicates that the two disorders are independent. Currently, in the DSM-5, oppositional defiant disorder and conduct disorder are considered distinct, but they can coexist. Many children with oppositional defiant disorder do not develop conduct disorder, and conduct disorder emerging in adolescence is not necessarily preceded by oppositional defiant disorder. The main distinguishing clinical feature between these two disorders is that in conduct disorder, the youths violate the fundamental rights of others, whereas, in oppositional defiant disorder, hostility and negativism fall short of seriously violating the rights of others.

Mood disorders are often present in children who exhibit irritability and aggressive behavior. We should rule out both major depressive disorder and bipolar disorder, but the full syndrome of conduct disorder can occur during the onset of a mood disorder. Substantial comorbidity exists between conduct disorder and depressive disorders. A recent report concludes that the high correlation between the two disorders arises from shared risk factors for both disorders rather than a causal relation. Thus, a series of factors, including family conflict, adverse life events, an early history of conduct disturbance, level of parental involvement, and affiliation with delinquent peers, contribute to the development of affective disorders and conduct disorder. This comorbidity is not the case with oppositional defiant disorder, which we cannot diagnose if it occurs exclusively during a mood disorder.

ADHD and learning disorders are commonly associated with conduct disorder. Usually, the symptoms of these disorders predate the diagnosis of conduct disorder. Substance use disorders are also more common in adolescents with conduct disorder than in the general population. Evidence indicates an association between fighting behaviors as a child and substance use as an adolescent. Once there is a pattern of drug use, this pattern may interfere with the development of positive mediators, such as social skills and problem-solving, which could enhance the remission of the conduct disorder. Thus, once substance abuse develops, it may promote the continuation of the conduct disorder. OCD also frequently seems to coexist with disruptive behavior disorders. All the disorders described here should be noted when they co-occur. Children with ADHD often exhibit impulsive and aggressive behaviors that may not meet the full criteria for conduct disorder.

Damien, age 12 years, was referred for psychiatric evaluation after being picked up by police for truancy and running away from home. Damien explained that he just wanted to get out of his house and see his friends. He does not like to be at home because his mother tries to tell him what to do. Damien's mother says that he left and stayed out overnight multiple times in the past year, but that he usually returns the next morning. She complains that he is always in trouble. He has shoplifted on several occasions that she knows of, the first time at age 8 years. She suspects that he also steals from neighbors or school. The police have been involved on many occasions, including for truancy, staying out all night, stealing from a neighborhood store, and smoking marijuana. Damien has a quick temper, and his mother knows he was involved in several fights over the past year in the neighborhood. Damien is particularly cruel to his younger brother, continually taunting and teasing him.

Damien's mother stated that he continually lies, sometimes for no apparent reason. When he was 6 years of age, he was fascinated with fire and set several small fires at home, fortunately with no serious injury or damage. Damien's mother was tearful when she disclosed that Damien is just like his no-good father and that she wished she never had him. Damien initially refused to answer questions and turned away scowling, but gradually began to talk. Damien presented a tough image with an indifferent attitude toward the interviewer. Damien denied any abuse at home, saying that he ran off because he was bored. However, upon further questioning, Damien admitted that his mother's previous boyfriend, who was in the home when Damien was between 6 and 8 years of age, used to hit him with a belt when he got out of line. Damien justified his behaviors as just having fun. He said others provoked the fights. Damien also denied using weapons, although he bragged about breaking the nose of another youth.

Damien's school records indicate that he required an Individualized Educational Plan (IEP) when he was in the second grade and was evaluated for symptoms of ADHD when he was in first grade. His psychiatrist prescribed methylphenidate; however, the family did not continue with treatment, and he is currently on no medication. Damien is currently in sixth-grade special education classes, having failed and repeated fifth grade. Damien's grades are failing, and he may have to repeat sixth grade. Damien admits to truancy on several occasions this year in addition to his problems with completing schoolwork. His previous evaluation indicates that child protective services evaluated the family for possible neglect when he was 5 years of age after he and his brother were found barefoot on the street late one evening without his mother. Damien's family was referred for counseling and never

attended. Both Damien's parents have a history of drug and alcohol abuse. Damien's birth was unplanned, and his mother used drugs during pregnancy. His parents separated soon after his birth, and his mother returned to live with her parents briefly. Damien and his mother moved to live with her boyfriend when Damien was 1 year of age after she became pregnant with his younger brother. Damien's mother's relationship ended within a year, and only Damien, his mother, and his brother live in their apartment. Damien's mother has worked several different jobs, and Damien wonders if she has a drinking problem.

Comorbidity

ADHD and conduct disorder often coexist, with ADHD often predating the development of conduct disorder, and not infrequently substance abuse. CNS injury, dysfunction, or damage predispose a child to impulsivity and behavioral disturbances, which sometimes evolve into conduct disorder.

Course and Prognosis

Negative prognostic signs for conduct disorder include young age, high number of symptoms, and severe symptoms. This finding is true partly because those with severe conduct disorder seem to be most vulnerable to comorbid disorders later in life, such as mood disorders and substance use disorders. A longitudinal study found that, although assaultive behavior in childhood and parental criminality predict a high risk for incarceration later in life, the diagnosis of conduct disorder does not correlate with imprisonment. Mild symptoms, no coexisting psychopathology, and normal intellectual functioning are good prognostic signs.

Treatment

Psychosocial Interventions.   Early sustained preventive interventions (e.g., at a kindergarten age) can significantly alter the course and prognosis of aggressive behavior. A screening program used with kindergarteners predicted lifetime disruptive behavior disorder by age 18 years, with the highest risk group demonstrating an 82 percent chance of a disruptive behavior diagnosis without intervention. One prevention program, *the Fast Track Preventive Intervention,* randomized 891 kindergarteners to either a 10-year prevention program or a control condition. The 10-year intervention included parent behavior management, child social cognitive skills, reading, home visiting, mentoring, and classroom curricula. The children in the Fast Track Intervention were less likely to develop conduct disorder during those 10 years and for 2 years after that.

A meta-analysis of controlled trials of CBT programs indicates that CBT can result in significant reductions in conduct-disordered symptoms in children and adolescents. CBT treatment interventions that are proven to be efficacious include the following:

Kazdin's Problem-Solving Skills Training (PSST) in which a 12-week sequential program helps children develop problem-solving solutions when faced with conflictual situations. Assignments called "supersolvers" provide vignette situations in which children can practice these techniques. Therapists can add a companion program, Parent Management Training (PMT), to the intervention, but PSST can be useful even without the parent component. Another CBT-based intervention, the Incredible Years (IY), targeting young children from 3 to 8 years, is administered over 22 weeks and delivers sessions to the child and has a parent training component and a teacher training. Another CBT-based intervention is the Anger Coping Program, an 18-session intervention for school-age children in grades 4 to 6 focused on a child's increased development of emotion recognition and regulation, and managing anger. Anger coping strategies include distraction, self-talk, perspective taking, goal setting, and problem-solving.

Overall, treatment programs have been more successful in decreasing overt symptoms of conduct, such as aggression, than the covert symptoms, such as lying or stealing. Treatment strategies for young children that focus on increasing social behavior and social competence reduce aggressive behavior. In one study, 548 third graders were administered a school-based intervention instead of a regular health curriculum in several public schools in North Carolina, called *Making Choices: Social Problem Solving Skills for Children* (MC), along with supplemental teacher and parent components. Compared with third graders receiving the routine health curriculum, children exposed to the MC program were rated lower on the posttest social and overt aggression, and higher on social competence. Also, they scored higher on information-processing skills. These findings support the notion that school-based prevention programs have the potential to strengthen social and emotional skills and diminish aggressive behavior among normal populations of school-age children. School settings can also use behavioral techniques to promote socially acceptable behavior toward peers and to discourage covert antisocial incidents.

Psychopharmacologic Interventions. The efficacy of psychopharmacologic interventions includes several placebo-controlled studies of risperidone for aggression in youth associated with disruptive behavior disorders or mental retardation. Also, risperidone is superior to placebo in reducing aggressive behavior in a large 6-month placebo-substitution study. One randomized, double-blind placebo-controlled trial with quetiapine also showed efficacy for aggressive behavior. Early studies of antipsychotics, most notably haloperidol, reported decreased aggressive and assaultive behaviors in children with a variety of psychiatric disorders. Atypical antipsychotics risperidone, olanzapine, quetiapine, ziprasidone, and aripiprazole have generally replaced the older antipsychotics in clinical practice due to their comparable efficacy and improved side effect profiles. Side effects of second-generation antipsychotics include sedation, increased prolactin levels (with risperidone use), and extrapyramidal symptoms, including akathisia. In general, however, the atypical antipsychotics appear to be well tolerated. A study of sodium valproate in youth with conduct disorder showed that those who responded most robustly exhibited aggression characterized by agitation, dysphoria, and distress. Although early trials suggested that carbamazepine was useful to control aggression, a double-blind, placebo-controlled study did not show the superiority of carbamazepine over placebo in decreasing aggression. A pilot study found that clonidine may decrease aggression. The SSRIs, including fluoxetine, sertraline, paroxetine, and citalopram, are used clinically to target symptoms of impulsivity, irritability, and mood lability, which frequently accompany conduct disorder. Conduct disorder often coexists with ADHD, learning disorders, and, over time, mood disorders, and substance-related disorders; thus, we also need to treat concurrent disorders.

Epidemiology

In the United States, conduct disorder ranges from 6 to 16 percent for males, and from 2 to 9 percent for females. The ratio of conduct disorder in males compared to females ranges from 4:1 to as much as 12:1. Conduct disorder occurs with higher frequency in the children of parents with antisocial personality disorder and alcohol use disorder than in the general population. The prevalence of conduct disorder and antisocial behavior is associated with socioeconomic factors, as well as parental psychopathology.

Etiology

A meta-analysis of longitudinal studies indicates that the most critical risk factors that predict conduct disorder include impulsivity, physical or sexual abuse or neglect, poor parental supervision and harsh and punitive parental discipline, low IQ, and poor school achievement.

Parental Factors. Harsh, punitive parenting characterized by severe physical and verbal aggression is associated with the development of children's maladaptive aggressive behaviors. Chaotic home conditions are associated with conduct disorder and delinquency. Divorce itself is not necessarily a risk factor, but the persistence of hostility, resentment, and bitterness between divorced parents may be the more significant contributor to maladaptive behavior. Parental psychopathology, child abuse, and negligence often contribute to conduct disorder. Sociopathy, alcohol use disorder, and substance use disorder in the parents are associated with conduct disorder in their children. Parents may be so negligent that a child's care is shared by relatives or assumed by foster parents. Many such parents were scarred by their upbringing and tended to be abusive, negligent, or engrossed in getting their personal needs met.

Studies indicate that parents of children with conduct disorder have high rates of severe psychopathology, including psychotic disorders. Data show that children who exhibit a pattern of aggressive behavior often experience physically or emotionally harsh parenting.

Genetic Factors. A study of more than 6,000 male, female, and opposite-sex twins found that genetic and environmental factors accounted for proportionally the same amount of variance in males and females. Genetic or shared environmental factors exert different effects on males and females in childhood conduct disorder, but by adulthood, the gender-specific influences on antisocial behavior are no longer apparent. The sex-specific effects on antisocial behavior in youth along with the replicated finding of a potential role for the X-linked monoamine oxidase A gene in the etiology of antisocial behavior leads to the need for further genetic investigation of conduct disorder on the X chromosome and for analyses of these behaviors to be done separately by gender.

Sociocultural Factors. Youth living in population-dense areas have higher rates of aggression and delinquency. Unemployed parents, lack of a supportive social network, and lack of positive participation in community activities seem to predict conduct disorder. Associated findings that may influence the development of conduct disorder in urban areas are exposure to and prevalence of substance use. A survey of alcohol use and mental health in adolescents found that weekly alcohol use among adolescents is associated with increased delinquent and aggressive behavior. Significant interactions between frequent alcohol use and age indicated that those adolescents with weekly alcohol use at younger ages were most likely to exhibit aggressive behaviors and mood disorders. Although drug and alcohol use does not cause conduct disorder, it increases the risks associated with it. Drug intoxication itself can also aggravate the symptoms. Thus, all factors that increase the likelihood of regular substance use may promote and expand the disorder.

Violent Video Games and Violent Behavior.   Longitudinal studies corroborate the contribution of media violence, including video gaming in middle-school children, with the expression of aggression in those adolescents. A review of the literature on the effect of violent video games on children and adolescents revealed that violent video game playing is related to aggressive affect, physiologic arousal, and aggressive behaviors. It stands to reason that the degree of exposure to violent games and the more restriction of activity would be related to a greater preoccupation with violent themes.

Psychological Factors.   Poor emotion regulation among youth is associated with higher rates of aggression and conduct disorder. Emotion regulation is associated with social competence and can be observed even in children of preschool age—those children with greater degrees of emotion dysregulation exhibit higher levels of aggression. Poor modeling of impulse control and the chronic lack of having their own needs met leads to a less developed sense of empathy.

Neurobiologic Factors.   Neuroimaging studies utilizing MRI have used voxel-based morphometry methods to compare structural brain differences between children with conduct disorder compared to healthy controls. Studies have reported that children with conduct disorder had decreased gray matter in limbic brain structures and the bilateral anterior insula and left amygdala compared to healthy controls. A study investigated structural brain differences in children comorbid for oppositional defiant disorder or conduct disorder and ADHD compared to those with ADHD alone and healthy controls. Findings included decreased gray matter in ADHD and ADHD comorbid for oppositional defiant disorder or conduct disorder compared to controls in regions including bilateral temporal and occipital cortices and the left amygdala.

Neurotransmitter studies in children with conduct disorder suggest a low level of plasma dopamine β-hydroxylase, an enzyme that converts dopamine to norepinephrine, leading to a hypothesis of decreased noradrenergic functioning in conduct disorder. Other studies of conduct-disordered juvenile offenders have found high plasma serotonin levels in the blood. Evidence indicates that blood serotonin levels correlate inversely with levels of 5-HIAA in the CSF and that low 5-HIAA levels in CSF correlate with aggression and violence.

NEUROLOGIC FACTORS.   An EEG study investigating resting frontal brain electrical activity, emotional intelligence, aggression, and rule-breaking in 10-year-old children found that aggressive children had significantly higher relative right frontal brain activity at rest compared with nonaggressive children. Frontal resting brain electrical activity likely reflects the ability to regulate emotion. Boys tended to show lower emotional intelligence than girls and more significant aggressive behavior than girls. No relationship, however, was found between emotional intelligence and pattern of frontal EEG activation.

Child Abuse and Maltreatment.   Evidence shows that children chronically exposed to violence, physical or sexual abuse, and neglect, particularly at a young age, are at high risk for demonstrating aggression. A study of female caregivers exposed to intimate partner violence revealed a strong association with offspring aggression and mood disturbance. Severely abused children and adolescents tend to be hypervigilant; in some cases, they misperceive benign situations as directly threatening and respond

defensively with violence. Not all expressed aggressive behavior in adolescents is synonymous with conduct disorder; however, youth with a repetitive pattern of hypervigilance and violent responses are likely to violate the rights of others.

▲ 2.13 Anxiety Disorders of Infancy, Childhood, and Adolescence: Separation Anxiety Disorder, Generalized Anxiety Disorder, and Social Anxiety Disorder (Social Phobia)

Anxiety disorders are among the most common disorders in youth, affecting 10 to 20 percent of children and adolescents. Although observable anxiety behaviors mark normative development in infants, anxiety disorders in childhood predict a wide range of psychological difficulties in adolescence, including additional anxiety disorders, panic attacks, and depressive disorders. Fear is an expected response to a real or perceived threat; however, anxiety is the anticipation of future danger. The main characteristic of all the anxiety disorders is a recurrent emotional and physiologic arousal in response to excessive perceptions of perceived threat or danger. Anxiety disorders commonly found in youth include separation anxiety disorder, generalized anxiety disorder, social anxiety disorder, and selective mutism. We classify them by how the anxiety is experienced, the situations that trigger it, and the course that it tends to follow.

Separation anxiety disorder, generalized anxiety disorder, and social anxiety disorder in children are often considered together in the evaluation process and differential diagnosis, and in developing treatment strategies, because they are highly comorbid and have overlapping symptoms. A child with separation anxiety disorder, generalized anxiety disorder, or social anxiety disorder has a 60 percent chance of having at least one of the other two disorders as well. Of children with one of the above anxiety disorders, 30 percent have all three of them. Children and adolescents may also have additional comorbid anxiety disorders such as specific phobia or panic disorder. Separation anxiety disorder, generalized anxiety disorder, and social anxiety disorder are distinguished from each other by the types of situations that elicit excessive anxiety and avoidance behaviors.

SEPARATION ANXIETY DISORDER

Separation anxiety is a universal human developmental phenomenon emerging in infants younger than 1 year of age and marking a child's awareness of separation from his or her mother or primary caregiver. Normative separation anxiety peaks between 9 and 18 months and will diminish by about 2½ years of age, enabling young children to develop a sense of comfort away from their parents in preschool. Separation anxiety or stranger anxiety most likely evolved as a human response that has survival value. The expression of transient separation anxiety is also typical in young children entering school for the first time. Approximately 15 percent of young children display intense and persistent fear, shyness, and social withdrawal when faced with unfamiliar settings and people. Young children with this pattern of significant behavioral inhibition are at higher risk for the development of separation anxiety disorder, generalized anxiety disorder, and social anxiety disorder. Behaviorally inhibited children, as a group, exhibit characteristic physiologic traits, including higher than average resting heart rates, higher morning cortisol levels than average, and low heart rate variability. Separation anxiety disorder is developmentally inappropriate and excessive anxiety related to separation from the primary attachment figure. According to the DSM-5, separation anxiety disorder is a level of fear or anxiety regarding separation from their parents or primary caregiver which is beyond developmental expectations.

Furthermore, there may be a pervasive worry that harm will come to a parent upon separation, which leads to extreme distress and sometimes nightmares. The DSM-5 requires the presence of at least three symptoms related to excessive worry about separation from a significant attachment figure for at least 4 weeks. The worries often take the form of refusal to go to school, fears, and distress on separation, repeated complaints of physical symptoms such as headaches and stomachaches when anticipating separation, and nightmares related to separation issues.

GENERALIZED ANXIETY DISORDER

Children with generalized anxiety disorder have significant distress in activities of daily life, often focused on the child's fears of incompetence in many areas, including school performance and in social settings. Also, children with generalized anxiety disorder, according to DSM-5, experience at least one of the following symptoms: restlessness, being easily fatigued, "mind going blank," irritability, muscle tension, or sleep disturbance. Children with generalized anxiety disorder tend to feel fearful in multiple settings and expect more negative outcomes when faced with academic or social challenges, compared with peers. Children and adolescents with generalized anxiety disorder may experience symptoms of autonomic hyperarousal such as tachycardia, shortness of breath, or dizziness, and are more likely than nonanxious youth to experience sweating, nausea, or diarrhea when they become anxious. Children and adolescents with generalized anxiety disorder tend to be overly concerned about potential natural disasters such as earthquakes or floods, and these worries can interfere with their daily activities. Finally, children and adolescents with generalized anxiety disorder are continuously worried about the quality of their performance in academics, sports, and other activities, and often seek excessive reassurance about their performance.

SOCIAL ANXIETY DISORDER (SOCIAL PHOBIA)

Children who experience intense discomfort and distress in social situations and are impaired by their fear of scrutiny or humiliation have the diagnosis of social anxiety disorder. Their distress may be expressed in the form of crying, tantrums, avoidance, freezing, or even becoming "mute" in these situations. According to DSM-5, this disorder is characterized by consistent anxiety and distress in almost all social situations. Any situation in which the child feels exposed to possible scrutiny by others can provoke fear or anxiety, and the child will often try to avoid these feared social situations. Children must experience anxiety in the presence of peers, not only with adults, in order to receive the diagnosis. A child or adolescent with social anxiety disorder may exhibit the performance only type, which targets a specific type of performing, such as fear of public speaking. The performance-only type typically manifests in school or academic settings in which one must perform public presentations, such as in front of classmates in school.

Social anxiety disorder has significant implications for future accomplishments, since it is associated with lower levels of satisfaction in leisure activities, increased rates of school dropout, less productivity in the workplace as adults, and increased rates of remaining single. Despite the significant impairment caused by social anxiety disorder, up to half of the individuals with the disorder do not receive treatment.

DIAGNOSIS AND CLINICAL FEATURES

Separation anxiety disorder, generalized anxiety disorder, and social anxiety disorder are highly related in children and adolescence because, in most children, overlapping symptoms, as well as comorbid disorders, emerge. Generalized anxiety disorder is the most common anxiety disorder among youth, more common in adolescents than in younger children; in almost one-third of these cases, a child with generalized anxiety disorder also exhibits separation anxiety disorder and social anxiety disorder.

Diagnostic criteria for separation anxiety disorder, according to the DSM-5, include three of the following symptoms for at least 4 weeks: persistent and excessive worry about losing, or possible harm befalling, significant attachment figures; persistent and excessive worry that an untoward event can lead to separation from a significant attachment figure; persistent reluctance or refusal to go to school or elsewhere because of fear of separation; persistent and excessive fear or reluctance to be alone or without major attachment figures at home or without significant adults in other settings; persistent reluctance or refusal to go to sleep without being near a major attachment figure or to sleep away from home; repeated nightmares involving the theme of separation; repeated complaints of physical symptoms, including headaches and stomachaches, when separation from significant attachment figures is anticipated; and recurrent excessive distress when separation from home or significant attachment figures is anticipated or involved. Table 2-30 lists the criteria for separation anxiety disorder.

The following case history demonstrates separation anxiety disorder along with autonomic arousal symptoms.

Jake was a 9-year-old boy who was referred for outpatient evaluation by his family physician. He refused to sleep in his room alone at night and exhibited violent tantrums each morning in order to avoid going to school. Jake expressed recurrent fears that something terrible would happen to his mother. He worried that she would get into a car accident or that there would be a fire at home, and his mother would die. Developmental history revealed that Jake was anxious and irritable as an infant and toddler. He had trouble adjusting to babysitters in the preschool years. There was a history of panic disorder, agoraphobia in the mother, and major depression in his father. Jake became more concerned and territorial over his mother when his father left the family, and his mother became depressed. Jake always kept track of his mother's whereabouts and insisted that she stay at home.

Nighttime was a particularly difficult time at home. When Jake's mother tried to get Jake to remain in his room, Jake would whine and cry and insist that his mother lie in bed with him until he is asleep. He also expected his mother to sleep across the hall from his room throughout the evening. Jake's mother reported that each evening her son would get up and peek through the crack in her bedroom door, as frequently as every 10 minutes, to be sure that she was still there. Jake reported frequent nightmares that his mother died and that monsters prevented him from rescuing his mother, taking him away from his family forever.

Table 2-30
Separation Anxiety Disorder

	DSM-5	ICD-10
Diagnostic name	Separation Anxiety Disorder	Separation Anxiety Disorder of Childhood
Duration	Children: ≥4 wk Adults: ≥6 mo	
Symptoms	Inappropriate fear of separation from a loved one or attachment figure: • Distressed when separated or anticipating separation • Worries about losing them or harm coming to them • Worry about possible forced separation • Hesitant to leave person or home • Fears being alone, without the person • Needs to be near that person to sleep • Nightmares about separation • Physical symptoms of anxiety when separated or anticipating separation	• Fear of separation causes anxiety • Anxiety during early childhood • Severity is inappropriate to situations and stage of development
Required number of symptoms	≥3	
Psychosocial consequences of symptoms	Marked distress and/or psychosocial impairment	Impaired functioning
Exclusions (not result of):	Another mental disorder	
Comments		Note: classified as an Emotional disorder with onset specific to childhood

During the daytime, Jake would shadow his mother around the house. Jake would agree to play a game with his sister in the lower level of the house only if his mother was nearby. When Jake's mother went upstairs, he would interrupt the game and follow her upstairs. He refused to sleep at a friend's house. Frequently, at home, as the evening progressed, Jake described a queasy sensation in his stomach mixed with feelings of sadness.

On school days, Jake usually complained of stomachaches and tried to stay home. Jake appeared distressed and panicky and would become violent when his mother attempted to drop him off at school. Once at school, he seemed calmer and less distressed, but frequently was seen in the nurse's office, complaining of nausea and seeking to be sent home. (Adapted from case material from Gail A. Bernstein, M.D. and Anne E. Layne, Ph.D.)

The essential feature of separation anxiety disorder is extreme anxiety precipitated by separation from parents, home, or other familiar surroundings. In contrast, in generalized anxiety disorder, fears are extended to adverse outcomes for all kinds of events, including academics, peer relationships, and family activities. In generalized anxiety disorder, a child or adolescent experiences at least one recurrent physiologic symptom, such as restlessness, poor concentration, irritability, or muscle tension. In social anxiety disorder, the child's fears peak during performance situations involving exposure to unfamiliar people or situations. Children and adolescents with social anxiety disorder have extreme concerns about being embarrassed, humiliated, or negatively judged. In each of the preceding anxiety disorders, the child's experience can approach terror or panic. The distress is higher than that normally expected for the child's developmental level and is not otherwise explainable. Morbid fears, preoccupations, and ruminations characterize separation anxiety disorder. Children with anxiety disorders overestimate the probability of danger and the likelihood of a negative outcome. Children with separation anxiety disorder and generalized anxiety disorder become overly fearful that someone close to them will be hurt or that something terrible will happen to them or their families, especially when they are away from their families. Many children with anxiety disorders are preoccupied with health and worry that their families or friends will become ill. Fears of getting lost, being kidnapped, and losing the ability to be in contact with their families are predominant among children with separation anxiety disorder.

Adolescents with anxiety disorders may not directly express their worries; however, their behavioral patterns often reflect either separation anxiety or other anxiety if they exhibit discomfort about leaving home, engage in solitary activities because of fears about how they will perform in front of peers, or have distress when away from their families. Separation anxiety disorder in children is often manifested at the thought of travel or in the course of travel away from home. Children may refuse to go to camp, a new school, or even a friend's house. Frequently, a continuum exists between mild anticipatory anxiety before separation to pervasive anxiety after the separation has occurred. Premonitory signs include irritability, difficulty eating, whining, staying in a room alone, clinging to parents, and following a parent everywhere. Often, when a family moves, a child displays separation anxiety by intense clinging to the mother figure. Sometimes, geographical relocation anxiety causes feelings of acute homesickness or psychophysiological symptoms that break out when the child is away from home or is going to a new country. The child yearns to return home and becomes preoccupied with fantasies of how much better the old home was. Integration into the new life situation may become extremely difficult. Children with anxiety disorders may retreat from social or group activities and express feelings of loneliness because of their self-imposed isolation.

Sleep difficulties are frequent in children and adolescents with any anxiety disorder or in severe separation anxiety; a child or adolescent may require having someone remain with him or her until he or she falls asleep. An anxious child may awaken and go to a parent's bed or even sleep at the parents' door to diminish anxiety. Nightmares and morbid fears may be expressions of anxiety.

Associated features of most anxiety disorders include fear of the dark and imaginary worries. Children may have the feeling that eyes are staring at them and monsters are reaching out for them in their bedrooms. Children with separation anxiety disorder, generalized anxiety disorder, and social anxiety disorder often complain of somatic symptoms and may be more sensitive to changes in their bodies compared to youth without anxiety disorders. Children with separation anxiety disorder, generalized anxiety disorder, or social anxiety disorder are often more emotionally sensitive than peers and more easily brought to tears. Frequent somatic complaints accompanying anxiety disorders include gastrointestinal symptoms, nausea, vomiting, and stomachaches; unexplained pain in various parts of the body; sore throats; and flu-like symptoms. Older children and adolescents typically complain of somatic experiences classically reported by adults with anxiety, such as cardiovascular and respiratory symptoms—palpitations, dizziness, faintness, and feelings of strangulation. Physiologic signs of anxiety are a part of the diagnostic criteria for generalized anxiety disorder, but they are more often also experienced by children with separation anxiety and social anxiety disorder than the general population. The following case history demonstrates a young adolescent with generalized anxiety disorder.

Rachel was a 13-year-old girl referred for an evaluation by her pediatrician based on her chronic gastrointestinal complaints without any organic illness. In the interview, Rachel appeared withdrawn and meek but responsive to questions. She endorsed several worries that included concerns about her health, her parents' safety, her school performance, and her peer relationships. Rachel's most significant worries were related to her health and safety. Rachel's mother reported that Rachel had recently been very reluctant to play outside because she feared she would contract Lyme disease from a tick bite or West Nile virus from a mosquito bite. Rachel was also very distressed by news reports about catastrophic events locally and around the world (e.g., kidnapping, crime, terrorism). Her family and teachers described Rachel as overly conscientious about her schoolwork and as often being concerned about adult matters (e.g., finances, parents' job security). Symptoms that accompanied Rachel's worries primarily involved stomach pain and problems with falling asleep. Rachel tended to be quite perseverative, repetitively verbalizing her worries even after receiving reassurance. Rachel admitted that she worried for hours each day and could not "turn off" her worried thoughts.

Rachel was the product of a healthy pregnancy and delivery. Her medical history was unremarkable, except for frequent gastrointestinal pain since kindergarten. Rachel was described as irritable and difficult to soothe as an infant. Her developmental milestones were within normal limits. She was described as very obedient and had no history of externalizing behavior problems. She was very concerned about her academic performance from an early age and earned A's with an occasional B. Rachel was somewhat shy in social situations but well-liked by her peers. Family history included depression in her maternal grandmother and a maternal history of generalized anxiety disorder, social anxiety, and separation anxiety disorder as a child. Rachel had two younger siblings who were high achievers and without notable problems. (Adapted from case material from Gail A. Bernstein, M.D. and Ann E. Layne, Ph.D.)

The next case history demonstrates an adolescent with multiple anxiety and depressive disorders.

Kate is a 15-year-old tenth grader who lives with her biologic parents and two sisters, ages 9 and 14 years. Kate is a very articulate teen who has always been a good student, although she never volunteers answers in school unless her teachers call on her. She gets along well with her sisters when at home, but ever since she entered high school in the ninth-grade year, she declines invitations to go to friends' homes, has turned down opportunities to go to parties, and has even stopped going on outings with her sisters to the neighborhood mall and the movies. Kate reports that she gets too nervous and blushes when she is with friends outside of the classroom at school because she cannot think of anything to say to them. She reports that she is embarrassed to go shopping or to the movies with her sisters because they often run into neighborhood peers along the way and stop to chat, and this makes her feel "stupid," because even though she is the oldest, she does not say anything and believes that her sisters' friends will laugh at her shyness. Recently, one of her former best friends confronted her about why she had stopped "hanging out" with her friends. Kate had stopped eating lunch with her friends in school because she felt humiliated when they would talk about their weekend plans, and even when they invited her to join, she would just look the other way and ignore the conversation. Kate had become isolated, even in school, and admitted to her sister that she was lonely. Kate was brought for an evaluation after her younger sister commented to her mother that Kate spent all of her time alone whenever her sisters saw their friends and that she looked sad and stressed out whenever she was around peers. Kate was down, always in poor spirits, and had stopped interacting with her sisters. On rare occasions, Kate's younger sister had invited Kate to parties or friend's homes, but Kate had declined and burst into tears.

Kate was evaluated by a child psychiatrist who made the diagnoses of social anxiety disorder, generalized anxiety disorder, and major depression and recommended a combination of treatment options, including cognitive-behavioral therapy and a trial of fluoxetine. Kate and her family decided to try the medication first. Kate started 10 mg of fluoxetine, and over the next month was titrated to a dose of 20 mg. By the third week of the medication trial, Kate was noticeably less resistant to going out with her sisters to places where they were likely to encounter peers. Her sisters noticed that she did not seem as stressed and started to sit with peers at lunch in the school cafeteria occasionally. She stated that she did not feel as self-conscious as she used to in class and was willing to go to a friend's house. She still declined to go to a birthday party of a peer that she did not know very well. Kate continued on the same medication, and within 2 months, she was significantly less anxious in social situations. She occasionally complained of a stomachache but tolerated the medication well. Her family was impressed when she requested they plan a birthday party for her 16th birthday and decided to invite 10 friends.

Pathology and Laboratory Examination

No specific laboratory measures help in the diagnosis of separation anxiety disorder, generalized anxiety disorder, or social anxiety disorder.

DIFFERENTIAL DIAGNOSIS

The presence of separation anxiety is a developmentally expected feature in a young child and often does not represent an impairing condition. Thus clinical judgment must be used in distinguishing normal anxiety from separation anxiety disorder in this age group. In older school-age children, a child experiencing more than normal distress is apparent when refusing school regularly. For children who resist school, it is essential to distinguish whether fear

Table 2-31
Common Characteristics in Childhood Anxiety Disorders

Criteria	Separation Anxiety Disorder	Social Anxiety Disorder	Generalized Anxiety Disorder
Minimum duration to establish diagnosis	At least 4 wk	Persistent, typically at least 6 mo	At least 6 mo
Precipitating stressors	Separation from home or attachment figures	Social situations with peers or other specific situations	Pressure for any type of performance, activities which are scored, school performance
Peer relationships	Good when no separation is involved	Tentative, overly inhibited	May appear overly eager to please, peers sought out for reassurance
Sleep	Reluctance or refusal to sleep away from home or not near attachment figure	May experience insomnia	Often difficulty falling asleep
Psychophysiological symptoms	Stomachaches, headaches nausea, vomiting, palpitations, dizziness when anticipating separation	May exhibit blushing, inadequate eye contact, soft voice, or rigid posture	Stomachaches, nausea, lump in the throat, shortness of breath, dizziness, palpitations when anticipating performing an activity
Differential diagnosis	GAD, Soc AD, major depressive disorder, panic disorder with agoraphobia, PTSD, oppositional defiant disorder	GAD, SAD, major depressive disorder, dysthymic disorder, selective mutism, agoraphobia	SAD, Soc AD, attention-deficit/hyperactivity disorder, obsessive-compulsive disorder, major depressive disorder, PTSD

GAD, generalized anxiety disorder; Soc AD, social anxiety disorder; SAD, separation anxiety disorder; PTSD, posttraumatic stress disorder.
Adapted from Sidney Werkman, M.D.

of separation, general worry about performance, or more specific fears of humiliation in front of peers or the teacher are driving the resistance. In many cases in which anxiety is the primary symptom, all three of the above-feared scenarios come into play. In generalized anxiety disorder, the focus of the anxiety is not mainly separation.

When depressive disorders occur in children, we should evaluate for possible comorbidities, such as separation anxiety disorder, as well. We can make a comorbid diagnosis of separation anxiety disorder and depressive disorder when the patient meets both criteria; the two diagnoses often coexist. Panic disorder with agoraphobia is uncommon before 18 years of age; the fear is of being incapacitated by a panic attack rather than of separation from parental figures. School refusal is a frequent symptom in separation anxiety disorder but is not pathognomonic of it. Children with other diagnoses, such as specific phobias, or social anxiety disorder, or fear of failure in school because of learning disorder, may also lead to school refusal. When school refusal occurs in an adolescent, the severity of the dysfunction is generally higher than when it emerges in a young child. Table 2-31 presents similar and distinguishing characteristics of childhood separation anxiety disorder, generalized anxiety disorder, and social anxiety disorder.

COURSE AND PROGNOSIS

The course and the prognosis of separation anxiety disorder, generalized anxiety disorder, and social anxiety disorder are varied and are related to the age of onset, the duration of the symptoms, and the development of comorbid anxiety and depressive disorders. Young children who can maintain attendance in school, after-school activities and peer relationships generally have a better prognosis than children or adolescents who refuse to attend school and withdraw from social activities. The large multisite randomized

clinical trial Child/Adolescent Anxiety Multimodal Study (CAMS) provided acute treatment for children and adolescents with one or more anxiety disorders with sertraline medication alone, CBT alone, or both together. The investigators found that predictors of future remission included younger age of initiation of treatment, lower severity of anxiety, absence of a comorbid depressive or anxiety disorder, and the absence of social anxiety disorder as the primary anxiety disorder. A follow-up study of children and adolescents with mixed anxiety disorders over 3 years reported that up to 82 percent no longer met the criteria for the anxiety disorder at follow-up. Of the group followed, 96 percent of those with separation anxiety disorder were remitted at follow-up. Most children who recovered did so within the first year. Early age of onset and later age at diagnosis were factors in this study that predicted slower recovery. Close to one-third of the group studied, however, had developed another psychiatric disorder within the follow-up period, and 50 percent of these children developed another anxiety disorder. Studies have shown significant overlap between separation anxiety disorder and depressive disorders. In cases with multiple comorbidities, the prognosis is more guarded. Longitudinal data indicate that some children with severe school refusal continue to resist attending school into adolescence and remain impaired for many years.

TREATMENT

The treatment of child and adolescent separation anxiety disorder, generalized anxiety disorder, and social anxiety disorder are often considered together, given the frequent comorbidity and overlapping symptomatology of these disorders. A multimodal comprehensive treatment approach usually includes psychotherapy, most often CBT, family education, family psychosocial intervention, and pharmacologic interventions, such as SSRIs. The best evidence-based treatments for childhood anxiety disorders include CBT and SSRIs. The comparative efficacy of CBT, SSRI medication, and their combination (CBT + SSRI) in the treatment of childhood anxiety disorders was investigated in the NIMH-funded CAMS. This double-blind, placebo-controlled, multi-site study included 488 children and adolescents with separation anxiety disorder, generalized anxiety disorder, or social anxiety disorder. The investigators treated them with either CBT alone, SSRI medication (sertraline) alone, both CBT and sertraline, or placebo. After an acute treatment phase of 12 weeks, those in the combined CBT + sertraline group had an 80.7 percent response rate of much or very much improved on the clinical global improvement (CGI) rating. Response rates for the CBT-only and sertraline-only groups were 59.7 and 54.9 percent, respectively. The placebo response was 23.7 percent. Over time, during an open follow-up, the combination of CBT plus sertraline continued to provide the most efficacy. All three treatments—CBT, sertraline, and their combination—were superior to placebo and thus effective treatments in childhood anxiety, but combined treatment was most likely to help children and adolescents with anxiety disorders. A trial of CBT may be applied first, if available, when a child can function sufficiently to engage in daily activities while obtaining this treatment. For a child with severe impairment, however, a combination of treatments is recommended. CBT is a first-line evidence-based treatment for childhood anxiety disorders. A meta-analysis reviewed 16 RCTs of CBT for childhood anxiety disorders and found CBT to be consistently superior to a wait-list control group or a psychological placebo group. Exposure-based CBT has received the most empiric support among psychotherapeutic interventions for anxiety disorders in youth and is superior to wait-list control groups in reducing impairment and symptoms of anxiety.

Several psychosocial interventions have been designed specifically for anxiety disorders in young children. In a randomized clinical trial of CBT for 4- to 7-year-old children, the children received a manualized intervention called "Being Brave: A Program for Coping with Anxiety for Young Children and their Parents." The intervention used a combination of parent-only sessions and child-and-parent sessions. Response rate, measured as much or very much improved on the Clinical Global Improvement Scale for Anxiety, was 69 percent among completers versus 32 percent of the wait-list controls. The treated children showed significantly better CGI improvement on social anxiety disorder, separation anxiety disorder, and specific phobia, but not on generalized anxiety disorder. This treatment, a developmentally modified parent–child CBT, shows promise in young children.

Coaching Approach behavior and Leading by Modeling (the CALM program) is an intervention aimed at treating anxiety disorders in children younger than 7 years of age, who are too young for traditional CBT. The CALM program draws on previous work with children aged 2 to 7 years through interventions that target a child's undesired behavior by modifying parents' behavior, called PCIT. The CALM program is a 12-session manual-based intervention that provides live, individualized coaching via a bug-in-the-ear receiver worn by the parent during sessions. It incorporates exposure tasks and promotes "brave" behavior with parent coaching. A pilot study using the CALM program with nine patients with a mean age of 5.4 years found that all treatment completers (seven patients and families) were global responders, and all but one showed functional improvement. Adapting the PCIT model for anxiety disorders in young children appears to be a promising approach to treating anxiety in early childhood.

A meta-analysis of RCTs of antidepressant agents for childhood anxiety provides evidence that multiple SSRIs, including fluvoxamine, fluoxetine, sertraline, and paroxetine, are efficacious in the treatment of childhood anxiety. Based on this evidence, SSRIs are the first choice of medication in the treatment of anxiety disorders in children and adolescents.

A large, multisite investigation by the NIMH (Research Units in Pediatric Psychopharmacology [RUPP]) confirmed the safety and efficacy of fluvoxamine in the treatment of childhood separation anxiety disorder, generalized anxiety disorder, and social anxiety disorder. This double-blind, placebo-controlled study of 128 children and adolescents revealed that 76 percent of children in the group treated with fluvoxamine showed significant improvement compared with 29 percent of those in the placebo group. Response to medication was noticeable after only 2 weeks of treatment. Fluvoxamine dosages ranged from 50 to 250 mg/day in children and up to 300 mg/day in adolescents. Children and adolescents with less comorbid depressive symptoms had the best response. Youths who responded continued fluvoxamine for 6 months, and almost all of them continued to be responders at the 6-month mark.

Several other randomized clinical trials have also supported the efficacy of SSRIs in the treatment of child and adolescent anxiety disorders. A randomized, controlled trial found fluoxetine, at a dose of 20 mg/day, to be safe and effective for children with these disorders, with minor side effects including gastrointestinal distress, headache, and drowsiness. Also, a randomized clinical trial for the treatment of generalized anxiety disorder in children lends support for the efficacy of sertraline. Finally, a large industry randomized clinical trial of paroxetine in the treatment of children with social anxiety disorder found that paroxetine was associated with a response in 78 percent of children treated. The dose of paroxetine was 10 to 50 mg/day.

The FDA has placed a "black box" warning on antidepressants, including all of the SSRI agents, used in the treatment of any childhood disorder, because of concerns about increased suicidality; however, no individual childhood anxiety study has found a statistically significant increase in suicidal thoughts or behaviors.

Currently, we do not recommend using tricyclic drugs due to their potentially serious cardiac adverse effects. Other agents, including buspirone and β-adrenergic receptor antagonists such as propranolol, have been used clinically in children with anxiety disorders, but currently, no data support their efficacy. Diphenhydramine may be used in the short term to control sleep disturbances in children with anxiety disorders. Open trials and one double-blind, placebo-controlled study suggested that alprazolam, a benzodiazepine, may help to control anxiety symptoms in separation anxiety disorder. Clonazepam has been studied in open trials and may be useful in controlling symptoms of panic and other anxiety symptoms.

Although SSRIs and CBT alone and in combination have demonstrated efficacy in the treatment of anxiety disorders in youth, approximately 20 to 35 percent of children and adolescents with anxiety disorders do not appear to benefit. Several novel agents may be useful, some based on their effect on the NMDA system. For example, D-cycloserine (DCS), currently FDA approved in the treatment of pediatric tuberculosis, is a partial receptor agonist of the NMDA system and is hypothesized to augment the benefits of exposure treatment for phobias. Some evidence suggests that DCS may increase the speed of exposure interventions; however, there is no proof of long-term gains. Riluzole is an antiglutamatergic agent that decreases glutamatergic transmission by inhibiting glutamate release and inactivation of sodium channels in cortical neurons and blocking GABA reuptake. Due to its antiglutamatergic effects, riluzole may provide augmentation in the treatment of OCD and generalized anxiety disorder. Another agent, memantine, an

NMDA receptor antagonist with FDA approval in the treatment of Alzheimer's disease, has been hypothesized to decrease anxiety due to its influence on the glutamatergic system. Published case reports have provided mixed results.

Although most childhood anxiety disorders wax and wane over time, school refusal associated with separation anxiety disorder is a psychiatric emergency. A comprehensive treatment plan involves the child, the parents, and the child's peers and school. Family interventions are critical in the management of separation anxiety disorder, especially in children who refuse to attend school, so that firm encouragement of school attendance is maintained while providing appropriate support. When a return to a full school day is overwhelming, the treatment team and school should help arrange a program so the child can progressively increase the time spent at school. Graded contact with an object of anxiety is a form of behavior modification useful for any type of separation anxiety. Some severe cases of school refusal require hospitalization. Cognitive-behavioral modalities include exposure to feared separations and cognitive strategies, such as coping self-statements aimed at increasing a sense of autonomy and mastery.

In summary, evidence-based treatments for anxiety disorders have focused on SSRIs and CBT. SSRIs are both safe and efficacious in the treatment of childhood anxiety disorders; however, in severe disorders, the evidence suggests that optimal treatment is to provide both CBT and SSRI antidepressant agents simultaneously.

EPIDEMIOLOGY

The prevalence of anxiety disorders has varied with the age group of the children surveyed and the diagnostic instruments used. The lifetime prevalence of any anxiety disorder in children and adolescents ranges from 10 to 27 percent. Anxiety disorders are common in preschoolers as well, and follow a similar epidemiologic profile as in older children. An epidemiologic survey using the PAPA found that 9.5 percent of preschoolers met criteria for any anxiety disorder, with 6.5 percent exhibiting generalized anxiety disorder, 2.4 percent meeting criteria for separation anxiety disorder, and 2.2 percent meeting criteria for social anxiety disorder. Separation anxiety disorder is estimated to be about 4 percent in children and young adolescents. Separation anxiety disorder is more common in young children than in adolescents and occurs equally in boys and girls. The onset may occur during preschool years, but is most common in children 7 to 8 years of age. The rate of generalized anxiety disorder in school-age children is estimated to be approximately 3 percent, the rate of social anxiety disorder is 1 percent, and the rate of simple phobias is 2.4 percent. In adolescents, lifetime prevalence for panic disorder is 0.6 percent; the prevalence of generalized anxiety disorder is 3.7 percent.

ETIOLOGY

Biopsychosocial Factors

Multiple investigations have found evidence for the influences of parental psychopathology and parenting styles on the emergence of anxiety disorders in childhood. Longitudinal studies have found that parental overprotection correlates with an increased risk of the development of anxiety disorders in children, and insecure parent–child attachment is associated with higher-than-expected rates of anxiety disorders in childhood. It is also well known that maternal depression and anxiety have led to an increased risk of anxiety and depression in children. Psychosocial factors, in conjunction with

a child's temperament, influence the degree of separation anxiety evoked in situations of brief separation and exposure to unfamiliar environments. The temperamental trait of shyness and withdrawal in unfamiliar situations is associated with a higher risk of developing separation anxiety disorder, generalized anxiety disorder, social anxiety disorder, or all three during childhood and adolescence.

External life stresses often coincide with the development of the disorder. The death of a relative, a child's illness, a change in a child's environment, or a move to a new neighborhood or school is frequent in the histories of children with separation anxiety disorder. In a vulnerable child, these changes probably intensify anxiety.

Neurophysiologic correlations exist with behavioral inhibition (extreme shyness); children with this constellation have a higher resting heart rate and an acceleration of heart rate with tasks requiring cognitive concentration. Additional physiologic correlates of behavioral inhibition include elevated salivary cortisol levels, elevated urinary catecholamine levels, and more significant papillary dilation during cognitive tasks.

Neuroimaging studies of adolescents with anxiety show increased activation of the amygdala compared to nonanxious adolescents when presented with anxiety-provoking stimuli. Furthermore, anxious adolescents maintain the hyperactivation of the amygdala over time, rather than showing an attenuation of the effect as in nonanxious adolescents. Structural studies of the amygdala in adolescents with anxiety have led to conflicting results, with some studies finding increased amygdala volumes, whereas other studies are finding decreased amygdala volumes.

Social Learning Factors

Fear, in response to a variety of unfamiliar or unexpected situations, may be unwittingly communicated from parents to children by direct modeling. If a parent is fearful, the child will probably have a phobic adaptation to new situations, especially to a school environment. There are much data to suggest that overprotective parenting promotes increased interpersonal sensitivity in healthy children and increases the risk of social anxiety disorder in children with behavioral inhibition or other anxiety disorders such as separation anxiety disorder. Some parents appear to teach their children to be anxious by overprotecting them from expected dangers or by exaggerating the dangers. For example, a parent who cringes in a room during a lightning storm teaches a child to do the same. A parent who is afraid of mice or insects conveys the affect of fright to a child.

Conversely, a parent who becomes angry with a child when the child expresses fear of a given situation, for example, when exposed to animals, may promote a phobic concern in the child by exposing the child to the intensity of the anger expressed by the parent. When parents have anxiety disorders, this magnifies the social learning factors in the development of anxiety reactions. These factors may be pertinent in the development of separation anxiety disorder as well as in generalized anxiety disorder and social anxiety disorder. A recent study found no association between psychosocial hardships, such as ongoing family conflict, and behavioral inhibition among young children. It appears that temperamental predisposition to anxiety disorders emerges as a highly heritable constellation of traits and due to psychosocial stressors.

Genetic Factors

Genetic studies suggest that genes account for at least one-third of the variance in the development of anxiety disorders. Heritability for anxiety disorders in children and adolescents ranges from 36 to 65 percent, with the highest estimates found in younger children with anxiety disorders. Two heritable characteristics—behavioral inhibition (the tendency toward fear and withdrawal in new situations) and physiological hyperarousal—have both been found to impart significant risk factors for the future development of an anxiety disorder. However, although the temperamental constellation of behavioral inhibition, excessive shyness, the tendency to withdraw from unfamiliar situations, and the eventual emergence of anxiety disorders have a genetic contribution, one-third to two-thirds of young children with behavioral inhibition do not appear to go on to develop anxiety disorders.

Family studies have shown that the offspring of adults with anxiety disorders are at an increased risk of having an anxiety disorder themselves. Separation anxiety disorder and depression in children overlap, and the presence of an anxiety disorder increases the risk of a future episode of a depressive disorder. The current consensus on the genetics of anxiety disorders suggests that what is inherited is a general predisposition toward anxiety, causing heightened levels of arousal, emotional reactivity, and increased negative affect, all of which increase the risk of developing separation anxiety disorder, generalized anxiety disorder, and social anxiety disorder.

▲ 2.14 Selective Mutism

Selective mutism, believed to be related to social anxiety disorder, although an independent disorder, is characterized in a child by persistent lack of speaking in one or more specific social situations, most typically, the school setting. A child with selective mutism may remain wholly silent or near-silent, in some cases only whispering in a school setting. Although selective mutism often begins before age 5 years, it may not be apparent until the child should be reading or speaking aloud in school. The current conceptualization of selective mutism highlights a convergence of underlying social anxiety, along with an increased likelihood of speech and language

problems leading to the failure to speak in certain situations. Typically, children with the disorder are silent during stressful situations, whereas some may verbalize almost inaudibly single-syllable words. Despite an increased risk for delayed speech and language acquisition in children with selective mutism, children with this disorder are fully capable of speaking competently when not in a socially anxiety-producing situation. Some children with the disorder will communicate with eye contact or nonverbal gestures but not verbally when at school. Otherwise, children with selective mutism speak fluently at home and in many familiar settings. Selective mutism is believed to be related to social anxiety disorder because of its expression primarily in selective social situations.

DIAGNOSIS AND CLINICAL FEATURES

The diagnosis of selective mutism is not difficult to make after it is clear that a child has adequate language skills in some environments but not in others. The mutism may have developed gradually or suddenly after a disturbing experience. The age of onset can range from 4 to 8 years. Mute periods are most commonly manifested in school or outside the home; in rare cases, a child is mute at home but not in school. Children who exhibit selective mutism may also have symptoms of separation anxiety disorder, school refusal, and delayed language acquisition. Because social anxiety is almost always present in children with selective mutism, behavioral disturbances, such as temper tantrums and oppositional behaviors, may also occur in the home. Compared to children with other anxiety disorders, except social anxiety disorder, children with selective mutism tend to have less social competence and more social anxiety. Table 2-32 lists the criteria for selective mutism.

Janine is a 6-year-old Chinese American first-grade girl who lives with her biologic mother, father, and siblings. Janine's parents reported a 2-year history of not speaking at school, beginning in kindergarten, or to any children or adults outside of her family, despite speaking at

Table 2-32
Selective Mutism

	DSM-5	ICD-10
Diagnostic name	Selective Mutism	Elective Mutism
Duration	≥1 mo (not 1st month of school)	
Symptoms	Persistent lack of speech • In certain social situations • Occurs when expected to speak • Has ability to speak appropriately in other situations	Persistent lack of speech • In certain social situations • Has ability to speak appropriately in other situations • Related to specific emotions • For example: anxiety, social withdrawal, and sensitivity
Psychosocial consequences of symptoms	Presence of psychosocial impairment	
Exclusions (not result of):	Another mental disorder Communication disorder Lack of proficiency with the spoken language in a given situation	Pervasive developmental disorders Developmental disorders of speech and language Transient mutism as part of separation anxiety in young children
Comments		Note: classified under Disorders of social functioning with onset specific to childhood and adolescence

home. At home, she reportedly is animated and quite talkative with her immediate family and a few young cousins as well. Although she speaks to adult relatives outside of her immediate family, her communication is often limited to one-word responses to their questions. By her parents' report, Janine also exhibits extreme social anxiety, to the point of "freezing" in certain situations when the attention is on her. At the time of her evaluation, Janine had not received prior treatment. Janine speaks fluent English as well as Mandarin, and, according to her parents, met all developmental milestones on time and appeared to have above-average intelligence. They also reported that Janine enjoys dancing, singing, and imaginative play with her sisters.

During the initial evaluation, Janine failed to make eye contact or respond verbally to the intake clinician. Janine's parents reported that this behavior is typical of her when in a new situation but that she communicates nonverbally and makes eye contact with most people once she "gets to know them." On request, Janine's parents provided a videotaped recording of Janine playing at home with her sisters. In the video, Janine was animated and was speaking spontaneously and fluently without apparent impairment. Janine received diagnoses of selective mutism and social anxiety disorder. The psychiatrist recommended CBT, and Janine began to see a therapist.

The therapist instructed Janine and her mother to come up with lists of easy, medium, and most challenging "speaking" situations and lists of small, medium, and large rewards. These lists then became the basis for assignments for exposures and reinforcement for speaking tasks that gradually increased in difficulty. CBT sessions included time with Janine and her mother together to review past and future assignments and time with Janine and the therapist alone.

When treatment began, Janine did not communicate at all verbally or nonverbally with the therapist. The therapist gradually developed a rapport with Janine utilizing less stressful tasks such as whispering to her mother with the therapist in the corner, then nodding yes or no, pointing, whispering to a stuffed animal, whispering to her mother while facing the therapist, and eventually responding to the therapist directly. The therapist used animal puppets to enable Janine to "warm-up" without talking directly to the therapist. After three sessions, Janine began to speak to the therapist in a whisper. Janine received stickers for completing each speaking assignment, and, after filling up the sticker charts, she received rewards (a small toy or treat from the reward list).

The therapist gave Janine assignments that involved her teacher and classmates. These were implemented gradually and included waving to the teacher, playing an audiotape of her saying "hello" to the teacher, whispering "hello" to the teacher, speaking "hello" to the teacher in a regular voice, and so on. After 14 sessions, Janine could speak in complete sentences during class when called on. She also spoke to her teacher in front of several other students.

During the last few sessions, Janine's mother took an increasingly active role in assigning and following up on speaking assignments. When Janine entered the second grade, it took only a few days for her to speak to her teacher and most peers in class. After completion of therapy, Janine's mother continued to monitor Janine's speaking behaviors and to promote speaking in new situations by encouraging (and rewarding) Janine's gradual successes with novel people and situations. (Adapted from case material from Lindsey Bergman, Ph.D., and John Piacentini, Ph.D.)

Pathology and Laboratory Examination

No specific laboratory measures are useful in the diagnosis or treatment of selective mutism.

DIFFERENTIAL DIAGNOSIS

Differential diagnosis of children who are silent in social situations emphasizes ruling out communications disorder, autism spectrum disorder, and social anxiety disorder. Social anxiety disorder may be comorbid with selective mutism. Once confirming that the child is fully capable of speaking when comfortable, but not in stressful situations, we should consider an anxiety disorder. Shy children may exhibit a transient muteness in new, anxiety-provoking situations. These children often have histories of not speaking in the presence of strangers and of clinging to their mothers. Most children who are mute on entering school improve spontaneously and may be described as having transient adaptation shyness. We should distinguish between selective mutism and intellectual disabilities, pervasive developmental disorders, and expressive language disorder. In these disorders, the child may have an inability, rather than a refusal, to speak. In mutism secondary to conversion disorder, the mutism is pervasive. Children introduced into an environment which uses a different language may be reticent to begin using the new language. We should only diagnose selective mutism when children also refuse to converse in their native language and when they have gained communicative competence in the new language but refuse to speak it.

COURSE AND PROGNOSIS

Children with selective mutism are often excessively shy during the preschool years, but the onset of the full disorder is usually not evident until age 5 or 6 years. Many very young children with early symptoms of selective mutism in a transitional period when entering preschool have a spontaneous improvement over several months and never fulfill the criteria for the disorder. A typical pattern for a child with selective mutism is to speak almost exclusively at home with the nuclear family but not elsewhere, especially not at school. Consequently, a child with selective mutism may have academic difficulties or even failure due to a lack of participation. Children with selective mutism are typically shy, anxious, and at increased risk for a depressive disorder. Many children with early-onset selective mutism remit with or without treatment. Recent data suggest that fluoxetine may influence the course of selective mutism, and treatment enhances recovery. Children in whom the disorder persists often have difficulty forming social relationships. Teasing and scapegoating by peers may cause them to refuse to go to school. Some children with any form of severe social anxiety are rigid, compulsive, negativistic, and prone to temper tantrums and oppositional and aggressive behavior at home. Other children with the disorder tolerate the feared situation by communicating with gestures, such as nodding, shaking the head, and saying "Uh-huh" or "No." In one follow-up study, about one-half of children with selective mutism improved within 5 to 10 years. Children who do not improve by age 10 years appear to have a long-term course and a worse prognosis. As many as one-third of children with selective mutism, with or without treatment, may develop other psychiatric disorders, particularly other anxiety disorders and depression.

TREATMENT

The optimal treatment is a multimodal approach using psychoeducation for the family, CBT, and SSRIs as needed. Preschool children may also benefit from a therapeutic nursery. For school-age children, individual CBT is the first-line treatment. Family education and cooperation are beneficial. Published data on the successful treatment of children with selective mutism is scant. However, reasonable evidence indicates that children with social anxiety disorder respond to various SSRIs, and, currently, CBT treatments have also demonstrated efficacy in children with anxiety disorders.

A recent report of 21 children with selective mutism treated in an open trial with fluoxetine suggested that this medication may be useful for childhood selective mutism. Reports have confirmed the efficacy of fluoxetine in the treatment of adult social anxiety disorder and at least one double-blind, placebo-controlled study using fluoxetine with children with mutism. A large NIMH-funded study of anxiety disorders in children and adolescents called Research Units in Pediatric Psychopharmacology (RUPP), has shown distinct superiority of fluvoxamine over placebo in the treatment of a variety of childhood anxiety disorders. Children with selective mutism may benefit similarly to those with social anxiety disorder, given the current belief that it is a subgroup of social anxiety disorder. SSRI medications that have been shown in randomized, placebo-controlled trials to have benefit in the treatment of children with social anxiety disorder include fluoxetine (20 to 60 mg/day), fluvoxamine (50 to 300 mg/day), sertraline (25 to 200 mg/day), and paroxetine (10 to 50 mg/day).

EPIDEMIOLOGY

The prevalence of selective mutism varies with age, with younger children at increased risk for the disorder. According to the DSM-5, the point prevalence of selective mutism using clinic or school samples ranges between 0.03 and 1 percent, depending on whether a clinical or community sample is studied. A sizeable epidemiologic survey in the United Kingdom reported a prevalence rate of selective mutism to be 0.69 percent in children 4 to 5 years of age. Another survey in the United Kingdom identified 0.06 percent of 7-year-olds as having selective mutism. Young children are more vulnerable to the disorder than older ones. Selective mutism appears to be more common in girls than in boys. Clinical reports suggest that many young children spontaneously "outgrow" this disorder as they age; the longitudinal course of the disorder remains to be studied.

ETIOLOGY

Genetic Contribution

Selective mutism may have many of the same etiologic factors leading to the emergence of social anxiety disorder. In contrast to other childhood anxiety disorders, however, children with selective mutism are at higher risk for delayed onset of speech or speech abnormalities that may be contributory. However, in addition to the speech and language factor, one survey found that 90 percent of children with selective mutism met diagnostic criteria for social anxiety disorder. These children showed high levels of social anxiety without notable psychopathology in other areas, according to parent and teacher ratings. Thus, selective mutism may not represent a distinct disorder but may be a subtype of social anxiety disorder. Maternal anxiety, depression, and heightened dependence needs occur in families of children with selective mutism, similar to families with children who exhibit other anxiety disorders.

Parental Interactions

Maternal overprotection and anxiety disorders in parents may exacerbate interactions that unwittingly reinforce selective mutism behaviors. Children with selective mutism usually speak freely at home and only exhibit symptoms when under social pressure either in school or other social situations. Some children seem predisposed to selective mutism after early emotional or physical trauma;

thus, some clinicians refer to the phenomenon as *traumatic mutism* rather than selective mutism.

Speech and Language Factors

Selective mutism is conceptualized as an anxiety-based refusal to speak; however, a higher-than-expected proportion of children with the disorder have a history of speech delay. An intriguing finding suggests that children with selective mutism are at higher risk for a disturbance in auditory processing, which may interfere with the efficient processing of incoming sounds. For the most part, however, speech and language problems in children with selective mutism are subtle and cannot account for the diagnosis.

▲ 2.15 Obsessive-Compulsive Disorder in Childhood and Adolescence

Data suggest that up to 25 percent of cases of OCD have their onset by 14 years of age. The overall clinical presentation of OCD in youth is similar to that in adults; however, compared to adults, children and adolescents with OCD more often do not consider their obsessional thoughts or repetitive behaviors to be unreasonable. In milder cases of OCD, a trial of CBT is the initial intervention. OCD in youth is often treated successfully with SSRIs or CBT alone or in combination. The results of a large-scale, randomized, placebo-controlled study called the Pediatric OCD Treatment Study (POTS), demonstrated that the highest rates of remission in pediatric OCD are with a combination of both serotonergic agents and CBT treatment.

DIAGNOSIS AND CLINICAL FEATURES

Children and adolescents with obsessions or compulsions present for treatment due to the excessive time that they devote to their intrusive thoughts and repetitive rituals. Some children see their compulsive rituals as reasonable responses to their extreme fears and anxieties. Nevertheless, they are aware of their discomfort and inability to carry out usual daily activities promptly due to the compulsions, such as getting ready to leave their homes to go to school each morning.

The most commonly reported obsessions in children and adolescents include extreme fears of contamination—exposure to dirt, germs, or disease—followed by worries related to harm befalling themselves, family members, or fear of harming others due to losing control over aggressive impulses. Also commonly reported are obsessional needs for symmetry or exactness, hoarding, and excessive religious or moral concerns. Typical compulsive rituals among children and adolescents involve cleaning, checking, counting, repeating behaviors, or arranging items. Associated features in children and adolescents with OCD include avoidance, indecision, doubt, and slowness to complete tasks. In most cases of OCD among youth, obsessions and compulsions are present. According to the DSM-5, diagnosis of OCD is identical to that of adults, with the note that young children may not be able to articulate the aims of their compulsions in diminishing their anxiety. The DSM-5 has also added the following specifiers: with good, fair, poor, or absent insight; that is, the greater the belief in the OCD obsessions and compulsions, the weaker the insight. An additional specifier indicates whether the individual has a current or past history of a tic disorder. We discuss this disorder in Chapter 9, where Table 9-4 designates the DSM-5 diagnostic criteria for OCD.

Many children and adolescents who develop OCD have an insidious onset and may hide their symptoms as long as possible so that their rituals will not be challenged or disrupted. A minority of children, particularly males with early-onset, may have a rapid unfolding of multiple symptoms within a few months. OCD is often comorbid with anxiety disorders, ADHD, and tic disorders, especially Tourette syndrome. Children with comorbid OCD and tic disorders are more likely to exhibit counting, arranging, or ordering compulsions and less likely to manifest excessive washing and cleaning compulsions. The high comorbidity of OCD, Tourette syndrome, and ADHD has led investigators to postulate a shared genetic vulnerability to all three of these disorders. It is crucial to search for comorbidity in children and adolescents with OCD so that the treatments can be optimal.

Jason, a 12-year-old boy in the sixth grade, was brought for evaluation by his parents, who expressed concerns over his repeated questions and anxiety regarding developing acquired immunodeficiency syndrome (AIDS). Jason was a high-functioning and well-adjusted boy who abruptly began to exhibit extremely disruptive behaviors related to his fears of AIDS approximately 2 to 3 months before the evaluation. Jason's new behaviors included relentless concerns about contracting illness, washing rituals, repeated expressions of uncertainty over his behavior, seeking reassurance, repeating rituals, and avoidance.

Jason repeatedly expressed his fear and belief that he was at risk for human immunodeficiency virus (HIV) through exposure to multiple strangers who were infected. For example, while riding in the car, if Jason saw a stranger from the window who appeared to him to be ill-kempt, he experienced a surge of extreme anxiety and obsessively agonized about whether the stranger could have AIDS and had exposed him to it. Despite his parents' reassurances about his safety and lack of exposure to illness, Jason insisted on vigorously washing for approximately 1 hour each time he reached home after being out. Jason continually expressed doubts about his behavior. He often asked his parents, "Did I use the s___ word? Did I use the f___ word?" Reassurance was only slightly calming. Jason, previously an excellent student, began to lose the ability to focus on schoolwork. While reading passages from assigned materials, Jason frequently experienced severe anxiety, wondering if he had missed a word or misunderstood the sentence, and proceeded to reread the material. Completing a page of written material began to take Jason 30 to 60 minutes. Over several weeks, he was less and less able to complete assignments, following which he became very distressed over his deteriorating grades.

During Jason's evaluation, his family history suggested that Jason's older sister had experienced a period in which she, too, had similar but milder anxieties, with less interference in functioning, and she had never received any treatment for those symptoms.

At the intake interview, Jason presented as a preoccupied and sad boy who was cooperative with questioning. He did not volunteer much information, and he allowed his parents to recount the extent of his symptoms. Jason believed that his relentless concerns were reasonable and that he required repeated reassurance from his parents in order to continue his daily activities. Jason met full diagnostic criteria for OCD. Symptoms of depression were present but not sufficient for major depressive disorder.

He began CBT; however, Jason was so fearful of deviating from his rituals that he was unable to participate fully in his treatment, and he became despondent about his future. Jason refused to go to school due to his increasing distress associated with reading and his shame regarding his diminishing academic performance. Given his limited

---

progress during the first 2 months of CBT, his psychiatrist added fluoxetine, titrated to 40 mg/day. Over 3 weeks, there was some improvement, and Jason was more amenable to cooperating with his CBT treatment. CBT and SSRI treatment continued over the next 3 months regularly. Over time, Jason finally began to show some flexibility with his rituals, and he was able to decrease the amount of time he spent with rituals. Once he had found some relief from his symptoms, Jason was able to focus more on his schoolwork and his family life. Follow-up over the next year was positive; Jason had maintained his gains from treatment, with only minimal interference from residual OCD symptoms. Jason's academic achievement improved, he was able to engage in activities with friends, and he spent almost no time preoccupied with obsessional thoughts of illness and cleansing rituals. (Adapted from a case courtesy of James T. McCracken, M.D.)

Pathology and Laboratory Examination

No specific laboratory measures are useful in the diagnosis of OCD.

Even when the onset of obsessions or compulsions appears to be associated with a recent infection with GABHS, antigens and antibodies to the bacteria do not indicate a causal relationship between GABHS and OCD.

DIFFERENTIAL DIAGNOSIS

Developmentally appropriate rituals in the play and behavior of young children should not be confused with OCD in that age group. Preschoolers often engage in ritualistic play and request a predictable routine such as bathing, reading stories, or selecting the same stuffed animal at bedtime to promote a sense of security and comfort. These routines allay developmentally normal fears and lead to reasonable completion of daily activities. On the other hand, extreme fears drive the obsessions or compulsions, and this significantly interferes with daily function because of the excessive time that they consume and the extreme distress that ensues when they are interrupted. The rituals of preschoolers generally become less rigid by the time they enter grade school, and school-age children do not typically experience a surge of anxiety when they encounter small changes in their routine.

Children and adolescents with generalized anxiety disorder, separation anxiety disorder, and social anxiety disorder experience intense worries that they repeatedly express; however, these are mundane compared to obsessions, which are often so extreme that they appear bizarre. A child with generalized anxiety disorder typically worries repeatedly about performance on academic examinations, whereas a child with OCD may experience repeated intrusive thoughts that he may harm someone he loves. The compulsions of OCD are not present in other anxiety disorders; however, children with autism spectrum disorders often display repetitive behaviors that may resemble OCD. In contrast with the rituals of OCD, children with autism spectrum disorder are not responding to anxiety, but are more often exhibiting stereotyped behaviors that are self-stimulating or self-comforting.

Children and adolescents with tic disorders such as Tourette syndrome may display complex repetitive, compulsive behaviors similar to the compulsions seen in OCD. Children and adolescents with tic disorders are at higher risk for the development of concurrent OCD.

Severe OCD symptoms may be difficult to distinguish from delusional symptoms, especially when the obsessions and compulsions are bizarre. In most adults, and often in youth with OCD, despite an inability to control their obsessions or resist completing compulsions, insight into their lack of reasonableness is preserved. That is, an individual's conviction in their beliefs often does not reach delusional intensity. When insight is present and underlying anxiety can be described, even in the face of significant dysfunction due to bizarre obsessions and compulsions, the diagnosis of OCD is suspect.

COURSE AND PROGNOSIS

OCD with onset in childhood and adolescence is most often a chronic, waxing, and waning disorder with variability in severity and outcome. Follow-up studies suggest that up to 40 to 50 percent of children and adolescents recover from OCD with minimal residual symptoms. A study of childhood OCD treatment with sertraline resulted in close to 50 percent of participants experiencing complete remission and partial remission in another 25 percent with a follow-up time of 1 year. Predictors of the best outcome were in those children and adolescents without comorbid disorders, including tic disorders and ADHD. A study of 142 children and adolescents with OCD followed over 9 years at the Maudsley Hospital in England found 41 percent to have a persistence of OCD, with 40 percent exhibiting an additional psychiatric diagnosis at follow-up. The main predictor for persistent OCD was the duration of illness at the time of the initial assessment. Approximately half of the follow-up group was still receiving treatment, and half believed that they needed continued treatment.

Neuropsychological functioning may also play a role in outcome and prognosis. A study of 63 youth with OCD who completed the Rey-Osterrieth Complex Figure (ROCF) along with specific subtests of the Wechsler Intelligence Scale for Children, Third Edition (WISC-III), found that 5-minute recall accuracy from the ROCF was positively correlated with response to treatment, particularly CBT. These findings imply that poorer performance on the ROCF and poor response to therapy may be in part due to executive functioning difficulties and that treatment may need to be modified to account for these obstacles.

Overall, the prognosis is hopeful for most children and adolescents with mild to moderate OCD. In about 10 percent of cases, OCD may represent a prodrome of a psychotic disorder in children and adolescents. In youth with subthreshold OCD symptoms, there is a high risk of developing the full OCD disorder within 2 years. Childhood OCD is responsive to available treatments, resulting in improvement, if not complete remission, in the majority of cases.

TREATMENT

CBT and SSRIs are both efficacious treatments for OCD in youth. CBT geared toward children of varying ages is based on the principle of developmentally appropriate exposure to the feared stimuli coupled with response prevention, leading to diminishing anxiety over time on exposure to feared situations. CBT manuals can ensure that the therapist can make developmentally appropriate interventions and that the child and parents receive comprehensive education.

Treatment guidelines for children and adolescents with mild to moderate OCD recommend a trial of CBT before initiating medication. However, the POTS, a multi-site National Institute of Health (NIH)–funded investigation of sertraline and CBT, each alone and in combination, for the treatment of childhood-onset OCD, revealed that the combination was superior to either treatment alone. Each treatment alone also provided encouraging levels of response. The mean daily dose of sertraline was 133 mg/day in the group

administered the combination treatment, and 170 mg/day for the sertraline alone group. Improvement with the pharmacologic intervention of childhood OCD usually occurs within 8 to 12 weeks of treatment. Most children and adolescents who experienced remission with acute treatment using SSRIs were still responsive over a year. Among youth with OCD who obtain a partial response to a therapeutic trial of SSRI treatment, augmentation with a short-term OCD-specific CBT leads to a significantly greater response. Evidence shows that higher treatment expectations by patients and families link to better treatment response, greater compliance with home-based CBT assignments, less drop out of treatment, and reduced impairment.

In addition to individual CBT, both family and group CBT interventions are efficacious in the treatment of childhood OCD. Family CBT (FCBT) intervention in the treatment of OCD in youth increases the response rates. A controlled comparison of family CBT and psychoeducation and relaxation (PRT) in 71 families of children with OCD showed that clinical remission rates in the FCBT group were significantly higher than those in the PRT group. The FCBT treatment reduced parent involvement and accommodation in their affected child's symptoms, which led to decreased symptomatology.

A randomized controlled study investigating web-camera delivered FCBT (W-CBT) compared to a waitlist condition assigned 31 families to one of the above conditions. Assessments were conducted immediately before and after treatment and at a 3-month follow-up for the W-CBT group. The W-CBT group was superior to the waitlist control group on all primary outcome measures, with large effect sizes. Eighty-one percent of the W-CBT group responded, compared to 13 percent of the waitlist group. The children maintained the gains at the 3-month follow-up assessment. The authors conclude that W-CBT may be efficacious in the treatment of OCD in youth and may be a promising tool for future dissemination.

Exposure and response prevention (ERP) was studied in a group format in youth with OCD in a community-based program. Group-based ERP was effective in reducing OCD symptom severity and depressive symptoms, but not anxiety symptoms, in a naturalistic treatment setting for children with OCD and comorbid anxiety or depressive features.

Multiple randomized clinical trials establish the efficacy of SSRIs for OCD in youth. A meta-analysis of 13 studies of SSRIs, including sertraline, fluvoxamine, fluoxetine, and paroxetine, has provided evidence of the efficacy of SSRIs with a moderate effect size. A randomized controlled clinical trial of citalopram versus fluoxetine in youth with OCD found that citalopram was as safe and effective as fluoxetine for the treatment of OCD in children and adolescents. There have been no apparent differences in the rate of response for the individual SSRIs.

Currently, three SSRIs: sertraline (at least 6 years), fluoxetine (at least 7 years), and fluvoxamine (at least 8 years), as well as clomipramine (at least 10 years), have received FDA approval for the treatment of OCD in youth. The black-box warning for antidepressants used in children for any disorder, including OCD, is applicable so that close monitoring for suicidal ideation or behavior is mandated when using these agents in children.

Typical side effects that emerge with the use of SSRIs include insomnia, nausea, agitation, tremor, and fatigue. Dosage ranges for the various SSRIs found to have efficacy in randomized clinical trials are the following: fluoxetine (20 to 60 mg), sertraline (50 to 200 mg), fluvoxamine (up to 200 mg), and paroxetine (up to 50 mg).

Clomipramine was the first antidepressant studied in the treatment of OCD in childhood and the only tricyclic antidepressant that has FDA approval for the treatment of anxiety disorders in childhood. Clomipramine was efficacious in doses up to 200 mg, or 3 mg/kg, whichever is less. Nevertheless, clomipramine is not recommended as a first-line treatment due to its higher potential risks compared to other SSRIs, including the cardiovascular risk of hypotension and arrhythmia and seizure risk.

Pediatric patients with OCD who respond only partially to medications tend to have at least moderate to severe OCD symptoms, high ratings of global impairment, and significant comorbidity even after their partial response to an adequate trial of medication. Augmentation strategies with medications to enhance serotonergic effects, such as with atypical antipsychotics (e.g., risperidone), have demonstrated increased response when SSRIs yield a partial response. Aripiprazole augmentation in 39 adolescents with OCD who did not respond to two trials of monotherapy with SSRIs led to 59 percent of patients being rated as improved or very much improved. Patients who responded to aripiprazole were less impaired at baseline in functional impairment but not in the clinical severity of their OCD. Aripiprazole's final mean dose was 12.2 mg/day. This agent may be useful for pediatric OCD and warrants further controlled trials.

Given the lack of data on discontinuation, recommendations for maintaining medication such as stabilization, education about relapse risk, and tapering medication during the summer are likely in order to minimize academic compromise in case of relapse. For children and adolescents with more severe or multiple episodes of significant exacerbation of symptoms, treatment for more than a year is recommended. Overall, the efficacy of treatment for children and adolescents with OCD is high with choices of SSRIs and CBT.

EPIDEMIOLOGY

OCD is common among children and adolescents, with a point prevalence of about 0.5 percent and a lifetime prevalence of 2 to 4 percent. The rate of OCD among youth rises exponentially with increasing age, with rates of 0.3 percent in children between the ages of 5 and 7 years, rising to rates between 0.6 and 1 percent among teens. According to the DSM-5, the prevalence of OCD in the United States is 1.2 percent, with a slightly higher rate in females. Rates of OCD among adolescents are higher than those for schizophrenia or bipolar disorder. Among young children with OCD, there appears to be a slight male predominance, which diminishes with age.

ETIOLOGY

Genetic Factors

Genetic factors contribute significantly to the development of OCD in early-onset illness. The rate of OCD among first-degree relatives of children and adolescents who develop OCD is 10 times greater than for the general population. Twin studies have shown that the concordance rates for OCD are higher for monozygotic twins (0.57) than for dizygotic twins (0.22); however, nongenetic factors play a role that may be equal to or greater than genetic contributions in some cases. OCD is a heterogeneous disorder that has been recognized for decades to run in families. Also, the presence of subclinical symptom constellations in family members appears to breed true. Genetic linkage studies have revealed evidence of susceptibility loci on chromosomes 1q, 3q, 6q, 7p, 9p, 10p, and 15q. The OCD collaborative genetics study found that the *Sapap3* gene was associated with grooming disorders and may be a promising candidate gene for OCD. There is evidence that the glutamate receptor–modulating genes may also be associated with and play a role in the emergence of OCD. Family studies have suggested a relationship between OCD and tic disorders such as Tourette syndrome. OCD and tic disorders likely share susceptibility factors, which may include both genetic and nongenetic factors.

Neuroimmunology

Immunologic contributions to the emergence of OCD are likely related to an inflammatory process in the basal ganglia associated with an immune response to a systemic infection that may trigger OCD and tics. A prototype of this hypothesis has been the controversial association of OCD symptoms in a small subgroup of children and adolescents following documented exposure to or infection with *group A β-hemolytic streptococcus* (GABHS). Under this hypothesis, cases of infection-triggered OCD have been termed Pediatric Autoimmune Neuropsychiatric Disorders Associated with Streptococcus (PANDAS), and parallel an autoimmune process leading to a movement disorder much like Sydenham chorea following rheumatic fever. Some evidence from MRI studies has documented a proportional relationship between the size of the basal ganglia and the severity of OCD symptoms in a small sample. GABHS may be one of many physiologic stressors that can lead to an increase or emergence of OCD or tics; however, a prospective longitudinal study of youth with PANDAS followed over 2 years found no evidence of a temporal association between GABHS infections and OCD symptom exacerbations in children who met the criteria for PANDAS. The presentation of OCD in children and adolescents due to acute exposure to GABHS represents a minority of OCD cases in youth and remains controversial.

Neurochemistry

The evidence that SSRIs diminish symptoms of OCD, along with findings of altered sensitivity to the acute administration of 5-hydroxytryptamine (5-HT) agonists in individuals with OCD, supports the probability of serotonin's role in OCD. Also, the dopamine system is likely influential in OCD, especially in light of the frequent comorbidity of OCD with tic disorders in childhood. Clinical observations have indicated that obsessions and compulsions worsen with stimulants, as with patients who have comorbid ADHD. Dopamine antagonists, administered along with SSRIs, may augment the effectiveness of SSRIs in the treatment of OCD. Evidence suggests that multiple neurotransmitter systems may play a role in OCD.

Neuroimaging

Both CT and MRI of untreated children and adults with OCD have revealed smaller volumes of basal ganglia segments compared to healthy controls. A meta-analysis of voxel-based morphometry (VBM) to assess gray matter density compared 343 OCD patients with 318 healthy controls and found that gray matter density in OCD patients was smaller in parietofrontal cortical regions (including the supramarginal gyrus, the dorsolateral prefrontal cortex, and the orbitofrontal cortex), but larger in the basal ganglia (the putamen) and anterior prefrontal cortex, compared to healthy controls. Increased gray matter volume in the basal ganglia of patients with OCD has been reported in other studies as well. These structural abnormalities in the prefrontal-basal ganglia are likely to be integrally involved in the pathophysiology of OCD. It is not clear whether the increases in gray matter in individuals with OCD occur before or after the symptoms emerge. In children, there is evidence of increased thalamic volume. Adult studies have provided evidence of hypermetabolism of frontal cortical-striatal-thalamo-cortical networks in untreated individuals with OCD. Of interest, imaging studies of before and after treatment have revealed that both medication and behavioral interventions lead to a reduction of orbitofrontal and caudate metabolic rates in children and adults with OCD.

▲ 2.16 Early-Onset Schizophrenia

Early-onset schizophrenia comprises childhood-onset and adolescent-onset schizophrenia. Childhood-onset schizophrenia is a rare and virulent form of schizophrenia now recognized as a progressive neurodevelopmental disorder. Childhood-onset is characterized by a more chronic course, with severe social and cognitive consequences and increased negative symptoms compared to adult-onset schizophrenia. Childhood-onset schizophrenia is an onset of psychotic symptoms before 13 years, believed to represent a subgroup of patients with schizophrenia with an increased heritable etiology, and evidence of widespread abnormalities in the development of brain structures including the cerebral cortex, white matter, hippocampus, and cerebellum. Children diagnosed with childhood-onset schizophrenia have higher than average rates of premorbid developmental abnormalities that appear to be nonspecific markers of abnormal brain development. Early-onset schizophrenia is an onset of disease before 18 years, including childhood-onset as well as adolescent-onset schizophrenia. Early-onset schizophrenia is associated with severe clinical course, poor psychosocial functioning, and increased severity of brain abnormalities. Despite the more severe course, current evidence supports the efficacy of both psychosocial and pharmacologic interventions in the management of childhood-onset and, particularly, adolescent-onset schizophrenia.

Children with childhood-onset schizophrenia have more significant deficits in measures of IQ, memory, and tests of perceptuomotor skills compared with adolescent-onset schizophrenia. Increased impairment in childhood-onset schizophrenia of cognitive measures such as IQ, working memory, and perceptuomotor skills may be premorbid markers of illness rather than sequelae of the disorder. Although cognitive impairments are more considerable in younger patients with schizophrenia, the clinical presentation of schizophrenia remains remarkably similar across the ages, and the diagnosis of childhood-onset schizophrenia is continuous with that in adolescents and adults, with one exception: in childhood-onset schizophrenia, a failure to achieve expected social and academic functioning may replace a deterioration in functioning. Chapter 5 discusses the features of the disorder in detail.

DIAGNOSIS AND CLINICAL FEATURES

All of the symptoms included in adult-onset schizophrenia may be manifest in children and adolescents with the disorder. However, youth with schizophrenia are more likely to have a premorbid history of social rejection, poor peer relationships, clingy withdrawn behavior, and academic trouble than those with adult-onset schizophrenia. Some children with schizophrenia evaluated in middle childhood have early histories of delayed motor milestones and language acquisition similar to some symptoms of autism spectrum disorder.

The onset of schizophrenia in childhood is frequently insidious, starting with inappropriate affect or unusual behavior; it may take months or years for a child to meet all of the diagnostic criteria for schizophrenia.

Auditory hallucinations commonly occur in children with schizophrenia. The voices may reflect an ongoing critical commentary or command hallucinations may instruct children to harm or kill themselves or others. Hallucinatory voices may sound human or animal, or "bizarre," for example, identified as "a computer in my head," "Martians," or the voice of someone familiar, such as a relative. The childhood-onset schizophrenia project at the NIMH found high rates across all hallucination modalities. However, there were unexpectedly high rates of tactile, olfactory, and visual hallucinations among this study group of patients with childhood-onset schizophrenia. Visual hallucinations were associated with lower IQ and earlier age at onset of disease. Visual hallucinations are often frightening; affected children may "see" images of the devil, skeletons, scary faces, or space creatures. Transient phobic visual hallucinations occur in severely anxious or traumatized children who do not develop major psychotic disorders. Visual, tactile, and olfactory hallucinations may be a marker of more severe psychosis.

Delusions occur in up to half of children and adolescents with schizophrenia, in various forms, including persecutory, grandiose, and religious. Delusions increase in frequency with increased age. Blunted or inappropriate affect appears almost universally in children with schizophrenia. Children with schizophrenia may giggle inappropriately or cry without being able to explain why. Formal thought disorders, including loosening of associations and thought blocking, are common features among youth with schizophrenia. Illogic thinking and poverty of thought are also often present. Unlike adults with schizophrenia, children with schizophrenia do not have poverty of speech content, but they speak less than other children of the same intelligence and are ambiguous in the way they refer to persons, objects, and events. The communication deficits observable in children with schizophrenia include unpredictably changing the topic of conversation without introducing the new topic to the listener (loose associations). Children with schizophrenia also exhibit illogical thinking and speaking and tend to underuse self-initiated repair strategies to aid in their communication. When an utterance is unclear or vague, normal children attempt to clarify their communication with repetitions, revision, and more detail. Children with schizophrenia, on the other hand, fail to aid communication with revision, fillers, or starting over. These deficits are examples of negative symptoms in childhood schizophrenia.

Although core phenomena for schizophrenia seem to be universal across the age span, a child's developmental level significantly influences the presentation of the symptoms. Delusions of young children are less complex, therefore, than those of older children; for example, age-appropriate content, such as animal imagery and monsters, is likely to be a source of delusional fear in young children. According to the DSM-5, a child with schizophrenia may experience deterioration of function, along with the emergence of psychotic symptoms, or the child may never achieve the expected level of functioning.

A 12-year-old sixth-grade boy named Ian, with a longstanding history of social isolation, academic problems, and temper outbursts, began to develop concerns that his parents might be poisoning his food. Over the next year, his symptoms progressed with increased suspiciousness and fearfulness, preoccupation with food, and beliefs that Satan was trying to communicate with him. Ian also appeared to be responding to auditory hallucinations that he believed were coming from the radio and television, which he found frightening and commanded him to harm his parents. Ian had also been informing his mother that their food had a strange smell and that he thought someone had poisoned it. At night, Ian would see frightening figures in his room. During this time, his parents also observed bizarre behaviors, including talking and yelling to himself, perseverating about devils and demons, and finally, assaulting family members because he thought they were evil. On one occasion, Ian scratched himself with a kitchen knife to "please God." No predominant mood symptoms emerged, and there was no history of substance abuse found.

Developmentally, Ian was the product of a full-term pregnancy complicated by a difficult labor and forceps delivery. His milestones, both motor and speech, were delayed by about 6 months. However, his pediatrician reassured his parents that this was within the limits of healthy development. As a younger child, Ian tended to be quiet and socially awkward. His intellectual function was tested and was in the average range; however, academic achievement testing was consistently below grade level. Ian remained lonely and isolated, and he had great difficulty making friends.

Ian has had no medical problems, and his immunizations were up to date.

Ian's family psychiatric history was significant for depression in a maternal aunt and a completed suicide in a maternal great-grandparent.

Ian was sent by ambulance to the hospital for the first time from school when he tried to jump off a balcony on the second story of his school in response to auditory hallucinations commanding him to kill himself. During his hospitalization, his parents reluctantly consented to a risperidone trial. The psychiatrist titrated Ian to 3 mg/day. His auditory hallucinations improved moderately after 2 weeks of treatment. However, he continued to be suspicious and mistrustful of his physicians and family.

Ian's family was perplexed as to what had caused Ian's severe symptoms, and the hospital treatment team met with his parents multiple times during his hospitalization to reassure them that they had not caused his illness and that their continued support might improve his chances of improvement. After discharge from the hospital 30 days later, Ian was placed in a special education program in a nonpublic school, and he was assigned a psychotherapist who met regularly with him individually and with his family. At the time of discharge from the hospital, Ian's symptoms had moderately improved, although he still had auditory hallucinations intermittently. Over the next 5 years after the onset of his illness, Ian had many exacerbations of his psychosis, and he was hospitalized nine times, including placement in a long-term residential program. Ian had received trials of olanzapine, quetiapine, and aripiprazole, each of which seemed to lead to improvement for a while, after which he was no longer responsive to the medications. Ian continued to receive individual cognitive-behavioral therapy and family therapy, and his family was very supportive. Even with these interventions, Ian's mental status continued to display tangential and disorganized thinking, paranoid delusions, loose associations, perseverative speech patterns, and a flat, at times, inappropriate affect. He had periods in which he resorted to pacing and muttering to himself, with no social interaction with others unless initiated by adults. Finally, Ian achieved significant improvement after being placed on clozapine therapy, although he remained mildly symptomatic. (Adapted from a case by Jon M. McClellan, M.D.)

Pathology and Laboratory Examinations

No specific laboratory tests are diagnostically specific for childhood-onset schizophrenia.

DIFFERENTIAL DIAGNOSIS

Making a diagnosis of childhood-onset schizophrenia is challenging. Very young children who report hallucinations, apparent thought disorders, language delays, and an inability to differentiate reality from fantasy may be manifesting phenomena better accounted for by other disorders such as PTSD, or sometimes developmental immaturity.

Nevertheless, the differential diagnosis of childhood-onset schizophrenia includes autism spectrum disorder, bipolar disorders, depressive disorders, psychotic disorders, multicomplex developmental syndromes, drug-induced psychosis, and psychosis caused by organic disease states. Children with childhood-onset schizophrenia have frequent comorbidities, including ADHD, oppositional defiant disorder, and major depression. Children with schizotypal personality disorder have some traits in common with children who meet diagnostic criteria for schizophrenia. Blunted affect, social isolation, eccentric thoughts, ideas of reference, and bizarre behavior occur in both disorders; however, in schizophrenia, overt psychotic symptoms, such as hallucinations, delusions, and incoherence, must be present at some point. Hallucinations alone, however, are not evidence of schizophrenia; patients must show either a deterioration of function or an inability to meet an expected developmental level to warrant the diagnosis of schizophrenia. Auditory and visual hallucinations can appear as self-limited events in nonpsychotic young children who are experiencing extreme stress or anxiety related to unstable home lives, abuse, or neglect or in children experiencing a significant loss.

Psychotic phenomena are common among children with major depressive disorder, in which both hallucinations and, less commonly, delusions may occur. The congruence of mood with psychotic features is most pronounced in depressed children, although children with schizophrenia may also seem sad. The hallucinations and delusions of schizophrenia are more likely to have a bizarre quality than those of children with depressive disorders. In children and adolescents with bipolar I disorder, it often is challenging to distinguish a first episode of mania with psychotic features from schizophrenia if the child has no history of previous depressions. Grandiose delusions and hallucinations are typical of manic episodes, but clinicians often must follow the natural history of the disorder to confirm the presence of a mood disorder. Autism spectrum disorders share some features with schizophrenia, most notably difficulty with social relationships, an early history of delayed language acquisition, and ongoing communication deficits. However, hallucinations, delusions, and formal thought disorder are core features of schizophrenia and not the usual features of autism spectrum disorder. Autism spectrum disorder is usually diagnosed by 3 years of age, whereas schizophrenia with childhood-onset usually manifests after 5 years of age.

Among adolescents, alcohol and other substance abuse sometimes can result in a deterioration of function, psychotic symptoms, and paranoid delusions. Amphetamines, lysergic acid diethylamide (LSD), and phencyclidine (PCP) may lead to a psychotic state. Sudden, flagrant onset of paranoid psychosis may suggest substance-induced psychotic disorder. Medical conditions that can induce psychotic features include thyroid disease, systemic lupus erythematosus, and temporal lobe disease.

COURSE AND PROGNOSIS

Significant predictors of the course and outcome of childhood and early-onset schizophrenia include the child's premorbid level of functioning, the age of onset, IQ, response to psychosocial and pharmacologic interventions, degree of remission after the first psychotic episode, and degree of family support. Early age at onset and children with comorbid developmental delays, learning disorders, lower IQ, and premorbid behavioral disorders, such as ADHD and conduct disorder, are less treatment responsive and likely to have the most guarded prognoses. Predictors of a poorer course of childhood-onset schizophrenia include a family history of schizophrenia, young age and insidious onset, developmental delays and lower level of premorbid function, and chronicity or length of a first psychotic episode. Psychosocial and family stressors are known to influence the relapse rate in adults with schizophrenia, and high expression of negative emotion (EE) likely affects children with childhood-onset schizophrenia as well.

An essential factor in the outcome is the accuracy and stability of the diagnosis of schizophrenia. One study reported that one-third of children who received an initial diagnosis of schizophrenia later have bipolar disorder in adolescence. Children and adolescents with bipolar I disorder may have a better long-term prognosis than those with schizophrenia. The NIMH-funded Treatment of Early-Onset Schizophrenia reported the outcome of neurocognitive functioning in 8- to 19-year-old youth with schizophrenia or schizoaffective disorders who participated in a randomized, double-blind clinical trial comparing molindone, olanzapine, and risperidone. The three medication groups yielded no group differences in neurocognitive functioning over a year; however, when data from the three groups were combined, a significant modest improvement was observed in several domains of neurocognitive functioning. The authors concluded that antipsychotic intervention in youth with early-onset schizophrenia spectrum disorders led to modest improvement in neurocognitive function.

TREATMENT

The treatment of childhood-onset schizophrenia requires a multimodal approach, including psychoeducation for families, pharmacologic interventions, psychotherapeutic interventions, social skills interventions, and appropriate educational placement. A recent RCT investigated the effectiveness of several psychosocial interventions on youth in an early prodromal stage characterized by changes in cognitive and social behavior. The interventions, termed integrated psychological interventions, specifically included CBT, group skills training, cognitive remediation therapy, multifamily psychoeducation, and supportive counseling on the prevention of psychosis. Of interest, the integrated psychological intervention was more effective than standard treatments in delaying the onset of psychosis over a 2-year follow-up period. These results sparked interest in the potential utility of psychosocial interventions to mediate psychosis and to alter the relapse rate and severity of illness over time. Children with childhood-onset schizophrenia may have less robust responses to antipsychotic medications than adolescents and adults. Family education and ongoing therapeutic family interventions are critical to maintaining the maximum level of support for the patient. Monitoring the most appropriate educational setting for a child with childhood-onset schizophrenia is essential, especially given the frequent social skills deficits, attention deficits, and academic difficulties that often accompany childhood-onset schizophrenia.

Pharmacotherapy

Second-generation antipsychotics, serotonin-dopamine antagonists, are the current mainstay pharmacologic treatments for children and adolescents with schizophrenia. Current data include six randomized clinical trials in youth investigating the efficacy of second-generation antipsychotics for early-onset schizophrenia, with limited support for one agent over the others. Although clozapine, a serotonin receptor antagonist with some dopamine (D_2) antagonism, may be more effective in reducing positive and negative symptoms, it remains a choice of last resort in youth based on its side effects. To date, however, evidence from multisite randomized clinical trials supports some efficacy of risperidone, olanzapine, aripiprazole, and clozapine in the treatment of childhood- and adolescent-onset schizophrenia. Two randomized clinical trials using risperidone in adolescents with schizophrenia found risperidone at doses up to 3 mg/day to be superior to placebo. A multisite randomized 6-week controlled trial of olanzapine in adolescents with schizophrenia found that it was more efficacious than a placebo. An RCT of aripiprazole at two fixed doses found that it was superior to placebo in the treatment of positive symptoms of adolescent schizophrenia; however, more than 40 percent of subjects in the active medication group did not achieve remission. Finally, clozapine is more effective than haloperidol in improving both positive and negative symptoms in treatment-resistant schizophrenia in youth. More recently, a study compared clozapine to high doses of olanzapine and found that response rates were about twice as high for clozapine as olanzapine (66 percent vs. 33 percent) when the investigators defined response as 30 percent or better reduction in symptoms on the Brief Psychiatric Rating Scale and improvement on the Clinical Global Impression Scale. The Treatment of Early-Onset Schizophrenia Spectrum Disorders Study compared the efficacy of risperidone and olanzapine with those of molindone, a mid-potency first-generation antipsychotic. In this study, lacking a placebo group, each of these agents provided a similar therapeutic effect; however, fewer than half of the patients responded optimally. Despite the limited randomized controlled studies of second-generation antipsychotics for the treatment of schizophrenia in youth, the FDA is progressively approving the use of these agents for pediatric schizophrenia and bipolar illness. In 2007, the FDA approved the use of risperidone and aripiprazole for the treatment of schizophrenia in 13- to 17-year-olds. The FDA approved the use of olanzapine and quetiapine in 2009 for the treatment of schizophrenia in 13- to 17-year-olds. Lurasidone and paliperidone were approved by the FDA in 2017 for the treatment of schizophrenia in adolescents.

A double-blind, randomized 8-week controlled trial compared the efficacy and safety of olanzapine to clozapine in childhood-onset schizophrenia. Children with childhood-onset schizophrenia who were resistant to at least two previous treatments with antipsychotics were randomized to treatment for 8 weeks with either olanzapine or clozapine followed by a 2-year open-label follow-up. Using the *Clinical Global Impression of Severity of Symptoms Scale and Schedule for the Assessment of Negative/Positive Symptoms,* clozapine was associated with a significant reduction in all outcome measures. In contrast, olanzapine showed improvement on some measures but not on all. The only statistically significant measure in which clozapine was superior to olanzapine was in alleviating negative symptoms compared with baseline. Clozapine was associated with more adverse events, such as lipid abnormalities and a seizure in one patient.

Several studies have provided evidence that risperidone, a benzisoxazole derivative, is as effective as the older high-potency first-generation antipsychotics, such as haloperidol, and causes less frequent severe side effects in the treatment of schizophrenia in older adolescents and adults. Published case reports and limited more extensive controlled studies have supported the efficacy of risperidone in the treatment of psychosis in children and adolescents. Risperidone can cause weight gain and dystonic reactions and other extrapyramidal adverse effects in children and adolescents. Olanzapine is generally well tolerated for extrapyramidal adverse effects compared with first-generation antipsychotics and risperidone, but it is associated with moderate sedation and significant weight gain.

Psychosocial Interventions

Psychosocial interventions aimed at family education and patient and family support are critical components of the treatment plan for childhood-onset schizophrenia. Although there are not yet RCTs of psychosocial interventions in children and adolescents with schizophrenia, family therapy, psychoeducation, and social skills training have been shown to lead to improved clinical symptoms in young adults with a first episode of schizophrenia, and reviews of the adult literature support the benefit of CBT and cognitive remediation as adjunctive treatments to pharmacologic agents in adults. Psychotherapists who work with children with schizophrenia must take into account a child's developmental level in order to support the child's reality testing and be sensitive to the child's sense of self. Long-term supportive family interventions and cognitive-behavioral and remediation interventions, combined with pharmacotherapy, are likely to be the most effective approach to early-onset schizophrenia.

EPIDEMIOLOGY

Childhood-onset schizophrenia affects less than 1 in 40,000 children. For adolescents, this increases by at least 50-fold. Childhood-onset schizophrenia resembles the more severe forms of adult schizophrenia, although it has exceptionally high comorbidity rates. Comorbid disorders include ADHD, depressive disorders, anxiety disorders, speech and language disorders, and motor disturbances.

Boys seem to have a slight preponderance among children diagnosed with schizophrenia, with an estimated ratio of about 1.67 boys to 1 girl. Boys often become identified at a younger age than girls do. Schizophrenia rarely is diagnosed in children younger than 5 years of age. The prevalence of schizophrenia among the parents of children with schizophrenia is about 8 percent, which is about twice the prevalence in the parents of patients with adult-onset schizophrenia.

ETIOLOGY

Childhood-onset schizophrenia is a neurodevelopmental disorder in which complex interactions between genes and the environment result in abnormal early brain development. The consequences of the aberrant brain development in schizophrenia may not be fully evident until adolescence or early adulthood; however, data support the hypothesis that white matter abnormalities and disturbances in myelination in childhood lead to abnormal connectivity between brain regions. The aberrant connectivity in various regions of the brain is likely a significant contributing factor in the psychotic symptoms and cognitive deficits in childhood-onset schizophrenia.

Genetic Factors

Estimates of heritability for childhood-onset schizophrenia have been as high as 80 percent. Children with childhood-onset schizophrenia have higher rates of schizophrenia among their relatives than do patients with adult-onset schizophrenia.

Endophenotype Markers for Childhood-Onset Schizophrenia.   Currently, no reliable method can identify persons at the highest risk for schizophrenia in a given family. Neurodevelopmental abnormalities and higher-than-expected rates of neurologic soft signs and impairments in sustaining attention and in strategies for information processing appear among children at high risk. Increased rates of disturbed communication styles exist in family members of individuals with schizophrenia. Reports have documented higher-than-expected neuropsychological deficits in attention, working memory, and premorbid IQ among children who later develop schizophrenia and its spectrum disorders.

Magnetic Resonance Imaging (MRI) Studies

An NIMH prospective study of more than 100 patients with childhood-onset schizophrenia and their typically developing siblings has demonstrated progressive loss of gray matter, delayed and disrupted white matter growth, and a decline in cerebellar volume in those with childhood-onset schizophrenia. Although siblings of children with childhood-onset schizophrenia also showed some of these brain disruptions, the gray matter abnormalities were normalized over time in the siblings, indicating a protective mechanism in siblings that was not present in those children with childhood-onset schizophrenia. Furthermore, the hippocampal volume loss across the age span appears to be static among children with childhood-onset schizophrenia. An MRI NIMH study of more than 100 children with childhood-onset schizophrenia and their typically developing siblings, studied for about two decades, documented that in childhood-onset schizophrenia, progressive brain gray matter loss occurs continuously over time. This gray matter shrinkage occurs with ventricular increases, with a pattern of loss originating in the parietal region and proceeding frontally to dorsolateral prefrontal and temporal cortices, including superior temporal gyri. Studies of childhood-onset schizophrenia at the NIMH provided evidence that early loss of parietal gray matter followed by frontal and parietal gray matter loss is more pronounced in childhood-onset schizophrenia than in schizophrenia with later onset. Other research utilized diffusion tensor images from children with childhood-onset schizophrenia versus controls and found increased diffusivities in the posterior corona radiata in children with childhood-onset schizophrenia, which implicated abnormal connectivity with the parietal lobes. These results contrasted with findings among subjects with later onset of schizophrenia in whom there were more abnormalities in the frontal lobes.

ATTENUATED PSYCHOSIS SYNDROME

Attenuated Psychosis Syndrome (APS) is a new diagnostic category included in DSM-5 as a condition for further study. It is a syndrome characterized by subthreshold psychotic symptoms, less severe than those found in psychotic disorders, but which are often present in prodromal psychotic states.

Debate and controversy among clinicians and researchers have surrounded the inclusion of APS in the DSM-5. Some believe that the identification and treatment of a prodromal syndrome of a psychotic disorder would either delay or diminish the severity of the future psychotic illness. However, others believe that identification of a prodromal syndrome, which may rarely, if ever, progress to a full psychotic illness, would lead to unnecessary exposure to antipsychotic agents with unpredictable and possibly harmful effects. There is an agreement, however, that patients with subthreshold prodromal psychotic symptoms are often impaired and need psychological and psychiatric intervention.

A recent meta-analysis reported that the rate of onset of psychotic disorders in those patients with prodromal psychotic symptoms was 18 percent at 6 months, 22 percent at 1 year, 29 percent at 2 years, and 36 percent at 3 years. In a follow-up study, of those with prodromal symptoms who went on to develop a threshold psychotic illness, 73 percent met the criteria for schizophrenia.

In children and adolescents, psychotic symptoms are not necessarily a hallmark of a threshold psychotic disorder compared to adults. For example, in 50 percent of children with major depressive episodes, psychotic symptoms were present. Also, epidemiologic studies have found that globally, auditory hallucinations occur in 9 percent to 21 percent of children and 8.4 percent of adolescents. Thus, in youth, the association between subthreshold psychotic symptoms and the emergence of future psychotic illness may not be a reliable predictor. Nevertheless, identification and follow up of youth with APS may provide an increased understanding of the longitudinal significance of these symptoms.

Diagnosis

Attenuated psychosis syndrome, according to DSM-5, is based on the presence of at least one of the following: delusions, hallucinations, or disorganized speech, which causes functional impairment. Although the symptoms may not have progressed to full psychotic severity, they must have been present at least once per week for 1 month and must have emerged or worsened in the past year. The symptoms must cause impairment and warrant clinical attention.

Attenuated delusions are described as either suspiciousness, persecutory or grandiose, resulting in a lack of trust in others, and a sense of danger. Attenuated delusions, in contrast to delusions of threshold illness, may lead to loosely organized beliefs about hostile intentions of others or danger; however, the delusions are not as fixed as they become in full-blown psychotic illness. Attenuated hallucinations include altered sensory perceptions such as the perception of murmurs, rumblings, or shadows that are disturbing, but which youth may doubt and challenge. Disorganized communication or speech may present as vague or confusing explanations or circumstantial or tangential communication. When severe but still in the attenuated range, thought blocking or loose associations may emerge; however, in contrast to psychotic illness, redirection is possible, and one can usually achieve a logical conversation. Although impairment is present in APS, the individual retains awareness and insight into the mental changes that are occurring.

Treatment

A recent review of the literature on treatment trials with patients at ultra-high-risk for psychosis found that early intervention with both psychological interventions and pharmacologic agents can reduce symptoms and either delay or prevent the onset of a full psychotic illness. Other studies, however, found mixed results for early psychological or pharmacologic interventions to prevent the onset of psychotic illness. One study found that most patients who became frankly psychotic did so within a few months after joining the study, making it difficult to determine if these patients were already exhibiting early signs of the onset of schizophrenia when identified as prodromal.

A variety of treatment approaches exist, including treatment with risperidone, olanzapine, omega-3 polyunsaturated fatty acid (w-3PUFA), CBT, cognitive therapy (CT), and one using an integrated psychological intervention (IPI) including cognitive approaches, psychoeducation, and social skills intervention. A review of treatment effectiveness in APS found that receiving treatment was associated with a lower risk of psychotic illness at 1 year, 2 years, and 3 years. Given the limited data, however, it is not clear which interventions are most efficacious. Therefore, until additional treatment trials provide efficacy data, the safest choices for treatment of APS include psychological interventions rather than the use of antipsychotic agents. In summary, APS identifies a group of patients with psychotic-like phenomena that warrant interventions in order to improve their distress and functional levels. Further study is needed, however, to determine the relationship between APS and the development of schizophrenia and other psychotic illnesses.

Etiology

Genetic Factors. Family studies have demonstrated that genetic factors influence vulnerability for schizophrenia spectrum disorders and other psychotic disorders. To the extent that APS and schizophrenia are related, genetic contributions are likely to be significant. Adoption and twin studies have confirmed that monozygotic twins have about a 50 percent concordance rate for schizophrenia compared to dizygotic twins who have a concordance rate of about 10 percent. Also, adopted children of parents with schizophrenia do not have higher rates of schizophrenia; but biologic children of schizophrenic parents do. However, genetic factors do not account fully for the emergence of schizophrenia spectrum disorders, since there is only a 50 percent concordance of exhibiting these disorders among monozygotic twins. Environmental factors also play an essential role.

Environmental Factors. Early environmental factors that increase the risk of developing schizophrenia include fetal malnutrition, hypoxia at birth, and possibly prenatal infections. Other environmental factors include trauma, stress, social adversity, and isolation. Finally, gene-environment interactions may influence an individual's sensitivity to adverse environmental events.

▲ 2.17 Adolescent Substance Use Disorders

Substance use is a public health concern among American youth. The most common substances used by adolescents in the United States are tobacco, alcohol, and marijuana. There are many other substances that adolescents may abuse. These include cocaine, heroin, inhalants, phencyclidine (PCP), lysergic acid diethylamide (LSD), dextromethorphan, anabolic steroids, and various club drugs, including 3,4-methylenedioxymethamphetamine (MDMA or Ecstasy), flunitrazepam, gamma-hydroxybutyrate (GHB), and ketamine.

Approximately 20 percent of 8th graders in the United States have tried illicit drugs, and about 30 percent of 10th through 12th graders have used an illicit substance. Alcohol remains the most common substance used and abused by adolescents. Binge drinking occurs in about 6 percent of adolescents, and teens with alcohol use disorders are at higher risk of problems with other substances as well.

The DSM-5 combines abuse and dependence under the diagnosis of substance use disorder. It also contains diagnoses for intoxication, withdrawal, and substance-induced disorders. These apply to youths as well as adults. Some experts are concerned about the relevance of the criteria to adolescents, especially regarding tolerance and withdrawal. Some adolescents may develop tolerance to alcohol, for example, without any impairment. Withdrawal may have clinical significance. However, it does not correlate well with the level of severity.

Many risk and protective factors influence the age of onset and severity of substance use among adolescents. Psychosocial risk factors mediating the development of substance use disorders include parent modeling of substance use, family conflict, lack of parental supervision, peer relationships, and individual stressful life events. Protective factors that mitigate substance use among adolescents include variables such as stable family life, strong parent–child bond, consistent parental supervision, investment in academic achievement, and a peer group that models prosocial family and school behaviors. Interventions that diminish risk factors are likely to mitigate substance use.

Approximately one of five adolescents has used marijuana or hashish. Approximately one-third of adolescents have used cigarettes by age 17 years. Studies of alcohol use among adolescents in the United States have shown that by 13 years of age, one-third of boys and almost one-fourth of girls have tried alcohol. By 18 years of age, 92 percent of males and 73 percent of females reported trying alcohol, and 4 percent reported using alcohol daily. Of high school seniors, 41 percent reported using marijuana; 2 percent reported using the drug daily.

Drinking among adolescents follows adult demographic drinking patterns: The highest proportion of alcohol use occurs among adolescents in the northeast; whites are more likely to drink than are other groups; among whites, Roman Catholics are the least likely nondrinkers. The four most common causes of death in persons between the ages of 10 and 24 years are motor vehicle accidents (37 percent), homicide (14 percent), suicide (12 percent), and other injuries or accidents (12 percent). In pediatric trauma centers, more than one-third of adolescents need treatment for alcohol or drug use.

Studies considering alcohol and illicit drug use by adolescents as psychiatric disorders have demonstrated a higher prevalence of substance use, particularly alcoholism, among biologic children of alcoholics than among adopted youth. This finding is supported by family studies of genetic contributions, by adoption studies, and by observing children of substance users reared outside the biologic home.

Numerous risk factors influence the emergence of adolescent substance abuse. These include parental belief in the harmlessness of substances, lack of anger control in families of substance abusers, lack of closeness and involvement of parents with children's activities, maternal passivity, academic difficulties, comorbid psychiatric disorders such as conduct disorder and depression, parental and peer substance use, impulsivity, and early onset of cigarette smoking. The higher the number of risk factors, the more likely it is that an adolescent will be a substance user.

DIAGNOSIS AND CLINICAL FEATURES

Chapter 4 discusses the substance-related disorders and their diagnoses, including substance use, substance intoxication, and substance withdrawal disorder.

We should make a diagnosis of alcohol or drug use in adolescents through a careful interview, observations, laboratory findings, and history provided by reliable sources. Many nonspecific signs may point to alcohol or drug use, and clinicians must be careful to corroborate hunches before jumping to conclusions. Substance use exists on a continuum with experimentation (the mildest use), regular use without visible impairment, abuse, and, finally, dependence. Changes in academic performance, nonspecific physical ailments, changes in relationships with family members, changes in one's peer group, unexplained phone calls, or changes in personal hygiene may indicate substance use in an adolescent. Many of these also occur with depression, prodromal psychotic disorders, and adjustment issues, for example, to a new school.

Substance use is related to a variety of behaviors, including early sexual experimentation, risky driving, destruction of property, stealing, "heavy metal" or electronic dance music (EDM), and, occasionally, preoccupation with cults or Satanism. Although none of these behaviors necessarily predicts substance use, at the extreme, many of these behaviors reflect alienation from the mainstream of developmentally expected social behavior. Adolescents with inadequate social skills may use a substance as a modality to join a peer group. In some cases, adolescents begin their substance use at home with their parents, who also use substances to enhance their social interactions. Although no evidence indicates what determines a typical adolescent user of alcohol or drugs, many substance users seem to have underlying social skills deficits, academic difficulties, and less than optimal peer relationships.

Nicotine

Nicotine is one of the most addictive substances known; it involves cholinergic receptors and enhancing acetylcholine, serotonin, and β-endorphin release. Young teens who smoke cigarettes are also exposed to other drugs more frequently than nonsmoking peers.

Alcohol

Alcohol use in adolescents rarely results in the sequelae observed in adults with chronic use of alcohol, such as withdrawal seizures, Korsakoff syndrome, Wernicke aphasia, or cirrhosis of the liver. One report, however, has stated that adolescent exposure to alcohol may result in diminished hippocampal brain volume. Because the hippocampus is involved with attention, it is conceivable that adolescent alcohol use could result in compromised cognitive function, especially concerning attention.

Marijuana

The short-term effects of the active ingredient in marijuana, tetrahydrocannabinol (THC), include impairment in memory and learning, distorted perception, diminished problem-solving ability, loss of coordination, increased heart rate, anxiety, and panic attacks. Abrupt cessation of heavy marijuana use by adolescents can result in a withdrawal syndrome characterized by insomnia, irritability, restlessness, drug craving, depressed mood, and nervousness followed by anxiety, tremors, nausea, muscle twitches, increased sweating, myalgia, and general malaise. Typically, the withdrawal syndrome begins 24 hours after the last use, peaks at 2 to 4 days, and diminishes after 2 weeks. Marijuana use correlates with an increased risk of psychiatric disorders. Poor cognitive functioning has been associated with chronic marijuana use, although it is not clear whether marijuana impairs cognitive function. Deficits in verbal learning, memory, and attention occur in chronic marijuana users, and both acute and chronic marijuana use is associated with changes in cerebral blood flow to specific brain regions, which can be detected by PET. Functional imaging studies suggest that there is less activity in brain regions involved with attention and memory in chronic marijuana users. A 15-year follow-up of 50,465 Swedish males in the military reported that participants who had used marijuana by 18 years of age were 2.4 times more likely to develop schizophrenia. Risks associated with chronic marijuana use include higher rates of motor vehicle accidents, impaired respiratory function, increased risk of cardiovascular disease, and potential increased risk for psychotic symptoms and disorders.

Cocaine

Cocaine can be sniffed or snorted, injected, or smoked. *Crack* is the term given to cocaine that has been changed to a free base for smoking. Cocaine's effects include constriction of peripheral blood vessels, dilated pupils, hyperthermia, increased heart rate, and hypertension. High doses or prolonged use of cocaine can induce paranoid thinking. There is an immediate risk of death secondary to cardiac arrest or from seizures followed by respiratory arrest. In contrast to stimulants used to treat ADHD, such as methylphenidate, cocaine quickly crosses the blood-brain barrier and moves off the dopamine transporter within 20 minutes; methylphenidate remains bound to dopamine for long periods.

Heroin

Heroin, a derivative of morphine, is produced from a poppy plant. Heroin usually appears as a white or brown powder that users can snort, but more commonly, they take it intravenously. Withdrawal symptoms include restlessness, muscle and bone pain, insomnia, diarrhea and vomiting, cold flashes with goosebumps, and kicking movements. Withdrawal occurs within a few hours after use; symptoms peak between 48 and 72 hours later and remit within about a week.

Club Drugs

Adolescents who frequent nightclubs, raves, bars, or music clubs also frequently use MDMA, GHB, flunitrazepam (Rohypnol), and ketamine. GHB, flunitrazepam (a benzodiazepine), and ketamine (an anesthetic) are primarily depressants and can be added to drinks without detection because they are often colorless, tasteless, and odorless. Congress passed The Drug-Induced Rape Prevention and Punishment Act after finding that these drugs were used in date rapes. MDMA is a derivative of methamphetamine, a synthetic with both stimulant and hallucinogenic properties. MDMA can inhibit serotonin and dopamine reuptake. MDMA can result in dry mouth, increased heart rate, fatigue, muscle spasm, and hyperthermia.

Lysergic Acid Diethylamide

LSD is odorless, colorless, and has a slightly bitter taste. Higher doses of LSD can produce visual hallucinations and delusions and, in some cases, panic. The sensations experienced after the ingestion of LSD usually diminish after 12 hours. Flashbacks can occur up to 1 year after use. LSD can produce tolerance; that is, after multiple uses, one needs more to feel the same degree of intoxication.

COMORBIDITY

Rates of alcohol and marijuana use are reportedly higher in relatives of youth with depression and anxiety disorders. On the other hand, mood disorders are common among those with alcoholism. Evidence indicates another strong link between early antisocial behavior, conduct disorder, and substance abuse. Substance abuse is a form of behavioral deviance that, unsurprisingly, is associated with other forms of social and behavioral deviance. Early intervention with children who show early signs of social deviance and antisocial behavior may conceivably impede the processes that contribute to later substance abuse.

It is essential to know about all comorbid disorders, which may show differential responses to treatment. Surveys of adolescents with alcoholism show rates of 50 percent or higher for additional psychiatric disorders, especially mood disorders. A recent survey of adolescents who used alcohol found that more than 80 percent met the criteria for another disorder. The disorders most frequently present were depressive disorders, disruptive behavior disorders, and drug use disorders. These rates of comorbidity are even higher than those for adults. The diagnosis of alcohol use disorder was likely to follow, rather than precede, other disorders; that a large proportion of adolescents with alcoholism have a previous childhood disorder may have both etiologic and treatment implications. In this survey, the onset of alcohol use disorders did not systematically precede other substance use disorders. In 50 percent of cases, alcohol use followed drug use. Alcohol use may be a gateway to drug use but is not in most cases. The presence of other psychiatric disorders was associated with an earlier onset of alcohol use disorder, but it did not seem to indicate a more protracted course of alcoholism.

TREATMENT

Interventions for substance use disorders in adolescents first require effective screening and identification of those teens in need of treatment. Once identifying a substance use disorder in a teen, we have a variety of treatment options.

Per the goals of the U.S. Substance Abuse Mental Health Services Administration (SAMHSA), a school-based alcohol and drug Screening, Brief Intervention, and Referral to Treatment (SBIRT) has been initiated in a study with 629 adolescents ages 14 to 17 years in 13 participating high schools in New Mexico. Initially, school-based health centers provided substance use screenings for all students seen in the clinic for any reason. Once identified, substance-using adolescents were offered either brief intervention by clinic staff (85.1 percent of those identified), whereas 14.9 percent received brief treatment or referral to treatment. The brief intervention was based on motivational interviewing to help the student to gain motivation for behavioral change, with referral for more intensive treatment if needed. Students who received the intervention, regardless of the severity of their substance use, reported decreases in self-reported drinking to intoxication at the 6-month follow-up.

The students reporting drug use self-reported using less at follow-up. Forty-two percent of the students reported alcohol use, and 37 percent reported intoxication. Eighty-five percent of study participants who reported drug use reported only marijuana use in the month before entering the study. The frequency of alcohol and marijuana as the most predominant substances in this age group is consistent with epidemiologic data. Overall, this school-based intervention had the advantage of being easily accessible to adolescents and provided a graded option for treatment according to the severity of substance use. This study suggests that school-based programs for identifying and providing brief interventions for high school students is viable and merits further study.

Treatment of substance use disorders in adolescents can directly prevent the substance use behaviors, provide education for the patient and family, and address cognitive, emotional, and psychiatric factors that influence the substance use in a variety of settings such as a residential milieu, group, and individual psychosocial session.

One validated instrument used as a guide for clinicians in the treatment of adolescent substance use designates levels of care appropriate for the symptoms. This instrument, called the *Child and Adolescent Levels of Care Utilization Services* (CALOCUS), outlines six levels of care:

0: Basic services (prevention)
1: Recovery maintenance (relapse prevention)
2: Outpatient (once per week visits)
3: Intensive outpatient (2 or more visits per week)
4: Intensive integrated services (day treatment, partial hospitalization, wraparound services)
5: Nonsecure, 24-hour medically monitored service (group home, residential treatment facility)
6: Secure 24-hour medical management (inpatient psychiatric or highly programmed residential facility)

Treatment settings that serve adolescents with alcohol or drug use disorders include inpatient units, residential treatment facilities, halfway houses, group homes, partial hospital programs, and outpatient settings. Components of adolescent alcohol or drug use treatment include individual psychotherapy, drug-specific counseling, self-help groups (Alcoholics Anonymous [AA], Narcotics Anonymous [NA], Alateen, Al-Anon), substance abuse education and relapse prevention programs, and random urine drug testing. Family therapy and psychopharmacologic intervention are also useful to add.

Before deciding on the most appropriate treatment setting for a particular adolescent, a screening process must take place in which structured and unstructured interviews help to determine the types of substances they are using as well as the quantities and frequencies. Determining coexisting psychiatric disorders is also critical. Rating scales can document pretreatment and posttreatment severity of abuse. The *Teen Addiction Severity Index* (T-ASI), the *Adolescent Drug and Alcohol Diagnostic Assessment* (ADAD), and the *Adolescent Problem Severity Index* (APSI) are several severity-oriented rating scales. The T-ASI is broken down into dimensions that include family function, school or employment status, psychiatric status, peer social relationships, and legal status.

After obtaining most of the information about substance use and the patient's overall psychiatric status, we must choose a treatment strategy, and an appropriate setting must be determined. Two very different approaches to the treatment of substance use disorders are the Minnesota model and the multidisciplinary professional model. The Minnesota model relies on the premise of AA; it is an intensive 12-step program with a counselor who functions as the primary therapist. The program uses self-help participation and group processes. Inherent in this treatment strategy is the need for adolescents to admit that substance use is problematic and that help is necessary. Furthermore, they must be willing to work toward altering their lifestyle to eradicate substance use.

The multidisciplinary professional model consists of a team of mental health professionals that usually is led by a physician.

Following a case-management model, each member of the team has specific areas of treatment for which he or she is responsible. Interventions may include CBT, family therapy, and pharmacologic intervention. This approach usually is suited for adolescents with comorbid psychiatric diagnoses.

Cognitive-behavioral approaches to psychotherapy for adolescents with substance use generally require that adolescents be motivated to participate in treatment and refrain from further substance use. The therapy focuses on relapse prevention and maintaining abstinence.

Psychopharmacological interventions for adolescent alcohol and drug users are still in their early stages. The presence of mood disorders indicates the need for antidepressants, and generally, the SSRIs are the first line of treatment. Occasionally, we might choose to substitute the illicit drug with another drug that is more amenable to the treatment situation; for example, using methadone instead of heroin. Adolescents are required to have documented attempts at detoxification and consent from an adult before they can enter such a treatment program.

Peter, a 16-year-old 11th grader, was admitted to substance abuse treatment for the second time, following a relapse and threats of suicide. Peter reported a longstanding history of ADHD, but he had been a good student and not had any difficulties until middle school. Peter reported an onset of substance use at age 13 years, a rapid progression in substance involvement since age 14 years, and current use of marijuana daily, drinking alcohol up to five times each week, and experimentation with a variety of substances, such as LSD and Ecstasy. After being discharged from the psychiatric hospital, Peter attended teen group sessions focusing on his substance use problems. Family sessions led to the realization that Peter's mother had been depressed for some time, and she entered into her own treatment. Peter was improving concerning his substance use; however, his depressive symptoms increased following 4 weeks of abstinence. His psychiatrist started him on fluoxetine. After titrating the medication to 30 mg, Perter remained on it for a month, at which time he showed improvement in mood and treatment compliance. Peter continued to attend teen AA meetings and outpatient therapy. The family conflict soon recurred, however, and Peter became noncompliant with outpatient treatment, medication, and meetings. He resumed old relationships with substance-using peers and relapsed into daily marijuana use and occasional alcohol use. (Courtesy of Oscar G. Bukstein, M.D.)

Efficacious treatments for cigarette smoking cessation include nicotine-containing gum, patches, or nasal spray or inhaler. Bupropion aids in diminishing cravings for nicotine and is beneficial in the treatment of smoking cessation.

Because comorbidity influences treatment outcome, it is essential to pay attention to other disorders, such as mood disorders, anxiety disorders, conduct disorder, or ADHD during the treatment of substance use disorders.

EPIDEMIOLOGY

Alcohol

The Centers for Disease Control and Prevention Youth Risk Behavior Survey found that 72.5 percent of high school students had tried at least one alcoholic drink, and 24.2 percent reported an episode of heavy drinking in the month preceding the survey. Findings from the Monitoring the Future Survey suggest that about 39 percent of adolescents have used alcohol before the eighth grade. Another survey found that drinking was a significant problem for 10 to

20 percent of adolescents. Seventy percent of eighth grade students reported drinking, and 54 percent reported drinking within the past year, 27 percent reported having gotten drunk at least once, and 13 percent reported binge drinking in the 2 weeks before the survey. By the 12th grade, 88 percent of high school students reported drinking, and 77 percent drank within the past year; 5 percent of 8th-grade students, 1.3 percent of 10th grade students, and 3.6 percent of 12th grade students reported daily alcohol use. In the age range of 13 to 17 years, in the United States, reports indicate there are 3 million problem drinkers and 300,000 adolescents with alcohol dependence. The gap between male and female alcohol consumers is narrowing.

Marijuana

For the last two decades, marijuana has been one of the most widely used drugs by young people in developed countries, and recently it has become highly used globally. The United Nations Office on Drugs and Crime estimated that 3.9 percent of people worldwide between ages 15 years and 64 use marijuana. Marijuana is the most commonly used illicit drug among high school students in the United States. About 10 percent of those who try marijuana become daily users and 20 to 30 percent become weekly users. Marijuana is a "gateway drug" because the strongest predictor of future cocaine use is frequent marijuana use during adolescence. Of 8th-, 10th-, and 12th-grade students, 10, 23, and 36 percent, respectively, report using marijuana, a slight decrease from the year preceding the survey. Of 8th-, 10th-, and 12th-grade students, 0.2, 0.8, and 2 percent, respectively, report daily marijuana use. Prevalence rates for marijuana are highest among Native American males and females; these rates are nearly as high in white males and females and Mexican American males. The lowest annual rates occur in Latin American females, African American females, and Asian American males and females.

Cocaine

The annual cocaine use reported by high school seniors decreased by more than 30 percent between 1990 and 2000. Currently, about 0.5 percent of 8th-grade students, 1 percent of 10th-grade students, and 2 percent of 12th-grade students are estimated to have used cocaine. Crack cocaine use, however, is increasing in prevalence and is most common among those between the ages of 18 and 25.

Crystal Methamphetamine

Crystal methamphetamine, or "ice," was at a relatively low level of use in adolescence about one decade ago of 0.5 percent, and has steadily increased to a recent rate of 1.5 percent among 12th graders.

Opioids

A survey of 7,374 high school seniors found that 12.9 percent reported nonmedical use of opioids. Of users, more than 37 percent reported intranasal administration of prescription opioids.

Lysergic Acid Diethylamide (LSD)

About 3 percent of 8th-grade students, 6 percent of 10th-grade students, and 9 percent of 12th-grade students used LSD. Of 12th-grade students, 0.1 percent report daily use. The current LSD rates are lower than the rates of LSD use during the past two decades.

3,4-Methylenedioxymethamphetamine (MDMA)

MDMA has increased in popularity over the last decade. In the United States, 5 percent of 10th graders and 8 percent of 12th graders use the drug. This is true even though its perceived danger has dramatically increased among adolescents. There have been accidental adolescent deaths due to MDMA.

Gamma-Hydroxybutyrate (GHB)

Gamma-hydroxybutyrate, a club drug, has been found in surveys to have an annual prevalence rate of 1.1 percent for 8th graders, 1.0 percent for 10th graders, and a 1.6 percent rate of use for 12th graders.

Ketamine

Ketamine, another club drug, was found recently to have a rate of 1.3 percent annual prevalence for 8th graders, 2.1 percent for 10th graders, and 2.5 percent rate for 12th graders.

Flunitrazepam (Rohypnol)

Flunitrazepam (Rohypnol), a third club drug, has been found to have an annual prevalence rate of about 1 percent for all high school grades combined.

Anabolic Steroids

Despite reported knowledge of the risks of anabolic steroids among high school students, surveys over the last 5 years found rates of anabolic steroid use to be 1.6 percent among 8th graders and 2.1 percent among 10th graders. Up to 45 percent of 10th and 12th graders reported knowledge of the risks of anabolic steroids; however, over the last decade, it appears that high school seniors reported less disapproval of their use.

Inhalants

The use of inhalants in the form of glue, aerosols, and gasoline is relatively more common among younger than older adolescents. Among 8th-, 10th-, and 12th-grade students, 17.6, 15.7, and 17.6 percent, respectively, report using inhalants; 0.2 percent of 8th-grade students, 0.1 percent of 10th-grade students, and 0.2 percent of 12th-grade students report daily use of inhalants.

Multiple Substance Use

Among adolescents enrolled in substance abuse treatment programs, 96 percent are polydrug users; 97 percent of adolescents who abuse drugs also use alcohol.

ETIOLOGY

Genetic Factors

The concordance for alcoholism is reportedly higher among monozygotic than dizygotic twins. Studies of children of alcoholics reared away from their biologic homes have shown that these children have about a 25 percent chance of becoming alcoholics.

Psychosocial Factors

Among adolescents, substance use, particularly marijuana use, is strongly influenced by peers, and especially for those adolescents who report using marijuana for relaxation, the drug is used to escape from stress and as a social activity. There are data to suggest, however, that marijuana use is also associated with both social anxiety disorder and depressive symptoms. Among young adolescents who start using alcohol, tobacco, and marijuana at an early age, data suggest that they often come from families with low parental supervision. The risk of early initiation of substances is most significant for children below 11 years of age. Increased parental supervision during middle childhood years may diminish drug and alcohol sampling and ultimately diminish the risk of using marijuana, cocaine, or inhalants in the future.

References

Intellectual Disabilities

American Association on Intellectual and Developmental Disabilities. Overview of intellectual disability: definition, classifications and systems of support. 2010.

Arnold LE, Farmer C, Kraemer HC, Davies M, Witwer A, Chuang S, DiSilvestro R, McDougle CJ, McCracken J, Vitello B, Aman M, Scahill L, Posey DJ, Swiezy NB. Moderators, mediators, and other predictors of risperidone response in children with autistic disorder and irritability. *J Child Adolesc Psychopharmacol.* 2010;20:83–93.

Boulet S, Boyle C, Schieve L. Trends in health care utilization and health impact of developmental disabilities, 1997–2005. *Arch Pediatr Adolesc Med.* 2009;163: 19–26.

Correia Filho AG, Bodanase R, Silva TL, Alvarez JP, Aman M, Rohde LA. Comparison of risperidone and methylphenidate for reducing ADHD symptoms in children and adolescents with moderate intellectual disability. *J Am Acad Child Adolesc Psychiatry.* 2005;44:748.

Ellison JW, Rosengeld JA, Shaffer LG. Genetic basis of intellectual disability. *Annu Rev Med.* 2013;64:441–450.

Fowler MG, Gable AR, Lampe MA, Etima M, Owor M. Perinatal HIV and its prevention: progress toward an HIV-free generation. *Clin Perinatol.* 2010;37:699–719.

Gothelf D, Furfaro JA, Penniman LC, Glover GH, Reiss AL. The contribution of novel brain imaging techniques to understanding the neurobiology of intellectual disability and developmental disabilities. *Ment Retard Dev Disabil Res Rev.* 2005;11:331.

Ismail S, Buckley S, Budacki R, Jabbar A, Gallicano GI. Screening, diagnosing and prevention of fetal alcohol syndrome: Is this syndrome treatable? *Dev Neurosci.* 2010;32:91–100.

Obi O, Braun KVN, Baio J, Drews-Botsch C, Devine O, Yeargin-Allsopp M. Effect of incorporating adaptive functioning scores on the prevalence of intellectual disability. *Am J Intellect Dev Disabil.* 2011;116:360–370.

Reyes M, Croonenberghs J, Augustyns I, Eerdekens M. Long-term use of risperidone in children with disruptive behavior disorders and subaverage intelligence: efficacy, safety, and tolerability. *J Child Adolesc Psychopharmacol.* 2006;16:260–272.

Rowles BM, Findling RL. Review of pharmacotherapy options for the treatment of attention-deficit/hyperactivity disorder (ADHD) and ADHD-like symptoms in children and adolescents with developmental disorders. *Dev Disabil Res Rev.* 2010;16:273–282.

Stuart H. United Nations convention on the rights of persons with disabilities: a roadmap for change. *Curr Opin Psychiatry.* 2012;25:365–369.

Sturgeon X, Le T, Ahmed MM, Gardiner KJ. Pathways to cognitive deficits in Down syndrome. *Prog Brain Res.* 2012;197:73–100.

United Nations General Assembly. Convention on the Rights of Persons with Disabilities (CRPD). Geneva: United Nations; December 13, 2006.

Wijetunge LS, Chatterji S, Wyllie DJ, Kind PC. Fragile X syndrome: from targets to treatments. *Neuropharmacology.* 2013;68:83–96.

Willen EJ. Neurocognitive outcomes in pediatric HIV. *Ment Retard Dev Disabil Res Rev.* 2006;12:223–228.

Communication Disorders

Adams C, Lockton E, Freed J, Gaile J, Earl G, McBean K, Nash J, Green J, Vail A, Law J. The Social Communication Intervention Project: a randomized controlled trial of the effectiveness of speech and language therapy for school-age children who have pragmatic and social communication problems with or without autism spectrum disorder. *Int J Lang Commun Disord.* 2012;47:233–244.

Blumgart E, Tran Y, Craig A. Social anxiety in adults who stutter. *Depress Anxiety.* 2010;27:687–692.

Boulet SL, Boyle CA, Schieve LA. Health care use and health and functional impact of developmental disabilities among US children 1997–2005. *Arch Pediatr Adolesc Med.* 2009;163:19–26.

Bressman T, Beitchman JH. Communication disorder not otherwise specified. In: Sadock BJ, Sadock VA, eds. *Kaplan & Sadock's Comprehensive Textbook of Psychiatry.* 9th ed. Philadelphia, PA: Lippincott Williams & Wilkins; 2009:3534.

Cantwell DP, Baker LP. *Psychiatric and Developmental Disorders in Children with Communication Disorders.* Washington, DC: American Psychiatric Press; 1991.

Cone-Wessen B. Prenatal alcohol and cocaine exposure: influences on cognition, speech, language and hearing. *J Commun Disord.* 2005;38:279.

Gibson J, Adams C, Lockton E, Green J. Social communication disorder outside autism? A diagnostic classification approach to delineating pragmatic language impairment, high functioning autism and specific language impairment. *J Child Psychol Psychiatry.* 2013;54:1186–1197.

Huerta M, Bishop SL, Duncan A, Hus V, Lord C. Application of DSM-5 criteria for autism spectrum disorder to three samples of children with DSM-IV diagnoses of pervasive developmental disorders. *Am J Psychiatry.* 2012;169:1056–1064.

Jones M, Onslow M, Packman A, O'Brian S, Hearne A, Williams S, Ormond T, Schwarz I. Extended follow-up of a randomised controlled trial of the Lidcombe Program of early stuttering intervention. *Int J Lang Commun Disord.* 2008;43: 649–661.

Kefalianos E, Onslow M, Block S, Menzies R, Reilly S. Early stuttering, temperament and anxiety: two hypotheses. *J Fluency Disord.* 2012;37:151–163.

Koyama E, Beitchman JH, Johnson CJ. Expressive language disorder. In: Sadock BJ, Sadock VA, Ruiz P, eds. *Kaplan & Sadock's Comprehensive Textbook of Psychiatry.* 9th ed. Vol. II. Philadelphia, PA: Lippincott Williams & Wilkins; 2009:3509.

Koyama E, Beitchman JH, Johnson CJ. Mixed receptive-expressive language disorder. In: Sadock BJ, Sadock VA, eds. *Kaplan & Sadock's Comprehensive Textbook of Psychiatry.* 9th ed. Vol. II. Philadelphia, PA: Lippincott Williams & Wilkins; 2009:3516.

Koyama E, Johnson CJ, Beitchman JH. Phonological disorder. In: Sadock BJ, Sadock VA, Ruiz P, eds. *Kaplan & Sadock's Comprehensive Textbook of Psychiatry.* 9th ed. Vol. II. Philadelphia, PA: Lippincott Williams & Wilkins; 2009:3522.

Kroll R, Beitchman JH. Stuttering. In: Sadock BJ, Sadock VA, Ruiz P, eds. *Kaplan & Sadock's Comprehensive Textbook of Psychiatry.* 9th ed. Vol. II. Philadelphia, PA: Lippincott Williams & Wilkins; 2009:3528.

Latterman C, Euler HA, Neumann K. A randomized control trial to investigate the impact of the lidcombe program on early stuttering in German-speaking preschoolers. *J Fluency Disord.* 2008;33:52–65.

Law J, Garrett Z, Nye C. Speech and language therapy interventions for children with primary speech and language delay or disorder. *Cochrane Database Syst Rev.* 2003;(3):CD00410.

Leevers HJ, Roesler CP, Flax J, Benasich AA. The Carter Neurocognitive Assessment for children with severely compromised expressive language and motor skills. *J Child Psychol Psychiatry.* 2005;46:287.

Marshall AJ. Parent-Child Interaction Therapy (PCIT) in school-aged children with specific language impairment. *Int J Lang Commun Disord.* 2011;46:397–410.

McLaughlin MR. Speech and language delay in children. *Am Fam Physician.* 2011; 83:1183–1188.

McPartland JC, Reichow B, Volkmar FR. Sensitivity and specificity of the proposed DMS-5 diagnostic criteria for autism spectrum disorder. *J Am Acad Child Adolesc Psychiatry.* 2012;51:368–383.

Millard SK, Nicholas A, Cook FM. Is parent-child interaction therapy effective in reducing stuttering? *J Speech Hearing Res.* 2008;51:636–650.

Nass RD, Trauner D. Social and affective impairments are important recovery after acquired stroke in children. *CNS Spectr.* 2004;9(6):420.

Norbury CF. Practitioner Review: social (pragmatic) communication disorder conceptualization, evidence and clinical implications. *J Child Psychol Psychiatry.* 2014; 55(3):204–216.

Onslow M, O'Brien S. Management of childhood stuttering. *J Paediatr Child Health.* 2013;49:E112–E115.

Packman A, Onslow M. Searching for the cause of stuttering. *Lancet.* 2002;360:655–656.

Petursdottir AI, Carr JE. A review of recommendations for sequencing receptive and expressive language instruction. *J Appl Behav Anal.* 2011;44:859–876.

Ramus F, Marshall DR, Rosen S, van der Lely HK. Phonological deficits in specific language impairment and developmental dyslexia: towards a multidimensional model. *Brain.* 2012;136:630–645.

Reilly S, Wake M, Ukoumunne OC, Bavin E, Prior M, Cini E, Conway L, Eadie P, Bretherton L. Predicting language outcomes at 4 years of age: findings from early language in Victoria study. *Pediatrics.* 2010;126:e1530–e1537.

Reisinger LM, Cornish KM, Fombonne E. Diagnostic differentiation of autism spectrum disorders and pragmatic language impairment. *J Autism Dev Disord.* 2011;41:1694–1704.

Ripley K, Yuill N. Patterns of language impairment and behavior in boys excluded from school. *Br J Educ Psychol.* 2005;75:37.

Rvachew S, Grawburg M. Correlates of phonological awareness in preschoolers with speech sound disorders. *J Speech Lang Hear Res.* 2006;49:74–87.

Smith BL, Smith TD, Taylor L, Hobby M. Relationship between intelligence and vocabulary. *Percept Mot Skills.* 2005;100:101.

Snowling MJ, Hulme C. Interventions for children's language and literacy difficulties. *Int J Commun Dis.* 2012;47:27–34.

Somerville MJ, Mervis CB, Young EJ, Seo EJ, Del Campo M, Bamforth S, Peregrine E, Loo W, Lilley M, Perez-Jurado LA, Morris CA, Scherer SW, Osborne LR. Severe expressive-language delay related to duplication of the Williams-Beuren locus. *N Engl J Med.* 2005;353:1655.

Trajkovski N, Andrews C, Onslow M, O'Brian S, Packman A, Menzies R. A phase II trial of the Westmead Program: syllable-timed speech treatment for preschool children who stutter. *Int J Speech Lang Pathol.* 2011;13:500–509.

Verhoeven L, van Balkom H, eds. *Classification of Developmental Language Disorders. Theoretical Issues and Clinical Implications.* Mahwah, NJ: Erlbaum; 2004:xii+450.

Wake M, Levickis P, Tobin S, Zens N, Law J, Gold L, Ukoumunne OC, Goldfield S, Le Ha ND, Skeat J, Reilly S. Improving outcomes of preschool language delay in the community: protocol for the language for learning randomized controlled trial. *BMC Pediatr*. 2012;12:96–107.

Wake M, Tobin S, Girolametto L, Ukomunne OC, Gold L, Levickis P, Sheehan J, Goldfeld S, Reilly S. Outcomes of population based language promotion for slow to talk toddlers at ages 2 and 3 years: let's learn language cluster randomised clinical trial. *BMJ*. 2011;343:d4741.

Yaruss JS, Coleman CE, Quesal RW. Stuttering in school-age children: a comprehensive approach to treatment. *Lang Speech Hear Serv Sch*. 2012;43:536–548.

Autism

Akins RS, Angkustiri K, Hansen RL. Complementary and alternative medicine in autism: an evidence-based approach to negotiating safe and efficacious interventions with families. *Neurotherapeutics*. 2010;7:307–319.

Aman MG, Arnold LE, McDougle CJ, Vitiello B, Scahill L, Davies M, McCracken JT, Tierney E, Nash PL, Posey DJ, Chuang S, Martin A, Shah B, Gonzalez HM, Swiezy NB, Ritz L, Koenig K, McGough J, Ghuman JK, Lindsay RL. Acute and long-term safety and tolerability of risperidone in children with autism. *J Child Adolesc Psychopharmacol*. 2005;15:869.

Autism and Developmental Disabilities Monitoring Network Surveillance Year 2006 Principal Investigators; Centers for Disease Control and Prevention (CDC). Prevalence of autism spectrum disorders—autism and developmental disabilities monitoring network, United States, 2006. *MMWR Surveill Summ*. 2009;58:1–20.

Baron-Cohen S, Knickmeyer RC, Belmonte MK. Sex differences in the brain: implications for explaining autism. *Science*. 2005;310:819.

Bishop DV, Mayberry M, Wong D, Maley A, Hallmayer J. Characteristics of the broader phenotype in autism: a study of siblings using the children's communication checklist-2. *Am J Med Genet B Neuropsychiatr Genet*. 2006;141B:117–122.

Boyd BA, McDonough SG, Bodfish JW. Evidence-based behavioral interventions for repetitive behaviors in autism. *J Autism Dev Disord*. 2012;1236–1248.

Canitano R, Scandurra V. Psychopharmacology in autism: an update. *Prog Neuropsychopharmacol Biol Psychiatry*. 2011;35:18–28.

Carminati GG, Deriaz N, Bertschy G. Low-dose venlafaxine in three adolescents and young adults with autistic disorder improves self-injurious behavior and attention deficit/hyperactivity disorder (ADHD)-like symptoms. *Prog Neuropsychopharmacol Biol Psychiatry*. 2006;30:312.

Constantino JN, Lajonchere C, Lutz M, Gray T, Abbacchi A, McKenna K, Singh D, Todd RD. Autistic social impairment in the siblings of children with pervasive developmental disorders. *Am J Psychiatry*. 2006;163:294–296.

Danfors T, von Knorring AL, Hartvig P, Langstrom B, Moulder R, Stromberg B, Tortenson R, Wester U, Watanabe Y, Eeg-Olofsson O. Tetrahydrobiopterin in the treatment of children with autistic disorder: a double-blind placebo-controlled crossover study. *J Clin Psychopharmacol*. 2005;25:485.

Gadow KD, DeVincent CJ, Pomeroy J. ADHD symptom subtypes in children with pervasive developmental disorder. *J Autism Dev Disord*. 2006;36(2):271–283.

Gardener H, Spiegelman D, Buka SL. Perinatal and neonatal risk factors for autism: a comprehensive meta-analysis. *Pediatrics*. 2011;128:344–355.

Hazlett HC, Poe, M, Gerig C, Smith RG, Provenzale J, Ross A, Gilmore J, Piven J. Magnetic resonance imaging and head circumference study of brain size in autism: birth through age 2 years. *Arch Gen Psychiatry*. 2005;62:1366.

Huffman LC, Sutcliffe TL, Tanner ISD, Feldman HM. Management of symptoms in children with autism spectrum disorders: a comprehensive review of pharmacologic and complementary-alternative medicine treatments. *J Dev Behav Pediatr*. 2011;32:56–68.

Kasari C, Lawton K. New directions in behavioral treatment of autism spectrum disorders. *Curr Opin Neurol*. 2010;23:137–143.

Ke JY, Chen CL, Chen YJ, Chen CH, Lee LF, Chiang TM. Features of developmental functions and autistic profiles in children with fragile X syndrome. *Chang Gung Med J*. 2005;28:551.

Koyama T, Tachimori H, Osada H, Kurita H. Cognitive and symptom profiles in high-functioning pervasive developmental disorder not otherwise specified and attention-deficit/hyperactivity disorder. *J Autism Dev Disord*. 2006;36(3):373–380.

Lehmkuhl, HD, Storch E, Bodfish JW, Geffken GR. Brief Report: exposure and response prevention for obsessive compulsive disorder in a 12-year-old with autism. *J Autism Dev Disord*. 2008;38:977–981.

Mandell DS, Novak MM, Zubritsky CD. Factors associated with age of diagnosis among children with autism spectrum disorders. *Pediatrics*. 2005;116:1480.

Miano S, Ferri R. Epidemiology and management of insomnia in children with autistic spectrum disorders. *Pediatr Drugs*. 2010;12:75–84.

Nazeer A. Psychopharmacology of autistic spectrum disorders in children and adolescents. *Pediatr Clin N Am*. 2011;58:85–97.

Owley T, Walton L, Salt J, Guter SJ, Winnega M, Leventhal BL, Cook EH. An open-label trial of escitalopram in pervasive developmental disorders. *J Am Acad Child Adolesc Psychiatry*. 2005;44:343.

Research Units on Pediatric Psychopharmacology Autism Network. Randomized, controlled crossover trial of methylphenidate in pervasive developmental disorders with hyperactivity. *Arch Gen Psychiatry*. 2005;62:1266–1274.

Research Units on Pediatric Psychopharmacology Autism Network. Risperidone treatment of autistic disorder: longer-term benefits and blinded discontinuation after 6 months. *Am J Psychiatry*. 2005;162:1361–1369.

Robinson EB, Koenen KC, McCormick MC, Munir K, Hallet V, Happe F, Plomin R, Ronald A. Evidence that autistic traits show the same etiology in the general population an at the quantitative extremes (5 percent, 2.5 percent, and 1 percent). *Arch Gen Psychiatry*. 2011;68:1113–1121.

Rogers SJ, Vismara LA. Evidence-based comprehensive treatments for early autism. *J Clin Child Adolesc Psychol*. 2008;37:8–38.

Ronald A, Hoekstra RA. Autism spectrum disorders and autistic traits: a decade of new twin studies. *Am J Med Genet Part B*. 2011;156:255–274.

Stigler KA, McDonald BC, Anand A, Saykin AJ, McDougle CJ. Structural and functional magnetic resonance imaging of autism spectrum disorders. *Brain Res*. 2011;1380:146–161.

Sugie Y, Sugie H, Fukuda T, Ito M. Neonatal factors in infants with autistic disorder and typically developing infants. *Autism*. 2005;5:487–494.

Tanaka JW, Wolf JM, Klaiman C, Koenig K, Cockburn J, Herlihy L, Brown C, Stahl S, Kaiser MD, Schultz RT. Using computerized games to teach face recognition skills to children with autism spectrum disorder: the Let's Face it! Program. *J Child Psychol Psychiatry*. 2010;51:944–952.

Vanderbuilt Evidence-Based Practice Center, Nashville TN. Therapies for children with autism spectrum disorders. *Comparative Effectiveness Review*. 2011;26:1–13.

Veenstra-VanderWeele J, Blakely RD. Networking in Autism: leveraging genetic, biomarker and model system findings in the search for new treatments. *Neuropsychopharmacology*. 2012;37:196–212.

Volkmar FR, Klin A, Schultz RT, State M. Pervasive developmental disorders. In: Sadock BJ, Sadock VA, Ruiz P, eds. *Kaplan & Sadock's Comprehensive Textbook of Psychiatry*. 9th ed. Vol. 2. Philadelphia, PA: Lippincott Williams & Wilkins; 2009:540.

Wang M, Reid D. Virtual reality in pediatric neurorehabilitation: attention deficit hyperactivity disorder, autism and cerebral palsy. *Neuroepidemiology*. 2011;36:2–18.

Wink LK, Erickson CA, McDougle CJ. Pharmacologic treatment of behavioral symptoms associated with autism and other pervasive developmental disorders. *Curr Treat Options Neurol*. 2010;12:529–538.

Zuddas A, Zanni R, Usala T. Second generation antipsychotics (SGAs) for nonpsychotic disorders in children and adolescents: a review of the randomized controlled trials. *Eur Neuropsychopharmacol*. 2011;21:600–620.

Attention Deficit Hyperactivity Disorder

Antshel KM, Hargrave TM, Simonescu M, Kaul P, Hendricks K, Faraone SV. Advances in understanding and treating ADHD. *BMC Med*. 2011;9:7.

Clarke AR, Barry RJ, Dupuy FE, Heckel LD, McCarthy R, Selikowitz M, Johnstone SJ. Behavioural differences between EEG-defined subgroups of children with attention-deficit/hyperactivity disorder. *Clin Neurophysiol*. 2011;122:1333–1341.

Cortese S, Kelly C, Chabernaud C, Proal E, Di Martino A, Milham MP, Castellanos FX. Toward systems neuroscience of ADHD: a meta-analysis of 55 fMRI studies. *Am J Psychiatry*. 2012;169:1038–1055.

Elbe D, MacBride A, Reddy D. Focus on lisdexamfetamine: a review of its use in child and adolescent psychiatry. *J Can Acad Child Adolesc Psychiatry*. 2010;19: 303–314.

Greenhill LL, Hechtman L. Attention-deficit disorders. In: Sadock BJ, Sadock VA, Ruiz P, eds. *Kaplan & Sadock's Comprehensive Textbook of Psychiatry*. 9th ed. Vol. 2. Philadelphia, PA: Lippincott Williams & Wilkins; 2009:3560.

Hammerness PG, Perrin JM, Shelley-Abrahamson R, Wilens TE. Cardiovascular risk of stimulant treatment in pediatric attention-deficit/hyperactivity disorder: update and clinical recommendations. *J Am Acad Child Adolesc Psychiatry*. 2011;50: 978–990.

Hechtman L. Comorbidity and neuroimaging in attention-deficit hyperactivity disorder. *Can J Psychiatry*. 2009;54:649–650.

Kratochvil CJ, Lake M, Pliszka SR, Walkup JT. Pharmacologic management of treatment-induced insomnia in ADHD. *J Am Acad Child Adolesc Psychiatry*. 2005;44:499.

McGough J. Adult manifestations of attention-deficit/hyperactivity disorder. In: Sadock BJ, Sadock VA, Ruiz P, eds. *Kaplan & Sadock's Comprehensive Textbook of Psychiatry*. 9th ed. Vol. 2. Philadelphia, PA: Lippincott Williams & Wilkins; 2009:3572.

Molina BSG, Hinshaw SP, Swanson JM, Arnold LE, Vitiello B, Jenson PS, Epstien JN, Hoza BM, Hechtman L, Abikoff HB, Elliot GR, Greenhill LL, Newcorn JH, Wells KC, Wigal T, Gibbons RD, Hur K, Houck PR, The MTA Cooperative Group. The MTA at 8 years: prospective follow-up of children treated for combined type ADHD in a multisite study. *J Am Acad Child Adolesc Psychiatry*. 2009;48:484–500.

MTA Cooperative Group. A 14-month randomized clinical trial of treatment strategies for attention-deficit/hyperactivity disorder. Multimodal treatment study of children with ADHD. *Arch Gen Psychiatry*. 1999;56:1073–1086.

Pelham WE, Manos MJ, Ezzell CE, Tresco KE, Gnagy EM, Hoffman MT, Onyango AN, Fabiano GA, Lopez-Williams A, Wymbs BT, Caserta D, Chronis AM, Burrows-Maclean L, Morse G. A dose-ranging study of a methylphenidate transdermal system in children with ADHD. *J Am Acad Child Adolesc Psychiatry*. 2005;44:522.

Ratner A, Laor N, Bronstein Y, Weizman A, Toren P. Six-week open-label reboxetine treatment in children and adolescents with attention-deficit/hyperactivity disorder. *J Am Acad Child Adolesc Psychiatry*. 2005;44:428.

Sassi RB. In this issue/Abstract thinking: from pixels to voxels: television, brain, and behavior. *J Am Acad Child Adolesc Psychiatry*. 2013;52:665–666.

Stevens LJ, Kuczek T, Burgess JR, Hurt E, Arnold LE. Dietary sensitivities and ADHD symptoms: thirty-five years of research. *Clin Pediatr*. 2011;50:279–293.

Tresco KE, Lefler EK, Power TJ. Psychosocial interventions to improve the school performance of students with attention-deficit/hyperactivity disorder. *Mind Brain*. 2011;1:69–74.

Weiss M, Tannock R, Kratochvil C, Dunn D, Velez-Borras J, Thomason C, Tamura R, Kelsey D, Stevens L, Allen AJ. A randomized, placebo-controlled study of once-daily atomoxetine in the school setting in children with ADHD. *J Am Acad Child Adolesc Psychiatry*. 2005;44:647.

Learning Disorders

Archibald LMD, Cardy JO, Joanisse MF, Ansari D. Language, reading, and math learning profiles in an epidemiological sample of school age children. *PLoS One.* 2013;8:e77463.

Badian NA. Persistent arithmetic, reading, or arithmetic and reading disability. *Ann Dyslexia.* 1999;49:43–70.

Bergstrom KM, Lachmann T. Does noise affect learning? A short review on noise effects on cognitive performance in children. *Front Psychol.* 2013;4:578.

Bernstein S, Atkinson AR, Martimianakis MA. Diagnosing the learner in difficulty. *Pediatrics.* 2013;132:210–212.

Bishop DV. Genetic influences on language impairment and literacy problems in children: same or different? *J Child Psychol Psychiatry.* 2001;42:189–198.

Butterworth B, Kovas Y. Understanding neurocognitive developmental disorders can improve education for all. *Science.* 2013;340:300–305.

Catone WV, Brady SA. The inadequacy of Individual Educational Program (IEP) goals for high school students with word-level reading difficulties. *Ann Dyslexia.* 2005;55:53.

Cragg L, Nation K. Exploring written narrative in children with poor reading comprehension. *Educ Psychol.* 2006;26:55–72.

Endres M, Toso L, Roberson R, Park J, Abebe D, Poggi S, Spong CY. Prevention of alcohol-induced developmental delays and learning abnormalities in a model of fetal alcohol syndrome. *Am J Obstet Gynecol.* 2005;193:1028.

Flax JF, Realpe-Bonilla T, Hirsch LS, Brzustowicz LM, Bartlett CW, Tallal P. Specific language impairment in families: evidence for co-occurrence with reading impairments. *J Speech Lang Hear Res.* 2003;46:530–543.

Fletcher JM. Predicting math outcomes: reading predictors and comorbidity. *J Learn Disabil.* 2005;38:308.

Gersten R, Jordan NC, Flojo JR. Early identification and interventions for students with mathematics difficulties. *J Learn Disabil.* 2005;38:305.

Gordon N. The "medical" investigation of specific learning disorders. *Pediatr Neurol.* 2004;2(1):3.

Hedges JH, Adolph KE, Amso D, Bavelier D, Fiez J, Krubitzer L, McAuley JD, Newcombe NS, Fitzpatrick SM, Ghajar J. Play, attention, and learning: how do play and timing shape the development of attention and influence classroom learning? *Ann N Y Acad Sci.* 2013;1292:1–20.

Jura MB, Humphrey LH. Neuropsychological and cognitive assessment of children. In: Sadock BJ, Sadock VA, eds. *Kaplan & Sadock's Comprehensive Textbook of Psychiatry.* 9th ed. Vol. 2. Philadelphia, PA: Lippincott Williams & Wilkins; 2005;895.

Lewis C, Hitch GJ, Peter W. The prevalence of specific arithmetic difficulties and specific reading difficulties in 9- to 10-year-old boys and girls. *J Child Psychol Psychiatry.* 1994;35:283–292.

Meeks J, Adler A, Kunert K, Floyd L. Individual psychotherapy of the learning-disabled adolescent. In: Flaherty LT, ed. *Adolescent Psychiatry: Developmental and Clinical Studies.* Vol. 28. Hillsdale, NJ: Analytic Press; 2004:231.

Plomin R, Kovas Y. Generalist genes and learning disabilities. *Psychol Bull.* 2005;131:592.

Tannock R. Disorder of written expression and learning disorder not otherwise specified. In: Sadock BJ, Sadock VA, eds. *Kaplan & Sadock's Comprehensive Textbook of Psychiatry.* 8th ed. Vol. 2. Philadelphia, PA: Lippincott Williams & Wilkins; 2005:3123.

Tannock R. Mathematics disorder. In: Sadock BJ, Sadock VA, eds. *Kaplan & Sadock's Comprehensive Textbook of Psychiatry.* 8th ed. Vol. 2. Philadelphia, PA: Lippincott Williams & Wilkins; 2005:3116.

Tannock R. Reading disorder. In: Sadock BJ, Sadock VA, eds. *Kaplan & Sadock's Comprehensive Textbook of Psychiatry.* 9th ed. Vol. 2. Philadelphia, PA: Lippincott Williams & Wilkins; 2005:3107.

Vadasy PF, Sanders EA, Peyton JA. Relative effectiveness of reading practice or word-level instruction in supplemental tutoring: how text matters. *J Learn Disabil.* 2005;38:364.

Motor Coordination Disorders

Blank R, Smits-Engelman B, Polatajko H, Wilson P, European Academy for Childhood Disability. European Academy of Childhood Disability: recommendations on the definition, diagnosis and intervention of developmental coordination disorder (long version). *Dev Med Child Neurol.* 2012;54:54–93.

Cairney J, Veldhuizen S, Szatmari P. Motor coordination and emotional-behavioral problems in children. *Curr Opin Psychiatry.* 2010;23:324–329.

Deng S, Li WG, Ding J, Wu J, Shang Y, Li F, Shen X. Understanding the mechanisms of cognitive impairments in developmental coordination disorder. *Pediatr Res.* 2014;75:210–216.

Dewey D, Bottos S. Neuroimaging of developmental motor disorders. In: Dewey D, Tupper DE, eds. *Developmental Motor Disorders: A Neuropsychological Perspective.* New York: Guilford Press; 2004:26.

Edwards J, Berube M, Erlandson K. Developmental coordination disorder in school-aged children born very preterm and/or at very low birth weight: a systematic review. *J Dev Behav Pediatr.* 2011;32:678–687.

Geuze RH. Postural control in children with developmental coordination disorder. *Neural Plast.* 2005;12:183.

Groen SE, de Blecourt ACE, Postema K, Hadders-Algra M. General movements in early infancy predict neuromotor development at 9 to 12 years of age. *Dev Med Child Neurol.* 2005;47(11):731.

Kargerer FA, Cfontreras-Vidal JL, Bo J, Clark JE. Abrupt, but not gradual visuomotor distortion facilitates adaptation in children with developmental coordination disorder. *Hum Mov Sci.* 2006;25:622–633.

Liberman L, Ratzon N, Bart O. The profile of performance skills and emotional factors in the context of participation among young children with developmental coordination disorder. *Res Dev Disabil.* 2013;34:87–94.

Pataki CS, Mitchell WG. Motor skills disorder: developmental coordination disorder. In: Sadock BJ, Sadock VA, Ruiz P, eds. *Kaplan & Sadock's Comprehensive Textbook of Psychiatry.* 9th ed. Vol. II. Philadelphia, PA: Lippincott Williams & Wilkins; 2009:3501.

Williams J, Thomas PR, Maruff P, Butson M, Wilson PH. Motor, visual and egocentric transformations in children with developmental coordination disorder. *Child Care Health Dev.* 2006;32:633–647.

Wilson PH, Ruddock S, Smits-Engelsman B, Polatajko H. Understanding performance deficits in developmental coordination disorder: a meta-analysis of recent research. *Dev Med Child Neurol.* 2013;55:217–228.

Zwicker JG, Harris SR, Klassen AF. Quality of life domains affected in children with developmental coordination disorder: a systematic review. *Child Care Health Dev.* 2013;39:562–580.

Zwicker JG, Missiuna C, Harris SR, Boyd LA. Brain activation associated with motor skill practice in children with developmental motor coordination disorder: an fMRI study. *Int J Dev Neurosci.* 2011;29:145–152.

Zwicker JG, Missiuna C, Harris SR, Boyd LA. Developmental coordination disorder: a review and update. *Eur J Paediatr Neurol.* 2012;6:573–581.

Movement Disorders

Barry S, Baird G, Lascelles K, Bunton P, Hedderly T. Neurodevelopmental movement disorders—an update on childhood motor stereotypies. *Dev Med Child Neurol.* 2011;53:979–985.

Doyle RL. Stereotypic movement disorders. In: Sadock BJ, Sadock VA, Ruiz P, eds. *Kaplan & Sadock's Comprehensive Textbook of Psychiatry.* 9th ed. Vol. II. Philadelphia, PA: Lippincott Williams & Wilkins; 2009:3642.

Edwards MJ, Lang AE, Bhatia KP. Stereotypies: a critical appraisal and suggestion of a clinically useful definition. *Mov Disord.* 2012;27:179–185.

Fernandez AE. Primary versus secondary stereotypic movements. *Rev Neurol.* 2004; 38(Suppl 1):21.

Freeman KA, Duke DC. Power of magic hands: parent-driven application of habit reversal to treat complex stereotypy in a 3-year-old. *Health Psychol.* 2013;32:915–920.

Freeman RD, Soltanifar A, Baer S. Stereotypic movement disorder: easily missed. *Dev Med Child Neurol.* 2010;52:733–738.

Harris KM, Mahone EM, Singer HS. Nonautistic motor stereotypies: clinical features and longitudinal follow-up. *Pediatr Neurol.* 2008;38:267–272.

Luby JL. Disorders of infancy and early childhood not otherwise specified. In: Sadock BJ, Sadock VA, eds. *Kaplan & Sadock's Comprehensive Textbook of Psychiatry.* 8th ed. Vol. 2. Philadelphia, PA: Lippincott Williams & Wilkins; 2005:3257.

Mahone EM, Bridges D, Prahme C, Singer HS. Repetitive arm and hand movements (complex motor stereotypies) in children. *J Pediatr.* 2004;145:391.

Melnick SM, Dow-Edwards DL. Correlating brain metabolism with stereotypic and locomotor behavior. *Behav Res Methods Instrum Comput.* 2003;35:452.

Miller JM, Singer HS, Bridges DD, Waranch HR. Behavioral therapy for treatment of stereotypic movements in nonautistic children. *J Child Neurol.* 2006;21:119.

Muehlmann AM, Lewis MH. Abnormal repetitive behaviours: shared phenomenology and pathophysiology. *J Intellect Disabil Res.* 2012;56:427–440.

Presti MF, Watson CJ, Kennedy RT, Yang M, Lewis MH. Behavior-related alterations of striatal neurochemistry in a mouse model of stereotyped movement disorder. *Pharmacol Biochem Behav.* 2004;77:501.

Stein DJ, Grant JE, Franklin ME, Keuthen N, Lochner C, Singer HS, Woods DW. Trichotillomania (hair pulling disorder) skin picking disorder, and stereotypic movement disorder: toward DSM-V. *Dep Anxiety.* 2010;27:611–626.

Zinner SH, Mink JW. Movement disorders I: Tics and stereotypies. *Pediatr Rev.* 2010;31:223–232.

Tic Disorders

Debes NM, Hansen A, Skov L, Larsson H. A functional magnetic resonance imaging study of a large clinical cohort of children with Tourette syndrome. *J Child Neurol.* 2011;26:560–569.

Du YS, Li HF, Vance A, Zhong YQ, Jiao FY, Wang HM. Randomized double-blind multicentre placebo-controlled clinical trial of the clonidine adhesive patch for the treatment of tic disorders. *Aust N Z J Psychiatry.* 2008;42:807–813.

Eddy CM, Rickards HE, Cavanna AE. Treatment strategies for tics in Tourette syndrome. *Ther Adv Neurol Disord.* 2011;4:25–45.

Hartmann A, Worbe Y. Pharmacological treatment of Gilles de la Tourette syndrome. *Neurosci Biobehav Rev.* 2013;37:1157–1161.

Janovic J, Jimenez-Shahed J, Brown L. A randomized, double-blind, placebo-controlled study of topiramate in the treatment of Tourette syndrome. *J Neurol Neurosurg Psychiatry.* 2010;81:70–73.

Jummani R, Coffey BJ. Tic disorders. In: Sadock BJ, Sadock VA, Ruiz P, eds. *Kaplan & Sadock's Comprehensive Textbook of Psychiatry.* 9th ed. Vol. 2. Philadelphia, PA: Lippincott Williams & Wilkins; 2009:3609.

Knight T, Stevvers T, Day L, Lowerison M, Jette N, Pringsheim T. Prevalence of tic disorders: a systematic review and meta-analysis. *Pediatr Neurol.* 2012;47:77–90.

Kraft JT, Dalsgaard S, Obel C, Thomsen PH, Henriksen TB, Scahill L. Prevalence and clinical correlates of tic disorders in a community sample of school-age children. *Eur Child Adolesc Psychiatry.* 2012;21:5–13.

Liu ZS, Chen YH, Zhong YQ, Zou LP, Wang H, Sun D. A multicentre controlled study on aripiprazole treatment for children with Tourette syndrome in China. *Zhonghua Er Ke Za Zhi.* 2011;49:572–576.

Paschou P. The genetic basis of Gilles de la Tourette syndrome. *Neurosci Biobehav Rev.* 2013;37:1026–1039.

Piacentini J, Woods DW, Scahill L, Wilhelm S, Peterson AL, Chang S. Behavior therapy for children with Tourette disorder. A randomized controlled trial. *JAMA.* 2010;303:1929–1937.

Porta M, Sassi M, Cavallazzi M, Fornari M, Brambilla A, Servello D. Tourette's syndrome and the role of tetrabenzine: review and personal experience. *Clin Drug Investig.* 2008;28:443–459.

Roessner V, Plessen KJ, Rothenberger A, Ludolph AG, Rizzo R, Skov L. European clinical guidelines for Tourette syndrome and other tic disorders. Part II: pharmacologic treatment. *Eur Child Adolesc Psychiatry.* 2011;20:173–196.

Rothenbertger A, Roessner V. Functional neuroimaging investigations of motor networks in Tourette syndrome. *Behav Neurol.* 2013;27:47–55.

Scharf JM, Miller LL, Mathews CA, Ben-Shlomo Y. Prevalence of Tourette syndrome and chronic tics in the population-based Avon longitudinal study of parents and children cohort. *J Am Acad Child Adolesc Psychiatry.* 2012;51:192–201.

Spencer TJ, Sallee FR, Gilbert DL, Dunn DW, McCracken JT, Coffey BJ. Atomoxetine treatment of ADHD in children with comorbid Tourette syndrome. *J Atten Disord.* 2008;11:470–481.

Steeves T, McKinlay BD, Gorman D, Billinghurst L, Day L, Carrol A, Dion Y, Doja A, Luscombe S, Sandor P, Pringsheim T. Canadian guidelines for the evidence-based treatment of tic disorders: behavioural therapy, deep brain stimulation and transcranial magnetic stimulation. *Can J Psychiatry.* 2012;57:144–151.

Storch EA, Murphy TK, Geffken GR, Sajid M, Allen P, Roberti JW, Goodman WK. Reliability and validity of the Yale Global Tic Severity Scale. *Psychol Assess.* 2005;17:486.

Thomas R, Cavanna AE. The pharmacology of Tourette syndrome. *J Neural Transm.* 2013;120(4):689–694.

Verdellen C, Griendt JVD, Hartmann A, Murphy T, the ESSTS Guidelines Group. European clinical guidelines for Tourette syndrome and other tic disorders. Part III: behavioural and psychosocial interventions. *Eur Child Adolesc Psychiatry.* 2011;20:97–207.

Weisman H, Qureshi IA, Leckman JF, Scahill L, Bloch MH. Systematic review: pharmacological treatment of tic disorders—Efficacy of antipsychotic and alpha-2 adrenergic agonist agents. *Neurosci Biobehav Rev.* 2013;37(6):1162–1171.

Woods DW, Piacentini JC, Scahill L, Peterson AL, Wilhelm S, Chang S. Behavior therapy for tics in children: acute and long-term effects on psychiatric and psychosocial functioning. *J Child Neurol.* 2011;7:858–865.

Feeding Disorders

Araujo CL, Victora CG, Hallal PC, Gigante DP. Breastfeeding and overweight in childhood: evidence from the Pelotas 1993 birth cohort study. *Int J Obes.* 2005;30(3):500.

Berger-Gross P, Colettoi DJ, Hirschkorn K, Terranova E, Simpser EF. The effectiveness of risperidone in the treatment of three children with feeding disorders. *J Child Adolesc Psychopharmacol.* 2004;14:621.

Bryant-Waugh R. Avoidant restrictive food intake disorder: an illustrative case example. *Int J Eat Disord.* 2013;46:420–423.

Bryant-Waugh R. Feeding and eating disorders in children. *Curr Opin Psychiatry.* 2013;26:537–542.

Call C, Walsh BT, Attia E. From DSM-IV to DSM-5: changes to eating disorder diagnoses. *Curr Opin Psychiatry.* 2013;26:532–536.

Chatoor I. Feeding and eating disorders of infancy or early childhood. In: Sadock BJ, Sadock VA, eds. *Kaplan & Sadock's Comprehensive Textbook of Psychiatry.* 9th ed. Vol. II. Philadelphia, PA: Lippincott Williams & Wilkins; 2009:3597.

Chial HJ, Camilleri M, Williams DE, Litzinger K, Perrault J. Rumination syndrome in children and adolescents: diagnosis, treatment, and prognosis. *Pediatrics.* 2003;111:158–162.

Cohen E, Rosen Y, Yehuda B, Iancu I. Successful multidisciplinary treatment in an adolescent case of rumination. *Isr J Psychiatry Relat Sci.* 2004;41:222.

DeMatteo C, Matovich D, Hjartarson A. Comparison of clinical and videofluoroscopic evaluation of children with feeding and swallowing difficulties. *Dev Med Child Neurol.* 2005;47:149.

Equit M, Palmke M, Beckner N, Moritz AM, Becker S, von Gontard A. Eating problems in young children: a population based study. *Acta Paediatr.* 2013:102(2):149–155.

Esparo G, Canals J, Ballespi S, Vinas F, Domenech E. Feeding problems in nursery children: prevalence and psychosocial factors. *Acta Pediatr* 2004;93:663.

Feldaman R, Keren M, Gross-Rozval O, Tyano S. Mother-child touch patterns in infant feeding disorders: relation to maternal, child, and environmental factors. *J Am Acad Child Adolesc Psychiatry.* 2004;43:1089.

Hughes SO, Anderson CB, Power TG, Micheli N, Jaramillo S, Nicklas TA. Measuring feeding in low-income African-American and Hispanic parents. *Appetite.* 2006;46(2):215.

Jacobi C, Agras WS, Bryson S, Hammer LD. Behavioral validation, precursors, and concomitants of picky eating in childhood. *J Am Acad Child Adolesc Psychiatry.* 2003;42:76.

Lewinsohn PM, Holm-Denoma JM, Gau JM, Joiner TE Jr, Striegel-Moore R, Bear P, Lamoureux B. Problematic eating and feeding behaviors of 36-month-old children. *Int J Eat Disord.* 2005;38(3):208–219.

Linscheid TN. Behavioral treatments for pediatric feeding disorders. *Behav Modif.* 2006;30:6–23.

Liu YL, Malik N, Sanger GJ, Friedman MI, Andrews PL. Pica—A model of nausea? Species differences in response to cisplatin. *Physiol Behav.* 2005;85(3):271–277.

Ornstein RM, Rosen DS, Mammel K, Callahan ST, Forman S. Distribution of eating disorders in children and adolescents using the proposed DSM-5 criteria for feeding and eating disorders. *J Adolesc Health.* 2013;53:303–305.

Rajindrajith S, Devanarayana NM, Perera BJC. Rumination syndrome in children and adolescents: a school survey assessing prevalence and symptomatology. *BMC Gastroenterol.* 2012;12:163–169.

Rastam M, Taljemark J, Tajnia A. Eating problems and overlap with ADHD and autism spectrum disorders in a nationwide twin study of 9- and 12-year-old children. *Sci World J.* 2013;15:315429.

Tack J, Blondeau K, Boecxstaens V, Rommel N. Review article: the pathophysiology, differential diagnosis and management of rumination syndrome. *Ailment Pharmacol Ther.* 2011;33:782–788.

Uher R, Rutter M. Classification of feeding and eating disorders: review of evidence and proposals for ICD-11. *World Psychiatry.* 2012;11:80–92.

Williams DE, McAdam D. Assessment, behavioral treatment, and prevention of pica: clinical guidelines and recommendations for practitioners. *Res Develop Disab.* 2012;33:2050–2057.

Attachment Disorders

Bernard K, Dozier M, Carlson E, Bick J, Lewis-Morrarty, Lindheim O. Enhancing attachment organization among maltreated children: results of a randomized clinical trial. *Child Dev.* 2012;83:623–636.

Boris NW, Zeanah CH. Reactive attachment disorder of infancy, childhood and adolescence. In: Sadock BJ, Sadock VA, Ruiz P, eds. *Kaplan & Sadock's Comprehensive Textbook of Psychiatry.* 9th ed. Vol. II. Philadelphia, PA: Lippincott Williams & Wilkins; 2009:3636.

Boris NW, Zeanah CH, Work Group on Quality Issues. Practice parameter for the assessment and treatment of children and adolescents with reactive attachment disorder of infancy and early childhood. *J Am Acad Child Adolesc Psychiatry.* 2005;44:1206.

Chaffin M, Hanson R, Saunders BE, Nichols T, Barnett D, Zeanah C, Berliner L, Egeland B, Newman E, Lyon T, LeTourneau E, Miller-Perrin C. Report of the APSAC task force on attachment therapy, reactive attachment disorder, and attachment problems. *Child Maltreat.* 2006;11:76.

Heller SS, Boris NW, Fuselier SH, Pate T, Koren-Karie N, Miron D. Reactive attachment disorder in maltreated twins follow-up: from 18 months to 8 years. *Attach Hum Dev.* 2006;8:63.

Kay C, Green J. Reactive attachment disorder following maltreatment: systematic evidence beyond the institution. *J Abnorm Child Psychol.* 2013;41:571–581.

Kocovska E, Puckering C, Follan M, Smillie M, Gorski C. Neurodevelopmental problems in maltreated children referred with indiscriminate friendliness. *Res Dev Disabil.* 2012;33:1560–1565.

Kocovska E, Wilson P, Young D, Wallace AM, Gorski C. Cortisol secretion in children with symptoms of reactive attachment disorder. *Psychiatr Res.* 2013;209:74–77.

Minnis H, Macmillan S, Pritchett R, Young D, Wallace B. Prevalence of reactive attachment disorder in a deprived population. *Br J Psychiatry.* 2013;202:342–346.

O'Connor TG, Marvin RS, Rutter M, Olrick J, Britner PA. The ERA Study Team. Child–parent attachment following early institutional deprivation. *Dev Psychopathol.* 2003;15:19–38.

O'Connor TG, Zeanah CH. Attachment disorders: assessment strategies and treatment approaches. *Attach Hum Dev.* 2003;5:223–244.

Pritchett R, Pritchett J, Marshall E, Davidson C, Minnis H. Reactive attachment disorder in the general population: a hidden ESSENCE disorder. *Sci World J.* 2013;2013:818157.

Task Force on Research Diagnostic Criteria: Infancy Preschool. Research diagnostic criteria for infants and preschool children. *J Am Acad Child Adolesc Psychiatry.* 2003;42:1504–1512.

Zeanah CH, Scheeringa MS, Boris NW, Heller SS, Smyke AT, Trapani J. Reactive attachment disorder in maltreated toddlers. *Child Abuse Negl.* 2004;28:877.

Zeanah CH, Smyke T, Dumitrescu A. Attachment disturbances in young children II: indiscriminate behavior and institutional care. *J Am Acad Child Adolesc Psychiatry.* 2002;41:983.

Zilberstein K. Clarifying core characteristics of attachment disorders: a review of current research and theory. *Am J Orthopsychiatry.* 2006;76:55.

Post Traumatic Stress Disorder

Breslau N. The epidemiology of trauma, PTSD, and other posttraumatic disorders. *Trauma Violence Abuse.* 2009;10:198–210.

Cohen JA. Posttraumatic stress disorder in children and adolescents. In: Sadock BJ, Sadock VA, Ruiz P, eds. *Kaplan & Sadock's Comprehensive Textbook of Psychiatry.* 9th ed. Vol. 2. Philadelphia, PA: Lippincott Williams and Wilkins; 2009:3678.

Cohen JA, Mannarino AP, Deblinger E. *Treating Trauma and Traumatic Grief in Children and Adolescents.* New York: The Guilford Press; 2009.

Cohen JA, Mannarino AP, Perel JM, Staron V. A pilot randomized controlled trial of combined trauma-focused CBT and sertraline for childhood PTSD symptoms. *J Am Acad Child Adolesc Psychiatry.* 2007;46:811–819.

Davis TE III, May A, Whiting SE. Evidence-based treatments of anxiety and phobia in children and adolescents: current status and effects on the emotional response. *Clin Psychol Rev.* 2011;31:592–602.

Dorsey S, Briggs EC, Woods BA. Cognitive behavioral treatment for posttraumatic stress disorder in children and adolescents. *Child Adolesc Psychiatr Clin N Am.* 2011;20:255–269.

Finkelhor D, Ormrod RK, Turner HA. The developmental epidemiology of childhood victimization. *J Interpers Violence.* 2009;24:711–731.

Finkelhor D, Turner H, Omrod R, Hamby SL. Violence, abuse, and crime exposure in a national sample of children and youth. *Pediatrics.* 2009;124:1–13.

Ford JD, Steinberg KL, Hawke J, Levine J, Xhang W. Randomized trial comparison of emotion regulation and relational psychotherapies for PTSD in girls involved in delinquency. *J Clin Child Adolesc Psychol*. 2012;41:27–37.

Huemer J, Erhart F, Steiner H. Posttraumatic stress disorder in children and adolescents: a review of psychopharmacological treatment. *Child Psychiatry Hum Dev*. 2010;41:624–640.

Jaycox LH, Cohen JA, Mannarino AP, Walker DW, Langley AK, Gegenheimer KL, Children's mental health care following Hurricane Katrina: a field trial of trauma-focused psychotherapies. *J Traum Stress*. 2010;23:223–231.

Jaycox, LH, Langley AK, Dean KL. Support for students exposed to trauma: the SSET program: group leader training manual, lesson plans and lesson materials and worksheets. *Santa Monica, CA: RAND Health*. 2009.

Meighen KG, Hines LA, Lagges AM. Risperidone treatment of preschool children with thermal burns and acute stress disorder. *J Child Adolesc Psychopharmacol*. 2007;17:223–232.

Robb AS, Cueva JE, Sporn J, Vanderberg DG. Sertraline treatment of children and adolescents with posttraumatic stress disorder: a double-blind placebo-controlled trial. *J Child Adolesc Psychopharmacol*. 2010;20:463–471.

Rynn M, Puliafico A, Heleniak C, Rikhi P, Ghalib K, Vidair H. Advances in pharmacotherapy for pediatric anxiety disorders. *Depress Anxiety*. 2011;28:76–87.

Depression and Suicide

Bayer JK, Rapee RM, Hiscock H, Ukoumunne OC, Mihalopoulos C, Wake M. Translational research to prevent internalizing problems in early childhood. *Depress Anxiety*. 2011;28:50–57.

Brent D, Emslie E, Clarke G, Wagner KD, Asarnow JR, Keller M, Ritz, L, Iyengar S, Abebe K, Birmaher B, Ryan N, Kennard B, Hughes C, DeBar L, McCracken J, Strober M, Suddath R, Spirito A, Leonard H, Meham N, Pora G, Onorato M, Zelazny J. Switching to another SSRI or to venlafaxine with or without cognitive behavioral therapy for adolescents with SSRI-resistant depression: the TORIDA randomized controlled trial. *JAMA*. 2008;299:901–913.

Christiansen E, Larsen KJ. Young people's risk of suicide attempts after contact with a psychiatric department—A nested case-control design using Danish register data. *J Child Psychol Psychiatry*. 2011;52:102.

Correll CU, Kratocvil CJ, March J. Developments in pediatric psychopharmacology: focus on stimulants, antidepressants and antipsychotics. *J Clin Psychiatry*. 2011;72:655–670.

Field T. Prenatal depression effects on early development: a review. *Infant Behav Dev*. 2011;34:1–14.

Frodl T, Reinhold E, Koutsoulieris N, Donohoe G, Bondy B, Reiser M, Moller Hj, Meisenzahl EM. Childhood stress, serotonin transporter gene and brain structures in major depression. *Neuropsychopharmacology*. 2010;35:1383–1390.

Gould MS, Greenberg T, Velting DM, Shaffer D. Youth suicide risk and preventive interventions: a review of the past ten years. *J Am Acad Child Adolesc Psychiatry*. 2003;42:386.

Hall WD. How have the SSRI antidepressants affected suicide risk? *Lancet*. 2006; 367(9527):1959.

Harro J, Kiive E. Droplets of black bile? Development of vulnerability and resilience to depression in young age. *Psychoneuroendocrinology*. 2011;36:380–392.

Heiligenstein JH, Hoog SL, Wagner KD, Findling RL, Galil N, Kaplan S, Busner J, Nilsson ME, Brown EB, Jacobson JG. Fluoxetine 40–60 mg versus fluoxetine 20 mg in the treatment of children and adolescents with a less-than-complete response to nine-week treatment with fluoxetine 10–20 mg: a pilot study. *J Child Adolesc Psychopharmacol*. 2006;16(1–2):207.

Hughes CW, Emslie GJ, Crimson ML, Posner K, Birmaher B, Ryan N, Jensen P, Curry J, Vitiello B, Lopez M, Shon SP, Piszka SR, Trivedi MH, The Texas Consensus Conference Panel on Medication Treatment of Childhood Major Depressive Disorder. Texas Children's Medication Algorithm Project: update from Texas Consensus Conference Panel on medication treatment of childhood major depressive disorder. *J Am Acad Child Adolesc Psychiatry*. 2007;46:667–686.

Kaess M, Parzer P, Haffner J, Steen R, Roos J, Klett M, Brunner R, Resch F. Explaining gender differences in non-fatal suicidal behavior among adolescents: a population-based study. *BMC Public Health*. 2011;11:597–603.

Luby J, Lenze S, Tillman R. A novel early intervention for preschool depression: findings from a pilot randomized controlled trial. *J Child Psychol Psychiatry*. 2012;53:313–322.

March J, Silva S, Petrycki S. The TADS Team. The Treatment for Adolescents with Depression Study (TADS): long-term effectiveness and safety outcomes. *Arch Gen Psychiatry*. 2007;64:1132–1143.

Newton AS, Hamm MP, Bethell J, Rhodes AE, Bryan CJ, Tjosvold L, Ali S, Logue E, Manion ID. Pediatric suicide-related presentations: a systematic review of mental health care in the emergency room department. *Ann Emerg Med*. 2010;56: 649–659.

Nock MK, Hwang I, Sampson N, Kessler RC, Angermeyer M, Beautrais A, Borges G, Bromet E, Bruffaerts R, de Girolamo G, de Graaf R, Florescu S, Gureje O, Haro JM, Hu C, Huang Y, Karam EG, Kawakami N, Kovess V, Levinson D, Postada-Villa J, Sagar R, Tomov T, Viana MC, Williams DR. Cross-national analysis of the associations among mental disorders and suicidal behavior: findings from the WHO World Mental Health Surveys. *PLoS Med*. 2009;6:1–13.

Olfson M, Shaffer D, Marcus SC, Greenberg T. Relationship between antidepressant medication treatment and suicide in adolescents. *Arch Gen Psychiatry*. 2003;60:978.

Rosso IM, Cintron CM, Steingard RJ, Renshaw PF, Young AD, Yurgelun-Todd DA. Amygdala and hippocampus volumes in pediatric major depression. *Biol Psychiatry*. 2005;57(1):21.

Von Knorring AL, Olsson GI, Thomson PH, Lemming OM, Hulten A. A randomized, double-blind, placebo-controlled study of citalopram in adolescents with major depressive disorder. *J Clin Psychopharmacol*. 2006;26:311.

Wagner KD. Pharmacotherapy for major depression in children and adolescents. *Prog Neuropsychopharmacol Biol Psychiatry*. 2005;29:819.

Wagner KD, Brent DA. Depressive disorders and suicide in children and adolescents. In: Sadock BJ, Sadock VA, Ruiz P, eds. *Kaplan & Sadock's Comprehensive Textbook of Psychiatry*. 9th ed. Vol. 2. Philadelphia, PA: Lippincott Williams & Wilkins; 2009:3652.

Whittington CJ, Kendall T, Fonagy P, Cotrell D, Cotgrove A, Boddington E. Selective serotonin reuptake inhibitors in childhood depression: systematic review of published versus unpublished data. *Lancet*. 2004;363:1341.

Zalsman G. Timing is critical: gene, environment and timing interactions in genetics of suicide in children and adolescents. *Eur Psychiatry*. 2010;25:284–286.

Bipolar Disorder

Axelson DA, Birmaher B, Strober M, Goldstein BI, Ha W, Gill MK, Goldstein TR, Yen S, Hower H, Hunt JI, Liao F, Iyengar S, Dickstein D, Kim E, Ryan ND, Frankel E, Keller MB. Course of subthreshold bipolar disorder in youth: diagnostic progression from bipolar disorder not otherwise specified. *J Am Acad Child Adolesc Psychiatry*. 2011;50:1001–1016.

Carlson GA. Bipolar disorder and mood dysregulation. *Proceedings; AACAP 2011 Psychopharmacology Update Institute: Controversies in Child and Adolescent Psychopharmacology*. 2011;257–284.

Carlson GA, Myer SE. Early-onset bipolar disorder. In: Sadock BJ, Sadock VA, Ruiz P, eds. *Kaplan & Sadock's Comprehensive Textbook of Psychiatry*. 9th ed. Vol. 2. Philadelphia, PA: Lippincott Williams & Wilkins; 2009:3663.

Correll CU, Kratochvil CJ, March JS. Developments in pediatric psychopharmacology: focus on stimulants, antidepressants and antipsychotics. *J Clin Psychiatry*. 2011;72:655–670.

Correll CU, Sheridan EM, DelBello MP. Antipsychotic and mood stabilizer efficacy and tolerability in pediatric and adult patients with bipolar I mania: a comparative analysis of acute, randomized, placebo-controlled trials. *Bipolar Disord*. 2010;12:116–141.

Findling RL, Landersdorfer CB, Kafantaris V, Pavulari M, McNamara NK, McClellan J, Frazier JA, Sikich L, Kowatch R, Lingler J, Faber J, Taylor-Zapata P, Jusko WJ. First-dose pharmacokinetics of lithium carbonate in children and adolescents. *J Clin Psychopharmacol*. 2010;30:404–410.

Larsky T, Krieger A, Elixhauser A, Vitiello B. Children's hospitalizations with a mood disorder diagnosis in general hospitals in the United States 2000–2006. *Child Adolesc Psychiatry Mental Health*. 2011;5:27–34.

Mathieu F, Dizier M-H, Etain B, Jamain S, Rietschel M, Maier W, Albus M, McKeon P, Roche S, Blackwood D, Muir W, Henry C, Malafosse A, Preisig M, Ferrero F, Cichon S, Schumacher J, Ohlraun S, Propping P, Jamra RA, Schulze TG, Zelenica D, Charon C, Marusic A, Dernovsek MC, Gurling H, Nothen M, Lathrop M, Leboyer M, Bellivier F. European collaborative study of early-onset bipolar disorder: evidence for heterogeneity on 2q14 according to age at onset. *Am J Med Genet Part B*. 2010;153B:1425–1433.

McNamara RK, Nandagopal JJ, Strakowski SM, DelBello M. Preventive strategies for early-onset bipolar disorder. Toward a clinical staging model. *CNS Drugs*. 2010;24:983–996.

Miklowitz DJ, Chang KD, Taylor DO, George EL, Singh MK, Schneck CD, Dickinson LM, Howe ME, Garber J. Early psychosocial intervention for youth at risk for bipolar I or II disorder: a one-year treatment development trial. *Bipolar Disord*. 2011;13:67–75.

Moreno C, Laje G, Blancvo C, Jiang H, Schmidtg AB, Olfson M. National trends in the outpatient diagnosis and treatment of bipolar disorder in youth. *Arch Gen Psychiatry*. 2007;64:1032–1039.

Nieto RG, Castellanos FX. A meta-analysis of neuropsychological functioning in patients with early onset schizophrenia and pediatric bipolar illness. *J Clin Child Adolesc Psychol*. 2011;40:266–280.

Nurnberger JI, McInnis M, Reich SW, Kastelic E, Wilcox HC, Glowinski A, Mitchell P, Fisher C, Erpe M, Gershon E, Berrettini W, Laite G, Schweitzer R, Rhoadarmer K, Coleman VV, Cai X, Azzouz F, Liu H, Kamali M, Brucksch C, Monahan PO. A high-risk study of bipolar disorder. Childhood clinical phenotypes as precursors of major mood disorders. *Arch Gen Psychiatry*. 2011;68:1012–1020.

Pavulari MN, Henry DB, Findling RL, Parnes S, Carbray JA, Mohammed T, Janicak PG, Sweeney JA. Double-blind randomized trial of risperidone versus sodium valproate in pediatric bipolar disorder. *Bipolar Disord*. 2010;12:593–605.

Pavulari MN, Passarotti AM, Lu LH, Carbray JA, Sweeney JA. Double-blind randomized trial of risperidone versus sodium valproate in pediatric bipolar disorder: fMRI outcomes. *Psychiatry Res*. 2011;193:28–37.

Stringaris A, Baroni A, Haimm C, Brotman M, Lowe CH, Myers F, Rustgi E, Wheeler W, Kayser R, Towbin K, Leibenluft E. Pediatric bipolar disorder versus severe mood dysregulation: risk for manic episodes on follow-up. *J Am Acad Child Adolesc Psychiatry*. 2010;49:397–405.

Versace Am Ladouceur CD, Romero S, Birmaher B, Axelson DA, Kupfer DJ, Phillips ML. Altered development of white matter in youth at high familial risk for bipolar disorder: a diffusion tensor imaging study. *J Am Acad Child Adolesc Psychiatry*. 2010;49:1249–1259.

Mood Dysregulation Disorder

Blader JC, Schooler NR, Jensen PS, Pliszka SR, Kafantaris V. Adjunctive sodium valproate versus placebo for children with ADHD and aggression refractory to stimulant monotherapy. *Am J Psychiatry*. 2009;166:1392–1401.

Brotman MA, Schmajuk M, Rich BA, Dickstein DP, Guyer AE, Costello EJ, Egger HL, Angold A, Pine DS, Leibenluft E. Prevalence, clinical correlates, and longitudinal course of severe mood dysregulation in children. *Biol Psychiatry*. 2006;60:991–997.

Copeland WE, Angold A, Costello J, Egger H. Prevalence, comorbidity, and correlates of DSM-5 proposed disruptive mood dysregulation disorder. *Am J Psychiatry*. 2013;170:173.

Fristad MA, Verducci JS. Walters K, Young ME. Impact of multifamily psychoeducational psychotherapy in treating children aged 8 to 12 years with mood disorder. *Arch Gen Psychiatry*. 2009;66:1013–1021.

Leibenluft E. Severe mood dysregulation, irritability, and the diagnostic boundaries of bipolar disorder in youths. *Am J Psychiatry*. 2011;168:129.

Leibenluft E, Cohen P, Gorrindo T, Brook JS, Pine DS. Chronic versus episodic irritability in youth: a community based longitudinal study of clinical and diagnostic associations. *J Child Adolesc Psychopharmacol*. 2006;16:456–466.

Margulies DM, Weintraub S, Basile J, Grover PJ, Carlson GA. Will disruptive mood dysregulation disorder reduce false diagnosis of bipolar disorder in children? *Bipolar Disord*. 2012;14:488.

Stringaris A, Barona A, Haimm C, Brotman MA, Lowe CH, Myers F, Rustgi E, Wheeler W, Kayser R, Towbin K, Leibenluft E. Pediatric bipolar disorder versus severe mood dysregulation: risk for manic episodes on follow-up. *J Am Acad Child Adolesc Psychiatry*. 2010;49:397.

West AE, Pavuluri MN. Psychosocial treatments for childhood and adolescent bipolar disorder. *Child Adolesc Psychiatr Clin N Am*. 2009;18:471–482.

Yearwood EL, Meadows-Oliver M. Mood dysregulation disorders. In: Yearwood EL, Pearson GS, Newland JA, eds. *Child and Adolescent Behavioral Health: A Resource for Advance Practice Psychiatric and Primary Care Practitioners in Nursing*. Hoboken, NJ: John Wiley & Sons Inc.; 2012:165.

Zonneyvlle-Bender MJ, Matthys W, van de Wiel NM, Lochman JE. Preventive effects of treatment of disruptive behavior disorder in middle childhood on substance use and delinquent behavior. *J Am Acad Child Adolesc Psychiatry*. 2007;46:33.

Conduct and Oppositional Defiant Disorder

Boxer P, Huesmann LR, Bushman BJ, O'Brien M, Moceri D. The role of violent media preference in cumulative developmental risk for violence and general aggression. *J Youth Adolesc*. 2009;38:417–428.

Canino G, Polanczyk G, Bauermeister JJ, Rhode LA, Frick P. Does the prevalence of CD and ODD vary across cultures? *Soc Psychiatry Psychiatr Epidemiol*. 2010;45:695–704.

Correll CU, Kratochvil CJ, March J. Developments in pediatric psychopharmacology: focus on stimulants, antidepressants, and antipsychotics. *J Clin Psychiatry*. 2011;72:655–670.

Dodge KA, Conduct Problems Prevention Research Group. The effects of the Fast Track Preventive Intervention on the development of conduct disorder across childhood. *Child Develop*. 2011;82:331–345.

Harden KP, D'Onofrio BM, Van Hulle C, Turkheimer E, Rodgers JL, Waldman ID, Lahey BB. Population density and youth antisocial behavior. *J Child Psychol Psychiatry*. 2009;50:999–1008.

Huebner T, Vloet TD, Marx I, Konrad K, Fink GR, Herpetz SC, Herpetz-Dahlmann B. Morphometric brain abnormalities in boys with conduct disorder. *J Am Acad Child Adolesc Psychiatry*. 2008;47:540–547.

Kim HW, Cho SC, Kim BN, Kim JW, Shin MS, Yeo JY. Does oppositional defiant disorder have temperament and psychopathological profiles independent of attention deficit/hyperactivity disorder? *Compr Psychiatry*. 2010;51:412–418.

LeBlanc JC, Binder CE, Armenteros JL, Aman MG, Want JS, Hew H, Kusumakar V. Risperidone reduces aggression in boys with a disruptive behavior disorder and below average intelligence quotient: analysis of two placebo-controlled randomized trials. *Int Clin Psychopharmacol*. 2005;20:275.

Lochman JE, Powell NP, Boxmeyer CL, Jimenez-Camargo L. Cognitive-behavioral therapy for externalizing disorders in children and adolescents. *Child Adolesc Psychiatric Clin N Am*. 2011;20:305–318.

Meier MH, Slutske WS, Heath AC, Martin NG. Sex differences in the genetic and environmental influences on childhood conduct disorder and adult antisocial behavior. *J Abnorm Psychol*. 2011;120:377–388.

Murray J, Farrington DP. Risk factors for conduct disorder and delinquency: key findings from longitudinal studies. *Can J Psychiatry*. 2010;55:633–642.

Padhy R, Saxena K, Remsing L, Heumer J, Plattner B, Steiner H. Symptomatic response to sodium valproate in subtypes of conduct disorder. *Child Psychiatry Hum Dev*. 2011;42:584–593.

Patel NC, Crismon ML, Hoagwood K, Jensen PS. Unanswered questions regarding atypical antipsychotic use in aggressive children and adolescents. *J Child Adolesc Psychopharmacol*. 2005;15:270.

Pelletier J, Collett B, Gimpel G, Crowley S. Assessment of disruptive behaviors in preschoolers: psychometric properties of the disruptive behavior disorders rating scale and school situations questionnaire. *J Psychoeduc Assess*. 2006;24:3–18.

Reyes M, Buitelaar J, Toren P, Augustyns I, Eerdekens M. A randomized, double-blind, placebo-controlled study of risperidone maintenance treatment in children and adolescents with disruptive behavior disorders. *Am J Psychiatry*. 2006;163:402–410.

Rutter M. Research review: child psychiatric diagnosis and classification: concepts, finding, challenges and potential. *J Child Psychol Psychiatry*. 2011;52:647–660.

Santesso DL, Reker DL, Schmidt LA, Segalowitz SJ. Frontal electroencephalogram activation asymmetry, emotional intelligence, and externalizing behaviors in 10-year-old children. *Child Psychiatr Hum Dev* 2006;36:311–328.

Sasayam D, Hayashida A, Yamasue H, Yuzuru H, Kaneko T, Kasai K, Washizuka S, Amano N. Neuroanatomical correlates of attention-deficit-hyperactivity disorder

accounting for comorbid oppositional defiant disorder and conduct disorder. *Psychiatry Clin Neurosci*. 2010:64:394–402.

Van Huylle CA, Waldman ID, D'Onofrio BM, Rodgers JL, Rthouz PJ, Lahey BB. Developmental structure of genetic influences on antisocial behavior across childhood and adolescence. *J Abnorm Psychol*. 2009;118:711–734.

Webster-Stratton C, Reid JM. The Incredible Years parents, teachers and children training series. In: Weisz JR, Kadin AE, eds. *Evidence-Based Psychotherapies for Children and Adolescents*. 2nd ed. New York: Guildford; 2010:194–210.

Zahrt DM, Melzer-Lange MD. Aggressive behavior in children and adolescents. *Pediatr Rev*. 2011;32:325–331.

Zuddas A, Zanni R, Usala T. Second generation antipsychotics (SGAs) for nonpsychotic disorders in children and adolescents: a review of the randomized controlled studies. *Eur Neuropsychopharmacol*. 2011;21:600–620.

Anxiety Disorders

Bittner A, Egger HL, Erkanli A. What do childhood anxiety disorders predict? *J Child Psychol Psychiatry*. 2007;48:1174–1183.

Comer JS, Puliafico AC, Ascenbrand SG, McKnight K, Robin JA, Goldfine ME, Albano AM. A pilot feasibility evaluation of the CALM Program for anxiety disorders in early childhood. *J Anxiety Disord*. 2012;26:40–49.

Compton SN, Walkup JT, Albano AM, Piacentini JC, Birmaher B, Sherrill JT, Ginsburg GS, Rynn MA, McCracken JT, Waslick BD, Iyengar S, Kendall PC, March JS. Child/Adolescent Anxiety Multimodal Study (CAMS): rationale, design, and methods. *Child Adolesc Psychiatry Ment Health*. 2010;4:1.

Connolly SC, Suarez L, Sylvester C. Assessment and treatment of anxiety disorders in children and adolescents. *Curr Psychiatry Rep*. 2011;13:99–110.

Davis TE III, May A, Whiting SE. Evidence-based treatment of anxiety and phobia in children and adolescents: current status and effects on the emotional response. *Clin Psychol Rev*. 2011;31:592–602.

Ginsburg GS, Kendall PC, Sakolsky D, Compton SN, Piacentini J, Albano AM, Walkup JT, Sherrill J, Coffey KA, Rynn MA, Keeton CP, McCracken JT, Bergman L, Iyengar S, Birmaher B, March J. Remission after acute treatment in children and adolescents with anxiety disorders: findings from The CAMS. *J Consult Clin Psychol*. 2011;79:806–813.

Hanna GL, Fischer DJ, Fluent TE. Separation anxiety disorder and school refusal in children and adolescents. *Pediatr Rev*. 2006;27:56–63.

Hirshfeld-Becker DR, Masek B, Henin A, Blakely LR, Pollock-Wurman RA, McQuade J, DePetrillo L, Briesch J, Ollendick TH, Rosenbaum JF, Biederman J. Cognitive behavioral therapy for 4- to 7-year-old children with anxiety disorders: a randomized clinical trial. *J Consult Clin Psychol*. 2010;78:498–510.

Otani K, Suzuki A, Matsumoto Y, Kamata M. Parental overprotection increases interpersonal sensitivity in healthy subjects. *Compr Psychiatry*. 2009;50:54–57.

Reinblatt SP, Walkup JT. Psychopharmacologic treatment of pediatric anxiety disorders. *Child Adolesc Psychiatric Clin N Am*. 2005;14:877.

Rockhill C, Kodish I, DiBassisto C, Macias M, Varley C, Ryan S. Anxiety disorders in children and adolescents. *Curr Prob Pediatr Adolesc Health Care*. 2010;40:A1–A4;65–100.

Rynn M, Puliafico A, Heleniak C, Rikhi P, Ghalib K, Vidair H. Advances in pharmacotherapy for pediatric anxiety disorders. *Depress Anxiety*. 2011;28:76–87.

Schneider S, Blatter-Meunier J, Herren C, Adornetto C, In-Albon T, Lavallee K. Disorder-specific cognitive-behavioral therapy for separation anxiety disorder in young children: a randomized waiting-list–controlled group. *Psychother Psychosom*. 2011;80:206–215.

Vanderwerker LC, Jacobs SC, Parkes CM, Prigerson HG. An exploration of associations between separation anxiety in childhood and complicated grief in later life. *J Nerv Ment Dis*. 2006;194(2):121–123.

Walkup JT, Albano AM, Piacentini J. Cognitive behavioral therapy, sertraline, or a combination in childhood anxiety. *N Engl J Med*. 2008;359:2753–2766.

Selective Mutism

Bergman RL, Lee JC. Selective mutism. In: Sadock BJ, Sadock VA, Ruiz P, eds. *Kaplan & Sadock's Comprehensive Textbook of Psychiatry*. 9th ed. Vol. 2. Philadelphia, PA: Lippincott Williams & Wilkins; 2009:3694.

Carbone D, Schmidt LA, Cunningham CC, McHolm AE, Edison S, St. Pierre J, Boyle JH. Behavioral and socio-emotional functioning in children with selective mutism: a comparison with anxious and typically developing children across multiple informants. *J Abnorm Child Psychol*. 2010;38:1057–1067.

Davis TE III, May A, Whiting SE. Evidence-based treatment of anxiety and phobia in children and adolescents: current status and effects on the emotional response. *Clin Psychol Rev*. 2011;31:592–602.

Kehle TJ, Bray MA, Theodore LA. Selective mutism. In: Bear GG, Minke KM, eds. *Children's Needs III: Development, Prevention, and Intervention*. Washington, DC: National Association of School Psychologists; 2006:293.

Rynn M, Puliafico A, Heleniak C, Rikhi P, Ghalib K, Vidair H. Advances in pharmacotherapy for pediatric anxiety disorders. *Depress Anxiety*. 2011;28:76–87.

Schwartz RH, Freedy AS, Sheridan MJ. Selective mutism: are primary care physicians missing the silence? *Clin Pediatr (Phila)*. 2006;45:43–48.

Scott S, Beidel DC. Selective mutism: an update and suggestions for future research. *Curr Psychiatry Rep*. 2011;13:251–257.

Toppelberg CO, Tabors P, Coggins A, Lum K, Burger C. Differential diagnosis of selective mutism in bilingual children. *J Am Acad Child Adolesc Psychiatry*. 2005;44(6):592–595.

Wagner KD, Berard R, Stein MB, Wetherhold E, Carpenter DJ, Perera P, Gee M, Davy K, Machin A. A multicenter, randomized, double-blind, placebo controlled trial of paroxetine in children and adolescents with social anxiety disorder. *Arch Gen Psychiatry*. 2004;61:1153.

Waslick B. Psychopharmacology intervention for pediatric anxiety disorders: a research update. *Child Adolesc Psychiatr Clin N Am*. 2006;1:51.

Yeganeh R, Beidel DC, Turner SM. Selective mutism: more than social anxiety? *Depress Anxiety*. 2006;23(3):117.

Obsessive-Compulsive Disorder

Alaghband-Rad J, Hakimshooshtary M. A randomized controlled clinical trial of citalopram versus fluoxetine in children and adolescents with obsessive-compulsive disorder (OCD). *Eur Child Adolesc Psychiatry*. 2009;18:131–135.

American Academy of Child and Adolescent Psychiatry. Practice parameter for the assessment and treatment of children and adolescent with obsessive-compulsive disorder. *J Am Acad Child Adolesc Psychiatry*. 2012;51:98–113.

Bienvenu OJ, Wany Y, Shugart YY, Welch JM, Fyer AJ, Rauch SL, McCracken JT, Rasmussen SA, Murphy DL, Cullen B, Valle D, Hoen-Saric R, Greenberg BD, Pinto A, Knowles JA, Piacentini J, Pauls DL, Liang KY, Willour VL, Riddle M, Samuels JF, Feng G, Nestadt G. Sapap3 and pathological grooming in humans: results from the OCD collaborative genetics study. *Am J Med Genet B Neuropsychiatry Genet*. 2009;150B:710–720.

Flessner CA, Allgair A, Garcia A, Freeman J, Sapyta J, Franklin ME, Foa E, March J. The impact of neuropsychological functioning on treatment outcome in pediatric obsessive-compulsive disorder. *Depress Anxiety*. 2010;27:365–371.

Franklin ME, Sapyta J, Freeman JB, Khanna M, Compton S, Almirall D, Moore P, Choate-Summers M, Garcia A, Edson AL, Foa EB, March JS. Cognitive behavior therapy augmentation of pharmacotherapy in pediatric obsessive-compulsive disorder: the Pediatric OCD Treatment Study II (POTS II) randomized controlled trial. *JAMA*. 2011;306:1224–1232.

Freeman J, Sapyta J, Garcia A, Fitzgerald D, Khanna M, Choate-Summers M, Moore P, Chrisman A, Haff N, Naeem A, March J, Franklin M. Still struggling: characteristics of youth with OCD who are partial responders to medication treatment. *Child Psychiatry Hum Dev*. 2011;42:424–441.

Leckman JF, King RA, Gilbert DL, Coffey BJ, Singer HS, Dure LS 4th, Grantz H, Katsovich L, Lin H, Lombroso PJ, Kawikova I, Johnson DR, Kurlan RM, Kaplan EL. Streptococcal upper respiratory tract infections and exacerbations of tic and obsessive-compulsive symptoms: a prospective longitudinal study. *J Am Acad Child Adolesc Psychiatry*. 2011;50:108–118.

Lewin AB, Peris TS, Bergman L, McCracken JT, Piacentini J. The role of treatment expectancy in youth receiving exposure-based CBT for obsessive compulsive disorder. *Behav Res Ther*. 2011;49:536–543.

Lewin AB, Piacentini J. Obsessive-compulsive disorder in children. In: Sadock BJ, Sadock VA, Ruiz P, eds. *Kaplan & Sadock's Comprehensive Textbook of Psychiatry*. 9th ed. Vol. 2. Philadelphia, PA: Lippincott Williams & Wilkins; 2009:3671.

Masi G, Pfanner C, Millepiedi S, Berloffa S. Aripiprazole augmentation in 39 adolescents with medication-resistant obsessive-compulsive disorder. *J Clin Psychopharmacol*. 2010;30:688–693.

Micali N, Hayman I, Perez M, Hilton K, Nakatani E, Turner C, Mataix-Cois D. Long-term outcomes of obsessive-compulsive disorder: follow-up of 142 children and adolescents. *Br J Psychiatry*. 2010;197:128–134.

Olino TM, Gillo S, Rowe D, Palermo S, Nuhfer EC, Birmaher B, Gilbert AR. Evidence for successful implementation of exposure and response prevention in a naturalistic group format for pediatric OCD. *Depress Anxiety*. 2011;4:342–348.

Pediatric OCD Treatment Study Team. Cognitive-behavior therapy, sertraline, and their combination for children and adolescents with obsessive-compulsive disorder: the Pediatric OCD Treatment Study (POTS) randomized controlled trial. *JAMA*. 2004;292:1969.

Piacentini J, Bergman RL, Chang S, Langley A, Peris T, Wood JJ, McCracken J. Controlled comparison of family cognitive behavioral therapy and psychoeducation/relaxation training for child obsessive-compulsive disorder. *J Am Acad Child Adolesc Psychiatry*. 2011;50:1149–1161.

Radua J, Mataix-Cois D. Voxel-wise meta-analysis of grey matter changes in obsessive-compulsive disorder. *Br J Psychiatry*. 2009;195:393–402.

Rotge JY, Langbour N, Guehl D, Bioulac B, Jaafari N, Allard M, Aouizerate B, Burbaud P. Gray matter alterations in obsessive-compulsive disorder: an anatomical likelihood estimation meta-analysis. *Neuropsychopharmacology*. 2010;35:686–691.

Storch EA, Caporino NE, Morgan JR, Lewin AB, Rojas A, Brauer L, Larson MJ, Murphy TK. Preliminary investigation of web-camera delivered cognitive-behavioral therapy for youth with obsessive-compulsive disorder. *Psychiatry Res*. 2011;189:407–412.

Szeszko PR, MacMillan S, McMeniman M, Chen S, Baribault K, Lim KO, Ivey J, Rose M, Banerjee SP, Bhandari R, Moore GJ, Rosenberg DR. Brain structural abnormalities in psychotropic drug-naive pediatric patients with obsessive-compulsive disorder. *Am J Psychiatry*. 2004;161:1049–1056.

Waslick B. Psychopharmacology intervention for pediatric anxiety disorders: a research update. *Child Adolesc Psychiatr Clin N Am*. 2006;1:51.

Psychotic Disorders

Addington J, Epstein I, Liu L, French P, Boydell KM. A randomized controlled trial of cognitive behavioral therapy for individuals at clinical high risk of psychosis. *Schizophr Res*. 2011;125:54–61.

Amminger GP, Schafer MR, Papageorgiou K, Klier CM, Cotton SM. Long-chain w-3 fatty acids for indicated prevention of psychotic disorder: a randomized placebo-controlled trial. *Arch Gen Psychiatry*. 2010;67:146–154.

Arango C. Attenuated psychotic symptoms syndrome: how it may affect child and adolescent psychiatry. *Eur Child Adolesc Psychiatry*. 2011;20:67–70.

Bechdolf A, Wagner M, Ruhrman S, Harrigan S, Putzfeld V, Pukrop R, Brockhaus-Dumke A, Berning J, Janssen B, Decker P, Bottlender R, Maurer K, Möller HJ, Gaebel W, Häfner H, Maier W, Klosterkötter J. Preventing progression to first episode psychosis in early initial prodromal states. *Br J Psychiatry*. 2012;200:22–29.

Biswas P, Malhotra S, Malhotra A, Gupta N. Comparative study of neuropsychological correlates in schizophrenia with childhood onset, adolescence and adulthood. *Eur Child Adolesc Psychiatry*. 2006;15:360.

Clark C, Narr KL, O'Neill J, Levitt J, Siddarth P, Phillips O, Toga A, Caplan R. White matter integrity, language, and childhood onset schizophrenia. *Schizophrenia Res*. 2012;138:150–156.

Correll CU. Symptomatic presentation and initial treatment for schizophrenia in children and adolescents. *J Clin Psychiatry*. 2010;71:11.

David CN, Greenstein D, Clasen L, Gochman P, Miller R, Tossell JW, Mattai AA, Gogtay N, Rapoport JL. Childhood onset schizophrenia: high rate of visual hallucinations. *J Am Acad Child Adolesc Psychiatry*. 2011;50:681–686.

Fagerlund B, Pagsberg AK, Hemmingsen RP. Cognitive deficits and levels of IQ in adolescent onset schizophrenia and other psychotic disorders. *Schizophr Res*. 2006; 85(1–3):30.

Findling RL, Johnson JL, McClellan J, Frazier JA, Vitiello B, Hamer RM, Lieberman JA, Ritz L, McNamara NK, Lingler J, Hlastala S, Pierson L, Puglia M, Maloney AE, Kaufman EM, Noyes N, Sikich L. Double-blind maintenance safety and effectiveness findings from the treatment of Early-Onset Schizophrenia Spectrum Disorders (TEOSS) study. *J Am Acad Child Adolesc Psychiatry*. 2010;49:583–594.

Findling RL, Robb A, Nyilas M, Forbes RA, Jin N, Ivanova S, Marcus R, McQuade RD, Iwamoto T, Carson WH. A multiple-center, randomized, double-blind, placebo-controlled study of oral aripiprazole for treatment of adolescents with schizophrenia. *Am J Psychiatry*. 2008;165:1432–1441.

Frazier JA, Giuliano AJ, Johnson JL, Yakutis L, Youngstrom EA, Breiger D, Sikich L, Findling RL, McClellan J, Hamer RM, Vitiello B, Lieberman JA, Hooper SR. Neurocognitive outcomes in the Treatment of Early-Onset Schizophrenia Spectrum Disorders study. *J Am Acad Child Adolesc Psychiatry*. 2012;51:496–505.

Fusar-Poli P, Bechdolf A, Taylor M, Carpenter W, Yung A, McGuire P. At risk for schizophrenia or affective psychosis? A meta-analysis of DSM/ICD diagnostic outcomes in individuals at high clinical risk. *Schizophr Bull*. 2013;39:923–932.

Fusar-Poli P, Bonoldi I, Yung AR. Predicting psychosis: a meta-analysis of transition outcomes in individuals at high clinical risk. *Arch Gen Psychiatry*. 2012;69: 220–229.

Fusar-Poli P, Borgwardt S, Bechdolf A, Addington J, Riecher-Rossler A, Schultze-Lutter F, Keshavan M, Wood S, Ruhrmann S, Seidman LJ, Valmaggia L, Cannon T, Velthorst E, De Haan L, Cornblatt B, Bonoldi I, Birchwood M, McGlashan T, Carpenter W, McGorry P, Klosterkötter J, McGuire P, Yung A. The psychosis high-risk state. A comprehensive state-of-the-art review. *JAMA Psychiatry*. 2013;70:107–120.

Gentile S. Clinical usefulness of second-generation antipsychotics in treating children and adolescents diagnosed with bipolar or schizophrenic disorders. *Pediatr Drugs*. 2011;13:291–302.

Haas M, Eerdekens M, Kushner SF, Singer J, Augustyns I, Quiroz J, Pandina G, Kusumakar V. Efficacy, safety and tolerability of two risperidone dosing regimens in adolescent schizophrenia: a double-blind study. *Br J Psychiatry*. 2009;194:158–164.

Haas M, Unis AS, Armenteros J, Copenhaver MD, Quiroz JA, Kushner SF. A 6-week randomized double-blind placebo-controlled study of the efficacy and safety of risperidone in adolescents with schizophrenia. *J Child Adolesc Psychopharmacol*. 2009;19:611–621.

Jacobs E, Kline E, Schiffman J. Defining treatment as usual for attenuated psychosis syndrome: a survey of community practitioners. *Psychiatr Serv*. 2012;63:1252–1256.

Jacquet H, Rapoport JL, Hecketsweiler B, Bobb A, Thibaut F, Frebourg T, Campion D. Hyperprolinemia is not associated with childhood onset schizophrenia. *Am J Med Genet B Neuropsychiatr Genet*. 2006;141:192.

Kryzhanovskaya L, Schulz SC, McDougle C, Frazier J, Dittmann R, Robertson-Plouch C, Bauer T, Xu W, Wang W, Carlson J, Tohen M. Olanzapine versus placebo in adolescents with schizophrenia: a 6-week, randomized, double-blind, placebo-controlled trial. *J Am Acad Child Adolesc Psychiatry*. 2009;48:60–70.

Kumra S, Kranzler H, Gerbine-Rosen G, Kester HM, De Thomas C, Kafantaris V, Correll C, Kane J. Clozapine and 'high-dose' olanzapine in refractory early-onset schizophrenia: a 12-week randomized and double-blind comparison. *Biol Psychiatry*. 2008;63:524–529.

McGlashan TH, Zipursky RB, Perkins D, Addington J, Miller T, Woods SW, Hawkins KA, Hoffman RE, Preda A, Epstein I, Addington D, Lindborg S, Trzaskoma Q, Tohen M, Breier A. Randomized, double-blind trial of olanzapine versus placebo in patients prodromally symptomatic for psychosis. *Am J Psychiatry*. 2006;163:790–799.

McGorry PD, Nelson B, Amminger GP, Bechdolf A, Francey SM, Berger G, Riecher-Rössler A, Klosterkötter J, Ruhrmann S, Schultze-Lutter F, Nordentoft M, Hickie I, McGuire P, Berk M, Chen EY, Keshavan MS, Yung AR. Intervention in individuals at ultra-high risk for psychosis: a review and future directions. *J Clin Psychiatry*. 2009;70:1206–1212.

McGorry PD, Yung AR, Phillips LJ, Yuen HP, Francey S, Cosgrave EM, Germano D, Bravin J, McDonald T, Blair A, Adlard S, Jackson H. Randomized controlled trial of interventions designed to reduce the risk of progression to first episode psychosis in a clinical sample with subthreshold symptoms. *Arch Gen Psychiatry*. 2002;59:921–928.

McGurk SR, Twamlety EW, Sitezer DL, McHugo JG, Mueser KT. A meta-analysis of cognitive remediation in schizophrenia. *Am J Psychiatry*. 2007;164: 1791–1802.

Morrison AP, French P, Walford L, Lewis SW, Kilcommons A, Green J, Parker S, Bentall R. Cognitive therapy for the prevention of psychosis in people at ultra-high risk: randomised controlled trial. *Br J Psychiatry*. 2004;185:291–297.

Peterson L, Jeppesen P, Thorup A, Abel MB, Øhlenschlaeger J, Christenson TØ, Krarup G, Jørgensen P, Nordentoft M. A randomised multicentre trial of integrated verus standard treatment of patients with a first episode of psychotic illness. *BMJ*. 2005;331:602.

Phillips LJ, Nelson B, Yuen HP, Francey SM, Simmons M. Randomized controlled trial of interventions for young people at ultra-high risk of psychosis; study design and baseline characteristics. *Aust N Z J Psychiatry*. 2009;43:818–829.

Preti A, Cella M. Randomized-controlled trails in people at ultra high risk of psychosis: a review of treatment effectiveness. *Schizophr Res*. 2010;123:30–36.

Rapoport JL, Gogtay N. Childhood onset schizophrenia: support for a progressive neurodevelopmental disorder. *Int J Dev Neurosci*. 2011;29:251–258.

Remschmidt J, Theisen FM. Early-onset schizophrenia. *Neuropsychobiology*. 2012;66:63–69.

Schimmelmann BG, Schmidt AJ, Carbon M, Correll CU. Treatment of adolescents with early-onset schizophrenia spectrum disorders: in search of a rational, evidence-informed approach. *Curr Opin Psychiatry*. 2013;26:219–230.

Seal JL, Gornick MC, Gotgay N, Shaw P, Greenstein DK, Coffee M, Gochman PA, Stromberg T, Chen Z, Merriman B, Nelson SF, Brooks J, Arepalli S, Wavrant-De Vrieze F, Hardy J, Rapoport JL, Addington AM. Segmental uniparental isodisomy on 5q32-qter in a patient with childhood-onset schizophrenia. *J Med Genet*. 2006;43(11):887–892.

Shaw P, Sporn A, Gogtay N, Overman GP, Greenstein D, Gochman P, Tossell JW, Lenane M, Rapoport JL. Childhood onset schizophrenia: a double-blind clozapine-olanzapine comparison. *Arch Gen Psychiatry*. 2006;63:721–730.

Shrivastava A, McGorry PD, Tsuang M, Woods SW, Cornblatt BA, Corcoran C, Carpenter W. "Attenuated psychotic symptoms syndrome" as a risk syndrome of psychosis, diagnosis in DSM-V: the debate. *Indian J Psychiatry*. 2011;53: 57–65.

Sikich L. Early onset psychotic disorders. In: Sadock BJ, Sadock VA, Ruiz P, eds. *Kaplan & Sadock's Comprehensive Textbook of Psychiatry*. 9th ed. Vol. 2. Philadelphia, PA: Lippincott Williams & Wilkins; 2009:3699.

Sikich L, Frazier JA, McClellan J, Findling RL, Vitiello B, Ritz L, Ambler D, Puglia M, Maloney AE, Michael E, De Jong S, Slifka K, Noyes N, Hlastala S, Pierson L, McNamara NK, Delporto-Bedoya D, Anderson R, Hamer RM, Lieberman JA. Double-blind comparison of first-and second-generation antipsychotics in early-onset schizophrenia and schizoaffective disorder: findings from the treatment of early-onset schizophrenia spectrum disorders (TEOSS) study. *Am J Psychiatry*. 2008;165:1420–1431.

Starling J, Williams LM, Hainsworth C, Harris AW. The presentation of early-onset psychotic disorders. *Aust N Z J Psychiatry*. 2013;47:43–50.

Vyas NS, Gogtay N. Treatment of early onset of schizophrenia: recent trends, challenges and future considerations. *Front Psychiatry*. 2012;3:1–5.

Vyas NS, Patel NH, Puri BK. Neurobiology and phenotypic expression in early-onset schizophrenia. *Early Interv Psychiatry*. 2011;5:3–14.

Yung AR, Phillips LJ, Nelson B, Francey SM, Panyuen H, Simmons MB, Ross ML, Kelly D, Baker K, Amminger GP, Berger G, Thompson AD, Thampi A, McGorry PD. Randomized controlled trial of interventions for young people at ultra-high risk for psychosis: 6-month analysis. *J Clin Psychiatry*. 2011;72:430–440.

Yung AR, Woods SW, Ruhrmann S, Addington J, Schultze-Lutter F. Wither the attenuated psychosis syndrome? *Schizophr Bull*. 2012;38:1130–1134.

Substance Use Disorders

Buckner JD, Heimberg RG, Schneier FR, Liu SM, Want S, Blanco C. The relationship between cannabis use disorder and social anxiety disorder in the National Epidemiologic Study of Alcohol and Related Conditions (NESARC). *Drug Alcohol Depend*. 2012;124:128–134.

Bukstein O. Adolescent substance abuse. In: Sadock BJ, Sadock VA, Ruiz P, eds. *Kaplan & Sadock's Comprehensive Textbook of Psychiatry*. 9th ed. Vol. II. Philadelphia, PA: Lippincott Williams & Wilkins; 2009:3818.

Eaton DK, Kann L, Kinchen S, Shanklin S, Ross J, Hawkins J, Harris WA, Lowry R, McManus T, Chyen D, Lim C, Whittle L, Brener ND, Wechsler H; Centers for Disease Control and Prevention (CDC). Youth risk behavior surveillance—United States, 2009. *MMWR Surveill Summ*. 2010;59(5):1–142.

Fiorentini A, Volunteri LS, Draogna F, Rovera C, Maffini M, Mauri MC, Altamura CA. Substance-induced psychoses: a critical review of the literature. *Curr Drug Abuse Rev*. 2011;4:228–240.

Fraser S, Hides L, Philips L, Proctor D, Lubman DI. Differentiating first episode substance induced primary psychotic disorders with concurrent substance use in young people. *Schizophr Res*. 2012;136:110–115.

Giedd J, Stocvkman M, Weele C. Anatomic magnetic resonance imaging of the developing child and adolescent brain. In: Reyna VF; Chapman SB, Dougherty MR, Copnfrey J, eds. *The Adolescent Brain: Learning, Reasoning, and Decision Making*. Washington, DC: American Psychological Association; 2012.

Harrow BS, Tompkins CP, Mitchell PD, Smith KW, Soldz S, Kasten L, Fleming K. The impact of publicly funded managed care on adolescent substance abuse treatment outcomes. *Am J Drug Alcohol Abuse*. 2006;32(3):379.

Johnston LD, O'Malley PM, Bachman JG, Schulenberg JE. Monitoring the Future: National Survey Results on Drug Use. 1975–2007. Vol 3 Secondary School Students. Bethesda, MD. National Institute on Drug Abuse; 2008.

Kaminer Y, Winters KC. Proposed DSM-5 substance use disorders for adolescents: If you build it, will they come? *Am J Addict*. 2012;21:280–281.

Lenk KM, Erickson DJ, Wonters KC, Nelson TF, Toomey TL. Screening services for alcohol misuse and abuse at four-year colleges in the U.S. *J Subst Abuse Treat*. 2012;43:352–358.

McCabe SE, West BT, Teter CJ, Boyd CJ. Medical and nonmedical use of prescription opioids among high school seniors in the United States. *Arch Pediatr Adolesc Med*. 2012;166:797–802.

Mitchell SG, Gryczynski J, Gonzales A, Moseley A, Peterson T, O'Grady KE, Schwartz RP. Screening, brief intervention, and referral to treatment (SBIRT) for substance use in a school-based program: services and outcomes. *Am J Addict*. 2012;21:S5–S13.

Tavolacci MP, Ladner J, Grigioni S, Richard L, Villet H, Dechelotte P. Prevalence and association of perceived stress, substance use and behavioral addictions: a cross-sectional study among university students in France, 2009–2011. *BMC Public Health*. 2013;13:724–732.

Winters KC. Advances in the science of adolescent drug involvement: implications for assessment and diagnosis—experience from the United States. *Curr Opin Psychiatry*. 2013;26:318–324.

Winters KC, Martim CS, Chung T. Substance use disorders in DSM-V. When applied to adolescents. *Addiction*. 2011;106:882–884.

Yuma-Guerrero PJ, Lawson KA, Velasquez MM, von Sternberg K, Maxson T, Garcia N. Screening, brief intervention, and referral for alcohol use in adolescents: a systematic review. *Pediatrics*. 2012;130:115–122.

## 3

Neurocognitive Disorders

Advances in molecular biology diagnostic techniques and medication management have significantly improved the ability to recognize and treat cognitive disorders. Cognition includes memory, language, orientation, judgment, conducting interpersonal relationships, performing actions (praxis), and problem-solving. Cognitive disorders reflect disruption in one or more of these domains. Frequently, behavioral symptoms complicate the disorder. Cognitive disorders exemplify the complex interface among neurology, medicine, and psychiatry in that medical or neurologic conditions often lead to cognitive disorders that, in turn, are associated with behavioral symptoms. Of all psychiatric conditions, cognitive disorders best demonstrate how biologic insults result in behavioral symptomatology. The clinician must carefully assess the history and context of the presentation of these disorders before arriving at a diagnosis and treatment plan.

Cognitive disorders tend to defy Occam's razor, challenging clinicians and nosologists with multiplicity, comorbidity, and unclear boundaries. These are most concerning for elderly adults, the demographic group most at risk for cognitive disorders. Dementias of late-life are particularly problematic in this regard. Existing, although often unrecognized, dementia is a significant risk factor for superimposed delirium. Moreover, certain dementias, such as dementia with Lewy bodies or late stages of Alzheimer disease, may have chronic clinical presentations virtually indistinguishable from delirium except for temporal onset and the lack of an identifiable acute source.

Similarly, behavioral syndromes complicate the course of nearly all subjects developing progressive dementia. These syndromes include anxiety, depression, sleep problems, psychosis, and aggression. These symptoms can be as distressing and disabling as the primary cognitive disorder. Some of these behavioral syndromes, such as psychosis, may themselves result from independent underlying biologies and may be additive with the primary neurodegenerative process.

The boundaries between types of dementia and between dementia and healthy aging can be similarly diffuse. Neuropathologic studies of both clinical and population samples have revealed a surprising truth. The most common neuropathologic presentation associated with dementia reveals mixtures of Alzheimer disease, vascular, and Lewy body pathologies. Pure syndromes are relatively less common, although often the dementia is ascribed to one of the coexisting pathologies. Strategies regarding how to understand or reconcile multiple pathologies in the clinic are needed, although they lag.

DEFINITION

The definitions of cognitive disorders follow. We will then describe each separately.

Delirium

Delirium describes a condition of short-term confusion and changes in cognition. There are four subcategories based on several causes: (1) general medical condition (e.g., infection), (2) substance-induced (e.g., cocaine, opioids, phencyclidine [PCP]), (3) multiple causes (e.g., head trauma and kidney disease), and (4) other or multiple etiologies (e.g., sleep deprivation, medications).

Dementia (Major Neurocognitive Disorder)

Dementia, also referred to as major neurocognitive disorder, in the fifth edition of DSM (DSM-5), is marked by severe impairment in memory, judgment, orientation, and cognition. The subcategories are (1) dementia of the Alzheimer type (Alzheimer Dementia), which usually occurs in persons older than 65 years of age and is manifested by progressive intellectual disorientation and dementia, delusions, or depression; (2) vascular dementia, caused by vessel thrombosis or hemorrhage; (3) human immunodeficiency virus (HIV) disease; (4) head trauma; (5) Pick disease or frontotemporal lobar degeneration; (6) prion disease such as Creutzfeldt–Jakob disease (CJD), which is caused by a slow-growing transmittable virus; (7) substance-induced, caused by toxin or medication (e.g., gasoline fumes, atropine); (8) multiple etiologies; and (9) not specified (if the cause is unknown).

In DSM-5, mild neurocognitive disorder describes a less severe form of dementia.

Amnestic Disorder

Amnestic disorders are *major neurocognitive disorders caused by other medical conditions*. They are marked primarily by memory impairment in addition to other cognitive symptoms. The causes include (1) medical conditions (hypoxia), (2) toxins or medications (e.g., marijuana, diazepam), and (3) unknown causes.

CLINICAL EVALUATION

During history taking, the clinician seeks to elicit the development of the illness. Subtle cognitive disorders, fluctuating symptoms, and progressing disease processes may be tracked effectively. The clinician should obtain a detailed rendition of changes in the patient's daily routine involving such factors as self-care, job responsibilities, and work habits; meal preparation; shopping and personal support; interactions with friends; hobbies and sports; reading interests; religious, social, and recreational activities; and ability to maintain personal finances. Understanding the past life of each patient provides an invaluable source of baseline data regarding changes in function, such as attention and concentration, intellectual abilities, personality, motor skills, and mood and perception. The examiner explores what the patient considers essential to their

Table 3-1
Neuropsychiatric Mental Status Examination

A. General Description
  1. General appearance, dress, sensory aids (glasses, hearing aid)
  2. Level of consciousness and arousal
  3. Attention to environment
  4. Posture (standing and seated)
  5. Gait
  6. Movements of limbs, trunk, and face (spontaneous, resting, and after instruction)
  7. General demeanor (including evidence of responses to internal stimuli)
  8. Response to examiner (eye contact, cooperation, ability to focus on interview process)
  9. Native or primary language
B. Language and Speech
  1. Comprehension (words, sentences, simple and complex commands, and concepts)
  2. Output (spontaneity, rate, fluency, melody or prosody, volume, coherence, vocabulary, paraphasic errors, complexity of usage)
  3. Repetition
  4. Other aspects
    a. Object naming
    b. Color naming
    c. Body part identification
    d. Ideomotor praxis to command
C. Thought
  1. Form (coherence and connectedness)
  2. Content
    a. Ideational (preoccupations, overvalued ideas, delusions)
    b. Perceptual (hallucinations)

D. Mood and Affect
  1. Internal mood state (spontaneous and elicited; sense of humor)
  2. Future outlook
  3. Suicidal ideas and plans
  4. Demonstrated emotional status (congruence with mood)
E. Insight and Judgment
  1. Insight
    a. Self-appraisal and self-esteem
    b. Understanding of current circumstances
    c. Ability to describe personal, psychological, and physical status
  2. Judgment
    a. Appraisal of major social relationships
    b. Understanding of personal roles and responsibilities
F. Cognition
  1. Memory
    a. Spontaneous (as evidenced during interview)
    b. Tested (incidental, immediate repetition, delayed recall, cued recall, recognition; verbal, nonverbal; explicit, implicit)
  2. Visuospatial skills
  3. Constructional ability
  4. Mathematics
  5. Reading
  6. Writing
  7. Fine sensory function (stereognosis, graphesthesia, two-point discrimination)
  8. Finger gnosis
  9. Right–left orientation
  10. "Executive functions"
  11. Abstraction

Courtesy of Eric D. Caine, M.D., and Jeffrey M. Lyness, M.D.

lifestyle and how the clinical condition affects these. This helps to assess both the disease and the success of future therapies.

Mental Status Examination

After taking a thorough history, the clinician's primary tool is the assessment of the patient's mental status. As with the physical examination, the mental status examination is a means of surveying functions and abilities to allow a definition of personal strengths and weaknesses. It is a repeatable, structured assessment of symptoms and signs that promotes effective communication among clinicians. It also establishes the basis for future comparison, essential for documenting therapeutic effectiveness, and it allows comparisons between different patients, with a generalization of findings from one patient to another. Table 3-1 lists the components of a comprehensive neuropsychiatric mental status examination.

Cognition

When testing cognitive functions, the clinician should evaluate memory; visuospatial and constructional abilities; and reading, writing, and mathematical abilities. The assessment of abstraction ability is also practical. However, many things can affect proverb interpretation, such as culture and education, and any interpretation should happen in that context.

PATHOLOGY AND LABORATORY EXAMINATION

As with all medical tests, we should interpret psychiatric evaluations in the context of thorough clinical and laboratory assessments.

Psychiatric and neuropsychiatric patients require a careful physical examination, particularly when issues exist that involve etiologically related or comorbid medical conditions. When consulting internists and other medical specialists, the clinician must ask specific questions to focus on the differential diagnostic process and use the consultation most effectively. In particular, most systemic medical or primary cerebral diseases that lead to psychopathological disturbances also manifest with a variety of peripheral or central abnormalities.

A screening laboratory evaluation is sought initially and may be followed by a variety of ancillary tests to increase the diagnostic specificity. Table 3-2 lists such procedures, some of which we also describe below.

Electroencephalography

Electroencephalography (EEG) is an easily accessible, noninvasive test of brain dysfunction that has a high sensitivity for many disorders but relatively low specificity. Beyond its recognized uses in epilepsy, EEG's highest utility is in detecting altered electrical rhythms associated with mild delirium, space-occupying lesions, and continuing complex partial seizures (in which the patient remains conscious, although behaviorally impaired). EEG is also sensitive to metabolic and toxic states, often showing a diffuse slowing of brain activity. We discuss the EEG in more detail in Chapter 1.

Computed Tomography and Magnetic Resonance Imaging

Computed tomography (CT) and magnetic resonance imaging (MRI) have proved to be powerful neuropsychiatric research tools.

Table 3-2
Screening Laboratory Tests

General Tests
Complete blood cell count
Erythrocyte sedimentation rate
Electrolytes
Glucose
Blood urea nitrogen and serum creatinine
Liver function tests
Serum calcium and phosphorus
Thyroid function tests
Serum protein
Levels of all drugs
Urinalysis
Pregnancy test for women of childbearing age
Electrocardiography

Ancillary Laboratory Tests
Blood
   Blood cultures
   Rapid plasma reagin test
   Human immunodeficiency virus (HIV) testing (enzyme-linked
      immunosorbent assay [ELISA] and Western blot)
   Serum heavy metals
   Serum copper
   Ceruloplasmin
   Serum B$_{12}$, red blood cell (RBC) folate levels
Urine
   Culture
   Toxicology
   Heavy metal screen
Electrography
   Electroencephalography
   Evoked potentials
   Polysomnography
   Nocturnal penile tumescence
Cerebrospinal fluid
   Glucose, protein
   Cell count
   Cultures (bacterial, viral, fungal)
   Cryptococcal antigen
   Venereal Disease Research Laboratory (VDRL) test
Radiography
   Computed tomography
   Magnetic resonance imaging
   Positron emission tomography
   Single photon emission computed tomography

Courtesy of Eric D. Caine, M.D., and Jeffrey M. Lyness, M.D.

Recent developments in MRI allow the direct measurement of structures such as the thalamus, basal ganglia, hippocampus, and amygdala, as well as temporal and apical areas of the brain and the structures of the posterior fossa. MRI has mostly replaced CT as the most utilitarian and cost-effective method of imaging in neuropsychiatry. CT is still the test of choice for patients with acute cerebral hemorrhages or hematomas, but these patients infrequently present in psychiatric settings. MRI better discriminates the interface between gray and white matter and is useful in detecting a variety of white matter lesions in the periventricular and subcortical regions. The pathophysiologic significance of such findings remains to be defined. White matter abnormalities occur in younger patients with multiple sclerosis or HIV infection and older patients with hypertension, vascular dementia, or dementia of the Alzheimer type. The prevalence of these abnormalities increases in healthy, aging individuals who have no defined disease process. In general, the highest utility of neuroimaging in the evaluation of patients with dementia arises from what it may exclude (tumors, vascular disease) rather than what it can demonstrate specifically.

Brain Biopsy

A brain needle biopsy can diagnose a variety of disorders: Alzheimer disease, autoimmune encephalopathy, and tumors. It is conducted stereotactically and indicated when no other investigative techniques such as MRI or lumbar puncture have been sufficient to make a diagnosis. The procedure is not without risk in that seizures may occur if scar tissue forms at the biopsy site.

Neuropsychologic Testing

Neuropsychologic testing provides a standardized, quantitative, reproducible evaluation of a patient's cognitive abilities. Such procedures may be useful for initial evaluation and periodic assessment. Tests are available that assess abilities across the broad array of cognitive domains, and many offer comparative normative groups or adjusted scores based on normative samples. The clinician seeking neuropsychologic consultation should understand enough about the strengths and weaknesses of selected procedures to benefit fully from the results obtained.

▲ 3.1 Delirium

Delirium is an acute decline in both the level of consciousness and cognition with particular impairment in attention. A life-threatening yet potentially reversible disorder of the central nervous system (CNS), delirium often involves perceptual disturbances, abnormal psychomotor activity, and sleep cycle impairment. Health care workers often underrecognize delirium. Part of the problem is that the syndrome has a variety of other names (Table 3-3).

The hallmark symptom of delirium is an impairment of consciousness, usually occurring in association with global impairments of cognitive functions. Abnormalities of mood, perception, and behavior are common psychiatric symptoms. Tremor, asterixis, nystagmus, incoordination, and urinary incontinence are common neurologic symptoms. Classically, delirium has a sudden onset (hours or days), a brief and fluctuating course, and rapid improvement when we can identify the cause and eliminate it, but each of these characteristic features can vary in individual patients. Physicians must recognize delirium to identify and treat the underlying cause and to avert the development of delirium-related complications such as accidental injury because of the patient's clouded consciousness.

Table 3-3
Delirium by Other Names

Intensive care unit psychosis
Acute confusional state
Acute brain failure
Encephalitis
Encephalopathy
Toxic metabolic state
Central nervous system toxicity
Paraneoplastic limbic encephalitis
Sundowning
Cerebral insufficiency
Organic brain syndrome

Table 3-4
Delirium

	DSM-5	ICD-10
Name	Delirium	Delirium, not induced by alcohol and other psychoactive substances Delirium, not superimposed on dementia Delirium, superimposed on dementia Other delirium Delirium, unspecified
Symptoms	Impaired attention/awareness Acute onset, change from baseline. May fluctuate throughout the day Symptoms develop acutely, represent a change from baseline, and may fluctuate Impairment of other cognitive functions • Memory • Language • Orientation • Perception Evidence for physiologic cause of the impairment (from history, examination, laboratory or other data)	Nonspecific organic cognitive syndrome with disturbed consciousness, awareness, memory, motor function, sleep, and emotion, with variable duration and severity; it can be acute or subacute
Required number of symptoms	All the above categories	
Exclusions (not result of):	A neurocognitive disorder Coma or other cause of reduced arousal	
Symptom specifiers	Hyperactive Hypoactive Mixed level of activity Based on cause: • Substance intoxication delirium, with or without use disorder (specify severity of use: mild/moderate/severe) • Substance withdrawal delirium, with or without use disorder (specify severity of use: mild/moderate/severe) • Medication-induced delirium • Delirium due to another medical condition • Delirium due to multiple etiologies	
Course Specifiers	**Acute:** hours to days **Persistent:** weeks to months	
Comments		If due to substance use, use "mental and behavioral disorders due to psychoactive substances"

DIAGNOSIS AND CLINICAL FEATURES

Table 3-4 compares the diagnostic approaches to delirium. Usually, the cause is one or more systemic or cerebral derangements that affect brain function.

A 70-year-old woman, Mrs. K, was brought to the emergency department by the police. The police had responded to complaints from neighbors that Mrs. K was wandering the neighborhood and was not taking care of herself. When the police found Mrs. K in her apartment, she was dirty, foul-smelling, and wearing nothing but a bra. Her apartment was also filthy with garbage and rotting food everywhere.

When interviewed, Mrs. K would not look at the interviewer and was confused and unresponsive to most of the questions asked. She knew her name and address but not the date. She was unable to describe the events that led to her admission.

The next day, the supervising psychiatrist attempted to interview Mrs. K. Her facial expression was still unresponsive, and she still did not know the month or the name of the hospital. She explained that the neighbors called the police because she was "sick" and that she did indeed feel sick and weak, with pains in her shoulder. She also

reported not eating for three days. She denied ever being in a psychiatric hospital or hearing voices but acknowledged seeing a psychiatrist at one point because she had trouble sleeping. She said the doctor had prescribed medication, but she could not remember the name.

Table 3-5 lists the core features of delirium.

Associated clinical features are often present and may be prominent. The EEG usually shows diffuse slowing of background activity, although patients with delirium caused by alcohol or sedative-hypnotic withdrawal have low-voltage fast activity.

The primary neurotransmitter hypothesized to be involved in delirium is acetylcholine, and the major neuroanatomical area is the reticular formation. The reticular formation of the brainstem is the principal area regulating attention and arousal; the major pathway implicated in delirium is the dorsal tegmental pathway, which projects from the mesencephalic reticular formation to the tectum and thalamus. Several studies have reported that a variety of delirium-inducing factors result in decreased acetylcholine activity in the brain. One of the most common causes of delirium is toxicity from too many prescribed medications with anticholinergic activity. Researchers

Table 3-5
Core Features of Delirium

- Altered consciousness (usually decreased level)
- Altered attention (diminished ability to focus, sustain, or shift attention)
- Other cognitive dysfunctions:
  - Disorientation (especially to time and space)
  - Impaired memory
- Typical course:
  - Relatively rapid onset (usually hours to days)
  - Brief duration (usually days to weeks)
  - Marked, unpredictable fluctuations in severity
  - Sometimes worse at night (sundowning), ranging from periods of lucidity to severe cognitive impairment and disorganization

have suggested other pathophysiologic mechanisms for delirium. In particular, the delirium associated with alcohol withdrawal correlates with hyperactivity of the locus ceruleus and its noradrenergic neurons. Serotonin and glutamate are also likely involved.

PHYSICAL AND LABORATORY EXAMINATIONS

Delirium is usually diagnosed at the bedside and presents as a sudden onset of symptoms. A bedside mental status examination—such as the Mini-Mental State Examination—can be used to document the cognitive impairment and to provide a baseline from which to measure the patient's clinical course. The physical examination often reveals clues to the cause of the delirium (Table 3-6). The presence of a known physical illness or a history of head trauma or alcohol or other substance use disorder increases the likelihood of the diagnosis.

The laboratory workup of a patient with delirium should include standard tests and additional studies indicated by the clinical situation (Table 3-7). In delirium, the EEG characteristically shows a generalized slowing of activity and may be useful in differentiating delirium from depression or psychosis. The EEG of a delirious patient sometimes shows focal areas of hyperactivity. In rare cases, it may be challenging to differentiate delirium related to epilepsy from delirium related to other causes.

DIFFERENTIAL DIAGNOSIS

Delirium versus Dementia

Several clinical features help distinguish delirium from dementia (Table 3-8). The major differential points between dementia and delirium are the time to development of the condition and the fluctuation in the level of attention in delirium compared with relatively consistent attention in dementia. The time to development of symptoms is usually short in delirium, and except for vascular dementia caused by stroke, it is usually gradual and insidious in dementia. Although both conditions include cognitive impairment, the changes in dementia are more stable over time and, for example, usually do not fluctuate over a day. A patient with dementia is usually alert; a patient with delirium has episodes of decreased consciousness. Occasionally, delirium occurs in a patient with dementia, a condition known as *beclouded dementia*. A dual diagnosis of delirium exists when there is a definite history of preexisting dementia.

Delirium versus Schizophrenia or Depression

We should differentiate delirium from schizophrenia and depressive disorder. Some patients with psychotic disorders, usually schizophrenia or manic episodes, can have periods of extremely disorganized behavior challenging to distinguish from delirium. In general, however, the hallucinations and delusions of patients with schizophrenia are more constant and better organized than those of patients with delirium. Patients with schizophrenia usually experience no change in their level of consciousness or their orientation. Patients with hypoactive symptoms of delirium may appear somewhat similar to severely depressed patients, but their confusion can help differentiate, as can an EEG. Other psychiatric diagnoses to consider in the differential diagnosis of delirium are brief psychotic disorder, schizophreniform disorder, and dissociative disorders. Patients with factitious disorders may attempt to simulate the symptoms of delirium but usually reveal the factitious nature of their symptoms by inconsistencies on their mental status examinations, and an EEG can easily separate the two diagnoses.

COURSE AND PROGNOSIS

Although the onset of delirium is usually sudden, prodromal symptoms (e.g., restlessness and fearfulness) can occur in the days preceding the onset of florid symptoms. The symptoms of delirium usually persist as long as the causally relevant factors are present, although delirium generally lasts less than 1 week. After identification and removal of the causative factors, the symptoms of delirium usually recede over a 3- to 7-day period, although some symptoms may take up to 2 weeks to resolve completely. The older the patient and the longer the patient has been delirious, the longer the delirium takes to resolve. Recall of what transpired during a delirium, once it is over, is characteristically spotty; a patient may refer to the episode as a bad dream or a nightmare only vaguely remembered. As stated in the discussion on epidemiology, the occurrence of delirium is associated with a high mortality rate in the ensuing year, primarily because of the severe nature of the associated medical conditions that lead to delirium.

Whether delirium progresses to dementia has not been demonstrated in carefully controlled studies, although many clinicians believe that they have seen such a progression. A clinical observation that has been validated by some studies, however, is that depression or posttraumatic stress may follow a delirium.

TREATMENT

In treating delirium, the primary goal is to treat the underlying cause. When the underlying condition is anticholinergic toxicity, physostigmine salicylate, 1 to 2 mg intravenously or intramuscularly, may help. We may have to repeat the dose every 15 to 30 minutes. The other important goal of treatment is to provide physical, sensory, and environmental support. Physical support is necessary so that delirious patients do not get into situations in which they may have accidents. Patients with delirium should be neither sensory deprived nor overly stimulated by the environment. A familiar person staying in the room, such as a friend or relative, may help. Familiar pictures and decorations; the presence of a clock or a calendar; and regular orientations to person, place, and time help make patients with delirium comfortable. Delirium can sometimes occur in older patients wearing eye patches after cataract surgery ("black-patch delirium"). Such patients can be helped by placing pinholes in the patches to let in some stimuli or by occasionally removing one patch at a time during recovery.

Pharmacotherapy

The three significant delirium symptoms that may require pharmacologic treatment are psychosis, agitation, and insomnia. A commonly

Table 3-6
Physical Examination of the Delirious Patient

Parameter	Finding	Clinical Implication
1. Pulse	Bradycardia	Hypothyroidism
		Stokes–Adams syndrome
		Increased intracranial pressure
	Tachycardia	Hyperthyroidism
		Infection
		Heart failure
2. Temperature	Fever	Sepsis
		Thyroid storm
		Vasculitis
3. Blood pressure	Hypotension	Shock
		Hypothyroidism
		Addison disease
	Hypertension	Encephalopathy
		Intracranial mass
4. Respiration	Tachypnea	Diabetes
		Pneumonia
		Cardiac failure
		Fever
		Acidosis (metabolic)
	Shallow	Alcohol or other substance intoxication
5. Carotid vessels	Bruits or decreased pulse	Transient cerebral ischemia
6. Scalp and face	Evidence of trauma	
7. Neck	Evidence of nuchal rigidity	Meningitis
		Subarachnoid hemorrhage
8. Eyes	Papilledema	Tumor
		Hypertensive encephalopathy
	Pupillary dilatation	Anxiety
		Autonomic overactivity (e.g., delirium tremens)
9. Mouth	Tongue or cheek lacerations	Evidence of generalized tonic–clonic seizures
10. Thyroid	Enlarged	Thyroid dysfunction
11. Heart	Arrhythmia	Inadequate cardiac output, possibility of emboli
	Cardiomegaly	Heart failure
		Hypertensive disease
12. Lungs	Congestion	Primary pulmonary failure
		Pulmonary edema
		Pneumonia
13. Breath	Alcohol	
	Ketones	Diabetes
14. Liver	Enlargement	Cirrhosis
		Liver failure
15. Nervous system		
a. Reflexes—muscle stretch	Asymmetry with Babinski signs	Mass lesion
		Cerebrovascular disease
		Preexisting dementia
	Snout	Frontal mass
		Bilateral posterior cerebral artery occlusion
b. Abducent nerve (sixth cranial nerve)	Weakness in lateral gaze	Increased intracranial pressure
c. Limb strength	Asymmetrical	Mass lesion
		Cerebrovascular disease
d. Autonomic	Hyperactivity	Anxiety
		Delirium

From Strub RL, Black FW. *Neurobehavioral Disorders: A Clinical Approach*. Philadelphia: FA Davis; 1981:121, with permission.

used drug for psychosis is haloperidol. Depending on a patient's age, weight, and physical condition, the initial dose may range from 2 to 5 mg intramuscularly, repeated in an hour if the patient remains agitated. As soon as the patient is calm, oral medication in liquid concentrate or tablet form should begin. Two daily oral doses should suffice, mostly at bedtime. The oral equivalent is about 1.5 times the parenteral dose. The effective total daily dose of haloperidol may range from 5 to 40 mg for most patients with delirium. Haloperidol may cause a prolonged QT interval. Clinicians should evaluate baseline and periodic electrocardiograms as well as monitor the cardiac status of the patient. Droperidol is a butyrophenone available as an alternative intravenous (IV) formulation, although careful monitoring of the electrocardiogram may be prudent with this treatment. The U.S. Food and Drug Administration (FDA) issued a Black Box

Table 3-7
Laboratory Workup of the Patient with Delirium

Standard studies
    Blood chemistries (including electrolytes, renal and hepatic
        indexes, and glucose)
    Complete blood count with white cell differential
    Thyroid function tests
    Serologic tests for syphilis
    Human immunodeficiency virus (HIV) antibody test
    Urinalysis
    Electrocardiogram
    Electroencephalogram
    Chest radiograph
    Blood and urine drug screens
Additional tests when indicated
    Blood, urine, and cerebrospinal fluid cultures
    B$_{12}$, folic acid concentrations
    Computed tomography or magnetic resonance imaging brain scan
    Lumbar puncture and CSF examination

Warning because of cases of patients with QT prolongation and torsades de pointes receiving droperidol. Because of its potential for serious proarrhythmic effects and death, it should be used only in patients who do not respond well to other treatments. Phenothiazines should be avoided in delirious patients because these drugs are associated with significant anticholinergic activity.

Agitation is a poorly defined symptom that can range from distressed anxiety to physical aggression. Because of the ambiguity of the term, agitation is challenging to study. However, some scales are available to aid research, such as the Richmond Agitation-Sedation Scale. Many medications have anecdotal support. However, studies on the pharmacologic treatment of agitation in delirium are disappointing. The antipsychotics are most commonly used. The approach is analogous to the above approach for psychosis in delirium, with adjustments for the severity and prolongation of the delirium. Sodium valproate given IV may be useful when antipsychotics fail. For severe agitation, dexmedetomidine, an α$_2$-adrenoreceptor agonist that is used as a sedative, can help sedate a patient, mainly a mechanically ventilated patient, without the deliriogenic effects of many other sedatives.

Second-generation antipsychotics, such as risperidone, clozapine, olanzapine, quetiapine, ziprasidone, and aripiprazole, may be considered for delirium management, but clinical trial experience with these agents for delirium is limited. Ziprasidone appears to have an activating effect and may not be appropriate in delirium management. Olanzapine is available for intramuscular (IM) use and as a rapidly disintegrating oral preparation. These routes of administration may be preferable for some patients with delirium who are poorly compliant with medications or who are too sedated to swallow medications safely.

Insomnia is difficult to treat. Benzodiazepines might be helpful; however, they risk worsening a patient's confusion. Also, there is no conclusive evidence to support the use of benzodiazepines in non–alcohol-related delirium. If pain is the cause, a physician should not hesitate to prescribe opioids for both their analgesic and sedative effects (Table 3-9). Melatonin is occasionally used but with mixed support and low-quality studies.

Treatment in Special Populations

Parkinson Disease.   In Parkinson disease, antiparkinsonian agents can cause delirium. If coexistent dementia is present, delirium is twice as likely to develop in patients with Parkinson

Table 3-8
Frequency of Clinical Features of Delirium Contrasted with Dementia

Symptom	Delirium	Dementia
Mental Status Examination		
Memory	Impaired, more short-term than long-term	Impaired, more long-term than short-term
Attention	Poor	Impaired although usually to a lesser degree
Orientation	Grossly disorganized	Varies
Sensorium	Prominent hallucinations (esp. visual or tactile)	Rare hallucinations
Thought content	May be paranoid	May be paranoid
Judgment, social skills and behavior	Grossly impaired	Initially relatively intact, worsens with time (depending on areas affected with frontal cortical damage causing more impairment)
Physical Examination		
Vital signs	Often abnormal	Dependent on cause
Neurologic examination	May be abnormal	Dependent on cause
Comorbid medical illnesses	Acute illnesses	Dependent on cause
Course		
Onset	Acute	Usually insidious
Short-term course	Fluctuates throughout day	Varies, but generally more stable
Long-term course	May improve (depending on underlying cause)	Usually chronic and progressive. May be gradual or stepwise depending on cause
Associated Features		
Comorbid medical illnesses	Acute illnesses	Dependent on cause
Most likely associated illnesses	Metabolic, toxic, or infectious illnesses	Neurodegenerative or vascular disorders

disease with dementia receiving antiparkinsonian agents than in those without dementia. Decreasing the dosage of the antiparkinsonian agent has to be weighed against a worsening of motor symptoms. If we cannot reduce the antiparkinsonian agents, or if the delirium persists after we do, an antipsychotic may help. However, this risks worsening the disorder. The FDA has approved pimavanserin for psychosis in Parkinson's. It appears to be an inverse agonist and antagonist activity of serotonin 5-HT$_{2A}$ and possibly 5-HT$_{2C}$, with no appreciable affinity for dopamine. Clozapine may also help and has empirical support. Quetiapine has not been as rigorously studied as clozapine and may have parkinsonian side effects, but it is used in clinical practice to treat psychosis in Parkinson disease.

Terminally Ill Patients.   When delirium occurs in the context of a terminal illness, issues about advanced directives and the

Table 3-9
Pharmacologic Treatment of Delirium

Pharmacologic Agent	Dosage	Side Effects	Comments
Typical Antipsychotics			
Haloperidol	0.5–1 mg p.o. twice a day (may be given every 4–6 hr as needed, too)	Extrapyramidal side (EPS) effects Prolonged QTc	Most commonly used Can be given intramuscularly
Atypical Antipsychotics		All can prolong QTc duration	
Risperidone	0.5–1 mg a day	EPS concerns	Limited data in delirium
Olanzapine	5–10 mg a day	Metabolic syndrome	Higher mortality in dementia patients
Quetiapine	25–150 mg a day	More sedating	
Benzodiazepine			
Lorazepam	0.5–3 mg a day and as needed every 4 hr	Respiratory depression, paradoxical agitation	Best use in delirium secondary to alcohol or benzodiazepine withdrawal Can worsen other types of delirium

existence of a health care proxy become more significant. This scenario emphasizes the importance of early development of advance directives for health care decision making while a person can communicate the wishes regarding the extent of aggressive diagnostic tests at life's end. The focus may change from an aggressive search for the etiology of the delirium to one of palliation, comfort, and assistance with dying.

EPIDEMIOLOGY

Delirium is a common disorder, with most incidence and prevalence rates reported in elderly adults. In community studies, 1 percent of elderly persons age 55 years or older have delirium (13 percent in the age 85 years and older group in the community). Among elderly emergency department patients, 5 to 10 percent have delirium. At the time of admission to medical wards, between 15 and 21 percent of older patients meet the criteria for delirium-prevalent cases. Of patients free of delirium at the time of hospital admission, 5 to 30 percent reported subsequent incidences of delirium during hospitalization. Delirium occurs in 10 to 15 percent of general surgical patients, 30 percent of open-heart surgery patients, and more than 50 percent of patients treated for hip fractures. Delirium occurs in 70 to 87 percent of intensive care unit patients and up to 83 percent of all patients receiving end of life care. Sixty percent of patients

in nursing homes or post-acute care settings have delirium. An estimated 21 percent of patients with severe burns and 30 to 40 percent of patients with acquired immune deficiency syndrome (AIDS) have episodes of delirium during hospitalization. Delirium develops in 80 percent of terminally ill patients. The causes of postoperative delirium include the stress of surgery, postoperative pain, insomnia, pain medication, electrolyte imbalances, infection, fever, and blood loss. Table 3-10 shows the incidence and prevalence rates for delirium across settings.

The risk for delirium could be conceptualized into two categories, predisposing and precipitating factors (Tables 3-11 and 3-12). Current approaches to delirium focus primarily on the precipitation factors and

Table 3-10
Delirium Incidence and Prevalence in Multiple Settings

Population	Prevalence Range (%)	Incidence Range (%)
General medical inpatients	10–30	3–16
Medical and surgical inpatients	5–15	10–55
General surgical inpatients	N/A	9–15 postoperatively
Critical care unit patients	16	16–83
Cardiac surgery inpatients	16–34	7–34
Orthopedic surgery patients	33	18–50
Emergency department	7–10	N/A
Terminally ill cancer patients	23–28	83
Institutionalized elderly	44	33

N/A, not available.

Table 3-11
Predisposing Factors for Delirium

Demographic characteristics
　Age 65 years and older
　Male sex
Cognitive status
　Dementia
　Cognitive impairment
　History of delirium
　Depression
Functional status
　Functional dependence
　Immobility
　History of falls
　Low level of activity
Sensory impairment
　Hearing
　Visual
Decreased oral intake
　Dehydration
　Malnutrition
Drugs
　Treatment with psychoactive drugs
　Treatment with drugs with anticholinergic properties
　Alcohol abuse
Coexisting medical conditions
　Severe medical diseases
　Chronic renal or hepatic disease
　Stroke
　Neurologic disease
　Metabolic derangements
　Infection with human immunodeficiency virus
　Fractures or trauma
　Terminal diseases

Adapted from Inouye SK. Delirium in older persons. *N Engl J Med.* 2016; 354(11):1157.

Table 3-12
Precipitating Factors for Delirium

Drugs
  Sedative–hypnotics
  Narcotics
  Anticholinergic drugs
  Treatment with multiple drugs
  Alcohol or drug withdrawal
Primary neurologic diseases
  Stroke, nondominant hemispheric
  Intracranial bleeding
  Meningitis or encephalitis
Intercurrent illnesses
  Infections
  Iatrogenic complications
  Severe acute illness
  Hypoxia
  Shock
  Anemia
  Fever or hypothermia
  Dehydration
  Poor nutritional status
  Low serum albumin levels
  Metabolic derangements
Surgery
  Orthopedic surgery
  Cardiac surgery
  Prolonged cardiopulmonary bypass
  Noncardiac surgery
Environmental
  Admission to intensive care unit
  Use of physical restraints
  Use of bladder catheter
  Use of multiple procedures
  Pain
  Emotional stress
  Prolonged sleep deprivation

Adapted from Inouye SK. Delirium in older persons. *N Engl J Med.* 2016; 354(11):1157.

do little to address the predisposing factors. Managing predisposing factors for delirium becomes essential in decreasing future episodes of delirium and the morbidity and mortality associated with it.

Advanced age is a significant risk factor for the development of delirium. Approximately 30 to 40 percent of hospitalized patients older than age 65 years have an episode of delirium, and another 10 to 15 percent of elderly persons exhibit delirium on admission to the hospital. Of nursing home residents older than age 75 years, 60 percent have repeated episodes of delirium. Male gender is also an independent risk factor for delirium.

Delirium is a poor prognostic sign. Rates of institutionalization are increased threefold for patients 65 years and older who exhibit delirium while in the hospital. The 3-month mortality rate of patients who have an episode of delirium is estimated to be 23 to 33 percent. The 1-year mortality rate for patients who have an episode of delirium may be as high as 50 percent. Elderly patients who experience delirium while hospitalized have a 21 to 75 percent mortality rate during that hospitalization. After discharge, up to 15 percent of these persons die within 1 month, and 25 percent die within 6 months.

ETIOLOGY

The significant causes of delirium are CNS disease (e.g., epilepsy), systemic disease (e.g., sepsis, cardiac failure), and either intoxication or withdrawal from pharmacologic or toxic agents (Table 3-13). When evaluating patients with delirium, clinicians should assume that any drug that a patient has taken could be a cause for delirium.

Table 3-13
Common Causes of Delirium

Central nervous system disorder	Seizure (postictal, nonconvulsive status, status)
	Migraine
	Head trauma, brain tumor, subarachnoid hemorrhage, subdural, epidural hematoma, abscess, intracerebral hemorrhage, cerebellar hemorrhage, nonhemorrhagic stroke, transient ischemia
Metabolic disorder	Electrolyte abnormalities
	Diabetes, hypoglycemia, hyperglycemia, or insulin resistance
Systemic illness	Infection (e.g., sepsis, malaria, erysipelas, viral, plague, Lyme disease, syphilis, or abscess)
	Trauma
	Change in fluid status (dehydration or volume overload)
	Nutritional deficiency
	Burns
	Uncontrolled pain
	Heat stroke
	High altitude (usually >5,000 m)
Medications	Pain medications (e.g., postoperative meperidine or morphine)
	Antibiotics, antivirals, and antifungals
	Steroids
	Anesthesia
	Cardiac medications
	Antihypertensives
	Antineoplastic agents
	Anticholinergic agents
	Neuroleptic malignant syndrome
Serotonin syndrome	
Over-the-counter preparations	Herbals, teas, and nutritional supplements
Botanicals	Jimsonweed, oleander, foxglove, hemlock, dieffenbachia, and *Amanita phalloides*
Cardiac	Cardiac failure, arrhythmia, myocardial infarction, cardiac assist device, cardiac surgery
Pulmonary	Chronic obstructive pulmonary disease, hypoxia, SIADH, acid–base disturbance
Endocrine	Adrenal crisis or adrenal failure, thyroid abnormality, parathyroid abnormality
Hematologic	Anemia, leukemia, blood dyscrasia, stem cell transplant
Renal	Renal failure, uremia, SIADH
Hepatic	Hepatitis, cirrhosis, hepatic failure
Neoplasm	Neoplasm (primary brain, metastases, paraneoplastic syndrome)
Drugs of abuse	Intoxication and withdrawal
Toxins	Intoxication and withdrawal
	Heavy metals and aluminum

SIADH, syndrome of inappropriate secretion of antidiuretic hormone.

▲ 3.2 Dementia (Major Neurocognitive Disorder)

Dementia refers to a disease process marked by progressive cognitive impairment in clear consciousness. Dementia does not refer to low intellectual functioning or mental retardation because these are developmental and static conditions, and the cognitive deficits in dementia represent a decline from a previous level of functioning. Dementia involves multiple cognitive domains, and cognitive deficits cause significant impairment in social and occupational functioning. There are several types of dementias based on etiology: Alzheimer disease, dementia of Lewy bodies, vascular dementia, frontotemporal dementia, traumatic brain injury (TBI), HIV, prion disease, Parkinson disease, and Huntington disease. Other medical and neurologic conditions can cause dementia, as can various substances.

The critical clinical points of dementia are the identification of the syndrome and the clinical workup of its cause. The disorder can be progressive or static, permanent, or reversible. We always assume an underlying cause, although, in rare cases, it is impossible to determine a specific cause. The potential reversibility of dementia is related to the underlying pathologic condition and the availability and application of effective treatment. Approximately 15 percent of people with dementia have reversible illnesses if we can initiate treatment before irreversible damage takes place.

DIAGNOSIS AND CLINICAL FEATURES

Table 3-14 compares the approaches to the general diagnosis of dementia. DSM-5 makes a distinction between major and minor cognitive disorders based upon levels of functioning, but the underlying etiology is similar.

DSM-5 specifics a variety of types of dementia based on their cause. Tables 3-15 to 3-24 compare the diagnostic approaches to the major etiologies.

We make a diagnosis of dementia from the clinical examination, including a mental status examination, and on information from the patient's family, friends, and employers. Complaints of a personality change in a patient older than age 40 years suggest that we should consider a diagnosis of dementia.

Clinicians should note patients' complaints about intellectual impairment and forgetfulness as well as evidence of patients' evasion, denial, or rationalization aimed at concealing cognitive deficits. Excessive orderliness, social withdrawal, or a tendency to relate events in minute detail can be characteristic, and sudden outbursts of anger or sarcasm can occur. We should observe the patient's appearance and behavior. Lability of emotions, sloppy grooming, uninhibited remarks, silly jokes, or a dull, apathetic, or vacuous facial expression and manner suggest the presence of dementia, especially when coupled with memory impairment.

Memory impairment is typically an early and prominent feature in dementia, especially in dementias involving the cortex, such as dementia of the Alzheimer type. Early in the course of dementia, memory impairment is mild and usually most marked for recent events; people forget telephone numbers, conversations, and events of the day. As the course of dementia progresses, memory impairment becomes severe, and the patient can only retain the earliest learned information (e.g., a person's place of birth).

Since memory is vital for orientation to person, place, and time, orientation can be progressively affected during a dementing illness. For example, patients with dementia may forget how to get back to their rooms after going to the bathroom. No matter how

Table 3-14
Approaches to the General Diagnosis of Dementia

	DSM-5	ICD-10
	Major and Mild Neurocognitive Disorders	**Dementias**
Symptoms	Significant (**Major**) or moderate (**Minor**) decline in cognitive functioning: • Attention • Executive function • Learning/Memory • Language • Perceptual–motor • Social cognition (For each of the specific diagnoses, one should specify whether major or minor in the diagnosis [i.e., minor neurocognitive disorder with Lewy bodies])	Defined by the specific cause of Dementia
Required number of symptoms	≥1; see above criteria	
Exclusions (not result of):	• Delirium • Another mental disorder	
Psychosocial Impact	Some impairments in ability to independently perform activities of daily living	
Symptom Specifiers	See specifiers for the specific disorders With or without behavioral disturbance	See specifiers for the specific disorders
Severity Specifiers	Based on what is impaired and level of impairment and this refers to the current level: **Mild:** instrumental activities of daily life (e.g., cooking, paying bills) impaired **Moderate:** basic activities of daily life impaired (e.g., eating, dressing) **Severe:** impaired in all activities, fully dependent on others	

Table 3-15
Neurocognitive Disorder due to Alzheimer Disease

DSM-5		ICD-10
Neurocognitive Disorder due to Alzheimer Disease		**Dementia in Alzheimer Disease**
Mild **Symptoms** • ↓ memory/learning • Progressive decline, no significant periods of stability • No evidence of mixed causes **Probable:** evidence of a genetic cause (family history/genetic testing) **Possible:** Above not met, all three symptoms present	**Major** **Symptoms** • ↓ memory/learning + ≥1 other cognitive domain • Progressive decline, no significant periods of stability • No evidence of mixed causes **Probable:** evidence of a genetic cause (family history/genetic testing) OR all three symptoms **Possible:** Some but not all the probable criteria met	**Dementia in Alzheimer disease with early onset** **Dementia in Alzheimer disease with late onset** **Dementia in Alzheimer disease, atypical or mixed type** **Dementia in Alzheimer disease, unspecified** **Early onset:** begins < age 65, rapid progression of functioning, involves higher levels of cognition **Late onset:** begins ≥ age 65, with slower progression, preferentially affects memory Symptoms presenting with insidious onset, progressive decline over years, and include characteristic neuropathology and neurochemical features

Table 3-16
Frontotemporal Neurocognitive Disorder

DSM-5		ICD-10
Frontotemporal Neurocognitive Disorder		**Dementia in Picks Disease** **Circumscribed Brain Atrophy**
Behavioral Variant **Affected:** social cognition/executive function **Spared:** learning/memory/perceptual–motor function **Associated Symptoms (≥3):** • Disinhibition • Apathy • ↓ sympathy/empathy • Perseveration/stereotypies • Hyperorality/dietary changes **Probable:** • evidence of a genetic cause (family history/ genetic testing) • Neuroimaging evidence of frontal/temporal pathology **Possible:** • Some but not all the probable criteria met	**Language Variant** **Affected:** language (word finding, naming, grammar, less spontaneous speech) **Spared:** learning/memory/perceptual–motor function **Probable:** • evidence of a genetic cause (family history/genetic testing) • Neuroimaging evidence of frontal/ temporal pathology **Possible:** Some but not all the probable criteria met	Progressive dementia Onset middle age **Affected:** personality/social skills **Later:** memory/mood/neurologic function

Table 3-17
Neurocognitive Disorder with Lewy Bodies

DSM-5	ICD-10
Neurocognitive Disorder with Lewy Bodies	**Dementia in Other Specified Diseases Classified Elsewhere**

Core:
• Fluctuating:
  • cognition
  • attention
  • alertness
• Recurrent well-formed visual hallucinations
• Parkinsonian symptoms (after cognitive decline)
Suggestive:
• REM sleep behavior disorder
• Severe neuroleptic sensitivity
Probable: ≥2 core features or 1 core/1 suggestive
Possible: 1 core feature
	Disorder is listed but not defined.

Table 3-18
Vascular Neurocognitive Disorder

DSM-5	ICD-10
Vascular Neurocognitive Disorder	**Vascular Dementia**
History + imaging/physical findings of cerebrovascular (CV) disease **Cognitive decline typical of vascular pathology (≥1):** • Cognitive decline after CV event • Cognitive areas mainly complex attention/frontal-executive function **Probable (≥1):** • Neuroimaging evidence of CV disease in brain • Neurocognitive symptoms are associated with the CV events • Clinical/genetic evidence of CV disease **Possible:** • No neuroimaging • No documented temporal relationship between CV events and cognitive changes	**Vascular dementia of acute onset: cognitive symptoms** develop after stroke(s) **Multi-infarct dementia:** progressive symptoms after repeated transient ischemic attacks **Subcortical Vascular dementia:** H/O hypertension, mainly white matter injury **Mixed cortical and subcortical vascular dementia** **Other vascular dementia** **Vascular dementia, unspecified**

Table 3-19
Neurocognitive Disorder due to Traumatic Brain Injury

DSM-5	ICD-10
Neurocognitive Disorder due to Traumatic Brain Injury	**Dementia in Other Specified Diseases Classified Elsewhere**
H/O traumatic brain injury, with associated noncognitive symptoms **Neurocognitive symptoms (≥1):** • Loss of consciousness • Amnesia following trauma • Confusion/disorientation • Neuroimaging evidence of injury/ Neurologic symptoms	Disorder is listed but not defined.

Table 3-20
Neurocognitive Disorder due to HIV Infection

DSM-5	ICD-10
Neurocognitive Disorder due to HIV Infection	**Dementia in Human Immunodeficiency Virus (HIV)**
HIV diagnosis Associated cognitive symptoms	HIV diagnosis Associated cognitive symptoms

Table 3-21
Neurocognitive Disorder due to Prion Disease

DSM-5	ICD-10
Neurocognitive Disorder due to Prion Disease	**Dementia in Creutzfeldt-Jakob Disease**
Cognitive impairment: Subtle onset Rapid progression **Additional features:** Motor symptoms, such as myoclonus/ataxia Biochemical marker on testing	Significant neurologic symptoms Subacute course Progressive rapid decline

Table 3-22
Neurocognitive Disorder due to Parkinson Disease

DSM-5	ICD-10
Neurocognitive Disorder due to Parkinson Disease	**Dementia in Parkinson Disease**
Occurring in the context of Parkinson disease Subtle onset Gradual progression **Probable** (both of the following:) **Possible** (one of the following:) • No evidence of mixed etiology • Parkinson disease precedes cognitive symptoms	Occurring in the context of Parkinson's disease

Table 3-23
Neurocognitive Disorder due to Huntington Disease

DSM-5	ICD-10
Neurocognitive Disorder due to Huntington Disease	**Huntington Disease**
Occurring in the context of Huntington disease Subtle onset Gradual progression	Occurring in the context of Huntington disease Caused by autosomal dominant gene Slow progression Motor symptom (chorea)

severe the disorientation seems, however, patients show no impairment in their level of consciousness.

Dementing processes that affect the cortex, primarily dementia of the Alzheimer type and vascular dementia, can affect patients' language abilities.

Psychiatric and Neurologic Changes

Personality. Changes in the personality of a person with dementia are especially disturbing for their families. Preexisting personality traits may accentuate during the development of dementia. Patients with dementia may also become introverted and seem to be less concerned than they previously were about the effects of their behavior on others. Persons with dementia who have paranoid delusions are generally hostile to family members and caretakers. Patients with frontal and temporal involvement are likely to have marked personality changes and may be irritable and explosive.

Hallucinations and Delusions. An estimated 20 to 30 percent of patients with dementia (primarily patients with dementia of the Alzheimer type) have hallucinations, and 30 to 40 percent have delusions, primarily of a paranoid or persecutory and unsystematized nature, although complex and sustained. Some patients also report well-systematized delusions. Physical aggression and other forms of violence are common in demented patients who also have psychotic symptoms.

Mood. In addition to psychosis and personality changes, depression and anxiety are significant symptoms in an estimated 40 to 50 percent of patients with dementia, although the full syndrome of depressive disorder may be present in only 10 to 20 percent. Patients with dementia also may exhibit pathologic laughter or crying—that is, extremes of emotions—with no apparent provocation.

Cognitive Change. In addition to the aphasias in patients with dementia, apraxias and agnosias are common. Other neurologic signs that can be associated with dementia are seizures, seen in approximately 10 percent of patients with dementia of the

Table 3-24
Additional Diagnosis Types of Dementia in DSM-5

Neurocognitive disorder due to another medical condition:
In the context of some other disorder not listed among the neurocognitive disorders
Neurocognitive disorder due to multiple etiologies
Substance/medication-induced neurocognitive disorder
Unspecified neurocognitive disorder

Alzheimer type and 20 percent of patients with vascular dementia, and atypical neurologic presentations, such as nondominant parietal lobe syndromes. Primitive reflexes, such as the grasp, snout, suck, tonic-foot, and palmomental reflexes, may be present on neurologic examination, and myoclonic jerks are present in 5 to 10 percent of patients.

Patients with vascular dementia may have additional neurologic symptoms, such as headaches, dizziness, faintness, weakness, focal neurologic signs, and sleep disturbances, possibly attributable to the location of the cerebrovascular disease. Pseudobulbar palsy, dysarthria, and dysphagia are also more common in vascular dementia than in other dementing conditions.

Abstractions and the Catastrophic Reaction. Patients with dementia also exhibit a reduced ability to apply what Kurt Goldstein called the "abstract attitude." Patients have difficulty generalizing from a single instance, forming concepts, and grasping similarities and differences among concepts. Furthermore, the ability to solve problems, to reason logically, and to make sound judgments is compromised. Goldstein also described a catastrophic reaction marked by agitation secondary to the subjective awareness of intellectual deficits under stressful circumstances. Persons usually attempt to compensate for defects by using strategies to avoid demonstrating failures in intellectual performance; they may change the subject, make jokes, or otherwise divert the interviewer. Lack of judgment and poor impulse control appear commonly, particularly in dementias that primarily affect the frontal lobes. Examples of these impairments include coarse language, inappropriate jokes, neglect of personal appearance and hygiene, and a general disregard for the conventional rules of social conduct.

Sundowner Syndrome. Sundowner syndrome is characterized by drowsiness, confusion, ataxia, and accidental falls. It occurs in older people who are overly sedated and in patients with dementia who react adversely to even a small dose of a psychoactive drug. The syndrome also occurs in demented patients when external stimuli, such as light and interpersonal orienting cues, are diminished.

Vascular Dementia

The general symptoms of vascular dementia are the same as those for dementia of the Alzheimer type, but the diagnosis of vascular dementia requires either clinical or laboratory evidence in support of a vascular cause of dementia. Vascular dementia is more likely to show a decremental, stepwise deterioration than is Alzheimer disease.

Substance-Induced Persisting Dementia

DSM lists substance-induced persisting dementia in two places, with the dementias, and with the substance-related disorders. The specific substances it cross-references are alcohol, inhalants, sedatives, hypnotics, or anxiolytics, and other or unknown substances.

Alcohol-Induced Persisting Dementia. For alcohol-induced persisting dementia, the patient must meet the criteria for dementia. Because amnesia can also occur in the context of Korsakoff psychosis, it is essential to distinguish between memory impairment accompanied by other cognitive deficits (i.e., dementia) and amnesia caused by thiamine deficiency. To complicate matters, however, evidence also suggests that other cognitive functions, such as attention and concentration, may also be impaired in Wernicke–Korsakoff syndrome. Also, alcohol abuse is frequently associated with mood changes, so poor concentration and other cognitive symptoms often

observed in the context of major depression must also be ruled out. Prevalence rates differ considerably according to the population studied and the diagnostic criteria used, although alcohol-related dementia roughly accounts for 4 percent of dementias.

Pathology, Physical Findings, and Laboratory Examination

We should perform a comprehensive laboratory workup when evaluating a patient with dementia. The purposes of the workup are to detect reversible causes of dementia and to provide the patient and family with a definitive diagnosis. The range of possible causes of dementia mandates selective use of laboratory tests. The evaluation should follow informed clinical suspicion based on the history and physical and mental status examination results. The continued improvements in brain imaging techniques, particularly MRI, have made the differentiation between dementia of the Alzheimer type and vascular dementia, in some cases, somewhat more straightforward than in the past. Single-photon emission computed tomography (SPECT) can be a useful adjunctive test to detect patterns of brain metabolism in various types of dementias.

A general physical examination is a routine component of the workup for dementia. It may reveal evidence of systemic disease causing brain dysfunction, such as an enlarged liver and hepatic encephalopathy, or it may demonstrate systemic disease related to particular CNS processes. The detection of Kaposi sarcoma, for example, should alert the clinician to the probable presence of AIDS and the associated possibility of AIDS dementia complex. Focal neurologic findings, such as asymmetrical hyperreflexia or weakness, are seen more often in vascular than in degenerative disease. Frontal lobe signs and primitive reflexes occur in many disorders and often point to more significant progression.

DIFFERENTIAL DIAGNOSIS

Dementia of the Alzheimer Type versus Vascular Dementia

Classically, vascular dementia has been distinguished from dementia of the Alzheimer type by the decremental deterioration that can accompany cerebrovascular disease over time. Although the discrete, stepwise deterioration may not be apparent in all cases, focal neurologic symptoms are more common in vascular dementia than in dementia of the Alzheimer type, as are the standard risk factors for cerebrovascular disease.

Vascular Dementia versus Transient Ischemic Attacks

Transient ischemic attacks (TIAs) are brief episodes of focal neurologic dysfunction lasting less than 24 hours (usually 5 to 15 minutes). Although a variety of mechanisms may be responsible, the episodes are frequently the result of microembolization from a proximal intracranial arterial lesion that produces transient brain ischemia, and the episodes usually resolve without significant pathologic alteration of the parenchymal tissue. Approximately one-third of persons with untreated TIAs experience a brain infarction later; therefore, recognition of TIAs is an essential clinical strategy to prevent brain infarction.

Clinicians should distinguish episodes involving the vertebrobasilar system from those involving the carotid arterial system. In general, symptoms of vertebrobasilar disease reflect a transient functional disturbance in either the brainstem or the occipital lobe;

carotid distribution symptoms reflect unilateral retinal or hemispheric abnormality. Anticoagulant therapy, antiplatelet agglutinating drugs such as aspirin, and extracranial and intracranial reconstructive vascular surgery are effective in reducing the risk of infarction in patients with TIAs.

Delirium

In general, delirium has a rapid onset, brief duration, cognitive impairment fluctuation during the day; nocturnal exacerbation of symptoms; marked disturbance of the sleep–wake cycle; and prominent disturbances in attention and perception (Table 3-8).

Depression

Some patients with depression have symptoms of cognitive impairment challenging to distinguish from symptoms of dementia. The clinical picture is sometimes referred to as *pseudodementia,* although the term *depression-related cognitive dysfunction* is preferable and more descriptive (Table 3-25). Patients with depression-related cognitive dysfunction generally have prominent depressive symptoms, more insight into their symptoms than do demented patients, and

often a history of depressive episodes. Fortunately, memory impairment from depression usually responds to antidepressant medication.

Malingering and Factitious Disorder

Persons who attempt to simulate memory loss, as in factitious disorder, do so erratically and inconsistently. In true dementia, one loses memory for time and place before memory for person, and recent memory before remote memory.

Schizophrenia

Although schizophrenia can be associated with some acquired intellectual impairment, its symptoms are much less severe than are the related symptoms of psychosis and thought disorder.

Normal Aging

Aging is not necessarily associated with any significant cognitive decline, but minor memory problems can occur as a normal part of aging. We sometimes call these normal occurrences *benign senescent forgetfulness, age-associated memory impairment,* or *normal*

Table 3-25
Major Clinical Features Differentiating Depression-Related Cognitive Dysfunction from Dementia

Depression	Dementia
Clinical Course and History	
Family always aware of dysfunction and its severity	Family often unaware of dysfunction and its severity
Onset can be dated with some precision	Onset can be dated only within broad limits
Symptoms of short duration before medical help is sought	Symptoms usually of long duration before medical help is sought
Rapid progression of symptoms after onset	Slow progression of symptoms throughout course
History of previous psychiatric dysfunction common	History of previous psychiatric dysfunction unusual
Complaints and Clinical Behavior	
Patients usually complain much of cognitive loss	Patients usually complain little of cognitive loss
Patients' complaints of cognitive dysfunction usually detailed	Patients' complaints of cognitive dysfunction usually vague
Patients emphasize disability	Patients conceal disability
Patients highlight failures	Patients delight in accomplishments, however trivial
Patients make little effort to perform even simple tasks	Patients struggle to perform tasks
	Patients rely on notes, calendars, and so on to keep up
Patients usually communicate strong sense of distress	Patients often appear unconcerned
Affective change often pervasive	Affect labile and shallow
Loss of social skills often early and prominent	Social skills often retained
Behavior often incongruent with severity of cognitive dysfunction	Behavior usually compatible with severity of cognitive dysfunction
Nocturnal accentuation of dysfunction uncommon	Nocturnal accentuation of dysfunction common
Clinical Features Related to Memory, Cognitive, and Intellectual Dysfunctions	
Attention and concentration often well preserved	Attention and concentration usually faulty
"Don't know" answers typical	Near-miss answers frequent
On tests of orientation, patients often give "don't know" answers	On tests of orientation, patients often mistake unusual for usual
Memory loss for recent and remote events usually severe	Memory loss for recent events usually more severe than for remote events
Memory gaps for specific periods or events common	Memory gaps for specific periods unusual[a]
Marked variability in performance on tasks of similar difficulty	Consistently poor performance on tasks of similar difficulty

[a]Except when caused by delirium, trauma, seizures, and so on.
Reprinted with permission from Wells CE. Pseudodementia. *Am J Psychiatry.* 1979;136:898.

benign age-related senescence. They are distinguished from dementia by their minor severity and because they do not interfere significantly with a person's social or occupational behavior.

Other Disorders

Intellectual disability, which does not include memory impairment, occurs in childhood. Amnestic disorder is a circumscribed loss of memory and no deterioration. We should rule out a pituitary disorder, but they are a rare cause.

COURSE AND PROGNOSIS

The classic course of dementia is onset in the patient's 60s (although there may be subtle earlier signs), with gradual deterioration over 5 to 10 years, leading eventually to death. The age of onset and the rapidity of deterioration vary among different types of dementia and within individual diagnostic categories. The average survival expectation for patients with dementia of the Alzheimer type is approximately 8 years, with a range of 1 to 20 years. Data suggest that in persons with an early onset of dementia or with a family history of dementia, the disease is likely to have a rapid course. In a recent study of 821 persons with Alzheimer disease, the median survival time was 3.5 years. After diagnosing dementia, patients must have a complete medical and neurologic workup because 10 to 15 percent of all patients with dementia have a potentially reversible condition if we initiate treatment before permanent brain damage occurs.

The most common course of dementia begins with several subtle signs that may, at first, be ignored by both the patient and the people closest to the patient. Gradual onset of symptoms is most commonly associated with dementia of the Alzheimer type, vascular dementia, endocrinopathies, brain tumors, and metabolic disorders. Conversely, the onset of dementia resulting from head trauma, cardiac arrest with cerebral hypoxia, or encephalitis can be sudden. Although the symptoms of the early phase of dementia are subtle, they become conspicuous as dementia progresses, and family members may then bring a patient to a physician's attention. People with dementia may be sensitive to the use of benzodiazepines or alcohol, which can precipitate agitated, aggressive, or psychotic behavior. In the terminal stages of dementia, patients become empty shells of their former selves—profoundly disoriented, incoherent, amnestic, and incontinent of urine and feces.

With psychosocial and pharmacologic treatment and possibly because of the self-healing properties of the brain, the symptoms of dementia may progress slowly for a time or may even recede somewhat. Symptom regression is certainly a possibility in reversible dementias (dementias caused by hypothyroidism, normal pressure hydrocephalus [NPH], and brain tumors) after initiating treatment. The course of dementia varies from a steady progression (commonly seen with dementia of the Alzheimer type) to an incrementally worsening dementia (commonly seen with vascular dementia) to stable dementia (as may be seen in dementia related to head trauma).

Psychosocial Determinants

The severity and course of dementia can be affected by psychosocial factors. The higher a person's premorbid intelligence and education, the better they can compensate for intellectual deficits. People who have a rapid onset of dementia use fewer defenses than do those who experience an insidious onset. Anxiety and depression can intensify and aggravate the symptoms.

TREATMENT

The first step in the treatment of dementia is the verification of the diagnosis. Accurate diagnosis is imperative because the progression may be halted or even reversed if one provides appropriate therapy. Preventive measures are essential, particularly in vascular dementia. Such measures might include changes in diet, exercise, and control of diabetes and hypertension. Pharmacologic agents might include antihypertensive, anticoagulant, or antiplatelet agents. Blood pressure control should aim for the higher end of the normal range because it may improve cognitive function in patients with vascular dementia. Blood pressure below the normal range can worsen cognitive function in patients with dementia. The choice of an antihypertensive agent can be significant in that β-adrenergic receptor antagonists are associated with exaggeration of cognitive impairment. Angiotensin-converting enzyme (ACE) inhibitors and diuretics have not been linked to exaggeration of cognitive impairment and may lower blood pressure without affecting cerebral blood flow, which presumably correlates with cognitive function. Surgical removal of carotid plaques may prevent subsequent vascular events in carefully selected patients. The general treatment approach to patients with dementia is to provide supportive medical care; emotional support for the patients and their families; and pharmacologic treatment for specific symptoms, including disruptive behavior.

Psychosocial Therapies

The deterioration of mental faculties has significant psychological meaning for patients with dementia. The experience of a sense of continuity over time depends on memory. Patients lose recent memory before remote memory in most cases of dementia, and many patients are profoundly distressed by clearly recalling how they used to function while observing their noticeable deterioration. At the most fundamental level, the self is a product of brain functioning. Patients' identities begin to fade as the illness progresses, and they can recall less and less of their past. Emotional reactions ranging from depression to severe anxiety to catastrophic terror can stem from the realization that the sense of self is disappearing.

Patients often benefit from supportive and educational psychotherapy in which the clinician clearly explains the nature and course of their illness. They may also benefit from assistance in grieving and accepting the extent of their disability and from attention to self-esteem issues. We should try to maximize any areas of intact functioning by helping patients identify activities in which successful functioning is possible. A psychodynamic assessment of defective functions and cognitive limitations can also be useful. Clinicians can help patients find ways to deal with the defective functions, such as keeping calendars for orientation problems, making schedules to help structure activities, and taking notes for memory problems.

Psychodynamic interventions with family members of patients with dementia may be of great assistance. Those who take care of a patient struggle with feelings of guilt, grief, anger, and exhaustion as they watch a family member gradually deteriorate. A common problem that develops among caregivers involves their self-sacrifice in caring for a patient. They often suppress any developing resentment from this self-sacrifice because of the guilt feelings it produces. Clinicians can help caregivers understand the complex mixture of feelings associated with seeing a loved one decline and can provide understanding as well as permission to express these feelings. Clinicians must also be aware of the caregivers' tendencies to blame themselves or others for patients' illnesses and must appreciate the role that patients with dementia play in the lives of family members.

Pharmacotherapy

Clinicians may prescribe sedative-hypnotics for insomnia and anxiety, antidepressants for depression, and antipsychotic drugs for delusions and hallucinations, but they should be aware of the possible adverse drug effects that may be worse in older people (e.g., disinhibition, confusion, and oversedation). In general, we should avoid drugs with high anticholinergic activity.

Donepezil, rivastigmine, galantamine, and tacrine are cholinesterase inhibitors used to treat mild to moderate cognitive impairment in Alzheimer disease. They reduce the inactivation of the neurotransmitter acetylcholine and thus potentiate the cholinergic neurotransmitter, which in turn produces a modest improvement in memory and goal-directed thought. These drugs are most useful for persons with mild to moderate memory loss who have sufficient preservation of their basal forebrain cholinergic neurons to benefit from augmentation of cholinergic neurotransmission.

Donepezil is well tolerated and widely used. We rarely use tacrine because of its potential for hepatotoxicity. Fewer clinical data are available for rivastigmine and galantamine, which appear more likely to cause gastrointestinal (GI) and neuropsychiatric adverse effects than does donepezil. None of these medications prevent the progressive neuronal degeneration of the disorder.

Memantine protects neurons from excessive amounts of glutamate, which may be neurotoxic. Sometimes we may combine the drug with donepezil. It appears to improve dementia sometimes.

Other Treatment Approaches.   There are many drugs under development for cognitive-enhancing activity and this is a very active area of drug research. Novel strategies are focusing on the β-amyloid plaques and neurofibrillary tangles associated with Alzheimer and some other neurodegenerative disorders. In the case of amyloid plaques, attempts to reduce their formation, aggregation and to increase their clearance are underway, and several monoclonal and polyclonal antibody vaccines are being tested.

Estrogen replacement therapy may reduce the risk of cognitive decline in postmenopausal women. However the data is correlational and clinical trials to date are largely disappointing. A variety of other interventions have been proposed to improve cognitive outcomes in dementia, including cognitive stimulation, music therapy, reminiscence therapy, omega 3 fish oil, statins, ginkgo biloba, aromatherapy, or nonsteroidal anti-inflammatory drugs; however, all lack sufficient evidence to make any recommendation. Exercise improves cognition in healthy adults, and there is some evidence of benefit in dementia, particularly in the early stages.

EPIDEMIOLOGY

With the aging population, the prevalence of dementia is rising. The prevalence of moderate to severe dementia in different population groups is approximately 5 percent in the general population older than 65 years of age, 20 to 40 percent in the general population older than 85 years of age, 15 to 20 percent in outpatient general medical practices, and 50 percent in chronic care facilities.

Of all patients with dementia, 50 to 60 percent have the most common type of dementia, dementia of the Alzheimer type (Alzheimer disease). Dementia of the Alzheimer type increases in prevalence with increasing age. For persons age 65 years, the

prevalence for men is 0.6 percent and women, 0.8 percent. These rates increase with age, and at age 90, about one-fifth of people have the disorder. For all of these figures, 40 to 60 percent of cases are moderate to severe. The rates of prevalence (men to women) are 11 and 14 percent at age 85 years, 21 and 25 percent at age 90 years, and 36 and 41 percent at age 95 years. Patients with dementia of the Alzheimer type occupy more than 50 percent of nursing home beds. More than 2 million persons with dementia live at home. By 2050, current predictions suggest that there will be 14 million Americans with Alzheimer disease and, therefore, more than 18 million people with dementia.

The second most common type of dementia is vascular dementia, which is causally related to cerebrovascular diseases. Hypertension predisposes a person to the disease. Vascular dementias account for 15 to 30 percent of all dementia cases. Vascular dementia is most common in persons between the ages of 60 and 70 and is more common in men than in women. Approximately 10 to 15 percent of patients have coexisting vascular dementia and dementia of the Alzheimer type.

Other common causes of dementia, each representing 1 to 5 percent of all cases, include head trauma; alcohol-related dementias; and various movement disorder-related dementias, such as Huntington disease and Parkinson disease. Because dementia is a reasonably general syndrome, it has many causes, and clinicians must embark on a careful clinical workup of a patient with dementia to establish its cause.

ETIOLOGY

The most common causes of dementia in individuals older than 65 years of age are (1) Alzheimer disease, (2) vascular dementia, and (3) mixed vascular and Alzheimer disease. Other illnesses that account for approximately 10 percent include Lewy body dementia, Pick disease, frontotemporal dementias, NPH, alcoholic dementia, infectious dementia, such as HIV or syphilis, and Parkinson disease. Many types of dementias evaluated in clinical settings can be attributable to reversible causes, such as metabolic abnormalities (e.g., hypothyroidism), nutritional deficiencies (e.g., vitamin B_{12} or folate deficiencies), or dementia syndrome caused by depression. See Table 3-26 for a review of possible etiologies of dementia.

Dementia of the Alzheimer Type

In 1907, Alois Alzheimer first described the condition that later assumed his name. He described a 51-year-old woman with a 4½-year course of progressive dementia. The final diagnosis of Alzheimer disease requires a neuropathologic examination of the brain; nevertheless, we can diagnose dementia of the Alzheimer type in the clinical setting after excluding other causes of dementia.

Genetic Factors.   Although the cause of dementia of the Alzheimer type remains unknown, researchers have made impressive progress toward understanding the molecular basis of the amyloid deposits that are a hallmark of the disorder's neuropathology. Studies suggest as many as 40 percent of patients have a family history of dementia of the Alzheimer type. Thus, genetic factors are likely to play some part in the development of the disorder. Additional support for a genetic influence is the concordance rate for monozygotic twins, which is higher than the rate for dizygotic twins (43 percent vs. 8 percent, respectively). In several well-documented cases, the disorder has been transmitted in families

Table 3-26
Possible Etiologies of Dementia

Degenerative dementias
  Alzheimer disease
  Frontotemporal dementias (e.g., Pick disease)
  Parkinson disease
  Lewy body dementia
  Idiopathic cerebral ferrocalcinosis (Fahr disease)
  Progressive supranuclear palsy
Miscellaneous
  Huntington disease
  Wilson disease
  Metachromatic leukodystrophy
  Neuroacanthocytosis
Psychiatric
  Pseudodementia of depression
  Cognitive decline in late-life schizophrenia
Physiologic
  Normal pressure hydrocephalus
Metabolic
  Vitamin deficiencies (e.g., vitamin B$_{12}$, folate)
  Endocrinopathies (e.g., hypothyroidism)
  Chronic metabolic disturbances (e.g., uremia)
Tumor
  Primary or metastatic (e.g., meningioma or metastatic breast or
    lung cancer)
Traumatic
  Dementia pugilistica, posttraumatic dementia
  Subdural hematoma
Infection
  Prion diseases (e.g., Creutzfeldt–Jakob disease, bovine
    spongiform encephalitis, Gerstmann–Sträussler syndrome)
  Acquired immune deficiency syndrome (AIDS)
  Syphilis
Cardiac, vascular, and anoxia
  Infarction (single or multiple or strategic lacunar)
  Binswanger disease (subcortical arteriosclerotic encephalopathy)
  Hemodynamic insufficiency (e.g., hypoperfusion or hypoxia)
Demyelinating diseases
  Multiple sclerosis
Drugs and toxins
  Alcohol
  Heavy metals
  Irradiation
  Cognitive dysfunction due to medications (e.g., anticholinergics)
  Carbon monoxide

through an autosomal dominant gene, although such transmission is rare. Alzheimer-type dementia has shown linkage to chromosomes 1, 14, and 21.

AMYLOID PRECURSOR PROTEIN.   The gene for amyloid precursor protein (APP) is on the long arm of chromosome 21. The process of differential splicing yields four forms of the APP. The β/A4 protein, the principal constituent of senile plaques, is a 42-amino acid peptide that is a breakdown product of APP. Down syndrome (trisomy 21) has three copies of the *APP* gene, and with a mutation at codon 717 in the *APP* gene, a pathologic process results in the excessive deposition of β/A4 protein. Whether the processing of abnormal APP is of primary causative significance in Alzheimer disease is unknown. However, many research groups are studying both the standard metabolic processing of APP and its processing in patients with dementia of the Alzheimer type in an attempt to answer this question.

MULTIPLE E4 GENES.   One study implicated gene E4 in the origin of Alzheimer disease. People with one copy of the gene have Alzheimer disease three times more frequently than do those with no E4 gene, and people with two E4 genes have the disease eight times more frequently than do those with no E4 gene. Diagnostic

testing for this gene is not contributory because it is found in persons without dementia and not found in all cases of dementia.

Neuropathology.   The classic gross neuroanatomical observation of a brain from a patient with Alzheimer disease is diffuse atrophy with flattened cortical sulci and enlarged cerebral ventricles. The classic and pathognomonic microscopic findings are senile plaques, neurofibrillary tangles, neuronal loss (particularly in the cortex and the hippocampus), synaptic loss (perhaps as much as 50 percent in the cortex), and granulovascular degeneration of the neurons. Neurofibrillary tangles (Fig. 3-1) are composed of cytoskeletal elements, primarily phosphorylated tau protein, although other cytoskeletal proteins are also present. Neurofibrillary tangles are not unique to Alzheimer disease; they also occur in Down syndrome, dementia pugilistica (punch-drunk syndrome), Parkinson–dementia complex of Guam, Hallervorden–Spatz disease, and the brains of healthy people as they age. Neurofibrillary tangles are common in the cortex, the hippocampus, the substantia nigra, and the locus ceruleus.

Senile plaques, also referred to as *amyloid plaques*, more strongly indicate Alzheimer disease, although they are also seen in Down syndrome and, to some extent, in healthy aging. Senile plaques are composed of a particular protein, β/A4, and astrocytes, dystrophic neuronal processes, and microglia. The number and the density of senile plaques present in postmortem brains correlate with the severity of the disease.

Neurotransmitters.   The neurotransmitters usually implicated in the pathophysiologic condition of Alzheimer disease are acetylcholine and norepinephrine, both of which are likely hypoactive in Alzheimer disease. Several studies have reported data consistent with the hypothesis that specific degeneration of cholinergic neurons is present in the nucleus basalis of Meynert in persons with Alzheimer disease. Other data supporting a cholinergic deficit in Alzheimer disease demonstrate decreased acetylcholine and choline acetyltransferase concentrations in the brain. Choline acetyltransferase is the critical enzyme for the synthesis of acetylcholine, and a reduction in choline acetyltransferase concentration suggests a decrease in the number of cholinergic neurons present. Additional support for the cholinergic deficit hypothesis comes from the observation that cholinergic antagonists, such as scopolamine and atropine, impair cognitive abilities, whereas cholinergic agonists, such as physostigmine and arecoline, enhance cognitive abilities. The decrease in norepinephrine-containing neurons in the locus ceruleus found in some pathologic examinations of Alzheimer disease brains suggests decreased norepinephrine activity in the disease. Two other neurotransmitters implicated in the pathophysiologic condition of Alzheimer disease are the neuroactive peptides somatostatin and corticotropin; there are decreased concentrations of both in persons with Alzheimer disease.

Other Causes.   Another theory to explain the development of Alzheimer disease is that an abnormality in the regulation of membrane phospholipid metabolism results in membranes that are less fluid—that is, more rigid—than usual. Several investigators are using molecular resonance spectroscopic imaging to assess this hypothesis directly in patients with dementia of the Alzheimer type. Some have suggested that aluminum toxicity is a causative factor because of the high levels of aluminum found in the brains of some patients with Alzheimer disease, but this is no longer considered a significant etiologic factor. Excessive stimulation by the transmitter glutamate that may damage neurons is another theory of causation.

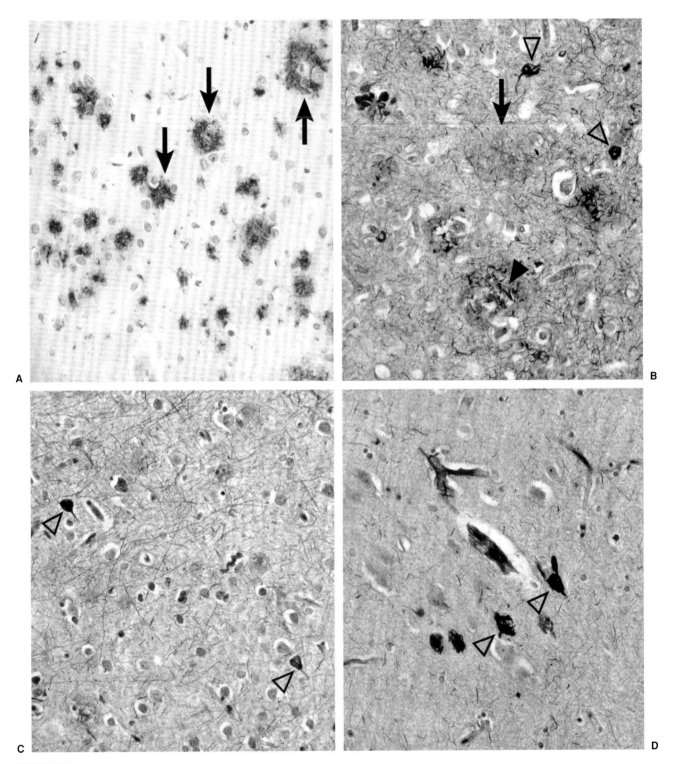

FIGURE 3-1

Photomicrographs of Alzheimer disease neuropathology. **A:** Deposition of insoluble fibrillar Aβ into plaques begins in the neocortex, labeled here using an antibody against Aβ and appearing as reddish-brown deposits (*arrows*). **B:** Bielchowsky stain of neocortex from an individual who died in advanced stages of Alzheimer disease (Braak stage VI). The Aβ plaques appear as dark brown in this preparation (*arrows*) and can be seen to be associated with dystrophic neuronal processes (*arrowheads*) in which insoluble microtubule-associated protein τ (MAPT) aggregates appear as black deposits. This neurofibrillary pathology also appears extensively throughout the neuropil, and several neurofibrillary tangles can be seen (*open arrowheads*). **C:** Bielchowsky stain of neocortex from an individual who died in a less advanced disease stage (Braak stage IV). Although some neurofibrillary tangles are still evident (*open arrowheads*), the degree of neurofibrillary pathology in the neuropil is substantially diminished. **D:** Isolated neurofibrillary tangles (*open arrowheads*) in entorhinal cortex that can be seen in normal aging (Bielchowsky stain). Notice the lack of Aβ plaques and limited neuropil involvement. Aβ, Beta amyloid. (All images obtained at 200× magnification and provided courtesy of Dr. Ronald L. Hamilton, Department of Pathology, Division of Neuropathology, University of Pittsburgh School of Medicine.)

FIGURE 3-2

Gross appearance of the cerebral cortex on coronal section from a patient with vascular dementia. The multiple bilateral lacunar infarcts involve the thalamus, the internal capsule, and the globus pallidus. (Courtesy of Daniel P. Perl, M.D.)

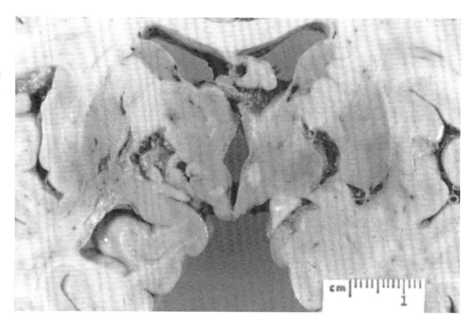

Familial Multiple System Tauopathy with Presenile Dementia.

A recently discovered type of dementia, familial multiple system tauopathy, shares some brain abnormalities found in people with Alzheimer disease. The gene that causes the disorder is likely on chromosome 17. The symptoms of the disorder include short-term memory problems and difficulty maintaining balance and walking. The onset of the disease is in the 40s and 50s. Persons with the disease live an average of 11 years after the onset of symptoms.

As in patients with Alzheimer disease, tau protein builds up in neurons and glial cells of persons with familial multiple system tauopathy. Eventually, the protein buildup kills brain cells. The disorder is not associated with the senile plaques seen with Alzheimer disease.

Mr. J, a 70-year-old retired businessman, was brought to psychiatric services on referral by the family physician. His wife claimed that Mr. J had become so forgetful that she was afraid to leave him alone, even at home. Mr. J retired at age 62 years after experiencing a decline in work performance during the previous 5 years. He also slowly gave up hobbies he once enjoyed (photography, reading, golf) and became increasingly quiet. However, his growing forgetfulness went unnoticed at home. Then one day, while walking in an area he knew well, he could not find his way home. From then on, his memory failure began to increase. He would forget appointments, misplace things, and lose his way around the neighborhood he resided in for 40 years. He failed to recognize people, even those he knew for many years. His wife had to start bathing and dressing him because he forgot how to do so himself.

On examination, Mr. J could not recall the time or place. He was only able to recall his name and place of birth. Mr. J seemed lost during the interview, only responding to questions with an occasional shrug of his shoulders. When asked to name objects or to recall words or numbers, Mr. J appeared tense and distressed. Mr. J had difficulty following instructions and was unable to dress or undress. His general medical condition was good. Laboratory examinations showed abnormalities on Mr. J's EEG and CT scans.

Vascular Dementia

The primary cause of vascular dementia, formerly referred to as *multi-infarct dementia,* is presumed to be multiple areas of cerebral vascular disease, resulting in a symptom pattern of dementia.

Vascular dementia is most common in men, especially those with preexisting hypertension or other cardiovascular risk factors. The disorder affects primarily small- and medium-sized cerebral vessels, which undergo infarction and produce multiple parenchymal lesions spread over wide areas of the brain (Fig. 3-2). The causes of the infarctions can include occlusion of the vessels by arteriosclerotic plaques or thrombemboli from distant origins (e.g., heart valves). An examination of a patient may reveal carotid bruits, funduscopic abnormalities, or enlarged cardiac chambers.

Binswanger Disease.

Binswanger disease, also known as *subcortical arteriosclerotic encephalopathy,* is characterized by the presence of many small infarctions of the white matter that spare the cortical regions (Fig. 3-3). Although Binswanger disease was

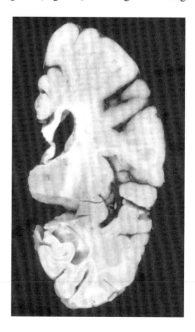

FIGURE 3-3

Binswanger disease. Cross-section demonstrating extensive subcortical white matter infarction, with sparing of the overlying gray matter. (Courtesy of Dushyant Purohit, M.D., Neuropathology Division, Mount Sinai School of Medicine, New York, NY.)

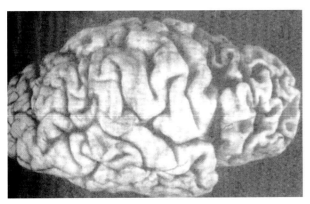

FIGURE 3-4
Pick disease gross pathology. This demonstrates the marked frontal and temporal atrophy seen in frontotemporal dementias, such as Pick disease. (Courtesy of Dushyant Purohit, M.D., Neuropathology Division, Mount Sinai School of Medicine, New York, NY.)

previously considered a rare condition, the advent of sophisticated and powerful imaging techniques, such as MRI, has revealed that the condition is more common than previously thought.

Frontotemporal Dementia (Pick Disease)

In contrast to the parietal–temporal distribution of pathologic findings in Alzheimer disease, Pick disease is a preponderance of atrophy in the frontotemporal regions. These regions also have neuronal loss, gliosis, and neuronal Pick bodies, which are masses of cytoskeletal elements. Pick bodies are seen in some postmortem specimens but are not necessary for the diagnosis. The cause of Pick disease is unknown, but the disease constitutes approximately 5 percent of all irreversible dementias. It is most common in men, especially those who have a first-degree relative with the condition. Pick disease is difficult to distinguish from dementia of the Alzheimer type. However, the early stages of Pick disease are more often characterized by personality and behavioral changes, with relative preservation of other cognitive

Table 3-27
Clinical Criteria for Dementia with Lewy Bodies (DLB)

The patient must have sufficient cognitive decline to interfere with social or occupational functioning. Of note, early in the illness, memory symptoms may not be as prominent as attention, frontosubcortical skills, and visuospatial ability. Probable DLB requires two or more core symptoms, whereas possible DLB only requires one core symptom.

Core features
 Fluctuating levels of attention and alertness
 Recurrent visual hallucinations
 Parkinsonian features (cogwheeling, bradykinesia, and resting tremor)
Supporting features
 Repeated falls
 Syncope
 Sensitivity to neuroleptics
 Systematized delusions
 Hallucinations in other modalities (e.g. auditory, tactile)

Adapted from McKeith LG, Galasko D, Kosaka K. Consensus guidelines for the clinical and pathologic diagnosis of dementia with Lewy bodies (DLB): Report of the consortium on DLB international workshop. 1996;47:1113–1124, with permission.

functions, and it typically begins before 75 years of age. Familial cases may have an earlier onset, and some studies have shown that approximately half of the cases of Pick disease are familial (Fig. 3-4). Features of Klüver–Bucy syndrome (e.g., hypersexuality, placidity, hyperorality) are much more common in Pick disease than in Alzheimer disease.

Lewy Body Disease

Lewy body disease is clinically similar to Alzheimer disease. However, it commonly presents with hallucinations, parkinsonian features, and extrapyramidal signs (Table 3-27). Lewy inclusion bodies are in the cerebral cortex (Fig. 3-5). The exact incidence is unknown. These patients often have Capgras syndrome (reduplicative paramnesia) as part of the clinical picture.

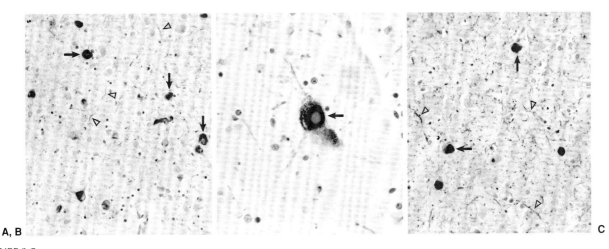

A, B   C

FIGURE 3-5
Photomicrographs of Lewy body pathology. **A:** Abnormal accumulation of α-synuclein aggregates demonstrated by immunocytochemistry in the amygdala of a subject with dementia. Lewy bodies appear as dense intracellular inclusions (*arrows*), but staining of neuronal processes can be seen throughout the neuropil (*arrowheads*). In individuals in whom Lewy body pathology occurs concurrently with Alzheimer disease, the amygdala is often the only region affected. **B:** Classic appearance of a Lewy body (*arrow*) in a large pigmented neuron of the substantia nigra. **C:** Lewy body pathology in the neocortex. Both Lewy bodies (*arrows*) and substantial labeling of neuronal processes in the neuropil (*arrowheads*) are evident. (Magnification for [A] and [B] 200×, for [C] 400×. All images provided courtesy of Dr. Ronald L. Hamilton, Department of Pathology, Division of Neuropathology, University of Pittsburgh School of Medicine.)

Table 3-28
Distinguishing Features of Subcortical and Cortical Dementias

Characteristic	Subcortical Dementia	Cortical Dementia	Recommended Tests
Language	No aphasia (anomia, if severe)	Aphasia early	FAS test Boston Naming test WAIS-R vocabulary test
Memory	Impaired recall (retrieval) > recognition (encoding)	Recall and recognition impaired	Wechsler memory scale; Symbol Digit Paired Associate Learning (Brandt)
Attention and immediate recall	Impaired	Impaired	WAIS-R digit span
Visuospatial skills	Impaired	Impaired	Picture arrangement, object assembly and block design; WAIS subtests
Calculation	Preserved until late	Involved early	Mini-Mental State
Frontal system abilities (executive function)	Disproportionately affected	Degree of impairment consistent with other involvement	Wisconsin Card Sorting Test; Odd Man Out test; Picture Absurdities
Speed of cognitive processing	Slowed early	Normal until late in disease	Trail making A and B: Paced Auditory Serial Addition Test (PASAT)
Personality	Apathetic, inert	Unconcerned	MMPI
Mood	Depressed	Euthymic	Beck and Hamilton depression scales
Speech	Dysarthric	Articulate until late	Verbal fluency (Rosen, 1980)
Posture	Bowed or extended	Upright	
Coordination	Impaired	Normal until late	
Motor speed and control	Slowed	Normal	Finger-tap; grooved pegboard
Adventitious movements	Chorea, tremor, tics, dystonia	Absent (Alzheimer dementia— some myoclonus)	
Abstraction	Impaired	Impaired	Category test (Halstead Battery)

From Pajeau AK, Román GC. HIV encephalopathy and dementia. In: J Biller, RG Kathol, eds. *The Psychiatric Clinics of North America: The Interface of Psychiatry and Neurolgy*. Vol. 15. Philadelphia, PA: WB Saunders; 1992:457.

Huntington Disease

Huntington disease is classically associated with the development of dementia. The dementia seen in this disease is the subcortical type of dementia, characterized by more motor abnormalities and fewer language abnormalities than in the cortical type of dementia (Table 3-28). The dementia of Huntington disease exhibits psychomotor slowing and difficulty with complex tasks, but memory, language, and insight remain relatively intact in the early and middle stages of the illness. As the disease progresses, however, the dementia becomes complete; the features distinguishing it from dementia of the Alzheimer type are the high incidence of depression and psychosis in addition to the classic choreoathetoid movement disorder.

Parkinson Disease

As with Huntington disease, parkinsonism is a disease of the basal ganglia, commonly associated with dementia and depression. An estimated 20 to 30 percent of patients with Parkinson disease have dementia, and an additional 30 to 40 percent have measurable impairment in cognitive abilities. The slow movements of persons with Parkinson disease parallel the slow thinking of some affected patients, a feature that clinicians may refer to as *bradyphrenia*.

Mr. M, 77 years of age, came for a neurologic examination because he noticed his memory was slipping, and he was having difficulty

concentrating, which interfered with his work. He complained of slowness and losing his train of thought. His wife stated that he was becoming withdrawn and was more reluctant to participate in activities he usually enjoyed. He denied symptoms of depression other than feeling mildly depressed about his disabilities. Two years prior, Mr. M developed an intermittent resting tremor in his right hand and a shuffling gait. Although a psychiatrist considered a diagnosis of Parkinson disease, the neurologist did not confirm it.

During an initial neurologic examination, Mr. M's spontaneous speech was hesitant and unclear (dysarthric). Cranial nerve examination was normal. Motor tone was increased slightly in the neck and all limbs. He performed alternating movements in his hands slowly. He had a slight intermittent tremor of his right arm at rest. Reflexes were symmetrical. Three weeks later, the patient had a neuropsychologic examination. On the examination, Mr. M had impairment of memory, naming, and constructional abilities.

HIV-Related Dementia

Encephalopathy in HIV infection is associated with dementia and is called *acquired immune deficiency syndrome* (AIDS) *dementia complex*, or *HIV dementia*. Patients infected with HIV experience dementia at an annual rate of approximately 14 percent. An estimated 75 percent of patients with AIDS have involvement of the CNS at the time of autopsy. The development of dementia in people infected with HIV parallels the appearance of parenchymal abnormalities in MRI scans. *Cryptococcus* or *Treponema pallidum* can cause other infectious dementias.

Table 3-29
Criteria for Clinical Diagnosis of HIV Type 1-Associated Dementia Complex

Laboratory evidence for systemic human immunodeficiency virus (HIV) type 1 infection with confirmation by Western blot, polymerase chain reaction, or culture.

Acquired abnormality in at least *two* cognitive abilities for a period of at least 1 mo: attention and concentration, speed of processing information, abstraction and reasoning, visuospatial skills, memory and learning, and speech and language. The decline should be verified by reliable history and mental status examination. History should be obtained from an informant, and examination should be supplemented by neuropsychological testing.

Cognitive dysfunction causes impairment in social or occupational functioning. Impairment should not be attributable solely to severe systemic illness.

At least *one* of the following:
Acquired abnormality in motor function verified by clinical examination (e.g., slowed rapid movements, abnormal gait, incoordination, hyperreflexia, hypertonia, or weakness), neuropsychological tests (e.g., fine motor speed, manual dexterity, or perceptual motor skills), or both.
Decline in motivation or emotional control or a change in social behavior. This may be characterized by a change in personality with apathy, inertia, irritability, emotional lability, or a new onset of impaired judgment or disinhibition.

This does not exclusively occur in the context of a delirium.

Evidence of another etiology, including active central nervous system opportunistic infection, malignancy, psychiatric disorders (e.g., major depression), or substance abuse, if present, is *not* the cause of the previously mentioned symptoms and signs.

Adapted from Working Group of the American Academy of Neurology AIDS Task Force. Nomenclature and research case definitions for neurologic manifestations of human immunodeficiency virus–type 1 (HIV-1) infection. *Neurology.* 1991;41:778–785, with permission.

The diagnosis of AIDS dementia complex is made by confirmation of HIV infection and exclusion of alternative pathology to explain cognitive impairment. The American Academy of Neurology AIDS Task Force developed research criteria for the clinical diagnosis of CNS disorders in adults and adolescents (Table 3-29). The AIDS Task Force criteria for AIDS dementia complex require laboratory evidence for systemic HIV, at least two cognitive deficits, and the presence of motor abnormalities or personality changes. Personality changes manifest with apathy, emotional lability, or behavioral disinhibition. The AIDS Task Force criteria also require the absence of clouding of consciousness or evidence of another etiology that could produce cognitive impairment. We should assess for cognitive, motor, and behavioral changes using physical, neurologic, and psychiatric examinations, in addition to neuropsychologic testing.

Head Trauma–Related Dementia

Dementia can be a sequela of head trauma. The so-called punch-drunk syndrome (dementia pugilistica) occurs in boxers after repeated head trauma over many years. The symptoms include emotional lability, dysarthria, and impulsivity. It also occurs in professional football players who developed dementia after repeated concussions over many years.

Mrs. S, 75 years of age, was brought to the emergency department after being found wandering her neighborhood in a confused and disoriented state. She was in good health until a few months before, when her husband had minor surgery, requiring 10-day hospitalization.

About a month after her husband returned home, he and their two adult children, who do not reside with them, reported a noticeable change in Mrs. S's mental status. Mrs. S became hyperactive and appeared to have excessive energy, was agitated and irritable, and had difficulty sleeping at night.

At the examination, Mrs. S was disoriented to time and place, agitated, and confused. Her husband revealed upon an interview that Mrs. S has for many years suffered from dizziness and lightheadedness upon standing and occasionally suffered from falls, none of which caused any significant damage. Not long before her confused symptoms began, Mrs. S had suffered a fall one night, and her husband found her the next morning lying next to the bed in a confused state. Because of her history of falls, neither Mr. S nor Mrs. S thought much of the incident. A CT scan revealed the presence of a subdural hematoma, which was surgically evacuated. Afterward, Mrs. S's confusion and disorientation cleared, and she returned to her normal state of functioning.

▲ 3.3 Major or Minor Neurocognitive Disorder due to Another Medical Condition (Amnestic Disorders)

The amnestic disorders cause impairment in memory as the primary sign and symptom, although other signs of cognitive decline may coexist. The authors of *Synopsis* believe amnestic disorder to be a clinically useful descriptive category of illness, but they are coded in DSM-5 as a neurocognitive disorder due to another medical condition with the specific medical condition noted.

The amnestic disorders are a broad category that results from a variety of diseases and conditions that have amnesia as the primary complaint. The syndrome is defined primarily by impairment in the ability to create new memories. Three different etiologies exist: amnestic disorder caused by a general medical condition (e.g., head trauma), substance-induced persisting amnestic disorder (e.g., caused by carbon monoxide poisoning or chronic alcohol consumption), and amnestic disorder not otherwise specified for cases in which the etiology is unclear.

DIAGNOSIS

The recognition of amnestic disorder occurs when there is impairment in the ability to learn new information or the inability to recall previously learned information, as a result of which there is significant impairment in social or occupational functioning and which is caused by a general medical condition (including physical trauma). Amnestic disorder may be transient, lasting for hours or days, or chronic, lasting weeks or months. We can make a diagnosis of substance-induced persisting amnestic disorder when evidence suggests that the symptoms are causatively related to the use of a substance. The DSM-5 refers clinicians to specific diagnoses within substance-related disorders: alcohol-induced disorder, sedative, hypnotic, or anxiolytic-induced disorder, and other (or unknown) substance-induced disorder.

CLINICAL FEATURES AND SUBTYPES

The central symptom of amnestic disorders is the development of a memory disorder characterized by an impairment in the ability to learn new information (anterograde amnesia) and an inability to recall previously remembered knowledge (retrograde amnesia). The symptom must result in significant problems for patients in their social or occupational functioning. The time in which a patient is amnestic can begin directly at the point of trauma or include a period before the trauma. The patient can also lose memory for the time during the physical insult (e.g., during a cerebrovascular event).

Short-term and recent memory is usually impaired. Patients cannot remember what they had for breakfast or lunch, the name of the hospital, or their doctors. In some patients, the amnesia is so profound that the patient cannot orient themselves to place and time, although the patient rarely loses orientation to person. Overlearned information or remote events usually remain intact, but there can be amnesia for even the less remote past (over the past decade). Immediate memory (tested, for example, by asking a patient to repeat six numbers) remains intact. With improvement, patients may experience a gradual shrinking of the time for which they lose memory, although some patients experience a gradual improvement in memory for the entire period.

The onset of symptoms can be sudden, as in trauma, cerebrovascular events, and neurotoxic chemical assaults, or gradual, as in nutritional deficiency and cerebral tumors. The amnesia can be of short duration.

A variety of other symptoms can be associated with amnestic disorders. For patients with other cognitive impairments, a diagnosis of dementia or delirium is more appropriate than a diagnosis of an amnestic disorder. Both subtle and gross changes in personality can accompany the symptoms of memory impairment in amnestic disorders. Patients may be apathetic, lack initiative, have unprovoked episodes of agitation, or appear to be overly friendly or agreeable. Patients with amnestic disorders can also appear bewildered and confused and may attempt to cover their confusion with confabulatory answers to questions. Characteristically, patients with amnestic disorders do not have good insight into their neuropsychiatric conditions.

A local nursing home transferred a 73-year-old survivor of the Holocaust to the psychiatric unit. She was born in Germany to a middle-class family. Her internment in a concentration camp cut short her education. She immigrated to Israel after liberation from the concentration camp and later to the United States, where she married and raised a family. Premorbidly, she was described as a quiet, intelligent, and loving woman who spoke several languages. At 55 years of age, she had a significant carbon monoxide exposure when a gas line leaked while she and her husband slept. Her husband died of carbon monoxide poisoning, but the patient survived after a period of coma. After being stabilized, she displayed significant cognitive and behavioral problems. She had difficulty with learning new information and making appropriate plans. She retained the ability to perform activities of daily living but could not be relied on to pay bills, buy food, cook, or clean, despite appearing to have retained the intellectual ability to do these tasks. She moved to a nursing home after several difficult years at home and in the homes of relatives. In the nursing home, she was able to learn her way about the facility. She displayed little interest in scheduled group activities, hobbies, reading, or television. She had frequent behavioral problems. She repeatedly pressed staff to get her sweets and snacks and cursed them vociferously with racial epithets and disparaging comments on their weight and dress. On one occasion, she scratched the cars of several staff members with a key. Neuropsychological testing demonstrated severe deficits in her delayed recall, intact performance on language and general knowledge measures, and moderate deficits in domains of executive function, such as concept formation and cognitive flexibility. She responded immediately to firmly set

limits and rewards, but deficits in memory prevented long-term incorporation of these boundaries. Management involved the development of a behavioral plan and empirical trials of medications aimed at the amelioration of irritability.

Although one might suggest this is not a pure amnestic disorder, by far the most disabling symptom for this patient was her memory loss.

Cerebrovascular Diseases

Cerebrovascular diseases affecting the hippocampus involve the posterior cerebral and basilar arteries and their branches. Infarctions are rarely limited to the hippocampus; they often involve the occipital or parietal lobes. Thus, common accompanying symptoms of cerebrovascular diseases in this region are focal neurologic signs involving vision or sensory modalities. Cerebrovascular diseases affecting the bilateral medial thalamus, particularly the anterior portions, are often associated with symptoms of amnestic disorders. A few case studies report amnestic disorders from the rupture of an aneurysm of the anterior communicating artery, resulting in infarction of the basal forebrain region.

Multiple Sclerosis

The pathophysiologic process of multiple sclerosis involves the seemingly random formation of plaques within the brain parenchyma. When the plaques occur in the temporal lobe and the diencephalic regions, symptoms of memory impairment can occur. The most common cognitive complaints in patients with multiple sclerosis involve impaired memory, which occurs in 40 to 60 percent of patients. Characteristically, digit span memory is normal, but immediate recall and delayed recall of information are impaired. Memory impairment can affect both verbal and nonverbal material.

Korsakoff Syndrome

Korsakoff syndrome is an amnestic syndrome caused by thiamine deficiency, most commonly associated with the poor nutritional habits of people with chronic alcohol use disorder. Other causes of poor nutrition (e.g., starvation), gastric carcinoma, hemodialysis, hyperemesis gravidarum, prolonged IV hyperalimentation, and gastric plication can also result in thiamine deficiency. Korsakoff syndrome is often associated with Wernicke encephalopathy, which is the associated syndrome of confusion, ataxia, and ophthalmoplegia. In patients with these thiamine deficiency–related symptoms, the neuropathologic findings include hyperplasia of the small blood vessels with occasional hemorrhages, hypertrophy of astrocytes, and subtle changes in neuronal axons. Although the delirium clears up within a month or so, the amnestic syndrome either accompanies or follows untreated Wernicke encephalopathy in approximately 85 percent of all cases.

Patients with Korsakoff syndrome typically demonstrate a change in personality as well, such that they display a lack of initiative, diminished spontaneity, and a lack of interest or concern. These changes appear frontal lobe–like, similar to the personality change ascribed to patients with frontal lobe lesions or degeneration. Indeed, such patients often demonstrate *executive function* deficits on neuropsychological tasks involving attention, planning, set-shifting, and inferential reasoning consistent with frontal pattern injuries. For this reason, Korsakoff syndrome is not a pure memory disorder, although it certainly is a useful paradigm of the more common clinical presentations for the amnestic syndrome.

The onset of Korsakoff syndrome can be gradual. Recent memory tends to be affected more than is remote memory, but this feature is variable. Confabulation, apathy, and passivity are often prominent symptoms in the syndrome. With treatment, patients may remain amnestic for up to 3 months and then gradually improve over the ensuing year. Administration of thiamine may prevent the development of additional amnestic symptoms, but the treatment seldom reverses severe amnestic symptoms when they are present. Approximately one-third to one-fourth of all patients recover completely, and approximately one-fourth of all patients have no improvement in their symptoms.

Alcoholic Blackouts

Some persons with severe alcohol abuse may exhibit the syndrome commonly referred to as an alcoholic blackout. Characteristically, these persons awake in the morning with a conscious awareness of being unable to remember a period the night before during which they were intoxicated. Sometimes specific behaviors (hiding money in a secret place, and provoking fights) are associated with the blackouts.

Electroconvulsive Therapy

Electroconvulsive therapy treatments are usually associated with retrograde amnesia for several minutes before the treatment and anterograde amnesia after the treatment. The anterograde amnesia usually resolves within 5 hours. Mild memory deficits may remain for 1 to 2 months after a course of ECT treatments, but the symptoms are entirely resolved 6 to 9 months after treatment.

Head Injury

Head injuries (both closed and penetrating) can result in a wide range of neuropsychiatric symptoms, including dementia, depression, personality changes, and amnestic disorders. Amnestic disorders caused by head injuries are commonly associated with a period of retrograde amnesia leading up to the traumatic incident and amnesia for the traumatic incident itself. The severity of the brain injury correlates somewhat with the duration and severity of the amnestic syndrome. However, the best correlate of eventual improvement is the degree of clinical improvement in the amnesia during the first week after the patient regains consciousness.

Transient Global Amnesia

Transient global amnesia is the abrupt loss of the ability to recall recent events or to remember new information. The syndrome includes mild confusion and a lack of insight into the problem, a clear sensorium, and, occasionally, the inability to perform some well-learned complex tasks. Episodes last from 6 to 24 hours. Studies suggest that transient global amnesia occurs in 5 to 10 cases per 100,000 persons per year, although for patients older than age 50 years, the rate may be as high as 30 cases per 100,000 persons per year. The pathophysiology is unknown, but it likely involves ischemia of the temporal lobe and the diencephalic brain regions. Several studies of patients with SPECT have shown decreased blood flow in the temporal and parietotemporal regions, particularly in the left hemisphere. Patients with transient global amnesia almost universally experience complete improvement, although one study found that approximately 20 percent of patients may have a recurrence of the episode, and another study found that approximately 7 percent of patients may have epilepsy. Patients with transient global amnesia differ from patients with TIAs in that fewer patients have diabetes, hypercholesterolemia, and hypertriglyceridemia, but more have hypertension and migrainous episodes.

PATHOLOGY AND LABORATORY EXAMINATION

Quantitative neuropsychologic testing can aid the diagnosis of amnestic disorder. Standardized tests also are available to assess recall of well-known historical events or public figures to characterize an individual's inability to remember previously learned information. Performance on such tests varies among individuals with amnestic disorder. Subtle deficits in other cognitive functions may occur in individuals with amnestic disorder. Memory deficits, however, constitute the predominant feature of the mental status examination and account largely for any functional deficits. No specific or diagnostic features are detectable on imaging studies such as MRI or CT. Damage of midtemporal lobe structures is typical, however, and may reflect enlargement of the third ventricle or temporal horns or in structural atrophy detected by MRI.

DIFFERENTIAL DIAGNOSIS

Table 3-30 lists the significant causes of amnestic disorders. To make the diagnosis, clinicians must obtain a patient's history, conduct a complete physical examination, and order all appropriate laboratory tests. Other diagnoses, however, can be confused with amnestic disorders.

Dementia and Delirium

Amnestic disorders can be distinguished from delirium because they occur in the absence of a disturbance of consciousness and are striking for the relative preservation of other cognitive domains.

Table 3-30
Major Causes of Amnestic Disorders

Thiamine deficiency (Korsakoff syndrome)
Hypoglycemia
Primary brain conditions
  Seizures
  Head trauma (closed and penetrating)
  Cerebral tumors (especially thalamic and temporal lobe)
  Cerebrovascular diseases (especially thalamic and temporal lobe)
  Surgical procedures on the brain
  Encephalitis due to herpes simplex
  Hypoxia (including nonfatal hanging attempts and carbon
    monoxide poisoning)
  Transient global amnesia
  Electroconvulsive therapy
  Multiple sclerosis
Substance-related causes
  Alcohol use disorders
  Neurotoxins
  Benzodiazepines (and other sedative-hypnotics)
  Many over-the-counter preparations (particularly anticholinergic
    or antihistaminic drugs)

Table 3-31
Comparison of Syndrome Characteristics in Dementia of the Alzheimer Type (DAT) and Amnestic Disorder

Characteristic	DAT	Amnestic Disorder
Onset	Insidious	Can be abrupt
Course	Progressive deterioration	Static or improvement
Anterograde memory	Impaired	Impaired
Retrograde memory	Impaired	Temporal gradient
Episodic memory	Impaired	Impaired
Semantic memory	Impaired	Intact
Language	Impaired	Intact
Praxis or function	Impaired	Intact

Table 3-31 outlines the critical distinctions between Dementia of the Alzheimer type (DAT) and amnestic disorders. Both disorders can have an insidious onset with slow progression, as in a Korsakoff psychosis in a chronic drinker. Amnestic disorders, however, can also develop precipitously, as in Wernicke encephalopathy, transient global amnesia, or anoxic insults. Although DAT progresses relentlessly, amnestic disorders tend to remain static or even improve after removing the offending cause. In terms of the actual memory deficits, the amnestic disorder and DAT still differ. DAT has an impact on retrieval in addition to encoding and consolidation. The deficits in DAT extend beyond memory to general knowledge (semantic memory), language, praxis, and general function. This is not the case for amnestic disorders. The dementias associated with Parkinson disease, AIDS, and other subcortical disorders demonstrate disproportionate impairment of retrieval, but relatively intact encoding and consolidation. The subcortical pattern dementias are also likely to display motor symptoms, such as bradykinesia, chorea, or tremor, that are not components of the amnestic disorders.

Normal Aging

Some minor impairment in memory may accompany healthy aging, but the requirement that the memory impairment causes significant impairment in social or occupational functioning should exclude normal aging from the diagnosis.

Dissociative Disorders

The dissociative disorders can sometimes be challenging to differentiate from amnestic disorders. Patients with dissociative disorders, however, are more likely to have lost their orientation to self and may have more selective memory deficits than do patients with amnestic disorders. For example, patients with dissociative disorders may not know their names or home addresses, but they are still able to learn new information and remember selected memories. Dissociative disorders are also often associated with emotionally stressful life events involving money, the legal system, or troubled relationships.

Factitious Disorders

Patients with factitious disorders who are mimicking an amnestic disorder often have inconsistent results on memory tests and have no evidence of an identifiable cause. These findings, coupled with evidence of primary or secondary gain for a patient, should suggest a factitious disorder.

COURSE AND PROGNOSIS

The course of an amnestic disorder depends on its etiology and treatment, particularly acute treatment. Generally, amnestic disorder has a static course. We see little improvement over time, but also no progression of the disorder. The exceptions are the acute amnesias, such as transient global amnesia, which resolves entirely over hours to days, and the amnestic disorder associated with head trauma, which improves steadily in the months after the trauma. Amnesia secondary to processes that destroy brain tissue, such as stroke, tumor, and infection, are irreversible, although it is, static once the disease process is halted.

TREATMENT

The primary approach to treating amnestic disorders is to treat the underlying cause. Although a patient is amnestic, supportive prompts about the date, the time, and the patient's location can be helpful and can reduce the patient's anxiety. After the resolution of the amnestic episode, psychotherapy of some type (cognitive, psychodynamic, or supportive) may help patients incorporate the amnestic experience into their lives.

Psychotherapy

Psychodynamic interventions may be of considerable value for patients who have amnestic disorders that result from insults to the brain. Understanding the course of recovery in such patients helps clinicians to be sensitive to the narcissistic injury inherent in damage to the CNS.

The first phase of recovery, in which patients are incapable of processing what happened because the ego defenses are overwhelmed, requires clinicians to serve as a supportive auxiliary ego who explains to a patient what is happening and provides missing ego functions. In the second phase of recovery, as the realization of the injury sets in, patients may become angry and feel victimized by the malevolent hand of fate. They may view others, including the clinician, as harmful or destructive, and clinicians must contain these projections without becoming punitive or retaliatory. Clinicians can build a therapeutic alliance with patients by explaining slowly and clearly what happened and by explaining the patient's internal experience. The third phase of recovery is integrative. As a patient accepts what has happened, a clinician can help the patient form a new identity by connecting current experiences of the self with past experiences. Grieving over the lost faculties may be an essential feature of the third phase.

Most patients who are amnestic because of brain injury engage in denial. Clinicians must respect and empathize with the patient's need to deny the reality of what has happened. Insensitive and blunt confrontations destroy any developing therapeutic alliance and can cause patients to feel attacked. In a sensitive approach, clinicians help patients accept their cognitive limitations by exposing them to these deficits bit by bit over time. When patients fully accept what has happened, they may need assistance in forgiving themselves and any others involved, so that they can get on with their lives. Clinicians must also be wary of being seduced into thinking that all of the patient's symptoms are directly related to the brain insult. An evaluation of preexisting personality disorders, such as borderline, antisocial, and narcissistic personality disorders, must be part of the overall assessment; many patients with personality disorders place themselves in situations that predispose them to injuries. These personality features may become a crucial part of the psychodynamic psychotherapy.

Centers for cognitive rehabilitation have rehabilitation-oriented therapeutic milieu designed to promote recovery from brain injury, especially that from traumatic causes. Despite the high cost of extended care at these sites, which provide both long-term institutional and daytime services, there is limited data to define therapeutic effectiveness for the heterogeneous groups of patients who participate in such tasks as memory retaining.

EPIDEMIOLOGY

No adequate studies have reported on the incidence or prevalence of amnestic disorders. We are most likely to see them with alcohol use disorders and head injury. In general practice and hospital settings, the frequency of amnesia related to chronic alcohol abuse has decreased, and the frequency of amnesia related to head trauma has increased.

ETIOLOGY

The major neuroanatomical structures involved in memory and the development of an amnestic disorder are particular diencephalic structures such as the dorsomedial and midline nuclei of the thalamus and midtemporal lobe structures such as the hippocampus, the mamillary bodies, and the amygdala. Although amnesia is usually the result of bilateral damage to these structures, some cases of unilateral damage result in an amnestic disorder, and evidence indicates that the left hemisphere may be more critical than the right hemisphere in the development of memory disorders. Many studies of memory and amnesia in animals have suggested that other brain areas may also be involved in the symptoms accompanying amnesia. Frontal lobe involvement can result in such symptoms as confabulation and apathy, which occurs in patients with amnestic disorders.

Amnestic disorders have many potential causes (see Table 3-30). Thiamine deficiency, hypoglycemia, hypoxia (including carbon monoxide poisoning), and herpes simplex encephalitis all have a predilection for damaging the temporal lobes, particularly the hippocampi, and thus can be associated with the development of amnestic disorders. Similarly, when tumors, cerebrovascular diseases, surgical procedures, or multiple sclerosis plaques involve the diencephalic or temporal regions of the brain, the symptoms of an amnestic disorder may develop. General insults to the brain, such as seizures, ECT, and head trauma, can also result in memory impairment. Transient global amnesia is presumed to be a cerebrovascular disorder involving transient impairment in blood flow through the vertebrobasilar arteries.

Many drugs are associated with the development of amnesia, and clinicians should review all drugs taken, including nonprescription drugs, in the diagnostic workup of a patient with amnesia. Benzodiazepines are the most commonly used prescription drugs associated with amnesia. All benzodiazepines can be associated with amnesia, especially if combined with alcohol. Triazolam has a reputation for causing amnesia. However, at standard doses, it is no more likely to cause memory loss than the other benzodiazepines. When using higher doses or combining it with alcohol, it can cause anterograde amnesia.

▲ 3.4 Neurocognitive and Other Psychiatric Disorders due to a General Medical Condition

Increasingly, scientific views of mental illness recognize that, whether caused by an identifiable anomaly (e.g., brain tumor), a neurotransmitter disturbance of unclear origin (e.g., schizophrenia), or a consequence of deranged upbringing or environment (e.g., personality disorder), all mental disorders ultimately share one common underlying theme: aberration in brain function. The treatments for those conditions, whether psychological or biologic, attempt to restore normal brain functioning.

The differential diagnosis for a mental syndrome in a patient should always include consideration of (1) any general medical condition that a patient may have and (2) any prescription, nonprescription, or illegal substances that a patient may be taking. Although some specific medical conditions are classically associated with mental syndromes, a much larger number of general medical conditions may occasionally cause mental syndromes.

The mental disorders caused by a general medical condition span the entire spectrum of diagnostic categories. Thus, one can have a cognitive disorder, mood disorder, sleep disorder, anxiety disorder, and psychotic disorder to mention but a few that are caused or aggravated by a medical condition. In this section, neurocognitive disorders due to a general medical condition are described, including epilepsy, autoimmune disorders, and AIDS, of which psychiatrists should be aware.

SPECIFIC DISORDERS

Epilepsy

Epilepsy is the most common chronic neurologic disease in the general population and affects approximately 1 percent of the population in the United States. For psychiatrists, the significant concerns about epilepsy are consideration of an epileptic diagnosis in psychiatric patients, the psychosocial ramifications of a diagnosis of epilepsy for a patient, and the psychological and cognitive effects of commonly used anticonvulsant drugs. Concerning the first of these concerns, 30 to 50 percent of all persons with epilepsy have psychiatric difficulties sometime during their illness. The most common behavioral symptom of epilepsy is a change in personality. Psychosis and violence occur much less often than was previously believed.

Definitions. A seizure is a transient paroxysmal pathophysiologic disturbance of cerebral function caused by a spontaneous, excessive discharge of neurons. Patients are said to have epilepsy if they have a chronic condition characterized by recurrent seizures. The ictus, or ictal event, is the seizure itself. The nonictal periods include the preictal, postictal, and interictal periods. The ictal symptoms depend mainly on the brain origin for the seizure and how the activity spreads in the brain. The ictal event influences the interictal symptoms as do other neuropsychiatric and psychosocial factors, such as coexisting psychiatric or neurologic disorders, the presence of psychosocial stressors, and premorbid personality traits.

Classification. The two major categories of seizures are partial and generalized. Partial seizures involve epileptiform activity

FIGURE 3-6

Electroencephalographic recording during generalized tonic–clonic seizure showing rhythmic sharp waves and muscles artifact during tonic phase, spike-and-wave discharges during clonic phase, and attenuation of activity during postictal state. (Courtesy of Barbara F. Westmoreland, M.D.)

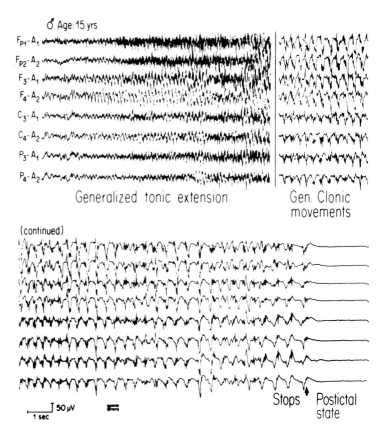

in localized brain regions. Generalized seizures involve the entire brain (Fig. 3-6). Table 3-32 outlines the classification system.

GENERALIZED SEIZURES. Generalized tonic–clonic seizures exhibit the classic symptoms of loss of consciousness, generalized tonic–clonic movements of the limbs, tongue biting, and incontinence. Although the diagnosis of the ictal events of the seizure is relatively straightforward, the postictal state, characterized by a slow, gradual recovery of consciousness and cognition, occasionally presents a diagnostic dilemma for a psychiatrist in an emergency department. The recovery period from a generalized tonic–clonic seizure ranges from a few minutes to many hours, and the clinical picture is that of a gradually clearing delirium. The most common psychiatric problems associated with generalized seizures involve helping patients adjust to a chronic neurologic disorder and assessing the cognitive or behavioral effects of anticonvulsant drugs.

Absence Seizure (Petit Mal). A complicated type of generalized seizure for a psychiatrist to diagnose is an absence or petit mal seizure. The epileptic nature of the episodes may go unrecognized because the characteristic motor or sensory manifestations of epilepsy may be absent or so slight that they do not arouse suspicion. Petit mal epilepsy usually begins in childhood between the ages of 5 and 7 years and ceases by puberty. Brief disruptions of consciousness, during which the patient suddenly loses contact with the environment, are characteristic of petit mal epilepsy, but the patient has no actual loss of consciousness and no convulsive movements during the episodes. The EEG produces a characteristic pattern of three-per-second spike-and-wave activity (Fig. 3-7). In rare instances, petit mal epilepsy begins in adulthood. Adult-onset petit mal epilepsy can present as sudden, recurrent psychotic episodes or deliriums that appear and disappear

Table 3-32
International Classification of Epileptic Seizures

I. Partial seizures (seizures beginning locally)
  A. Partial seizures with elementary symptoms (generally without impairment of consciousness)
    1. With motor symptoms
    2. With sensory symptoms
    3. With autonomic symptoms
    4. Compound forms
  B. Partial seizures with complex symptoms (generally with impairment of consciousness; temporal lobe or psychomotor seizures)
    1. With impairment of consciousness only
    2. With cognitive symptoms
    3. With affective symptoms
    4. With psychosensory symptoms
    5. With psychosensory symptoms (automatisms)
    6. Compound forms
  C. Partial seizures secondarily generalized

II. Generalized seizures (bilaterally symmetrical and without local onset)
  A. Absence (petit mal) seizures
  B. Myoclonus
  C. Infantile spasms
  D. Clonic seizures
  E. Tonic seizures
  F. Tonic–clonic seizures (grand mal)
  G. Atonic seizures
  H. Akinetic seizures

III. Unilateral seizures

IV. Unclassified seizures (because of incomplete data)

Adapted from Gastaut H. Clinical and electroencephalographical classification of epileptic seizures. *Epilepsia.* 1970;11:102, with permission.

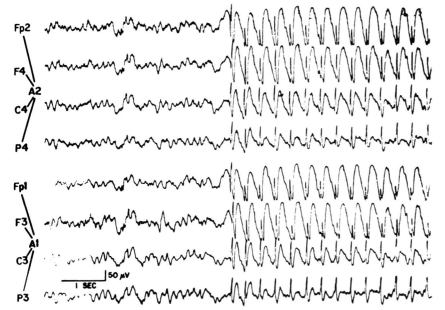

FIGURE 3-7
Petit mal epilepsy characterized by bilaterally synchronous, 3-Hz spike and slow-wave activity.

abruptly. The symptoms may include a history of falling or fainting spells.

PARTIAL SEIZURES. Partial seizures can be simple (without alterations in consciousness) or complex (with an alteration in consciousness). Somewhat more than half of all patients with partial seizures have complex partial seizures. Other terms used for complex partial seizures are temporal lobe epilepsy, psychomotor seizures, and limbic epilepsy; these terms, however, are not accurate descriptions of the clinical situation. Complex partial epilepsy, the most common form of epilepsy in adults, affects approximately 3 of 1,000 persons. About 30 percent of patients with complex partial seizures have a major mental illness such as depression.

Symptoms

PREICTAL SYMPTOMS. Preictal events (auras) in complex partial epilepsy include autonomic sensations (e.g., fullness in the stomach, blushing, and changes in respiration); cognitive sensations (e.g., *déjà vu, jamais vu,* forced thinking, dreamy states); affective states (e.g., fear, panic, depression, elation); and, classically, automatisms (e.g., lip-smacking, rubbing, chewing).

ICTAL SYMPTOMS. Brief, disorganized, and uninhibited behavior characterizes the ictal event. Although some defense attorneys may claim otherwise, rarely does a person exhibit organized, directed violent behavior during an epileptic episode. The cognitive symptoms include amnesia for the time during the seizure and a period of resolving delirium after the seizure. A seizure focus can be found on an EEG in 25 to 50 percent of all patients with complex partial epilepsy (Fig. 3-8). The use of sphenoidal or anterior temporal electrodes and sleep-deprived EEGs may increase the likelihood of finding an EEG abnormality. We might obtain multiple normal EEGs for a patient with complex partial epilepsy; therefore, we cannot use normal EEGs to exclude a diagnosis of complex partial epilepsy. The use of long-term EEG recordings (usually 24 to 72 hours) can help clinicians detect a seizure focus in some patients. Nasopharyngeal leads probably do not add much to the sensitivity of an EEG and cause discomfort for the patient.

INTERICTAL SYMPTOMS

Personality Disturbances. The most frequent psychiatric abnormalities reported in patients with epilepsy are personality disorders, and they are especially likely to occur in patients with epilepsy of temporal lobe origin. The most common features are religiosity, a heightened experience of emotions—a quality usually called *viscosity of personalit*y—and changes in sexual behavior. The syndrome in its complete form is relatively rare, even in those with complex partial seizures of temporal lobe origin. Many patients are not affected by personality disturbances; others have a variety of disturbances that differ strikingly from the classic syndrome.

A striking religiosity may be manifested not only by increased participation in overtly religious activities but also by unusual concern for moral and ethical issues, preoccupation with right and wrong, and heightened interest in global and philosophical concerns. The hyperreligious features can sometimes seem like the prodromal symptoms of schizophrenia and can result in a diagnostic problem in an adolescent or a young adult.

The symptom of viscosity of personality is usually most noticeable in a patient's conversation, which is likely to be slow, serious, ponderous, pedantic, overly replete with nonessential details, and often circumstantial. The listener may grow bored but be unable to find a courteous and successful way to disengage from the conversation. The speech tendencies are often mirrored in the patient's writing and result in a symptom known as *hypergraphia,* which some clinicians consider virtually pathognomonic for complex partial epilepsy.

Changes in sexual behavior can include hypersexuality, deviations in sexual interest, such as fetishism and transvestism, and, most commonly, hyposexuality. The hyposexuality is characterized both by a lack of interest in sexual matters and by reduced sexual arousal. Some patients with the onset of complex partial epilepsy before puberty may fail to reach an average level of sexual interest after puberty, although this characteristic may not disturb the patient. For patients with the onset of complex partial epilepsy after puberty, the change in sexual interest may be bothersome and worrisome.

Psychotic Symptoms. Interictal psychotic states are more common than ictal psychoses. Schizophrenia-like interictal episodes can

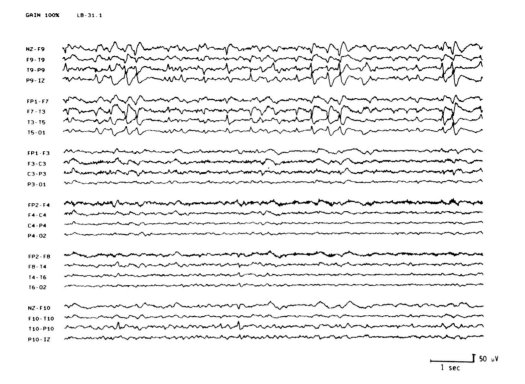

GAIN 100%   LB-31.1

FIGURE 3-8
An interictal encephalograph in a patient with complex partial seizures reveals frequent left temporal spike discharges and rare, independent right temporal sharp-wave activity. (From Cascino GD. Complex partial seizures: Clinical features and differential diagnosis. *Psychiatr Clin North Am*. 1992;15:377, with permission.)

occur in patients with epilepsy, particularly those with temporal lobe origins. An estimated 10 percent of all patients with complex partial epilepsy have psychotic symptoms. Risk factors for the symptoms include female gender, left-handedness, the onset of seizures during puberty, and a left-sided lesion.

The onset of psychotic symptoms in epilepsy is variable. Classically, psychotic symptoms appear in patients who have had epilepsy for a long time, and the development of personality changes related to the epileptic brain activity precedes the onset of psychotic symptoms. The most characteristic symptoms of psychoses are hallucinations and paranoid delusions. Patients usually remain warm and appropriate in affect, in contrast to the abnormalities of affect commonly seen in patients with schizophrenia. The thought disorder symptoms in patients with psychotic epilepsy are most commonly those involving conceptualization and circumstantiality rather than the classic schizophrenic symptoms of blocking and looseness.

Violence. Episodic violence has been a problem in some patients with epilepsy, especially epilepsy of temporal and frontal lobe origin. Whether the violence is a manifestation of the seizure itself or is of interictal psychopathological origin is uncertain. Most evidence points to the extreme rarity of violence as an ictal phenomenon. Only in rare cases should violence in the patient with epilepsy be attributed to the seizure itself.

Mood Disorder Symptoms. Mood disorder symptoms, such as depression and mania, are seen less often in epilepsy than are schizophrenia-like symptoms. The mood disorder symptoms that do occur tend to be episodic and appear most often when the epileptic foci affect the temporal lobe of the nondominant cerebral hemisphere. The importance of mood disorder symptoms may be attested to by the increased incidence of attempted suicide in people with epilepsy.

Diagnosis. A correct diagnosis of epilepsy can be particularly tricky when the ictal and interictal symptoms of epilepsy are severe manifestations of psychiatric symptoms in the absence of significant changes in consciousness and cognitive abilities. Psychiatrists, therefore, must maintain a high level of suspicion during the evaluation of a new patient and must consider the possibility of an epileptic disorder even in the absence of the classic signs and symptoms. Another differential diagnosis to consider is *psychogenic nonepileptic seizures* (previously called *pseudoseizures*), in which a patient has some conscious control over mimicking the symptoms of a seizure (Table 3-33).

For patients who have previously received a diagnosis of epilepsy, we should consider the appearance of new psychiatric symptoms as possibly representing an evolution in their epileptic symptoms. The appearance of psychotic symptoms, mood disorder symptoms, personality changes, or symptoms of anxiety (e.g., panic attacks) should cause a clinician to evaluate the control of the patient's epilepsy and to assess the patient for the presence of an independent mental disorder. In such circumstances, the clinician should evaluate the patient's compliance with the anticonvulsant drug regimen and should consider whether the psychiatric symptoms could be adverse effects from the antiepileptic drugs themselves. When psychiatric symptoms appear in a patient who has had epilepsy diagnosed or considered as a diagnosis in the past, the clinician should obtain results of one or more EEG examinations.

In patients who have not previously received a diagnosis of epilepsy, four characteristics should cause a clinician to be suspicious of the possibility: the abrupt onset of psychosis in a person previously regarded as psychologically healthy, the abrupt onset of delirium without a recognized cause, a history of similar episodes with an abrupt onset and spontaneous recovery, and a history of previous unexplained falling or fainting spells.

Table 3-33
Differentiating Features of Psychogenic Nonepileptic Seizures (PNES) and Epileptic Seizures

Feature	Epileptic Seizures	PNES
Clinical Features		
Nocturnal seizure	Common	Uncommon
Stereotyped aura	Usually	None
Cyanotic skin changes during seizures	Common	None
Self-injury	Common	Rare
Incontinence	Common	Rare
Postictal confusion	Present	None
Body movements	Tonic or clonic or both	Nonstereotyped and asynchronous
Affected by suggestion	No	Yes
EEG Features		
Spike and waveforms	Present	Absent
Postictal slowing	Present	Absent
Interictal abnormalities	Variable	Variable

EEG, electroencephalogram.
From Stevenson JM, King JH. Neuropsychiatric aspects of epilepsy and epileptic seizures. In: Hales RE, Yodofsky SC, eds. *American Psychiatric Press Textbook of Neuropsychiatry*. Washington, DC: American Psychiatric Press; 1987:220.

Treatment. First-line drugs for generalized tonic–clonic seizures are valproate and phenytoin. First-line drugs for partial seizures include carbamazepine, oxcarbazepine, and phenytoin. Ethosuximide and valproate are first-line drugs for absence (petit mal) seizures. Table 3-34 lists the drugs used for various types of seizures. Carbamazepine and valproic acid may help control the symptoms of irritability and outbursts of aggression, as do the typical antipsychotic drugs. Psychotherapy, family counseling, and group therapy may be useful in addressing the psychosocial issues associated with epilepsy. Also, clinicians should be aware that many antiepileptic drugs cause mild to moderate cognitive impairment, and we should consider an adjustment of the dosage or a change in medications if symptoms of cognitive impairment are a problem in a patient.

Brain Tumors

Brain tumors and cerebrovascular diseases can cause virtually any psychiatric symptom or syndrome, but cerebrovascular diseases, by the nature of their onset and symptom pattern, are rarely misdiagnosed as mental disorders. In general, tumors cause fewer psychopathological signs and symptoms than cerebrovascular diseases affecting a similar volume of brain tissue. The two critical approaches to the diagnosis of either condition are a comprehensive clinical history and a complete neurologic examination. The performance of the appropriate brain imaging technique is usually the final diagnostic procedure; the imaging should confirm the clinical diagnosis.

Clinical Features, Course, and Prognosis. Mental symptoms occur at some time during the illness in approximately 50 percent of patients with brain tumors. In approximately 80 percent of these patients with mental symptoms, the tumors are located in frontal or limbic brain regions rather than in parietal or temporal regions. Whereas meningiomas are likely to cause focal symptoms by compressing a limited region of the cortex, gliomas are likely to cause diffuse symptoms. Delirium is most often a component of rapidly growing, large, or metastatic tumors. If a patient's history and a physical examination reveal bowel or bladder incontinence, a frontal lobe tumor should be suspected; if the history and examination reveal abnormalities in memory and speech, we should suspect a temporal lobe tumor.

COGNITION. Impaired intellectual functioning often accompanies the presence of a brain tumor, regardless of its type or location.

LANGUAGE SKILLS. Disorders of language function may be severe, mainly if tumor growth is rapid. Defects of language function often obscure all other mental symptoms.

Table 3-34
Commonly Used Anticonvulsant Drugs

Drug	Use	Maintenance Dosage (mg/day)
Carbamazepine	Generalized tonic–clonic, partial	600–1,200
Clonazepam	Absence, atypical myoclonic	2–12
Ethosuximide	Absence	1,000–2,000
Gabapentin	Complex partial seizures (augmentation)	900–3,600
Lamotrigine	Complex partial seizures, generalized (augmentation)	300–500
Oxcarbazepine	Partial	600–2,400
Phenobarbital	Generalized tonic–clonic	100–200
Phenytoin	Generalized tonic–clonic, partial, status epilepticus	300–500
Primidone	Partial	750–1,000
Tiagabine	Generalized	32–56
Topiramate	Complex partial seizures (augmentation)	200–400
Valproate	Absence, myoclonic, generalized tonic–clonic, akinetic, partial seizures	750–1,000
Zonisamide	Generalized	400–600

MEMORY.   Loss of memory is a frequent symptom of brain tumors. Patients with brain tumors exhibit an amnestic syndrome and retain no memory of events that occurred since the illness began. Events of the immediate past, even painful ones, are lost. Patients, however, retain old memories and are unaware of their loss of recent memory.

PERCEPTION.   Prominent perceptual defects are often associated with behavioral disorders, mainly because patients must integrate tactile, auditory, and visual perceptions to function normally.

AWARENESS.   Alterations of consciousness are common late symptoms of increased intracranial pressure caused by a brain tumor. Tumors arising in the upper part of the brainstem can produce a unique symptom called *akinetic mutism,* or *vigilant coma.* The patient is immobile and mute yet alert.

Colloid Cysts.   Although they are not brain tumors, colloid cysts located in the third ventricle can exert physical pressure on structures within the diencephalon and produce such mental symptoms as depression, emotional lability, psychotic symptoms, and personality changes. The classic associated neurologic symptoms are position-dependent intermittent headaches.

Head Trauma

Head trauma can result in an array of mental symptoms and lead to a diagnosis of dementia due to head trauma or to mental disorder not otherwise specified due to a general medical condition (e.g., postconcussional disorder). The postconcussive syndrome remains controversial because it focuses on the full range of psychiatric symptoms, some serious, that can follow what seems to be minor head trauma.

Pathophysiology.   Head trauma is a common clinical situation; an estimated 2 million incidents involve head trauma each year. Head trauma most commonly occurs in people 15 to 25 years of age and has a male-to-female predominance of approximately 3 to 1. Gross estimates based on the severity of the head trauma suggest that virtually all patients with severe head trauma, more than half of patients with moderate head trauma, and about 10 percent of patients with mild head trauma have ongoing neuropsychiatric sequelae resulting from the head trauma. Head trauma can be divided grossly into penetrating head trauma (e.g., trauma produced by a bullet) and blunt trauma, in which there is no physical penetration of the skull. Blunt trauma is far more common than penetrating head trauma. Motor vehicle accidents account for more than half of all the incidents of blunt CNS trauma; falls, violence, and sports-related head trauma account for most of the remaining cases (Fig. 3-9).

Whereas brain injury from penetrating wounds localizes to the areas directly affected by the missile, brain injury from blunt trauma involves several mechanisms. During the actual head trauma, the head usually moves back and forth violently, so that the brain repeatedly hits against the skull as it and the skull mismatch their rapid deceleration and acceleration. This crashing results in focal contusions, and the stretching of the brain parenchyma produces diffuse axonal injury. Later developing processes, such as edema and hemorrhaging, can result in further damage to the brain.

Symptoms.   The two significant clusters of symptoms related to head trauma are those of cognitive impairment and behavioral sequelae. After a period of posttraumatic amnesia, there is usually

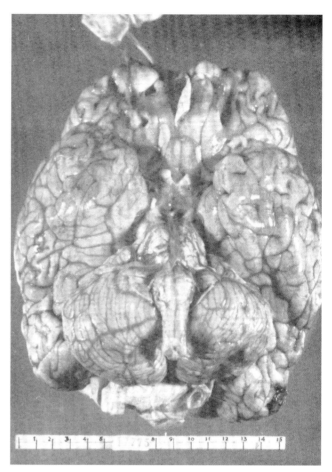

FIGURE 3-9

Severe contusion of the frontal poles has resulted in their atrophy and distortion. (Courtesy of Dr. H. M. Zimmerman.)

a 6- to 12-month period of recovery, after which the remaining symptoms are likely to be permanent. The most common cognitive problems are decreased speed in information processing, decreased attention, increased distractibility, deficits in problem-solving and in the ability to sustain an effort, and problems with memory and learning new information. A variety of language disabilities can also occur.

Behaviorally, the significant symptoms involve depression, increased impulsivity, increased aggression, and changes in personality. Alcohol can exacerbate these symptoms, and it is often involved in the head trauma event itself. A debate has ensued about how preexisting character and personality traits affect the development of behavioral symptoms after head trauma. We do not have the critical studies needed to answer the question definitively, but the weight of opinion is leaning toward a biologically and neuroanatomically based association between the head trauma and the behavioral sequelae.

Treatment.   The treatment of the cognitive and behavioral disorders in patients with head trauma is similar to the treatment approaches used in other patients with these symptoms. One difference is that patients with head trauma may be particularly susceptible to the side effects associated with psychiatric drugs; therefore, we should initiate treatment with these agents in lower dosages than usual, and they should be titrated upward more slowly than usual. We can use standard antidepressants to treat depression and

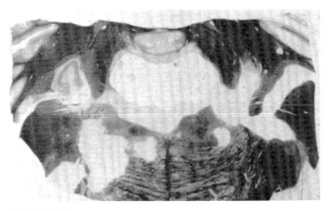

FIGURE 3-10
Multiple sclerosis. Irregular, seemingly punched out zones of demyelination are evident in this section through the level of the fourth ventricle. Myelin stain. 2.6×. (Courtesy of Dr. H. M. Zimmerman.)

either anticonvulsants or antipsychotics for aggression and impulsivity. Other approaches to the symptoms include lithium, calcium channel blockers, and β-adrenergic receptor antagonists.

Clinicians must support patients through individual or group psychotherapy and should support the primary caretakers through couples and family therapy. Patients with minor and moderate head trauma often rejoin their families and restart their jobs; therefore, all involved parties need help to adjust to any changes in the patient's personality and mental abilities.

Demyelinating Disorders

Multiple sclerosis (MS) is a major demyelinating disorder. Other demyelinating disorders include amyotrophic lateral sclerosis (ALS), metachromatic leukodystrophy, adrenoleukodystrophy, gangliosidoses, subacute sclerosing panencephalitis, and Kufs disease. All of these disorders can be associated with neurologic, cognitive, and behavioral symptoms.

Multiple Sclerosis.   MS consists of multiple episodes of symptoms, pathophysiologically related to multifocal lesions in the white matter of the CNS (Fig. 3-10). The cause remains unknown, but studies have focused on slow viral infections and disturbances in the immune system. The estimated prevalence of MS in the Western Hemisphere is 50 per 100,000 people. The disease is much more frequent in cold and temperate climates than in the tropics and subtropics and more common in women than in men; it is predominantly a disease of young adults. In most patients, the onset occurs between the ages of 20 and 40 years.

The neuropsychiatric symptoms of MS include cognitive and behavioral types. Research reports have found that 30 to 50 percent of patients with MS have mild cognitive impairment (MCI) and that 20 to 30 percent of them have severe cognitive impairments. Although evidence indicates that patients with MS experience a decline in their general intelligence, memory is the most commonly affected cognitive function. The severity of the amnesia and the neurologic symptoms do not correlate well. Nor do they correlate with the duration of the illness.

The behavioral symptoms associated with MS are varied and can include euphoria, depression, and personality changes. Psychosis is a rare complication. Approximately 25 percent of persons with MS exhibit a euphoric mood. This mood is not hypomanic but somewhat more cheerful than their situation warrants and not

necessarily in character with their disposition before the onset of MS. Only 10 percent of patients with MS have a sustained and elevated mood, although it is still not genuinely hypomanic. Depression, however, is common; it affects 25 to 50 percent of patients with MS and results in a higher rate of suicide than is seen in the general population. Risk factors for suicide in patients with MS are male sex, the onset of MS before age 30 years, and a relatively recent diagnosis of the disorder. Personality changes are also frequent in patients with MS; they affect 20 to 40 percent of patients and often include irritability or apathy.

Amyotrophic Lateral Sclerosis.   ALS is a progressive, noninherited disease of asymmetrical muscle atrophy. It begins in adult life and progresses over months or years to involve all the striated muscles except the cardiac and ocular muscles. In addition to muscle atrophy, patients have signs of pyramidal tract involvement. The illness is rare and occurs in approximately 1.6 persons per 100,000 annually. A few patients have concomitant dementia. The disease progresses rapidly, and death generally occurs within 4 years of onset.

Infectious Diseases

Herpes Simplex Encephalitis.   Herpes simplex encephalitis, the most common type of focal encephalitis, most commonly affects the frontal and temporal lobes. The symptoms often include anosmia, olfactory and gustatory hallucinations, and personality changes and can also involve bizarre or psychotic behaviors. Complex partial epilepsy may also develop in patients with herpes simplex encephalitis. Although the mortality rate for the infection has decreased, many patients exhibit personality changes, symptoms of memory loss, and psychotic symptoms.

Rabies Encephalitis.   The incubation period for rabies ranges from 10 days to 1 year, after which symptoms of restlessness, overactivity, and agitation can develop. Hydrophobia, present in up to 50 percent of patients, is characterized by an intense fear of drinking water. The fear develops from the severe laryngeal and diaphragmatic spasms that the patients experience when they drink water. When rabies encephalitis develops, the disease is fatal within days or weeks.

Neurosyphilis.   Neurosyphilis (also known as general paresis) appears 10 to 15 years after the primary *Treponema* infection. Since the advent of penicillin, neurosyphilis has become a rare disorder, although AIDS is associated with reintroducing neurosyphilis into medical practice in some urban settings. Neurosyphilis generally affects the frontal lobes and results in personality changes, the development of poor judgment, irritability, and decreased care for self. Delusions of grandeur develop in 10 to 20 percent of affected patients. The disease progresses with the development of dementia and tremor until patients are paretic. The neurologic symptoms include Argyll Robertson pupils, which are small, irregular, and unequal and have light-near reflex dissociation, tremor, dysarthria, and hyperreflexia. Cerebrospinal fluid (CSF) examination shows lymphocytosis, increased protein, and a positive result on a Venereal Disease Research Laboratory (VDRL) test.

Chronic Meningitis.   Chronic meningitis is becoming more common than earlier because of the immunocompromised condition of people with AIDS. The usual causative agents are *Mycobacterium tuberculosis*, *Cryptococcus* spp., and *Coccidioides* spp. The usual symptoms are headache, memory impairment, confusion, and fever.

Subacute Sclerosing Panencephalitis.

Subacute sclerosing panencephalitis is a disease of childhood and early adolescence, with a 3-to-1 male-to-female ratio. The onset usually follows either an infection with measles or vaccination for measles. The initial symptoms may be behavioral change, temper tantrums, sleepiness, and hallucinations, but the classic symptoms of myoclonus, ataxia, seizures, and intellectual deterioration eventually develop. The disease progresses relentlessly to coma and death in 1 to 2 years.

Lyme Disease.

Lyme disease is caused by infection with the spirochete *Borrelia burgdorferi* transmitted through the bite of the deer tick (*Ixodes scapularis*), which feeds on infected deer and mice. About 16,000 cases are reported annually in the United States.

A characteristic bull's eye rash occurs at the site of the tick bite followed shortly after that by flulike symptoms. Impaired cognitive functioning and mood changes are associated with the illness and may be the presenting complaint. These include memory lapses, difficulty concentrating, irritability, and depression.

No clear-cut diagnostic test is available. About 50 percent of patients become seropositive to *B. burgdorferi*. The prophylaxis vaccine is not always effective and is controversial. Treatment consists of a 14- to 21-day course of doxycycline, which results in a 90 percent cure rate. Specific psychiatric drugs can help treat the psychiatric sign or symptom (e.g., a benzodiazepine for anxiety). Left untreated, about 60 percent of persons develop a chronic condition. Such patients may get an erroneous diagnosis of a primary depression rather than one secondary to the medical condition. Support groups for patients with chronic Lyme disease are essential. Group members provide each other with emotional support that helps improve their quality of life.

Prion Disease.

Prion disease is a group of related disorders caused by a transmissible infectious protein known as a *prion*. Included in this group are Creutzfeldt–Jakob disease (CJD), Gerstmann–Sträussler–Scheinker disorder (GSS), fatal familial insomnia (FFI), and kuru. A variant of CJD (vCJD), also called "mad cow disease," appeared in 1995 in the United Kingdom and is attributed to the transmission of bovine spongiform encephalopathy (BSE) from cattle to humans. Collectively, these disorders are also known as *subacute spongiform encephalopathy* because of shared neuropathologic changes that consist of (1) spongiform vacuolization, (2) neuronal loss, and (3) astrocyte proliferation in the cerebral cortex. Amyloid plaques may or may not be present.

ETIOLOGY.   Prions are transmissible agents but differ from viruses in that they lack nucleic acid. Prions are mutated proteins generated from the human prion protein gene (PrP), located on the short arm of chromosome 20.

The PrP mutates into a disease-related isoform PrP-Super-C (PrP^{Sc}), which can replicate and is infectious. The neuropathologic changes that occur in prion disease are presumed to be caused by direct neurotoxic effects of PrP^{Sc}.

The specific prion disease that develops depends on the mutation of PrP that occurs. Mutations at PrP 178N/129V cause CJD, mutations at 178N/129M cause FFI, and mutations at 102L/129M cause GSS and kuru. Other mutations of PrP occur, and research continues in this vital area of genomic identification. Some mutations are both fully penetrant and autosomal dominant and account for inherited forms of prion disease. For example, both GSS and FFI are inherited disorders, and about 10 percent of cases of CJD are also inherited. Prenatal testing for the abnormal PrP gene is available; whether or not we should do routine testing is an open question.

CREUTZFELDT–JAKOB DISEASE.   First described in 1920, CJD is an invariably fatal, rapidly progressive disorder that occurs mainly in middle-aged or older adults. It manifests initially with fatigue, flu-like symptoms, and cognitive impairment. As the disease progresses, focal neurologic findings such as aphasia and apraxia occur. Psychiatric manifestations are protean and include emotional lability, anxiety, euphoria, depression, delusions, hallucinations, or marked personality changes. The disease progresses over months, leading to dementia, akinetic mutism, coma, and death.

The rates of CJD range from one to two cases per 1 million persons a year worldwide. The infectious agent self-replicates and can be transmitted to humans by inoculation with infected tissue and sometimes by ingestion of contaminated food. Iatrogenic transmission has been reported via transplantation of contaminated cornea or dura mater or to children via contaminated supplies of human growth hormone derived from infected persons. Neurosurgical transmission also occurs. Household contacts are not at higher risk for developing the disease than the general population unless there is direct inoculation.

Diagnosis requires a pathologic examination of the cortex, which reveals the classic triad of spongiform vacuolation, loss of neurons, and astrocyte cell proliferation. The cortex and basal ganglia are most affected. An immunoassay test for CJD in the CSF shows promise in supporting the diagnosis; however, this needs more testing. Although not specific for CJD, EEG abnormalities are present in nearly all patients, consisting of a slow and irregular background rhythm with periodic complex discharges. CT and MRI studies may reveal cortical atrophy later in the course of the disease. SPECT and positron emission tomography (PET) reveal heterogeneously decreased uptake throughout the cortex.

No known treatment exists for CJD. Death usually occurs within 6 months after diagnosis.

VARIANT CJD.   In 1995, a vCJD appeared in the United Kingdom. The patients affected all died; they were young (younger than age 40 years), and none had risk factors of CJD. At autopsy, pathologists found a prion disease. The disease was transmitted between cattle and cattle to humans in the 1980s. BSE appears to have originated from sheep scrapie–contaminated feed given to cattle. Scrapie is a spongiform encephalopathy found in sheep and goats that does not cause human disease; however, it is transmissible to other animal species.

There have been more than 200 reported cases of vCJD to date, with the majority in the United Kingdom. Four cases have been reported in the United States. Clinicians must be alert to the diagnosis in young people with behavioral and psychiatric abnormalities in association with cerebellar signs such as ataxia or myoclonus. The psychiatric presentation of vCJD is not specific. Most patients have reported depression, withdrawal, anxiety, and sleep disturbance. Paranoid delusions have occurred. Neuropathologic changes are similar to those in CJD, with the addition of amyloid plaques.

Epidemiologic data gathering is ongoing. The incubation period for vCJD and the number of infected meat products required to cause infection is unknown. One patient had been a vegetarian for 5 years before contracting the disease. vCJD can be diagnosed antemortem by examining the tonsils with Western blot immunostains to detect PrP^{Sc} in lymphoid tissue. Diagnosis relies on the development of progressive neurodegenerative features in persons who have ingested contaminated meat or brains. No cure exists, and death usually occurs within 2 to 3 years after diagnosis. Prevention is dependent on careful monitoring of cattle for disease and feeding them grain instead of meat byproducts.

KURU. Kuru is an epidemic prion disease found in New Guinea that is caused by cannibalistic funeral rituals in which the practitioners eat the brains of the deceased. Women are more affected by the disorder than men, presumably because they participate in the ceremony to a greater extent. Death usually occurs within 2 years after symptoms develop. Neuropsychiatric signs and symptoms consist of ataxia, chorea, strabismus, delirium, and dementia. Pathologic changes are similar to those with other prion diseases: neuronal loss, spongiform lesions, and astrocytic proliferation. The cerebellum is most affected. Iatrogenic transmission of kuru has occurred when doctors transplanted infected dura mater and corneas into normal recipients. Since the cessation of cannibalism in New Guinea, the incidence of the disease has decreased drastically.

GERSTMANN–STRÄUSSLER–SCHEINKER DISEASE. First described in 1928, GSS is a neurodegenerative syndrome characterized by ataxia, chorea, and cognitive decline leading to dementia. The cause is a mutation in the PrP gene that is fully penetrant and autosomal dominant; thus, the disease is inherited, and affected families have been identified over several generations. Genetic testing can confirm the presence of abnormal genes before onset. Pathologic changes characteristic of prion disease are present: spongiform lesions, neuronal loss, and astrocyte proliferation. Amyloid plaques occur in the cerebellum. The onset of the disease occurs between 30 and 40 years of age. The disease is fatal within 5 years of onset.

FATAL FAMILIAL INSOMNIA. FFI is an inherited prion disease that primarily affects the thalamus. A syndrome of insomnia and autonomic nervous system dysfunction consisting of fever, sweating, labile blood pressure, and tachycardia occurs that is debilitating. Onset is in middle adulthood, and death usually occurs in 1 year. No treatment currently exists.

FUTURE DIRECTIONS. Determining how prions mutate to produce disease phenotypes and determining how they transmit between different mammalian species are essential areas of research. Public health measures to prevent transmission of animal disease to humans are ongoing and must be relentless, mainly because these disorders are invariably fatal within a few years of onset. Developing genetic interventions that prevent or repair damage to the normal prion gene offers the best hope of a cure. Psychiatrists must manage cases of persons who have the disease and those with hypochondriacal fears of having contracted the disease. In some patients, such fears can reach delusional proportions. Treatment is symptomatic and involves anxiolytics, antidepressants, and psychostimulants, depending on symptoms. Supportive psychotherapy may be of use in early stages to help patients and families cope with the illness.

Preventing unintentional human-to-human or animal-to-human transmission of prions remains the best way to limit the scope of these diseases. Sporadic cases of CJD will still appear, however, because of the rare spontaneous mutation of the normal prion protein into the abnormal form. At present, little exists to offer patients with prion disease other than supportive treatment and emotional support.

Immune Disorders

The primary immune disorder in contemporary society is HIV and AIDS, but other immune disorders such as lupus erythematosus and autoimmune disorders that affect brain neurotransmitters (discussed below) can also present diagnostic and treatment challenges to mental health clinicians.

HIV Infection and AIDS. HIV is a retrovirus related to the human T-cell leukemia viruses (HTLV) and to retroviruses that infect animals, including nonhuman primates. At least two types of HIV exist, HIV-1 and HIV-2. HIV-1 is the causative agent for most HIV-related diseases; HIV-2, however, seems to be causing an increasing number of infections in Africa. Other types of HIV may exist, currently classified as HIV-O. HIV is present in the blood, semen, cervical and vaginal secretions, and, to a lesser extent, in saliva, tears, breast milk, and the CSF of those who are infected. HIV usually transmits through sexual intercourse or the transfer of contaminated blood from one person to another. Health providers should be aware of the guidelines for safe sexual practices and should advise their patients to practice safe sex (Table 3-35). The Centers for Disease Control and Prevention guidelines for the prevention of HIV from infected to uninfected persons is listed in Table 3-36.

After infection with HIV, AIDS develops in 8 to 11 years, although this time is gradually increasing because of early treatment. When a person is infected with HIV, the virus primarily targets T4 (helper) lymphocytes, so-called CD4+ lymphocytes, to which the virus binds because a glycoprotein (gp120) on the viral surface has a high affinity for the CD4 receptor on T4 lymphocytes. After binding, the virus can inject its ribonucleic acid (RNA) into the infected lymphocyte, where the RNA is transcribed into deoxyribonucleic acid (DNA) by the action of reverse transcriptase. The resultant DNA can then be incorporated into the host cell's genome and translated and eventually transcribed when the lymphocyte divides. After lymphocytes have produced viral proteins, the various components of the virus assemble, and new mature viruses bud off from the host cell.

Table 3-35
AIDS Safe-Sex Guidelines

Safe Sexual Behaviors and Risk-Reduction Strategies for patients with HIV
- Adhering to ART and ongoing medical care, even if viral load is undetectable.
- Communicating HIV status with others.
- Correctly and consistently using condoms (to prevent STDs) and appropriate non–oil-based lubricants, even when negotiation of use occurs in the heat of the moment.
- Assessing relative risk of HIV transmission associated with various sexual activities (e.g., oral sex is less risky than receptive anal sex).
- Discussing how alcohol and/or drug use can impair judgment.
- Using PrEP for some HIV-negative partners, including women planning to become pregnant.
- Using PEP for emergencies for HIV-negative or unknown status partners (e.g., if a condom breaks or is not used and the patient is not virally suppressed).

Source: Centers for Disease Control and Prevention. Safer sexual behavior. https://www.cdc.gov/hiv/clinicians/treatment/safer-sex.html#discussion-topics

Table 3-36
Centers for Disease Control and Prevention Guidelines for the Prevention of HIV Transmission from Infected to Uninfected Persons

Infected persons should be counseled to prevent the further transmission of HIV by:

1. Informing prospective sex partners of their infection with HIV so they can take appropriate precautions. Abstention from sexual activity with another person is one option that would eliminate any risk of sexually transmitted HIV infection.
2. Protecting a partner during any sexual activity by taking appropriate precautions to prevent that person's coming into contact with the infected person's blood, semen, urine, feces, saliva, cervical secretions, or vaginal secretions. Although the efficacy of using condoms to prevent infections with HIV is still under study, the consistent use of condoms should reduce the transmission of HIV by preventing exposure to semen and infected lymphocytes.
3. Informing previous sex partners and any persons with whom needles were shared of their potential exposure to HIV and encouraging them to seek counseling and testing.
4. For IV drug abusers, enrolling or continuing in programs to eliminate the abuse of IV substances. Needles, other apparatus, and drugs must never be shared.
5. Never sharing toothbrushes, razors, or other items that could become contaminated with blood.
6. Refraining from donating blood, plasma, body organs, other tissue, or semen.
7. Avoiding pregnancy until more is known about the risks of transmitting HIV from the mother to the fetus or newborn.
8. Cleaning and disinfecting surfaces on which blood or other body fluids have spilled in accordance with previous recommendations.
9. Informing physicians, dentists, and other appropriate health professionals of antibody status when seeking medical care, so that the patient can be appropriately evaluated.

HIV, human immunodeficiency virus; IV, intravenous.
From Centers for Disease Control (CDC). Additional recommendations to reduce sexual and drug abuse-related transmission of human T-lymphotropic virus type III/lymphadenopathy-associated virus. *MMWR Morb Mortal Wkly Rep.* 1986;35:152.

DIAGNOSIS

Serum Testing. Techniques are now widely available to detect the presence of anti-HIV antibodies in humans. The conventional test uses blood (time to result, 3 to 10 days), and the rapid test uses an oral swab (time to result, 20 minutes). Both tests are 99.9 percent sensitive and specific. Health care workers and their patients must understand that the presence of HIV antibodies indicates infection, not immunity to infection. Those who test positive have been exposed to the virus, have the virus within their bodies, have the potential to transmit the virus to another person, and will almost certainly eventually develop AIDS. Those who test negative either have not been exposed to HIV or were exposed but have not yet developed antibodies; the latter is possible if the exposure was less than a year prior. Seroconversion most commonly occurs 6 to 12 weeks after infection, although in rare cases, seroconversion can take 6 to 12 months.

COUNSELING. Although specific groups of persons who are at high risk for contracting HIV are a priority, anyone who wants a test should have it. We should try to ascertain the reason for the request, to detect unspoken concerns and motivations that may merit psychotherapeutic intervention.

Counseling should include a discussion of past practices that may have put the testee at risk for HIV infection and safe sexual practices. During posttest counseling, counselors should

explain that a negative test finding implies that the person should espouse safe sexual behavior and avoid shared needles to remain free of infection. Those with positive results must receive counseling about safe practices and potential treatment options. They may need additional psychotherapeutic interventions if anxiety or depressive disorders develop after they discover that they are infected. A person may react to a positive HIV test finding with a syndrome similar to posttraumatic stress disorder. Adjustment disorder with anxiety or depressed mood may develop in as many as 25 percent of those informed of a positive HIV test result.

CONFIDENTIALITY. No one should be given an HIV test without previous knowledge and consent, although various jurisdictions and organizations, such as the military, now require HIV testing for all inhabitants or members. The results of an HIV test can be shared with other members of a medical team, although no one else should have the information except for exceptional circumstances. We should advise the patient against disclosing the result of HIV testing too readily to employers, friends, and family members; the information could result in discrimination in employment, housing, and insurance.

The major exception to restriction of disclosure is the need to notify potential and past sexual or IV substance use partners. If a treating physician knows that a patient who is HIV infected is putting another person at risk of becoming infected, the physician may try either to hospitalize the infected person involuntarily (to prevent danger to others) or to notify the potential victim. Clinicians should be aware of the laws about such issues, which vary among the states. These guidelines also apply to inpatient psychiatric wards when a patient with HIV infection may have had sex with other patients.

CLINICAL FEATURES

Nonneurologic Factors. About 30 percent of persons infected with HIV experience a flulike syndrome 3 to 6 weeks after becoming infected; most never notice any symptoms immediately or shortly after their infection. The flulike syndrome includes fever, myalgia, headaches, fatigue, GI symptoms, and sometimes a rash. The syndrome may include splenomegaly and lymphadenopathy.

The most common infection in persons affected with HIV who have AIDS is *Pneumocystis carinii* pneumonia, which is characterized by a chronic, nonproductive cough and dyspnea, sometimes sufficiently severe to result in hypoxia and its resultant cognitive effects. For psychiatrists, the importance of these nonneurologic, nonpsychiatric complications lies in their biologic effects on patients' brain function (e.g., hypoxia in *P. carinii* pneumonia) and their psychological effects on patients' moods and anxiety states.

Neurologic Factors. An extensive array of disease processes can affect the brain of a patient infected with HIV (Table 3-37). The most important diseases for mental health workers to be aware of are *HIV mild neurocognitive disorder* and *HIV-associated dementia.*

Psychiatric Syndromes. HIV-associated dementia presents with the typical triad of symptoms seen in other subcortical dementias—memory and psychomotor speed impairments, depressive symptoms, and movement disorders. Patients may initially notice slight problems with reading, comprehension, memory, and mathematical skills, but these symptoms are subtle and may be overlooked or discounted as fatigue and illness. The Modified HIV Dementia

Table 3-37
Conditions Associated with Human Immunodeficiency Virus (HIV) Infection

Bacterial infections, multiple or recurrent[a]
Candidiasis of bronchi, trachea, or lungs
Candidiasis, esophageal
Cervical cancer, invasive[b]
Coccidioidomycosis, disseminated or extrapulmonary
Cryptococcosis, extrapulmonary
Cryptosporidiosis, chronic intestinal (>1 mo duration)
Cytomegalovirus disease (other than liver, spleen, or nodes)
Cytomegalovirus retinitis (with loss of vision)
Encephalopathy, HIV-related
Herpes simplex, chronic ulcers (>1 mo duration); or bronchitis, pulmonitis, or esophagitis
Histoplasmosis, disseminated or extrapulmonary
Isosporiasis, chronic intestinal (>1 mo duration)
Kaposi sarcoma
Lymphoid interstitial pneumonia or pulmonary lymphoid hyperplasia[a]
Lymphoma, Burkitt's (or equivalent term)
Lymphoma, immunoblastic (or equivalent term)
Lymphoma, primary, of brain
Mycobacterium avium complex or *Mycobacterium kansasii,* disseminated or extrapulmonary
Mycobacterium tuberculosis, any site (pulmonary[b] or extrapulmonary)
Mycobacterium, other species or unidentified species, disseminated or extrapulmonary
Pneumocystis carinii pneumonia
Pneumonia, recurrent[b]
Progressive multifocal leukoencephalopathy
Salmonella septicemia, recurrent
Toxoplasmosis of brain
Wasting syndrome due to HIV

[a]Children younger than 13 years old.
[b]Added in the 1993 expansion of the AIDS surveillance case definition for adolescents and adults.
Adapted from 1993 revised classification system for HIV infection and expanded surveillance, case definition for AIDS among adolescents and adults. *MMWR Recomm Rep.* 1992:41.

Scale is a useful bedside screen and can document disease progress with serial administration. The development of dementia in HIV-infected patients is generally a poor prognostic sign, and 50 to 75 percent of patients with dementia die within 6 months.

HIV-associated neurocognitive disorder (also known as HIV encephalopathy) involves impaired cognitive functioning and reduced mental activity that interferes with work, domestic, and social functioning. No laboratory findings are specific to the disorder, and it occurs independently of depression and anxiety. Progression of HIV-associated dementia usually occurs but may be prevented by early treatment.

Delirium can result from the same causes that lead to dementia in patients with HIV. Clinicians have classified delirious states characterized by both increased and decreased activities. Delirium in patients infected with HIV is probably underdiagnosed, but it should always precipitate a medical workup of a patient infected with HIV to determine whether a new CNS-related process has begun.

Patients with HIV infection may have any of the anxiety disorders, but generalized anxiety disorder, posttraumatic stress disorder, and obsessive-compulsive disorder (OCD) are particularly common.

Adjustment disorder with anxiety or depressed mood occurs in 5 to 20 percent of HIV-infected patients. The incidence of adjustment disorder in HIV-infected patients is higher than usual in some special populations, such as military recruits and prison inmates.

Depression is a significant problem in HIV and AIDS. Approximately 4 to 40 percent of HIV-infected patients meet the criteria for depressive disorders. Major depression is a risk factor for HIV infection by its impact on behavior, intensification of substance abuse, exacerbation of self-destructive behaviors, and promotion for poor partner choice in relationships. The pre-HIV infection prevalence of depressive disorders may be higher than usual in some groups who are at risk for contracting HIV. Depression can hinder effective treatment in infected persons. Patients with major depression are at increased risk of disease progression and death. HIV increases the risk of developing major depression through a variety of mechanisms, including direct injury to subcortical areas of the brain, chronic stress, worsening social isolation, and intense demoralization. Depression is higher in women than in men.

Mania can occur at any stage of HIV infection for individuals with preexisting bipolar disorder. AIDS mania is a type of mania that most commonly occurs in late-stage HIV infections and is associated with cognitive impairment. AIDS mania has a somewhat different clinical profile than bipolar mania. Patients tend to have cognitive slowing or dementia, and irritability is more characteristic than euphoria. AIDS mania is usually quite severe in its presentation and malignant in its course. It seems to be more chronic than episodic, has infrequent spontaneous remissions, and usually relapses with the cessation of treatment. One clinically significant presentation is the delusional belief that one has discovered the cure for HIV or has been cured, which may result in high-risk behaviors and the spread of the HIV infection.

Substance abuse is a primary vector for the spread of HIV. This is true not only for IV drug users and their partners but others impaired by substances. All addictions tend to increase impulsive and unsafe behaviors. Ongoing substance abuse has grave medical implications for HIV-infected patients. The accumulation of medical sequelae from chronic substance abuse can accelerate the process of immunocompromise and amplify the progressive burdens of the HIV infection itself. In addition to the direct physical effects caused by drugs, active substance use is highly associated with both nonadherence and reduced access to antiretroviral medication.

Suicidal ideation and suicide attempts may increase in patients with HIV infection and AIDS. The risk factors for suicide among persons infected with HIV include having friends who died from AIDS, recent notification of HIV seropositivity, relapses, complicated social issues relating to homosexuality, inadequate social and financial support, and the presence of dementia or delirium.

Psychotic symptoms are usually later-stage complications of HIV infection. They require an immediate medical and neurologic evaluation and often require management with antipsychotic medications.

The worried well are people in high-risk groups who, although they tested negative and are disease-free, are anxious about contracting the virus. Repeated negative test results reassure some, but others cannot be reassured. Their worry well status can progress quickly to generalized anxiety disorder, panic attacks, OCD, and a somatic symptom and related disorder.

TREATMENT. Prevention is the primary approach to HIV infection. Primary prevention involves protecting persons from getting the disease; secondary prevention involves modification of the disease's course. All persons with any risk of HIV infection should be informed about safe-sex practices and about the necessity to avoid sharing contaminated hypodermic needles. The assessment of patients infected with HIV should include a complete sexual and substance use history, a psychiatric history, and an evaluation of the support systems available to them.

Pharmacotherapy.   A growing list of agents that act at different points in viral replication has raised the hope that HIV might be permanently suppressed or eradicated from the body. These agents divide into five major drug classes. Reverse transcriptase inhibitors (RTIs) interfere with the critical step during the HIV life cycle known as reverse transcription. There are two types of RTIs: nucleoside/nucleotide RTIs (NRTIs), which are faulty DNA building blocks, and nonnucleoside RTIs (NNRTIs), which bind to RT, interfering with its ability to convert the HIV RNA into HIV DNA. Protease inhibitors interfere with the protease enzyme that HIV uses to produce infectious viral particles. Fusion or entry inhibitors interfere with the virus's ability to fuse with the cellular membrane, thereby blocking entry into the host cell. Integrase inhibitors block integrase, the enzyme HIV uses to integrate the genetic material of the virus into its target host cell. Multidrug combination products combine drugs from more than one class into a single product. The most common of this class of drugs is the highly active antiretroviral therapy (HAART). Table 3-38 lists the available agents in each of these categories.

Antiretroviral agents have many adverse effects. Of importance to psychiatrists is that protease inhibitors can increase levels of certain psychotropic drugs such as bupropion, meperidine, various benzodiazepines, and selective serotonin reuptake inhibitors (SSRIs). We should take caution when prescribing psychiatric drugs to persons taking protease inhibitors.

Psychotherapy.   Major psychodynamic themes for patients infected with HIV involved self-blame, self-esteem, and issues regarding death. The entire range of psychotherapeutic approaches may be appropriate for patients with HIV-related disorders. Both individual and group therapy can be useful. Individual therapy may be either short term or long term and may be supportive, cognitive, behavioral, or psychodynamic. Group therapy techniques can range from psychodynamic to completely supportive. It is crucial to include direct counseling regarding substance use and its potential adverse effects on the health of the patient. Specific treatments for particular substance-related disorders should be initiated if necessary for the total well-being of the patient.

Systemic Lupus Erythematosus.
Systemic lupus erythematosus (SLE) is an autoimmune disease that involves inflammation of multiple organ systems. The officially accepted diagnosis of SLE requires a patient to have 4 of 11 criteria that have been defined by the American Rheumatism Association. Between 5 and 50 percent of patients with SLE have mental symptoms at the initial presentation, and approximately 50 percent eventually show neuropsychiatric manifestations. The primary symptoms are depression, insomnia, emotional lability, nervousness, and confusion. Treatment with steroids commonly induces further psychiatric complications, including mania and psychosis.

Autoimmune Disorders Affecting Brain Neurotransmitters.
A group of autoimmune receptor-seeking disorders exists that causes encephalitis that mimics schizophrenia. Among those is anti-NMDA (N-methyl D-aspartate)-receptor encephalitis that

Table 3-38
Antiretroviral Agents

Generic Names	Trade Name	Usual Abbreviation
Reverse Transcriptase Inhibitors		
Nucleoside/nucleotide reverse transcriptase inhibitors		
Lamivudine and zidovudine	Combivir	
Emtricitabine	Emtriva	FTC
Lamivudine	Epivir	3TC
Abacavir and lamivudine	Epzicom	
Zidovudine, azidothymidine	Retrovir	ZDV or AZT
Abacavir, zidovudine, and lamivudine	Trizivir	
Tenofovir disoproxil fumarate and emtricitabine	Truvada	
Didanosine, dideoxyinosine	Videx	ddl
Enteric-coated didanosine	Videx EC	ddl EC
Tenofovir disoproxil fumarate	Viread	TDF
Stavudine	Zerit	d4t
Abacavir sulfate	Ziagen	ABC
Nonnucleoside Reverse Transcriptase Inhibitors		
Rilpivirine	Edurant	
Etravirine	Intelence	
Delavirdine	Rescriptor	DLV
Efavirenz	Sustiva	EFV
Nevirapine	Viramune	NVP
Protease Inhibitors		
Amprenavir	Agenerase	APV
Tipranavir	Aptivus	TPV
Indinavir	Crixivan	IDV
Saquinavir mesylate	Invirase	SQV
Lopinavir and ritonavir	Kaletra	LPV/RTV
Fosamprenavir calcium	Lexiva	FOS-APV
Ritonavir	Norvir	RTV
Darunavir	Prezista	
Atazanavir sulfate	Reyataz	ATV
Delfinavir mesylate	Viracept	NFV
Fusion/Entry Inhibitors		
Enfuvirtide	Fuzeon	T-20
Maraviroc	Selzentry	
Multi-Class Combination Products		
Efavirenz, emtricitabine, and tenofovir disoproxil fumarate	Atripla	
Emtricitabine, rilpivirine, and tenofovir disoproxil fumarate	Complera	

causes dissociative symptoms, amnesia, and vivid hallucinations. The disorder occurs mostly in women; the memoir *Brain on Fire* vividly chronicled the writer's experience with it. There is no treatment, although intravenous immunoglobulins have proved useful. Recovery does occur, but some patients might require prolonged intensive care.

Endocrine Disorders

Thyroid Disorders.
Hyperthyroidism includes symptoms of confusion, anxiety, and an agitated, depressive syndrome. Patients may also complain of being easily fatigued and of feeling generally weak. Insomnia, weight loss despite increased appetite, tremulousness, palpitations, and increased perspiration are also common symptoms. Serious psychiatric symptoms include impairments in

memory, orientation, and judgment, manic excitement, delusions, and hallucinations.

In 1949, Irvin Asher named hypothyroidism "myxedema madness." In its most severe form, hypothyroidism includes symptoms of paranoia, depression, hypomania, and hallucinations. Slowed thinking and delirium can also be symptoms. The physical symptoms include weight gain, a deep voice, thin and dry hair, loss of the lateral eyebrow, facial puffiness, cold intolerance, and impaired hearing. Approximately 10 percent of all patients have residual neuropsychiatric symptoms after hormone replacement therapy.

Parathyroid Disorders.   Dysfunction of the parathyroid gland results in the abnormal regulation of calcium metabolism. Excessive secretion of parathyroid hormone causes hypercalcemia, which can result in delirium, personality changes, and apathy in 50 to 60 percent of patients and cognitive impairments in approximately 25 percent of patients. Neuromuscular excitability, which depends on proper calcium ion concentration, is reduced, and muscle weakness may appear.

Hypocalcemia can occur with hypoparathyroidism and can result in neuropsychiatric symptoms of delirium and personality changes. If the calcium level decreases gradually, clinicians may see the psychiatric symptoms without the characteristic tetany of hypocalcemia. Other symptoms of hypocalcemia are cataract formation, seizures, extrapyramidal symptoms, and increased intracranial pressure.

Adrenal Disorders.   Adrenal disorders disturb the normal secretion of hormones from the adrenal cortex and produce significant neurologic and psychological changes. Chronic adrenocortical insufficiency (Addison's disease) is usually the result of adrenocortical atrophy or granulomatous invasion caused by tuberculous or fungal infection. Patients with this disorder exhibit mild mental symptoms, such as apathy, easy fatigability, irritability, and depression. Occasionally, confusion or psychotic reactions develop. Cortisone or one of its synthetic derivatives is effective in correcting such abnormalities.

Excessive quantities of cortisol produced endogenously by an adrenocortical tumor or hyperplasia (Cushing syndrome) lead to a secondary mood disorder, a syndrome of agitated depression, and often suicide. Decreased concentration and memory deficits may also be present. Psychotic reactions, with schizophrenia-like symptoms, are seen in a few patients. The administration of high doses of exogenous corticosteroids typically leads to a secondary mood disorder similar to mania. Severe depression can follow the termination of steroid therapy.

Pituitary Disorders.   Patients with total pituitary failure can exhibit psychiatric symptoms, particularly postpartum women who have hemorrhaged into the pituitary, a condition known as *Sheehan syndrome*. Patients have a combination of symptoms, especially of thyroid and adrenal disorders, and can show virtually any psychiatric symptom.

Metabolic Disorders

A common cause of organic brain dysfunction, metabolic encephalopathy can produce alterations in mental processes, behavior, and neurologic functions. We should consider the diagnosis whenever recent and rapid changes in behavior, thinking, and consciousness occur. The earliest signals are likely to be impairment of memory, particularly recent memory, and impairment of orientation. Some patients become agitated, anxious, and hyperactive; others become quiet, withdrawn, and inactive. As metabolic encephalopathies

progress, confusion or delirium gives way to decreased responsiveness, stupor, and, eventually, death.

Hepatic Encephalopathy.   Severe hepatic failure can result in hepatic encephalopathy, characterized by asterixis, hyperventilation, EEG abnormalities, and alterations in consciousness. The alterations in consciousness can range from apathy to drowsiness to coma. Associated psychiatric symptoms are changes in memory, general intellectual skills, and personality.

Uremic Encephalopathy.   Renal failure is associated with alterations in memory, orientation, and consciousness. Restlessness, crawling sensations on the limbs, muscle twitching, and persistent hiccups are associated symptoms. In young people with brief episodes of uremia, the neuropsychiatric symptoms tend to be reversible; in older people with prolonged episodes of uremia, the neuropsychiatric symptoms can be irreversible.

Hypoglycemic Encephalopathy.   Hypoglycemic encephalopathy can be caused either by excessive endogenous production of insulin or by excessive exogenous insulin administration. The premonitory symptoms, which do not occur in every patient, include nausea, sweating, tachycardia, and feelings of hunger, apprehension, and restlessness. As the disorder progresses, disorientation, confusion, and hallucinations, as well as other neurologic and medical symptoms, can develop. Stupor and coma can occur, and residual and persistent dementia can sometimes be a serious neuropsychiatric sequela of the disorder.

Diabetic Ketoacidosis.   Diabetic ketoacidosis begins with feelings of weakness, easy fatigability, and listlessness and increasing polyuria and polydipsia. Headache and, sometimes, nausea and vomiting appear. Patients with diabetes mellitus have an increased likelihood of chronic dementia with general arteriosclerosis.

Acute Intermittent Porphyria.   The porphyrias are disorders of heme biosynthesis that result in excessive accumulation of porphyrins. The triad of symptoms is acute, colicky abdominal pain, motor polyneuropathy, and psychosis. Acute intermittent porphyria is an autosomal dominant disorder that affects more women than men and has its onset between ages 20 and 50 years. The psychiatric symptoms include anxiety, insomnia, lability of mood, depression, and psychosis. Some studies have found that between 0.2 and 0.5 percent of chronic psychiatric patients may have undiagnosed porphyrias. Barbiturates precipitate or aggravate the attacks of acute porphyria, and we should never use them in this disorder (less a concern in modern treatments, however some headache treatments, e.g., Fioricet and Fiorinal, remain popular). We should also avoid those or similar medications in relatives or people with the disease.

Nutritional Disorders

Niacin Deficiency.   Dietary insufficiency of niacin (nicotinic acid) and its precursor tryptophan are associated with pellagra, a globally occurring nutritional deficiency disease seen in association with alcohol abuse, vegetarian diets, and extreme poverty and starvation. The neuropsychiatric symptoms of pellagra include apathy, irritability, insomnia, depression, and delirium; the medical symptoms include dermatitis, peripheral neuropathies, and diarrhea. Traditionally, some refer to the course of pellagra as the "five Ds": dermatitis, diarrhea, delirium, dementia, and death. The response to treatment with nicotinic acid is rapid, but dementia from prolonged illness may improve only slowly and incompletely.

Thiamine Deficiency.   Thiamine (vitamin B$_1$) deficiency leads to beriberi, characterized chiefly by cardiovascular and neurologic changes, and to Wernicke–Korsakoff syndrome, which is most often associated with chronic alcohol abuse. Beriberi occurs primarily in Asia and areas of famine and poverty. The psychiatric symptoms include apathy, depression, irritability, nervousness, and poor concentration; severe memory disorders can develop with prolonged deficiencies.

Cobalamin Deficiency.   Deficiencies in cobalamin (vitamin B$_{12}$) arise because of the failure of the gastric mucosal cells to secrete a specific substance, intrinsic factor, required for the normal absorption of vitamin B$_{12}$ in the ileum. The deficiency state is characterized by the development of a chronic macrocytic megaloblastic anemia (pernicious anemia) and by neurologic manifestations resulting from degenerative changes in the peripheral nerves, the spinal cord, and the brain. Neurologic changes occur in approximately 80 percent of all patients. These changes are commonly associated with megaloblastic anemia, but they occasionally precede the onset of hematologic abnormalities.

Mental changes, such as apathy, depression, irritability, and moodiness, are frequent. In a few patients, encephalopathy and its associated delirium, delusions, hallucinations, dementia, and sometimes paranoid features are prominent and are sometimes called *megaloblastic madness.* The neurologic manifestations of vitamin B$_{12}$ deficiency can be rapidly and entirely arrested by early and continued administration of parenteral vitamin therapy.

Toxins

Environmental toxins are becoming an increasingly severe threat to physical and mental health in contemporary society.

Mercury.   Either inorganic or organic mercury can cause mercury poisoning. Inorganic mercury poisoning results in the "mad hatter" syndrome (previously seen in workers in the hat industry who softened mercury-containing felt by putting it in their mouths), with depression, irritability, and psychosis. Associated neurologic symptoms are headache, tremor, and weakness. Contaminated fish or grain can cause organic mercury poisoning and result in depression, irritability, and cognitive impairment. Associated symptoms are sensory neuropathies, cerebellar ataxia, dysarthria, paresthesias, and visual field defects. Mercury poisoning in pregnant women causes abnormal fetal development. No specific therapy is available, although chelation therapy with dimercaprol may help with acute poisoning.

Lead.   Lead poisoning occurs when the amount of lead ingested exceeds the body's ability to eliminate it. It takes several months for toxic symptoms to appear.

The signs and symptoms of lead poisoning depend on the level of lead in the blood. When lead reaches levels above 200 mg/L, symptoms of severe lead encephalopathy occur, with dizziness, clumsiness, ataxia, irritability, restlessness, headache, and insomnia. Later, an excited delirium occurs, with associated vomiting and visual disturbances, and progresses to convulsions, lethargy, and coma.

Treatment of lead encephalopathy should be instituted as rapidly as possible, even without laboratory confirmation, because of the high mortality rate. The treatment of choice to facilitate lead excretion is intravenous administration of calcium disodium edetate (calcium disodium versenate) daily for 5 days.

Manganese.   Early manganese poisoning (sometimes called *manganese madness*) causes symptoms of headache, irritability, joint pains, and somnolence. An eventual picture appears of emotional lability, pathologic laughter, nightmares, hallucinations, and compulsive and impulsive acts associated with periods of confusion and aggressiveness. Lesions involving the basal ganglia and pyramidal system result in gait impairment, rigidity, monotonous or whispering speech, tremors of the extremities and tongue, masked facies (manganese mask), micrographia, dystonia, dysarthria, and loss of equilibrium. The psychological effects tend to clear 3 or 4 months after the patient's removal from the site of exposure, but neurologic symptoms tend to remain stationary or to progress. No specific treatment exists for manganese poisoning, other than removal from the source of poisoning. The disorder occurs in persons working in refining ore, brick workers, and those making steel casings.

Arsenic.   Chronic arsenic poisoning most commonly results from prolonged exposure to herbicides containing arsenic or from drinking water contaminated with arsenic. Silicon-based computer chip manufacturing also uses arsenic. Early signs of toxicity are skin pigmentation, GI complaints, renal and hepatic dysfunction, hair loss, and a characteristic garlic odor to the breath. Encephalopathy eventually occurs, with generalized sensory and motor loss. Chelation therapy with dimercaprol can help successfully treat arsenic poisoning.

▲ 3.5 Mild Cognitive Impairment

The past decade has seen the emergence of a new concept, *mild cognitive impairment* (MCI), which is defined as the presence of mild cognitive decline not warranting the diagnosis of dementia but with preserved basic activities of daily living.

DSM-5 classifies MCI as *mild neurocognitive disorder due to multiple etiologies or unspecified neurocognitive disorder.* It will most likely receive more attention in future revisions of the DSM.

DEFINITION

Although the term *mild cognitive impairment* has been in use for more than 25 years, it became a diagnostic category because of the need to fill the gap between cognitive changes associated with aging and cognitive impairment suggestive of dementia. The criteria proposed by the Mayo Clinic Alzheimer's Disease Research Center (MCADRC) are listed in Table 3-39. At this time, there are no international diagnostic criteria for MCI.

Table 3-39
Mild Cognitive Impairment Original Criteria

1. Memory complaint, preferably qualified by an informant
2. Memory impairment for age and education
3. Preserved general cognitive function
4. Intact activities of daily living
5. Not demented

Table 3-40
Terms Related to Mild Cognitive Impairment

Term	Author(s)	Year	Inclusion Criteria	Observations
Malignant senescent forgetfulness (MSF)	VA Kral	1962	Memory difficulties for recent events Lack of awareness regarding the memory deficit	Two-year follow-up showed a faster evolution of patients with MSF toward dementia
Age-associated memory impairment (AAMI)	NIMH (Crook, Bartus, and Ferris)	1986	Age-related memory disturbances leading to (1) subjective concern; (2) functional problem No underlying neurologic illness	Memory tests were validated on young populations, leading to high rates of AAMI in elderly adults
Age-associated cognitive decline (AACD)	International Psychogeriatric Association and World Health Organization (Levy)	1994	Cognitive deficits not meeting the criteria for dementia	Does not include prognosis regarding evolution to dementia Includes several kinds of cognitive decline (not exclusive memory decline)
Cognitively impaired no dementia (CIND)	Canadian Study of Health and Aging	1997	Age 65 yr and older	Includes static encephalopathies

Historical Perspective

The imprecise border between normal aging-related cognitive decline and dementia-related cognitive impairment has been described for several decades. Thus, in 1962, Kral introduced the terms *benign senescent forgetfulness* (forgetfulness for less essential facts and awareness of problems) and *malignant senescent forgetfulness* (memory problems for recent events and lack of awareness). In 1986, the National Institutes of Mental Health (NIMH) recommended the term *age-associated memory impairment* for age-related normal memory changes. In 1994, the International Psychogeriatrics Association presented the concept of *age-associated cognitive decline,* which described cognitive deficits, including but not limited to memory impairment, in the absence of dementia or other affecting cognitive conditions. *Cognitive impairment no dementia* was introduced in 1997 by the Canadian Study of Health and Aging to describe the presence of nondemented cognitive impairment regardless of the underlying process (neurologic, psychiatric, medical). Several other classifications, including age-consistent memory impairment and late-life forgetfulness, are defined on the bases of performance on various cognitive tests (Table 3-40).

The exact place of MCI in the psychiatric nosology will be challenging. Based on the current definition of MCI, functional impairment is an exclusion criterion for MCI, but the same "functional impairment" is one of the standard criteria for defining psychiatric disorders. Further developments in finding biologic markers for MCI will probably contribute to a more solid conceptualization and, hopefully, treatment of patients with prodromal dementia.

CLINICAL PRESENTATION

The clinical picture of MCI is a function of the criteria used to define it. Memory impairment is necessary but has been challenging to quantify. One measure has been an objective loss of memory or other cognitive domain that is more than 1.5 standard deviations below the mean for individuals of similar age and education. Some have suggested subjective complaints of memory loss be a marker, but this runs the risk of many false-positive diagnoses.

Assessment

Neuropsychological Assessment. Most experts agree that earlier deficits occur in episodic (vs. semantic) memory. There is no consensus among experts concerning which memory tests and which cutoffs to use. There is a lack of norms, test scores do not have normal distributions, and multiple demographic characteristics influence test performance. Several experts have proposed that a scale such as the delayed recall task from the Consortium to Establish a Registry for Alzheimer Disease might be useful in detecting Alzheimer disease in the earliest stages. Brief mental status instruments (e.g., the Mini-Mental State Examination) are relatively insensitive for the detection of memory problems in MCI.

Biomarkers. In the past decade, researchers have studied several markers of progression from MCI to dementia of the Alzheimer type. Among these, apolipoprotein E4 (APOE4) allele carrier status has been one of the most prominent variables. For the amnestic MCI, APOE4 is a risk factor for a more rapid progression to Alzheimer disease. Several CSF markers are also possible predictors of disease progression: Pathologic low concentrations of $A\beta_{42}$ (the 42 amino acid form of β-amyloid), as well as pathologic high concentrations of total tau (t-tau) and phospho tau (p-tau), may differentiate early Alzheimer disease from normal aging. Locating alterations in the expression of proteins involved in the pathogenetic pathways of Alzheimer disease (proteomic approach) is another approach used to help early detection of Alzheimer disease. We can identify several proteins (cystatin C, β-2 microglobulin, and BEGF polypeptides) through new techniques, and currently, there are several proteins from both CSF and blood that correlate with Alzheimer disease pathology.

Genetics. Because MCI is likely a prodromal stage for several disorders (dementia of the Alzheimer type frontotemporal or vascular dementia), different genes are probably related to MCI. Four genes have a relationship with Alzheimer disease: the *APP* gene, presenilin-1 (*PSEN1*), presenilin-2 (*PSEN2*), and the apolipoprotein E (*APOE*) gene. Because the first three genes are involved in rare autosomal dominant forms of Alzheimer disease, screening for each of these mutations will have minimal value for the diagnosis of MCI in the general population. The *APOE* gene, a common genetic

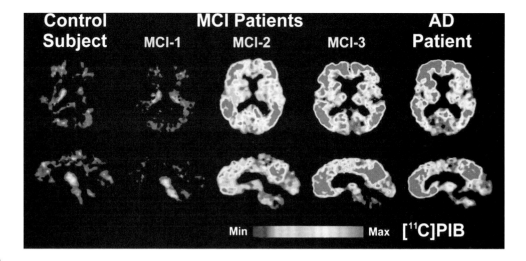

FIGURE 3-11

Positron emission tomography images obtained with the amyloid-imaging agent Pittsburgh Compound-B ([carbon-11]-PIB) in a normal individual with mild cognitive impairment (MCI; *center images*) and a patient with mild Alzheimer disease (AD) (*far right*). Some MCI patients have control-like levels of amyloid, some have Alzheimer disease–like levels of amyloid, and some have intermediate levels. (Courtesy of William E. Klunk, M.D., University of Pittsburgh, Department of Psychiatry, Pittsburgh, PA. All rights retained.)

risk factor for early as well as for late-onset Alzheimer disease, has been studied more thoroughly in relationship to MCI, but the results have been inconsistent. Because the etiology of MCI is heterogeneous, a very large number of different genes likely underlie the pathology of MCI. We have not discovered many of these genes.

Neuroimaging. Advances in neuroimaging studies aim to develop measures allowing the differentiation between MCI and healthy aging as well as within MCI among subjects who will convert to dementia of the Alzheimer type or will remain stable over time.

Structural studies of volumetric MCI showed early changes in the medial temporal structures, including neuronal atrophy, decreased synaptic density, and overall neuronal loss. Atrophy of the hippocampal volume and entorhinal cortex occur in MCI. Hippocampal formation atrophy predicts the rate of progression from MCI to dementia of the Alzheimer type. Three-dimensional modeling techniques have localized shape alteration and specific regions of atrophy within the hippocampus. Other methods, such as tensor-based morphometry, allow tracking brain changes in detail, quantifying tissue growth or atrophy throughout the brain and indicating the local rate at which one loses tissue. Other innovations in neuroimaging include MR relaxometry, imaging of iron deposition, diffusion tensor imaging, and high-field MRI scanning.

Perhaps the most promising development has been the advent of PET tracer compounds that visualize amyloid plaques and neurofibrillary tangles. These new compounds—Pittsburgh Compound B (carbon-11-PIB) and fluorine-18-FDDNP—track pathology changes in the preclinical stages of Alzheimer disease. These specific tracers allow investigators to visualize the pathologic process and are also used to monitor progression from MCI to Alzheimer disease. However, the burden of β-amyloid plaques does not always correlate with the clinical stages, because some MCI subjects can present with a minimal burden similar to healthy control participants, but others have amyloid burden comparable to Alzheimer disease participants. A single biomarker will probably be insufficient to identify incipient Alzheimer disease. Thus, the combination of several markers further increases the accuracy of the prediction and will probably become the norm as described by recent studies

(the combination of decreased parietal rCBF and CSF biomarkers as Aβ42, t-tau, and p-tau) (Fig. 3-11).

Diagnostic Differential

The Cognitive Continuum. The cognitive continuum describes the subtle pathway from age-related cognitive decline to MCI to dementia. Per this model, there is an overlap at both ends of MCI, which indicates that it can be quite challenging to identify the transition points (Fig. 3-12). In practice, differentiating MCI from age-related cognitive decline resides mainly on neuropsychological testing, showing a cognitive decline more severe for age and less education. The primary differentiation between MCI and dementia of the Alzheimer type resides in the lack of functional impairment in MCI.

COURSE AND PROGNOSIS

The typical rate at which MCI patients progress to dementia of the Alzheimer type is 10 to 15 percent per year and is associated with progressive loss of function. However, several studies have

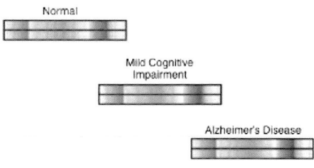

FIGURE 3-12

Cognitive continuum showing the overlap in the boundary between normal aging and the mild cognitive impairment and Alzheimer disease. (Reprinted with permission from Petersen RC, ed. *Mild Cognitive Impairment: Aging to Alzheimer's Disease.* New York: Oxford University Press, 2003.)

indicated that the diagnosis is not stable in both directions; patients can either convert to dementia of the Alzheimer type or revert to normal. This variability in course relates to the heterogeneous source of the subjects (clinical vs. community) as well as to the heterogeneous definition criteria used by different studies. Amnestic MCI occurs with increased morbidity compared with reference subjects.

TREATMENT

There are no FDA-approved treatments for MCI at this time. MCI treatment involves adequate screening and diagnosis. Ideally, MCI treatment would also include improvement of memory loss, together with the prevention of further cognitive decline to dementia. Cognitive training programs may be mildly beneficial for compensating memory difficulties in MCI. Most likely, controlling vascular risk factors (high blood pressure, hypercholesterolemia, diabetes mellitus) helps to prevent the progression of MCI cases with underlying vascular pathology. Currently, sensitive tools (imaging techniques or biomarkers) are not available for MCI screening in the general population.

In the primary care setting, clinicians should maintain a high suspicion for subjective cognitive complaints and should corroborate these complaints with collateral information whenever possible. Also, identifying reversible causes of cognitive impairment (hypothyroidism, vitamin B_{12} deficiency, medication-induced cognitive impairment, depression) can further benefit some of the prodromal dementia MCI cases.

Currently, there is no evidence for the long-term efficacy of pharmacotherapies in reversing MCI. Several epidemiologic studies indicated a reduced risk of dementia in persons taking antihypertensive medications, cholesterol-lowering drugs, antioxidants, and anti-inflammatory and estrogen therapy, but no randomized controlled trials verify these data. Concerning cognitive enhancers, most trials have ambiguous results (Table 3-41). Most of these studies had several problems, including (1) obtaining homogeneous samples and identifying potential beneficiaries

of treatment; (2) treating a broader population, which led to large percentages of negative responses and problematic side effects; and (3) translation of the MCI construct into multiple cultures and languages and using dementia of the Alzheimer type diagnosis as the primary outcome, given the variability of this diagnosis in different countries.

Advances in MCI detection will be paramount for early detection and treatment of patients with Alzheimer disease; experts agree that disease-modifying treatments for Alzheimer disease will focus on cognitively intact individuals at increased risk. The field of identifying sensitive and specific biomarkers (biologic and neuroimaging markers) will probably witness exponential development in the coming years.

EPIDEMIOLOGY AND ETIOLOGY OF MCI

The recognition that Alzheimer disease pathology may exist in the brain long before the presence of clinical symptoms led to the focus on preclinical stages to characterize initial impairments that are associated with an increased risk of progression to Alzheimer disease.

The clinical expression of MCI is a result of the interaction among several risk factors and several protective factors. The most significant risk factors are related to the different types of neurodegeneration witnessed in dementias. There are different subtypes of MCI, most notably ones associated with amnesia. Other risk factors include the APOE4 allele status and cerebrovascular events in the form of either cerebrovascular accident or lacunar disease. The role of chronic exposure to high levels of cortisol, as seen in late-life depression, is also hypothesized to increase the risk for cognitive impairment through hippocampal volume reduction. The notion of "brain reserve" suggests that effects of brain size and neuron density may be protective against dementia despite the presence of neurodegeneration (a more significant number of neurons and synaptic connections and a bigger brain volume would protect against clinical manifestations of Alzheimer disease, despite the presence of neurodegeneration) (Fig. 3-13).

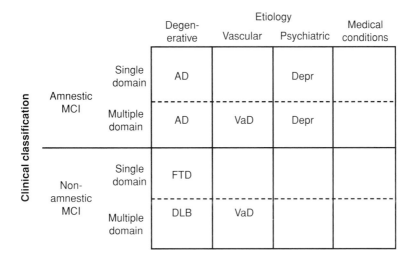

MCI Subtypes

FIGURE 3-13

Outcome of clinical phenotypes of mild cognitive impairment (MCI) according to presumed etiology. AD, Alzheimer disease; Depr, depression; DLB, dementia with Lewy bodies; FRD, frontotemporal dementia; VaD, vascular dementia. (Adapted with permission from Petersen RC, ed. *Mild Cognitive Impairment: Aging to Alzheimer's Disease.* New York: Oxford University Press; 2003.)

Table 3-41
Treatment Trials for MCI

Study	N	Duration	Primary Outcome	Results	OBS	Sponsor
Donepezil + vitamin E (Thall et al., 1999)	769	3 yr	Conversion to AD	Partially positive (reduced risk of developing AD in the active arm group for the first 12 mo)	Amnestic MCI status and the presence of APOE4 allele– predictive of rate of progression to AD	ADCS
Donepezil (Salloway et al., 2004)	269	24 wk	ADAS-Cog total score; NYU PTIR	Negative	Positive results in secondary outcome measures (ADAS-Cog13)	Pfizer (The Donepezil "401" Study Group)
Donepezil (Doody et al., 2009)	821	48 wk	ADAS-Cog cognitive subscale; CDR-SB	Minimally positive with small decrease in ADAS-Cog score in donepezil group. No significant change in CDR-SB	On secondary measures only global assessment differed significantly in favor of donepezil	Eisai and Pfizer
Rivastigmine (Feldman et al., 2007)	1,018	48 mo	Conversion to AD	Negative		Novartis
Galantamine (Winbald et al., 2008) Two studies	2,048		Progression of CDR score (from .5 to 1) Incident dementia	Negative	Attention assessed by DSST favored galantamine in both studies	Janssen-Cilag and Johnson & Johnson
Piribedil (Nagaraja et al., 2001)	60	12 wk	MMSE score	Favored piribedil	Mean MMSE change from baseline also favored intervention group	NIMH
Rofecoxib (Thall et al., 2005)	1,457	3–4 yr	Conversion to AD	Negative	Primary outcome favored placebo while secondary outcomes (ADS-cog, CDR) did not differentiate between rofecoxib and placebo	Merck
Nicotine patch (Newhouse et al., 2012)	74	6 mo	Attention on CCPT and global functioning on CGIC	Nicotine improved attention but not global functioning	Secondary outcome measures showed improvements in attention, memory, and psychomotor speed	
Piracetam	675	12 mo	Composite score extracted from eight tests	Negative		UCB Pharma
Ginkgo biloba (DeKosky et al., 2008) (Snitz et al., 2009)	3,069	6.1 yr	Incident dementia	Negative	No effect noted in normal cognitive either	NCCAM and NIH
		6.1 yr	Rates of change in MMSE, ADAS-Cog, and other cognitive domains	Negative		
B Vitamins (B$_{12}$, B$_6$, folic acid) (van Uffelen et al., 2008)	152	1 yr	Cognitive function at 6 and 12 mo	Negative	Moderate intensity walking improved memory in men and memory and attention in women	TNO-VU University Medical Center

MCI, mild cognitive impairment; AD, Alzheimer disease; ADCS, Alzheimer Disease Cooperative Study; CDR, Clinical Dementia Rating; NYU PTIR, New York University Paragraph Test Immediate Recall; DSST, Digit Symbol Substitution test; CCPT, Connors Continuous Performance Test; NCCAM, National Center for Complimentary Medicine.

References

Delirium

Caraceni A, Grassi L. *Delirium: Acute Confusional States in Palliative Medicine.* 2nd ed. New York: Oxford University Press; 2011.

Franco JG, Trzepacz PT, Meagher DJ, Kean J, Lee Y, Kim J-L, Kishi Y, Furlanetto LM, Negreiros D, Huang M-C, Chen C-H, Leonard M, de Pablo J. Three core domains of delirium validated using exploratory and confirmatory factor analyses. *Psychosomatics.* 2013;54(3):227–238.

Hosie A, Davidson PM, Agar M, Sanderson CR, Philips J. Delirium prevalence, incidence, and implications for screening in specialist palliative care inpatient settings: A systematic review. *Palliat Med.* 2013;27(6):486–498.

Juliebö V, Björo K, Krogseth M, Skovlund E, Ranhoff AH, Wyller TB. Risk factors for preoperative and postoperative delirium in elderly patients with hip fracture. *J Am Geriatr Soc.* 2009;57(8):1354–1361.

Kiely DK, Marcantonio ER, Inouye SK, Shaffer ML, Bergmann MA, Yang FM, Fearing MA, Jones RN. Persistent delirium predicts greater mortality. *J Am Geriatr Soc.* 2009;57(1):55–61.

Maldonado JR, Wysong A, van der Starre PJA, Block T, Miller C, Reitz BA. Dexmedetomidine and the reduction of postoperative delirium after cardiac surgery. *Psychosomatics.* 2009;50(3):216–217.

Morandi A, McCurley J, Vasilevskis EE. Tools to detect delirium superimposed on dementia: A systematic review. Erratum. *J Am Ger Soc.* 2113;61:174.

O'Mahony R, Murthy L, Akunne A, Young J, Guideline Development Group. Synopsis of the National Institute for Health and Clinical Excellence guideline for prevention of delirium. *Ann Intern Med.* 2011;154(11):746–711.

Pisani MA, Kong SYJ, Kasl SV, Murphy TE, Araujo KLB, Van Ness PH. Days of delirium are associated with 1-year mortality in an older intensive care unit population. *Am J Respir Crit Care.* 2009;180(11):1092–1097.

Popeo DM. Delirium in older adults. *MT Sinai J Med.* 2011;78(4):571–582.

Singh Joy, Subhashni D. Delirium directly related to cognitive impairment. *Am J Nurs.* 2011;111(1):65.

Solai LKK. Delirium. In: Sadock BJ, Sadock VA, Ruiz P, eds. *Kaplan & Sadock's Comprehensive Textbook of Psychiatry.* 9th ed. Philadelphia, PA: Lippincott Williams & Wilkins; 2109:1153.

Thomas E, Smith JE, Forrester DA, Heider G, Jadotte YT, Holly C. The effectiveness of non-pharmacological multi-component interventions for the prevention of delirium in non-intensive care unit older adult hospitalized patients: A systematic review. *JBI Database Syst Rev Implement Rep.* 2014;12(4):180–232.

Witlox J, Eurelings LSM, de Jonghe JFM, Kalisvaart KJ, Eikelenboom P, van Gool WA. Delirium in elderly patients and the risk of postdischarge mortality, institutionalization, and dementia: A meta-analysis. *JAMA.* 2010;304(4):443–451.

Yang FM, Marcantonio ER, Inouye SK, Kiely DK, Rudolph JL, Fearing MA, Jones RN. Phenomenological subtypes of delirium in older persons: Patterns, prevalence, and prognosis. *Psychosomatics.* 2009;50(3):248–254.

Dementia (Major Neurocognitive Disorder)

Balzer D. Neurocognitive disorders in DSM-5. *Am J Psych.* 2013;170(6):585–587.

Blanc-Lapierre A, Bouvier G, Gruber A, Leffondré K, Lebailly P, Fabrigoule C, Baldi I. Cognitive disorders and occupational exposure to organophosphates: Results from the PHYTONER study. *Am J Epidemiol.* 2013;177(10):1086–1096.

Bondi MW, Salmon DP, Kaszniak AW. The neuropsychology of dementia. In: Grant I, Adams KM, eds. *Neuropsychological Assessment of Neuropsychiatric and Neuromedical Disorders.* 3rd ed. New York: Oxford University Press; 2009:159.

Brand BL, Stadnik R. What contributes to predicting change in the treatment of dissociation: Initial levels of dissociation, PTSD, or overall distress? *J Trauma Dissociation.* 2013;14(3):328–341.

Bugnicourt J-M, Godefroy O, Chillon J-M, Choukroun G, Massy ZA. Cognitive disorders and dementia in CKD: The neglected kidney-brain axis. *J Am Soc Nephrol.* 2013;24(3):353–363.

Bugnicourt J-M, Guegan-Massardier E, Roussel M, Martinaud O, Canaple S, Triquenot-Bagan A, Wallon D, Lamy C, Leclercq C, Hannequin D, Godefroy O. Cognitive impairment after cerebral venous thrombosis: A two-center study. *J Neurol.* 2013;260(5):1324–1331.

Clare L, Whitaker CJ, Nelis SM, Martyr A, Markova IS, Roth I, Woods RT, Morris RG. Self-concept in early stage dementia: Profile, course, correlates, predictors and implications for quality of life. *Int J Geriatr Psychiatry.* 2013;28(5):494–503.

Craft S. The role of metabolic disorders in Alzheimer disease and vascular dementia: Two roads converged. *Arch Neurol.* 2009;66(3):300–305.

Elvish R, Lever S-J, Johnstone J, Cawley R, Keady J. Psychological interventions for carers of people with dementia: A systematic review of quantitative and qualitative evidence. *Counsel Psychother Res.* 2013;13(2):106–125.

Fields J, Dumaop W, Langford TD, Rockenstein E, Masliah E. Role of neurotrophic factor alterations in the neurodegenerative process in HIV associated neurocognitive disorders. *J Neuroimmune Pharmacol.* 2014;9(2):102–116.

Goldman J, Stebbins G, Merkitch D, Dinh V, Bernard D, DeToledo-Morrell L, Goetz C. Hallucinations and dementia in Parkinson's disease: Clinically related but structurally distinct (P5. 257). *Neurology.* 2014;82(10 Suppl):P5-257.

Graff-Radford NR, Woodruff BK. Frontotemporal dementia. *Semin Neurol.* 2007; 27:48.

Hansen KF, Karenlina K, Sakamoto K, Wayman GA, Impey S, Obrietan K. miRNA-132: A dynamic regulator of cognitive capacity. *Brain Struct Funct.* 2013;218(3): 817–831.

Insausti R, Annese J, Amaral DG, Squire LR. Human amnesia and the medial temporal lobe illuminated by neuropsychological and neurohistological findings for patient E.P. *Proc Natl Acad Sci U S A.* 2013;110(21):E1953–E1962.

Jack CR Jr, Lowe VJ, Senjem ML, Weigand SD, Kemp BJ, Shiung MM, Knopman DS, Boeve BF, Klunk WE, Mathis CA, Petersen RC. ¹¹C PiB and structural MRI provide complementary information in imaging of Alzheimer's disease and amnestic mild cognitive impairment. *Brain.* 2008;131(Pt 3):665–680.

Kemp PM, Holmes C. Imaging in dementia with Lewy bodies: A review. *Nucl Med Commun.* 2007;28(7):511–519.

Launer LJ. Epidemiologic insight into blood pressure and cognitive disorders. In: Yaffe K, ed. *Chronic Medical Disease and Cognitive Aging: Toward a Healthy Body and Brain.* New York: Oxford University Press; 2013:1.

Mayeux R, Reitz C, Brickman AM, Haan MN, Manly JJ, Glymour MM, Weiss CC, Yaffe K, Middleton L, Hendrie HC, Warren LH, Hayden KM, Welsh-Bohmer KA, Breitner JCS, Morris JC. Operationalizing diagnostic criteria for Alzheimer's disease and other age-related cognitive impairment—Part 1. *Alzheimers Dement.* 2011; 7(1):15–34.

McLaren AN, LaMantia MA, Callahan CM. Systematic review of non-pharmacologic interventions to delay functional decline in community-dwelling patients with dementia. *Aging Ment Health.* 2013;17(6):655–666.

Mitchell SL, Teno JM, Kiely DK, Shaffer ML, Jones RN, Prigerson HG, Volicer L, Given JL, Hamel MB. The clinical course of advanced dementia. *N Engl J Med.* 2009;361(16):1529–1538.

Nervi A, Reitz C, Tang MX, Santana V, Piriz A, Reyes D, Lantigua R, Medrano M, Jiménez-Velázquez IZ, Lee JH, Mayeux R. Familial aggregation of dementia with Lewy bodies. *Arch Neurol.* 2011;68(1):90–93.

Nguyen TP, Soukup VM, Gelman BB. Persistent hijacking of brain proteasomes in HIV-associated dementia. *Am J Pathol.* 2010;176(2):893–902.

Panza F, Frisardi V, Capurso C, D'Introno A, Colacicco AM, Imbimbo BP, Santamato A, Vendemiale G, Seripa D, Pilotto A, Capurso A, Solfrizzi V. Late-life depression, mild cognitive impairment, and dementia: Possible continuum? *Am J Geriatr Psychiatry.* 2010;18(2):98–116.

Richards SS, Sweet RA. Dementia. In: Sadock BJ, Sadock VA, Ruiz P, eds. *Kaplan & Sadock's Comprehensive Textbook of Psychiatry.* 9th ed. Philadelphia, PA: Lippincott Williams & Wilkins; 2009:1167.

Schneider JA, Arvanitakis Z, Bang W, Bennett DA. Mixed brain pathologies account for most dementia cases in community-dwelling older persons. *Neurology.* 2007;69(24):2197–2204.

Sonnen JA, Larson EB, Crane PK, Haneuse S, Li G, Schellenberg GD, Craft S, Leverenz JB, Montine TJ. Pathological correlates of dementia in a longitudinal, population-based sample of aging. *Ann Neurol.* 2007;62(4):406–413.

Sweet RA. Cognitive disorders: Introduction. In: Sadock BJ, Sadock VA, Ruiz P, eds. *Kaplan & Sadock's Comprehensive Textbook of Psychiatry.* 9th ed. Philadelphia, PA: Lippincott Williams & Wilkins; 2009:1152.

Verdelho A, Madureira S, Moleiro C, Ferro JM, Santos CO, Erkinjuntti T, Pantoni L, Fazekas F, Visser M, Waldemar G, Wallin A, Hennerici M, Inzitari D; LADIS Study. White matter changes and diabetes predict cognitive decline in the elderly: The LADIS study. *Neurology.* 2010;75(2):160–167.

Watson PD, Voss JL, Warren DE, Tranel D, Cohen NJ. Spatial reconstruction by patients with hippocampal damage is dominated by relational memory errors. *Hippocampus.* 2013;23(7):570–580.

Weiner MF. Cognitive disorders as psychobiological processes. In: Weiner MF, Lipton AM. *The American Psychiatric Publishing Textbook of Alzheimer Disease and Other Dementias.* Arlington, VA: American Psychiatric Publishing; 2009:137.

Zarit SH, Zarit JM. Disorders of aging: Delirium, dementia and other cognitive problems. In: Zarit SH, Zarit JM. *Mental Disorders in Older Adults: Fundamentals of Assessment and Treatment.* 2nd ed. New York: Guilford Press; 2007:40.

Major or Minor Neurocognitive Disorder due to Another Medical Condition (Amnestic Disorders)

Andreescu C, Aizenstein HJ. Amnestic disorders and mild cognitive impairment. In: Sadock BJ, Sadock VA, Ruiz P, eds. *Kaplan & Sadock's Comprehensive Textbook of Psychiatry.* 9th ed. Philadelphia, PA: Lippincott Williams & Wilkins; 2009:1198.

Auyeunga M, Tsoi TH, Cheung CM, Fong DYT, Li R, Chan JKW, Lau KY. Association of diffusion weighted imaging abnormalities and recurrence in transient global amnesia. *J Clin Neurosci.* 2011;18(4):531–534.

Gerridzen IJ, Goossensen MA. Patients with Korsakoff syndrome in nursing homes: Characteristics, comorbidity, and use of psychotropic drugs. *Int Psychogeriatr.* 2014;26(1):115–121.

Kearney H, Mallon P, Kavanagh E, Lawler L, Kelly P, O'Rourke K. Amnestic syndrome due to meningovascular neurosyphilis. *J Neurol.* 2010;257(4):669–671.

McLaren AN, LaMantia MA, Callahan CM. Systematic review of non-pharmacologic interventions to delay functional decline in community-dwelling patients with dementia. *Aging Ment Health.* 2013;17(6):655–666.

Purohit V, Rapaka R, Frankenheim J, Avila A, Sorensen R, Rutter J. National Institute on Drug Abuse symposium report: Drugs of abuse, dopamine, and HIV-associated neurocognitive disorders/HIV-associated dementia. *J Neurovirol.* 2013;19(2):119–122.

Race E, Verfaellie M. Remote memory function and dysfunction in Korsakoff's syndrome. *Neuropsychol Rev.* 2012;22(2):105–116.

Rogalski EJ, Rademaker A, Harrison TM, Helenowski I, Johnson N, Bigio E, Mishra M, Weintraub S, Mesulam MM. ApoE E4 is a susceptibility factor in amnestic but not aphasic dementias. *Alzheimer Dis Assoc Disord.* 2011;25(2):159–163.

Tannenbaum C, Paquette A, Hilmer S, Holroyd-Leduc J, Carnahan R. A systematic review of amnestic and non-amnestic mild cognitive impairment induced by anticholinergic, antihistamine, GABAergic and opioid drugs. *Drugs Aging*. 2012; 29(8):639–658.

van Geldorp B, Bergmann HC, Robertson J, Wester AJ, Kessels RPC. The interaction of working memory performance and episodic memory formation in patients with Korsakoff's amnesia. *Brain Res*. 2012;1433:98–103.

Neurocognitive and Other Disorders due to a General Medical Condition

Boyd AD, Riba M. Depression and pancreatic cancer. *J Natl Compr Canc Netw*. 2007; 5(1):113–116.

Cahalan S. *Brain on Fire*. New York: Simon & Schuster; 2013.

Carrico AW, Riley ED, Johnson MO, Charlebois ED, Neilands TB, Remien RH, Lightfoot MA, Steward WT, Weinhardt LS, Kelly JA, Rotheram-Borus MJ, Morin SF, Chesney MA. Psychiatric risk factors for HIV disease progression: The role of inconsistent patterns of antiretroviral therapy utilization. *J Acquir Immune Defic Syndr*. 2011;56(2):146–150.

Clare L, Whitaker CJ, Nelis SM, Martyr A, Markova IS, Roth I, Woods RT, Morris RG. Self-concept in early stage dementia: Profile, course, correlates, predictors and implications for quality of life. *Int J Geriatr Psychiatry*. 2013;28(5):494–503.

Cohen MA, Goforth HW, Lux JZ, Batista SM, Khalife S, Cozza KL, Soffer J, eds. *Handbook of AIDS Psychiatry*. New York: Oxford University Press; 2010.

Dalmau J, Lancaster E, Martinez-Hernandez E, Rosenfeld MR, Balice-Gordon R. Clinical experience and laboratory investigations in patients with anti-NMDAR encephalitis. *Lancet Neurol*. 2011;10(1):63–74.

Elvish R, Lever S-J, Johnstone J, Cawley R, Keady J. Psychological interventions for carers of people with dementia: A systematic review of quantitative and qualitative evidence. *Counsel Psychother Res*. 2013;13:106.

Goldstein BI, Fagiolini A, Houck P, Kupfer DJ. Cardiovascular disease and hypertension among adults with bipolar I disorder in the United States. *Bipolar Disord*. 2009;11(6):657–662.

Grossman CI, Gordon CM. Mental health considerations in secondary HIV prevention. *AIDS Behav*. 2010;14(2):263–271.

Gur RE, Yi JJ, McDonald-McGinn DM, Tang SX, Calkins ME, Whinna D, Souders MC, Savitt A, Zackai EH, Moberg PJ, Emanuel BS, Gur RC. Neurocognitive development in 22q11.2 deletion syndrome: Comparison with youth having developmental delay and medical comorbidities. *Mol Psychiatry*. 2014;21.

Iudicello JE, Woods SP, Cattie JE, Doyle K, Grant I; HIV Neurobehavioral Research Program Group. Risky decision-making in HIV-associated neurocognitive disorders (HAND). *Clin Neuropsychol*. 2013;27(2):256–275.

Kennedy CA, Hill JM, Schleifer SJ. HIV/AIDS and substance use disorders. In: Frances RJ, Miller SI, Mack AH, eds. *Clinical Textbook of Addictive Disorders*. 3rd ed. New York: The Guildford Press; 2011:411.

Lavery LL, Whyte EM. Other cognitive and mental disorders due to a general medical condition. In: Sadock BJ, Sadock VA, Ruiz P, eds. *Kaplan & Sadock's Comprehensive Textbook of Psychiatry*. 9th ed. Philadelphia, PA: Lippincott Williams & Wilkins; 2009:1207.

Lippmann S, Perugula ML. Delirium or dementia? *Innov Clin Neurosci*. 2016;13 (9–10):56–57.

Martins IP, Lauterbach M, Luis H, Amaral H, Rosenbaum G, Slade PD, Townes BD. Neurological subtle signs and cognitive development: astudy in late childhood and adolescence. *Child Neuropsychol*. 2013;19(5):466–478.

Pressler SJ, Subramanian U, Kareken D, Perkins SM, Gradus-Pizlo I, Sauve MJ, Ding Y, Kim JS, Sloan R, Jaynes H, Shaw RM. Cognitive deficits in chronic heart failure. *Nurs Res*. 2010;59(2):127–139.

Price CC, Tanner JJ, Monk TG. Postoperative cognitive disorders. In: Mashour GA, Lydic R, eds. *Neuroscientific Foundations of Anesthesiology*. New York: Oxford University Press; 2011:255.

Rao V, Bertrand M, Rosenberg P, Makley M, Schretlen DJ, Brandt J, Mielke MM. Predictors of new-onset depression after mild traumatic brain injury. *J Neuropsychiatry Clin Neurosci*. 2010;22(1):100–104.

Simioni S, Cavassini M, Annoni JM, Abraham AR, Bourquin I, Schiffer V, Calmy A, Chave JP, Giacobini E, Hirschel B, Du Pasquier RA. Cognitive dysfunction in HIV patients despite long-standing suppression of viremia. *AIDS*. 2010;24(9): 1243–1250.

Mild Cognitive Impairment

Aggarwal NT, Wilson RS, Beck TL, Bienias JL, Berry-Kravis E, Bennett DA. The apolipoprotein E epsilon4 allele and incident Alzheimer's disease in persons with mild cognitive impairment. *Neurocase*. 2005;11(1):3–7.

Andreescu C, Aizenstein HJ. Amnestic disorders and mild cognitive impairment. In: Sadock BJ, Sadock VA, Ruiz P, eds. *Kaplan & Sadock's Comprehensive Textbook of Psychiatry*. 9th ed. Philadelphia, PA: Lippincott Williams & Wilkins; 2009:1198.

Birks J, Flicker L. Donepezil for mild cognitive impairment. *Cochrane Database Syst Rev*. 2006;(3):CD006104.

Breitner JCS. Mild cognitive impairment and progression to dementia: New findings. *Neurology*. 2014;82(4):e34–e35.

Doody RS, Ferris SH, Salloway S, Meuser TM, Murthy AK, Li C, Goldman R: Identifying amnestic mild cognitive impairment in primary care: A feasibility study. *Clin Drug Investig*. 2011;31(7):483–491.

Edwards ER, Spira AP, Barnes DE, Yaffe K. Neuropsychiatric symptoms in mild cognitive impairment: Differences by subtype and progression to dementia. *Int J Geriatr Psychiatry*. 2009;24(7):716–722.

Gallagher D, Coen R, Kilroy D, Belinski K, Bruce I, Coakley D, Walsh B, Cunningham C, Lawlor BA. Anxiety and behavioural disturbance as markers of prodromal Alzheimer's disease in patients with mild cognitive impairment. *Int J Geriatr Psychiatry*. 2011;26(2):166–172.

Goldberg TE, Koppel J, Keehlisen L, Christen E, Dreses-Werringloer U, Conejero-Goldberg C, Gordon ML, Davies P. Performance-based measures of everyday function in mild cognitive impairment. *Am J Psychiatry*. 2010;167(7):845–853.

Hendrix SB, Welsh-Bohmer KA. Separation of cognitive domains to improve prediction of progression from mild cognitive impairment to Alzheimer's disease. *Alzheimers Res Ther*. 2013;5(3):22.

Mecocci P, Polidori MC, Praticó D. Antioxidant clinical trials in mild cognitive impairment and Alzheimer's disease. In: Praticó D, Mecocci P, eds. *Studies on Alzheimer's disease*. New York: Springer Science+Business Media; 2013:223.

Pedersen KF, Larsen JP, Tysnes O-B, Alves G. Prognosis of mild cognitive impairment in early Parkinson disease: The Norwegian ParkWest study. *JAMA Neurol*. 2013;70(5):580–586.

Roberts JS, Karlawish JH, Uhlmann WR, Petersen RC, Green RC. Mild cognitive impairment in clinical care: A survey of American Academy of Neurology members. *Neurology*. 2010;75(5):425–431.

Rog LA, Fink JW. Mild cognitive impairment and normal aging. In: Ravdin LD, Katzen HL, eds. *Handbook on the Neuropsychology of Aging and Dementia*. New York: Springer Science+Business Media; 2013:239.

Smith CN, Frascino JC, Hopkins RO, Squire LR. The nature of anterograde and retrograde memory impairment after damage to the medial temporal lobe. *Neuropsychologia*. 2013;51(13):2709–2714.

Wang L, Goldstein FC, Veledar E, Levey AI, Lah JJ, Meltzer CC, Holder CA, Mao H. Alterations in cortical thickness and white matter integrity in mild cognitive impairment measured by whole-brain cortical thickness mapping and diffusion tensor imaging. *AJNR Am J Neuroradiol*. 2009;30(5):893–899.

Zola SM, Manzanares CM, Clopton P, Lah JJ, Levey AI. A behavioral task predicts conversion to mild cognitive impairment and Alzheimer's disease. *Am J Alzheimers Dis Other Demen*. 2013;28(2):179–184.

4

Substance Use and Addictive Disorders

▲ 4.1 General Features of the Substance-Related Disorders

This chapter covers substance use disorders with descriptions of the clinical phenomena associated with the following: alcohol; caffeine; cannabis; hallucinogens (including phencyclidine [PCP]); inhalants; opioids; sedatives, hypnotics, and anxiolytics; stimulants (including cocaine); tobacco; anabolic-androgenic steroids (AAS); and other substances, such as nitrous oxide and γ-hydroxybutyrate. We also discuss gambling disorder, as DSM-5 reclassified this as a non–substance-related addictive disorder in the most recent (fifth) edition of the Diagnostic and Statistical Manual of Mental Disorders (DSM-5).

The substance use disorders share many features; however, the range of substances is broad in that there are differences in the pharmacology, intoxication, and associated behaviors that make for unique effects with many of the substances. For that reason, we begin with a general description of the substance use disorders in this section and discuss the features of each specific disorder in the following subsections of the chapter.

THE CLINICAL PRESENTATION

Behavioral, physical, and psychological dependence (see terminology below) are the hallmark of substance use disorders. While the direct effects of a substance on behavioral, physical, and psychological function will vary depending on the particular substance used, the overall impact of the substance in causing impaired functioning has a similar pattern, regardless of substance. The symptoms typically fall within one of four categories, including pharmacologic symptoms, symptoms of impaired use, impairment in social domains, and use in risky or hazardous situations.

Terminology

Various terms have been used over the years to refer to drug abuse. For example, the term *dependence* has been and is used in one of two ways when discussing substance use disorders. In *behavioral dependence,* the emphasis is on substance-seeking activities and related evidence of pathologic use patterns, whereas *physical dependence* refers to the physical (physiologic) effects of multiple episodes of substance use. Psychological dependence, also referred to as habituation, is characterized by a continuous or intermittent craving (i.e., intense desire) for the substance to avoid a dysphoric state.

Somewhat related to dependence are the words addiction and addict. The word *addict* has acquired a pejorative connotation that ignores the concept of substance abuse as a medical disorder. The

internet and other popular mediums have trivialized *Addiction*, as in the terms *TV addiction* and *chocolate addiction (or more commonly, "chocoholic");* however, the term still has value. There are common neurochemical and neuroanatomical substrates found among all addictions, whether it is to substances or gambling, sex, stealing, or eating. These various addictions may have similar effects on the activities of specific reward areas of the brain.

DIAGNOSIS

There are three major diagnostic categories in the DSM-5: (1) Substance Use Disorder; (2) Substance Intoxication; (3) Substance Withdrawal. Also, DSM includes a category of Substance-Induced Mental Disorder, to account for presentations of a psychiatric disorder that are likely due to a substance. This possibility is among the standard rule out criteria for most DSM-5 and ICD-10 mental disorders.

For both DSM-5 and ICD-10, the diagnoses are generic and do not differ among substances. Thus, we believe it is preferable to understand the overall diagnostic criteria, with the understanding that we can then apply them to each of the substances discussed in later sections. In DSM-5, the disorders are substance-specific. Therefore, when diagnosing a disorder, the clinician should indicate the specific substance or drug used or that caused intoxication or withdrawal.

Substance Use Disorder

Substance use disorder is the diagnostic term for the prolonged use and abuse of a substance. When used, the specific substance is identified, for example, "alcohol use disorder" or "opioid use disorder."

Table 4-1 lists the diagnostic approaches to substance use disorder in DSM-5 and ICD-10.

Substance Intoxication

Substance intoxication is the diagnosis used to describe a syndrome characterized by specific signs and symptoms resulting from recent ingestion or exposure to the substance. As with substance use disorder, in practice, the specific substance is identified, for example, "alcohol intoxication" or "opioid intoxication." Table 4-2 lists the diagnostic approaches to substance intoxication in DSM-5 and ICD-10.

Substance Withdrawal

Substance withdrawal is the diagnosis used to describe a substance-specific syndrome that results from the abrupt cessation of heavy and prolonged use of a substance. As with substance use disorder, in

Table 4-1
Substance Use Disorder

	Substance Use Disorder	
Disorder	**DSM-5**	**ICD-10**
Diagnostic name	Alcohol use disorder Cannabis use disorder Hallucinogen use disorder Inhalant use disorder Opioid use disorder Sedative/hypnotic/anxiolytic use disorder Stimulant use disorder Tobacco use disorder	Mental and behavioral disorders due to • Use of alcohol • Use of opioids • Use of cannabinoids • Use of sedatives or hypnotics • Use of cocaine • Use of other stimulants, including caffeine • Use of hallucinogens • Use of tobacco • Use of volatile solvents Indicate if includes a dependence syndrome
Duration	Symptoms occur within 12 mo	

Symptoms	*Physiologic Symptoms:*
	  1. Tolerance
	  2. Withdrawal (does not apply to inhalants and hallucinogens)
	Symptoms typical of addiction or obsessive use
	  3. Craving to use
	  4. Using more than intended
	  5. Difficulty stopping or reducing use
	  6. Spending significant time devoted to the substance (using, obtaining, recovering)
	  7. Use despite acknowledging health problems (physical, mental) because of use
	Psychosocial sequelae of use
	  8. Using despite social, occupational or other adverse consequences
	  9. Neglecting other responsibilities because of use
	  10. Neglecting other activities because of use
	  11. Risky or dangerous behaviors or situations because of use
		Tolerance and withdrawal states
		Adverse health effects of use: physiologic, cognitive or behavioral
		Craving or difficulty controlling substance use
		Use despite acknowledging adverse consequences of use
		Prioritizing the substance over other psychosocial obligations

Required number of symptoms	Two or more of the above	
Psychosocial consequences of symptoms	Marked impairment and/or distress	
Exclusions		*Psychotic state* *Nonalcoholic Korsakoff psychosis or syndrome*

Symptom specifiers	***In a controlled environment:*** (i.e., access to the substance is restricted)
	On maintenance therapy: (tobacco or opioids)
	For hallucinogens or inhalants, specify the specific substance
		Associated specifiers:
		  Psychotic disorder (following substance use)
		  Amnesic syndrome (chronic memory loss because of use)

Course specifiers	**In early remission:** no symptoms for 3–12 mo (craving may still be present) **In sustained remission:** no symptoms for >12 mo (craving may still be present)	
Severity specifiers	Severity is measured by the number of symptoms present. See DSM-5 for ranges.	
Comments	Applies to the following substances: • Alcohol • Cannabis • Opioids • Sedatives, hypnotics, anxiolytics • Stimulants • Hallucinogens • Inhalants • Tobacco	Note: ICD additionally defines "harmful use" as pattern of use causing harm to health, both physical and/or mental. This classification is independent of presence of a dependence syndrome.

Table 4-2
Substance Intoxication

Disorder	Substance Intoxication	
	DSM-5	**ICD-10**
Diagnostic name	Alcohol intoxication Caffeine intoxication Cannabis intoxication Hallucinogen intoxication Inhalant intoxication Opioid intoxication Sedative/hypnotic/anxiolytic intoxication Stimulant intoxication	Mental and behavioral disorders due to • Use of alcohol • Use of opioids • Use of cannabinoids • Use of sedatives or hypnotics • Use of cocaine • Use of other stimulants, including caffeine • Use of hallucinogens • Use of tobacco • Use of volatile solvents Indicate if acute intoxication
Duration	Not specified	Not specified
Symptoms	Recent use of substance Mood or behavioral problems resulting from that use One or more substance-specific symptoms of intoxication (see individual substances for descriptions of the intoxication state)	Some mental change resulting from substance use: cognitive, psychological or behavioral Symptoms due to the substance resolve when stopped
Required number of symptoms	Specific to substance: Stimulants: ≥2 Caffeine: ≥5 or more symptoms Sedative/hypnotic/anxiolytics: ≥1 Opioids: ≥1 Inhalants: ≥2 Hallucinogens: ≥2 plus change in perception or alertness Cannabis: ≥2 Alcohol: ≥1	
Exclusions	Medical condition Other mental disorder Intoxication with another substance	Intoxication due to poisoning
Symptom specifiers	For cannabis, opioids, or stimulants: *with perceptual disturbance:* hallucinations but no loss or reality testing and not delirious	
Comments	Applies to the following substances: • Alcohol • Cannabis • Opioids • Sedatives, hypnotics, anxiolytics • Stimulants • Hallucinogens • Inhalants • Caffeine	

practice, the specific substance is identified, for example, "alcohol withdrawal" or "opioid withdrawal." Table 4-3 lists the diagnostic approaches to substance withdrawal in DSM-5 and ICD-10.

COMORBIDITY

Comorbidity is the occurrence of two or more psychiatric disorders in a single patient at the same time. People seeking treatment for alcohol, cocaine, or opioid dependence have a high prevalence of additional psychiatric disorders; some studies have shown that up to 50 percent of addicts have a comorbid psychiatric disorder. Although opioid, cocaine, and alcohol abusers with current psychiatric problems are more likely to seek treatment, those who do not seek treatment are not necessarily free of comorbid psychiatric problems; such persons may have social supports that enable them

to deny the impact that drug use is having on their lives. Two extensive epidemiologic studies have shown that even among representative samples of the population, those who meet the criteria for alcohol or drug abuse and dependence (excluding tobacco dependence) are also far more likely to meet the criteria for other psychiatric disorders.

In various studies, a range of 35 to 60 percent of patients with substance abuse or substance dependence also meet the diagnostic criteria for antisocial personality disorder. The range is even higher when investigators include persons who meet all the antisocial personality disorder diagnostic criteria, except the requirement that the symptoms started at an early age. That is, a high percentage of patients with substance abuse or substance dependence diagnoses have a pattern of antisocial behavior, whether it was present before the substance use started or developed during substance

Table 4-3
Substance Withdrawal

Disorder	Withdrawal	
	DSM-5	ICD-10
Diagnostic name	Alcohol withdrawal Caffeine withdrawal Cannabis withdrawal Opioid withdrawal Sedative/hypnotic/anxiolytic withdrawal Stimulant withdrawal Tobacco withdrawal	Mental and behavioral disorders due to • Use of alcohol • Use of opioids • Use of cannabinoids • Use of sedatives or hypnotics • Use of cocaine • Use of other stimulants, including caffeine • Use of hallucinogens • Use of tobacco • Use of volatile solvents Indicate withdrawal state

Duration	Onset is specific to substance:
	    sedatives/hypnotics/anxiolytics, stimulants:
	      hours to days
	    alcohol and cannabis: none listed
	    opioids: minutes to days
	    caffeine, tobacco: within 24 hr	

Symptoms	No or reduced use after prolonged or heavy use
	Substance-specific symptoms (see individual
	    substances for typical symptoms of
	    withdrawal)
		• Group of symptoms occurring with cessation
		  or reduction of a substance following period of
		  prolonged and/or regular use
		• Symptoms are time limited and substance-
		  specific

Required number of symptoms	Specific to substance:
	    sedatives/hypnotics/anxiolytics: ≥2
	    alcohol: ≥2
	    stimulants: ≥2 plus dysphoric mood
	    opioids: ≥3
	    caffeine: ≥3
	    cannabis: ≥3
	    tobacco: ≥4	

Psychosocial consequences of symptoms	Distress and/or impairment in functioning	
Exclusions	Medical condition Other mental disorder Intoxication with or withdrawal from another substance	

Symptom specifiers	For alcohol and sedative/hypnotic/anxiolytic
	    withdrawal: *with perceptual disturbance:*
	    hallucinations but no loss or reality testing
	    and not delirious
		Withdrawal state with delirium

Comments	Applies to the following substances: • Alcohol • Cannabis • Opioids • Sedatives, hypnotics, anxiolytics • Stimulants • Tobacco • Caffeine	

use. Patients with substance abuse or substance dependence diagnoses who have antisocial personality disorder are likely to use more illegal substances; to have more psychopathology; to be less satisfied with their lives; and to be more impulsive, isolated, and depressed than patients with antisocial personality disorders alone.

Depression and Suicide

Depressive symptoms are common among persons diagnosed with substance abuse or substance dependence. About one-third to one-half of all those with opioid abuse or opioid dependence and about 40 percent of those with alcohol abuse or alcohol dependence meet the criteria for major depressive disorder sometime during their lives. Substance use is also a major precipitating factor for suicide. Persons who abuse substances are about 20 times more likely to die by suicide than the general population. About 15 percent of persons with alcohol abuse or alcohol dependence commit suicide. This frequency of suicide is second only to the frequency in patients with major depressive disorder.

TREATMENT APPROACH

Some persons who develop substance-related problems recover without formal treatment, especially as they age. For those patients with less severe disorders, such as nicotine addiction, relatively brief interventions are often as effective as more intensive treatments. Because these brief interventions do not change the environment, alter drug-induced brain changes, or provide new skills, a change in the patient's motivation (cognitive change) probably has the best impact on the drug-using behavior. For those individuals who do not respond or whose dependence is more severe, a variety of interventions described below appear to be effective.

It is useful to distinguish among specific procedures or techniques (e.g., individual therapy, family therapy, group therapy, relapse prevention, and pharmacotherapy) and treatment programs. Most programs use several specific procedures and involve a variety of professional disciplines as well as nonprofessionals who have special skills or personal experience with the specific substance problem. The best treatment programs combine specific procedures and disciplines with meeting the needs of the individual patient after a careful assessment.

There is no generally accepted classification system for either the specific procedures used in treatment or programs using various combinations of procedures. This lack of standardized terminology for categorizing procedures and programs presents a problem, even when we narrow the field of interest to treatment for a single substance, such as alcohol, tobacco, or cocaine. Except in carefully monitored research projects, even the definitions of specific procedures (e.g., individual counseling, group therapy, and methadone maintenance) tend to be so imprecise that usually just what transactions occur cannot be inferred. Nevertheless, for descriptive purposes, programs are often broadly grouped based on one or more of their salient characteristics: whether the program aims to merely control acute withdrawal and consequences of recent drug use (detoxification) or focuses on longer-term behavioral change (rehabilitation); whether the program makes extensive use of pharmacologic interventions; and whether the program mainly uses individual therapy, Alcoholics Anonymous (AA) or other 12-step principles, or therapeutic community principles. For example, the National Institute on Drug Abuse suggested the following categories of treatment: long-term residential treatment, short-term residential treatment, outpatient treatment programs, individualized drug counseling, group counseling, and treatments for individuals involved in the criminal justice system.

Selecting a Treatment

Not all interventions apply to all types of substance use disorders, and some of the more coercive interventions used for illicit drugs do not apply to legal substances, such as tobacco. Addictive behaviors do not change abruptly but through a series of stages. Experts propose five stages in this gradual process: precontemplation, contemplation, preparation, action, and maintenance. For some types of addictions, the therapeutic alliance improves when the treatment approach is tailored to the patient's stage of readiness to change. Interventions for some drug use disorders may have a specific pharmacologic agent as a critical component; for example, disulfiram, naltrexone, or acamprosate for alcoholism; methadone, levomethadyl acetate, or buprenorphine for heroin addiction; and nicotine delivery devices, varenicline, or bupropion for tobacco dependence.

In general, brief interventions (e.g., a few weeks of detoxification, whether in or out of a hospital) used for persons who are severely dependent on illicit opioids have limited effect on outcome measured a few months later. Substantial reductions in illicit drug use, antisocial behaviors, and psychiatric distress among patients dependent on cocaine or heroin are much more likely following treatment lasting at least 3 months. Such a time-in-treatment effect occurs across very different modalities, from residential therapeutic communities to ambulatory methadone maintenance programs. Although some patients appear to benefit from a few days or weeks of treatment, a substantial percentage of users of illicit drugs drop out (or are dropped) from treatment before they have achieved significant benefits.

Treatment outcomes vary widely; this is partly due to the great variety of patients that enter treatment as well as their circumstances. Programs based on similar philosophical principles and using what seem to be similar therapeutic procedures vary greatly in effectiveness, however. Some of the differences among programs that seem to be similar reflect the range and intensity of services offered. Programs with a professionally trained staff that provide more comprehensive services to patients with more severe psychiatric difficulties are more likely able to retain those patients in treatment and help them make positive changes. Differences in the skills of individual counselors and professionals can strongly affect outcomes.

Such generalizations concerning programs serving illicit drug users may not hold for programs dealing with those seeking treatment for alcohol, tobacco, or even cannabis problems uncomplicated by heavy use of illicit drugs. In such cases, relatively brief periods of individual or group counseling can produce long-lasting reductions in substance use. The outcomes usually considered in programs dealing with illicit drugs have typically included measures of social functioning, employment, and criminal activity, as well as decreased drug-using behavior.

Treatment of Comorbidity

Treatment of the severely mentally ill (primarily those with schizophrenia and schizoaffective disorders) who are also drug-dependent continues to pose problems for clinicians. Although some specialized facilities use both antipsychotic drugs and therapeutic community principles, for the most part, specialized addiction agencies have difficulty treating these patients. Generally, integrated treatment in which the same staff can treat both the psychiatric disorder and the addiction is more effective than either parallel treatment (mental health and a specialty addiction program providing care concurrently) or sequential treatment (treating either the addiction or the psychiatric disorder first and then dealing with the comorbid condition).

Services and Outcome

The extension of managed care into the public sector has produced a significant reduction in the use of hospital-based detoxification and the virtual disappearance of residential rehabilitation programs for alcoholics. Managed-care organizations, however, tend to assume that the relatively brief courses of outpatient counseling that are effective with private-sector alcoholic patients are also useful with patients who are dependent on illicit drugs and who have minimal social supports. For the present, the trend is to provide the care that costs the least over the short term and to ignore studies showing that more services can produce better long-term outcomes.

Treatment is often a worthwhile social expenditure. For example, the treatment of antisocial illicit drug users in outpatient settings can decrease antisocial behavior and reduce rates of human immunodeficiency virus (HIV) seroconversion that more than offset the treatment cost. Treatment in a prison setting can decrease postrelease costs associated with drug use and rearrests. Despite such evidence, problems exist in maintaining public support for the treatment of substance dependence in both the public and private sectors. This lack of support suggests that these problems continue to be viewed, at least in part, as moral failings rather than as medical disorders.

The Epidemiology of Substance Use Disorders

The National Institute of Drug Abuse (NIDA) and other agencies, such as the National Survey of Drug Use and Health (NSDUH), conduct periodic surveys of the use of illicit drugs in the United States. As of 2017, more than 19 million persons older than the age of 12 years (about 7 percent of the total US population) had a substance-related disorder in the past year.

In general, more men than women abuse substances. Those who use substances earlier are more likely to develop a disorder. Among ethnic and racial groups in the United States, the highest lifetime rate is among American Indian or Alaska Natives; whites are more affected than blacks or African Americans. There is a sociodemographic effect as well. For example, those with some college education use more substances than those with less education, and the unemployed have higher rates than those with either part-time or full-time employment.

We will discuss the specific epidemiology of various substances in the appropriate section. Also, a comprehensive survey of drug use and trends in the United States is available at www.samhsa.gov.

ETIOLOGY

Substance use disorders are complicated psychiatric conditions, and, like other psychiatric disorders, both biologic factors and environmental circumstances are etiologically significant.

The model of substance use disorders is the result of a process in which multiple interacting factors influence drug-using behavior and the loss of judgment for decisions about using a given drug. Although the actions of a given drug are critical in the process, we cannot assume that all drug-dependent people experience the effects of a particular drug similarly, or have the same set of motivating factors. Furthermore, different factors may be more or less important at different stages of the process. Thus, drug availability, social acceptability, and peer pressures may be the significant determinants of initial experimentation with a drug. However, other factors, such as personality and individual biology, probably are more important in how the effects of a given drug are perceived and the degree to which repeated drug use produces changes in the central nervous system (CNS). Still, other factors, including the particular actions of the drug, may represent primary determinants of whether drug use progresses to drug dependence. In contrast, others may still be valuable influences on the likelihood that drug use (1) leads to adverse effects or (2) to successful recovery from dependence.

We often hear the assertion that addiction is a "brain disease," meaning that the critical processes that transform voluntary drug-using behavior to compulsive drug use are changes in the structure and neurochemistry of the brain of the drug user. Sufficient evidence now indicates that such changes in relevant parts of the brain do occur. The perplexing and unanswered question is whether these changes are both necessary and sufficient to account for the drug-using behavior. Many argue that they are not, that the capacity of drug-dependent individuals to modify their drug-using behavior in response to positive reinforcers or aversive contingencies indicates that the nature of addiction is more complex and requires the interaction of multiple factors.

The central element of drug dependence is the drug-using behavior itself. The decision to use a drug is influenced by immediate social and psychological situations as well as by the person's more remote history. The use of the drug initiates a sequence of consequences that can be rewarding or aversive and which, through a process of learning, can result in a greater or lesser likelihood that the drug-using behavior will repeat. For some drugs, use also initiates the biologic processes associated with tolerance, physical dependence, and sensitization. In turn, tolerance can reduce some of the adverse effects of the drug, permitting or requiring the use of larger doses, which then can accelerate or intensify the development of physical dependence. Above a certain threshold, the aversive qualities of a withdrawal syndrome provide a distinct recurrent motive for further drug use. Sensitization of motivational systems can increase the salience of drug-related stimuli.

The Neurobiology of Substance Use Disorders

Genetic Factors.   Strong evidence from studies of twins, adoptees, and siblings brought up separately indicates that the cause of alcohol abuse has a genetic component. Many less conclusive data show that other types of substance abuse or substance dependence have a genetic pattern in their development. Researchers have used restriction fragment length polymorphism (RFLP) in the study of substance use disorders, and preliminary results show associations with genes that affect dopamine production.

Neurochemical Factors
RECEPTORS AND RECEPTOR SYSTEMS.   Except for alcohol, researchers have identified particular neurotransmitters or neurotransmitter receptors involved with most substances of abuse. Some researchers base their studies on such hypotheses. The opioids, for example, act on opioid receptors. A person with too little endogenous opioid activity (e.g., low concentrations of endorphins) or with too much activity of an endogenous opioid antagonist may be at risk for developing an opioid use disorder. Even in a person with completely normal endogenous receptor function and neurotransmitter concentration, the long-term use of a particular substance of abuse may eventually modulate receptor systems in the brain so that the presence of the exogenous substance is needed to maintain homeostasis. Such a receptor-level process may be the mechanism for developing tolerance within the CNS. Demonstrating modulation of neurotransmitter release and neurotransmitter receptor function has proved difficult, however, and recent research focuses on the effects of substances on the second-messenger system and gene regulation.

Pathways and Neurotransmitters.   The primary neurotransmitters possibly involved in developing substance use disorders are the opioid, catecholamine (mainly dopamine), and γ-aminobutyric acid (GABA) systems. The dopaminergic neurons in the ventral tegmental area (VTA) are particularly important. These neurons project to the cortical and limbic regions, especially the nucleus accumbens. This pathway is probably involved in the sensation of reward and may represent the primary mediator of the effects of such substances as amphetamine and cocaine. The locus ceruleus, the largest group of adrenergic neurons, probably mediates the effects of the opiates and the opioids. These pathways have collectively been called the *brain-reward circuitry.*

The Psychology of Substance Use Disorders

Psychodynamic Factors.   The range of psychodynamic theories about substance abuse reflects the various popular theories during the last 100 years. According to classic theories, substance abuse is a masturbatory equivalent (some heroin users describe the initial "rush" as similar to a prolonged sexual orgasm), a defense against anxious impulses, or a manifestation of oral regression (i.e., dependency). New psychodynamic formulations relate substance use as a reflection of disturbed ego functions (i.e., the inability to deal with reality). As a form of self-medication, alcohol may control panic, opioids may diminish anger, and amphetamines may alleviate depression. Some addicts have great difficulty recognizing their inner emotional states, a condition called *alexithymia* (i.e., being unable to find words to describe their feelings).

Learning and Conditioning.   Drug use, whether occasional or compulsive, can be viewed as behavior maintained by its consequences. Drugs can reinforce antecedent behaviors by terminating some noxious or aversive state such as pain, anxiety, or depression. In some social situations, drug use, apart from its pharmacologic effects, can be reinforced if it results in special status or the approval of friends. Each use of the drug evokes rapid positive reinforcement, either as a result of the rush (the drug-induced euphoria), alleviation of disturbed affects, alleviation of withdrawal symptoms, or any combination of these effects. Also, some drugs may sensitize neural systems to the reinforcing effects of the drug. Eventually, the paraphernalia (needles, bottles, cigarette packs) and behaviors associated with substance use can become secondary reinforcers, as well as cues signaling the availability of the substance, and in their presence, craving or a desire to experience the effects increases.

Drug users respond to the drug-related stimuli with increased activity in limbic regions, including the amygdala and the anterior cingulate. A variety of drugs can have this effect, including cocaine, opioids, and cigarettes (nicotine). Of interest, cocaine-related stimuli can activate the same regions that are affected by sexual stimuli in both healthy controls and cocaine users.

In addition to the operant reinforcement of drug-using and drug-seeking behaviors, other learning mechanisms probably play a role in dependence and relapse. Opioid and alcohol withdrawal phenomena can be conditioned (in the Pavlovian or classical sense) to environmental or interoceptive stimuli. For a long time after withdrawal (from opioids, nicotine, or alcohol), the addict exposed to environmental stimuli previously linked with substance use or withdrawal may experience conditioned withdrawal, conditioned craving, or both. The feeling of craving may be independent of feelings of withdrawal. Conditions associated with the availability or use of a substance, such as watching someone else use heroin or light a cigarette or being offered some drug by a friend, bring about the most intense craving. Preexisting pathologies may superimpose on those learning and conditioning phenomena; however, the development of powerfully reinforced substance-seeking behavior does not require preexisting difficulties.

▲ 4.2 Alcohol-Related Disorders

Alcohol is a potent drug that causes both acute and chronic changes in almost all neurochemical systems. Thus alcohol abuse can produce severe, temporary psychological symptoms including depression, anxiety, and psychoses. Increasing levels of regular alcohol consumption can cause tolerance. Chronic use can cause such intense adaptation of the body that stopping drinking can precipitate withdrawal syndromes, including insomnia, autonomic nervous system hyperactivity, and anxiety. Therefore, in an adequate evaluation of life problems and psychiatric symptoms in a patient, the clinician must consider the possibility that the clinical situation reflects the effects of alcohol.

DIAGNOSIS AND CLINICAL FEATURES

The DSM-5 and ICD-10 include several diagnoses related to alcohol, they generally follow the template for all substance use disorders (see Section 4.1 and Tables 4-1 through 4-3). A need for daily use of large amounts of alcohol for adequate functioning, a regular pattern of heavy drinking limited to weekends, and long periods of sobriety interspersed with binges of heavy alcohol intake lasting for weeks or months strongly suggest an alcohol use disorder. The drinking patterns are often associated with certain behaviors: the inability to cut down or stop drinking; repeated efforts to control or reduce excessive drinking by "going on the wagon" (periods of temporary abstinence) or by restricting drinking to certain times of the day; binges (e.g., remaining intoxicated throughout the day for at least 2 days); occasional consumption of large amounts of alcohol in a sitting (e.g., a fifth of spirits or the equivalent in wine or beer); amnestic periods for events occurring while intoxicated (blackouts); the continuation of drinking despite a severe physical disorder that the person knows the alcohol is exacerbating; and drinking nonbeverage alcohol, such as fuel and commercial products containing alcohol. Also, persons with alcohol use disorders show impaired social or occupational functioning because of alcohol use (e.g., violence while intoxicated, absence from work, job loss), legal difficulties (e.g., arrest for intoxicated behavior and traffic accidents while intoxicated), and arguments or difficulties with family members or friends about excessive alcohol consumption.

Mark, a 45-year-old divorced man, was examined in a hospital emergency room because he had been confused and unable to care for himself for the preceding 3 days. His brother, who brought him to the hospital, reported that the patient had consumed large quantities of beer and wine daily for more than 5 years. His home life and job were reasonably stable until his divorce 5 years prior. The brother indicated that Mark's drinking pattern since the divorce had been approximately five beers and a fourth of wine a day. Mark often experienced blackouts from drinking and missed days of work frequently. As a result, Mark has lost several jobs in the past 5 years. Although he usually provides for himself marginally with small jobs, 3 days earlier, he ran out of money and alcohol and resorted to panhandling on the streets for cash to buy food. Mark had been poorly nourished, having one meal per day at best, and was relying on beer as his prime source of nourishment.

On examination, Mark alternates between apprehension and chatty, superficial warmth. He is keyed up and continually talks in a rambling and unfocused manner. His recognition of the physician varies; at times, he recognizes him, and other times he becomes confused and believes the doctor to be his other brother who lives in another state. On two occasions, he referred to the physician by said brother's name and asked when he arrived in town, evidently having lost track of the interview up to that point. He has a gross hand tremor at rest and is confused about the time. He believes he is in a parking lot rather than a hospital. Efforts at memory and calculation testing fail because Mark's attention shifts so rapidly.

Table 4-4
Levels of Impairment at Different Blood Alcohol Concentrations

Level (mg/dL)	Likely Impairment
20–30	Slowed motor performance and decreased thinking ability
30–80	Increases in motor and cognitive problems
80–200	Increases in incoordination and judgment errors Mood lability Deterioration in cognition
200–300	Nystagmus, marked slurring of speech, and alcoholic blackouts
>300	Impaired vital signs and possible death

Alcohol Intoxication

The DSM-5 diagnostic criteria for alcohol intoxication use the standard approach for all substance intoxications (see Section 4.1 and Table 4-3) and include evidence of recent ingestion of ethanol, maladaptive behavior, and at least one of several possible physiologic correlates of intoxication. As a conservative approach to identifying blood levels that are likely to have significant effects on driving abilities, the legal definition of intoxication in most states in the United States requires a blood concentration of 80- or 100-mg ethanol per deciliter of blood (mg/dL), which is the same as 0.08 to 0.10 g/dL. Table 4-4 lists the rough estimates of the levels of impairment likely to be seen at various blood alcohol concentrations for most people. Anyone who does not show significant levels of impairment in motor and mental performance at approximately 150 mg/dL probably has significant pharmacodynamic tolerance.

Alcohol Withdrawal

Alcohol withdrawal, even without delirium, can be severe; it can include seizures and autonomic hyperactivity. Conditions that may predispose to, or aggravate, withdrawal symptoms include fatigue, malnutrition, physical illness, and depression. The DSM-5 criteria for alcohol withdrawal require the cessation or reduction of alcohol use that was heavy and prolonged as well as the presence of specific physical or neuropsychiatric symptoms. The diagnosis also allows for the specification "with perceptual disturbances."

The classic sign of alcohol withdrawal is tremulousness. However, the spectrum of symptoms can expand to include psychotic and perceptual symptoms (e.g., delusions and hallucinations), seizures, and the symptoms of delirium tremens (DTs), called alcohol delirium in DSM-5.

Table 4-5 outlines the progression of alcohol withdrawal from mild to life threatening symptoms. These are rough approximates,

Table 4-5
The Progression of Alcohol Withdrawal Symptoms

	Symptoms	Usual Time to Present
Mild	Tremulousness	6–8 hr
Moderate	Perceptual disturbances	8–12 hr
Severe	Seizures	12–24 hr
Life threatening	Delirium tremens	Within 72 hr

and there is great variation, for example, the syndrome of withdrawal sometimes skips the usual progression and, for example, goes directly to DTs.

The tremor of alcohol withdrawal can be similar to either physiologic tremor, with a continuous tremor of high amplitude and of more than 8 Hz, or familial tremor, with bursts of tremor activity slower than 8 Hz. Other symptoms of withdrawal include general irritability and gastrointestinal (GI) symptoms (e.g., nausea and vomiting). Also standard are symptoms of autonomic hyperactivity, including anxiety, arousal, sweating, facial flushing, mydriasis, tachycardia, and mild hypertension. Patients experiencing alcohol withdrawal are generally alert but may startle easily.

Twenty-nine-year-old Mr. F had been a heavy drinker for 8 years. One evening after work, he started drinking with friends and drank throughout the evening. He fell asleep in the early morning hours and, upon awakening, had a strong desire to drink and decided not to attend work. He had several Bloody Mary's instead of food because the food did not appeal to him. He went to a local bar in the afternoon and consumed large quantities of beer. That evening he met with some friends and continued to drink.

This drinking pattern continued for the next week. At the beginning of the following week, Mr. F attempted to have a cup of coffee but found his hands too shaky to hold the cup. He eventually managed to pour himself some wine in a glass and drank as much as he could. His hands then became less shaky, but he now felt nauseous and began having dry heaves. He tried to drink repeatedly, but he could not keep the alcohol down. He felt very ill and anxious, so he contacted his physician, who recommended he report to a hospital.

Upon evaluation, Mr. F was alert. He had a marked resting and intention tremor of the hands, and his tongue and eyelids were tremulous. He was oriented and had no memory impairment. When inquired about his drinking, Mr. F admitted to drinking several drinks each day for the past 8 years but claimed that his drinking never interfered with his work or his relations with colleagues or friends. He denied having any aftereffects from his drinking other than mild hangovers. He denied ever having a binge such as this before and denied ever needing to drink daily to function adequately. He admitted, however, that he has never tried to reduce or stop drinking.

Withdrawal Seizures.   Seizures associated with alcohol withdrawal are stereotyped, generalized, and tonic–clonic in character. Patients often have more than one seizure 3 to 6 hours after the first seizure. Status epilepticus is relatively rare and occurs in less than 3 percent of patients. Seizure activity in patients with known alcohol abuse histories should still prompt clinicians to consider other causative factors, such as head injuries, CNS infections, CNS neoplasms, and other cerebrovascular diseases. Long-term severe alcohol abuse can result in hypoglycemia, hyponatremia, and hypomagnesemia—all of which can also be associated with seizures.

Delirium.   We should always carefully monitor patients with recognized alcohol withdrawal symptoms to prevent progression to alcohol withdrawal delirium, the most severe form of the withdrawal syndrome, also known as DTs. Alcohol withdrawal delirium is a medical emergency that can result in significant morbidity and mortality. Patients with delirium are a danger to themselves and others. Because of the unpredictability of their behavior, patients with delirium may be assaultive or suicidal. They may act on hallucinations or delusional thoughts as if they were genuine dangers. Untreated, DTs have a mortality rate of 20 percent. This high rate of mortality is usually a result of an intercurrent medical illness such as pneumonia, renal disease, hepatic insufficiency, or heart failure.

Table 4-6
Delirium Tremens Symptoms

Delirium
  Confusion
  Disorientation
  Hallucinations (tactile common)
  Delusions
Autonomic hyperactivity
  Tachycardia
  Diaphoresis
  Fever
  Hypertension
Anxiety
Insomnia
Fluctuating levels of psychomotor activity (ranging from lethargy to agitation)

Although withdrawal seizures commonly precede the development of alcohol withdrawal delirium, delirium can also appear unheralded. The essential feature of the syndrome is delirium occurring within 1 week after a person stops drinking or reduces the intake of alcohol. In addition to the symptoms of delirium, the features of alcohol intoxication delirium include a variety of symptoms, including autonomic symptoms, perceptual, and psychomotor. We list these in Table 4-6.

About 5 percent of hospital patients with alcohol-related disorders have DTs. Because the syndrome usually develops on the third hospital day, a patient admitted for an unrelated condition may unexpectedly have an episode of delirium; this may be the first sign of a previously undiagnosed alcohol-related disorder. Episodes of DTs usually begin in a patient's 30s or 40s after 5 to 15 years of heavy drinking, typically of the binge type. Physical illness (e.g., hepatitis or pancreatitis) predisposes to the syndrome; a person in good physical health rarely has DTs during alcohol withdrawal.

R, a 40-year-old man, was admitted to the orthopedic department of a general hospital after experiencing a fall down his stairs and breaking his leg. On the third day of his hospital stay, he became increasingly nervous and started to tremble. He was unable to sleep at night, talked incoherently, and was very anxious. Mr. R, when asked, denied an alcohol problem other than an occasional glass of wine.

When asked directly, his wife admitted that Mr. R drank large quantities of wine for over 4 years. During the previous year, his drinking would begin every evening when he came home from work and would not end until he fell asleep. On the evening of admission, the fall occurred before he was able to consume any alcohol.

During the few weeks before his admission, Mr. R had eaten very little. On several occasions, Mrs. R noticed that Mr. R was unable to recall even essential events from the previous day. He had a car accident 3 years prior but without significant injury. Mr. R had no other major health problems. His relationship with Mrs. R became problematic after he began drinking, and Mrs. R was seriously contemplating divorce. Mr. R had a tense relationship with his four children, and he often argued with them. Recently, the children have been trying to avoid Mr. R as much as possible.

On examination, Mr. R's speech was rambling and incoherent. He believed that he was still at work and that he had a job to finish. At times he thought the physicians and nurses were his coworkers. At times he picked at bugs that he could see on his bedsheets. He was disoriented in time and was startled easily by sounds from outside the room. He was sweating profusely and could not hold a glass without spilling some of the contents.

Alcohol-Induced Disorders

Alcohol-Induced Persisting Dementia. Alcohol-induced persisting dementia is a poorly studied, heterogeneous long-term cognitive problem that can develop in the course of alcoholism. Patients have decreased intellectual functioning, cognitive abilities, and memory. Recent memory difficulties are consistent with global cognitive impairment, an observation that helps to distinguish this from alcohol-induced persisting amnestic disorder. Brain functioning tends to improve with abstinence, but perhaps half of all affected patients have long-term and even permanent disabilities in memory and thinking. Approximately 50 to 70 percent of these patients have increased brain ventricles and shrinkage of the cerebral sulci. However, these changes appear to be wholly or partially reversible after a year of abstinence.

Alcohol-Induced Persisting Amnestic Disorder. The essential feature of alcohol-induced persisting amnestic disorder is a disturbance in short-term memory caused by prolonged heavy use of alcohol. Because the disorder usually occurs in persons who have been drinking heavily for many years, it is rare in persons younger than age 35.

WERNICKE–KORSAKOFF SYNDROME.   The classic names for alcohol-induced persisting amnestic disorder are Wernicke encephalopathy (a set of acute symptoms) and Korsakoff syndrome (a chronic condition). Whereas Wernicke encephalopathy is entirely reversible with treatment, only about 20 percent of patients with Korsakoff syndrome recover. The pathophysiologic connection between the two syndromes is thiamine deficiency, caused either by poor nutritional habits or by malabsorption problems. Thiamine is a cofactor for several critical enzymes and may also be involved in the conduction of the axon potential along the axon and synaptic transmission. The neuropathologic lesions are symmetrical and paraventricular, involving the mammillary bodies, the thalamus, the hypothalamus, the midbrain, pons, medulla, fornix, and cerebellum.

Wernicke encephalopathy, also called *alcoholic encephalopathy,* is an acute neurologic disorder characterized by ataxia (affecting the gait primarily), vestibular dysfunction, confusion, and a variety of ocular motility abnormalities, including horizontal nystagmus, lateral orbital palsy, and gaze palsy. These eye signs are usually bilateral but not necessarily symmetrical. Other eye signs may include a sluggish reaction to light and anisocoria (unequal pupillary size). Wernicke encephalopathy may clear spontaneously in a few days or weeks or may progress to Korsakoff syndrome.

Korsakoff syndrome is the chronic amnestic syndrome that can follow Wernicke encephalopathy. The cardinal features of Korsakoff syndrome are impaired mental syndrome (especially recent memory) and anterograde amnesia in an alert and responsive patient. The patient may or may not have the symptom of confabulation.

Blackouts.   Blackouts are similar to episodes of transient global amnesia in that they are discrete episodes of anterograde amnesia that occur in association with alcohol intoxication. The periods of amnesia can be particularly distressing when persons fear that they have unknowingly harmed someone or behaved imprudently while intoxicated. During a blackout, persons have relatively intact remote memory but experience a specific short-term memory deficit in which they are unable to recall events that happened in the previous 5 or 10 minutes. Because their other intellectual faculties are well preserved, they can perform complicated tasks and appear normal to casual observers. This deficit is directly caused by alcohol, which can block the consolidation of new memories into old memories, a process that likely involves the hippocampus and related temporal lobe structures.

Alcohol-Induced Psychotic Disorder.

Approximately 3 percent of alcoholic persons experience auditory hallucinations or paranoid delusions in the context of heavy drinking or withdrawal. The most common auditory hallucinations are voices, but they are often unstructured. The voices are characteristically maligning, reproachful, or threatening, although some patients report that the voices are pleasant. The hallucinations usually last less than a week, but during that week, impaired reality testing is frequent. After the episode, most patients realize the hallucinatory nature of the symptoms.

Hallucinations after alcohol withdrawal are considered rare, and the syndrome is distinct from alcohol withdrawal delirium in that the patient has a clear sensorium. The hallucinations can occur at any age but usually, appear in persons abusing alcohol for a long time. Although the hallucinations usually resolve within a week, some linger; in these cases, clinicians must consider other psychotic disorders in the differential diagnosis.

Mr. G was a 40-year-old unemployed man living alone in a studio apartment and was brought to the hospital by the police. He contacted them, complaining that he heard voices of men on the street below his window talking about him and threatening to kill him. He stated that every time he looked out the window, the men had always disappeared.

Mr. G had a 15-year history of almost daily alcohol use. He was intoxicated each day and often experienced shakes upon awakening in the morning. On the previous day, he had only one glass of beer instead of his usual four because of gastrointestinal problems. He was fully alert and oriented.

Alcohol-Induced Mood Disorder.

Heavy intake of alcohol over several days results in many of the symptoms observed in major depressive disorder, but the intense sadness markedly improves within several days to 1 month of abstinence. Eighty percent of people with alcoholism report having histories of intense depression, including 30 to 40 percent who were depressed for two or more weeks at a time. However, only 10 to 15 percent of alcoholic persons have ever had depression that meets the criteria for major depressive disorder when they have not been drinking heavily.

Even severe substance-induced depressions are likely to improve fairly rapidly with abstinence, without specific treatment for the depression. A logical approach for these substance-induced conditions is to teach the patient how to best view and deal with the temporary sadness through education and cognitive-behavioral treatment and to watch and wait at least 2 to 4 weeks before starting antidepressant medications.

A primary care doctor requested a consult for a 42-year-old woman with alcohol use disorder who complained of persisting severe depressive symptoms despite 5 days of abstinence. In the initial stage of the interview, she noted that she had "always been depressed" and felt that she "drank to cope with the depressive symptoms." Her current complaint included a prominent sadness that had persisted for several weeks, difficulties concentrating, initial and terminal insomnia, and a feeling of hopelessness and guilt.

From a detailed discussion of the patient's history, it became clear that there had been no major depressive episodes before her mid-20s when alcohol use disorder began. During 1 year of abstinence

related to the birth and infancy of her son, her mood had significantly improved. The psychiatrist made a provisional diagnosis of an alcohol-induced mood disorder.

The psychiatrist offered the patient education, reassurance, and cognitive therapy to help her to deal with the depressive symptoms but did not prescribe antidepressant medications. The depressive symptoms remained at their original intensity for several additional days and then began to improve. After 3 weeks of abstinence, the patient was no longer significantly depressed, although she had some minor mood swings for several additional weeks. (Courtesy of Marc A. Shuckit, M.D.)

Alcohol-Induced Anxiety Disorder.

Anxiety symptoms fulfilling the diagnostic criteria for alcohol-induced anxiety disorder are also common in the context of acute and protracted alcohol withdrawal. Almost 80 percent of alcoholic persons report panic attacks during at least one acute withdrawal episode; their complaints can, at times, be sufficiently intense for the clinician to consider diagnosing panic disorder. Similarly, during the first 4 weeks or so of abstinence, people with severe alcohol problems are likely to avoid some social situations for fear of being overwhelmed by anxiety (i.e., they have symptoms resembling social phobia); their problems can at times be severe enough to resemble agoraphobia. However, when patients only show symptoms of anxiety in the context of heavy drinking, or shortly after abstinence, then the symptoms are likely to diminish and disappear over time.

A primary care physician referred a 48-year-old woman for evaluation and treatment of her recent onset of panic attacks. These episodes occurred two to three times per week over the preceding 6 months, with each lasting typically between 10 and 20 minutes. Panic symptoms occurred regardless of levels of life stress and were not due to any medications or medical conditions. The workup included an evaluation of her laboratory test values, which revealed a carbohydrate-deficient transferrin (CDT) level of 28 U/L and a γ-glutamyltransferase value of 47. All other blood tests were within normal limits.

The atypical age of onset of the panic attacks, along with the blood results, encouraged the clinician to probe further regarding the pattern of alcohol-related life problems with both the patient and, separately, her spouse. This approach revealed a history of alcohol use disorder with an onset at approximately 35 years of age, with no evidence of panic disorder before that date. During her periods of abstinence, the patient had no significant panic attacks after about 2 weeks. A working diagnosis of an alcohol use disorder, severe with an alcohol-induced anxiety disorder characterized by panic attacks, was made, and the patient was encouraged to abstain. The psychiatrist also recommended that the primary care doctor appropriately treat the patient for possible withdrawal symptoms. Over the subsequent 3 weeks after a taper of benzodiazepines used for the treatment of withdrawal, the panic symptoms diminished in intensity and subsequently disappeared. (Courtesy of Marc A. Schuckit, M.D.)

Alcohol-Induced Sexual Dysfunction.

The formal diagnosis of symptoms of sexual dysfunction associated with alcohol intoxication is alcohol-induced sexual dysfunction, and we discuss this in the chapter on sexual dysfunctions (see Chapter 16).

Alcohol-Induced Sleep Disorder.

We discuss alcohol-induced sleep disorders in the sleep disorders chapter (see Chapter 15).

Unspecified Alcohol-Related Disorder.

The DSM-5 uses the diagnosis of unspecified alcohol-related disorder for alcohol-related disorders that do not meet the diagnostic criteria for any of the other diagnoses.

Table 4-7
Neurologic and Medical Complications of Alcohol Use

Alcohol intoxication
  Acute intoxication
  Pathologic intoxication (atypical, complicated, unusual)
  Blackouts
Alcohol withdrawal syndromes
  Tremulousness (the shakes or the jitters)
  Alcoholic hallucinosis (horrors)
  Withdrawal seizures (rum fits)
  Delirium tremens (shakes)
Nutritional diseases of the nervous system secondary to alcohol abuse
  Wernicke–Korsakoff syndrome
  Cerebellar degeneration
  Peripheral neuropathy
  Optic neuropathy (tobacco–alcohol amblyopia)
  Pellagra
Alcoholic diseases of uncertain pathogenesis
  Central pontine myelinolysis
  Marchiafava–Bignami disease
  Fetal alcohol syndrome
  Myopathy
  Alcoholic dementia
  Alcoholic cerebral atrophy
Systemic diseases due to alcohol with secondary neurologic
  complications
  Liver disease
    Hepatic encephalopathy
    Acquired (non-Wilsonian) chronic hepatocerebral degeneration
  Gastrointestinal diseases
  Malabsorption syndromes
  Postgastrectomy syndromes
  Possible pancreatic encephalopathy

Cardiovascular diseases
  Cardiomyopathy with potential cardiogenic emboli and
    cerebrovascular disease
  Arrhythmias and abnormal blood pressure leading to
    cerebrovascular disease
Hematologic disorders
  Anemia, leukopenia, thrombocytopenia (could possibly lead to
    hemorrhagic cerebrovascular disease)
Infectious disease, especially meningitis (especially pneumococcal
  and meningococcal)
Hypothermia and hyperthermia
Hypotension and hypertension
Respiratory depression and associated hypoxia
Toxic encephalopathies, including alcohol and other substances
Electrolyte imbalances leading to acute confusional states and,
  rarely, local neurologic signs and symptoms
  Hypoglycemia
  Hyperglycemia
  Hyponatremia
  Hypercalcemia
  Hypomagnesemia
  Hypophosphatemia
Increased incidence of trauma
  Epidural, subdural, and intracerebral hematoma
  Spinal cord injury
  Posttraumatic seizure disorders
  Compressive neuropathies and brachial plexus injuries (Saturday
    night palsies)
  Posttraumatic symptomatic hydrocephalus (normal pressure
    hydrocephalus)
  Muscle crush injuries and compartmental syndromes

Other Alcohol-Related Neurologic Disorders. We are restricting our discussion to the significant neuropsychiatric syndromes associated with alcohol use. The complete list of neurologic syndromes is lengthy, Table 4-7 provides an example list of some neurologic and medical complications of alcohol use.

Alcoholic pellagra encephalopathy is one diagnosis of potential interest to psychiatrists presented with a patient who appears to have Wernicke–Korsakoff syndrome but who does not respond to thiamine treatment. We list the symptoms of alcoholic pellagra in Table 4-8.

Fetal Alcohol Syndrome. Data indicate that women who are pregnant or are breast-feeding should not drink alcohol. Fetal alcohol syndrome, the leading cause of intellectual disability in the United States, occurs when mothers who drink alcohol expose fetuses to alcohol in utero. The alcohol inhibits intrauterine growth and postnatal development. Microcephaly, craniofacial malformations, and limb and heart defects are common in affected infants.

Table 4-8
Possible Symptoms of Alcohol Pellagra

Confusion, ranging from mild to full delirium
Clouding of consciousness
Myoclonus
Oppositional hypertonias
Fatigue
Apathy
Irritability
Anorexia
Insomnia

Short adult stature and development of a range of adult maladaptive behavior are also associated with fetal alcohol syndrome.

Women with alcohol-related disorders have a 35 percent risk of having a child with defects. Although the precise mechanism of the damage to the fetus is unknown, the damage seems to result from exposure in utero to ethanol or its metabolites; alcohol may also cause hormone imbalances that increase the risk of abnormalities.

Laboratory Tests

The adverse effects of alcohol appear in standard laboratory tests, which can be useful diagnostic aids in identifying persons with alcohol-related disorders. Table 4-9 lists some of the more useful tests, all of which are related to the damaging effects of alcohol.

Table 4-9
Laboratory Test Associated with Heavy Drinking

State Markers of Heavy Drinking Useful in Screening for AUDs	
Test	**Relevant Range of Results**
γ-glutamyltransferase (GGT)	>35.0 U/L
Carbohydrate-deficient transferrin (CDT)	>3.0%
Mean corpuscular volume (MCV)	>91.0 μm^3
Serum glutamic oxaloacetic transaminase (aspartate aminotransferase)	>45.0 IU/L
Serum glutamic pyruvic transaminase (alanine aminotransferase)	>45.0 IU/L

COMORBIDITY

The psychiatric diagnoses most associated with alcohol-related disorders are other substance-related disorders, antisocial personality disorder, mood disorders, and anxiety disorders. Although the data are somewhat controversial, most suggest that persons with alcohol-related disorders have a markedly higher suicide rate than the general population.

Antisocial Personality Disorder

Researchers and clinicians have frequently reported a relation between antisocial personality disorder and alcohol-related disorders. Some studies suggest that antisocial personality disorder is particularly common in men with an alcohol-related disorder and can precede the development of an alcohol-related disorder. Other studies, however, suggest that antisocial personality disorder and alcohol-related disorders are entirely distinct entities that are not causally related.

Mood Disorders

About 30 to 40 percent of persons with an alcohol-related disorder meet the diagnostic criteria for major depressive disorder sometime during their lifetimes. Depression is more common in women than in men with these disorders. Several studies reported that depression is likely to occur in patients with alcohol-related disorders who have a high daily consumption of alcohol and a family history of alcohol abuse. Persons with alcohol-related disorders and major depressive disorder are at significant risk for attempting suicide and are likely to have other substance-related disorder diagnoses. Some clinicians recommend antidepressant drug therapy for depressive symptoms that remain after 2 to 3 weeks of sobriety. Patients with bipolar disorder are at risk of developing an alcohol-related disorder; they may use alcohol to self-medicate their manic episodes.

Anxiety Disorders

Many persons use alcohol for its efficacy in alleviating anxiety. Although the comorbidity between alcohol-related disorders and mood disorders is widely recognized, perhaps 25 to 50 percent of all persons with alcohol-related disorders also meet the diagnostic criteria for an anxiety disorder. Phobias and panic disorder are particularly frequent comorbid diagnoses in these patients. Persons with anxiety may use alcohol to self-medicate symptoms of agoraphobia or social phobia. Still, an alcohol-related disorder is likely to precede the development of panic disorder or generalized anxiety disorder.

Suicide

Most estimates of the prevalence of suicide among persons with alcohol-related disorders range from 10 to 15 percent, although alcohol use itself may be involved in a much higher percentage of suicides. Some investigators have questioned whether the suicide rate among persons with alcohol-related disorders is as high as the numbers suggest. Table 4-10 lists factors associated with suicide among persons with alcohol-related disorders.

COURSE AND PROGNOSIS

Between 10 and 40 percent of alcoholic persons enter some formal treatment program. Several prognostic signs are favorable. Table 4-11

Table 4-10
Factors Associated with Suicide in Persons with Alcohol Use Disorder

Presence of a major depressive episode
Weak psychosocial support systems
A serious coexisting medical condition
Unemployment
Living alone

lists some of the most predictive factors, and the combination of these predicts at least a 60 percent chance for one or more years of abstinence. Few studies have documented the long-term course, but researchers agree that 1 year of abstinence is associated with a good chance for continued abstinence over an extended period. Alcoholic persons with severe drug problems (especially intravenous drug use or cocaine or amphetamine use disorders) and those who are homeless may have only a 10 to 15 percent chance of achieving 1 year of abstinence, however.

Accurately predicting whether any specific person will achieve or maintain abstinence is impossible, but the prognostic factors listed earlier are associated with an increased likelihood of abstinence. The factors reflecting life stability, however, probably explain only 20 percent or less of the course of alcohol use disorders. Many other factors, some that may be hard to measure, also affect the clinical course significantly. These somewhat intangible factors are likely to include motivational levels and the quality of the patient's social support system.

In general, alcoholic persons with preexisting independent major psychiatric disorders—such as antisocial personality disorder, schizophrenia, and bipolar disorder—are likely to run the course of their independent psychiatric illness. Clinicians should treat the patient with bipolar disorder who has alcoholism with appropriate pharmacotherapy and psychotherapy. The same can be said for an antisocial personality disorder, schizophrenia, or other psychiatric disorders. The goal is to minimize the symptoms of the independent psychiatric disorder in the hope that better life stability will be associated with a better prognosis for the patient's alcohol problems.

TREATMENT OF ALCOHOL USE DISORDERS

Three general steps are involved in treating the alcoholic person: intervention, detoxification, and rehabilitation. These approaches assume that we have already addressed the patient's medical functioning and addressed any psychiatric emergencies. Thus, for example, an alcoholic person with symptoms of depression sufficiently severe to be suicidal requires inpatient hospitalization for at least several days until the suicidal ideation disappears. Similarly, a person presenting with cardiomyopathy, liver difficulties, or GI bleeding first needs adequate treatment of the medical emergency.

The patient with alcohol use disorder must then be brought face-to-face with the reality of the disorder (intervention), be

Table 4-11
Alcohol Use Disorders: Positive Prognostic Signs

No premorbid antisocial personality disorder
Good psychosocial functioning
    Stable job
    Stable family
    No legal problems
Adherence to treatment

detoxified if needed, and begin rehabilitation. The essentials of these three steps for an alcoholic person with independent psychiatric syndromes closely resemble the approaches used for the primary alcoholic person without independent psychiatric syndromes. In the former case, however, we should apply these treatments after stabilizing the psychiatric disorder as much as possible.

Intervention

The goal of intervention is to use the principles of motivational interviewing and brief interventions to help patients recognize the adverse consequences likely to occur if they do not stop drinking. A discussion of the presenting complaint (e.g., insomnia or depression) is a useful way to both show empathy and enhance motivation for change. As part of an intervention, we would emphasize how alcohol either created or contributed to these problems and reassure the patient that abstinence is possible. If the person does not respond to the first brief intervention or motivational interview, we can use the same nonjudgmental but persistent approach each time an alcohol-related problem arises. It is the persistence rather than exceptional interpersonal skills that usually gets results. A single intervention is rarely sufficient. Most alcoholic persons need a series of reminders of how alcohol contributed to each developing crisis before they seriously consider abstinence as a long-term option.

> JP, a 47-year-old physician, was confronted regarding his alcohol-related behaviors by his wife and 21-year-old daughter. They told him about his slurred speech on several recent occasions when the daughter called home, as well as a large number of wine bottles in the trash each week. JP's wife complained of the hours he spent alone in his study and his practice of staying up after she went to bed, retiring later with alcohol on his breath. She also related her concern about his consumption of about 10 or 12 drinks at a recent party. He also tended to isolate himself from the other guests. She then reminded him of his need to pack liquor when they go on trips where alcohol may not be readily available, and the tremor of his hands some mornings after being drunk the night before. The family shared their concern directly with JP at a time when he was not actively intoxicated, emphasizing specific times and events when his impairment with alcohol occurred. They had also made an appointment with the clinician at an alcohol and drug treatment program to facilitate the next step if the intervention was successful. (Adapted from Marc A. Schuckit, M.D.)

Detoxification

Most persons with alcohol use disorder have relatively mild symptoms when they stop drinking. If the patient is in relatively good health, is adequately nourished, and has a sound social support system, the depressant withdrawal syndrome usually resembles a mild case of the flu. Even intense withdrawal syndromes rarely approach the severity of symptoms described by some early textbooks in the field.

The essential first step in detoxification is a thorough physical examination. In the absence of a severe medical disorder or combined drug abuse, severe alcohol withdrawal is unlikely. The second step is to offer rest, adequate nutrition, and multiple vitamins, especially those containing thiamine.

Seizures.   Seizures can occur suddenly and without other signs of withdrawal. About 1 percent of patients may have a single grand

mal convulsion; the rare person has multiple fits, with the peak incidence on the second day of withdrawal.

Such patients require neurologic evaluation to rule out an independent seizure disorder. Assuming no other cause for the seizures is found, benzodiazepines are the treatment of choice for managing alcohol-related seizures. Anticonvulsants, although often used (particularly before the cause of the seizure is known), do not appear to offer additional benefit.

Mild or Moderate Withdrawal.   Withdrawal develops because the brain has physically adapted to the presence of a brain depressant and cannot function adequately in the absence of the drug. Giving sufficient brain depressant on the first day to diminish symptoms and then weaning the patient off the drug over the next 5 days offers most patients optimal relief. It also minimizes the possibility that severe withdrawal will develop. Any CNS depressant (including benzodiazepines, barbiturates, or even alcohol) can work, but most clinicians choose a benzodiazepine for its relative safety. Many studies have found that benzodiazepines control most of the symptoms associated with alcohol withdrawal. We can give adequate treatment with either short-acting drugs (e.g., lorazepam), or long-acting substances (e.g., chlordiazepoxide and diazepam). We may choose to give benzodiazepines orally or parenterally; however, we should not give intramuscular (IM) diazepam or chlordiazepoxide as their IM absorption is erratic. We should titrate the dosage of the benzodiazepine, starting with a high dosage and lowering the dosage as the patient recovers. We should aim to give sufficient benzodiazepines to keep patients calm and sedated but not so sedated that we cannot arouse them for procedures and examinations.

Although benzodiazepines are the standard treatment for alcohol withdrawal, studies have shown that carbamazepine in daily doses of 800 mg is as effective as benzodiazepines and has the added benefit of minimal abuse liability. Carbamazepine use is gradually becoming common in the United States and Europe.

Table 4-12 gives an example of withdrawal treatment using chlordiazepoxide. When giving a long-acting agent, such as chlordiazepoxide, the clinician must avoid producing excessive sleepiness through overmedication; if the patient is sleepy, it is best to omit the next scheduled dose. When taking a short-acting drug, such as lorazepam, the patient must not miss any dose because rapid changes in benzodiazepine concentrations in the blood can precipitate severe withdrawal.

A social model program of detoxification saves money by avoiding medications while using social supports. This less-expensive regimen can be helpful for mild or moderate withdrawal syndromes. Some clinicians also use β-adrenergic receptor antagonists (e.g., propranolol) or α-adrenergic receptor agonists

Table 4-12
An Example Treatment for Alcohol Withdrawal

Day 1: chlordiazepoxide 25 mg by mouth 3–4 times daily, hold if sedated
   1–2 additional doses if
     The patient is jittery
     Has increased tremor
     Has autonomic dysfunction
Day 2: give the total dose used on day 1 minus 20% divided across 3–4 doses
Following days: continue a 20% decrease until no further medication is needed (4–5 days)

(e.g., clonidine) to block the symptoms of sympathetic hyperactivity. However, these medications do not appear to be superior to benzodiazepines. Unlike the brain depressants, these other agents are not effective treatments for seizures or delirium.

Severe Withdrawal.   For the approximately 1 percent of alcoholic patients with extreme autonomic dysfunction, agitation, and confusion—that is, those with alcohol withdrawal delirium, or DTs—no optimal treatment has yet been developed. The best treatment for DTs is prevention. When that is not possible, the first step is to ask why such a severe and relatively uncommon withdrawal syndrome has occurred. The answer often relates to a severe concomitant medical problem that needs immediate treatment.

Once a delirium appears, the treatment remains similar to that for the standard withdrawal but with higher doses. Example regimens are 50 to 100 mg of chlordiazepoxide given every 4 hours orally, or lorazepam, given intravenously (IV) if oral medication is not possible. A high-calorie, high-carbohydrate diet supplemented by multivitamins is also essential.

Physically restraining patients with the DTs is risky; they may fight against the restraints to a dangerous level of exhaustion. When patients are disorderly and uncontrollable, it may be preferable to use a seclusion room. Adjunctive antipsychotic medications, such as haloperidol, are sometimes used to control severe agitation and hallucinations. However, antipsychotic medications may reduce the seizure threshold in patients. Dehydration, often exacerbated by diaphoresis and fever, can be corrected with fluids given by mouth or IV. Anorexia, vomiting, and diarrhea often occur during withdrawal. The emergence of focal neurologic symptoms, lateralizing seizures, increased intracranial pressure, or evidence of skull fractures or other indications of CNS pathology should prompt clinicians to examine a patient for neurologic disease.

Warm, supportive psychotherapy in the treatment of DTs is essential. Patients are often bewildered, frightened, and anxious because of their tumultuous symptoms, and skillful verbal support is imperative.

Protracted Withdrawal.   Symptoms of anxiety, insomnia, and mild autonomic overactivity are likely to continue for 2 to 6 months after the acute withdrawal has disappeared. These protracted withdrawal symptoms may enhance the probability of relapse. Although there is little evidence that medications are helpful, it is possible that some of the medications used for the rehabilitation phase, especially acamprosate, may work by diminishing some of these symptoms. The clinician should warn the patient that some level of sleep problems or feelings of nervousness might remain after acute withdrawal and discuss cognitive and behavioral approaches that might be appropriate to help the patient feel comfortable.

Rehabilitation

For most patients, rehabilitation includes three major components, which are listed in Table 4-13. These components happen

Table 4-13
Three Components of Alcohol Rehabilitation

Continued efforts to increase and maintain high levels of
  motivation for abstinence
Work to help the patient readjust to a lifestyle free of alcohol
Relapse prevention

Table 4-14
Stages of Alcohol Rehabilitation Treatment

Early intensive period (2–4 wk)
Intervention (withdrawal treatment, preventing craving)
Optimizing physical and psychological functioning
Enhancing motivation
Reaching out to the family

Long term (3–6 mo)
Individual and group counseling
Judicious avoidance of psychotropic medications unless needed for
  independent disorders
Involvement in self-help groups such as AA

at a difficult time: the patient may still be experiencing withdrawal symptoms as well as life crises. Repetition will be necessary, with frequent reminders of how vital abstinence is, and that it helps the patient develop new day-to-day support systems and coping styles.

No single major life event, traumatic life period, or identifiable psychiatric disorder is known to be the sole cause of alcoholism. Regardless of any possible cause, after years of alcohol use, it develops a life of its own. Many alcoholic persons believe that the cause was depression, anxiety, life stress, or pain syndromes. However, usually, the reality is that alcohol contributed to the mood disorder, accident, or life stress, not vice versa.

The treatment approach remains the same regardless of setting, including both inpatient and outpatient treatments. The selection of the more intensive (and expensive) inpatient mode often depends on several factors. These include whether there are additional severe medical or psychiatric syndromes, what other options are available, and whether the patient has previously failed outpatient treatment.

The treatment process in either setting involves an intensive early phase, which lasts 2 to 4 weeks, followed by longer-term care. Table 4-14 lists some of the approaches used in these phases.

Counseling

Counseling efforts in the first several months should focus on day-to-day life issues to help patients maintain a high level of motivation for abstinence and to enhance their functioning. Psychotherapy techniques that provoke anxiety or that require deep insights are not likely to be of benefit during the early months of recovery and, at least theoretically, may impair efforts to maintain abstinence. Thus, this discussion focuses on the efforts likely to characterize the first 3 to 6 months of care.

Both individual and group counseling is an option, and few data suggest that either approach is superior. The technique used is not likely to matter much and usually boils down to simple day-to-day counseling or almost any behavioral or psychotherapeutic approach focusing on the here and now. Treatment sessions should explore the consequences of drinking, the likely future course of alcohol-related life problems, and the marked improvement that results from abstinence. Whether in an inpatient or an outpatient setting, individual or group counseling is usually offered a minimum of three times a week for the first 2 to 4 weeks, followed by less intense efforts, perhaps once a week, for the subsequent 3 to 6 months.

Much time in counseling deals with how to build a lifestyle free of alcohol. Discussions cover the need for a sober peer group, a plan for social and recreational events without drinking, and approaches for reestablishing communication with family members and friends.

The third major component, relapse prevention, first identifies situations in which the risk for relapse is high. The counselor must help the patient develop modes of coping for when the craving for alcohol increases or when an event or emotional state makes a return to drinking likely. An essential part of relapse prevention is reminding the patient about the appropriate attitude toward slips. Short-term experiences with alcohol should not be an excuse for returning to regular drinking. Recovery is not an "all or none" game. Instead, it is a process of trial and error; patients use slips as information to identify high-risk situations and to develop more appropriate coping techniques.

Most treatment efforts recognize the effects that alcoholism has on the significant persons in the patient's life, and an essential aspect of recovery involves helping family members and close friends understand alcoholism and realize that rehabilitation is an ongoing process that lasts for 6 to 12 or more months. Couples and family counseling and support groups for relatives and friends help the persons involved to rebuild relationships, to learn how to avoid protecting the patient from the consequences of any drinking in the future, and to be as supportive as possible of the alcoholic patient's recovery program.

Medication Treatment

Following detoxification, there is little reason to prescribe antidepressant or anxiety medications if the patient does not have an independent psychiatric disorder. Lingering levels of anxiety and insomnia as part of a reaction to life stresses and protracted abstinence should be treated with behavior modification approaches and reassurance. Medications for these symptoms are likely to lose their effectiveness much faster than the symptoms will disappear, and the patient may increase the dose, leading to subsequent problems. Similarly, sadness and mood swings can linger at low levels for several months. Controlled clinical trials, however, indicate no benefit in prescribing antidepressant medications or lithium to treat the average alcoholic person who has no independent or long-lasting psychiatric disorder. The mood disorder will clear before the medications can take effect, and patients who resume drinking while on the medications face significant potential dangers. With little or no evidence that the medications are effective, the dangers significantly outweigh any potential benefits from their routine use.

Data from double-blind trials support modest effects for two medications offered in the context of cognitive-behavioral therapy (CBT). The first involves the opioid antagonist naltrexone, which appears to decrease the craving for alcohol or blunt the rewarding effects of drinking. The COMBINE study (Combined Pharmacotherapies and Behavioral Interventions) demonstrated that naltrexone improves clinical outcomes, and a Cochrane review of naltrexone concluded that naltrexone was effective in reducing heavy drinking days. The typical dose is 50 mg/day, and side effects include mild GI upset and lethargy.

The second medication, acamprosate, antagonizes neuronal overactivity related to the excitatory neurotransmitter glutamate, at least in part, by acting as an antagonist to N-methyl-D-aspartate (NMDA) receptors. Acamprosate may diminish mild anxiety, mood swings, and other sleep difficulties associated with the protracted withdrawal syndrome observed after the first 4 to 5 days of abstinence. The typical dose is about 2,000 mg divided into three doses per day and is associated with relatively mild side effects of GI problems such as diarrhea.

A third possible drug of interest is the alcohol-sensitizing agent disulfiram. Disulfiram is given in daily doses of 250 mg before discharging the patient from the intensive first phase of outpatient rehabilitation or inpatient care. The goal is to place the patient in a condition in which drinking alcohol precipitates an uncomfortable physical reaction, including nausea, vomiting, and a burning sensation in the face and stomach. Few data support disulfiram's effectiveness, most likely because patients stop it when they resume drinking. Many clinicians have stopped routinely prescribing the agent, partly in recognition of the dangers associated with the drug itself: mood swings, rare instances of psychosis, the possibility of increased peripheral neuropathies, the relatively rare occurrence of other significant neuropathies, and potentially fatal hepatitis. Moreover, we should not give disulfiram to patients with preexisting heart disease, cerebral thrombosis, diabetes, and some other conditions, because an alcohol reaction to the disulfiram could be fatal.

Table 4-15 gives a summary of medications used for alcohol dependence.

Two other medications, while not yet approved for the treatment of alcohol use disorders, are worth brief mention. Several studies using the anticonvulsant topiramate have reported improvement in drinking patterns. Additionally, some data suggest that the 5-HT$_3$ ondansetron might be beneficial in alcohol use disorder treatment. No evidence exists that antidepressant medications, such as selective serotonin reuptake inhibitors (SSRIs), lithium, or antipsychotic medications, are significantly effective in the treatment of alcoholism.

Alcoholics Anonymous

Clinicians must recognize the potential importance of self-help groups such as AA. Members of AA have help available 24 hours a day, associate with a sober peer group, learn that it is possible to participate in social functions without drinking, and are given a model of recovery by observing the accomplishments of sober members of the group.

Learning about AA usually begins during inpatient or outpatient rehabilitation. The clinician can play a significant role in helping patients understand the differences between specific groups. Some groups are single gender, others are mixed. Certain groups may differ by socioeconomic level as well, or place great emphasis on religion. Such specialized groups may be a practical approach. Anyone can suffer from alcoholism, but a person may be more likely to stick with a group toward which they feel some affinity. Patients with coexisting psychiatric disorders may need some additional education about AA. The clinician should remind them that some members of AA may not understand their unique needs for medications and should arm the patients with ways of coping when group members inappropriately advise against medications. Although challenging to evaluate using double-blind controls, most studies indicate that participation in AA is associated with improved outcomes, as well as being cost-efficient.

Treatment of Alcohol-Related Disorders

Treatment of Alcohol-Induced Amnestic Disorders. In the early stages, Wernicke encephalopathy responds rapidly to large doses of parenteral thiamine, which is likely effective at preventing the progression to Korsakoff syndrome. The dosage of thiamine is usually initiated at 100 mg by mouth two to three times daily and continued for 1 to 2 weeks. In patients with alcohol-related disorders who are receiving IV administration of glucose solution, it is good practice to include 100 mg of thiamine in each liter of the glucose solution.

Table 4-15
Medications for Treating Alcohol Dependence

	Naltrexone	Acamprosate	Disulfiram
Action	Blocks opioid receptors, resulting in reduced craving and reduced reward in response to drinking	Not well understood. Likely an NMDA receptor antagonist and positive allosteric modulator of GABA$_a$ receptors	Inhibits intermediate metabolism of alcohol, causing a buildup of acetaldehyde and a reaction of flushing, sweating, nausea, and tachycardia if a patient drinks alcohol
Contraindications	Currently using opioids or in acute opioid withdrawal; anticipated need for opioid analgesics; acute hepatitis or liver failure	Severe renal impairment (CrCl ≤30 mL/min)	Concomitant use of alcohol or alcohol-containing preparations or metronidazole; coronary artery disease; severe myocardial disease
Precautions	Other hepatic disease; renal impairment; history of suicide attempts. If opioid analgesia is required, larger doses may be required, and respiratory depression may be deeper and more prolonged	Moderate renal impairment (dose adjustment for CrCl between 30 and 50 mL/min); depression or suicidality	High impulsivity—likely to drink while using it; psychoses (current or history); diabetes mellitus; epilepsy; hepatic dysfunction; hypothyroidism; renal impairment; rubber contact dermatitis
Serious adverse reactions	Will precipitate severe withdrawal if patient is dependent on opioids; hepatotoxicity (uncommon at usual doses). Pregnancy Category C.	Anxiety; depression. Rare events include the following: suicide attempt, acute kidney failure, heart failure, mesenteric arterial occlusion, cardiomyopathy, deep thrombophlebitis, and shock. Pregnancy Category C.	Hepatitis; optic neuritis; peripheral neuropathy; psychotic reactions. Pregnancy Category C.
Common side effects	Nausea; abdominal pain; constipation; dizziness; headache; anxiety; fatigue	Diarrhea; flatulence; nausea; abdominal pain; headache; back pain; infection; flu syndrome; chills; somnolence; decreased libido; amnesia; confusion	Metallic aftertaste; dermatitis
Examples of drug interactions	Opioid analgesics (blocks action); yohimbine (use with naltrexone increases negative drug effects)	No clinically relevant interactions known	Amitriptyline; anticoagulants such as warfarin; diazepam; isoniazid; metronidazole; phenytoin; theophylline; warfarin; any nonprescription drug-containing alcohol
Usual adult dosage	*Oral dose:* 50 mg daily *before prescribing:* evaluate for possible current opioid use; consider a urine toxicology screen for opioids, including synthetic opioids. Obtain liver function tests *Follow-up:* monitor liver function tests periodically	*Oral dose:* 666 mg (two 333-mg tablets) three times daily *or,* for patients with moderate renal impairment (CrCl 30–50 mL/min), reduce to 333 mg (one tablet) three times daily *before prescribing:* establish abstinence	*Oral dose:* 250 mg daily (range 125–500 mg) *before prescribing:* (1) warn that the patient should not take disulfiram for at least 12 hr after drinking and that a disulfiram-alcohol reaction can occur up to 2 wk after the last dose; and (2) warn about alcohol in the diet (e.g., sauces and vinegars) and in medications and toiletries *Follow-up:* monitor liver function tests periodically

CrCl, creatinine clearance; GABA, γ-aminobutyric acid.

Treatment of Korsakoff syndrome is also thiamine given 100 mg by mouth two to three times daily; the treatment regimen should continue for 3 to 12 months. Few patients who progress to Korsakoff syndrome ever fully recover, although many have some improvement in their cognitive abilities with thiamine and nutritional support.

In a patient who appears to have Wernicke–Korsakoff syndrome but who does not respond to thiamine treatment, one should consider the diagnosis of alcoholic pellagra encephalopathy (see Other Alcohol-Related Neurologic Disorders). Such patients have a niacin (nicotinic acid) deficiency, and the specific treatment is 50 mg of niacin by mouth four times daily or 25 mg parenterally two to three times daily.

Treatment of Alcohol Withdrawal-Related Hallucinations.
The treatment of alcohol withdrawal-related hallucinations is much like the treatment of DTs—benzodiazepines, adequate nutrition, and fluids, if necessary. If this regimen fails or for long-term cases, clinicians may add antipsychotics.

Treatment of Idiosyncratic Alcohol Intoxication.   In treating idiosyncratic alcohol intoxication, clinicians must help protect

Table 4-16
Alcohol Epidemiology

Condition	Population (%)
Ever had a drink	90
Current drinker	60–70
Temporary problems	40+
Alcohol use disorder (AUD) lifetime	Male: 15+ Female: 10+
AUDs in psychiatric patients	30

The percentages listed here are approximations generated across studies.
From *Kaplan and Sadock's Comprehensive Textbook of Psychiatry.* 10th ed. 2017.

patients from harming themselves and others. Physical restraint may be necessary, but it is difficult because of the abrupt onset of the condition. Once restraining the patient, it may be helpful to inject an antipsychotic, such as haloperidol, to control assaultiveness. We should differentiate this condition from other causes of abrupt behavioral change, such as complex partial epilepsy. Some persons with the disorder reportedly showed temporal lobe spiking on an EEG after ingesting small amounts of alcohol.

Epidemiology

Alcohol use disorder is among the most common psychiatric disorders observed in the Western world. Alcohol-related problems in the United States contribute to 88,000 deaths each year, with nearly 10,000 deaths as a result of alcohol-impaired driving. According to data from the World Health Organization (WHO), alcohol is the fifth leading risk factor for premature death and disability across the world. Table 4-16 lists some composite epidemiologic data on alcohol use.

Prevalence of Drinking. At some time during life, 90 percent of the population in the United States drinks, with most people beginning their alcohol intake in the early to middle teens. By the end of high school, 80 percent of students have consumed alcohol, and more than 60 percent have been intoxicated. At any time, two of three men are drinkers, with a ratio of persisting alcohol intake of approximately 1.3 men to 1.0 women, and the highest prevalence of drinking from the middle or late teens to the mid-20s.

Men and women with higher education and income are most likely to imbibe, and, among religious denominations, Jewish persons have the highest proportion who consume alcohol but among the lowest rates of alcohol use disorders. Other ethnicities, such as the Irish, have higher rates of severe alcohol problems, but they also have significantly higher rates of abstentions. Some estimates show that more than 60 percent of men and women in some Native American and Inuit tribes have at some time had an alcohol use disorder. In the United States, the average adult consumes 2.4 gallons of absolute alcohol a year, a considerable decrease from 5 gallons of absolute alcohol yearly intake in the 1700s.

Drinking alcohol-containing beverages is generally considered an acceptable habit in the United States. About 90 percent of all US residents have consumed alcohol at least once in their lives. About 56 percent of all US adults used alcohol in the past month. Alcohol is the third leading preventable cause of death in the United States, behind tobacco use and poor diet/physical inactivity. Excessive alcohol use is associated with 2.5 million years of potential life lost in the United States each year and causes 10 percent of all deaths among working adults. Although persons involved in automotive fatalities do not always meet the diagnostic criteria for an alcohol-related disorder, drunk drivers are involved in about 31 percent of all automotive fatalities. Alcohol use and alcohol-related disorders are associated with about 25 percent of all suicides.

PATHOLOGY

Effects of Alcohol

The term *alcohol* refers to a large group of organic molecules that have a hydroxyl group (–OH) attached to a saturated carbon atom. Ethyl alcohol, also called *ethanol,* is the standard form of drinkable alcohol, sometimes referred to as *beverage alcohol.* The chemical formula for ethanol is $CH_3–CH_2–OH$.

The characteristic tastes and flavors of alcohol-containing beverages result from their methods of production, which produce various congeners in the final product, including methanol, butanol, aldehydes, phenols, tannins, and trace amounts of various metals. Although the congeners may confer some differential psychoactive effects on the various alcohol-containing beverages, these differences are minimal compared with the effects of ethanol itself. A single drink typically contains about 12 g of ethanol, which is the content of 12 oz of beer (7.2 proof, 3.6 percent ethanol in the United States), one 4-oz glass of nonfortified wine, or 1 to 1.5 oz of an 80-proof (40 percent ethanol) liquor (e.g., whiskey or gin). In calculating patients' alcohol intake, however, clinicians should be aware that beers vary in their alcohol content, that beers are available in small and large cans and mugs, that glasses of wine range from 2 to 6 oz, and that mixed drinks at some bars and in most homes contain 2 to 3 oz of liquor. Nonetheless, using the moderate sizes of drinks, clinicians can estimate that a single drink increases the blood alcohol level of a 150-lb man by 15 to 20 mg/dL, which is about the concentration of alcohol that an average person can metabolize in 1 hour.

The possible beneficial effects of alcohol have been publicized, especially by the makers and the distributors of alcohol. Some epidemiologic data suggest that one or two glasses of red wine each day lower the incidence of cardiovascular disease; these findings, however, are highly controversial.

Absorption. The stomach absorbs about 10 percent of consumed alcohol, and the small intestine absorbs the rest. It takes about 30 to 90 minutes to reach peak blood concentration, depending on whether the alcohol was ingested on an empty stomach (which enhances absorption) or with food (which delays absorption). Also, rapid drinking reduces the time to peak concentration; slower drinking increases it. Absorption is most rapid, with beverages containing 15 to 30 percent alcohol (30 to 60 proof). There is some dispute about whether carbonation (e.g., in champagne and drinks mixed with seltzer) enhances the absorption of alcohol.

The body has protective devices against inundation by alcohol. For example, if the concentration of alcohol in the stomach becomes too high, mucus is secreted, and the pyloric valve closes. These actions slow the absorption and keep the alcohol from passing into the small intestine, where there are no significant restraints on absorption. Thus, a large amount of alcohol can remain unabsorbed in the stomach for hours. Furthermore, pylorospasm often results in nausea and vomiting.

Once the bloodstream absorbs the alcohol, it distributes to all body tissues. Alcohol uniformly dissolves in the body's water, so tissues containing a high proportion of water receive a high concentration of alcohol. The intoxicating effects are more significant for a given blood alcohol concentration when the concentration is rising than when it is falling (the Mellanby effect). For this reason, the rate of absorption bears directly on the intoxication response.

Metabolism. Hepatic oxidation accounts for about 90 percent of alcohol metabolism. The remaining 10 percent is excreted unchanged by the kidneys and lungs. The rate of oxidation by the liver is constant and independent of the body's energy requirements. The body can metabolize about 15 mg/dL per hour, with a range of 10 to 34 mg/dL per hour. That is, the average person oxidizes three-fourths of an ounce of 40 percent (80 proof) alcohol in an hour. In persons with a history of excessive alcohol consumption, upregulation of the necessary enzymes results in rapid alcohol metabolism.

Two enzymes metabolize alcohol: alcohol dehydrogenase (ADH) and aldehyde dehydrogenase. ADH catalyzes the conversion of alcohol into acetaldehyde, which is a toxic compound; aldehyde dehydrogenase catalyzes the conversion of acetaldehyde into acetic acid. Disulfiram inhibits aldehyde dehydrogenase. Some studies have shown that women have a lower ADH blood content than men; this fact may account for woman's tendency to become more intoxicated than men after drinking the same amount of alcohol. The decreased function of alcohol-metabolizing enzymes in some Asian persons can also lead to more rapid intoxication and toxic symptoms.

Alcohol's Effects on the Brain

Biochemistry. Alcohol has prominent effects on almost all neurochemical systems, with different actions during intoxication versus withdrawal. Perhaps the most potent effects are on GABA complexes in the brain, especially on the GABA-A receptor ($GABA_A$), contributing to the sedating, sleep-inducing, anticonvulsant, and muscle-relaxing properties of alcohol. Ethanol also impacts NMDA receptors, with dampened stimulatory effects during intoxication and heightened activity during withdrawal. Alcohol acutely increases dopamine and its metabolites, and chronic drinking changes dopamine receptor numbers and sensitivity, with related effects on intoxication and craving, in part through changes in the pleasure centers in the VTA of the brain. Alcohol also increases serotonin in the synapses and upregulates serotonin receptors, and acutely enhances the functioning of the opioid-related brain systems and impacts adenosine, acetylcholine, and cannabinoid 1 (CB1) receptors.

Behavioral Effects. Alcohol is a depressant, much like the barbiturates and the benzodiazepines, with which alcohol has some cross-tolerance and cross-dependence. At a level of 0.05 percent alcohol in the blood, thought, judgment, and restraint are loosened and sometimes disrupted. At a concentration of 0.1 percent, voluntary motor actions usually become perceptibly clumsy. Most states define legal intoxication as a 0.08 percent blood alcohol level. At 0.2 percent, the function of the entire motor area of the brain is measurably depressed, and the parts of the brain that control emotional behavior are also affected. At 0.3 percent, a person is commonly confused or may become stuporous; at 0.4 to 0.5 percent, the person falls into a coma. At higher levels, the primitive centers of the brain that control breathing and heart rate are affected, and death ensues secondary to direct respiratory depression or the aspiration of vomitus. Persons with long-term histories of alcohol use disorders, however, can tolerate much higher concentrations of alcohol than can alcohol-naïve persons; their alcohol tolerance may cause them to appear less intoxicated than they are.

Sleep Effects. Although alcohol consumed in the evening usually increases the ease of falling asleep (decreased sleep latency), alcohol also has adverse effects on sleep architecture. Specifically, alcohol use is associated with a decrease in rapid eye movement sleep (REM or dream sleep) and deep sleep (stage 4) and more sleep fragmentation, with more and longer episodes of awakening. Therefore, the idea that drinking alcohol improves a person's sleep is a myth.

Other Physiologic Effects

LIVER.   The most significant adverse effects of alcohol use are related to liver damage. Alcohol use, even as short as week-long episodes of increased drinking, can result in an accumulation of fats and proteins, which produce the appearance of a fatty liver, sometimes found on physical examination as an enlarged liver. The association between fatty infiltration of the liver and severe liver damage remains unclear. Alcohol use, however, is associated with the development of alcoholic hepatitis and hepatic cirrhosis.

GASTROINTESTINAL SYSTEM.   Long-term heavy drinking is associated with developing esophagitis, gastritis, achlorhydria, and gastric ulcers. The development of esophageal varices can accompany particularly heavy alcohol use; the rupture of the varices is a medical emergency often resulting in death by exsanguination. Disorders of the small intestine occasionally occur, and pancreatitis, pancreatic insufficiency, and pancreatic cancer are also associated with heavy alcohol use. Heavy alcohol intake can adversely affect the normal processes of food digestion and absorption. Alcohol use disorders also appear to inhibit the intestine's capacity to absorb various nutrients, such as vitamins and amino acids. This effect, coupled with the often poor dietary habits of those with alcohol-related disorders, can cause serious vitamin deficiencies, particularly of the B vitamins.

OTHER BODILY SYSTEMS.   A significant intake of alcohol is associated with increased blood pressure, dysregulation of lipoprotein and triglyceride metabolism, and increased risk for myocardial infarction and cerebrovascular disease. Alcohol can affect the hearts of nonalcoholic persons who do not usually drink, increasing the resting cardiac output, the heart rate, and the myocardial oxygen consumption. Evidence indicates that alcohol intake can adversely affect the hematopoietic system and can increase the incidence of cancer, particularly head, neck, esophageal, stomach, hepatic, colonic, and lung cancer. Acute intoxication may also be associated with hypoglycemia, which, when unrecognized, may be responsible for some of the sudden deaths of persons who are intoxicated. Muscle weakness is another side effect of alcohol use disorders.

Alcohol intake also raises the blood concentration of estradiol in women. The increase in estradiol correlates with the blood alcohol level.

DRUG INTERACTIONS.   The interaction between alcohol and other substances can be dangerous, even fatal. Certain substances, such as alcohol and phenobarbital, are metabolized by the liver, and their prolonged use can lead to the acceleration of their metabolism. When persons with alcohol-related disorders are sober, this accelerated metabolism makes them unusually tolerant to many drugs such as sedatives and hypnotics; when they are intoxicated, however, these drugs compete with the alcohol for the same detoxification mechanisms, and potentially toxic concentrations of all involved substances can accumulate in the blood.

The effects of alcohol and other CNS depressants are usually synergistic. Sedatives, hypnotics, and drugs that relieve pain, motion sickness, head colds, and allergy symptoms must be used with caution by persons with alcohol-related disorders. Narcotics depress the sensory areas of the cerebral cortex and can produce pain relief, sedation, apathy, drowsiness, and sleep; high doses can result in respiratory failure and death. Increasing the dosages of sedative–hypnotic drugs, such as chloral hydrate and benzodiazepines, especially when combining them with alcohol, produces a range of effects from sedation to motor and intellectual impairment to stupor, coma, and death. Because sedatives and other psychotropic drugs can potentiate the effects of alcohol, it is important to warn patients about the dangers of combining CNS depressants and alcohol, particularly when they are driving or operating machinery.

ETIOLOGY

Many factors affect the decision to drink, the development of temporary alcohol-related difficulties, and the development of alcohol use disorders. The initiation of drinking probably depends mainly on social, religious, and personality characteristics, although genetic characteristics might also contribute. The reasons for beginning to drink may differ from the factors that later lead to an alcohol use disorder.

A similar interplay between genetic and environmental influences contributes to many medical and psychiatric conditions, and, thus, a review of these factors in alcohol use disorders offers information about complex genetic disorders overall. Dominant or recessive genes, although relevant, explain only rare conditions. Most disorders have some level of genetic predisposition that usually relates to a series of different genetically influenced characteristics, each of which increases or decreases the risk for the disorder.

A series of genetic influences likely combine to explain approximately 60 percent of the proportion of risk for alcohol use disorders, with the environment responsible for the remaining proportion of the variance. The divisions offered in this section, therefore, are more heuristic than real, because it is the combination of a series of psychological, sociocultural, biologic, and other factors that are responsible for the development of severe, repetitive alcohol-related life problems.

Psychological Theories

A variety of theories assume that we use alcohol to reduce tension, increase feelings of power, and decrease the effects of psychological pain. Perhaps the most considerable interest has been paid to the observation that people with alcohol-related problems often report that alcohol decreases their feelings of nervousness and helps them cope with the day-to-day stresses of life. The psychological theories are built, in part, on the observation among nonalcoholic people that the intake of low doses of alcohol in a tense social setting or after a stressful day enhances feelings of well-being and improved ease of interactions. In high doses, especially at falling blood alcohol levels, however, most measures of muscle tension and psychological feelings of nervousness and tension are increased. Thus, the tension-reducing effects of this drug might have an impact most on light to moderate drinkers or add to the relief of withdrawal symptoms, but play a minor role in causing

alcohol use disorders. The theories that focus on alcohol's potential to enhance one's esteem are challenging to evaluate definitively.

Psychodynamic Theories.   Related to the disinhibiting or anxiety-lowering effects of lower doses of alcohol is the hypothesis that some people may use this drug to help them deal with self-punitive harsh superegos and unconscious stress. Also, classic psychoanalytical theory hypothesizes that at least some people with alcohol use disorders may have become fixated at the oral stage of development and use alcohol to relieve their frustrations by taking the substance by mouth. Hypotheses regarding arrested phases of psychosexual development, although heuristically useful, have had little effect on the usual treatment approaches and are not the focus of extensive ongoing research.

Similarly, most studies have not been able to document an "addictive personality" present in most individuals with alcohol use disorders and associated with a propensity to lack control of the intake of a wide range of substances and foods. Although patients often have pathologic scores on personality during intoxication, withdrawal, and early recovery, many of these characteristics predate alcoholism, and most disappear with abstinence. Similarly, prospective studies of children of alcoholics without any co-occurring psychiatric disorders show a high risk for alcohol use disorders. As elsewhere described, one exception is the extreme impulsivity seen in the 15 to 20 percent of alcoholic men with an antisocial personality disorder, because they have high risks for criminality, violence, and multiple substance use disorders.

Behavioral Theories.   Expectations about the rewarding effects of drinking, cognitive attitudes toward responsibility for one's behavior, and subsequent reinforcement after alcohol intake all contribute to the decision to drink again after the first experience with alcohol and to continue to imbibe despite problems. These issues are critical in efforts to modify drinking behaviors in the general population, and they contribute to some important aspects of rehabilitation of alcohol use disorders.

Sociocultural Theories.   Sociocultural theories often extrapolate from social groups that have high and low rates of alcohol use disorders. Theorists hypothesize that ethnic groups, such as Jews, who introduce children to modest levels of drinking during religious rituals and eschew drunkenness, have low rates of alcohol use disorders. However, other groups have similar practices, such as French Catholics, but have higher rates of alcohol use disorders. Recent studies have found little evidence to suggest that introducing children to modest drinking in the home impacts the risks for heavy drinking and alcohol problems. So, it is likely that cultural attitudes toward drinking, drunkenness, and personal responsibility for consequences are essential contributors to the rates of alcohol-related problems in a society. In the final analysis, social and psychological theories are probably highly relevant because they outline factors that contribute to the onset of drinking, the development of temporary alcohol-related life difficulties, and even alcohol use disorders. The problem is how to gather relatively definitive data to support or refute the theories.

Childhood History.   Researchers have identified several factors in the childhood histories of persons with later alcohol-related disorders and in children at high risk for having an alcohol-related disorder because one or both of their parents are affected. In experimental studies, children at high risk for alcohol-related disorders possess, on average, a range of deficits on neurocognitive testing.

Table 4-17
Evidence that Alcohol Has a Genetic Influence

Close relatives have a 3–4 times increased risk for severe alcohol
  problems
The rate of alcohol problems increases with:
  The number of relatives with AUDs
  The severity of their illness
  The closeness of their genetic relationship to the person studied
Higher concordance for severe AUDs identical twins than fraternal
  twins in most investigations, which estimate that genes explain
  40–60% of the variance
Adoption studies show increased risk for children of patients with
  AUDs even when separated from their biologic parents since
  birth and raised without any contact
The risk is not enhanced when the adoptive parents have AUD
Animals studies support the role of genes

These deficits include a low amplitude of the P300 wave on evoked potential testing and a variety of abnormalities on electroencephalography (EEG) recordings. Studies of high-risk offspring in their 20s have also shown a generally blunted effect of alcohol compared with that seen in persons whose parents lacked an alcohol-related disorder. These findings suggest that a heritable biologic brain function may predispose a person to an alcohol-related disorder. A childhood history of attention-deficit/hyperactivity disorder (ADHD), conduct disorder, or both, increases a child's risk for an alcohol-related disorder as an adult. Personality disorders, especially antisocial personality disorder, as noted earlier, also predispose a person to an alcohol-related disorder.

Genetic Factors

Table 4-17 lists some lines of evidence that support the conclusion that genes have an essential influence on alcoholism. Twin studies suggest that genes explain 60 percent of the variance, with the remainder relating to nonshared, probably adult environmental influences. Animal studies support the importance of a variety of yet-to-be-identified genes in the free-choice use of alcohol, subsequent levels of intoxication, and some consequences.

▲ 4.3 Cannabis-Related Disorders

Cannabis is the most widely used illegal drug in the world. Over the past 40 years, cannabis use has become a standard part of youth culture in most developed societies, with first use now occurring in the mid-to-late teens. In the United States, there is a movement to legalize cannabis at the state level, with some states allowing the use of cannabis for medical purposes only and others for recreational use.

CLINICAL FEATURES

Most young people use cannabis to experience a "high," characterized by feelings of mild euphoria, relaxation, and perceptual alterations. Cognitive changes include impaired short-term memory and attention that makes it easy for the user to become lost in pleasant reverie and have difficulty sustaining goal-directed mental activity. Motor skills, reaction time, motor coordination, and many forms of skilled psychomotor activity are impaired while the user is intoxicated.

DIAGNOSIS

The DSM-5 and ICD-10 include several diagnoses related to cannabis, and they generally follow the template for all substance use disorders (see Section 4.1 and Tables 4-1 through 4-3). The DSM-5 includes the diagnoses of cannabis intoxication, cannabis intoxication delirium, cannabis withdrawal, cannabis use disorder, cannabis-induced psychotic disorder, cannabis-induced anxiety disorder, cannabis-induced sleep disorder, and unspecified cannabis-related disorder. The ICD-10 includes cannabis-related disorders under the general heading of "Mental and behavioral disorders due to psychoactive substance use."

Cannabis Intoxication

Cannabis intoxication commonly heightens users' sensitivities to external stimuli and subjectively slows the appreciation of time. In high doses, users may experience depersonalization and derealization. Cannabis use impairs motor skills, and this effect remains after the euphoriant effects have resolved. For 8 to 12 hours after using cannabis, users' impaired motor skills interfere with the operation of motor vehicles and other heavy machinery. Moreover, these effects are additive to those of alcohol.

> Mr. M was an unemployed 20-year-old man who lived with his parents. He was brought to a hospital by some friends in a state of anxiety and agitation. He had been out at a restaurant, and after a couple of beers, he decided to have some cannabis. He had smoked cannabis on previous occasions; however, this time, he ate a lump of cannabis despite warnings from his friends. After about half an hour, Mr. M appeared tense and anxious and complained that everything was changing. He could see the faces of his friends increasing to about three times their original size. The room became distorted, and its proportions and colors kept altering. He felt that the other guests in the restaurant were talking about him and his friends menacingly, so he suddenly rushed outside because he felt that he was in danger. He became increasingly agitated and started running down the middle of the street, dodging in and out among the traffic. Eventually, his friends were able to catch him. They were unable to quiet his anxiety, however, and had a hard time persuading him to go with them to the hospital.
>
> On examination, Mr. M appeared tense and apprehensive, looking around the room as if he felt uneasy with the surroundings. He denied perceptual symptoms and did not believe that he was the subject of persecution. He was fully aware of his surroundings, but his attention was fleeting, and he did not always answer questions. There was no marked impairment of memory, and he was fully oriented.
>
> Physical examination revealed conjunctival injection and an increased pulse rate of 120 beats/min, but otherwise, there were no abnormalities. The neurologic examination also revealed no abnormalities. In the course of a few hours, Mr. M quieted down and eventually left the hospital with his friends.

Cannabis Intoxication Delirium.   Cannabis intoxication can markedly impair cognition and performance. Even modest doses of cannabis impair memory, reaction time, perception, motor coordination, and attention. High doses that also impair users' levels of consciousness have marked effects on cognitive measures.

Cannabis Withdrawal

Studies have shown that cessation of use in daily cannabis users results in withdrawal symptoms within 1 to 2 weeks of cessation. Table 4-18 lists typical cannabis withdrawal symptoms.

Table 4-18
Cannabis Withdrawal Symptoms

Irritability
Cannabis cravings
Nervousness
Anxiety
Insomnia
Disturbed or vivid dreaming
Decreased appetite
Weight loss
Depressed mood
Restlessness
Headache
Chills
Stomach pain
Sweating
Tremors

Cannabis Use Disorder

People who use cannabis daily for weeks to months are most likely to develop a cannabis use disorder. The risk of developing cannabis use disorder is around one in ten for anyone who uses cannabis. The earlier the age of first use, the more often cannabis has been used, and the longer it is used, the higher the risk of developing the disorder.

Cannabis-Induced Psychotic Disorder

Cannabis-induced psychotic disorder, in which there is a genuine psychotic process, is rare; transient paranoid ideation, however, is common.

Florid psychosis is somewhat commonplace in countries in which some persons have long-term access to high potency cannabis. The psychotic episodes are sometimes called "hemp insanity." Cannabis use rarely causes the "bad-trip" experience we associate with hallucinogen intoxication. When cannabis-induced psychotic disorder does occur, the affected person is likely to have a preexisting personality disorder.

Cannabis-Induced Anxiety Disorder

Cannabis-induced anxiety disorder is common during acute intoxication, which in many persons, induces short-lived anxiety states often provoked by paranoid thoughts. In such circumstances, ill-defined and disorganized fears may induce a panic attack. Anxiety symptoms are the most common adverse effect of moderate cannabis use and correlate with the dose taken. Inexperienced users are much more likely to experience anxiety symptoms than are experienced users.

A friend gave a 35-year-old married man who was naïve to cannabis two "joints." The man smoked the first of the two in the same manner that he usually smoked a cigarette (in about 3 to 5 minutes). Noting no significant effects, he proceeded immediately to smoke the second in the same amount of time. Within 30 minutes, he began to experience rapid heartbeat, dry mouth, mounting anxiety, and the delusional belief that his throat was closing up and that he was going to die. That belief induced further panic, and the patient was brought to the emergency department of a local hospital during the experience. There, the emergency team could not reassure him that he would not die. After sedating him with diazepam, some of his anxiety diminished. He eventually went to sleep, and on awakening after 5 hours, he was asymptomatic with full recall of previous events.

Unspecified Cannabis-Related Disorders

DSM-5 includes the category unspecified cannabis-related disorders for cannabis disorders that do not fit into the other diagnoses. Examples could be episodes of depressive or hypomanic symptoms, although these symptoms may suggest long-term cannabis use.

When either sleep disorder or sexual dysfunction symptoms are related to cannabis use, they almost always resolve within days or a week after cessation.

Flashbacks. There are case reports of persons who have experienced sensations related to cannabis intoxication after the short-term effects of the substance have disappeared. Whether flashbacks are related to cannabis use alone or the concomitant use of other substances (intended or tainted) remains a subject of debate.

Cognitive Impairment. Clinical and experimental evidence indicates that the long-term use of cannabis may produce subtle forms of cognitive impairment in the higher cognitive functions of memory, attention, and organization and the integration of complex information. This evidence suggests that the longer the period of heavy cannabis use, the more pronounced the cognitive impairment. Nonetheless, because the impairments in performance are subtle, it remains to be determined how significant they are for everyday functioning. It also remains to be investigated whether these impairments resolve after an extended period of abstinence from cannabis.

Amotivational Syndrome. A controversial cannabis-related syndrome is *amotivational syndrome*. Whether the syndrome is related to cannabis use or reflects characterologic traits in a subgroup of persons regardless of cannabis use is under debate. Traditionally, a person's unwillingness to persist in a task—be it at school, at work, or in any setting that requires prolonged attention or tenacity—characterizes the syndrome, which is associated with long-term heavy use. People with the syndrome become apathetic and anergic, may gain weight, or appear slothful.

COMORBIDITY

Cannabis is often referred to as a "gateway drug," meaning that cannabis users are at high risk for other substance use disorders. Also, cannabis use may be comorbid with depression, anxiety, conduct disorder, and suicidality.

TREATMENT AND REHABILITATION

Treatment of cannabis use rests on the same principles as the treatment of other substances of abuse—abstinence and support. Abstinence involves direct interventions, such as hospitalization, or careful monitoring on an outpatient basis by the use of urine drug screens, which can detect cannabis for up to 4 weeks after use. We can use individual, family, and group psychotherapies to support the patient. Education should be a cornerstone of both abstinence and support programs. A patient who does not understand the intellectual reasons for addressing a substance use disorder has little motivation to stop. For some patients, an antianxiety drug may be useful for short-term relief of withdrawal symptoms. For other patients, cannabis use may be due to an underlying depressive disorder that may respond to specific antidepressant treatment.

Medical Use of Marijuana

People have used marijuana as a medicinal herb for centuries, and cannabis was listed in the US Pharmacopeia until the end of the 19th century as a remedy for anxiety, depression, and GI disorders, among others.

Cannabis is currently a controlled substance, and the Drug Enforcement Agency (DEA) does not recognize any medical use for the substance. Despite this, patients and doctors have used the drug, sometimes illegally, to treat a variety of disorders, including nausea secondary to chemotherapy, HIV-associated weight loss, multiple sclerosis (MS) chronic pain, epilepsy, and glaucoma. We currently live in a time of differing views and conflicting laws regarding the use of cannabis. The US federal government continues to consider the drug to be illegal under any circumstances; the Supreme Court confirmed this in 2001. However, as of 2020, 15 states have legalized the recreational and medicinal use of marijuana, along with the District of Columbia, and several US territories. Many other states have some degree of medical exemption or have decriminalized the drug. Table 4-19 lists the status of cannabis laws in the United States and territories as of 2020, however this remains a rapidly changing field.

Dronabinol, a synthetic form of THC, has been approved by the US Food and Drug Administration (FDA) for the treatment of anorexia-associated weight loss in HIV and nausea and vomiting associated with chemotherapy; dronabinol is also under investigation for the treatment of obstructive sleep apnea. Nabilone, which is a synthetic cannabinoid, has been approved for the treatment of nausea and vomiting associated with chemotherapy. In 2013, cannabidiol was granted orphan drug status for the treatment of certain rare, intractable types of epilepsy in children. Additionally, nabiximols, an oral spray consisting of natural cannabis extracts, is currently being investigated for the treatment of cancer pain. A 2019 study found that nabiximols reduced cannabis use among individuals with cannabis use disorder when used along with concurrent behavioral therapy. Nabiximols is currently available by prescription in several countries outside of the United States for patients with neuropathic pain, MS, and other conditions.

EPIDEMIOLOGY

Cannabis is the most widely used illegal drug in the United States, with an estimated 24 million users aged 12 and older in 2016 (approximately 9 percent of the population). Of those individuals, roughly 4 million met criteria for a marijuana use disorder in the past year.

Prevalence and Recent Trends

The *Monitoring the Future* survey of adolescents in school indicates that 36 percent of twelfth graders used marijuana in the past year, which is slightly lower than the most recent peak in the 1990s (39 percent in 1997). Annual marijuana use by eighth and tenth graders is significantly lower than the corresponding rates in the 1990s; in 2018, the prevalence of marijuana use was 28 percent in tenth graders (compared to 35 percent in 1997) and 11 percent in eighth-graders (compared to 18 percent in 1997).

Demographic Correlates

Rates of cannabis use in the user's lifetime, the past year, and the past week are consistently higher among males than females, as are daily use and long-term daily use.

Table 4-19
The Legal Status of Cannabis as of 2020

Illegal
Alabama
Idaho
Kansas
Nebraska[a]
North Carolina[a]
South Carolina
Tennessee
Wyoming

Fully Legal
Alaska
California
Colorado
District of Columbia
Illinois
Maine
Massachusetts
Michigan
Nevada
Oregon
Vermont
Washington
Arizona[b]
Montana[b]
New Jersey[b]
South Dakota[b]

Medicinal Use
Arkansas
Connecticut[a]
Delaware[a]
Florida
Hawaii[a]
Louisiana
Maryland[a]
Minnesota[a]
Missouri[a]
New Hampshire[a]
New Mexico[a]
New York[a]
North Dakota[a]
Ohio[a]
Oklahoma
Pennsylvania
Rhode Island[a]
Utah
West Virginia
Mississippi[a]

CBD Oil Only
Georgia
Indiana
Iowa
Kentucky
Texas
Virginia[a]
Wisconsin

[a]Decriminalized.
[b]As of 2020 election, enactment is pending as of this date.

Information on the relationship between ethnicity and cannabis use is limited. Even in the extensive Monitoring the Future survey, samples from several years have to be combined to make reliable comparisons between the three largest ethnic groups. These show that African American students have lower rates of use in all grades than white or Hispanic students.

PATHOLOGY

Cannabis Preparations

The plant *Cannabis sativa* is the source for cannabis preparations. It has been used in China, India, and the Middle East for approximately 8,000 years, primarily for its fibers and secondarily for its medicinal properties. The plant occurs in male and female forms. The female plant contains the highest concentrations of cannabinoids. Delta-9-tetrahydrocannabinol (Δ9-THC) is primarily responsible for the psychoactive effects of cannabis. The most potent forms of cannabis come from the flowering tops of the plants or from the dried, black-brown, resinous exudate from the leaves, called *hashish* or *hash*. The cannabis plant is usually cut, dried, chopped, and rolled into cigarettes (commonly called "joints"). The common names for cannabis are marijuana, grass, pot, weed, tea, and Mary Jane, although there are many other names. The potency of marijuana preparations has increased in recent years because of improved agricultural techniques used in cultivation so that plants may contain up to 15 or 20 percent THC.

Physical Effects of Cannabis Use

Table 4-20 lists the most common physical effects of cannabis use. There is no documented case of death caused by cannabis intoxication alone; this reflects the substance's lack of effect on the respiratory rate. The most serious potential adverse effects of cannabis use are those caused by inhaling the same carcinogenic hydrocarbons present in conventional tobacco, and some data indicate that heavy cannabis users are at risk for chronic respiratory disease and lung cancer. The practice of smoking cannabis-containing cigarettes to their very ends, so-called "roaches," further increases the intake of tar (particulate matter).

Many reports indicate that long-term cannabis use is associated with other serious effects, also listed in Table 4-20. These reports,

Table 4-20
Physical Effects of Cannabis Use

Common
Dilation of the conjunctival blood vessels (red eyes)
Mild tachycardia
Increased appetite
Dry mouth
Orthostatic hypotension (higher doses)

Heavy chronic use (some of these are controversial)
Chronic respiratory disease
Lung cancer
Cerebral atrophy
Seizure susceptibility
Chromosomal damage
Birth defects
Impaired immune reactivity
Alterations in testosterone concentrations
Dysregulation of menstrual cycles

however, have not been conclusively replicated, and the association between these findings and cannabis use is uncertain.

Neuropharmacology

As stated above, the principal component of cannabis is Δ9-THC; however, the cannabis plant contains more than 400 chemicals, of which about 60 are chemically related to Δ9-THC. In humans, Δ9-THC rapidly converts to 11-hydroxy-Δ9-THC, the metabolite that is active in the CNS.

A specific receptor for the cannabinols has been identified, cloned, and characterized. The cannabinoid receptor, a member of the G-protein–linked family of receptors, is linked to the inhibitory G protein (G_i), which inhibits adenylyl cyclase. The highest concentrations of the cannabinoid receptor are in the basal ganglia, hippocampus, and cerebellum, with lower concentrations in the cerebral cortex. The brainstem lacks this receptor, explaining the drug's minimal effects on respiratory and cardiac functions. Studies in animals have shown that cannabinoids affect monoamine and GABA neurons.

According to most studies, animals do not self-administer cannabinoids as they do most other substances of abuse. It is not clear whether the cannabinoids stimulate the so-called reward centers of the brain, such as the dopaminergic neurons of the VTA. Tolerance to cannabis does develop, however, as does psychological dependence. The evidence for physiologic dependence is not as strong. Withdrawal symptoms in humans are limited to modest increases in irritability, restlessness, insomnia, and anorexia and mild nausea; all these symptoms appear only when a person abruptly stops taking high doses of cannabis.

When smoking cannabis, the euphoric effects appear within minutes, peak in about 30 minutes, and last 2 to 4 hours. Some motor and cognitive effects last 5 to 12 hours. Oral cannabis is also frequent, usually as an additive in baked goods, such as brownies and cakes. It requires about two to three times as much oral cannabis to be as potent as smoked cannabis. Many variables affect the psychoactive properties of cannabis, including the potency of the cannabis used, the route of administration, the smoking technique, the effects of pyrolysis on the cannabinoid content, the dose, the setting, and the user's experience, expectations, and unique biologic vulnerability to the effects of cannabinoids.

▲ 4.4 Opioid-Related Disorders

The word *opioid* describes a class of psychoactive compounds, both naturally occurring and chemically synthesized, that are related to opiates: alkaloid compounds found as natural products in the opium poppy plant, *Papaver somniferumi*.

Many synthetic opioids have been manufactured, including meperidine, methadone, pentazocine, and propoxyphene.

Humans have used opioids for analgesic and other medicinal purposes for thousands of years, but they also have a long history of misuse for their psychoactive effects. Continued opioid misuse can result in abuse and dependence and cause disturbances in mood, behavior, and cognition that can mimic other psychiatric disorders. In developed countries, the opioid drug most frequently associated with abuse and dependence is heroin; however, there is growing public health concern about prescription opioids, which are widely

Table 4-21
Opioids Available in the United States

Proprietary Name	Trade Name
Morphine	
Heroin (diacetylmorphine)	
Hydromorphone (dihydromorphinone)	Dilaudid
Oxymorphone (dihydrohydroxymorphinone)	Numorphan
Levorphanol	Levo-Dromoran
Methadone	Dolophine
Meperidine (pethidine)	Demerol, Pethadol
Fentanyl	Sublimaze
Codeine	
Hydrocodone (dihydrocodeinone)	Hycodan, Others
Drocode (dihydrocodeine)	Synalgos-Dc, Compal
Oxycodone (dihydrohydroxycodeinone)	Roxicodone, Oxycontin, Percodan, Percocet, Vicodin
Propoxyphene	Darvon, Others
Buprenorphine	Buprenex (parenteral), Sublocade (subcutaneous, extended-release)
Pentazocine	Talwin
Nalbuphine	Nubain
Butorphanol	Stadol

available and have significant abuse liability. Opioid addiction affects the young and the old, the wealthy and the poor, and the professional and the unemployed. Over the last few decades, there have been significant advances in treatment and understanding of opioid use disorder. Opioid use disorder is often a chronic, relapsing disorder amenable to medical treatment and intervention. Table 4-21 lists various opioids that are used therapeutically in the United States, except for heroin.

CLINICAL FEATURES

Opioids can be taken orally, snorted intranasally, and injected intravenously or subcutaneously. Opioids are subjectively addictive because of the euphoric high (the rush) that users experience, especially those who take the substances intravenously. The associated symptoms include a feeling of warmth, heaviness of the extremities, dry mouth, itchy face (especially the nose), and facial flushing. A period of sedation follows the initial euphoria, known in street parlance as "nodding off." Opioid use can induce dysphoria, nausea, and vomiting in opioid-naive persons.

Diagnosis

The DSM-5 and ICD-10 include several diagnoses related to opioids, and they generally follow the template for all substance use disorders (see Section 4.1 and Tables 4-1 through 4-3). These include opioid use disorder, opioid intoxication, opioid withdrawal, opioid-induced sleep disorder, and opioid-induced sexual

dysfunction. Opioid intoxication delirium can occur in hospitalized patients. Opioid-induced psychotic disorder, opioid-induced mood disorder, and opioid-induced anxiety disorder, by contrast, are uncommon with μ-agonist opioids but can occur with some mixed agonist–antagonist opioids acting at other receptors. The diagnosis of opioid-related disorder not elsewhere classified is for situations that do not meet the criteria for any of the other opioid-related disorders.

Opioid Use Disorder

Opioid use disorder is a pattern of maladaptive use of an opioid drug, leading to clinically significant impairment or distress and occurring within 12 months.

A surgeon referred a 42-year-old public relations executive to psychiatry after discovering the executive sneaking large quantities of a codeine-containing cough medicine into the hospital. The patient had been a heavy cigarette smoker for 20 years and had a chronic, hacking cough. He had come into the hospital for a hernia repair and found the pain from the incision unbearable when he coughed.

A back operation 5 years previously had led his doctors to prescribe codeine to help relieve the incisional pain at that time. Over the intervening 5 years, however, the patient had continued to use codeine-containing tablets and had increased his intake to 60 to 90 mg daily. He stated that he often "just took them by the handful—not to feel good, you understand, just to get by." He spent considerable time and effort developing a circle of physicians and pharmacists to whom he would "make the rounds" at least three times a week to obtain new supplies of pills. He had tried several times to stop using codeine but had failed. During this period, he lost two jobs because of lax work habits, and his wife of 11 years divorced him.

Opioid Intoxication

Opioid intoxication includes maladaptive behavioral changes and specific physical symptoms of opioid use. In general, altered mood, psychomotor retardation, drowsiness, slurred speech, and impaired memory and attention in the presence of other indicators of recent opioid use strongly suggest a diagnosis of opioid intoxication.

Opioid Withdrawal

Opioid withdrawal develops after the cessation of or reduction in opioid use that has been heavy and prolonged. The withdrawal syndrome also occurs when administering an opioid partial agonist such as buprenorphine or an opioid antagonist such as naloxone or naltrexone to a patient who is regularly taking an opioid agonist. The withdrawal symptoms are usually the physiologic opposite of the intoxication symptoms. The withdrawal syndrome consists of severe muscle cramps and bone aches, profuse diarrhea, abdominal cramps, rhinorrhea, lacrimation, piloerection or gooseflesh (from which derives the term *cold turkey* for the abstinence syndrome), yawning, fever, pupillary dilation, hypertension, tachycardia, and temperature dysregulation, including hypothermia and hyperthermia. Persons with opioid dependence seldom die from opioid withdrawal unless they have a severe preexisting physical illness such as cardiac disease. Residual symptoms—such as insomnia, bradycardia, temperature dysregulation, and a craving for opioids—can persist for months after withdrawal. Associated features of opioid withdrawal include restlessness, irritability, depression, tremor, weakness, nausea, and vomiting. At any time during the abstinence syndrome, a single injection of morphine or heroin eliminates all the symptoms.

The general rule about the onset and duration of withdrawal symptoms is that substances with short durations of action tend to produce short, intense withdrawal syndromes, and substances with long durations of action produce prolonged but mild withdrawal syndromes. An exception to the rule, narcotic antagonist-precipitated withdrawal after long-acting opioid misuse can be severe. See Section 4.1, Table 4-3 for the diagnostic criteria for substance withdrawal.

When an opioid antagonist precipitates an abstinence syndrome, the symptoms begin within seconds of such an intravenous injection and peak in about 1 hour. Opioid craving rarely occurs in the context of analgesic administration for pain from physical disorders or surgery. The full withdrawal syndrome, including an intense craving for opioids, usually occurs only secondary to abrupt cessation of use in persons with longstanding opioid misuse.

Morphine and Heroin.   The morphine and heroin withdrawal syndrome begin 6 to 8 hours after the last dose, usually after a 1- to 2-week period of continuous use or after the administration of a narcotic antagonist. The withdrawal syndrome reaches its peak intensity during the second or third day and subsides during the next 7 to 10 days, but some symptoms may persist for 6 months or longer.

Methadone.   Methadone withdrawal usually begins 1 to 3 days after the last dose and ends in 10 to 14 days.

Opioid Intoxication Delirium.   Opioid intoxication delirium is most likely to happen when using opioids in high doses, or mixing them with other psychoactive compounds, or when a person with preexisting CNS disorder (e.g., brain damage or epilepsy) uses them.

Opioid-Induced Psychotic Disorder.   The opioid-induced psychotic disorder can begin during opioid intoxication. Clinicians can specify whether hallucinations or delusions are the predominant symptoms.

Opioid-Induced Mood Disorder.   An opioid-induced mood disorder can begin during opioid intoxication. Opioid-induced mood disorder symptoms can have a manic, depressed, or mixed nature, depending on a person's response to opioids. A person who comes to psychiatric attention with opioid-induced mood disorder usually has mixed symptoms, combining irritability, expansiveness, and depression.

Opioid-Induced Sleep Disorder and Opioid-Induced Sexual Dysfunction.   Opioid-induced sleep disorder and opioid-induced sexual dysfunction are common, and both hypersomnia and insomnia are common complaints of patients who either have opioid use disorder or use opioids regularly for therapeutic purposes. Common sexual dysfunctions for chronic opioid users include erectile dysfunction and orgasmic difficulties.

Unspecified Opioid-Related Disorder.   The DSM-5 includes diagnoses for other opioid-related disorders with symptoms of delirium, abnormal mood, psychosis, abnormal sleep, and sexual dysfunction. Clinical situations that do not fit into these categories exemplify appropriate cases for the use of the DSM-5 diagnosis of an unspecified opioid-related disorder.

COMORBIDITY

Nearly 70 percent of men and 75 percent of women with opioid use disorder in their lifetimes have an additional psychiatric disorder. The most common comorbid disorders include mood disorders, antisocial personality disorder, anxiety disorders, and alcohol use disorder. Table 4-22 highlights the need to develop a broad-based treatment program that also addresses patients' associated psychiatric disorders.

In addition to the morbidity and mortality associated directly with the opioid-related disorders, the association between the transmission of both hepatitis and the HIV with intravenous opioid and opiate use is recognized as a leading national health concern.

TREATMENT AND REHABILITATION

Methadone is the current gold standard in the treatment of opioid use disorder with physiologic dependence. Methadone is used for detoxification and as a maintenance agent.

The opioid partial agonist buprenorphine binds to the receptor but activates it only partially. Due to buprenorphine's high affinity (binding strength) to the receptor and a low dissociation from the receptor, it often functions as an antagonist (blocker), preventing compounds with lower receptor affinity from activating the receptor. If a patient is actively using an agonist at the time they receive a dose of buprenorphine, the buprenorphine will abruptly displace the agonist from the receptor. Since the buprenorphine only has a partial effect at the receptor, it will cause a sudden drop in the level of agonist effect, resulting in a precipitated withdrawal. Buprenorphine is used to assist detoxification and as a maintenance agent.

Opioid antagonists (e.g., naloxone, nalmefene, and naltrexone) bind to the receptor but do not exert any activity. These medications function as antagonists—they compete for binding at the receptor with agonists and partial agonists, and if the dose of the antagonist is high enough, they may displace the agonist from the receptor and prevent the agonist from binding to the receptor and exerting any effect. Naloxone reverses an overdose; as it is a short-acting agent, it can be dosed very accurately without the risk of an unnecessarily prolonged effect. Naltrexone is a long-acting agent used following detoxification as a strategy to prevent recurrent physiologic dependence and relapse.

Overdose Treatment

The first task in overdose treatment is to ensure an adequate airway. Tracheopharyngeal secretions should be aspirated, and it may be necessary to insert an airway. The patient should be ventilated mechanically until the clinicians can give naloxone. Naloxone is administered intravenously at a slow rate—initially about 0.8 mg per 70 kg of body weight. Signs of improvement (increased respiratory rate and pupillary dilation) should occur promptly. In patients physiologically dependent on opioids, too much naloxone may produce signs of withdrawal. If no response to the initial dosage occurs, clinicians can repeat the naloxone administration after intervals of a few minutes. If there is no response after 4 to 5 mg, some think that nonopioid substances may be contributing to the CNS depression. The duration of action of naloxone is short compared with that of many opioids, such as methadone and levomethadyl acetate, and repeated administration may be required to prevent recurrence of opioid toxicity.

Table 4-22
Substance and Non–Substance-Related Psychiatric Disorders in Opioid Users

Mood, Anxiety, and Personality Disorders Among Individuals with Lifetime Opioid Use Disorders in NESARC by Gender

(N = 355)	Men (%) (N = 223)	Women (%) (N = 578)	Total (%)	Odds Ratio (95% Confidence Interval)
Heroin/other opioids				
Abuse	75.6	67.5	73	0.67 (0.43, 1.04)
Dependence	24.4	32.5	27	1.49 (0.96, 2.31)
Cocaine				
Abuse	37.6	17	30.9	0.34 (0.20, 0.58)***
Dependence	17.4	20.5	18.4	1.22 (0.73, 2.03)
Marijuana				
Abuse	56.2	39.3	50.7	0.51 (0.33, 0.78)**
Dependence	19.4	19.9	19.6	1.03 (0.62, 1.72)
Alcohol				
Abuse	22.6	20.4	21.8	0.88 (0.55, 1.41)
Dependence	67.1	54.5	63	0.59 (0.40, 0.86)**
Sedatives				
Abuse	37.7	23.3	33	0.50 (0.30, 0.85)*
Dependence	9.1	12.9	10.3	1.48 (0.77, 2.87)
Amphetamine				
Abuse	35.9	28	33.3	0.70 (0.45, 1.08)
Dependence	13.3	18.5	15	1.47 (0.80, 2.72)
Hallucinogen				
Abuse	37.4	27.5	34.2	0.63 (0.40, 1.01)
Dependence	9	9.5	9.1	1.06 (0.51, 2.20)
Tranquilizers				
Abuse	37.7	22.7	32.9	0.49 (0.30, 0.78)**
Dependence	8.7	12.4	9.9	1.49 (0.80, 2.81)
Inhalants				
Abuse	13	6.7	10.9	0.48 (0.24, 0.95)*
Dependence	1.7	2.1	1.9	1.22 (0.30, 4.99)
Any other substance				
Abuse	23.1	21.6	22.6	0.92 (0.60, 1.41)
Dependence	72.4	62.3	69.1	0.63 (0.43, 0.91)*
Any mood or anxiety disorder	68.5	73.8	70.3	1.30 (0.84, 2.00)
Any mood disorder	54.1	71.2	59.7	2.10 (1.35, 3.26)**
Major depression	45.7	63.5	51.5	2.07 (1.38, 3.12)**
Dysthymia	15.3	25.3	18.6	1.88 (1.20, 2.93)**
Manic disorder	16.7	27.1	20.1	1.86 (1.17, 2.94)*
Hypomanic disorder	9	10.9	9.6	1.24 (0.61, 2.50)
Any anxiety disorder	33.6	50.1	39	1.98 (1.35, 2.92)***
Panic disorder w/o agoraphobia	13.2	18.3	14.9	1.46 (0.88, 2.45)
Panic disorder w/ agoraphobia	4.1	6.6	4.9	1.65 (0.63, 4.33)
Social phobia	9.3	19.8	12.7	2.42 (1.36, 4.30)**
Specific phobia	12.9	30.1	18.5	2.91 (1.69, 5.02)***
Generalized anxiety disorder	9.7	17.7	12.3	2.01 (1.13, 3.56)*
Any personality disorder	49.2	50.7	49.7	1.06 (0.74, 1.52)
Paranoid	12.9	22.2	15.9	1.93 (1.17, 3.21)*
Avoidant	9.5	12.4	10.4	1.35 (0.71, 2.57)
Dependent	3	2.3	2.8	0.77 (0.25, 2.37)
Obsessive compulsive	16	23	18.3	1.56 (0.95, 2.57)
Schizoid	11.5	12.8	11.9	1.13 (0.61, 2.11)
Histrionic	9.8	8.5	9.4	0.86 (0.42, 1.76)
Antisocial	34.1	22.4	30.3	0.56 (0.36, 0.87)*

Asterisks indicate significance level for *p*-values. **indicates *p* ≤0.05; ***indicates *p* ≤0.01; ****indicates *p* ≤0.001.
Adapted from Grella CE, Karno MP, Wards US, Niv N, Moore AA. Gender and comorbidity among individuals with opioid use disorders in the NESARC study. *Addict Behav.* 2009;34(6–7):498–504.

Medically Supervised Withdrawal and Detoxification

Opioid Agents for Treating Opioid Withdrawal

METHADONE. Methadone is a synthetic narcotic (an opioid) that substitutes for heroin. When given to addicts to replace their typical substance of abuse, the drug suppresses withdrawal symptoms. The initial dose of methadone is usually 20 to 30 mg orally; if objective signs of withdrawal persist after the first dose, clinicians can repeat the dose after approximately 2 to 4 hours. As a general rule, initial stabilization does not require more than 40 mg during the first 24 hours, although it can be higher in the inpatient setting if clear signs of moderate or severe withdrawal are present after the first 6 to 10 hours of the observation period. After 24 to 48 hours of dose stabilization, the patient's methadone dose can be gradually reduced by 10 to 20 percent or by 5 mg/day. Most patients can complete inpatient detoxification within 1 week.

In the case of detoxification with methadone in an outpatient setting, the first-day dose should not exceed 40 mg. Over the next few days, clinicians may titrate the dose (generally by no more than 10-mg increments every 2 to 3 days) until the patient has no discernible withdrawal symptoms. In most cases, the dose of 40 to 60 mg/day is sufficient to prevent any opioid withdrawal; however, this dose may not be adequate to eliminate craving. If the patient continues to use opioids, the dose of methadone can increase. In that case, clinicians should postpone detoxification and the goal becomes stabilization—no withdrawal symptoms, craving, or opioid use. Generally, a period of dose stabilization, at a minimum of 4 weeks in duration, is necessary before a slow dose reduction schedule. In the outpatient setting, gradual dose reductions (e.g., 3 percent per week), have a higher likelihood of success, with even slower reductions once the total daily dose is down to 20 to 30 mg/day.

BUPRENORPHINE. As with methadone, buprenorphine is an opioid agonist used for treating opioid withdrawal. Physicians can dispense it on an outpatient basis, but they must demonstrate that they have received specialized training in its use. Buprenorphine is available in several formulations, including as monotherapy or combination therapy with buprenorphine plus naloxone. The monotherapy versions include a parenteral formulation and an extended-release subcutaneous injection. The combination product is preferred, as it carries a lower risk of diversion and misuse.

Buprenorphine can be used for detoxification in an inpatient setting under direct monitoring. The first dose of buprenorphine begins when the patient experiences at least moderate severity of withdrawal, with several, preferably objective, signs present. The first dose of buprenorphine is generally 2 mg, and subsequent 2-mg doses are given every 2 to 4 hours until the successful elimination of withdrawal. Usually, the total daily dose needed to suppress withdrawal on the first day effectively is 8 to 12 mg. Buprenorphine taper is usually started on the second day, while the daily dose is decreased by 2 mg every day, with 1 mg decreases on the last 2 days of taper. The complete taper usually takes 5 to 7 days, and the long elimination half-life of buprenorphine (31 to 35 hours) helps to extend the effect after discontinuation.

Buprenorphine can also assist detoxification in the outpatient setting. The strategy is generally similar to the methadone-assisted detoxification. Ideally, the first day's dosing should occur under medical supervision to minimize the risk of buprenorphine-precipitated withdrawal. The physician usually instructs patients to arrive in withdrawal, which typically starts 12 hours after the last dose of a short-acting opioid or 24 hours after a long-acting opioid like methadone. The first dose of buprenorphine is usually 2 mg, and if there are no signs of precipitated withdrawal, subsequent 2-mg doses are given at the clinic every 2 hours, with additional doses given to take at home, until the elimination of withdrawal. If withdrawal worsens after the first buprenorphine dose, it is best to wait for 4 to 6 hours before giving the next buprenorphine dose while the precipitated withdrawal can be treated symptomatically with medications such as clonidine. Usually, the total daily dose needed on the first day is 8 to 12 mg. Clinicians can use subsequent daily dose increases of 2 to 4 mg to relieve opioid withdrawal and initiate opioid abstinence. Once establishing a period of stabilization, slow dose reductions can begin, usually in 2-mg dose increments and usually at weekly intervals. As with methadone, slower dosage reduction schedules are usually better tolerated and less likely to prompt relapse.

Symptomatic Treatment of Opioid Withdrawal. It is also possible to treat an opioid withdrawal with nonopioid medications, primarily targeting several uncomfortable withdrawal symptoms. Table 4-23 lists some of these medications and their uses.

Medications for the Treatment of Opioid Use Disorder

For some individuals, opioid detoxification is not successful, and others may not feel ready for detoxification, although they may desire freedom from the daily struggle associated with opioid use and the associated psychosocial problems. In these individuals, opioid substitution therapy with either methadone or buprenorphine may be appropriate. For patients who can complete opioid detoxification, antagonist therapy can help them to maintain abstinence.

Opioid Substitution Therapy. Opioid substitution therapy has several advantages. First, it frees persons with opioid use disorder from using injectable heroin or other illicit opioids and, thus,

Table 4-23
Nonopioid Medications Used to Treat Withdrawal

Target Symptom	Medication Class	Example
Autonomic symptoms (e.g., sweating, restlessness, tremor, and rhinorrhea)	α_2-agonist	Clonidine
Anxiety and psychomotor agitation	Benzodiazepines (usually reserved for the inpatient setting)	Lorazepam
Insomnia	Hypnotics	Zolpidem, zopiclone
	Sedating antidepressants	Trazodone
	Atypical antipsychotics	Quetiapine
Musculoskeletal pain	Nonsteroidal anti-inflammatory drugs	Ibuprofen
	Antispasmodic agents	Cyclobenzaprine
GI distress and diarrhea	Antiemetic agents	Prochlorperazine
	Peripheral μ-opioid receptor agonists	Loperamide

reduces the chance of spreading HIV or hepatitis through contaminated needles. Second, opioid agonists produce minimal euphoria and rarely cause drowsiness or depression when taken for a long time. Third, opioid agonists allow patients to engage in gainful employment instead of criminal activity. The major disadvantage of opioid agonist use is that patients remain dependent on a narcotic.

METHADONE. Meta-analytical studies show methadone's clear superiority over treatments without medication on improving treatment retention and reducing heroin or other illicit opioid use. The majority of patients treated in methadone programs also show decreased nonopioid drug use, criminal behavior, symptoms of depression, and increased gainful employment.

The effectiveness of opioid maintenance treatment depends on the dose and the quality of the additional services provided. The optimal dose is generally in the 80 to 120 mg/day range, with some patients requiring higher doses to achieve an optimal clinical response. Among the most common side effects of methadone are constipation, excessive sweating, decreased libido, and sexual dysfunction. In the United States, methadone can be dispensed only at an outpatient opioid treatment program (OTP) certified by SAMHSA and registered with the DEA or to a hospitalized patient in an emergency. SAMHSA-certified OTP facilities provide daily doses of methadone under direct supervision until the patient is stable enough to receive take-home doses.

BUPRENORPHINE/NALOXONE COMBINATION. Buprenorphine is a high-affinity partial μ-opioid receptor agonist, κ-receptor antagonist, and ORL-1 agonist. At lower doses of up to 16 mg, buprenorphine has a dose-dependent opiate-like effect, but at higher doses, there is progressively less increase in opiate-like effects. There is a ceiling to the μ-opioid agonist effects of buprenorphine, which limits respiratory depression and other adverse effects, increasing its safety profile. Buprenorphine has poor bioavailability and is usually administered sublingually as a tablet or as a film.

Naloxone is mixed with the buprenorphine in a four to one ratio; this is to decrease the risk of abuse. Because naloxone has poor sublingual bioavailability, it exerts minimal effect when taking the preparation as prescribed, but if it is dissolved and injected by an opioid-dependent person, it blocks some of the effects of buprenorphine and may precipitate withdrawal.

Treatment with buprenorphine is best suited for individuals who present with at least mild withdrawal symptoms. Unlike methadone, there is little concern about overdose during treatment initiation. However, combining buprenorphine with benzodiazepines or other sedative–hypnotics can produce excessive sedation, and there are case reports of fatalities associated with parenteral misuse of buprenorphine and a benzodiazepine. Common side effects of buprenorphine include constipation, nausea, headache, upset stomach, excessive sweating, somnolence, and decreased interest in sex. In the United States, to prescribe buprenorphine, physicians must complete a training course and receive a waiver granted by the DEA.

OPIOID ANTAGONISTS. Opioid antagonists block or antagonize the effects of opioids. Unlike methadone, they do not exert narcotic effects and do not cause dependence. Opioid antagonists include naloxone, which is used in the treatment of opioid overdose because it reverses the effects of narcotics, and naltrexone, the longest-acting (72 hours) antagonist. The theory for using an antagonist for opioid-related disorders is that blocking opioid agonist effects, particularly euphoria, discourages persons with physiologic dependence on opioids from substance-seeking behavior and,

thus, deconditions this behavior. The major weakness of the antagonist treatment model is the lack of any mechanism that compels a person to continue to take the antagonist. Naltrexone can be taken orally or in a long-acting injectable formulation.

Psychotherapy

The entire range of psychotherapeutic modalities is appropriate for treating opioid-related disorders. Individual psychotherapy, behavioral therapy, CBT, family therapy, support groups (e.g., Narcotics Anonymous [NA]), and social skills training may all prove useful for specific patients. Patients with few social skills should receive social skills training. Most patients living with family members should also receive family therapy.

Therapeutic Communities

Therapeutic communities are residences in which all members have a substance abuse problem.

Abstinence is the rule; to be admitted to such a community, a person must show a high level of motivation. The goals are to effect a complete change of lifestyle, including abstinence from substances; to develop personal honesty, responsibility, and useful social skills; and to eliminate antisocial attitudes and criminal behavior.

Education and Needle Exchange

Although the essential treatment of opioid use disorders is encouraging persons to abstain from opioids, education about the transmission of HIV must receive equal attention. It is essential to teach persons with opioid use disorders who use intravenous or subcutaneous routes of administration safe-sex practices. Free needle-exchange programs are often subject to intense political and societal pressures but, where allowed, should be made available to persons with opioid use disorders. Several studies have indicated that unsafe needle sharing is common when it is difficult to obtain enough clean needles and is also common in persons with legal difficulties, severe substance problems, and psychiatric symptoms.

Narcotic Anonymous

NA is a self-help group of abstinent drug addicts modeled on the 12-step principles of AA. Such groups now exist in most large cities and can provide useful group support. Although the scientific evidence supportive of the usefulness of such groups has been very limited, observational studies support its effectiveness, and therefore, patients receiving pharmacologic treatments should be encouraged to participate in the self-help groups.

Pregnant Women with Opioid Use Disorders

Illicit opioid use during pregnancy is associated with adverse effects for both the pregnant woman and the fetus but is not associated with any specific teratogenic effects. However, there is a higher risk of infections, preeclampsia, miscarriage, premature rupture of membranes, and premature labor as well as stillbirths, premature infants, and infants with low birth weight and neonatal opioid withdrawal (also called the neonatal abstinence syndrome). Infants who survive may be infected with HIV and other diseases as a result of maternal high-risk behavior and are at risk of sudden infant death syndrome (SIDS). Most of these risks can be substantially reduced with methadone or buprenorphine maintenance treatment.

EPIDEMIOLOGY

The use and dependence rates derived from national surveys do not accurately reflect fluctuations in drug use among opioid-dependent and previously opioid-dependent populations. When the supply of illicit heroin increases in purity or decreases in price, use among that vulnerable population tends to increase, with subsequent increases in adverse consequences (emergency department visits) and requests for treatment. The number of current (past month) heroin users in the United States is about 475,000 in those ages 12 and up. That number grows to 3.3 million, or approximately 1.2 percent of the population, for current (past month) pain relievers. The majority (53 percent) of individuals who misuse pain relievers report obtaining them from friends or family. When considering all opioid use over the past year, the number is staggering: 11.8 million individuals 12 years old and older used opioids in the past year, representing approximately 4.4 percent of the population.

PATHOLOGY

Effects of Opioids

The physical effects of opioids include respiratory depression, pupillary constriction, smooth muscle contraction (including the ureters and the bile ducts), constipation, and changes in blood pressure, heart rate, and body temperature. The brainstem mediates the respiratory depressant effects.

Adverse Effects

The most common and most serious adverse effect associated with opioid-related disorders is the potential transmission of hepatitis and HIV through the use of contaminated needles by more than one person. Persons can experience idiosyncratic allergic reactions to opioids, which result in anaphylactic shock, pulmonary edema, and death if they do not receive prompt and adequate treatment. Another serious adverse effect is an idiosyncratic drug interaction between meperidine and monoamine oxidase inhibitors (MAOIs), which can produce gross autonomic instability, severe behavioral agitation, coma, seizures, and death. Opioids and MAOIs should not be given together for this reason.

Opioid Overdose

Death from an overdose of an opioid is usually attributable to respiratory arrest from the respiratory depressant effect of the drug. The symptoms of overdose include marked unresponsiveness, coma, slow respiration, hypothermia, hypotension, and bradycardia. When presented with the clinical triad of coma, pinpoint pupils, and respiratory depression, clinicians should consider opioid overdose as a primary diagnosis. They can also inspect the patient's body for needle tracks in the arms, legs, ankles, groin, and even the dorsal vein of the penis.

Neuropharmacology

The primary effects of the opioid drugs are mediated via the opioid receptors, discovered in the early 1970s. The μ-opioid receptors are involved in the regulation and mediation of analgesia, respiratory depression, constipation, and drug dependence; the κ-opioid receptors, with analgesia, diuresis, and sedation; and the Δ-opioid receptors, with analgesia.

In 1975, the enkephalins, two endogenous pentapeptides with opioid-like actions, were identified. This discovery led to the identification of three classes of endogenous opioids within the brain. These include the endorphins, the dynorphins, and the enkephalins. Eric Simon was one of the discoverers, and he coined the term "endorphin," which was a contraction of "endogenous" and "morphine." Endorphins are involved in neural transmission and pain suppression. They are released naturally in the body when a person is physically hurt or severely stressed, and they may account for the absence of pain during acute injuries.

The endogenous opioids also have significant interactions with other neuronal systems, such as the dopaminergic and noradrenergic neurotransmitter systems. Several types of data indicate that the VTA dopaminergic neurons (which project to the cerebral cortex and the limbic system) mediate the rewarding properties of opioids.

Heroin, the most commonly abused opioid, is more lipid-soluble than morphine. It crosses the blood–brain barrier faster and has a more rapid and pleasurable onset than morphine. First introduced as a treatment for morphine addiction, heroin is more dependence-producing than morphine. Codeine, which occurs naturally as about 0.5 percent of the opiate alkaloids in opium, is absorbed quickly through the GI tract and is subsequently transformed into morphine in the body. Results of at least one study using positron emission tomography (PET) have suggested that one effect of all opioids is decreased cerebral blood flow (CBF) in selected brain regions in persons with opioid dependence. There is compelling evidence indicating that the endorphins are involved in other addictions, such as alcoholism, cocaine, and cannabinoid addiction. The opioid antagonist, naltrexone, has shown value in mitigating alcohol addiction.

Tolerance and Dependence. Tolerance to all actions of opioid drugs does not develop uniformly. Tolerance to some actions of opioids can be so high that a 100-fold increase in dose is required to produce the original effect. For example, terminally ill cancer patients may need 200 to 300 mg a day of morphine, whereas a dose of 60 mg can easily be fatal to an opioid-naive person. The symptoms of opioid withdrawal do not appear unless a person has been using opioids for a long time or when cessation is particularly abrupt, as occurs when a person takes an opioid antagonist. The long-term use of opioids results in changes in the number and sensitivity of opioid receptors, which mediate at least some of the effects of tolerance and withdrawal. Although long-term use is associated with increased sensitivity of dopaminergic, cholinergic, and serotonergic neurons, the effect of opioids on the noradrenergic neurons is probably the primary mediator of the symptoms of opioid withdrawal. Short-term use of opioids appears to decrease the activity of the noradrenergic neurons in the locus ceruleus; long-term use activates a compensatory homeostatic mechanism within the neurons, and opioid withdrawal results in rebound hyperactivity. This hypothesis also explains why clonidine, an α$_2$-adrenergic receptor agonist that decreases the release of norepinephrine, is useful in the treatment of opioid withdrawal symptoms.

ETIOLOGY

Psychosocial Factors

Social attitudes, peer pressure, individual temperament, and drug availability all predispose people to problematic opioid use. Social stigma is less with prescription opioids than heroin, and prescription opioids are believed to be safer in comparison to heroin and are more widely available. As prescription opioid users develop some functional impairments, their opioid use often transitions to heroin and the IV route of administration due to lower cost and increasing tolerance for slower-acting agents. The presence of a significant number of opioid users in a geographic area can also create a subculture of opioid experimentation. In the United States, areas in which the prevalence of opioid use disorder is high also often have associated high crime rates, unemployment rates, and poorly performing school systems. While correlation does not equal causation, these factors can all be conceptualized as contributing to reduced resistance to opioid use and may worsen the prognosis and treatment efficacy. Most urban heroin users are children of single parents or divorced parents and are from families in which at least one other member has a substance-related disorder. Children from such settings are at high risk for opioid use disorder, especially if they also evidence behavioral problems in school or other signs of conduct disorder.

Biologic and Genetic Factors

Evidence now exists for common and drug-specific, genetically transmitted vulnerability factors that increase the likelihood of developing drug dependence. Individuals who abuse a substance from any category are more likely to abuse substances from other categories. Twin studies estimate that around 50 to 60 percent of the liability for heroin addiction is genetic.

Ongoing linkage and genome-wide association studies continue to investigate promising targets for understanding the genetics and genomics of opioid use disorder.

▲ 4.5 Sedative-, Hypnotic-, or Anxiolytic-Related Disorders

Anxiolytic or sedative–hypnotic drugs are on a continuum with their hypnotic or sleep-inducing effects. In addition to their psychiatric indications, clinicians also use these drugs as antiepileptics, muscle relaxants, anesthetics, and anesthetic adjuvants. Alcohol and all drugs of this class are cross-tolerant, and their effects are additive. Physical and psychological dependence develops to these drugs, and all are associated with withdrawal symptoms. In the practice of psychiatry and addiction medicine, the drug class that is most important clinically is the benzodiazepines.

The three major groups of drugs associated with this class of substance-related disorders are benzodiazepines, barbiturates, and barbiturate-like substances. We discuss each below.

Clinical Features

Specific Agents

BENZODIAZEPINES. Many benzodiazepines, differing primarily in their half-lives, are available in the United States. Examples of benzodiazepines are diazepam, flurazepam, oxazepam, and chlordiazepoxide. Benzodiazepines are used primarily as anxiolytics, hypnotics, antiepileptics, and anesthetics, as well as for alcohol withdrawal. After their introduction in the United States in the 1960s, benzodiazepines rapidly became the most prescribed drugs; about 15 percent of all persons in the United States have had a benzodiazepine prescribed by a physician. Increasing awareness of

the risks for dependence on benzodiazepines and increased regulatory requirements, however, have decreased the number of benzodiazepine prescriptions. The DEA classifies all benzodiazepines as Schedule IV controlled substances.

Flunitrazepam, a benzodiazepine used in Mexico, South America, and Europe but not available in the United States, has become a drug of abuse. When taken with alcohol, it may lead to promiscuous sexual behavior and rape. It is illegal to bring flunitrazepam into the United States. Although misused in the United States, it remains a standard anxiolytic in many countries.

Nonbenzodiazepine sedatives such as zolpidem, zaleplon, and eszopiclone—the so-called Z drugs—have clinical effects similar to the benzodiazepines and are also subject to misuse and dependence.

BARBITURATES. Barbiturates were popular before the introduction of benzodiazepines, but because of their high abuse potential, their use is much rarer today. Secobarbital was popular in the 1960s through the 1980s. It acquired many nicknames, including "reds," "red devils," "seggies," and "downers," among many others. Pentobarbital was also popular, and its nicknames included "yellow jackets," "yellows," and "nembies." A secobarbital–amobarbital combination was also widely available, and was called "reds and blues," "rainbows," "double-trouble," and "tooies." Pentobarbital, secobarbital, and amobarbital are now under the same federal legal controls as morphine.

The first barbiturate, barbital, was introduced in the United States in 1903. Barbital and phenobarbital, introduced shortly after that, are long-acting drugs with half-lives of 12 to 24 hours. Amobarbital is an intermediate-acting barbiturate with a half-life of 6 to 12 hours. Pentobarbital and secobarbital are short-acting barbiturates with half-lives of 3 to 6 hours. Although barbiturates are useful and effective sedatives, they are highly lethal, with only ten times the standard dose producing coma and death.

BARBITURATE-LIKE SUBSTANCES. The most commonly abused barbiturate-like substance is methaqualone. Various manufacturers produced it in the United States until being discontinued in 1985. It is often used by young persons who believe that the substance heightens the pleasure of sexual activity. The street names for methaqualone include "mandrakes" (from the United Kingdom preparation Mandrax) and "soapers" (from the brand name Sopor). "Luding out" (from the brand name Quaalude) means getting high on methaqualone, often along with alcohol.

Other barbiturate-like substances include meprobamate, a carbamate derivative that has weak efficacy as an antianxiety agent but has muscle-relaxant effects, chloral hydrate, a hypnotic that is highly toxic to the GI system and when combined with alcohol, is known as a "Mickey Finn"; and ethchlorvynol, a rapidly acting sedative agent with anticonvulsant and muscle-relaxant properties. All are subject to abuse.

Patterns of Abuse

Oral Use. Sedatives and hypnotics are usually taken orally, either occasionally to achieve a time-limited specific effect or regularly to obtain a constant, usually mild, intoxication state. The occasional use pattern is associated with young persons who take the substance to achieve specific effects—relaxation for an evening, intensification of sexual activities, and a short-lived period of mild euphoria. The user's personality and expectations about the substance's effects, as well as the setting, also affect the substance-induced experience. The regular use pattern is associated with middle-aged, middle-class persons who usually obtain the substance from a family physician as a prescription for insomnia or anxiety. Abusers of this type may have prescriptions from several physicians, and the pattern of abuse may go undetected until apparent signs of a substance use disorder are noticed by the person's family, coworkers, or physicians.

Intravenous Use.

A severe form of misuse involves the intravenous use of this class of substances. The users are mainly young adults who are intimately involved with illegal substances. Intravenous barbiturate use is associated with a pleasant, warm, drowsy feeling, and users may be inclined to use barbiturates more than opioids because barbiturates are less costly. The physical dangers of injection include transmission of HIV, cellulitis, vascular complications from accidental injection into an artery, infections, and allergic reactions to contaminants. Intravenous use is associated with rapid and profound tolerance and dependence and severe withdrawal syndrome.

Overdose

Benzodiazepines.

In contrast to the barbiturates and the barbiturate-like substances, the benzodiazepines have a large margin of safety when taken in overdoses, a feature that has contributed significantly to their rapid acceptance. The ratio of the lethal dose to effective dose is about 200 to 1 or higher, because of the minimal degree of respiratory depression associated with the benzodiazepines. Table 4-24 lists the equivalent therapeutic doses of benzodiazepines. Even when users take grossly excessive amounts (more than 2 g) in suicide attempts, the symptoms include only drowsiness, lethargy, ataxia, some confusion, and mild depression of the user's vital signs. The most lethal overdoses occur when the user takes a benzodiazepine in combination with other sedatives, such as alcohol. In such cases, small doses of benzodiazepines can cause death. The availability of flumazenil, a specific benzodiazepine antagonist, has reduced the lethality of the benzodiazepines.

Table 4-24
Approximate Therapeutic Equivalent Doses of Benzodiazepines

Generic Name	Trade Name	Dose (mg)
Alprazolam	Xanax	1
Chlordiazepoxide	Librium	25
Clonazepam	Klonopin	0.5–1.0
Clorazepate	Tranxene	15
Diazepam	Valium	10
Estazolam	Prosom	1
Flurazepam	Dalmane	30
Lorazepam	Ativan	2
Oxazepam	Serax	30
Temazepam	Restoril	20
Triazolam	Halcion	0.25
Quazepam	Doral	15
Zolpidem	Ambien	10
Zaleplon	Sonata	10

Flumazenil can be used in emergency departments to reverse the effects of benzodiazepines.

Barbiturates.

Barbiturates are lethal when taken in an overdose because they induce respiratory depression. In addition to intentional suicide attempts, accidental or unintentional overdoses are common. Barbiturates in home medicine cabinets are a common cause of fatal drug overdoses in children. As with benzodiazepines, the lethal effects of the barbiturates are additive to those of other sedatives or hypnotics, including alcohol and benzodiazepines. Barbiturate overdose can induce coma, respiratory arrest, cardiovascular failure, and death.

The lethal dose varies with the route of administration and the degree of tolerance for the substance. For the most commonly abused barbiturates, the ratio of the lethal dose to effective dose ranges between 3:1 and 30:1. Dependent users often take an average daily dose of 1.5 g of a short-acting barbiturate, and some take as much as 2.5 g a day for months.

The lethal dose is not much higher for the long-term abuser than for the neophyte. Tolerance develops quickly, to the point at which withdrawal in a hospital becomes necessary to prevent accidental death from overdose.

Barbiturate-Like Substances.

The barbiturate-like substances vary in their lethality and are usually intermediate between the relative safety of the benzodiazepines and the high lethality of the barbiturates. An overdose of methaqualone, for example, can result in restlessness, delirium, hypertonia, muscle spasms, convulsions, and, in very high doses, death. Unlike barbiturates, methaqualone rarely causes severe cardiovascular or respiratory depression, and most fatalities result from combining methaqualone with alcohol.

DIAGNOSIS

Sedative, Hypnotic, or Anxiolytic Use Disorder

The DSM-5 and ICD-10 include several diagnoses related to sedatives, and they generally follow the template for all substance use disorders (see Section 4.1 and Tables 4-1 through 4-3).

Sedative, Hypnotic, or Anxiolytic Intoxication

The intoxication syndromes induced by all these drugs are similar. Table 4-25 lists some of the common symptoms. Blood toxicology is the best way to confirm the diagnosis.

Benzodiazepines.

Behavioral disinhibition is a typical result of benzodiazepine intoxication. It can potentially result in hostile or aggressive behavior in users, most commonly when they also take alcohol. Benzodiazepine intoxication is associated with less euphoria than is intoxication by other drugs in this class. This characteristic is the basis for the lower abuse and dependence potential of benzodiazepines than of barbiturates.

Barbiturates and Barbiturate-Like Substances.

The clinical syndrome of barbiturate (and barbiturate-like substance) intoxication is indistinguishable from alcohol intoxication, at least in lower doses. Table 4-25 lists both symptoms common to all sedative–hypnotics as well as additional symptoms associated with barbiturates. Sluggishness usually resolves after a few hours, but, depending primarily on the half-life of the abused substance, the

Table 4-25
Sedative–Hypnotic Intoxication Symptoms

Common symptoms
Incoordination
Dysarthria
Nystagmus
Impaired memory
Gait disturbance
Severe cases: stupor, coma, or death

Barbiturate intoxication (additional symptoms)
Sluggishness
Slow speech
Slow comprehension
Faulty judgment
Disinhibited sexual aggressive impulses
Narrowed range of attention
Emotional lability
Exaggerated basic personality traits
Hostility
Argumentativeness
Moroseness
Paranoid and suicidal ideation
Neurologic symptoms: nystagmus, diplopia, strabismus, ataxic gait, positive Romberg sign, hypotonia, and decreased superficial reflexes

---

effects on judgment, mood, and motor skills may remain for 12 to 24 hours.

Sedative, Hypnotic, or Anxiolytic Withdrawal

Benzodiazepines. The severity of the withdrawal syndrome associated with the benzodiazepines varies with the average dose and the duration of use, but a mild withdrawal syndrome can follow even short-term use of relatively low doses of benzodiazepines. A significant withdrawal syndrome is likely to occur at the cessation of dosages in the range of 40 mg a day for diazepam, for example, although 10 to 20 mg a day, taken for a month, can also result in a withdrawal syndrome when stopping it. The onset of withdrawal symptoms usually occurs 2 to 3 days after the cessation of use, but with long-acting drugs, such as diazepam, the latency before onset can be 5 or 6 days. The symptoms include anxiety, dysphoria, intolerance for bright lights and loud noises, nausea, sweating, muscle twitching, and sometimes seizures (generally at dosages of 50 mg a day or more of diazepam). Table 4-26 lists the signs and symptoms of benzodiazepine withdrawal.

Barbiturates and Barbiturate-Like Substances. The withdrawal syndrome for barbiturate and barbiturate-like substances range from mild symptoms (e.g., anxiety, weakness, sweating, and insomnia) to severe symptoms (e.g., seizures, delirium, cardiovascular collapse, and death). Persons who have been abusing phenobarbital in the range of 400 mg a day may experience mild withdrawal symptoms; those who have been abusing the substance in the range of 800 mg a day can experience orthostatic hypotension, weakness, tremor, and severe anxiety. About 75 percent of these persons have withdrawal-related seizures. Users of dosages higher than 800 mg a day may experience anorexia, delirium, hallucinations, and repeated seizures.

Most symptoms appear in the first 3 days of abstinence, and seizures generally occur on the second or third day, when the

Table 4-26
Signs and Symptoms of the Benzodiazepine Discontinuation Syndrome

The following signs and symptoms may be seen when benzodiazepine therapy is discontinued; they reflect the return of the original anxiety symptoms (recurrence), worsening of the original anxiety symptoms (rebound), or emergence of new symptoms (true withdrawal):
* *Disturbances of mood and cognition*
  anxiety, apprehension, dysphoria, pessimism, irritability, obsessive rumination, and paranoid ideation
* *Disturbances of sleep*
  insomnia, altered sleep–wake cycle, and daytime drowsiness
* *Physical signs and symptoms*
  tachycardia, elevated blood pressure, hyperreflexia, muscle tension, agitation/motor restlessness, tremor, myoclonus, muscle and joint pain, nausea, coryza, diaphoresis, ataxia, tinnitus, and grand mal seizures
* *Perceptual disturbances*
  hyperacusis, depersonalization, blurred vision, illusions, and hallucinations

---

symptoms are worst. If seizures do occur, they always precede the development of delirium. The symptoms rarely occur more than a week after stopping the substance. A psychotic disorder, if it develops, starts on the third to the eighth day. The various associated symptoms generally run their course within 2 to 3 days but can last as long as 2 weeks.

Other Sedative-, Hypnotic-, or Anxiolytic-Induced Disorders

Delirium. Delirium that is indistinguishable from DTs associated with alcohol withdrawal is seen more commonly with barbiturate withdrawal than with benzodiazepine withdrawal. Delirium associated with intoxication can be seen with either barbiturates or benzodiazepines if the dosages are sufficiently high.

Neurocognitive Disorders. The diagnosis of this disorder is complex because it is difficult to know whether a neurocognitive disorder is due to the substance use itself or associated features of substance use.

Psychotic Disorders. The psychotic symptoms of barbiturate withdrawal can be indistinguishable from those of alcohol-associated DTs. Agitation, delusions, and hallucinations are usually visual, but sometimes tactile or auditory features develop after about 1 week of abstinence. Psychotic symptoms associated with intoxication or withdrawal are more common with barbiturates than with benzodiazepines. DSM-5 diagnoses them as sedative, hypnotic, or anxiolytic withdrawal with perceptual disturbances when reality testing is intact (the individual is aware the drug is causing the psychotic symptoms). If reality testing is not intact (the individual believes the hallucinations are real), a diagnosis of substance/medication-induced psychotic disorder is more appropriate. Clinicians can further specify whether delusions or hallucinations are the predominant symptoms, including the type (e.g., auditory, visual, or tactile).

Other Disorders. Sedative, hypnotic, and anxiolytic use may also cause mood disorders, anxiety disorders, sleep disorders, and sexual dysfunctions.

Unspecified Sedative-, Hypnotic-, or Anxiolytic-Related Disorder. When none of the previously discussed diagnostic categories is appropriate for a person with sedative-, hypnotic-, or anxiolytic-related disorder, and he or she does not meet the diagnostic criteria for any general substance-related disorder, the appropriate diagnosis is an unspecified sedative-, hypnotic-, or anxiolytic-related disorder.

TREATMENT AND REHABILITATION

Withdrawal

Benzodiazepines.   Because some benzodiazepines are eliminated from the body slowly, symptoms of withdrawal can continue to develop for several weeks. To prevent seizures and other withdrawal symptoms, clinicians should gradually reduce the dosage. Table 4-27 lists guidelines for treating benzodiazepine withdrawal.

Barbiturates.   To avoid sudden death during barbiturate withdrawal, clinicians must follow conservative clinical guidelines. Clinicians should not give barbiturates to a comatose or grossly intoxicated patient. A clinician should attempt to determine a patient's usual daily dose of barbiturates and then verify the dosage clinically. For example, a clinician can give a test dose of 200 mg of pentobarbital every hour until a mild intoxication occurs, but withdrawal symptoms are absent (Table 4-28). The clinician can then taper the total daily dose at a rate of about 10 percent of the total daily dose. Once the correct dosage is determined, the clinician can

Table 4-27
Guidelines for Treatment of Benzodiazepine Withdrawal

1. Evaluate and treat concomitant medical and psychiatric conditions.
2. Obtain drug history and urine and blood samples for drug and ethanol assay.
3. Determine required dose of benzodiazepine or barbiturate for stabilization, guided by history, clinical presentation, drug–ethanol assay, and (in some cases) challenge dose.
4. Detoxification from supratherapeutic dosages:
   a. Hospitalize if there are medical or psychiatric indications, poor social supports, or polysubstance dependence, or the patient is unreliable.
   b. Some clinicians recommend switching to longer-acting benzodiazepine for withdrawal (e.g., diazepam, clonazepam); others recommend stabilizing on the drug that patient was taking or on phenobarbital.
   c. After stabilization reduce dosage by 30% on the second or third day and evaluate the response, keeping in mind that symptoms that occur after decreases in benzodiazepines with short elimination half-lives (e.g., lorazepam) appear sooner than with those with longer elimination half-lives (e.g., diazepam).
   d. Reduce dosage further by 10–25% every few days if tolerated.
   e. Use adjunctive medications if necessary—carbamazepine, β-adrenergic receptor antagonists, valproate, clonidine, and sedative antidepressants have been used but their efficacy in the treatment of the benzodiazepine abstinence syndrome has not been established.
5. Detoxification from therapeutic dosages:
   a. Initiate 10–25% dose reduction and evaluate response.
   b. Dose, duration of therapy, and severity of anxiety influence the rate of taper and need for adjunctive medications.
   c. Most patients taking therapeutic doses have uncomplicated discontinuation.
6. Psychological interventions may assist patients in detoxification from benzodiazepines and in the long-term management of anxiety.

Courtesy of Domenici A. Ciraulo, M.D., and Ofra Sarid-Segal, M.D.

Table 4-28
Pentobarbital Test Dose Procedure for Barbiturate Withdrawal

Symptoms After Test Dose of 200 mg Oral Pentobarbital	Estimated 24-Hr Oral Pentobarbital Dose (mg)	Estimated 24-Hr Oral Phenobarbital Dose (mg)
Level I: asleep but arousable; withdrawal symptoms not likely	0	0
Level II: mild sedation; patient may have slurred speech, ataxia, nystagmus	500–600	150–200
Level III: patient is comfortable: no evidence of sedation; may have nystagmus	800	250
Level IV: no drug effect	1,000–1,200	300–600

use a long-acting barbiturate for the detoxification period. During this process, the patient may begin to experience withdrawal symptoms, in which case the clinician should halve the daily decrement.

In the withdrawal procedure, phenobarbital can substitute for the more commonly abused short-acting barbiturates. The effects of phenobarbital last longer, and because barbiturate blood levels fluctuate less, phenobarbital does not cause observable toxic signs or a severe overdose. An adequate dose is 30 mg of phenobarbital for every 100 mg of the short-acting substance. Clinicians should maintain the user for at least 2 days at that level before reducing the dose further. The regimen is analogous to the substitution of methadone for heroin.

After withdrawal is complete, the patient must overcome the desire to start retaking the substance. Although clinicians sometimes try to substitute a nonbarbiturate sedative or hypnotic for a barbiturate, this often replaces one substance dependence with another. If a user is to remain substance-free, follow-up treatment, usually with psychiatric help and community support, is vital. Otherwise, a patient will almost certainly return to barbiturates or a substance with similar hazards.

EPIDEMIOLOGY

According to the NSDUH, approximately 500,000 individuals aged 12 and older used sedatives in the past month. Persons older than 26 years have the highest use. In 2016, more than 600,000 individuals met the criteria for a tranquilizer use disorder in the past year. Benzodiazepines are probably not abused as frequently as other substances to get "high," or inducing a euphoric feeling. Instead, people use them to experience a general relaxed feeling.

PATHOLOGY

Neuropharmacology

The benzodiazepines, barbiturates, and barbiturate-like substances all have their primary effects on the GABA$_A$ receptor complex, which contains a chloride ion channel, a binding site for GABA, and a well-defined binding site for benzodiazepines. The barbiturates and barbiturate-like substances probably bind somewhere on the GABA$_A$ receptor complex. When one of these substances binds to the complex, the effect is to increase the affinity of the receptor for its endogenous neurotransmitter, GABA. GABA then increases the flow of chloride ions through the channel into the neuron. The influx of negatively charged chloride ions into the neuron is inhibitory and hyperpolarizes the neuron relative to the extracellular space.

Although all the substances in this class induce tolerance and physical dependence, we best understand the mechanisms for the benzodiazepines. Long-term benzodiazepine use attenuates the usual agonist effects on the receptor. Specifically, GABA stimulation of the GABA$_A$ receptors results in less chloride influx than was caused by GABA stimulation before the benzodiazepine administration. This downregulation of receptor response is not caused by a decrease in receptor number or by a decreased affinity of the receptor for GABA. The basis for the downregulation seems to be in the coupling between the GABA binding site and the activation of the chloride ion channel. This decreased efficiency in coupling may be regulated within the GABA$_A$ receptor complex itself or by other neuronal mechanisms.

Misuse Liability and Other Risks of Long-Term Use

Surveys of prescribing practices, patient-initiated dosage changes, and recreational or nonmedical benzodiazepine use along with reports from emergency departments, medical examiners, and law enforcement agencies provide a complex picture of the public health implications of the benzodiazepines. The vast majority of medical and psychiatric patients use benzodiazepines appropriately, although rates of misuse by patients dependent on alcohol and other drugs may be higher than individuals with anxiety or insomnia without a history of substance use problems. Furthermore, long-term use is high among patients with psychiatric disorders and the elderly, with the latter group being sensitive to drug toxicity.

Also, long-term use of benzodiazepines may increase the risk of developing dementia. A recent meta-analysis found that this risk is higher for those taking benzodiazepines with a longer half-life and for those who have been taking benzodiazepines for a longer duration (more than 3 years), although other data suggest that there may not be an increased risk for dementia.

▲ 4.6 Stimulant-Related Disorders

CLINICAL FEATURES

Types of Stimulants

Amphetamines.   The racemic amphetamine sulfate (Benzedrine) was first synthesized in 1887, and Smith, Kline, and French marketed it as a decongestant in the early 1930s. In 1930, benzedrine sulfate was introduced for the treatment of narcolepsy, postencephalitic parkinsonism, depression, and lethargy. In the 1970s, a variety of social and regulatory factors began to curb widespread amphetamine distribution. The current US FDA–approved indications for amphetamine are limited to ADHD; however, they are used for many symptoms, some of which we list in Table 4-29.

Table 4-29
Some Indications for Amphetamines

FDA approved
Attention-deficit/hyperactivity disorder
Narcolepsy

Off label uses
Obesity
Depression and dysthymia
Chronic fatigue syndrome
Acquired immunodeficiency syndrome (AIDS)
Cancer-related fatigue
End-of-life care (depressive symptoms)
Dementia
Multiple sclerosis
Fibromyalgia
Neurasthenia

PREPARATIONS.   The main amphetamines currently available and used in the United States are dextroamphetamine, methamphetamine, a mixed dextroamphetamine-amphetamine salt, and the amphetamine-like compound methylphenidate. These drugs go by such street names as ice, crystal, crystal meth, and speed. As a general class, the amphetamines also called analeptics, sympathomimetics, stimulants, and psychostimulants. The typical amphetamines are used to increase performance and to induce a euphoric feeling, for example, by students studying for examinations, by long-distance truck drivers on trips, by business people with pressing deadlines, by athletes in competition, and by soldiers during wartime. Although not as addictive as cocaine, amphetamines are nonetheless addictive drugs.

Other amphetamine-like substances are ephedrine, pseudoephedrine, and phenylpropanolamine (PPA). These drugs, PPA in particular, can dangerously exacerbate hypertension, precipitate a toxic psychosis, cause an intestinal infarction, or result in death. The safety margin for PPA is particularly narrow, and three to four times the standard dose can result in life-threatening hypertension. In 2005, the FDA recalled medications containing PPA, and in 2006, they prohibited the sale of over-the-counter (OTC) medications containing ephedrine and regulated the sale of OTC medications containing pseudoephedrine, which was used illegally to make methamphetamine.

Amphetamine-type drugs with abuse potential also include phendimetrazine (which is Schedule II of the Controlled Substance Act [CSA]), and diethylpropion, benzphetamine, and phentermine (which are Schedules III or IV of the CSA). All of these drugs, most likely, are capable of causing all of the listed amphetamine-induced disorders. Modafinil, used in the treatment of narcolepsy, also has stimulant and euphorigenic effects in humans, but its toxicity and likelihood of producing amphetamine-induced disorders are unknown.

Methamphetamine is a potent form of amphetamine that abusers of the substance inhale, smoke, or inject intravenously. Its psychological effects last for hours and are particularly powerful. Unlike cocaine (see discussion later in this section), which is imported, methamphetamine is a synthetic drug that can be manufactured domestically in illicit laboratories.

Other agents called *substituted,* or *designer amphetamines* are discussed separately later in this section.

Cocaine.   People have used cocaine in its raw form for more than 15 centuries. In the United States, cycles of widespread stimulant misuse and associated problems have occurred for more than 100 years. Cocaine and cocaine use disorders became a major public health issue in the 1980s when an epidemic of use spread throughout the country. Due to education and intervention, cocaine use has since declined. However, high rates of legal, psychiatric, medical, and social problems related to cocaine use still exist; thus, cocaine-related disorders remain a significant public health issue.

Cocaine is an alkaloid derived from the shrub *Erythroxylum coca,* which is indigenous to South America, where the leaves of the shrub are chewed by local inhabitants to obtain the stimulating effects. The cocaine alkaloid was first isolated in 1855 and first used as a local anesthetic in 1880. It continues to be used, especially for eye, nose, and throat surgery, for which its vasoconstrictive and analgesic effects are helpful. In 1884, Sigmund Freud made a study of cocaine's general pharmacologic effects, and, for some time, according to his biographers, he was addicted to the drug. In the 1880s and 1890s, cocaine was widely touted as a cure for many ills, and the 1899 *Merck Manual* listed it. It was the active ingredient in the beverage Coca-Cola until 1903. In 1914, as its addictive effects became known, cocaine was classified as a narcotic, alongside morphine and heroin.

METHODS OF USE. Because drug dealers often dilute cocaine powder with sugar or procaine, street cocaine varies greatly in purity. Amphetamines are occasionally combined with cocaine. The most common method of using cocaine is inhaling the finely chopped powder into the nose; a practice referred to as "snorting" or "tooting." Other methods of ingesting cocaine are subcutaneous or intravenous injection and smoking (freebasing). Freebasing involves mixing street cocaine with chemically extracted pure cocaine alkaloid (the freebase) to get an increased effect. Smoking is also the method used to ingest crack cocaine. Inhaling is the least dangerous method of cocaine use; intravenous injection and smoking are the most dangerous. The most direct methods of ingestion are often associated with cerebrovascular diseases, cardiac abnormalities, and death. Although users can take cocaine orally, they rarely do this as it is the least effective route.

Crack. Crack, a freebase form of cocaine, is extremely potent. Dealers sell it in small, ready-to-smoke amounts, often called "rocks." Crack cocaine is highly addictive; even one or two experiences with the drug can cause an intense craving for more. Users may resort to extremes of behavior to obtain the money to buy more crack. Reports from urban emergency departments have also associated extremes of violence with crack abuse.

Substituted Amphetamines.
MDMA (3,4-methylenedioxymethamphetamine) is one of a series of substituted amphetamines that also includes MDEA, MDA (3,4-methylenedioxyamphetamine), DOB (2,5-dimethoxy-4-bromoamphetamine), PMA (paramethoxyamphetamine), and others. These drugs produce subjective effects resembling those of amphetamine and lysergic acid diethylamide (LSD), and in that sense, MDMA and similar analogs may represent a distinct category of drugs.

A methamphetamine derivative that came into use in the 1980s, MDMA was not technically subject to legal regulation at the time. Although a considered "designer drug," meaning synthesized to evade legal regulation, in reality, it was synthesized and patented in 1914. At one time, it was legal and used as an aid for psychotherapy. However, the FDA never approved the drug. Its use raised questions of both safety and legality, because the related amphetamine derivatives MDA, DOB, and PMA had caused several overdose deaths, and MDA was known to cause extensive destruction

of serotonergic nerve terminals in the CNS. Using emergency scheduling authority, the DEA made MDMA a Schedule I drug under the CSA, along with LSD, heroin, and marijuana. Despite its illegal status, MDMA continues to be manufactured, distributed, and used in the United States, Europe, and Australia. Its use is frequent at extended dances ("raves") popular with adolescents and young adults.

Currently, no established clinical uses exist for MDMA, although before its regulation, there were several reports of its beneficial effects as an adjunct to psychotherapy.

After taking usual doses (100 to 150 mg), MDMA users experience an elevated mood and, according to various reports, increased self-confidence and sensory sensitivity, peaceful feelings coupled with insight, empathy, and closeness to persons, and decreased appetite. The effect on concentration varies with both increased and decreased concentration reported. Users also report dysphoric reactions, psychotomimetic effects, and even psychosis. Higher doses seem more likely to produce psychotomimetic effects. Sympathomimetic effects of tachycardia, palpitation, increased blood pressure, sweating, and bruxism are common. The subjective effects are prominent for about 4 to 8 hours, but that can vary widely depending on the dose and route of administration. The drug is usually taken orally but is also snorted and injected. Users report both tachyphylaxis and some tolerance.

Although not as toxic as MDA, MDMA can cause various toxicities as well as fatal overdoses. It does not appear to be neurotoxic when injected into the brains of animals, but humans and animals do metabolize it to MDA. In animals, MDMA produces selective, long-lasting damage to serotonergic nerve terminals. It is not clear whether the levels of the MDA metabolite reached in humans after the usual doses of MDMA suffice to produce lasting damage.

"Bath Salts".
Catha edulis, or "Khat," is a plant indigenous to Eastern Africa and Southern Arabia. It releases a variety of psychoactive chemicals, including the stimulants cathinone and cathine. Khat is chewed like tobacco and held between the cheek and gums after chewing. The National Institute on Drug Abuse estimates that as many as 10 million people worldwide use Khat, including many in Eastern Africa and the Middle East, as well as an unknown number of immigrants to the United States.

In the mid-2000s, synthetic cathinones began to appear, marketed as "legal high" chemicals. They were packaged under labels including "screen cleaner," "jewelry cleaner," and most notoriously "bath salts." Produced as powders (generally marked "not for human consumption"), users can ingest them by oral, intranasal, inhaled (smoked) or intravenous routes. These compounds are substituted cathinones that are chemically modified to avoid regulatory control. There are a large number of specific compounds in the class, and a given package often contains a mix of agents, further increasing the risk of toxicity. Generally, substituted cathinones increase synaptic catecholamine levels by inhibiting the dopamine, serotonin, and norepinephrine reuptake transporters in a fashion similar to cocaine. Most also facilitate catecholamine release, similar to methamphetamine. Animal models indicate strong reinforcing properties of these compounds, suggesting that they are highly addictive.

"Club Drugs".
Club drugs is a generic term for drugs associated with dance clubs, bars, and all-night dance parties (raves). They include LSD, γ-hydroxybutyrate (GHB), ketamine, methamphetamine, MDMA (ecstasy), and Rohypnol or "roofies" (flunitrazepam). These represent various classes of drugs, with different

chemical structures and a range of physical and subjective effects. GHB, ketamine, and Rohypnol are sometimes called *date rape drugs* because they produce disorienting and sedating effects, and often users cannot recall what occurred during all or part of an episode under the influence of the drug. These drugs may be given surreptitiously, such as slipped into a beverage, or a person might be convinced to take the drug, not understanding its effect.

Emergency department mentions of GHB, ketamine, and Rohypnol are relatively few. Of the club drugs, methamphetamine is the substance that accounts for the largest share of treatment admissions.

DIAGNOSIS

Stimulant Use Disorder

The DSM-5 and ICD-10 include several diagnoses related to stimulant use disorder, and they generally follow the template for all substance use disorders (see Section 4.1 and Tables 4-1 through 4-3).

Amphetamine dependence can result in a rapid downward spiral of a person's abilities to cope with work- and family-related obligations and stresses. A person who abuses amphetamines requires increasingly high doses of amphetamine to obtain the usual high, and physical signs of chronic amphetamine use (e.g., decreased weight and paranoid ideas) almost always develop with continued use.

Mr. H, a 35-year-old married man, was admitted to a psychiatric hospital because he felt persecuted by gang members who were out to kill him. He could not explain why they wished to kill him, but he heard voices from people whom he suspected to be mob drug dealers, and they were discussing that they should kill him. He used methamphetamine for several years, so he had dealt with drug dealers before. He began using at age 27 at the persuasion of a friend to try it. After injecting 20 mg, he felt euphoric and powerful, and his sleepiness and fatigue disappeared. After a few tries, Mr. H found that he could not stop using it. He always thought about how he would obtain the drug and started increasing the dosage he used. During times that he could not get methamphetamine, he felt lethargic and sleepy and became irritable and dysphoric. Mr. H's wife learned of his drug use and attempted to persuade him to stop using it. He lost his job 2 months before his admission as he was repeatedly abusive to work colleagues because he felt that they were trying to harm him. With no income, Mr. H had to cut down his use of methamphetamine to only occasional usage. He finally decided to quit when his wife threatened to divorce him. Once he stopped using, he felt fatigued, seemed gloomy, and often sat in his favorite chair and did nothing. After a few weeks, Mr. H told his wife that he did not wish to leave the house because he had heard dealers on the street talking about him. He wanted all doors and windows locked, and he refused to eat in fear that the people were poisoning his food.

On examination, Mr. H seemed withdrawn, only giving short answers to questions. He was in clear consciousness and fully oriented and showed no marked impairment of cognitive functions. Physical and neurologic testing showed no abnormalities except needle scars on his arms from methamphetamine injections. An EEG was normal.

Clinically and practically, clinicians may suspect cocaine use disorder in patients with unexplained changes in personality. Frequent changes associated with cocaine use are irritability, impaired ability to concentrate, compulsive behavior, severe insomnia, and weight loss. Colleagues at work and family members may notice a person's general and increasing inability to perform the expected tasks associated with work and family life. The patient may show new evidence of increased debt or inability to pay bills on time because of the vast sums used to buy cocaine. Individuals with cocaine use disorder often excuse themselves from work or social situations every 30 to 60 minutes to find a secluded place to inhale more cocaine. Because of the vasoconstricting effects of cocaine, users almost always develop nasal congestion, which they may attempt to self-medicate with decongestant sprays.

Mr. D, a 45-year-old married man, was referred by his therapist to a private outpatient substance use treatment program for evaluation and treatment of a possible cocaine problem. According to the therapist, Mr. D's wife expressed concern for a possible substance use problem on several occasions. A few days prior, Mr. D admitted to the therapist and his wife that he "occasionally" used cocaine for the past year. His wife insisted that he obtain treatment for his drug problem or else she would file for divorce. Mr. D reluctantly conceded to treatment but insisted that his cocaine use was not a problem and that he felt capable of stopping without entering a treatment program.

During the initial evaluation interview, Mr. D reported that he currently used cocaine, intranasally, 3 to 5 days a week and that this pattern has been continuing for a year and a half. On average, he consumes a total of 1 to 2 g of cocaine weekly. He mostly uses cocaine at work, in his office, or the bathroom. He usually started thinking about cocaine during his drive to work in the morning and once at work, was unable to avoid thinking about the cocaine in his desk drawer. Despite his attempts at distraction and postponing use, he usually takes his first line of cocaine within an hour of arriving at work. On some days, he will take another two to three lines during the day, but, on days where he is frustrated and stressed, he may take a line or two every hour from morning until late afternoon. He rarely uses cocaine at home and never uses it in front of his wife or his three daughters. He occasionally takes a line or two during a weekday evening or weekends at home when everyone else is out of the house. He denies using alcohol or any other illicit drugs. He denies any history of alcohol or drug abuse and any history of emotional or marital problems.

Stimulant Intoxication

The diagnostic criteria for stimulant intoxication emphasize behavioral and physical signs and symptoms of stimulant use (Table 4-30). Persons use stimulants for their characteristic effects of elation, euphoria, heightened self-esteem, and perceived improvement on mental and physical tasks. With high doses, symptoms of intoxication include agitation, irritability, impaired judgment, impulsive and potentially dangerous sexual behavior, aggression, a generalized increase in psychomotor activity, and potentially, symptoms of mania. The significant associated physical symptoms are tachycardia, hypertension, and mydriasis.

Table 4-30
Signs and Symptoms of Stimulant Intoxication

- Mydriasis
- Psychomotor agitation or retardation
- Tachycardia or bradycardia
- Perspiration or chills
- Cardiac arrhythmias or chest pain
- Elevated or lowered blood pressure
- Dyskinesias
- Dystonias
- Weight loss
- Nausea or vomiting
- Muscular weakness
- Respiratory depression
- Confusion, seizures, or coma

Mrs. T, a 38-year-old married businesswoman, was admitted to the psychiatric service after a 3-month period in which she became increasingly mistrustful of others and suspicious of business associates. She took statements from others out of context, twisting their words and making inappropriately hostile and accusatory comments. On one occasion, Mrs. T physically attacked a coworker in a bar, accusing the coworker of having an affair with her husband and plotting with other coworkers to kill her.

One year previously, Mrs. T's physician prescribed her methylphenidate for narcolepsy due to daily irresistible sleep attacks and episodes of a sudden loss of muscle tone when she became emotionally excited. After taking the medication, Mrs. T became asymptomatic and was able to work effectively and have an active social life with family and friends.

In the 5 months before admission, Mrs. T had been using increasingly large doses of methylphenidate to maintain alertness late at night because of an increased amount of work that she could not complete during the day. She reported that during this time, she often could feel her heart racing and that she had trouble sitting still.

Mr. P, an 18-year-old man, was brought to a hospital emergency department via ambulance in the middle of the night. He was accompanied by a friend who called the ambulance as he felt that Mr. P was going to die. Mr. P was agitated and argumentative, his breathing was irregular and rapid, his pulse was rapid, and he had dilated pupils. His friend eventually admitted that they had used much cocaine that evening.

When his mother arrived at the hospital, Mr. P's condition had somewhat improved, although his loud singing created a commotion in the emergency department. His mother states that Mr. P has some disciplinary problems; he is disobedient, resentful, and violently argumentative. He was arrested on a few occasions for shoplifting and for driving while intoxicated. His mother suspected that Mr. P was using drugs due to his behavior and because she heard him talk to his friends about drugs. However, she has no direct proof of his use.

Within 24 hours, Mr. P was well and willing to talk. He boastfully stated that he had been using alcohol and various drugs regularly since he was 13. It started with just alcohol and marijuana, but once he entered high school and became acquainted with older teenagers, he experimented with other drugs such as speed and cocaine. By the time he was 16, he was using combinations of alcohol, speed, marijuana, and cocaine. He settled on just cocaine after a year of mixing drugs.

Mr. P frequently skipped school, and, when he attended school, he was usually intoxicated. To support his habit, he acquired money in various schemes, such as borrowing money from friends that he had no intention of paying back or stealing car radios or stealing from his mother.

Despite his blatant admission of drug use, Mr. P denies having a problem. When asked about his ability to control his drug use, he defensively replied that, of course, he could, but as he does not see a problem, he has not tried.

Stimulant Withdrawal

After stimulant intoxication, a "crash" occurs with symptoms of anxiety, tremulousness, dysphoric mood, lethargy, fatigue, nightmares (accompanied by rebound REM sleep), headache, profuse sweating, muscle cramps, stomach cramps, and insatiable hunger. The withdrawal symptoms generally peak in 2 to 4 days and are resolved in 1 week. The most serious withdrawal symptom is depression, which can be particularly severe after the sustained use of high doses of stimulants and which can be associated with suicidal ideation or behavior. A person in the state of withdrawal can experience powerful and intense cravings for cocaine, mainly because taking cocaine can eliminate unpleasant withdrawal symptoms. Persons experiencing cocaine withdrawal often attempt to

self-medicate with alcohol, sedatives, hypnotics, or antianxiety agents such as diazepam.

Stimulant Intoxication Delirium

Delirium associated with stimulant use generally results from high doses of a stimulant or sustained use, and so sleep deprivation affects the clinical presentation. The combination of stimulants with other substances and the use of stimulants by a person with preexisting brain damage can also cause delirium. It is not uncommon for university students who are using amphetamines to cram for examinations to exhibit this type of delirium.

Stimulant-Induced Psychotic Disorder

The hallmark of stimulant-induced psychotic disorder is the presence of paranoid delusions and hallucinations, which occurs in up to 50 percent of those who misuse stimulants. Auditory hallucinations are also common, but visual and tactile hallucinations are less common than paranoid delusions. Cocaine can also cause the sensation of bugs crawling beneath the skin (formication). The presence of these symptoms depends on the dose, duration of use, and the user's sensitivity to the substance. Cocaine-induced psychotic disorders are most familiar with intravenous use and crack users, and the psychotic symptoms are more common in men than in women. The treatment of choice for amphetamine-induced psychotic disorder is the short-term use of an antipsychotic medication such as haloperidol.

Mr. H is a 20-year-old college student who was functioning well until the weeks of his finals when he began taking large amounts of cocaine because he felt he was unprepared for his tests. He began having delusional beliefs that the police were following him at the request of his parents to spy on him. He also believed that his roommate would give reports to them about his study habits and social life. He was brought to the emergency department after he threatened to harm his roommate if he continued to report on him.

During his evaluation, Mr. P reported sleeplessness and auditory hallucinations that told him that his roommate was conspiring against him. He was very agitated and paced continuously. After admission to the hospital, Mr. P was given antipsychotics and sleeping medications and recovered in 3 days.

Stimulant-Induced Mood Disorder

Stimulant-induced mood disorder includes the diagnoses of stimulant-induced bipolar disorder and stimulant-induced depressive disorder, either of which can begin during either intoxication or withdrawal. In general, intoxication is associated with manic or mixed mood features, whereas withdrawal is associated with depressive mood features.

Stimulant-Induced Anxiety Disorder

The onset of stimulant-induced anxiety disorder can occur during intoxication or withdrawal. Stimulants can induce symptoms similar to those seen in panic disorder and phobic disorders, in particular.

Stimulant-Induced Obsessive-Compulsive Disorder

The onset of stimulant-induced obsessive-compulsive disorder (OCD) can occur during intoxication or withdrawal. After high doses of stimulants, some individuals develop time-limited stereotyped behaviors or rituals (i.e., picking at clothing, and arranging and rearranging items purposelessly) that share some features with the type of compulsions seen in OCD.

Stimulant-Induced Sexual Dysfunction

People sometimes use amphetamines as an antidote to the sexual side effects of serotonergic agents such as fluoxetine, but stimulants are often misused by persons to enhance sexual experiences. High doses and long-term use are associated with erectile disorder and other sexual dysfunctions.

Stimulant-Induced Sleep Disorder

Stimulant-induced sleep disorder can begin during either intoxication or withdrawal, and sleep dysfunction can vary depending on the onset. Stimulant intoxication can produce insomnia and sleep deprivation, whereas persons undergoing stimulant withdrawal can experience hypersomnolence and nightmares.

COMORBIDITY

Studies of the prevalence of non–substance-related psychiatric disorders among individuals with stimulant use disorders have consistently found elevated levels of psychiatric disorders in this population. Results from the community-based Epidemiological Catchment Area (ECA) Study demonstrated elevated rates of non–substance-related mental disorders in those with cocaine use disorders. In this study, the estimated lifetime prevalence rate for mental disorders was 76 percent or 11 times that found in the general population; nearly 85 percent of those with cocaine use disorders also had co-occurring alcohol use disorders. Studies that have compared treatment-seeking individuals with cocaine use disorders to those who do not seek treatment have demonstrated higher rates of major depression and ADHD among the former group. Likewise, most studies report high levels of co-occurring other substance use disorders in individuals with amphetamine-type stimulant use disorders. Mood disorders, psychotic disorders, and anxiety disorders are also common. While psychotic symptoms are most commonly methamphetamine-induced, mood and anxiety disorders are often not substance-induced.

TREATMENT AND REHABILITATION

Detoxification and Early Treatment

The stimulant withdrawal syndrome is distinct from that of opioids, alcohol, or sedative–hypnotic agents as the physiologic effects are not severe enough to require inpatient or residential drug withdrawal. Thus, it is generally possible to engage in a therapeutic trial of outpatient withdrawal before deciding whether the patient will need a more intensive or controlled setting to stop the drug. Patients withdrawing from stimulants typically experience fatigue, dysphoria, disturbed sleep, and some craving; some may experience depression. No pharmacologic agents reliably reduce the intensity of withdrawal, but recovery over a week or two is generally uneventful. It may take longer, however, for sleep, mood, and cognitive function to recover fully.

Most stimulant users do not come to treatment voluntarily. Their experience with the substance is too positive, and the adverse effects are perceived as too minimal to warrant seeking treatment.

The major hurdle to overcome in the treatment of cocaine-related disorders is the user's intense craving for the drug. Although animal studies have shown that cocaine is a potent inducer of self-administration, these studies have also shown that animals limit their use of cocaine when investigators add negative reinforcers to the cocaine intake. In humans, negative reinforcers may take the form of work and family-related problems brought on by cocaine use. Therefore, clinicians must take a broad treatment approach and include social, psychological, and perhaps biologic strategies in the treatment program.

Attaining abstinence from stimulants in patients may require complete or partial hospitalization to remove them from the social settings in which they had obtained or used stimulants. Frequent, unscheduled urine testing is almost always necessary to monitor patients' continued abstinence, especially in the first weeks and months of treatment. Relapse prevention therapy (RPT) relies on cognitive and behavioral techniques in addition to hospitalization and outpatient therapy to achieve the goal of abstinence.

Psychosocial Therapies

Psychological intervention usually involves individual, group, and family modalities. In individual therapy, therapists should focus on the dynamics leading to stimulant use, the perceived positive effects of the stimulant, and other ways to achieve these effects. Group therapy and support groups, such as NA, often focus on discussions with other persons who use stimulants and on sharing experiences and effective coping methods. Family therapy is often an essential component of the treatment strategy. Typical issues discussed in family therapy are the ways the patient's past behavior has harmed the family and the responses of family members to these behaviors. Therapy should also focus, however, on the future and on changes in the family's activities that may help the patient stay off the drug and direct energies in different directions. Clinicians can use this approach for outpatient treatment.

Network Therapy. Network therapy is a specialized type of combined individual and group therapy designed to ensure greater success in the office-based treatment of addicted patients. Network therapy uses both psychodynamic and cognitive-behavioral approaches to individual therapy while engaging the patient in a group support network. The group, composed of the patient's family and peers, is used as a therapeutic network joining the patient and therapist at intervals in therapy sessions. The approach promotes group cohesiveness as a vehicle for engaging patients in this treatment. This network is managed by the therapist to provide cohesiveness and support and to promote compliance with treatment. Although network therapy has not received systematic, controlled evaluation, it is frequently applied in the psychiatric practice because it is one of the few manualized approaches designed for use by individual practitioners in an office setting.

Pharmacologic Adjuncts

Presently, no pharmacologic treatments produce decreases in stimulant use. However, investigators have explored several agents, and those are summarized below.

Amphetamines. Multiple medications have been investigated as potential treatment options for amphetamine-type stimulant disorders, though the results have been mostly disappointing. Most serotonergic medications studied have not demonstrated efficacy, though mirtazapine has shown some effectiveness in a small sample of men who have sex with men. The opioid-receptor antagonist naltrexone and the dopamine antidepressant bupropion have both shown promise in those with less severe amphetamine use disorders, but little effect on more dependent individuals. Other medications, including topiramate, aripiprazole, baclofen, gabapentin, and modafinil, have demonstrated little effectiveness in this population.

Cocaine.   A variety of pharmacologic agents, most approved for other uses, have been, and are being tested clinically for the treatment of cocaine use disorder and relapse.

Cocaine users presumed to have preexisting ADHD or mood disorders have been treated with methylphenidate and lithium, respectively. Those drugs are of little or no benefit in patients without the disorders, and clinicians should adhere strictly to diagnostic criteria before using either of them in the treatment of cocaine use disorder. In patients with ADHD, slow-release forms of methylphenidate may be less likely to trigger cocaine craving, but the impact of such pharmacotherapy on cocaine use is not clear.

Investigators have explored many pharmacologic agents on the premise that chronic cocaine use alters the function of multiple neurotransmitter systems, especially the dopaminergic and serotonergic transmitters regulating hedonic tone, and that cocaine induces a state of relative dopaminergic deficiency. Although the evidence for such alterations in dopaminergic function has been growing, it has been challenging to demonstrate that agents theoretically capable of modifying dopamine function can alter the course of treatment.

Tricyclic antidepressant drugs yielded some positive results when used early in treatment with minimally drug-dependent patients; however, they are of little or no use inducing abstinence in moderate or severe cases.

Also tried but not confirmed effective in controlled studies are other antidepressants, such as bupropion, MAOIs, SSRIs, antipsychotics, lithium, several different calcium channel inhibitors, and anticonvulsants. Several studies have found increased rates of abstinence with the use of topiramate for cocaine use disorders; however, there are also negative trials of topiramate in this population.

Disulfiram has demonstrated potential benefits in the pharmacotherapy of cocaine use disorder. Disulfiram has long been used in the treatment of alcohol use disorder because it inhibits an enzyme involved in the metabolism of ethanol. Though disulfiram was initially considered a potential treatment option for individuals with both alcohol and cocaine use disorders, studies demonstrated that disulfiram appears to have a direct effect on the metabolism of dopamine and cocaine itself; it acts as an inhibitor of dopamine β-hydroxylase, thereby slowing the breakdown of synaptic dopamine and increasing dopamine levels. Individuals who are co-administered cocaine and disulfiram describe more negative responses to cocaine, including anxiety, restlessness, and paranoia. These reactions may, in part, explain the effects of disulfiram in decreasing cocaine use. Issues affecting treatment response to disulfiram include challenges with treatment nonadherence, risks of inducing psychotic symptoms with combined cocaine and disulfiram use, and risks of serious medical consequences if a patient were to consume alcohol, given the frequent co-occurrence of alcohol and cocaine use disorders.

EPIDEMIOLOGY

Amphetamines

According to the 2017 National Survey on Drug Use and Health (NSDUH), 0.3 percent of persons 12 years or older were current users of methamphetamine, and 5.4 percent have a lifetime history of methamphetamine use. In 2016, 684,000 individuals older than 12 years met the criteria for a methamphetamine use disorder, representing 0.3 percent of the population.

Cocaine

Cocaine Use.   In 2016, 1.9 million (0.7 percent) persons aged 12 years or older used cocaine in the past month. Persons aged 18 to 25 (1.6 percent) had a higher rate of past-month cocaine use than persons aged 26 or older (0.6 percent) and youths aged 12 to 17 (0.1 percent). The lifetime rate of cocaine use by persons aged 12 years and older is 14.9 percent.

Cocaine Use Disorder.   In 2016, more than 850,000 (0.3 percent) persons aged 12 or older met the criteria for a cocaine use disorder. Persons aged 18 to 25 (0.6 percent) had the highest rate of meeting criteria for cocaine use disorder in the past year, followed by persons aged 26 or older (0.3 percent) and youths aged 12 to 17 (0.1 percent).

PATHOLOGY

As a result of actions in the CNS, stimulants can produce a sense of alertness, euphoria, and well-being. Users may experience decreased hunger and less need for sleep. Performance impaired by fatigue is usually improved. Some users believe that cocaine enhances sexual performance.

Adverse Effects

Stimulant use can cause medical complications both as a result of direct toxic effects and because of complications related to methods of preparation and administration. Stimulants are potent sympathomimetic drugs, causing physiologic effects, including vasoconstriction, increased heart rate, and elevated blood pressure through adrenergic stimulation. The combination of increased myocardial demand with constriction of coronary blood vessels can precipitate angina pectoris and even myocardial infarction. Acute hypertension associated with stimulant use can also predispose to arterial hemorrhages, such as hemorrhagic stroke or aortic dissection. Vasoconstriction can involve damage to other end organs, including the brain, kidneys, or intestines. With intranasal use, decreased blood flow to the nasal mucosa frequently causes nasal symptoms (e.g., rhinorrhea, nosebleeds) and mucosal ulceration. A combination of vasoconstriction and bruxism associated with the use of methamphetamine causes markedly poor dentition, or "meth mouth." Grand mal seizures are frequent with stimulant overdose and may occur with routine use as well. Furthermore, individuals who misuse stimulants regularly may develop neuropsychological deficits, including problems with attention, learning, and memory. In many cases, these abnormalities persist during periods of abstinence.

Stimulant misuse can also precipitate behaviors that place an individual at increased risk of harm by violence or accidental injury. Unsafe sexual behaviors may lead to the transmission of HIV or other sexually transmitted diseases. The drugs can cause accidental injury, for example, driving while intoxicated. The associated illegal behaviors involved in obtaining cocaine or methamphetamine can also increase one's risk of violent injury.

Neuropharmacology

Amphetamines.   All the amphetamines are rapidly absorbed orally and have a rapid onset of action, usually within 1 hour, when taken orally. The classic amphetamines are also taken intravenously and have an almost immediate effect by this route. Users can also inhale ("snort") nonprescribed amphetamines or designer amphetamines. Tolerance develops with both classic and designer amphetamines, although amphetamine users respond by taking more of the drug. Amphetamine is less addictive than cocaine, as evidenced by experiments on rats in which not all animals spontaneously self-administered low doses of amphetamine.

The classic amphetamines (i.e., dextroamphetamine, methamphetamine, and methylphenidate) produce their primary effects by causing the release of catecholamines, particularly dopamine, from presynaptic terminals. The effects are particularly potent for the dopaminergic neurons projecting from the VTA to the cerebral cortex and the limbic areas. Some neuroscientists call this the *reward circuit pathway,* and its activation is probably the primary addicting mechanism for the amphetamines. The designer amphetamines cause the release of catecholamines (dopamine and norepinephrine) and serotonin, the neurotransmitter implicated as the significant neurochemical pathway for hallucinogens. Therefore, the clinical effects of designer amphetamines are a blend of the effects of classic amphetamines and those of hallucinogens.

Cocaine.   In vitro animal studies using radiolabeled cocaine or cocaine analogs demonstrate high amounts of binding in dopamine-rich brain regions, including the caudate-putamen and the VTA. Moderate levels of cocaine binding also occur in the substantia nigra, amygdala, hypothalamus, and locus coeruleus. In humans, cocaine rapidly permeates the striatum, then quickly redistributes out of it with a half-life of about 20 minutes. The time course of self-reported "high" closely follows this pattern of rapid uptake and clearance.

Drug-related reinforcement is most strongly related to the dopaminergic projections from the VTA to the nucleus accumbens. Cocaine administration causes transient increases in extracellular dopamine levels in these regions by binding to the presynaptic dopamine transporter (DAT), thereby inhibiting dopamine reuptake. Subjective euphoria appears to be a function of both DAT occupancy (with a threshold of 50 percent occupancy to be detectable) and rapidity of onset, with the most robust responses occurring when dopaminergic neurotransmission is increasing dynamically.

ETIOLOGY

Genetic Factors

The most convincing evidence to date of a genetic influence on cocaine use disorder comes from studies of twins. Monozygotic twins have higher concordance rates for stimulant use disorder (cocaine, amphetamines, and amphetamine-like drugs) than dizygotic twins. The analyses indicate that genetic factors and unique (unshared) environmental factors contribute equally to the development of stimulant dependence.

Sociocultural Factors

Social, cultural, and economic factors are potent determinants of initial use, continuing use, and relapse. Excessive use is far more likely in countries where cocaine is readily available. Different economic opportunities may influence certain groups more than others to engage in selling illicit drugs, and selling is more likely to be carried out in familiar communities than in communities where the seller runs a high risk of arrest.

Learning and Conditioning

Learning and conditioning are also considered important in perpetuating cocaine use. Each inhalation or injection of cocaine yields a "rush" and a euphoric experience that reinforces the antecedent drug-taking behavior. Also, the environmental cues associated with substance use become associated with the euphoric state so that, long after a period of cessation, such cues (e.g., white powder and paraphernalia) can elicit memories of the euphoric state and reawaken craving for cocaine.

In cocaine abusers (but not in healthy controls), cocaine-related stimuli activate brain regions subserving episodic and working memory and produce EEG arousal (desynchronization). Increased metabolic activity in the limbic-related regions, such as the amygdala, parahippocampal gyrus, and dorsolateral prefrontal cortex, reportedly correlates with reports of craving for cocaine, but the degree of EEG arousal does not.

▲ 4.7 Tobacco-Related Disorders

Tobacco use disorder is among the most prevalent, deadly, and costly of substance use disorders. It is also one of the most ignored, particularly by psychiatrists. Despite recent research that shows commonalities between tobacco use disorder and other substance use disorders, tobacco use disorder differs from other substance use disorders in unique ways. Tobacco does not cause behavioral problems; therefore, few tobacco-dependent persons seek psychiatric treatment, nor are they referred. Tobacco is a legal drug, and most persons who stop tobacco use have done so without treatment. Thus a common but erroneous view is that, unlike alcohol and other illicit drugs, most smokers do not need treatment.

Several trends may change the reluctance of psychiatrists to play a role in treating tobacco use disorders: (1) the growing recognition that most psychiatric patients smoke and many die from the consequences of tobacco use disorders; (2) remaining smokers will be more and more likely to have psychiatric problems, which suggests that many need intensive treatments; and (3) the development of multiple pharmacologic agents to aid smokers in quitting.

CLINICAL FEATURES

Behaviorally, the stimulatory effects of nicotine produce improved attention, learning, reaction time, and problem-solving ability. Tobacco users also report that cigarette smoking lifts their mood, decreases tension, and lessens depressive feelings. Results of studies of the effects of nicotine on CBF suggest that short-term nicotine exposure increases CBF without changing cerebral oxygen metabolism, but long-term nicotine exposure decreases CBF. In contrast to its stimulatory CNS effects, nicotine acts as a skeletal muscle relaxant.

DIAGNOSIS

Tobacco Use Disorder

The DSM-5 includes a diagnosis for tobacco use disorder characterized by craving, persistent and recurrent use, tolerance, and withdrawal when stopping tobacco. Dependence on tobacco develops quickly, probably because nicotine activates the VTA dopaminergic system, the same system affected by cocaine and amphetamine. The development of dependence is enhanced by substantial social factors that encourage smoking in some settings and by the powerful effects of tobacco company advertising. Persons are likely to smoke if their parents or siblings smoke and serve as role models. Several recent studies have also suggested a genetic diathesis toward tobacco dependence. Most persons who smoke want to quit and have tried many times to quit but have been unsuccessful.

Tobacco Withdrawal

The DSM-5 does not have a diagnostic category for tobacco intoxication, but it does have a diagnostic category for nicotine withdrawal. Withdrawal symptoms can develop within 2 hours of smoking the last cigarette; they generally peak in the first 24 to 48 hours and can last for weeks or months. The common symptoms include an intense craving for tobacco, tension, irritability, difficulty concentrating, drowsiness and paradoxical trouble sleeping, decreased heart rate and blood pressure, increased appetite and weight gain, decreased motor performance, and increased muscle tension. A mild syndrome of tobacco withdrawal can appear when a smoker switches from regular to low-nicotine cigarettes.

TREATMENT

For those who already smoke, psychiatrists should advise them to quit smoking. For patients who are ready to stop smoking, it is best to set a "quit date." Most clinicians and smokers prefer abrupt cessation, but because no good quality data indicate that abrupt cessation is better than gradual cessation, patient preference for gradual cessation should be respected. Brief advice should focus on the need for medication or group therapy, weight gain concerns, high-risk situations, making cigarettes unavailable, and so forth. Because relapse is often rapid, the first follow-up phone call or visit should be 2 to 3 days after the quit date. These strategies may double self-initiated quit rates. Table 4-31 presents a model, "The 5 A's" for helping tobacco cessation that uses a motivational interviewing approach.

> Ms. H was a 45-year-old patient with schizophrenia who smoked 35 cigarettes per day. She began her cigarette use at approximately 20 years of age during the prodromal stages of her first psychotic break. During the first 20 years of treatment, no psychiatrist or physician advised her to stop smoking.
>
> When the patient was 43 years of age, her primary physician recommended smoking cessation. Ms. H attempted to stop on her own but lasted only 48 hours, partly because her housemates and friends smoked. During a routine medication check, her psychiatrist recommended that she stop smoking, and Ms. H described her prior attempts. The psychiatrist and Ms. H discussed ways to avoid smokers and had the patient announce her intent to quit and request that her friends try not to smoke around her and to offer encouragement for her attempt to quit. The psychiatrist also noted that Ms. H became irritable, slightly depressed, and restless and that she had insomnia during prior cessation attempts, and thus recommended medications. Ms. H chose to use a nicotine patch plus nicotine gum as needed.
>
> The psychiatrist had Ms. H call 2 days after she attempted to quit smoking. At this point, Ms. H stated that the patch and gum were helping. One week later, the patient returned after having relapsed back to smoking. The psychiatrist praised Ms. H for not smoking for 4 days. He suggested that Ms. H contact him again if she wished to try to stop again. Seven months later, during another medication check, the psychiatrist again asked Ms. H to consider cessation, but she was reluctant.
>
> Two months later, Ms. H called and said she wished to try again. This time, the psychiatrist and Ms. H listed several activities that she could do to avoid being around friends who smoked, phoned Ms. H's boyfriend to ask him to assist her in stopping, asked the nurses on the inpatient ward to call Ms. H to encourage her, plus enrolled Ms. H in a support group for the next 4 weeks. This time the psychiatrist prescribed the non-nicotine medication varenicline and followed her with 15-minute visits for each of the first 3 weeks. She had two "slips" but did not go back to smoking and remained an ex-smoker. (Adapted from John R. Hughes, M.D.)

Psychosocial Therapies

Behavior therapy is the most widely accepted and well-proved psychological therapy for smoking. Skills training and relapse prevention identify high-risk situations and plan and practice behavioral or cognitive coping skills for those situations in which smoking occurs. Stimulus control involves eliminating cues for smoking in the environment. Aversive therapy has smokers smoke repeatedly and rapidly to the point of nausea, which associates smoking with unpleasant, rather than pleasant, sensations. Aversive therapy appears to be effective but requires a good therapeutic alliance and patient compliance.

Hypnosis. Some patients benefit from a series of hypnotic sessions. The hypnotist gives suggestions about the benefits of not smoking, which the patient assimilates into their cognitive framework. The clinician can also use posthypnotic suggestions that cause cigarettes to taste unpleasant or to produce nausea.

Psychopharmacological Therapies

Table 4-32 lists the pharmacotherapies typically used for tobacco use disorder.

Table 4-31
The 5 Major Steps to Intervention (The 5 A's)

1. **Ask:** Identify and document tobacco use status for every patient at every visit.
2. **Advise:** In a clear, strong, and personalized manner, urge every tobacco user to quit.
3. **Assess:** Is the tobacco user willing to make a quit attempt at this time?
4. **Assist:** For the patient willing to make a quit attempt, use counseling and pharmacotherapy to help him or her quit. (See https://www.ahrq.gov/prevention/guidelines/tobacco/clinicians/index.html for materials to help).
5. **Arrange:** Schedule follow-up contact, in person or by telephone, preferably within the first week after the quit date.

Source: Five Major Steps to Intervention (The "5 A's"). Agency for Healthcare Research and Quality, Rockville, MD. Content last reviewed: December 2012. Accessed November 30, 2020. https://www.ahrq.gov/prevention/guidelines/tobacco/5steps.html

Table 4-32
FDA-Approved Medications for Smoking Cessation

Product	Route of Administration	Availability	Usual Dose
Nicotine Replacement Medications			
NicoDerm, Habitrol, Generic versions	Patch	OTC	Varies by product and amount a person has smoked. See manufacturer guidelines for specific instructions
Nicorette, Commit, Generic versions	Oral (Gum, Lozenge)	OTC	
Nicotrol	Inhaled (Nasal Spray, Inhaler)	Prescription	
Non-Nicotine Medications			
Bupropion (marketed as Zyban, however brand discontinued by manufacturer, in US)	Pill	Prescription	Starting: 150 mg × 3 days After 3 days increase to 150 twice a day Begin 1 wk before quitting
Varenicline Tartrate (Chantix)	Pill	Prescription	Days 1–3: 0.5 mg once daily Days 4–7: 0.5 mg twice daily Day 8–End of treatment: 1 mg twice daily

Source: US Food and Drug Administration, www.fda.gov

Nicotine Replacement Therapies. All nicotine replacement therapies double cessation rates, presumably because they reduce nicotine withdrawal. Hospitals may use these therapies on the wards to reduce withdrawal. Replacement therapies use a short period of maintenance of 6 to 12 weeks, often followed by a gradual reduction period of another 6 to 12 weeks.

Nicotine polacrilex gum is an OTC product that releases nicotine via chewing and buccal absorption. A 2 mg variety for those who smoke fewer than 25 cigarettes a day and a 4 mg variety for those who smoke more than 25 cigarettes a day are available. Smokers are to use one to two pieces of gum per hour up to a maximum of 24 pieces per day after abrupt cessation. Venous blood concentrations from the gum are one-third to one-half between-cigarette levels. Acidic beverages (coffee, tea, soda, and juice) should not be used before, during, or after gum use because they decrease absorption. Compliance with the gum has often been a problem. Adverse effects are minor and include unpleasant taste and sore jaws. About 20 percent of those who quit take the gum for long periods, but 2 percent use it for longer than a year; long-term use does not appear to be harmful. The significant advantage of nicotine gum is its ability to provide relief in high-risk situations.

Nicotine lozenges deliver nicotine and are also available in 2- and 4-mg forms; they are useful, especially for patients who smoke a cigarette immediately on awakening. Generally, 9 to 20 lozenges a day are used during the first 6 weeks, with a decrease in dosage after that. Lozenges offer the highest level of nicotine of all nicotine replacement products. Users must suck the lozenge until dissolved and not swallow it. Side effects include insomnia, nausea, heartburn, headache, and hiccups.

Nicotine patches also sold over the counter, are available in a 16-hour, no-taper preparation and a 24- or 16-hour tapering preparation. Patches are administered each morning and produce blood concentrations about half those of smoking. Compliance is high, and the only significant adverse effects are rashes and, with 24-hour wear, insomnia. Using gum and patches in high-risk situations increases quit rates by another 5 to 10 percent. After 6 to 12 weeks, patients should discontinue the patch.

Nicotine nasal spray, available only by prescription, produces nicotine concentrations in the blood that are more similar to those

from smoking a cigarette, and it appears to be especially helpful for heavily dependent smokers. The spray, however, causes rhinitis, watering eyes, and coughing in more than 70 percent of patients.

The nicotine inhaler, also available only by prescription, was designed to deliver nicotine to the lungs, but the nicotine is absorbed in the upper throat. It delivers 4 mg per cartridge, and resultant nicotine levels are low. The primary asset of the inhaler is that it provides a behavioral substitute for smoking. The inhaler doubles quit rates. These devices require frequent puffing—about 20 minutes to extract 4 mg of nicotine—and have minor adverse effects.

Non-Nicotine Medications. Non-nicotine therapy may help smokers who object philosophically to the notion of replacement therapy and smokers who fail replacement therapy. Bupropion is an antidepressant medication that has both dopaminergic and adrenergic actions. Bupropion SR started at 150 mg/day for 3 days and increased to 150 mg twice a day for 6 to 12 weeks. Daily dosages of 300 mg double quit rates in smokers with and without a history of depression. In one study, a combined bupropion and nicotine patch had higher quit rates than either alone. Adverse effects include insomnia and nausea, but these are rarely significant. Contraindications to use of bupropion include a seizure disorder (the risk of seizures in those appropriately screened is less than 1 in 1,000), current/past bulimia or anorexia nervosa, rennet/concurrent MAOI, or other bupropion use. Though bupropion at one point carried a black box warning regarding neuropsychiatric adverse events during smoking cessation, the FDA has since removed this warning. This medication can be started 1 to 2 weeks before a quit date and used for up to 6 months post quit. Of interest, another antidepressant, nortriptyline, appears to be useful for smoking cessation as well.

Varenicline is a partial agonist at the $\alpha_4\beta_2$ neuronal nicotinic acetylcholine receptor; it both relieves craving and withdrawal and, unlike other medications, reduces the reinforcing effects of nicotine by blocking dopaminergic stimulation responsible for smoking reinforcement/reward. While there were concerns about the FDA-issued black box warnings for neuropsychiatric adverse events (depressed mood, agitation, changes in behavior, suicidal ideation, and suicide), more recent research of varenicline in psychiatric patients has found that psychiatric symptoms do not worsen nor does the risk of suicide increase. The FDA has removed the black box warning associated with neuropsychiatric adverse events from varenicline. There is also a concern for potential cardiovascular adverse events in patients taking varenicline ("a small, increased risk of certain cardiovascular adverse events in people who have a cardiovascular disease"). Clinicians should counsel patients on these risks and monitor for symptoms related to mental status and cardiac status.

Combined Psychosocial and Pharmacologic Therapy

Several studies have shown that combining nicotine replacement and behavior therapy increases quit rates over either therapy alone.

EPIDEMIOLOGY

The *2018 Monitoring the Future Survey* reported that nicotine use via cigarettes is currently at a historic low. Thirty-day smoking rates among eighth, tenth and twelfth graders were 2.2 percent, 4.2 percent, and 7.6 percent, respectively. However, vaping, which involves the use of a battery-powered device to heat a liquid to or other substances until it aerosolizes chemicals for inhalation, increased significantly in 2018. Popular manufacturers of vaping liquids commonly sell them in flavors that are especially appealing to adolescents. Thirty-day nicotine vaping prevalence rates in the eighth, tenth, and twelfth graders were 6 percent, 16 percent, and 21 percent, respectively, and were substantially higher than cigarette use. The increase in nicotine vaping was particularly high for tenth and twelfth graders (increasing by 9 and 11 percent for these grades).

The WHO estimates that there are 1 billion smokers worldwide, and more men than women smoke. Although the prevalence of smoking is decreasing overall, the number of persons smoking in the Eastern Mediterranean and African regions is increasing.

Tobacco is commonly smoked in cigarettes, as well as in cigars, snuff, chewing tobacco, and pipes. Additionally, there is an increasing prevalence of vaping and the use of e-cigarettes.

Currently, about 14 percent of Americans smoke. Dependence features appear to develop quickly. Classroom and other programs to prevent initiation are only mildly effective, but increased taxation does decrease initiation.

Nearly 70 percent of smokers indicate that they want to quit, and, as of 2015, more than 50 percent reported that they tried to quit in the past year. On a given attempt, only 30 percent remain abstinent for even 2 days, and only 5 to 10 percent stop permanently. Most smokers make 5 to 10 attempts, however, so eventually 50 percent of "ever smokers" quit. In the past, 90 percent of successful attempts to quit involved no treatment. With the advent of OTC and non-nicotine medications in 1998, about one-third of all attempts involved the use of medication.

In terms of the diagnosis of tobacco use disorder per se, about 20 percent of the population develop tobacco dependence at some point, making it one of the most prevalent psychiatric disorders. Approximately 85 percent of current daily smokers are tobacco-dependent. Tobacco withdrawal occurs in about 50 percent of smokers who try to quit.

According to the Centers for Disease Control and Prevention (CDC), regional differences exist in smoking throughout the United States. The 11 states with the highest prevalence of current smoking are Kentucky, West Virginia, Louisiana, Ohio, Indiana, Missouri, Oklahoma, Arkansas, Mississippi, Tennessee, and Alabama. Those states with the lowest prevalence are Utah and California.

Education

Level of education attainment correlated with tobacco use. Of adults who had not completed high school, 23 percent smoked cigarettes (and of those with a GED, 37 percent smoked), whereas only 7 percent of college graduates smoked.

Psychiatric Patients

Psychiatrists must be particularly concerned and knowledgeable about tobacco use disorders because of the high proportion of psychiatric patients who smoke. Approximately 50 percent of all psychiatric outpatients, 70 percent of outpatients with bipolar I disorder, almost 90 percent of outpatients with schizophrenia, and 70 percent of patients with substance use disorder smoke. Moreover, data indicate that patients with depressive disorders or anxiety disorders are less successful in their attempts to quit smoking than other persons; thus, a holistic health approach for these patients probably includes helping them address their smoking habits in addition to the primary mental disorder. The high percentage of patients with schizophrenia who smoke may be due to tobacco's ability to reduce their extraordinary sensitivity to outside sensory stimuli and to increase their concentration. In that sense, such patients are self-monitoring to relieve distress.

Death

Death is the primary adverse effect of cigarette smoking. Tobacco use is associated with more than 400,000 premature deaths each year in the United States, which is 20 percent of all deaths. Individuals who smoke tend to die 10 years earlier than nonsmokers. Cancer causes chronic obstructive pulmonary disease, other lung diseases, cancer, heart disease, stroke, and diabetes. The increased use of chewing tobacco and snuff (smokeless tobacco) is associated with the development of oropharyngeal cancer.

Researchers have found that tobacco smoke causes nearly 30 percent of cancer deaths in the United States, making tobacco the single most lethal carcinogen in the United States. Smoking (mainly cigarette smoking) causes cancer of the lung, upper respiratory tract, esophagus, bladder, and pancreas and probably of the stomach, liver, and kidney. Smokers are 15 to 30 times more likely than nonsmokers to develop lung cancer, and lung cancer has surpassed breast cancer as the leading cause of cancer-related deaths in women. Despite these staggering statistics, smokers can dramatically lower their chances of developing smoke-related cancers by merely quitting.

PATHOLOGY

Neuropharmacology

The psychoactive component of tobacco is nicotine, which affects the CNS by acting as an agonist at the nicotinic subtype of acetylcholine receptors. About 25 percent of the nicotine inhaled during smoking reaches the bloodstream, through which nicotine reaches the brain within 15 seconds. The half-life of nicotine is about 2 hours. Nicotine likely produces its positive reinforcing and addictive properties by activating the dopaminergic pathway projecting from the VTA to the cerebral cortex and the limbic system. In addition to activating this dopamine reward system, nicotine causes an increase in the concentrations of circulating norepinephrine and epinephrine and an increase in the release of vasopressin, β-endorphin, adrenocorticotropic hormone (ACTH), and cortisol. These hormones contribute to the primary stimulatory effects of nicotine on the CNS.

Adverse Effects of Nicotine

Nicotine is a highly toxic alkaloid. Doses of 60 mg in an adult are fatal secondary to respiratory paralysis; doses of 0.5 mg are delivered by smoking an average cigarette. In low doses, the signs and symptoms of nicotine toxicity include nausea, vomiting, salivation, pallor (caused by peripheral vasoconstriction), weakness, abdominal pain (caused by increased peristalsis), diarrhea, dizziness, headache, increased blood pressure, tachycardia, tremor, and cold sweats. Toxicity is also associated with an inability to concentrate, confusion, and sensory disturbances. Nicotine is further associated with a decrease in the user's amount of REM sleep. Tobacco use during pregnancy is associated with an increased incidence of low–birth-weight babies and an increased incidence of newborns with persistent pulmonary hypertension.

Health Benefits of Smoking Cessation

Smoking cessation has significant and immediate health benefits for persons of all ages and provides benefits for persons with and without smoking-related diseases. Former smokers live longer than those who continue to smoke. Smoking cessation decreases the risk of lung cancer and other cancers, myocardial infarction, cerebrovascular diseases, and chronic lung diseases. Women who stop smoking before pregnancy or during the first 3 to 4 months of pregnancy reduce their risk of having low–birth-weight infants to that of women who never smoked. The health benefits of smoking cessation substantially exceed any risks from the average 5-lb (2.3-kg) weight gain or any adverse psychological effects after quitting.

▲ 4.8 Caffeine-Related Disorders

Caffeine affects various neurobiologic and physiologic systems and produces significant psychological effects. Caffeine is not associated with any life-threatening illnesses, but its use can result in psychiatric symptoms and disorders. The habitual use of caffeine and its widely accepted integration into daily customs can lead to an underestimation of the role that caffeine may play in one's daily life and can make the recognition of caffeine-associated disorders particularly challenging. Hence, the clinician should be familiar with caffeine, its effects, and associated problems.

CLINICAL FEATURES AND DIAGNOSIS

Caffeine use is associated with five disorders: caffeine intoxication, caffeine withdrawal, caffeine use disorder, caffeine-induced anxiety disorder, and caffeine-induced sleep disorder. The diagnosis of caffeine intoxication or other caffeine-related disorders depends primarily on a comprehensive history of a patient's intake of caffeine-containing products. The history should cover whether a patient had experienced any symptoms of caffeine withdrawal during periods when caffeine consumption was either stopped or severely reduced. Table 4-33 lists some essential diagnoses to consider in the

**Table 4-33
Differential Diagnosis for Caffeine-Related Disorders**

Generalized anxiety disorder
Panic disorder with or without agoraphobia
Bipolar II disorder
Attention-deficit/hyperactivity disorder (ADHD)
Sleep disorders

differential for caffeine-related disorders. The differential diagnosis should include the abuse of caffeine-containing OTC medications, anabolic steroids, and other stimulants, such as amphetamines and cocaine. A urine sample may be needed to screen for these substances. The differential diagnosis should also include hyperthyroidism and pheochromocytoma.

Caffeine Intoxication

After the ingesting 50 to 100 mg of caffeine, the common symptoms can be pleasant (e.g., alertness) or only mildly annoying (diuresis). As the dose increases, the symptoms become more concerning; Table 4-34 lists these. Caffeine intoxication generally occurs above 250 mg. The annual incidence of intoxication is about 10 percent

**Table 4-34
Symptoms and Signs of Caffeine Use**

Mild to Moderate Use (50–100 mg)
Alertness
A mild sense of well-being
A sense of improved verbal and motor performance
Diuresis
Cardiac muscle stimulation
Increased intestinal peristalsis
Increased gastric acid secretion
Increased (usually mildly) blood pressure

250 mg or More ("Caffeine Intoxication")
Anxiety
Psychomotor agitation
Restlessness
Irritability
Psychophysiological complaints:
    Muscle twitching
    Flushed face
    Nausea
    Diuresis
    Gastrointestinal distress
    Excessive perspiration
    Tingling in the fingers and toes
    Insomnia

1 g or More
Rambling speech
Confused thinking
Cardiac arrhythmias
Inexhaustibleness
Marked agitation
Tinnitus
Mild visual hallucinations (light flashes)

More than 10 g
Generalized tonic-clonic seizures
Respiratory failure
Death

Table 4-35
Symptoms of Caffeine Withdrawal

Headache
Fatigue
Anxiety
Irritability
Mild depressive symptoms
Impaired psychomotor performance
Nausea
Vomiting
Craving for caffeine
Muscle pain and stiffness

of the population. Above 10 g of caffeine—almost impossible to achieve with usual caffeinated beverages but possible with pills or other supplements—caffeine can be fatal.

> Ms. B, a 30-year-old, went for consultation due to "anxiety attacks." The attacks occurred mid- to late afternoon when Ms. B became restless, nervous, and quickly excited and sometimes was noticed to be flushed, sweating, and, according to coworkers, "talking a mile a minute." In response to questioning, Ms. B admitted to consuming six to seven cups of coffee each day before the time the attacks usually occurred.

Caffeine Withdrawal

The appearance of withdrawal symptoms reflects the tolerance and physiologic dependence that develop with continued caffeine use. Several epidemiologic studies have reported symptoms of caffeine withdrawal in 50 to 75 percent of all caffeine users studied.

Table 4-35 lists the symptoms of caffeine withdrawal; the most common ones are headache and fatigue. The amount of caffeine and the abruptness of stopping it correlate with the number and severity of the withdrawal symptoms. Caffeine withdrawal symptoms begin about 12 to 24 hours after the last dose, peak in 24 to 48 hours, and resolve within 1 week.

The induction of caffeine withdrawal can sometimes be iatrogenic. Physicians often ask their patients to discontinue caffeine intake before specific medical procedures, such as endoscopy, colonoscopy, and cardiac catheterization. Also, physicians often recommend that patients with anxiety symptoms, cardiac arrhythmias, esophagitis, hiatal hernias, fibrocystic disease of the breast, and insomnia stop caffeine intake. Some persons decide that it would be good for them to stop using caffeine-containing products. In all these situations, caffeine users should taper the use of caffeine-containing products over a 7- to 14-day period rather than stop abruptly.

> Mr. F was a 43-year-old attorney whose wife brought him for a psychiatric consultation. Mr. F had been complaining of fatigue, loss of motivation, sleepiness, headache, nausea, and difficulty concentrating. His symptoms occurred mostly over the weekends. He withdrew from weekend social activities due to his symptoms, which worried Mrs. F because he seems fine during the week. Mr. F is in good health with no recent history of medical disorders.
>
> Mr. F worked in hectic law practice, many times working 60-hour weeks, and barely sees his family during the week. At work, he is often anxious, restless, and always busy. He worries about his job so much that he has difficulty sleeping on weeknights. He denies any marital or family problems, apart from those related to his insisting on working on the weekend.

At work, Mr. F regularly consumes approximately four to five cups of coffee per day. He cut out coffee on the weekends because he felt that it might be contributing to his anxiety and sleeplessness.

Caffeine Use Disorder

Some people with problematic caffeine consumption might have a caffeine use disorder. DSM-5 includes this diagnosis in Section III, meant for conditions requiring further study. No studies have examined the course and prognosis for patients with a diagnosis of caffeine use disorder. Subjects with caffeine use disorder have reported continued use of caffeine despite repeated efforts to discontinue their caffeine use.

> Ms. G was a 35-year-old married homemaker with three children aged 8, 6, and 2. She took no prescription medications, took a multivitamin and vitamins C and E daily, did not smoke, and had no history of psychiatric problems. She drank moderate amounts of alcohol on the weekends, had smoked marijuana in college but had not used it since, and had no other history of illicit drug use.
>
> She had started consuming caffeinated beverages while in college, and her current beverage of choice was caffeinated diet cola. Ms. G had her first soft drink early in the morning, shortly after getting out of bed, and she jokingly called it her "morning hit." She spaced out her bottles of soft drinks over the day, with her last bottle at dinnertime. She typically drank four to five 20-oz bottles of caffeinated diet cola each day.
>
> She and her husband had argued about her caffeinated soft drink use in the past, and her husband had believed she should not drink caffeinated soft drinks while pregnant. However, she had continued to do so during each of her pregnancies. Despite a desire to stop drinking caffeinated soft drinks, she was unable to do so. She described having a strong desire to drink caffeinated soft drinks, and if she resisted this desire, she found that she could not think of anything else. She drank caffeinated soft drinks in her car, which had a manual transmission, and noted that she fumbled while shifting and holding the soft drink and spilled it in the car. She also noted that her teeth had become yellowed, and she suspected this was related to her tendency to swish the soft drink in her mouth before swallowing it. When asked to describe a time when she stopped using soft drinks, Ms. G reported that she ran out of it on the day one of her children was to have a birthday party, and she did not have time to leave her home to buy more. In the early afternoon of that day, a few hours before the scheduled start of the party, she felt extreme lethargy, a severe headache, irritability, and craving for a soft drink. She called her husband and told him she planned to cancel the party. She then went to the grocery store to buy soft drinks, and after drinking two bottles, she felt well enough to host the party.
>
> Although initially expressing interest in decreasing or stopping her caffeinated soft drink use, Ms. G did not attend scheduled follow-up appointments after her first evaluation. When finally contacted at home, she reported she had only sought help initially at her husband's request, and she had decided to try to cut down on her caffeine use on her own. (Courtesy of Eric Strain, M.D.)

Caffeine-Induced Disorders

Caffeine-Induced Anxiety Disorder. The anxiety related to caffeine use can resemble that of generalized anxiety disorder. Patients with the disorder may be perceived as "wired," overly talkative, and irritable; they may complain of not sleeping well and of having too much energy. Caffeine can induce and exacerbate panic attacks in persons with a panic disorder. Although there is no conclusive proof of a causative relation between caffeine and panic disorder, it is prudent to advise patients with panic disorder to avoid caffeine.

Mr. B was a 28-year-old male graduate student who was in good health and had no history of previous psychiatric evaluation or treatment. He took no medications, did not smoke or consume alcohol, and had no current or past history of illicit drug use.

His chief complaint was that he had begun feeling mounting "anxiety" when working in the laboratory where he was pursuing his graduate studies. His work had been progressing well, and he felt his relationship with his advisor was excellent and supportive, and he could not identify any problems with staff or peers that might explain his anxiety. He had been working long hours, but found the work exciting and had recently had his first paper accepted for publication.

Despite these successes, he reported feeling "crescendoing anxiety" as his day would progress. He noted that by the afternoon, he would be experiencing palpitations, bursts of his heart racing, tremors in his hands, and an overall feeling of "being on edge." He also noted nervous energy in the afternoons. These experiences were occurring daily and seemed confined to the laboratory (although he admitted he was in the laboratory every day of the week).

During the history-taking, it became clear that Mr. B consumed large amounts of coffee. The staff made a large urn of caffeinated coffee each morning, and Mr. B routinely started with a large mug of coffee. Throughout the morning, he would consume three to four mugs of coffee (the equivalent of about six or eight 6-oz cups of coffee) and continued this for the afternoon. He occasionally had a single can of a caffeinated soft drink and used no other forms of caffeine regularly. Mr. B estimated that he drank a total of six to eight or more mugs of coffee per day (which was estimated to be at least 1,200 mg of caffeine per day). Once pointed out to him, he realized that this level of caffeine consumption was considerably higher than at any other time in his life. He admitted he liked the taste of coffee and felt a burst of energy in the morning when he drank coffee that helped him start his day.

Mr. B and his physician developed a plan to decrease his caffeine use by tapering off caffeine. Mr. B was successful in decreasing his caffeine use and had a reasonable resolution of his anxiety symptoms once his daily coffee use had markedly decreased. (Courtesy of Laura M. Juliano, Ph.D., and Roland R. Griffiths, Ph.D.)

Caffeine-Induced Sleep Disorder. Caffeine is associated with a delay in falling asleep, inability to remain asleep, and early morning awakening.

Caffeine-Related Disorder Not Elsewhere Classified. This category includes caffeine-related disorders that do not meet the criteria for caffeine use disorder, caffeine intoxication, caffeine withdrawal, caffeine-induced anxiety disorder, or caffeine-induced sleep disorder.

COMORBIDITY

Persons with caffeine-related disorders are more likely to have additional substance-related disorders than are those without diagnoses of caffeine-related disorders. About two-thirds of those who consume large amounts of caffeine daily also use sedative and hypnotic drugs. Significant caffeine consumption is associated with major depression, generalized anxiety disorder, panic disorder, antisocial personality disorder, and other substance use disorders, including alcohol, cannabis, and cocaine.

Caffeine Use and Nonpsychiatric Illnesses

Despite a great deal of research, no one has conclusively demonstrated a significant health risk from routine caffeine use. Nonetheless, caffeine use is considered relatively contraindicated for various conditions; Table 4-36 lists these. Some of these are very controversial; for example, there may be a mild association between

Table 4-36
Possible Contraindications to Caffeine Use

Generalized anxiety disorder
Panic disorder
Primary insomnia
Gastroesophageal reflux
Cardiovascular disease (particularly hypertension and hypercholesterolemia)
Pregnancy
Infertility

higher-daily caffeine use in women and delayed conception and slightly lower birth weight. Studies, however, have not found such associations, and effects, when found, are usually with relatively high daily dosages of caffeine (e.g., the equivalent of five cups of brewed coffee per day). For a woman who is considering pregnancy, especially if there is some difficulty in conceiving, it may be useful to counsel stopping caffeine use. Similarly, for a woman who becomes pregnant and has moderate- to high-daily caffeine consumption, a discussion about decreasing her daily caffeine use may be warranted.

TREATMENT

Analgesics, such as aspirin, usually control the headaches and muscle aches that may accompany caffeine withdrawal. Rarely do patients require benzodiazepines to relieve withdrawal symptoms. When using benzodiazepines, we should restrict them to small doses and short durations, about 7 to 10 days at the longest.

The first step to reducing or eliminating caffeine is to have the patient determine their daily consumption of caffeine. A daily food diary can help determine an accurate dose. We may have to educate the patient about the many sources of caffeine in the diet. After several days of diet tracking, we can review the diary with the patient and determine the average-daily caffeine dose.

After obtaining an accurate accounting of all caffeine use, we can work with the patient to decide on a reasonable taper. A typical schedule would be a decrease of 10 percent every few days. Because most of the caffeine usually comes from beverages, gradually substituting decaffeinated beverages for caffeinated ones can be a simple strategy. The diary should be maintained, and the progress monitored. The tapering should be individualized for each patient so that the rate of caffeine decrease minimizes withdrawal symptoms. Although abrupt withdrawal is possible, most patients find the withdrawal too uncomfortable.

EPIDEMIOLOGY

Caffeine is the most widely consumed psychoactive substance in the world. In the United States, 87 percent of children and adults consume foods and beverages containing caffeine. Caffeine is found in more than 60 species of plants and belongs to the methylxanthine class of alkaloids, which also includes theobromine (found in chocolate) and theophylline (often used in the treatment of asthma).

Many drinks, foods, prescription medicines, and OTC medicines contain caffeine (Table 4-37). The mean caffeine intake among adults (over age 22) in the United States was estimated to be 300 mg/day, although, among coffee drinkers, the mean intake was 375 mg/day. A cup of coffee generally contains 100 to 150 mg of caffeine; tea contains about one-third as much. Many OTC medications contain one-third to one-half as much caffeine as a cup of

Table 4-37
Caffeine Content of Common Foods and Medications

Product	Serving Size (Volume or Weight)	Typical Caffeine Content (mg)	Range (mg)
BEVERAGES			
Coffee			
Brewed/Drip	12 oz	200	107–420
Instant	12 oz	140	40–260
Espresso	1 oz	70	60–95
Decaffeinated	12 oz	8	0–20
Starbucks drip	12 oz	260	
Starbucks cappuccino	12 oz	75	
Starbucks espresso	1 oz	75	
Starbucks bottled Frappuccino	9.5 oz	90	
Starbucks decaffeinated	12 oz	20	
Tea			
Brewed	6 oz	40	30–90
Instant	6 oz	30	10–35
Canned or Bottled	12 oz	20	8–32
Soft drinks			
Typical caffeinated soft drink	12 oz	40	22–69
Mountain Dew/Diet Mt. Dew	12 oz	54	
Diet Coke	12 oz	47	
Sunkist/Diet Sunkist	12 oz	41	
Dr. Pepper/Diet Dr. Pepper	12 oz	41	
Pepsi	12 oz	38	
Diet Pepsi	12 oz	36	
Pepsi Max	12 oz	69	
Coke Classic	12 oz	35	
A & W Cream Soda	12 oz	29	
Barq's Root Beer	12 oz	23	
A & W Diet Cream Soda	12 oz	22	
A & W Root Beer	12 oz	0	
7UP/Diet 7UP	12 oz	0	
Fanta Orange	12 oz	0	
Sprite/Diet Sprite	12 oz	0	
Canada Dry Ginger Ale	12 oz	0	
Cocoa/Hot Chocolate	6 oz	7	2–10
Chocolate Milk	6 oz	4	2–7
Caffeinated water			
Typical amount	16.9 oz	60	60–200
Water Joe	16.9 oz	60	
Buzzwater	16.9 oz	100 or 200	
Energy drinks			
Typical amount	varies	varies	50–500
AMP	16 oz	142	
Red Bull	8.4 oz	80	
Full Throttle	16 oz	160	
Monster	16 oz	160	
Rockstar	16 oz	160	
Spike Shooter	8.4 oz	300	
VPX Redline Energy	8 oz	316	
Wired-X-344	16 oz	344	
Rage inferno	24 oz	375	
Energy Shots			
Typical	varies	varies	
5-hour energy	2 oz	200	
5-hour energy extra strength	2 oz	230	
10-hour energy shot	1.93 oz	422	

(continued)

Table 4-37
Caffeine Content of Common Foods and Medications (*Continued*)

Product	Serving Size (Volume or Weight)	Typical Caffeine Content (mg)	Range (mg)
FOODS			
Chocolate			
Hershey's Chocolate Bar	1.55 oz	9	
Hershey's Special Dark	1.45 oz	18	
Kit Kat Wafer Bar	1.5 oz	6	
Reese's Peanut Butter Cups	1.6 oz	4	
Miscellaneous Foods			
Penguin Peppermints	1 mint	7	
Starbucks Classic Coffee Ice Cream	4 oz	30	
Dannon Coffee Yogurt	6 oz	30	
Jolt Caffeinated Gum	1 stick	33	
Powerbar Tangerine Powergel	41 g	50	
Stay-Alert Caffeinated Gum	1 stick	100	
PRESCRIPTION MEDICATIONS			
Headache/Migraine/Pain			
Fiorinal	2 capsules	80	
Fioricet/Esgic/Many others	2 tablets	80	
Cafergot	2 tablets	200	
Norgesic	2 tablets	60	
OVER-THE-COUNTER MEDICATIONS			
Stimulants			
Typical	1 tablet	100 or 200	100–200
Vivarin	1 tablet	200	
No-Doz/No-Doz Maximum Strength	1 tablet	100 or 200	
Ultra Pep-Back	1 tablet	200	
Analgesics			
Goody's Headache Powder	1 powder packet	32.5	
BC Fast Pain Relief	1 powder packet	33.3	
BC Arthritis Pain and Influenza	1 powder packet	38	
Anacin Advanced Headache	2 tablets	130	
Excedrin Extra Strength	2 tablets	130	
Menstrual Pain Relief/Diuretics			
Diurex Water Pills	2 tablets	100	
Midol Menstrual Complete	2 caplets	120	
Pamprin Max	2 caplets	130	
DIETARY SUPPLEMENTS/WEIGHT LOSS PRODUCTS			
Typical	1 or 2 tablets	varies	50–300
Dexatrim Max	1 caplet	50	
Metabolife Weight Management	2 tablets	101	
Metabolife Ultra	2 caplets	150	
Hydroxycut Weight Loss Formula	2 caplets	200	
Leptopril	2 capsules	220	
Stacker 2	1 capsule	253	
Stacker 3	1 capsule	254	
Twinlab Ripped Fuel	2 capsules	220	
Swarm Extreme Energizer	1 capsule	300	
Xenadrine EFX	2 capsules	200	

Caffeine values for all brand name products were obtained directly from product labels, the manufacturer's website, or customer service department.
Data from Juliano LM, Ferre S, Griffiths RR. The pharmacology of caffeine. In: Ries RK, Fiellin DA, Miller SC, Saitz R, eds. *ASAM Principles of Addiction Medicine.*
   5th ed. Baltimore, MD: Lippincott Williams & Wilkins; 2014:180–200; McCusker RR, Fuehrlein B, Goldberger BA, Gold MS, Cone EJ. Caffeine content of decaffeinated coffee. *J Anal Toxicol.* 2006;30(8):611; McCusker RR, Goldberger BA, Cone EJ. Caffeine content of specialty coffees. *J Anal Toxicol.* 2003;27(7):520.

coffee, and some migraine medications and OTC stimulants contain more caffeine than a cup of coffee. Cocoa, chocolate, and soft drinks contain significant amounts of caffeine, enough to cause some symptoms of caffeine intoxication in small children when they ingest a candy bar and a 12-oz cola drink.

Special Populations

Cigarette smokers consume more caffeine than nonsmokers. This observation may reflect a shared genetic vulnerability to caffeine use and cigarette smoking. It may also be related to increased rates of caffeine elimination in cigarette smokers. Preclinical and clinical studies indicate that regular caffeine use can potentiate the reinforcing effects of nicotine.

Heavy use and clinical dependence on alcohol are associated with heavy use and clinical dependence on caffeine as well. Individuals with anxiety disorders tend to report lower levels of caffeine use, although one study showed that a more significant proportion of heavy caffeine consumers also use benzodiazepines. Several studies have also shown high-daily amounts of caffeine use in psychiatric inpatients. For example, several studies have found that such patients consume the equivalent of an average of five or more cups of brewed coffee each day. Finally, high-daily caffeine consumption occurs in prisoners.

PATHOLOGY AND ETIOLOGY

After exposure to caffeine, several factors influence continued consumption, such as the pharmacologic effects of caffeine, caffeine's reinforcing effects, genetic predispositions to caffeine use, and personal attributes of the consumer.

Neuropharmacology. Caffeine, a methylxanthine, is more potent than the other methylxanthine, theophylline. The half-life of caffeine in the human body is 3 to 10 hours, and the time of peak concentration is 30 to 60 minutes. Caffeine readily crosses the blood–brain barrier. Caffeine acts primarily as an antagonist of adenosine receptors. Adenosine receptors activate an inhibitory G protein (G_i), which then inhibits the formation of the second-messenger cyclic adenosine monophosphate (cAMP). Caffeine intake, therefore, results in an increase in intraneuronal cAMP concentrations in neurons with adenosine receptors.

Three cups of coffee are estimated to deliver enough caffeine to the brain caffeine to occupy about 50 percent of the adenosine receptors. Several experiments indicate that caffeine, especially at high doses or concentrations, can affect dopamine and noradrenergic neurons. Specifically, caffeine may enhance dopamine activity, a hypothesis that could explain clinical reports associating caffeine intake with an exacerbation of psychotic symptoms in patients with schizophrenia. Activation of noradrenergic neurons may be involved in the mediation of some symptoms of caffeine withdrawal.

Subjective Effects and Reinforcement. The subjective effect of single low to moderate doses of caffeine (i.e., 20 to 200 mg) is usually pleasurable. Studies have shown that these doses result in increased ratings on measures such as well-being, energy and concentration, and motivation to work. Also, these doses of caffeine produce decreases in ratings of feeling sleepy or tired. In the range of 300 to 800 mg (the equivalent of several cups of brewed coffee ingested at once), subjects tend to rate the effects of caffeine as more unpleasant, with feelings of anxiety and nervousness. Animal studies have generally found it difficult to demonstrate that

caffeine functions as a reinforcer. However, well-controlled studies in humans have shown that people choose caffeine over placebo when given a choice under controlled experimental conditions. In habitual users, caffeine's ability to suppress withdrawal symptoms also reinforces the effects of caffeine. Thus, the profile of caffeine's subjective effects and its ability to function as a reinforcer contribute to the regular use of caffeine.

Genetics and Caffeine Use. Some genetic predisposition may exist to continued coffee use after exposure to coffee. Some studies have shown higher concordance rates for monozygotic twins for total caffeine consumption, heavy use, caffeine tolerance, caffeine withdrawal, and caffeine intoxication, with heritabilities ranging between 35 and 77 percent. Multivariate structural equation modeling of caffeine use, cigarette smoking, and alcohol use suggest that a common genetic factor—polysubstance use—underlies the use of these three substances.

Effects on Cerebral Blood Flow. Most studies have found that caffeine results in global cerebral vasoconstriction, with a resultant decrease in CBF, although this effect may not occur in persons over 65 years of age. According to one study, tolerance does not develop to these vasoconstrictive effects, and the CBF shows a rebound increase after withdrawal from caffeine. Some clinicians believe that caffeine use can cause a similar constriction in the coronary arteries and produce angina in the absence of atherosclerosis.

▲ 4.9 Hallucinogen-Related Disorders

CLINICAL FEATURES

Hallucinogens, by definition, are intoxicants. Table 4-38 lists some of the psychological effects of hallucinogenic drugs. Hallucinations are usually visual, often of geometric forms and figures, but

Table 4-38
Psychological Effects of Hallucinogens

Heightened perceptions (richer colors, sharpened contours, richer responses to music, smells or tastes)
Synesthesia
Changes in body image
Alterations in time and space
Intense, labile emotions
Suggestibility
Either sensitivity or detachment from others
Awareness of internal organs
The recovery of lost early memories
The release of unconscious material in symbolic form
Regression and the apparent reliving of past events, including birth
Introspective reflection and feelings of religious and philosophical insight
Depersonalization
Derealization
Anxiety, panic attacks
Flashbacks (hallucinogen-persisting perception disorder)
Mood disorders
Anxiety disorders
Psychosis
Delirium

Table 4-39
Overview of Representative Hallucinogens

Agent	Locale	Chemical Classification	Biologic Sources	Common Route	Typical Dose	Duration of Effects	Adverse Reactions
Lysergic acid diethylamide (LSD)	Globally distributed, semisynthetic	Indolealkylamine	Fungus in rye yields lysergic acid	Oral	100 µg	6–12 hr	Extensive, including pandemic 1965–1975
Mescaline	Southwestern US	Phenethylamine	Peyote cactus, *l. Williamsii*	Oral	200–400 mg or 4–6 cactus buttons	10–12 hr	Little or none verified
Methylenedioxyamphetamine (MDA)	US, synthetic	Phenethylamine	Synthetic	Oral	80–160 mg	8–12 hr	Documented
Methylenedioxymethamphetamine (MDMA)	US, synthetic	Phenethylamine	Synthetic	Oral	80–150 mg	4–6 hr	Documented
Psilocybin	Southern US, Mexico, south America	Phosphorylated hydroxylated DMT	Psilocybin mushrooms	Oral	4–6 mg or 5–10 g of dried mushroom	4–6 hr	Psychosis
Ibogaine	West central Africa	Indolealkylamine	Tabernanthe iboga	Eating powdered root	200–400 mg	8–48 hr	CNS excitation, death?
Ayahuasca	South American tropics	Harmine, other β-carbolines	Bark or leaves of *Banisteriopsis Caapi*	As a tea	300–400 mg	4–8 hr	None reported
Dimethyltryptamine	South America, synthetic	Substituted tryptamine	leaves of *Virola Calophylla*	As a snuff, iv	0.2 mg/kg iv	30 min	None reported
Morning glory	American tropics and warm zones	D-lysergic acid alkaloids	Seeds of *Ipomoea Violacea, Turbina Corymbosa*	Orally as infusion	7–13 seeds	3 hr	Toxic delirium
Nutmeg and mace	Warm zones of Europe, Africa, Asia	Myristicin and aromatic ethers	Fruit of *m. Fragrans*, commercial species	Orally or as a snuff	1 teaspoon, 5–15 g	Unknown	Similar to atropinism, with seizures, death
Yopo/Cohoba	Northern South America, Argentina	β-carbolines and tryptamines	Beans of *Anadenanthera Peregrina*	Smoked or as a snuff	Unknown	Unknown	Ataxia, hallucinations, seizures?
Bufotenin	Northern south America, Argentina	5-OH-dimethyl-tryptamine	Skin glands of toads; seeds of *A. Peregrina*	As a snuff or IV	Unknown	15 min	None reported
Phencyclidine (PCP)	US, synthetic	1-phenylcyclohexylpiperidine	Synthetic	Oral, smoked, as a snuff, IV	5–10 mg	4–6 hr	Psychotic
Ketamine	US, synthetic	(+/−)-2-(2-chlorophenyl)-2-(methylamino)-cyclohexanone	Synthetic	Oral, snorted, IV	Unknown	1–2 hr	Psychotic

Adapted from Henry David Abraham, MD.

318

auditory and tactile hallucinations can occur. The sense of self is much changed, sometimes to the point of depersonalization, merging with the external world to the point of feeling separation of oneself from one's body.

Specific Substances

Hallucinogens are natural and synthetic substances that are variously called *psychedelics* or *psychotomimetics*. The hallucinogens are classified as Schedule I controlled substances; the US FDA has decreed that they have no medical use and high abuse potential.

Table 4-39 lists some natural and synthetic hallucinogens. The most common naturally occurring hallucinogens are psilocybin, derived from certain mushrooms, and mescaline, derived from peyote cactus. The classic synthetic hallucinogen is LSD, synthesized in 1938 by Albert Hoffman, who accidentally ingested the drug and experienced the first LSD trip. Some researchers include some of the so-called designer amphetamines, such as 3,4-methylenedioxyamphetamine (MDMA), as hallucinogens, but we include them among the stimulants.

Phencyclidine and Ketamine. Phencyclidine (PCP; 1-1 [phenylcyclohexyl] piperidine), also known as *angel dust,* was developed as a novel anesthetic in the late 1950s. This drug and the closely related compound ketamine were called *dissociative anesthetics,* because subjects taking them were awake but insensitive to, or dissociated from, the environment. Phencyclidine and ketamine exert their unique behavioral effects by blocking NMDA-type receptors for the excitatory neurotransmitter glutamate. They can cause a variety of symptoms, from anxiety to psychosis. Phencyclidine and ketamine are classified as Schedule II and Schedule III controlled substances, respectively. Although somewhat different from standard hallucinogens, both DSM-5 and we include among the hallucinogens given their psychological effects.

LSD. LSD is the prototype for a large class of hallucinogenic compounds with well-studied structure–activity relationships. LSD is a synthetic base derived from the lysergic acid nucleus from the ergot alkaloids. That family of compounds was discovered in rye fungus and was responsible for lethal outbreaks of St. Anthony's fire in the Middle Ages. The compounds are also present in morning glory seeds in low concentrations. Researchers have studied many homologs and analogs of LSD, but none more potent than LSD.

Table 4-40 lists the physiologic symptoms from LSD, which are typically few and mild. Usually, somatic symptoms appear first, then mood and perceptual changes, and, finally, psychological changes. The effects may overlap, and depending on the particular hallucinogen, the time of onset and offset varies. The intensity of LSD effects in a nontolerant user generally is proportional to dose, with 25 μg as an approximate threshold dose.

The significant difference between LSD, psilocybin, and mescaline is potency. A 100-μg dose of LSD is roughly equivalent to 10 to 15 mg of psilocybin, which is equivalent to 300 to 400 mg of mescaline. With mescaline, the onset of symptoms is slower and more nausea and vomiting occur, but in general, the perceptual effects are more similar than different.

Tolerance, particularly to the sensory and other psychological effects, is evident as soon as the second or third day of repeated LSD use. Four to 6 days free of LSD is necessary to lose significant

Table 4-40
Physiologic Symptoms of LSD

Common:
Dilated pupils
Increased deep tendon motor reflexes
Muscle tension
Mild motor incoordination
Ataxia

Occasional:
Increased heart rate
Increased respiration
Hypertension
Nausea
Decreased appetite
Salivation
Sweating
Blurred vision

tolerance. Tolerance is associated with frequent use of any of the hallucinogens.

Cross-tolerance among these hallucinogens occurs, but not between amphetamine and LSD, despite the chemical similarity of amphetamine and mescaline. Previously distributed as tablets, liquid, powder, and gelatin squares, in recent years, LSD has been commonly distributed as "blotter acid." Sheets of paper are soaked with LSD, and dried and perforated into small squares. Manufacturers stamp popular designs on the paper. Each sheet contains as many as a few hundred squares; one square containing 30 to 75 μg of LSD is one chewed dose, more or less. Planned massive ingestion is uncommon but massive ingestion happens by accident.

The onset of action of LSD occurs within an hour, peaks in 2 to 4 hours, and lasts 8 to 12 hours. LSD is a sympathomimetic, and death caused by cardiac or cerebrovascular pathology related to hypertension or hyperthermia can occur. Some reports suggest that LSD can cause a syndrome similar to neuroleptic malignant syndrome. Death can also result from physical injury when LSD impairs a person's judgment: people may run into traffic or attempt to fly. The psychological effects are usually well tolerated, but when persons cannot recall experiences or appreciate that the experiences are substance-induced, they may fear the onset of insanity.

There is no clear evidence that LSD causes drastic personality changes or chronic psychosis. Some heavy users of hallucinogens, however, may experience chronic anxiety or depression.

Many persons maintain that a single experience with LSD has given them an increased creative capacity, new psychological insights, relief from neurotic or psychosomatic symptoms, or a desirable change in personality. In the 1950s and 1960s, researchers were interested in the possible pharmacologic effects of LSD. However, results have been inconsistent. The principal value of these drugs for science has been for the basic neurosciences.

Phenethylamines. Phenethylamines are compounds with chemical structures similar to those of the neurotransmitters dopamine and norepinephrine. Mescaline (3,4,5-trimethoxyphenethylamine), a classic hallucinogen in every sense of the term, was the first hallucinogen and is described below.

Another series of phenethylamine analogs with hallucinogenic properties is the 3,4-methylenedioxyamphetamine (MDA)–related amphetamines. MDMA or ecstasy is the currently most popular and, to society, the most troublesome member of this large family of drugs. It is more a relatively mild stimulant than a hallucinogen. MDMA produces an altered state of consciousness with sensory changes and, most notable for some users, a feeling of enhanced personal interactions.

MESCALINE. Mescaline derives from the peyote cactus, which grows in the southwestern United States and northern Mexico. Mescaline human pharmacology was characterized in 1896 and synthesized 23 years later. Although we have recognized many psychoactive plants since antiquity, only mescaline's structure was understood, until we discovered LSD.

People usually take mescaline as peyote "buttons," picked from the small blue-green cacti *Lophophora williamsii* and *Lophophora diffusa*. The buttons are the dried, round, fleshy cacti tops. Mescaline is the active hallucinogenic alkaloid in the buttons. The use of peyote is legal for the Native American Church members in some states. Adverse reactions to peyote are rare during structured religious use. Peyote usually is not consumed casually because of its bitter taste and sometimes severe nausea and vomiting that precede the hallucinogenic effects.

The many structural variations of mescaline are relatively well characterized. One analog, 2,5-dimethoxy-4-methylamphetamine (DOM), also known as STP, an unusually potent amphetamine with hallucinogen properties, had a relatively brief period of illicit popularity in the 1960s. However, it appears to have disappeared from the illicit market.

Psilocybin and Its Analogs.   An unusual collection of tryptamines has its origin in the world of fungi. The natural prototype is psilocybin itself. As many as 100 species of mushroom, mainly of the *Psilocybe* genus contain psilocybin or related homologs.

People usually ingest psilocybin as mushrooms. Many species of psilocybin-containing mushrooms exist worldwide. In the United States, large *Psilocybe cubensis* (gold caps) grow in Florida and Texas and are easily grown with cultivation kits advertised in drug-oriented magazines and on the internet. The tiny *Psilocybe semilanceata* (liberty cap) grows in lawns and pastures in the Pacific Northwest. Psilocybin remains active when the mushrooms are dried or cooked into foods.

Psilocybin mushrooms are used in religious activities by Mexican Indians. They are valued in Western society by users who prefer to ingest a mushroom rather than a synthetic chemical. Of course, one danger of eating wild mushrooms is misidentification and ingestion of a poisonous variety.

Although not originating from mushrooms, another analog of psilocybin is N,N-dimethyltryptamine (DMT). Many plants contain this substance, which is also found normally in human biofluids at very low concentrations. When DMT is taken parenterally or by sniffing, a brief, intense hallucinogenic episode can result. As with mescaline, DMT is one of the oldest, best documented, but least potent of the tryptamine hallucinogens. Researchers have evaluated synthesized homologs of DMT in humans, and have described the structure–activity relationships.

Phencyclidine.   Phencyclidine and its related compounds are sold as a crystalline powder, paste, liquid, or drug-soaked paper (blotter). Most commonly, drug dealers add PCP to a cannabis- or parsley-containing cigarette. Experienced users report that the effects of 2 to 3 mg of smoked PCP occur in about 5 minutes and plateau in 30 minutes. The bioavailability of PCP is about 75 percent when taken by intravenous administration and about

**Table 4-41
Effects of PCP**

Physical
Nystagmus
Hypertension
Hyperthermia
Less common:
    Head-rolling movements
    Stroking
    Grimacing
    Muscle rigidity on stimulation
    Vomiting

Psychological
Euphoria
Labile emotions
Bodily warmth
Tingling
Peaceful floating sensations
Depersonalization
Feelings of isolation and estrangement
Auditory and visual hallucinations
Alterations of body image
Distortions of space and time perception
Paranoia
Delusions
Intensified dependence
Confusion
Disorganization of thought
Irritability
Depression
Behavioral
Repetitive chanting speech
Aggressive behavior

30 percent when smoked. The half-life of PCP in humans is about 20 hours, and the half-life of ketamine in humans is about 2 hours.

The amount of PCP varies greatly from PCP-laced cigarette to cigarette; 1 g can make as few as four or as many as several dozen cigarettes. Less than 5 mg of PCP is considered a low dose, and doses above 10 mg are considered high. Dose variability makes it difficult to predict the effect, although smoking PCP is the easiest and most reliable way for users to titrate the dose.

Persons who have just taken PCP are frequently uncommunicative, appear to be oblivious, and report active fantasy production. They can have a range of side effects, such as those listed in Table 4-41.

The short-term effects last 3 to 6 hours and sometimes give way to a mild depression in which the user becomes irritable, somewhat paranoid, and occasionally belligerent or assaultive. The effects can last for several days. Users sometimes find that it takes 1 to 2 days to recover completely; laboratory tests show that PCP can remain in the patient's blood and urine for more than a week.

Ketamine.   Ketamine is a dissociative anesthetic agent, derived initially from PCP, which is available for use in human and veterinary medicine. It has become a drug of abuse, with sources primarily from stolen supplies. It is available as a powder or in a solution for intranasal, oral, inhalational, or (rarely) intravenous use. Ketamine functions by working at the NMDA receptor and, as with PCP, can cause hallucinations and a dissociated state in which the patient has an altered sense of the body and reality and little concern for the environment.

Ketamine causes cardiovascular stimulation and no respiratory depression. On physical examination, the patient may be hypertensive and tachycardic, have increased salivation and bidirectional or rotary nystagmus, or both. The onset of action is within seconds when used intravenously, and analgesia lasting 40 minutes and dissociative effects lasting for hours may occur. Clinicians should monitor a patient's cardiovascular status and administer supportive care. There have been reports of dystonic reactions and flashbacks, but a more common complication is a lack of concern for the environment or personal safety.

Ketamine has a briefer duration of effect than PCP. Peak ketamine levels occur approximately 20 minutes after intramuscular injection. After intranasal administration, the duration of effect is approximately 1 hour. Ketamine is N-demethylated by liver microsomal cytochrome P450 (CYP), especially CYP3A, into norketamine. Ketamine, norketamine, and dehydronorketamine are detectable in urine, with half-lives of 3, 4, and 7 hours, respectively. Urinary ketamine and norketamine levels vary widely from individual to individual and can range from 10 to 7,000 ng/mL after intoxication. As of yet, there are no formal studies of the relationship between serum ketamine levels and clinical symptoms. Often, Ketamine is combined with other drugs of abuse, especially cocaine. Ketamine may enhance cocaine metabolism. Recent years have seen a growing number of ketamine infusion clinics for the treatment of depression, along with the FDA approval of esketamine nasal spray for treatment-resistant depression.

Additional Hallucinogens

CANTHINONES. Canthinones are alkaloids similar to amphetamines naturally found in the khat plant and synthetically made and known as "bath salts." They are CNS stimulants that cause a massive release of dopamine, and a single dose can last up to 8 hours. They produce profound toxic effects that can lead to seizures, strokes, or death. Hallucinations and delusions are common. They are swallowed, injected, or "snorted" to produce the desired euphoric effect.

IBOGAINE. Ibogaine is a complex alkaloid found in the African shrub *Tabernanthe iboga*. Ibogaine is a hallucinogen at the 400-mg dose range. The plant originates in Africa, where it is used in traditional ceremonies. It has not been a popular hallucinogen because of its unpleasant somatic effects when taken at hallucinogenic doses. However, psychiatrists may encounter patients exposed to ibogaine because of therapeutic claims.

AYAHUASCA. Ayahuasca, currently a popular subject of internet hallucinogen websites, initially referred to a decoction from one or more South American plants. The substance contains the alkaloids harmaline and harmine. Both of those β-carboline alkaloids have hallucinogenic properties, but it also causes significant nausea. Amazon tribes discovered that adding leaves from plants containing substantial amounts of DMT enhanced the visual and sacramental impact of ayahuasca. Thus, when people use ayahuasca, it is often in combination with other drugs.

In recent years, the term *ayahuasca* has evolved to a less specific term to refer to any mixture of two things that are hallucinogenic when taken in combination. For example, harmine and harmaline are available as fine chemicals and, when taken along with many botanicals containing DMT, result in a mixture with hallucinogen properties, initially intense but usually of brief duration.

SALVIA DIVINORUM. American Indians in northern Oaxaca, Mexico, have used *Salvia divinorum* as a medicine and as a sacred sacrament, which is now widely discussed, advertised, and sold on the internet. Chewing the plant or smoking dried leaves can produce hallucinogen effects. Salvinorin-A, an active component in the plant, is parenterally potent, active at 250-μg doses when smoked, and of scientific and potential medical interest because it binds to the opioid κ-receptor.

DIAGNOSIS

Hallucinogen Use Disorder

Long-term hallucinogen use is uncommon. Some long-term users of PCP are said to be "crystallized," a syndrome characterized by dulled thinking, decreased reflexes, loss of memory, loss of impulse control, depression, lethargy, and impaired concentration. Although psychological dependence occurs, it is rare, in part because each LSD experience is different and in part because there is no reliable euphoria.

> B, a 16-year-old boy from divorced parents, was admitted to the psychiatric unit of a local hospital. During the previous night, he slashed his wrists, severing nerves and tendons in his left hand, and drifted in and out of consciousness during the night. He finally contacted the mother of a friend who lived nearby in the morning who immediately brought him to the hospital.
>
> B had a history of juvenile delinquency from the age of 13 when he began hanging out with some older boys at his junior high school. He and his friends shoplifted, stole, smoked marijuana, and took LSD. B's grades dropped, and he got in trouble at school on two occasions for getting into fights with other students.
>
> On admission, B stated that he did not intend to commit suicide when he slashed his wrist. After some questioning, he revealed that he had been "dropping acid" with some friends, and after they left, he thought he heard the sirens of police cars approaching his home. He did not wish to get arrested, so he slashed his wrist and then lost consciousness. He denies feeling depressed, although he claims his life is pointless and felt it made no difference whether he lived or died.

Hallucinogen Intoxication

The hallmarks of hallucinogen intoxication are maladaptive behavioral and perceptual changes, along with particular physiologic signs (Table 4-42). The differential diagnosis for hallucinogen intoxication includes anticholinergic and amphetamine intoxication and alcohol withdrawal. The preferred treatment for hallucinogen intoxication is talking down the patient; during this process, guides can reassure patients that the symptoms are drug-induced, that they are not going crazy, and that the symptoms will resolve shortly. In the most severe cases, dopaminergic antagonists—for example, haloperidol—or benzodiazepines—for example, diazepam—can be used for a limited time. Hallucinogen intoxication usually lacks a withdrawal syndrome.

Table 4-42
Physiologic Changes from Hallucinogens

1. Pupillary dilation
2. Tachycardia
3. Sweating
4. Palpitations
5. Blurring of vision
6. Tremors
7. Incoordination

Short-term PCP intoxication can have potentially severe complications and should be considered a psychiatric emergency. Some patients may present within hours of ingesting PCP, but often 2 to 3 days elapse before they seek psychiatric help. Persons who lose consciousness are brought for help earlier than those who remain conscious. Most patients recover completely within a day or two, but some remain psychotic for as long as 2 weeks. Patients presenting in a coma often exhibit disorientation, hallucinations, confusion, and difficulty communicating on regaining consciousness. These symptoms may also occur in noncomatose patients, but their symptoms appear to be less severe. Behavioral disturbances sometimes are severe; they can include public masturbation, stripping off clothes, violence, urinary incontinence, crying, and inappropriate laughing. Patients frequently have amnesia for the entire period of the psychosis.

Police brought a 17-year-old male patient to the emergency room after finding him disoriented on the street. As the police attempted to question him, he became increasingly agitated; when they attempted to restrain him, he became assaultive. Attempts to question or to examine him in the emergency department evoked increased agitation.

Initially, it was impossible to determine vital signs or to draw blood. Based on the observation of horizontal, vertical, and rotatory nystagmus, clinicians made a preliminary diagnosis of PCP intoxication. Within a few minutes of being placed in a darkened examination room, his agitation markedly decreased. Blood pressure was 170/100; other vital signs were within normal limits. The patient agreed to take 20 mg of diazepam orally. Thirty minutes later, he was less agitated and could be interviewed, although he responded to questions in a fragmented fashion and was slightly dysarthric. He stated that he must have inadvertently taken a larger-than-usual dose of "dust," which he reported having used once or twice a week for several years. He denied using any other substance and any history of mental disorder. He was confused and disoriented to time and place. The qualitative toxicology screen revealed PCP and no other drugs. Results of neurologic examination were within normal limits, but he had brisk deep tendon reflexes. Some 90 minutes after arrival, his temperature, initially normal, was elevated to 38°C, his blood pressure had increased to 182/110, and he was poorly responsive to stimulation. He was admitted to a medical bed. His blood pressure and level of consciousness continued to fluctuate over the ensuing 18 hours. Results of hematologic and biochemical analyses of blood, as well as urinalyses, remained within normal limits. A history obtained from his family revealed that the patient had had multiple emergency room visits for complications from PCP use during the previous several years. He had completed a 30-day residential treatment program and had participated in several outpatient programs but had consistently relapsed. The doctors discharged the patient, with a referral to an outpatient treatment program, after his vital signs and level of consciousness had been within normal limits for 8 hours. At discharge, nystagmus and dysarthria were no longer present. (Courtesy of Daniel C. Javitt, M.D., Ph.D., and Stephen R. Zukin, M.D.)

Hallucinogen-Persisting Perception Disorder

Long after ingesting a hallucinogen, a person can experience a flashback of hallucinogenic symptoms. The DSM-5 calls this syndrome *hallucinogen-persisting perception disorder* and ICD-10 refers it as post hallucinogen perception disorder. Table 4-43 lists the comparative criteria for each disorder.

According to studies, from 15 to 80 percent of users of hallucinogens report having experienced flashbacks. They can be triggered by emotional stress, sensory deprivation (e.g., monotonous driving), or use a psychoactive substance, such as alcohol or marijuana.

Flashbacks are spontaneous, transitory recurrences of the substance-induced experience. Table 4-44 gives some examples of flashbacks. The episodes usually last a few seconds to a few minutes, but sometimes last longer. Most often, even in the presence of distinct perceptual disturbances, the person has insight into the pathologic nature of the disturbance. Suicidal behavior, major depressive disorder, and panic disorder are potential complications.

When diagnosing this disorder several other similar syndromes should be considered in the differential. Migraines and seizures can cause flashback-like experiences. Posttraumatic stress disorder (PTSD) can also cause flashbacks. In addition, a variety of visual system abnormalities can cause perceptual problems that may resemble flashbacks.

Table 4-43
Flashbacks

	Flashbacks Due to Hallucinogen Use	
Disorder	**DSM-5**	**ICD-10**
Diagnostic name	Hallucinogen-Persisting Perception Disorder	Post hallucinogen perception disorder
Symptoms	1. Reexperiencing, following cessation of use, of perceptual symptoms that were present during intoxication 2. Symptoms cause distress or functional impairment	• Substance-induced changed in cognition, personality, affect, behavior persisting beyond generally accepted period, with onset of symptoms directly related to use of substance • Flashbacks are episodic, short duration, and frequently identical or similar to perceptual distortions experienced during acute intoxication
Required number of symptoms	Both of the above	
Psychosocial consequences of symptoms	Significant distress and/or impairment	
Exclusions	**Result of:** • Medical condition • Another mental disorder	**Result of:** • Alcohol- or psychoactive substance-induced Korsakov syndrome • Alcohol- or psychoactive substance-induced psychotic state

Table 4-44
Examples of Flashbacks

Visual distortion
Geometric hallucinations
Hallucinations of sounds or voices
False perceptions of movement in peripheral fields
Flashes of color
Trails of images from moving objects
Positive afterimages and halos
Macropsia
Micropsia
Time expansion
Physical symptoms
Relived intense emotions

A 20-year-old undergraduate presented with a chief complaint of "seeing the air." The visual disturbance consisted of perception of white pinpoint specks too numerous to count in both the central and peripheral visual fields. They were always present along with the perception of trails of moving objects left behind as they passed through the patient's visual field. Attending a hockey game was difficult, as the brightly dressed players left streaks of their images against the white of the ice for seconds at a time. The patient also described the false perception of movement in stable objects, usually in his peripheral visual fields, halos around objects, and positive and negative afterimages. Other symptoms included mild depression, daily bitemporal headache, and a loss of concentration in the last year.

The visual syndrome had gradually emerged over the last 3 months following experimentation with the hallucinogenic drug LSD-25 on three separate occasions. He feared he had sustained "brain damage" from the drug experience. He denied using any other agents. He had smoked marijuana twice a week for 7 months at age 17.

The patient had consulted two ophthalmologists, who found no visual abnormality. A neurologist's examination also proved negative. A therapeutic trial of an anticonvulsant medication resulted in a 50 percent improvement in the patient's visual symptoms and remission of his depression.

Hallucinogen Intoxication Delirium

Hallucinogen intoxication delirium is a relatively rare disorder beginning during intoxication in those who have ingested pure hallucinogens. An estimated 25 percent of all PCP-related emergency room patients may meet the criteria for hallucinogen intoxication delirium. Hallucinogens are often mixed with other substances, however, and those other substances or the subsequent drug–drug interactions can also cause delirium.

Hallucinogen-Induced Psychotic Disorders

If a patient using a hallucinogen has psychotic symptoms and inadequate reality testing, a diagnosis of a hallucinogen-induced psychotic disorder may be warranted. The course of this can be variable. Occasionally, a protracted psychotic episode is difficult to distinguish from a classic psychosis, such as from schizophrenia. Whether a chronic psychosis after drug ingestion is the result of drug ingestion, is unrelated, or is a combination of both the drug ingestion and predisposing factors is currently unanswerable. In some cases, however, the person had some predisposing disorder, such as schizoid personality disorder.

A 22-year-old photography student presented to the hospital with an inappropriate mood and bizarre thinking. She had no prior psychiatric history. Nine days before admission, she ingested one or two psilocybin mushrooms. Following the immediate ingestion, the patient began to giggle. She then described euphoria, which progressed to auditory hallucinations and belief in the ability to broadcast her thoughts on the media. Two days later, she repeated the ingestion and continued to exhibit psychotic symptoms to the day of admission. When examined, she heard voices telling her she could be president and reported the sounds of "lambs crying." She continued to giggle inappropriately, bizarrely turning her head from side to side ritualistically. She continued to describe euphoria, but with an intermittent sense of hopelessness in a context of thought blocking. Her self-description was "feeling lucky." She received haloperidol, 10 mg twice a day, benztropine 1 mg three times a day, and lithium carbonate 300 mg twice a day. On this regimen, her psychosis improved after 5 days.

Hallucinogen-Induced Mood Disorder

Unlike cocaine-induced mood disorder and amphetamine-induced mood disorder, in which the symptoms are somewhat predictable, mood disorder symptoms accompanying hallucinogen abuse can vary. Abusers may experience manic-like symptoms with grandiose delusions or depression-like feelings and ideas or mixed symptoms. As with the hallucinogen-induced psychotic disorder symptoms, the symptoms of hallucinogen-induced mood disorder usually resolve after elimination from the body.

Hallucinogen-Induced Anxiety Disorder

Hallucinogen-induced anxiety disorder also varies in its symptom pattern, but few data about symptom patterns are available. Anecdotally, emergency department physicians who treat these patients frequently find that the syndrome resembles panic disorder. Anxiety is probably the most common symptom causing a PCP-intoxicated person to seek help in an emergency room.

Unspecified Hallucinogen-Related Disorder

When a patient with a hallucinogen-related disorder does not meet the criteria for any of the standard hallucinogen-related disorders, this diagnosis may apply. An example would be a withdrawal syndrome associated with a hallucinogen, which has been occasionally reported, although DSM-5 does not include this diagnosis.

TREATMENT

Hallucinogen Intoxication

The most necessary treatment is reassurance and supportive care. Patients experiencing intense and unpleasant hallucinogen intoxication can be helped by a quiet environment, verbal reassurance, and the passage of time. More rapid relief of severe anxiety is likely after oral administration of 20 mg of diazepam or a parenteral benzodiazepine if oral use is not practical. Anxiety and other symptoms generally diminish within 20 minutes of medication administration, compared to hours with only psychological and environmental support; however, perceptual symptoms may persist. Patients may need gentle restraint if they present a danger to themselves or others, but clinicians should avoid restraints if possible. Antipsychotic medications, particularly if given at excessive doses, may worsen symptoms and are best avoided unless the diagnosis remains unclear and the behavior is unmanageable. The marketing of lower doses of LSD and a more sophisticated approach to the treatment of casualties by drug users themselves have combined to reduce the appearance of this once-common disorder in psychiatric treatment facilities.

Phencyclidine. Treatment of PCP intoxication aims to reduce systemic PCP levels and to address significant medical, behavioral, and psychiatric issues. For intoxication and PCP-induced psychotic disorder, although the resolution of current symptoms and signs is paramount, the long-term goal of treatment is to prevent relapse to PCP use. PCP levels can fluctuate over many hours or even days, especially after oral administration. A prolonged period of clinical observation is, therefore, mandatory before concluding that no severe or life-threatening complications will ensue.

Trapping of ionized PCP in the stomach has led to the suggestion of continuous nasogastric suction as a treatment for PCP intoxication. This strategy, however, can be needlessly intrusive and can induce electrolyte imbalances. The preferred treatment is to administer activated charcoal, which binds PCP and diminishes its toxic effects in animal studies.

Trapping of ionized PCP in urine has led to the suggestion of urinary acidification as an aid to drug elimination. This strategy, however, may be ineffective and is potentially dangerous. The urine only excretes a small portion of PCP, metabolic acidosis itself carries significant risks, and acidic urine can increase the risk of renal failure secondary to rhabdomyolysis.

Hemodialysis and hemoperfusion are also ineffective, given the substantial volume of distribution of PCP.

No drug is known to function as a direct PCP antagonist. Any compound binding to the PCP receptor, located within the ion channel of the NMDA receptor, would block NMDA receptor-mediated ion fluxes, as PCP does. NMDA receptor mechanisms predict that pharmacologic strategies promoting NMDA receptor activation (e.g., administration of a glycine site agonist drug) would promote rapid dissociation of PCP from its binding sites. To date, there have been no clinical trials of NMDA agonists for PCP or ketamine intoxication in humans.

Because PCP disrupts sensory input, environmental stimuli can cause unpredictable, exaggerated, distorted, or violent reactions. A cornerstone of treatment, therefore, is to minimize sensory inputs. Patients should be evaluated and treated in a quiet and calm environment. Precautionary physical restraint is recommended by some authorities, with the risk of rhabdomyolysis from struggling against the restraints balanced by the avoidance of violent or disruptive behavior. Both antipsychotics and benzodiazepines are useful as sedatives, and neither is demonstrably superior. As PCP is an anticholinergic at high doses, drugs with anticholinergic properties (including some antipsychotics) should be avoided.

Hallucinogen-Persisting Perception Disorder. Treatment for hallucinogen-persisting perception disorder is palliative. The first step in the process is to identify the disorder; it is not uncommon for the patient to consult several specialists before receiving a diagnosis. Pharmacologic approaches include long-acting benzodiazepines, such as clonazepam and, to a lesser extent, anticonvulsants, including valproic acid and carbamazepine. No drug is entirely adequate. Antipsychotics should only be used for psychotic symptoms because their side effects could exacerbate symptoms.

The second dimension of treatment is behavioral. We should instruct the patient to avoid gratuitous stimulation in the form of OTC drugs, caffeine, and alcohol, and avoidable physical and emotional stressors. Marijuana smoke is a particularly strong intensifier of the disorder, even when passively inhaled.

Finally, three comorbid conditions are associated with hallucinogen-persisting perception disorder: panic disorder, major depression, and alcohol use disorder. All these conditions require primary prevention and early intervention.

Hallucinogen-Induced Psychosis. Treatment of hallucinogen-induced psychosis does not differ from conventional treatment for other psychoses. In addition to antipsychotic medications, several agents are reportedly effective, including lithium carbonate, carbamazepine, and electroconvulsive therapy. Antidepressant drugs, benzodiazepines, and other anticonvulsants may have a role as well. Unlike schizophrenia, patients with this disorder lack negative symptoms—they have positive symptoms of psychosis but can still relate well to the psychiatrist. Also important are supportive, educational, and family therapies. The goals of treatment are the control of symptoms, minimal use of hospitals, daily work, the development and preservation of social relationships, and the management of comorbid illnesses such as alcohol use disorder.

EPIDEMIOLOGY

People have used hallucinogens for thousands of years, and drug-induced hallucinogenic states have been part of social and religious rituals. The discovery of LSD in 1943 increased the use and misuse of hallucinogens because it is easy and inexpensive to make such synthetic hallucinogens. They are also more potent than their botanical counterparts, and the development of synthetic hallucinogens is mostly responsible for the psychiatric disorders associated with these drugs.

The incidence of hallucinogen use has had two notable periods of increase. Between 1965 and 1969, there was a 10-fold increase in the estimated annual number of initiates. This increase was driven primarily by the use of LSD. The second peak in first-time hallucinogen use occurred from around 1992 until 2000, fueled mainly by ecstasy (MDMA). Decreases in the initiation of both LSD and ecstasy were evident between then and 2013, coinciding with an overall drop in hallucinogen incidence from 1.6 to 1.1 million.

The NSDUH found that approximately 0.5 percent of persons age 12 years or older reported current use of hallucinogens. In 2016, the NSDUH added questions about the use of ketamine, DMT/AMT (α-methyltryptamine)/"Foxy" (5-methoxy-N,N-dimethyltryptamine [5-MeO-DMT]), and *Salvia divinorum*; for this reason, it is not possible to compare current rates of use with past rates. The lifetime prevalence of hallucinogen use disorder is about 0.6 to 1.7 percent. Approximately 5 percent of those with a lifetime history of hallucinogen use may develop hallucinogen dependence.

Hallucinogen use is most common among young (15 to 35 years of age) white men. About 60 percent of hallucinogen users are men. Persons 26 to 34 years of age show the highest use of hallucinogens, with 16 percent having used a hallucinogen at least once. Persons 18 to 25 years of age have the highest recent use of a hallucinogen. The ratio of whites to blacks who have used a hallucinogen is 2:1; the white to Hispanic ratio is about 1.5:1.

Cultural factors influence the use of hallucinogens; their use in the western United States is significantly higher than in the southern United States.

Hallucinogen use is associated with less morbidity and less mortality than many other substances of abuse. For example, one study found that only 1 percent of substance-related emergency department visits were related to hallucinogens, compared with 40 percent for cocaine-related problems. Of persons visiting the emergency department for hallucinogen-related reasons, however, more than 50 percent were younger than 20 years of age. Currently, there may be a resurgence in the popularity of hallucinogens among youths.

Phencyclidine

Phencyclidine and some related substances are relatively easy to synthesize in illegal laboratories and relatively inexpensive to buy on the street. The variable quality of the laboratories, however, results in a range of potency and purity. PCP use varies most markedly with geography. Most users of PCP also use other substances, particularly alcohol, but also opiates, opioids, marijuana, amphetamines, and cocaine. Marijuana products often include PCP, with severe untoward effects on users. The actual rate of PCP use disorder is not known, but PCP is associated with 3 percent of substance abuse deaths and 32 percent of substance-related emergency department visits nationally.

PATHOLOGY

Neuropharmacology

LSD is a reasonable prototype for this group, although there is considerable variation. LSD probably acts on the serotonergic system—but exactly how, and in what direction, is not clear. Data at this time suggest that LSD acts as a partial agonist at postsynaptic serotonin receptors.

Most hallucinogens are well absorbed after oral ingestion, although some are inhaled, smoked, or injected. Tolerance to hallucinogens develops rapidly and is virtually complete after 3 or 4 days of continuous use. Tolerance also reverses quickly, usually in 4 to 7 days. Most people do not experience physical dependence or withdrawal, but they can develop psychological dependence, especially if they find the hallucinations pleasant or useful.

Phencyclidine and Ketamine.   PCP and ketamine antagonize the NMDA subtype of glutamate receptors. PCP binds to a site within the NMDA-associated calcium channel and prevents the influx of calcium ions. PCP also activates the dopaminergic neurons of the VTA, which project to the cerebral cortex and the limbic system. Activation of these neurons is usually involved in mediating the reinforcing qualities of PCP.

Tolerance for the effects of PCP occurs in humans, although physical dependence generally does not occur. In animals that are administered more PCP per pound for longer times than most humans, PCP does induce physical dependence. Physical withdrawal in humans is rare, likely because the doses and durations are much lower. Although the physical dependence on PCP is rare in humans, psychological dependence on both PCP and ketamine is common.

PCP usually comes from illicit laboratories, so impurities are likely. One such contaminant is 1-piperidenocyclohexane carbonitrite, which releases hydrogen cyanide in small quantities when ingested. Another contaminant is piperidine, which can be recognized by its strong, fishy odor.

▲ 4.10 Inhalant-Related Disorders

Inhalant drugs (also called *volatile substances* or *solvents*) are volatile hydrocarbons that vaporize to gaseous fumes at room temperature and are inhaled through the nose or mouth to enter the bloodstream via the transpulmonary route. These compounds are commonly found in many household products and are divided into four commercial classes: (1) solvents for glues and adhesives; (2) propellants (e.g., for aerosol paint sprays, hair sprays, and shaving cream); (3) thinners (e.g., for paint products and correction fluids); and (4) fuels (e.g., gasoline, propane). These drugs likely share some similar pharmacologic properties despite their chemical differences.

CLINICAL FEATURES

Persons, especially adolescents, like to inhale these products for their intoxicating effect. Inhalants are associated with several problems, including conduct disorder, mood disorders, suicidality, and physical abuse or neglect and sexual abuse. In some cases, early time-limited use of inhalants may signal a lifelong problem with externalizing behaviors and risk-taking propensity. A smaller subgroup uses inhalants chronically, and such use can cause multiple sequelae, including significant behavioral and organ pathology from the drugs' toxicity.

In small initial doses, inhalants can be disinhibiting and produce feelings of euphoria and excitement as well as pleasant floating sensations, the effects for which persons presumably use the drugs. High doses of inhalants can cause psychological symptoms of fearfulness, sensory illusions, auditory and visual hallucinations, and distortions of body size. The neurologic symptoms can include slurred speech, decreased speed of talking, and ataxia. Long-term use can be associated with irritability, emotional lability, and impaired memory.

Tolerance for the inhalants does develop for some users; a withdrawal syndrome can accompany the cessation of inhalant use. The withdrawal syndrome does not occur frequently; when it does, it includes sleep disturbances, irritability, jitteriness, sweating, nausea, vomiting, tachycardia, and (sometimes) delusions and hallucinations.

DIAGNOSIS

The DSM-5 describes several disorders related to inhalants, including inhalant use disorder, inhalant intoxication, inhalant intoxication delirium, inhalant-induced neurocognitive disorder, inhalant-induced psychotic disorder, inhalant-induced mood and anxiety disorders, and other inhalant-induced disorders. The DSM-5 excludes anesthetic gases (e.g., nitrous oxide and ether) and short-acting vasodilators (e.g., amyl nitrite) from the inhalant-related disorders, these are classified within the generic category of "other (or unknown) substance-related disorders." ICD-10 follows a similar approach.

Inhalant Use Disorder

Most persons probably use inhalants for a short time without developing dependence or abuse. Nonetheless, dependence and abuse of inhalants occur.

Inhalant Intoxication

The diagnostic criteria for inhalant intoxication specify the presence of maladaptive behavioral changes and at least two physical symptoms. People who become intoxicated on inhalants may have apathy, diminished social and occupational functioning, impaired judgment, and impulsive or aggressive behavior. They can also have nausea, anorexia, nystagmus, depressed reflexes, and diplopia. With high doses and long exposures, a user's neurologic status can progress to stupor and unconsciousness, and a person may later be amnestic for the period of intoxication. Clinicians can sometimes identify a recent user of inhalants by rashes around the patient's nose and mouth; unusual breath odors; the residue of the inhalant substances on the patient's face, hands, or clothing; and irritation of the patient's eyes, throat, lungs, and nose. The disorder can be chronic, as in the following case.

> A 16-year-old single Hispanic female came to a university substance-treatment program for evaluation. The patient had been convicted for auto theft, using a weapon, and being out of control by her family. By age 15, she had regularly been using inhalants and drinking alcohol heavily. She had tried typewriter-erasing fluid, bleach, tile cleaner, hairspray, nail polish, glue, and gasoline, but preferred spray paint. She had sniffed paint many times each day for about 6 months at age 15, using a maximum of eight paint cans per day. The patient said, "It blacks out everything." Sometimes she had lost consciousness, and she believed that the paint had impaired her memory and made her "dumb." (Courtesy of Thomas J. Crowley, M.D.)

Inhalant Intoxication Delirium. The inhalants can directly cause delirium. Also, their interactions with other substances or the hypoxia caused by their use can cause delirium. If the delirium results in severe behavioral disturbances, short-term treatment with a dopamine receptor antagonist, such as haloperidol, may be necessary. Clinicians should avoid benzodiazepines because of the possibility of increasing the patient's respiratory depression.

Inhalant-Induced Neurocognitive Disorder. Inhalant-induced neurocognitive disorder, as with delirium, may result from the neurotoxic effects of the inhalants themselves, the neurotoxic effects of the metals (e.g., lead) commonly used in inhalants; or the impact of frequent and prolonged periods of hypoxia. Dementia caused by inhalants is likely to be irreversible in all but the mildest cases.

Inhalant-Induced Psychotic Disorder. Clinicians can specify hallucinations or delusions as predominant symptoms. Paranoid states are probably the most common psychotic syndromes during inhalant intoxication.

Inhalant-Induced Mood Disorder and Inhalant-Induced Anxiety Disorder. Inhalant-induced mood disorder and inhalant-induced anxiety disorder allow the classification of inhalant-related disorders characterized by prominent mood and anxiety symptoms. Depressive disorders are the most common mood disorders associated with inhalant use, and panic disorders and generalized anxiety disorder are the most common anxiety disorders.

Other Inhalant-Induced Disorders. Other Inhalant-Induced Disorder is the recommended DSM-5 diagnosis for inhalant-related disorders that do not fit into one of the diagnostic categories discussed earlier.

TREATMENT

Inhalant intoxication, as with alcohol intoxication, usually requires no medical attention and resolves spontaneously. However, possible effects of the intoxication, such as coma, bronchospasm, laryngospasm, cardiac arrhythmias, trauma, or burns, need treatment. Otherwise, care primarily involves reassurance, quiet support, and attention to vital signs and level of consciousness. Sedative drugs, including benzodiazepines, are contraindicated because they worsen inhalant intoxication.

No established treatment exists for the cognitive and memory problems of inhalant-induced neurocognitive disorder. Severely deteriorated, inhalant-dependent, homeless adults could benefit from street outreach and extensive social service. Patients may require comprehensive support within their families or in foster or domiciliary care.

The course and treatment of inhalant-induced psychotic disorder are like those of inhalant intoxication. The disorder is brief, lasting a few hours to (at most) a very few weeks beyond the intoxication. Vigorous treatment of such life-threatening complications as respiratory or cardiac arrest is indicated, together with conservative management of the intoxication itself. Symptoms such as confusion, panic, and psychosis require special attention to patient safety. Severe agitation may require cautious control with haloperidol (5 mg intramuscularly per 70 kg body weight). Clinicians should avoid sedative drugs because they may aggravate psychosis. Inhalant-induced anxiety and mood disorders may precipitate suicidal ideation, and we should carefully evaluate patients for that possibility. Antianxiety medications and antidepressants are not useful in the acute phase of the disorder; they may be of use in cases of coexisting anxiety or depressive illness.

Day Treatment and Residential Programs

Day treatment and residential programs have been used successfully, especially for adolescent abusers with combined substance use disorders and other psychiatric disorders. Treatment addresses the comorbid state, which, in most cases, is conduct disorder or, in some other cases, may be ADHD, major depressive disorder, persistent depressive disorder (dysthymia), and PTSD. Treatment for abuse or neglect, both very common in these patients, is also important. Both group and individual therapy that are behaviorally oriented are employed, with immediate rewards for progress toward objectively defined goals in treatment and consequences for lapses to previous behaviors. Patients attend on-site schools with special education teachers, together with planned recreational activities, and the programs provide birth control consultations. The patients' families, often very chaotic, are engaged in modifications of structural family therapy or multisystemic therapy, both of which have reasonable empirical support. Participation in 12-step programs is required. Treatment interventions are coordinated carefully with interventions by community social workers and probation officers. We can monitor progress with urine and breath samples analyzed for alcohol and other drugs at intake and frequently during treatment.

Treatment usually lasts 3 to 12 months. Table 4-45 lists some goals for treatment.

EPIDEMIOLOGY

Inhalant substances are readily available, legal, and inexpensive. These three factors contribute to the high use of inhalants among

Table 4-45
Goals of Treatment for Inhalant Disorder

Has practiced a plan to stay abstinent
Is showing fewer antisocial behaviors
Has a plan to continue any needed psychiatric treatment (e.g.,
    treatment for comorbid depression)
Has a plan to live in a supportive, drug-free environment
Is interacting with the family in a more productive way
Is working or attending school
Is associating with drug-free, nondelinquent peers

poor persons and young persons. Approximately 0.2 percent of persons age 12 and older in the United States are current users of inhalants. Adolescents (ages 12 to 17) are more likely to use inhalants than individuals in other age groups. According to the NSDUH, in 2016, only 0.2 percent of adults were using inhalants. In contrast, twice to three times as many adolescents were using inhalants. In adolescents, males and females use inhalants almost equally (with a slight increase in use for females), while in adults, inhalant use is rare in females.

Inhalant use among adolescents may be most common in those whose parents or older siblings use illegal substances, or among adolescents who have experienced childhood trauma or maltreatment. Inhalant use among adolescents is also associated with an increased likelihood of conduct disorder or antisocial personality disorder.

Pathology

Neuropharmacology. Inhalants most used by American adolescents are gasoline, glue (which usually contains toluene), spray paint, solvents, cleaning fluids, and assorted other aerosols. Sniffing vapor through the nose or huffing (taking deep breaths) through the mouth leads to transpulmonary absorption with very rapid drug access to the brain. Breathing through a solvent-soaked cloth, inhaling fumes from a glue-containing bag, huffing vapor sprayed into a plastic bag, or breathing vapor from a gasoline can are common. Approximately 15 to 20 breaths of 1 percent gasoline vapor produce several hours of intoxication. Inhaled toluene concentrations from a glue-containing bag may reach 10,000 ppm, and people may inhale fumes from several tubes each day. By comparison, one study of just 100 ppm of toluene showed that a 6-hour exposure produced a temporary neuropsychological performance decrement of approximately 10 percent.

Inhalants generally act as a CNS depressant. Tolerance for inhalants can develop, although withdrawal symptoms are usually relatively mild.

Inhalants are rapidly absorbed through the lungs and quickly delivered to the brain. The effects appear within 5 minutes and can last for 30 minutes to several hours, depending on the inhalant substance and the dose. The concentrations of many inhalant substances in the blood increase when combined with alcohol, perhaps because of the competition for hepatic enzymes.

Although about one-fifth of an inhalant substance is excreted unchanged by the lungs, the liver metabolizes the remainder. Inhalants are detectable in the blood for 4 to 10 hours after use, and blood samples should be taken in the emergency department when inhalant use is suspected.

Much like alcohol, inhalants have specific pharmacodynamic effects that are not well understood. Because their effects are generally similar and additive to the effects of other CNS depressants

(e.g., ethanol, barbiturates, and benzodiazepines), some investigators have suggested that inhalants operate by enhancing the GABA system. Other investigators have suggested that inhalants work through membrane fluidization, which may also be a pharmacodynamic effect of ethanol.

Organ Pathology and Neurologic Effects. Inhalants are associated with many potentially dangerous adverse effects. The most serious of these is death, which can result from respiratory depression, cardiac arrhythmias, asphyxiation, aspiration of vomitus, or accident or injury (e.g., driving while intoxicated with inhalants).

Placing an inhalant-soaked rag and one's head into a plastic bag, a standard procedure for inhalant users can cause coma and suffocation.

Chronic inhalant users may have numerous neurologic problems. Computed tomography (CT) and magnetic resonance imaging (MRI) reveal diffuse cerebral, cerebellar, and brainstem atrophy with white matter disease, a leukoencephalopathy. Single-photon emission CT (SPECT) of former solvent-abusing adolescents showed both increases and decreases in blood flow in different cerebral areas. Several studies of house painters and factory workers exposed to solvents for long periods also have found evidence of brain atrophy on CT scans, with decreased CBF.

Neurologic and behavioral signs and symptoms can include hearing loss, peripheral neuropathy, headache, paresthesias, cerebellar signs, persisting motor impairment, parkinsonism, apathy, poor concentration, memory loss, visual–spatial dysfunction, impaired processing of linguistic material, and lead encephalopathy. White matter changes, or pontine atrophy on MRI, have been associated with worse intelligence quotient (IQ) test results. The combination of organic solvents with high concentrations of copper, zinc, and heavy metals can cause brain atrophy, temporal lobe epilepsy, decreased IQ, and a variety of EEG changes.

Other serious adverse effects associated with long-term inhalant use include irreversible hepatic disease or renal damage (tubular acidosis) and permanent muscle damage associated with rhabdomyolysis. Additional adverse effects include cardiovascular and pulmonary symptoms (e.g., chest pain and bronchospasm) as well as GI symptoms (e.g., pain, nausea, vomiting, and hematemesis). There are several clinical reports of *toluene embryopathy,* with signs such as those of fetal alcohol syndrome. These include low birth weight, microcephaly, shortened palpebral fissures, small face, low-set ears, and other dysmorphic signs. These babies reportedly develop slowly, show hyperactivity, and have cerebellar dysfunction. No convincing evidence indicates, however, that toluene, the best-studied inhalant, produces genetic damage in somatic cells.

▲ 4.11 Anabolic-Androgenic Steroid Use

The anabolic-androgenic steroids (AAS) are a family of hormones that includes testosterone, the natural male hormone, which, together with numerous synthetic analogs of testosterone, have been developed over the last 70 years (Table 4-46). These drugs exhibit various degrees of anabolic (muscle building) and androgenic (masculinizing) effects; none of these drugs display purely anabolic effects in the absence of androgenic effects. It is important not to confuse the AAS (testosterone-like hormones) with corticosteroids (cortisol-like hormones such as hydrocortisone and prednisone).

Table 4-46
Examples of Commonly Used Anabolic Steroids

Compounds Usually Administered Orally Department:
Fluoxymesterone (Halotestin, Android-F, Ultandren)
Methandienone (formerly called Methandrostenolone; Dianabol)
Methyltestosterone (Android, Testred, Virilon)
Mibolerone (Cheque Drops[a])
Oxandrolone (Anavar)
Oxymetholone (Anadrol, Hemogenin)
Mesterolone (Mestoranum, Proviron)
Stanozolol (Winstrol)

Compounds Usually Administered Intramuscularly:
Nandrolone decanoate (Deca-Durabolin)
Nandrolone phenpropionate (Durabolin)
Methenolone enanthate (Primobolan Depot)
Boldenone undecylenate (Equipoise[a])
Stanozolol (Winstrol-V[a])
Testosterone esters blends (Sustanon, Sten)
Testosterone cypionate
Testosterone enanthate (Delatestryl)
Testosterone propionate (Testoviron, Androlan)
Testosterone undecanoate (Andriol, Restandol)
Trenbolone acetate (Finajet, Finaplix[a])
Trenbolone hexahydrobencylcarbonate (Parabolan)

---

[a]Veterinary compound.
Note: Many of the brand names listed in this table are from other countries, but they are included because of the widespread illicit use of foreign steroid preparations in the United States.

Corticosteroids are hormones secreted by the adrenal gland, rather than by the testes. Corticosteroids have no muscle-building properties and, hence, little abuse potential; they treat many inflammatory conditions such as poison ivy or asthma. AAS, by contrast, have only limited legitimate medical applications, such as in the treatment of hypogonadal men and diseases associated with muscle wasting, such as acquired immunodeficiency syndrome (AIDS) and cancer. AAS, however, are widely used illicitly, especially by boys and young men seeking to gain increased muscle mass and strength, either for athletic purposes or to improve personal appearance.

AAS do not have a diagnostic category in the DSM-5; instead, it is coded as one of the other or unknown substance-related disorders. ICD-10 includes the diagnosis in the category "Abuse of non–dependence-producing substances," which also includes antacids, herbal remedies, and vitamins.

CLINICAL FEATURES AND DIAGNOSIS

Steroids may initially induce euphoria and hyperactivity. After relatively short periods, however, their use can become associated with less desirable symptoms. Studies have reported that 2 to 15 percent of anabolic steroid abusers experience hypomanic or manic episodes, and a smaller percentage may have psychotic symptoms. Also disturbing is a correlation between steroid abuse and violence ("roid rage" in the parlance of users). Steroid abusers with no record of antisocial behavior or violence have committed murders and other violent crimes.

Steroids are addictive substances. When abusers stop taking steroids, they can become depressed, anxious, and concerned about the physical state of their bodies. Some male and female weight lifters may have muscle dysmorphia, a form of body dysmorphic disorder in which the individual feels that he or she is not sufficiently muscular and lean. There are some similarities between an athlete's

and a patient with anorexia nervosa's self-perception; to an observer, both groups seem to distort the realistic assessment of the body.

Iatrogenic addiction is a consideration given the increasing number of geriatric patients who are receiving testosterone from their physicians in an attempt to increase libido and reverse some aspects of aging.

> Mr. A is a 26-year-old single man. He is 69 in tall and presently weighs 204 lb, with a body fat of 11 percent. He reports that he began lifting weights at age 17, at which time he weighed 155 lb. About 2 years after beginning his weight lifting, he began taking AAS, which he obtained through a friend at his gymnasium. His first "cycle" (course) of AAS, lasting for 9 weeks, involved methandienone, 30 mg a day, orally, and testosterone cypionate, 600 mg a week, intramuscularly. During these 9 weeks, he gained 20 lb of muscle mass. He was so pleased with these results that he took five further cycles of AAS over the next 6 years. During his most ambitious cycle, approximately 1 year ago, he used testosterone cypionate, 600 mg/wk; nandrolone decanoate, 400 mg a week; stanozolol, 12 mg a day; and oxandrolone, 10 mg a day.
>
> During each of the cycles, Mr. A has noted euphoria, irritability, and grandiose feelings. These symptoms were most prominent during his most recent cycle when he felt "invincible." During this cycle, he also noted a decreased need for sleep, racing thoughts, and a tendency to spend excessive amounts of money. For example, he impulsively purchased a $2,700 stereo system when he could not afford to spend more than $500. He also became uncharacteristically irritable with his girlfriend, and on one occasion, put his fist through the side window of her car during an argument, an act inconsistent with his normally mild-mannered personality. After this cycle of AAS ended, he became mildly depressed for about 2 months.
>
> Mr. A has used several drugs to lose weight in preparation for bodybuilding contests. These include ephedrine, amphetamine, triiodothyronine, and thyroxin. Recently, he has also begun to use the opioid agonist–antagonist nalbuphine intravenously (IV) to treat muscle aches from weight lifting. He also used oral opioids, such as controlled-release oxycodone, at least once a week. He uses oral opioids sometimes to treat muscle aches, but often to get high. He reports that the use of nalbuphine and other opioids is widespread among other AAS users of his acquaintance.
>
> Mr. A exhibits characteristic features of muscle dysmorphia. He regularly checks his appearance, including his reflection in windows or even in the back of a spoon. He becomes anxious if he misses even one day of working out at the gym, and acknowledges that his preoccupation with weight lifting has cost him both social and occupational opportunities. Although he has a 48-in chest and 19-in biceps, he has frequently declined invitations to go to the beach or a swimming pool for fear that he would look too small when seen in a bathing suit. He is anxious because he has lost some weight since the end of his previous cycle of AAS and is eager to resume another cycle of AAS soon. (Adapted from Harrison G. Pope, Jr., M.D., and Kirk J. Brower, M.D.)

Anabolic Steroid–Induced Mood Disorders

Table 4-47 lists some typical symptoms associated with anabolic steroid use. Although athletes using these drugs have long recognized that syndromes of anger and irritability could be associated with AAS use, the scientific literature did not recognize this syndrome until the late 1980s and 1990s. Since then, a series of observational field studies of athletes have suggested that some AAS users develop prominent hypomanic or even manic symptoms during AAS use.

A possible severe consequence of AAS-induced mood disorders may be violent or even homicidal behavior. Several published reports have anecdotally described individuals with no apparent history of psychiatric disorder, no criminal record, and no history of violence, who committed violent crimes, including murder, while under the

Table 4-47
Symptoms Associated with Anabolic Steroid Use

Euphoria
Hyperactivity
Irritability
Anger
Aggressiveness
Hypomania
Mania
Violent behavior ("Roid Rage")
Homicidal behavior
Suicide
Psychosis
Withdrawal symptoms: somatization, depression

influence of AAS. Although a causal link is difficult to establish in these cases, lawyers have presented evidence of AAS use in forensic settings as a possible mitigating factor in criminal behavior.

Depressive syndromes induced by AAS have occurred, and suicide is a risk. A brief and self-limited syndrome of depression occurs upon AAS withdrawal, probably as a result of the depression of the hypothalamic–pituitary–gonadal axis after exogenous AAS administration.

Anabolic Steroid–Induced Psychotic Disorder

Psychotic symptoms are rare in association with anabolic steroid use, but they occasionally occur, primarily in individuals who were using the equivalent of more than 1,000 mg of testosterone a week. Usually, these symptoms consist of grandiose or paranoid delusions, generally occurring in the context of a manic episode, although occasionally occurring in the absence of a frank manic syndrome. In most cases reported, psychotic symptoms have disappeared promptly (within a few weeks) after the discontinuation of the offending agent, although temporary treatment with antipsychotic agents was sometimes required.

Other Anabolic Steroid–Related Disorders

Symptoms of anxiety disorders, such as panic disorder and social phobia, can occur during AAS use. AAS use may serve as a "gateway to the use of opioid agonists or antagonists, such as nalbuphine, or to use of frank opioid agonists, such as heroin."

TREATMENT

Abstinence is the treatment goal of choice for patients manifesting AAS use disorders. To the extent that users of AAS abuse other addictive substances (including alcohol), traditional treatment approaches for substance-related disorders may be used. Nevertheless, AAS users may differ from other addicted patients in several ways that have implications for treatment. First, the euphorigenic and reinforcing effects of AAS may only become apparent after weeks or months of use in conjunction with intensive exercising. When compared with immediately and passively reinforcing drugs, such as cocaine, heroin, and alcohol, AAS use may entail more delayed gratification. Second, AAS users may manifest a more significant commitment to culturally endorsed values of physical fitness, success, victory, and goal directedness than users of other illicit drugs. Finally, AAS users are often preoccupied with their physical attributes and may rely excessively on these attributes for

self-esteem. Treatment, therefore, depends on a therapeutic alliance and a thorough and nonjudgmental understanding of the patient's values and motivations for using AAS.

Though there are no controlled trials of treatment for AAS-related disorders, following the generally recommended approaches for the related idiopathic syndrome may be appropriate. For example, muscle dysmorphia may improve with CBTs or the use of SSRIs.

AAS Withdrawal

Supportive therapy and monitoring are essential for treating AAS withdrawal because suicidal depressions can occur. Hospitalization may be required when suicidal ideation is severe. Patients should be educated about the possible course of withdrawal and reassured that symptoms are time-limited and manageable. Clinicians should reserve antidepressant agents for patients whose depressive symptomatology persists for several weeks after AAS discontinuation and who likely have a comorbid depressive disorder. SSRIs are the preferred agents because of their favorable adverse effect profile and their effectiveness in a reported case series of treated AAS users with major depressive disorder. Physical withdrawal symptoms are not life threatening and do not ordinarily require pharmacotherapy. Nonsteroidal anti-inflammatory drugs (NSAIDs) may be useful to treat musculoskeletal pain and headaches. AAS-induced hypogonadism, including loss of libido, erectile dysfunction, and possible major depression, may begin during AAS withdrawal and can sometimes be prolonged, requiring treatment by an endocrinologist. Patients with AAS-induced hypogonadism may benefit from physiologic exogenous doses of testosterone, gradually tapered over time, as well as clomiphene (to restore hypothalamic–pituitary–testicular [HPT] function) and HCG (to stimulate the testis to resume production of testosterone and spermatozoa).

EPIDEMIOLOGY

It is difficult to estimate the lifetime prevalence of illicit AAS use in the United States because most available data rely on anonymous surveys of students, particularly students of high school age. There are two serious problems with the use of these data. First, the median age of onset of AAS use, both in the United States and other countries, is approximately 23 years of age—older than for any other major category of illicit drugs. Second, anonymous surveys are vulnerable to serious errors in the opposite direction as a result of false-positive responses to the survey questions about "steroids." When asking students a typical survey question, such as whether they have used "steroid pills or shots without a doctor's prescription," they may falsely respond in the affirmative when in fact they have taken only corticosteroids, or have purchased nutritional supplements OTC that they mistakenly believed were steroids. After allowing for these sources of error, the true prevalence of AAS in high school girls is close to 0 percent and in boys about 1 percent. However, by adulthood, perhaps 3 to 4 percent of American men have used AAS at some time in their lives, and approximately 1.8 percent of American women have used AAS. In general, males are more likely to take AAS than females, and athletes are more likely to take AAS than nonathletes.

The current high rates of steroid use among younger individuals appear to represent an essential shift in the epidemiology of steroid use. In the 1970s, most users were competition bodybuilders or other elite athletes. Since then, however, it appears that an increasing number of young men, and occasionally even young women may use these drugs purely to enhance personal appearance rather than for any athletic purpose.

PATHOLOGY

Pharmacology

All steroid drugs—including AAS, estrogens, and corticosteroids—are synthesized in vivo from cholesterol and resemble cholesterol in their chemical structure. Testosterone has a four-ring chemical structure containing 19 carbon atoms.

Average testosterone plasma concentrations for men range from 300 to 1,000 ng/dL. Generally, 200 mg of testosterone cypionate taken every 2 weeks restores physiologic testosterone concentrations in a hypogonadal male. A eugonadal male who initiates physiologic dosages of testosterone has no net gain in testosterone concentrations because exogenously administered AAS shut down endogenous testosterone production via feedback inhibition of the hypothalamic–pituitary–gonadal axis. Consequently, illicit users take higher than therapeutic dosages to achieve supraphysiologic effects. The dose–response curve for anabolic effects may be logarithmic, which could explain why illicit users generally take 10 to 100 times the therapeutic dosages. Doses in this range usually require combinations of oral and injected AAS, which illicit AAS users often do. Transdermal testosterone, available by prescription for testosterone replacement therapy, may also be used.

Therapeutic Indications. The AAS are indicated primarily for testosterone deficiency (male hypogonadism), hereditary angioedema (a congenital skin disorder), and some rare forms of anemia caused by bone marrow or renal failure. Women may use AAS for metastatic breast cancer, osteoporosis, endometriosis, and adjunctive treatment of menopausal symptoms. However, these are not first-line treatments. In men, they have been used experimentally as a male contraceptive and for treating major depressive disorder and sexual disorders in eugonadal men. Recently, they have been used to treat wasting syndromes associated with AIDS. Controlled studies have also suggested that testosterone has antidepressant effects in some men infected with HIV with major depressive disorder and is also a supplementary (augmentation) treatment in some depressed men with low endogenous testosterone levels who are refractory to conventional antidepressants.

Adverse Reactions

The most common adverse medical effects of AAS involve the cardiovascular, hepatic, reproductive, and dermatologic systems.

The AAS produce an adverse cholesterol profile by increasing levels of low-density lipoprotein cholesterol and decreasing levels of high-density lipoprotein cholesterol. High-dose use of AAS can also activate hemostasis and increase blood pressure. Isolated case reports of myocardial infarction, cardiomyopathy, left ventricular hypertrophy, and stroke among users of AAS, including fatalities, have appeared.

Among the AAS-induced endocrine effects in men are testicular atrophy and sterility, both usually reversible after discontinuing AAS, and gynecomastia, which may persist until surgical removal. In women, shrinkage of breast tissue, irregular menses (diminution or cessation), and masculinization (clitoral hypertrophy, hirsutism, and deepened voice) can occur. Masculinizing effects in women may be irreversible. Androgens taken during pregnancy could cause the masculinization of a female fetus. Dermatologic effects include acne and male pattern baldness. Abuse of AAS by children has led to concerns that AAS-induced premature closure of bony epiphyses could cause shortened stature. Other uncommon adverse effects include edema of the extremities caused by water retention, exacerbation of tic disorders, sleep apnea, and polycythemia.

ETIOLOGY

The primary reason for taking illicit AAS is to enhance either athletic performance or physical appearance. Taking AAS is reinforced because they can produce the athletic and physical effects that users desire, especially when combined with proper diet and training. Further reinforcement derives from winning competitions and from social admiration for physical appearance. AAS users also perceive that they can train more intensively for longer durations with less fatigue and with decreased recovery times between workouts.

Although the anabolic or muscle-building properties of AAS are important to those seeking to enhance athletic performance and physical appearance, psychoactive effects may also be valuable in the persistent and dependent use of AAS. Anecdotally, some AAS users report feelings of power, aggressiveness, and euphoria, which become associated with and can reinforce AAS taking.

▲ 4.12 Gambling Disorder

Although not related to a substance, gamblers share many features in common with other addictive disorders.

CLINICAL FEATURES

Pathologic gamblers often appear overconfident, somewhat abrasive, energetic, and free-spending. They often show apparent signs of personal stress, anxiety, and depression. They commonly have the attitude that money is both the cause of and the solution to all their problems. As their gambling increases, they may lie to obtain money and to continue gambling while hiding the extent of their gambling. They make no serious attempt to budget or save money. When without borrowing resources, they are likely to engage in antisocial behavior to obtain money for gambling. Their criminal behavior is typically nonviolent, such as forgery, embezzlement, or fraud, and they consciously intend to return or repay the money.

Complications include alienation from family members and acquaintances, the loss of life accomplishments, suicide attempts, and association with fringe and illegal groups. Arrest for nonviolent crimes may lead to imprisonment.

DIAGNOSIS

DSM-5 refers to this disorder as gambling disorder, whereas ICD-10 calls it pathologic gambling; Table 4-48 lists their comparative approaches to the disorder.

Previous editions of the DSM include pathologic gambling disorder in the impulse-control disorder category because of the patient's preoccupation or compulsion to gamble. However, the criteria for the disorder are more similar to substance-related disorders, given the compulsive behavior, tolerance, and withdrawal effects that develop. Substance use is often comorbid with gambling. Thus, in DSM-5, gambling disorder is included in the section on substance use and addictive disorders and is diagnosed as a non–substance-related disorder. ICD-10 continues to include it among the habit and impulse disorders, referring to it as pathologic gambling.

Gerry was a 35-year-old former auto dealership owner. Two of his uncles were compulsive gamblers, and his paternal grandfather had major depressive disorder. He played poker and had been a racecourse habitué since the age of 15 years. He had dropped out of college after

Table 4-48
Gambling Disorder

Disorder	DSM-5	ICD-10
	Gambling Disorder	
Diagnostic Name	Gambling Disorder	Pathologic Gambling
Duration	Symptoms present within a 12-month period	
Symptoms	• Needing higher stakes to achieve the same thrill • Becomes irritable when trying to stop • Unsuccessful attempts at reducing gambling • Preoccupation with thoughts about gambling • Gambling in response to distress • Gambling to recoup prior losses • Lies to hide gambling • Losses due to gambling: jobs, relationships, other opportunities • Borrows or steals money from others for gambling	Pattern of gambling that is dominant in the patient's life and resulting in adverse consequences in social, occupational, family, and other areas of life
Required number of symptoms	Four or more of the above	
Psychosocial consequences of symptoms	Marked impairment and/or distress	
Exclusions	Manic episode	• Excessive gambling by manic patients • Gambling and betting NOS • Gambling in dissocial personality disorder
Course specifiers	**Episodic:** meets criteria more than once over time, separated by at least several months **Persistent:** continuous over several years **In early remission:** no symptoms for 3–12 mo **In sustained remission:** no symptoms for >12 mo	
Severity specifiers	Severity is measured by the number of symptoms present See DSM-5 for ranges	

a few months and became a car sales representative. Soon he was promoted to showroom manager and then went out on his own. By age 32 years, he was a multimillionaire owner of a dealership chain, happily married with two children.

Gerry continued to gamble frequently. He was a successful weekend sports bettor, as well as a consistent winner at weekly gin rummy and poker games and occasional jaunts to Las Vegas and Atlantic City.

In the context of his wife giving birth to a stillborn child, Gerry started going to casinos more often, gradually increasing the size of bets at blackjack and craps. His sports wagers also escalated. His games at home gradually became boring—"there was zilch action." He began frequenting an illegal local poker parlor that featured high-stake action.

Over several years, Gerry slipped into a typical gambling spiral. He accumulated several million dollars in debts and lied to family and colleagues about his whereabouts. He raided his business and personal accounts, including his children's college funds, maxed out credit cards, and borrowed from loan sharks at exorbitant rates. He grew profoundly depressed and seriously thought of killing himself in a car crash so that his insurance would "take care of my family after I am gone."

Gerry's dire situation was unmasked when his Porsche was repossessed one Sunday morning. Initially, his wife threatened to divorce him. However, a wealthy relative intervened and bailed him out. He swore never to gamble again, entered Gamblers Anonymous, and within 2 months, resumed his frantic gambling.

Over the next decade, Gerry underwent four more episodes of recovery and relapse. His wife divorced him, he lost his dealerships, and he had to declare bankruptcy. Gerry finally enrolled in a pilot dual-diagnostic recovery program, where he was diagnosed with atypical bipolar disorder. His treatment included Gamblers Anonymous

meetings, individual and family counseling, and pharmacotherapy with bupropion and lamotrigine.

Gerry eventually reconciled with his wife and family. He returned to selling cars, started living modestly, and continued to attend Gamblers Anonymous meetings regularly. However, he declared emphatically that he always considers himself one step away from becoming a "degenerate gambler" again. (Courtesy of Harvey Roy Greenberg, M.D.)

DIFFERENTIAL DIAGNOSIS

Social gambling is distinguished from pathologic gambling in that the former occurs with friends, on special occasions, and with predetermined acceptable and tolerable losses. Gambling that is symptomatic of a manic episode can usually be distinguished from pathologic gambling by the history of a marked mood change and the loss of judgment preceding the gambling.

Manic-like mood changes are frequent in pathologic gambling, but they always follow winning and are usually succeeded by depressive episodes because of subsequent losses. Persons with an antisocial personality disorder may have problems with gambling. When both disorders are present, clinicians should diagnose both.

COMORBIDITY

Significant comorbidity occurs between pathologic gambling and mood disorders (especially major depression and bipolarity) and other substance use and addictive disorders (notably, alcohol, stimulant, caffeine, and tobacco use disorders). Comorbidity also exists

Table 4-49
The Four Phases of Pathologic Gambling

1. The winning phase, ending with a big win, equal to about a year's salary, which hooks patients. Women usually do not have a big win but use gambling as an escape from problems.
2. The progressive-loss phase, in which patients structure their lives around gambling and then move from being excellent gamblers to being stupid ones who take considerable risks, cash in securities, borrow money, miss work, and lose jobs.
3. The desperate phase, with patients frenziedly gambling with large amounts of money, not paying debts, becoming involved with loan sharks, writing bad checks, and possibly embezzling.
4. The hopeless stage of accepting that losses can never be made up, but the gambling continues because of the associated arousal or excitement. The disorder may take up to 15 yr to reach the last phase, but then, within a year or two, patients have totally deteriorated.

with ADHD (particularly in childhood), various personality disorders (notably, narcissistic, antisocial, and borderline personality disorders), and disruptive, impulse control, and conduct disorders. Although many pathologic gamblers have obsessive personality traits, full-blown OCD is uncommon in this group.

COURSE AND PROGNOSIS

Pathologic gambling usually begins in adolescence for men and late in life for women. The disorder waxes and wanes and tends to be chronic. Table 4-49 lists the four phases of pathologic gambling.

TREATMENT

Gamblers seldom come forward voluntarily to be treated. Legal difficulties, family pressures, or other psychiatric complaints bring gamblers to treatment. Gamblers Anonymous (GA) was founded in Los Angeles in 1957 and modeled on AA. It is accessible, at least in large cities, and is an effective treatment for gambling in some patients. GA is a method of inspirational group therapy that involves public confession, peer pressure, and the presence of reformed gamblers (as with sponsors in AA) available to help members resist the impulse to gamble. The dropout rate from GA is high, however. Hospitalization may sometimes help by removing patients from their environments. Clinicians should not start insight-oriented psychotherapy until patients have been away from gambling for 3 months. At this point, patients who are pathologic gamblers may become excellent candidates for this form of psychotherapy. Family therapy is often valuable. CBT (e.g., relaxation techniques combined with visualization of gambling avoidance) has had some success.

Psychopharmacological treatment, once largely unsuccessful, now plays a significant role in the management of pathologic gamblers. Useful agents include antidepressants, notably SSRIs and bupropion; mood stabilizers, including sustained-release lithium and antiepileptics such as lamotrigine; atypical antipsychotics; and opioid agents such as naltrexone. In many patients, it is difficult to determine whether an antidepressant or mood stabilizer alleviates gambling cravings directly or via treatment of a comorbid condition, particularly depressive or bipolar disorders.

EPIDEMIOLOGY

Although we lack comprehensive worldwide statistics, available information indicates that 1 to 2 percent of the general population are problem gamblers. Problem gambling is more common in men and

young adults than in women and older adults; however, escalation has been noted in the poor, notably poor minorities, adolescents, elderly retirees, and women. Pathologic gambling is associated with intimate partner violence—both as a perpetrator (for both men and women) and as a victim (typically women only). However, this violence is also due to comorbid psychiatric and substance use disorders.

ETIOLOGY

Psychosocial Factors

Several factors have been described as predisposing persons to develop the disorder: loss of a parent by death, separation, divorce, or desertion before a child is 15 years of age; inappropriate parental discipline (absence, inconsistency, or harshness); exposure to, and availability of, gambling activities for adolescents; a family emphasis on material and financial symbols; and a lack of family emphasis on saving, planning, and budgeting.

Psychoanalytic theory has focused on several core character difficulties. Edmund Bergler suggested that compulsive gamblers have an unconscious desire to lose and gamble to relieve unconscious feelings of guilt, though these ideas are questionable. Another suggestion is that the gamblers are narcissists whose grandiose and omnipotent fantasies lead them to believe they can control events and even predict their outcome. Learning theorists view uncontrolled gambling as resulting from erroneous perceptions about control of impulses.

Biologic Factors

Many studies indicate that pathologic gamblers suffer from complex neurotransmitter dysregulation, similar to the abnormalities found in substance use disorders and patients with other behavioral/impulsive problems. Most major neurotransmitters have, at some point, been implicated as a significant factor in the dysfunction of cerebral sites and pathways mediating behavioral arousal, inhibition/disinhibition, reward/reinforcement, and psychophysiological stress.

The particular focus on the role of increased dopaminergic activity in pathologic gambling arose from the serendipitous discovery that approximately one-third of patients receiving dopamine agonists for Parkinson disease develop the illness without any previous history. The gambling excesses of these patients usually disappear upon withdrawal of the offending drug.

▲ 4.13 Other Disorders Related to the Addictive Disorders

INTERNET GAMING DISORDER

Also called *Internet Addiction,* such persons spend almost all their waking hours at their computer. Their patterns of use are repetitive and constant, and they are unable to resist intense urges to use the computer or to "surf" the internet. Internet addicts may gravitate to certain sites that meet specific needs (e.g., shopping, sex, and interactive games, among others). In DSM-5, there is a condition proposed for further study called "internet gaming disorder," which refers to persons who continually use the internet to play games to the extent that it interferes with social relations and work performance. However, as mentioned earlier, the disorder need not be limited to games. Other activities may be involved. General population surveys show a

Table 4-50
Symptoms of Internet Gaming Disorder

Activities associated with Gaming
  Preoccupation w/ gaming
  Withdrawal (discomfort when deprived of gaming)
  Tolerance (spending more time to achieve same enjoyment from the game)

Compulsive Behavior
  Lack of control around gaming

Social or Occupational Dysfunction
  Decreased alternative activities
  Negative effects on personal relationships, occupational or school performance due to gaming
  Lying to loved ones or clinicians about the frequency of gaming
  Relying on gaming to improve mood
  Continued use despite recognize the harmful effects of compulsive gaming

wide range of reported prevalence, from 0 to almost 50 percent, with some of the highest percentages reported in South Asian countries.

Table 4-50 lists some of the common symptoms and effects of the disorder. They are organized so as to be consistent with the DSM-5 approach to substance use disorder (see Section 4.1).

Internet Use and Victims

The combination of anonymity, convenience, and escape (the ACE model) promotes the internet as a focus of psychopathology. It can be easy to conceal one's identity and even create alternate identities using various internet platforms. The resulting deception can take a malignant turn as sexual predators deceive their victims with false identities only to exploit and harm them when they meet. These contacts are unregulated and difficult to detect except by monitoring and checking the computers used. There are frequent reports of minors having been lured into sometimes lethal situations by sexual predators. Occasionally there is a report of a couple that met to marry only to discover they had missed verifying crucial details, such as each other's sex.

Some people who make little use of the internet nonetheless become victims and enter treatment. The suicide of one teenager after reading untruths entered by a peer's malicious mother ("cyberbullying") has inspired laws to criminalize such behavior. Internet identity theft is also rampant. An underreported and growing problem, medical identity theft, is harder to detect and remedy, often requiring painstaking record correction.

MOBILE OR CELL PHONE COMPULSION

Some persons compulsively use mobile or smartphones. Often these individuals find themselves engaging in many of the same patterns of behavior as those with the proposed internet gaming disorder, though the focus is not specifically on the internet or gaming. These individuals may be preoccupied with checking for new messages (text or email), new social media posts, or other smartphone-related activities.

REPETITIVE SELF-MUTILATION

Persons who repeatedly cut themselves or do damage to their bodies may do so in a compulsive manner. Parasuicidal behavior is typical in, but not limited to, borderline personality disorder. Compulsive body piercing or tattooing may be a symptom of a paraphilia or a depressive equivalent.

In DSM-5, there is a proposed diagnosis called "non-suicidal self-injury" to refer to persons who repeatedly damage their bodies, who, however, do not wish to die, contrasted with those persons who harm themselves with real suicidal intent. Most individuals who engage in this behavior do so to obtain relief from dysphoric states or to resolve a conflict. Cutting the skin or inflicting bodily pain may release endorphins or raise dopamine levels in the brain, both of which contribute to a euthymic or elated mood, thus alleviating depressed states of mind in those who practice self-mutilation.

COMPULSIVE SEXUAL BEHAVIOR

Some persons repeatedly seek out sexual gratification, often in perverse ways (e.g., exhibitionism). They are unable to control their behavior and may not experience feelings of guilt after an episode of acting-out behavior. Sometimes called *sexual addiction,* we discuss this condition in the chapter on sexual disorders (Chapter 16).

References

Achar S, Rostamian A, Narayan SM. Cardiac and metabolic effects of anabolic-androgenic steroid abuse on lipids, blood pressure, left ventricular dimensions, and rhythm. *Am J Cardiol.* 2010;106(6):893.

Agrawal A, Wetherill L, Dick DM, Xuei X, Hinrichs A, Hesselbrock V, Kramer J, Nurnberger JI Jr, Schuckit M, Bierut LJ, Edenberg HJ, Foroud T. Evidence for association between polymorphisms in the cannabinoid receptor 1 (CNR1) gene and cannabis dependence. *Am J Med Genet.* 2009;150B:736.

"Alcohol Facts and Statistics." Alcohol Facts and Statistics, National Institute on Alcohol Abuse and Alcoholism, August 2018. www.niaaa.nih.gov/alcohol-facts-and-statistics.

American Psychiatric Association. *Diagnostic and Statistical Manual of Mental Disorders.* 5th ed. Arlington, VA: American Psychiatric Association; 2013.

Anton RF, O'Malley SS, Ciraulo DA, Cisler RA, Couper D, Donovan DM, Gastfriend DR, Hosking JD, Johnson BA, LoCastro JS, Longabaugh R, Mason BJ, Mattson ME, Miller WR, Pettinati HM, Randall CL, Swift R, Weiss RD, Williams LD, Zweben A; COMBINE Student Research Group. Combined pharmacotherapies and behavioral interventions for alcohol dependence: the COMBINE study: a randomized controlled trial. *JAMA.* 2006;295:2003–2017.

Arehart-Treichel J. Smoking high on list of suicide-risk factors. *Psychiatr News.* 2011;46:16.

Ashley LL, Boehlke KK. Pathological gambling: A general overview. *J Psychoactive Drugs.* 2012;44:27.

Auta J, Kadriu B, Giusti P, Costa E, Guidotti A. Anticonvulsant, anxiolytic, and nonsedating actions of imidazenil and other imidazo-benzodiazepine carboxamide derivatives. *Pharmacol Biochem Behav.* 2010;95(4):383.

Baggish AL, Weiner RB, Kanayama G, Hudson JI, Picard MH, Hutter AM Jr, Pope HJ Jr. Long-term anabolic-androgenic steroid use is associated with left ventricular dysfunction. *Circ Heart Fail.* 2010;3:472.

Baillie AJ, Sannibale C, Stapinski LA, Teesson M, Rapee RM, Haber PS. An investigator-blinded randomized study to compare the efficacy of combined CBT for alcohol use disorders and social anxiety disorder versus CBT focused on alcohol alone in adults with comorbid disorders: The Combined Alcohol Social Phobia (CASP) trial protocol. *BMC Psychiatry.* 2013;13:199.

Balster RL, Cruz SL, Howard MO, Dell CA, Cottler LB. Classification of abused inhalants. *Addiction.* 2009;104:878.

Baltazar A, Hopkins G, McBride D, Vanderwaal C, Pepper S, Mackey S. Parental influence on inhalant use. *J Child Adolesc Subst Abuse.* 2013;22(1):25–37.

Barceloux DG. Amphetamines and phenethylamine derivatives. In: *Medical Toxicology of Drug Abuse: Synthesized Chemicals and Psychoactive Plants.* Hoboken, NJ: John Wiley & Sons; 2012:3.

Barceloux DG. Barbiturates (amobarbital, butalbital, pentobarbital, secobarbital). In: *Medical Toxicology of Drugs Abuse: Synthesized Chemicals and Psychoactive Plants.* Hoboken, NJ: John Wiley & Sons Inc.; 2012:467.

Barnett SR, Riddle MA. Anxiolytics and sedative/hypnotics: Benzodiazepines, buspirone, and other. In: Martin A, Scahill L, Kratochvil C, eds. *Pediatric Psychopharmacology: Principles and Practice.* New York: Oxford University Press Inc.; 2011:338.

Barry DT, Beitel M, Cutter CJ, Joshi D, Falcioni J, Schottenfeld RS. Conventional and nonconventional pain treatment utilization among opioid dependent individuals with pain seeking methadone maintenance treatment: A needs assessment study. *J Addict Med.* 2010;4:81.

Basile JR, Binmadi NO, Zhou H, Yang Y-H, Paoli A, Proia P. Supraphysiological doses of performance enhancing anabolic-androgenic steroids exert direct toxic effects on neuron-like cells. *Front Cell Neurosci.* 2013;7:69.

Bender E. Troubling trends found in teen inhalant use. *Psychiatr News.* 2009;44:6.

Benowitz NL. Neurobiology of nicotine addiction: Implications for smoking cessation treatment. *Am J Med.* 2008;121:S3.

Bhargava S, Arora RR. Cocaine and cardiovascular complications. *Am J Ther.* 2011;18(4):e95.

Bhorkar AA, Dandekar MP, Nakhate KT, Subhedar NK, Kokare DM. Involvement of the central melanocortin system in the effects of caffeine on anxiety-like behavior in mice. *Life Sci*. 2014;95(2):72–80.

Blazer DG, Wu LT. Patterns of tobacco use and tobacco-related psychiatric morbidity and substance use among middle-aged and older adults in the United States. *Aging Ment Health*. 2012;16:296.

Bogenschutz MP, Ross S. Hallucinogen-related disorders. In: Sadock BJ, Sadock VA, Ruiz P, eds. *Kaplan & Sadock's Comprehensive Textbook of Psychiatry*. 10th ed. Philadelphia, PA: Wolters Kluwer; 2017:1312–1327.

Bohnert ASB, Valenstein M, Bair MJ, Ganoczy D, McCarthy JF, Ilgen MA, Blow FC. Association between opioid prescribing patterns and opioid overdose-related deaths. *JAMA*. 2011;305:1315.

Bokor G, Anderson PD. Ketamine: An update on its abuse. *J Pharm Pract*. 2014; 27:582–586.

Bonder BR. Substance-related disorders. In: Bonder BR, ed. *Psychopathology and Function*. 4th ed. Thorofare, NJ: SLACK Inc.; 2010:103.

Bosco D, Plastino M, Colica C, Bosco F, Arianna S, Vecchio A, Galati F, Cristiano D, Consoli A, Consoli D. Opioid antagonist naltrexone for the treatment of pathological gambling in Parkinson Disease. *Clin Neuropharmacol*. 2012;35:118.

Buckner JD, Silgado J, Schmidt NB. Marijuana craving during a public speaking challenge: Understanding marijuana use vulnerability among women and those with social anxiety disorder. *J Behav Ther Exp Psychiatry*. 2011;42:104.

Butt MS, Sultan MT. Coffee and its consumption: Benefits and risks. *Crit Rev Food Sci Nutr*. 2011;51:363.

Cairney S, O'Connor N, Dingwall KM. A prospective study of neurocognitive changes 15 years after chronic inhalant abuse. *Addiction*. 2013;108(6):1107–1114.

Callaghan RC, Cunningham JK, Sajeev G, Kish SJ. Incidence of Parkinson's disease among hospital patients with methamphetamine-use disorders. *Mov Disord*. 2010;25(14):2333.

Caraci F, Pistarà V, Corsaro A, Tomasello F, Giuffrida ML, Sortino MA, Nicoletti F, Copani A. Neurotoxic properties of the anabolic androgenic steroids nandrolone and methandrostenolone in primary neuronal cultures. *J Neurosci Res*. 2011;89(4):592.

Carter GT, Flanagan AM, Earleywine M, Abrams DI, Aggarwal SK, Grinspoon L. Cannabis in palliative medicine: Improving care and reducing opioid-related morbidity. *Am J Hosp Palliat Care*. 2011;28:297.

Cash MS, Rae CD, Steel AH, Winkler A. Internet addiction: A brief summary of research and practice. *Curr Psychiatry Rev*. 2012;8:292–298.

Catts VS, Catts SV. Psychotomimetic effects of PCP, LSD, and ecstasy: Pharmacological models of schizophrenia? In: Sachdev PS, Keshavan MS, eds. *Secondary Schizophrenia*. New York: Cambridge University Press; 2010:141.

Choo ED, McGregor AJ, Mello MJ, Baird J. Gender, violence and brief interventions for alcohol in the emergency department. *Drug Alcohol Depend*. 2013;127:115.

Clark CT, Richards EM, Antoine DG II, Chisolm MS. Perinatal toluene use: Associated risks and considerations. *Addict Disord Treat*. 2011;10:1.

Clark R, Samnaliev M, McGovern MP. Impact of substance disorders on medical expenditures for Medicaid beneficiaries with behavioral health disorders. *Psychiatr Serv*. 2009;60:35.

Cohen AS, Buckner JD, Najolia GM, Stewart DW. Cannabis and psychometrically-defined schizotypy: Use, problems and treatment considerations. *J Psychiatr Res*. 2011;45:548.

Colfax GN, Santos GM, Das M, Santos DM, Matheson T, Gasper J, Shoptaw S, Vittinghoff E. Mirtazapine to reduce methamphetamine use: a randomized controlled trial. *Arch Gen Psychiatry*. 2011;68:1168–1175.

Comer SD, Sullivan MA, Whittington RA, Vosburg SK, Kowalczyk WJ. Abuse liability of prescription opioids compared to heroin in morphine-maintained heroin abusers. *Neuropsychopharmacology*. 2008;33(5):1179.

Connery HS. Medication-assisted treatment of opioid use disorder: review of the evidence and future directions. *Harv Rev Psychiatry*. 2015;23:63–75.

Crane CA, Easton CJ, Devine S. The association between phencyclidine use and partner violence: An initial examination. *J Addict Dis*. 2013;32:150.

Crean RD, Crane NA, Mason BJ. An evidence-based review of acute and long-term effects of cannabis on executive cognitive functions. *J Addict Med*. 2011;5:1.

Crean RD, Tapert SF, Minassian A, MacDonald K, Crane NA, Mason BJ. Effects of chronic, heavy cannabis use on executive functions. *J Addict Med*. 2011;5:9.

Cunningham-Williams RM, Gattis MN, Dore PM, Shi P, Spitznagel EL. Towards DSM-V: Considering other withdrawal-like symptoms of pathological gambling disorder. *Int J Methods Psychiatr Res*. 2009;18:13.

"Current Cigarette Smoking Among Adults in the United States." Smoking & Tobacco Use, Centers for Disease Control and Prevention, February 4, 2019. https://www.cdc.gov/tobacco/data_statistics/fact_sheets/adult_data/cig_smoking/index.htm.

Dome P, Lazary J, Kalapos MP, Rihmer Z. Smoking, nicotine and neuropsychiatric disorders. *Neurosci Biobehav Rev*. 2010;34:295.

Driscoll MD, Arora A, Brennan ML. Intramuscular anabolic steroid injection leading to life-threatening clostridial myonecrosis: A case report. *J Bone Joint Surg Am*. 2011;93(16):e92 1–3.

Ehlers CL, Gizer IR, Vieten C, Wilhelmsen KC. Linkage analyses of cannabis dependence, craving, and withdrawal in the San Francisco family study. *Am J Med Genet*. 2010;153B:802.

Ersche KD, Jones PS, Williams GB, Turton AJ, Robbins TW, Bullmore ET. Abnormal brain structure implicated in stimulant drug addiction. *Science*. 2012;335:601.

"Fact Sheets—Alcohol Use and Your Health." Alcohol and Public Health, Centers for Disease Control and Prevention, January 3, 2018. www.cdc.gov/alcohol/fact-sheets/alcohol-use.htm.

Fantegrossi WE, Murnane KS, Reissig CJ. The behavioral pharmacology of hallucinogens. *Biochem Pharmacol*. 2008;75:17.

Fazel S, Långström N, Hjern A, Grann M, Lichtenstein P. Schizophrenia, substance abuse, and violent crime. *JAMA*. 2009;301(19):2016.

Fiore M, Jean C, Baker T, Bailey W, Benowitz N. *Treating Tobacco Use and Dependence: Clinical Practice Guideline*. Washington, DC: US Public Health Service; 2008.

Fontanilla D, Johannessen D, Hajipour AR, Cozzi NV, Jackson MB, Ruoho AE. The hallucinogen N,N-dimethyltryptamine (DMT) is an endogenous sigma-1 receptor regulator. *Science*. 2009;323:934.

Frances RJ, Miller SI, Mack AH, eds. *Clinical Textbook of Addictive Disorders*. 3rd ed. New York: The Guildford Press; 2011.

Fridberg DJ, Skosnik PD, Hetrick WP, O'Donnell BF. Neural correlates of performance monitoring in chronic cannabis users and cannabis-naïve controls. *J Psychopharmacol*. 2013;27:515.

Garland EL, Howard MO. Adverse consequences of acute inhalant intoxication. *Exp Clin Psychopharmacol*. 2011;19:134.

Garland EL, Howard MO. Phenomenology of adolescent inhalant intoxication. *Exp Clin Psychopharmacol*. 2010;18:498.

Geraci MJ, Peele J, McCoy SL, Elias B. Phencyclidine false positive induced by lamotrigine (Lamictal) on a rapid urine toxicology screen. *Int J Emerg Med*. 2010;3(4):327.

Grant JE, Kim SW, Potenza MN. Advances in the pharmacological treatment of pathological gambling. *J Gambl Stud*. 2003;19:85.

Greenberg HR. Pathological gambling. In: Sadock BJ, Sadock VA, Ruiz P, eds. *Kaplan & Sadock's Comprehensive Textbook of Psychiatry*. 10th ed. Philadelphia, PA: Wolters Kluwer; 2017:1799–1811.

Grella CE, Karno MP, Warda US, Niv N, Moore AA. Gender and comorbidity among individuals with opioid use disorders in the NESARC study. *Addict Behav*. 2009;34:498–504.

Griffin O, Fritsch AL, Woodward VH, Mohn RS. Sifting through the hyperbole: One hundred year of marijuana coverage in The New York Times. *Deviant Behav*. 2013;34:767.

Gros DF, Milanak ME, Brady KT, Back SE. Frequency and severity of comorbid mood and anxiety disorders in prescription opioid dependence. *Am J Addict*. 2013; 22(3):261–265.

Gunderson EW, Kirkpatrick MG, Willing LM, Holstege CP. Substituted cathinone products: A new trend in "bath salts" and other designer stimulant drug use. *J Addict Med*. 2013;7(3):153–162.

Hall WD, Degenhardt L. Cannabis-related disorders. In: Sadock BJ, Sadock VA, Ruiz P, eds. *Kaplan & Sadock's Comprehensive Textbook of Psychiatry*. 10th ed. Philadelphia, PA: Wolters Kluwer; 2017:1303–1312.

Hall MT, Edwards JD, Howard MO. Accidental deaths due to inhalant misuse in North Carolina: 2000–2008. *Subst Use Misuse*. 2010;45:1330.

Hall MT, Howard MO, McCabe SE. Subtypes of adolescent sedative/anxiolytic misusers: A latent profile analysis. *Addict Behav*. 2010;35(10):882.

Haller DL, Acosta MC. Characteristics of pain patients with opioid-use disorder. *Psychosomatics*. 2010;51:257.

Haney M. Neurobiology of stimulants. In: Galantar M, Kleber HD, eds. *Textbook of Substance Abuse Treatment*. 3rd ed. Washington, DC: American Psychiatric Publishing; 2008:143.

Harper AD. Substance-related disorders. In: Thornhill J, ed. *NMS Psychiatry*. 6th ed. Baltimore, MD: Lippincott Williams & Wilkins; 2011:109.

Hasin DS, O'Brien CP, Auriacombe M. DSM-5 criteria for substance use disorders: Recommendations and rationale. *Am J Psychiatry*. 2013;170:834.

Hatsukami DK, Benowitz NL, Donny E, Henningfield J, Zeller M. Nicotine reduction: Strategic research plan. *Nicotine Tob Res*. 2013;15(6):1003–1013.

He Q, Chen X, Wu T, Li L, Fei X. Risk of dementia in long-term benzodiazepine users: Evidence from a meta-analysis of observational studies. *J Clin Neurol*. 2019;15:9–19.

Herlitz LC, Markowitz GS, Farris AB, Schwimmer JA, Stokes MB, Kunis C, Colvin RB, D'Agati VD. Development of focal segmental glomerulosclerosis after anabolic steroid abuse. *J Am Soc Nephrol*. 2010;21:163.

Hoblyn JC, Balt SL, Woodard SA, Brooks JO. Substance use disorders as risk factors for psychiatric hospitalization in bipolar disorder. *Psychiatr Serv*. 2009;60:55.

Hodgins DC. Reliability and validity of the Sheehan Disability Scale modified for pathological gambling. *BMC Psychiatry*. 2013;13:177.

Hodgins DC, Fick GH, Murray R, Cunningham JA. Internet-based interventions for disordered gamblers: Study protocol for a randomized controlled trial of online self-directed cognitive-behavioral motivational therapy. *BMC Public Health*. 2013;13:10.

Hoque R, Chesson AL Jr. Zolpidem-induced sleepwalking, sleep related eating disorder, and sleep-driving: Fluorine-18-flouorodeoxyglucose positron emission tomography analysis, and a literature review of other unexpected clinical effects of zolpidem. *J Clin Sleep Med*. 2009;5(5):471.

Houston CM, McGee TP, MacKenzie G, Troyano-Cuturi K, Rodriguez PM, Kutsarova E, Diamanti E, Hosie AM, Frank NP, Brickley SG. Are extrasynaptic GABAA receptors important targets for sedative/hypnotic drugs? *J Neurosci*. 2012;32:3887.

Howard MO, Bowen SE, Garland EL. Inhalant-related disorders. In: Sadock BJ, Sadock VA, Ruiz P, eds. *Kaplan & Sadock's Comprehensive Textbook of Psychiatry*. 10th ed. Philadelphia, PA: Wolters Kluwer; 2017:1328–1342.

Howard MO, Bowen SE, Garland EL, Perron BE, Vaughn MG. Inhalant use and inhalant use disorders in the United States. *Addict Sci Clin Pract*. 2011;6:18.

Howe CQ, Sullivan MD. The missing 'P' in pain management: how the current opioid epidemic highlights the need for psychiatric services in chronic pain care. *Gen Hosp Psychiatry*. 2014;36(1):99–104.

Hurd YL, Michaelides M, Miller ML, Jutras-Aswad D. Trajectory of adolescent cannabis use on addiction vulnerability. *Neuropharmacology*. 2014;76:416–424.

Husten CG, Deyton LR. Understanding the Tobacco Control Act: Efforts by the US Food and Drug Administration to make tobacco-related morbidity and mortality part of the USA's past, not its future. *Lancet*. 2013;381(9877):1570–1580.

Iannucci RA, Weiss RD. Stimulant-related disorders. In: Sadock BJ, Sadock VA, Ruiz P, eds. *Kaplan & Sadock's Comprehensive Textbook of Psychiatry*. 10th ed. Philadelphia, PA: Wolters Kluwer; 2017:1280–1291.

Incerti M, Vink J, Roberson R, Benassou I, Abebe D, Spong CY. Prevention of the alcohol-induced changes in brain-derived neurotrophic factor expression using neuroprotective peptides in a model of fetal alcohol syndrome. *Am J Obstet Gynecol*. 2010;202(5):457.

Jackson KM, Bucholz KK, Wood PK, Steinley D, Grant JD, Sher KJ. Towards the characterization and validation of alcohol use disorder subtypes: integrating consumption and symptom data. *Psychol Med*. 2014;44(01):143–159.

Jann M, Kennedy WK, Lopez G. Benzodiazepines: a major component in unintentional prescription drug overdoses with opioid analgesics. *J Pharm Pract*. 2014; 27(1):5–16.

Johnson BA. Medication treatment of different types of alcoholism. *Am J Psychiatry*. 2010;167:630.

Johnson BA, Marzani-Nissen G. Alcohol. Clinical Aspects. In: Johnson BA, ed. *Addiction Medicine: Science and Practice*. New York: Springer; 2011:381.

Jones HE. Treating opioid use disorders during pregnancy: Historical, current, and future directions. *Subst Abus*. 2013;34(2):89–91.

Jones RT. Hallucinogen-related disorders. In: Sadock BJ, Sadock VA, Ruiz P, eds. *Kaplan & Sadock's Comprehensive Textbook of Psychiatry*. 9th ed. Philadelphia, PA: Lippincott Williams & Wilkins; 2009:1331.

Jonjev ZS, Bala G. High-energy drinks may provoke aortic dissection. *Coll Antropol*. 2013;37:227.

Juliano LM, Griffiths RR. Caffeine-related disorders. In: Sadock BJ, Sadock VA, Ruiz P, eds. *Kaplan & Sadock's Comprehensive Textbook of Psychiatry*. 10th ed. Philadelphia, PA: Wolters Kluwer; 2017:1291–1303.

Kanayama G, Brower KJ, Wood RI, Hudson JI, Pope HG Jr. Issues for DSM-V: Clarifying the diagnostic criteria for anabolic-androgenic steroid dependence. *Am J Psychiatry*. 2009;166:642.

Kanayama G, Hudson JI, Pope HG Jr. Illicit anabolic-androgenic steroid use. *Horm Behav*. 2010;58:111.

Kanayama G, Hudson JI, Pope HG Jr. Long-term psychiatric and medical consequences of anabolic-androgenic steroid abuse: a looming public health concern? *Drug Alcohol Depend*. 2008;98:1.

Kanayama G, Hudson JI, Pope HG. Demographic and psychiatric features of men with anabolic-androgenic steroid dependence: a comparative study. *Drug Alcohol Depend*. 2009;102:130.

Kanayama G, Kean J, Hudson JI, Pope HG Jr. Cognitive deficits in long-term anabolic-androgenic steroid users. *Drug Alcohol Depend*. 2013;130(1–3):208–214.

Karoly HC, Harlaar N, Hutchison KE. Substance use disorders: A theory-driven approach to the integration of genetics and neuroimaging. *Ann N Y Acad Sci*. 2013;1282:71.

Kendler KS, Myers J, Gardner CO. Caffeine intake, toxicity, and dependence and lifetime risk for psychiatric and substance use disorders: an epidemiologic and co-twin control analysis. *Psychol Med*. 2006;36:1717–1725.

Kennedy DO, Haskell CF. Cerebral blood flow and behavioural effects of caffeine in habitual and non-habitual consumers of caffeine: A near infrared spectroscopy study. *Biol Psychol*. 2011;86:298.

Kessler RC, Hwang I, LaBrie R, Petuhova M, Sampson NA, Winters KC, Shaffer HJ. DSM-IV pathological gambling in the National Comorbidity Survey Replication. *Psychol Med*. 2008;38:1351.

Kohmura K, Iwamoto K, Aleksic B, Sasada K, Kawano N, Katayama H, Noda Y, Noda A, Lidaka T, Ozaki N. Effects of sedative antidepressants on prefrontal cortex activity during verbal fluency task in healthy subjects: A near-infrared spectroscopy study. *Psychopharmacology*. 2013;226(1):75–81.

Kosten TR, Newton TF, De La Garza R II, Haile CN, eds. *Cocaine and Methamphetamine Dependence: Advances in Treatment*. Arlington, VA: American Psychiatric Association; 2012.

Krenek M, Maisto SA. Life events and treatment outcomes among individuals with substance use disorders: A narrative review. *Clin Psychol Rev*. 2013;33:470.

Lakhan SE, Kirchgessner A. Anti-inflammatory effects of nicotine in obesity and ulcerative colitis. *J Transl Med*. 2011;9:129.

Larance B, Degenhardt L, Copeland J, Dillon P. Injecting risk behaviour and related harm among men who use performance- and image-enhancing drugs. *Drug Alcohol Rev*. 2008;27:679.

Lee NK, Pohlman S, Baker A, Ferris J, Kay-Lambkin F. It's the thought that counts: Craving metacognitions and their role in abstinence from methamphetamine use. *J Subst Abuse Treat*. 2010;38(3):245.

Leeman RF, Potenza MN. Similarities and differences between pathological gambling and substance use disorders: a focus on impulsivity and compulsivity. *Psychopharmacology*. 2012;219:469.

Lieberman JA III, Sylvester L, Paik S. Excessive sleepiness and self-reported shift work disorder: an internet survey of shift workers. *Postgrad Med*. 2013;125:162.

Ling W, Casadonte P, Bigelow G, Kampman KM, Patkar A, Bailey GL, Rosenthal RN, Beebe KL. Buprenorphine implants for treatment of opioid dependence. *JAMA*. 2010;304:1576.

Lintzeris N, Bhardwaj A, Mills L, Dunlop A, Copeland J, McGregor I, Bruno R, Gugusheff J, Phung N, Montebello M, Chan T, Kirby A, Hall M, Jefferies M, Luksza J, Shanahan M, Kevin R, Allsop D; Agonist Replacement for Cannabis Dependence (ARCD) study group. Nabiximols for the treatment of cannabis dependence: a randomized clinical trial. *JAMA Intern Med*. 2019;179(9):1242–1253.

Liu S, Lane SD, Schmitz JM, Waters AJ, Cunningham KA, Moeller FG. Relationship between attentional bias to cocaine-related stimuli and impulsivity in cocaine-dependent subjects. *Am J Drug Alcohol Abuse*. 2011;37(2):117.

López-Muñoz F, Álamo C, García-García P. The discovery of chlordiazepoxide and the clinical introduction of benzodiazepines: Half a century of anxiolytic drugs. *J Anxiety Disord*. 2011;25(4):554.

Ludden AB, Wolfson AR. Understanding adolescent caffeine use: Connecting use patterns with expectancies, reasons, and sleep. *Health Educ Behav*. 2010;37:330.

Luo SX, Bisaga A. Opioid use and related disorders: From neuroscience to treatment. In: Sadock BJ, Sadock VA, Ruiz P, eds. *Kaplan & Sadock's Comprehensive Textbook of Psychiatry*. 10th ed. Philadelphia, PA: Wolters Kluwer; 2017:1352–1373.

Luoma JB, Kohlenberg BS, Hayes SC, Fletcher L. Slow and steady wins the race: A randomized clinical trial of acceptance and commitment therapy targeting shame in substance use disorders. *J Consult Clin Psychol*. 2012;80:43.

MacKillop J, Miranda R Jr, Monti PM, Ray LA, Murphy JG, Rohsenow DJ, McGeary JE, Swift RM, Tidey JW, Gwaltney CJ. Alcohol demand, delayed reward discounting, and craving in relation to drinking and alcohol use disorders. *J Abnorm Psychol*. 2010;11:106.

MacLean KA, Johnson MW, Griffiths RR. Mystical experiences occasioned by the hallucinogen Psilocybin lead to increases in the personality domain of openness. *J Psychopharmacol*. 2011;25:1453.

Magdum SS. An overview of Khat. *Addict Disord Treat*. 2011;10(2):72.

Mahler SV, Hensley-Simon M, Tahsili-Fahadan P, LaLumiere RT, Thomas C, Fallon RV, Kalivas PW, Aston-Jones G. Modafinil attenuates reinstatement of cocaine seeking: role for cystine-glutamate exchange and metabotropic glutamate receptors. *Addict Biol*. 2014;19(1):49–60.

Mahoney CR, Brunyé TT, Giles GE. Caffeine effects on aggression and risky decision making. In: Kanarek RB, Lieberman HR, eds. *Diet, Brain, Behavior: Practical Implications*. Boca Raton: Taylor & Frances Group, LLC; 2012:293.

Mahoney JJ III, Hawkins RY, De La Garza R II, Kalechstein AD, Newton TF. Relationship between gender and psychotic symptoms in cocaine-dependent and methamphetamine-dependent participants. *Gend Med*. 2010;7(5):414.

Maisto SA, Galizo M, Conner GJ. Hallucinogens. In: *Drug Use and Abuse*. 6th ed. Belmont, CA: Wadsworth; 2011:283.

Margerison-Zilko C, Cubbin C. Socioeconomic disparities in tobacco-related health outcomes across racial/ethnic groups in the United States: National Health Interview Survey 2010. *Nicotine Tob Res*. 2013;15(6):1161–1165.

Mariani JJ. Chapter 24: Sedative-, hypnotic-, or anxiolytic-related disorders. In: Sadock BJ, Sadock VA, Ruiz P, eds. *Kaplan & Sadock's Comprehensive Textbook of Psychiatry*. 10th ed. Philadelphia, PA: Wolters Kluwer; 2017:1374–1390.

Marino EN, Rosen KD, Gutierrez A, Eckmann M, Ramamurthy S, Potter JS. Impulsivity but not sensation seeking is associated with opioid analgesic misuse risk in patients with chronic pain. *Addict Behav*. 2013;38(5):2154–2157.

Martins SS, Keyes KM, Storr CL, Zhu H, Chilcoat HD. Pathways between nonmedical opioid use/dependence and psychiatric disorders: Results from the National Epidemiologic Survey on Alcohol and Related Conditions. *Drug Alcohol Depend*. 2009;103:16.

McCann UD. Amphetamine, methylphenidate, and excessive sleepiness. In: Thropy MJ, Billiard M, eds. *Sleepiness: Causes, Consequences, and Treatment*. New York: Cambridge University Press; 2011:401.

Mędraś M, Brona A, Jóźków P. The central effects of androgenic-anabolic steroid use. *J Addict Med*. 2018;2(3):184–192.

Miller PM, Anton RF. Biochemical alcohol screening in primary health care. *Addict Behav*. 2004;29:1427–1437.

Minozzi S, Cinquini M, Amato L, Davoli M, Farrell MF, Pani PP, Vecchi S. Anticonvulsants for cocaine dependence. *Cochrane Database Syst Rev*. 2015;CD006754.

Moberg CA, Curtin JJ. Alcohol selectively reduces anxiety but not fear: startle response during unpredictable versus predictable threat. *J Abnorm Psychol*. 2009;118(2):335.

Mojtabai R, Chen LY, Kaufmann CN, Crum RM. Comparing barriers to mental health treatment and substance use disorder treatment among individuals with comorbid major depression and substance use disorders. *J Subst Abuse Treat*. 2014;46(2): 268–273.

Moore EA. *The Amphetamine Debate: The Use of Adderall, Ritalin, and Related Drugs for Behavior Modification, Neuroenhancement, and Anti-Aging Purposes*. Jefferson, NC: McFarland & Co Inc.; 2011.

Morgan T, White H, Mun E. Changes in drinking before a mandated brief intervention with college students. *J Stud Alcohol Drugs*. 2008;69:286.

Mushtaq N, Beebe LA, Vesely SK, Neas BR. A multiple motive/multi-dimensional approach to measure smokeless tobacco dependence. *Addict Behav*. 2014;39(3):622–629.

Nickerson LD, Ravichandran C, Lundahl LH, Rodolico J, Dunlap S, Trksak GH, Lukas SE. Cue reactivity in cannabis-dependent adolescents. *Psychol Addict Behav*. 2011;25:168.

NIDA. "Principles of Drug Addiction Treatment: A Research-Based Guide (Third Edition)." National Institute on Drug Abuse, January 17, 2018. https://www.drugabuse.gov/publications/principles-drug-addiction-treatment-research-based-guide-third-edition. Accessed August 24, 2019.

Nilsen P. Brief alcohol intervention—where to from here? Challenges remain for research and practice. *Addiction*. 2010;105(6):954.

NSDUH, Monitoring the Future. https://www.drugabuse.gov/related-topics/trends-statistics/monitoring-future.

Odlaug BL, Marsh PJ, Kim SW, Grant JE. Strategic vs. nonstrategic gambling: Characteristics of pathological gamblers based on gambling preference. *Ann Clin Psychiatry*. 2011;3:105.

Oleski J, Cox BJ, Clara I, Hills A. Pathological gambling and the structure of common mental disorders. *J Nerv Ment Dis*. 2011;199:956.

Oreskovich MR, Kaups KL, Balch CM, Hanks JB, Satele D, Sloan J, Meredith C, Buhl A, Dyrbye LN, Shanafelt TD. Prevalence of alcohol use disorders among American surgeons. *Arch Surg*. 2012;147(2):168.

Oviedo-Joekes E, Brissette S, Marsh DC, Lauzon P, Guh D, Anis A, Schechter MT. Diacetylmorphine versus methadone for the treatment of opioid addiction. *N Engl J Med.* 2009;361:777.

Pacek LR, Martins SS, Crum RM. The bidirectional relationships between alcohol, cannabis, co-occurring alcohol and cannabis use disorders with major depressive disorder: results from a national sample. *J Affect Disord.* 2013;148:188.

Perron BE, Glass JE, Ahmedani BK, Vaughn MG, Roberts DE, Wu LT. The prevalence and clinical significance of inhalant withdrawal symptoms among a national sample. *Subst Abuse Rehabil.* 2011;2:69.

Perron BE, Howard MO, Maitra S, Vaughn MG. Prevalence, timing, and predictors of transitions from inhalant use to inhalant use disorders. *Drug Alcohol Depend.* 2009;100:277.

Perron BE, Mowbray O, Bier S, Vaughn MG, Krentzman A, Howard MO. Service use and treatment barriers among inhalant users. *J Psychoactive Drugs.* 2011;43:69.

Petry NM. Discounting of probabilistic rewards is associated with gambling abstinence in treatment-seeking pathological gamblers. *J Abnorm Psychol.* 2012;121:151.

Pope HG, Brower KJ. Treatment of anabolic-androgenic steroid-related disorders. In: Galanter M, Kleber H, eds. *The American Psychiatric Publishing Textbook of Substance Abuse Treatment.* 4th ed. Washington, DC: American Psychiatric Publishing; 2008:237.

Pope HG Jr, Kanayama G. Anabolic-androgenic steroid abuse. In: Sadock BJ, Sadock VA, Ruiz P, eds. *Kaplan & Sadock's Comprehensive Textbook of Psychiatry.* 10th ed. Philadelphia, PA: Wolters Kluwer; 2017:1390–1404.

Pope HG Jr, Kanayama G, Hudson JI. Risk Factors for illicit anabolic-androgenic steroid use in male weightlifters: A cross-sectional cohort study. *Biol Psychiatry.* 2012;71:254.

Rasmussen C, Bisnaz J. Executive functioning in children with Fetal Alcohol Spectrum Disorders: Profiles and age-related differences. *Child Neuropsychol.* 2009;15(3):201.

Reissig CJ, Strain EC, Griffiths RR. Caffeinated energy drinks—A growing problem. *Drug Alcohol Depend.* 2009;99:1.

Renner JA, Suzuki J. Opiates and prescription drugs. In: Johnson BA, ed. *Addiction Medicine: Science and Practice.* Vol. 1. New York: Springer, LLC; 2011:463.

Rich BA, Webster LR. A review of forensic implications of opioid prescribing with examples from malpractice cases involving opioid-related overdose. *Pain Med.* 2011;12:S59.

Roberts A, Landon J, Sharman S, Hakes J, Suomi A, Cowlishaw S. Gambling and physical intimate partner violence: results from the national epidemiologic survey on alcohol and related conditions (NESARC). *Am J Addict.* 2018;27:7–14.

Rodrigues R, Ramos S, Almeida N. Anabolic androgenic steroids in psychiatric practice. *Eur Neuropsychopharmacol.* 2012;22:S403.

Roman J. Nicotine-induced fibronectin expression might represent a common mechanism by which tobacco promotes lung cancer progression and obstructive airway disease. *Proc Am Thorac Soc.* 2012;9:85.

Rösner S, Hackl-Herrwerth A, Leucht S, Vecchi S, Srisurapanont M, Soyka M. Opioid antagonists for alcohol dependence. *Cochrane Database Syst Rev.* 2010; (12):CD001867.

Ruiz P, Strain EC. *The Substance Abuse Handbook.* 2nd ed. Philadelphia, PA: Lippincott Williams & Wilkins, 2014.

Sagoe D, Molde H, Andreassen CS, Torsheim T, Pallesen S. The global epidemiology of anabolic-androgenic steroid use: A meta-analysis and meta-regression analysis. *Ann Epidemiol.* 2014;24(5):383–398.

Saland SK, Rodefer JS. Environmental enrichment ameliorates phencyclidine-induced cognitive deficits. *Pharmacol Biochem Behav.* 2011;98(3):455.

Saleh T, Badshah A, Afzal K. Spontaneous acute subdural hematoma secondary to cocaine abuse. *South Med J.* 2010;103(7):714.

Sanchez ZM, Ribeiro LA, Moura YG, Noto AR, Martins SS. Inhalants as intermediate drugs between legal and illegal drugs among middle and high school students. *J Addict Dis.* 2013;32(2):217–226.

Santamarina RD, Besocke AG, Romano LM, Ioli PL, Gonorazky SE. Ischemic stroke related to anabolic abuse. *Clin Neuropharmacol.* 2008;31(2):80.

Schatzberg AF, Cole JO, DeBattista C. Phencyclidine. In: *Manual of Clinical Psychopharmacology.* 7th ed. Arlington, VA: American Psychiatric Publishing; 2010:588.

Schuckit MA. Alcohol-related disorders. In: Sadock BJ, Sadock VA, Ruiz P, eds. *Kaplan & Sadock's Comprehensive Textbook of Psychiatry.* 10th ed. Philadelphia, PA: Wolters Kluwer; 2017:1264–1279.

Scott KD, Scott AA. Adolescent inhalant use and executive cognitive functioning. *Child Care Health Dev.* 2014;40(1):20–28.

Sepkowitz KA. Energy drinks and caffeine-related adverse effects. *JAMA.* 2013;309:243.

Shaffer HJ, Martin R. Disordered gambling: Etiology, trajectory, and clinical considerations. *Annu Rev Clin Psychol.* 2011;7:483.

Smetaniuk P. A preliminary investigation into the prevalence and prediction of problematic cell phone use. *J Behav Addict.* 2014;3:41–53.

Smith HS, Kirsh KL, Passik SD. Chronic opioid therapy issues associated with opioid abuse potential. *J Opioid Manag.* 2009;5:287.

Spiegel D. Trance formations: Hypnosis in brain and body. *Depress Anxiety.* 2013; 30(4):342–352.

Stafford LD, Wright C, Yeomans MR. The drink remains the same: Implicit positive associations in high but not moderate or non-caffeine users. *Psychol Addict Behav.* 2010;24:274.

Strain EC. Chapter 11: Substance-related disorders: Introduction. In: Sadock BJ, Sadock VA, Ruiz P, eds. *Kaplan & Sadock's Comprehensive Textbook of Psychiatry.* 10th ed. Philadelphia, PA: Wolters Kluwer; 2017:1262–1264.

Suh JJ, Pettinati HM, Kampman KM, O'Brien CP. The status of disulfiram: a half of a century later. *J Clin Psychopharmacol.* 2006;26:290–302.

Svrakic DM, Lustman PJ, Mallya A, Lynn TA, Finney R, Svrakic NM. Legalization, decriminalization & medicinal use of cannabis: A scientific and public health perspective. *Mo Med.* 2012;109:90.

Tavares H, Zilberman ML, el-Guebaly N. Are there cognitive and behavioural approaches specific to the treatment of pathological gambling? *Can J Psychiatry.* 2003;48:22.

Testa A, Giannuzzi R, Sollazzo F, Petrongolo L, Bernardini L, Dain S. Psychiatric emergencies (part II): psychiatric disorders coexisting with organic diseases. *Eur Rev Med Pharmacol Sci.* 2013;17:65.

Todd G, Noyes C, Flavel SC, Della Vedova CB, Spyropoulos P, Chatterton B, Berg D, White JM. Illicit stimulant use is associated with abnormal substantia nigra morphology in humans. *PLoS One.* 2013;8(2):e56438.

Toneatto T, Brands B, Selby P. A randomized, double-blind, placebo-controlled trial of naltrexone in the treatment of concurrent alcohol use disorder and pathological gambling. *Am J Addict.* 2009;18:219.

Unger A, Jung E, Winklbaur B, Fischer G. Gender issues in the pharmacotherapy of opioid-addicted women: Buprenorphine. *J Addict Dis.* 2010;29:217.

Unger JB. The most critical unresolved issues associated with race, ethnicity, culture, and substance use. *Subst Use Misuse.* 2012;47:390.

Vallée M, Vitiello S, Bellocchio L, Hébert-Chatelain E, Monlezun S, Martin-Garcia E, Kasanetz F, Baillie GL, Panin F, Cathala A, Roullot-Lacarrière V, Fabre S, Hurst DP, Lynch DL, Shore DM, Deroche-Gamonet V, Spampinato U, Revest JM, Maldonado R, Reggio PH, Ross RA, Marsicano G, Piazza PV. Pregnenolone can protect the brain from cannabis intoxication. *Science.* 2014;343(6166):94–98.

Van der Pol P, Liebregts N, de Graaf R, Ten Have M, Korf DJ, van den Brink W, van Laar M. Mental health differences between frequent cannabis users with and without dependence and the general population. *Addiction.* 2013;108:1459.

Vergés A, Jackson KM, Bucholz KK, Grant JD, Trull TJ, Wood PK, Sher KJ. Deconstructing the age-prevalence curve of alcohol dependence: Why "maturing out" is only a small piece of the puzzle. *J Abnorm Psychol.* 2012;121:511.

Vilar-Lopez R, Takagi M, Lubman DI. The effects of inhalant misuse on attentional networks. *Dev Neuropsychol.* 2013;38(2):126–136.

Vinkers CH, Klanker M, Groenink L, Korte SM, Cook JM, Van Linn ML, Hopkins SC, Olivier B. Dissociating anxiolytic and sedative effects of GABAAergic drugs using temperature and locomotor responses to acute stress. *Psychopharmacology.* 2009;204(2):299.

Vogel M, Knopfli B, Schmid O, Prica M, Strasser J, Prieto L, Wiesbeck GA, Dursteler-Macfarland KM. Treatment or "high": Benzodiazepine use in patients on injectable heroin or oral opioids. *Addict Behav.* 2013;38(10):2477.

Warbrick T, Mobascher A, Brinkmeyer J, Musso F, Stoecker T, Shah NJ, Vossel S, Winterer G. Direction and magnitude of nicotine effects on the fMRI BOLD response are related to nicotine effects on behavioral performance. *Psychopharmacology.* 2011;215:333.

Weaver MF, Schnoll SH. Ketamine and phencyclidine. In: Johnson BA, ed. *Addiction Medicine: Science and Practice.* Vol. 1. New York: Springer, LLC; 2011:603.

Webster LR, Dasgupta N. Obtaining adequate data to determine causes of opioid-related overdose deaths. *Pain Med.* 2011;12:S86.

Weinberger AH, Desai RA, McKee SA. Nicotine withdrawal in U.S. smokers with current mood, anxiety, alcohol use, and substance use disorders. *Drug Alcohol Depend.* 2010;108:7.

Weinberger AH, Sofuoglu M. The impact of cigarette smoking on stimulant addiction. *Am J Drug Alcohol Abuse.* 2009;35:12.

Weinstein A, Lejoyeux M. Internet addiction or excessive internet use. *Am J Drug Alcohol Abuse.* 2010;36:277–283.

Weiss RD, Iannucci RA. Cocaine-related disorders. In: Sadock BJ, Sadock VA, Ruiz P, eds. *Kaplan & Sadock's Comprehensive Textbook of Psychiatry.* 9th ed. Philadelphia, PA: Lippincott Williams & Wilkins; 2009:1318.

Wilson D, da Silva Lobo DS, Tavares H, Gentil V, Vallada H. Family-based association analysis of serotonin genes in pathological gambling disorder: Evidence of vulnerability risk in the 5HT-2A receptor gene. *J Mol Neurosci.* 2013;49(3):550–553.

Winhusen T, Lewis D, Adinoff B, Brigham G, Kropp F, Donovan DM, Seamans CL, Hodgkins CC, Dicenzo JC, Botero CL, Jones DR, Somoza E. Impulsivity is associated with treatment non-completion in cocaine- and methamphetamine-dependent patients but differs in nature as a function of stimulant-dependence diagnosis. *J Subst Abuse Treat.* 2013;44(5):541–547.

Witton J, Reed KD. Cannabis and mental health. *Int J Clin Rev.* 2010;11:7.

Wood KE. Exposure to bath salts and synthetic tetrahydrocannabinol from 2009 to 2012 in the United States. *J Pediatr.* 2013;163:213.

Wu LT, Ringwalt CL, Yang C, Reeve BB, Pan JJ, Blazer DG. Construct and differential item functioning in the assessment of prescription opioid use disorders among American adolescents. *J Am Acad Child Adolesc Psychiatry.* 2009;48:563.

Wu LT, Woody GE, Yang C, Li JH, Blazer DG. Recent national trends in Salvia divinorum use and substance-use disorders among recent and former Salvia divinorum users compared with nonusers. *Subst Abuse Rehabil.* 2011;2:53.

Wynn J, Hudyma A, Hauptman E, Houston TN, Faragher JM. Treatment of problem gambling: development, status, and future. *Drugs and Alcohol Today.* 2014;14(1):6.

Yang A, Palmer AA, de Wit H. Genetics of caffeine consumption and responses to caffeine. *Psychopharmacology.* 2010;211:245.

Ziedonis DM, Tonelli ME, Das S. Tobacco-related disorders. In: Sadock BJ, Sadock VA, Ruiz P, eds. *Kaplan & Sadock's Comprehensive Textbook of Psychiatry.* 10th ed. Philadelphia, PA: Wolters Kluwer; 2017:1342–1352.

## 5

Schizophrenia Spectrum and Other Psychotic Disorders

Although we tend to discuss schizophrenia as if it is a single disease, it likely comprises a group of disorders with heterogeneous etiologies, which includes patients whose clinical presentations, treatment response, and courses of illness vary. Signs and symptoms are variable and include changes in perception, emotion, cognition, thinking, and behavior. The expression of these symptoms varies across patients and over time, but the effect of the illness is always severe and is usually long-lasting. The disorder usually begins before age 25 years, persists throughout life, and affects persons of all social classes. Both patients and their families often suffer from inadequate care and social ostracism because of widespread ignorance about the disorder. Schizophrenia is one of the most common of the severe mental disorders, but its essential nature remains to be clarified. Thus, it is sometimes referred to as a syndrome, as a group of disorders, or, as in the fifth edition of the Diagnostic and Statistical Manual of Mental Disorders (DSM-5), the schizophrenia spectrum disorders. Clinicians should appreciate that the diagnosis of schizophrenia is based entirely on psychiatric history and mental status examination. There is no laboratory test for schizophrenia.

Because schizophrenia begins early in life, causes significant and long-lasting impairments, makes heavy demands for hospital care, and requires ongoing clinical care, rehabilitation, and support services, the financial cost of the illness in the United States likely exceeds that of all cancers combined. Patients with a diagnosis of schizophrenia account for 15 to 45 percent of homeless Americans, and about 5% of patients with schizophrenia per year are homeless. Worldwide, schizophrenia is one of the top 25 leading causes of disability. This fact is striking, given its relatively low prevalence. However, this disorder affects not only individuals but families, caregivers, and societies overall. For this reason, indirect costs are enormous and often underestimated.

THE CLINICAL PRESENTATION

No clinical sign or symptom is pathognomonic for schizophrenia; every sign or symptom seen in schizophrenia occurs in other psychiatric and neurologic disorders. Therefore, a patient's history is essential for the diagnosis of schizophrenia; clinicians cannot diagnose schizophrenia only by results of a single mental status examination, as symptoms change with time. For example, a patient may have intermittent hallucinations and a varying ability to perform adequately in social situations, or significant symptoms of a mood disorder may come and go. The clinician should also take into account the patient's educational level, intellectual ability, and cultural and subcultural membership. An impaired ability to understand abstract concepts, for example, may reflect either the patient's

education or intelligence. Religious organizations and cults may have customs that seem strange to outsiders but are typical to those within the cultural setting.

The appearance of a patient with schizophrenia can range from that of a completely disheveled, screaming, agitated person to an obsessively groomed, completely silent, and immobile person. Between these two extremes, patients may be talkative and may exhibit bizarre postures. Their behavior may become agitated or violent, apparently in an unprovoked manner, but usually in response to hallucinations. Patients with schizophrenia are often poorly groomed, fail to bathe, and dress too warmly for the prevailing temperatures. Other odd behaviors include tics, stereotypies, mannerisms, and, occasionally, echopraxia, in which patients imitate the posture or the behavior of the examiner.

Patient AB, a 32-year-old woman, began to lose weight and became careless about her work, which deteriorated in quality and quantity. She believed that other women at her place of employment were circulating slanderous stories concerning her and complained that a young man employed in the same plant had put his arm around her and insulted her. Her family demanded that the charge be investigated, which showed not only that the charge was without foundation but also that the man in question had not spoken to her for months. One day she returned home from work, and as she entered the house, she laughed loudly, watched her sister-in-law suspiciously, refused to answer questions, and at the sight of her brother began to cry. She refused to go to the bathroom, saying that a man was looking in the windows at her. She ate no food, and the next day she declared that her sisters were "bad women," that everyone was talking about her, and that someone had been having sexual relations with her, and although she could not see him, he was "always around."

The patient was admitted to a public psychiatric hospital. As she entered the admitting office, she laughed loudly and repeatedly screamed in a loud tone, "She cannot stay here; she's got to go home!" She grimaced and performed various stereotyped movements of her hands. When seen on the ward an hour later, she paid no attention to questions, although she talked to herself in a childish tone. She moved about constantly, walked on her toes in a dancing manner, pointed aimlessly about, and put out her tongue and sucked her lips in the manner of an infant. At times she moaned and cried like a child but shed no tears. As the months passed, she remained silly, childish, preoccupied, and inaccessible, grimacing, gesturing, pointing at objects in a stereotyped way, and usually chattering to herself in a peculiar high-pitched voice, with little of what she said being understood. Her condition continued to deteriorate, she remained unkempt, and she presented a picture of extreme introversion and regression, with no interest either in the activities of the institution or in her relatives who visited her. (Adapted from case of Arthur P. Noyes, M.D., and Lawrence C. Kolb, M.D.)

Catatonic stupor, often referred to simply as catatonia, is a condition in which patients seem completely lifeless and may exhibit such signs as muteness, negativism, and automatic obedience. Waxy flexibility, once a common sign in catatonia, has become rare, as has manneristic behavior. A person with a less extreme subtype of catatonia may show marked social withdrawal and egocentricity, a lack of spontaneous speech or movement, and an absence of goal-directed behavior. Patients with catatonia may sit immobile and speechless in their chairs, respond to questions with only short answers, and only move when directed. Other overt behavior may include odd clumsiness or stiffness in body movements.

Localizing and nonlocalizing neurologic signs (also known as hard and soft signs, respectively) are more common in patients with schizophrenia than in other psychiatric patients. Nonlocalizing signs include dysdiadochokinesis, astereognosis, primitive reflexes, and diminished dexterity. The presence of neurologic signs and symptoms correlates with increased severity of illness, affective blunting, and a poor prognosis. Other abnormal neurologic signs include tics, stereotypies, grimacing, impaired fine motor skills, abnormal motor tone, and abnormal movements. Most patients are not aware of their abnormal involuntary movements.

In addition to the disorder of smooth ocular pursuit (saccadic movement), patients with schizophrenia have an elevated blink rate. The elevated blink rate may reflect hyperdopaminergic activity.

The inability of schizophrenia patients to perceive the prosody of speech or to inflect their speech is characteristic of disorders of the nondominant parietal lobe. Other parietal lobe–like symptoms in schizophrenia include the inability to carry out tasks (i.e., apraxia), right–left disorientation, and a lack of concern about the disorder.

Mood

Two common affective symptoms in schizophrenia are reduced emotional responsiveness, sometimes severe enough to warrant the label of anhedonia, and overly active and inappropriate emotions such as extremes of rage, happiness, and anxiety. A flat or blunted affect can be a symptom of the illness itself, of the parkinsonian adverse effects of antipsychotic medications, or depression, and differentiating these symptoms can be a clinical challenge. Overly emotional patients may describe exultant feelings of omnipotence, religious ecstasy, terror at the disintegration of their souls, or paralyzing anxiety about the destruction of the universe. Other feeling tones include perplexity, a sense of isolation, overwhelming ambivalence, and depression.

Thoughts

Psychotic disorders are, first and foremost, thought disorders and the disorder may affect either the process or content of their thought or both. A schizophrenia patient's thoughts may be challenging to understand and elicit. However, this is essential, as thought symptoms may represent the core symptoms of schizophrenia.

Disorders of thought concern the way we formulate ideas and languages. We sometimes call these *formal thought disorders*. The examiner infers a disorder from what and how the patient speaks, writes, or draws. The examiner may also assess the patient's thought process by observing their behavior, especially in carrying out discrete tasks (e.g., in occupational therapy).

When mild, thought disorders might present as stilted or vague. As it worsens, associations become looser. The patient may display circumstantiality, tangential thinking, perseverative thinking, neologisms, echolalia, verbigeration, word salad, and mutism.

Delusions

Delusions, the most obvious example of a disorder of thought content, are varied in schizophrenia and may assume persecutory, grandiose, religious, or somatic forms.

Patients may believe that an outside entity controls their thoughts or behavior or, conversely, that they extraordinarily control outside events (such as causing the sun to rise). Patients may have an intense and consuming preoccupation with esoteric, abstract, symbolic, psychological, or philosophic ideas. Patients may also worry about allegedly life-threatening but bizarre and implausible somatic conditions, such as the presence of aliens inside the patient's testicles affecting his ability to father children.

The phrase *loss of ego boundaries* describes the lack of a clear sense of where the patient's own body, mind, and influence end and where those of other animate and inanimate objects begin. For example, patients may think that other persons, the television, or the newspapers are referring to them (ideas of reference). Thought control, in which outside forces are controlling what the patient thinks or feels, is common, as is thought broadcasting, in which patients think others can read their minds or that they can broadcast their thoughts through televisions.

Other signs of a loss of ego boundaries include the sense that the patient has physically fused with an external object (e.g., a tree or another person) or that the patient has disintegrated and fused with the entire universe (cosmic identity). With such a state of mind, some patients with schizophrenia doubt their gender or their sexual orientation. These symptoms should not be confused with gender identity problems.

Hallucinations

Any of the five senses may be affected by hallucinatory experiences in patients with schizophrenia. The most common hallucinations, however, are auditory, with voices that are often threatening, obscene, accusatory, or insulting. Two or more voices may converse among themselves, or a voice may comment on the patient's life or behavior.

A 48-year-old man, who had been diagnosed with schizophrenia while in the army at age 21 years, led an isolated and often frightened existence, living alone and supported by disability payments. Although he would confirm that he had chronic auditory hallucinations, he was never comfortable with discussing the content of these hallucinations, and a review of records showed this was a long-term pattern for the patient. Otherwise the patient had good rapport with his psychiatrist and was enthusiastic about the possibility of participating in a study of a novel antipsychotic agent. During the informed consent procedure, the patient asked about the possibility that the new medication might decrease his chronic auditory hallucinations. When it was acknowledged that any response was possible, including decreases in his hallucinations, the patient broke off the discussion abruptly and left the office. At a later visit, he reported that his most reliable pleasure in life was nightly discussions of gossip with hallucinations of voices he believed belonged to 17th-century French courtiers, and the chance that he might lose these conversations and the companionship they offered was too frightening for him to consider. (Adapted from Stephen Lewis, M.D., P. Rodrigo Escalona, M.D., and Samuel J. Keith, M.D.)

Visual hallucinations are common, but tactile, olfactory, and gustatory hallucinations are unusual; their presence should prompt the clinician to consider the possibility of an underlying medical or neurologic disorder that is causing the entire syndrome.

Psychotic disorders can affect other senses, as well. For example, *cenesthetic hallucinations* are unfounded sensations of altered states in bodily organs. Examples of cenesthetic hallucinations include a burning sensation in the brain, a pushing sensation in the blood vessels, and a cutting sensation in the bone marrow. Bodily distortions may also occur.

Cognition

Patients with schizophrenia are usually oriented to person, time, and place. The lack of such orientation should prompt clinicians to investigate the possibility of a medical or neurologic brain disorder. Some patients with schizophrenia may give incorrect or bizarre answers stemming from their delusions, such as "I am Christ; this is heaven, and it is AD 35."

Memory, as tested in the mental status examination, is usually intact, but there can be minor cognitive deficiencies. It may not be possible, however, to get the patient to attend closely enough to the memory tests for the ability to be assessed adequately.

A significant development in the understanding of the psychopathology of schizophrenia is the appreciation of subtle cognitive impairment. In outpatients, cognitive impairment is a better predictor of the level of function than is the severity of psychotic symptoms. Patients with schizophrenia typically exhibit subtle cognitive dysfunction in the domains of attention, executive function, working memory, and episodic memory. Although a substantial percentage of patients have average intelligence quotients, every person who has schizophrenia may have cognitive dysfunction compared with what he or she would be able to do without the disorder. Although these impairments cannot function as diagnostic tools, they are strongly related to the functional outcome of the illness and, for that reason, have clinical value as prognostic variables, as well as for treatment planning.

The cognitive impairment seems already to be present when patients have their first episode and appear largely to remain stable throughout the early illness. There may be a small subgroup of patients who have true dementia in late life that is not due to other cognitive disorders, such as Alzheimer disease. Cognitive impairments are also present in attenuated forms in nonpsychotic relatives of schizophrenia patients.

The cognitive impairments of schizophrenia have become the target of pharmacologic and psychosocial treatment trials. Hopefully, effective treatments for these impairments will become available soon.

Insight and Judgment and Reliability

Classically, patients with schizophrenia have poor insight into the nature and severity of their disorder. The so-called lack of insight is associated with poor compliance with treatment. When examining schizophrenia patients, clinicians should carefully define various aspects of insight, such as awareness of symptoms, trouble getting along with people, and the reasons for these problems. Such information can be clinically useful in tailoring a treatment strategy and theoretically useful in postulating what areas of the brain contribute to the observed lack of insight (e.g., the parietal lobes).

A patient with schizophrenia is no less reliable than any other psychiatric patient. The nature of the disorder, however, requires the examiner to verify relevant information through additional sources.

Safety Concerns

Patients with schizophrenia may be agitated and have little impulse control when ill. They may also have decreased social sensitivity and appear to be impulsive when, for example, they grab another patient's cigarettes, change television channels abruptly, or throw food on the floor. Some impulsive behavior, including suicide and homicide attempts, may be in response to hallucinations commanding the patient to act.

Violent behavior (excluding homicide) is common among untreated schizophrenia patients, and the increased odds of a patient with schizophrenia committing acts of violence, compared to the general population, is 49% to 68%. Delusions of a persecutory nature, previous episodes of violence, and neurologic deficits are risk factors for violent or impulsive behavior. If a clinician feels fearful in the presence of a schizophrenic patient, they should take this as an internal clue that the patient may be on the verge of acting out violently. In such cases, the clinician should terminate the interview or conduct it with an attendant at the ready.

Suicide.   Suicide is the single leading cause of premature death among people with schizophrenia. The lifetime prevalence of suicidality in patients with schizophrenia is about 34.5 percent. Suicide attempts are made by 20 to 50 percent of the patients, with long-term rates of suicide estimated to be 10 to 13 percent. According to DSM-5, approximately 5 to 6 percent of schizophrenic patients die by suicide, but this is probably an underestimation. Often, suicide in schizophrenia seems to occur "out of the blue," without prior warnings or expressions of verbal intent. The most crucial factor is the presence of a major depressive episode. Epidemiologic studies indicate that up to 80 percent of schizophrenia patients may have a major depressive episode at some time in their lives. Some data suggest that those patients with the best prognosis (few negative symptoms, preservation of capacity to experience affects, better abstract thinking) can paradoxically also be at the highest risk for suicide. The profile of the patient at most significant risk is a young man who once had high expectations, declined from a higher level of functioning, realizes that his dreams are not likely to come true, and has lost faith in the effectiveness of treatment. Other possible contributors to the high rate of suicide include command hallucinations and drug abuse. Two-thirds or more of schizophrenic patients who commit suicide have seen an unsuspecting clinician within 72 hours of death. A large pharmacologic study suggests that clozapine may have particular efficacy in reducing suicidal ideation in schizophrenia patients with prior hospitalizations for suicidality. Adjunctive antidepressant medications may be effective for alleviating cooccurring major depression in schizophrenia.

Homicide.   Despite the sensational attention that the news media provides when a patient with schizophrenia murders someone, the available data indicate that these patients are no more likely to commit homicide than is a member of the general population. When a patient with schizophrenia does commit homicide, it may be for unpredictable or bizarre reasons based on hallucinations or delusions. Possible predictors of homicidal activity are a history of previous violence, dangerous behavior while hospitalized, and hallucinations or delusions involving violence.

The Symptoms of Schizophrenia Can be Divided into Three Groupings

We can divide the symptoms of schizophrenia into three groups: positive, negative, and cognitive.

Positive Symptoms Are Abnormal Behaviors. Positive symptoms are symptoms that are present and usually observable. These are the symptoms associated with an acute psychotic episode and are primarily disorders of thought and presentation. They include hallucinations, delusions, and other bizarre behaviors. Table 5-1 lists examples of positive symptoms.

Negative Symptoms Are the Absence of Normal Behaviors. Negative symptoms are defined by their absence and sometimes also called deficit symptoms. They are commonly associated with the progression of the illness. These include the absence of affect, the absence of thought, the absence of motivation, the absence of pleasure, and the absence of attention. Table 5-2 lists examples of negative symptoms.

Cognitive Symptoms Are Impairments in Normal Cognitive Functions. The cognitive symptoms of schizophrenia may be subtle, particularly early in the disease process, but are very impairing and account for much of the disability associated with this disorder. They include impairments of attention, working memory, and executive functioning.

Table 5-1
Positive Symptoms

Hallucinations
　　Auditory hallucinations
　　Voices commenting
　　Voices conversing
　　Somatic or tactile hallucinations
　　Olfactory hallucinations
　　Visual hallucinations
Delusions
　　Persecutory delusions
　　Delusions of jealousy
　　Delusions of guilt or sin
　　Grandiose delusions
　　Religious delusions
　　Somatic delusions
　　Delusions of reference
　　Delusions of being controlled
　　Delusions of mind reading
　　Thought broadcasting
　　Thought insertion
　　Thought withdrawal
Bizarre behavior
　　Clothing and behavior
　　Social and sexual behavior
　　Aggressive behavior
　　Repetitive or stereotyped behavior
Positive formal thought disorder
　　Derailment
　　Tangentiality
　　Incoherence
　　Illogicality
　　Circumstantiality
　　Pressure of speech
　　Distractible speech
　　Clanging

Table 5-2
Negative Symptoms

Affective flattening or blunting
　　Unchanging facial expressions
　　Decreased spontaneous movement
　　Paucity of expressive gesture
　　Poor eye contact
　　Affective nonresponsivity
　　Inappropriate affect
　　Lack of vocal inflections
Alogia
　　Poverty of speech
　　Poverty of content of speech
　　Blocking
　　Increased latency of response
Avolition—apathy
　　Grooming and hygiene
　　Impersistence at work or school
　　Physical anergia
Anhedonia—asociality
　　Recreational interests and activities
　　Sexual interest and activities
　　Intimacy and closeness
　　Relationships with friends
Attention
　　Social inattentiveness
　　Inattentiveness during testing

Presentation in Special Populations

The Disorder in Children and Adolescents. A small minority of patients manifest schizophrenia in childhood. Such children may at first present diagnostic problems, particularly with differentiation from mental retardation and autistic disorder. Recent studies have established that we should base our diagnosis of childhood schizophrenia on the same symptoms used for adult schizophrenia. Its onset is usually insidious, its course tends to be chronic, and the prognosis is mostly unfavorable.

The Disorder in Older People. Late-onset schizophrenia is clinically indistinguishable from schizophrenia but has an onset after age 45 years. This condition tends to appear more frequently in women and tends to be characterized by a predominance of paranoid symptoms. The prognosis is favorable, and these patients usually do well on antipsychotic medication.

DIAGNOSIS

Schizophrenia

Table 5-3 compares the different approaches to diagnosing schizophrenia. The patient should have evidence of a psychotic disorder. However, the presence of hallucinations or delusions is not necessary for a diagnosis of schizophrenia; the patient's disorder is diagnosed as schizophrenia when the patient demonstrates any two of the several symptoms included under the broad category of "psychotic symptoms." These symptoms should persist for an extended time: 6 months for DSM-5 and 1 month for ICD-10. The DSM-5 diagnostic criteria include course specifiers (i.e., prognosis) that offer clinicians several options and describe actual clinical situations.

Catatonic Type. The catatonic type of schizophrenia, which was prevalent several decades ago, has become rare in Europe and North America. The classic feature of the catatonic type is a marked

Table 5-3
Schizophrenia

	DSM-5	ICD-10
Diagnostic name	Schizophrenia	Schizophrenia
Duration	Symptoms present continuously for at least 6 mo	
Symptoms	Delusions Hallucinations Disorganization of speech Disorganization of behavior or catatonia Negative symptoms	Thought distortions Perceptual disorders Negative affect, often blunted Possible cognitive dysfunction Other possible symptoms: • Thought echo • Thought insertion or withdrawal • Thought broadcasting • Delusional perception • Delusions of control, influence, or passivity • Hallucinatory voices • Disordered/disorganized thinking • Negative symptoms
Required number of symptoms	≥2, including at least 1 of the first 3 listed	Defined by the first three listed, although the other symptoms are considered common
Psychosocial consequences of symptoms	Functional impairment	
Exclusions (not better explained by):	Substances Other medical conditions Other psychiatric conditions	Other neurologic diseases Schizoaffective disorder Epilepsy Psychoactive substances
Symptom Specifiers	**With catatonia,** defined as presence of three or more of the following: • ↓ psychomotor activity/stupor • Catalepsy (holding a posture for an extended period) • Waxy flexibility (hold a position but movable to a new posture as if made of wax) • Mutism • Negativism • Posturing • Odd mannerisms • Stereotypic behaviors • Agitation • Grimacing • Echolalia (imitating another's speech) • Echopraxia (imitating another's movements)	**Paranoid schizophrenia**—primarily defined by delusions. Less or no disturbance of affect or volition **Hebephrenic schizophrenia**—negative affect with inappropriate mood, social isolation and unpredictable behavior **Catatonic schizophrenia**—psychomotor changes, such as posturing, odd mannerisms/affect, stupor vs. agitation **Undifferentiated Schizophrenia** **Residual schizophrenia**—chronic illness and cognitive changes resulting from a prolonged psychotic illness **Simple schizophrenia**—slow progressive development of changes in behavior and functioning, affective blunting without preceding psychotic symptoms **Other Schizophrenia** **Schizophrenia unspecified**
Course specifiers	**First episode, currently in acute episode** **First episode, currently in partial remission:** currently less symptoms than needed for diagnosis **First episode, currently in full remission:** 0 symptoms **Multiple episodes, currently in acute episode:** ≥2 episodes **Multiple episodes, currently in partial remission** **Multiple episodes, currently in full remission** **Continuous** **Unspecified**	

disturbance in motor function; this disturbance may involve stupor, negativism, rigidity, excitement, or posturing.

AC, age 32 years, was admitted to the hospital. On arrival, he was noted to be an asthenic, poorly nourished man with dilated pupils, hyperactive tendon reflexes, and a pulse rate of 120 beats/min. He showed many mannerisms, laid down on the floor, pulled at his foot, made undirected violent striking movements, struck attendants, grimaced, assumed rigid and strange postures, refused to speak, and appeared to be having auditory hallucinations. When seen later in the day, he

was found to be in a stuporous state. His face was without expression, he was mute and rigid, and he paid no attention to those about him or to their questions. His eyes were closed, and his eyelids could be separated only with effort. There was no response to pinpricks or other painful stimuli.

He gradually became accessible, and when asked concerning himself, he referred to his stuporous period as sleep and maintained that he had no recollection of any events occurring during it. He said, "I didn't know anything. Everything seemed to be dark as far as my mind is concerned. Then I began to see a little light, like the shape of a star. Then my head got through the star gradually. I saw more and more light until I saw everything in a perfect form a few days ago." He explained his mutism by saying that he had been afraid he would "say the wrong thing" and that he "didn't know exactly what to talk about." From his obviously inadequate emotional response and his statement that he was "a scientist and an inventor of the most extraordinary genius of the 20th century," it was plain that he was still far from well. (Adapted from case of Arthur P. Noyes, M.D., Lawrence C. Kolb, M.D.)

Sometimes the patient shows a rapid alternation between extremes of excitement and stupor. Associated features include stereotypies, mannerisms, and waxy flexibility. Mutism is particularly common. During catatonic excitement, patients need careful supervision to prevent them from hurting themselves or others. Patients also often require medical care because of malnutrition, exhaustion, hyperpyrexia, or self-inflicted injury.

Subtypes from Previous Versions of DSM. Previous versions of the DSM described subtypes of schizophrenia based predominantly on the clinical features. These were: paranoid, disorganized, catatonic, undifferentiated, and residual subtype. DSM-5 no longer includes these as experts in the field frequently questioned their validity. ICD-10 does continue to include them. Although having some face validity for clinicians, they have only a weak relationship to biologic variables, poor long-term stability, and poor predictive value.

Schizoaffective Disorder

Schizoaffective disorder has features of both schizophrenia and mood disorders. In current diagnostic systems, patients can receive the diagnosis of schizoaffective disorder if they fit into one of the following six categories: (1) patients with schizophrenia who have mood symptoms, (2) patients with a mood disorder who have symptoms of schizophrenia, (3) patients with both mood disorder and schizophrenia, (4) patients with a third psychosis unrelated to schizophrenia and mood disorder, (5) patients whose disorder is on a continuum between schizophrenia and mood disorder, and (6) patients with some combination of the above. Clinicians frequently use a preliminary diagnosis of schizoaffective disorder when they are uncertain of the diagnosis.

It remains unclear whether the disorder is a subtype of schizophrenia, a mood disorder, or the simultaneous expression of each. It is unlikely that this represents a simultaneous expression of both disorders, as it appears to be more common than would be expected for coincidental co-occurrence. Schizoaffective disorder may also be a third distinct type of psychosis, one that is unrelated to either schizophrenia or a mood disorder. The most likely possibility is that schizoaffective disorder is a heterogeneous group of disorders encompassing all of these possibilities. As will be discussed below, the genetic abnormalities in schizophrenia overlap with that for mood disorders, making an overlap between the disorders more likely.

In the DSM-5 criteria for schizoaffective disorder, the clinician must accurately diagnose the mood disorder, making sure it meets the criteria of either a manic or depressive episode but also determining the exact length of each episode (not always easy or even possible). Table 5-4 compares the diagnostic approaches to schizoaffective disorder.

The length of each episode is critical for two reasons. First, to meet the requirement that the psychotic symptoms must also occur independently of the mood symptoms, it is essential to know when the affective episode ends, and the psychosis continues. Second, the relative lengths of the mood and psychotic episodes should be roughly equal, which requires us to know the course of the episodes.

Mrs. P is a 47-year-old, divorced, unemployed woman who lived alone and who experienced chronic psychotic symptoms despite treatment with olanzapine 20 mg per day and citalopram 20 mg per day. She believed that she was getting messages from God and the police department to go on a mission to fight against drugs. She also believed that an organized crime group was trying to stop her in this pursuit. The onset of her illness began at age 20 years when she experienced the first of several depressive episodes. She also described periods when she felt more energetic and talkative, had a decreased need for sleep, and was more active, sometimes cleaning her house throughout the night. About 4 years after the onset of her symptoms, she began to hear "voices" that became stronger when she was depressed but were still present and disturbed her even when her mood was euthymic. About 10 years after her illness began, she developed the belief that policemen were everywhere and that the neighbors were spying on her. She was hospitalized voluntarily. Two years later, she had another depressive episode, and the auditory hallucinations told her she could not live in her apartment. She was tried on lithium, antidepressants, and antipsychotic medications but continued to be chronically symptomatic with mood symptoms as well as psychosis.

Mrs. P demonstrates a "classic" presentation of schizoaffective disorder in which clear depressive and hypomanic episodes are present in combination with continuous psychotic illness and first-rank symptoms. Her course is typical of many individuals with schizoaffective disorder.

Schizophreniform Disorder

The symptoms of schizophreniform are similar to those of schizophrenia. However, with schizophreniform disorder, the symptoms are short term, lasting at least 1 month but less than 6 months. Patients with schizophreniform disorder should then return to their baseline level of functioning.

Like schizoaffective disorder, schizophreniform disorder appears to be a heterogeneous disorder. Many patients seem to have a disorder that is similar to schizophrenia, while others may have a disorder more like a mood disorder.

Table 5-5 compares the diagnostic approaches to schizophreniform disorder.

The disorder is an acute psychotic disorder with a rapid onset. It lacks a long prodromal phase. Although many patients with schizophreniform disorder may experience functional impairment at the time of an episode, they are unlikely to report a progressive decline in social and occupational functioning. The initial symptom profile is the same as for schizophrenia in that two or more psychotic symptoms must be present.

By definition, patients with schizophreniform disorder have the symptoms for at least a month and return to their baseline state within 6 months. In some instances, the illness is episodic, with more than one episode occurring after long periods of full remission. If the combined duration of symptomatology exceeds 6 months, however, then schizophrenia should be considered.

Mr. C, a 28-year-old accountant, was brought to the emergency department by the police in handcuffs. He was disheveled and shouted and struggled with the police officers. It was apparent that he was hearing voices because he would respond to them with shouts such as, "Shut up! I told you I won't do it!" However, when confronted about the voices, he denied hearing anything. Mr. C had a hypervigilant stare and

Table 5-4
Schizoaffective Disorder

	DSM-5	ICD-10
Diagnostic name	Schizoaffective Disorder	Schizoaffective disorders
Duration	Mood symptoms present majority of time during the illness However, there is also a 2-wk period of psychotic symptoms without mood symptoms	
Symptoms	Meets criteria for a major depressive or manic episode Meets criteria for Schizophrenia	Symptoms of affective episode and schizophrenic symptoms
Required number of symptoms	See criteria for the individual disorders	
Psychosocial consequences of symptoms	Functional impairment	
Exclusions (not better explained by):	Substance use Another mental illness Another medical condition	Schizophrenia Depressive/manic episodes
Symptom Specifiers	**Bipolar Type:** manic episode **Depressive Type:** depressive episode **With catatonia:** See Table 5-3 for catatonia symptoms	**Schizoaffective disorder, manic type** **Schizoaffective disorder, depressive type** **Schizoaffective disorder, mixed type** **Schizoaffective disorder, unspecified** **Other schizoaffective disorder**
Course specifiers	**First episode, currently in acute episode** **First episode, currently in partial remission:** currently less symptoms than needed for diagnosis **First episode, currently in full remission:** 0 symptoms **Multiple episodes, currently in acute episode:** ≥2 episodes **Multiple episodes, currently in partial remission** **Multiple episodes, currently in full remission** **Continuous** **Unspecified**	

Table 5-5
Schizophreniform Disorder

	DSM-5	ICD-10
Diagnostic name	Schizophreniform Disorder	Acute and Transient psychotic disorder
Duration	≥1 mo, but <6 mo	<1 mo on average

Symptoms	Same as schizophrenia (see Table 5-3)	Symptoms of schizophrenia, including:
		  Thought echo
		  Thought insertion or withdrawal
		  Thought broadcasting
		  Delusional perception
		  Delusions of control, influence, or passivity
		  Hallucinatory voices
		  Disordered/disorganized thinking
		  Negative symptoms
		May or may not be associated with polymorphic (unstable, frequently changing) delusions, hallucinations and/or behavioral symptoms

Required number of symptoms	Same as schizophrenia (see Table 5-3)	
Exclusions (not better explained by):	Same as schizophrenia (see Table 5-3)	If symptoms persist, diagnosis should be changed to schizophrenia
Symptom Specifiers	**With catatonia:** See Table 5-3 for catatonia symptoms	

Course specifiers	**With good prognostic features:**
	≥2 of following:
	  Psychotic symptoms within 4 wk of initial behavioral changes
	  Confusion
	  Good premorbid function
	  No negative symptoms
	Without good prognostic features	

jumped at the slightest noise. He stated that he must run away quickly because he knew he would be killed shortly otherwise.

Mr. C was functioning well until 2 months before hospitalization. He was an accountant at a prestigious company and had close friends and a live-in girlfriend. Most people who knew him would describe him as friendly, but he was occasionally quarrelsome.

When his girlfriend suddenly broke off the relationship and moved out of their apartment, Mr. C was distressed. However, he was convinced that he could win her back, so he began to "accidentally" run into her at her job or her new apartment with flowers and various gifts. When she strongly told him that she wanted nothing more to do with him and requested that he leave her alone, Mr. C was convinced that she wanted him dead. He became so preoccupied with this notion that his work began to suffer. Out of fear for his life, Mr. C took off from work frequently, and when he did report to work, he was often tardy and did subpar work, making many errors. His supervisor confronted Mr. C about his behavior, threatening termination if it continued. Mr. C was embarrassed and resented his supervisor for the confrontation. He believed that his ex-girlfriend had hired the supervisor to kill him.

His beliefs were confirmed by a voice that would mock him. The voice told him time and again that he should quit his job, relocate to another city, and forget about his ex-girlfriend, but Mr. C refused, believing it would give them "more satisfaction than they deserved." He continued working, albeit cautiously, all the while fearing for his life.

Through it all, Mr. C believed himself to be the lone victim. He would awake abruptly at night from nightmares but would be able to fall right back to sleep. He had not lost any weight and had no other vegetative symptoms. His affect alternated between rage and terror. His mind was unusually alert and active, but he was not otherwise hyperactive, excessively energetic, or expansive. He did not display any formal thought disorder.

Mr. C was hospitalized and treated with antipsychotic medication. His symptoms remitted after several weeks of treatment, and he was well and able to return to work shortly after discharge.

Perhaps 60 to 80 percent of patients with this disorder will later develop schizophrenia. The remaining may have relapses of similar time-limited episodes of the disease, whereas some, although unfortunately only a few patients, will have only a single episode.

Brief Psychotic Disorder

Brief psychotic disorder is defined as a psychotic condition that involves the sudden onset of psychotic symptoms, which lasts 1 day or more but less than 1 month. Remission is full, and the individual returns to the premorbid level of functioning. Brief psychotic disorder is an acute and transient psychotic syndrome. The exact incidence and prevalence of brief psychotic disorder is not known, but it is generally considered uncommon. The disorder occurs more often among younger patients (20s and 30s) than among older patients. Brief psychotic disorder is more common in women than in men. Such epidemiologic patterns are sharply distinct from those of schizophrenia. Some clinicians indicate that the disorder may be seen most frequently in patients from low socioeconomic classes and in those who have experienced disasters or major cultural changes (e.g., immigrants). The age of onset in industrialized settings may be higher than in developing countries. Table 5-6 compares the diagnostic approaches to brief psychotic disorder.

The cause of the disorder is not known, however it is common in patients with personality disorders. Persons who have gone through major psychosocial stressors may be at greater risk for subsequent brief psychotic disorder.

The symptoms of brief psychotic disorder always include at least one major symptom of psychosis, such as hallucinations, delusions, and disorganized thoughts, usually with an abrupt onset, but do not always include the entire symptom pattern seen in schizophrenia. Some clinicians have observed that labile mood, confusion, and impaired attention may be more common at the onset of brief psychotic disorder than at the onset of eventually chronic psychotic disorders. Characteristic symptoms in brief

Table 5-6
Brief Psychotic Disorder

	DSM-5	ICD-10
Diagnostic name	Brief Psychotic Disorder	See Table 5-5 definition of Acute and Transient psychotic disorder—ICD 10 does not distinguish between these two disorders
Duration	≥1 day, <1 mo with return to baseline	
Symptoms	Same as for schizophrenia (see Table 5-3) except negative symptoms not included	
Required number of symptoms	1 of first 3 symptoms (delusions, hallucinations or disorganized speech) +/− behavioral symptoms	
Exclusions (not better explained by):	Culturally sanctioned response/behavior Another mental illness Substance use Another medical condition	
Symptom Specifiers	**With marked stressors** **Without marked stressors** **With catatonia:** See Table 5-3 for catatonia symptoms	
Course specifiers	**With peripartum onset:** during pregnancy or ≤4 wk after delivery	

psychotic disorder include emotional volatility, strange or bizarre behavior, screaming or muteness, and impaired memory of recent events. Some of the symptoms suggest a diagnosis of delirium and warrant a medical workup, especially to rule out adverse reactions to drugs.

A 20-year-old man was admitted to the psychiatric ward of a hospital shortly after starting military duty. During the first week after his arrival to the military base, he thought the other recruits looked at him in a strange way. He watched the people around him to see whether they were out "to get" him. He heard voices calling his name several times. He became increasingly suspicious and after another week had to be admitted for psychiatric evaluation. There he was guarded, scowling, skeptical, and depressed. He gave the impression of being very shy and inhibited. His psychotic symptoms disappeared rapidly when he was treated with an antipsychotic drug. However, he had difficulties in adjusting to hospital life. Transfer to a long-term medical hospital was considered, but after 3 months, a decision was made to discharge him to his home. He was subsequently judged unfit to return to military services.

The patient was the eldest of five siblings. His father was an intemperate drinker who became angry and brutal when drunk. The family was poor, and there were constant fights between the parents. As a child, the patient was inhibited and fearful and often ran into the woods when troubled. He had academic difficulties.

When the patient got older, he preferred to spend time alone and disliked being with people. He occasionally took part in local parties. Although he was never a heavy drinker, he often got into fights when he had a drink or two.

The patient was reinterviewed by hospital personnel at 4 years, 7 years, and 23 years after his admission. He has had no recurrences of any psychotic symptoms and has been fully employed since 6 months after he left the hospital. He married, and at the last follow-up, he had two grown children.

After leaving the hospital, the patient worked for 2 years in a factory. For the past 20 years, he has managed a small business, and it has run well. He has been very happy at work and in his family life. He has made an effort to overcome his tendency toward isolation and has several friends.

The patient believes that his natural tendency is to be socially isolated and that his disorder was connected with the fact that in the military, he was forced to deal with other people. (Adapted from Laura J. Fochtmann, M.D., Ramin Mojtabai, M.D., Ph.D., M.P.H., and Evelyn J. Bromet, Ph.D.)

Delusional Disorder

The diagnosis of delusional disorder is made when a person exhibits one or more delusions of at least 1 month's duration that cannot be attributed to other psychiatric disorders. The delusions are often nonbizarre, meaning that the delusions are about situations that can occur in real life, such as being followed, infected, loved at a distance, and so on; that is, they usually have to do with phenomena that, although not real, are nonetheless possible. Several types of delusions may be present. Table 5-7 compares the diagnostic approaches to delusional disorder.

Table 5-7
Delusional Disorder

	DSM-5	ICD-10
Diagnostic name	Delusional Disorder	Delusional Disorder
Duration	≥1 mo	
Symptoms	Delusions (see symptom specifiers for examples)	Delusions Persistent +/− hallucinations
Required number of symptoms	≥1	≥1 delusions
Psychosocial consequences of symptoms	No marked functional impairment	
Exclusions (not better explained by):	Schizophrenia Another medical condition Substance use Another mental illness	Personality disorder Psychosis Psychogenic reaction Schizophrenia
Symptom Specifiers	**Erotomanic type** **Grandiose type** **Jealous type** **Persecutory type** **Somatic type** **Mixed type** **Unspecified type** **With bizarre content:** if not related to reality or a life experience or not possible, include this specifier	
Course specifiers	**First episode, currently in acute episode** **First episode, currently in partial remission:** currently less symptoms than needed for diagnosis **First episode, currently in full remission:** 0 symptoms **Multiple episodes, currently in acute episode:** ≥2 episodes **Multiple episodes, currently in partial remission** **Multiple episodes, currently in full remission** **Continuous** **Unspecified**	

Patients are usually well groomed and well dressed, without evidence of gross disintegration of personality or of daily activities, yet they may seem eccentric, odd, suspicious, or hostile. They are sometimes litigious and may make this inclination clear to the examiner. The most remarkable feature of patients with delusional disorder is that the mental status examination shows them to be quite normal except for a markedly abnormal delusional system. Patients may attempt to engage clinicians as allies in their delusions, but a clinician should not pretend to accept the delusion; this collusion further confounds reality and sets the stage for eventual distrust between the patient and the therapist.

Patients' moods are consistent with the content of their delusions. A patient with grandiose delusions is euphoric; one with persecutory delusions is suspicious. Whatever the nature of the delusional system, the examiner may sense some mild depressive qualities.

By definition, patients with delusional disorder do not have prominent or sustained hallucinations. A few delusional patients have other hallucinatory experiences—virtually always auditory rather than visual. They also have generally normal cognition apart from their delusion.

The disorders can be of several types, and in the diagnosis the clinician should specify the type. The types include: persecutory (believing others are trying to harm them), jealous (believing that a lover or partner is unfaithful), erotomanic (believing that another person, often of higher status, is in love with them), somatic (believing the person has some physical disorder), and grandiose (a "delusion of grandeur"). There is also a mixed and unspecified type, for delusions that are a combination of types or not described by one of the categories. Of these types, persecutory and jealous are probably the most common.

Mrs. S, a 62-year-old-woman, was referred to a psychiatrist because of reports of being unable to sleep. She had previously worked full time taking care of children, and she played tennis almost every day and managed her household chores. However, she had now become preoccupied with the idea that her downstairs neighbor was doing a variety of things to harass her and wanted to get her to move away. At first, Mrs. S based her belief on certain looks that he gave her and damage done to her mailbox, but later she felt he might be leaving empty bottles of cleaning solutions in the basement so she would be overcome by fumes. As a result, the patient was fearful of falling asleep, convinced that she might be asphyxiated and unable to awaken in time to get help. She felt somewhat depressed and thought her appetite might be decreased from the stress of being harassed. However, she had not lost weight and still enjoyed playing tennis and going out with friends. At one point she considered moving to another apartment but then decided to fight back. The episode had gone on for 8 months when her daughter persuaded her to have a psychiatric assessment. In the interview, Mrs. S was pleasant and cooperative. Except for mild depressive symptoms and the specific delusion about being harassed by her neighbor, her mental status was normal.

Mrs. S had a past history of depression 30 years before, which followed the death of a close friend. She saw a counselor for several months and found this helpful, but she was not treated with medication. For the current episode, she agreed to take medications, although she believed her neighbor was more in need of treatment than she was. Her symptoms improved somewhat with risperidone 2 mg at bedtime and clonazepam 0.5 mg every morning and at bedtime.

This patient presented with a single delusion regarding her neighbor that was within the realm of possibility (i.e., not bizarre). Other areas of her functioning were normal. Although mild depressive symptoms

---

were present, she did not meet criteria for major depressive disorder. Her prior symptoms of depression appeared to be related to a normal bereavement reaction and had not required pharmacotherapy or hospitalization. Thus, her current presentation is one of delusional disorder, persecutory type and not major depressive disorder with psychotic features. In terms of treatment, the ability to create a working alliance with the patient, avoiding the discussion of the veracity of her delusion, and focusing on her anxiety, depression, and difficulty falling asleep enabled her psychiatrist to introduce the medications with beneficial results. (Courtesy of Laura J. Fochtmann, M.D., Ramin Mojtabai, M.D., Ph.D., M.P.H., and Evelyn J. Bromet, Ph.D.)

Mr. M was a 51-year-old married white man who lived with his wife in their own home and who worked full time driving a sanitation truck. Before his hospitalization, he became concerned that his wife was having an affair. He began to follow her, kept notes on his observations, and badgered her constantly about this, often waking her up in the middle of the night to make accusations. Shortly before admission, these arguments led to physical violence, and he was brought to the hospital by police. In addition to concerns about his wife's fidelity, Mr. M reported feelings of depression over his wife's "betrayal of [their] marriage vows," but he noted no changes in sleep, appetite, or work-related functioning. He was treated with a low dose of an antipsychotic medication and described being less concerned about his wife's behavior. After discharge, he remained on medications and was seen by a psychiatrist monthly, but 10 years later, he continued to believe that his wife was unfaithful. His wife noted that he sometimes became upset about the delusion but that he had not become aggressive or required readmission.

This patient experienced a fixed, encapsulated delusion of jealousy that did not interfere with his other activities and that showed a partial response to antipsychotic medications. Although he initially reported feeling somewhat depressed over his wife's perceived infidelity, he did not have other symptoms suggestive of a major depressive episode. (Courtesy of Laura J. Fochtmann, M.D., Ramin Mojtabai, M.D., Ph.D., M.P.H., and Evelyn J. Bromet, Ph.D.)

Little is known about the epidemiology of delusional disorder as it is rare, and is, likely, a heterogeneous group of disorders that manifest as delusions. Despite many theories, the causes are not known. Many patients with the disorder can function well in society and never come to psychiatric attention. Psychiatrists may only meet them when they are evaluating them for another disorder, such as major depressive disorder. Other times, a physician may request a psychiatric consult for a patient they are evaluating for some other medical disorder and notice some odd responses. The disorder appears to be stable over time. Although reliable data are limited, patients with persecutory, somatic, and erotomanic delusions are thought to have a better prognosis than patients with grandiose and jealous delusions.

Other Psychotic Disorders

Patients may present with psychotic symptoms that are not easily described by one of the psychotic disorders. Some examples include patients with persistent auditory hallucination but no other symptoms, or delusions that present with significant mood symptoms. In some cases a clinician may consider the symptoms that seem psychotic to be so minor as not to deserve a diagnosis of a typical disorder; these can include very transient symptoms or presentations where the patient seems to have full insight into their delusions or hallucinations.

One pattern of psychosis that deserves mention is the presence of delusional symptoms in a partner of an individual with delusional disorder, commonly called "shared psychosis," or *folie á deux*. It is probably rare, but incidence and prevalence figures are lacking, and the literature consists almost entirely of case reports.

The disorder is characterized by the transfer of delusions from one person to another. Both persons are closely associated for a long time and typically live together in relative social isolation. In its most common form (and the one recognized in DSM-5), the individual who first has the delusion (the primary case) is often chronically ill and typically is the influential member of a close relationship with a more suggestible person (the secondary case) who also develops the delusion. The person in the secondary case is frequently less intelligent, more gullible, more passive, or more lacking in self-esteem than the person in the primary case. If the pair separates, the secondary person may abandon the delusion, but this outcome is not seen uniformly. The occurrence of the delusion is attributed to the strong influence of the more dominant member. Old age, low intelligence, sensory impairment, cerebrovascular disease, and alcohol abuse are among the factors associated with this peculiar form of psychotic disorder. A genetic predisposition to idiopathic psychoses has also been suggested as a possible risk factor.

Other special forms have been reported, such as *folie simultanée*, in which two persons become psychotic simultaneously and share the same delusion. Occasionally, more than two individuals are involved (e.g., *folie á trois, quatre, cinq*; also *folie á famille*), but such cases are especially rare. The most common relationships in shared psychotic disorder are sister–sister, husband–wife, and mother–child, but other combinations have also been described. Almost all cases involve members of a single family.

A 52-year-old man was referred by the court for inpatient psychiatric examination, charged with disturbing the peace. He had been arrested for disrupting a trial, complaining of harassment by various judges. He had walked into a courtroom, marched to the bench, and begun to berate the probate judge. While in the hospital, he related a detailed account of conspiratorial goings-on in the local judiciary. A target of certain judges, he claimed he had been singled out for a variety of reasons for many years: he knew what was going on; he had kept records of wrongdoings; and he understood the significance of the whole matter. He refused to elaborate on the specific nature of the conspiracy. He had responded to it with frequent letters to newspapers, the local bar association, and even to a Congressional subcommittee. His mental state, apart from his story and a mildly depressed mood, was entirely normal.

A family interview revealed that his wife and several grown children shared the belief in a judicial conspiracy directed against the patient. There was no change in delusional thinking in the patient or the family after 10 days of observation. The patient refused follow-up.

In this case, protection is provided by others who share the delusion and believe in the reasonableness of the response; such cases are uncommon, if not rare. (Courtesy of TC Manschreck, M.D.)

OBJECTIVE TESTS FOR THE DISORDER

Schizophrenia and the other psychotic disorders remain clinical diagnoses and no tests are sensitive or specific enough for diagnostic purposes. Most tests, such as serologic testing, are mainly used to rule out other causes of psychosis (such as syphilis or anti-NMDA receptor encephalitis). However, some tests are abnormal on average when comparing groups of patients with schizophrenia to patients without the disorder. Examples include computerized electroencephalogram (EEG), which show differences in event-related potentials.

Diagnostic and Rating Scales for Schizophrenia

Several diagnostic interviews and rating scales exist for schizophrenia. Some are useful for diagnosing the disorder, although they are mainly used in research settings.

Most scales measure the outcomes of various interventions, not the presence of a diagnosis. They focus on measuring clinical symptoms associated with the disorder. These include the Positive and Negative Syndrome Scale (PANSS), and the Brief Psychiatric Rating Scale (BPRS), both of which can track the significant symptoms of the disorder. We can assess for extrapyramidal symptoms with a variety of instruments, but the Simpson Angus Scale (SAS), the Abnormal Involuntary Movement Scale (AIMS) and Barnes Akathisia Rating Scale (BARS) are most common.

Psychological Testing

Patients with schizophrenia generally perform poorly on a wide range of neuropsychological tests. Vigilance, memory, and concept formation are most affected and consistent with pathologic involvement in the frontotemporal cortex.

Objective measures of neuropsychological performance, such as the Halstead–Reitan battery and the Luria–Nebraska battery, often give abnormal findings, such as bilateral frontal and temporal lobe dysfunction, including impairments in attention, retention time, and problem-solving ability. Motor ability is also impaired, possibly related to brain asymmetry.

Intelligence Tests. When comparing groups of patients with schizophrenia with groups of psychiatric patients without schizophrenia or from the general population, schizophrenia patients tend to score lower on intelligence tests. Statistically, the evidence suggests that low intelligence is often present at the onset, and intelligence may continue to deteriorate with the progression of the disorder.

Projective and Personality Tests. Projective tests, such as the Rorschach test and the Thematic Apperception Test, may indicate bizarre ideation. Personality inventories, such as the Minnesota Multiphasic Personality Inventory, often give abnormal results in schizophrenia, but the contribution to diagnosis and treatment planning is minimal.

DIFFERENTIAL DIAGNOSIS FOR PSYCHOTIC DISORDERS

Secondary Psychotic Disorders

A wide range of nonpsychiatric medical conditions and a variety of substances can induce symptoms of psychosis and catatonia (Table 5-8). The most appropriate diagnosis for such symptoms is a psychotic disorder due to a general medical condition, catatonic disorder due to a general medical condition, or substance-induced psychotic disorder.

When evaluating a patient with psychotic symptoms, clinicians should follow the general guidelines for assessing nonpsychiatric conditions. First, clinicians should aggressively pursue an undiagnosed nonpsychiatric medical condition when a patient exhibits any unusual or rare symptoms or any variation in the level of

Table 5-8
Potential Medical Etiologies of Delusional Syndromes

Disease or Disorder Class	Examples
Neurodegenerative disorders	Alzheimer disease, Pick disease, Huntington disease, basal ganglia calcification, multiple sclerosis, metachromatic leukodystrophy
Other central nervous system disorders	Brain tumors, especially temporal lobe and deep hemispheric tumors; epilepsy, especially complex partial seizure disorder; head trauma (subdural hematoma); anoxic brain injury; fat embolism
Vascular disease	Atherosclerotic vascular disease, especially when associated with diffuse, temporoparietal, or subcortical lesions; hypertensive encephalopathy; subarachnoid hemorrhage, temporal arteritis
Infectious disease	HIIV/AIDS encephalitis lethargica, Creutzfeldt–Jakob disease, syphilis, malaria, acute viral encephalitis
Metabolic disorder	Hypercalcemia, hyponatremia, hypoglycemia, uremia, hepatic encephalopathy, porphyria
Endocrinopathies	Addison disease, Cushing syndrome, hyper- or hypothyroidism, panhypopituitarism
Vitamin deficiencies	Vitamin B_{12} deficiency, folate deficiency, thiamine deficiency, niacin deficiency
Medications	Adrenocorticotropic hormones, anabolic steroids, corticosteroids, cimetidine, antibiotics (cephalosporins, penicillin), disulfiram, anticholinergic agents
Substances	Amphetamines, cocaine, alcohol, cannabis, hallucinogens
Toxins	Mercury, arsenic, manganese, thallium

consciousness. Second, clinicians should attempt to obtain a complete family history, including a history of medical, neurologic, and psychiatric disorders. Third, clinicians should consider the possibility of a nonpsychiatric medical condition, even in patients with previous diagnoses of schizophrenia. A patient with schizophrenia is just as likely to have a brain tumor that produces psychotic symptoms, as is a patient without schizophrenia.

Mood Disorders

A patient with a major depressive episode may present with delusions and hallucinations, as can a patient with bipolar disorder. Delusions seen with psychotic depression are typically mood-congruent and involve themes such as guilt, self-depreciation, deserved punishment, and incurable illnesses. In mood disorders, psychotic symptoms resolve entirely with the resolution of depression. A depressive episode that is this severe may also result in loss of functioning, a decline in self-care, and social isolation, but these are secondary to the depressive symptoms and should not be confused with the negative symptoms of schizophrenia.

A full-blown manic episode often presents with delusions and sometimes hallucinations. Delusions in mania are most often mood-congruent and typically involve grandiose themes. The flight of ideas seen in mania may, at times, be confused with the thought disorder of schizophrenia. Special attention during the mental status examination of a patient with a flight of ideas is required to note whether the associative links between topics are conserved. However, the conversation is awkward for the observer to follow because of the patient's accelerated rate of thinking.

Personality Disorders

Various personality disorders may have some features of schizophrenia. Schizotypal, schizoid, and borderline personality disorders are personality disorders with several overlapping symptoms. A severe obsessive-compulsive personality disorder may mask an underlying schizophrenic process. Personality disorders, unlike schizophrenia, have mild symptoms and a history of occurring throughout a patient's life; they also lack an identifiable date of onset.

Malingering and Factitious Disorders

For a patient who imitates the symptoms of schizophrenia but does not have the disorder, either malingering or factitious disorder may be an appropriate diagnosis. Although truly mimicking the symptoms of schizophrenia is difficult, especially in front of an experienced clinician, persons have faked schizophrenic symptoms and have been admitted into and treated at psychiatric hospitals. The condition of patients who are entirely in control of their symptom production may qualify for a diagnosis of malingering; such patients usually have some apparent financial or legal reason to want to be considered mentally ill. The condition of patients who are less in control of their falsification of psychotic symptoms may qualify for a diagnosis of factitious disorder. Some patients with schizophrenia, however, may falsely complain of an exacerbation of psychotic symptoms to obtain increased assistance benefits or to gain admission to a hospital.

COMORBIDITY

Substance Use Disorders

Comorbid substance use disorders in patients with schizophrenia are widespread, with a lifetime prevalence of 74%. Tobacco, alcohol, cannabis, and cocaine use disorders are most common, and almost half of the patients with schizophrenia will have a severe problem with drugs or alcohol during their lifetime.

The link between the two disorders is not clear, and experts in the field have proposed several explanations. The diathesis-stress model suggests that a biologically vulnerable person, when encountering external stress (of which a substance may be one), is more likely to develop schizophrenia. The self-medication hypothesis suggests that patients use substances to lessen their symptoms or side effects. The shared vulnerability model suggests that both schizophrenia and substance use disorders share a common etiology and pathology. More research is required. However, the available evidence supports a shared vulnerability, in which a shared genetic risk or environmental insult leads to dysfunctions in specific key circuits, such as reward pathways. The result is the increased use of substances during adolescence, as well as the development of schizophrenia.

Complex Partial Epilepsy

Schizophrenia-like psychoses occur more frequently than expected in patients with complex partial seizures, especially seizures involving the temporal lobes. Factors associated with the development of psychosis in these patients include a left-sided seizure focus, medial temporal location of the lesion, and an early onset of seizures. Some psychotic symptoms are similar to symptoms of patients with complex partial epilepsy and may reflect the presence of a temporal lobe disorder when seen in patients with schizophrenia.

Obesity

Patients with schizophrenia appear to be more obese, with higher body mass indexes (BMIs) than age- and gender-matched cohorts in the general population. This obesity is due, at least in part, to the effect of many antipsychotic medications, as well as poor nutritional balance and decreased motor activity. This weight gain, in turn, contributes to an increased risk of cardiovascular morbidity and mortality, an increased risk of diabetes, and other obesity-related conditions such as hyperlipidemia and obstructive sleep apnea.

Diabetes Mellitus

Schizophrenia is associated with an increased risk of type II diabetes mellitus. This comorbidity is probably due, in part, to the association with obesity noted above, but there is also evidence that some antipsychotic medications cause diabetes through a direct mechanism.

Cardiovascular Disease

Many antipsychotic medications have direct effects on cardiac electrophysiology. Also, obesity, increased rates of smoking, diabetes, and hyperlipidemia, and a sedentary lifestyle all independently increase the risk of cardiovascular morbidity and mortality.

HIV

Patients with schizophrenia appear to have a risk of HIV infection that is 1.5 to 2 times that of the general population. This association is likely due to increased risk behaviors, such as unprotected sex, multiple partners, and increased drug use.

Chronic Obstructive Pulmonary Disease

Rates of chronic obstructive pulmonary disease are increased in schizophrenia compared with the general population. The increased prevalence of smoking is a prominent contributor to this problem; it is not clear whether this is the only one.

Rheumatoid Arthritis

Patients with schizophrenia have a reduced risk of rheumatoid arthritis than is found in the general population. Researchers have replicated this inverse association several times, the significance of which is unknown. GWAS studies also indicate negative genetic correlations, suggesting that they may have shared pathogenesis but differential risks. The exact nature of this relationship remains a mystery and is an ongoing subject of investigation.

COURSE

Onset of Schizophrenia

Premorbid Signs and Symptoms. In theoretical formulations of the course of schizophrenia, premorbid signs and symptoms appear before the prodromal phase of the illness. The differentiation implies that premorbid signs and symptoms exist before the disease process evidences itself and that the prodromal signs and symptoms are parts of the evolving disorder. In the typical, but not invariable, premorbid history of schizophrenia, patients had schizoid or schizotypal personalities characterized as quiet, passive, and introverted; as children, they had few friends. Preschizophrenic adolescents may have no close friends and no dates and may avoid team sports. They may enjoy watching movies and television, listening to music, or playing computer games to the exclusion of social activities. Some adolescent patients may show a sudden onset of obsessive-compulsive behavior as part of the prodromal picture.

A premorbid pattern of symptoms may be the first evidence of illness, although the importance of the symptoms is usually recognized only retrospectively. Nevertheless, although the family members often believe the disorder began with the first hospitalization, signs and symptoms have often been present for months or even years. The signs may have started with complaints about somatic symptoms, such as headache, back and muscle pain, weakness, and digestive problems. The initial diagnosis may be malingering, chronic fatigue syndrome, or somatic symptom disorder. Family and friends may eventually notice that the person has changed and is no longer functioning well in occupational, social, and personal activities. During this stage, a patient may begin to develop an interest in abstract ideas, philosophy, and the occult or religious questions (Fig. 5-1). Additional prodromal signs and

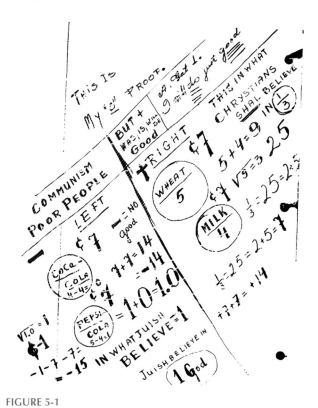

FIGURE 5-1
Schizophrenia patient schema. This illustrates his fragmented, abstract, and overly inclusive thinking and preoccupation with religious ideologies and mathematical proofs. (Courtesy of Heinz E. Lehmann.)

symptoms can include markedly peculiar behavior, abnormal affect, unusual speech, bizarre ideas, and strange perceptual experiences.

Emergence of Symptoms.   Characteristically, the symptoms begin in adolescence and are followed by the development of prodromal symptoms in days to a few months. Social or environmental changes, such as going away to college, using a substance, or a relative's death, may precipitate the disturbing symptoms, and the prodromal syndrome may last a year or more before the onset of overt psychotic symptoms.

Duration.   The classic course of schizophrenia is one of exacerbations and remissions. After the first psychotic episode, a patient gradually recovers and may then function relatively normally for a long time. Patients usually relapse, however, and the pattern of illness during the first 5 years after the diagnosis generally indicates the patient's course. Further deterioration in the patient's baseline functioning follows each relapse of psychosis. This failure to return to baseline functioning after each relapse was historically thought to be the primary distinction between schizophrenia and mood disorders. Sometimes a clinically observable postpsychotic depression follows a psychotic episode, and the schizophrenia patient's vulnerability to stress is usually lifelong. Positive symptoms tend to become less severe with time, but the socially debilitating negative or deficit symptoms may increase in severity.

An unmarried man, 27 years old, was brought to the mental hospital because he had on several occasions become violent toward his father. For a few weeks, he had hallucinations and heard voices. The voices eventually ceased, but he then adopted a strange way of life. He would sit up all night, sleep all day, and become very angry when his father tried to get him out of bed. He did not shave or wash for weeks, smoked continuously, ate very irregularly, and drank enormous quantities of tea.

In the hospital, he adjusted rapidly to the new environment and was found to be generally cooperative. He showed no marked abnormalities of mental state or behavior, except for his lack of concern for just about anything. He kept to himself as much as possible and conversed little with patients or staff. His personal hygiene had to be supervised by the nursing staff; otherwise, he would quickly become dirty and untidy.

Six years after his admission to the hospital, he is described as shiftless and careless, sullen and unreasonable. He lies on a couch all day long. Although many efforts have been made to get the patient to accept therapeutic work assignments, he refuses to consider any kind of regular occupation. In the summer, he wanders about the hospital grounds or lies under a tree. In the winter, he wanders through the tunnels connecting the various hospital buildings and is often seen stretched out for hours under the warm pipes that carry the steam through the tunnels. (Courtesy of Heinz E. Lehmann, M.D.)

Although about one-third of all schizophrenia patients have some marginal or integrated social existence, most have lives characterized by aimlessness, inactivity, frequent hospitalizations, and, in urban settings, homelessness and poverty.

Other Disorders

Schizoaffective Disorder.   The course of schizoaffective disorder is intermediate between schizophrenia and mood disorders, with a better course and prognosis than for schizophrenia and a worse one than for bipolar disorder or major depressive disorder.

Schizophreniform Disorder.   Patients with schizophreniform disorder who do not develop schizophrenia have a better outcome than do patients with schizophrenia.

PROGNOSIS

Having a diagnosis of schizophrenia is associated with a reduction of life expectancy by as much as 20 percent. Persons with schizophrenia have a higher mortality rate from accidents and natural causes than the general population. Institution- or treatment-related variables do not explain the increased mortality rate. However, the higher rate may be related to the fact that the diagnosis and treatment of medical and surgical conditions in schizophrenia patients can be clinical challenges, and in some cases, clinical neglect may be a factor.

Reported remission rates range from 10 to 60 percent, and a reasonable estimate is that 20 to 30 percent of all schizophrenia patients can lead somewhat normal lives. About 20 to 30 percent of patients continue to experience moderate symptoms, and 40 to 60 percent of patients remain significantly impaired by their disorder for their entire lives. Patients with schizophrenia do much poorer than patients with mood disorders, although 20 to 25 percent of mood disorder patients are also severely disturbed at long-term follow-up.

Prognostic Indicators

Several studies have shown that over the 5- to 10-year period after the first psychiatric hospitalization for schizophrenia, only about 10 to 20 percent of patients can be described as having a good outcome. More than 50 percent of patients can be described as having a poor outcome, with repeated hospitalizations, exacerbations of symptoms, episodes of major mood disorders, and suicide attempts. Despite these glum figures, schizophrenia does not always run a deteriorating course, and several factors have been associated with a good prognosis (Table 5-9).

Negative symptoms are rare for schizophreniform disorder, but when they occur, they are considered a poor prognostic feature, and many patients with negative symptoms will later develop schizophrenia.

TREATMENT APPROACH

Although antipsychotic medications are the mainstay of the treatment for schizophrenia, research has found that psychosocial interventions, including psychotherapy, can augment clinical improvement. The complexity of schizophrenia usually renders any single therapeutic approach inadequate to deal with the multifaceted disorder. Psychosocial modalities should be integrated into the drug

    Table 5-9
**Positive and Negative Prognostic Factors
for Schizophrenia**

Positive Prognostic Factors
Acute onset
Female sex
Living in a developed country

Poor Prognostic Factors
Insidious onset
Childhood or adolescent onset
Poor premorbid functioning
Cognitive impairment

treatment regimen and should support it. Patients with schizophrenia benefit more from the combined use of antipsychotic drugs and psychosocial treatment than from either treatment used alone.

Hospitalization

The development of effective antipsychotic drugs and changes in political and popular attitudes toward the treatment and the rights of persons who are mentally ill have dramatically changed the patterns of hospitalization for schizophrenia patients since the mid-1950s. Despite these changes, readmissions after the first hospitalization are frequent, perhaps 40 to 60 percent within 2 years. Patients with schizophrenia occupy about 50 percent of all psychiatric hospital beds and account for about 16 percent of all psychiatric patients who receive any treatment.

In current practice, hospitalization is indicated for diagnostic purposes, for stabilization of medications, for patients' safety because of suicidal or homicidal ideation, and for grossly disorganized or inappropriate behavior, including the inability to take care of basic needs such as food, clothing, and shelter. Establishing an active association between patients and community support systems is also a primary goal of hospitalization.

Short stays of 4 to 6 weeks are just as effective as long-term hospitalizations, and hospital settings with active behavioral approaches produce better results than do custodial institutions. Hospital treatment plans should orient toward practical issues of self-care, quality of life, employment, and social relationships. During hospitalization, clinicians should coordinate with aftercare facilities, including family homes, foster families, board-and-care homes, and halfway houses. Daycare centers and home visits by therapists or nurses can help patients remain out of the hospital for long periods and can improve the quality of their daily lives.

Pharmacotherapy

Patients usually first present for the treatment of acute psychotic symptoms, which require immediate attention. Treatment during the acute phase focuses on alleviating the most severe psychotic symptoms. This phase usually lasts from 4 to 8 weeks.

Antipsychotic medications are considered the mainstay of treatment, both in the acute and maintenance phases of the illness. Table 5-10 lists the second-generation and commonly used first generation antipsychotics.

Most guidelines recommend starting with a second-generation antipsychotic. Although they are likely the most effective for patients with severe symptoms, and predominantly positive symptoms, they are useful across a broad range of symptoms and severity. There is little guidance for choosing a specific medication: some studies suggest they have individual differences in efficacy. However, the most significant difference between the drugs is in their side effects, and we should consider these carefully when choosing a treatment.

Agitation is a typical symptom in the acute phase. Clinicians have several options for managing agitation that results from psychosis. Antipsychotics and benzodiazepines can result in a relatively rapid calming of patients. With highly agitated patients, intramuscular administration of antipsychotics produces a more rapid effect. An advantage of an antipsychotic is that a single intramuscular injection of a first- or second-generation antipsychotic can often calm the patient without excessive sedation. Low-potency antipsychotics are often associated with sedation and postural hypotension, mainly when administering them intramuscularly.

Intramuscular ziprasidone and olanzapine are similar to their oral counterparts in not causing substantial extrapyramidal side effects during acute treatment. This can be a significant advantage over haloperidol or fluphenazine, which can cause frightening dystonias or akathisia in some patients. A rapidly dissolving oral formulation of olanzapine may also be helpful as an alternative to an intramuscular injection.

Benzodiazepines are also useful for agitation during acute psychosis. Lorazepam has the advantage of reliable absorption when administering it either orally or intramuscularly. The use of benzodiazepines may also reduce the amount of antipsychotic that is needed to control psychotic patients.

Treating Side Effects.   Patients frequently experience the side effects of an antipsychotic before they experience clinical improvement. Whereas a clinical response may take days or weeks after starting a drug, side effects may begin almost immediately. First-generation antipsychotics most commonly cause extrapyramidal side effects, and in the case of low potency, first-generation antipsychotics, sedation and postural hypotension, whereas second-generation antipsychotics cause weight gain and metabolic derangements.

EXTRAPYRAMIDAL SIDE EFFECTS.   Most first-generation antipsychotics cause extrapyramidal side effects, including parkinsonian symptoms, dystonias, and akathisia. Although less common in second-generation antipsychotics, extrapyramidal effects can still occur.

Clinicians have several alternatives for treating these side effects. These include reducing the dose of the antipsychotic, adding an antiparkinson medication, and changing the patient to a medication that is less likely to cause extrapyramidal side effects. The most effective antiparkinson medications are anticholinergic antiparkinson drugs. However, these medications have additional side effects, including dry mouth, constipation, blurred vision, and, often, memory loss. Also, these medications are often only partially effective, leaving patients with substantial amounts of lingering extrapyramidal side effects. Centrally acting β-blockers, such as propranolol, may help treat akathisia. Most patients respond to dosages between 30 and 90 mg per day.

If prescribing conventional antipsychotics, clinicians may consider prescribing prophylactic antiparkinson medications for patients who are likely to experience disturbing extrapyramidal side effects. These include patients who have a history of extrapyramidal side effect sensitivity and those treated with relatively high doses of high-potency drugs. Prophylactic antiparkinson medications may help when prescribing high-potency drugs for young men, who tend to have an increased vulnerability for developing dystonias. Again, these patients should be candidates for newer drugs.

Some individuals are highly sensitive to extrapyramidal side effects at the dose that is necessary to control their psychosis. For many of these patients, medication side effects may seem worse than the illness itself. These patients should be treated routinely with a medication less likely to cause extrapyramidal side effects. Risperidone may cause extrapyramidal side effects even at low doses—for example, 0.5 mg—but the severity and risk are increased at higher doses—for example, more than 6 mg. Olanzapine and ziprasidone are also associated with dose-related parkinsonism and akathisia.

TARDIVE DYSKINESIA.   About 20 to 30 percent of patients on long-term treatment with a first-generation antipsychotic will exhibit symptoms of tardive dyskinesia. About 3 to 5 percent of young patients receiving a first-generation drug develop tardive

Table 5-10
Pharmacologic, Formulation and Dosing Information for Second-Generation Antipsychotics and Selected First-Generation Antipsychotics

Antipsychotic	Principal Liver Enzyme Target	Protein Binding	Bio-Availability	Time to Peak Level	Half-Life	CPZ Dose Equivalent, mg[a]	Typical Starting Dose, mg[b]	Typical Dose Range, mg[b]	Maximum Approved Dose, mg[b]	Dose Strength, mg	Route of Administration/ Formulation
Second-Generation Antipsychotics											
Partial Dopamine D2 Agonists											
Aripiprazole	2D6 >3A4	>99%	87%	PO: 3–5 hr; IM short: 1–3 hr; IM long: 5–7 hr	PO: 75 hr; IM long: 30–47 days	7.5	PO: 10–15; IM long (gluteal): 400 with 2 wk oral aripiprazole 10–20	PO: 10–30; IM long (gluteal): 400 every 4 wk	PO: 30; IM long: 400	Tablets: 2, 5, 10, 15, 20, 30; Diss: 10, 15; Liquid: 1 mg/mL (except: 30 mg = 25 mL); IM short: 9.75/1.3 mL; IM long q4wk (monohydrate): 300/1.5 mL, 400/1.9 mL IM long q4 or 6 (882 mg) wk (lauroxil): 441/1.6 mL, 662/2.4 mL, 882/3.2 mL	PO, diss, liquid; IM short, IM long
Brexpiprazole	2D6, 3A4	>99%	95%	4 hr	91 hr	N/A	0.5–1	2–4	4	0.25, 0.5, 1, 2, 3, 4	PO
Cariprazine	3A4 >2D6	91–97%	52% (1 mg)	3–6 hr	2–5 days (didesmethyl-cariprazine: 1–3 wk)	N/A	1.5	1.5–6	6	1.5, 3, 4.5, 6	PO
Dopamine D2—Serotonin 2A Antagonists											
Asenapine	1A2 >3A4	98	35% (≤2% if swallowed)	0.5–1.5 hr	First: 6 hr, terminal: 24 hr	7.5	5 bid	10–20	20	Tablets: 5, 10	Sublingual (avoid eating or drinking for 10 min after administration)
Clozapine	1A2 (30%) >2C19 (24%) >3A4 (22%) >2C9 (12%) >2D6 (6%)	97%	50–60%	1.5–2.5 hr	12 hr	50	12.5	50–600	900	Tablets: 25, 50, 100, 200; Diss: 12.5, 25, 100, 150, 200; Liquid: 50 mg/mL	PO, diss, liquid
Iloperidone	2D6 >3A4 >1A2	95%	96%	2–4 hr	18 hr	5	1 mg bid × 1 day, 2 mg × 1 day, then increase 2 mg/d daily to therapeutic dose	12–24	24	Tablets: 1, 2, 4, 6, 8, 10, 12	PO
Lurasidone	3A4	99%	9–19%	1–3 hr	18 hr	25	40–80	40–120	160	Tablets: 20, 40, 80, 120	PO (with ≥350 kcal meal)
Olanzapine	1A2, 2D6, 3A4	93%	60%	PO: 6 hr; IM short: 15–45 min; IM long: 7 days	PO: 30 hr; IM short: 30 hr; IM long: 30 days	5	PO: 5–10; IM long (gluteal): 210/2 wk or 405/4 wk (= oral 10), 300/2 wk (= oral 15 or 20)	PO: 10–20; IM long (gluteal): 150/2 wk or 300/4 wk (= oral 10), 210/2 wk or 405/2 wk (= oral 15), 300/2 wk (= oral 20)	20	Tablets: 2.5, 5, 7.5, 10, 15, 20; Diss: 5, 10, 15, 20; IM short: 10/2 mL; IM long q2 or 4 wk: 150/1.3 mL, 210/1.3 mL, 300/1.8 mL, 405/2.3 mL	PO, diss; IM short, IM long

Paliperidone	<10% first-pass hepatic clearance	74%	28%	PO: 24 hr; IM long: 13 days	PO: 23 hr; IM long; 25–49 days	3	PO: 6; IM long: 234 mg into deltoid day 1, then 156 mg day 8, then 39–234 into deltoid or gluteus every 4 wk	PO: 3–12; IM long (deltoid or gluteal): 117–234 every 4 wk	12	Tablets: 1.5, 3, 6, 9; IM long q4wk: 39 0.25 mL, 78/0.5 mL, 117/0.75 mL, 156/1 mL, 234/1.5 mL; IM long q12wk: 273 0.875 mL, 410/1.315 mL, 546/1.75 mL, 819/2.625 mL	PO (ER); IM long
Quetiapine	3A4	83%	100%	IR: 1.5 hr; XR: 6 hr	IR: 6–7 hr	75	IR: 25–100; XR: 200–300	IR: 150–750; XR: 400–800	800	Tablets IR: 25, 50, 100, 200, 300, 400; XR: 50, 150, 200, 300, 400	PO (IR, XR)
Risperidone	2D6 >3A4	90%	70%	3 hr	3 hr	2	PO: 2; IM long (deltoid or gluteal): 25 with 3 wk oral risperidone	PO: 2–8; IM long (deltoid or gluteal): 12.5–50 into deltoid or gluteal muscle every 2 wk	16	Tablets: 0.25, 0.5, 1, 2, 3, 4; Diss: 0.5, 1, 2, 3, 4; Liquid: 1 mg/mL; IM long q2w: 12.5/1 mL, 25/2 mL, 37.5/2 mL, 50/2 mL	PO, diss, liquid; IM long
Ziprasidone	Aldehyde oxidase (2/3) >3A4 (1/3)	>99%	60%	PO: 6–8 hr; IM short: ≤60 min	PO: 7 hr; IM short: 2–5 hr	60	20–40 bid	80–160	160	Tablets: 20, 40, 60, 80 IM short: 20/1 mL	PO (with ≥500 kcal meal), IM short

First-Generation Antipsychotics (Dopamine D2 Antagonists)

Chlorpromazine	2D6	>90	20%	2–4 hr	30 hr	100	PO: 25–100 mg; IM short: 25, followed by 25–50 mg as needed after 1–4 hr	PO: 200–800; IV/IM short: 400 mg every 4–6 hr	2,000	Tablets: 10, 25, 50, 100, 200; Spansule: 30, 75, 150; Syrup: 5 mL = 10 mg; Liquid: 25 mg/5 mL; IM short: 25/mL; Supp: 25, 100	PO, syrup; IM short; IV; rectal suppository
Fluphenazine	1A2	>90	<50%	PO: 2 hr; IM long: 8–10 hr	PO: 14–16 hr; IM long: 14 days	2	PO: 2.5–10 in 2–3 divided doses	PO: 1–5 in 2–3 divided doses; IM long (deltoid or gluteal): 12.5–25 mg every 2–4 wk	40	Tablets: 1, 2.5, 5, 10; Liquid: 2.5 or 5/mL; IM long: 25 mg/mL	PO; IM long
Haloperidol	3A4	92%	60%–70%	PO: 2–6 hr; IM short: 10–20 min; IM long: 6–7 days	PO: 18 hr; IM short: 10–20 hr; IM long: 3 wk	2	PO: 1–2; IM short: 2–5 mg every 4–8 hr as needed; IM long (deltoid or gluteal): 10–20 times the oral dose every 4 wk (≤100)	PO: 2–10; IM long (deltoid or gluteal): 10–15 times the oral dose every 4 wk (≤100)	PO: 60; IM long: 100	Tablets: 0.5, 1, 2, 5, 10, 20 Liquid: 2 or 10 mg/mL IM short: 5; IM long q4wk: 50 mg/mL, 100 mg/mL	PO; IM short, IM long
Perphenazine	2D6	>90%	40%	1–3 hr	9–12 hr	10	Inpatient: 8–16 divided in 2–3 doses; Outpatient: 4–8 divided in 3 doses	8–32	64	2, 4, 8, 16	PO

[a] Chlorpromazine dose equivalents (i.e., dose given in the table is equivalent to 100 mg of chlorpromazine).

[b] Doses need to be individualized based on efficacy and tolerability.

CPZ, chlorpromazine; Diss, dissolvable tablet; ER, extended release; IM, intramuscular; IR, immediate release; IV, intravenous; N/A, not available; q, every; PO, oral; Supp, suppository; XR, extended release.

Source: Package insert information for each medication.

dyskinesia each year. The risk in elderly patients is much higher. Although severely disabling dyskinesia is uncommon, it can affect walking, breathing, eating, and talking when it occurs. Individuals who are more sensitive to acute extrapyramidal side effects appear to be more vulnerable to developing tardive dyskinesia. Patients with comorbid cognitive or mood disorders may also be more vulnerable to tardive dyskinesia than those with only schizophrenia.

The abnormal movements usually begin while the patient is receiving an antipsychotic or within 4 weeks of discontinuing an oral antipsychotic or 8 weeks after the withdrawal of a depot antipsychotic.

There is a lower risk of tardive dyskinesia with new-generation drugs. However, there still is some risk of tardive dyskinesia with newer drugs.

Recommendations for preventing and managing tardive dyskinesia include: (1) using the lowest effective dose of antipsychotics; (2) prescribing cautiously with children, elderly patients, and patients with mood disorders; (3) examining patients regularly for evidence of tardive dyskinesia; (4) considering alternatives to the current antipsychotic and considering dosage reduction when observing tardive dyskinesia; and (5) considering several options if the tardive dyskinesia worsens, including discontinuing the antipsychotic or switching to a different drug. Clozapine is effective in reducing severe tardive dyskinesia or tardive dystonia.

OTHER SIDE EFFECTS.   Sedation and postural hypotension can be significant side effects for patients treated with low-potency first-generation drugs, such as perphenazine. These effects are often most severe during the initial dosing of these medications. As a result, patients treated with these medications—or with clozapine—may require weeks to reach a therapeutic dose. Although most patients develop tolerance to sedation and postural hypotension, sedation may continue to be a problem. In these patients, daytime drowsiness may interfere with a patient's attempts to return to community life.

All antipsychotics elevate prolactin levels, which can result in galactorrhea and irregular menses. Long-term elevations in prolactin and the resultant suppression in gonadotropin-releasing hormone can cause suppression in gonadal hormones. These, in turn, may have effects on libido and sexual functioning. There is also concern that elevated prolactin may cause decreases in bone density and lead to osteoporosis. The concerns about hyperprolactinemia, sexual functioning, and bone density are based on experiences with prolactin elevations related to tumors and other causes. It is unclear if these risks are also associated with the lower elevations that occur with prolactin-elevating drugs.

HEALTH MONITORING IN PATIENTS RECEIVING ANTIPSYCHOTICS. Because of the effects of the second-generation antipsychotics on insulin metabolism, psychiatrists should monitor several health indicators, including BMI, fasting blood glucose, and lipid profiles. We should weigh patients and calculate their BMIs for every visit for at least 6 months after a medication change.

Clozapine.
Clozapine is considered the most effective of antipsychotics, particularly in patients who have been unresponsive to other treatments. However, it is a challenging drug to administer, given its risk of both severe side effects (agranulocytosis in approximately 0.3 percent of those taking it, seizures in as high as 5 percent of those on doses above 600 mg, and, more rarely, myocarditis) and common ones (hypersalivation, sedation, tachycardia, weight gain, and postural hypotension). The concerns over agranulocytosis have resulted in a monitoring system in the United States in which

patients who receive clozapine must be in a program of weekly blood monitoring for the first 6 months and biweekly monitoring for the next 6 months, and monthly after that.

These limitations have relegated clozapine to a later treatment option, and most guidelines recommend considering it after a patient has failed at least two other antipsychotic trials.

Duration and Prophylaxis

In the stable or maintenance phase, the illness is in a relative stage of remission. The goals during this phase are to prevent psychotic relapse and to assist patients in improving their level of functioning. Newer medications, with a substantially reduced risk of tardive dyskinesia, have diminished one of the major concerns about long-term treatment. During this phase, patients are usually in a relative state of remission with only minimal psychotic symptoms. Stable patients who are maintained on an antipsychotic have a much lower relapse rate than patients who have their medications discontinued. Data suggest that 16 to 23 percent of patients receiving treatment will experience a relapse within 1 year, and 53 to 72 percent will relapse without medications.

We should maintain patients experiencing a first episode of psychosis for at least a year. However, such patients still have a high chance of relapsing at least once over the following 5 years, and some experts believe that 1 year is inadequate. This is a particular concern when patients have achieved functional employment status or are involved in educational programs because they have a lot to lose if they experience another psychotic decompensation.

For patients experiencing two or more episodes, most experts recommend that we consider indefinite treatment.

Acute Treatment Failures

Addressing Noncompliance.   Noncompliance with long-term antipsychotic treatment is very high. An estimated 40 to 50 percent of patients become noncompliant within 1 or 2 years. Long-acting injectable antipsychotics were developed to help improve adherence, particularly in patients likely to discontinue daily oral medications. Although there is some controversy in the literature, the weight of data suggests that long-term depot formulations do help adherence and decrease relapse, mainly when considered in real-world settings.

When beginning long-acting drugs, some oral supplementation is necessary while achieving peak plasma levels. Fluphenazine, haloperidol, risperidone, paliperidone, aripiprazole, and olanzapine have long-acting injectable formulations.

There are several advantages to using long-acting injectable medication. Clinicians quickly know when noncompliance occurs and have some time to initiate appropriate interventions before the medication effect dissipates. Also, there is less day-to-day variability in blood levels, making it easier to establish a minimum effective dose. Finally, many patients prefer it to managing daily dosage schedules.

Selecting Second Treatment Options.   When giving patients with acute schizophrenia an antipsychotic medication, approximately 60 percent will improve to the extent that they will achieve a complete remission or experience only mild symptoms. The remaining 40 percent of patients will improve but still demonstrate variable levels of positive symptoms that are resistant to the medications. One meta-analysis of available studies found that patients who did not show at least some response to treatment by the second week were less likely to benefit from the drug, and a treatment change may be the best option.

Rather than categorizing patients into responders and nonresponders, it is more accurate to consider the degree to which the illness improves with medication. Some resistant patients are so severely ill that they require chronic institutionalization. Others respond to an antipsychotic with substantial suppression of their psychotic symptoms but demonstrate persistent symptoms, such as hallucinations or delusions.

Before considering a patient a poor responder to a particular drug, it is vital to assure that they received an adequate trial of the medication. A 4- to 6-week trial on an adequate dose of an antipsychotic represents a reasonable trial for most patients. Patients who demonstrate even a mild amount of improvement during this period may continue to improve at a steady rate for 3 to 6 months. It may be helpful to confirm that the patient is receiving an adequate amount of the drug by monitoring the plasma concentration; that said, most of the accepted levels pertain to first-generation drugs, and there is less rationale for obtaining levels in patients who receive second-generation drugs. However, in any patient, a deficient plasma concentration may indicate that the patient has been noncompliant or, more commonly, only partially compliant. It may also suggest that the patient is a rapid metabolizer of the antipsychotic or is not absorbing the drug adequately. Under these conditions, raising the dose may be helpful. If the level is relatively high, clinicians should consider whether side effects may be interfering with therapeutic response.

If the patient is responding poorly, one may increase the dose above the usual therapeutic level; however, higher than recommended doses usually do not improve response. Changing to another drug is preferable.

As discussed earlier, clozapine is useful for patients who respond poorly to other antipsychotics. Double-blind studies comparing clozapine with other antipsychotics indicated that clozapine had the most evident advantage over conventional drugs in patients with the most severe psychotic symptoms, as well as in those who had previously responded poorly to other antipsychotics.

Researchers and clinicians have tried several adjunctive medications, most with mixed success. These include lamotrigine, mirtazapine, donepezil, D-alanine, D-serine, estradiol, memantine, and allopurinol.

Other Somatic Treatments

Researchers have studied electroconvulsive therapy (ECT) in both acute and chronic schizophrenia. Studies in recent-onset patients indicate that ECT is about as effective as antipsychotic medications and more effective than psychotherapy. Other studies suggest that supplementing antipsychotic medications with ECT is more effective than antipsychotic medications alone. Antipsychotic medications should be administered during and after ECT treatment.

Some initial studies have suggested neuromodulation, using transcranial magnetic stimulation (TMS) or transcranial direct current stimulation (tDCS), may be useful for treating hallucinations or negative symptoms.

Although we no longer consider psychosurgery to be appropriate treatment, some research centers practice it on a limited experimental basis for severe, intractable cases.

Psychosocial Therapy

Psychotherapy is considered an essential part of treatment for schizophrenia, and patients who receive psychotherapy along with medications tend to have better adherence to therapy, less negative symptoms, and better overall functioning.

Currently, there is no convincing evidence to suggest that any single psychotherapeutic approach is preferable to another, although all tend to emphasize structured approaches rather than open-ended, exploratory methods. Psychosocial therapies include a variety of methods to increase social abilities, self-sufficiency, practical skills, and interpersonal communication in schizophrenia patients. The goal is to enable persons who are severely ill to develop social and vocational skills for independent living. Many sites use these approaches, including hospitals, outpatient clinics, mental health centers, day hospitals, and home or social clubs.

Cognitive Behavioral Therapy.   Cognitive-behavioral therapy (CBT) has been used in schizophrenia patients to improve cognitive distortions, reduce distractibility, and correct errors in judgment. There are reports of ameliorating delusions and hallucinations in some patients using this method. Patients who might benefit generally have some insight into their illness, and clinicians usually use this approach after treating an acute psychotic episode. The approach generally incorporates cognitive restructuring, self-monitoring, and graded coping skills. Although at least one randomized controlled study showed a benefit for CBT as a sole treatment, most experts recommend it in combination with antipsychotic treatment.

Social Skills Training.   Social skills training, also called behavioral skills therapy, can be directly supportive and useful for a patient. In addition to the psychotic symptoms seen in patients with schizophrenia, other noticeable symptoms involve the way the person relates to others, including poor eye contact, unusual delays in response, odd facial expressions, lack of spontaneity in social situations, and inaccurate perception or lack of perception of emotions in other people. Behavioral skills training addresses these behaviors through the use of videotapes of others and the patient, role-playing in therapy, and homework assignments for practicing the specific skills. Social skills training can reduce relapse rates and the need for hospitalization.

Group Therapy.   Group psychotherapy for patients with schizophrenia can help improve social functioning and decrease negative symptoms. Group therapy for persons with schizophrenia generally focuses on real-life plans, problems, and relationships. Groups may be behaviorally oriented, psychodynamically or insight-oriented, or supportive. Some investigators doubt that dynamic interpretation and insight therapy are valuable for typical patients with schizophrenia. However, group therapy is effective in reducing social isolation, increasing the sense of cohesiveness, and improving reality testing for patients with schizophrenia. Groups led in a supportive manner appear to be most helpful for schizophrenia patients.

Family-Oriented Therapies.   Family therapy can be a significant adjunct to treatment and reduces relapse and rehospitalization rates compared to patients receiving standard care. Such therapy generally includes practical approaches such as psychoeducation and problem-solving training. Because patients with schizophrenia are often discharged in an only partially remitted state, a family to which a patient returns can often benefit from a brief but intensive (as often as daily) course of family therapy. The therapy should focus on the immediate situation and should include identifying and avoiding potentially troublesome situations. When problems do emerge with the patient in the family, the aim of the therapy should be to resolve the problem quickly.

In wanting to help, family members often encourage a relative with schizophrenia to resume regular activities too quickly, both from ignorance about the disorder and from denial of its severity. Without being overly discouraging, therapists must help both the family and the patient understand and learn about schizophrenia and must encourage discussion of the psychotic episode and the events leading up to it. Ignoring the psychotic episode, a common occurrence, often increases the shame associated with the event and does not exploit the freshness of the episode to understand it better. Psychotic symptoms often frighten family members, and talking openly with the psychiatrist and with the relative with schizophrenia often eases all parties. Therapists can direct later family therapy toward the long-range application of stress-reducing and coping strategies and the patient's gradual reintegration into everyday life.

Therapists must control the emotional intensity of family sessions with patients with schizophrenia. The excessive expression of emotion during a session can damage a patient's recovery process and undermine potentially successful future family therapy. Several studies have shown that family therapy is especially useful in reducing relapses.

Case Management and Assertive Community Treatment.
Because a variety of professionals with specialized skills, such as psychiatrists, social workers, and occupational therapists, among others, are involved in a treatment program, it is helpful to have one person aware of all the forces acting on the patient. The case manager helps coordinate this and ensures that the patient keeps appointments and complies with treatment plans. The case manager may also make home visits and even accompany the patient to work. The success of the program depends on the educational background, training, and competence of the individual case manager, which vary. Most important is maintaining a small caseload (less than 20 cases per manager), which can be challenging for overtaxed and underfunded systems.

The Assertive Community Treatment (ACT) program was initially developed by researchers in Madison, Wisconsin, in the 1970s, for the delivery of services for persons with chronic mental illness. Patients are assigned to one multidisciplinary team (e.g., case manager, psychiatrist, nurse, general physicians). The team has a fixed caseload of patients and delivers all services when and where needed by the patient, 24 hours a day, 7 days a week. ACT is a mobile and intensive intervention that provides treatment, rehabilitation, and support activities. These include home delivery of medications, monitoring of mental and physical health, in vivo social skills, and frequent contact with family members. There is a high staff-to-patient ratio (1:12). ACT programs can effectively decrease the risk of rehospitalization for persons with schizophrenia, but they are labor-intensive and expensive programs to administer.

Although the evidence is low in quality, there is some evidence to suggest that intensive case management can reduce hospitalization time and increase adherence to treatment. Intensive case management approaches seem to be most effective when they incorporate ACT.

Individual Psychotherapy.
Studies of the effects of individual psychotherapy in the treatment of schizophrenia suggest that therapy is helpful and that the effects are additive to those of pharmacologic treatment. In psychotherapy with a schizophrenia patient, developing a therapeutic relationship that the patient experiences as safe is critical. The therapist's reliability, the emotional distance between the therapist and the patient, and the genuineness of the therapist as interpreted by the patient all affect the therapeutic experience. When considering psychotherapy for a patient with schizophrenia, we should think in decades, rather than sessions, months, or even years.

The best predictor of psychotherapy outcome is probably the strength of the therapeutic alliance. Schizophrenia patients who can form a positive therapeutic alliance are likely to remain in psychotherapy, to remain compliant with their medications, and to have good outcomes at 2-year follow-up evaluations.

The relationship between clinicians and patients differs from that encountered in the treatment of nonpsychotic patients. Establishing a relationship is often challenging. Persons with schizophrenia are desperately lonely, yet defend against closeness and trust; they are likely to become suspicious, anxious, or hostile or to regress when someone attempts to draw close.

Therapists should scrupulously respect a patient's distance and privacy and should demonstrate simple directness, patience, sincerity, and sensitivity to social conventions in preference to premature informality and the condescending use of first names. The patient is likely to perceive exaggerated warmth or professions of friendship as attempts at bribery, manipulation, or exploitation. In the context of a professional relationship, however, flexibility is essential in establishing a working alliance with the patient.

Vocational Therapy and Supported Employment.
A variety of methods and settings can help patients regain old skills or develop new ones. These include sheltered workshops, job clubs, and part-time or transitional employment programs. Enabling patients to become gainfully employed is both a means toward and a sign of recovery. Many schizophrenia patients are capable of performing high-quality work despite their illness. Others may exhibit exceptional skill or even brilliance in a limited field as a result of some distinctive aspects of their disorder.

Supported employment focuses on helping patients to obtain competitive employment as opposed to sheltered workshops. It has strong data for helping patients to find and maintain jobs; it also is associated with less need for treatment and improved self-esteem. It is less consistently associated with overall disease outcomes.

Art Therapy.
Many schizophrenia patients benefit from art therapy, which provides them with an outlet for their constant bombardment of imagery. It helps them communicate with others and share their inner, often frightening world with others.

Cognitive Remediation.
Cognitive remediation or cognitive training is a behavioral therapy that attempts to improve cognitive processes. It uses computer-generated exercises to influence neural networks to improve cognition, including working memory. This can then improve social functioning. One metanalysis determined that its effect size is in the medium range.

National Alliance on Mental Illness (NAMI).
The NAMI and similar organizations offer support groups for family members and friends of patients who are mentally ill and for patients themselves. These organizations offer emotional and practical advice about obtaining care in the sometimes complex health care delivery system and are useful sources to which to refer family members. NAMI has also waged a campaign to destigmatize mental illness and to increase government

awareness of the needs and rights of persons who are mentally ill and their families.

THE EPIDEMIOLOGY OF THE DISORDERS

Incidence and Prevalence

The worldwide lifetime prevalence of schizophrenia is about 0.7 percent. One meta-analysis of 101 prevalence rates published between 1990 and 2015 found that the mean global lifetime prevalence of psychotic disorders worldwide was 7.49 per 1,000 individuals. However, there was an extensive range across studies representing an approximately five-fold difference. These variations could largely be accounted for by the different methodologic approaches of different studies, including

different populations and settings studied, different diagnostic criteria and diagnoses included, and differences in the study quality.

Table 5-11 lists some of the major epidemiologic studies of schizophrenia.

In the United States, about 0.05 percent of the total population is treated for schizophrenia in any single year. Perhaps only one-half of all patients with schizophrenia will obtain treatment, despite the severity of the disorder.

Sex

Schizophrenia is equally prevalent in men and women. The two sexes differ in the onset and course of illness. The onset of schizophrenia is earlier for men. Also, more than half of all male schizophrenia

Table 5-11
Selected Prevalence Studies of Schizophrenia

Author	Country	Population	Method	Prevalence per 1,000 Population at Risk
Brugger (1931)	Germany	Area in Thuringia (*n* = 37,561); age 10+ yr	Census; interview of sample	2.4
Strömgren (1938); Bøjholm and Strömgren (1989)	Denmark	Island population (*n* = 50,000)	Census interviews; repeat census	3.9 → 3.3
Böök (1953); Böök et al. (1978)	Sweden	Genetic isolate (*n* = 9,000); age 15–50 yr	Census interviews; repeat census	9.5 → 17.0
Essen–Möller et al. (1956); Hagnell (1966)	Sweden	Community in southern Sweden	Census interviews; repeat census	6.7 → 4.5
Rin and Lin (1962); Lin et al. (1989)	Taiwan	Population sample	Census interviews; repeat census	2.1 → 1.4
Crocetti et al. (1971)	Croatia	Sample of 9,201 households	Census based on hospital records and interviews	5.9
Dube and Kumar (1972)	India	4 areas in Agra (*n* = 29,468)	Census based on hospital and clinic records	2.6
Rotstein (1977)	Russia	Population sample (*n* = 35,590)	Census based on hospital and clinic records	3.8
Keith et al. (1991)	USA	Aggregated data across 5 ECA sites	Sample survey; interviews	7.0 (point) 15.0 (lifetime)
Jeffreys et al. (1997)	UK	London health district (*n* = 112,127)	Census; interview of sample (*n* = 172)	5.1
Kebede et al. (1999)	Ethiopia	25 districts of Addis Ababa (*n* = 2,228,490)	Screening by self-report questionnaire, interviews of sample (*n* = 2,042)	7.0 (point) 9.0 (lifetime)
Jablensky et al. (2000)	Australia	4 urban areas (*n* = 1,084,978)	Census, screen for psychosis; interviews of sample (*n* = 980)	3.1–5.9 (point)[a] 3.9–6.9 (period, 1 yr)[b]
Waldo et al. (1999)	Micronesia	Island of Kosrae Genetic isolate	Screen of hospital records, interviews	6.8 (point)
Arajärvi et al. (2005)	Finland	Birth cohort (*n* = 14,817) Genetic isolate	Case register data; interviews of 55% of register cases	15.0 (lifetime) 19.0[c] (lifetime)
Wu et al. (2006)	USA (California)	Medicaid/Medicare health insurance data	20% random sample of insured subjects	5.1 (period, 1 yr)
Perälä et al. (2007)	Finland	National sample (*n* = 8,028)	Screen for psychosis, interviews of sample; register and case note data also used	10.0 (lifetime) 22.9[d] (lifetime)

[a]All psychoses.
[b]Schizophrenia and other nonaffective psychotic disorders.
[c]Schizophrenia spectrum disorders.
[d]Nonaffective psychotic disorders.
→ Changes in prevalence found in repeat surveys of the same population.

patients, but only one-third of all female schizophrenia patients, will be hospitalized for the disorder before age 25 years. Some studies have indicated that men are more likely to be impaired by negative symptoms than are women and that women are more likely to have better social functioning than are men before disease onset. In general, the outcome for female schizophrenia patients is better than that for male schizophrenia patients.

Age

In the United States, the peak ages of onset are between 10 and 25 years for men and 25 and 35 years for women. Unlike men, women display a bimodal age distribution, with a second peak occurring in middle age—approximately 3 to 10 percent of women with schizophrenia present with disease onset after age 40 years. About 90 percent of patients in treatment for schizophrenia are between 15 and 55 years old. The onset of schizophrenia before age 10 years or after age 60 years is scarce. Late-onset schizophrenia refers to the occurrence of the disorder after age 45 years.

Other Factors Affecting Epidemiology

Seasonality of Birth.   Persons who develop schizophrenia are more likely to have been born in the winter or early spring. In the Northern Hemisphere, including the United States, persons with schizophrenia are more often born in the months from January to April. In the Southern Hemisphere, persons with schizophrenia are more often born in the months from July to September.

Maternal Factors Affecting the Fetus.   Complications during delivery, maternal malnutrition during pregnancy, as well as other illnesses, appear to be risk factors for schizophrenia.

Early Life Experiences.   Childhood trauma, social isolation, and other types of deprivation also seem to be risk factors.

Urban Upbringing.   Several studies, mainly from the 1990s, have suggested that being born or living in a city is a risk for schizophrenia. This has been reported in various countries. The relationship appears to be more convincing for being raised in rather than being born in a city. The relationship may be "dose-related," meaning that the larger the city, the higher the risk.

Cannabis.   There is an association between cannabis use and psychosis, and the use of cannabis may increase the risk of schizophrenia by as much as 40%, particularly in heavy users.

Cognitive Deficits May also be a Risk Factor.   More recent research has suggested that cognitive deficits, such as poor verbal learning and memory and slower processing speed, can be a predictor of impending psychosis.

Other Psychotic Disorders

Schizoaffective disorder is less common than schizophrenia, possibly in the range of 0.5 to 0.8 percent, although the varying criteria used in different studies limits the findings. The sex differences are more typical of mood disorders in which there is a higher ratio of women than men having the depressed subtype but a similar ratio with the bipolar subtype. The bipolar subtype may be more common in younger persons than in adults, who are more commonly depressed. As with schizophrenia, women tend to get it later than men.

We know little about the incidence, prevalence, and sex ratio of schizophreniform disorder. It appears to be about half as common as schizophrenia, more common in men, and most common in adolescents and young adults. The relatives of patients with schizophreniform disorder are more likely to have mood disorders than are the relatives of patients with schizophrenia. Many of those mood disorders include psychotic symptoms, however.

THE NEUROBIOLOGY OF THE DISORDER

Anatomic Findings

In the 19th century, neuropathologists failed to find a neuropathologic basis for schizophrenia, and thus they classified schizophrenia as a functional disorder. By the end of the 20th century, however, researchers had better tools and made significant strides in revealing a potential neuropathologic basis for schizophrenia.

Cerebral Ventricles.   Computed tomography (CT) scans of patients with schizophrenia have consistently shown lateral and third ventricular enlargement and some reduction in cortical volume. Reduced volumes of cortical gray matter have been demonstrated during the earliest stages of the disease. Several investigators have attempted to determine whether the abnormalities detected by CT are progressive or static. Some studies have concluded that the lesions observed on CT scan are present at the onset of the illness and do not progress. Other studies, however, have concluded that the pathologic process visualized on CT scan continues to progress during the illness. Thus, whether an active pathologic process is continuing to evolve in schizophrenia patients is still uncertain.

Reduced Symmetry.   There is a reduced symmetry in several brain areas in schizophrenia, including the temporal, frontal, and occipital lobes. This reduced symmetry is believed by some investigators to originate during fetal life and to be indicative of a disruption in brain lateralization during neurodevelopment.

Limbic System.   Because of its role in controlling emotions, researchers believe that the limbic system is involved in the pathophysiology of schizophrenia. Studies of postmortem brain samples from schizophrenia patients have shown a decrease in the size of the region, including the amygdala, the hippocampus, and the parahippocampal gyrus. This neuropathologic finding agrees with the observation made by magnetic resonance imaging studies of patients with schizophrenia. The hippocampus is not only smaller in size in schizophrenia but is also functionally abnormal, as indicated by disturbances in glutamate transmission. Brain tissue sections also show the disorganization of the neurons within the hippocampus in some patients with schizophrenia.

Prefrontal Cortex.   There is considerable evidence from postmortem brain studies that support anatomical abnormalities in the prefrontal cortex in schizophrenia. Functional deficits in the prefrontal brain imaging region have also been demonstrated. Of interest, several symptoms of schizophrenia mimic those found in persons with prefrontal lobotomies or frontal lobe syndromes.

Thalamus.   Some studies of the thalamus show evidence of volume shrinkage or neuronal loss in particular subnuclei. The medial dorsal nucleus of the thalamus, which has reciprocal connections with the prefrontal cortex, has been reported to contain a reduced number of neurons. The total number of neurons, oligodendrocytes, and astrocytes is reduced by 30 to 45 percent in schizophrenia patients. This putative finding does not appear to be due to the effects of antipsychotic drugs, because the volume of the thalamus is similar in size between patients with schizophrenia treated chronically with medication and neuroleptic-naive subjects.

Basal Ganglia and Cerebellum. The basal ganglia and cerebellum have been of theoretical interest in schizophrenia for at least two reasons. First, many patients with schizophrenia show odd movements, even in the absence of medication-induced movement disorders. The odd movements can include an awkward gait, facial grimacing, and stereotypies. Because the basal ganglia and cerebellum are involved in the control of movement, disease in these areas is implicated in the pathophysiology of schizophrenia. Second, the movement disorders involving the basal ganglia (e.g., Huntington disease, Parkinson disease) are the ones most commonly associated with psychosis. Neuropathologic studies of the basal ganglia have produced variable and inconclusive reports about cell loss or the reduction of volume of the globus pallidus and the substantia nigra. Studies have also shown an increase in the number of D_2 receptors in the caudate, putamen, and the nucleus accumbens. The question remains, however, whether the increase is secondary to the patient having received antipsychotic medications. Some investigators have begun to study the serotonergic system in the basal ganglia; the clinical usefulness of antipsychotic drugs that are serotonin antagonists suggests a role for serotonin in psychotic disorders.

Physiologic Findings

Functional Imagining. PET studies have shown a variety of neurotransmitter abnormalities, including increased dopamine levels in the ventral striatum and reduced levels in the frontal cortex.

Studies using magnetic resonance spectroscopy have demonstrated increased glutamate levels, particularly in the prefrontal and medial temporal areas. Furthermore, concentrations of N-acetyl aspartate, a marker of neurons, were lower in the hippocampus and frontal lobes of patients with schizophrenia.

Electrophysiologic Findings. Electroencephalographic studies indicate that many schizophrenia patients have abnormal records, increased sensitivity to activation procedures (e.g., frequent spike activity after sleep deprivation), decreased alpha activity, increased theta and delta activity, possibly more epileptiform activity than usual, and possibly more left-sided abnormalities than usual. Schizophrenia patients also exhibit an inability to filter out irrelevant sounds and are extremely sensitive to background noise. The flooding of sound that results makes concentration difficult and may be a factor in the production of auditory hallucinations. This sound sensitivity may be associated with a genetic defect.

Evoked Potentials. A large number of abnormalities are seen in the evoked potential of patients with schizophrenia. The P300 is most studied; it is a large, positive evoked-potential wave that occurs about 300 milliseconds after a sensory stimulus is detected. The primary source of the P300 wave is likely in the limbic system structures of the medial temporal lobes. In patients with schizophrenia, the P300 is statistically smaller than in comparison groups. Abnormalities in the P300 wave are also common in children who,

because they have affected parents, are at high risk for schizophrenia. Whether the characteristics of the P300 represent a state or a trait phenomenon remains controversial. Other evoked potentials reported to be abnormal in patients with schizophrenia are the N100 and the contingent negative variation. The N100 is a negative wave that occurs about 100 milliseconds after a stimulus, and the contingent negative variation is a slowly developing, negative-voltage shift following the presentation of a sensory stimulus that is a warning for an upcoming stimulus. The evoked-potential data likely indicates that, although patients with schizophrenia are unusually sensitive to a sensory stimulus (larger early evoked potentials), they compensate for the increased sensitivity by blunting the processing of information at higher cortical levels (indicated by smaller late evoked potentials).

Eye Movement Dysfunction. The inability to follow a moving visual target accurately is the defining basis for the disorders of smooth visual pursuit and disinhibition of saccadic eye movements seen in patients with schizophrenia. Eye movement dysfunction may be a trait marker for schizophrenia; it is independent of drug treatment and clinical state and also occurs in first-degree relatives of probands with schizophrenia. Various studies have reported abnormal eye movements in 50 to 85 percent of patients with schizophrenia compared with about 25 percent in psychiatric patients without schizophrenia and fewer than 10 percent in nonpsychiatrically ill control participants.

Prepulse Inhibition Deficits. Prepulse inhibition refers to a dysfunction of sensorimotor gating. Usually, a prepulse or weak stimulus, such as a noise, can decrease the startle reaction to a subsequent more substantial stimulus, such as a louder noise. As early as the 1970s, researchers found that patients with schizophrenia lacked this normal inhibition, and this was later found in the relatives of schizophrenia patients as well. Dopamine regulates sensorimotor gating, which adds additional support for the importance of dopamine in schizophrenia.

Neurotransmitters and Receptors

Excessive dopamine release in patients with schizophrenia is associated with the severity of positive psychotic symptoms. Positron emission tomography studies of dopamine receptors have shown that patients with schizophrenia have increases in subcortical synaptic dopamine content and increased subcortical synthesis capacity. These appear localized to the area of the associative striatum. These abnormalities, particularly increased subcortical synaptic dopamine content, are associated with the positive symptoms of schizophrenia and positive treatment response. However, the dopamine abnormalities are not merely due to the symptoms, as these abnormalities precede the onset of illness. They also occur in individuals considered to be at high risk for schizophrenia.

In addition to dopamine, there are increased levels of glutamate and decreased levels of γ-aminobutyric acid (GABA). Some patients with schizophrenia show a loss of GABAergic neurons in the hippocampus.

Postmortem studies in schizophrenia have demonstrated decreased muscarinic and nicotinic receptors in the caudate-putamen, hippocampus, and selected regions of the prefrontal cortex. These receptors play a role in the regulation of neurotransmitter systems involved in cognition, which is impaired in schizophrenia.

As a result of these neurotransmitter alterations, there are alterations in a variety of receptors. For example, N-methyl-D-aspartate

(NMDA) receptors appear to hypofunction as a result of glutamate and dopamine excesses.

Psychoneuroimmunology

Several immunologic abnormalities are associated with patients who have schizophrenia. The abnormalities include decreased T-cell interleukin-2 production, reduced number and responsiveness of peripheral lymphocytes, abnormal cellular and humoral reactivity to neurons, and the presence of brain-directed (antibrain) antibodies. The data can be interpreted variously as representing the effects of a neurotoxic virus or an endogenous autoimmune disorder.

The observation further strengthens the hypothesis that several autoimmune diseases can cause psychosis, such as systemic lupus encephalitis. Similarly, some types of immune encephalitis, such as anti-NMDA receptor encephalitis, can cause a psychotic illness that resembles schizophrenia, at least early in the illness.

Psychoneuroendocrinology

Many reports describe neuroendocrine differences between groups of patients with schizophrenia and groups of control subjects. For example, the results of the dexamethasone-suppression test are abnormal in various subgroups of patients with schizophrenia, although the test lacks practical or predictive value.

Some data suggest decreased concentrations of luteinizing hormone or follicle-stimulating hormone, perhaps correlated with age of onset and length of illness. Two additional reported abnormalities may correlate with the presence of negative symptoms: a blunted release of prolactin and growth hormone on gonadotropin-releasing hormone or thyrotropin-releasing hormone stimulation and a blunted release of growth hormone on apomorphine stimulation.

Infections

The support for infections being operative in schizophrenia is mostly indirect. As already mentioned, persons with schizophrenia may be more likely to be born in the winter months, thus suggesting a season-specific risk factor such as a virus (there are other explanations, however, such as changes in diet).

Epidemiologic data show a high incidence of schizophrenia after prenatal exposure to influenza during several epidemics of the disease. Some studies show that the frequency of schizophrenia increases after exposure to influenza during the second trimester of pregnancy. Influenza is, of course, more prevalent during the winter than other seasons. Other data supporting a viral hypothesis are an increased number of physical anomalies at birth, an increased rate of pregnancy and birth complications, seasonality of birth consistent with a viral infection, geographical clusters of adult cases, and seasonality of hospitalizations.

Viral theories stem from the fact that several specific viral theories have the power to explain the particular localization of pathology necessary to account for a range of manifestations in schizophrenia without overt febrile encephalitis.

Environmental Factors

In addition to infections, a variety of other factors, particularly in the prenatal period, can contribute a small but significant risk for schizophrenia. These include birth complications, trauma after delivery, nutritional deficiencies, and other factors that may negatively affect healthy development.

Our Understanding of the Genetics of Schizophrenia

Studies of Inheritance Patterns. At least as early as the 1930's, twin and family studies demonstrated that schizophrenia was an inherited disorder. The heritability of schizophrenia is estimated to be about 60 to 80 percent.

The likelihood of a person having schizophrenia correlates with the closeness of the relationship to an affected relative (e.g., first- or second-degree relative). In the case of monozygotic twins who have an identical genetic endowment, there is an approximately 50 percent concordance rate for schizophrenia. This rate is four to five times the concordance rate in dizygotic twins or the rate of occurrence found in other first-degree relatives (i.e., siblings, parents, or offspring). The role of genetic factors is further reflected by the drop-off in the occurrence of schizophrenia among second- and third-degree relatives, in whom one would hypothesize a decreased genetic loading. The finding of a higher rate of schizophrenia among the biologic relatives of an adopted-away person who develops schizophrenia, compared with the adoptive, nonbiologic relatives who raise the patient, provides further support to the genetic contribution to the etiology of schizophrenia.

Nevertheless, the monozygotic twin data demonstrate the fact that individuals who are genetically vulnerable to schizophrenia do not inevitably develop schizophrenia; other factors (e.g., environment) must be involved in determining a schizophrenia outcome. If a vulnerability–liability model of schizophrenia is correct in its postulation of an environmental influence, then other biologic or psychosocial environmental factors may prevent or cause schizophrenia in genetically vulnerable individuals.

Some data indicate that the age of the father correlates with the development of schizophrenia. In studies of schizophrenia patients with no history of illness in either the maternal or paternal line, those born from fathers older than the age of 60 years were vulnerable to developing the disorder. Presumably, spermatogenesis in older men is subject to more significant epigenetic damage than in younger men.

Genetic Studies. The modes of genetic transmission in schizophrenia are unknown, but many genes are associated with schizophrenia. Newer studies using more direct methods, such as comparative genomic hybridization, small nucleotide polymorphism (SNP) chips, next generation sequencing (NGS), GWAS, and the Clustered Regularly Interspaced Short Palindromic Repeats-associated Nuclease 9 (CRISPR/Cas9) genomic editing have revolutionized the genetic research of schizophrenia, and the number of genes associated with schizophrenia continues to rise. Many of these are likely chance findings. However, at least some are plausible candidates for contributing to schizophrenia vulnerability.

Linkage and association genetic studies have provided strong evidence for several specific candidate genes. The best candidates are those involved in synaptic transmission, including those for various monoamine receptors and those involved in glutamate release and signaling.

Given the role dopamine plays in schizophrenia, it is no surprise that many genetic studies have concentrated on genes involved in dopamine regulation. For example, some studies implicate catecholamine O-methyltransferase (COMT) polymorphism, which is involved in dopamine metabolism (as well as other catecholamines).

Copy number variation (CNV) studies suggest that perhaps between 2 to 5 percent of schizophrenia may be due, in part, to genetic variants that are highly penetrant but very rare. These included genes that were involved in regulating synaptic function and neurodevelopment. An example of a rare variant that is associated with psychosis is the 22q11.2 microdeletion, which causes 22q11.2 deletion or velocardiofacial syndrome (also called DiGeorge syndrome), which occurs in about 1 in 4,000 live births.

However, most of the risk is explained by common alleles, numbering in the hundreds, each having a small effect on risk. GWAS studies have yielded several loci of interest, including the DRD genes which encode the dopamine receptors, as well as several other loci involved in functions thought essential to the pathogenesis of schizophrenia. These include genes involved with glutamate, calcium signaling, dendritic spine formation, and other aspects of neuronal and neurodevelopmental function. As will be described in greater detail below, subsequent research has focused on genes related to the immune system and involved in synaptic pruning.

Many implicated genes do not code for proteins such as those described above, but have a role in genetic processing, affecting transcription and various epigenetic factors.

The extensive and sometimes conflicting findings are likely related to the heterogeneity of the disorder, and researchers are working to develop endophenotypes that more closely map to the genetics of the disorder. For example, prepulse inhibition is a likely candidate for a schizophrenia endotype. Researchers have identified several other endophenotype traits. These have the benefit of being measurable and lend themselves to quantitative analysis.

THE PSYCHOLOGY OF THE DISORDER

Family Dynamics

In a classic early study of 4-year old British children, children rated as having a poor mother–child relationship had a six-fold increase in the risk for schizophrenia. However, this leaves open the question of which came first, the poor relationship or the child's disease-related inability to form close relationships. It is telling that those who were adopted away from their mothers were more likely to develop schizophrenia if raised in adverse circumstances. In another study, children of schizophrenic mothers raised in a kibbutz (a type of commune) were more likely to develop schizophrenia than children raised in a family home. Nevertheless, no well-controlled evidence indicates that a specific family pattern plays a causative role in the development of schizophrenia. Some patients with schizophrenia do come from dysfunctional families, just as do many nonpsychiatrically ill persons. It is crucial, however, not to overlook pathologic family behavior that can significantly increase the emotional stress with which a vulnerable patient with schizophrenia must cope.

ETIOLOGY

Biologic Theories

The Dopamine Hypothesis. The simplest formulation of the dopamine hypothesis of schizophrenia posits that schizophrenia results from too much dopaminergic activity. The theory evolved from two observations. First, the efficacy and the potency of many antipsychotic drugs (i.e., the dopamine receptor antagonists [DRAs]) correlate with their ability to act as antagonists of the dopamine type 2 (D_2) receptor. Second, drugs that increase dopaminergic activity, notably cocaine and amphetamine, are psychotomimetic. There is also support from the fact that certain functions that are regulated by dopamine (e.g., prepulse inhibition) are abnormal in patients with schizophrenia.

The basic theory does not comment on whether dopaminergic hyperactivity results from too much dopamine, too many dopamine receptors, hypersensitivity of the receptors to dopamine, or a combination of these.

Which dopamine tracts in the brain are involved is also not specified. Historically, models of schizophrenia suggested that dysfunctions in the mesolimbic pathway were responsible for the positive symptoms of schizophrenia. This was due to a variety of observations, including that seizures and tumors in these regions produced schizophrenia-like symptoms. Also, amphetamines, which can induce psychosis, seemed to affect the nucleus accumbens, and antipsychotics injected in this area seemed to reverse this effect.

However, subsequent research suggests that the striatum (usually thought to be involved in motor function) plays an important role. This is suggested by functional neuroimaging studies, which found that the most significant differences in dopamine function found for schizophrenic patients were in the dorsal striatum and associated projections. This relation is also true for people at high risk for schizophrenia. This area has an integrative role, and dysfunctions in this area could explain the associative deficits that occur in schizophrenia. Also, as this area has a vital role in habit formation, it may argue for a model of psychosis as a habitual or rigid type of thinking, in which a person has difficulty considering alternative explanations for an experience.

Serotonin. Current hypotheses posit serotonin excess as a cause of both positive and negative symptoms in schizophrenia. The robust serotonin antagonist activity of clozapine and other second-generation antipsychotics coupled with the effectiveness of clozapine to decrease positive symptoms in chronic patients has contributed to the validity of this proposition.

GABA. Some have implicated the inhibitory amino acid neurotransmitter γ-aminobutyric acid (GABA) in the pathophysiology of schizophrenia based on the finding that some patients with schizophrenia have a loss of GABAergic neurons in the hippocampus. GABA has a regulatory effect on dopamine activity, and the loss of inhibitory GABAergic neurons could lead to the hyperactivity of dopaminergic neurons.

Neuropeptides. Neuropeptides, such as substance P and neurotensin, are localized with the catecholamine and indoleamine neurotransmitters and influence the action of these neurotransmitters. Alteration in neuropeptide mechanisms could facilitate, inhibit, or otherwise alter the pattern of firing in these neuronal systems.

Glutamate. Glutamate is also of interest, as ingestion of phencyclidine, a glutamate antagonist, produces an acute syndrome similar to schizophrenia. The hypotheses proposed about glutamate include those of hyperactivity, hypoactivity, and glutamate-induced neurotoxicity.

Acetylcholine and Nicotine. As noted, some studies suggest deficits in muscarinic and nicotinic receptors. These receptors play a role in the regulation of neurotransmitter systems involved in cognition, which is impaired in schizophrenia.

Neural Circuits (The Disconnect Hypothesis).   There has been a gradual evolution from conceptualizing schizophrenia as a disorder that involves discrete areas of the brain to a perspective that views schizophrenia as a disorder of brain neural circuits. For example, as mentioned previously, the basal ganglia and cerebellum are reciprocally connected to the frontal lobes, and the abnormalities in frontal lobe function seen in some brain imaging studies may be due to disease in either area rather than in the frontal lobes themselves. It is possible that an early developmental lesion of the dopaminergic tracts to the prefrontal cortex results in the disturbance of the prefrontal and limbic system function and leads to the positive and negative symptoms and cognitive impairments observed in patients with schizophrenia.

Of particular interest in the context of neural circuit hypotheses linking the prefrontal cortex and limbic system are studies demonstrating a relationship between hippocampal morphologic abnormalities and disturbances in prefrontal cortex metabolism or function (or both). Data from functional and structural imaging studies in humans suggest that whereas dysfunction of the anterior cingulate basal ganglia thalamocortical circuit underlies the production of positive psychotic symptoms, dysfunction of the dorsolateral prefrontal circuit underlies the production of primary, enduring negative or deficit symptoms. There is a neural basis for cognitive functions that are impaired in patients with schizophrenia. The observation of the relationship among impaired working memory performance, disrupted prefrontal neuronal integrity, altered prefrontal, cingulate, and inferior parietal cortex, and altered hippocampal blood flow provides strong support for disruption of the normal working memory neural circuit in patients with schizophrenia. The involvement of this circuit, at least for auditory hallucinations, has been documented in several functional imaging studies that contrast hallucinating and nonhallucinating patients.

Viruses, Neurotoxicity, and Neuroinflammation.   Most carefully conducted investigations that have searched for evidence of neurotoxic viral infections in schizophrenia have had negative results. However, as noted, indirect epidemiologic data support a viral role. Nonetheless, the inability to detect genetic evidence of viral infection reduces the significance of all circumstantial data. The possibility of autoimmune brain antibodies has some data to support it; the pathophysiologic process, if it exists, however, probably explains only a subset of the population with schizophrenia.

The neurotoxicity hypothesis suggests that psychosis can be toxic, increasing stress levels and associated cortisol, leading to brain changes. Also, the use of exogenous toxins such as cannabis and alcohol may further contribute. There is also some evidence that antipsychotic medications could contribute as well. As described below, however, the lack of evidence for neurodegeneration argues against this process.

Many studies have suggested that neuroinflammation plays a role in the pathogenesis of schizophrenia. Schizophrenia and certain autoimmune diseases have overlapping clinical, epidemiologic, and genetic features. Furthermore, at least a subset of patients with schizophrenia has laboratory findings indicating immune activation. These findings may be particularly prominent in patients with structural brain changes, although these results are inconsistent.

Several GWAS studies have found implicated genes that regulate the immune response, particularly the major histocompatibility complex (MHC) region and specific genes involved in synaptic pruning, lending more support for the neurodevelopmental hypothesis, discussed next.

Increasing Evidence Suggests that Schizophrenia Is a Neurodevelopmental Disorder.   Schizophrenia is likely a disorder of neurodevelopment, in which the standard neural structure does not develop properly. Earlier researchers speculated that this would be the case based on the observation that many patients who developed schizophrenia in early adulthood had motor and cognitive impairments as younger persons. Also, as discussed above, obstetrical complications are a risk factor for schizophrenia. Furthermore, for many patients with schizophrenia, cognitive deficits do not deteriorate significantly after illness onset. Evidence for this includes the lack of gliosis found in the brains of schizophrenia patients, as well as no consistent evidence of neurodegeneration, which suggests that the significant deficits are not due to cell death but rather the lack of proper cell growth. Also, many of the genes implicated in schizophrenia have relatively higher expression before birth and are likely involved in early brain development. Some of the genes may even affect the placenta, making it more sensitive to environmental stress.

As noted, one of the strongest genetic associations found to date for schizophrenia has been with variations in the MHC. These genes, particularly the C4 alleles, are involved in synaptic pruning during critical developmental periods, which occur during adolescence and adulthood, and may explain why symptoms of schizophrenia only become apparent during this period.

Schizophrenia Likely Involves Multiple Dysfunctions at Various Levels.   We know from neurologic patients suffering various focal lesions that the lesions causing hallucinations are often in the networks associated with that sensory system; thus, visual hallucinations are associated with occipital lesions as well as other areas along the visual pathway, such as the striatum and thalamus. Similarly, auditory hallucinations can be caused by lesions in the auditory cortex, hippocampus, amygdala, or thalamus. However, most patients with these focal lesions retain insight and recognize their hallucinations for what they are. Lesions in the corticostriatal networks can cause loss of insight, and the dopamine-related dysfunctions in this network likely account for the delusional beliefs about the hallucinations and other disordered thoughts. Still, other circuits are involved in the affective reaction to these abnormal experiences. In this way, the symptoms of schizophrenia are probably due to multiple dysfunctions along several networks.

This approach to understanding schizophrenia helps account for why antipsychotics are only partly useful for treating schizophrenia. By normalizing the dopamine dysfunction, antipsychotics decrease the abnormally high dopamine signaling in the associative striatum, and reduce the psychotic symptoms associated with the disorder. However, they are acting only on this particular circuit, and therefore have little effect on the negative and cognitive symptoms of the disorder.

Psychosocial Theories

If schizophrenia is a disease of the brain, it is likely to parallel diseases of other organs (e.g., myocardial infarctions, diabetes) whose courses are affected by psychosocial stress. Thus, clinicians should consider both psychosocial and biologic factors affecting schizophrenia.

The disorder affects individual patients, each of whom has a unique psychological makeup. Although many psychodynamic theories about the pathogenesis of schizophrenia seem outdated, perceptive clinical observations can help contemporary clinicians understand how the disease may affect a patient's psyche.

Psychoanalytic Theories. Sigmund Freud thought that schizophrenia resulted from developmental fixations early in life. These fixations produce defects in ego development, and he postulated that such defects contributed to the symptoms of schizophrenia. Margaret Mahler and Paul Federn concentrated on distortions in the mother–infant relationship, and Harry Stack Sullivan viewed schizophrenia as a disturbance in interpersonal relatedness. To Sullivan, schizophrenia is an adaptive method used to avoid panic, terror, and disintegration of the sense of self. The source of pathologic anxiety results from cumulative experiential traumas during development.

THE OBJECT RELATIONS DEFICIT MODEL OF SCHIZOPHRENIA. Object relationship theory posits that relations with other people are "introjected" and applied to new relationships. One can approach the challenge of new relationships by drawing on the internal models one collects from past relationships. In the case of schizophrenia, this normal process is disrupted, presumably due to errors in neurodevelopment that affect the filters that interpret information from the environment. Thus, the introjects one collects are distorted and incomplete, and interpreted as dangerous and threatening. As a result, the patient avoids relationships, thus having less chance for corrective experiences. Reality becomes terrifying, and the reaction is to create an alternate reality through psychotic thinking.

This theory has the benefit of accounting for both the positive and negative symptoms of schizophrenia. It also points at potential treatments. For example, the job of the therapist is to provide positive experiences that the patient can introject to help correct their distorted world view.

Regardless of the theoretical model, all psychodynamic approaches rely on the premise that psychotic symptoms have meaning in schizophrenia. Patients, for example, may become grandiose after an injury to their self-esteem. Similarly, all theories recognize that human relatedness may be terrifying for persons with schizophrenia. Although research on the efficacy of psychotherapy with schizophrenia shows mixed results, concerned persons who offer compassion and a sanctuary in the confusing world of schizophrenia must be a cornerstone of any overall treatment plan. Long-term follow-up studies show that some patients who bury psychotic episodes do not benefit from exploratory psychotherapy, but those who can integrate the psychotic experience into their lives may benefit from some insight-oriented approaches. There is renewed interest in the use of long-term individual psychotherapy in the treatment of schizophrenia, especially when combined with medication.

Learning Theories. According to learning theorists, children who later have schizophrenia learn irrational reactions and ways of thinking by imitating parents who have significant emotional problems. In learning theory, the poor interpersonal relationships of persons with schizophrenia develop because of poor models for learning during childhood.

References

Barnes TR. A rating scale for drug-induced akathisia. *Br J Psychiatry*. 1989;154: 672–676.

Bearden CE, Forsyth JK. The many roads to psychosis: Recent advances in understanding risk and mechanisms. *F1000Res*. 2018;7:F1000 Faculty Rev-1883.

Braff D, Stone C, Callaway E, Geyer M, Glick I, Bali L. Prestimulus effects on human startle reflex in normals and schizophrenics. *Psychophysiology*. 1978;15(4): 339–343.

Bramon E, Murray RM. A plausible model of schizophrenia must incorporate psychological and social, as well as neuro developmental, risk factors. *Dialogues Clin Neurosci*. 2001;3(4):243–256.

Chong HY, Teoh SL, Wu DBC, Kotirum S, Chiou CF, Chaiyakunapruk N. Global economic burden of schizophrenia: A systematic review. *Neuropsychiatr Dis Treat*. 2016;12:357–373.

Dewan MJ. The psychology of schizophrenia: Implications for biological and psychotherapeutic treatments. *J Nerv Ment Dis*. 2016;204(8):564–569.

DiLalla LF, McCrary M, Diaz E. A review of endophenotypes in schizophrenia and autism: The next phase for understanding genetic etiologies. *Am J Med Genet C Semin Med Genet*. 2017;175(3):354–361.

Fischer M. Psychoses in the offspring of schizophrenic monozygotic twins and their normal co-twins. *Br J Psychiatry*. 1971;118(542):43–52.

Furukawa TA, Levine SZ, Tanaka S, Goldberg Y, Samara M, Davis JM, Cipriani A, Leucht S. Initial severity of schizophrenia and efficacy of antipsychotics: Participant-level meta-analysis of 6 placebo-controlled studies. *JAMA Psychiatry*. 2015;72(1): 14–21.

Guy W. *ECDEU Assessment Manual for Psychopharmacology (Rev. 1976.).* Rockville, MD: U.S. Dept. of Health, Education, and Welfare, Public Health Service, Alcohol, Drug Abuse, and Mental Health Administration, National Institute of Mental Health, Psychopharmacology Research Branch, Division of Extramural Research Programs; 1976.

Jones C, Hacker D, Cormac I, Meaden A, Irving CB, Xia J, Shi C, Chen J. Cognitive behavioral therapy plus standard care versus standard care plus other psychosocial treatments for people with schizophrenia. *Schizophr Bull*. 2019;45(2):284–286.

Jones P, Rodgers B, Murray R, Marmot M. Child development risk factors for adult schizophrenia in the British 1946 birth cohort. *Lancet*. 1994;344(8934):1398–1402.

Kay SR, Fiszbein A, Opler LA. The positive and negative syndrome scale (PANSS) for schizophrenia. *Schizophr Bull*. 1987;13(2):261–276.

Kendell RE, Cooper JE, Gourlay AJ, Copeland JR, Sharpe L, Gurland BJ. Diagnostic criteria of American and British psychiatrists. *Arch Gen Psychiatry*. 1971;25(2): 123–130.

Kesby J, Eyles D, McGrath J, Scott J. Dopamine, psychosis and schizophrenia: The widening gap between basic and clinical neuroscience. *Transl Psychiatry*. 2018;8(1):30.

Khokhar JY, Dwiel LL, Henricks AM, Doucette WT, Green AI. The link between schizophrenia and substance use disorder: A unifying hypothesis. *Schizophr Res*. 2018;194:78–85.

Kirson NY, Weiden PJ, Yermakov S, Huang W, Samuelson T, Offord SJ, Greenberg PE, Wong BJO. Efficacy and effectiveness of depot versus oral antipsychotics in schizophrenia: Synthesizing results across different research designs. *J Clin Psychiatry*. 2013;74(6):568–575.

Kishimoto T, Robenzadeh A, Leucht C, Leucht S, Watanabe K, Mimura M, Borenstein M, Kane JM, Correll CU. Long-acting injectable vs oral antipsychotics for relapse prevention in schizophrenia: A meta-analysis of randomized trials. *Schizophr Bull*. 2014;40(1):192–213.

Kondej M, Stępnicki P, Kaczor AA. Multi-target approach for drug discovery against schizophrenia. *Int J Mol Sci*. 2018;19(10):3105.

Kumari V, Das M, Zachariah E, Ettinger U, Sharma T. Reduced prepulse inhibition in unaffected siblings of schizophrenia patients. *Psychophysiology*. 2005;42(5): 588–594.

Leucht C, Heres S, Kane JM, Kissling W, Davis JM, Leucht S. Oral versus depot antipsychotic drugs for schizophrenia—A critical systematic review and meta-analysis of randomised long-term trials. *Schizophr Res*. 2011;127(1–3):83–92.

Leucht S, Cipriani A, Spineli L, Mavridis D, Orey D, Richter F, Samara M, Barbui C, Engel RR, Geddes JR, Kissling W, Stapf MP, Lässig B, Salanti G, Davis JM. Comparative efficacy and tolerability of 15 antipsychotic drugs in schizophrenia: A multiple-treatments meta-analysis. *Lancet*. 2013;382(9896):951–962.

Lieberman JA, First MB. Psychotic disorders. *N Engl J Med*. 2018;379(3):270–280.

Malavia T, Chaparala S, Wood J, Chowdari K, Prasad KM, McClain L, Jegga AG, Ganapathiraju MK, Nimgaonkar VL. Generating testable hypotheses for schizophrenia and rheumatoid arthritis pathogenesis by integrating epidemiological, genomic, and protein interaction data. *NPJ Schizophr*. 2017;3:11.

McCutcheon RA, Abi-Dargham A, Howes OD. Schizophrenia, dopamine and the striatum: From biology to symptoms. *Trends Neurosci*. 2019;42(3):205–220.

Mirsky AF, Silberman EK, Latz A, Nagler S. Adult outcomes of high-risk children: Differential effects of town and kibbutz rearing. *Schizophr Bull*. 1985;11(1): 150–154.

Moreno-Küstner B, Martín C, Pastor L. Prevalence of psychotic disorders and its association with methodological issues. A systematic review and meta-analyses. *PLoS One*. 2018;13(4):e0195687.

Morrison AP, Turkington D, Pyle M, Spencer H, Brabban A, Dunn G, Christodoulides T, Dudley R, Chapman N, Callcott P, Grace T, Lumley V, Drage L, Tully S, Irving K, Cummings A, Byrne R, Davies LM, Hutton P. Cognitive therapy for people with schizophrenia spectrum disorders not taking antipsychotic drugs: A single-blind randomised controlled trial. *Lancet*. 2014;383(9926):1395–1403.

National Collaborating Centre for Mental Health (UK). Psychosis and Schizophrenia in Adults: Treatment and Management: Updated Edition 2014; 2014. Available at http://www.ncbi.nlm.nih.gov/books/NBK248060/

Orfanos S, Banks C, Priebe S. Are group psychotherapeutic treatments effective for patients with schizophrenia? A systematic review and meta-analysis. *Psychother Psychosom*. 2015;84(4):241–249.

Overall JE, Gorham DR. The Brief Psychiatric Rating Scale (BPRS): Recent developments in ascertainment and scaling. *Psychopharmacol Bull*. 1988;24(1):97–99.

Pharoah F, Mari J, Rathbone J, Wong W. Family intervention for schizophrenia. *Cochrane Database Syst Rev*. 2010;(12):CD000088.

Poloni N, Ielmini M, Caselli I, Lucca G, Gasparini A, Gasparini A, Lorenzoli G, Callegari C. Oral antipsychotic versus long-acting injections antipsychotic in schizophrenia spectrum disorder: A mirror analysis in a real-world clinical setting. *Psychopharmacol Bull*. 2019;49(2):17–27.

Samara MT, Leucht C, Leeflang MM, Anghelescu IG, Chung YC, Crespo-Facorro B, Elkis H, Hatta K, Giegling I, Kane JM, Kayo M, Lambert M, Lin CH, Möller HJ, Pelayo-Terán JM, Riedel M, Rujescu D, Schimmelmann BG, Serretti A, Correll CU, Leucht S. Early improvement as a predictor of later response to antipsychotics in schizophrenia: A diagnostic test review. *Am J Psychiatry*. 2015;172(7): 617–629.

Sampson S, Mansour M, Maayan N, Soares-Weiser K, Adams CE. Intermittent drug techniques for schizophrenia. *Cochrane Database Syst Rev*. 2013;(7): CD006196.

Schizophrenia Working Group of the Psychiatric Genomics Consortium. Biological insights from 108 schizophrenia-associated genetic loci. *Nature*. 2014;511(7510): 421–427.

Sekar A, Bialas AR, de Rivera H, Davis A, Hammond TR, Kamitaki N, Tooley K, Presumey J, Baum M, Van Doren V, Genovese G, Rose SA, Handsaker RE; Schizophrenia Working Group of the Psychiatric Genomics Consortium, Daly MJ, Carroll MC, Stevens B, McCarroll SA. Schizophrenia risk from complex variation of complement component 4. *Nature*. 2016;530(7589):177–183.

Simpson GM, Angus JW. A rating scale for extrapyramidal side effects. *Acta Psychiatr Scand Suppl*. 1970;212:11–19.

Tomasik J, Rahmoune H, Guest PC, Bahn S. Neuroimmune biomarkers in schizophrenia. *Schizophr Res*. 2016;176(1):3–13.

Volkow ND. Substance use disorders in schizophrenia—Clinical implications of comorbidity. *Schizophr Bull*. 2009;35(3):469–472.

Walsh T, McClellan JM, McCarthy SE, Addington AM, Pierce SB, Cooper GM, Nord AS, Kusenda M, Malhotra D, Bhandari A, Stray SM, Rippey CF, Roccanova P, Makarov V, Lakshmi B, Findling RL, Sikich L, Stromberg T, Merriman B, Gogtay N, Butler P, Eckstrand K, Noory L, Gochman P, Long R, Chen Z, Davis S, Baker C, Eichler EE, Meltzer PS, Nelson SF, Singleton AB, Lee MK, Rapoport JL, King MC, Sebat J. Rare structural variants disrupt multiple genes in neurodevelopmental pathways in schizophrenia. *Science*. 2008;320(5875):539–543.

Weinberger DR. Future of days past: Neurodevelopment and schizophrenia. *Schizophr Bull*. 2017;43(6):1164–1168.

Wójciak P, Rybakowski J. Clinical picture, pathogenesis and psychometric assessment of negative symptoms of schizophrenia. *Psychiatr Pol*. 2018;52(2):185–197.

Zareifopoulos N, Bellou A, Spiropoulou A, Spiropoulos K. Prevalence of comorbid chronic obstructive pulmonary disease in individuals suffering from schizophrenia and bipolar disorder: A systematic review. *COPD*. 2018;15(6):612–620.

Zhuo C, Hou W, Li G, Mao F, Li S, Lin X, Jiang D, Xu Y, Tian H, Wang W, Cheng L. The genomics of schizophrenia: Shortcomings and solutions. *Prog Neuropsychopharmacol Biol Psychiatry*. 2019;93:71–76.

The bipolar disorders include bipolar disorder type I, commonly referred to as manic depression, bipolar type II disorder, and cyclothymia. Historically, we considered these mood disorders to be on a continuum with depressive disorders—hence the concept of polarity, with depression at one end and mania the other. Since the 1980s and the introduction of DSM-III, we separated the bipolar disorders from depressive disorders mainly because the disorders have different epidemiologic characteristics, courses, and treatments. However, at various times experts in mood disorders have reconsidered this separation, noting that many patients with major depressive disorder have past episodes of at least some manic symptoms. Many authorities see considerable continuity between recurrent depressive and bipolar disorders. There continues to be widespread discussion and debate about the bipolar spectrum, which incorporates classic bipolar disorder, bipolar II, and recurrent depressions.

THE CLINICAL PRESENTATION

Manic Episodes

Manic patients are excited, talkative, sometimes amusing, and frequently hyperactive. Their speech is usually rapid and loud and challenging to interrupt. It is commonly referred to as *pressured*, appearing as if driven by some unknown urgency. Pressured speech is considered a hallmark of mania.

An elevated, expansive, or irritable mood is the hallmark of a manic episode. The elevated mood is euphoric and often infectious and can even cause a countertransferential denial of illness by an inexperienced clinician. Although uninvolved persons may not recognize the unusual nature of a patient's mood, those who know the patient recognize it as abnormal. Alternatively, the mood may be irritable, especially when someone prevents a patient from some unrealistic plan. Patients often exhibit a change of predominant mood from euphoria early in the course of the illness to later irritability. They also have a low frustration tolerance, which can lead to feelings of anger and hostility. Manic patients may be emotionally labile, switching from laughter to irritability to depression in minutes or hours.

Manic patients describe rapid thoughts, as inferred from their speech. As the manic state increases, their speech contains puns, jokes, rhymes, or plays on words. They may seem clever, even brilliant. Manic patients are often easily distracted, and their cognitive functioning in the manic state is unrestrained, with an accelerated flow of ideas. At a still higher activity level, associations become loosened, the ability to concentrate fades, and flight of ideas, clanging, and neologisms appear. In acute manic excitement, speech can be incoherent and indistinguishable from that of a person with schizophrenia.

The manic patient's thought content includes themes of self-confidence and self-aggrandizement.

At times, manic patients are grossly psychotic and disorganized and require physical restraints and the intramuscular injection of sedating drugs.

A 37-year-old engineer had experienced three manic episodes for which he had been hospitalized; all three episodes were preceded by several weeks of moderate psychomotor retardation. Although he had responded to lithium each time, once outside the hospital, he had been reluctant to take it and eventually refused to do so. Now that he was "euthymic," after his third and most disruptive episode during which he had badly beaten his wife, he could more accurately explain how he felt when manic. He experienced mania as "God implanted in him," so he could serve as "testimony to man's communication with God." He elaborated as follows: "Ordinary mortals will never, never understand the supreme manic state which I'm privileged to experience every few years. It is so vivid, so intense, so compelling. When I feel that way, there can be no other explanation: To be manic is, ultimately, to be God. God himself must be supermanic: I can feel it when mania enters through my left brain like laser beams, transforming my sluggish thoughts, recharging them, galvanizing them. My thoughts acquire such momentum, they rush out of my head, to disseminate knowledge about the true nature of mania to psychiatrists and all other ordinary mortals. That's why I will never accept lithium again—to do so is to obstruct the divinity in me." Although he was on the brink of divorce, he would not yield to his wife's plea to go back on lithium.

Delusions occur in 75 percent of all manic patients. Mood-congruent manic delusions are often concerned with great wealth, extraordinary abilities, or power. Bizarre and mood-incongruent delusions and hallucinations also appear in mania.

A 29-year-old female college graduate, mother of two children, and wife of a bank president, had experienced several manic and retarded depressive episodes that had responded to lithium carbonate. She was referred because she had developed the delusion that she had been involved in an international plot. Careful probing revealed that the delusion represented further elaboration, in a rather fantastic fashion, of a grandiose delusion that she had experienced during her last postpartum manic episode. She believed that she had played an important role in uncovering the plot, thereby becoming a national hero. Nobody knew about it, she contended, because the circumstances of the plot were top secret. She further believed that she had saved her country from the international scheme and suspected that she was singled out for persecution by the perpetrators of the plot. At one point, she had even entertained the idea that the plotters sent special radio communications to intercept and to interrupt her thoughts. As is typical in such cases, she was on a heavy dosage of a lithium–antipsychotic combination. The consultation was requested because the primary mood symptoms were under control, yet, she had not given up her grandiose delusion. She flippantly remarked, "I must be crazy to believe in my involvement in an international plot," but she could not help but believe in it. Over several months, seen typically in 60-minute sessions weekly, the patient had developed sufficient trust that the psychiatrist could gently challenge her beliefs.

She was, in effect, told that her self-professed role in the international scheme was highly implausible and that someone with her superior education and high social standing could not entertain a belief, to use her own words, "as crazy as that." She eventually broke into tears, saying that everyone in her family was so accomplished and famous that to keep up with them she had to be involved in something grand; in effect, the international scheme, she said, was her only claim to fame: "Nobody ever gives me credit for raising two kids, and throwing parties for my husband's business colleagues: My mother is a dean, my older brother holds high political office; my sister is a medical researcher with five discoveries to her credit [all true], and who am I? Nothing. Now, do you understand why I need to be a national hero?" As she alternated, over subsequent months, between such momentary flashes of insight and delusional denial, antipsychotic medication was gradually discontinued. Maintained on lithium, she now only makes passing reference to the grand scheme. She was encouraged to pursue her career goal toward a master's degree in library science. (Courtesy of HS Akiskal, M.D.)

Grossly, orientation and memory are intact, although some manic patients may be so euphoric that they answer questions testing orientation incorrectly. Emil Kraepelin called the symptom delirious mania.

We know less about the cognitive deficits associated with bipolar disorder than such chronic disorders like schizophrenia. However, there is some evidence to suggest they share some common deficits.

Impaired judgment is a hallmark of manic patients. They may break laws about credit cards, sexual activities, and finances and sometimes involve their families in financial ruin. Manic patients also have little insight into their disorder. Their disinhibition may result in other examples of poor judgment, such as making phone calls during inappropriate times of the day. Pathologic gambling, a tendency to disrobe in public places, wearing clothing and jewelry of bright colors in unusual or outlandish combinations, and inattention to small details (e.g., forgetting to hang up the telephone) are also symptomatic of the disorder. Patients act impulsively, and at the same time, with a sense of conviction and purpose. They are sometimes preoccupied with religious, political, financial, sexual, or persecutory ideas that can evolve into complex delusional systems. Occasionally, manic patients become regressed and play with their urine and feces.

About 75 percent of all manic patients are assaultive or threatening at some time. Manic patients are at increased risk for suicide. However, the most significant risk seems to be when bipolar patients are depressed. Manic patients often drink alcohol excessively, perhaps in an attempt to self-medicate.

Depressive Episodes

The depressive episodes in bipolar disorder are similar to those described for depressive disorders. Many experts in the field feel that there are qualitative differences in the depressive episodes experienced by bipolar patients, and researchers have attempted to find reliable differences between bipolar I disorder depressive episodes and episodes of major depressive disorder, but the differences are elusive. Although the data are inconsistent and controversial, some clinicians report that the depressed patients who we later diagnose as having bipolar disorder often have hypersomnia, psychomotor retardation, psychotic symptoms, a history of postpartum episodes, a family history of bipolar I disorder, and a history of antidepressant-induced hypomania. Table 6-1 lists some differences between the depressive disorder seen in bipolar disorder and major depression.

Table 6-1
Differentiating Characteristics of Bipolar and Unipolar Depressions

	Bipolar	Unipolar
History of mania or hypomania (definitional)	Yes	No
Temperament and personality	Cyclothymic and extroverted	Dysthymic and introverted
Sex ratio	Equal	More women than men
Age of onset	Teens, 20s, and 30s	30s, 40s, and 50s
Postpartum episodes	More common	Less common
Onset of episode	Often abrupt	More insidious
Number of episodes	Numerous	Fewer
Duration of episode	3–6 mo	3–12 mo
Psychomotor activity	Retardation > agitation	Agitation > retardation
Sleep	Hypersomnia > insomnia	Insomnia > hypersomnia
Family History		
Bipolar disorder	Yes	±
Unipolar disorder	Yes	Yes
Alcoholism	Yes	Yes
Pharmacologic Response		
Most antidepressants	Induce hypomania–mania	±
Lithium carbonate	Prophylaxis	±

Bipolar Disorder in Children and Adolescents

It is easy to misdiagnose mania in adolescents as a conduct disorder, antisocial personality disorder, or schizophrenia. Symptoms of mania in adolescents may include psychosis, alcohol or other substance abuse, suicide attempts, academic problems, philosophical brooding, OCD symptoms, multiple somatic complaints, marked irritability resulting in fights, and other antisocial behaviors. Although we can see many of these symptoms in healthy adolescents, severe or persistent symptoms should cause clinicians to consider bipolar I disorder in the differential diagnosis.

DIAGNOSIS

Patients with both manic and depressive episodes or patients with manic episodes alone are said to have *bipolar disorder*. The terms unipolar mania and pure mania are sometimes used for patients who are bipolar but who do not have depressive episodes.

Three additional categories of mood disorders are hypomania, cyclothymia, and dysthymia. Hypomania is an episode of manic symptoms that do not meet the criteria for a manic episode. Cyclothymia and dysthymia are disorders that represent less severe forms of bipolar disorder and major depression, respectively.

Bipolar I Disorder

Bipolar I patients have at least one manic episode. It is what most people mean when they refer to bipolar as a disorder. Table 6-2 compares the different approaches to diagnosing bipolar I disorder.

Table 6-2
Bipolar I Disorder

Bipolar I Disorder		
	DSM-5	**ICD-10**
Name	Bipolar I Disorder	Bipolar Affective Disorder ***NOTE:** ICD-10 does not distinguish between Bipolar I and II, requiring only history of discrete episodes of mania, hypomania and/or depression, with episodes demarcated by switches in mood/affect.*
Duration	• Manic episode: 1 wk+ • Hypomanic episode: 4 days+ • Major depressive episode: 2 wk+	
Symptoms	**Manic or hypomanic episodes** • Abnormally ↑ or irritable mood (required) • Grandiose thoughts • ↓ Need for sleep • Pressured speech • Racing and expansive thoughts • Distractibility • Hyperactivity • Impulsivity/high-risk activities **Depressive episodes** • Similar to that for major depressive disorder	• History of episodes of mania, hypomania and/or depression • Switches in mood/affect **Mania** • Abnormally ↑ or irritable mood (required) • ↑ Activity • ↑ Talkativeness • Flight of ideas/racing thoughts • Social disinhibition • ↓ Need for sleep • Grandiose thoughts • Distractibility • Impulsivity/recklessness • Hypersexuality **Hypomania** • Abnormally ↑ mood (required) • Psychomotor agitation • ↑ Talkativeness • Poor concentration/distractibility • ↓ Need for sleep • Hypersexuality • Impulsivity or ↑ spending • Over-familiarity **Depressive episode** • Depressed mood • Loss of interest or pleasure • Decreased energy *Additional symptoms:* • Low self-esteem • Excessive guilt or shame • Recurrent thoughts of death or suicide • Poor concentration • Psychomotor changes • Sleep disturbance • Change in appetite and/or weight
Required number of symptoms	At least 1 manic episode • Abnormally ↑ or irritable mood (required) ≥3 of the other symptoms (4 if irritable mood)	**Bipolar affective disorder, current episode hypomanic** • Hypomania • History of a prior affective episode (manic, hypomanic, depressed, mixed) **Bipolar affective disorder, current episode manic** • Mania • History of prior affective episode (manic, hypomanic, depressed, mixed) **Bipolar disorder, current episode mild/moderate/severe depression** • Depressive episode • History of prior affective episode (manic, hypomanic, depressed, mixed) **Bipolar disorder, current episode mixed** • Mixture or rapid alternation of hypomanic, manic and/or depressive symptoms • History of prior affective episode (manic, hypomanic, depressed, mixed)
Exclusions (not better explained by):	Drug abuse Medication effect Other medical condition Other psychiatric illness	Psychoactive substance use Another mental disorder

(continued)

Table 6-2
Bipolar I Disorder (*Continued*)

	Bipolar I Disorder	
	DSM-5	**ICD-10**
Psychosocial Impact	**Manic episode:** impaired functioning or needing hospitalization **Hypomanic episode:** No impairment or need for hospitalization **Depressive episode:** marked distress and/or psychosocial impairment	

Symptom Specifiers	**With mixed features:**
	• Either depressive or manic/hypomanic episode
	• Additional symptoms of depressive or manic/hypomanic period (not full criteria)
	With rapid cycling:
	• ≥4 mood episodes in 1 yr
	• ≥2-mo period of partial/full remission between episodes
	With melancholic features:
	Similar to that for major depressive disorder
	With atypical features:
	Similar to that for major depressive disorder
	With anxious distress:
	≥2 symptoms among the following:
	• Feeling tense
	• Restlessness
	• Difficulty with concentration due to worrying
	• ↑ fear without cause
	• Fear of loss of control
	With mood-congruent psychotic features
	With mood-incongruent psychotic features
	With catatonia
		Current episode hypomanic
		Current episode manic without psychotic symptoms
		Current episode manic with psychotic symptoms
		    mood congruent
		    mood incongruent
		Current episode of depression
		Current episode mixed
		Currently in remission—no symptoms. History of previous episodes.

Severity Specifiers	**Mild**—minimal symptoms, no to minimal impairment and/or distress
	Moderate—moderate symptomatology and impairment
	Severe—maximal symptoms, marked distress and impairment
		For current episode of depression
		    Mild: 2–3 symptoms
		    Moderate: ≥4 symptoms, including ≥2 among loss of pleasure, depressed mood, and low energy
		    Severe: symptoms are marked and distressing, suicidal thoughts are common
		        without psychotic symptoms
		        with psychotic symptoms
		            mood congruent
		            mood incongruent

Course Specifiers	**With peripartum onset:** • Episode occurs during pregnancy or within 4 wk after delivery **With seasonal pattern** • Pattern present for ≥2 yr **In partial remission** **In full remission**	

Patients with this disorder may have a single or recurrent episode. We consider manic episodes as distinct when they are separated by at least 2 months without significant symptoms of mania or hypomania. The episodes should not be due to another apparent cause, such as medication (including an antidepressant).

Bipolar II Disorder

Bipolar patients have hypomania rather than mania—manic-type symptoms that are not as severe or as impairing as full mania. Table 6-3 compares the different approaches to diagnosing bipolar II disorder.

It is easy to confuse other disorders, including dramatic but normal moods, with hypomania. For example, some patients with depression may be thrilled and very euphoric once emerging from a depressive episode. Many medications, including antidepressants, can induce hypomanic symptoms. The diagnostic approaches attempt to help distinguish hypomania from these other causes of a heightened mood.

Diagnostic Specifiers

Rapid Cycling. Some patients experience frequent manic episodes. When a patient has at least four such episodes in a year, we diagnose them with the rapid cycling subtype of bipolar I

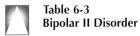

Table 6-3
Bipolar II Disorder

	Bipolar II Disorder	
	DSM-5	**ICD-10**
Name	Bipolar II Disorder	Bipolar Affective Disorder ***NOTE:*** ICD-10 does not distinguish between Bipolar I and II, requiring only history of discrete episodes of mania, hypomania and/or depression, with episodes demarcated by switches in mood/affect.
Duration	See Table 6-2 for hypomanic and depressive episodes	See Table 6-2

Symptoms	**Hypomanic episodes**
	  (see Table 6-2)
	Depressive episodes
	  (see Table 6-2)
		See Table 6-2

Required number of symptoms	≥1 hypomanic episode ≥1 depressive episode	
Exclusions (not better explained by):	Drug abuse Medication effect Other medical condition Another psychiatric illness Diagnose bipolar I if h/o manic episode	Psychoactive substance use Better explained by another mental disorder
Psychosocial Impact	• Hypomanic episode: NO marked impairment in functioning and NO hospitalization necessitated • Depressive episode: marked distress and/or impairment in psychosocial functioning	

Symptom Specifiers	**Current episode (see Table 6-2 for definitions)**
	  Depressed
	  Hypomanic
	With anxious distress
	With mixed features
	With rapid cycling
	With melancholic features
	With atypical features
	With mood-congruent psychotic features
	With mood-incongruent psychotic features
	With catatonia
		See Table 6-2

Severity Specifiers	**Mild**—minimal symptoms, no to minimal impairment and/or distress **Moderate**—moderate symptomatology and impairment **Severe**—maximal symptoms, marked distress and impairment (note, impairment occurs during depressive episode)	See Table 6-2
Course Specifiers	**With peripartum onset**—see Table 6-2 **With seasonal pattern**—see Table 6-2 **In partial remission** **In full remission**	

disorder. Patients with rapid cycling bipolar I disorder are likely to be female and to have had depressive and hypomanic episodes. No data indicate that rapid cycling has a familial pattern of inheritance; thus, an external factor such as stress or drug treatment may provoke rapid cycling.

With Seasonal Pattern.   As with depressive disorders, mania can occur primarily during certain seasons. Some studies have found a higher prevalence of manic episodes in the spring and summer months. However, available research is most convincing for the seasonality of depressive episodes.

With Peripartum Onset.   Mania occurring after pregnancy is a critical issue given the potential risk to the child.

Catatonia.   Clinicians often do not associate catatonic symptoms with bipolar I disorder because of the marked contrast between the symptoms of stuporous catatonia and the classic symptoms of mania. They are associated with depressive episodes, however.

Other Bipolar Disorders

Cyclothymia.   Cyclothymic disorder has also been appreciated clinically for some time as a less severe form of bipolar disorder. Patients with cyclothymic disorder have at least 2 years of frequently occurring hypomanic symptoms that cannot fit the diagnosis of a manic episode and of depressive symptoms that cannot fit the diagnosis of a major depressive episode. Table 6-4 compares the different approaches to diagnosing cyclothymia.

Table 6-4
Cyclothymic Disorder

	Cyclothymic Disorder	
	DSM-5	**ICD-10**
Name	Cyclothymic Disorder	Cyclothymia
Duration	≥2 yr (≥1 for children) with depressive and hypomanic symptoms present ≥50% of the time	2-yr w/ periods of depression and elevated mood, without ever meeting criteria for a depressive episode or manic episode
Symptoms	Hypomanic episodes (see Table 6-2) Depressive episodes (see Table 6-2)	Unstable moods, many periods of depression or mild elation which are insufficient to be called hypomania or mild major depressive disorder
Required number of symptoms	Symptoms of hypomania and depression present, without ever meeting full criteria for a depressive episode or manic episode	Several episodes, symptoms are insufficient for a diagnosis of hypomania, major depression or another bipolar affective disorder
Exclusions (not better explained by):	• Substance use • Medication effect • Other medical condition • Other mental illness (i.e., Bipolar I or II)	Bipolar affective disorder (though history of bipolar affective disorder may be present)
Psychosocial Impact	Marked distress or impairment in areas of functioning	
Symptom Specifiers	**With anxious distress:** including at least two symptoms among feeling tense, restlessness, difficulty with concentration due to worrying, excessive fear without identifiable cause, fear of loss of control	Affective personality disorder Cycloid personality Cyclothymic personality

Mr. B, a 25-year-old single man, came for evaluation due to irritability, insomnia, jumpiness, and excessive energy. He reported that such episodes lasted from a few days to a few weeks and alternated with longer periods of feeling hopeless, dejected, and worn out with thoughts of suicide. Mr. B reported having been this way for as long as he could remember. He had never been treated for his symptoms. He denied using drugs and said he had "only the occasional drink to relax."

As a child, Mr. B went from one foster family to another and was an irresponsible and trouble-making child. He frequently ran away from home, was absent from school, and committed minor crimes. He ran away from his last foster family at the age of 16 years and drifted ever since, taking occasional odd jobs. When he became restless at one location or job, he quickly moved on to the next. He did not have close friends because he would form and end friendships quickly.

DIFFERENTIAL DIAGNOSIS

When a patient with bipolar I disorder has a depressive episode, the differential diagnosis is the same as that for a patient with major depressive disorder. However, when a patient is manic, there is a broad differential, including other mood disorders, psychiatric disorders, medical disorders, and substances. We list some of these in Table 6-5.

Psychotic Disorders

It can be tough to distinguish a manic episode from the acute psychosis of a patient experiencing a psychotic episode. Although challenging, a differential diagnosis is possible. Merriment, elation, and infectiousness of mood are much more common in manic episodes than in schizophrenia. The combination of a heightened mood, rapid speech, and hyperactivity weighs toward mania. Mania often begins rapidly and is a marked change from previous behavior. Family history is also helpful.

When evaluating patients with catatonia, clinicians should look carefully for a history of manic or depressive episodes and a family history of mood disorders. There is an unfortunate tendency to misdiagnose manic symptoms in persons from minority groups (mainly Black and Hispanic) as schizophrenic symptoms.

Personality Disorders

Hypomania can frequently be confused with the mood lability of personality disorders, particularly borderline personality disorder.

Table 6-5
Differential Diagnosis of Mania

Medical
    AIDS/HIV
    Delirium
    Hyperthyroidism
    Postencephalitic syndrome

Substance induced
    Antidepressant-induced mania
    Steroid-induced mania
    Amphetamine-induced mania
    Cocaine-induced mania
    Phencyclidine-induced mania
    Alcohol intoxication
    L-Dopa–induced mania
    Bronchodilator-induced mania
    Decongestant-induced mania

Psychiatric
    Atypical psychosis
    Bipolar disorder
    Catatonic schizophrenia
    Schizoaffective disorder

Patients with a borderline personality disorder often have a severely disrupted life, similar to that of patients with bipolar II disorder, because of the multiple episodes of significant mood disorder symptoms.

A 19-year-old single woman presented with the chief complaint that "all men are bastards." Since her early teens, with the onset of her menses, she had complained of extreme variability in her moods on a nearly daily basis; irritability with hostile outbursts was her main affect, although more-protracted hypersomnic depressions with multiple overdoses and wrist slashings had led to at least three hospitalizations. She also had migrainous headaches that, according to her mother, had motivated at least one of those overdoses. Despite her tempestuous and suicidal moods that led to these hospitalizations, she complained of "inner emptiness and a bottomless void." She had used heroin, alcohol, and stimulants to overcome this troubling symptom. She also gave history of ice cream craving and frequent purging. She was talented in English and wrote much-acclaimed papers on the American confessional poet Anne Sexton. She said that she was mentally disturbed because of a series of stepfathers who had all forced "oral rape" on her when she was between 11 and 15 years of age. She subsequently gave herself sexually to any man that she met in bars, no longer knowing whether she was a "prostitute" or a "nice little girl." On two occasions, she had inflicted cigarette burns inside her vagina "to feel something." She had also engaged in a "brief lesbian relationship" that ultimately left her "emptier" and guilt ridden; nonetheless, she now believed that she should burn in hell because she could not get rid of "obsessing" about the excitement of mutual cunnilingus with her much older female partner. The patient's mother, who owned an art gallery, had been married five times and gave a history of unmistakable hypomanic episodes; a maternal uncle had died from alcohol-induced cirrhosis. The patient's father, a prominent lawyer known for his "temper and wit," had committed suicide. The patient was given phenelzine, eventually raised to 75 mg/day, at which point the mother described her as "the sweet daughter she was before age 13." At her next premenstrual phase, the patient developed insomnia, ran away from home at night, started "dancing like a go-go girl, met an incredibly handsome man" of 45 years of age (a pornography shop owner), and had a clandestine marriage to him. After many dose adjustments, she is now maintained on a combination of lithium (900 mg/day) and divalproex 750 mg/day. The patient now attends college and has completed four semesters in art history. In addition to control of her irritable and suicidal moods, bulimic and migraine attacks have abated considerably. Her marriage has been annulled on the basis that she was not mentally competent at the time of the wedding. She is no longer promiscuous and now expresses fear of intimacy with men that she is attracted to. She is receiving individual psychotherapy for this problem.

Medical Conditions

In contrast to depressive symptoms, which are present in almost all psychiatric disorders, manic symptoms are more distinctive. However, a wide range of medical disorders and substances can cause manic symptoms. Antidepressant treatment can also be associated with the precipitation of mania in some patients.

COMORBIDITY

Whereas men more frequently present with substance use disorders, women more frequently present with comorbid anxiety and eating disorders. In general, patients with bipolar disorder more frequently show comorbidity of substance use and anxiety disorders than do patients with unipolar major depression. In the Epidemiologic Catchment Area (ECA) study, the lifetime history of substance use disorders, panic disorder, and OCD was approximately twice as high among patients with bipolar I disorder (61 percent, 21 percent, and 21 percent, respectively) than in patients with unipolar major depression (27 percent, 10 percent, and 12 percent, respectively). Comorbid substance use disorders and anxiety disorders worsen the prognosis of the illness and markedly increase the risk of suicide.

Although cyclothymic disorder is sometimes diagnosed retrospectively in patients with bipolar I disorder, no identified personality traits are associated explicitly with bipolar I disorder.

COURSE

The natural history of bipolar I disorder is such that it is often useful to make a graph of a patient's disorder and to keep it up to date as the treatment progresses (Fig. 6-1).

Onset

About 5 to 10 percent of patients with an initial diagnosis of major depressive disorder have a manic episode 6 to 10 years after the first depressive episode. The mean age for this switch is 32 years, and it often occurs after two to four depressive episodes.

Bipolar I disorder most often starts with depression (75 percent of the time in women, 67 percent in men) and is a recurring disorder. Most patients experience both depressive and manic episodes, although 10 to 20 percent experience only manic episodes.

The incidence of bipolar I disorder in children and adolescents is about 1 percent, and the onset can be as early as age 8 years.

Manic symptoms are common in older persons, although the range of causes is broad and includes nonpsychiatric medical conditions, dementia, and delirium, as well as bipolar I disorder. The onset of true bipolar I disorder in older persons is relatively uncommon.

Duration

The manic episodes typically have a rapid onset (hours or days) but may evolve over a few weeks. An untreated manic episode lasts about 3 months; therefore, clinicians should not discontinue giving drugs before that time. Depressive episodes are generally similar to those for depressive disorders.

Of persons who have a single manic episode, 90 percent are likely to have another. As the disorder progresses, the time between episodes often decreases. After about five episodes, however, the interepisode interval often stabilizes at 6 to 9 months. Of persons with bipolar disorder, 5 to 15 percent have four or more episodes per year and are classified as rapid cyclers.

Bipolar II Disorder

The course and prognosis of bipolar II disorder indicate that the diagnosis is stable because there is a high likelihood that patients with bipolar II disorder will have the same diagnosis up to 5 years later. Bipolar II disorder is a chronic disease that warrants long-term treatment strategies.

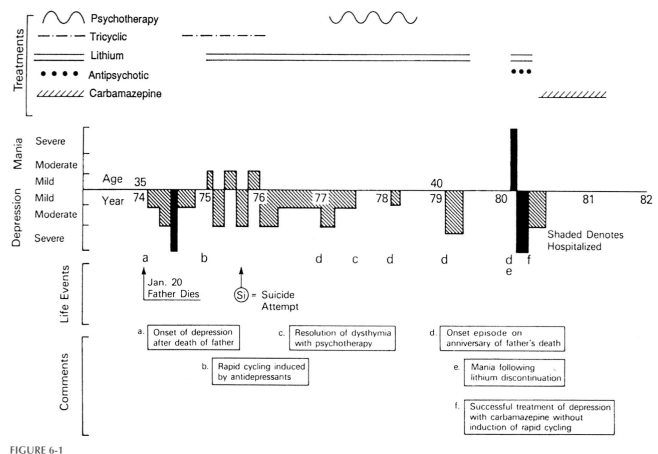

FIGURE 6-1

Graphing the course of a mood disorder. Prototype of a life chart. (Courtesy of Robert M. Post, M.D.)

PROGNOSIS

Patients with bipolar I disorder have a poorer prognosis than do patients with major depressive disorder. About 40 to 50 percent of patients with bipolar I disorder may have a second manic episode within 2 years of the first episode. Although lithium prophylaxis improves the course and prognosis of bipolar I disorder, probably only 50 to 60 percent of patients achieve significant control of their symptoms with lithium. About 7 percent of patients with bipolar I disorder do not have a recurrence of symptoms; 45 percent have more than one episode, and 40 percent have a chronic disorder. Patients may have from 2 to 30 manic episodes, although the mean number is about 9. About 40 percent of all patients have more than 10 episodes. On long-term follow-up, 15 percent of all patients with bipolar I disorder are well, 45 percent are well but have multiple relapses, 30 percent are in partial remission, and 10 percent are chronically ill. One-third of all patients with bipolar I disorder have chronic symptoms and evidence of significant social decline.

Prognostic Indicators

One 4-year follow-up study of patients with bipolar I disorder found that a premorbid poor occupational status, alcohol dependence, psychotic features, depressive features, interepisode depressive features, and male gender were all factors that contributed to a poor prognosis. A short duration of manic episodes, advanced age of onset, few suicidal thoughts, and few coexisting psychiatric or medical problems predict a better outcome.

TREATMENT APPROACH

Hospitalization

It is best to treat patients with severe mania in the hospital where aggressive dosing is possible, and it is possible to achieve an adequate response relatively quickly. Manic patients may test the limits of ward rules, shift responsibility for their acts onto others, or exploit the weaknesses of others, and they can create conflicts among staff members.

Choosing a Treatment

Medications are the treatments of choice for patients with bipolar disorders. However, psychotherapies can offer an essential adjunct to treatment.

Somatic Treatments

Pharmacotherapy

GENERAL CLINICAL GUIDELINES. We can divide the pharmacologic treatment of bipolar disorders into acute and maintenance phases. Bipolar treatment, however, also involves the formulation of different strategies for the patient who is experiencing mania or

Table 6-6
Recommendations for Pharmacologic Treatment of Acute Mania

First line	Monotherapy: lithium, divalproex, divalproex ER, olanzapine, risperidone, quetiapine, quetiapine XR, aripiprazole, ziprasidone, asenapine, paliperidone ER, cariprazine
	Adjunctive therapy with lithium or divalproex: risperidone, quetiapine, olanzapine, aripiprazole, asenapine
Second line	Monotherapy: carbamazepine, carbamazepine ER, ECT, haloperidol
	Combination therapy: lithium + divalproex
Third line	Monotherapy: chlorpromazine, clozapine, tamoxifen
	Combination therapy: lithium or divalproex + haloperidol, lithium + carbamazepine, adjunctive tamoxifen
Not recommended	Monotherapy: gabapentin, topiramate, lamotrigine, verapamil, tiagabine
	Combination therapy: risperidone + carbamazepine, olanzapine + carbamazepine

ECT, electroconvulsive therapy; XR or ER, extended release.
Modified from CANMAT/ISBD Guidelines.

hypomania or depression. Lithium and its augmentation by antidepressants, antipsychotics, and benzodiazepines have been the principal approach to the illness. However, three anticonvulsant mood stabilizers—carbamazepine, valproate, and lamotrigine—are commonly used options, as well as a series of atypical antipsychotics. Often, it is necessary to try different medications before finding an optimal treatment. Furthermore, although one strives for monotherapy, in the case of bipolar disorder, polypharmacy is common.

Table 6-6 lists some recommended medications for treating acute mania.

Adherence to treatment, however, is often a problem because patients with mania frequently lack insight into their illness and refuse to take medication. Because impaired judgment, impulsivity, and aggressiveness combine to put the patient or others at risk, we must medicate patients when we need to protect themselves and others from harm.

INITIAL MEDICATION SELECTION. Figure 6-2 diagrams a strategy for selecting and preparing a bipolar patient for pharmacotherapy.

Acute Mania. The treatment of acute mania, or hypomania, usually is the most straightforward phase to treat. We can use agents alone or in combination to bring the patient down from a high.

Lithium Carbonate. Lithium carbonate is considered the prototypical mood stabilizer. However, because the onset of antimanic action with lithium can be slow, we often supplement it in the early phases of treatment by atypical antipsychotics, mood-stabilizing anticonvulsants, or high-potency benzodiazepines. Therapeutic lithium levels are between 0.6 and 1.2 mEq/L. The acute use of lithium has been limited in recent years by its unpredictable efficacy, problematic side effects, and the need for frequent laboratory tests. The introduction of newer drugs with more favorable side effects, lower toxicity, and less need for frequent laboratory testing has resulted in a decline in lithium use. For many patients, however, its clinical benefits can be remarkable.

Anticonvulsants. Valproate (valproic acid or divalproex sodium) has surpassed lithium in use for acute mania. Unlike lithium, valproate is only indicated for acute mania, although most experts agree it also has prophylactic effects. Normal dose levels of valproic acid are 750 to 2,500 mg/day, achieving blood levels between 50 and 120 µg/mL. Rapid oral loading with 15 to 20 mg/kg of divalproex sodium from day 1 of treatment has been well tolerated and associated with a rapid onset of response. Some laboratory testing is required during valproate treatment.

Carbamazepine has been used worldwide for decades as a first-line treatment for acute mania. The FDA approved it for acute mania in the United States in 2004. Typical doses of carbamazepine to treat acute mania range between 600 and 1,800 mg/day associated with blood levels of between 4 and 12 µg/mL. The keto congener of carbamazepine, oxcarbazepine, is better tolerated than carbamazepine, but the data for its efficacy are conflicting. A Cochrane review concluded there is insufficient evidence for this medication in acute mania.

Antipsychotics. The FDA approved many of the atypical antipsychotics for use in bipolar disorder. We list them in Table 6-7. Compared with older agents, such as haloperidol and chlorpromazine, atypical antipsychotics have a lesser liability for excitatory postsynaptic potential and tardive dyskinesia; many do not increase prolactin. However, many of them have the risk of weight gain with its associated medical problems. Some patients, however, require maintenance treatment with antipsychotic medication.

Acute Bipolar Depression
Lithium. There is limited evidence for lithium in bipolar depression. Early studies were promising, but later placebo-controlled studies did not confirm lithium's efficacy. More extensive studies that included lithium did suggest that lithium was at least as useful as other mood stabilizers for bipolar depression.

Anticonvulsants. The most promising anticonvulsant has been lamotrigine, which has several reasonable studies showing efficacy for bipolar depression. Its major limitation is that it must be titrated gradually to prevent a severe skin rash. Evidence for valproate and other anticonvulsants is limited. Gabapentin and levetiracetam appear to be ineffective.

Antipsychotics. Several of the atypical antipsychotics have shown efficacy for bipolar depression. Quetiapine has the best evidence. It appears that quetiapine, in a modest dose (300 mg/day), is sufficient to improve symptoms. Olanzapine, lurasidone, and cariprazine also have positive studies, and the FDA approved lurasidone for this indication. Ziprasidone and aripiprazole do not appear to be effective.

Antidepressants. It remains controversial whether antidepressants are useful for the depressive phase of bipolar disorder. This is particularly true in patients with rapid cycling and mixed states. They seem to be less effective than for major depressive disorder and may induce cycling, mania, or hypomania. The risk of inducing mania seems highest for tricyclic antidepressants, monoamine oxidase inhibitors, and perhaps the serotonin norepinephrine reuptake inhibitors such as venlafaxine. Most experts agree that antidepressants are not appropriate as monotherapy for patients with bipolar disorder.

Whether we can use them as adjuncts is also controversial. Some antidepressants have some evidence of efficacy for adjunctive therapy, such as fluoxetine. On the whole, the available evidence suggests they may have some usefulness when combined with a mood stabilizer.

"Basic" parameters for all patients prior to treatment implementation

History: medical comorbidities (including CVD risk factors), smoking status, alcohol use, pregnancy status, family history of CVD risk factors

Investigations: waist circumference and/or BMI (weight & height), BP, FBC, EUC, LFTs, fasting glucose, fasting lipid profile

---

Manage any identified medical conditions as appropriate

Selection of medication, taking into consideration overall health risk profile

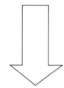

"Add-on" parameters according to treatment selected

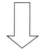 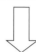 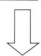

Lithium

Baseline: TSH, Ca

Serum level: 2 levels to establish therapeutic dose, then every 3–6 months, after dose increases and as clinically indicated

Longitudinal monitoring
- EUC every 3–6 months
- Ca, TSH, and weight after 6 months, then annually

Valproate and carbamazepine

Baseline: Hematologic and hepatic history

Serum level: 2 levels to establish therapeutic dose (4 weeks apart for carbamazepine), then as clinically indicated

Longitudinal monitoring
- *Valproate:* Weight, FBC, LFT, menstrual history every 3 months for the first year, then annually; BP, fasting glucose, and lipid profile if risk factors; bone densitometry if risk factors
- *Carbamazepine:* FBC, LFT, EUC monthly for first 3 months, then annually; alert to rash especially in first few months of treatment; bone densitometry if risk factors; review contraceptive efficacy where applicable

Lamotrigine
- Alert to rash

Atypical antipsychotics[a]

Longitudinal monitoring
- Weight monthly for first 3 months, then every 3 months
- BP and fasting glucose every 3 months for first year, then annually
- Fasting lipid profile after 3 months, then annually
- ECG and prolactin level as clinically indicated

[a]Clozapine an exception

CVD, cardiovascular disease; BMI, body mass index; BP, blood pressure; FBC, full blood count; EUC, electrolytes, urea, and creatinine; LFTs, liver function tests; TSH, thyroid stimulating hormone; Ca, calcium; ECG, electrocardiogram.

FIGURE 6-2
Recommendations for treatment monitoring in bipolar disorder. (Used with permission from ISBD safety monitoring guidelines.)

Electroconvulsive Therapy. Electroconvulsive therapy may also be useful for patients with bipolar depression who do not respond to lithium or other mood stabilizers and their adjuncts, particularly in cases in which strong suicidal tendency presents as a medical emergency.

Other Agents. Various clinicians and researchers have tried many other agents in an attempt to find more options for treatment. Most studies have not been promising. Dopamine agonists, including modafinil and armodafinil, have some preliminary evidence. Omega-3-fatty acid adjunctive therapy has conflicting evidence. N-acetylcysteine (a glutathione precursor) has some preliminary evidence. Ketamine and other glutamatergic modulators may have a role in treatment-resistant patients.

Table 6-7
Atypical Antipsychotics for Bipolar Disorder: Efficacy Summary and Dose Ranges

Drug	Dose Range (mg)	Acute Mania	Acute Bipolar Depression	Mood Episodes	Mania	Depression	Comments
				Prophylaxis			
Olanzapine	5–20	Yes	Yes (see comments)	Yes	Yes	Yes	Improvement was seen mostly in sleep, appetite, and inner tension but not in core depressive symptoms. Magnitude of benefit for depression less than for mania
Risperidone	1–6	Yes	No data	Yes	Yes	No	Prophylactic efficacy was demonstrated with Risperdal Consta but no studies with oral risperidone
Quetiapine	300–800	Yes	Yes	Yes	Yes	Yes	For bipolar depression, 300 mg/day is as effective as 600 mg/day (see text for guidance). Appears to have equal efficacy in preventing both mania and depression
Ziprasidone	80–160	Yes	No	Yes	Yes	No	Prophylaxis demonstrated for adjunctive therapy but no data for monotherapy
Aripiprazole	15–30	Yes	No	Yes	Yes	No	
Paliperidone	6–12	Yes	No data	Yes	Yes	No	Less effective than olanzapine in preventing mood episodes
Asenapine	10–20	Yes	No data	Yes	Yes	Yes	Numerically fewer patients in the asenapine group had relapse of manic and depressive episodes but the differences were not significant
Lurasidone	40–120	No data	Yes	Studies underway	Studies underway	Studies underway	Effective in depressed patients with mixed features
Cariprazine	3–12	Yes	Yes	No data	No data	No data	For bipolar depression, 1.5–3 mg/day is recommended, while for mania, up to 12 mg/day is appropriate

DURATION AND PROPHYLAXIS

Maintenance Treatment.   Preventing recurrences of mood episodes is the greatest challenge facing clinicians. Not only must the chosen regimen achieve its primary goal—sustained euthymia—but the medications should not produce unwanted side effects that affect functioning. Sedation, cognitive impairment, tremor, weight gain, and rash are some side effects that lead to treatment discontinuation.

Lithium, carbamazepine, and valproic acid, alone or in combination, are the most widely used agents for the long-term treatment of patients with bipolar disorder. For patients treated with long-term lithium, thyroid supplementation is often necessary to treat lithium-induced hypothyroidism.

Lamotrigine has prophylactic antidepressant and, potentially, mood-stabilizing properties. Lamotrigine appears to be superior at the acute and prophylactic treatment of the depressive phase of illness compared to the manic.

ACUTE TREATMENT FAILURES.   Most patients will respond to treatment within 2 weeks. When they do not respond, we should consider using a different approach. When patients do not respond to initial treatment, it makes sense to try another first-line treatment as there are several from which to choose. Most patients will respond to one of these treatments, at least during their manic phase; depression may be more difficult.

SELECTING SECOND TREATMENT OPTIONS.   In the rare case that first-line treatment fails, other options include haloperidol, carbamazepine, and combination treatment with lithium and valproate. If those fail, other antipsychotics could be considered.

Other Somatic Treatments.   In addition to ECT (discussed above), transcranial magnetic stimulation and magnetic seizure therapy have limited, although promising, data.

Psychosocial Therapy

Psychotherapy can be a crucial adjunct for patients. The goals of this therapy include helping treatment adherence, promoting stability, and avoiding risk factors for the disorder. Cognitive-behavioral therapy, interpersonal and social rhythm therapy, and family focused therapy are all reasonable therapies to use. Table 6-8 summarizes psychotherapeutic treatments for bipolar disorder, including the presumed underlying mechanism and sample interventions.

Table 6-8
Efficacious Psychotherapeutic Treatments for Bipolar Disorder

Treatment	Conceptualization of Disorder Etiology	Sample Interventions
Cognitive-behavioral therapy	Biologic vulnerability interacting with stress Skills deficits limit ability to manage symptoms	Identify and challenge automatic thoughts that interfere with treatment adherence Engage in rewarding activities that provide increased routine and stability Practice communication skills with providers
Interpersonal and social rhythm therapy	Interpersonal vulnerabilities arising from early attachment and learned relationship patterns, plus disruption of social rhythms	Develop awareness of patterns in primary relationships and the therapeutic relationship Track and stabilize social rhythms Interpersonal skills training Communication analysis
Family-focused therapy	Biologic vulnerability exacerbated by negative expressed emotion in family environment	Education regarding the disorder, including precipitants, risk factors, and effective treatment Establish relapse prevention plan, agreed upon by all involved family members Communication skills training Problem-solving skills training

THE EPIDEMIOLOGY OF THE DISORDER(S)

Incidence and Prevalence

We show the US prevalence rates of different clinical forms of bipolar disorder in Figure 6-3. The annual incidence of bipolar illness is usually estimated to be less than 1 percent. Worldwide it is estimated to vary from 0.3 to 1.2 percent by country. However, it is difficult to estimate because it is easy to miss milder forms of bipolar disorder.

Sex

In contrast to major depressive disorder, bipolar I disorder has a roughly equal prevalence among men and women. Manic episodes are more common in men, and depressive episodes are more common in women. When manic episodes occur in women, they are more likely than men to present a mixed picture (e.g., mania and depression). Women also have a higher rate of having the rapid cycling subtype of bipolar I disorder.

Age

The onset of bipolar I disorder is earlier than that of major depressive disorder. The age of onset for bipolar I disorder ranges from childhood (as early as age 5 or 6 years) to 50 years or even older in rare cases, with a mean age of 30 years. The overall prevalence of bipolar disorder in adolescents is similar to adults. However, it increases with age; that is, the prevalence is about 2 percent in 13- and 14-year-olds, but it doubles by age 18.

Other Factors

Bipolar I disorder is more common in divorced and single persons than among married persons, but this difference may reflect the early onset and the resulting marital discord characteristic of the disorder.

There is a higher than average incidence of bipolar I disorder in upper socioeconomic groups. Bipolar I disorder is more common in persons who did not graduate from college than in college graduates. This may also reflect the relatively early age of onset for the disorder.

THE NEUROBIOLOGY OF THE DISORDER

Similar to the depressive disorders, the most consistent abnormality observed in bipolar disorders is an increased frequency of abnormal hyperintensities in subcortical regions, such as periventricular regions, the basal ganglia, and the thalamus. We find this more commonly in bipolar I disorder than in depressed adults. These hyperintensities likely reflect the deleterious neurodegenerative effects of recurrent episodes.

Our Understanding of the Genetics of Bipolar Disorder

Studies of Inheritance Patterns. A family history of bipolar disorder conveys a higher risk for mood disorders in general and, specifically, a much greater risk for bipolar disorder. Unipolar depression is typically the most common form of mood disorder in families of bipolar probands. One large study found a threefold increase in the rate of bipolar disorder and a twofold increase in unipolar disorder in the biologic relatives of bipolar probands. First-degree relatives have an approximately 10-fold risk of developing the disorder. Twin studies suggest that the heritability is between 0.7 and 0.8.

Genetic Studies. Linkage studies have historically implicated several regions, most notably chromosomes 18q and 22q. Several linkage studies have found evidence for the involvement of specific genes in clinical subtypes. For example, the linkage evidence on 18q mainly derived from bipolar II–bipolar II sibling pairs and families that had panic symptoms.

GWAS studies report an ever-growing list of associated loci. Current evidence suggests a pattern of polygenic risk—many susceptible loci, each with a small effect that contributes to the disorder. These genes do not appear to be specific to bipolar disorder but rather overlap with other severe psychiatric disorders, particularly schizophrenia. Studies have tended to focus on genes that could give clues to etiology, such as genes involved in neurodevelopment, or genes encoding for voltage-dependent calcium channels.

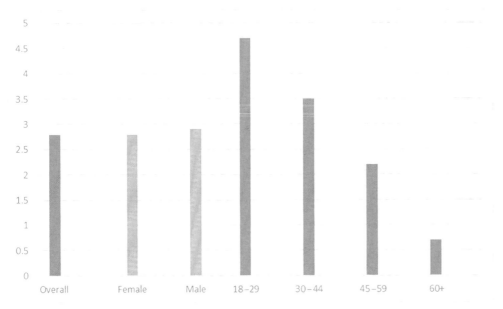

FIGURE 6-3
Past year prevalence of bipolar disorder in US Adults. (Data from the National Comorbidity Survey Replication [2001–2003].)

Perhaps the most important finding from genetic studies is that of the many genes found to be associated with bipolar disorder, most of them are also associated with schizophrenia.

Pathologic Imaging Findings

Structural Imaging.   Individual studies have reported various areas of the brain with variations in gray matter volume, including the striatum, thalamus, amygdala, hippocampus, and pituitary—potentially meaningful findings as these are traditionally regions of interest in this disorder given their presumed functions. However, many of these are small studies with findings with conflicting results. At least one meta-analysis concluded that the evidence taken as a whole did not support morphologic differences in these areas.

There have been some consistent structural findings in other brain regions, including the inferior frontal gyrus, left insula, cerebellum, and left orbitofrontal gyrus, which are seen both in affected individuals and first-degree relatives. Although the significance of these findings is not well understood, many of these areas seem involved in emotional regulation, and the inferior frontal gyrus may have a particular role in executive function, particularly response inhibition. In several cases, the differences are of increased thickness in bipolar patients, suggesting that these brain changes may represent compensatory reactions to the disorder rather than etiologic risk factors.

Functional Imaging.   There are fewer fMRI or PET studies than there are MRI studies; the majority examine the brain during the performance of various cognitive or emotional tasks and suggest either increased or decreased activations along various circuits. Consistent findings include abnormalities along a network that includes the superior and medial frontal cortex and insula, which showed increased activation compared with controls. As many of the areas are involved in executive functioning and working memory, this appears to be consistent with neuropsychological studies of the disorder. Other areas may show decreased activation, including the amygdala, basal ganglion, and limbic system. These findings may be evidence for downregulation of specific circuits, perhaps in response to the abnormal activity in the other circuits.

Inflammatory Markers

Some inflammatory markers, most notably interleukin-6, are elevated in bipolar patients. Markers of inflammation may be particularly evident during adolescence and become less evident in adulthood.

Other Neurochemical Findings.   Some studies have found alterations in brain-derived neurotrophic factor, and in at least one study, this alteration may predict lithium responsiveness. Similarly, some studies of measures of oxidative stress in bipolar patients showed abnormalities that related to lithium response, however these findings are preliminary.

Assessment of the hypothalamic–pituitary–adrenal (HPA) axis suggests a dysregulated system, as evidenced by increased ACTH and cortisol levels in bipolar patients. However, these findings appear only to occur after individuals become symptomatic, suggesting that this is a result of the disorder.

THE PSYCHOLOGY OF THE DISORDER

Psychological studies have focused on neuropsychological findings, particularly of cognitive deficits associated with the disorder. Most commonly reported are deficits of executive functioning and verbal memory and learning. A variety of other related deficits, including deficits of cognitive flexibility, psychomotor speed, and attention, are also reported, although not consistently. Response inhibition is the executive function focused on the ability to prevent one's impulsive response to a situation when such a response would be inappropriate in the environmental context. This inhibition is often deficient in bipolar patients, as well as in first-degree relatives without bipolar disorder. It is particularly deficient in individuals who have bipolar disorder with psychotic features. Other executive function deficits include general impulsivity and risk-taking behavior. We see some of these same deficits with schizophrenia. However, they are less severe in schizophrenia and less likely to be recognized before the disorder appears. It may be that the cognitive deficits are indicative of a broader disorder that crosses traditional diagnostic lines and represents a spectrum of disorders defined by psychotic symptoms.

ETIOLOGY

Biologic Theories

As noted, several pathologic findings point at specific disrupted systems in the brain, particularly areas involved in the regulation of emotions and executive functioning. What remains unclear are which findings are the results of the disorder and which are causative. For example, the significant disruptions seen in the HPA axis in patients with bipolar disorder seem to represent a neurobiologic scar that is seen only after symptoms occur.

As discussed above, converging evidence suggests that calcium signaling may be, at least in part, implicated in the disorder. The genetic abnormalities found in genes associated with voltage-gated calcium channels noted above, as well as the clinical observation that certain drugs have mechanisms of action involving calcium channels (e.g., antiepileptic drugs) lend support for such a theory. Furthermore, preclinical cellular studies show some evidence for increased intracellular calcium signaling in the neurons of bipolar patients. The evidence for calcium channel abnormalities in high risk but asymptomatic individuals, as well as first-degree relatives of patients with the disorder, suggests that this may be involved in the etiology of the disorder.

Neurodevelopment likely plays a role as well, like schizophrenia, and the fact that immunologic markers are more prevalent in bipolar individuals during adolescence than adulthood appears to support a developmental etiology for the disorder.

Psychosocial Theories

Most psychodynamic theories of mania view manic episodes as a defense against underlying depression.

Ms. G, a 42-year-old housewife and mother of a 4-year-old boy, developed symptoms of hypomania and later of frank mania without psychosis, when her only son was diagnosed with acute lymphocytic leukemia. A profoundly religious woman who had experienced 10 years of difficulty with conception, Ms. G was a devoted mother. She reported that she was usually rather down. Before her son's illness, she used to joke that she had become pregnant with him by divine intervention. When her son was diagnosed and subsequently hospitalized, he required painful medical tests and emergency chemotherapy, which made him very ill. The doctors regularly barraged Ms. G with bad news about his prognosis during the first few weeks of his illness.

Ms. G was ever present with her son at the hospital, never sleeping, always caring for him, yet the pediatricians noted that as the child became more debilitated and the prognosis more grim, she seemed to bubble over with renewed cheerfulness, good humor, and high spirits. She could not seem to stop herself from cracking jokes to the hospital staff during her son's painful procedures, and as the jokes became louder and more inappropriate, the staff grew more concerned. During her subsequent psychiatric consultation (requested by the pediatric staff), Ms. G reported that her current "happiness and optimism" were justified by her sense of "oneness" with Mary, the mother of God. "We are together now, she and I, and she has become a part of me. We have a special relationship," she winked. Despite these statements, Ms. G was not psychotic and said that she was "speaking metaphorically, of course, only as a good Catholic would." Her mania resolved when her son achieved remission and was discharged from the hospital. (Courtesy of JC Markowitz, M.D. and BL Milrod, M.D.)

However, such approaches to understanding bipolar disorder have become less accepted as the biologic evidence has mounted. The role of the environment, particularly psychosocial stress, is likely crucial in the etiology. Karl Abraham, for example, believed that the manic episodes might reflect an inability to tolerate a developmental tragedy, such as the loss of a parent. The manic state may also result from a tyrannical superego, which produces excessive self-criticism that is then replaced by euphoric self-satisfaction. Bertram Lewin regarded the manic patient's ego as overwhelmed by pleasurable impulses, such as sex, or by feared impulses, such as aggression. Melanie Klein also viewed mania as a defensive reaction to depression, using manic defenses such as omnipotence, in which the person develops delusions of grandeur.

References

Akiskal HS. Mood disorders. In: Sadock BJ, Sadock VA, Ruiz P, eds. *Kaplan & Sadock's Comprehensive Textbook of Psychiatry*. 10th ed. Philadelphia, PA: Wolters Kluwer; 2017.

Belvederi Murri M, Prestia D, Mondelli V, Pariante C, Patti S, Olivieri B, Arzani C, Masotti M, Respino M, Antonioli M, Vassallo L, Serafini G, Perna G, Pompili M, Amore M. The HPA axis in bipolar disorder: systematic review and meta-analysis. *Psychoneuroendocrinology*. 2016;63:327–342.

Craddock N, Sklar P. Genetics of bipolar disorder. *Lancet*. 2013;381(9878):1654–1662.

Fava GA, Rafanelli C, Tomba E, Guidi J, Grandi S. The sequential combination of cognitive behavioral treatment and well-being therapy in cyclothymic disorder. *Psychother Psychosom*. 2011;80(3):136–143.

Fusar-Poli P, Howes O, Bechdolf A, Borgwardt S. Mapping vulnerability to bipolar disorder: a systematic review and meta-analysis of neuroimaging studies. *J Psychiatry Neurosci*. 2012;37(3):170–184.

Geoffroy PA, Bellivier F, Scott J, Boudebesse C, Lajnef M, Gard S, Kahn JP, Azorin JM, Henry C, Leboyer M, Etain B. Bipolar disorder with seasonal pattern: clinical characteristics and gender influences. *Chronobiol Int*. 2013;30(9):1101–1107.

Gitlin M, Frye MA. Maintenance therapies in bipolar disorders. *Bipolar Disord*. 2012;14(Suppl 2):51–65.

Harrison PJ, Geddes JR, Tunbridge EM. The emerging neurobiology of bipolar disorder. *Trends Neurosci*. 2018;41(1):18–30.

Helseth V, Samet S, Johnsen J, Bramness JG, Waal H. Independent or substance-induced mental disorders? An investigation of comorbidity in an acute psychiatric unit. *J Dual Diagn*. 2013;9(1):78–86.

Mason BL, Brown ES, Croarkin PE. Historical underpinnings of bipolar disorder diagnostic criteria. *Behav Sci (Basel)*. 2016;6(3):14.

Mechri A, Kerkeni N, Touati I, Bacha M, Gassab L. Association between cyclothymic temperament and clinical predictors of bipolarity in recurrent depressive patients. *J Affect Disord*. 2011;132(1–2):285–288.

Merikangas KR, He JP, Burstein M, Swanson SA, Avenevoli S, Cui L, Benjet C, Georgiades K, Swendsen J. Lifetime prevalence of mental disorders in U.S. adolescents: results from the National Comorbidity Survey Replication–Adolescent Supplement (NCS-A). *J Am Acad Child Adolesc Psychiatry*. 2010;49(10):980–989.

Ng F, Mammen OK, Wilting I, Sachs GS, Ferrier IN, Cassidy F, Beaulieu S, Yatham LN, Berk M, International Society for Bipolar Disorders. The International Society for Bipolar Disorders (ISBD) consensus guidelines for the safety monitoring of bipolar disorder treatments. *Bipolar Disord*. 2009;11(6):559–595.

Özerdem A, Ceylan D, Can G. Neurobiology of risk for bipolar disorder. *Curr Treat Options Psychiatry*. 2016;3(4):315–329.

Perugi G, Popovic D. Practical management of cyclothymia. In: Young AH, Ferrier IN, Michalak EE, eds. *Practical Management of Bipolar Disorders*. New York: Cambridge University Press; 2010:139.

Serretti A, Chiesa A, Calati R, Linotte S, Sentissi O, Papageorgiou K, Kasper S, Zohar J, De Ronchi D, Mendlewicz J, Amital D, Montgomery S, Souery D. Influence of family history of major depression, bipolar disorder, and suicide on clinical features in patients with major depression and bipolar disorder. *Eur Arch Psychiatry Clin Neurosci*. 2013;263(2):93–103.

Tomba E, Rafanelli C, Grandi S, Guidi J, Fava GA. Clinical configuration of cyclothymic disturbances. *J Affect Disord*. 2012;139(3):244–249.

Totterdell P, Kellett S, Mansell W. Cognitive behavioural therapy for cyclothymia: cognitive regulatory control as a mediator of mood change. *Behav Cogn Psychother*. 2012;40(4):412–424.

Vaingankar JA, Rekhi G, Subramaniam M, Abdin E, Chong SA. Age of onset of lifetime mental disorders and treatment contact. *Soc Psychiatry Psychiatr Epidemiol*. 2013;48(5):835–843.

Van Meter AR, Youngstrom EA, Findling RL. Cyclothymic disorder: a critical review. *Clin Psychol Rev*. 2012;32(4):229–243.

Depressive Disorders

THE CLINICAL PRESENTATION

A depressed mood and a loss of interest or pleasure are the key symptoms of depression. Patients may say that they feel blue, hopeless, in the dumps, or worthless. For a patient, the depressed mood often has a distinct quality that differentiates it from the normal emotion of sadness or grief. Patients often describe the symptom of depression as one of agonizing emotional pain. Alternately they perceive it as a physical illness in which they feel exhausted and unmotivated. Others report feeling little, being unable to cry, and finding it difficult to experience any pleasure.

The classic presentation of a depressed patient is a person with a stooped posture, decreased movement, and a downward averted gaze. In practice, there is a considerable range of behaviors ranging from persons with no observable symptoms to the catatonically depressed patient. Among observable signs of depression, generalized psychomotor retardation is the most often described, in which patients show little spontaneous movement. At times it may be so severe as to be challenging to differentiate from catatonia.

> Ms. A, a 34-year-old literature professor, presented to a mood clinic with the following complaint: "I am in a daze, confused, disoriented, staring. My thoughts do not flow, my mind is arrested.... I seem to lack any sense of direction, purpose.... I have such an inertia, I cannot assert myself. I cannot fight; I have no will."

Psychomotor agitation may occur, including such behaviors as hand wringing and hair pulling. Many depressed patients have a decreased rate and volume of speech; they respond to questions with single words and exhibit delayed responses to questions.

When present, observable symptoms are helpful in the diagnosis; however, the lack of such symptoms does not imply that a patient has no disorder. It is not abnormal, for example, to encounter patients who can maintain a measure of social appropriateness, even smiling and laughing when with others, despite feeling internally miserable.

The most typical somatic symptoms of depression are called the *neurovegetative symptoms of depression* and typically include a variety of physical symptoms. Table 7-1 lists typical neurovegetative symptoms.

Almost all depressed patients (97 percent) complain about reduced energy; they have difficulty finishing tasks, are impaired at school and work, and have less motivation to undertake new projects. About 80 percent of patients complain of trouble sleeping, especially early morning awakening (i.e., terminal insomnia) and multiple awakenings at night, during which they ruminate about their problems. Many patients have decreased appetite and weight loss, but others experience increased appetite and weight gain and sleep longer than usual. These are sometimes called *reversed neurovegetative symptoms* or *atypical features*.

Depression is, by definition, a mood disorder, and disturbances of mood are at the core. Patients feel "bad" and may use words such as "sad," "depressed," "blue," "down," or similar words to describe this feeling. Here we use the term *dysphoria* to encompass these various depressive feelings as a way to avoid the confusion inherent in using the word "depressed" to mean both the diagnosis and the core symptom. Also, many patients are reluctant to use the word "depressed" as they may have difficulty coming to terms with their diagnosis. In such cases, other synonyms, including those above, may seem less threatening to the patient.

Some patients deny dysphoria altogether, but instead, describe feeling unable to enjoy things that are usually enjoyable to them. We call this *anhedonia* or a lack of pleasure. In addition to dysphoria and anhedonia, many depressed patients also report feeling anxious.

The critical point is that although sadness and even depression may be, in themselves, normal reactions, when encountered in the context of a depressive disorder, patients do not experience them as normal. Patients will often feel genuinely ill and be able to distinguish their emotional state from "normal" feelings of sadness. Many will first interpret this as indicative of medical illness and present to their primary care doctor complaining of feeling "sick" rather than depressed.

Depressed patients customarily have negative views of the world and themselves. Their thought content often includes nondelusional ruminations about loss, guilt, suicide, and death. About 10 percent of all depressed patients have marked symptoms of a thought disorder, usually thought blocking and profound poverty of content.

> A 42-year-old civil servant said that she was so paralyzed by depression that she felt that she had no personal initiative and volition left; she believed that some malignant force had taken over her actions and that it was commenting on every action that she was undertaking. The patient recovered fully with thymoleptic medication. There is no reason to believe that, in this patient, the feelings of somatic passability and running commentary indicated a schizophrenic process.

Depressed patients may complain of either delusions or hallucinations associated with their depressive episode: such patients may have a major depressive episode with psychotic features, often called psychotic depression. Delusions and hallucinations that are consistent with a depressed mood are said to be mood-congruent. Mood-congruent delusions in a depressed person include those of guilt, sinfulness, worthlessness, poverty, failure, persecution, and terminal somatic illnesses (such as cancer and a "rotting" brain). The content of mood-incongruent delusions or hallucinations is not

Table 7-1
Neurovegetative Symptoms of Depression

Common:
　Fatigue, low energy
　Inattention
　Insomnia, early morning awakening
　Poor appetite, associated weight loss
Sometimes included:
　Decreased libido and sexual performance
　Menstrual irregularities
　Worse depression in the AM

consistent with a depressed mood. For example, a mood-incongruent delusion in a depressed person might involve grandiose themes of exaggerated power, knowledge, and worth.

About two-thirds of all depressed patients contemplate suicide, and 10 to 15 percent commit suicide. Those recently hospitalized with a suicide attempt or suicidal ideation have a higher lifetime risk of successful suicide than those never hospitalized for suicidal ideation.

Depressed patients with psychotic features occasionally consider killing a person as a result of their delusional systems, but the most severely depressed patients often lack the motivation or the energy to act impulsively or violently. Patients with depressive disorders are at increased risk of suicide as they begin to improve and regain the energy needed to plan and carry out suicide (paradoxical suicide).

About 50 to 75 percent of all depressed patients have some measure of cognitive impairment. Cognitive symptoms include subjective reports of an inability to concentrate (84 percent of patients in one study) and impairments in thinking (67 percent of patients in another study).

Most depressed patients are oriented, although some may not have sufficient energy or interest to answer questions about these subjects during an interview. Memory can be challenging to disentangle from concentration difficulties. However, some patients appear to have genuine memory difficulties in addition to other cognitive deficits.

Some depressed patients sometimes seem unaware of their depression and do not complain of a mood disturbance even though they exhibit withdrawal from family, friends, and activities that previously interested them. Other depressed patients, particularly those with disordered thoughts, may be overly negative, hyperbolic in their symptomatic description, and hopeless about their future. It may be difficult to convince such patients that improvement is possible.

We can assess judgment by reviewing patients' actions in the recent past and their behavior during the interview. Patients with particularly negative outlooks should be cautioned not to make important life decisions (e.g., around a relationship or job) until they are "thinking normally" again.

In interviews and conversations, depressed patients may emphasize the bad and minimize the good. They may be pessimistic about past treatment trials. A common clinical mistake is to unquestioningly believe a depressed patient who states that a previous trial of antidepressant medications did not work. Such statements may be false, and they require a confirmation from another source. Psychiatrists should not view patients' misinformation as an intentional fabrication; the admission of any hopeful information may be impossible for a person in a depressed state of mind.

Other patients, particularly those with poor insight, may have difficulty reporting symptoms or past episodes. Asking about changes in functioning rather than emotional states may be helpful ("have there been times that you felt unable to work, or care for your children?").

Presentation in Special Populations

Depression in Children and Adolescents.   School phobia and excessive clinging to parents may be symptoms of depression in children. Poor academic performance, substance abuse, antisocial behavior, sexual promiscuity, truancy, and running away may be symptoms of depression in adolescents.

Depression in Older People.   Depression is more common in older persons than it is in the general population. Various studies have reported prevalence rates ranging from 25 to almost 50 percent, although the percentage of these cases that are caused by major depressive disorder is uncertain. Several studies indicate that depression in older persons correlates with low socioeconomic status, the loss of a spouse, a concurrent physical illness, and social isolation. Other studies have indicated that depression in older persons is underdiagnosed and undertreated, perhaps particularly by general practitioners. The underrecognition of depression in older persons may occur because the disorder appears more often with somatic complaints in older than in younger, age groups. Further, ageism may influence and cause clinicians to accept depressive symptoms as usual in older patients.

DIAGNOSIS

Depressive disorders can take many forms, depending on their severity and chronicity. The disorder that we most associate with "classic" depression is major depressive disorder, and this is the disorder most often referred to when someone reports that they suffer from depression. However, it is essential to understand the different varieties of depressive disorders, including those not included in some formal classifications, as all are significant sources of morbidity.

Major Depressive Disorder

The primary feature of major depressive disorder is the occurrence of at least one episode of major depression, which is significant depressive symptoms that last for a significant time. Table 7-2 compares the different approaches to diagnosing major depressive disorder.

With Psychotic Features.   The presence of psychotic features in major depressive disorder reflects severe disease and is a poor prognostic indicator. We often categorize psychotic symptoms as either mood-congruent, that is, in harmony with the mood disorder ("I deserve punishment because I am so bad"), or mood-incongruent, not in harmony with the mood disorder. Patients with mood-incongruent psychotic symptoms may be more likely to have a comorbid primary psychotic disorder, such as schizoaffective disorder or schizophrenia.

With Melancholic Features.   Melancholia is one of the oldest terms used in psychiatry, dating back to Hippocrates in the 4th century to describe the dark mood of depression. We still use it to refer to a depression characterized by severe anhedonia, early morning awakening, weight loss, and profound feelings of guilt (often over trivial events). It is not uncommon for patients who are melancholic

Table 7-2
Major Depressive Disorder

	DSM-5	ICD-10
Diagnostic name	Major Depressive Disorder	Major Depressive Episode
Duration	2 wk	
Symptoms	• Dysphoria or feeling depressed • Anhedonia • ↑ or ↓ weight or appetite • ↑ or ↓ sleep • ↑ or ↓ activity • ↓ energy • Depressing thoughts: worthlessness, guilt • ↓ concentration • Suicidal ideation/plan	• ↓ mood • ↓ energy • ↓ activity • ↓ capacity for enjoyment • ↓ interest • ↓ concentration • Fatigue after even minimal effort • Disturbed sleep/early morning awakening • Disturbed appetite/ ↓ weight • ↓ self esteem • ↓ self-confidence • Guilt or worthlessness • Mood unreactive to circumstances • Anhedonia • Worse symptoms in the AM • Psychomotor disturbance: agitation or retardation • ↓ libido
Required number of symptoms	5 (1 has to be one of the first two listed)	
Psychosocial consequences of symptoms	Distress or impaired functioning (social, occupational, or other significant areas)	Depends on severity
Exclusions (Not better explained by):	Medical illness Substance Other psychiatric disorder History of mania or hypomania	Adjustment disorder Conduct disorder Recurrent depressive disorder (which is considered a separate diagnosis)

Symptom specifiers	**With anxious distress**
	• 2+ symptoms of anxiety
	With mixed features
	• 3+ manic/hypomanic symptoms *during* the depressive episode (if occur independently, diagnose bipolar disorder)
	With melancholic features
	• Loss of pleasure or reactivity to pleasure
	• 3+ of the following
	  • Severe depression/despair
	  • Mood worse in AM
	  • Early morning awakening
	  • Psychomotor disturbance
	  • Anorexia/weight loss
	  • Guilt
	With atypical features
	• Mood reactivity
	• 2+ of following
	  • Increased appetite/weight
	  • Hyposomnia
	  • Leaden paralysis
	  • Rejection sensitivity
	With mood-congruent psychotic features
	With mood-incongruent psychotic features
	With catatonia
	• Must be present during most of depressive episode
	With peripartum onset
	With seasonal pattern
	• Usually occurs during a specific season
		Depressive reaction
		Psychogenic depression
		Reactive depression

Course specifiers	**With psychotic features**
	• Psychotic symptoms occurring only during the depressive episode
	  • Mood-congruent
	  • Mood-incongruent
	In partial remission
	• Full criteria no longer met
	In full remission
	• 0 symptoms for 2 mo
		Recurrent Depressive Disorder (Coded as separate disorder): Repeated episodes of the above symptoms. No mania.

(continued)

Table 7-2
Major Depressive Disorder (*Continued*)

	DSM-5	ICD-10
Severity specifiers	**Mild:** minimal symptoms **Moderate:** between mild and severe **Severe:** # of symptoms and severity/dysfunction well beyond that required for diagnosis	**Mild** • 2–3 symptoms • Functions normal despite distress **Moderate** • 4+ symptoms • Difficulty with functioning **Severe** • Several symptoms marked and distressing • Loss of self-esteem/feels worthless and guilty • Suicidal ideation/acts • Somatic symptoms of depression **Severe with psychotic symptoms** • As above but with psychosis **Other** • Atypical depression • Single episodes of "masked depression" **Unspecified**

to have suicidal ideation. Melancholia is associated with changes in the autonomic nervous system and endocrine functions. For that reason, we sometimes refer to melancholia as "endogenous depression" or depression that arises in the absence of external life stressors or precipitants.

With Atypical Features.   Patients with major depressive disorder with atypical features have specific, predictable characteristics. As described above, these tend to be the reverse of the neurovegetative symptoms. They may, for example, overeat or oversleep. Patients with atypical features have a younger age of onset and more severe psychomotor slowing. They also are more likely to have comorbid disorders, including anxiety disorders, substance use disorder, or somatic symptom disorder. They are easy to misdiagnose as having an anxiety disorder rather than a mood disorder. Patients with atypical features may also have a long-term course, a diagnosis of bipolar I disorder, or a seasonal pattern to their disorder.

> Kevin, a 15-year-old adolescent, was referred to a sleep center to rule out narcolepsy. His main complaints were fatigue, boredom, and a need to sleep all the time. Although he had always started the day somewhat slowly, he now could not get out of bed to go to school. That alarmed his mother, prompting sleep consultation. Formerly a B student, he had been failing most of his courses in the 6 months before referral. Psychological counseling, predicated on the premise that his family's recent move from another city had led to Kevin's isolation, had not been beneficial. Extensive neurologic and general medical workup findings had also proven negative. He slept 12 to 15 hours per day but denied cataplexy, sleep paralysis, and hypnagogic hallucinations. During psychiatric interview, he denied being depressed but admitted that he had lost interest in everything except his dog. He had no drive, participated in no activities, and had gained 30 lb in 6 months. He believed that he was "brain damaged" and wondered whether it was worth living like that. The question of suicide disturbed him because it was contrary to his religious beliefs. These findings led to the prescription of an antidepressant. Not only did the antidepressant reverse the presenting complaints, but it also pushed him to the brink of a manic episode. (Courtesy of HS Akiskal, M.D.)

With Catatonic Features.   As a symptom, catatonia can be present in several mental disorders, most commonly, schizophrenia

and mood disorders. The hallmark symptoms of catatonia are stupor, blunted affect, extreme withdrawal, negativism, and marked psychomotor retardation. The presence of catatonic features in patients with mood disorders may have prognostic and treatment significance.

Postpartum Onset.   We diagnose the postpartum subtype if the onset of symptoms is within 4 weeks postpartum. Postpartum mental disorders commonly include psychotic symptoms.

Seasonal Pattern.   Patients with a seasonal pattern to their mood disorders tend to experience depressive episodes during a particular season, most commonly winter. The pattern has become known as seasonal affective disorder (SAD), although DSM-5 does not use this term. There is some controversy regarding whether this represents a subtype of major depressive disorder or a distinct entity. Either way, the presence of the disorder has implications for treatment, as patients with a seasonal pattern to their depression may preferentially respond to light therapy.

Dysthymic Disorder

Dysthymic disorder (also called dysthymia) is the presence of depressive symptoms that are less severe than those of major depressive disorder. Although less severe than a major depressive disorder, it is often more chronic. Table 7-3 compares the different approaches to diagnosing.

The most typical feature of dysthymia, also known as persistent depressive disorder, is the presence of a depressed mood that lasts most of the day and is present almost continuously. There are associated feelings of inadequacy, guilt, irritability, and anger; withdrawal from society; loss of interest; and inactivity and lack of productivity. The term dysthymia, which means "ill-humored," was introduced in 1980. Before that time, we tended to classify patients having dysthymia as having "neurotic depression."

Dysthymia is distinguished from major depressive disorder by the fact that patients complain that they have always been depressed. Thus, most cases are of early-onset, beginning in childhood or adolescence, and, almost always, by a patient's 20s.

Table 7-3
Dysthymic Disorder

	DSM-5	ICD-10
Diagnostic name	Persistent Depressive Disorder	Dysthymia [F43.1]
Duration	2+ yr (1+ yr for children) ≤2-mo symptom free during illness	
Symptoms	Depressed mood most of the time ↓ appetite ↓ or ↑ sleep ↓ energy ↓ self-esteem ↓ concentration/decision-making ability Hopelessness	Chronically depressed mood that does not meet criteria for a depressive episode, though criteria may have been met in the past
Required number of symptoms	First symptom and 2+ of rest	
Psychosocial consequences of symptoms	Distress and functional impairment	
Exclusions	History of bipolar disorder Another mental illness Substance Another medical illness	Anxiety Depression Bereavement Schizophrenia
Symptom specifiers	**With pure dysthymic syndrome:** criteria for depressive episode not met in the last 2 yr **With persistent major depressive episode:** has met diagnostic criteria for a depressive episode for entire 2-yr period **With intermittent major depressive episode, with current episode:** in current episode, 8 wk+ in last 2 yr with subdiagnostic symptoms episode **With intermittent major depressive episode, without current episode:** Not currently in episode, 1+ depressive episode in past 2 yr **With anxious distress** *≥2 of following:* • Feeling tense • Restlessness • ↓ concentration due to worrying • ↑ fear without apparent cause • Fear of loss of control **With mixed features**—depressive or manic/hypomanic episode, + with additional symptoms of other episode but subdiagnostic **With melancholic features:** see Table 7-2 **With atypical features:** see Table 7-2 **With psychotic features** • Mood-congruent • Mood-incongruent	
Course specifiers	**With peripartum onset**—episode is during pregnancy or ≤4 wk after delivery	
Severity specifiers	**Mild:** minimal symptoms **Moderate:** between mild and severe **Severe:** # of symptoms and severity/dysfunction well beyond that required for diagnosis	

A 27-year-old male grade-school teacher presented with the chief complaint that life was a painful duty that had always lacked luster for him. He said that he felt "enveloped by a sense of gloom" that was nearly always with him. Although he was respected by his peers, he felt "like a grotesque failure, a self-concept I have had since childhood." He stated that he merely performed his responsibilities as a teacher and that he had never derived any pleasure from anything he had done in life. He said that he had never had any romantic feelings; sexual activity, in which he had engaged with two different women, had involved pleasureless orgasm. He said that he felt empty, going through life without any sense of direction, ambition, or passion, a realization that itself was tormenting. He had bought a pistol to put an end to what he called his "useless existence" but did not carry out suicide, believing that it would hurt his students and the small community in which he lived. (Courtesy of HS Akiskal, M.D.)

A late-onset subtype, much less prevalent and not well characterized clinically, has been identified among middle-aged and geriatric populations, mainly through epidemiologic studies in the community.

The family history of patients with dysthymia is typically replete with both depressive and bipolar disorders, which is one of the more robust findings supporting its link to primary mood disorder.

Other Diagnoses

Minor Depressive Disorder. Minor depressive disorder consists of episodes of depressive symptoms that are less severe than those seen in major depressive disorder. The difference between dysthymia and minor depressive disorder is primarily the episodic nature of the symptoms in the latter. Between episodes, patients with minor depressive disorder have a euthymic mood, but patients with dysthymia have virtually no euthymic periods. DSM-5 does not include this diagnosis. However, ICD-10 includes it as a mild type of depressive episode. DSM-5 would diagnose it as an "Other Specified Depressive Disorder."

Recurrent Brief Depressive Disorder. Recurrent brief depressive disorder consists of brief periods (less than 2 weeks) during which depressive episodes are present. Patients with the disorder would meet the diagnostic criteria for a major depressive disorder if their episodes lasted longer. Patients with recurrent brief depressive disorder differ from patients with dysthymia on two counts: they have an episodic disorder, and their symptoms are more severe. ICD-10 lists this as an "Other Recurrent Mood Disorder," whereas DSM-5 would diagnose it as an "Other Specified Depressive Disorder."

Double Depression. An estimated 40 percent of patients with major depressive disorder also meet the criteria for dysthymia, a combination often referred to as a double depression. Available data support the conclusion that patients with double depression have poorer prognoses than patients with major depressive disorder alone. The treatment of patients with double depression should be directed toward both disorders because the resolution of the symptoms of major depressive episode still leaves these patients with significant psychiatric impairment.

Objective Rating Scales for Depression

There is a growing literature suggesting that the use of objective scales can significantly improve the reliability of depressive diagnoses. They can also be useful for tracking the course of an episode. Several validated scales exist.

Clinician Administered Scales. The Hamilton Rating Scale for Depression (HAM-D) is a widely used depression scale. It contains up to 24 items, each rated on a 0 to 4 or 0 to 2 scale. The clinician evaluates the patient's answers to questions about feelings of guilt, thoughts of suicide, sleep habits, and other symptoms of depression, and derives the ratings from that interview. The usual scoring cutoffs are 10 to 13 for mild depression, 14 to 17 for mild-to-moderate depression, and >17 for moderate-to-severe depression.

Self-Administered Scales. The Zung Self-Rating Depression Scale is a 20-item report scale. A normal range is 34 or less; a depressed score is 50 or more. The scale provides a global index of the intensity of a patient's depressive symptoms, including the affective expression of depression.

The Raskin Depression Scale is a clinician-rated scale that measures the severity of a patient's depression, as reported by the patient and as observed by the physician, on a 5-point scale of three dimensions: verbal report, displayed behavior, and secondary symptoms. The scale has a range of 3 to 13; a normal score is 3, and a depressed score is 7 or more.

DIFFERENTIAL DIAGNOSIS

The symptoms of depressive disorders commonly overlap with other syndromes and disorders. As a result, the differential is wide.

Often a careful history and examination will make the differential clear. In other cases, one may have to observe the disorder over time before the diagnosis becomes clear.

General Medical Disorders

It is essential to consider whether a patient's depression is due to a general medical condition. Failure to obtain a good clinical history or to consider the context of a patient's current life situation can lead to diagnostic errors. Clinicians should have depressed adolescents tested for mononucleosis, and we should test patients who are markedly overweight or underweight for adrenal and thyroid dysfunctions. We should test patients with appropriate risk factors for HIV, and older patients for viral pneumonia and other medical conditions.

Table 7-4 lists some pharmacologic and medical conditions that can cause depression.

Table 7-4
Pharmacologic Factors and Physical Diseases Associated with Onset of Depression

Pharmacologic
   Steroidal contraceptives
   Reserpine, methyldopa
   Anticholinesterase insecticides
   Amphetamine or cocaine withdrawal
   Alcohol or sedative–hypnotic withdrawal
   Cimetidine, indomethacin
   Phenothiazine antipsychotic drugs
   Thallium, mercury
   Cycloserine
   Vincristine, vinblastine
   Interferon

Endocrine–metabolic[a]
   Hypothyroidism and hyperthyroidism
   Hyperparathyroidism
   Hypopituitarism
   Addison disease
   Cushing syndrome
   Diabetes mellitus

Infectious
   General paresis (tertiary syphilis)
   Toxoplasmosis
   Influenza, viral pneumonia
   Viral hepatitis
   Infectious mononucleosis
   Acquired immune deficiency syndrome

Collagen
   Rheumatoid arthritis
   Lupus erythematosus

Nutritional
   Pellagra
   Pernicious anemia

Neurologic
   Multiple sclerosis
   Parkinson disease
   Head trauma
   Complex partial seizures
   Sleep apnea
   Cerebral tumors
   Cerebrovascular infarction (and disease)

Neoplastic
   Abdominal malignancies
   Disseminated carcinomatosis

[a]Cholesterol is not mentioned because low levels as a factor in depression have been inconsistently reported.

Many neurologic and medical disorders and pharmacologic agents can produce symptoms of depression. Patients with depressive disorders often first visit their general practitioners with somatic complaints. We can detect most medical causes of depressive disorders with a comprehensive medical history, a complete physical and neurologic examination, and routine blood and urine tests. The workup should include tests for thyroid and adrenal functions because disorders of both of these endocrine systems can appear as depressive disorders. In substance-induced mood disorder, a reasonable rule of thumb is that any drug a depressed patient is taking should be considered a potential factor in the mood disorder. Cardiac drugs, antihypertensives, sedatives, hypnotics, antipsychotics, antiepileptics, antiparkinsonian drugs, analgesics, antibacterials, and antineoplastics are all commonly associated with depressive symptoms.

Neurologic Conditions

The most common neurologic problems that manifest depressive symptoms are Parkinson disease, dementing illnesses, epilepsy, cerebrovascular diseases, and tumors. About 50 to 75 percent of all patients with Parkinson disease have marked symptoms of depressive disorder that do not correlate with the patient's physical disability, age, or duration of illness but do correlate with the presence of abnormalities found on neuropsychological tests. The motor symptoms of Parkinson disease can mask a depressive disorder as the motor symptoms are similar. Depressive symptoms often respond to antidepressant drugs or ECT. The interictal changes associated with temporal lobe epilepsy can mimic a depressive disorder, especially if the epileptic focus is on the right side. Depression is a frequent complicating feature of cerebrovascular diseases, particularly in the 2 years after the episode. Depression is more common in anterior brain lesions than in posterior brain lesions and, in both cases, often responds to antidepressant medications. Tumors of the diencephalic and temporal regions are particularly likely to be associated with depressive disorder symptoms.

Dementia.   Major depressive disorder can have a profound effect on concentration and even memory, and can occasionally be confused with a neurodegenerative illness such as Alzheimer disorder. At times the term "pseudodementia" has been used to describe this. However, that may be ill-advised as it implies that the cognitive symptoms are not genuine, which is not the case. Clinicians can usually differentiate cognitive symptoms of a major depressive disorder from the dementia of a disease, such as dementia of the Alzheimer type, on clinical grounds. The cognitive symptoms in major depressive disorder have a sudden onset, and other symptoms of the disorder, such as self-reproach, are also present. A diurnal variation in the cognitive problems, not seen in primary dementias, may occur. Whereas depressed patients with cognitive difficulties often do not try to answer questions, patients with dementia may confabulate. During an interview, depressed patients can sometimes be coached and encouraged into remembering, an ability that demented patients lack.

Other Mental Disorders

Depression can be a feature of virtually any mental disorder.

Other Mood Disorders.   Clinicians must consider a range of diagnostic categories before arriving at a final diagnosis. We should

Table 7-5
Features of a Depressive Episode that Are More Predictive of Bipolar Disorder

Early age at onset
Psychotic depression before 25 yr of age
Postpartum depression, especially one with psychotic features
Rapid onset and offset of depressive episodes of short duration (less than 3 mo)
Recurrent depression (more than five episodes)
Depression with marked psychomotor retardation
Atypical features (reverse vegetative signs)
Seasonality
Bipolar family history
High-density three-generation pedigrees
Trait mood lability (cyclothymia)
Hyperthymic temperament
Hypomania associated with antidepressants
Repeated (at least three times) loss of efficacy of antidepressants after initial response
Depressive mixed state (with psychomotor excitement, irritable hostility, racing thoughts, and sexual arousal *during* major depression)

From Akiskal. Mood disorders. In: Sadock BJ, Sadock VA, Ruiz P, eds. *Kaplan & Sadock's Comprehensive Textbook of Psychiatry*. 10th ed. Philadelphia, PA: Wolters Kluwer; 2017.

determine whether a patient has had episodes of mania-like symptoms, which might indicate any one of the bipolar disorders. The depressive episode of a bipolar disorder may be identical to that of a major depressive disorder. However, there may be certain features that are more predictive of a bipolar disorder, and we list these in Table 7-5.

If a patient's symptoms are solely depressive, the patient most likely has a depressive disorder. Even then, we must differentiate between the various depressive disorders discussed in this chapter. To do this, we must understand the severity and the course of the disorder in detail.

Other Mental Disorders.   Substance-related disorders, psychotic disorders (Table 7-6), eating disorders, adjustment disorders, and somatoform disorders are all commonly associated with depressive symptoms and should be considered in the differential diagnosis of a patient with depressive symptoms.

Perhaps the most challenging differential is that between anxiety disorders with depression and depressive disorders with marked

Table 7-6
Common Causes of Misdiagnosis of Mood Disorder as Schizophrenia

Reliance on cross-sectional rather than longitudinal picture
Incomplete interepisodic recovery equated with schizophrenic defect
Equation of bizarreness with schizophrenic thought disorder
Ascribing irritable and cantankerous mood to paranoid delusions
Mistaking depressive anhedonia and depersonalization for schizophrenic emotional blunting
Flight of ideas perceived as loose associations
Lack of familiarity with the phenomenologic approach in assessing affective delusions and hallucinations
Heavy weight given to incidental Schneiderian symptoms

Adapted from Akiskal HS, Puzantian VR. Psychotic forms of depression and mania. *Psychiatr Clin North Am*. 1979;2:419.

Table 7-7
Unique Cross-Sectional Profiles of Clinical Anxiety and Depression

Anxiety	Depression
Hypervigilance	Psychomotor retardation
Severe tension and panic	Severe sadness
Perceived danger	Perceived loss
Phobic avoidance	Loss of interest—anhedonia
Doubt and uncertainty	Hopelessness—suicidal
Insecurity	Self-deprecation
Performance anxiety	Loss of libido
	Early-morning awakening
	Weight loss

Reprinted with permission from Akiskal HS. Toward a clinical understanding of the relationship of anxiety and depressive disorders. In: Maser JP, Cloninger CR, eds. *Comorbidity of Mood and Anxiety Disorders*. Washington, DC: American Psychiatric Press; 1990.

anxiety. Table 7-7 compares the unique features of depression with those of anxiety.

Uncomplicated Bereavement. Uncomplicated bereavement is not a mental disorder even though about one-third of all bereaved spouses for a time meet the diagnostic criteria for major depressive disorder. Some patients with uncomplicated bereavement do develop a major depressive disorder, but we do not make this diagnosis unless the grief does not resolve. The severity and course of symptoms are significant differences. Table 7-8 lists features that would indicate that normal bereavement has progressed to a depressive disorder.

> A 75-year-old widow was brought to treatment by her daughter because of severe insomnia and total loss of interest in daily routines after her husband's death 1 year before. She had been agitated for the first 2 to 3 months and thereafter "sank into total inactivity—not wanting to get out of bed, not wanting to do anything, not wanting to go out." According to her daughter, she was married at 21 years of age, had four children, and had been a housewife until her husband's death from a heart attack. Her past psychiatric history was negative; premorbid adjustment had been characterized by compulsive traits. During the interview, she was dressed in black; appeared moderately slowed; and sobbed intermittently, saying "I search everywhere for him.... I don't find him." When asked about life, she said, "Everything I see is black." Although she expressed no interest in food, she did not seem to have lost an appreciable amount of weight. The patient declined psychiatric care, stating that she "preferred to join her husband rather than get well." She was too religious to commit suicide, but by refusing treatment, she felt that she would "pine away... find relief in death and reunion." (Courtesy of HS Akiskal, M.D.)

In cases of severe bereavement, regardless of diagnosis, some suggest that it would be clinically unwise to withhold antidepressants from many persons experiencing such intense mourning.

COMORBIDITY

Individuals with major depressive disorders are at an increased risk of having one or more additional comorbid disorders. The most

Table 7-8
Signs that a Bereaved Person Has Progressed to a Depressive Disorder

Beliefs. Grieving persons and their relatives perceive bereavement as a normal reaction, whereas those with depressive disorder often view themselves as sick and may actually believe they are losing their minds.

Emotional reactivity. Unlike the melancholic person, the grieving person reacts to the environment and tends to show a range of positive effects.

Psychomotor activity. Marked psychomotor retardation is not observed in normal grief.

Guilt. Although bereaved persons often feel guilty about not having done certain things that they believe might have saved the life of the deceased loved one (guilt of omission), they typically do not experience guilt of commission.

Delusions. Delusions of worthlessness or sin and psychotic experiences in general point toward mood disorder.

Suicidal ideation. Active suicidal ideation is rare in grief but common in major depressive disorder.

Behaviors. "Mummification" (i.e., keeping the belongings of the deceased person exactly as they were before his or her death) indicates serious psychopathology.

Anniversaries. Severe anniversary reactions should alert the clinician to the possibility of psychopathology.

From Akiskal. Mood disorders. In: Sadock BJ, Sadock VA, Ruiz P, eds. *Kaplan & Sadock's Comprehensive Textbook of Psychiatry*. 10th ed. Philadelphia, PA: Wolters Kluwer; 2017.

frequent disorders are alcohol abuse or dependence, panic disorder, obsessive-compulsive disorder (OCD), and social anxiety disorder. Conversely, individuals with substance use disorders and anxiety disorders also have an elevated risk of lifetime or current comorbid depressive disorders.

Anxiety

In anxiety disorders, DSM-5 notes the existence of mixed anxiety–depressive disorder. Significant symptoms of anxiety can and often do coexist with significant symptoms of depression. Whether patients who exhibit significant symptoms of both anxiety and depression are affected by two distinct disease processes or by a single disease process that produces both sets of symptoms are not yet resolved. Patients of both types may constitute a group of patients with mixed anxiety–depressive disorder.

Substance Use Disorder

Alcohol dependence frequently coexists with mood disorders. Both patients with major depressive disorder and those with bipolar I disorder are likely to meet the diagnostic criteria for an alcohol use disorder. The available data indicate that alcohol dependence is more strongly associated with a coexisting diagnosis of depression in women than in men. In contrast, the genetic and family data about men who have both a mood disorder and alcohol dependence indicate that they are likely to have two genetically distinct disease processes.

Substance-related disorders other than alcohol dependence are also commonly associated with mood disorders. The abuse of substances may be involved in precipitating an episode of illness or, conversely, may represent patients' attempts to treat their illnesses.

Although manic patients seldom use sedatives to dampen their euphoria, depressed patients often use stimulants, such as cocaine and amphetamines, to relieve their depression.

Patients with dysthymia commonly meet the diagnostic criteria for a substance-related disorder. This comorbidity can be logical; patients with dysthymia tend to develop coping methods for their chronically depressed state that involve substance abuse. Therefore, they are likely to use alcohol, stimulants such as cocaine, or marijuana, the choice perhaps depending primarily on a patient's social context. The presence of a comorbid diagnosis of substance abuse presents a diagnostic dilemma for clinicians; the long-term use of many substances can result in a symptom picture indistinguishable from that of dysthymia.

Medical Conditions

Depression commonly coexists with medical conditions, especially in older persons. When depression and medical conditions coexist, clinicians must try to determine whether the underlying medical condition is pathophysiologically related to the depression or whether any drugs that the patient is taking for the medical condition are causing the depression. Many studies indicate that the treatment of a coexisting major depressive disorder can improve the course of the underlying medical disorder, including cancer.

COURSE

Studies of the course and prognosis of mood disorders have generally concluded that mood disorders tend to have long courses and that patients tend to have relapses.

Major Depressive Disorder

Onset.   About 50 percent of patients having their first episode of major depressive disorder exhibited significant depressive symptoms before the first identified episode. Therefore, early identification and treatment of early symptoms may prevent the development of a full depressive episode. Although symptoms may have been present, patients with major depressive disorder usually have not had a premorbid personality disorder. The first depressive episode occurs before age 40 years in about 50 percent of patients. Later onset is associated with the absence of a family history of mood disorders, antisocial personality disorder, and alcohol abuse.

Duration.   An untreated depressive episode lasts 6 to 13 months; most treated episodes last about 3 months. The withdrawal of antidepressants before 3 months has elapsed almost always results in the return of the symptoms. As the course of the disorder progresses, patients tend to have more frequent episodes that last longer. Over 20 years, the mean number of episodes is five or six.

Other Depressive Disorders

About 50 percent of patients with dysthymia experience an insidious onset of symptoms before age 25 years. Despite the early onset, patients often suffer from the symptoms for a decade before seeking psychiatric help and may consider early-onset dysthymia part of life. Patients with an early onset of symptoms are at risk for either major depressive disorder or bipolar I disorder in the course of their disorder. Studies of patients with the diagnosis of

dysthymia indicate that about 20 percent progressed to major depressive disorder, 15 percent to bipolar II disorder, and fewer than 5 percent to bipolar I disorder.

The prognosis for patients with dysthymia varies. Antidepressive agents and specific types of psychotherapies (e.g., cognitive and behavior therapies) have positive effects on the course and prognosis of dysthymia. The available data about previously available treatments indicate that only 10 to 15 percent of patients are in remission 1 year after the initial diagnosis. About 25 percent of all patients with dysthymia never attain complete recovery. Overall, however, the prognosis is good with treatment.

PROGNOSIS

Major depressive disorder is not a benign disorder. It tends to be chronic, and patients tend to relapse. Patients hospitalized for the first episode of major depressive disorder have about a 50 percent chance of recovering in the first year. The percentage of patients recovering after repeated hospitalization decreases with time. Many unrecovered patients remain affected by a dysthymic disorder. About 25 percent of patients have a recurrence in the first 6 months after leaving the hospital. Another 30 to 50 percent recur in the following 2 years. About 50 to 75 percent of all patients will have a recurrence within 5 years. The incidence of relapse is lower than these figures in patients who continue prophylactic psychopharmacological treatment and in patients who have had only one or two depressive episodes. In general, as a patient experiences more and more depressive episodes, the time between the episodes decreases, and the severity of each episode increases.

Prognostic Indicators

Many studies have focused on identifying both good and bad prognostic indicators in the course of major depressive disorder. Table 7-9 lists some of the positive and negative predictors.

TREATMENT APPROACH

The treatment of mood disorders is rewarding for psychiatrists. Specific treatments are available for depressive episodes, and data indicate that prophylactic treatment is also useful. We should be optimistic, as the prognosis for each episode is excellent. This fact tends to be welcome news for patients and families. Mood disorders are chronic, however, and the psychiatrist must educate the patient and the family about future treatment strategies.

Historically, patients with dysthymia either received no treatment or received long-term, insight-oriented psychotherapy. Contemporary data suggest that the treatments for dysthymia are similar to those for major depressive disorder.

There are several treatment goals. First, the patient's safety must be guaranteed. Second, a complete diagnostic evaluation of the patient is necessary. Third, we should initiate a treatment plan that addresses not only the immediate symptoms but also the patient's prospective well-being. Although current treatment emphasizes pharmacotherapy and psychotherapy addressed to the individual patient, stressful life events increase the chance of relapse. Thus, treatment should address the number and severity of stressors in patients' lives.

Table 7-10 lists the phases of treatment and the typical goals and activities for each phase.

Table 7-9
Prognostic Indicators for Depression

Positive Indicators
Clinical
  Mild severity
  No psychotic symptoms
  Short hospital stay
  No comorbid disease (medical/psychiatric)
  No more than 1 hospitalization
  Advanced age of onset

Psychosocial
  Solid friendships during adolescence
  Stable family functioning
  Good social/occupational functioning in previous 5 yr

Negative Indicators
Comorbid dysthymic disorder and major depressive disorder
Substance use disorder
Anxiety symptoms
>1 previous episodes
Male

Hospitalization

The first and most critical decision a physician must make is whether to hospitalize a patient or attempt outpatient treatment. Definite indications for hospitalization are the risk of suicide or homicide, a patient's grossly reduced ability to get food and shelter, and the need for diagnostic procedures. A history of rapidly progressing symptoms and the rupture of a patient's natural support systems are also indications for hospitalization.

A physician may safely treat dysthymia and other forms of milder depression in the office, seeing the patient frequently. Clinical signs of impaired judgment, weight loss, or insomnia should be minimal. The patient's support system should be reliable, neither overinvolved nor withdrawing from the patient. Any adverse changes in the patient's symptoms or behavior or the attitude of the patient's support system may suffice to warrant hospitalization.

Patients with mood disorders are often unwilling to enter a hospital voluntarily, and we may have to commit them involuntarily. These patients often cannot make decisions because of their slowed thinking, negative *Weltanschauung* (world view), and hopelessness.

Choosing a Treatment

Combined Treatments May Offer the Best Option.
We often combine medication and psychotherapy. If physicians view mood disorders as fundamentally evolving from psychodynamic issues, their ambivalence about the use of drugs may result in a poor response, noncompliance, and probably inadequate dosages for too short a treatment period. Alternatively, if physicians ignore the psychosocial needs of a patient, the outcome of pharmacotherapy may be compromised. Several trials of a combination of pharmacotherapy and psychotherapy for chronically depressed outpatients have shown a higher response and higher remission rates for the combination than for either treatment used alone.

Although combination remains the general—and our—recommendation—we should point out that there are other views. Some have argued that most data suggest that single treatment, either psychopharmacological or psychotherapeutic, alone is sufficient for most people, and that combining treatments exposes patients to unnecessary costs and adverse effects.

Somatic Treatments

Pharmacotherapy.
The efficacy of pharmacotherapy for major depressive disorder has been well established in more than 500 randomized controlled studies. In general, all available antidepressants show an at least modest effect compared with placebo. Efficacy is broadly similar across agents, at least when compared against placebo. However, tolerability and acceptability vary.

After establishing a diagnosis, we can formulate a pharmacologic treatment strategy. Accurate diagnosis is crucial because unipolar and bipolar spectrum disorders require different treatment regimens.

The objective of pharmacologic treatment is symptom remission, not just symptom reduction. Patients with residual symptoms, as opposed to full remission, are more likely to experience a relapse or recurrence of mood episodes and to experience ongoing impairment of daily functioning.

The use of specific pharmacotherapy approximately doubles the chances that a depressed patient will recover in 1 month. All currently available antidepressants may take up to 3 to 4 weeks to exert significant therapeutic effects, although they may begin to show their effects earlier. The choice of antidepressants partly depends on the side effect profile that is least objectionable to a given patient's physical status, temperament, and lifestyle. Chapter 21 discusses the many classes of antidepressants. Although most antidepressants

Table 7-10
Phases of Treatment

Treatment Phase	Duration	Goals	Activities
Acute and continuation	8–12 wk	Achieve symptomatic remission Monitor side effects Restore function	Establish therapeutic alliance Provide psychoeducation Select optimal antidepressant treatment(s) Supportive and measurement-based care Monitor progress
Maintenance	6–24 mo or longer	Return to full function and quality of life Prevention of recurrence	Continue psychoeducation Rehabilitate Manage comorbidities Monitor for recurrence

Modified from Lam RW, McIntosh D, Wang J, Enns MW, Kolivakis T, Michalak EE, Sareen J, Song WY, Kennedy SH, MacQueen GM, Milev RV, Parikh SV, Ravindran AV; CANMAT Depression Work Group. Canadian Network for Mood and Anxiety Treatments (CANMAT) 2016 clinical guidelines for the management of adults with major depressive disorder: section 1. Disease burden and principles of care. *Can J Psychiatry*. 2016;61(9):510–523.

Table 7-11
SSRI and SNRI Antidepressant Medications and Their Side Effect Profiles

Drug Class	Recommended Dose Range (mg)	Side Effect Frequency	
		10–30%	>30%
SSRI			
Citalopram	20–40	Nausea, dry mouth, sweating	None
Escitalopram	10–20	Male sexual dysfunction and nausea	None
Fluoxetine	20–60	Nausea, dry mouth, somnolence, nervousness, anxiety, insomnia, tremor, anorexia	None
Fluvoxamine	100–300	Dry mouth, headaches, somnolence, agitation, insomnia, sweating, tremor, anorexia, dizziness, constipation	Nausea
Paroxetine	20–60	Nausea, diarrhea, dry mouth, headaches, somnolence, insomnia, sweating, asthenia, male sexual dysfunction, dizziness	None
Sertraline	50–200	Nausea, diarrhea, dry mouth, headaches, somnolence, insomnia, fatigue, tremor, male sexual dysfunction, dizziness	None
SNRI			
Venlafaxine	75–375	Headaches, somnolence, dry mouth, dizziness, nervousness, insomnia, sweating, male sexual dysfunction	Nausea
Desvenlafaxine	50–100	Dry mouth, dizziness, nausea, sweating	None
Duloxetine	30–120	Nausea, dry mouth, constipation, insomnia, male sexual dysfunction	None
Levomilnacipran	20–80	Nausea, dry mouth, headaches, male sexual dysfunction	None
Other Second-Generation and Novel Antidepressants			
Agomelatine[a]	25–50	None	None
Bupropion	150–450	Insomnia, dry mouth, nausea	Headaches
Mirtazapine	15–60	Dry mouth, constipation, increased appetite, weight gain	Somnolence
Moclobemide[a]	300–600	None	None
Vilazodone	10–40	Diarrhea, nausea, headaches	None
Vortioxetine	10–20	Nausea	None

[a]Not routinely available in the United States.
Data from Kennedy SH, Lam RW, McIntyre RS, Tourjman SV, Bhat V, Blier P, Hasnain M, Jollant F, Levitt AJ, MacQueen GM, McInerney SJ, McIntosh D, Milev RV, Müller DJ, Parikh SV, Pearson NL, Ravindran AV, Uher R; CANMAT Depression Work Group. Canadian Network for Mood and Anxiety Treatments (CANMAT) 2016 clinical guidelines for the management of adults with major depressive disorder: section 3. Pharmacological treatments. *Can J Psychiatry*. 2016;61(9):540–560; Kennedy SH, Rizvi SJ. Chapter 246: SSRIs and related compounds. In: Stolerman I, ed. *Encyclopedia of Pharmacology*. New York: Springer; 2010.

seem to have similar mechanisms of action and hence similar efficacy, there are some variations across classes. This variation gives us some diversity of choice. Although the first antidepressant drugs, the monoamine oxidase inhibitors (MAOIs) and tricyclic antidepressants (TCAs), are still in use, newer compounds have made the treatment of depression more "clinician and patient-friendly."

Table 7-11 lists selective serotonin reuptake inhibitors (SSRIs) and serotonin-norepinephrine reuptake inhibitors (SNRIs) by class as well as their side-effect profiles.

GENERAL CLINICAL GUIDELINES. The most common clinical mistake leading to an unsuccessful trial of an antidepressant drug is the use of too low a dosage for too short a time. Unless adverse events prevent it, the dosage of an antidepressant should be raised to the maximum recommended level and maintained at that level for at least 4 or 5 weeks before a drug trial is considered unsuccessful. Alternatively, if a patient is improving clinically on a low dosage of the drug, this dosage should not be raised unless clinical improvement stops before obtaining a maximal benefit. When a patient does not begin to respond to appropriate dosages of a drug after 2 or 3 weeks, clinicians may decide to obtain a plasma

concentration of the drug if such a test is available. The test may indicate either noncompliance or a particularly unusual pharmacokinetic disposition of the drug and may thereby suggest an alternative dosage.

INITIAL MEDICATION SELECTION. The available antidepressants do not differ in overall efficacy, speed of response, or long-term effectiveness. Antidepressants, however, do differ in their pharmacology, drug–drug interactions, short- and long-term side effects, the likelihood of discontinuation symptoms, and ease of dose adjustment. Most often, we start with second- and third-generation antidepressants. Among them, the selective serotonin reuptake inhibitors (SSRIs) remain the most commonly used medications for depression.

Selection of the initial treatment depends on the chronicity of the condition, course of illness (a recurrent or chronic course increases the likelihood of subsequent depressive symptoms without treatment), family history of illness and treatment response, symptom severity, concurrent general medical or other psychiatric conditions, prior treatment responses to other acute-phase treatments, potential drug–drug interactions, and patient preference.

In general, approximately 45 to 60 percent of all outpatients with uncomplicated (i.e., minimal psychiatric and general medical comorbidity), nonchronic, nonpsychotic major depressive disorder who begin treatment with medication respond (i.e., achieve at least a 50 percent reduction in baseline symptoms); however, only 35 to 50 percent achieve remission (i.e., the virtual absence of depressive symptoms).

DURATION AND PROPHYLAXIS. We should maintain antidepressant treatment for at least 6 months or the length of a previous episode, whichever is greater. When discontinuing antidepressant treatment, the drug dose should be tapered gradually over 1 to 2 weeks, depending on the half-life of the particular compound.

Prophylactic treatment with antidepressants is effective in reducing the number and severity of recurrences. One study concluded that when episodes are less than $2^{1}/_{2}$ years apart, we should recommend prophylactic treatment. Another factor suggesting prophylactic treatment is the seriousness of previous depressive episodes. Episodes that have involved significant suicidal ideation or impairment of psychosocial functioning may indicate that the risk of stopping treatment is too considerable.

Prevention of new mood episodes (i.e., recurrences) is the aim of the maintenance phase of treatment. Only patients with recurrent or chronic depressions are candidates for maintenance treatment. Several studies indicate that maintenance antidepressant medication appears to be safe and effective for the treatment of chronic depression.

TREATMENT OF SPECIFIC DEPRESSIVE DISORDERS. Clinical types of major depressive episodes may have varying responses to particular antidepressants or drugs other than antidepressants. Antidepressants with dual action on both serotonergic and noradrenergic receptors may have greater efficacy in melancholic depressions. We can treat patients with seasonal winter depression with light therapy.

Treatment of major depressive episodes with psychotic features may require a combination of an antidepressant and an atypical antipsychotic. Several studies have also shown that ECT is useful for this indication—perhaps more effective than pharmacotherapy.

For those with atypical symptom features, strong evidence exists for the effectiveness of MAOIs. SSRIs and bupropion are also of use in atypical depression.

COMORBID DISORDERS. The simultaneous presence of another disorder can affect initial treatment selection. For example, the successful treatment of an OCD associated with depressive symptoms usually results in remission of the depression. Similarly, when panic disorder occurs with major depression, medications with demonstrated efficacy in both conditions are preferred (e.g., tricyclics and SSRIs). In general, the nonmood disorder dictates the choice of treatment in comorbid states.

Concurrent substance abuse raises the possibility of a substance-induced mood disorder, which must be evaluated by history or by requiring abstinence for several weeks. Abstinence often results in remission of depressive symptoms in substance-induced mood disorders. For those with continuing significant depressive symptoms, even with abstinence, an independent mood disorder is diagnosed and treated.

General medical conditions are established risk factors in the development of depression. The presence of a major depressive episode is associated with increased morbidity or mortality of many general medical conditions (e.g., cardiovascular disease, diabetes, cerebrovascular disease, and cancer).

THERAPEUTIC USE OF SIDE EFFECTS. Choosing more sedating antidepressants (such as mirtazapine or paroxetine) for more anxious, depressed patients or more activating agents (bupropion) for more psychomotor-retarded patients is not as helpful as one might think. For example, any short-term benefits with paroxetine or mirtazapine on symptoms of anxiety or insomnia may become liabilities over time. These drugs often continue to be sedating in the longer run, which can lead to patients prematurely discontinuing medication and increase the risk of relapse or recurrence. Some practitioners use adjunctive medications, such as hypnotics or anxiolytics, combined with antidepressants to provide more immediate symptom relief or to cover those side effects to which most patients ultimately adapt.

Understanding a patient's prior treatment history is essential because an earlier response typically predicts future responses. A documented failure on a properly conducted trial of a particular antidepressant class is grounds to choose an agent from an alternative class. The history of a first-degree relative responding to a particular drug is associated with a positive response to the same class of agents in the patient.

ACUTE TREATMENT FAILURES. Patients may not respond to medication, because (1) they cannot tolerate the side effects, even in the face of an excellent clinical response; (2) an idiosyncratic adverse event may occur; (3) the clinical response is not adequate; or (4) the wrong diagnosis has been made. Acute phase medication trials should last 4 to 6 weeks to allow for adequate time for meaningful symptom reduction. Most (but not all) patients who ultimately respond fully show at least a partial response by the fourth week, assuming an adequate dose. A "partial response" is defined as at least a 20 to 25 percent reduction in pretreatment depressive symptom severity. Patients who have not even a partial response in that time likely need a change of treatment. More extended periods—8 to 12 weeks or longer—are needed to define the ultimate degree of symptom reduction achievable with a medication. Approximately half of patients require a second medication treatment trial because the initial treatment is poorly tolerated or ineffective.

Selecting Second Treatment Options. When the initial treatment is unsuccessful, switching to an alternative treatment or augmenting the current treatment is a standard option. The choice between switching from the single initial treatment to a new single treatment (as opposed to adding a second treatment to the first one) rests on the patient's prior treatment history, the degree of benefit achieved with the initial treatment, and patient preference. As a rule, switching rather than augmenting is preferred after an initial medication failure. On the other hand, augmentation strategies are helpful with patients who have gained some benefit from the initial treatment but who have not achieved remission. A review of the different strategies suggested there is some evidence suggesting that both strategies do confer some benefit. However, the evidence is inadequate to suggest one strategy over another.

When switching from one monotherapy to another, the usual suggestion is to pick a medication in a different class. For example, we might switch from an SSRI to an SNRI. However, when putting these assumptions to the test, it is difficult to find any advantage for any particular strategy. For example, in the landmark STAR*D study, which remains one of the most extensive studies of treatment strategies following initial failure, although medication switches were modestly helpful, both switches within and outside a class were equally effective.

Among augmentation options, several approaches have reasonable evidence. Several antipsychotics, most notably quetiapine and aripiprazole, are effective for augmentation. Lithium augmentation is also effective for augmenting both SSRIs and TCAs. There are also positive studies of thyroid hormone. However, this strategy is rarely used in clinical practice owing to the need for ongoing monitoring and potential adverse effects. Several other agents have been studied, including bupropion, buspirone, lamotrigine, methylphenidate, and pindolol; however, these have limited placebo-controlled data. One meta-analysis of the available data on switching strategies concluded that quetiapine and aripiprazole have the best evidence as augmentation agents. However, we should use these cautiously given their side effect profile.

NOVEL PHARMACOLOGIC AGENTS

Ketamine. The anesthetic agent ketamine is effective in treatment-resistant depression. It has a mechanism of action that inhibits the postsynaptic glutamate-binding protein N-methyl-D-aspartate (NMDA) receptor. Because abnormalities in glutamatergic signaling seem to have a role in major depressive disorder, this may account for its efficacy. Until recently, ketamine was only available intravenously, limiting its use as we had to monitor patients while they received an infusion of the drug over 30 minutes in a clinical setting. The most common side effects are dizziness, headache, and poor coordination, which are transitory. Dissociative symptoms, including hallucinations, may also occur. A positive response is usually seen within 24 hours, making this a genuinely novel substance in that it appears to act much more rapidly than standard antidepressants. However, the effect seems to be short-lived, and wears off after between 2 and 7 days, again limiting its use. There are little data on longer-term treatment as well as concern over associated adverse effects, particularly the psychogenic effect. Also, the agent has an abuse potential, making it less attractive as a long-term option.

More recently, esketamine in a nasal spray formulation was approved by the FDA for treatment-resistant depression. Given the abuse risk, it is only available through a restricted distribution system. Most of the supportive evidence for the agent is from short-term use. However, one longer-term study suggested that continuation treatment could be effective for some patients.

Brexanolone. Brexanolone is an intravenous formulation of allopregnanolone, which was approved by the FDA in 2019 for the treatment of postpartum depression. It is a neuroactive steroid that also has a neuroactive effect, functioning as an allosteric modulator of GABA$_A$, which may be central to the mechanism of postpartum depression. It is also only available in the United States through a restricted program that requires administrating the drug in a clinical setting over 60 hours. The most common adverse effects are sleepiness, dry mouth, loss of consciousness, and flushing. As with ketamine, brexanolone differs from standard antidepressants in its apparent rapid effect, reducing depressive symptoms as early as 24 hours after administration. In trials, the effect continued for at least 30 days. As of this writing, phase 3 trials for an oral version of the medication have promising results.

Other Somatic Treatments

NEUROSTIMULATION

Vagal Nerve Stimulation. Experimental stimulation of the vagus nerve in several studies designed for the treatment of epilepsy found that patients showed improved mood. This observation led to the use of left vagal nerve stimulation (VNS) using an electronic device implanted in the skin, similar to a cardiac pacemaker. Preliminary studies have shown that many patients with chronic, recurrent major depressive disorder went into remission when treated with VNS. The mechanism of action of VNS to account for improvement is unknown. The vagus nerve connects to the enteric nervous system and, when stimulated, may cause the release of peptides that act as neurotransmitters.

Transcranial Magnetic Stimulation. Transcranial magnetic stimulation (TMS) shows promise as a treatment for depression. It involves the use of very short pulses of magnetic energy to stimulate nerve cells in the brain. The FDA has indicated this treatment for depression in adult patients who have failed to achieve satisfactory improvement from one prior antidepressant medication at or above the minimal effective dose and duration in the current episode.

Repetitive transcranial magnetic stimulation (rTMS) produces focal secondary electrical stimulation of targeted cortical regions. It is nonconvulsive, requires no anesthesia, has a safe side effect profile, and is not associated with cognitive side effects.

The patients do not require anesthesia or sedation and remain awake and alert. It is a 40-minute outpatient procedure that is prescribed by a psychiatrist and performed in a psychiatrist's office. The treatment is typically administered daily for 4 to 6 weeks. The most common adverse event related to treatment was scalp pain or discomfort.

TMS therapy is contraindicated in patients with implanted metallic devices or nonremovable metallic objects in or around the head.

PHOTOTHERAPY. Phototherapy (light therapy) was introduced in 1984 as a treatment for SAD (mood disorder with seasonal pattern). In this disorder, patients typically experience depression as the photoperiod of the day decreases with advancing winter. Women represent at least 75 percent of all patients with seasonal depression, and the mean age of presentation is 40 years. Patients rarely present older than the age of 55 years with SAD.

Phototherapy typically involves exposing the affected patient to bright light in the range of 1,500 to 10,000 lux or more, typically with a lightbox that sits on a table or desk. Patients sit in front of the box for approximately 1 to 2 hours before dawn each day. Some patients may also benefit from exposure after dusk. Alternatively, some manufacturers have developed light visors, with a light source built into the brim of the hat. These light visors allow mobility, but recent controlled studies have questioned the use of this type of light exposure. Trials have typically lasted 1 week, but longer treatment durations may be associated with a more significant response.

Phototherapy is usually well tolerated. Newer light sources tend to use lower light intensities and come equipped with filters; patients are instructed not to look directly at the light source. As with any effective antidepressant, phototherapy, on rare occasions, has been implicated in switching some depressed patients into mania or hypomania.

In addition to seasonal depression, the other significant indication for phototherapy may be in sleep disorders. Phototherapy can decrease the irritability and diminished functioning associated with shift work. Sleep disorders in geriatric patients have reportedly improved with exposure to bright light during the day. Likewise, some evidence suggests that jet lag might respond to light therapy. Preliminary data indicate that phototherapy may benefit some patients with OCD that has a seasonal variation.

SLEEP DEPRIVATION. Sleep disturbances are common in depression. Depression can be associated with either hypersomnia or insomnia. Sleep deprivation may temporarily relieve depression in those who have unipolar depression. Approximately 60 percent of

Table 7-12
Evidence-Based Psychotherapies for Major Depressive Disorder

Treatment	Conceptualization of Disorder Etiology	Sample Interventions
Behavioral therapy	Deficit of reinforcers, including pleasant activities and positive interpersonal contacts	Increase activity level Structured goal setting Interpersonal skills training
Cognitive-behavioral therapy	Interaction of beliefs with matching stressor	Identify and challenge automatic thoughts Engage in activities that provide evidence disproving dysfunctional beliefs Modify core beliefs by reviewing evidence
Interpersonal psychotherapy	Interpersonal vulnerabilities arising from early attachment and learned relationship patterns	Develop awareness of patterns in primary relationships and the therapeutic relationship Interpersonal skills training Communication analysis
Behavioral marital therapy	Marital distress increases stress while impairing support resources	Assertive communication training Active listening exercises Problem-solving skills Increasing reinforcing behaviors toward spouse

patients with depressive disorders exhibit significant but transient benefits from total sleep deprivation. The positive results usually reverse by the next night of sleep. Several strategies have been used in an attempt to achieve a more sustained response to sleep deprivation. One method used serial total sleep deprivation with a day or two of normal sleep in between. This method does not achieve a sustained antidepressant response because the depression tends to return during the "normal sleep" days. Another approach used phase delay in the time patients go to sleep each night, or partial sleep deprivation. In this method, patients may stay awake from 2 AM to 10 PM daily. Up to 50 percent of patients get same-day antidepressant effects from partial sleep deprivation, but this benefit also tends to wear off in time. In some reports, however, serial partial sleep deprivation has been used successfully to treat insomnia associated with depression. The third, and probably most useful strategy combines sleep deprivation with pharmacologic treatment of depression. Several studies have suggested that total and partial sleep deprivation followed by immediate treatment with an antidepressant or lithium sustains the antidepressant effects of sleep deprivation. Likewise, several reports have suggested that sleep deprivation accelerates the response to antidepressants. Sleep deprivation may also improve premenstrual dysphoria.

Psychosocial Therapy

Three types of short-term psychotherapies—cognitive therapy, interpersonal therapy, and behavior therapy—have extensive studies for the treatment of major depressive disorder. In addition to these individual therapies, there are positive studies for behavioral marital therapy as well. Table 7-12 lists the evidence-based psychotherapies for major depressive disorder.

There are no generally accepted guidelines for choosing one therapy over another. The National Institute of Mental Health (NIMH) Treatment of Depression Collaborative Research Program did find some possible predictors of good response to specific treatments. Table 7-13 summarizes those findings.

Cognitive Therapy.   Cognitive therapy, originally developed by Aaron Beck, focuses on the cognitive distortions postulated to be present in major depressive disorder. Such distortions include selective

attention to the negative aspects of circumstances and unrealistically morbid inferences about consequences. For example, apathy and low energy result from a patient's expectation of failure in all areas. The goal of cognitive therapy is to alleviate depressive episodes and prevent their recurrence by helping patients identify and test negative cognitions; develop alternative, flexible, and positive ways of thinking; and rehearse new cognitive and behavioral responses.

> In this example, the therapist takes a cognitive approach when a patient shows up late to an appointment.
>
> Therapist: You mentioned that you were upset because you were late. Can you tell me what you were thinking when you realized you were late?
> Patient: I figured you'd be angry.
> Therapist: Okay, and when you thought I'd be angry, how did you feel?
> Patient: Pretty nervous.
> Therapist: So that is what we will focus on in here, how your thinking in different situations influences how you feel. In this case, you were late, thought "he'll be angry," and felt nervous. Our goal is to test out the beliefs, like "he'll be angry," and change them when they aren't healthy or accurate. The great thing is that you sort of implicitly tested out the belief that I'll be angry by showing up. Was I angry?
> Patient: You didn't seem angry.

Table 7-13
Predictors of Response to Several Therapies for Depression

Treatment	Predictors
Interpersonal psychotherapy	Low social dysfunction High depression severity
Cognitive-behavioral therapy	Low cognitive dysfunction
Pharmacotherapy	Low cognitive dysfunction High depression severity High work dysfunction

Data from Sotsky SM, Glass DR, Shea MT, Pilkonis PA, Collins JF, Elkin I, Watkins JT, Imber SD, Leber WR, Moyer J, Oliveri ME. Patient predictors of response to psychotherapy and pharmacotherapy: findings in the NIMH Treatment of Depression Collaborative Research Program. *Am J Psychiatry.* 1991;148:997–1108.

Therapist: How anxious did you feel once we started talking?

Patient: Well, I'm feeling more comfortable.

Therapist: What thoughts do you have now about me being angry?

Patient: I don't think you're angry.

Therapist: So, this is an example of what we're going to be doing in therapy—I'll be helping you to identify thoughts that make you feel bad. We're then going to work together to come up with ways to check them out and change them if they're not true or accurate. You checked out whether I was angry by observing me, and you changed your thought, and, now, I get the impression that you feel better.

Studies have shown that cognitive therapy is useful in the treatment of major depressive disorder. Most studies found that cognitive therapy is equal in efficacy to pharmacotherapy and is associated with fewer adverse effects and better follow-up than pharmacotherapy. Some of the best-controlled studies have indicated that the combination of cognitive therapy and pharmacotherapy is more efficacious than either therapy alone, although other studies have not found that additive effect.

Interpersonal Therapy.   Interpersonal therapy, developed by Gerald Klerman, focuses on one or two of a patient's current interpersonal problems. This therapy has two assumptions. First, current interpersonal problems are likely to have their roots in early dysfunctional relationships. Second, current interpersonal problems are likely to be involved in precipitating or perpetuating the current depressive symptoms. Controlled trials have indicated that interpersonal therapy is effective for treatment of major depressive disorder and, not surprisingly, may be specifically helpful in addressing interpersonal problems. Some studies indicate that interpersonal therapy may be the most effective method for severe major depressive episodes when the treatment choice is psychotherapy alone.

The interpersonal therapy program usually consists of 12 to 16 weekly sessions and is characterized by an active therapeutic approach. Intrapsychic phenomena, such as defense mechanisms and internal conflicts, are not addressed. Discrete behaviors—such as lack of assertiveness, impaired social skills, and distorted thinking—may be addressed but only in the context of their meaning in, or their effect on, interpersonal relationships.

Behavior Therapy.   Behavior therapy rests on the hypothesis that maladaptive behavioral patterns result in a person's receiving little positive feedback and perhaps outright rejection from society. By addressing maladaptive behaviors in therapy, patients learn to function in the world in such a way that they receive positive reinforcement. Behavior therapy for major depressive disorder has not yet been the subject of many controlled studies. The limited data indicate that it is an effective treatment for major depressive disorder.

Psychoanalytically Oriented Therapy.   Although not as well researched as those three therapies, many clinicians use psychoanalytically oriented psychotherapy as their primary method. What differentiates the short-term psychotherapy methods from the psychoanalytically oriented approach are the active and directive roles of the therapist, the directly recognizable goals, and the endpoints for short-term therapy.

The psychoanalytic approach to mood disorders uses psychoanalytic theories about depression. The goal of psychoanalytic psychotherapy is to effect a change in a patient's personality structure or character, not merely to alleviate symptoms. Improvements in interpersonal trust, capacity for intimacy, coping mechanisms, the capacity to grieve, and the ability to experience a wide range of emotions are some of the aims of psychoanalytic therapy. Treatment often requires the patient to experience periods of heightened anxiety and distress during therapy, which may continue for several years.

Accumulating evidence is encouraging about the efficacy of dynamic therapy. In a randomized, controlled trial comparing psychodynamic therapy with cognitive-behavioral therapy, the outcome of the depressed patients was the same in the two treatments.

Family Therapy.   Family therapy is usually the first-line treatment for major depressive disorder, but increasing evidence indicates that helping a patient with a mood disorder to reduce and cope with stress can lessen the chance of a relapse. We should consider family therapy if the disorder jeopardizes a patient's marriage or family functioning or if the mood disorder is promoted or maintained by the family situation. Family therapy examines the role of the mood-disordered member in the overall psychological well-being of the whole family; it also examines the role of the entire family in the maintenance of the patient's symptoms. Patients with mood disorders have a high rate of divorce, and about 50 percent of all spouses report that they would not have married or had children if they had known that the patient was going to develop a mood disorder.

THE EPIDEMIOLOGY OF DEPRESSION

Research on the epidemiology of depression, both in the United States and worldwide, has considerably broadened our understanding of the disorder. We have discovered that depression is much more common than once thought. It is also one of the more debilitating disorders known to humanity, as it often affects individuals during what should be their most productive years. Hence the depressive disorders are one of the most costly disorders in society.

Measuring the Incidence and Prevalence of Major Depressive Disorder Is Challenging

Measuring the true incidence of major depressive disorder is complicated and highly dependent on the methods used to collect the sample, definitions of the disorder, and the particular instruments used to measure depression. For example, studies that use self-assessment tend to report higher incidences than studies using clinician-rated instruments. The timing of a study likely affects the results as well. As depressive illness become less stigmatized, persons may be more willing to endorse symptoms of the disorder to the well-meaning strangers who knock at their door, call their phone, or email them and identify themselves as researchers.

Incidence and Prevalence

In a reasonably recent meta-analysis, which included 90 studies from 30 countries done from 1994 to 2014, with combined data on more than 1 million participants, the point prevalence for depression was 12.9 percent, the 1-year prevalence was 7.2 percent, and the lifetime prevalence was 10.8 percent. There was significant heterogeneity among the different studies.

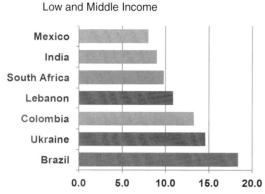
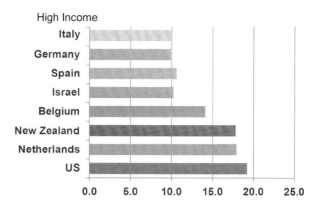

FIGURE 7-1

Lifetime prevalence of major depression across the world.

In the United States, the most recent epidemiologic data is from the National Survey on Drug Use and Health (NSDUH), sponsored by the Substance Abuse and Mental Health Services Administration (SAMHSA). Using a definition of a major depressive episode based on DSM-5, they found the overall 1-year prevalence of a major depressive episode to be 7.1 percent, hence very similar to the international data. Figure 7-1 summarizes some of the international prevalence data as it related to per capita income.

Sex

An almost universal observation, independent of country or culture, is that depression is more common in women than men. In the international meta-analysis, the aggregate prevalence for women was 14.4 percent versus 11.5 percent in men. In the United States, women were more likely to report a major depressive episode in the past year (8.7 percent) than men (5.3 percent).

There are various possible explanations, both biologic, psychological, and social, for this difference. A women's unequal status in many societies may make women more vulnerable to depression. Although this remains a valid hypothesis, it is notable that in societies where women have gained a better level of status, such as many Western societies, the ratio has not significantly changed. Although the explanation is undoubtedly complex and multifactorial, the weight of existing evidence suggests that biologic differences between men and women, such as variations in hormonal levels, do account for at least part of this difference.

Age

The mean age of onset for major depressive disorder is about 40 years, with 50 percent of all patients having an onset between the ages of 20 and 50 years. Major depressive disorder can also begin in childhood or old age. Some epidemiologic data suggest that the incidence of major depressive disorder may be increasing among younger persons. For example, in the SAMHSA study, major depressive disorder was almost twice as prevalent in adolescents as it was in adults, the most substantial difference being seen in adolescent females who reported a 1-year prevalence of major depression of 20 percent. The highest 1-year prevalence for major depressive disorder was in younger adults (adults ages 18 to 25).

Marital Status

Major depressive disorder occurs most often in persons without close interpersonal relationships and in those who are divorced or separated.

Socioeconomic and Cultural Factors

There is no proven correlation between socioeconomic status and major depressive disorder. Depression may be more common in rural areas than in urban areas. However, the most recent international meta-analysis described above did not find such a difference. It may be that technology and globalization have been able to narrow the differences between rural and urban settings.

Racial and ethnic differences may be particularly challenging to measure and may be highly dependent on method, approach, and locale. In the SAMSHA study, the highest prevalence was seen in White and Native American respondents.

THE NEUROBIOLOGY OF DEPRESSION

Since the time of Kraepelin, researchers have examined the brains, bodies, and behaviors of depressed patients in the search for clues of the underlying pathology of depression. This search is complicated by the fact that most experts on depression agree what we call major depressive disorder is not a single disease, but rather a collection of disorders with overlapping phenomenology but different etiologies and pathologies. Although this assumption seems likely, we have yet to find definitive subtypes or distinct patterns that we can confidently group into separate disorders. This area of research is a rapidly changing field, and improvements in technology, including higher-resolution imaging, more efficient genotyping, and more powerful computing power are getting us closer to the search for valid "biotypes" of depression.

What follows here are examples of pathologic findings, most of which have been reasonably replicated by different investigators. Some are long known, others are recent. However, the growing collection of pathologic findings is helping us to understand what is happening when a patient says that they are "depressed."

Depression as a Disorder of Homeostasis

Depression and the Hypothalamic–Pituitary–Adrenal Axis.

We have known for more than 50 years that, on average, depressed patients have an overactive hypothalamic–pituitary–adrenal (HPA) axis. Compared with controls, depressed patients have increased cortisol levels over 24 hours. We have documented elevated HPA activity in depression via excretion of urinary-free cortisol (UFC), 24-hour (or shorter time segments) intravenous (IV) collections of plasma cortisol levels, salivary cortisol levels, and tests of the integrity of feedback inhibition. Evidence of increased HPA activity is apparent in 20 to 40 percent of depressed outpatients and 40 to 60 percent of depressed inpatients.

This hypercortisolemia is due to increased corticotropin-releasing hormone (CRH) from the hypothalamus, along with decreased feedback inhibition. We can test for a disturbance of feedback inhibition using the dexamethasone test (DST). The DST was devised in the 1980s—patients were given dexamethasone—a synthetic steroid. This should create a negative feedback loop, and serum cortisol should decrease. However, depressed patients show an initial decrease but then "escape" from the suppression and return to abnormally high levels of cortisol. Although this is a replicable finding, it is not useful enough to be a diagnostic test, as it is neither sensitive (many patients diagnosed with depression have a normal DST) nor specific (many other conditions, such as Cushing syndrome, or simple environmental stress, can cause an abnormal DST).

Postmortem studies have shown increased neurons in the hypothalamus, which is likely what is driving the increased activity. This neuronal increase is likely in response to chronic stress.

Elevated HPA activity is a hallmark of the mammalian stress responses and one of the most unambiguous links between depression and the biology of chronic stress. Hypercortisolema in depression suggests one or more of the following central disturbances: decreased inhibitory serotonin tone, increased drive from norepinephrine, acetylcholine (ACh), or CRH; or decreased feedback inhibition from the hippocampus. Some studies in depressed humans indicate that a history of early trauma is associated with increased HPA activity accompanied by structural changes (i.e., atrophy or decreased volume) in the cerebral cortex.

DEPRESSION ALSO AFFECTS OTHER ENDOCRINE AND RELATED REGULATORY SYSTEMS

Thyroid Axis Activity. Approximately 5 to 10 percent of people evaluated for depression have previously undetected thyroid dysfunction, as reflected by an elevated basal thyroid-stimulating hormone (TSH) level or an increased TSH response to a 500-mg infusion of the hypothalamic neuropeptide thyroid-releasing hormone (TRH). Such abnormalities are often associated with elevated antithyroid antibody levels and, unless corrected with hormone replacement therapy, can compromise response to treatment. An even more significant subgroup of depressed patients (e.g., 20 to 30 percent) shows a blunted TSH response to TRH challenge. To date, the major therapeutic implication of a blunted TSH response is evidence of an increased risk of relapse despite preventive antidepressant therapy. Of note, unlike the dexamethasone-suppression test (DST), blunted TSH response to TRH does not usually normalize with effective treatment.

Growth Hormone. Growth hormone (GH) is secreted from the anterior pituitary after stimulation by NE and dopamine. Somatostatin, a hypothalamic neuropeptide, and CRH inhibit this secretion. Decreased CSF somatostatin levels occur in depression, as do increased levels in mania.

Prolactin. Prolactin is released from the pituitary by serotonin stimulation and inhibited by dopamine. Most studies have not found significant abnormalities of basal or circadian prolactin secretion in depression, although some see a blunted prolactin response to various serotonin agonists. This response is uncommon among premenopausal women, suggesting that estrogen has a moderating effect.

Brain-Derived Neurotrophic Factor. Various growth factor proteins, of which brain-derived neurotrophic factor (or BDNF) is best understood, are responsible for the ongoing maintenance of neurons in the brain, and disruption of it causes a reduction in neuronal number and size. It is challenging to measure BDNF in the living subjects, but postmortem studies have suggested deficits in BDNF may correlate with psychopathology. For example, some studies have found that in postmortem examination of persons who died from suicide, the average BDNF in the prefrontal cortex (PFC) and hippocampus was lower than for control subjects. Indirect studies in live patients, looking at BDNF in plasma rather than the brain (the correlation between the two is not clear), found increases in serum BDNF in depressed patients who responded to antidepressants.

BDNF may provide clues to the relationship between chronic stress and depression as the activity of the gene coding for this growth factor decreases with chronic stress, as does neurogenesis.

Similarly, animal studies show that a variety of factors, including antidepressants, estrogen, lithium, and neurostimulation, all increase BDNF in the brain, suggesting a possible common link between known treatments for depression.

DEPRESSION ALSO DISRUPTS CIRCADIAN RHYTHM. It has also long been known that depression is associated with a premature loss of deep (slow-wave) sleep and an increase in nocturnal arousal. Four types of disturbance reflect the latter: (1) an increase in nocturnal awakenings, (2) a reduction in total sleep time, (3) increased phasic rapid eye movement (REM) sleep, and (4) increased core body temperature. The combination of increased REM drive and decreased slow-wave sleep results in a significant reduction in the first period of non-REM (NREM) sleep, a phenomenon referred to as *reduced REM latency.* Blunted secretion of GH may cause this reduction in latency, which usually increases with sleep onset. It is very persistent, often lasting beyond recovery from depression. Some patients manifesting a characteristically abnormal sleep profile are known to be less responsive to psychotherapy and to have a higher risk of relapse or recurrence and may benefit preferentially from pharmacotherapy.

As with the HPA access, the association between sleep disturbances and depression is common, but it is neither sensitive nor specific enough for clinical use. About 40 percent of outpatients and 80 percent of inpatients show a typical pattern of reduced REM latency, increased REM density, and decreased sleep maintenance. False-negative findings are common in younger, hypersomnolent patients, who may experience an increase in slow-wave sleep during episodes of depression. Approximately 10 percent of otherwise healthy individuals have abnormal sleep profiles, as do many patients suffering from other medical or psychiatric disorders.

Neurotransmitter Deficits Are Involved.
Much of the research into the neurobiology of depression has centered on the role played by neurotransmitters. This approach was understandable, given that most somatic treatments for depression appear to act by influencing neurotransmission. In the 1950s, researchers found that reserpine, an antihypertensive that acts by inhibiting the release of monoamine neurotransmitters, sometimes induced depression. During the same decade, others discovered the earliest antidepressants. Although the discoveries were serendipitous, it eventually became clear that they all interfered with the catabolism of monoamine neurotransmitters, and researchers presumed that this must be

their mechanism of action. It was reasonable, then, to assume that depression was due to abnormally low levels of these monoamines. Early theories of depression explained the disorder as a deficit or imbalance in neurotransmitters: hence depressed patients were often told that they had a "chemical imbalance." Such a simplistic theory was, of course, overly optimistic, and subsequent neurochemical research did not find such simple relationships. However, neurotransmitters do play an essential role in the disorder, and subsequent findings have helped to clarify this role.

NOREPINEPHRINE.   Perhaps the most compelling evidence for the central role of the noradrenergic system in depression is the well-replicated finding that antidepressant response is correlated with the downregulation or decreased sensitivity of β-adrenergic receptors. Also, presynaptic β_2-receptors appear to have a role, as activation of these receptors results in a decrease in the amount of norepinephrine released. Presynaptic β_2-receptors are also located on serotonergic neurons and regulate the amount of serotonin released.

SEROTONIN.   Most modern antidepressants act on serotonin, rather than norepinephrine, and as a result, serotonin has become the biogenic amine neurotransmitter most commonly associated with depression. The identification of multiple serotonin receptor subtypes has also increased the excitement within the research community about the development of even more specific treatments for depression. Besides treatment studies, other data indicate that serotonin is involved in the pathophysiology of depression. Depletion of serotonin may precipitate depression, and some patients with suicidal impulses have low cerebrospinal fluid (CSF) concentrations of serotonin metabolites and low concentrations of serotonin uptake sites on platelets.

DOPAMINE.   Although norepinephrine and serotonin are the biogenic amines most often associated with the pathophysiology of depression, dopamine may also play a role. Dopamine activity may be reduced in depression and increased in mania. The discovery of new subtypes of the dopamine receptors and an increased understanding of the presynaptic and postsynaptic regulation of dopamine function have further enriched research into the relationship between dopamine and mood disorders. Drugs that reduce dopamine concentrations, including the reserpine mentioned above, as well as diseases that deplete dopamine such as Parkinson disease, all may cause depressive symptoms. In contrast, drugs that increase dopamine concentrations, such as tyrosine, amphetamine, and bupropion, reduce the symptoms of depression.

OTHER NEUROTRANSMITTER DISTURBANCES.   Acetylcholine (ACh) is found in neurons that are distributed diffusely throughout the cerebral cortex. Cholinergic neurons have reciprocal or interactive relationships with all three monoamine systems. Abnormal levels of choline, which is a precursor to ACh, have been found at autopsy in the brains of some depressed patients. Cholinergic agonists can cause symptoms of lethargy, anergia, and psychomotor retardation. In an animal model of depression, strains of mice that are super- or subsensitive to cholinergic agonists have been found susceptible or more resistant to animal models of depression. Cholinergic agonists can induce changes in HPA activity and sleep that mimic those associated with severe depression. Some patients with mood disorders in remission, as well as their never-ill first-degree relatives, have a trait-like increase in sensitivity to cholinergic agonists.

γ-Aminobutyric acid (GABA) has an inhibitory effect on ascending monoamine pathways, particularly the mesocortical and mesolimbic systems. Reductions of GABA occur in plasma, CSF, and brain GABA levels in depression. Animal studies have also found that chronic stress can reduce and eventually can deplete GABA levels. By contrast, antidepressants upregulate GABA receptors, and some GABAergic medications have weak antidepressant effects.

The amino acids glutamate and glycine are the primary excitatory and inhibitory neurotransmitters in the CNS. Glutamate and glycine bind to sites associated with the NMDA receptor and an excess of glutamatergic stimulation can cause neurotoxic effects. Importantly, a high concentration of NMDA receptors exists in the hippocampus. Glutamate, thus, may work in conjunction with hypercortisolemia to mediate the deleterious neurocognitive effects of severe recurrent depression. Emerging evidence suggests that drugs that antagonize NMDA receptors have antidepressant effects.

SECOND MESSENGERS AND INTRACELLULAR CASCADES.   The binding of a neurotransmitter and a postsynaptic receptor triggers a cascade of membrane-bound and intracellular processes mediated by second messenger systems. Second messengers regulate the function of neuronal membrane ion channels. Increasing evidence also indicates that mood-stabilizing drugs act on these second messengers.

Immunologic Disturbance.

Depressive disorders are associated with several immunologic abnormalities, including decreased lymphocyte proliferation in response to mitogens and other forms of impaired cellular immunity. These lymphocytes produce neuromodulators, such as corticotropin-releasing factor (CRF), and cytokines, peptides known as interleukins. There appears to be an association with clinical severity, hypercortisolism, and immune dysfunction, and the cytokine interleukin-1 may induce gene activity for glucocorticoid synthesis.

Findings from Brain Imaging

STRUCTURAL IMAGING.   The most consistent abnormality observed in depressive disorders is the increased frequency of abnormal hyperintensities in subcortical regions, such as periventricular regions, the basal ganglia, and the thalamus. More common among elderly adults, these hyperintensities appear to reflect the deleterious neurodegenerative effects of recurrent affective episodes. Ventricular enlargement, cortical atrophy, and sulcal widening also have been reported in some studies. Some depressed patients also may have reduced hippocampal or caudate nucleus volumes, or both, suggesting more focal defects in relevant neurobehavioral systems. Diffuse and focal areas of atrophy are associated with increased illness severity, bipolarity, and increased cortisol levels.

Also, specific structures appear reduced in volume in patients with depression, for example, the hippocampus. This reduction may be due to neuronal loss due to the neurotoxic effects of the increased cortisol found in depressed patients. Although many areas of the brain are susceptible to this toxic effect, the hippocampus is particularly vulnerable, as it is rich in glutaminergic neurons. Other areas with reported brain loss include the PFC, cingulate gyrus, and cerebellum.

FUNCTIONAL IMAGINING.   The most widely replicated positron emission tomography (PET) finding in depression is decreased anterior brain metabolism, which is generally more pronounced on the left side. From a different vantage point, depression may cause a relative increase in nondominant hemispheric activity. Furthermore, a reversal of hypofrontality occurs after shifts from depression into hypomania, such that higher left hemisphere reductions occur in depression compared with more significant right hemisphere reductions in mania. Other studies have observed more specific reductions of reduced cerebral blood flow or metabolism, or

Representation and Regulation of Emotion in Depression

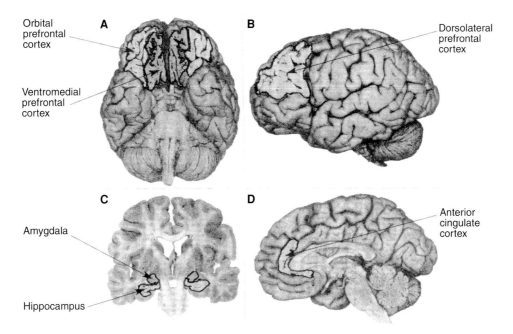

FIGURE 7-2

Key brain regions involved in affect and mood disorders. **A:** Orbital prefrontal cortex and the ventromedial prefrontal cortex. **B:** Dorsolateral prefrontal cortex. **C:** Hippocampus an˙˙d amygdala. **D:** Anterior cingulate cortex. (From Thase ME. Mood disorders neurobiology. In: Sadock BJ, Sadock VA, Ruiz P. (eds.). *Kaplan & Sadock's Comprehensive Textbook of Psychiatry*. 10th ed. Philadelphia, PA: Lippincott Williams & Wilkins, 2017.)

both, in the dopaminergically innervated tracts of the mesocortical and mesolimbic systems in depression. Evidence suggests that antidepressants at least partially normalize these changes.

In addition to a global reduction of anterior cerebral metabolism, increased glucose metabolism occurs in several limbic regions, particularly among patients with relatively severe recurrent depression and a family history of mood disorder. During episodes of depression, increased glucose metabolism correlates with intrusive ruminations.

One meta-analysis found three consistent differences when comparing fMRI studies of depressed patients with healthy controls. They found activation of the pulvinar nucleus of the thalamus, more significant response to negative stimuli in the amygdala, insula and anterior cingulate, and lesser response in the dorsal striatum and dorsal lateral PFC.

Figure 7-2 illustrates some of the brain regions thought to be most critical to mood regulation.

Our Understanding of the Genetics of Depressive Disorders

Numerous family, adoption, and twin studies have long documented the heritability of mood disorders. Recently, however, the primary focus of genetic studies has been to identify specific susceptibility genes using molecular genetic methods.

Studies of Inheritance Patterns. Depression aggregates within families and meta-analytic studies suggest that first-degree relatives of persons with major depressive disorder have an increased odds ratio of 2.84 for developing the disease. Only limited adoption studies have been done, of varying quality and with mixed results, and most of what we know about the genetic contribution to the disorder comes from twin studies, which estimate

the heritability to be 37 percent. It appears that this heritability is higher in women. The twin studies also concluded that shared environmental factors did not play a significant role in the familial aggregation of the disorder.

Genetic Studies. Genome-wide association studies have not found significant associations. Although there are various explanations for the lack of replicated findings, it likely relates to the fact that GWAS is powered to detect common variants, and that the genes relevant to depression risk are rare.

Candidate gene studies, which instead focus on specific genes of interest, have resulted in many reported findings. However, few of these are replicated. The most considerable focus has been on genes that might have a role in the proposed mechanism of depression, such as the gene involved in the encoding of serotonin (HTR1A), the serotonin transporter (5HTTP/SLC6A4), or the dopamine receptor (DRD4), and transporter (SLC6A3). Although some have replicated the most significant associations for these genes (most often for the 5HTTP/SLC6A4 gene), the effect size are small, and the sample sizes are smaller than those using GWAS, leading some experts to question the role of statistical error in the positive and negative findings. If some or all of the candidate gene studies are significant, the most likely interpretation of available findings is that much, or most of the genetic heritability for depression is the result of many genes each contributing a small effect, which only becomes meaningful when combined across thousands of genes. It is also possible, however, that there is some rare, still undetected genetic variant.

THE PSYCHOLOGY OF DEPRESSION

A great deal of psychological and sociologic research has also shed light on the pathology of depression. Perhaps the most meaningful contributions come from research on the role of stress and depression.

Stress and Depression

Some clinicians believe that life events play the primary or principal role in depression; others suggest that life events have only a limited role in the onset and timing of depression. The most compelling data indicate that the life event most often associated with the development of depression is losing a parent before age 11 years. The environmental stressor most often associated with the onset of an episode of depression is the loss of a spouse. Another risk factor is unemployment; persons out of work are three times more likely to report symptoms of an episode of major depression than those who are employed.

Personality

No single personality trait or type uniquely predisposes a person to depression; all humans, of whatever personality pattern, can and do become depressed under appropriate circumstances. Persons with certain personality disorders—OCPD, histrionic, and borderline—may be at higher risk for depression than persons with an antisocial or paranoid personality disorder. The latter can use projection and other externalizing defense mechanisms to protect themselves from their inner rage.

ETIOLOGY

As we can see, there is a great deal of data accumulating on various pathologies and dysregulations in the brain and body that are associated with depression. Many experts in the field have attempted to combine various lines of research into a coherent explanation of what causes us to suffer from a depressive disorder. Although there is no single unifying theory, several theories have emerged over the last century that attempt to account for the various clinical, psychological, and biologic findings in depression.

Biologic Theories

The Monoamine Hypothesis.   As already noted, the fact that all known antidepressants acted on the monoamines (particularly catecholamines as noted above) coupled with the fact that drugs and diseases that deplete monoamines (e.g., reserpine and Parkinson disease) can cause depressive symptoms led to the supposition that depression is the result of some deficiency or dysregulation in brain monoamines.

Although the theory became, and to a point remains, prevalent, several lines of evidence suggested it was an inadequate explanation for the etiology of depression. Most notably, antidepressants take weeks to work, even though their presumed action of increasing monoamine levels happens quickly, often within hours after administration. Also, there is no convincing evidence of any neurochemical imbalance, for example, in studies of the CSF of depressed patients or postmortem brain tissue.

As noted in our discussion of the pathology of depression, there is good evidence to suggest that neurotransmitters do play an important role, and that receptor or second messenger relationships may explain some of the inconsistent findings. Some have attempted to modify the monoamine hypothesis, suggesting that it remains true, but is more complicated than initially thought. However, a consistent and coherent explanation of the role of neurotransmitters remains elusive, and we still do not know whether their relationship to depression is one of causation or a later effect of the disease.

Brain Dysfunction.   Theories of brain dysregulation attempt to incorporate both findings of dysregulation with the increased and decreased responses to various negative stimuli observed in studies. Areas of interest include:

The amygdala. Part of the limbic system, the amygdala appears to be a crucial way station for processing novel stimuli of emotional significance and coordinating or organizing cortical responses.

The hippocampus. Adjacent to the amygdala, the hippocampus is most associated with learning and memory. Emotional or contextual learning appears to involve a direct connection between the hippocampus and the amygdala. Also, the hippocampus regulates the HPA axis by inhibiting activity.

The Prefrontal Cortex (PFC). We think of the PFC as the structure that holds representations of goals and appropriate responses to obtain these goals. There are areas of specialization. For example, whereas left-sided activation of regions of the PFC is more involved in goal-directed or appetitive behaviors, regions of the right PFC are implicated in avoidance behaviors and inhibition of appetitive pursuits. Subregions in the PFC appear to localize representations of behaviors related to reward and punishment.

The anterior cingulate cortex (ACC). The ACC is involved in attention, motivation, and environmental exploration and appears to help integrate attentional and emotional inputs. The more rostral and ventral region has an affective subdivision that connects extensively with limbic regions of the brain. Activation of the ACC may facilitate control of emotional arousal, particularly when thwarting goal when attainment encountering novel problems.

There are various theories that attempt to integrate various pathologic findings into an understanding of the etiology of depression. Although there are many approaches and variations, many theories broadly fall into one of two categories: neurogenesis hypotheses and neuroplastic hypotheses.

Neurogenesis Hypotheses.   Neurogenesis hypotheses suppose that the brain abnormalities leading to depression are the result of abnormalities in development such that there is a deficit in the number of newborn neurons in the brain.

There are several explanations for the cause of this deficit. Some versions attempt to link the role of stress, particularly chronic stress, in causing depression. Stress can cause increased activity in the HPA axis, which results in increased glucocorticoid production. Glucocorticoids are known to decrease neurogenesis. As neurogenesis continues in the adult hippocampus, this may be an area preferentially affected by stress. The hippocampus is then unable to adequately regulate the HPA axis, leading to continued elevated glucocorticoid levels in the brain and further inhibition of neurogenesis.

Neuroplasticity Hypotheses.   Neuroplasticity hypotheses propose that the atrophy of already developed neurons causes depression. In this version, rather than a deficit of nerve growth, atrophy occurs in already mature neurons. As noted, chronic stress can increase glucocorticoid levels, which can cause atrophy. It can also decrease the expression of BDNF, which is essential for the survival, growth, and differentiation of neurons in the brain; the result is atrophy. As this preferentially happens in the hippocampus, this can account for the finding of decreased hippocampal volume in depressed patients.

Psychosocial Theories

Life Events and Environmental Stress.   A long-standing clinical observation is that stressful life events more often precede first, rather than subsequent, episodes of mood disorders. One theory proposed to explain this observation is that the stress accompanying the first episode results in long-lasting changes in the brain's biology. As a result, a person has a high risk of undergoing subsequent episodes of a mood disorder, even without an external stressor.

> Ms. C, a 23-year-old woman, became acutely depressed when she was accepted to a prestigious graduate school. Ms. C had been working diligently toward this acceptance for the past 4 years. She reported being "briefly happy, for about 20 minutes" when she learned the good news but rapidly slipped into a hopeless state in which she recurrently pondered the pointlessness of her aspirations, cried constantly, and had to physically stop herself from taking a lethal overdose of her roommate's insulin. In treatment, she focused on her older brother, who had regularly insulted her throughout the course of her life, and how "he's not doing well." She found herself very worried about him. She mentioned that she was not used to being the "successful" one of the two of them. In connection with her depression, it emerged that Ms. C's brother had had a severe, life-threatening, and disfiguring pediatric illness that had required much family time and attention throughout their childhood. Ms. C had become "used to" his insulting manner toward her. In fact, it seemed that she required her brother's abuse of her in order not to feel overwhelmed by survivor guilt about being the "healthy, normal" child. "He might insult me, but I look up to him. I adore him. Any attention he pays to me is like a drug," she said. Ms. C's acceptance to graduate school had challenged her defensive and essential compensatory image of herself as being less successful, or damaged, in comparison with her brother, thereby overwhelming her with guilt. Her depression remitted in psychodynamic psychotherapy as she better understood her identification with and fantasy submission to her brother. (Courtesy of J. C. Markowitz, M.D. and B. L. Milrod, M.D.)

Psychodynamic Theories of Depression.   The psychodynamic understanding of depression defined by Sigmund Freud and expanded by Karl Abraham is known as the classic view of depression. That theory involves four key points: (1) disturbances in the infant–mother relationship during the oral phase (the first 10 to 18 months of life) predispose to subsequent vulnerability to depression; (2) depression can be linked to real or imagined object loss; (3) introjection of the departed objects is a defense mechanism invoked to deal with the distress connected with the object's loss; and (4) because the lost object is regarded with a mixture of love and hate, feelings of anger are directed inward at the self.

> Ms. E, a 21-year-old college student, presented with major depression and panic disorder since early adolescence. She reported hating herself, crying constantly, and feeling profoundly hopeless in part because of the chronicity of her illness. Even at the time of presentation, she noted her sensitivity to her mother's moods. "My mother's just always depressed, and it makes me so miserable. I just don't know what to do," she said. "I always want something from her, I don't even know what, but I never get it. She always says the wrong thing, talks about how disturbed I am, stuff like that, makes me feel bad about myself." In one session, Ms. E poignantly described her childhood: "I spent a lot of time with my mother, but she was always too tired, she never wanted to do anything or play with me. I remember building a house with blankets over the coffee table and peeking out, spying on her. She was always depressed and negative, like a negative sink in the room, making it empty and sad. I could never get her to do anything." This patient experienced extreme guilt in her psychotherapy when she began to talk about her mother's depression. "I feel so bad," she sobbed. "It's like I'm saying bad things about her. And I love her so much, and I

know she loves me. I feel it's so disloyal of me." Her depression remitted in psychodynamic psychotherapy as she became more aware of and better able to tolerate her feelings of rage and disappointment with her mother. (Courtesy of J. C. Markowitz M.D. and B. L. Milrod, M.D.)

Cognitive Theory.   According to cognitive theory, depression results from specific cognitive distortions present in persons susceptible to depression. These distortions, referred to as depressogenic schemata, are cognitive templates that perceive both internal and external data in ways that are altered by early experiences. Aaron Beck postulated a cognitive triad of depression that consists of (1) views about the self—a negative self-precept, (2) about the environment—a tendency to experience the world as hostile and demanding, and (3) about the future—the expectation of suffering and failure. Therapy consists of modifying these distortions. We summarize the elements of cognitive theory in Table 7-14.

Learned Helplessness.   The learned helplessness theory of depression connects depressive phenomena to the experience of uncontrollable events. For example, when dogs in a laboratory are exposed to electrical shocks from which they cannot escape, they showed behaviors that differentiate them from dogs not exposed to such uncontrollable events. The dogs exposed to the shocks would not cross a barrier to stop the flow of electric shock when put in a new learning situation. They remained passive and did not move. According to the learned helplessness theory, the shocked dogs learned that outcomes were independent of responses, so they had both cognitive motivational deficits (i.e., they would not attempt to escape the shock) and emotional deficits (indicating decreased reactivity to the shock). In the reformulated view of learned helplessness as applied to human depression, internal causal explanations may produce a loss of self-esteem after adverse external events. Behaviorists who subscribe to this theory often stress that

Table 7-14
Elements of Cognitive Theory

Element	Definition
Cognitive triad	Beliefs about oneself, the world, and the future
Schemas	Ways of organizing and interpreting experiences
Cognitive distortions	Persistent ways of thinking that are inaccurate and usually negatively biased
Arbitrary inference	Drawing a specific conclusion without sufficient evidence
Specific abstraction	Focus on a single detail while ignoring other, more important aspects of an experience
Overgeneralization	Forming conclusions based on too little and too narrow experience
Magnification and minimization	Over- or undervaluing the significance of a particular event
Personalization	Tendency to self-reference external events without basis
Absolutist, dichotomous thinking	Tendency to place experience into all-or-none categories

Courtesy of Robert M.A. Hirschfeld, M.D. and M. Tracie Shea, Ph.D.

improvement of depression is contingent on the patient's learning a sense of control and mastery of the environment.

Evolutionary Theory.   Some theorists take an evolutionary perspective toward depression. From this perspective, depression is an adaptive response to perceived threats in the environment. From this perspective, depression is an adaptive response to perceived threats in the environment, and the tendency for depressed persons to withdraw from the environment in the face of possible threats could be protective. Beyond threats of bodily harm, social threats (e.g.,of exclusion or defeat) could also be considered threats in that such social threats can reduce one's perceived fitness, and hence, the desirability of a mate. The depressive response in which one decreases activity, withdraws from social situations, and approaches novel situations with a negative bias ("that person will think I am a loser") could be interpreted as adaptive ways to reduce risk and avoid further social failures. There are many varieties of evolutionary theory, some of which stress the adaptive benefit of depression, others which see it as an outmoded response which may have had a benefit in ancient societies, but is counterproductive in our modern world. Other versions see the basic ability to vary mood as adaptive but suggest depression is a dysregulation of that normal function. These theories are difficult to test, as it is challenging to test the fitness of a particular trait that is very common in a population.

Integrative Approaches

It remains difficult, if not impossible, to incorporate all the various observations and research findings on depression into one grand unified theory. However, the various attempts by investigators and theoreticians to incorporate these findings have certain common features.

It seems clear that there exists some genetic vulnerability that puts persons at risk for depression. Such persons who then encounter stress, either external or internal, have epigenetic changes that differ from normal responses to stress; for example, they may be less able to transcribe certain growth factors in response to stress. This deficit results in subtle neuronal loss, and this loss is particularly apparent in some vulnerable areas (e.g., the hippocampus). The result is a disruption of the usual regulatory systems in the brain, causing changes in the expressions of transmitters, hormones, and other regulatory systems. This causes the physical changes that we associate with depression, and our behavioral response to this is the subjective feeling of depression.

References

Akiskal. Mood disorders. In: Sadock BJ, Sadock VA, Ruiz P, eds. *Kaplan & Sadock's Comprehensive Textbook of Psychiatry*. 10th ed. Philadelphia, PA: Wolters Kluwer; 2017.

Albert PR. Why is depression more prevalent in women? *J Psychiatry Neurosci*. 2015;40(4):219–221.

Badcock PB, Davey CG, Whittle S, Allen NB, Friston KJ. The depressed brain: an evolutionary systems theory. *Trends Cogn Sci*. 2017;21(3):182–194.

Boku S, Nakagawa S, Toda H, Hishimoto A. Neural basis of major depressive disorder: beyond monoamine hypothesis. *Psychiatry Clin Neurosci*. 2018;72(1):3–12.

Cipriani A, Furukawa TA, Salanti G, Chaimani A, Atkinson LZ, Ogawa Y, Leucht S, Ruhe HG, Turner EH, Higgins JPT, Egger M, Takeshima N, Hayasaka Y, Imai H, Shinohara K, Tajika A, Ioannidis JPA, Geddes JR. Comparative efficacy and acceptability of 21 antidepressant drugs for the acute treatment of adults with major depressive disorder: a systematic review and network meta-analysis. *Lancet*. 2018;391(10128):1357–1366.

Flint J, Kendler KS. The genetics of major depression. *Neuron*. 2014;81(3):484–503.

Hamilton JP, Etkin A, Furman DJ, Lemus MG, Johnson RF, Gotlib IH. Functional neuroimaging of major depressive disorder: a meta-analysis and new integration of base line activation and neural response data. *Am J Psychiatry*. 2012;169(7):693–703.

Krause JS, Reed KS, McArdle JJ. Factor structure and predictive validity of somatic and nonsomatic symptoms from the patient health questionnaire-9: a longitudinal study after spinal cord injury. *Arch Phys Med Rehabil*. 2010;91(8):1218–1224.

Lim GY, Tam WW, Lu Y, Ho CS, Zhang MW, Ho RC. Prevalence of depression in the community from 30 countries between 1994 and 2014. *Sci Rep*. 2018;8(1):2861.

Results from the 2017 National Survey on Drug Use and Health: Detailed Tables, SAMHSA, CBHSQ. https://www.samhsa.gov/data/sites/default/files/cbhsq-reports/NSDUHDetailedTabs2017/NSDUHDetailedTabs2017.htm#tab8-56A. n.d. Accessed April 1, 2019.

Rush AJ, Trivedi MH, Wisniewski SR, Stewart JW, Nierenberg AA, Thase ME, Ritz L, Biggs MM, Warden D, Luther JF, Shores-Wilson K, Niederehe G, Fava M; STAR*D Study Team. Bupropion-SR, sertraline, or venlafaxine-XR after failure of SSRIs for depression. *N Engl J Med*. 2006;354(12):1231–1242.

Santaguida P (Lina), MacQueen G, Keshavarz H, Levine M, Beyene J, Raina P. Treatment for Depression After Unsatisfactory Response to SSRIs. In AHRQ Comparative Effectiveness Reviews. 2012. http://www.ncbi.nlm.nih.gov/books/NBK97406/.

Schildkraut JJ. The catecholamine hypothesis of affective disorders: a review of supporting evidence. *Am J Psychiatry*. 1965;122(5):509–522.

Sullivan PF, Neale MC, Kendler KS. Genetic epidemiology of major depression: review and meta-analysis. *Am J Psychiatry*. 2000;157(10):1552–1562.

Zhou X, Ravindran AV, Qin B, Del Giovane C, Li Q, Bauer M, Liu Y, Fang Y, da Silva T, Zhang Y, Fang L, Wang X, Xie P. Comparative efficacy, acceptability, and tolerability of augmentation agents in treatment-resistant depression: systematic review and network meta-analysis. *J Clin Psychiatry*. 2015;76(4):e487–e498.

## 8

Anxiety Disorders

Everyone experiences anxiety. The experience of anxiety has two components: the awareness of the physiologic sensations (e.g., palpitations and sweating) and the awareness of being nervous or frightened. It is a diffuse, unpleasant, vague sense of apprehension, usually accompanied by autonomic symptoms. Although the physical and emotional symptoms of anxiety are similar to "fear," it differs from fear in that it is not a response to an overt danger, but rather an impending one. Both fear and anxiety are normal adaptive responses to a potentially dangerous environment. They make us better prepared to survive a danger, either through fight, flight, or freezing, as the situation may warrant.

Much of psychology research and psychoanalytic thought is devoted to understanding what we would consider being normal anxiety. This chapter will concentrate, however, on pathologic anxiety: when it is inappropriately triggered and maladaptive, hence an anxiety disorder.

Anxiety disorders are the most prevalent psychiatric syndromes in the U.S. population. Nearly one-fifth of adults report a lifetime history of one of the major anxiety disorders, and 1 in 10 suffer from a current anxiety disorder. Anxiety disorders are associated with social impairment and, when occurring in childhood, can interfere with healthy development, having consequences for later social and occupational functioning. Worldwide, they are the sixth most significant contributor to nonfatal health loss globally, and they explain 10 percent of the disability-adjusted life years for all mental, neurologic, and substance use disorders, second only to major depression.

THE CLINICAL PRESENTATION

The anxious patient has a variety of symptoms, particularly cognitive and physical. Some of the symptoms, particularly the autonomic ones, are observable and quantifiable, making it easier to develop objective measures. It also makes research on these disorders somewhat more straightforward.

Anxiety can have a variety of physical manifestations. The most common is its effect on the autonomic system, including such symptoms as headache, perspiration, palpitations, tightness in the chest, and mild stomach discomfort. It can also produce motor symptoms, such as restlessness, indicated by an inability to sit or stand still for long. The particular constellation of symptoms present during anxiety tends to vary among persons.

The anxious individual may describe themselves as "nervous" or "frightened." Their mood is frequently observable, particularly in patients who are experiencing a panic attack, as a classically fearful expression: eyes and mouth open, eyebrows raised. In patients with more chronic forms of anxiety, the expression may be more blunted and more akin to a depressed affect.

Thoughts may be more rapid, and in cases of severe anxiety, may become more disorganized. In extreme forms, a person may have great difficulty thinking clearly. For example, during a panic attack, a patient may ruminate or stammer.

In the setting of acute anxiety, the thoughts are focused on the perceived cause of the anxiety. Patients may catastrophize and overestimate the danger they are facing. In the case of a panic attack, somatic concerns of death from a cardiac or respiratory problem may be the primary focus of patients' attention during panic attacks. Patients may believe that the palpitations and chest pain indicate that they are about to die. As many as 20 percent of such patients have syncopal episodes during a panic attack. The patients may present in emergency departments as young, physically healthy persons who nevertheless insist that they are about to die from a heart attack. As anxiety becomes chronic, thoughts may take the form of more negative thinking.

Although hallucinations are rare, patients with severe anxiety may have distortions in perception, not only of time and space but also of persons and the meanings of events.

In the proper dose, anxiety can help attention by increasing our alertness and focusing our attention. However, in excess, it can impair cognition. Patients with severe anxiety can become confused. They can have difficulty focusing their attention, and as a result, may have trouble with recall.

Usually, anxiety does not reach a level where it significantly affects insight or judgment. However, patients can become selective in their interpretation of the environment, focusing on specific aspects and neglecting others to prove that they are justified in their reactions.

Although the patients do not tend to talk about suicidal ideation, they are at increased risk of committing suicide. Some studies have found that the lifetime risk of suicide in persons with panic disorder is higher than it is in persons with no mental disorder.

Presentation in Special Populations

Anxiety has many possible disorders, and different populations can present differently. For example, children or the elderly may present more with somatic symptoms than adults.

Certain cultural groups may have syndromes unique to their group, some of which represent culturally specific understandings of their body. Examples include the multiple anxiety syndromes related to the fear of "wind attacks" in Cambodians, or the syndrome *of Ataque de Nervios* (attack of nerves) in Puerto Rican and Dominican patients. In most cases, anxiety symptoms do not differ from those in other cultures. However, the emphasis may be on the specific ones relevant to beliefs about the underlying cause. In most cases, a full history and examination can elucidate the problem. It is often helpful to seek a cultural consultation for an understanding of the particular syndrome. In the past, there have been some broad overgeneralizations about different ethnic or cultural groups. However, these often reflect a bias and are usually not helpful.

DIAGNOSIS

Within this category, there are several disorders, including panic disorder (with and without agoraphobia), agoraphobia (without a history of panic disorder), specific phobia, social phobia, and generalized anxiety disorder.

Panic Disorder

Panic disorder is an acute intense attack of anxiety (a panic attack) accompanied by feelings of impending doom. The anxiety occurs during discrete periods of intense fear that can vary from several attacks during 1 day to only a few attacks during a year. Patients with panic disorder present with several comorbid conditions, most commonly agoraphobia, which refers to a fear of or anxiety regarding places from which escape might be difficult.

A panic attack is a sudden period of intense fear or apprehension that may last from minutes to hours. It is a symptom, and many disorders and situations besides panic disorder can cause panic attacks.

Mrs. K was a 35-year-old woman who initially presented for treatment at the medical emergency department at a large university-based medical center. She reported that while sitting at her desk at her job, she had suddenly experienced difficulty breathing, dizziness, tachycardia, shakiness, and a feeling of terror that she was going to die of a heart attack. A colleague drove her to the emergency department, where she received a full medical evaluation, including electrocardiography and routine blood work, which revealed no sign of cardiovascular, pulmonary, or other illness. She was subsequently referred for psychiatric evaluation, where she revealed that she had experienced two additional episodes over the past month, once when driving home from work and once when eating breakfast. However, she had not presented for medical treatment because the symptoms had resolved relatively quickly each time, and she worried that if she went to the hospital without ongoing symptoms, "people would think I'm crazy." Mrs. K reluctantly took the phone number of a local psychiatrist but did not call until she experienced the fourth episode of a similar nature. (Courtesy of Erin B. McClure-Tone, Ph.D. and Daniel S. Pine, M.D.)

Table 8-1 compares the different approaches to diagnosing panic disorder.

Table 8-1
Panic Disorder

	DSM-5	ICD-10
Diagnostic name	Panic Disorder	Panic disorder (episodic paroxysmal anxiety)
Duration	1 mo of worry after 1 panic attack Panic attacks occur during a discrete period	
Symptoms	Panic attacks: *Cardiopulmonary:* • Feeling short of breath • Palpitations • Chest discomfort *Gastrointestinal:* • Nausea or GI discomfort *Skin and systemic:* • Sweating • Chills or feeling flushed *Neurologic:* • Tremulousness • Dizziness • Numbness or tingling *Psychiatric:* • Derealization or depersonalization • Fear of losing control • Fear of dying Symptoms are abrupt and unpredictable Persistent symptoms between attacks, including: *Anticipatory anxiety:* fearing further attacks *Avoidance behaviors:* trying to avoid real or imagined triggers to prevent another attack	Recurrent attacks of severe anxiety or panic Unpredictable *Physiologic symptoms:* • Chest pain • Palpitations • Difficulty breathing • Sweating • Dizziness *Additional symptoms* • Depersonalization • Derealization • Fear of losing control • Fear of dying
Required number of symptoms	*Panic attack:* 4+ symptoms ≥1 attack Avoidance behavior or anticipatory anxiety: 1+ month	
Exclusions (not result of):	Substance use Another medical condition Another mental disorder	Another mental illness

Comments	DSM-5 also includes a "Panic Attack Specifier" for
	  discrete panic attacks without the additional criteria
	  for a full panic disorder	

The diagnosis includes a variety of symptoms, including somatic, cognitive, and mood. Patients can feel the physical symptoms in many organs and systems, including cardiorespiratory, gastrointestinal, and otoneurologic. Panic attacks can occur as a part of another mental disorder, particularly the phobias and PTSD. They may or may not be associated with an identifiable situational stimulus and unexpected panic attacks are not uncommon. Some panic attacks do not fit easily into the distinction between unexpected and expected. We call these *situationally predisposed panic attacks*. They may or may not occur when encountering a specific trigger, or they may occur either immediately after exposure or after a considerable delay.

In the DSM-5, to be diagnosed with a panic disorder, a patient must have recurrent, unexpected attacks. This requirement is to help distinguish the disorder from the phobias and other possible causes of panic attacks.

Agoraphobia

Agoraphobia refers to a fear of or anxiety regarding places from which escape might be difficult. It can be the most disabling of the phobias because it can significantly interfere with a person's ability to function in work and social situations outside the home. Although agoraphobia often coexists with panic disorder, in that patients are afraid to leave the safety of home lest they have a panic attack in a public place, DSM-5 considers agoraphobia a separate condition that may or may not be comorbid with panic disorder. Often patients with agoraphobia alone still have some measure of anxiety, "panic-like" symptoms, although those symptoms may not reach the level of an actual panic attack.

> Mrs. W was a 33-year-old married woman. She visited an anxiety clinic, reporting that she felt like she was having a heart attack whenever she left her home. Her disorder began 8 years earlier while attending a yoga class when she suddenly noticed a dramatic increase in her heartbeat, felt stabbing pains in her chest, and had difficulty breathing. She began sweating and trembling and felt dizzy. She immediately went to the emergency department, where they performed an electrocardiogram. No abnormalities were detected. Over the next few months, Mrs. W experienced similar attacks of 15 to 30 minutes' duration about four times per month. She often sought medical advice after each episode, and each time no physical abnormalities were detected. After experiencing a few of these attacks, Mrs. W became afraid of having an attack away from home and would not leave her home unless necessary, in which case she needed to have her cell phone or be accompanied by someone. Even so, she avoided crowded places such as malls, movie theaters, and banks, where rapid escape is sometimes blocked. Her symptoms and avoidance dominated her life, although she was aware that they were irrational and excessive. She experienced mild depression and restlessness and had difficulty sleeping.

Patients with agoraphobia rigidly avoid situations in which it would be challenging to obtain help. They prefer to be accompanied by a friend or a family member when leaving home, especially if their destination is crowded or closed-in. Severely affected patients may simply refuse to leave the house. Patients may be terrified that they are going "crazy."

Table 8-2 compares the different approaches to diagnosing agoraphobia. Several situations might cause anxiety, some involving confining spaces (public transportation, elevators, stores), open spaces (parks, shopping centers), or crowds. What they have in common is the fact that a person is away from home and safety and cannot quickly return to it.

Specific Phobia

The term *phobia* refers to excessive fear of a specific object, circumstance, or situation. A *specific phobia* is an intense, persisting

Table 8-2
Agoraphobia

	DSM-5	ICD-10
Diagnostic name	Agoraphobia	Agoraphobia
Duration	≥6 mo	

Symptoms	Fear or anxiety from:
	  Public transportation
	  Open spaces
	  Confined spaces
	  Being in a line or in a crowd
	  Being alone outside of home
	Avoidance of the situations, due to:
	  Fear of having a panic attack while there
	  Or, no access to a companion to help
	    withstand the situation
	Fear and avoidance is out of proportion to the
	  potential threat
		Fear of:
		  Leaving home
		  Going to a public place
		  Going to a crowded place
		  Traveling alone
		Avoidance of anxiety-provoking situations
		Frequently associated with panic disorders

Required number of symptoms	At least 1 of the above sources of fear	
Psychosocial consequences of symptoms	Marked distress or impairment	
Exclusions (not result of):	Another medical condition Another mental disorder	

Comments	This is for cases in which the above occurs
	  without a panic disorder, despite the fear of
	  having one	

Table 8-3
Specific Phobia

	DSM-5	ICD-10
Diagnostic name	Specific Phobia	Specific (Isolated) Phobias
Duration	Persistent and lasting ≥6 months	
Symptoms	Fear/anxiety about an object or situation Exposure to the object/situation causes immediate fear/anxiety Avoidance behaviors: of the object or situation The fear/anxiety is out of proportion to the likely threat	Phobias, restricted to highly specific situations, objects, or activities Exposure to the above causes panic
Required number of symptoms	All the above	
Psychosocial consequences of symptoms	Marked distress or impairment	
Exclusions (not result of):	Another mental disorder	

Symptom specifiers	Animals
	Natural environment
	Blood–injection–injury
	   Fear of blood
	   Fear of injections and transfusions
	   Fear of other medical care
	   Fear of injury
	Situational
	Other	

Comments		Also contains categories for "Other phobic anxiety disorder" and an unspecified type

fear of an object or situation, considered dangerous. The fear should be out of proportion to the actual threat. The diagnosis of specific phobia requires the development of intense anxiety, even to the point of panic, when exposed to the feared object. Persons with specific phobias may anticipate harm, such as being bitten by a dog, or may panic at the thought of losing control; for instance, if they fear elevators, they may also worry about fainting after the door closes.

> Mr. S was a successful lawyer who presented for treatment after his firm, to which he had previously been able to walk from home, moved to a new location that he could only reach by driving. Mr. S reported that he was "terrified" of driving, particularly on highways. Even the thought of getting into a car led him to worry that he would die in a fiery crash. His thoughts were associated with intense fear and numerous somatic symptoms, including a racing heart, nausea, and sweating. Although the thought of driving was terrifying in and of itself, Mr. S became nearly incapacitated when he drove on busy roads, often having to pull over to vomit. (Courtesy of Erin B. McClure-Tone, Ph.D. and Daniel S. Pine, M.D.)

Table 8-3 compares the different approaches to diagnosing specific phobia. There are many possible objects of the fear, including things (animals), environments (storms, dark rooms), situations (driving, flying, blood injections), and many other things that do not fit into these categories. What they have in common is the irrational fear that the object of one's fear is harmful or dangerous.

In each case, the anxiety usually occurs immediately after exposure to the object or situation. The result is either avoidance or painful endurance. It should last for at least 6 months.

Social Anxiety Disorder

Social anxiety disorder (also referred to as *social phobia*) involves the fear of social situations, including situations that involve scrutiny or contact with strangers. The term social anxiety reflects the distinct differentiation of social anxiety disorder from a specific phobia, which is the intense and persistent fear of an object or situation. Persons with social anxiety disorder are fearful of embarrassing themselves in social situations (i.e., social gatherings, oral presentations, meeting new people). They may have specific fears about performing specific activities such as eating or speaking in front of others, or they may experience a vague, nonspecific fear of "embarrassing oneself." In either case, the fear in social anxiety disorder is of the embarrassment that may occur in the situation, not the situation itself.

> Ms. B was a 29-year-old computer programmer who presented for treatment after she was offered a promotion to a managerial position at her firm. Although she wanted the raise and the increased responsibility that would come with the new job, which she had agreed to try on a probationary basis, Ms. B reported that she was reluctant to accept the position because it required frequent interactions with employees from other divisions of the company, as well as occasional public speaking. She stated that she had always felt nervous around new people, whom she worried would ridicule her for "saying stupid things" or committing a social faux pas. She also reported feeling "terrified" to speak before groups. These fears had not previously interfered with her social life and job performance. However, since starting her probationary job, Ms. B reported that they had become problematic. She noted that when she had to interact with others, her heart started racing, her mouth became dry, and she felt sweaty. At meetings, she had sudden thoughts that she would say something very foolish or commit a terrible social gaffe that would cause people to laugh. As a consequence, she had skipped several important meetings and left others early. (Courtesy of Erin B. McClure-Tone, Ph.D. and Daniel S. Pine, M.D.)

Table 8-4 compares the different approaches to diagnosing social anxiety disorder. Many people feel anxiety in social situations, and

Table 8-4
Social Anxiety Disorder

	DSM-5	ICD-10
Diagnostic name	Social anxiety disorder	Social anxiety disorder
Duration	≤6 mo	
Symptoms	Fear of being judged/scrutinized in social situation Fear that others will notice the anxiety, causing additional judgment, embarrassment, or rejection Avoidance behaviors: of the feared social situations The fear/anxiety is out of proportion to the social risk	Fear of being judged/scrutinized by others Avoidance behaviors: of the feared social situations May be associated with low self-esteem May cause panic attacks
Required number of symptoms	All the above	
Psychosocial consequences of symptoms	Marked distress and/or impairment	
Exclusions (not result of):	Another mental illness Another medical illness	
Symptom specifiers	Performance only (performance anxiety)	

it is rare to find the person who feels no anxiety over speaking in public or attending a party where they will not know anyone. The key feature in social anxiety disorder is that this anxiety is significant to the point of being disabling, meaning that it is sufficient to cause clinically significant distress or impairment. It also occurs while one is scrutinized, and includes a fear of negative judgment. Furthermore, DSM-5 emphasizes that the fear should occur in situations in which the individual is under scrutiny and that the fear is of being "negatively evaluated" (embarrassed or rejected).

DSM-5 includes a specifier for performance anxiety ("performance only"), in which the fear is limited to public speaking or performance.

Generalized Anxiety Disorder

Generalized anxiety disorder is defined as excessive anxiety and worries about several events or activities most of the time for at least 6 months. The worry is difficult to control and is associated with somatic symptoms, such as muscle tension, irritability, difficulty sleeping, and restlessness. The worry usually involves a broad swath of everyday life, such as simple daily activities, timeliness, finances, or health. These are ordinary worries for many people. However, patients with a generalized anxiety disorder worry about them to the point where catastrophe seems possible, likely, and imminent. Another feature is that these concerns cannot be prioritized or put aside to deal with more pressing matters that may pop up. This inability to prioritize is a key feature that contributes to the pathologic effect that this disorder has on functioning.

Mr. G was a successful, married, 28-year-old teacher who presented for a psychiatric evaluation to treat mounting symptoms of worry and anxiety. Mr. G noted that for the preceding year, he had become more and more worried about his job performance. For example, although he had always been a respected and popular lecturer, he found himself worrying about his ability to engage students and convey the material effectively. Similarly, although he had always been financially secure, he increasingly worried that he was going to lose his wealth due to unexpected expenses. Mr. G noted frequent somatic symptoms that

accompanied his worries. For example, he often felt tense and irritable while he worked and spent time with his family, and he had difficulty distracting himself from worries about the upcoming challenges for the next day. He reported feeling increasingly restless, especially at night, when his worries kept him from falling asleep. (Courtesy of Erin B. McClure-Tone, Ph.D. and Daniel S. Pine, M.D.)

Table 8-5 compares the different approaches to diagnosing generalized anxiety disorder. The distinction between generalized anxiety disorder and normal anxiety is that the worry is excessive, difficult to control, and causes impairment.

Objective Rating Scales for the Disorder

There are many scales for measuring anxiety. Some popular examples are the Beck Anxiety Inventory (BAI), Hospital Anxiety and Depression Scale (HADS), and the Generalized Anxiety Disorder scale (GAD-7), but there are many more. Many other broader scales include measures of anxiety. Some scales measure anxiety per se, while others help to identify a specific disorder. Scales may also differentiate between state and trait anxiety, which is situational anxiety versus anxiety that seems characteristic for a person and independent of the situation. An example for the latter is the State-Trait Anxiety Inventory.

DIFFERENTIAL DIAGNOSIS

Distinguishing Between the Anxiety Disorders

Anxiety disorders have overlapping symptoms. Sometimes it is difficult to distinguish between panic disorder, on the one hand, and specific and social phobias, on the other hand. Some patients who experience a single panic attack in a specific setting (e.g., an elevator) may go on to have long-lasting avoidance of the specific setting, regardless of whether they ever have another panic attack. These patients meet the diagnostic criteria for a specific phobia, and clinicians must use their judgment about what is the most appropriate diagnosis. In another example, a person who

Table 8-5
Generalized Anxiety Disorder

	DSM-5	ICD-10
Diagnostic name	Generalized Anxiety Disorder	Generalized Anxiety Disorder
Duration	≤6 mo	
Symptoms	Excessive anxiety/worry Difficulty controlling/ managing worry *Anxiety characterized by:* • Restlessness • Fatigue • Poor concentration • Irritability • Muscle tension • Insomnia	Persistent anxiety *Anxiety characterized by:* • Shaking • Muscle tension • Sweating • Lightheadedness • Palpitations • GI symptoms
Required number of symptoms	First two criteria and 3+ of the specific symptoms	
Psychosocial consequences of symptoms	Marked distress and/or impairment	
Exclusions (not result of):	• Another mental disorder • Substance use • Another medical condition	Anxiety not associated with an object, event, or situation

experiences one or more panic attacks may then fear to speak in public. Although the clinical picture is almost identical to the clinical picture in social anxiety disorder, we would not diagnose a social anxiety disorder because the avoidance of the public situation is based on fear of having a panic attack rather than on fear of the public speaking itself.

Other Psychiatric Disorders

The differential diagnosis for agoraphobia includes all the psychiatric disorders that can cause anxiety or depression. A panic disorder is the most common cause of agoraphobia, and a separate diagnosis of agoraphobia is not necessary. Other disorders include major depressive disorder, schizophrenia, paranoid personality disorder, avoidant personality disorder, and dependent personality disorder.

Medical Disorders

Many medical disorders can cause anxiety or have symptoms that overlap with anxiety disorders.

Several medical conditions produce symptoms that are similar to panic disorder. Panic attacks are associated with a variety of endocrinologic disorders, including both hypo- and hyperthyroid states, hyperparathyroidism, and pheochromocytomas. Episodic hypoglycemia associated with insulinomas can also produce panic-like states, as can primary neuropathologic processes. These include seizure disorders, vestibular dysfunction, neoplasms, or the effects of both prescribed and illicit substances on the CNS. Finally, disorders of the cardiac and pulmonary systems, including arrhythmias, chronic obstructive pulmonary disease, and asthma, can produce autonomic symptoms and accompanying crescendo anxiety that can be difficult to distinguish from panic disorder. Clues of an underlying medical etiology to panic-like symptoms include the presence of atypical features during panic attacks, such as ataxia, alterations in consciousness, or bladder dyscontrol, onset of panic disorder relatively late in life, and physical signs or symptoms indicative of a medical disorder.

COMORBIDITY

Depressive symptoms are often present in panic disorder, and in some patients, a depressive disorder coexists with the panic disorder, and depression can complicate the symptom picture in anywhere from 40 to 80 percent of all patients, as estimated by various studies.

In addition to agoraphobia, other phobias and OCD can coexist with panic disorder.

Alcohol and other substance use disorders occur in about 20 to 40 percent of all patients, and OCD may also develop.

COURSE

Panic attacks, by definition, have a sudden onset and relatively short duration. The first panic attack is often completely spontaneous, although panic attacks occasionally follow excitement, physical exertion, sexual activity, or moderate emotional trauma.

The attack often begins with 10 minutes of rapidly increasing symptoms. The significant mental symptoms are extreme fear and a sense of impending death and doom. Patients usually cannot name the source of their fear; they may feel confused and have trouble concentrating. The physical signs often include tachycardia, palpitations, dyspnea, and sweating. Patients often try to leave whatever situation they are in to seek help. The attack generally lasts 20 to 30 minutes and rarely more than an hour.

Panic disorder usually has its onset in late adolescence or early adulthood, although onset during childhood, early adolescence, and midlife do occur. Some data implicate increased psychosocial stressors with the onset of panic disorder, although in most cases, there are no identifiable psychosocial stressors.

Panic disorder is a chronic disorder, although its course is variable, both among patients and within a single patient. The available long-term follow-up studies of panic disorder are difficult to interpret because they have not controlled for the effects of treatment. Nevertheless, about 30 to 40 percent of patients seem to be symptom-free at long-term follow-up, about 50 percent have symptoms that are sufficiently mild not to affect their lives significantly, and about 10 to 20 percent continue to have significant symptoms.

After the first one or two panic attacks, patients may be relatively unconcerned about their condition; with repeated attacks, however, the symptoms may become a significant concern. Between attacks, patients may have anticipatory anxiety about having another attack. Patients may attempt to keep the panic attacks secret and thereby cause their families and friends concern about unexplained changes in behavior. The frequency and severity of the attacks can fluctuate. Panic attacks can occur several times in a day or less than once a month. Excessive intake of caffeine or nicotine can exacerbate the symptoms.

When agoraphobia is part of a panic disorder, improving panic symptoms often also improves agoraphobia. For rapid and complete reduction of agoraphobia, behavior therapy is useful. Agoraphobia without a history of panic disorder is often incapacitating and chronic, and depressive disorders and alcohol use disorder often complicate its course.

The presence of comorbid disorders, particularly alcohol and substance use disorders, complicates the course of anxiety disorders. Patients with good premorbid functioning and symptoms of brief duration tend to have a favorable prognosis.

Most of the other anxiety disorders also have long-term courses with multiple relapses. Overall these are all chronic disorders. Generalized anxiety disorder commonly has multiple relapses, although some may occur long after the initial episode, sometimes giving a false sense of security. Clinicians should regularly monitor the symptoms.

Most of these disorders also have an increased risk of suicide, and clinicians should monitor this as well.

TREATMENT APPROACH

With treatment, most patients exhibit dramatic improvement in their anxiety symptoms. Treatments include pharmacologic, psychologic, and combined treatments for all anxiety disorders. Meta-analyses generally suggest that pharmacologic treatment has the largest effect size of the various options. However, depending on the anxiety disorder, there are many pharmacologic, psychotherapeutic, and combined options available.

Hospitalization

Patients rarely require hospitalization unless they need a diagnostic workup, for example, to rule out a medical cause. Also, we may hospitalize patients with comorbid disorders such as substance use or those who are suicidal.

Pharmacotherapy

Among the medication options, selective serotonin reuptake inhibitors are the first-line agents for most anxiety disorders, including panic disorder, generalized anxiety disorder, and social anxiety disorder. Some non-SSRIs are also useful, for example, venlafaxine for panic disorder, generalized anxiety disorder, and social anxiety disorder. Tricyclic antidepressants are useful for panic disorder as well, although less popular due to their side effects. Many clinicians consider mirtazapine to be useful for anxiety disorders, owing to its sedative effect. However, there are few studies of its use for anxiety disorder.

Benzodiazepines remain one of the most popular medications used for anxiety disorder, perhaps the most popular. Most treatment guidelines suggest that they be mostly limited to short-term use, either as an adjunct to SSRIs during the initial treatment phase or for acute use during exacerbations of the anxiety. Generally, most guidelines recommend that we should only consider long-term benzodiazepines for patients who do not respond or cannot tolerate the SSRIs. The main concerns are the potential for dependence, as well as the cognitive and other side effects. Tolerance to the anxiolytic effects does not seem to develop.

Antipsychotics and anticonvulsants are not recommended as initial therapy but may have some role for treatment-resistant patients. Among them, quetiapine is popular and may be useful as a second-line treatment for generalized anxiety disorder.

Buspirone is an azapirone, and effective for the treatment of generalized anxiety disorders. It is given in three divided doses during the day. The time to effect is similar to that for antidepressants, several weeks, and may take as long as several months. It may be useful as an adjunct to antidepressants for other anxiety disorders; however, most of the evidence is anecdotal.

β-Blockers, such as propranolol, are sometimes used for anxiety disorders, particularly social anxiety disorder. However, the available evidence does not support this use. Anecdotally, many consider it useful for social anxiety, particularly performance anxiety. The presumed mechanism is the drug's ability to block many of the physiologic symptoms of anxiety. However, there is little data to support this, and at least one study showed no effect. One study concluded it might be useful for performance anxiety—specifically musical performances—however, it also had significant side effects that could impair performance.

Antihistamines, such as hydroxyzine, are also used, particularly as alternatives to benzodiazepines for acute treatment. It has some evidence for its use in generalized anxiety disorder. We know little about its long-term effect.

Table 8-6 lists the common classes of drugs used for anxiety disorders and the evidence supporting their use.

Treatment Approach. Table 8-7 gives some pointers for using medications to treat patients with anxiety.

For most anxiety disorders, a conservative approach is, to begin with, an SSRI. Benzodiazepines are most useful when a patient requires rapid control of severe anxiety symptoms. In those cases, a short-term benzodiazepine, such as lorazepam or alprazolam, is helpful in the short term. Concurrently, an SSRI should be started and slowly increased.

For panic disorder, SSRIs or the serotonin–norepinephrine reuptake inhibitor (SNRI) venlafaxine are first-line options. Tricyclic antidepressants or MAOIs are effective but less preferably given their side effects. Other agents, such as mirtazapine, are other second-line options. As mentioned, the benzodiazepines are effective options but mainly used for short-term use or exacerbations. Long-term antidepressant therapy is useful for preventing relapse, with studies suggesting that the beneficial effects last for up to 1 to 3 years. When appropriate, maintenance therapy should be discontinued very slowly.

For generalized anxiety disorder, the approach is similar, with SSRIs and SNRIs being the first-line treatments. Reasonable alternatives if those are not effective include agomelatine, pregabalin, buspirone, and quetiapine.

For social anxiety disorder, the approach is similar to those already described, with SSRIs and SNRIs being the first-line choice. Pregabalin and clonazepam also have strong evidence, although the same caveats for other benzodiazepines apply to clonazepam. Phenelzine is effective as well but is rarely used because of the side effects. Tricyclic antidepressants, buspirone, and quetiapine are not recommended owing to their side effects. As noted above,

Table 8-6
Evidence-Based Recommendations for Monotherapy of Anxiety Disorders

Classes and Agents	Anxiety Disorders		
	GAD	PD	SAD
SSRIs	First line	First line	First line
SNRIs	First line	First line	First line
TCAs	Second line	Second line	Not recommended
MAOIs	Insufficient evidence	Second line	Second line
RIMA-Moclobemide	Insufficient evidence	Insufficient evidence	Second Line
Other Psychotropics—Agomelatine, Buspirone, Mirtazapine	Second line	Second line	Second line
Benzodiazepines	Second line	Second line	Second line
Atypical Antipsychotics—Quetiapine	Second line	Insufficient evidence	Not recommended
Anticonvulsant—Pregabalin	Second line	Insufficient evidence	Second line

Note: Beta-adrenergic blocking agents are recommended only for performance anxiety.
RIMA, reversible monoamine oxidase inhibitor; GAD, generalized anxiety disorder; PD, panic disorder; SAD, social anxiety disorder.

β-blockers may be useful for performance anxiety. However, their use does not appear to generalize to other types of social anxiety.

In the case of specific phobia, psychotherapies, particularly behavioral therapies, are the first-line choice. SSRIs may be helpful, although there are few studies of SSRIs for this disorder.

For agoraphobia, the main goal of pharmacotherapy is to treat the panic attacks that are usually comorbid. Early studies did not support the use of medications for "pure" agoraphobia; however, there has been little research since.

Psychosocial Therapies

There is strong support for a variety of psychosocial therapies for anxiety disorders, including cognitive-behavioral therapy (CBT), behavioral therapies, and interpersonal therapy. Studies of CBT suggest it has a substantial effect on generalized anxiety disorder, panic disorder, and social anxiety disorder, although this evidence is tempered by concerns about treatment bias in the studies. Some treatment guidelines consider individual CBT to be a first-line treatment for social anxiety disorder. Group psychotherapy, mainly using CBT techniques, is also useful for social anxiety disorder. In vivo exposure therapy is the treatment of choice for specific phobia.

Cognitive Therapy. The two major foci of cognitive therapy for panic disorder are instruction about a patient's false beliefs and information about panic attacks. The instruction about false beliefs centers on the patient's tendency to misinterpret mild bodily

Table 8-7
Pharmacotherapy of Anxiety Disorders: Key Pointers

- SSRIs are the first-line option.
- Start low and go slow.
- Routine increase to higher doses not recommended, but a subgroup might benefit.
- Concomitant benzodiazepines as initial therapy in the short term may be useful.
- 8–12 weeks of pharmacotherapy at optimum doses may be needed to assess efficacy.
- Good evidence for the benefit of maintenance treatment at least up to 6 months.

sensations as indicating impending panic attacks, doom, or death. The information about panic attacks includes explanations that when panic attacks occur, they are time-limited and not life-threatening.

Behavioral Therapies. In behavior therapy, the underlying assumption is that change can occur without the development of psychologic insight into underlying causes. Techniques include positive and negative reinforcement, systematic desensitization, flooding, implosion, graded exposure, response prevention, thought stopping, relaxation techniques, panic control therapy, self-monitoring, and hypnosis. For patients with specific phobias, the approach usually involves gradually increasing the patient's exposure to the feared stimulus (e.g., climbing to increasingly higher floors in a building for a patient with a fear of heights) while practicing relaxation techniques until the patient masters each successive step.

Interpersonal Psychotherapy. There is good evidence for interpersonal psychotherapy, particularly interpersonal skills training for social anxiety disorder. The assumption is that such patients have interpersonal deficits that contribute to their anxiety and lack the skills to interact with others effectively. The result is that patients experience more of the "punishments" and less of the rewards from social interaction than most other people.

Virtual Therapy. Computer programs exist that allow us to treat a variety of anxiety disorders, including agoraphobia, specific phobia, and social anxiety disorder. As an example, patients with agoraphobia may experience a virtual environment in which they are in a crowded space (e.g., a supermarket). As they identify with the avatars in repeated computer sessions, they can learn to master their anxiety until they are ready to try the exposure in real life. This approach is particularly useful for situations that are not easily reproduced inside or near a clinician's office (i.e., flying).

Supportive Psychotherapy. Supportive psychotherapy involves the use of psychodynamic concepts and a therapeutic alliance to promote adaptive coping. Adaptive defenses are encouraged and strengthened, and maladaptive ones are discouraged. The therapist assists in reality testing and may offer behavioral advice. Although lacking empirical support, clinicians frequently incorporate some degree of supportive psychotherapy as an adjunct to medication.

Insight-Oriented Psychotherapy. In insight-oriented psychotherapy, the goal is to increase the patient's development of insight into psychologic conflicts that, if unresolved, can manifest as symptomatic behavior. For a time, it was the classic treatment for many types of anxiety, with the assumption that the anxiety represented an underlying psychodynamic conflict. Some studies suggest that psychodynamic psychotherapy can help decrease anxiety symptoms, and may have a lasting effect. However, the studies tend to have methodologic problems, and we lack the large, comparative studies needed to determine efficacy.

THE EPIDEMIOLOGY OF THE DISORDER(S)

Incidence and Prevalence

Anxiety disorders make up one of the most common groups of psychiatric disorders. The National Comorbidity Study reported that one of four persons met the diagnostic criteria for at least one anxiety disorder and that there is a 12-month prevalence rate of 17.7 percent.

Most epidemiologic studies of panic disorder suggest a 12-month prevalence between 0.2 and 1.1 percent. The lowest rate reported rate was 0.1 percent (Nigeria), and the highest was 6.9 percent (Italy), with a median of 2.3 percent.

Most epidemiologic studies of generalized anxiety disorder suggest a 12-month prevalence between about 2.1 and 3.1 percent in the United States. The ranges vary widely, with ranges from 0 percent (Nigeria) to 2.6 percent (Germany).

The 12-month prevalence of social anxiety disorder varies widely across regions. The United States has the highest reported rates (6.8 percent), and China the lowest (0.2 percent). The median is about 4 percent to 5 percent. It may be that these differences involve differing cultural concepts of social fears or even difficulties in translating this concept to different cultures.

The 12-month prevalence of agoraphobia is mostly consistent across regions, with a range from 0 (China) to 0.8 percent (U.S.). An exception is South Africa, with a reported rate of 4.8 percent.

The rates of specific phobias vary widely, with a range of 1.9 percent (China) to 8.7 percent (U.S.).

Table 8-8 compares the 12-month and lifetime prevalence of anxiety disorders across different countries.

Sex

Women have higher rates of almost all anxiety disorders than do men. The difference is twofold for most disorders. The exception is social anxiety disorder, where the ratio is about equal. This difference is true across all ages but is most evident during early and mid-adulthood.

Age

The anxiety disorders have one of the earliest onsets of all psychiatric disorders. Most of the disorders begin in childhood or adolescence; the median age is 12.

In general, phobic disorders are the most stable of the disorders over time. Panic and generalized anxiety disorder are much like major depressive disorder in that they tend to have exacerbations and remissions over the life span.

Sociocultural and Ethnic Variables

Anxiety disorders appear to be common in persons of lower socioeconomic status and educational level. However, these relationships are very complex.

Some studies have reported higher rates of anxiety disorders in African Americans and lower rates in Hispanics.

THE NEUROBIOLOGY OF THE DISORDER

Genetics

Like most psychiatric disorders, anxiety disorders are complex disorders. Studying anxiety disorders has an advantage over many, as fear and anxiety are common to animals and are easily observed, at least compared to other mental phenomena. Thus, animal models have much informed the research on genetics and other aspects of the disorder. Here, we will, however, concentrate on human studies.

Studies of Inheritance Patterns. A relatively large number of family studies have supported the familial aggregation of the major anxiety disorders, including panic disorder, generalized anxiety disorder, phobias, and agoraphobia. For panic disorder, the familial risk was highest for early-onset panic disorder. In the case of social anxiety disorder, it was strongest for the generalized subtype.

Several large twin studies have demonstrated higher inheritance for monozygotic than dizygotic twins, suggesting a genetic component. The genetic contribution appears to be about 30 percent or more, perhaps as high as 60 percent for the phobias.

Genetic Studies. Among candidate gene studies, linkage studies have had inconsistent results, which is not a surprise, given the assumption that this is a complex disorder. Thus we are unlikely to find highly penetrant genes. Association studies usually rely on candidate genes, usually chosen for their presumed relevance to the disorder or because of prior studies suggesting an association. Most studied are the genes for the neurotransmitter systems and the stress response. Again, the results have been inconsistent.

Genome-wide studies (GWAS) do not require the same a priori assumptions or degree of penetrance. A limitation is the large sample sizes needed, and this limits many of the genetic studies in psychiatry. The most studied has been panic disorder. One study found support for immune-related involvement for the disorder. Another study found two associated single nucleotide polymorphisms (SNPs), a finding later replicated in another study. The genes are involved in mRNA expression in the frontal cortex. Although intriguing, the results remain preliminary. A large research collaboration, the Psychiatric Genetics Consortium, has found several possible novel risk genes; again, these results are tentative.

To date, there is little data on gene–environment interactions, given the substantial sample sizes needed. However, with converging evidence suggesting a role for both cumulative and specific life events, this is an essential area for investigation. There is also limited but compelling evidence for the role of epigenetics in anxiety disorders. However, this area is just emerging.

Neuroimaging Studies

Preclinical data on fear circuitry has guided the search for neuroanatomical associations with anxiety. Thus, the amygdala,

Table 8-8
Lifetime and 12-Month Prevalence Rates of DSM-IV Anxiety Disorders in International Community Studies of Adults

Study	GAD 12 mo	GAD LT	Panic Disorder 12 mo	Panic Disorder LT	Separation Anxiety 12 mo	Separation Anxiety LT	Agoraphobia 12 mo	Agoraphobia LT	Social Phobia 12 mo	Social Phobia LT	Specific Phobia 12 mo	Specific Phobia LT	All Anxiety 12 mo	All Anxiety LT
U.S. (NESARC)[a]	2.1	4.1	2.1	5.1	—	—	0.1	0.2	2.8	5.0	7.1	9.4	11.1[h]	17.2[h]
Iran[b]	—	1.3	—	1.3	—	—	—	0.7	—	0.8	—	—	—	8.4
Australia (NSMHWB)[c]	2.6	—	1.1	—	—	—	0.5	—	1.3	—	—	—	5.6	—
Germany (GHS-MHS)[d]	1.5	—	2.3	—	—	—	12.6[i]	—	12.6[i]	—	12.6[i]	—	14.5	—
Italy, Sesto Fiorentino[e]	—	6.9	—	6.9	—	—	—	0.4	—	3.7	—	1.5	—	16.9
Korea (KECA-R)[f]	0.8	1.6	0.1	1.6	—	—	0.2	0.2	0.4	0.5	3.4	3.8	5.3	6.9
WHO WMH Surveys[g]														
U.S.	3.1	5.7	2.7	4.7	1.9	9.2	0.8	1.4	6.8	12.1	8.7	12.5	18.1	28.8
Mexico	—	0.9	—	1.0	0.9	4.5	—	1.0	—	2.9	—	7.0	—	14.3
Belgium	—	1.9	—	16	0.1	1.4	—	—	—	2.0	—	6.8	—	13.1
Italy	0.5	1.9	0.6	16	0.0	1.5	0.4	1.2	1.0	2.1	2.7	5.7	5.1	11.1
Ukraine	1.2	1.9	1.3	1.9	—	—	0.2	0.3	1.5	2.6	—	—	6.1	3.8
Lebanon	1.3	—	0.2	—	1.9	6.9	0.3	—	1.1	—	8.2	—	11.2	—
Nigeria	0.0	0.1	0.1	0.2	0.0	0.2	0.2	0.4	0.3	0.3	3.5	5.4	4.1	5.7
New Zealand	—	6.0	—	2.7	—	—	—	1.2	—	9.4	—	10.8	—	24.9
Japan	1.2	—	0.5	—	—	—	0.3	—	0.8	—	2.7	—	4.8	—
China	0.8	—	0.2	—	0.4	1.3	0.0	0.0	0.2	0.5	1.9	2.6	2.7	4.8
South Africa	1.4	—	0.8	—	—	—	4.8	—	1.9	—	—	—	8.1	—

[a]From Hasin DS, Grant BF. The National Epidemiologic Survey on Alcohol and Related Conditions (NESARC) Waves 1 and 2: Review and summary of findings. *Soc Psychiatry Psychiatr Epidemiol*. 2015;50(11):1609–1640.
[b]Mohammadi MR, Davidian H, Noorbala AA, Malekafzali H, Naghavi HR, Pouretemad HR, Yazdi SAB, Rahgozar M, Alaghebandrad J, Amini H, Razzaghi EM, Mesgarpour B, Soori H, Mohammadi M, Ghanizadeh A. An epidemiological survey of psychiatric disorders in Iran. *Clin Pract Epidemol Ment Health*. 2005;26;1:16.
[c]Oakley Browne MA, Wells JE, Scott KM, McGee MA; New Zealand Mental Health Survey Research Team. Lifetime prevalence and projected lifetime risk of DSM-IV disorders in Te Rau Hinengaro: the New Zealand Mental Health Survey. *Aust N Z J Psychiatry*. 2006;40(10):865–874.
[d]Jacobi F, Wittchen HU, Holting C, Höfler M, Pfister H, Müller N, Lieb R. Prevalence, co-morbidity and correlates of mental disorders in the general population: Results from the German Health Interview and Examination Survey (GHS). *Psychol Med*. 2004;34(4):597–611.
[e]Faravelli C, Abrardi L, Bartolozzi D, Cecchi C, Cosci F, D'Adamo D, Iacono BL, Ravaldi C, Scarpato MA, Truglia E, Rosi S. The Sesto Fiorentino study: background, methods and preliminary results. Lifetime prevalence of psychiatric disorders in an Italian community sample using clinical interviewers. *Psychother Psychosom*. 2004;73(4):216–225.
[f]Cho MJ, Chang SM, Lee YM, Bae A, Ahn JH, Son J, Hong JP, Bae JN, Lee DW, Cho SJ, Park JI, Lee JY, Kim JY, Jeon HJ, Sohn JH, Kim BS. Prevalence of DSM-IV major mental disorders among Korean adults: A 2006 National Epidemiologic Survey (KECA-R). *Asian J Psychiatr*. 2010;3(1):26–30.
[g]The WHO World Mental Health Survey Consortium. Prevalence, severity, and unmet need for treatment of mental disorders in the World Health Organization World Mental Health Surveys. *JAMA*. 2004;291:2581–2590.
[h]Not including PTSD.
[i]Any phobia, including social phobia, specific phobia, and agoraphobia.

and the other components of the frontoamygdala connections (the perirhinal cortex, ventrolateral prefrontal cortex (vlPFC), and anterior insula) have been the most studied. Another focus is the hippocampus, which plays a critical role in fear learning and extinction. Other areas include the posterior and lateral orbitofrontal cortex (OFC), anterior insula, and vlPFC, which show increased neurophysiologic activity in patients with phobias.

Neurochemical systems are also a focus, including central noradrenergic systems, central serotonergic and dopaminergic, and GABA systems.

Studies of fear conditioning in healthy humans are similar to those of animals, confirming that the fear circuitry is conserved across species. The amygdala, ventromedial PFC (vmPFC), and hippocampus have been implicated in both PET and fMRI studies.

Studies of panic disorder suggest that there are abnormalities both when patients are at rest and during an acute panic attack. In the resting state, hippocampal and parahippocampal areas are implicated, whereas during panic, the associations are in the insular and striatal regions, with reduced activity in other regions such as the PFC. MRI studies also suggest abnormalities of the gray matter volume in the parahippocampal and temporal regions. Also interesting are MRI studies of brain lactate, which suggest an exaggerated response to hypocapnia, suggesting a suffocation response. Receptor-binding studies show abnormalities in GABA and serotonergic, particularly 5-HT$_{1A}$, binding.

Studies in specific phobias suggest activation of anterior paralimbic regions and sensory association cortices related to the particular phobia (be it visual, auditory, or other senses). These suggest hypersensitivity to specific threat-related cues. Also, the amygdala is again implicated.

In social anxiety disorder, functional neuroimaging studies show an exaggerated response to social stimuli, particularly in the medial temporal lobe structures. Most commonly, investigators find amygdala hyperresponsivity to social threats.

Unlike the other disorders, generalized anxiety disorder does not show clear findings of amygdala hyperactivity. The core features are more typical of emotional dysregulation, with disruptions of the functional connections between the anterior cingulate and the amygdala, as well as the uncinate fasciculus. This may suggest weaker frontoamygdala connectivity and fear overgeneralization. Preliminary evidence suggests that effective treatments target these areas, including CBT and pharmacotherapies.

Psychological Studies.   Behavioral scientists have helped to elucidate the psychology of fear and anxiety through both animal and human studies. A full discussion of the psychological research is well beyond the scope of this chapter, but most relevant to anxiety disorders are the work of Pavlov and later scientists on the nature of conditioning. In the classic studies, the scientist exposes an animal to an neutral stimulus, such as an auditory tone, and then presents the tone while introducing an aversive stimulus, such as an electric shock. With the repeated pairing of the two stimuli, the neutral stimulus becomes associated with the aversive one, to the point where it alone can elicit the same response even when removing the aversive stimulus. The result is that the animal has been conditioned or learned to fear the neutral stimuli. In behavioral science, the neutral stimulus is called the conditioned stimulus and the aversive one the unconditioned stimulus. If the scientist presents the conditioned stimulus without the unconditioned one and repeats this often enough, the animal will no longer associate the two stimuli; this is called extinction. How long extinction learning takes will depend on the particular stimuli and the individual animal. It also can depend on context, and a different setting can change the response. Behavioral studies suggest that the animal does not forget the conditioning. Instead, it is now competing with a new memory. Under appropriate circumstances, the pairing, and associated fear response, can be reinstated.

As humans are animals, they experience conditioning and extinction as well. The relevance to anxiety disorders, particularly phobias, should be obvious. Research in conditioning has gone well beyond this simplified description to identify and elaborate the many subtleties of conditioned learning.

ETIOLOGY

Biologic Theories

Neurochemicals and the Fight-or-Flight Reaction.   When we perceive stress, our bodies activate certain neurotransmitters and neuropeptides. The result is the "fight-or-flight" reaction. This response is adaptive in specific contexts. However, overgeneralization of their reaction can be disabling and underlies many of the anxiety disorders.

Chronic activation can cause alterations in a variety of systems. Some evidence suggests that early-life stressors can cause this, making us predisposed to anxiety disorders later in life. Why some of us are more susceptible than others, under similar circumstances, is an area of active investigation.

Several neurochemicals and systems are thought to be most relevant to the mechanism between anxiety disorders, including the monoamines, the hypothalamic–pituitary–adrenal (HPA) axis, corticotropin-releasing hormone (CRH) and other chemicals. Broadly put, patients with anxiety disorders have symptoms that

Table 8-9
Neurochemical Systems Involved in Anxiety Disorders and Related Treatment Approaches

Neurochemical	Brain Regions	Association with Anxiety Disorders	Treatment Approaches (Current and Future)
Noradrenergic system	Locus coeruleus, amygdala, hippocampus, hypothalamus, prefrontal cortex	Unrestrained, excessive system activation	SNRIs first-line therapy for anxiety disorders (along with SSRIs) Propranolol for performance anxiety
Hypothalamic–pituitary–adrenal (HPA) axis	Hippocampus, amygdala, hypothalamus, prefrontal cortex	Dysregulated HPA axis function (excessive cortisol release, abnormal feedback) in some studies	Cortisol administration under study for SAD and spider phobia Mifepristone under study for GAD and PD
Corticotropin-releasing hormone (CRH)	Prefrontal and cingulate cortices, amygdala, hippocampus, hypothalamus, bed nucleus of stria terminalis, nucleus accumbens, periaqueductal gray matter, locus coeruleus, dorsal raphe nuclei	Persistently increased CRH concentration	To date, CRH-1 receptor antagonists have failed to demonstrate efficacy in clinical trials
Neurosteroids	Hippocampus, amygdala, cortex	Abnormal peripheral levels of neurosteroids in PD; possibly also in GAD and SAD (inconsistent findings)	Paroxetine found to increase peripheral levels of allopregnanolone in one study of PD patients, but not in a second study Synthetic analogs of neurosteroids under development

(continued)

Table 8-9
Neurochemical Systems Involved in Anxiety Disorders and Related Treatment Approaches (*Continued*)

Neurochemical	Brain Regions	Association with Anxiety Disorders	Treatment Approaches (Current and Future)
Arginine vasopressin (AVP)	Paraventricular nucleus of hypothalamus, septum, hippocampus, cortex	Single nucleotide polymorphism in AVP V1b receptor gene linked to PD	AVP V1b receptor antagonist (SSR149415) failed to demonstrate efficacy for GAD in a clinical trial New AVP V1b receptor antagonists currently under study
Dopaminergic system	Amygdala, nucleus accumbens, prefrontal cortex	Excessive mesocortical dopamine release, persistently high levels of dopamine in prefrontal cortex	Bupropion is an NDRI used primarily to treat depression, sometimes as an adjunct for anxiety disorders
Serotonergic system	Dorsal raphe nuclei, amygdala, hippocampus, prefrontal cortex	Low activity of postsynaptic 5-HT1A receptors in PD and SAD	SSRIs and SNRIs first-line therapy for anxiety disorders
γ-amino butyric acid (GABA)	Substantia nigra, globus pallidus, hypothalamus, periaqueductal gray matter, hippocampus, amygdala, anterior cingulate	Reduced GABA-A and benzodiazepine binding in PD Reduced GABA levels in PD, possible imbalance between tonic GABAergic inhibition and glutamate-mediated excitation	Tiagabine, an SGRI (selective GABA reuptake inhibitor) and vigabatrin (inhibitor of GABA transaminase) are potential treatments Tiagabine equivocal findings in GAD Topiramate (blocks voltage-sensitive sodium channels, potentiates GABA) mixed findings in PD Compounds selective for specific GABA-A receptor subtypes under development **Note:** Gabapentin and pregabalin, although structurally related to GABA, do not act on GABA receptors
Glutamate	Amygdala, hippocampus, frontal and cingulate cortices	Possible imbalance between tonic GABAergic inhibition and glutamate-mediated excitation in PD	Efficacy of DCS as adjunct to exposure therapy for acrophobia, SAD and PD Glycine transporter inhibitors under study Metabotropic receptor modulators under study NMDA receptor antagonism as potential anxiolytic—preliminary efficacy of riluzole for GAD
Neuropeptide Y (NPY)	Amygdala, hippocampus, brainstem, nucleus accumbens, locus coeruleus, hypothalamus	Low NPY levels in PTSD, less well studied in anxiety disorders	Intranasal NPY administration may reduce anxiety, under investigation Y1 and Y2 receptors potential targets for treatment
Galanin	Prefrontal cortex, amygdala, hippocampus, locus coeruleus	Very few studies in patients with anxiety disorders Galanin gene polymorphism associated with PD, only in women	Potential of galanin modulators as future approach; no known studies
Cholecystokinin (CCK)	Cerebral cortex, hippocampus, amygdala, caudate, putamen, thalamus, hypothalamus	Lower CSF levels of CCK in PD	To date, CCK-B receptor antagonists have failed to demonstrate efficacy for GAD or PD
Oxytocin	Hypothalamus, ventral tegmental area, amygdala	Oxytocin gene receptor polymorphism associated with increased risk for anxiety in individuals with early life stress	Intranasal oxytocin administration beneficial for SAD, under study; potential benefit for GAD
Endocannabinoid system	Prefrontal cortex, hypothalamus, amygdala, hippocampus	Dysregulation of endocannabinoid signaling	Cannabidiol reduced anxiety in patients with SAD during public speaking; under study
			Studies of FAAH inhibitors as potential treatment under way for PTSD (no longer classified as anxiety disorder); needed in anxiety disorders

GAD, generalized anxiety disorder; PD, panic disorder; SAD, social anxiety disorder; NMDA, *N*-methyl-D-aspartate; NDRI, norepinephrine–dopamine reuptake inhibitor; SSRI, selective serotonin reuptake inhibitor; SNRI, serotonin–norepinephrine reuptake inhibitor; DCS, D-cycloserine; FAAH, fatty acid amide hydrolase.

suggest an exaggerated noradrenergic system output, along with increased autonomic and sympathetic activation. Table 8-9 summarizes the major neurochemical systems thought to be relevant to anxiety disorders.

Preclinical Studies of Fear Learning. As we mentioned above, the ubiquity of fear and anxiety in many animals makes it relatively easy to study through animal models. Using conditioned models of fear, researchers can study the anatomical correlates of fear anxiety. It is daunting to summarize the many aspects of what we know about the etiology of fear and anxiety. In its broadest sense, one can imagine a stimulus, collected through afferent systems. That stimulus is then processed and evaluated to assess whether it is averse. This assessment involves including previous experiences and environmental contexts associated with the stimulus. What results is a fear or anxiety response, which employs a range of behavioral, endocrine, and autonomic responses to react to that stimulus.

Many areas of the brain and connections between those areas are involved in this response. For example, the amygdala plays a vital role. The amygdala has many subnuclei, called the amygdaloid complex, each with a unique function. The lateral nucleus of the amygdala (LA), for example, is the primary interface for visual, auditory, and somatic sensory information received from the thalamus and cortex. The connections between the thalamus and this

nucleus appear to be central to fear conditioning related to these particular stimuli.

Once entering the L.A., it sends the neural representation of the stimulus to various other amygdaloid nuclei. It is then modulated by an array of systems, including ones that supply context from memory, or about different homeostatic states in the body. Some of the most extensive projections are to the basal (BA) nuclei, which are involved in forming the long-lasting traces for fear conditioning. After much processing, including from other cortical regions, the output nuclei of the amygdala organize the behavioral responses that reflect the sum of the activity of the many nuclei. The central nucleus of the amygdala then outputs this to various motor, autonomic, and neuroendocrine systems involved in expressing fear. This includes the hypothalamus, midbrain, and medulla. For example, the hypothalamus can then activate the CRH to start the associated stress response. The hippocampus, among other structures, also has a critical role in fear learning and extinction and helps in the development of the emotional responses associated with fear.

This discussion is just a brief introduction into what we know and theorize about the neurobiology of anxiety disorders. Our *Comprehensive Textbook of Psychiatry* has a much expanded discussion as well as references to many of the relevant articles. Figure 8-1 summarizes the stages of the fear response, as well as some of the brain regions involved in these stages.

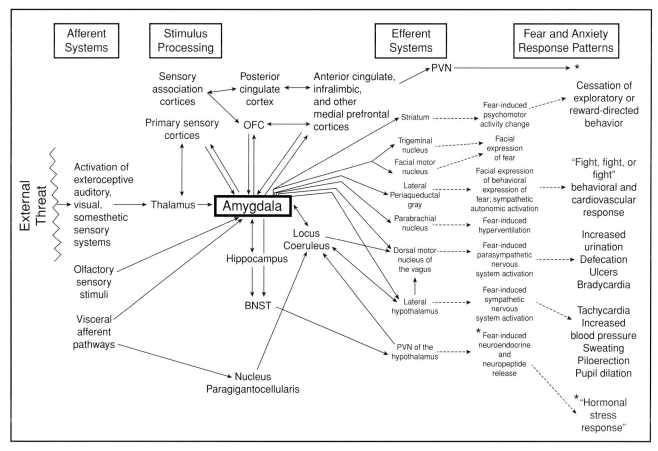

FIGURE 8-1

Neuroanatomical circuitry underlying fear and anxiety, organized by systems that evaluate the salience of potentially threatening stimuli (to the left) and systems that organize and mediate the expression of fear and anxiety behaviors (to the right). BNST, bed nucleus of the stria terminalis; OFC, orbitofrontal cortex; PVN, paraventricular nucleus. (From Charney DS, Drevets WC. The neurobiological basis of anxiety disorders. In: Davis K, Charney DS, Coyle J, Nemeroff CB, eds. *Psychopharmacology. The Fifth Generation of Progress.* New York: Lippincott Williams & Wilkins; 2002:901.)

References

Baldwin DS, Anderson IM, Nutt DJ, Allgulander C, Bandelow B, den Boer JA, Christmas DM, Davies S, Fineberg N, Lidbetter N, Malizia A, McCrone P, Nabarro D, O'Neill C, Scott J, van der Wee N, Wittchen HU. Evidence-based pharmacological treatment of anxiety disorders, post-traumatic stress disorder and obsessive-compulsive disorder: a revision of the 2005 guidelines from the British Association for Psychopharmacology. *J Psychopharmacol*. 2014;28(5):403–439.

Bandelow B, Reitt M, Röver C, Michaelis S, Görlich Y, Wedekind D. Efficacy of treatments for anxiety disorders: A meta-analysis. *Int Clin Psychopharmacol*. 2015;30(4):183–192.

Bandelow B, Sher L, Bunevicius R, Hollander E, Kasper S, Zohar J, Möller HJ; WFSBP Task Force on Mental Disorders in Primary Care; WFSBP Task Force on Anxiety Disorders, OCD and PTSD. Guidelines for the pharmacological treatment of anxiety disorders, obsessive-compulsive disorder and posttraumatic stress disorder in primary care. *Int J Psychiatry Clin Pract*. 2012;16(2):77–84.

Beck AT, Epstein N, Brown G, Steer RA. An inventory for measuring clinical anxiety: Psychometric properties. *J Consult Clin Psychol*. 1988;56(6):893–897.

Craske MG, Rauch SL, Ursano R, Prenoveau J, Pine DS, Zinbarg RE. What is an anxiety disorder? *Depress Anxiety*. 2009;26:1066–1085.

Crocq M-A. A history of anxiety: From Hippocrates to DSM. *Dialogues Clin Neurosci*. 2015;17(3):319–325.

Dell'Osso B, Buoli M, Baldwin DS, Altamura AC. Serotonin norepinephrine reuptake inhibitors (SNRIs) in anxiety disorders: A comprehensive review of their clinical efficacy. *Hum Psychopharmacol*. 2010;25(1):17–29.

Depping AM, Komossa K, Kissling W, Leucht S. Second-generation antipsychotics for anxiety disorders. *Cochrane Database Syst Rev*. 2010;(12):CD008120.

Dresler T, Guhn A, Tupak SV, Ehlis A-C, Herrmann MJ, Fallgatter AJ, Deckert J, Domschke K. Revise the revised? New dimensions of the neuroanatomical hypothesis of panic disorder. *J Neural Transm (Vienna)*. 2013;120(1):3–29.

Fentz HN, Hoffart A, Jensen MB, Arendt M, O'Toole MS, Rosenberg NK, Hougaard E. Mechanisms of change in cognitive behaviour therapy for panic disorder: The role of panic self-efficacy and catastrophic misinterpretations. *Behav Res Ther*. 2013; 51:579–587.

Funayama T, Furukawa TA, Nakano Y, Noda Y, Ogawa S, Watanabe N, Chen J, Noguchi Y. In-situation safety behaviors among patients with panic disorder: Descriptive and correlational study. *Psych Clin Neurosci*. 2013;67:332–339.

Generoso MB, Trevizol AP, Kasper S, Cho HJ, Cordeiro Q, Shiozawa P. Pregabalin for generalized anxiety disorder: An updated systematic review and meta-analysis. *Int Clin Psychopharmacol*. 2017;32(1):49–55.

Goodwin RD, Stein DJ. Anxiety disorders and drug dependence: Evidence on sequence and specificity among adults. *Psych Clin Neurosci*. 2013;67:167–173.

Gorman JM, Kent JM, Sullivan GM, Coplan JD. Neuroanatomical hypothesis of panic disorder, revised. *Am J Psychiatry*. 2000;157(4):493–505.

Gorman JM, Liebowitz MR, Fyer AJ, Stein J. A neuroanatomical hypothesis for panic disorder. *Am J Psychiatry*. 1989;146(2):148–161.

Hamm AO. Specific phobias. *Psychiatr Clin North Am*. 2009;32(3):577.

Hasin DS, Grant BF. The National Epidemiologic Survey on Alcohol and Related Conditions (NESARC) Waves 1 and 2: Review and summary of findings. *Soc Psychiatry Psychiatr Epidemiol*. 2015;50(11):1609–1640.

Hofmann SG, Hinton DE. Cross-cultural aspects of anxiety disorders. *Curr Psychiatry Rep*. 2014;16(6):450.

Julian LJ. Measures of anxiety. *Arthritis Care Res (Hoboken)* [Internet]. 2011 Nov [cited November 24, 2019];63(0 11):5467–5472. Available from: https://www.ncbi.nlm.nih.gov/pmc/articles/PMC3879951/

Khalsa SS, Feinstein JS, Li W, Feusner JD, Adolphs R, Hurlemann R. Panic anxiety in humans with bilateral amygdala lesions: Pharmacological induction via cardiorespiratory interoceptive pathways. *J Neurosci*. 2016;36(12):3559–3566.

Klein DF. Historical aspects of anxiety. *Dialogues Clin Neurosci*. 2002;4(3):295–304.

Lovibond PF, Lovibond SH. The structure of negative emotional states: comparison of the Depression Anxiety Stress Scales (DASS) with the Beck Depression and Anxiety Inventories. *Behav Res Ther*. 1995;33(3):335–343.

Marteau TM, Bekker H. The development of a six-item short-form of the state scale of the Spielberger State-Trait Anxiety Inventory (STAI). *Br J Clin Psychol*. 1992;31(3):301–306.

McLean CP, Asnaani A, Litz BT, Hofmann SG. Gender differences in anxiety disorders: Prevalence, course of illness, comorbidity and burden of illness. *J Psychiatr Res*. 2011;45:1027–1035.

Meyerbroker K, Morina N, Kerkhof G, Emmelkamp PM. Virtual reality exposure treatment of agoraphobia: A comparison of computer automatic virtual environment and head-mounted display. *Stud Health Technol Inform*. 2011;167:51–56.

Naragon-Gainey K, Gallagher MW, Brown TA. A longitudinal examination of psychosocial impairment across the anxiety disorders. *Psycholog Med*. 2013;43:1475.

Perna G, Daccò S, Menotti R, Caldirola D. Antianxiety medications for the treatment of complex agoraphobia: Pharmacological interventions for a behavioral condition. *Neuropsychiatr Dis Treat*. 2011;7:621–637.

Practice Guideline for the Treatment of Patients With Panic Disorder. In: *APA Practice Guidelines for the Treatment of Psychiatric Disorders: Comprehensive Guidelines and Guideline Watches [Internet]*. 1st ed. Arlington, VA: American Psychiatric Association; 2006 [cited July 26, 2020]. Available from: http://www.psychiatryonline.com/content.aspx?aID=51396

Sanchez C, Reines EH, Montgomery SA. A comparative review of escitalopram, paroxetine, and sertraline: Are they all alike? *Int Clin Psychopharmacol*. 2014;29(4):185–196.

Shear MK, Vander Bilt J, Rucci P, Endicott J, Lydiard B, Otto MW, Pollack MH, Chandler L, Williams J, Ali A, Frank DM. Reliability and validity of a structured interview guide for the Hamilton Anxiety Rating Scale (SIGH-A). *Depress Anxiety*. 2001;13(4):166–178.

Spitzer RL, Kroenke K, Williams JBW, Löwe B. A brief measure for assessing generalized anxiety disorder: The GAD-7. *Arch Intern Med*. 2006;166(10):1092–1097.

Steenen SA, van Wijk AJ, van der Heijden GJ, van Westrhenen R, de Lange J, de Jongh A. Propranolol for the treatment of anxiety disorders: Systematic review and meta-analysis. *J Psychopharmacol*. 2016;30(2):128–139.

Stein DJ, Nesse RM. Threat detection, precautionary responses, and anxiety disorders. *Neurosci Biobehav Rev*. 2011;35:1075–1079.

Vinkers CH, Olivier B. Mechanisms underlying tolerance after long-term benzodiazepine use: A future for subtype-selective GABAA receptor modulators? *Adv Pharmacol Sci* [Internet]. 2012;2012:416864 [cited July 26, 2020]. Available from: https://www.ncbi.nlm.nih.gov/pmc/articles/PMC3321276/

World Health Organization. Depression and other common mental disorders: Global health estimates. 2017 [cited September 26, 2019]. Available from: https://apps.who.int/iris/handle/10665/254610

Zigmond AS, Snaith RP. The hospital anxiety and depression scale. *Acta Psychiatr Scand*. 1983;67(6):361–370.

Zimmerman M, Clark H, McGonigal P, Harris L, Holst CG, Martin J. Reliability and validity of the DSM-5 anxious distress specifier interview. *Compr Psychiatry*. 2017;76:11–17.

Zimmerman M, Martin J, Clark H, McGonigal P, Harris L, Holst CG. Measuring anxiety in depressed patients: A comparison of the Hamilton anxiety rating scale and the DSM-5 Anxious Distress Specifier Interview. *J Psychiatr Res*. 2017;93:59–63.

## 9

Obsessive-Compulsive and Related Disorders

This chapter includes disorders characterized by repetitive, intrusive thoughts and/or repeated mental acts or behaviors. These disorders include obsessive-compulsive disorder (OCD), body dysmorphic disorder (BDD), hoarding disorder (HD), hair-pulling disorder (trichotillomania), and excoriation (skin-picking) disorder, as well as some related disorders.

THE CLINICAL PRESENTATION

Obsessive-Compulsive Disorder

OCD is a diverse group of symptoms that include intrusive thoughts, rituals, preoccupations, and compulsions. Obsessions are intrusive and unwanted repetitive thoughts, urges, or impulses that often lead to a marked increase in anxiety or distress. Compulsions are repetitive behaviors or mental acts that are done in response to obsessions, or in a rigid, rule-bound way. These recurrent obsessions or compulsions cause severe distress to the person. The obsessions or compulsions are time-consuming and interfere significantly with the person's routine, occupational functioning, usual social activities, or relationships. A patient with OCD may have only obsessions or only compulsions, but in most cases, both obsessions and compulsions are present.

Obsessions and compulsions are the essential features of OCD. An idea or an impulse intrudes itself insistently and persistently into a person's conscious awareness. Typical obsessions associated with OCD include thoughts about contamination ("My hands are dirty") or doubts ("I forgot to turn off the stove").

The typical patterns of OCD symptoms cluster within several limited dimensions, including contamination/cleansing, forbidden thoughts/checking, symmetry/ordering, and hoarding symptoms (see below). Most patients with OCD typically have good insight into the fact that their OCD beliefs are not real. However, some patients have poor insight, and a small number lack any insight—their obsessions are delusional. Such patients may be misdiagnosed with a psychotic disorder and receive inappropriate treatment.

The presentation of obsessions and compulsions is heterogeneous in adults (Table 9-1) and children and adolescents (Table 9-2). The symptoms of an individual patient can overlap and change with time, but OCD has four major symptom patterns, as outlined below.

Contamination/Cleansing. The most common pattern is an obsession of contamination, followed by washing or accompanied by compulsive avoidance of the presumably contaminated object. The feared object is often hard to avoid (e.g., feces, urine, dust, or germs). Patients may rub the skin off their hands by excessive handwashing or may be unable to leave their homes because of fear of germs. Although anxiety is the most common emotional response to the feared object, obsessive shame and disgust are also common. Patients with contamination obsessions usually believe that the contamination is spread from object to object or person to person by the slightest contact.

Pathologic Doubt/Checking. The second most common pattern is an obsession of doubt, followed by compulsions of checking. The obsession often implies some danger of violence (e.g., forgetting to turn off the stove or not locking a door). The checking may involve multiple trips back into the house to check the stove, for example. These patients have obsessional self-doubt and always feel guilty about having forgotten or committed something.

Intrusive/Forbidden Thoughts. In the third most common pattern, there are intrusive obsessional thoughts without a compulsion. Patients usually experience thoughts of a sexual or aggressive act that is reprehensible to the patient. Patients obsessed with thoughts of aggressive or sexual acts may report themselves to the police or confess to a priest. Suicidal ideation may also be obsessive (and unlikely to be acted on), but we should assess for actual risk.

Symmetry/Ordering. The fourth most common pattern is the need for symmetry or precision, which can lead to a compulsion of slowness. Patients can take hours to eat a meal or shave their faces.

Other Symptom Patterns. Religious obsessions and compulsive hoarding are common in patients with OCD. Compulsive hairpulling and nail-biting are behavioral patterns related to OCD. Masturbation may also be compulsive.

Ms. K was referred for psychiatric evaluation by her general practitioner. In the interview, Ms. K described a long history of checking rituals that had caused her to lose several jobs and had damaged numerous relationships. She reported, for example, that she often had the thought that she had not locked the door to the car. It was difficult for her to leave her car until she had repeatedly checked that it was secure. She had broken several car door handles with the vigor of her checking and had been up to an hour late to work because she spent too much time checking her car door.

Similarly, she had recurrent thoughts that she had left the door to her apartment unlocked. She returned several times to check her door before she left for work. She reported that checking doors decreased her anxiety about security. Ms. K reported that she had occasionally tried to leave her car or apartment without checking the door (e.g., when she was already late for work). However, she found that she became so worried that someone would steal her car or break into her apartment that she had difficulty going anywhere. Ms. K reported that her obsessions about security had become so extreme over the past 3 months

---

Table 9-1
Obsessive-Compulsive Symptoms in Adults

Variable	%
Obsessions (N = 200)	
Contamination	45
Pathologic doubt	42
Somatic	36
Need for symmetry	31
Aggressive	28
Sexual	26
Other	13
Multiple obsessions	60
Compulsions (N = 200)	
Checking	63
Washing	50
Counting	36
Need to ask or confess	31
Symmetry and precision	28
Hoarding	18
Multiple comparisons	48
Course of illness (N = 100)[a]	
Type	
Continuous	85
Deteriorative	10
Episodic	2
Not present	71
Present	29

[a]Age at onset: men, 17.5 ± 6.8 years; women, 20.8 ± 8.5 years.
From Rasmussen SA, Eisen JL. The epidemiology and differential diagnosis of obsessive compulsive disorder. *J Clin Psychiatry*. 1992;(53 Suppl):4–10, with permission.

Table 9-2
Reported Obsessions and Compulsions for 70 Consecutive Child and Adolescent Patients

Major Presenting Symptom	No. (%) Reporting Symptom at Initial Interview[a]
Obsession	
Concern or disgust with bodily wastes or secretions (urine, stool, saliva), dirt, germs, environmental toxins	30 (43)
Fear something terrible may happen (fire, death or illness of loved one, self, or others)	18 (24)
Concern or need for symmetry, order, or exactness	12 (17)
Scrupulosity (excessive praying or religious concerns out of keeping with patient's background)	9 (13)
Lucky and unlucky numbers	6 (8)
Forbidden or perverse sexual thoughts, images, or impulses	3 (4)
Intrusive nonsense sounds, words, or music	1 (1)
Compulsion	
Excessive or ritualized handwashing, showering, bathing, toothbrushing, or grooming	60 (85)
Repeating rituals (e.g., going in and out of door, up and down from chair)	36 (51)
Checking doors, locks, stove, appliances, car brakes	32 (46)
Cleaning and other rituals to remove contact with contaminants	16 (23)
Touching	14 (20)
Ordering and arranging	12 (17)
Measures to prevent harm to self or others (e.g., hanging clothes a certain way)	11 (16)
Counting	13 (18)
Hoarding and collecting	8 (11)
Miscellaneous rituals (e.g., licking, spitting, special dress pattern)	18 (26)

[a]Multiple symptoms recorded, so total exceeds 70.
From Rapoport JL. The neurobiology of obsessive-compulsive disorder. *JAMA*. 1988;260:2889, with permission.

that she had lost her job due to recurrent tardiness. She recognized the irrational nature of her obsessive concerns but could not bring herself to ignore them. (Courtesy of Erin B. McClure-Tone, Ph.D., and Daniel S. Pine, M.D.)

Body Dysmorphic Disorder

Persons with BDD have persistent preoccupations about one or more perceived defects or flaws in one's appearance. The defects or flaws appear slight or are not observable to others. Their concerns about their appearance result in a range of mental acts or behaviors, including comparing themselves with others, checking in the mirror, or camouflaging their perceived flaws.

The most common concerns (Table 9-3) involve the face and head, particularly those involving specific parts (e.g., the skin, nose shape and size, hair), although symptoms may focus on any area of the body. Sometimes the concern is vague and confusing to understand, such as extreme concern over a "scrunchy" chin. Throughout their illness, patients worry about five to seven different body areas. More than a quarter of patients are concerned with the symmetry of their appearance.

Commonly associated symptoms include ideas or delusions of reference, frequent mirror checking or avoidance of reflective surfaces, and attempts to hide the presumed deformity. The ideas or delusions of reference are usually about others noticing the alleged flaw. The effects on a person's life can be significant, and it is essential to assess for avoidance due to BDD symptoms, which can range from minor social avoidance to being housebound. Patients

with BDD have less insight into the truth of their beliefs than those with OCD. Only a quarter of BDD patients have reasonable insight, and around one-third have absent insight.

Ms. R, a 28-year-old single woman, presented with the complaint that she is "ugly" and that she feels others are laughing at her, despite family telling her she was attractive. She first became preoccupied with her appearance when she was 13. She became obsessed with her "facial defects," feeling, for example, that her nose was fat, or her eyes were too far apart. Up until this point, Ms. R was confident, a good student, and socially active. However, her fixation on her face caused her to withdraw socially and have difficulty concentrating in school, which in turn hurt her grades.

Ms. R dropped out of high school and went for her GED due to her preoccupation. She began to frequently pick at "blemishes" and hairs on her face. She frequently checked herself in mirrors and other reflective surfaces (e.g., spoons, windows), and found herself thinking about her defects almost daily. Her family and others could not convince her that there was nothing wrong with her appearance.

Table 9-3
Location of Imagined Defects in 30 Patients with Body Dysmorphic Disorder[a]

Location	N	%
Hair[b]	19	63
Nose	15	50
Skin[c]	15	50
Eyes	8	27
Head, face[d]	6	20
Overall body build, bone structure	6	20
Lips	5	17
Chin	5	17
Stomach, waist	5	17
Teeth	4	13
Legs, knees	4	13
Breasts, pectoral muscles	3	10
Ugly face (general)	3	10
Ears	2	7
Cheeks	2	7
Buttocks	2	7
Penis	2	7
Arms, wrists	2	7
Neck	1	3
Forehead	1	3
Facial muscles	1	3
Shoulders	1	3
Hips	1	3

[a]Total is greater than 100% because most patients had "defects" in more than one location.
[b]Involved head hair in 15 cases, beard growth in 2 cases, and other body hair in 3 cases.
[c]Involved acne in 7 cases, facial lines in 3 cases, and other skin concerns in 7 cases.
[d]Involved concerns with shape in 5 cases and size in 1 case.
From Phillips KA, McElroy SL, Keck PE Jr., Pope HG, Hudson JL. Body dysmorphic disorder: 30 cases of imagined ugliness. *Am J Psychiatry*. 1993;150:303, with permission.

Hoarding Disorder

Persons with HD have persistent and profound difficulty discarding or parting with their possessions. The disorder leads to significant congestion and clutter and substantive distress or impairment, differentiating it from regular collecting. Compulsive hoarding is a common and often disabling phenomenon associated with impairment in such functions as eating, sleeping, and grooming. Hoarding may result in health problems and poor sanitation, particularly when hoarding of animals is involved. It may also lead to injuries from fire or falling. As a rule, people with the disorder acquire things of little or no value and cannot throw them away.

What drives the behavior appears to be the fear of losing items that the patient believes will be needed later and a distorted belief about or an emotional attachment to possessions. Most hoarders do not perceive their behavior to be a problem. Many perceive their behavior to be reasonable and part of their identity. Most hoarding

patients accumulate possessions passively rather than intentionally, thus clutter accumulates gradually. Commonly hoarded items include newspapers, mail, magazines, old clothes, bags, books, lists, and notes. Hoarding poses risks to not only the patient but also to those around them. Clutter accumulated from hoarding has caused deaths from fire or other accidents. It can also attract pest infestations that can pose a health risk both to the patient and residents around them. Many sufferers have been evicted from their homes or threatened with eviction as a result of their hoarding. In severe cases, hoarding can interfere with work, social interaction, and necessary activities such as eating or sleeping.

The pathologic nature of hoarding comes from the inability to organize possessions and keep them organized. Many patients hoard rather than make decisions about discarding items. Patients with HD also overemphasize the importance of recalling information and possessions. For example, a hoarder will keep old newspapers and magazines because they believe that important information may be lost. Patients may believe that forgetting the information will lead to severe consequences and prefer to keep their possessions within sight so as not to forget them.

> Ms. T, a 55-year-old single woman, presented to a therapist accompanied by her adult son, who expressed concern about Ms. T's inability to "throw things away." He reported that Ms. T's home was extremely cluttered with "needless things." Whenever he attempted to help her "organize things," however, Ms. T would become agitated and argumentative. Ms. T confirmed her son's complaint and reported having this difficulty for as long as she could remember, but never really viewed it as a problem.
>
> Over the past 5 years, Ms. T's home had become increasingly cluttered to the point that it became more and more challenging to move around within it. She was able to keep the kitchen and bathroom relatively clutter-free. However, boxes and bags filled with papers, magazines, clothes, and miscellaneous gifts and trinkets filled the rest of her home. Her living room was the most affected. Her son could no longer visit his mother as so uncomfortable at her home. Ms. T admits that his avoidance of her home has been a significant source of depression for her. Ms. T had enjoyed entertaining her family and friends but had not done so in years as she felt that her home was no longer suitable. She had made a few attempts to clean out her home but was unable to discard most items. When asked why she was keeping them, she replied, "I may need them later."

Hair-Pulling Disorder (Trichotillomania)

Hair-pulling disorder is a chronic disorder characterized by repetitive hairpulling, leading to variable hair loss that may be visible to others. It is also known as *trichotillomania*, from the Greek *trich* (hair) and *tillein* (to pull or pluck), a term coined by a French dermatologist Francois Hallopeau in 1889. Although once considered rare, it appears to be relatively common. It resembles both obsessive-compulsive and impulse control disorder: increased tension before the hairpulling leads to the behavior and then subsequent relief or satisfaction.

Hair-pulling disorder, or trichotillomania, is characterized by pulling out one's hair. The pulling is not for cosmetic reasons, but instead, individuals often describe an irresistible urge to pull out their hair. This hairpulling results in noticeable hair loss and is associated with repeated attempts to decrease or stop hairpulling. Patients with hair-pulling disorder may experience an increasing sense of tension before engaging in the behavior and achieve a sense of release or gratification from pulling out their hair. All areas of the body may be affected, most commonly the scalp (Fig. 9-1).

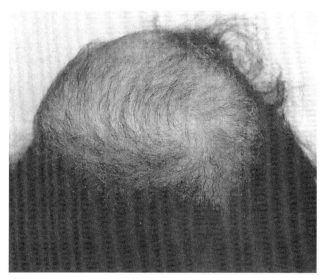

FIGURE 9-1

Hair-pulling disorder (trichotillomania). Note the typical findings of an area of incomplete alopecia involving the frontal and vertex scalp. (From Sadock BJ, Sadock VA, Ruiz P, eds. *Kaplan & Sadock's Comprehensive Textbook of Psychiatry*. 9th ed. Philadelphia, PA: Lippincott Williams & Wilkins; 2009, with permission.)

Other areas involved are eyebrows, eyelashes, and beard; trunk, armpits, and pubic areas are less commonly involved.

There are (at least) two types of hairpulling. *Focused pulling* is the use of an intentional act to control unpleasant personal experiences, such as an urge, bodily sensation (e.g., itching or burning), or thought. In contrast, *automatic pulling* occurs outside the person's awareness and, most often, during sedentary activities. Most patients have a combination of these types.

The hair loss usually appears as short, broken strands near long, healthy hairs in the affected areas. No abnormalities of the skin or scalp are present. The hairpulling is usually painful, although pruritus and tingling may occur in the affected area. *Trichophagy,* mouthing of the hair, may follow the hair plucking. Complications of trichophagy include trichobezoars, malnutrition, and intestinal obstruction. Patients usually deny the behavior and often try to hide the resultant alopecia. The patients may also self-mutilate in other ways, such as headbanging, nail-biting, scratching, gnawing, or excoriation.

Ms. C, a 27-year-old single woman, came to a local clinic complaining of persistent hairpulling. She first started at age 11 when she began to pick the hairs at the nape of her neck. She would persistently pick at the hair until there was almost none left. Fortunately, her hair was long, so no one noticed the lack of hair at the back of her neck. Over the years, her hair picking progressed until she began picking hair from her entire head, leaving noticeable small bald patches. She strategically hid the bald patches by brushing over the remainder of her hair or with carefully placed scarves and hats. Despite her habit, Ms. C's daily functioning was average. She earned good grades in school and was a year away from getting her master's degree.

Ms. C's habit was constant, occurring every day, often without her noticing it. She could only be reading an assignment for school, and eventually, her hand would find its way into her hair to find hair to pull. Soon she would notice a small pile of hairs in her book or on her lap, indicating that she had been pulling her hair out for a while. Whenever she tried to stop herself from pulling her hair, she would become increasingly nervous and anxious until she resumed the hairpulling. Her hair-pulling sessions lasted anywhere from 10 minutes to an hour.

Excoriation (Skin-Picking) Disorder

People with excoriation disorder repeatedly pick their skin, sufficiently to cause lesions. Individuals with skin-pulling attempt to decrease or stop skin-picking; however, they are unable to do so. While some picking of scabs is likely universal, in the case of excoriation disorder, the behavior causes clinically significant distress or impairment. The historical literature describes cases of "neurotic excoriation" or "psychogenic excoriation," however, it was only with *Diagnostic and Statistical Manual of Mental Disorders* (DSM-5) that the disorder became a separate diagnosis.

Skin-picking may be from any area of the body but is most commonly from the face, followed by the hands, fingers, arms, and legs (Fig. 9-2). Patients may pick from multiple sites. In severe cases, skin-picking can result in physical disfigurement and medical consequences that require medical or surgical interventions (e.g., skin grafts or radiosurgery).

Patients may experience tension before picking and relief or gratification after picking. Patients may pick to relieve stress, tension, and other negative feelings. Despite the feeling of relief felt from picking, patients often feel guilty or embarrassed at their behavior. Up to 87 percent of patients report feeling embarrassed by the picking and 58 percent report avoiding social situations. Many patients use bandages, makeup, or clothing to hide their picking. Of skin-picking patients, 15 percent report suicidal ideation due to their behavior, and about 12 percent have attempted suicide.

Ms. J, a 22-year-old single woman, presented to a psychiatrist at the urging of her dermatologist because of compulsively picking her facial skin. She picked at it every day up to three times a day in sessions lasting from 20 minutes to over an hour. She had massive scarring and lesions on her face. She went to a physician 6 months prior when one of the lesions had become infected.

Ms. J began picking her face at age 11 at the onset of puberty. At first, she only picked at acne that formed on her face, but as the urge to pick became greater, she started picking at clear patches of skin as well. Due to the scaring and lesions, Ms. J became increasingly withdrawn and avoided all social engagements. She reported feeling great tension before picking, and only felt relief after she began picking.

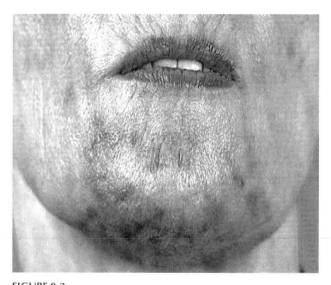

FIGURE 9-2

Skin-picking disorder. Multiple erythematous and pigmented maculae and crusted erosions on chin. (From Sadock BJ, Sadock VA, Ruiz P. *Kaplan & Sadock's Comprehensive Textbook of Psychiatry*. 9th ed. Philadelphia, PA: Lippincott Williams & Wilkins; 2009, with permission.)

Obsessive-Compulsive or Related Disorder due to Another Medical Condition

As with most psychiatric disorders, when OCD (or another disorder in this category) is due to some other medical condition, we use a different diagnosis. We include a discussion of medical causes of obsessive and compulsive symptoms in our section on differential diagnosis.

Substance-Induced Obsessive-Compulsive or Related Disorder

Sometimes the symptoms described in this chapter may be due to a substance, including drugs, medications, and alcohol (either during use or during withdrawal), and is not part of a delirium. In such cases, we would use this separate diagnosis.

Other Specified Obsessive-Compulsive or Related Disorder

This category is for patients who have symptoms characteristic of obsessive-compulsive and related disorder but do not meet the full criteria for any specific obsessive-compulsive or related disorder. This diagnosis is appropriate under three situations: (1) an atypical presentation, (2) another specific syndrome not listed in DSM-5 (such as Olfactory Reference Syndrome, described next), and (3) the information presented is insufficient to make a full diagnosis of an obsessive-compulsive or related disorder.

Olfactory Reference Syndrome.   People with olfactory reference syndrome have a false belief that they have a foul body odor that is not perceived by others. The preoccupation leads to repetitive behaviors such as washing the body or changing clothes. Patients with the disorder may have good, fair, poor, or absent insight into the behavior. The syndrome is predominant in males and single persons. The mean age of onset is 25 years of age. The belief of a subjective sense of smell that does not exist externally may rise to the level of a somatic delusion, in which a diagnosis of a delusional disorder may be more appropriate. The syndrome has been frequently described in the psychiatric literature, usually classified as a delusion of perception. Whether or not it deserves a unique diagnosis remains controversial.

In assessing a patient with olfactory reference syndrome, it is essential to exclude other medical causes. Some patients with temporal lobe epilepsy may complain of smelling foul odors. Local irritations of the hippocampus from pituitary tumors may also cause olfactory sensations. Patients with inflammation of the frontal, ethmoidal, or sphenoidal sinuses may also have a subjective sense of offensive odors. DSM-5 includes olfactory reference syndrome in the "other specified" designation for the obsessive-compulsive and related disorder of DSM-5.

DIAGNOSIS

Obsessive-Compulsive Disorder

Table 9-4 lists the diagnostic approaches to OCD in DSM-5 and ICD-10. We can usually diagnose OCD with a thorough psychiatric history and examination. Patients often attempt to neutralize obsessions with compulsions. These compulsions are usually not credibly connected to the thoughts, or they are excessive. When assessing the negative impact of OCD symptoms, it is important also to address avoidance of triggers of obsessions and compulsions.

Body Dysmorphic Disorder

Table 9-5 lists the diagnostic approaches to BDD in DSM-5 and ICD-10. The DSM-5 diagnostic criteria for BDD stipulate preoccupation with a perceived defect in appearance or overemphasis of a slight defect. It also requires that at some point during the disorder, the patient has compulsive behaviors or mental acts related to the preoccupation. These compulsions may include mirror checking, excessive grooming, or comparing their appearance to that of others. The preoccupation causes patients significant emotional distress or markedly impairs their ability to function in important areas.

Hoarding Disorder

Table 9-6 lists the diagnostic approaches to HD in DSM-5 and ICD-10. We diagnose HD using the significant features of the disorder: patients acquire large amounts of useless or valueless possessions, they cannot throw them away, and this leads to significant clutter in living areas. If their space is not cluttered, it is because others have stepped in to clean it. Finally, it should cause significant distress or functional impairment. The fifth edition of the DSM-5 includes diagnostic specifiers that relate to insight, which may be rated poor, fair, or good. Some patients are completely unaware of the full extent of the problem and resistant to treatment. At times, delusional beliefs about hoarded items are present.

Hair-Pulling Disorder (Trichotillomania)

Table 9-7 lists the diagnostic approaches to hair-pulling disorder in DSM-5 and ICD-10. It emphasizes the repetitive and compulsive nature of the behavior as well as the fact that it is not motivated by cosmetic reasons.

Excoriation (Skin-Picking) Disorder

Table 9-8 lists the diagnostic approaches to excoriation (skin-picking) disorder in DSM-5 and ICD-10. DSM-5 diagnostic criteria for skin-picking disorder require recurrent skin-picking resulting in skin lesions and repeated attempts to decrease or stop picking. The skin-picking must cause clinically relevant distress or impairment in functioning. The skin-picking behavior cannot be attributed to another medical or mental condition and cannot be a result of a substance use disorder (e.g., cocaine or methamphetamine use). A thorough physical examination is crucial before a psychiatric diagnosis.

DIFFERENTIAL DIAGNOSIS

Medical Conditions

Several primary medical disorders can produce syndromes bearing a striking resemblance to OCD.

OCD-like symptoms have been reported in children following group A beta-hemolytic streptococcal infection and have been called *pediatric autoimmune neuropsychiatric disorders associated with streptococcus* (PANDAS). They may result from an autoimmune process that leads to inflammation of the basal ganglia that disrupts cortical–striatal–thalamic axis functioning.

The current conceptualization of OCD as a disorder of the basal ganglia derives from the phenomenologic similarity between idiopathic OCD and OCD-like disorders that are associated with

Table 9-4
Obsessive-Compulsive Disorder

	Obsessive-Compulsive Disorder	
Disorder	**DSM-5**	**ICD-10**
Diagnostic name	Obsessive-Compulsive Disorder	Obsessive-Compulsive Disorder

Symptoms	1. Obsessions (Intrusive thoughts that accompany behaviors and that individuals may attempt to ignore or counteract through action)
	2. Compulsions (repetitive actions, commonly driven by an obsessive thought, performed to relieve anxiety or fear)
		• Recurrent obsessional thoughts and/or compulsive acts
		  • Obsessions: ideas, images, or impulses occurring recurrently
		  • Compulsions: repeated stereotyped behaviors meant to neutralize a thought/anxiety or prevent a perceived adverse event
		• Attempts at resisting thoughts and behaviors are frequently unsuccessful and cause worsening anxiety

Required number of symptoms	Obsessive thoughts, compulsions, or both	Presence of obsessions, compulsions, or both
Psychosocial consequences of symptoms	Symptoms and behaviors consume at least 1 hr/day or cause significant distress and impairment	
Exclusions (not result of):	Medical illness Substance Other psychiatric disorder	Obsessive-compulsive personality disorder
Symptom specifiers	**Tic related** • current or prior tic disorder **With good or fair insight** • understanding that beliefs surrounding actions may not be true **With poor insight** • feeling that beliefs surrounding actions are likely true **With absent insight and/or delusional beliefs** • strong conviction that beliefs surrounding actions are true	• Predominantly obsessional thoughts or ruminations • Predominantly compulsive acts (obsessional rituals) • Mixed obsessional thoughts and acts
Severity specifiers	With or without insight (per above)	

basal ganglia diseases, such as Sydenham chorea and Huntington disease. It is essential to search for the neurologic signs of these disorders when assessing a patient with presumed OCD. Also, OCD often develops before age 30 years, and new-onset OCD in an older individual should raise questions about potential neurologic contributions to the disorder.

Many medical disorders can cause alopecia. A biopsy may be necessary to distinguish hair-pulling disorder from alopecia areata and tinea capitis.

Many dermatologic conditions can cause skin-picking. Conditions associated with itching (such as scabies) can cause picking, as well as other medical conditions (such as in Prader–Willi syndrome).

Tourette Disorder. OCD is closely related to Tourette disorder, as the two conditions frequently co-occur, both in individuals over time and within families. About 90 percent of persons with Tourette disorder have compulsive symptoms, and as many as two-thirds meet the diagnostic criteria for OCD.

Classically, patients with Tourette disorder have recurrent vocal and motor tics that bear only a slight resemblance to OCD. The premonitory urges that precede tics often strikingly resemble obsessions, however, and many of the more complicated motor tics are very similar to compulsions.

Other Psychiatric Conditions

Many other psychiatric disorders include obsessive-compulsive symptoms, and we must also rule out these conditions when diagnosing OCD. OCD exhibits a superficial resemblance to obsessive-compulsive personality disorder, which is associated with an obsessive concern for details, perfectionism, and other similar personality traits. However, only OCD is associated with genuine obsessions and compulsions. Worries in generalized anxiety disorder are about real-life concerns, and they tend to be less irrational and ego-dystonic than in OCD. Similarly, the ruminations of depression and preoccupations of mania are typically mood-congruent and ego-syntonic; in neither case are symptoms neutralized by compulsions.

Psychotic symptoms often lead to obsessive thoughts and compulsive behaviors, bodily preoccupations, or hoarding behaviors that can be difficult to distinguish from the obsessive-compulsive and related disorder. Patients with psychotic disorders, however, cannot acknowledge the unreasonableness of their behavior. Also, psychotic patients typically have a host of other features that are not characteristic of OCD.

In some patients with BDD, their preoccupations have a delusional intensity. In such cases, delusional disorder, somatic type can be made, generally in addition to BDD, to capture the true nature of the patient's presentation.

Table 9-5
Body Dysmorphic Disorder

Disorder	Body Dysmorphic Disorder	
	DSM-5	ICD-10
Diagnostic name	Body Dysmorphic Disorder	Body Dysmorphic Disorder
Symptoms	1. Preoccupation with physical appearance and subjective flaws 2. Presence of repetitive behaviors at some point during the disorder • Checking • Grooming • Skin-picking • Recurrent thoughts/perseveration on comparing physical appearance to that of others	Excessive preoccupation with image or appearance
Required number of symptoms	Both of the above, causing significant impairment and/or distress and excluding other causes of symptoms	
Psychosocial consequences of symptoms	Symptoms and behaviors cause significant distress and impairment	Significant distress or impairment in areas of functioning
Exclusions (not result of):	Medical illness Substance Eating disorder Other psychiatric disorder	
Symptom specifiers	**With muscle dysmorphia** • preoccupation with perceived low muscle mass or small body build **With good or fair insight** • understanding that beliefs may not be true **With poor insight** • feeling that beliefs are likely true **With absent insight and/or delusional beliefs** • strong conviction that beliefs are true	
Severity specifiers	With or without insight (per above)	

Similarly, major depression is often associated with obsessive thoughts that, at times, border on actual obsessions. However, in the case of major depression, the obsessive symptoms are only found during a depressive episode.

Individuals with an avoidant personality disorder or social phobia may worry about being embarrassed by imagined or real defects in appearance. However, this concern is usually not prominent, persistent, distressing, or impairing.

Other psychiatric disorders may cause hoarding symptoms, including autism spectrum disorders (where collections may reflect a specific interest) and psychotic disorders. We should only diagnose HD if the hoarding symptoms are independent of these other disorders.

Neurodevelopmental and neurodegenerative conditions may be associated with hoarding. For example, in Prader–Willi Syndrome, individuals are characterized by hoarding of food, obesity, and skin-picking. Alzheimer disease is another example. Damage to specific brain regions (anterior ventromedial prefrontal and cingulate cortices) may cause excessive and indiscriminate hoarding activity.

Patients with anorexia nervosa have a bodily preoccupation, but the focus is on weight. In gender dysphoria, it is a discomfort with, or a sense of wrongness about, one's primary and secondary sex characteristics. In major depressive disorder, there may be mood-congruent cognitions involving appearance that occur exclusively during a major depressive episode.

Olfactory reference syndrome may result in other compulsive or repetitive behaviors such as washing or changing one's clothes.

Individuals with BDD have obsessional preoccupations about their appearance and may have associated compulsive behaviors (e.g., mirror checking). We should only include multiple diagnoses when the specific focus of concerns of the obsessions extends beyond the usual focus of that disorder.

Some patients with OCD may hoard as a response to an unwanted obsession. This situation is most familiar with obsessions around symmetry, incompleteness, or fears of harm or contamination (e.g., keeping an object in case discarding that object leads to harm). In contrast, in HD, there is no associated obsession; instead, the individual wishes to retain saved items and is distressed by the thought of discarding them. In some cases, both OCD and HD may be comorbid. Skin-picking may also occur in response to obsessions about contamination. Skin-picking is also common in BDD, but in these individuals, it is a response to concerns about body appearance, and a second diagnosis is not necessary.

Patients with factitious dermatitis or *dermatitis artefacta* pick their skin as a type of self-inflicted injury and use more elaborate methods than simple excoriation to self-induce skin lesions. It is seen in 0.3 percent of dermatology patients and has a female:male ratio of 8:1. It can present at any age but occurs most frequently in adolescents and young adults. It may include a variety of skin lesions, such as blisters, ulcers, erythema, edema, purpura, and sinuses. The morphology of factitious dermatitis lesions is often bizarre and linear, with clear-cut, angulated, or geometric edges. The presence of entirely healthy, unaffected skin adjacent to the horrific-looking lesions is a clue to the diagnosis of factitious dermatitis (Fig. 9-3). Also, the patient's

Table 9-6
Hoarding Disorder

| Disorder | Hoarding Disorder | |
	DSM-5	ICD-10
Diagnostic name	Hoarding Disorder	Hoarding Disorder
Symptoms	1. Excessive attachment to possessions 2. Distress related to being separated from items 3. Excessive accumulation of possessions 4. Accumulation results in significant distress, impairment, and/or safety/health compromise	• Difficulty parting with objects due to perceived need to save possessions • Distress and functional impairment associated with being separated from possessions
Required number of symptoms	All of the above	
Psychosocial consequences of symptoms	Symptoms and behaviors cause significant distress and impairment	Symptoms and behaviors cause significant distress and impairment
Exclusions (not result of):	Medical illness Neurocognitive disorder Other psychiatric disorder	
Symptom specifiers	**With excessive acquisition** • hoarding accompanied by excessive acquisition of additional possessions **With good or fair insight** • understanding that actions are problematic **With poor insight** • belief that actions may not be problematic **With absent insight and/or delusional beliefs** • strong conviction that actions are not problematic	
Severity specifiers	**With or without insight (per above)**	

description of the history of the lesions is usually vague and lacks detail about the appearance and evolution of the lesions.

Normal Behaviors

Certain normal behaviors can become more prominent in specific individuals without being a disorder. We live in a society concerned with appearance; some persons are more concerned than others.

Some of us are more careful about avoiding contamination or germs and may wash or avoid touching potentially infected persons or items. Living during a global pandemic naturally blurs the line between contamination phobia and understandable caution. We expect this overlap between pathologic and prudent to continue long after the pandemic. Many of us occasionally remove stray hair, often for cosmetic reasons. We may bite at a fingernail or pick at a scab. Collecting is an enjoyable and sometimes lucrative hobby for many people.

Table 9-7
Hair-Pulling Disorder (Trichotillomania)

| Disorder | Trichotillomania | |
	DSM-5	ICD-10
Diagnostic name	Trichotillomania (Hair-Pulling Disorder)	Trichotillomania
Symptoms	1. Recurrent hairpulling causing hair loss 2. Hairpulling despite repeated attempts to change/ end behaviors 3. Actions cause distress and/or impaired functioning	• Presence of noticeable hair loss due to recurrent hairpulling • Hair-pulling behavior preceded by increased anxiety that is relieved by hairpulling
Required number of symptoms	All of the above	
Psychosocial consequences of symptoms	Symptoms and behaviors cause significant distress and impairment	
Exclusions (not result of):	Medical illness Other psychiatric disorder	Pre-existing inflammation of skin Response to delusion or hallucination Stereotyped movement disorder

Table 9-8
Excoriation (Skin-Picking)

| | Excoriation Disorder | |
Disorder	DSM-5	ICD-10
Diagnostic name	Excoriation (Skin-Picking) Disorder	Excoriation (Skin-Picking) Disorder
Symptoms	1. Recurrent skin-picking causing lesions to the skin 2. Ongoing skin-picking despite repeated attempts to change/end behaviors 3. Actions cause distress and/or impaired functioning	See criteria for obsessive-compulsive disorders
Required number of symptoms	All of the above	
Psychosocial consequences of symptoms	Symptoms and behaviors cause significant distress and impairment	
Exclusions (not result of):	Other psychiatric disorder	Factitious dermatitis

In each case, the behavior is desired, usually restricted (e.g., a collector may only collect certain toys) and often enjoyable. These disorders, however, represent impulsive behaviors that cause distress and impairment.

COMORBIDITY

Obsessive-Compulsive Disorder

Persons with OCD are commonly affected by other mental disorders. The lifetime prevalence for major depressive disorder in persons with OCD is about 67 percent and for social phobia about 25 percent. Suicide is a risk for all patients with OCD. Other common comorbid psychiatric diagnoses in patients with OCD include alcohol use disorders, generalized anxiety disorder, specific phobia, panic disorder, eating disorders, and personality disorders. OCD exhibits a superficial resemblance to obsessive-compulsive personality disorder, which is associated with an obsessive concern for details, perfectionism, and other similar personality traits. The incidence of Tourette disorder in patients with OCD is 5 to 7 percent, and 20 to 30 percent of patients with OCD have a history of tics.

Body Dysmorphic Disorder

Of the various obsessive-compulsive and related disorders, it appears that BDD is the one most associated with comorbid depression with a lifetime rate of 75 percent, as well as with suicidality, with 80 percent having experienced suicidal ideation. About one-third of BDD patients have a lifetime history of OCD, and around 30 percent of BDD patients experience panic attacks triggered by appearance concerns. BDD is also associated with high levels of rejection sensitivity and low self-esteem. Many patients with BDD use substances to self-medicate symptoms of social anxiety or emotional pain.

Hoarding Disorder

Comorbid OCD is common in patients with HD. Other prevalent comorbid disorders include generalized anxiety disorder and major depressive disorder.

Hair-Pulling Disorder

Comorbid conditions include other body-focused repetitive behavior disorders, with excoriation disorder the most common. OCD is also more prevalent in hair-pulling disorder than in the general population. More than half of treatment-seeking individuals with hair-pulling disorder have a comorbid psychiatric disorder, with mood and anxiety disorders the most common. Also, hair-pulling disorder can result in medical sequelae (e.g., trichobezoars) and decreased quality of life.

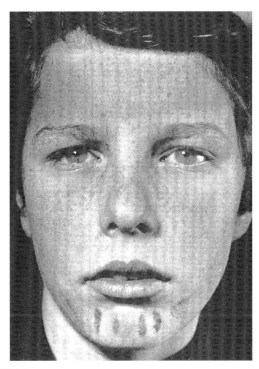

FIGURE 9-3
Typical self-produced lesions with scabbing. (From Douthwaite AH, ed. *French's Index of Differential Diagnosis*. 7th ed. Baltimore, MD: Williams & Wilkins; 1954, with permission.)

Excoriation Disorder

Comorbid conditions in excoriation disorder include other body-focused repetitive behavior disorders, with hair-pulling disorder the most common. OCD and BDD are also more prevalent in excoriation disorder than in the general population. Other common comorbid psychiatric disorders in excoriation disorder include mood and anxiety disorders.

COURSE AND PROGNOSIS

Obsessive-Compulsive Disorder

The course of OCD is generally chronic, and in the absence of intervention, symptoms may persist for decades. Nevertheless, recent data emphasize that long-term outcomes can be positive. Thus, patients should be encouraged to remain hopeful and to try a range of different evidence-based treatments.

Body Dysmorphic Disorder

The course of BDD is generally chronic, and in the absence of intervention, symptoms may persist for decades. Earlier age of onset and more severe symptoms at intake may predict a worse course.

Hoarding Disorder

HD has a somewhat later course than most obsessive-compulsive and related disorders. In the absence of intervention, its course appears to be often chronic and progressive. Hoarding symptoms often begin in childhood and adolescence, with diagnostic criteria met only in the 30s, and worsening of symptoms in each subsequent decade.

Hair-Pulling Disorder

There are relatively little data on the long-term course of hair-pulling disorder. In the absence of intervention, its course is likely often chronic. However, some data indicate that in a proportion of cases, remission does occur.

Excoriation Disorder

Those data which exist on the long-term course of excoriation disorder suggest that, without intervention, this is often chronic, albeit with fluctuations in severity over time. As is the case in other obsessive-compulsive and related disorders, individuals often report that they have not sought medical attention because they are embarrassed by their symptoms, feel that they should stop the symptoms by themselves, or because they are unaware that the symptoms may be part of a known condition or that there are efficacious treatments.

TREATMENT

Obsessive-Compulsive Disorder

Pharmacotherapy. Effective medications include clomipramine and selective serotonin reuptake inhibitors (SSRIs, which, along with clomipramine and other serotonergic medications, are sometimes called serotonin reuptake inhibitor [SRIs]). Head-to-head comparisons of clomipramine and SSRIs show equal efficacy but better tolerability of the SSRIs. In general, clinicians must use higher doses to achieve an optimal effect. Examples are doses of 80 mg of fluoxetine or 200 mg of sertraline. Some patients respond to even higher doses. Exceeding the recommended doses is not, however, advisable for clomipramine or citalopram, due to safety

concerns. There is also some evidence that response to SRIs is slower in OCD than in depression; clinicians are therefore encouraged to prescribe an SRI for at least 12 weeks before deciding to switch agents or augment with another psychotropic. A general rule of thumb is that we should continue to use the dose that was required to obtain a response for at least 1 to 2 years. When discontinuing medication, there is a real risk of relapse, so this should be done very gradually, with small adjustments made every few months.

Patients who fail to respond to one SRI may respond to another.

The most extensive evidence base is for antipsychotics in adult OCD. Among those, risperidone and aripiprazole are best supported as adjuncts. Some studies have indicated that these are particularly useful in patients with tics, but not all data are consistent. When a response to these agents occurs, it typically happens relatively quickly (e.g., 4 weeks). When using dopamine receptor blockers, it is crucial to monitor adverse events.

Memantine, riluzole, ketamine, lamotrigine, and *N*-acetylcysteine (NAC) are other promising augmentation agents.

Psychotherapy.   There is a long history of understanding OCD symptoms from a psychodynamic perspective, but there is no rigorous evidence that a psychodynamic approach is useful in the treatment of OCD. Instead, empirical research on the psychotherapy of OCD has emerged from behavioral and cognitive perspectives. Exposure and response prevention (ERP) has proven to be a particularly effective component of treatment, with more recent work also focusing on the potential role for cognitive and mindfulness approaches. The essential principle of ERP is to minimize avoidance of distressing cues, and instead to encourage in vivo exposure to feared situations and imaginal exposure to feared consequences. After such exposures, it is important not to engage in the usual compulsive response. The therapist and patient then develop a hierarchy of gradual exposure to more distressing cues and follow it. As in the case of pharmacotherapy, it is essential to ensure that the dose and duration of ERP are sufficient.

Other cognitive approaches to OCD focus on thought distortions (e.g., inflated responsibility). The therapist and patient collaborate to test such distortions and replace them with more adaptive thinking patterns. More recently, mindfulness techniques have supplemented these approaches. Family sessions may also be helpful, particularly with younger patients, to better understand OCD and the principles of ERP.

Combined Treatment.   Clinical guidelines indicate that either pharmacotherapy or psychotherapy is a reasonable first-line intervention for the management of OCD. In younger patients, it seems reasonable to begin cognitive-behavioral therapy (CBT) first. In patients with more severe symptoms or comorbid depression, it seems reasonable to begin pharmacotherapy first. There is some evidence that the combination of CBT and pharmacotherapy is particularly useful.

Other Somatic Therapies.   Targeted neurosurgical lesions to cortico-striatal-thalamic-cortical (CSTC) tracts have been shown efficacious in a proportion of highly treatment-refractory patients. Approaches have included anterior cingulotomy and capsulotomy, among other techniques. The more recent focus on neurosurgical work has been on deep brain stimulation, with implantation of electrodes to stimulate specific brain regions. Transcranial magnetic stimulation has also been studied for OCD, although data are not yet sufficiently strong to motivate for routine clinical use. Electroconvulsive therapy does not seem to be useful for OCD.

Body Dysmorphic Disorder

SSRIs are efficacious in the treatment of BDD, including delusional BDD. There is some evidence that, as in the case of OCD, doses higher than those ordinarily used in the treatment of depression are beneficial in BDD, as are longer durations. Again, the duration of treatment should be longer, with gradual tapering of dosage and close monitoring of emergent symptoms.

Patients who do not respond to one SRI may respond to another. There is anecdotal evidence that buspirone augmentation of SRIs is useful in partial responders. There is little controlled data on using dopamine receptor blockers as augmenting agents; what exists is not encouraging. However, clinicians have reported anecdotal evidence for using aripiprazole as an augmenting agent. Also, irreversible MAOIs have some positive, although experiential, reports.

Relation to Plastic Surgery.   Few data exist about the number of patients seeking plastic surgery who have BDD. One study found that only 2 percent of the patients in a plastic surgery clinic had the diagnosis, but DSM-5 reports the figure to be 7 to 8 percent. The overall percentage may be much higher, however. Surgical requests are varied: removal of facial sags, jowls, wrinkles, or puffiness; rhinoplasty; breast reduction or enhancement; and penile enlargement. Men who request penile enlargements and women who request cosmetic surgery of the labia of the vagina or the lips of the mouth may be suffering from this disorder. Commonly associated with the belief about appearance is an unrealistic expectation of how much surgery will correct the defect. As reality sets in, the person realizes they have not solved their problems by merely altering a perceived cosmetic defect. These patients, hopefully, will explore their feelings of inadequacy using psychotherapy. The patients may take out their unfulfilled expectations and anger by taking legal action against their plastic surgeons or becoming depressed.

Hoarding Disorder

HD is challenging to treat. Although it shows similarities to OCD, effective treatments for OCD have shown little benefit for patients with HD. In one study, only 18 percent of patients responded to medication and CBT. The challenges posed by hoarding patients to typical CBT treatment include poor insight into the behavior and low motivation and resistance to treatment.

The most effective treatment for the disorder is a cognitive-behavioral model that includes training in decision making and categorizing; exposure and habituation to discarding; and cognitive restructuring. Treatment includes both office and in-home sessions. The role of the therapist in this model is to assist in the development of decision-making skills, to provide feedback about normal saving behavior, and to identify and challenge the patient's erroneous beliefs about possessions. The goal in treatment is to get rid of a significant amount of possessions and make the living space livable. Also, treatment can provide the patients with the skills to maintain a positive balance between the number of possessions and livable space.

Evidence for pharmacologic treatment relies on limited and uncontrolled data that support the use of SSRIs or venlafaxine.

Hair-Pulling Disorder

Early data indicated that hair-pulling disorder, like OCD and BDD, responded more robustly to clomipramine than to desipramine.

Unfortunately, subsequent trials of SSRIs and venlafaxine in hair-pulling disorder have not consistently demonstrated efficacy. The most significant positive clinical trial to date is with NAC (1200 to 2400 mg/day), a nutraceutical that acts on the glutamatergic system. However, a trial of NAC in pediatric hair-pulling disorder was negative. There are small controlled trials indicating that dopamine receptor blockers may also be useful in these conditions. Given their favorable side-effect profile, it may be reasonable to use NAC as a first-line agent in adults with hair-pulling disorder, to use SSRIs when patients have comorbid conditions for which these agents are efficacious, and to consider low-dose dopamine receptor blockers in more treatment-refractory cases.

Habit reversal training (HRT) is a set of cognitive-behavioral techniques that have been shown efficacious in the treatment of childhood and adult hair-pulling disorder. Components of HRT include awareness training, competing for response training, and social support. Also, therapists use stimulus control (SC) to change the patient's environment so that hairpulling is more effortful or less reinforcing. Controlled trials of augmentation of HRT/SC with acceptance and commitment therapy, dialectical behavior therapy, or cognitive therapy, have also suggested efficacy in hair-pulling disorder.

Excoriation Disorder

Excoriation disorder is challenging to treat, and there are few data on effective treatments. Most patients do not actively seek treatment due to embarrassment or because they believe their condition is untreatable. There is support for the use of SSRIs. Studies comparing fluoxetine against placebo have shown fluoxetine to be superior in reducing skin-picking.

Other agents have limited data. Lamotrigine has demonstrated inconsistent results. Glutamatergic agents, such as the nutraceutical NAC, have some positive, although anecdotal reports, as do dopamine receptor blockers. Nonpharmacologic treatments include HRT and brief CBT.

EPIDEMIOLOGY

Obsessive-Compulsive Disorder

The rates of OCD are relatively consistent, with a lifetime prevalence in the general population estimated at 2 to 3 percent. Community studies indicate a higher prevalence of OCD in females, but in clinical contexts, there are roughly equal numbers of male and female patients. The mean age of onset is about 19 years, with early-onset more common in males. The onset of the disorder typically occurs in adolescence or childhood, and onset after age 30 is rare.

Body Dysmorphic Disorder

Point prevalence estimates in the United States and elsewhere have ranged from 1.7 to 2.4 percent, indicating that this is one of the more common obsessive-compulsive and related disorders. Furthermore, clinical studies have found high rates of BDD in general adult psychiatric inpatients, in cosmetic surgery clinics, and in dermatology clinics.

The mean age of onset is in adolescence. As in the case of OCD, community studies indicate a higher prevalence of females with BDD, while clinical reports indicate a roughly even male:female ratio.

Hoarding Disorder

Most prevalence studies of HD have not used DSM-5 diagnostic criteria. Available data indicate that HD is remarkably prevalent in Western countries, with one study that employed DSM-5 criteria yielding a point prevalence of 1.5 percent. The male:female ratio is estimated to be about 1. In contrast, in clinics, females are more common than males, perhaps indicating greater insight. Unlike the picture seen in most obsessive-compulsive and related disorders, the prevalence of hoarding increases with age, and in clinical settings, the average age of first treatment is around 50.

Hair-Pulling Disorder

Studies of select populations, such as college students, indicate that the point prevalence of trichotillomania is around 0.5 to 2 percent. Age of onset is typically at menarche, and female:male ratio is about 4:1 in adults. Pediatric samples include an equal distribution between males and females.

Excoriation Disorder

Community-based prevalence studies of excoriation disorder have found a point prevalence of 1.4 to 5.4 percent. Age of onset is somewhat more variable than hair-pulling disorder, although the mean age is 12 years, typically coinciding with the onset of puberty. Although many more females than males have excoriation disorder, the ratio is more even than in the case of hair-pulling disorder.

ETIOLOGY

Obsessive-Compulsive Disorder

OCD is now primarily viewed as a neuropsychiatric disorder that is mediated by specific neurocircuits. From a cognitive-affective neuroscience perspective, OCD has several specific neuropsychological impairments, including cognitive inflexibility and alterations in the habit system. Early clinical work established that OCD could be precipitated by damage to striatal circuitry, as was seen in the global influenza epidemic in the early 20th century. More recent advances have delineated the role of neuroanatomy, neurocircuitry, neurotransmitters, and other molecules involved in the pathogenesis of OCD.

Cognitive and neuropsychological studies of OCD have found several alterations, including a range of impairments in executive function, and with evidence for cognitive inflexibility, motor impulsivity, and excessive habit formation. Such work is consistent with the hypothesis that OCD represents impaired control of automated, habitual behaviors.

Several brain regions, including the anterior cingulate, orbitofrontal cortex, and striatum, have consistently been implicated in OCD. There is, however, evidence that many other regions have an important role (Fig. 9-4). One hypothesis has been that cortico–striatal–thalamic–cortical (CSTC) circuitry plays a particularly important role in mediating the cognitive-affective impairments seen in OCD, with activation or inhibition of different components of this circuitry driving the compulsive and impulsive features of obsessive-compulsive and related disorders. Early imaging work was seminal in showing that both pharmacotherapy and CBT were able to normalize functional alterations in CSTC circuitry in OCD.

Also, data indicate that a range of neurotransmitter systems contribute to OCD, including serotonergic, dopaminergic, glutamatergic, and GABAergic systems. A serotonin hypothesis of OCD has been influential; a range of evidence points to the involvement of this system in OCD, and patients respond to treatment with SRIs but not to treatment with noradrenergic reuptake inhibitors. At the same time, there is relatively little evidence that serotonin plays a causal role in OCD. Furthermore, a range of evidence points to the involvement of the dopaminergic system in OCD, and, notably, augmentation of serotonin reuptake blockers with dopamine receptor blockers as a first-line intervention for treatment-refractory OCD. Most recently, there has been some interest in other systems, including the glutamatergic system, with evidence that some glutamatergic agents may be useful in this condition.

Genetic findings may increasingly influence future work on the cognitive-affective neuroscience of OCD. Twin and family studies indicate that genetic susceptibility plays a role in OCD, and more so in childhood-onset OCD.

Body Dysmorphic Disorder

There is some evidence that specific cognitive-affective impairments characterize BDD. For example, neuropsychological studies have suggested deficits in executive functioning and visual processing. Brain imaging and neurogenetic studies have provided some insights into the potential mechanisms that underlie such deficits, and into potential overlaps with other obsessive-compulsive and related disorders. For example, CSTC circuits may be involved, as well as circuits involved in visual processing. Family and twin data provide preliminary evidence for genetic susceptibility, as well as a relationship to OCD. However, the etiology of BDD is still far from clear.

Hoarding Disorder

Patients with HD may demonstrate impairment in various neuropsychological domains, including spatial planning, working memory, response inhibition, and set-shifting. Structural and functional brain imaging studies have indicated that the relevant neurocircuitry overlaps only partially with that involved in OCD. Research on patients with neurologic disorders has suggested that ventromedial prefrontal/anterior cingulate cortices and medial temporal regions are involved in hoarding. Also, animal studies have pointed to a possible role for the dopaminergic system in hoarding, and twin studies indicate genetic susceptibility for developing pathologic hoarding.

Hair-Pulling Disorder

From a cognitive-affective neuroscience perspective, neuropsychological investigations of hair-pulling disorder have demonstrated some evidence of deficits in working memory and visual–spatial learning. Structural and functional brain imaging studies have suggested some involvement of CSTC circuits relevant to habit learning, although data is sparse. There is also evidence of the involvement of brain regions associated with reward processing and affect regulation. Family and twin studies provide evidence for genetic susceptibility, as well as a relationship to OCD and other body-focused repetitive behaviors. Several candidate genes may be associated with hair-pulling disorder, but the evidence is preliminary.

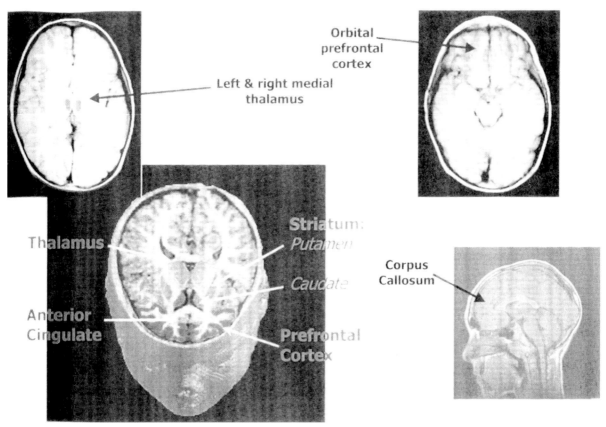

FIGURE 9-4
Brain regions implicated in the pathophysiology of obsessive-compulsive disorder. (From Rosenberg DR, MacMillan SN, Moore GJ. Brain anatomy and chemistry may predict treatment response in paediatric obsessive-compulsive disorder. *Int J Neuropsychopharmacol.* 2001;4(2):179–190, with permission.)

Excoriation Disorder

From a cognitive-affective neuroscience perspective, neuropsychological investigations of excoriation disorder have demonstrated some overlap with OCD regarding motor impulsivity. Brain imaging studies have similarly suggested some involvement of CSTC circuitry, although the data is sparse, and other regions also appear to be implicated. There is also some evidence that suggests that the dopaminergic system plays a role in excoriation disorder. Family and twin studies provide evidence for genetic susceptibility, as well as a relationship to OCD and other body-focused repetitive behaviors. As with hair-pulling disorder, preliminary evidence has identified several candidate genes.

References

American Psychiatric Association. *Diagnostic and Statistical Manual of Mental Disorders.* 5th ed. Arlington, VA: American Psychiatric Association; 2013.

Bloch MH. Trichotillomania and other impulsive-control disorders. In: Hudak R, Dougherty DD, eds. *Clinical Obsessive-Compulsive Disorders in Adults and Children.* New York: Cambridge University Press; 2011:207.

Cicek E, Cicek IE, Kayhan F, Uguz F, Kaya N. Quality of life, family burden and associated factors in relatives with obsessive-compulsive disorder. *Gen Hosp Psychiatry.* 2013;35(3):253–258.

Conrado LA, Hounie AG, Diniz JB, Fossaluza V, Torres AR, Miguel EC, Rivitti EA. Body dysmorphic disorder among dermatologic patients: Prevalence and clinical features. *J Am Acad Derm.* 2010;63:235.

Del Casale A, Sorice S, Padovano A, Simmaco M, Ferracuti S, Lamis DA, Rapinesi C, Sani G, Girardi P, Kotzalidis GD, Pompili M. Psychopharmacological treatment of obsessive-compulsive disorder (OCD). *Curr Neuropharmacol.* 2019;17(8):710–736.

DiMauro J, Genova M, Tolin DF, Kurtz MM. Cognitive remediation for neuropsychological impairment in hoarding disorder: A pilot study. *J Obsess Compul Relat Disord.* 2014;3(2):132–138.

Endrass T, Schuermann B, Kaufmann C, Spielberg R, Kniesche R, Kathmann N. Performance monitoring and error significance in patients with obsessive-compulsive disorder. *Biol Psychol.* 2010;84:257.

Fang A, Hofmann SG. Relationship between social anxiety disorder and body dysmorphic disorder. *Clin Psychol Rev.* 2010;30:1040.

Fang A, Matheny NL, Wilhelm S. Body dysmorphic disorder. *Psychiatr Clin North Am.* 2014;37(3):287–300.

Feusner JD, Arienzo D, Li W, Zhan L, Gadelkarim J, Thompson PM, Leow AD. White matter microstructure in body dysmorphic disorder and its clinical correlates. *Psychiatry Res.* 2013;211(2):132–140.

Frost RO, Steketee G, Tolin DF. Comorbidity in hoarding disorder. *Depress Anxiety.* 2011;28:876.

Frost RO, Tolin DF, Steketee G, Fitch KE, Selbo-Bruns A. Excessive acquisition in hoarding. *J Anxiety Disord.* 2009;23:632.

Gillan CM, Papmeyer M, Morein-Zamir S, Sahakian BJ, Fineberg NA, Robbins TW, de Wit S. Disruption in the balance between goal-directed behavior and habit learning in obsessive-compulsive disorder. *Am J Psychiatry.* 2011;168:718.

Goes F, McCusker M, Bienvenu O, Mackinnon DF, Mondimore FM, Schweizer B, National Institute of Mental Health Genetics Initiative Bipolar Disorder Consortium; Depaulo JR, Potash JB. Co-morbid anxiety disorders in bipolar disorder and major depression: Familial aggregation and clinical characteristics of co-morbid panic disorder, social phobia, specific phobia and obsessive-compulsive disorder. *Psychol Med.* 2012;42(7):1449–1459.

Grant JE, Chamberlain SR. Trichotillomania. *Am J Psychiatry.* 2016;173(9):868–874.

Grant JE, Odlaug BL, Chamberlain SR, Keuthen NJ, Lochner C, Stein DJ. Skin picking disorder. *Am J Psychiatry.* 2012;169(11):1143–1149.

Grant JE, Odlaug BL, Kim SW. A clinical comparison of pathologic skin picking and obsessive-compulsive disorder. *Compr Psychiatry.* 2010;51:347.

Grant JE, Stein DJ, Woods DW, Keuthen NJ, eds. *Trichotillomania, Skin Picking, and Other Body-Focused Repetitive Behaviors.* Arlington, VA: American Psychiatric Publishing; 2011.

Greenberg JL, Falkenstein M, Reuman L, Fama J, Marques L, Wilhelm S. The phenomenology of self-reported body dysmorphic disorder by proxy. *Body Image.* 2013;10(2):243–246.

Grisham JR, Norberg MM, Williams AD, Certoma SP, Kadib R. Categorization and cognitive deficits in compulsive hoarding. *Behav Res Ther.* 2010;48:886.

Hall BJ, Tolin DF, Frost RO, Steketee G. An exploration of comorbid symptoms and clinical correlates of clinically significant hoarding symptoms. *Depress Anxiety.* 2013;30(1):67–76.

Hirschtritt MW, Bloch MH, Mathews CA. Obsessive-compulsive disorder: Advances in diagnosis and treatment. *JAMA.* 2017;317(13):1358–1367.

Iervolino AC, Perroud N, Fullana MA, Guipponi M, Cherkas L, Collier DA, Mataix-Cols D. Prevalence and heritability of compulsive hoarding: A twin study. *Am J Psychiatry.* 2009;116:1156.

Kelly MM, Didie ER, Phillips KA. Personal and appearance-based rejection sensitivity in body dysmorphic disorder. *Body Image.* 2014;11(3):260–265.

Keuthen NJ, Rothbaum BO, Falkenstein MJ, Meunier S, Timpano KR, Jenike MA, Welch SS. DBT-enhanced habit reversal treatment for trichotillomania: 3- and 6-month follow-up results. *Depress Anxiety.* 2011;28:310.

Kumar B. The mind-body connection: An integrated approach to the diagnosis of colonic trichobezoar. *Int J Psychiatry Med.* 2011;41:263.

Lee HJ, Franklin SA, Turkel JE, Goetz AR, Woods DW. Facilitated attentional disengagement from hair-related cues among individuals diagnosed with trichotillomania: An investigation based on the exogenous cueing paradigm. *J Obsess Compul Relat Disord.* 2012;1:8.

Levy HC, McLean CP, Yadin E, Foa EB. Characteristics of individuals seeking treatment for obsessive-compulsive disorder. *Behav Ther.* 2013;44(3):408–416.

Lochner C, Seedat S, Stein DJ. Chronic hair-pulling: Phenomenology-based subtypes. *J Anxiety Disord.* 2010;24:196.

Mancuso SG, Knoesen NP, Castle DJ. Delusional versus nondelusional body dysmorphic disorder. *Compr Psychiatry.* 2010;51.177.

Markarian Y, Larson MJ, Aldea MA, Baldwin SA, Good D, Berkeljon A, Murphy TK, Storch EA, McKay D. Multiple pathways to functional impairment in obsessive-compulsive disorder. *Clin Psychol Rev.* 2010;30:78.

McDonald KE. Trichotillomania: Identification and treatment. *J Counsel Dev.* 2012;90:421.

Miller JL, Angulo M. An open-label pilot study of N-acetylcysteine for skin-picking in Prader–Willi syndrome. *Am J Med Gen.* 2014;164(2):421–424.

Nestadt G, Di C, Riddle M, Grados MA, Greenberg BD, Fyer AJ, McCracken JT, Rauch SL, Murphy DL, Rasmussen SA, Cullen B, Pinto A, Knowles JA, Piacentini J, Pauls DL, Bienvenu OJ, Wang Y, Liang KY, Samuels JF, Roche KB. Obsessive-compulsive disorder: Subclassification based on co-morbidity. *Psychol Med.* 2009;39(9):1491–1501.

Nordsletten AE, Reichenberg A, Hatch SL, Fernandez de la Cruz L, Pertusa A, Hotopf M, Mataix-Cols D. Epidemiology of hoarding disorder. *Br J Psychiatry.* 2013;203(6):445–452.

Odlaug BL, Grant JE. Pathological skin-picking. *Am J Drug Alcohol Abuse.* 2010;36:296.

Odlaug BL, Kim SW, Grant JE. Quality of life and clinical severity in pathological skin picking and trichotillomania. *J Anxiety Disord.* 2010;24:823.

Panza KE, Pittenger C, Bloch MH. Age and gender correlates of pulling in pediatric trichotillomania. *J Am Acad Child Adolesc Psychiatry.* 2013;52(3):241–249.

Park LE, Calogero RM, Young AF, Diraddo AM. Appearance-based rejection sensitivity predicts body dysmorphic disorder symptoms and cosmetic surgery acceptance. *J Soc Clin Psychol.* 2010;29:489.

Peng ZW, Xu T, Miao GD, He QH, Zhao Q, Dazzan P, Chan RC. Neurological soft signs in obsessive-compulsive disorder: The effect of comorbid psychosis and evidence for familiality. *Prog Neuropsychopharmacol Biol Psychiatry.* 2012;39(1):200–205.

Philips KA, Pinto A, Hart AS, Coles ME, Eisen JL, Menard W, Rasmussen SA. A comparison of insight in body dysmorphic disorder and obsessive-compulsive disorder. *J Psych Res.* 2012;46:1293.

Piallat B, Polosan M, Fraix V, Goetz L, David O, Fenoy A, Torres N, Quesada JL, Seigneuret E, Pollak P, Krack P, Bougerol T, Benabid AL, Chabardès S. Subthalamic neuronal firing in obsessive-compulsive disorder and Parkinson disease. *Ann Neurol.* 2011;69:793.

Pittenger C, Bloch MH. Pharmacological treatment of obsessive-compulsive disorder. *Psychiatr Clin North Am.* 2014;37(3):375–391.

Prazeres AM, Nascimento AL, Fontenelle LF. Cognitive-behavioral therapy for body dysmorphic disorder: A review of its efficacy. *Neuropsychiatr Dis Treat.* 2013;9:307–316.

Riesel A, Endrass T, Kaufmann C, Kathmann N. Overactive error-related brain activity as a candidate endophenotype for obsessive-compulsive disorder: Evidence from unaffected first-degree relatives. *Am J Psychiatry.* 2011;168:317.

Schuck K, Keijsers GP, Rinck M. The effects of brief cognitive-behaviour therapy for pathological skin picking: A randomized comparison to wait-list control. *Behav Res Ther.* 2011;49:11.

Smith AK, Mittal V. Delusions of body image in the prodrome. *Schizophr Res.* 2013;146(1–3):366–367.

Smith AH, Wetterneck CT, Hart JM, Short MB, Björgvinsson T. Differences in obsessional beliefs and emotion appraisal in obsessive-compulsive symptom presentation. *J Obsessive Compulsive Relat Disord.* 2012;1:54.

Snorrason I, Smari J, Ólafsson RP. Emotion regulation in pathological skin picking: Findings from a non-treatment seeking sample. *J Behav Ther Exp Psychiatry.* 2010;41:238.

Snorrason I, Stein D, Woods D. Classification of excoriation (skin picking) disorder: Current status and future directions. *Acta Psychiatr Scand.* 2013;128(5):406–407.

Stein DJ, Lochner C. Chapter 15: Obsessive-compulsive and related disorders. In: Sadock BJ, Sadock VA, Ruiz P, eds. *Kaplan & Sadock's Comprehensive Textbook of Psychiatry.* 10th ed. Philadelphia, PA: Wolters Kluwer; 2017:1785–1798.

Steketee G, Siev J, Fama JM, Keshaviah A, Chosak A, Wilhelm S. Predictors of treatment outcome in modular cognitive therapy for obsessive-compulsive disorder. *Depress Anxiety.* 2011;28:333.

Timpano KR, Rasmussen J, Exner C, Rief W, Schmidt NB, Wilhelm S. Hoarding and the multi-faceted construct of impulsivity: A cross-cultural investigation. *J Psychiatr Res.* 2013;47(3):363–370.

Tolin DF, Villavicencio A. Inattention, but not obsessive-compulsive disorder, predicts the core features of hoarding disorder. *Behav Res Ther.* 2011;49:120.

Via E, Cardoner N, Pujol J, Alonso P, López-Solà M, Real E, Contreras-Rodríguez O, Deus J, Segalàs C, Menchón J, Soriano-Mas C, Harrison BJ. Amygdala activation and symptom dimensions in obsessive-compulsive disorder. *Brit J Psychiatry.* 2014;204(1):61–68.

Wahl K, Huelle JO, Zurowski B, Kordon A. Managing obsessive thoughts during brief exposure: An experimental study comparing mindfulness-based strategies and distraction in obsessive-compulsive disorder. *Cogn Ther Res.* 2013;37(4):752–761.

Walther MR, Snorrason I, Flessner CA, Franklin ME, Burkel R, Woods DW. The Trichotillomania Impact Project in Young Children (TIP-YC): Clinical Characteristics, Comorbidity, Functional Impairment and Treatment Utilization. *Child Psychiatry & Hum Dev.* 2014;45(1):24–31.

Whittal ML, Robichaud M. Obsessive-compulsive disorder. In: Hofmann SG, Reinecke MA, eds. *Cognitive-Behavioral Therapy With Adults: A Guide to Empirically-Informed Assessment and Intervention.* New York: Cambridge University Press; 2010:92.

Wilhelm S, Philips KA, Steketee G. *Cognitive Behavioral Therapy for Body Dysmorphic Disorder: A Treatment Manual.* New York: Guilford; 2013.

Williams M, Powers MB, Foa EB. Obsessive-compulsive disorder. In: Sturmey P, Hersen M, eds. *Handbook of Evidence-Based Practice in Clinical Psychology.* Hoboken, NJ: Wiley; 2012:313.

Woods DW. Treating trichotillomania across the lifespan. *J Am Acad Child Adolesc Psychiatry.* 2013;52(3):223–224.

10 ▲

Trauma- and Stressor-Related Disorders

This chapter includes disorders characterized by exposure to significant stress or trauma. These disorders include posttraumatic stress disorder (PTSD), acute stress disorder, and adjustment disorders.

THE CLINICAL PRESENTATION

Persons suffering from one of these disorders develop emotional and behavioral symptoms in response to a significant stressor or traumatic event.

Posttraumatic Stress Disorder and Acute Stress Disorder

Persons who have PTSD or acute stress disorder have increased stress and anxiety following exposure to a traumatic or stressful event. Traumatic or stressful events may include experiencing a violent accident or crime, military combat, assault, being kidnapped, being involved in a natural disaster, being diagnosed with a life-threatening illness, or experiencing systematic physical or sexual abuse. A PTSD patient typically relives the trauma or tries to avoid reminders of it. They experience negative thoughts and moods about the event and feel hyperaroused or hyperactive. The patient may relive the trauma in their dreams or experience "flashbacks" or waking thoughts about the ordeal.

The stressors causing both acute stress disorder and PTSD are sufficiently overwhelming to affect almost everyone. They can arise from experiences in war, torture, natural catastrophes, assault, rape, and serious accidents.

Physicians have appreciated the link between acute mental syndromes and traumatic events for more than 200 years. After the American Civil War, physicians documented trauma-related syndromes, and early psychoanalytic writers, including Sigmund Freud, noted a relationship between neurosis and trauma. In World Wars I and II, these disorders were given various names, including "battle fatigue," "shell shock," and "soldier's heart." Moreover, increasing documentation of mental reactions to the Holocaust, to a series of natural disasters, and assault contributed to the growing recognition of a close relation between trauma and psychopathology.

> Mrs. M sought treatment for symptoms that she developed in the wake of an assault that had occurred about 6 weeks before her psychiatric evaluation. While leaving work late one evening, Mrs. M was attacked in a parking lot next to the hospital in which she worked. She was raped and badly beaten but was able to escape and call for help. On referral, Mrs. M reported frequent intrusive thoughts about the assault, including nightmares about the event and recurrent intrusive

visions of her assailant. She now took the bus to work to avoid the scene of the attack and changed her work hours to avoid leaving the building after dark. Also, she reported that she had difficulty interacting with men, particularly those who resembled her attacker, and that she consequently avoided such interactions whenever possible. Mrs. M described increased irritability, difficulty staying asleep at night, poor concentration, and an increased focus on her environment, particularly after dark. (Courtesy of Erin B. McClure-Tone, Ph.D., and Daniel S. Pine, M.D.)

Clinical Features. Individuals with PTSD relive distressing instances of the traumatic event, with vivid emotional proximity and high, imperative intensity. They organize their lives trying to contain and mitigate the persistent effects of the traumatic experience. For those traumatized in a war zone, they often feel as if the war never ended. Victims of rape, assault, or torture describe difficulties engaging and trusting other humans. Constantly reliving the trauma in the present, PTSD patients' lives become a series of effortful attempts to avoid reminders of the traumatic event. They scan the environment for threat signals, which they fearfully expect, and remain on guard, tense, restless, and exhausted. The persistence of symptoms despite the termination of the threat, combined with an inability to regain a sense of safety, are core features of PTSD. Another core feature is the involuntary, uncontrollable, and intense nature of symptoms.

Adjustment Disorders

People with adjustment disorders have an emotional response to a stressful event. It is one of the few diagnostic entities that directly links an external stressor to the development of symptoms. Typically, the stressor involves financial issues, a medical illness, or a relationship problem. The symptom complex that develops may involve anxious or depressive affect or may present with a disturbance of conduct. The symptoms must begin within 3 months of the stressor. The *Diagnostic and Statistical Manual of Mental Disorders* (DSM-5) includes a variety of subtypes of the disorder, including adjustment disorder with depressed mood, mixed anxiety and depressed mood, disturbance of conduct, mixed disturbance of emotions and conduct, and unspecified type.

Clinical Features. Patients with adjustment disorders develop intense emotional or behavioral symptoms in response to one or more external stressors. The intensity of the symptoms is subjectively considered beyond what one would expect in the given situation and impairs the patient's ability to function.

Other Specified or Unspecified Trauma- or Stressor-Related Disorder

As with other psychiatric diagnoses, the DSM-5 includes separate categories to account for persons whose symptoms do not meet the full criteria for another trauma- or stressor-related disorder.

DIAGNOSIS

Posttraumatic Stress Disorder and Acute Stress Disorder

The diagnosis includes several categories of symptoms, including symptoms of intrusion, avoidance, negative mood or cognitions, and hyperarousal. These symptoms cause significant functional impairment and are present for more than a month.

We outline the diagnostic approach to posttraumatic stress disorder in Table 10-1.

As with most disorders, substance use or a medical condition should not better explain the symptoms.

With acute stress disorder, the primary feature differentiating this disorder from PTSD is the time course, with the symptoms of acute stress disorder occurring 3 days to 1 month following a traumatic event. Acute stress disorder can have any of the symptoms of PTSD; however, they do not have to have all the domains. A person who experiences a minimum of nine symptoms from any of these domains within 3 days to 1 month of a traumatic event meets the criteria for acute stress disorder.

We outline the diagnostic approach to acute stress disorder in Table 10-2.

Three weeks after a train derailment, a 42-year-old budget analyst presented to the mental health clinic. He noted that he was embarrassed to seek care, as he was previously a firefighter, but felt he needed "some reassurance that what I'm experiencing is normal." He reported that, since the wreck, he had been feeling nervous and on edge. He experienced some difficulty focusing his attention at work, and he had occasional intrusive recollections of "the way the ground just shook; the tremendous 'bang' and then the screaming when the train rolled over." He noted that he had spoken with five business colleagues who were also on the train, and three acknowledged similar symptoms. However, they said that they were improving. He was more concerned about the frequency of tearful episodes, sometimes brought on by hearing the name of a severely injured friend, but, at other times, occurring "for no particular reason." Also, he noted that, when he evacuated the train, rescue workers gave him explicit directions about where to report, and, although the man complied, he now felt extremely guilty about not returning to the train to assist in the rescue of others. He reported a modest decrease in appetite and denied weight loss but noted that he had stopped jogging during his lunch break. He had difficulty initiating sleep, so he had begun consuming a "glass or two" of wine before bed to help with this. He did not feel rested on awakening. He denied suicidal ideation or any psychotic symptoms. His sister had taken an antidepressant several years ago, but he did not desire medication. He feared that side effects could further diminish his ability to function at the workplace and could cause him to gain weight. (Courtesy of D. M. Benedek, M.D., R. J. Ursano, M.D., and H. C. Holloway, M.D.)

Adjustment Disorders

Clinicians tend to use the diagnostic category of adjustment disorders liberally. Although this disorder must follow a stressor, the symptoms do not necessarily begin immediately. Up to 3 months

may elapse between a stressor and the development of symptoms. Symptoms do not always subside as soon as the stressor ceases; if the stressor continues, the disorder may be chronic. The disorder can occur at any age, and its symptoms vary considerably, with depressive, anxious, and mixed features most common in adults. Physical symptoms, which are most common in children and the elderly, can occur in any age group. Manifestations may also include impulsivity, violence, excessive alcohol consumption, and suspiciousness.

The clinical presentations of adjustment disorder can vary widely.

We outline the diagnostic approach to adjustment disorder in Table 10-3.

Adjustment Disorder with Depressed Mood. In adjustment disorder with depressed mood, symptoms may manifest as depression, hyposomnia, low self-esteem, or suicidal ideation. We should distinguish this disorder from a major depressive disorder and uncomplicated bereavement.

Adjustment Disorder with Anxiety. Symptoms such as generalized anxiety, increased motor activity, and situational anxiety are present in adjustment disorder with anxiety, which we should differentiate from anxiety disorders.

Adjustment Disorder with Mixed Anxiety and Depressed Mood. In adjustment disorder with mixed anxiety and depressed mood, patients exhibit features of both anxiety and depression that do not meet the criteria for an already established anxiety disorder or depressive disorder.

A 48-year-old married woman, in good health, with no previous psychiatric difficulties, presented to the emergency room, reporting that she had overdosed on a handful of antihistamines shortly before she arrived. She described her problems as having started 2 months earlier, soon after her husband unexpectedly requested a divorce. She felt betrayed after having devoted much of her 20-year marriage to being a wife, mother, and homemaker. She was sad and tearful at times, and she occasionally had difficulty sleeping. Otherwise, she had no vegetative symptoms and enjoyed time with family and friends. She felt desperate and suicidal after she realized that "he no longer loves me." After crisis intervention in the emergency setting, she responded well to individual psychotherapy for over 3 months. She occasionally required benzodiazepines for anxiety during the period of treatment. By the time of discharge, she had returned to her baseline function. She came to terms with the possibility of life after divorce and was exploring her best options under the circumstances. (Courtesy of Jeffrey W. Katzman, M.D., and C. M. A. Geppert, M.D., Ph.D., M.P.H.)

Adjustment Disorder with Disturbance of Conduct. In adjustment disorder with disturbance of conduct, symptoms include impulsivity, lack of insight, and violent behavior. We should differentiate this category from conduct disorder and antisocial personality disorder.

Adjustment Disorder with Mixed Disturbance of Emotions and Conduct. A combination of disturbances of emotions and conduct sometimes occurs. Examples include excessive alcohol ingestion, suspiciousness, hostility, defrauding behavior, and homicidal ideation. Clinicians are encouraged to try to make one or the other diagnosis in the interest of clarity.

Table 10-1
Posttraumatic Stress Disorder Diagnoses in DSM-5 and ICD-10

Disorder	Posttraumatic Stress Disorder	
	DSM-5	**ICD-10**
Diagnostic name	Posttraumatic Stress Disorder	Posttraumatic Stress Disorder
Duration	≥1 mo	Symptoms arise in weeks to months following traumatic event
Symptoms	1. History of exposure to (directly experiencing, repeated exposure witnessing in person, learning of occurrence in close acquaintance) actual threatened death, severe injury, or sexual trauma 2. Intrusive symptoms • Involuntary intrusive memories • In children <6 yr, may see reenactment of event through play • Recurrent nightmares/dreams of the event • In children <6 yr, frightening dreams without identifiable content may be present • Dissociative responses or reliving of prior experience (i.e., flashbacks) • In children <6 yr, may see reenactment of event through play • Psychological distress related to exposure to stimuli that are reminders of prior trauma • Presence of physiologic response to stimuli that are reminders of prior trauma 3. Pattern of avoidance of stimuli associated with prior experience of trauma • Avoidance of memories related to trauma • Avoidance of external reminders of trauma 4. Negative mood or cognitions related to trauma • Impairment in memories related to event • Negative perceptions of self and others • Cognitive distortions related to event • Excessive guilt, anger or fear • Diminished interest and social withdrawal • Subjective detachment from others • Difficulty experiencing positive feelings in response to previously pleasurable stimuli 5. Altered level of arousal • Irritability and/or anger • Risk taking • Hypervigilance • Increased startle response • Difficulties with concentration • Sleep disturbances	1. Symptoms arise as a delayed or prolonged response to a single or recurrent stressful experience that is life-threatening or catastrophic in severity 2. Traumatic event would cause distress in most individuals 3. Symptoms may include • Flashbacks • Dreams/nightmares • Emotional blunting and subjective numbness • Social withdrawal/detachment • Anhedonia • Avoidance • Hyperarousal/hypervigilance • Sleep disturbance 4. May or may not be associated with co-occurring anxiety and/or depression
Required number of symptoms	In addition to history of exposure to trauma, must have • at least one symptom of intrusion • at least one symptom of avoidance • at least two symptoms of negative mood/cognition • at least two symptoms of arousal alterations	Any of the above
Psychosocial consequences of symptoms	Marked distress and impairment in functioning	
Exclusions	• Exposure through media, electronics, movie, or photo • Related to substance use • Related to another medical condition	
Symptom specifiers	**With dissociative symptoms:** • **Depersonalization:** perception of feeling outside one's own body • **Derealization:** perception of surrounding environment being unreal or distorted	
Course specifiers	**With delayed expression:** • All diagnostic criteria not met until 6 mo or more after initial traumatic event	
Severity specifiers		

Table 10-2
Acute Stress Disorder Diagnoses in DSM-5 and ICD-10

Disorder	Acute Stress Disorder	
	DSM-5	**ICD-10**
Diagnostic name	Acute Stress Disorder	Acute Stress Reaction
Duration	3 days to <1 mo following exposure to trauma	Symptoms arise transiently in response to emotional or physical stress and usually resolve within hours or days
Symptoms	1. History of exposure to (directly experiencing, repeated exposure witnessing in person, learning of occurrence in close acquaintance) actual threatened death, severe injury, or sexual trauma 2. Presence of symptoms in the following categories (same as PTSD categories) • Intrusion • Negative mood/cognition • Dissociation • Avoidance • Arousal	1. Cognitive "daze" 2. Narrowed attention 3. Difficulties with comprehension 4. Disorientation 5. Autonomic symptoms of panic 6. May be followed by further withdrawal from the situation or possible agitation/excitability 7. May have partial or complete amnesia related to the event
Required number of symptoms	Nine symptoms from among the above five categories	
Psychosocial consequences of symptoms	Marked distress and impairment in functioning	
Exclusions (not result of):	Substance Other medical condition Brief psychotic disorder or other psychiatric illness	

Table 10-3
Adjustment Disorder Diagnoses in DSM-5 and ICD-10

Disorder	Adjustment Disorders	
	DSM-5	**ICD-10**
Diagnostic name	Adjustment Disorder	Adjustment Disorders
Duration	Occurring within 3 mo of an acute stressor and resolving within 6 mo of resolution of stressor	
Symptoms	1. Emotional or behavioral changes 2. Marked distress/impairment that is felt to be out of proportion to the stressor itself	1. Subjective distress/emotional disturbance 2. Arises during period of adaptation to a change or stress 3. Symptoms of depressed mood or anxiety may arise, and conduct disturbance may be noted in adolescents
Required number of symptoms	All of the above	
Psychosocial consequences of symptoms	Marked distress/functional impairment	Often result in impairment in social functioning
Exclusions (not result of):	Exacerbation of existing mental illness Normal bereavement Other psychiatric illness	
Symptom specifiers	**With depressed mood:** • Predominant low mood, hopelessness **With anxiety:** • Predominant anxiety, worry **With mixed anxiety and depressed mood:** • Both low mood and anxiety present **With mixed disturbance of emotions and conduct:** • Mood and conduct disturbance present **Unspecified**	

Adjustment Disorder Unspecified. Adjustment disorder unspecified is a residual category for atypical maladaptive reactions to stress. Examples include inappropriate responses to the diagnosis of physical illness, such as massive denial, severe noncompliance with treatment, and social withdrawal, without significant depressed or anxious mood.

Other Specified or Unspecified Trauma- or Stressor-Related Disorder

DSM-5 uses the categories of "other specified trauma- or stressor-related disorder" or "unspecified trauma- or stressor-related disorder" uses for patients who develop emotional or behavioral symptoms in response to an identifiable stressor, but do not meet the full criteria for any of the above disorders. The primary difference between these two categories is that "other specified trauma- or stressor-related disorder" is used when it is essential to convey the reason that the patient does not meet the full criteria for one of the other disorders.

DIFFERENTIAL DIAGNOSIS FOR THE TRAUMA- AND STRESSOR-RELATED DISORDERS

Generally, the time requirements and diagnostic criteria help to differentiate PTSD, acute stress disorder, and other psychiatric disorders. With adjustment disorder, one of the challenges is that there are no clear criteria that define the stressors that are required to make this diagnosis. PTSD and acute stress disorder have the nature of the stressor better characterized and include a defined constellation of affective, cognitive, and autonomic symptoms. In contrast, the stressor in adjustment disorder can be of any severity, with a wide range of possible symptoms. When the response to an extreme stressor does not meet the acute stress or posttraumatic disorder threshold, the adjustment disorder diagnosis would be appropriate.

We list some common disorders that can also cause posttraumatic symptomatology in Table 10-4.

Posttraumatic Stress Disorder and Acute Stress Disorder

Because patients often exhibit complex reactions to trauma, the clinician must be careful to exclude other syndromes as well when evaluating patients presenting in the wake of trauma. It is particularly important to recognize potentially treatable medical contributors to posttraumatic symptomatology, especially head injury during the trauma. A careful history and examination can help detect

medical contributors. Epilepsy, alcohol use disorders, and other substance-related disorders can also either cause or exacerbate the symptoms. Acute intoxication or withdrawal from some substances may also present a clinical picture that is difficult to distinguish from the disorder until the effects of the substance have worn off.

Symptoms of PTSD can be difficult to distinguish from both panic disorder and generalized anxiety disorder because all three syndromes are associated with prominent anxiety and autonomic arousal. Keys to correctly diagnosing PTSD include a careful review of the time course relating the symptoms to a traumatic event. PTSD is also associated with intrusion symptoms and avoidance of anything that reminds the person of the trauma, something not usually present in panic or generalized anxiety disorder. Major depression is also a frequent concomitant of PTSD. Although the two syndromes are not generally difficult to distinguish phenomenologically, it is essential to note the presence of comorbid depression because this can influence the treatment of PTSD. We also must differentiate PTSD from several related disorders that can look similar, including borderline personality disorder, dissociative disorders, and factitious disorders. Borderline personality disorder can be difficult to distinguish from PTSD. The two disorders can coexist or even be causally related. Patients with dissociative disorders do not usually have the same degree of avoidance and arousal that PTSD patients do. The time course can distinguish PTSD and acute stress disorder.

Adjustment Disorders

Although uncomplicated bereavement often produces temporarily impaired social and occupational functioning, the person's dysfunction remains within the expectable bounds of a reaction to the loss of a loved one and, thus, is not considered adjustment disorder. We discuss uncomplicated bereavement among the depressive disorders in Chapter 7.

We must differentiate adjustment disorder from many other disorders, and we list some of these in Table 10-5. Patients with an adjustment disorder are impaired in social or occupational functioning and show symptoms beyond the usual and expectable reaction to the stressor. Because no absolute criteria help to distinguish an adjustment disorder from another condition, clinical judgment is necessary. Some patients may meet the criteria for both an adjustment disorder and a personality disorder. If the adjustment disorder follows a physical illness, the clinician must make sure that the symptoms are not a continuation or another manifestation of the illness or its treatment.

COMORBIDITY

Posttraumatic Stress Disorder

Comorbidity rates are high among patients with PTSD, with about two-thirds having at least two other disorders. Common comorbid

Table 10-4
Differential Diagnosis of Posttraumatic Stress Disorder

Medical causes	Traumatic brain injury Epilepsy Alcohol use disorder Substance-related disorders Acute substance or alcohol withdrawal
Psychiatric diagnoses	Panic disorder Generalized anxiety disorder Major depressive disorder Dissociative identity disorder Borderline personality disorder Factitious disorders Acute stress disorder

Table 10-5
Differential Diagnosis of Adjustment Disorders

Major depressive disorder
Brief psychotic disorder
Generalized anxiety disorder
Somatic symptom disorder
Substance-related disorder
Conduct disorder
Antisocial personality disorder
Posttraumatic stress disorder

conditions include depressive disorders, substance-related disorders, anxiety disorders, and bipolar disorders. Comorbid disorders make persons more vulnerable to develop PTSD.

Adjustment Disorders

Most psychiatric disorders can co-occur with adjustment disorder. However, it is critical to ensure that another psychiatric disorder does not best explain the person's response to the stressor.

COURSE AND PROGNOSIS

Posttraumatic Stress Disorder

Immediately following exposure to a traumatic event, many people experience symptoms such as shock, nightmares, and intrusive thoughts about the event. However, we cannot make a diagnosis of PTSD unless enough symptoms persist for at least 1 month. Symptoms can fluctuate over time and may be most intense during periods of stress. Untreated, about 30 percent of patients recover completely, 40 percent continue to have mild symptoms, 20 percent continue to have moderate symptoms, and 10 percent remain unchanged or become worse. After 1 year, about 50 percent of patients will recover.

We list some predictors of good prognosis in Table 10-6.

In general, the very young and the very old have more difficulty with traumatic events than do those in midlife. For example, about 80 percent of young children who sustain a burn injury show symptoms of PTSD 1 or 2 years after the initial injury; only 30 percent of adults who suffer such an injury have symptoms of PTSD after 1 year. Presumably, young children do not yet have adequate coping mechanisms to deal with the physical and emotional insults of the trauma. Likewise, older persons are likely to have more rigid coping mechanisms than younger adults and to be less able to muster a flexible approach to dealing with the effects of trauma. Furthermore, physical disabilities typical of late life can exacerbate the symptoms. Examples include impairments of the nervous system and the cardiovascular system, such as reduced cerebral blood flow, failing vision, palpitations, and arrhythmias. Pre-existing psychiatric disability also increases the effects of stressors. PTSD that is comorbid with other disorders is often more severe and perhaps more chronic and may be challenging to treat. The availability of social supports may also influence the development, severity, and duration of PTSD. In general, patients who have a good network of social support are less likely to have the disorder and to experience it in its severe forms and are more likely to recover faster.

Adjustment Disorders

With appropriate treatment, the overall prognosis of an adjustment disorder is generally favorable. Most patients return to their previous level of functioning within 3 months. Some persons

(particularly adolescents) who receive a diagnosis of an adjustment disorder later have mood disorders or substance-related disorders. Adolescents usually require a longer time to recover than adults.

Research has disclosed a risk for suicide not previously fully appreciated. Some studies suggest that a high proportion of patients with adjustment disorders have had past suicide attempts and recent suicidality. This data is difficult to interpret, given the extensive and sometimes inconsistent use of this diagnosis; however, it is critical to evaluate for suicidality in patients with this disorder.

A 16-year-old high school senior's first relationship ended when his girlfriend rejected him. In the weeks after the end of the relationship, he began to exhibit dysphoric mood accompanied by anxiety and psychomotor agitation. He had received counseling in junior high school when his parents divorced, and he began using alcohol and marijuana. His school suspended him during his freshman year for fighting. A month after the breakup, he began to tell his parents that life was no longer worth living without his former girlfriend. Two months later, his parents came home from work and found him hanging in the garage with a note stating he could not go on alone. (Courtesy of J. W. Katzman, M.D., and C. M. A. Geppert, M.D., Ph.D., M.P.H.)

TREATMENT APPROACH

Posttraumatic Stress Disorder

We list some of the most common treatments for PTSD and related disorders in Table 10-7.

Pharmacotherapy. Currently, selective serotonin reuptake inhibitors (SSRIs), particularly sertraline and paroxetine, have the most robust evidence for efficacy. There are promising initial findings for the noradrenergic and serotonergic reuptake inhibitor venlafaxine, the atypical antipsychotic risperidone, and the anticonvulsant topiramate. We lack evidence for the effectiveness

Table 10-7
Treatments for PTSD

Pharmacologic interventions	Strong evidence
	SSRIs (sertraline, paroxetine)
	Promising initial evidence
	SNRI (venlafaxine)
	Atypical antipsychotic (risperidone)
	Anticonvulsant (topiramate)
	Limited evidence
	Alpha 1-adrenergic antagonist (prazosin)
	Lack of evidence
	Benzodiazepines
	Symptom-specific
	Prazosin (nightmares)
	Orexin (insomnia)
	Trazodone (insomnia)
Psychotherapeutic interventions	Trauma-focused cognitive-behavioral therapy (TFCBT),
	Prolonged exposure (PE) therapy
	Cognitive processing therapy (CPT)
	Eye movement desensitization and reprocessing therapy (EMDR)
	Present centered therapy (PCT)
	Cognitive processing therapy (CPT)
	Psychodynamic psychotherapy
	Group and family therapy

Table 10-6
Positive Prognostic Factors for PTSD

Rapid onset of the symptoms
Short duration of the symptoms (less than 6 mo)
Good premorbid functioning
Strong social supports
Absence of other psychiatric, medical, or substance-related
   disorders or other risk factors

of benzodiazepines, despite their continued use in practice; one meta-analysis went so far as to consider benzodiazepines relatively contraindicated in this population. Finally, the alpha 1-adrenergic antagonist prazosin and the atypical antipsychotics show some efficacy in treatment-resistant PTSD, and prazosin shows effectiveness for treating nightmares. Insomnia is prevalent and disabling in chronic PTSD, with low-dose trazodone preferable to benzodiazepines. The orexin antagonist suvorexant is promising for managing trauma-related insomnia.

Psychotherapy. Several therapies are effective for PTSD and related disorders; we list these in Table 10-7. Trauma-focused cognitive-behavioral therapy (TFCBT) includes prolonged exposure (PE) therapy, which focuses on reexperiencing the traumatic event through repeatedly engaging with the memories (imaginal exposure) and everyday reminders (in vivo exposure) rather than avoiding triggers. Eye movement desensitization and reprocessing therapy (EMDR) involves repeatedly recalling distressing images while receiving sensory inputs. Present centered therapy (PCT) focuses on the current relationship and work challenges rather than the trauma, and cognitive processing therapy (CPT) emphasizes correcting faulty attributions including posttraumatic overgeneralizations of the world as dangerous, uncontrollable, and unpredictable. Psychodynamic psychotherapy may also be useful in the treatment of many patients with PTSD. In some cases, reconstruction of the traumatic events with associated abreaction and catharsis may be therapeutic. Still, psychotherapy must be tailored to the individual, because reexperiencing the trauma overwhelms some patients.

In addition to individual therapy techniques, group therapy and family therapy are effective for PTSD. The advantages of group therapy include the sharing of traumatic experiences and support from other group members. Group therapy has been particularly successful with Vietnam veterans and survivors of catastrophic disasters such as earthquakes. Family therapy often helps sustain a marriage through periods of exacerbated symptoms. Hospitalization may be necessary when symptoms are particularly severe or when the risk of suicide or other violence exists.

Adjustment Disorders

Psychotherapy. Psychotherapy remains the treatment of choice for adjustment disorders. Group therapy can be particularly useful for patients who have had similar stresses—for example, a group of retired persons or patients having renal dialysis. Individual psychotherapy interventions include supportive psychological approaches, cognitive-behavioral, problem-solving techniques, and psychodynamic interventions. After successful therapy, patients sometimes emerge from an adjustment disorder stronger than in the premorbid period, although no pathology was evident during that period. Because there is an explicit stressor, some clinicians mistakenly deemphasize psychotherapy and believe that the disorder will remit spontaneously. This viewpoint, however, ignores the fact that many persons exposed to the same stressor experience different symptoms, and in adjustment disorders, the response is pathologic. Psychotherapy can help persons adapt to stressors that are not reversible or time-limited and can serve as a preventive intervention if the stressor does remit.

Crisis Intervention. Crisis intervention and case management are short-term treatments aimed at helping persons with adjustment disorders resolve their situations quickly by supportive techniques, suggestion, reassurance, environmental modification, and even

hospitalization, if necessary. The frequency and length of visits for crisis support vary according to patients' needs; daily sessions may be required, sometimes two or three times each day. Flexibility is essential in this approach.

Pharmacotherapy. There is limited evidence for the efficacy of pharmacologic interventions in persons with adjustment disorder. Still, it may be reasonable to use medication to treat specific symptoms for a brief time. The judicious use of medications can help patients with adjustment disorders, but we should only use them for short periods. Depending on the type of adjustment disorder, a patient may respond to an antianxiety agent or an antidepressant. It is often helpful and important to treat insomnia and severe anxiety with pharmacologic interventions in the short run. It is not as clear whether it helps to treat the depressive symptoms using medication. Clinicians have found some SSRIs to be useful for treating some subthreshold depressive symptoms and may benefit certain subtypes of adjustment disorders. Pharmacologic intervention in this population should mainly augment psychosocial strategies and not serve as the primary modality.

EPIDEMIOLOGY

Posttraumatic Stress Disorder

About 6.8 percent of the general population has a lifetime prevalence of PTSD, with a current past year prevalence estimated at 3.5 percent. The lifetime prevalence rate is 9.7 percent in women and 3.6 percent in men. According to the National Vietnam Veterans Readjustment Study (NVVRS), 30.9 percent of men developed full-blown PTSD after having served in the war, and 26.9 percent of women developed the disorder. A 25-year follow-up of the NVVRS, the National Vietnam Veteran Longitudinal Study (NVVLS), was conducted to assess the course of PTSD 40 years after the war. This study found that the current prevalence of war zone PTSD was 4.5 percent, and the lifetime prevalence of war zone PTSD was 17 percent.

Although PTSD can appear at any age, it is most prevalent in young adults because they tend to be more exposed to precipitating situations. Children can also have the disorder. The disorder is most likely to occur in those who are single, divorced, widowed, socially withdrawn, or of low socioeconomic level, but anyone can be affected, and no one is immune. The most important risk factors, however, for this disorder are the severity, duration, and proximity of a person's exposure to the actual trauma. A familial pattern seems to exist for this disorder, and first-degree biologic relatives of persons with a history of depression have an increased risk for developing PTSD following a traumatic event.

Adjustment Disorders

Few studies have examined the prevalence of adjustment disorder in community samples. One study that did assess for the presence of adjustment disorder was the European Outcome of Depression International Network (ODIN) study, which found that less than 1 percent of subjects had adjustment disorder. Another study examined the prevalence of adjustment disorder in a primary care setting and found that 2.94 percent of the sample met the criteria for adjustment disorder. There is a higher prevalence of adjustment disorder in the medical setting—especially patients with cancer and those receiving palliative care. For example, one study found that 11 percent of individuals with mixed cancer diagnoses had an adjustment disorder.

ETIOLOGY

Posttraumatic Stress Disorder

Risk Factors for PTSD.   Even when faced with overwhelming trauma, most persons do not experience PTSD symptoms. The National Comorbidity Study found that 60 percent of males and 50 percent of females had experienced some significant trauma. In contrast, the reported lifetime prevalence of PTSD, as mentioned earlier, was much lower. Similarly, events that may appear mundane or less than catastrophic to most persons can produce PTSD in some. Evidence indicates a dose–response relationship between the degree of trauma and the likelihood of symptoms.

A meta-analysis of risk factors for PTSD in the community found that female gender, age at trauma, race, lower education, childhood abuse, higher severity of trauma exposure, lack of social support, and additional life stress increased risk for PTSD. A second meta-analysis identified seven predictors: prior trauma, prior psychological adjustment, family history of psychopathology, more significant perceived life threat during the trauma, lower posttrauma social support, more considerable emotional distress during exposure, and higher dissociation during exposure. For combat-related PTSD, identified risk factors include lower education, non-officer ranks, army service, combat specialization, higher numbers of deployments, longer cumulative length of deployments, more adverse life events, prior trauma exposure, and previous psychological problems. Various aspects of the trauma period also constituted risk factors, including higher levels of combat exposure, discharging a weapon, witnessing someone being wounded or killed, severe trauma, and deployment-related stressors. Another study reported that killing enemy combatants, prisoners of war, and civilians in the war zone increased the risk of PTSD.

Table 10-8 summarizes vulnerability factors that appear to play etiologic roles in the disorder.

Genetics and Risk for PTSD.   Genes account for about 30 percent of the variance in the risk for PTSD. A study of Vietnam veteran twin pairs reported that monozygotic twins of veterans with combat-related PTSD had more significant mood disorder symptoms than monozygotic co-twins of combat controls or dizygotic co-twins of veterans with PTSD. The findings suggest a shared genetic vulnerability to PTSD and mood disorders. Other studies have indicated that PTSD symptoms are moderately heritable, with the remaining vulnerability accounted for by unique environmental experiences. Several common genetic variants are associated with PTSD, including polymorphisms in FKBP5, PACAP1, COMT, DRD2, GABA alpha-2 receptor, G-protein signaling 2 (RSG2), an SNP in an intergenic region of the fourth chromosome, and an estrogen response element on ADCYAP R1. Also, the s/s genotype

Table 10-8
Predisposing Vulnerability Factors in Posttraumatic Stress Disorder

Presence of childhood trauma
Borderline, paranoid, dependent, or antisocial personality disorder traits
Inadequate family or peer support system
Being female
Genetic vulnerability to psychiatric illness
Recent stressful life changes
Perception of an external locus of control (natural cause) rather than an internal one (human cause)
Recent excessive alcohol intake

of the serotonin transporter gene may interact with childhood adversity to increase PTSD risk.

Adjustment Disorders

By definition, a stressor precipitates an adjustment disorder. The severity of the stressor or stressors does not always predict the severity of the disorder; the stressor severity is a complex function of degree, quantity, duration, reversibility, environment, and personal context. For example, the loss of a parent is different for a child 10 years of age than for a person 40 years of age. Personality organization and cultural or group norms and values also contribute to the disproportionate responses to stressors.

Stressors may be single, such as the death of a loved one, divorce, losing a job, or medical illness. Alternatively, they can be a combination of any of these. Stressors may be recurrent, such as seasonal business difficulties, or continuous, such as chronic illness or poverty. A discordant intrafamilial relationship can produce an adjustment disorder that affects the entire family system, or the disorder may be limited to a patient who was perhaps the victim of a crime or who has a physical illness. Sometimes, adjustment disorders occur in a group or community setting, and the stressors affect several persons, as in a natural disaster or racial, social, or religious persecution. Specific developmental stages, such as beginning school, leaving home, getting married, becoming a parent, failing to achieve occupational goals, having the last child leave home, and retiring, are often associated with adjustment disorders.

Psychodynamic Factors.   Pivotal to understanding adjustment disorders is an understanding of three factors: the nature of the stressor, the conscious and unconscious meanings of the stressor, and the patient's pre-existing vulnerability. A concurrent personality disorder or organic impairment may make a person vulnerable to adjustment disorders. Vulnerability is also associated with the loss of a parent during infancy or growing up in a dysfunctional family. Actual or perceived support from crucial relationships can affect behavioral and emotional responses to stressors.

Clinicians must undertake a detailed exploration of a patient's experience of the stressor. Some patients commonly place all the blame on a particular event when a less apparent event may have had more significant psychological meaning for the patient. Current events may reawaken past traumas or disappointments from childhood, so patients should be encouraged to think about how the current situation relates to similar past events.

Throughout early development, each child develops a unique set of defense mechanisms to deal with stressful events. Because of higher amounts of trauma or greater constitutional vulnerability, some children have less mature defensive constellations than other children. This disadvantage may cause them as adults to react with substantially impaired functioning when facing a loss, divorce, or a financial setback; those who have developed mature defense mechanisms are less vulnerable and bounce back more quickly from the stressor. Resilience is also crucially determined by the nature of children's early relationships with their parents. Studies of trauma repeatedly indicate that supportive, nurturing relationships prevent traumatic incidents from causing permanent psychological damage.

Psychodynamic clinicians must consider the relationship between a stressor and the human developmental life cycle. When adolescents leave home for college, for example, they are at high developmental risk for reacting with a temporary symptomatic picture. Similarly, if the young person who leaves home is the last child in the family, the parents may be particularly vulnerable to a reaction of adjustment disorder. Moreover, middle-aged persons who are confronting their mortality may be especially sensitive to the effects of loss or death.

References

Alexander S, Kuntz S. PTSD-related sleep disturbances: Is there evidence-based treatment? *JAAPA*. 2012;25:44.

American Psychiatric Association. *Diagnostic and Statistical Manual of Mental Disorders*. 5th ed. Arlington, VA: American Psychiatric Association; 2013.

Barnes JB, Dickstein BD, Maguen S, Neria Y, Litz BT. The distinctiveness of prolonged grief and posttraumatic stress disorder in adults bereaved by the attacks of September 11th. *J Affect Disord*. 2012;136:366.

Benedek DM, Ursano RJ, Holloway HC. Disaster psychiatry: Disaster, terrorism, and war. In: Sadock BJ, Sadock VA, Ruiz P, eds. *Kaplan & Sadock's Comprehensive Textbook of Psychiatry*. 10th ed. Philadelphia, PA: Wolters Kluwer; 2017:2564–2576.

Biggs QM, Fullerton CS, Reeves JJ, Grieger TA, Reissman D, Ursano RJ. Acute stress disorder, depression, and tobacco use in disaster workers following 9/11. *Am J Orthopsychiatry*. 2010;80:586.

Bryant RA. Acute stress disorder as a predictor of posttraumatic stress disorder: A systematic review. *J Clin Psychiatry*. 2011;72:233.

Busch AB, Yoon F, Barry CL, Azzone V, Normand SL, Goldman HH, Huskamp HA. The effects of mental health parity on spending and utilization for bipolar, major depression, and adjustment disorders. *Am J Psychiatry*. 2013;170(2):180–187.

Casey P, Maracy M, Kelly BD, Lehtinen V, Ayuso-Mateos JL, Dalgard OS, Dowrick C. Can adjustment disorder and depressive episode be distinguished? Results from ODIN. *J Affective Disord*. 2006;92:291–297.

Chen PF, Chen CS, Chen CC, Lung FW. Alexithymia as a screening index for male conscripts with adjustment disorder. *Psychiatr Q*. 2011;82:139.

Cloitre M, Garvert DW, Brewin CR, Bryant RA, Maercker A. Evidence for proposed ICD-11 PTSD and complex PTSD: A latent profile analysis. *Eur J Psychotraumatol*. 2013;4.

Daniels J. The perils of "adjustment disorder" as a diagnostic category. *J Humanistic Counsel*. 2009;48:77.

Elklit A, Christiansen DM. Acute stress disorder and posttraumatic stress disorder in rape victims. *J Interper Viol*. 2010;25(8):1470–1488.

Fareed A, Eilender P, Haber M, Bremner J, Whitfield N, Drexler K. Comorbid posttraumatic stress disorder and opiate addiction: A literature review. *J Addict Dis*. 2013;32(2):168–179.

Fernández A, Mendive JM, Salvador-Carulla L, Rubio-Valera M, Luciano JV, Pinto-Meza A, Haro JM, Palao DJ, Bellón JA, Serrano-Blanco A; DASMAP investigators. Adjustment disorders in primary care: Prevalence, recognition and use of services. *Br J Psychiatry*. 2012;201:137–142.

Forneris CA, Gartlehner G, Brownley KA, Gaynes BN, Sonis J, Coker-Schwimmer E, Jonas DE, Greenblatt A, Wilkins TM, Woodell CL, Lohr KN. Interventions to prevent posttraumatic stress disorder: A systematic review. *Am J Prev Med*. 2013;44(6):635–650.

Fuina J, Rossetter SR, DeRhodes BJ, Nahhas RW, Welton RS. Benzodiazepines for PTSD: A systematic review and meta-analysis. *J Psychiatr Pract*. 2015;21:281–303.

Giltaij HP, Sterkenburg PS, Schuengel C. Psychiatric diagnostic screening of social maladaptive behaviour in children with mild intellectual disability: Differentiating disordered attachment and pervasive developmental disorder behaviour. *J Intellect Disabil Res*. 2015;59(2):138–149.

Jamieson JP, Mendes WB, Nock MK. Improving acute stress responses: The power of reappraisal. *Curr Dir Psychol Sci*. 2013;22(1):51–56.

Jovanovic T, Sakoman AJ, Kozarić-Kovačić D, Meštrović AH, Duncan EJ, Davis M, Norrholm SD. Acute stress disorder versus chronic posttraumatic stress disorder: Inhibition of fear as a function of time since trauma. *Depress Anxiety*. 2013;30(3):217–224.

Katzman JW, Geppert CMA. Adjustment disorders. In: Sadock BJ, Sadock VA, Ruiz P, eds. *Kaplan & Sadock's Comprehensive Textbook of Psychiatry*. 10th ed. Philadelphia, PA: Wolters Kluwer; 2017.

Kim-Cohen J, Turkewitz R. Resilience and measured gene-environment interactions. *Dev Psychopathol*. 2012;24(4):1297–1306.

Krystal JH, Pietrzak RH, Rosenheck RA, Cramer JA, Vessicchio J, Jones KM, Huang GD, Vertrees JE, Collins J, Krystal AD; Veterans Affairs Cooperative Study #504 Group. Sleep disturbance in chronic military-related PTSD: clinical impact and response to adjunctive risperidone in the Veterans Affairs Cooperative Study #504. *J Clin Psychiatry*. 2016;77:483–491.

Kryzhanovskaya L, Canterbury R. Suicidal behavior in patients with adjustment disorders. *Crisis*. 2001;22:152–131.

Le QA, Doctor JN, Zoellner LA, Feeny NC. Cost-effectiveness of prolonged exposure therapy versus pharmacotherapy and treatment choice in posttraumatic stress disorder (the optimizing PTSD treatment trial): A doubly randomized preference trial. *J Clin Psychiatry*. 2014;75(3):222–230.

Lederberg MS, Loscalzo MJ, McCorkle RS, eds. *Psycho-Oncology*. 2nd ed. New York: Oxford University Press; 2010:303.

Li M, Hales S, Rodin GM. Adjustment disorders. In: Holland JC, Breitbart WS, Jacobsen PB, Lederberg MS, Loscalzo MJ, McCorkle RS, eds. *Psycho-Oncology*. 2nd ed. New York: Oxford University Press; 2010.

Marmar CR, Schlenger W, Henn-Haase C, Qian M, Purchia E, Li M, Corry N, Williams CS, Ho C, Horesh D, Karstoft K, Shalev A, Kulka RA. Course of posttraumatic stress disorder 40 years after the Vietnam War: Findings from the National Vietnam Veterans Longitudinal Study. *JAMA Psychiatry*. 2015;72:875–881.

Mehnert A, Brahler E, Faller H, Härter M, Keller M, Schulz H, Wegscheider K, Weis J, Boehncke A, Hund B, Reuter K, Richard M, Sehner S, Sommerfeldt S, Szalai C, Wittchen HU, Koch U. Four-week prevalence of mental disorders in patients with cancer across major tumor entities. *J Clin Oncol*. 2014;32:3540–3546.

Panagioti M, Gooding PA, Tarrier N. Hopelessness, defeat, and entrapment in posttraumatic stress disorder: Their association with suicidal behavior and severity of depression. *J Nerv Ment Dis*. 2012;200:676.

Ponniah K, Hollon SD. Empirically supported psychological treatments for adult acute stress disorder and posttraumatic stress disorder: A review. *Depress Anxiety*. 2009;26:1086.

Regier DA, Kuhl EA, Kupfer DJ. The DSM-5: Classification and criteria changes. *World Psychiatry*. 2013;12(2):92–98.

Schuengel C, Schipper JC, Sterkenburg PS, Kef S. Attachment, intellectual disabilities and mental health: Research, assessment and intervention. *J Appl Res Intellect Dis*. 2013;26(1):34–46.

Schulze T, Maercker A, Horn AB. Mental health and multimorbidity: Psychosocial adjustment as an important process for quality of life. *Gerontology*. 2014;60(3):249–254.

Shalev AY, Marmar C. Posttraumatic stress disorder. In: Sadock BJ, Sadock VA, Ruiz P, eds. *Kaplan & Sadock's Comprehensive Textbook of Psychiatry*. 10th ed. Philadelphia, PA: Wolters Kluwer; 2017:1812–1826.

Shalev AY, Marmar CR. Posttraumatic stress disorder. In: Sadock BJ, Sadock VA, Ruiz P, eds. *Kaplan & Sadock's Comprehensive Textbook of Psychiatry*. 10th ed. Philadelphia, PA: Wolters Kluwer; 2017.

Simon NM. Treating complicated grief. *JAMA*. 2013;310(4):416–423.

Sones HM, Thorp SR, Raskind M. Prevention of posttraumatic stress disorder. *Psychiatr Clin North Am*. 2011;34:79.

Strain JJ, Diefenbache A. The adjustment disorders: The conundrums of the diagnoses. *Compr Psychiatry*. 2008;49:121.

Strain JJ, Friedman MJ. Considering adjustment disorders as stress response syndromes for DSM-5. *Depress Anxiety*. 2011;28:818.

Varma A, Moore MB, Miller CWT, Himelhoch S. Topiramate as monotherapy or adjunctive treatment for posttraumatic stressor disorder: A meta-analysis. *J Trauma Stress*. 2018;31:125–133.

Watts BV, Schnurr PP, Mayo L, Young-Xu Y, Weeks WB, Friedman MJ. Meta-analysis of the efficacy of treatments for posttraumatic stress disorder. *J Clin Psychiatry*. 2013;74:e541–e550.

Zantvoord JB, Diehle J, Lindauer RJ. Using neurobiological measures to predict and assess treatment outcome of psychotherapy in posttraumatic stress disorder: Systematic review. *Psychother Psychosom*. 2013;82(3):142–151.

Zimmerman M, Martinez JH, Dalrymple K, Chelminski I, Young D. "Subthreshold" depression: Is the distinction between depressive disorder not otherwise specified and adjustment disorder valid? *J Clin Psychiatry*. 2013;74(5):470–476.

11 ◢◣

Dissociative Disorders

In psychiatry, *dissociation* is an unconscious defense mechanism involving the segregation of any group of mental or behavioral processes from the rest of the person's psychic activity. Dissociative disorders involve this mechanism so that there is a disruption in one or more mental functions, such as memory, identity, perception, consciousness, or motor behavior. The disturbance may be sudden or gradual, transient or chronic, and psychological trauma is often the cause.

DIAGNOSTIC AND CLINICAL FEATURES

Dissociative Amnesia

The main feature of dissociative amnesia is the inability to recall important personal information, usually related to a significant trauma or stressor, that is too extensive to be explained by ordinary forgetfulness. The disorder cannot result from the direct physiologic effects of a substance or a neurologic or other general medical condition.

Table 11-1 lists the different types of dissociative amnesia.

> A 45-year-old, divorced, left-handed, male bus dispatcher was seen in psychiatric consultation on a medical unit. He had been admitted with an episode of chest discomfort, light-headedness, and left-arm weakness. He had a history of hypertension and had a medical admission in the past year for ischemic chest pain, although he had not suffered a myocardial infarction. Psychiatric consultation was called, because the patient complained of memory loss for the previous 12 years, behaving and responding to the environment as if it were 12 years previously (e.g., he did not recognize his 8-year-old son, insisted that he was unmarried, and denied recollection of current events, such as the name of the current president). Physical and laboratory findings were unchanged from the patient's usual baseline. Brain computed tomography (CT) scan was normal.
>
> On mental status examination, the patient displayed intact intellectual function but insisted that the date was 12 years earlier, denying recall of his entire subsequent personal history and of current events for the past 12 years. He was perplexed by the contradiction between his memory and current circumstances. The patient described a family history of brutal beatings and physical discipline. He was a decorated combat veteran, although he described amnestic episodes for some of his combat experiences. In the military, he had been a champion golden glove boxer noted for his powerful left hand.
>
> He was educated about his disorder and given the suggestion that his memory could return as he could tolerate it, perhaps overnight during sleep or perhaps over a longer time. If this strategy was unsuccessful, hypnosis or an amobarbital interview was proposed. (Adapted from a case of Richard J. Loewenstein, M.D., and Frank W. Putnam, M.D.)

Classic Presentation. The classic disorder is an overt, florid, dramatic clinical disturbance that quickly presents for medical attention. A history of extreme acute trauma is typical. It also commonly develops, however, in the context of profound intrapsychic conflict or emotional stress. Patients may present with physical symptoms, alterations in consciousness, depersonalization, derealization, trance states, spontaneous age regression, and even ongoing anterograde dissociative amnesia. There is a significant risk of depression and suicidal ideation. No single personality profile or antecedent history is consistently reported in these patients, although a prior personal or family history of somatoform or dissociative symptoms can predispose individuals to develop acute amnesia during traumatic circumstances. Many of these patients have histories of prior adult or childhood abuse or trauma. In wartime cases, as in other forms of combat-related posttraumatic disorders, the most crucial variable in the development of dissociative symptoms, however, appears to be the intensity of combat.

Table 11-2 presents the mental status evaluation of dissociative amnesia.

Nonclassic Presentation. These patients frequently come to treatment for a variety of symptoms, such as depression or mood swings, substance abuse, sleep disturbances, somatoform symptoms, anxiety and panic, suicidal or self-mutilating impulses and acts, violent outbursts, eating problems, and interpersonal problems. Self-mutilation and violent behavior in these patients may also occur. Amnesia may also occur for flashbacks or behavioral reexperiencing episodes related to trauma.

Dissociative Fugue. DSM-5 treats dissociative fugue as a subtype of dissociative amnesia, whereas it is a separate diagnosis in ICD-10. It can occur in patients with both dissociative amnesia and dissociative identity disorder.

Dissociative fugue is as sudden, unexpected travel away from home or one's customary place of daily activities. Also, the person cannot recall some or all of one's past. Along with the amnesia, the person is confused about their identity or may even assume a new identity. The disturbance is not due to the direct physiologic effects of a substance or a general medical condition.

Dissociative fugues have been described to last from minutes to months. Some patients report multiple fugues. In some extreme cases of posttraumatic stress disorder (PTSD), a person may awaken from a nightmare in a fugue state. Children or adolescents may be more limited than adults in their ability to travel. Thus, fugues in this population may be brief and involve only short distances.

> A teenage girl was continually sexually abused by her alcoholic father and another family friend. She was threatened with perpetration of sexual abuse on her younger siblings if she told anyone about the abuse. The girl became suicidal but felt that she had to stay alive to

Table 11-1
Types of Dissociative Amnesia

Localized amnesia: Inability to recall events related to a circumscribed period of time

Selective amnesia: Ability to remember some, but not all, of the events occurring during a circumscribed period of time

Generalized amnesia: Failure to recall one's entire life

Continuous amnesia: Failure to recall successive events as they occur

Systematized amnesia: Failure to remember a category of information, such as all memories relating to one's family or to a particular person

protect her siblings. She ran away from home after being raped by her father and several of his friends. She traveled to a part of the city where she had lived previously with the idea of finding her grandmother with whom she had lived before the abuse began. She traveled by public transportation and walked the streets, apparently without attracting attention. After approximately 8 hours, she was stopped by the police in a curfew check. When questioned, she could not recall recent events or give her current address, insisting that she lived with her grandmother. On initial psychiatric examination, she was aware of her identity, but she believed that it was 2 years earlier, giving her age as 2 years younger and insisting that none of the events of recent years had occurred. (Courtesy of Richard J. Loewenstein, M.D., and Frank W. Putnam, M.D.)

Table 11-2
Mental Status Examination Questions for Dissociative Amnesia

If answers are positive, ask the patient to describe the event. Make sure to specify that the symptom does not occur during an episode of intoxication.

1. Do you ever have blackouts? Blank spells? Memory lapses?
2. Do you lose time? Have gaps in your experience of time?
3. Have you ever traveled a considerable distance without recollection of how you did this or where you went exactly?
4. Do people tell you of things you have said and done that you do not recall?
5. Do you find objects in your possession (such as clothes, personal items, groceries in your grocery cart, books, tools, equipment, jewelry, vehicles, weapons, and so on) that you do not remember acquiring? Out-of-character items? Items that a child might have? Toys? Stuffed animals?
6. Have you ever been told or found evidence that you have talents and abilities that you did not know that you had? For example, musical, artistic, mechanical, literary, athletic, or other talents? Do your tastes seem to fluctuate a lot? For example, food preference, personal habits, taste in music or clothes, and so forth.
7. Do you have gaps in your memory of your life? Are you missing parts of your memory for your life history? Are you missing memories of some important events in your life? For example, weddings, birthdays, graduations, pregnancies, birth of children, and so on.
8. Do you lose track of or tune out conversations or therapy sessions as they are occurring? Do you find that, while you are listening to someone talk, you did not hear all or part of what was just said?
9. What is the longest period of time that you have lost? Minutes? Hours? Days? Weeks? Months? Years? Describe.

Adapted from Loewenstein RJ. An office mental status examination for chronic complex dissociative symptoms and multiple personality disorder. *Psychiatr Clin North Am.* 1991;14(3):567–604.

After the termination of a fugue, the patient may experience perplexity, confusion, trance-like behaviors, depersonalization, derealization, and conversion symptoms, in addition to amnesia. Some patients may terminate a fugue with an episode of generalized dissociative amnesia.

As the patient with dissociative fugue begins to become less dissociated, he or she may display mood disorder symptoms, intense suicidal ideation, and PTSD or anxiety disorder symptoms. In classic cases, the person has an alter identity under whose auspices the patient lives for a period. Many of these latter cases are better classified as dissociative identity disorder or, if using DSM-5, as other specified dissociative disorder with features of dissociative identity disorder.

Differential Diagnosis

Table 11-3 lists the differential diagnosis of dissociative amnesia.

Ordinary Forgetfulness and Nonpathologic Amnesia.
Ordinary forgetfulness is benign and unrelated to stressful events. In dissociative amnesia, memory loss is more extensive than in nonpathologic amnesia. There are other types of nonpathologic amnesia as well, including infantile and childhood amnesia, amnesia for sleep and dreaming, and hypnotic amnesia.

Dementia, Delirium, and Amnestic Disorders due to Medical Conditions.
In patients with dementia, delirium, and amnestic disorders due to medical conditions, memory loss is part of a more extensive set of cognitive, language, attentional, behavioral, and memory problems. Loss of memory for personal identity is usually not found without evidence of a marked disturbance in many domains of cognitive function. Causes of organic amnestic disorders include Korsakoff psychosis, cerebral vascular accident (CVA), postoperative amnesia, postinfectious amnesia, anoxic amnesia, and transient global amnesia (see below). Electroconvulsive therapy (ECT) may also cause marked temporary amnesia, as well as persistent memory problems in some cases. Here, however, memory loss for autobiographical experience is unrelated to traumatic or overwhelming experiences and seems to involve many different types of personal experiences, most commonly those occurring just before or during the ECT treatments.

Posttraumatic Amnesia.
In posttraumatic amnesia caused by brain injury, we usually find a history of a clear-cut physical trauma, a period of unconsciousness or amnesia, or both. Also, there is objective clinical evidence of brain injury.

Seizure Disorders.
In most seizure cases, the clinical presentation differs significantly from that of dissociative amnesia, with clear-cut ictal events and sequelae. In complex–partial seizures, patients may wander or show semipurposeful behavior, or both, during seizures or in postictal states, for which subsequent amnesia occurs. Rarely, patients with recurrent, complex–partial seizures present with ongoing bizarre behavior, memory problems, irritability, or violence, leading to a differential diagnostic puzzle. Seizure patients in an epileptic fugue often exhibit abnormal behavior, however, including confusion, perseveration, and abnormal or repetitive movements. Patients with pseudoepileptic seizures may also have dissociative symptoms, such as amnesia and an antecedent history of psychological trauma. In some of these cases, the diagnosis can be clarified only by telemetry or ambulatory electroencephalographic (EEG) monitoring.

Table 11-3
Differential Diagnosis of Dissociative Amnesia

Ordinary forgetfulness
   Age-related cognitive decline
Nonpathologic forms of amnesia
   Infantile and childhood amnesia
   Amnesia for sleep and dreaming
   Hypnotic amnesia
Dementia
Delirium
Amnestic disorders
Neurologic disorders with discrete memory loss episodes
   Posttraumatic amnesia
   Transient global amnesia
   Amnesia related to seizure disorders
Substance-related amnesia
   Alcohol
   Sedative–hypnotics
   Anticholinergic agents
   Steroids
   Marijuana
   Narcotic analgesics
   Psychedelics
   Phencyclidine
   Methyldopa (Aldomet)
   Pentazocine (Talwin)
   Hypoglycemic agents
   β-Blockers
   Lithium carbonate
   Many others
Other dissociative disorders
   Dissociative fugue
   Dissociative identity disorder
   Dissociative disorder not otherwise specified
	Acute stress disorder
	Posttraumatic stress disorder
	Somatization disorder
	Psychotic episode
	   Lack of memory for psychotic episode when returns to
	     nonpsychotic state
	Mood disorder episode
	   Lack of memory for aspects of episode of mania when depressed
	     and vice versa or when euthymic
	Factitious disorder
	Malingering
	Psychophysiologic symptoms or disorders
	   Asthma and breathing problems
	   Perimenstrual disorders
	   Irritable bowel syndrome
	   Gastroesophageal reflux disease
	   Somatic memory
	Affective symptoms
	   Depressed mood, dysphoria, or anhedonia
	   Brief mood swings or mood lability
	   Suicidal thoughts and attempts or self-mutilation
	   Guilt and survivor guilt
	   Helpless and hopeless feelings
	Obsessive-compulsive symptoms
	   Ruminations about trauma
	   Obsessive counting, singing
	   Arranging
	   Washing
	   Checking

Substance-Related Amnesia. A variety of substances and intoxicants can cause amnesia. Table 11-3 lists some common offending agents.

Transient Global Amnesia. Transient global amnesia can be mistaken for dissociative amnesia, especially because stressful life events may precede either disorder. In transient global amnesia, however, there is the sudden onset of complete anterograde amnesia and learning abilities; pronounced retrograde amnesia; preservation of memory for personal identity; anxious awareness of memory loss with repeated, often perseverative, questioning; overall normal behavior; lack of gross neurologic abnormalities in most cases; and rapid return of baseline cognitive function, with a persistent short retrograde amnesia. The patient usually is older than 50 years of age and shows risk factors for cerebrovascular disease, although epilepsy and migraine are also possible causes.

Dissociative Identity Disorder. Patients with dissociative identity disorder can present with acute forms of amnesia and fugue episodes. These patients, however, have symptoms beyond that found in dissociative amnesia. Concerning amnesia, most patients with dissociative identity disorder, and those with an unspecified dissociative disorder with dissociative identity disorder features, report multiple forms of complex amnesia, including recurrent blackouts, fugues, unexplained possessions, and fluctuations in skills, habits, and knowledge.

Acute Stress Disorder and Posttraumatic Stress Disorder. Many trauma spectrum disorders, including acute stress disorder and PTSD, are associated with dissociative amnesia. When

diagnoses of acute stress disorder or PTSD are appropriate, we should add the co-occurring diagnosis of dissociative amnesia if the amnesia persists beyond the immediate trauma.

Malingering and Factitious Amnesia. No absolute way exists to differentiate dissociative amnesia from factitious or malingered amnesia. Malingerers may continue their deception even during hypnotically or barbiturate-facilitated interviews. A patient who presents to psychiatric attention seeking to recover repressed memories as a chief complaint most likely has a factitious disorder or has been subject to suggestive influences. Most of these individuals do not describe bona fide amnesia when carefully questioned but are often insistent that they must have been abused in childhood to explain their unhappiness or dysfunction. Malingering of dissociative fugue can occur in individuals who are attempting to flee a situation involving legal, financial, or personal difficulties, as well as in soldiers who are attempting to avoid combat or unpleasant military duties. No test, battery of tests, or set of procedures exist that invariably distinguish actual dissociative symptoms from malingering. Many malingerers confess spontaneously or when confronted. In the forensic context, when a patient claims to have a fugue, the examiner should always carefully consider the diagnosis of malingering.

DEPERSONALIZATION/DEREALIZATION DISORDER

Depersonalization is the persistent or recurrent feeling of detachment or estrangement from one's self. The individual may report feeling like an automaton or watching himself or herself in a

Table 11-4
Depersonalization/Derealization Disorder

	DSM-5	ICD-10
Name	**Depersonalization/Derealization Disorder**	**Depersonalization/Derealization Syndrome**
Symptoms	Depersonalization: • Feeling detached from oneself • Feeling as if observing oneself • Sense of unreality • Sense of distorted time • Sense of distorted perceptions Derealization • Sense of unreality • Feeling detached from one's surroundings	Perceived change in mental activity, such that thoughts, body, or surroundings feel: Unreal Remote Automatized Loss of emotions Feeling estranged or detached
# Symptoms needed	Either depersonalization or derealization as above Intact reality testing	Any of above Intact reality testing
Exclusions (not result of):	Substance use Another medical condition Another mental disorder	Schizophrenic Depressive disorders Phobic disorders Obsessive-compulsive disorder
Psychosocial impact	Marked distress and/or impairment	

movie. Derealization is somewhat related and refers to feelings of unreality or of being detached from one's environment. The patient may describe his or her perception of the outside world as lacking lucidity and emotional coloring, as though dreaming or dead.

Table 11-4 compares the diagnostic approaches to depersonalization/derealization disorder.

Several distinct components comprise the experience of depersonalization, including a sense of (1) bodily changes, (2) duality of self as observer and actor, (3) feeling cut off from others, and (4) feeling cut off from one's own emotions. Patients experiencing depersonalization often have great difficulty expressing what they are feeling. Trying to express their subjective suffering with banal phrases, such as "I feel dead," "Nothing seems real," or "I'm standing outside of myself," depersonalized patients may not adequately convey to the examiner the distress they experience. While complaining bitterly about how this is ruining their life, they may nonetheless appear remarkably without distress.

Ms. R was a 27-year-old, unmarried, graduate student with a master's degree in biology. She complained about intermittent episodes of "standing back," usually associated with anxiety-provoking social situations. When asked about a recent episode, she described presenting in a seminar course. "All of a sudden, I was talking, but it didn't feel like it was me talking. It was very disconcerting. I had this feeling, 'Who's doing the talking?' I felt like I was just watching someone else talk. Listening to words come out of my mouth, but I wasn't saying them. It wasn't me. It went on for a while. I was calm, even sort of peaceful. It was as if I was very far away. In the back of the room somewhere—just watching myself. But the person talking didn't even seem like me really. It was like I was watching someone else." The feeling lasted the rest of that day and persisted into the next, during which time it gradually dissipated. She thought that she remembered having similar experiences during high school but was confident that they occurred at least once a year during college and graduate school.

As a child, Ms. R reported frequent intense anxiety from overhearing or witnessing the frequent violent arguments and periodic physical fights between her parents. In addition, the family was subject to many unpredictable dislocations and moves owing to the patient's father's intermittent difficulties with finances and employment. The patient's anxieties

did not abate when the parents divorced when she was a late adolescent. Her father moved away and had little further contact with her. Her relationship with her mother became increasingly angry, critical, and contentious. She was unsure if she experienced depersonalization during childhood while listening to her parents' fights. (Adapted from a case of Richard J. Loewenstein, M.D., and Frank W. Putnam, M.D.)

Differential Diagnosis

The variety of conditions associated with depersonalization complicates the differential diagnosis of depersonalization disorder. Depersonalization can result from a medical condition or neurologic condition, intoxication or withdrawal from illicit drugs, as a side effect of medications, or can be associated with panic attacks, phobias, PTSD, or acute stress disorder, major depression, schizophrenia, illness anxiety disorder, or another dissociative disorder. A thorough medical and neurologic evaluation is essential, including standard laboratory studies, an EEG, and any indicated drug screens. Drug-related depersonalization is typically transient. However, persistent depersonalization can follow an episode of intoxication with a variety of substances, including marijuana, cocaine, and other psychostimulants. A range of neurologic conditions, including seizure disorders, brain tumors, postconcussion syndrome, metabolic abnormalities, migraine, vertigo, and Ménière disease, have been reported as causes. Depersonalization caused by organic conditions tends to be primarily sensory without the elaborated descriptions and personalized meanings common to psychiatric etiologies.

DISSOCIATIVE IDENTITY DISORDER

Dissociative identity disorder, previously called multiple personality disorder, has been the most extensively researched of all the dissociative disorders. It is the presence of two or more distinct identities or personality states. The identities or personality states, sometimes called *alters, self-states, alter identities,* or *parts,* among other terms, differ from one another in that each presents as having its pattern of perceiving, relating to, and thinking about the environment and self, in short, its personality. It is the paradigmatic dissociative psychopathology in that the symptoms of all the other dissociative disorders occur in patients with dissociative identity disorder: amnesia, often with fugue, depersonalization, derealization, and similar symptoms.

Diagnostic Features

The critical feature in diagnosing this disorder is the presence of two or more distinct personality states. Also, individuals with this disorder often report losing time beyond what one would expect from ordinary forgetfulness. There are many other diverse signs and symptoms, making diagnosis difficult. Table 11-5 describes the many other associated symptoms commonly found in patients with dissociative identity disorder, and Table 11-6 compares the different diagnostic approaches to dissociative identity disorder.

Mental Status

A careful and detailed mental status examination is essential in making the diagnosis. It is easy to mistake patients with this disorder as suffering from schizophrenia, borderline personality disorder, or outright malingering. Table 11-7 lists the questions clinicians should ask to make the proper diagnosis.

Memory and Amnesia Symptoms

Dissociative disturbances of memory are manifest in several fundamental ways and are frequently observable in clinical settings. As part of the general mental status examination, clinicians should routinely inquire about experiences of losing time, blackout spells, and significant gaps in the continuity of recall for personal information. Dissociative time loss experiences are too extensive to be explained by normal forgetting and typically have sharply demarcated onsets and offsets.

Patients with dissociative identity disorder often report significant gaps in autobiographical memory, especially for childhood

Table 11-5
Associated Symptoms Commonly Found in Dissociative Identity Disorder

Posttraumatic stress disorder symptoms
    Intrusive symptoms
    Hyperarousal
    Avoidance and numbing symptoms
Somatic symptoms
    Conversion and pseudoneurologic symptoms
    Seizure-like episodes
    Pain symptoms
    Headache, abdominal, musculoskeletal, pelvic pain
    Psychophysiologic symptoms or disorders
    Asthma and breathing problems
    Perimenstrual disorders
    Irritable bowel syndrome
    Gastroesophageal reflux disease
    Somatic memory
Affective symptoms
    Depressed mood, dysphoria, or anhedonia
    Brief mood swings or mood lability
    Suicidal thoughts and attempts of self-mutilation
    Helpless and hopeless feelings
Obsessive-compulsive symptoms
    Ruminations about trauma
    Obsessive counting, singing
    Arranging
    Washing
    Checking

events. Dissociative gaps in the autobiographical recall are usually sharply demarcated and do not fit the usual decline in autobiographical recall for younger ages.

Ms. A, a 33-year-old married woman employed as a librarian in a school for disturbed children, presented to psychiatric attention after discovering her 5-year-old daughter "playing doctor" with several neighborhood children. Although this event was of little consequence, the

Table 11-6
Dissociative Identity Disorder

	DSM-5	ICD-10
Name	**Dissociative Identity Disorder**	**Other Dissociative (Conversion) Disorders**

Symptoms	Sense of one's identity is distorted
	Sense of having at least two personality states, each with unique
	    Sense of self-control
	    Affect
	    Behavior
	    Memory
	    Perception
	    Sensory motor function
	    Memory lapses about past events	

# Symptoms needed	All the above	
Exclusions (not result of):	Acceptable cultural beliefs Normal forgetting Substance use Another medical condition Fantasy play in children	
Psychosocial impact	Marked distress and/or impairment	
Comments		Listed among the other disorders, along with Ganser syndrome and psychogenic confusion/twilight state. Symptoms are not detailed.

Table 11-7
Mental Status Examination Questions for Dissociative Identity Disorder Process Symptoms

If answers are positive, ask the patient to describe the event. Make sure to specify that the symptom does not occur during an episode of intoxication.

1. Do you act so differently in one situation compared to another situation that you feel almost like you were two different people?
2. Do you feel that there is more than one of you? More than one part of you? Side of you? Do they seem to be in conflict or in a struggle?
3. Does that part (those parts) of you have its (their) own independent way(s) of thinking, perceiving, and relating to the world and the self? Have its (their) own memories, thoughts, and feelings?
4. Does more than one of these entities take control of your behavior?
5. Do you ever have thoughts or feelings, or both, that come from inside you (outside you) that you cannot explain? That do not feel like thoughts or feelings that you would have? That seem like thoughts or feelings that are not under your control (passive influence)?
6. Have you ever felt that your body was engaged in behavior that did not seem to be under your control? For example, saying things, going places, buying things, writing things, drawing or creating things, hurting yourself or others, and so forth? That your body does not seem to belong to you?
7. Do you ever feel that you have to struggle against another part of you that seems to want to do or to say something that you do not wish to do or to say?
8. Do you ever feel that there is a force (pressure, part) inside you that tries to stop you from doing or saying something?
9. Do you ever hear voices, sounds, or conversations in your mind? That seem to be discussing you? Commenting on what you do? Telling you to do or not do certain things? To hurt yourself or others? That seem to be warning you or trying to protect you? That try to comfort, support, or soothe you? That provide important information about things to you? That argue or say things that have nothing to do with you? That have names? Men? Women? Children?
10. I would like to talk with that part (side, aspect, facet) of you (of the mind) that is called the "angry one" (the Little Girl, Janie, that went to Atlantic City last weekend and spent lots of money, etc.). Can that part come forward now, please?
11. Do you frequently have the experience of feeling like you are outside yourself? Inside yourself? Beside yourself, watching yourself as if you were another person?
12. Do you ever feel disconnected from yourself or your body as if you (your body) were not real?
13. Do you frequently experience the world around you as unreal? As if you are in a fog or daze? As if it were painted? Two-dimensional?
14. Do you ever look in the mirror and not recognize who you see? See someone else there?

Adapted from Loewenstein RJ. An office mental status examination for chronic complex dissociative symptoms and multiple personality disorder. *Psychiatr Clin North Am.* 1991;14:567–604, with permission.

patient began to become fearful that her daughter would be molested. The patient was seen by her internist and was treated with antianxiety agents and antidepressants, but with little improvement. She sought psychiatric consultation from several clinicians but repeated, appropriate trials of antidepressants, antianxiety agents, and supportive psychotherapy resulted in limited improvement. After the death of her father from complications of an alcohol use disorder, the patient became more symptomatic. He was estranged from the family since the patient was approximately 12 years of age, owing to his drinking and associated antisocial behavior.

Psychiatric hospitalization was precipitated by the patient's arrest for disorderly conduct in a nearby city. She was found in a hotel, in revealing clothing, engaged in an altercation with a man. She denied knowledge of how she had come to the hotel, although the man insisted that she had come there under a different name for a voluntary sexual encounter.

On psychiatric examination, the patient described dense amnesia for the first 12 years of her life, with the feeling that her "life started at 12 years old." She reported that, for as long as she could remember, she had an imaginary companion, an elderly black woman, who advised her and kept her company. She reported hearing other voices in her head: several women and children, as well as her father's voice repeatedly speaking to her in a derogatory way. She reported that since age 12, she had episodes of amnesia: for work, for her marriage, for the birth of her children, and her sex life with her husband. She reported perplexing changes in skills; for example, people told her that she played the piano well but had no conscious awareness that she could do so. Her husband reported that she had always been "forgetful" of conversations and family activities. He also noted that, at times, she would speak like a child; at times, she would adopt a southern accent; and, at other times, she would be angry and provocative. She frequently had little recall of these episodes.

When questioned about her early life, the patient appeared to enter a trance and stated, "I just don't want to be locked in the closet"

in a childlike voice. Inquiry about this produced rapid shifts in a state between alter identities who differed in manifested age, facial expression, voice tone, and knowledge of the patient's history. One spoke in an angry, expletive-filled manner and appeared irritable and preoccupied with sexuality. She discussed the episode with the man in the hotel and stated that it was she who had arranged it. Gradually, the alters described a history of family chaos, brutality, and neglect during the first 12 years of the patient's life, until her mother, who also struggled with alcohol use disorder, achieved sobriety and fled her husband, taking her children with her. The patient, in the alter identities, described episodes of physical abuse, sexual abuse, and emotional torment by the father, her siblings, and her mother.

After an assessment of family members, the patient's mother also met diagnostic criteria for dissociative identity disorder, as did her older sister, who also had been molested. A brother met diagnostic criteria for PTSD, major depression, and alcohol use disorder. (Adapted from a case of Richard J. Loewenstein, M.D., and Frank W. Putnam, M.D.)

Dissociative Alterations in Identity

Clinically, dissociative alterations in identity may first manifest with odd first-person plural or third-person singular or plural self-references. Also, patients may refer to themselves using their first names or make depersonalized self-references, such as "the body," when describing themselves and others. Patients often describe a profound sense of concretized internal division or personified internal conflicts between parts of themselves. In some instances, these parts may have proper names, or the patient may refer to them by their predominate affect or function, for example, "the angry one" or "the wife." Patients may suddenly change how they refer to others, for example, "the son" instead of "my son."

Other Associated Symptoms

Most patients with dissociative identity disorder meet the criteria for a mood disorder, usually one of the depression spectrum disorders. Frequent, rapid mood swings are common but are usually part of posttraumatic and dissociative phenomena, not a cyclic mood disorder. Considerable overlap may exist between PTSD symptoms of anxiety, disturbed sleep, and dysphoria, and mood disorder symptoms.

Obsessive-compulsive personality traits are common in dissociative identity disorder, and intercurrent obsessive-compulsive disorder (OCD) symptoms occur in patients with dissociative identity disorder, with a subgroup manifesting severe OCD symptoms. OCD symptoms commonly have a posttraumatic quality: repeatedly checking to be sure that no one can enter the house or the bedroom, compulsive washing to relieve a feeling of being dirty because of abuse, and repetitive counting or singing in one's head to distract from anxiety over being abused, for example.

Child and Adolescent Presentations

Children and adolescents manifest the same core dissociative symptoms and secondary clinical phenomena as adults. Age-related differences in autonomy and lifestyle, however, may significantly influence the clinical expression of dissociative symptoms in youth. Younger children have a less linear and less continuous sense of time and often are not able to self-identify dissociative discontinuities in their behavior. Often additional informants, such as teachers and relatives, are available to help document dissociative behaviors.

Several normal childhood phenomena, such as imaginary companionship and elaborated daydreams, must be carefully differentiated from pathologic dissociation in younger children. The clinical presentation may be that of an elaborated or autonomous imaginary companionship, with the imaginary companions taking control of the child's behavior, often experienced through passive influence experiences or auditory pseudohallucinations, or both, that command the child to behave in specific ways.

Differential Diagnosis

Table 11-8 lists the most common differentials for dissociative identity disorder.

Factitious, Imitative, and Malingered Dissociative Identity Disorder.
Indicators of falsified or *imitative dissociative identity disorder* include those typical of other factitious or malingering

Table 11-8
Differential Diagnosis of Dissociative Identity Disorder

Comorbidity versus differential diagnosis
Affective disorders
Psychotic disorders
Anxiety disorders
Posttraumatic stress disorder
Personality disorders
Neurocognitive disorders
Neurologic and seizure disorders
Somatic symptom disorders
Factitious disorders
Malingering
Other dissociative disorders
Deep-trance phenomena

presentations. These include symptom exaggeration, lies, use of symptoms to excuse antisocial behavior (e.g., amnesia only for bad behavior), amplification of symptoms when under observation, refusal to allow collateral contacts, legal problems, and pseudologia fantastica. Patients with genuine dissociative identity disorder are usually confused, conflicted, ashamed, and distressed by their symptoms and trauma history. Those with the nongenuine disorder frequently show little dysphoria about their disorder.

OTHER SPECIFIED OR UNSPECIFIED DISSOCIATIVE DISORDER

The categories of specified or unspecified dissociative disorders cover all the conditions characterized by a primary dissociative response that does not meet diagnostic criteria for one of the other DSM-5 dissociative disorders. Specified dissociative disorders include chronic and recurrent syndromes of mixed dissociative symptoms; identity disturbance due to prolonged and intense coercive persuasion (e.g., brainwashing); acute dissociative reactions to stressful events; and dissociative trance.

Dissociative Trance

Dissociative trance is manifest by a temporary, marked alteration in the state of consciousness or by loss of the customary sense of personal identity without the replacement by an alternate sense of identity. A variant of this, possession trance, involves single or episodic alternations in the state of consciousness, characterized by the exchange of the person's customary identity with a new identity usually attributed to a spirit, divine power, deity, or another person. In this possessed state, the individual exhibits stereotypical and culturally determined behaviors or experiences an entity controlling them. There must be partial or full amnesia for the event. The trance or possession state must not be a commonly accepted part of cultural or religious practice and must cause significant distress or functional impairment in one or more of the usual domains. Finally, the dissociative trance state must not occur exclusively during a psychotic disorder and is not the result of any substance use or general medical condition.

Brainwashing

DSM-5 describes this dissociative disorder as "identity disturbance due to prolonged and intense coercive persuasion." Brainwashing occurs mostly in the setting of political reform, as has been described at length with the Cultural Revolution in communist China, war imprisonment, torture of political dissidents, terrorist hostages, and, more familiarly, in Western culture, totalitarian cult indoctrination. It implies that under conditions of adequate stress and duress, those in power can make individuals comply with their demands, thereby undergoing significant changes in their personality, beliefs, and behaviors. Persons subjected to such conditions can undergo considerable harm, including loss of health and life, and they typically manifest a variety of posttraumatic and dissociative symptoms.

Some have likened the first stage in coercive processes to the artificial creation of an identity crisis, with the emergence of a new pseudoidentity that manifests characteristics of a dissociative state. Under circumstances of extreme and malignant dependency, overwhelming vulnerability, and danger to one's existence, individuals develop a state characterized by an extreme idealization of their captors, with ensuing identification with the aggressor and externalization of their superego, regressive adaptation known as *traumatic infantilism,* paralysis of will, and a state of frozen fright. The coercive techniques include isolation of the subject, degradation, control of overall communications and essential daily functions, induction of fear and confusion, peer pressure, assignment of repetitive and monotonous routines, the unpredictability of environmental supplies, renunciation of past relationships and values, and various deprivations. Even though physical or sexual abuse, torture, and extreme sensory deprivation and physical neglect can be part of this process, they are not required to define a coercive process. As a result, victims manifest extensive posttraumatic and dissociative symptomatology, including drastic alteration of their identity, values, and beliefs; reduction of cognitive flexibility with regression to simplistic perceptions of good versus evil and dominance versus submission; numbing of experience and blunting of affect; trance-like states and diminished environmental responsiveness; and, in some cases, more severe dissociative symptoms such as amnesia, depersonalization, and shifts in identity.

Ganser Syndrome

Ganser syndrome is a poorly understood condition characterized by the giving of approximate answers (*paralogia*), together with a clouding of consciousness, and, often, hallucinations and other dissociative, somatoform, or conversion symptoms.

The symptom of *passing over* (*vorbeigehen*) the correct answer for a related but incorrect one is the hallmark of Ganser syndrome. The approximate answers often just miss the mark but bear an obvious relation to the question, indicating that the person must have understood. When asked how old she was, a 25-year-old woman answered, "I'm not five." If asked to do simple calculations (e.g., 2 + 2 = 5); for general information (the capital of the United States is New York); to identify simple objects (a pencil is a key); or to name colors (green is gray), the patient with Ganser syndrome gives erroneous but comprehensible answers. They may even answer incorrectly to rhetorical questions ("how many legs are on a three-legged stool?" "Four?")

A clouding of consciousness also occurs, usually manifest by disorientation, amnesias, loss of personal information, and some impairment of reality testing. Visual and auditory hallucinations occur in roughly one-half of the cases. Neurologic examination may reveal what Ganser called *hysterical stigmata,* for example, nonneurologic analgesia or shifting hyperalgesia. It must include other dissociative symptoms, such as amnesias, conversion symptoms, or trance-like behaviors.

Differential Diagnosis. The examiner should conduct a thorough neurologic and medical evaluation, given the reported frequent history of organic brain syndromes, seizures, head trauma, and psychosis in Ganser syndrome. Differential diagnoses include organic dementia, depressive pseudodementia, the confabulation of Korsakoff syndrome, organic dysphasia, and reactive psychoses. Patients with dissociative identity disorder occasionally may also exhibit Ganser-like symptoms.

COMORBIDITY

Common comorbidities found in dissociative disorders include depressive disorders, adjustment disorder, anxiety disorders, trauma and stress-related disorders, eating disorders, OCD, somatic symptom disorders, and conversion disorder. Individuals with dissociative disorders may also meet the criteria for personality disorders, with reports of co-occurring avoidant, borderline, dependent, and obsessive-compulsive personality disorders predominating.

COURSE AND PROGNOSIS

Dissociative Amnesia

We know little about the clinical course of dissociative amnesia. After removing the person to safety from traumatic or overwhelming circumstances, the acute dissociative amnesia frequently spontaneously resolves. At the other extreme, some patients do develop chronic forms of generalized, continuous, or severe localized amnesia and are profoundly disabled and require high levels of social support, such as nursing home placement or intensive family caretaking. Clinicians should try to restore patients' lost memories to consciousness as soon as possible; otherwise, the repressed memory may form a nucleus in the unconscious mind around which future amnestic episodes may develop.

In those who develop a dissociative fugue, most fugue states are relatively brief, lasting from hours to days. Most individuals appear to recover, although refractory dissociative amnesia may persist in rare cases. Some studies have described recurrent fugues in most individuals presenting with an episode of dissociative fugue.

Depersonalization/Derealization Disorder

Depersonalization after traumatic experiences or intoxication commonly remits spontaneously after removal from the traumatic circumstances or ending of the episode of intoxication. Depersonalization accompanying mood, psychotic, or other anxiety disorders commonly remit with the definitive treatment of these conditions.

Depersonalization disorder may have an episodic, relapsing and remitting, or chronic course. Many patients with chronic depersonalization may have a severe and chronic functional impairment. The mean age of onset is usually late adolescence or early adulthood.

Dissociative Identity Disorder

We know little about the natural history of untreated dissociative identity disorder. Some individuals with untreated dissociative identity disorder may continue in abusive relationships or violent subcultures, or both, that may result in the traumatization of their children, with the potential for additional family transmission of the disorder. Many authorities believe that some percentage of patients with undiagnosed or untreated dissociative identity disorder die by suicide or because of their risk-taking behaviors.

Prognosis is poorer in patients with comorbid medical disorders, psychotic disorders (*not* dissociative identity disorder pseudopsychosis), and severe medical illnesses. Refractory substance use and eating disorders also suggest a poorer prognosis. Other factors that usually indicate a poorer outcome include significant antisocial personality features, current criminal activity, ongoing perpetration of abuse, and current victimization, with the refusal to leave abusive relationships. Repeated adult traumas with recurrent episodes of acute stress disorder may severely complicate the clinical course.

TREATMENT

Dissociative Amnesia

Psychotherapy

PHASE-ORIENTED TREATMENT. Phase-oriented treatment is the current standard of care for the treatment of dissociative amnesia, although there are no systematic studies with large cohorts of dissociative amnesia patients. This phasic treatment follows the three-stage phasic treatment model developed for the treatment of complex PTSD and dissociative identity disorder, which is discussed extensively in the section on treatment of dissociative identity disorder, below. When applied to dissociative amnesia treatment, memory recall is a central issue, because the loss of memory for personal identity and gaps in current autobiographical memory are acutely disabling symptoms that require relatively rapid intervention.

COGNITIVE THERAPY.   Cognitive therapy may have specific benefits for individuals with trauma disorders. Identifying the specific cognitive distortions about the trauma may provide an entrée into autobiographical memory for which the patient experiences amnesia. As the patient becomes able to correct cognitive distortions, particularly about the meaning of prior trauma, a more detailed recall of traumatic events may occur.

HYPNOSIS.   Hypnotic interventions can help to contain, modulate, and titrate the intensity of symptoms; to facilitate controlled recall of dissociated memories; to provide support and ego strengthening for the patient; and, finally, to promote working through and integration of dissociated material. Also, the patient can learn self-hypnosis to apply containment and calming techniques in his or her everyday life. Successful use of containment techniques, whether hypnotically facilitated or not, also increases the patient's sense that he or she can more effectively be in control of alternations between intrusive symptoms and amnesia.

GROUP PSYCHOTHERAPY.   Time-limited and longer-term group psychotherapies can help combat veterans with PTSD and survivors of childhood abuse. During group sessions, patients may recover memories for which they have had amnesia. Supportive interventions by the group members or the group therapist, or both, may facilitate integration and mastery of the dissociated material.

Somatic Therapies.   No known pharmacotherapy exists for dissociative amnesia other than pharmacologically facilitated interviews. The interviews have used a variety of sedatives, including sodium amobarbital, thiopental, oral benzodiazepines, and amphetamines.

Pharmacologically facilitated interviews using intravenous amobarbital or diazepam are used primarily in working with acute amnesias and conversion reactions, among other indications, in general hospital medical and psychiatric services. This procedure is also occasionally useful in refractory cases of chronic dissociative amnesia when patients are unresponsive to other interventions. The material uncovered in a pharmacologically facilitated interview needs to be processed by the patient in his or her usual conscious state. The Joint Commission now considers pharmacologically facilitated interviews to be conscious sedation, requiring the presence of an anesthesiologist.

Depersonalization/Derealization Disorder

Clinicians working with patients with depersonalization/derealization disorder often find them to be a singularly clinically refractory group. However, benzodiazepines, serotonin reuptake inhibitors, and stimulants appear to be partially efficacious for some patients. There is absolutely no empirical evidence for the efficacy of typical or atypical antipsychotic medications in depersonalization/derealization disorder, and indeed these medications may increase a feeling of emotional deadness and lack of emotional response to oneself or the world. Also, opioid antagonists such as naltrexone and cognitive enhancers have had some benefit in the

clinical treatment of specific depersonalization/derealization disorder patients. Early data suggest the possible efficacy of repetitive transcranial magnetic stimulation (rTMS) treatment.

Many different types of psychotherapy may help depersonalization disorder: psychodynamic, cognitive, cognitive-behavioral, hypnotherapeutic, and supportive. However, the response is not robust for many patients. Stress management strategies, distraction techniques, reduction of sensory stimulation, relaxation training, and physical exercise may be somewhat helpful in some patients.

Dissociative Identity Disorder

Psychotherapy.   The current model of treatment of the dissociative identity disorder patient follows a phasic model that is the current standard of care for complex posttraumatic disorders. The phases include: (1) development of safety and symptom stabilization; (2) (optionally) focused, in-depth attention to traumatic material; and (3) integration or reintegration, in which the individual moves away from a life adaptation based on chronic traumatization and victimization. These phases are relatively heuristic, and aspects of each may be part of the others.

STAGE 1 PHASIC TRAUMA TREATMENT: STABILIZATION AND SAFETY.   Stabilization of the individual with dissociative identity disorder is vital to the successful negotiation of all aspects of treatment. Stabilization focuses on the safety and management of core dissociative identity disorder and comorbid symptoms. The majority of patients with dissociative identity disorder come to treatment because of overwhelming PTSD and dissociative symptoms and because of some form of self-destructive behavior or violence against others.

Before establishing safety, the patient in reality or symbolically lives in a world of ongoing trauma, whether perpetrated on the patient by others or by the patient on him/herself due to chronic forms of repeated self-destruction and high-risk behavior. The clinician must logically prioritize basic life and health over other interventions. The clinician may need to resort to many different levels and types of interventions to protect the patient, including hospitalization, specialized substance use or eating disorders programs, police assistance and shelter for victims of intimate partner violence, social service interventions to protect minor children, and assistance with housing, and access to medical care.

STAGE 2 PHASIC TRAUMA TREATMENT: WORK ON TRAUMATIC MEMORIES.   For patients who stabilize and form a reasonable working alliance in treatment, longer-term treatment goals involve the detailed, affectively intense, psychotherapeutic processing of life experiences, and the transformation of the meaning of these experiences for the individual. Authorities emphasize that, in most cases, intensive, detailed psychotherapeutic work with traumatic memories should only start after the patient has demonstrated the ability to use symptom management skills independently, after the self-state system can work together in a reasonably cooperative way, and after a stable therapeutic relationship has been established.

The patient should be able to give informed consent and have a realistic understanding of the potential risks and benefits of intensive focus on traumatic material. Potential risks may include temporary, acute worsening of PTSD, affective, somatoform, and self-destructive symptoms, and short-term interference with daily activities. Long-term benefits may include significant amelioration of dissociative and PTSD symptoms, decreases in subjective self-division, the fusion of identities, and freeing of psychological energy for daily life. The patient must be able to understand that the goal is the integration of dissociated thoughts, feelings, recollections, and perceptions, not the exhumation or expulsion of memories per se.

The patient should not be in the midst of an acute life crisis or significant life change. Also, we should first stabilize comorbid medical and psychiatric disorders. The patient should have the ego strength and psychosocial resources to withstand the rigors of the process, and there must be adequate resources, such as support by significant others, and, potentially, support for additional sessions.

Experienced clinicians attempt to carefully structure affectively intense sessions focused on traumatic material, with attention to affect modulation, restabilization of the patient before concluding the session, and reasonable availability to assist the patient supportively between sessions. It may require many sessions to fully explicate the cognitive and emotional meaning of traumatic events, so that they may become part of the patient's repertoire of nondissociated, ordinary memories for life experience.

STAGE 3 PHASIC TRAUMA TREATMENT: FUSION, INTEGRATION, RESOLUTION, AND RECOVERY. Throughout treatment, we may observe significant unification of dissociated mental processes. Self-states lose distinctness and decrease compartmentalization of thoughts, memories, and affects. The patient develops a more unified sense of self. Transference is modified, consistent with these changes. Amnesia and switching become less apparent than before. The fusion of states results in the psychological merging of two or more entities at a point in time, with a subjective experience of loss of all separateness. The term *integration* is sometimes used synonymously with *fusion* but is a more general term, describing the process of undoing all forms of dissociative division during treatment. Some patients seem to proceed to a complete fusion of all states. They may shift in self-representation, and develop a consistent and continuous sense of self. Many patients never attain a complete fusion of their personalities but achieve a therapeutic *resolution:* improved communication, collaboration, and cooperation among self-states leading to relative stability and adequate function.

HYPNOSIS. Hypnotherapeutic interventions can often alleviate self-destructive impulses or reduce symptoms, such as flashbacks, dissociative hallucinations, and passive-influence experiences. Teaching the patient self-hypnosis may help with crises outside of sessions. Hypnosis can be useful for accessing specific alter personality states, and their sequestered affects and memories. Hypnosis can create relaxed mental states in which the subject can examine adverse life events without overwhelming anxiety. Clinicians using hypnosis should obtain specialized training in trauma populations. Clinicians should be aware of current controversies over the impact of hypnosis on accurate reporting of recollections and should use appropriate informed consent for its use.

GROUP THERAPY. In therapy groups, including general psychiatric patients, the emergence of alter personalities can be disruptive to the group process by eliciting excess fascination or by frightening other patients. Therapy groups composed only of patients with dissociative identity disorder seem to be more successful, although the groups must be carefully structured, must provide firm limits, and should generally focus only on here-and-now issues of coping and adaptation.

FAMILY THERAPY. Family or couples therapy is often crucial for long-term stabilization and to address pathologic family and marital processes that are common in patients with dissociative identity disorder and their family members. Education of family and concerned others about dissociative identity disorder and its

treatment may help family members cope more effectively with dissociative identity disorder and PTSD symptoms in their loved ones. Group interventions for education and support of family members have also been found helpful. Sex therapy may be a critical part of couples' treatment, because patients with dissociative identity disorder may become intensely phobic of intimate contact for periods, and spouses may have little idea how to deal with this helpfully.

SELF-HELP GROUPS. Patients with dissociative identity disorder usually have a negative outcome to self-help groups or 12-step groups for incest survivors. A variety of problematic issues occur in these settings, including the intensification of PTSD symptoms because of discussion of trauma material without clinical safeguards, exploitation of the patient with dissociative identity disorder by predatory group members, contamination of the patient's recall by group discussions of trauma, and a feeling of alienation even from these other reputed sufferers of trauma and dissociation.

EXPRESSIVE AND OCCUPATIONAL THERAPIES. Expressive and occupational therapies, such as art and movement therapy, have proved particularly helpful in the treatment of patients with dissociative identity disorder. Art therapy may help with the containment and structuring of severe dissociative identity disorder and PTSD symptoms, as well as to permit these patients safer expression of thoughts, feelings, mental images, and conflicts that they have difficulty verbalizing. Movement therapy may facilitate the normalization of body sense and body image for these severely traumatized patients. Occupational therapy may help the patient with focused, structured activities that can be completed successfully and may help with grounding and symptom management.

EYE MOVEMENT DESENSITIZATION AND REPROCESSING. Eye movement desensitization and reprocessing (EMDR) is a treatment for PTSD. No systematic studies have been done in dissociative identity disorder patients using EMDR. Case reports suggest that some dissociative identity disorder patients may be destabilized by EMDR procedures, especially those with acutely increased PTSD and dissociative symptoms. Some authorities believe that EMDR can be a helpful adjunct for later phases of treatment in well-stabilized dissociative identity disorder outpatients. The International Society for the Study of Trauma and Dissociation dissociative identity disorder treatment guidelines suggest that EMDR only be used in this patient population by clinicians who have taken advanced EMDR training, are knowledgeable and skilled in phasic trauma treatment for dissociative disorders and have received supervision in the use of EMDR in dissociative identity disorder.

DIALECTICAL BEHAVIOR THERAPY. Dialectical behavior therapy (DBT) is a treatment developed by the psychologist Marsha Linehan for borderline personality disorder. Its concepts and techniques may be helpful to structure aspects of stabilization throughout dissociative identity disorder treatment since many patients with borderline personality disorder report significant trauma histories and fit the complex trauma construct. Helpfully for the patient with dissociative identity disorder, DBT focuses on the primacy of safety, therapy-interfering behaviors, affect regulation strategies, distress tolerance, and radical acceptance.

However, DBT may also have notable limitations for the patient with a dissociative identity disorder. It does not focus on stabilization and management of dissociative symptoms such as depersonalization/derealization and dissociative amnesia, flashbacks, and unconscious reenactments, traumatic transference, and related trauma-based symptoms.

Psychopharmacologic Interventions.   Guidelines for the use of medications with dissociative patients emphasize the need to identify specific treatment-responsive symptoms rather than attempting to treat the dissociation per se. Medications may help attenuate symptoms to assist the patient in stabilizing during treatment. We should advise patients that the medication response is likely to be partial, devising the best "shock-absorber" system for the patient at a given time. In general, success is more likely if the target symptoms are present across most or all personality states, rather than confined to one or a few. Because rapid symptom oscillations are characteristic in this population, it is not advisable to chase each symptom shift with a medication change.

The most robust medication treatment effect in this patient population is the response of nightmares to the α_1-adrenergic antagonist prazosin. If the patient tolerates the blood pressure effects, dosages of prazosin as high as 25 mg daily, in single or twice-daily doses, can be useful. Daytime dosing may also be effective for control of flashbacks and intrusive symptoms. Doxazosin, a longer-acting α_1-adrenergic antagonist, may also help with nightmares and intrusive symptoms in PTSD.

Antidepressant medications can reduce depression and stabilize mood. A variety of PTSD symptoms, especially intrusive and hyperarousal symptoms, are partially medication responsive. Clinicians report some success with SSRI, tricyclic, and monoamine oxidase (MAO) antidepressants, β-blockers, clonidine, anticonvulsants, and benzodiazepines in reducing intrusive symptoms, hyperarousal, and anxiety in patients with a dissociative identity disorder. Patients with obsessive-compulsive symptoms may respond to serotonergic antidepressants. Emerging data suggest that naltrexone may help ameliorate recurrent self-injurious behaviors in a subset of traumatized patients.

The atypical neuroleptics, such as risperidone, quetiapine, ziprasidone, aripiprazole, and olanzapine, may be more effective and better tolerated than typical neuroleptics for overwhelming anxiety and intrusive PTSD symptoms in patients with dissociative identity disorder. However, weight gain and metabolic syndrome may be a particularly problematic side effect for these nonpsychotic patients. Occasionally, an extremely disorganized, overwhelmed, chronically ill patient with dissociative identity disorder, who has not responded to trials of other neuroleptics, responds favorably to a trial of clozapine.

Electroconvulsive Therapy.   For some patients, ECT helps to ameliorate refractory mood disorders and does not worsen dissociative memory problems. Clinical experience in tertiary care settings for severely ill patients with dissociative identity disorder suggests that a clinical picture of major depression with persistent, refractory melancholic features across all alter states may predict a positive response to ECT. This response is usually only partial, however, as is typical for most successful somatic treatments in the dissociative identity disorder population.

Table 11-9 lists target symptoms and somatic treatments for dissociative identity disorder.

Dissociative Trance

There are no systematic studies of dissociative trance disorder in the absence of pathologic possession. In general, treatment should focus on the patient understanding the nature of trance states and their relationship to more ordinary phenomena such as daydreaming. Assessment of hypnotizability may also allow the

Table 11-9
Medications for Associated Symptoms in Dissociative Identity Disorder

Medications and somatic treatments for posttraumatic stress disorder (PTSD), affective disorders, anxiety disorders, and obsessive-compulsive disorder (OCD)
  Selective serotonin reuptake inhibitors (no preferred agent, except for OCD symptoms)
  Fluvoxamine (for OCD presentations)
  Clomipramine (for OCD presentations)
  Tricyclic antidepressants
  Monoamine oxidase inhibitors (if patient can reliably maintain diet safely)
  Electroconvulsive therapy (for refractory depression with persistent melancholic features across all dissociative identity disorder alters)
  Mood stabilizers (more useful for PTSD and anxiety than mood swings)
  Divalproex
  Lamotrigine
  Oral or intramuscular benzodiazepines
Medications for sleep problems
  Low-dose trazodone
  Low-dose mirtazapine
  Low-dose tricyclic antidepressants
  Low-dose neuroleptics
  Benzodiazepines (often less helpful for sleep problems in this population)
  Zolpidem
  Anticholinergic agents (diphenhydramine, hydroxyzine)
Medications for self-injury, addictions
  Naltrexone

clinician to produce the same symptoms the patient is experiencing with a hypnotic induction. This may lead to an increased sense of control and may be enough to assist the patient in recognizing autohypnotic states and having strategies to manage these. In more chronic cases, supportive–expressive psychotherapy, like that for conversion disorder, may be most successful.

Brainwashing

There are no empirical treatment studies of individuals subjected to extreme coercion applied in the service of indoctrination into a belief system or an attempt at identity alteration. The basic principles of phased trauma treatment would seem to provide an organizing framework for their care, as for victims of other forms of torture. Family and social interventions may be necessary because of the duress and disruption accompanying the precipitating events and the social effects of the profound changes in the patient's attitudes, behaviors, and beliefs, as well as sequestration from everyday events during the period of captivity.

Ganser Syndrome

No systematic treatment studies have been conducted, given the rarity of this condition. In most case reports, the patient has been hospitalized and provided with a protective and supportive environment. In some instances, low doses of antipsychotic medications may be beneficial. Confrontation or interpretations of the patient's approximate answers are not productive, but the exploration of possible stressors may be helpful. Hypnosis and amobarbital narcosynthesis can also help patients reveal the underlying stressors that preceded the development of the syndrome, with the concomitant cessation of the Ganser symptoms.

Usually, a relatively rapid return to normal function occurs within days, although some cases may take a month or more to resolve. The individual is typically amnesic for the period of the syndrome.

EPIDEMIOLOGY

Dissociative Amnesia

Dissociative amnesia is in a range of approximately 2 to 6 percent of the general population. There is no known difference in incidence between men and women. Cases generally begin to be reported in late adolescence and adulthood. Dissociative amnesia can be especially challenging to assess in preadolescent children because of their more limited ability to describe the subjective experience.

Depersonalization/Derealization Disorder

Transient experiences of depersonalization and derealization are prevalent in normal and clinical populations. They are the third most commonly reported psychiatric symptoms, after depression and anxiety. Transient symptoms are common in the general population, with a lifetime prevalence of 26 to 74 percent, and 31 to 66 percent at the time of a traumatic event. Symptoms can occur with the use of illicit drugs, especially marijuana, hallucinogens, ketamine, and 3,4-methylenedioxymethamphetamine (MDMA or Ecstasy). They have been described after certain types of meditation, deep hypnosis, extended mirror or crystal gazing, and sensory deprivation experiences. They are also common after mild to moderate head injury, wherein little or no loss of consciousness occurs, but they are significantly less likely if unconsciousness lasts for more than 30 minutes. Depersonalization/derealization symptoms also occur in patients with epilepsy, both as a manifestation of the aura as well as the seizure itself, particularly in complex–partial seizure patients. The prevalence of depersonalization/derealization disorder is approximately 2.5 percent, with no age or gender differences.

Dissociative Identity Disorder

Few systematic epidemiologic data exist for dissociative identity disorder. Based on community samples, the prevalence in the general population is approximately 1 to 1.5 percent. Developmental studies indicate that the ratio of female to male dissociative identity disorder cases steadily increases from 1 to 1 in early childhood to approximately 8 to 1 by late adolescence in North American samples.

Ganser Syndrome

The overall frequency of Ganser syndrome has declined with time. Men outnumber women by approximately 2 to 1, and cases have been reported in a variety of cultures. Three of Ganser's first four cases were convicts, leading some authors to consider it to be a disorder of penal populations and, thus, an indicator of potential malingering.

ETIOLOGY

Dissociative Amnesia

In many cases of acute dissociative amnesia, the psychosocial environment out of which the amnesia develops is massively conflictual, with the patient experiencing intolerable emotions of shame, guilt, despair, rage, and desperation. These usually result from conflicts over unacceptable urges or impulses, such as intense sexual, suicidal, or violent compulsions. Traumatic experiences such as physical or sexual abuse can induce the disorder. In some cases, the trauma is caused by a betrayal by a trusted, needed other (betrayal trauma). This betrayal may influence how the event is processed and remembered.

Depersonalization/Derealization Disorder

Psychodynamic. Traditional psychodynamic formulations have emphasized the disintegration of the ego or have viewed depersonalization as an affective response in defense of the ego. These explanations stress the role of overwhelming, painful experiences or conflictual impulses as triggering events.

Traumatic Stress. A substantial proportion—typically one-third to one-half—of patients in clinical depersonalization case series have histories of significant trauma. Several studies of accident victims find as many as 60 percent of those with a life-threatening experience report at least transient depersonalization during the event or immediately after that. Military training studies find that stress and fatigue can evoke symptoms of depersonalization and derealization and affect performance.

Neurobiologic Theories. There are several neurobiologic theories related to depersonalization and derealization symptoms. These include animal models of *submissive immobility* when an organism determines it is unable to defend itself from a predator, like the concept of "playing dead"; disturbances in inferior bilateral frontal, medial prefrontal, cingulate, insula, and temporoparietal cortex; and neurochemical dysregulation, with various studies implicating the NMDA glutamate receptor, neuropeptide Y, norepinephrine, serotonin, and the opioid system.

Dissociative Identity Disorder

Severe experiences of early childhood trauma are the likely cause of dissociative identity disorder. From 85 to 97 percent of dissociative identify disorder cases reported severe childhood trauma or maltreatment. Physical and sexual abuse are common sources of childhood trauma.

Ganser Syndrome

Some case reports identify precipitating stressors, such as personal conflicts and financial reverses, whereas others note organic brain syndromes, head injuries, seizures, and medical or psychiatric illness. Psychodynamic explanations are common in the older literature; in some cases, there are clear medical or neurologic causes. The physiologic insults from such a disorder may act as acute stressors, precipitating the syndrome in vulnerable individuals. Some patients have reported significant histories of childhood maltreatment and adversity.

References

American Psychiatric Association. *Diagnostic and Statistical Manual of Mental Disorders*. 5th ed. Arlington, VA: American Psychiatric Association; 2013.

Anderson MC, Ochsner KN, Kuhl B, Cooper J, Robertson E, Gabrieli SW, Glover GH, Gabrieli JDE. Neural systems underlying the suppression of unwanted memories. *Science*. 2004;303:232–235.

Biswas J, Chu JA, Perez DL, Gutheil TG. From the neuropsychiatric to the analytic: Three perspectives on dissociative identity disorder. *Harvard Rev Psychiatry*. 2013; 21(1):41–51.

Brown RJ, Schrag A, Trimble MR. Dissociation, childhood interpersonal trauma, and family functioning in patients with somatization disorder. *Am J Psychiatry*. 2005;162:899–905.

Farina B, Liotti G. Does a dissociative psychopathological dimension exist? A review on dissociative processes and symptoms in developmental trauma spectrum disorders. *Clin Neuropsychiatry*. 2013;10(1):11–18.

Foote B, Smolin Y, Kaplan M, Legatt ME, Lipschitz D. Prevalence of dissociative disorders in psychiatric outpatients. *Am J Psychiatry*. 2006;163(4):623–629.

Hunter ECM, Baker D, Phillips ML, Sierra M, David AS. Cognitive-behaviour therapy for depersonalization disorder: An open study. *Behav Res Ther*. 2005;43:1121–1130.

Isaac M, Chand PK. Dissociative and conversion disorder: Defining boundaries. *Curr Opin Psychiatry*. 2006;19:61–66.

Karris BC, Capobianco M, Wei X, Ross L. Treatment of depersonalization disorder with repetitive transcranial magnetic stimulation. *J Psychiatr Pract*. 2017;23:141–144.

Lanius RA, Williamson PC, Densmore M, Boksman K, Neufeld RWJ, Gati JS, Menon R. The nature of traumatic memories: A 4-T fMRI functional connectivity analysis. *Am J Psychiatry*. 2004;161:36–44.

Loewenstein RJ, Frewen P, Lewis-Fernandez R. Chapter 20: Dissociative disorders. In: Sadock BJ, Sadock VA, Ruiz P, eds. *Kaplan & Sadock's Comprehensive Textbook of Psychiatry*. 10th ed. Philadelphia, PA: Wolters Kluwer; 2017:1866–1952.

Maaranen P, Tanskanen A, Honkalampi K, Haatainen K, Hintikka J, Viinamaki H. Factors associated with pathological dissociation in the general population. *Aust N Z J Psychiatry*. 2005;39:387–394.

Markowitsch HJ. Psychogenic amnesia. *Neuroimage*. 2003;20:S132–S138.

Martinez-Taboas A, Dorahy M, Sar V, Middleton W, Kruger C. Growing not dwindling: International research on the worldwide phenomenon of dissociative disorders. *J Nerv Ment Dis*. 2013;201(4):353–354.

Middleton W. Owning the past, claiming the present: Perspectives on the treatment of dissociative patients. *Australas Psychiatry*. 2005;13:40–49.

Rachid F. Treatment of a patient with depersonalization disorder with low frequency repetitive transcranial magnetic stimulation of the right temporo-parietal junction in a private practice setting. *J Psychiatr Pract*. 2017;23:145–147.

Reinders AA, Nijenhuis ERS, Paans AMJ, Korf J, Willemsen ATM, den Boer JA. One brain, two selves. *Neuroimage*. 2003;20:2119–2125.

Simeon D, Knutelska M, Nelson D, Guralnik O. Feeling unreal: A depersonalization disorder update of 117 cases. *J Clin Psychiatry*. 2003;64:990–997.

Vermetten E, Spiegel D. Trauma and dissociation: Implications for borderline personality disorder. *Curr Psychiatry Rep*. 2014;16(2):1–10.

Somatic Symptom and Related Disorders

Everyone experiences somatic symptoms, and most can cope with them effectively. However, some people's lives are overwhelmed by their somatic concerns. Sometimes the somatic concerns stem from well-established major medical illnesses; sometimes, the origins of the concerns are never quite clear. What is common in both situations are the pervasive and overwhelming thoughts and behaviors centered on these sensations. DSM-5 incorporated this perspective because the older perspective (only counting or cataloging symptoms labeled as medically unexplained) embodied in the previous versions of the disorder was unreliable and such perspective often put the doctor and the patient at odds over the question of the legitimacy and "reality" of the patient's symptoms and personal suffering. ICD-10 continues the older approach. However, the planned revision will be more in line with DSM-5.

THE CLINICAL PRESENTATION

Persons suffering from one of these disorders have one or more somatic symptoms that become all-consuming or lead to notable impairment in their day-to-day lives. These symptoms are no longer required to be medically unexplained, as such a distinction in itself is unreliable, and because psychiatrists commonly treat patients with medically established diagnoses who are disproportionately troubled by or preoccupied with their physical symptoms.

Somatic Symptom Disorder

Patients with somatic symptom disorder believe that they have some severe yet undetected disease, and evidence to the contrary does not persuade them otherwise. They may maintain a belief that they have a particular disease or, over time, may transfer their belief to another disease. They are fixated on one or more somatic symptoms that they are convinced are evidence of illness. For some individuals, their convictions persist despite negative laboratory results, the benign course of the alleged disease over time, and appropriate reassurances from physicians. Others may have a genuine medical condition about which they develop excessive and unreasonable anxiety, and this is also a manifestation of somatic symptom disorder. Patients with somatic symptom disorder often experience symptoms of depression and anxiety, in addition to their somatic symptoms.

Illness Anxiety Disorder

Patients with illness anxiety disorder, like those with somatic symptom disorder, believe they have a serious but undiagnosed disease despite evidence to the contrary. They may maintain a belief that they have a particular disease or, as time progresses, they may transfer their belief to another disease. Their convictions

persist despite negative laboratory results, the benign course of the alleged disease over time, and appropriate reassurances from physicians. Their preoccupation with illness interferes with their interaction with family, friends, and coworkers. They are often addicted to internet searches about their feared illness, inferring the worst from information (or misinformation) they find there. Unlike somatic symptom disorder, however, these individuals do not have significant physical symptoms. Sometimes people with this disorder develop a fear of going to medical appointments, while other times, they seek excessive reassurance about their health from medical providers.

Conversion Disorder (Functional Neurologic Symptom Disorder)

Persons with conversion disorder (also called functional neurologic symptom disorder) present with what appears to be a neurologic condition. The symptoms may be motor or sensory but are incompatible with known neurologic conditions. Often the illness is preceded by conflicts or other stressors and may seem to be associated with apparent psychological factors. Individuals with conversion disorder do not intentionally produce these symptoms or deficits. Conversion motor symptoms mimic syndromes such as paralysis, ataxia, dysphagia, or seizure disorder (nonepileptic seizures [NESs]), and the sensory symptoms mimic neurologic deficits such as blindness, deafness, or anesthesia. There can also be disturbances of consciousness (e.g., amnesia, fainting spells).

Psychological Factors Affecting Other Medical Conditions

Patients with this disorder have physical disorders caused by or adversely affected by emotional or psychological factors. A medical condition must always be present to make the diagnosis. Common clinical examples include denial and refusal of treatment for an acute condition (such as myocardial infarct or abdominal emergencies) by individuals with certain personality styles (e.g., domineering or controlling), the exacerbation of asthma or irritable bowel attacks by anxiety, and the manipulation of insulin by an individual with diabetes, or diuretics in the case of hypertensive patients, in efforts to lose weight.

Factitious Disorder

Patients with factitious disorder feign, misrepresent, simulate, cause, induce, or aggravate illness to receive medical attention, regardless of whether or not they are ill. Thus, they may inflict painful, deforming, or even life-threatening injuries on themselves, their children, or other dependents. The primary motivation is not the avoidance of duties, financial gain, or anything concrete. The motivation is simply to receive medical care and to partake in the medical system.

Factitious disorders can lead to significant morbidity or even mortality. Therefore, even the patients falsify their presenting complaints, health professionals must take the medical and psychiatric needs of these patients seriously, as their self-induced symptoms can result in significant harm or even death. Historically this disorder was called "Munchausen syndrome," a reference to the Baron Munchausen, legendary for his outrageously exaggerated stories of his military career.

Other Specified and Unspecified Somatic Symptom and Related Disorders

Patients with other specified somatic symptom and related disorders present with somatic symptoms that do not meet the threshold for another disorder. For example, they may present with symptoms consistent with illness anxiety disorder, except that the symptoms do not meet the duration criterion; in this case, the diagnosis would be brief illness anxiety disorder.

When there is not enough information to make a specific diagnosis, then clinicians should use the unspecified somatic symptom and related disorder diagnosis.

DIAGNOSIS

Somatic Symptom Disorder

According to the DSM-5, individuals with somatic symptom disorder present with one or more somatic complaints that result in significant angst or functional impairment. Also, they must be anxious about their symptoms or be preoccupied with them. The analogous diagnosis in ICD-10, as well in the previous version of the DSM is somatization disorder. The biggest difference between the two concepts is whether there needs to be evidence that there is

no underlying medical cause for the disorder—ICD-10 does, and DSM-IV did require this whereas DSM-5 does not. Table 12-1 compares the approaches to this diagnosis.

Mr. K, a white man in his mid-50s, consulted a general medicine clinic complaining of gastrointestinal problems. He had a long list of physical symptoms and concerns, mostly related to the gastrointestinal system. These included abdominal pain, left lower quadrant cramps, bloating, persistent sense of fullness in stomach hours after eating, intolerance to foods, constipation, decrease in physical stamina, heart palpitations, and feelings that "skin is getting yellow" and "not getting enough oxygen." A review of systems disclosed disturbances from virtually every organ system, including tired eyes with blurred vision, sore throat and "lump" in the throat, heart palpitations, irregular heartbeat, dizziness, trouble breathing, and general weakness.

The patient reported that symptoms started more than 20 years ago. Over this time, psychiatrists, general practitioners, and other medical specialists evaluated him, including surgeons. He used the internet regularly and traveled extensively in search of expert evaluations, seeking new procedures and diagnostic assessments. He had undergone repeated colonoscopies, sigmoidoscopies, and computed tomographic (CT) scans, magnetic resonance imaging (MRI) studies, and ultrasound examinations of the abdomen that had revealed Barrett esophagus but no other pathology. He was on disability and had been unable to work for more than 2 years due to his condition.

About 3 years before his visit to the medical clinic, his abdominal complaints and his fixed belief that he had an intestinal obstruction led to an exploratory surgical intervention for the first time, apparently with negative findings. However, according to the patient, the surgery "got things even worse," and since then, he had undergone at least five more operations. During these surgeries, he has undergone subtotal colectomies and ileostomies due to possible "adhesions" to rule out "mechanical" obstruction. However, available records from some of the surgeries do not disclose any specific pathology other than "intractable constipation." Pathologic specimens were also inconclusive.

A complete physical and neurologic examination showed a well-developed, well-nourished male who was afebrile. A complete physical

Table 12-1
Somatic Symptom Disorder (DSM-5) and Somatization Disorder (ICD-10)

Name	DSM-5 **Somatic Symptom Disorder**	ICD-10 **Somatization Disorder**
Duration	≥6 mo	≥2 yr
Symptoms	• Preoccupied with symptoms and their potential seriousness. • Anxious about symptoms and health • Time and energy devoted to the symptoms	• Recurring symptoms • Symptoms frequently change • Prolonged involvement with the medical system • High use of healthcare services
# Symptoms needed	≥1	
Exclusion (not the result of):		Malingering Medical cause for symptoms on workup
Psychosocial impact	Distress or impairment	Social, interpersonal, and familial disruption
Symptom specifiers	With predominant pain	
Severity specifiers	**Mild:** 1 symptom **Moderate:** ≥2 symptoms **Severe:** ≥2 symptoms, with multiple symptomatic complaints or 1 that is severe	Undifferentiated somatoform disorder: <2 yr, less severe symptoms Somatoform autonomic dysfunction: autonomic arousal symptoms or other less specific complaints Persistent somatoform pain disorder (pain is the predominant symptom)
Course specifiers	**Persistent:** >6 mo of severe symptoms and impairment	

and neurologic examination was normal except for examination of the abdomen, which revealed multiple abdominal scars. Right ileostomy was present, with soft stool in the bag and active bowel sounds. There was no point tenderness and no abdominal distension. During the examination, the patient kept pointing to an area of "hardness" in the left lower quadrant that he thought was a "tight muscle strangling his bowels." However, the examination did not disclose any palpable mass. Skin and extremities were all within normal limits, and all joints had a full range of motion and no swelling. Musculature was well developed. Neurologic examination was within normal limits. His primary care physician scheduled brief monthly visits by, during which the doctor performed brief physicals, reassured the patient, and allowed the patient to talk about "stressors." The physician avoided invasive tests or diagnostic procedures, did not prescribe any medications and avoided telling the patient that the symptoms were mental or "all in his head." The primary care physician then referred the patient back to psychiatry.

The psychiatrist confirmed a long list of physical symptoms that started in his 20s, most of which remained medically unexplained. The psychiatric examination revealed some anxiety symptoms, including apprehension, tension, uneasiness, and somatic components such as blushing and palpitations that seemed particularly prominent in social situations. Possible symptoms of depression included mild dysphoria, low energy, and sleep disturbance, all of which the patient blamed on his "medical" problems. The mental status examination showed that Mr. K's mood was rather somber and pessimistic, although he denied feeling sad or depressed. Affect was irritable. He was somatically focused and had little if any, psychological insight. The examination revealed the presence of a few life stressors (unemployment, financial problems, and family issues) that the patient quickly discounted as unimportant. The psychiatrist diagnosed somatic symptom disorder, severe.

Although the patient continued to deny having any psychiatric problems or any need for psychiatric intervention or treatment, he agreed to a few regular visits to continue to assess his situation. He refused to have anyone from his family involved in this process. Efforts to engage the patient with formal therapy such as cognitive-behavioral therapy (CBT) or a medication trial were all futile, so he was seen only for "supportive psychotherapy," with the hope of developing rapport and preventing additional iatrogenic complications.

During the follow-up period, the patient was operated on at least one more time and continued to complain of abdominal bloating and constipation and to rely on laxatives. The patient continued to believe he had an obstruction of his intestines; this bordered on the delusional. However, he continued to refuse pharmacologic treatment. The only medication he accepted was a low-dose benzodiazepine for anxiety. He continued to monitor his intestinal function 24 hr/day and to seek evaluation by prominent specialists, traveling to high-profile specialty centers far from home in search of solutions. (Courtesy of J. I. Escobar, M.D.)

Although DSM-5 specifies that the symptoms must be present for at least 6 months, transient manifestations can occur after significant stresses, most commonly the death or severe illness of someone important to the patient. It can also occur after a severe illness that resolved but left the patient shaken by the experience. Such states that last fewer than 6 months are diagnosed as "Other Specified Somatic Symptom and Related Disorders" in DSM-5. Transient somatic symptom disorder responses to external stress generally remit with a resolution of the stress, but they can become chronic if friends or healthcare professionals reinforce the concerns.

Illness Anxiety Disorder

The primary DSM-5 diagnostic criteria for illness anxiety disorder are that patients be preoccupied with the false belief that they have or will develop a severe disease in the presence of few if any physical signs or symptoms. With illness anxiety disorder, patients have relatively minor somatic symptoms and instead focus on concerns that they will get sick or have an undiagnosed illness; on the other hand, with somatic symptom disorder, there are significant health concerns along with substantial somatic symptoms. The analogous disorder in ICD-10 and the earlier DSM-IV is hypochondriasis. Table 12-2 compares the two disorders.

Conversion Disorder (Functional Neurologic Symptom Disorder)

A conversion reaction is a rather acute and temporary loss or alteration in motor or sensory function that requires substantial discordance between the symptoms displayed and any neurologic condition,

Table 12-2
Illness Anxiety Disorder (DSM-5) and Hypochondriasis (ICD-10)

	DSM-5	ICD-10
Name	**Illness Anxiety Disorder**	**Hypochondriacal Disorder**
Duration	≥6 mo	
Symptoms	• Preoccupied with having or getting a serious illness without good reason • Anxious about the belief • Excess health-related behaviors related to the belief ("care-seeking"), maladaptive behaviors, or avoidance behaviors ("care-avoiding")	Preoccupied with having a serious medical illness Anxiety Somatic complaints Concerns about appearance Distress or depression associated with the above
# Symptoms needed	All the above	
Exclusion (not the result of):	Another mental disorder	
Symptom specifiers	Care-seeking type Care-avoidant type	
Comments		Body dysmorphic disorder is included with this diagnosis as a subtype

Table 12-3
Conversion Disorder

Name	DSM-5 Conversion Disorder (Functional Neurologic Symptom Disorder)	ICD-10 Dissociative (Conversion) Disorders
Symptoms	• ≥ Voluntary motor or sensory symptoms • No correlation between any medical or neurologic illness and the symptoms on examination	
Exclusion (not the result of):	Another mental illness Another medical condition	
Psychosocial impact	Marked distress and/or functional impairment	
Symptom specifiers	**With weakness or paralysis** **With abnormal movement** **With swallowing symptoms** **With speech symptom** **With attacks or seizures** **With anesthesia or sensory loss** **With special sensory symptoms** (i.e., vision, olfaction, hearing) **With mixed symptoms** **Can also specify with or without psychological stressor**	**Dissociative stupor** **Dissociative motor disorder** (limb, speech, or gait) **Dissociative convulsions** **Dissociative anesthesia and sensory loss** **Mixed dissociative (conversion) disorders**
Course specifiers	**Acute episode** (<6 mo) **Persistent** (≥6 mo)	

such that it would be impossible for the patient's presentation to be consistent with a neurologic disease. Because the onset frequently coincides with psychological issues (conflict), early theorists speculated that such issues were "converted" to neurologic symptoms. The problem is that stress is omnipresent in life, and many patients present with conversion without an obvious stressor. The classic syndromes represent neurologic syndromes such as paralysis, seizures, or blindness. In DSM-5, we can indicate the type of symptom the patient is experiencing. Table 12-3 compares the approaches to diagnosing this disorder in DSM-5 and ICD-10. Table 12-4 lists common symptoms of conversion disorder. Table 12-5 lists examples of significant physical examination findings often found in disorder.

Mr. J is a 28-year-old single man who works in a factory. He was brought to an emergency department by his father, complaining that he had lost his vision while sitting in the back seat on the way home from a family gathering. He had been playing volleyball at the gathering

Table 12-4
Common Symptoms of Conversion Disorder

Motor Symptoms	Sensory Deficits
Involuntary movements	Anesthesia, especially of extremities
Tics	Midline anesthesia
Blepharospasm	Blindness
Torticollis	Tunnel vision
Opisthotonos	Deafness
Seizures	**Visceral Symptoms**
Abnormal gait	Psychogenic vomiting
Falling	Pseudocyesis
Astasia–abasia	Globus hystericus
Paralysis	Swooning or syncope
Weakness	Urinary retention
Aphonia	Diarrhea

(Courtesy of Frederick G. Guggenheim, M.D.)

but had sustained no significant injury except for the volleyball hitting him in the head a few times. He was initially reluctant to play volleyball because of his mediocre athleticism and was a last-minute addition to the team. He recalls having some problems with seeing during the game, but his vision did not become ablated until he was in the car on the way home. By the time he got to the emergency department, his vision was improving, although he still complained of blurriness and mild diplopia. The physician could attenuate the double vision by having the patient focus on different items at different distances.

On examination, Mr. J was fully cooperative, somewhat uncertain about why this would have occurred, and rather nonchalant. Pupillary, oculomotor, and general sensorimotor examinations were routine. After being cleared medically, the physician referred the patient to a mental health center for further evaluation.

At the mental health center, the patient recounts the same story as he did in the emergency department. His father continued to accompany him. He said his vision improved when his father stopped the car, and they talked about the day's events. He spoke with his father about how he had felt embarrassed and somewhat conflicted about playing volleyball but felt pressure to play. Further history from the patient and his father revealed that this young man had been shy as an adolescent, particularly around athletic participation. He had never had another episode of visual loss. He did recount feeling anxious and sometimes not feeling well in his body during athletic activities.

Discussion with the patient at the mental health center focused on the potential role of psychological and social factors in acute vision loss. The patient was somewhat perplexed by this but was also amenable to discussion. He stated that he recognized that he began seeing and feeling better when his father pulled off to the side of the road and discussed things with him. Doctors stated that they did not know the cause of the vision loss and that it would likely not return. The patient and his father were satisfied with the medical and psychiatric evaluation and agreed to return for care if there were any further symptoms. The patient was appointed a follow-up time at the outpatient psychiatric clinic. (Courtesy of Michael A. Hollifield, M.D.)

Table 12-5
Distinctive Physical Examination Findings in Conversion Disorder

Condition	Test	Conversion Findings
Anesthesia	Map dermatomes	Sensory loss does not conform to recognized pattern of distribution
Hemianesthesia	Check midline	Strict half-body split
Astasia–abasia	Walking, dancing	With suggestion, those who cannot walk may still be able to dance; alteration of sensory and motor findings with suggestion
Paralysis, paresis	Drop paralyzed hand onto face	Hand falls next to face, not on it
	Hoover test	Pressure noted in examiner's hand under paralyzed leg when attempting straight leg raising
	Check motor strength	Give-away weakness
Coma	Examiner attempts to open eyes	Resists opening; gaze preference is away from doctor
	Ocular cephalic maneuver	Eyes stare straight ahead, do not move from side to side
Aphonia	Request a cough	Essentially normal coughing sound indicates cords are closing
Intractable sneezing	Observe	Short nasal grunts with little or no sneezing on inspiratory phase; little or no aerosolization of secretions; minimal facial expression; eyes open; stops when asleep; abates when alone
Syncope	Head-up tilt test	Magnitude of changes in vital signs and venous pooling do not explain continuing symptoms
Tunnel vision	Visual fields	Changing pattern on multiple examinations
Profound monocular blindness	Swinging flashlight sign (Marcus Gunn)	Absence of relative afferent pupillary defect
	Binocular visual fields	Sufficient vision in "bad eye" precludes plotting normal physiologic blind spot in good eye
Severe bilateral blindness	"Wiggle your fingers, I'm just testing coordination"	Patient may begin to mimic new movements before realizing the slip
	Sudden flash of bright light	Patient flinches
	"Look at your hand"	Patient does not look there
	"Touch your index fingers"	Even blind patients can do this by proprioception

(Courtesy of Frederick G. Guggenheim, M.D.)

Sensory Symptoms. In conversion disorder, anesthesia and paresthesia are common, especially of the extremities. All sensory modalities can be involved, and the distribution of the disturbance is usually inconsistent with either central or peripheral neurologic disease. Thus, clinicians may see the characteristic stocking-and-glove anesthesia of the hands or feet or the hemianesthesia of the body beginning precisely along the midline.

Conversion disorder symptoms may involve the organs of special sense and can produce deafness, blindness, and tunnel vision. These symptoms can be unilateral or bilateral, but neurologic evaluation reveals intact sensory pathways. In conversion disorder blindness, for example, patients walk around without collisions or self-injury, their pupils react to light, and their cortical-evoked potentials are normal.

Motor Symptoms. The motor symptoms of conversion disorder include abnormal movements, gait disturbance, weakness, and paralysis. Gross rhythmical tremors, choreiform movements, tics, and jerks may be present. The movements generally worsen when calling attention to them. One gait disturbance seen in conversion disorder is *astasia–abasia,* which is a wildly ataxic, staggering gait accompanied by gross, irregular, jerky truncal movements and thrashing and waving arm movements. Patients with the symptoms rarely fall; if they do, they are generally not injured.

Other common motor disturbances are paralysis and paresis involving one, two, or all four limbs, although the distribution of the involved muscles does not conform to the neural pathways. Reflexes remain normal; the patients have no fasciculations or muscle atrophy (except after long-standing conversion paralysis); electromyography findings are normal.

Seizure Symptoms. NESs are another symptom of conversion disorder. Clinicians may find it challenging to differentiate NESs from an actual seizure by clinical observation alone. Some patients with NESs also have a coexisting epileptic disorder, which may complicate the clinical picture. Tongue-biting, urinary incontinence, and injuries after falling can occur in NESs, although these symptoms are generally not present. Patients with NESs retain pupillary and gag reflexes after their seizure-like activity, and patients have no postseizure increase in prolactin concentrations.

Other Associated Features. Several psychological symptoms are also associated with conversion disorder.

PRIMARY GAIN. Patients achieve primary gain by keeping internal conflicts outside their awareness. Symptoms have symbolic value; they represent an unconscious psychological conflict.

SECONDARY GAIN. Patients accrue tangible advantages and benefits as a result of being sick; for example, being excused from obligations and difficult life situations, receiving support and assistance that might not otherwise be forthcoming, and controlling others' behavior.

LA BELLE INDIFFÉRENCE.   *La belle indifférence* ("beautiful indifference") is a patient's inappropriately cavalier attitude toward severe symptoms; that is, the patient seems to be unconcerned about what appears to be a significant impairment. That bland indifference may also occur in some seriously ill medical patients who develop a stoic attitude. The presence or absence of *la belle indifférence* is not pathognomonic of conversion disorder, but it is often associated with the condition.

IDENTIFICATION.   Patients with conversion disorder may unconsciously model their symptoms on those of someone important to them. For example, a parent or a person who has recently died may serve as a model for conversion disorder. During pathologic grief reaction, bereaved persons commonly have symptoms of the deceased.

Psychological Factors Affecting Other Medical Conditions

According to DSM-5, individuals with this condition have a medical illness that is significantly impacted by psychological influences or patterns of behavior. We should only make the diagnosis when the effect of the psychological issue on the medical condition is unambiguous and leads to documentable effects on the course and outcome of the medical condition. Psychological or behavioral factors include psychological distress, patterns of interpersonal interaction, coping styles, and maladaptive health behaviors such as denial of symptoms or poor adherence to medical recommendations.

The reverse situation, the psychiatric or psychological consequences of having a medical condition, is more appropriately classified as an adjustment disorder. Other ambiguous situations where psychological and physical symptoms coexist (the so-called "comorbidities") present particular challenges. For example, many somatic, anxiety, and mood disorders are associated with chronic medical conditions (diabetes, hypertension, hypercholesterolemia) or "functional" syndromes (irritable bowel, migraine headaches, and several others).

Mr. A, a 55-year-old man, was hospitalized in the intensive care unit following a cardiac arrest. He had been experiencing severe substernal chest pain but "ignored it." He became diaphoretic and reported reluctantly to a nearby emergency room where he had a cardiac arrest while awaiting evaluation. He was successfully resuscitated and transferred to the ICU. He emphatically rejected having had a heart attack, took his EKG leads off, and was preparing to leave the unit against medical advice. The psychiatric consultant obtained a history that the patient's father and his brother had died of coronary disease. At the time of the initial assessment, the patient was irritable and somewhat anxious. He agreed to stay in the ICU overnight after his wife insisted that he stay, and the psychiatrist explained the tests further. The psychiatrist prescribed a low dose of a benzodiazepine, and, on the next day, he was agreeable to remain in the hospital for further treatment.

Factitious Disorder

Factitious disorder is the faking of physical or psychological signs and symptoms. Symptoms can be imposed on self or imposed on another. Table 12-6 compares criteria for the disorder and Table 12-7 list some clues that should trigger suspicion of this disorder.

Factitious Disorder Imposed on Self.
We diagnose this condition when an individual feigns having a medical or psychiatric illness in order to achieve the sick role. Patients may simply misrepresent their symptoms, may cause injury to themselves, or may use other dishonest methods in order to appear as if they are sick.

Some patients show psychiatric symptoms judged to be fake. This determination can be difficult and is often made only after a prolonged investigation. The feigned symptoms frequently include depression, hallucinations, dissociative and conversion symptoms, and bizarre behavior. Because the patient's condition does not improve after routine therapeutic measures, he or she may receive large doses of psychoactive drugs and may undergo electroconvulsive therapy. Patients may appear depressed and may explain their depression by offering a false history of the recent death of a significant friend or relative. Elements of the history that may suggest factitious bereavement include a violent or bloody death,

Table 12-6
Factitious Disorder

Name	DSM-5 Factitious Disorder	ICD-10 Intentional Production or Feigning of Symptoms or Disabilities, Either Physical or Psychological (Factitious Disorder)
Symptoms	**Factitious disorder imposed on self:** • Fabricates their symptoms and clinical findings • Claims to be ill • Purposely misleads health professionals • No apparent external reward or motivation (outside of the illness role) **Factitious disorder imposed on another:** • As above except the object of the feigned illness or injury is another person.	Feigns symptoms No apparent external reward or motivation Aim is to take on the sick role
Exclusion (not the result of):	Another mental disorder	Factitious dermatitis Malingering
Course specifiers	**Single episode** **Recurrent episodes** (2 or more discrete events)	
Comments	*Note: In factitious disorder imposed on another, the perpetrator receives the diagnosis, not the victim.*	

Table 12-7
Clues That Should Trigger Suspicion of Factitious Disorder

1. The patient has sought treatment at various different hospitals or clinics
2. The patient is an inconsistent, selective, or misleading informant; he or she resists allowing the treatment team access to outside sources of information
3. The course of the illness is atypical and does not follow the natural history of the presumed disease
4. A remarkable number of tests, consultations, and medical and surgical treatments have been done to little or no avail
5. The magnitude of symptoms consistently exceeds objective pathology or symptoms have proved to be exaggerated by the patient
6. Some findings are discovered to have been self-induced or at least worsened through self-manipulation
7. The patient might eagerly agree to or request invasive medical procedures or surgery
8. Physical evidence of a factitious cause might be discovered during the course of treatment
9. The patient predicts deteriorations or there are exacerbations shortly before their scheduled discharge
10. A diagnosis of factitious disorder has been explicitly considered by at least one healthcare professional
11. The patient is noncompliant with diagnostic or treatment recommendations or is disruptive on the unit
12. Evidence from laboratory or other tests disputes information provided by the patient
13. The patient has a history of work in the healthcare field
14. The patient engages in gratuitous, self-aggrandizing lying
15. The patient has been prescribed (or obtained) opiate drugs when not indicated
16. While seeking medical or surgical intervention, the patient opposes psychiatric assessment

a death under dramatic circumstances, and the dead person being a child or a young adult. Other patients may describe either recent and remote memory loss or both auditory and visual hallucinations. Some patients may use psychoactive substances to produce symptoms, such as stimulants to produce restlessness or insomnia, or hallucinogens to produce distortions of reality. Combinations of psychoactive substances can produce very unusual presentations. Other psychological symptoms include pseudologia fantastica and impostorship.

In *pseudologia fantastica*, the patient mixes limited factual material with extensive and colorful fantasies. The listener's interest pleases the patient and, thus, reinforces the symptom. In addition to distortions of the history, patients often give false and conflicting accounts about other areas of their lives (e.g., they may claim the death of a parent, to play on the sympathy of others). Imposture is commonly related to lying in these cases. Many patients assume the identity of a prestigious person. They may, for example, report being war heroes and attribute their surgical scars to wounds received during battle or in other dramatic and dangerous exploits. Similarly, they may say that they have ties to accomplished or renowned figures.

Other patients may feign physical symptoms suggesting a disorder involving any organ system. They are familiar with the diagnoses of most disorders that usually require hospital admission or medication and can give excellent histories capable of deceiving even experienced clinicians. Clinical presentations are myriad and include hematoma, hemoptysis, abdominal pain, fever, hypoglycemia, lupus-like syndromes, nausea, vomiting, dizziness, and seizures. For example, the patient may contaminate urine with blood or feces or take anticoagulants to simulate bleeding disorders,

or insulin to produce hypoglycemia. Such patients often insist on surgery and claim adhesions from previous surgical procedures. They may acquire a "gridiron" or washboard-like abdomen from multiple procedures. Complaints of pain, especially that simulating renal colic, are common, with the patients wanting narcotics. In about half the reported cases, these patients demand treatment with specific medications, usually analgesics. Once in the hospital, they continue to be demanding and challenging. After each test result is negative, they may accuse doctors of incompetence, threaten litigation, and become generally abusive. Some may sign out abruptly shortly before they believe the healthcare team is going to confront them with their factitious behavior. They then go to another hospital in the same or another city and begin the cycle again. Specific predisposing factors are actual physical disorders during childhood, leading to extensive medical treatment. Other factors may include a grudge against the medical profession, employment in the healthcare industry, or a significant relationship with a physician in the past.

Table 12-8 provides a comprehensive overview of a variety of signs and symptoms that may be faked and mistaken for genuine illness. The table also includes the means of simulation and possible methods of detection.

Factitious Disorder Imposed on Another (formerly Factitious Disorder by Proxy). In this diagnosis, a person intentionally produces physical signs or symptoms in another person who is under the first person's care. One apparent purpose of the behavior is for the caretaker to assume the sick role indirectly; another is to be relieved of the caretaking role by having the child hospitalized. The most common cause of factitious disorder imposed on another involves a mother who deceives medical personnel into believing that her child is ill. The deception may involve a false medical history, contamination of laboratory samples, alteration of records, or induction of injury and illness in the child. Table 12-9 lists some clues that should trigger suspicion of this disorder.

BC, a 1-month-old girl, was admitted for the evaluation of fever. The medical team requested a psychiatric consult because of inconsistencies in the mother's reporting of medical information despite her presentation as a knowledgeable and caring mother who worked as an emergency medical technician. BC's mother reported her own diagnosis of ovarian cancer when she was 3 months pregnant with BC. She reported undergoing a hysterectomy during her cesarean section, and that she had been getting radiation therapy at a local hospital since BC's birth. The pediatrician called the local hospital with the mother's permission and learned that she had a corpus luteum cyst removed at 3 months' gestation and mild hydronephrosis but no cancer or hysterectomy. BC's mother, when confronted with this, replied that she might need a kidney transplant for the hydronephrosis.

On further exploration, the medical team discovered that the mother had brought her children to multiple emergency rooms, giving inaccurate histories that prompted excessive testing. At one visit, she told clinicians that her 2-year-old son had lupus and hypergammaglobulinemia, and at another visit, that he had asthma and seizures. She also pursued a minor cosmetic surgical procedure for him against his pediatrician's recommendation.

Clinicians suspected that BC's mother intentionally fabricated symptoms, such as by warming BC's thermometer, and that she did not actively induce symptoms in her children. She was faithful in keeping medical appointments, and her children appeared healthy and well cared for, despite her factitious behavior. The mother denied a psychiatric history but agreed to let the clinicians contact the local

Table 12-8
Methods of Factitious Symptom Production, Suggestive Signs, and Confirmatory Tests by Systems

Symptom	Method of Factitious Symptom Manufacture	Signs Suggestive of Factitiousness	Test for Factitious Method
Infectious Disease			
Fever	Injecting infectious material into vein/intravenous line	Higher than 41°C	Monitoring while temperature taken
	Ingesting thyroid hormone	Not accompanied by other vital sign abnormalities	Using electronic thermometer instead of mercury thermometer
	Drinking hot fluids	Does not follow diurnal pattern	Recording oral and rectal temperatures simultaneously
	Manipulating thermometers with lightbulb or heating pad	No diaphoresis with rapid defervescence	Noting thermometer brand names/serial numbers
	Substituting another thermometer		
	Warm wax/wet cotton in ears	Measuring fresh urine specimen temperature	
Bacteremia	Injection of contaminated substance	Polymicrobial bacteremia	Culture
		Absence of urologic/biliary/GI obstruction	
		Stool flora/pet flora noted	
HIV/AIDS	False history/reports	Normal CD4 count/undetectable viral load/Ab negative	Repeat HIV ELISA, western blot, viral load
			Confirm test results with laboratory
Gastrointestinal			
Diarrhea	Laxative abuse (magnesium, castor oil, phenolphthalein)	Metabolic alkalosis	Detection of laxative in urine or stool (usually need multiple tests)
		Acute hyperchloremic metabolic acidosis with normal anion gap	3-day stool collection
		Decreased serum bicarbonate with metabolic acidosis	Urine screen for phenolphthaleins, anthraquinones, bisacodyl
		High daily stool volume	Stool screen for magnesium >45 mmol/L, phosphate
		Melanosis coli on sigmoidoscopy	
		Cathartic colon on barium enema	
		Low urine potassium concentration	
		High fecal fluid potassium concentration	
		Fecal fluid osmolality <290 mOsm/kg	
	Adding water to stool sample	High stool osmolar gap >125 mOsmol/kg	
Vomiting	Ipecac/cathartic abuse	Hypokalemia	Detection of ipecac in stool by chromatography
		High urine potassium concentration	Serum/urine emetine levels
		Low urine chloride concentration	EKG with abnormalities c/w ipecac toxicity
		Metabolic alkalosis with increased serum bicarbonate	
Pancreatitis	Spitting into urine sample (salivary amylase)	Hyperamylasuria with normal serum amylase	Obtain monitored sample
GI bleeding	Injection of blood from transfusions	Nasogastric tube shows blood despite normal endoscopy	Radiolabeling transfusions
	Ingestion of NSAIDs/salicylates	Single-stripe sign on colonoscopy	
Obstruction	Ingestion of loperamide		HPLC of serum/stool for motility-slowing agent
Renal			
Diuresis	Diuretic abuse	High urine potassium concentration	Detection of diuretics by chromatography
Bartter syndrome	Loop diuretic abuse	Hypokalemia, urine chloride low or variable	Renal biopsy for juxtaglomerular hyperplasia
	Self-induced vomiting		Screen urine for diuretics

Table 12-8
Methods of Factitious Symptom Production, Suggestive Signs, and Confirmatory Tests by Systems (*Continued*)

Symptom	Method of Factitious Symptom Manufacture	Signs Suggestive of Factitiousness	Test for Factitious Method
Metabolic			
Hypervitaminosis A	Vitamin A abuse	Increased gamma-glutamyltransferase Increased bilirubin	Increased serum/tissue levels vitamin A, retinoic acid derivatives
Hypokalemia	Laxative abuse	See above	
Hyperkalemia	Injection of urine into blood sample	Potassium level incompatible with life	Monitoring sample gathering yields normal result
Hypernatremia	Salt load	Fractional excretion of sodium high Gastric aspirate salt concentration >200 mmol/L	
Urologic			
Hematuria	Adding blood from another wound/meat Traumatizing urethra Inserting foreign bodies into the bladder Ingestion of anticoagulants Addition of coloring to urine	Lack of red blood cell/hemoglobin casts Lack of distorted red blood cells	"3-tube" urinalysis (more blood in first tube if urethral trauma) Physical examination Radiography
Proteinuria	Injection of egg protein in bladder	Large day-to-day variations in urine protein concentration Serum albumin concentration remains in normal range Lack of other signs of nephrotic syndrome	Electrophoresis of urine protein/pure albumin Large albumin band on urine protein electrophoresis without transferrin increase Antibody confirmation of human albumin
Bacteriuria	Injecting bacteria into bladder or urine specimens		
Urinary calculi	Adding pepper grains to urine Inserting stones into bladder Submitting quartz, feldspar as samples		Infrared spectrophotometry Chemical analysis X-ray diffraction X-ray crystallography
Hematologic			
Anemia	Self-bloodletting	Decreased serum iron, ferritin, iron-binding capacity Decreased bone marrow iron concentration No evidence of bleeding	Iron-59 elimination studies Urine/stool iron levels Blood typing
Sickle cell crisis		Serum protein electrophoresis normal	Genetic testing Hemoglobin electrophoresis
Pancytopenia	Ingestion of chemotherapy		
Hemorrhage/purpura	Ingestion of anticoagulant (rodenticide/Coumadin) Heparin injection	Prolonged prothrombin time (PT) Prolonged partial thromboplastin time (PTT) with normal PT	Warfarin/brodifacoum/heparin assay PTT measured every 2 hours under observation Reversal with protamine sulfate Normal reptilase time Failure of PTT to correct in 1:1 mixture with normal plasma Correction of PTT with heparin removal measures
	Ingestion of quinidine	Purpura with thrombocytopenia	Detection of quinidine-dependent antiplatelet antibodies

(continued)

Table 12-8
Methods of Factitious Symptom Production, Suggestive Signs, and Confirmatory Tests by Systems (*Continued*)

Symptom	Method of Factitious Symptom Manufacture	Signs Suggestive of Factitiousness	Test for Factitious Method
Endocrine			
Hypoglycemia	Injection of insulin Ingestion of oral hypoglycemic (sulfonylurea) Ingestion of tolbutamide Manipulation of testing strips	Serum insulin concentration >100 mU/L	Normal proinsulin levels (increased in insulinoma) High insulin/low C-peptide levels Insulin/C-peptide ratio >1.0 Extreme elevations in insulin levels Insulin antibodies (less reliable with human recombinant insulin) Failure of glucagon to produce C-peptide Glyburide assay in serum/urine Tolbutamide assay in serum
Hyperglycemia	Insufficient administration of insulin		
Hyperthyroidism	Ingestion of thyroid hormone	Goiter/eye findings absent Increased thyroxine or liothyronine levels Low TSH in thyroid storm	Serum thyroglobulin low–normal or undetectable Radioactive iodine uptake low
Cushing syndrome	Injecting/ingesting glucocorticoid Adding glucocorticoid to urine	Plasma/urinary cortisol increased Plasma ACTH low/undetectable Normal corticosterone/high cortisol	Detection of synthetic glucocorticoids in serum/urine Serum cortisol and corticosterone levels
Pheochromocytoma	Injection of epinephrine, isoproterenol Ingestion of stimulant Injection of epinephrine into urine sample	Normal chromogranin A level Lack of metabolites of epinephrine (metanephrines) Lack of norepinephrine increase after glucagon Normal response to clonidine suppression test	Epinephrine/norepinephrine levels in serum/urine Metanephrine/normetanephrine levels in serum/urine Provocative (glucagon)/suppression (clonidine) tests 44-metaiodobenzylguanidine nuclear scan
Hyperaldosteronism	Ingestion of black licorice/glycyrrhizic acid	Treatment-resistant hypokalemia Metabolic alkalosis Hypernatremia	Serum glycyrrhizic acid level
Cardiovascular			
Arrhythmia	Rearranging of EKG leads Ingestion of digitalis, beta blockers, calcium channel blockers	Unusual pattern on EKG	Supervise placement of EKG leads Serum levels of drugs Electrochemiluminescence assays detect BBs in urine
Hypertension	Valsalva maneuver Ingestion of stimulants	Office BPs normal, home BPs high	Observe BP checks Serum/urine assay for pseudoephedrine
Infarction	Beating self with towel to raise creatine kinase	EKGs don't change Enzymes do not rise appropriately	Repeat EKGs Repeat troponins
Dermatologic			
Cheilitis granulomatosa	Self-inoculation with polyvinylpyrrolidone (PVP)		Liver/lymph node biopsies show PVP in histiocytes
Dermatitis artefacta	Self-mutilation	Distribution of lesions in reachable areas	Skin biopsy shows mechanical trauma, necrosis, blood
Erythematous lesion	Applying alcohol to lesion		
Nonhealing wounds	Injection of air/contaminants/foreign bodies	Heal when casted Resistant to treatment Subcutaneous emphysema	Apply fluorescein to wound, examine hands/nails for fluorescence

Table 12-8
Methods of Factitious Symptom Production, Suggestive Signs, and Confirmatory Tests by Systems (*Continued*)

Symptom	Method of Factitious Symptom Manufacture	Signs Suggestive of Factitiousness	Test for Factitious Method
Obstetrical			
Ectopic pregnancy	Injection of hCG	Negative urine b-hCG Widely varying b-hCG levels	Negative ultrasound
Vaginal discharge	Intravaginal insertion	Inconsistent pH Vaginal wall shows abrasion/denies intercourse	
Neurologic			
Movement disorders	Ingestion of neuroleptics to induce parkinsonism	MRI/EEG/EMG inconsistent Hoover sign/tremor entrainable/ distractible Prolactin elevated with antipsychotics	Serum levels of neuroleptic
Multiple sclerosis		Examination inconsistent	CSF protein electrophoresis
Pseudoseizures		History inconsistent Semiology inconsistent Never observed seizing by others	Video EEG
Pulmonary			
Asthma	Tape interfering with pulse oximeters Inhalation of irritant (talc) Ingestion of allergens	Intractable hypoxia Intractable status asthmaticus	Lung biopsy Serum salicylate level
Cystic fibrosis	Manipulation of sweat test	Normal x-rays Normal examination/lack of clubbing	Sweat potassium
Hemoptysis	Ingestion of anticoagulants Cough abrasion of lung Self-induced trauma to respiratory tract	Normal bronchoscopy/lack of blood	
Respiratory failure		Incongruous arterial blood gas Marked hypocapnia	
Rheumatologic			
Arthritis	Insertion of metal fragments in joints		X-rays Synovial aspirate analysis
Lupus	Feigned history/borderline positive ANA	Repeat serum autoimmune tests negative Normal complement in active flare	Repeat serum tests
Vasculitis	Injection of contaminants to create purpura		Tissue biopsy of lesions reveals foreign material
Ophthalmologic			
Conjunctivitis	Instillation of foreign substance	Purulent discharge purposely left on skin and eyelashes Severity of discharge greater than severity of redness Severity of swelling less than severity of redness Mainly inferior conjunctival involvement Cornea uninvolved	Corneal examination/conjunctival biopsy
Anisocoria	Instillation of atropine eye drops		

Table 12-9
Clues Triggering Suspicion for Factitious Disorder Imposed on Another Person

1. Diagnosis does not match the objective findings
2. Signs or symptoms are bizarre
3. Caregiver or suspected offender does not express relief or pleasure when told that dependent is improving or that dependent does not have a particular illness
4. Inconsistent histories of symptoms from different observers
5. Caregiver insists on invasive or painful procedures or hospitalizations
6. Caregiver's behavior does not match expressed distress or report of symptoms (e.g., unusually calm)
7. Signs and symptoms begin only in the presence of one caregiver
8. Sibling or another dependent has or had an unusual or unexplained illness or death
9. Sensitivity to multiple environmental substances or medicines
10. Failure of the dependent's illness to respond to its normal treatments or unusual intolerance to those treatments
11. Caregiver publicly solicits sympathy or donations or benefits because of the dependent's rare illness
12. Extensive unusual illness history in the caregiver or caregiver's family; caregiver's history of somatization disorders
13. Caregiver seeks other medical opinions when told the dependent does not have illness
14. Caregiver perseverates about borderline abnormal results of no clinical relevance despite repeated reassurance, or refutes the validity of normal results

psychiatric hospital. That hospital revealed her history of depression, anorexia, panic disorder, and a suicide attempt resulting in psychiatric hospitalization. After the hospitalization, she received psychotherapy and medication, which she stopped a few months before this presentation. During BC's admission for fever, her mother agreed to resume psychiatric treatment. The team made a referral to social services, and the pediatrician scheduled regular follow-up visits for the children.

Other Specified or Unspecified Somatic Symptom and Related Disorders

This DSM-5 category describes conditions characterized by one or more unexplained physical symptoms, which are below the threshold for a diagnosis of somatic symptom or a related disorder. The symptoms are not better explained solely by another medical, psychiatric, or substance use disorder, and they cause clinically significant distress or impairment. Disorders in this category generally have too few symptoms are too brief to meet the criteria for a full disorder.

EVALUATION OF SOMATIC SYMPTOM AND RELATED DISORDERS

Patients with severe and protracted somatic syndromes approach medical encounters with a mixture of unrealistic expectations, pessimism, and distrust of the medical profession. The patients base these attitudes on their previous experiences with physicians, in which the physicians showed a lack of interest or disbelief in the patient's complaints and suffering. Building a trusting alliance must begin with respect for the patient's symptoms and an acknowledgment of their validity. Active, receptive listening, tolerance for repetition, and a "neutral" approach (avoiding being dismissive, confrontational, or overly reassuring) are essential skills.

Many of these patients often bring "thick" charts that include descriptions of many clinical encounters and multiple tests and procedures that are redundant and ordered without a clear rationale. The prospect of reviewing these medical records is challenging and often leads to a negative attitude from the physician. The physician should keep an open mind, despite forewarnings in the medical records, and perform an independent assessment of the patient. Avoid an emphasis on psychological questioning and interpretations at this stage. The patient may perceive premature reassurance as disinterest or dismissiveness.

Many patients with somatic symptom and related disorders do not readily acknowledge or recognize "emotional" issues and will feel more comfortable dealing with questions related to their physical symptoms than questions related to psychological issues. Taking a history of multiple somatic complaints can be carried over into subsequent appointments. A thorough physical examination, including neurologic examination, should follow history-taking at the initial visit, and the clinician should perform briefer physical assessments at subsequent visits. An inclusive drug history, including prescription and nonprescription remedies, should also be completed. As history-taking moves along, attitudes, beliefs, and attributions should become more evident and patterns of interaction and illness behavior discernible.

In the case of conversion disorder, there should be careful attention to any history of trauma, sexual abuse, physical abuse, and family history of conversion symptoms. Additionally, a neurologic workup of suspected conversion disorder should include routine laboratory studies, electroencephalograms, and other special studies (such as MRI) to rule out organic causes.

In the case of factitious disorder, the psychiatric examination should emphasize securing information from any available friends, relatives, or other informants, because interviews with reliable outside sources often reveal the false nature of the patient's illness. Although time-consuming and tedious, corroborating all the facts presented by the patient about previous hospitalizations and medical care is essential. Psychiatric evaluation is requested on a consultation basis in about 50 percent of cases, usually after a simulated illness is suspected. Under these circumstances, it is necessary to avoid pointed or accusatory questioning that may provoke truculence, evasion, or flight from the hospital. A danger may exist in provoking frank psychosis when using vigorous confrontation. In some instances, the feigned illness serves an adaptive function and is a desperate attempt to ward off further disintegration.

DIFFERENTIAL DIAGNOSIS

Somatic Symptom Disorder

We should differentiate somatic symptom disorder from nonpsychiatric medical conditions, especially disorders that show symptoms that are not necessarily easily diagnosed. Such diseases include acquired immunodeficiency syndrome (AIDS), endocrinopathies, myasthenia gravis, multiple sclerosis, degenerative diseases of the nervous system, systemic lupus erythematosus, and occult neoplastic disorders.

Somatic symptom disorder is differentiated from illness anxiety disorder by the emphasis on illness anxiety disorder on fear of having a disease rather than a concern about many symptoms. Patients with illness anxiety disorder usually complain about fewer symptoms than patients with somatic symptom disorder; they are primarily concerned about being sick.

Conversion disorder is acute and generally transient and usually involves a symptom rather than a particular disease. The presence or absence of *la belle indifférence* is an unreliable feature with which to differentiate the two conditions.

Patients with body dysmorphic disorder wish to appear normal, but believe that others notice that they are not, whereas those with somatic symptom disorder seek out attention for their presumed diseases.

Somatic symptom disorder can also occur in patients with depressive disorders and anxiety disorders. Patients with panic disorder may initially complain that they are affected by a disease (e.g., heart trouble), but careful questioning during the medical history usually uncovers the classic symptoms of a panic attack. Delusional beliefs occur in schizophrenia and other psychotic disorders but can be differentiated from somatic symptom disorder by their delusional intensity and by the presence of other psychotic symptoms. Also, schizophrenic patients' somatic delusions tend to be bizarre, idiosyncratic, and out of keeping with their cultural milieus, as illustrated in the case below.

> A 52-year-old man complained, "my guts are rotting away." Even after an extensive medical workup, the physician could not reassure the man that he was not ill.

Somatic symptom disorder is distinguished from factitious disorder and from malingering in that patients with somatic symptom disorder experience and do not simulate the symptoms they report.

Illness Anxiety Disorder

Again, we must differentiate illness anxiety disorder from other medical conditions. Too often, doctors dismiss these patients as "chronic complainers" and do not perform a careful medical examination. Patients with an illness anxiety disorder are differentiated from those with somatic symptom disorder by the emphasis on illness anxiety disorder on fear of having a disease versus the emphasis on somatic symptom disorder on concern about many symptoms. However, both may exist to varying degrees in each disorder. Patients with illness anxiety disorder usually complain about fewer symptoms than patients with somatic symptom disorder. Conversion disorder is differentiated from illness anxiety disorder by the fact that it is acute, generally transient, and usually involves a symptom rather than a particular disease. The fear of illness can also occur in patients with depressive and anxiety disorders. If a patient meets the full diagnostic criteria for both illness anxiety disorder and another major mental disorder, such as major depressive disorder or generalized anxiety disorder, the patient should receive both diagnoses. Illness anxiety disorder can be differentiated from obsessive-compulsive disorder by the singularity of their beliefs and by the absence of compulsive behavioral traits, but there is often an obsessive quality to the patient's fear. Delusional beliefs can be differentiated from illness anxiety disorder by their delusional intensity and the presence of other psychotic symptoms.

Conversion Disorder (Functional Neurologic Symptom Disorder)

One of the significant problems in diagnosing conversion disorder is the difficulty in definitively ruling out a medical disorder. Concomitant nonpsychiatric medical disorders are common in hospitalized patients with conversion disorder, and evidence of a current or previous neurologic disorder or a systemic disease affecting the brain occurs in 18 to 64 percent of such patients. An estimated 25 to 50 percent of patients classified as having conversion disorder eventually receive diagnoses of neurologic or nonpsychiatric medical disorders that could have caused their earlier symptoms. Thus, a thorough medical and neurologic workup is essential in all cases. If the suggestion resolves the symptom, such as with hypnosis, or parenteral amobarbital or lorazepam, the symptoms are probably the result of conversion disorder.

Neurologic disorders (e.g., dementia and other degenerative diseases), brain tumors, and basal ganglia disease are part of the differential diagnosis. For example, weakness may be confused with myasthenia gravis, polymyositis, acquired myopathies, or multiple sclerosis. Optic neuritis can resemble conversion disorder blindness. Other diseases that can cause confusing symptoms are Guillain–Barré syndrome, Creutzfeldt–Jakob disease, periodic paralysis, and early neurologic manifestations of AIDS. Conversion disorder symptoms occur in schizophrenia, depressive disorders, and anxiety disorders, but these other disorders are associated with their distinct symptoms that eventually make differential diagnosis possible.

The demarcation between conversion disorder and somatic symptom disorder is not that clear, and conversion symptoms may form part of the constellation of symptoms seen in somatic symptom disorder. One differentiating feature is that conversion disorder requires that the presenting symptoms be inconsistent with neurologic conditions, whereas somatic symptom disorder does not require this inconsistency.

In both malingering and factitious disorder, the symptoms are under conscious, voluntary control. A malingerer's history is usually more inconsistent and contradictory than that of a patient with conversion disorder, and a malingerer's fraudulent behavior is goal-directed.

Psychological Factors Affecting Other Medical Conditions

Differential diagnosis can be complicated and should include other somatic symptom disorders (somatic symptom disorder, conversion disorder, factitious disorder) as well as personality disorders (e.g., borderline personality disorder).

Factitious Disorder

Any disorder in which physical signs and symptoms are prominent are part of the differential diagnosis, and the physician must explore the possibility of authentic or concomitant physical illness. Additionally, a history of many surgeries in patients with factitious disorder may predispose such patients to complications or actual diseases, necessitating even further surgery. Factitious disorder is on a continuum between somatic symptom and related disorders and malingering, the goal being to assume the sick role.

A factitious disorder is differentiated from conversion disorder by the voluntary production of factitious symptoms, the extreme course of multiple hospitalizations, and the seeming willingness of patients with a factitious disorder to undergo an extraordinary number of mutilating procedures. Patients with conversion disorder are not usually conversant with medical terminology and hospital routines, and their symptoms have a direct temporal relation or symbolic reference to specific emotional conflicts.

Illness anxiety disorder differs from factitious disorder in the lack of voluntary production of symptoms.

Because of their pathologic lying, lack of close relationships with others, hostile and manipulative manner, and associated substance use and criminal history, clinicians may think that patients with factitious disorder have an antisocial personality disorder. Antisocial persons, however, do not usually volunteer for invasive procedures or resort to a way of life marked by repeated or long-term hospitalization. Because of attention-seeking and an occasional flair for the dramatic, they may also be diagnosed with a histrionic personality disorder. However, not all such patients have a dramatic flair, and many are withdrawn and bland. Consideration of the patient's chaotic lifestyle, history of disturbed interpersonal relationships, identity crisis, substance abuse, self-damaging acts, and manipulative tactics may lead to the diagnosis of borderline personality disorder.

We should distinguish factitious disorders from malingering. Malingerers have a manifest, recognizable environmental goal in producing signs and symptoms. They may seek hospitalization to secure financial compensation, evade the police, avoid work, or merely obtain free bed and board for the night, but they always have some apparent end for their behavior. Moreover, these patients can usually stop producing their signs and symptoms when the symptoms are no longer useful to them or when the risk becomes too high.

COMORBIDITY

Somatic Symptom Disorder

Individuals with somatic symptom disorders often have co-occurring anxiety disorders and depressive disorders, as well as comorbid medical illnesses. It is possible to have a diagnosed medical condition and receive a co-occurring diagnosis of somatic symptom disorder when the individual experiences more considerable distress and anxiety about the illness than would be expected.

Illness Anxiety Disorder

Given that illness anxiety disorder is new to DSM-5, there is limited data on comorbidity. However, a 2017 study demonstrated comorbidity of illness anxiety disorder and both depressive and anxiety disorders, especially generalized anxiety disorder and panic disorder.

Conversion Disorder (Functional Neurologic Symptom Disorder)

Medical and, especially, neurologic disorders, frequently occur among patients with conversion disorders. What one typically sees in these comorbid neurologic or medical conditions is an elaboration of symptoms stemming from the original lesion.

Depressive disorders, anxiety disorders, and somatic symptom disorder often occur alongside conversion disorder. It is rarer with schizophrenia, however, it does occur. Personality disorders also frequently accompany conversion disorder, especially histrionic, dependent, and antisocial personality disorders, or individuals with passive–aggressive personality styling. Conversion disorders can occur, however, in persons with no predisposing medical, neurologic, or psychiatric disorder.

Psychological Factors Affecting Other Medical Conditions

All individuals with this diagnosis have at least one other medical condition that is comorbid, as per the DSM-5 diagnostic criteria.

Factitious Disorder

Many persons diagnosed with factitious disorder have comorbid psychiatric diagnoses (e.g., mood disorders, personality disorders, or substance-related disorders).

COURSE AND PROGNOSIS

Somatic Symptom Disorder

The course of the disorder is usually episodic; the episodes last from months to years with equally long quiescent periods. There may be an apparent association between exacerbations of somatic symptoms and psychosocial stressors. Although no well-conducted extensive outcome studies exist, an estimated one-third to one-half of all patients with somatic symptom disorder eventually improve significantly. A good prognosis is associated with high socioeconomic status, treatment-responsive anxiety or depression, sudden onset of symptoms, the absence of a personality disorder, the absence of childhood adversity, and the absence of a related nonpsychiatric medical condition. Most children with the disorder will recover by late adolescence or early adulthood.

Illness Anxiety Disorder

Because the disorder is a new diagnosis, there are no reliable data about the prognosis. One may extrapolate from the course of somatic symptom disorder, which is usually episodic; the episodes last from months to years and have equally long quiescent periods in between. A good prognosis is associated with high socioeconomic status, treatment-responsive anxiety or depression, sudden onset of symptoms, the absence of a personality disorder, and the absence of a related nonpsychiatric medical condition.

Conversion Disorder (Functional Neurologic Symptom Disorder)

The onset of conversion disorder is usually acute, but a crescendo of symptomatology may also occur. Symptoms or deficits are usually of short duration, and approximately 95 percent of acute cases remit spontaneously, usually within 2 weeks in hospitalized patients. If symptoms have been present for 6 months or longer, the prognosis for symptom resolution is less than 50 percent and diminishes further, the longer that conversion is present. Recurrence occurs in one-fifth to one-fourth of people within 1 year of the first episode. Thus, one episode is a predictor for future episodes. Acute onset, presence of clearly identifiable stressors at the time of onset, a short interval between onset and the institution of treatment, and above-average intelligence are all good prognostic indicators. Paralysis, aphonia, and blindness are associated with a good prognosis, whereas tremor and seizures are poor prognostic factors.

Psychological Factors Affecting Other Medical Conditions

This condition can occur at any age. Little has been reported about course and prognosis.

Factitious Disorder

Factitious disorders typically begin in early adulthood, although they can appear during childhood or adolescence. The onset of the disorder or of discrete episodes of seeking treatment may follow a real illness, loss, rejection, or abandonment. Usually, the patient or a close relative had a hospitalization in childhood or early adolescence for genuine physical illness. After that, a long pattern of successive hospitalizations begins insidiously and evolves. As the disorder progresses, the patient becomes knowledgeable about medicine and hospitals.

Factitious disorders are incapacitating to the patient and often produce severe trauma or untoward reactions related to treatment. A course of repeated or long-term hospitalization is incompatible with meaningful vocational work and sustaining interpersonal relationships. The prognosis, in most cases, is poor.

TREATMENT OF SOMATIC SYMPTOM AND RELATED DISORDERS

Treatment Approach

Reviews of controlled studies have shown a good efficacy of psychotherapy, particularly of the cognitive-behavioral therapy (CBT) type, and some evidence for the efficacy of pharmacotherapy in the treatment of several somatic syndromes. Kroenke and colleagues found 34 randomized controlled trials on somatoform disorders, which included more than 1,000 patients. Of these, 13 were CBT trials, 5 were antidepressant trials, and 16 involved other modalities. Overall, CBT showed the highest efficacy, with virtually all reported studies showing a significant effect of CBT on symptoms compared to no treatment. Antidepressants seem to work in painful syndromes, and the data favored older antidepressants (tricyclics) over newer ones (serotonin reuptake inhibitors [SSRIs]). Other interventions, including the use of a psychiatric consultation letter, brief psychodynamic psychotherapy, exercise, and more recently, biofeedback, have also shown beneficial effects on some of these symptoms. A more recent article reviewed 15 randomized controlled trials of the efficacy of CBT in somatoform disorders and found that CBT improved somatic, anxiety, and depressive symptoms and improved social functioning.

However, patients with somatic symptom and related disorders sometimes are not open to psychological explanations of their symptoms or psychological or psychiatric treatment. More specific treatment guidelines are listed for each diagnosis, below.

Somatic Symptom Disorder

Therapeutic goals should be modest at first and limited to small, attainable gains such as a decrease in medical visits, a commitment to a single primary care physician, and the avoidance of unnecessary tests and procedures. The physician should prepare for a long-term commitment to the patient. Physicians should limit specialist consultations unless there is evidence of comorbid physical conditions. Some of the elements of CBT, such as diary keeping, should be incorporated into the primary care physician's treatment strategy. Recommendations for exercise, yoga, relaxation, meditation, and massage may be useful and are generally better accepted by patients than psychological treatments.

The use of a brief "consultation letter" intended for primary care physicians has demonstrated effectiveness in improving patients' functional capacity and decreasing their utilization of health services. This consultation letter provides physicians with "do's and don'ts" regarding their encounters with patients with multiple medically unexplained physical symptoms and briefly instructs them on using of a few fundamental management techniques. The letter should urge the physicians to see these patients during regularly scheduled appointments, perform brief physical examinations focusing on the area of discomfort at each visit, avoid unnecessary diagnostic procedures, invasive treatments, and hospitalizations, avoid using statements such as "symptoms are all in your head," and briefly allow/encourage patients to talk about "stressors."

A body of research has demonstrated the efficacy of CBT for the treatment of somatic symptom disorder and related syndromes. CBT-type interventions appear to help patients by modifying thoughts and behaviors associated with somatization. In the typical CBT program, the therapist systematically introduces patients to several behavioral techniques, which include relaxation training and graded increases in activities. From a cognitive perspective, CBT helps patients to identify thoughts that contribute to increased stress, inactivity, and health concern. Often, patients with this condition tend to think catastrophically about their physical symptoms. Such thoughts lead them to conclude that they are sick and must limit physical activity, creating a cycle that perpetuates the somatic process. Reports indicate that brief psychodynamic therapy of unexplained somatic symptoms may be useful, although most of the recent evidence in terms of randomized controlled trials involves CBT.

In general, we should avoid medications when treating patients with somatic symptom disorder except in the presence of clearly delineated anxious, depressive, or psychotic symptoms. Despite the development of new pharmacologic agents such as dual (norepinephrine and serotonin) reuptake inhibitors and limited data on gabapentin, there is no evidence that a purely pharmacologic approach targeting the treatment of somatic symptom disorder will be sufficient.

Illness Anxiety Disorder

Various group and individual therapies, including CBT and psychodynamic therapy, have been proposed over the years to manage patients with health anxiety. Several controlled trials have demonstrated efficacy for CBT interventions, making CBT the prototype, first-line treatment for illness anxiety disorder. Other types of therapy, including mindfulness training, exposure therapy, and acceptance and commitment therapy, have also demonstrated some efficacy.

Limited data exist to guide pharmacologic treatment of illness anxiety disorder. There have been a few randomized, placebo-controlled trials that demonstrated benefit with SSRIs. Most reports have been anecdotal, single-blind studies. A recent randomized controlled trial of 195 patients with hypochondriasis demonstrated the efficacy and safety of fluoxetine in this patient population. Interestingly, the addition of CBT to fluoxetine conferred a slight added benefit.

Conversion Disorder (Functional Neurologic Symptom Disorder)

Many conversion syndromes have an acute, benign course and may remit spontaneously with understanding and support. Early intervention can forestall potential chronicity and the progression into a well-entrenched somatization disorder. Once chronicity has developed, intensive treatment may use all treatment modalities, including hospitalization, individual or group therapy, insight-oriented therapies, behavioral techniques, hypnosis, sodium amytal interview, physical therapy, biofeedback, relaxation training, and medication (primarily for comorbid anxiety, depression, or other somatoform disorders). Psychological interpretations or explanations do not work well early in the process, but reassuring patients that critical tests are normal and that symptoms will eventually improve may be helpful. Any implication to the patient that he or she is malingering is very counterproductive. Behavioral interventions should focus on improving self-esteem, the capacity for emotional expression and assertiveness, and the ability to communicate comfortably with others. With chronic conversion, muscle contractures can occur, and physical therapy is necessary. Even in the absence of such contractures, however, many conversion patients find that physical therapy can be helpful for muscular symptoms or balance problems. The process of slowly progressive exercises and activity can help restore functioning.

Psychological Factors Affecting Other Medical Conditions

Treatment frequently involves communication with the patient's primary medical team as well as family. The psychoeducational intervention clarifies the role that emotional and behavioral factors play in aggravating the underlying medical condition. Medication to treat another underlying psychiatric disorder may be necessary.

Factitious Disorder

No specific psychiatric therapy has been effective in treating factitious disorders. It is a clinical paradox that patients with the disorders simulate severe illness and seek and submit to unnecessary treatment while they deny to themselves and others their actual illness and thus avoid possible treatment for it. Ultimately, the patients elude meaningful therapy by abruptly leaving the hospital or failing to keep follow-up appointments.

Treatment, thus, is best focused on management rather than on cure. Table 12-10 lists the guidelines for treating and managing factitious disorder. The three primary goals in the treatment and management of factitious disorders are (1) to reduce the risk of morbidity and mortality, (2) to address the underlying emotional needs or psychiatric diagnosis underlying factitious illness behavior, and (3) to be mindful of legal and ethical issues. Perhaps the single most crucial factor in successful management is a physician's

Table 12-10
Guidelines for Management and Treatment of Factitious Disorder

Keep in mind that active pursuit of a prompt diagnosis can minimize the risk of morbidity and mortality.

Minimize harm. Avoid unnecessary tests and procedures, especially if they are invasive. Treat according to clinical judgment, keeping in mind that subjective complaints may be deceptive.

Arrange regular interdisciplinary meetings to reduce conflict and splitting among staff. Manage staff countertransference.

Steer the patient toward psychiatric treatment in an empathic, nonconfrontational, face-saving manner. Avoid aggressive direct confrontation.

Treat underlying psychiatric disturbances. In psychotherapy, address coping strategies and emotional conflicts.

Appoint a primary care provider as a gatekeeper for all medical and psychiatric treatment.

Consider involving risk management and bioethicists from an early point.

Consider appointing a guardian for medical and psychiatric decisions.

As a behavioral disincentive, consider prosecution for fraud.

Table 12-11
Pediatric Factitious Disorder Imposed on Another—Basic Principles of Management

Make sure the child is safe.

Make sure the child's future safety is also assured.

Allow treatment to occur in the least restrictive setting possible.

A pediatrician should serve as "gatekeeper" for medical care utilization.

All other physicians should coordinate care with the gatekeeper.

Child-protective services should be informed whenever a child is harmed.

Family psychotherapy and/or individual psychotherapy should be instituted for the perpetrating parent and the child.

Health insurance companies, school officials, and other nonmedical sources should be asked to report possible medical abuse to the physician gatekeeper. Permission of a parent or of child-protective services must first be obtained.

The possibility should be considered of admitting the child to an inpatient or partial hospital setting to facilitate diagnostic monitoring of symptoms and to institute a treatment plan.

The child may require placement in another family. The perpetrating parent may need to be removed from the child through criminal prosecution and incarceration.

early recognition of the disorder. In this way, physicians can forestall a multitude of painful and potentially dangerous diagnostic procedures for these patients. There must be a good liaison between psychiatrists and the medical or surgical staff. Although a few cases of individual psychotherapy exist in the literature, no consensus exists about the best approach. In general, working in concert with the patient's primary care physician is more effective than working with the patient in isolation.

The personal reactions of physicians and staff members are of great significance in treating and establishing a working alliance with these patients, who invariably evoke feelings of futility, bewilderment, betrayal, hostility, and even contempt. In essence, staff members must abandon a fundamental element of their relationship with patients—accepting the truthfulness of the patients' statements. One appropriate psychiatric intervention is to suggest to the staff ways of remaining aware that even though the patient's illness is factitious, the patient is ill. Physicians should try not to feel resentment when patients humiliate their diagnostic prowess, and they should avoid any unmasking ceremony that sets up the patients as adversaries and precipitates their flight from the hospital. The staff should not perform unnecessary procedures or discharge patients abruptly, both of which are manifestations of anger.

In cases of factitious disorder imposed on another, physicians have obtained a legal intervention in several instances, particularly with children. The senselessness of the disorder and the denial of false action by parents are obstacles to successful court action and often make conclusive proof unobtainable. In such cases, the treatment team should notify the child welfare and make arrangements for ongoing monitoring of the children's health (see Table 12-11 for interventions for pediatric factitious disorder imposed on another).

EPIDEMIOLOGY

Somatic Symptom Disorder

The prevalence of somatic symptom disorder is not yet known. Data do exist, however, for somatization disorder as defined by DSM-IV. Studies in the United States, Puerto Rico, Germany, and

Italy found lifetime prevalence rates of "full" somatization disorder ranging from 0.1 percent in the United States to 0.8 percent in Germany. In contrast, lifetime rates of "abridged" somatization disorder ranged from 5.6 percent in Germany to 19 percent in Puerto Rico. Much higher prevalence rates have been reported for more broadly defined somatic symptom clusters.

Illness Anxiety Disorder

The prevalence of this disorder is unknown, aside from using data that relate to hypochondriasis, which gives a prevalence of 4 to 6 percent in a general medical clinic population. In other surveys, up to 10 percent of persons in the general population worry about becoming sick and incapacitated as a result.

Conversion Disorder (Functional Neurologic Symptom Disorder)

The epidemiologic information on conversion disorder is limited. Estimates vary broadly: Less than 1 percent in the general population, 5 to 14 percent among general hospital medical/surgical referrals to psychiatry consultation services, and 5 to 25 percent in treated psychiatric outpatients. The disorder appears to be more frequent in females and can occur in children as young as 7 or 8 years old. It is rare after the age of 35 years.

Psychological Factors Affecting Other Medical Conditions

The prevalence of this condition is unknown. In mental health systems, it is most frequently diagnosed in consultation–liaison psychiatry settings.

Factitious Disorder

No comprehensive epidemiologic data on factitious disorder exist. However, it is estimated to comprise approximately 1 percent of the healthcare-seeking population. Factitious disorder imposed on another account for less than 0.04 percent of reported child abuse in the United States each year.

ETIOLOGY

Somatic Symptom Disorder

Early family studies suggested an association between hysteria/Briquet syndrome in females and antisocial personality in their male first-degree relatives. Also, studies of adopted-away children highlighted the presence of alcoholism and violence in biologic fathers of women with somatization disorder. However, since developing the new diagnostic criteria, there have been no major epidemiologic studies.

Some have postulated that persons with this disorder augment and amplify their somatic sensations; they have low thresholds for and low tolerance of physical discomfort. For example, what persons usually perceive as abdominal pressure, persons with somatic symptom disorder experience as abdominal pain. They may focus on bodily sensations, misinterpret them, and become alarmed by them because of a faulty cognitive scheme.

Others have proposed a social learning model. They see the symptoms of this disorder as a request for admission to the sick role made by a person facing seemingly insurmountable and unsolvable problems. The sick role offers an escape that allows a patient to avoid noxious obligations, to postpone unwelcome challenges, and to evade usual duties and obligations.

Illness Anxiety Disorder

The etiology is unknown. The social learning model described for somatic symptom disorder may apply to this disorder as well, with a similar dynamic to what we described above.

Conversion Disorder (Functional Neurologic Symptom Disorder)

Biologic Factors. The neuropsychologic conceptualization speaks of an inherent deficit in certain brain functions, especially those in the dominant hemisphere that may interfere with verbal associations. Also, functional MRI studies have shown differences in brain activation between patients with conversion disorder and controls.

Psychological Factors The behavioral theory attributes conversion disorder to faulty childhood learning, with the nonadaptive behavioral responses used for secondary gain and control of interpersonal relationships. The psychoanalytic theory, on the other hand, describes symptoms as compromise formations with primary gain of conflict resolution through a partial expression of the conflict without conscious awareness of its significance. Some have suggested a strong relationship between childhood traumatization by sexual or physical abuse and a later propensity for conversion disorder. Other studies, however, do not confirm such an association.

Factitious Disorder

Etiology is generally not clear, except that a common denominator is that these patients tend to be avid medical service seekers. The underlying motivations for the behaviors are likely unconscious. Two factors may underlie most cases of factitious disorder: (1) an affinity for the medical system, and (2) poor, maladaptive coping skills. In the case of factitious disorder imposed on another, psychodynamic theories predominately view the disorder as an objectification of the child to serve the parent's psychological needs.

References

Aduan RP, Fauci AS, Dale DD. Factitious fever and self-induced infection: A report of 32 cases and review of the literature. *Ann Intern Med*. 1979;90:230.

Alexander F. Psychosomatic medicine: Its principles and application. New York: Norton; 1950.

American Psychiatric Association. *Diagnostic and Statistical Manual of Mental Disorders*. 5th ed. Arlington, VA: American Psychiatric Association; 2013.

Ani C, Reading R, Lynn R, Forlee S, Garralda E. Incidence and 12-month outcome of non-transient childhood conversion disorder in the UK and Ireland. *Br J Psychiatry*. 2013;202(6):413–418.

Bass C, Taylor M. Recovery from chronic factitious disorder (Munchausen's syndrome): A personal account. *Personal Ment Health*. 2013;7(1):80–83.

Brody S. Hypochondriasis: Attentional, sensory, and cognitive factors. *Psychosomatics*. 2013;54(1):98.

Bryant RA, Das P. The neural circuitry of conversion disorder and its recovery. *J Abnorm Psychology*. 2012;121(1):289.

Cannon WB. *The Wisdom of the Body*. New York: Norton; 1932.

Carson AJ, Brown R, David AS, Duncan R, Edwards MJ, Goldstein LH, Grunewald R, Howlett S, Kanaan R, Mellers J, Nicholson TR, Reuber M, Schrag AE, Stone J, Voon V; UK-FNS. Functional (conversion) neurological symptoms: Research since the millennium. *J Neurol Neurosurg Psychiatry*. 2012;83(8):842–850.

Chaturvedi SK, Desai G. Measurement and assessment of somatic symptoms. *Int Rev Psychiatry*. 2013;25(1):31–40.

Daum C, Aybek S. Validity of the "drift without pronation" sign in conversion disorder. *BMC Neurol*. 2013;13:31.

Dimsdale JE, Creed F, Escobar J, Sharpe M, Wulsin L, Barsky A, Lee S, Irwin MR, Levenson J. Somatic symptom disorder: An important change in DSM. *J Psychosom Res*. 2013;75(3):223–228.

Eisendrath SJ. Factitious physical disorders: Treatment without confrontation. *Psychosomatics*. 1989;30:383.

El-Gabalawy R, Mackenzie CS, Thibodeau MA, Asmundson GJG, Sareen J. Health anxiety disorders in older adults: Conceptualizing complex conditions in late life. *Clin Psychol Rev*. 2013;33(8):1096–1105.

Escobar JI, Dimsdale JEE. Somatic symptom and related disorders. In: Sadock BJ, Sadock VA, Ruiz P, eds. *Kaplan & Sadock's Comprehensive Textbook of Psychiatry*. 10th ed. Philadelphia, PA: Wolters Kluwer; 2017:1827–1845.

Fallon BA, Ahern DK, Pavlicova M, Slavov I, Skritskya N, Barsky AJ. A randomized controlled trial of medication and cognitive-behavioral therapy for hypochondriasis. *Am J Psychiatry*. 2017;174(8):756–764.

Frances A. The new somatic symptom disorder in DSM-5 risks mislabeling many people as mentally ill. *BMJ*. 2013;346:f1580.

Frye EM, Feldman MD. Factitious disorder by proxy in educational settings: A review. *Educ Psychol Rev*. 2012;24(1):47–61.

Gropalis M, Bleichhardt G, Hiller W, Witthöft M. Specificity and modifiability of cognitive biases in hypochondriasis. *J Consult Clin Psychol*. 2013;81(3):558–565.

Guidi J, Rafanelli C, Roncuzzi R, Sirri L, Fava GA. Assessing psychological factors affecting medical conditions: Comparison between different proposals. *Gen Hosp Psychiatry*. 2013;35(2):141–146.

Guz H, Doganay Z, Ozkan A, Colak E, Tomac A, Sarisoy G. Conversion and somatization disorders: Dissociative symptoms and other characteristics. *J Psychosom Res*. 2004;56:287–291.

Hamilton JC, Eger M, Razzak S, Feldman MD, Hallmark N, Cheek S. Somatoform, factitious, and related diagnoses in the National Hospital Discharge Survey: Addressing the proposed DSM-5 revision. *Psychosomatics*. 2013;54(2):142–148.

Höfling V, Weck F. Assessing bodily preoccupations is sufficient: Clinically effective screening for hypochondriasis. *J Psychosom Res*. 2013;75(6):526–531.

Kinns H, Housley D, Freedman DB. Munchausen syndrome and factitious disorder: The role of the laboratory in its detection and diagnosis. *Ann Clin Biochem*. 2013;50(3):194–203.

Krasnik C, Grant C. Conversion disorder: Not a malingering matter. *Paediatr Child Health*. 2012;17(5):246.

Kroenke K. Efficacy of treatment for somatoform disorders: A review of randomized controlled trials. *Psychosom Med*. 2007;69:881–888.

Kroenke K, Sharpe M, Sykes R. Revising the classification of somatoform disorders: Key questions and preliminary recommendations. *Psychosomatics*. 2007;48:277–285.

Lee S, Lam IM, Kwok KP, Leung C. A community-based epidemiological study of health anxiety and generalized anxiety disorder. *J Anxiety Disord*. 2014;28(2):187–194.

Liu J, Gill NS, Teodorczuk A, Li Z-J, Jing S. The efficacy of cognitive behavioural therapy in somatoform disorders and medically unexplained physical symptoms: A meta-analysis of randomized controlled trials. *J Affect Disord*. 2019;245: 98–112.

McCormack R, Moriarty J, Mellers JD, Shotbolt P, Pastena R, Landes N, Goldstein L, Fleminger S, David AS. Specialist inpatient treatment for severe motor conversion disorder: A retrospective comparative study. *J Neurol Neurosurg Psychiatry*. 2014;85(8):895–900.

Newby JM, Hobbs MJ, Mahoney AEJ, Wong S, Andrews G. DSM-5 illness anxiety disorder and somatic symptom disorder: Comorbidity, correlates, and overlap with DSM-IV hypochondriasis. *J Psychosom Res*. 2017;101:31–37.

Nicholson TR, Aybek S, Kempton MJ, Daly EM, Murphy DG, David AS, Kanaan RA. A structural MRI study of motor conversion disorder: Evidence of reduction in thalamic volume. *J Neurol Neurosurg Psychiatry*. 2014;85(2):227–229.

Phillips MR, Ward NG, Ries RK. Factitious mourning: Painless patienthood. *Am J Psychiatry*. 1983;147:1057.

Prior KN, Bond MJ. Somatic symptom disorders and illness behaviour: Current perspectives. *Int Rev Psychiatry*. 2013;25(1):5–18.

Quinn DK, Wang D, Powsner S, Eisendrath SJ. Factitious disorder. In: Sadock BJ, Sadock VA, Ruiz P, eds. *Kaplan & Sadock's Comprehensive Textbook of Psychiatry*. 10th ed. Philadelphia, PA: Wolters Kluwer; 2017:1846–1865.

Rogers R, Bagby RM, Rector N. Diagnostic legitimacy of factitious disorder with psychological symptoms. *Am J Psychiatry*. 1989;146:1312.

Scarella TM, Boland RJ, Barsky AJ. Illness anxiety disorder: psychopathology, epidemiology, clinical characteristics, and treatment. *Psychosom Med*. 2019;81(5):398–407.

Scarella TM, Laferton JAC, Ahern DK, Fallon BA, Barsky A. The relationship of hypochondriasis to anxiety, depressive, and somatoform disorders. *Psychosomatics*. 2016;57(2):200–207.

Schrag AE, Mehta AR, Bhatia KP, Brown RJ, Frackowiak RS, Trimble MR, Ward NS, Rowe JB. The functional neuroimaging correlates of psychogenic versus organic dystonia. *Brain*. 2013;136(3):770–781.

Shorter E. From paralysis to fatigue: A history of psychosomatic illness in the modern era. New York: Free Press; 1992.

Sirri L, Fava GA. Diagnostic criteria for psychosomatic research and somatic symptom disorders. *Int Rev Psychiatry*. 2013;25(1):19–30.

Somashekar B, Jainer A, Wuntakal B. Psychopharmacotherapy of somatic symptoms disorders. *Int Rev Psychiatry*. 2013;25(1):107–115.

Starcevic V. Hypochondriasis and health anxiety: Conceptual challenges. *Br J Psychiatry*. 2013;202(1):7–8.

Stone J, Smyth R, Carson A, Lewis S, Prescott R, Warlow C, Sharpe M. Systematic review of misdiagnosis of conversion symptoms and "hysteria." *BMJ*. 2005; 331(7523):989.

Tomenson B, Essau C, Jacobi F, Ladwig KH, Leiknes KA, Lieb R, Meinlschmidt G, McBeth J, Rosmalen J, Rief W, Sumathipala A, Creed F; EURASMUS Population Based Study Group. Total somatic symptom score as a predictor of health outcome in somatic symptom disorders. *Br J Psychiatry*. 2013;203(5): 373–380.

Voigt K, Wollburg E, Weinmann N, Herzog A, Meyer B, Langs G, Löwe B. Predictive validity and clinical utility of DSM-5 somatic symptom disorder: Prospective 1-year follow-up study. *J Psychosom Res*. 2013;75(4):358–361.

13 △

Feeding and Eating Disorders

This chapter deals with several feeding and eating disorders, including anorexia nervosa, bulimia nervosa, binge-eating disorder, and other specified feeding and eating disorders. There are different feeding and eating disorders that are typically associated with childhood and adolescence (e.g., pica, rumination disorder, and avoidant/restrictive food intake disorder); Neurodevelopmental Disorders and Other Childhood Disorders (Chapter 2) covers those disorders.

CLINICAL FEATURES

Anorexia Nervosa

The term anorexia nervosa comes from the Greek term for "loss of appetite" and a Latin word implying nervous origin. Anorexia nervosa is a syndrome characterized by three essential criteria, one behavioral, one psychopathological, and the last, physiologic. The first is self-induced starvation, to a significant degree (behavioral). The second is a relentless drive for thinness or a morbid fear of fatness (psychopathological). The third criterion is the presence of medical signs and symptoms resulting from starvation (physiologic). Anorexia nervosa is often, but not always, associated with disturbances of body image, the perception that one is distressingly large despite evident medical starvation. The distortion of body image is disturbing when present; it is, however, not pathognomonic, invariable, or required for diagnosis. Two subtypes of anorexia nervosa exist: restricting and binge/purge. The theme in all anorexia nervosa subtypes is the highly disproportionate emphasis placed on thinness as a vital source of self-esteem, with weight, and to a lesser degree, shape, becoming the overriding and consuming daylong preoccupation of thoughts, mood, and behaviors.

Approximately half of anorexic persons will lose weight by drastically reducing their total food intake. The other half of these patients will not only diet but will also regularly engage in binge eating, followed by purging behaviors. Some patients routinely purge after eating small amounts of food. Anorexia nervosa is much more prevalent in females than in males and usually has its onset in adolescence. Hypotheses of an underlying psychological disturbance in young women with the disorder include conflicts surrounding the transition from girlhood to womanhood. Some have also suggested that psychological issues related to feelings of helplessness and difficulty establishing autonomy also contribute to the development of the disorder. Bulimic symptoms can occur as a separate disorder or as part of anorexia nervosa. Persons with either disorder are excessively preoccupied with weight, food, and body shape. The outcome of anorexia nervosa varies from spontaneous recovery to a waxing and waning course to death.

Bulimia Nervosa

People with bulimia nervosa have episodes of binge eating combined with inappropriate ways of stopping weight gain. Physical discomfort—for example, abdominal pain or nausea—terminates the binge eating, which is often followed by feelings of guilt, depression, or self-disgust. Unlike patients with anorexia nervosa, those with bulimia nervosa typically maintain average body weight.

The term bulimia nervosa derives from the terms for "ox-hunger" in Greek and "nervous involvement" in Latin. For some patients, bulimia nervosa may represent a failed attempt at anorexia nervosa, sharing the goal of becoming very thin, but occurring in an individual less able to sustain prolonged semistarvation or severe hunger as consistently as classic restricting anorexia nervosa patients. For others, eating binges represent "breakthrough eating" episodes of giving in to hunger pangs generated by efforts to limit eating to maintain a socially desirable level of thinness. Still, others use binge eating as a means to self-medicate during times of emotional distress. Regardless of the reason, eating binges provoke panic as individuals feel that their eating has been out of control. The unwanted binges lead to subsequent attempts to avoid the feared weight gain by a variety of compensatory behaviors, such as purging or excessive exercise.

Binge-Eating Disorder

Individuals with binge-eating disorder engage in recurrent binge eating during which they eat an abnormally large amount of food over a short time. Unlike bulimia nervosa, patients with binge-eating disorder do not compensate in any way after a binge episode (e.g., vomiting, laxative use). Binge episodes often occur in private, generally include foods of dense caloric content, and, during the binge, the person feels he or she cannot control his or her eating.

Other Specified Feeding or Eating Disorders

This diagnostic category also includes eating conditions that may cause significant distress but do not meet the full criteria for a classified eating disorder. Conditions included in this category include night-eating syndrome, purging disorder, and subthreshold forms of anorexia nervosa, bulimia nervosa, and binge-eating disorder.

Night-Eating Syndrome. Night-eating syndrome is characterized by the consumption of large amounts of food after the evening meal. Individuals generally have little appetite during the day and suffer from insomnia.

Purging Disorder. Purging disorder is characterized by recurrent purging behavior after consuming a small amount of food in persons of average weight who have a distorted view of their weight or body image. Purging behavior includes self-induced vomiting, laxative abuse, enemas, and diuretics. This behavior should not be associated with anorexia nervosa. Purging disorder is differentiated from bulimia nervosa because purging behavior occurs after eating small quantities of food or drink and does not occur as a result of a binge episode.

DIAGNOSIS AND CLINICAL FEATURES

Anorexia Nervosa

The onset of anorexia nervosa usually occurs between the ages of 10 and 30 years. We summarize the diagnostic criteria in DSM-5 and ICD-10 for the disorder in Table 13-1.

Intense fear of gaining weight and becoming obese is present in all patients with the disorder and undoubtedly contributes to their lack of interest in and even resistance to therapy. Most aberrant behavior directed toward losing weight occurs in secret. Patients with anorexia nervosa usually refuse to eat with their families or in public places. They lose weight by drastically reducing their total food intake, with a disproportionate decrease in high-carbohydrate and fatty foods.

The term anorexia is a misnomer because the loss of appetite is usually rare until late in the disorder. Evidence that patients are frequently thinking about food is their passion for collecting recipes and for preparing elaborate meals for others. Some patients cannot continuously control their voluntary restriction of food intake, and so have eating binges. These binges usually occur secretly, often

at night, and are frequently followed by self-induced vomiting. Patients abuse laxatives and even diuretics to lose weight, and ritualistic exercising, extensive cycling, walking, jogging, and running are everyday activities.

Patients with the disorder show peculiar behavior surrounding food. They hide food all over the house and frequently carry large quantities of candies in their pockets and purses. While eating meals, they try to dispose of food in their napkins or hide it in their pockets. They cut their meat into tiny pieces and spend a great deal of time rearranging these pieces on their plates. If someone confronts the patient about the behavior, they often deny that it is unusual or flatly refuse to discuss it.

Obsessive-compulsive behavior, depression, and anxiety are other psychiatric symptoms of anorexia nervosa most frequently noted clinically. Patients tend to be rigid and perfectionist, and somatic complaints, especially epigastric discomfort, are usual. Compulsive stealing, usually of candies and laxatives but occasionally of clothes and other items, may occur.

Patients with the disorder frequently have poor sexual adjustment. Many adolescent patients with anorexia nervosa have delayed psychosocial sexual development; in adults, a markedly decreased interest in sex often accompanies the onset of the disorder. A minority of anorexic patients have a premorbid history of promiscuity, substance abuse, or both, but during the disorder show a decreased interest in sex.

Patients usually come to medical attention when their weight loss becomes apparent. As the weight loss grows profound, physical signs such as hypothermia (as low as 35°C), dependent edema, bradycardia, hypotension, and lanugo (the appearance of

Table 13-1
Anorexia Nervosa Diagnoses

Disorder	Anorexia Nervosa	
	DSM-5	**ICD-10**
Diagnostic name	Anorexia nervosa	Anorexia nervosa

Symptom	• Food restriction leading to abnormally low weight
	• Fear of gaining weight and behaviors to prevent weight gain
	• Distorted body image
	  • Misperceiving weight or shape
	  • Self-evaluation based on thinness, lack of recognition of the seriousness of one's weight
		• Deliberate weight loss induced by the patient
		• Fear of being fat or flabby
		• Associated physiologic disturbances due to low weight
		• Specific behaviors:
		  • Restricted diet
		  • Excess exercise
		  • Binging behavior
		  • Use of appetite suppressants and diuretics

Required number of symptom	All	
Exclusions		Loss of appetite (physical or psychological)
Symptom specifiers	Restricting type: Primary behaviors are dieting, fasting, and exercise for last 3 mo Binge eating type: Binging and purging behavior for last 3 mo. Can include use of laxatives or other substances to aid purging	
Course specifiers	Partial remission: Symptoms present but no longer an abnormally low weight Full remission: No symptoms for a sustained period	
Severity specifiers	Severity is measured by BMI level See DSM-5 for ranges	
Comments		If lacking core symptoms, the diagnosis of "atypical anorexia nervosa" is made

Table 13-2
Medical Complications of the Eating Disorders

Disorder and System Affected	Consequence
Anorexia Nervosa	
Vital signs	Bradycardia, hypotension with marked orthostatic changes, hypothermia, poikilothermia
General	Muscle atrophy, loss of body fat
Central nervous system	Generalized brain atrophy with enlarged ventricles, decreased cortical mass, seizures, abnormal electroencephalogram
Cardiovascular	Peripheral (starvation) edema, decreased cardiac diameter, narrowed left ventricular wall, decreased response to exercise demand, superior mesenteric artery syndrome
Renal	Prerenal azotemia
Hematologic	Anemia of starvation, leukopenia, hypocellular bone marrow
Gastrointestinal	Delayed gastric emptying, gastric dilatation, decreased intestinal lipase and lactase
Metabolic	Hypercholesterolemia, nonsymptomatic hypoglycemia, elevated liver enzymes, decreased bone mineral density
Endocrine	Low luteinizing hormone, low follicle-stimulating hormone, low estrogen or testosterone, low/normal thyroxine, low triiodothyronine, increased reverse triiodothyronine, elevated cortisol, elevated growth hormone, partial diabetes insipidus, increased prolactin
Bulimia Nervosa and Binge Eating and Purging Type Anorexia Nervosa	
Metabolic	Hypokalemic alkalosis or acidosis, hypochloremia, dehydration
Renal	Prerenal azotemia, acute and chronic renal failure
Cardiovascular	Arrhythmias, myocardial toxicity from emetine (ipecac)
Dental	Lingual surface enamel loss, multiple caries
Gastrointestinal	Swollen parotid glands, elevated serum amylase levels, gastric distention, irritable bowel syndrome, melanosis coli from laxative abuse
Musculoskeletal	Cramps, tetany

neonatal-like hair) appear, and patients show a variety of metabolic changes. These and other medical complications are listed in Table 13-2.

Subtypes.   Anorexia nervosa has two clinical subtypes: food restricting and purging. In the food-restricting category, present in approximately 50 percent of cases, food intake is highly restricted (usually with attempts to consume fewer than 300 to 500 calories per day and no fat grams) and the patient may be relentlessly and compulsively overactive, with overuse athletic injuries. In the purging subtype, patients alternate attempts at rigorous dieting with intermittent binge or purge episodes. Purging represents a secondary compensation for the unwanted calories, most often accomplished by self-induced vomiting, frequently by laxative abuse, less frequently by diuretics, and occasionally with emetics. Sometimes, repetitive purging occurs without prior binge eating, after ingesting only relatively few calories. Both types may be socially isolated and have depressive disorder symptoms and diminished sexual interest. Overexercising and perfectionistic traits are also common in both types.

Those who practice binge eating and purging share many features with persons who have bulimia nervosa without anorexia nervosa. Those who binge eat and purge tend to have families in which some members are obese, and they have histories of heavier body weights before the disorder than do persons with the restricting type. Binge eating–purging persons are likely to be associated with substance abuse, impulse control disorders, and personality disorders. Persons with restricting anorexia nervosa often have obsessive-compulsive traits concerning food

and other matters. Some persons with anorexia nervosa may purge but not binge.

Patients with anorexia nervosa are often secretive, deny their symptoms, and resist treatment. In almost all cases, relatives or intimate acquaintances must confirm a patient's history. The mental status examination usually shows a patient who is alert and knowledgeable on the subject of nutrition and who is preoccupied with food and weight.

A young woman who weighed 10 percent above the average weight but was otherwise healthy, functioning well, and working hard as a university student joined a track team. She started training for hours a day, more than her teammates, began to perceive herself as fat, and thought that her performance would be enhanced if she lost weight. She started to diet and reduced her weight to 87 percent of the "ideal weight" for her age according to standard tables. At her point of maximum weight loss, her performance declined, and she pushed herself even harder in her training regimen. She started to feel apathetic and morbidly afraid of becoming fat. Her food intake became restricted, and she stopped eating anything containing fat. Her menstrual periods became skimpy and infrequent but did not cease. (Courtesy of Arnold E. Andersen, M.D. and Joel Yager, M.D.)

Bulimia Nervosa

People with bulimia nervosa have binge episodes with compensatory behaviors. Like persons with anorexia nervosa, they fear becoming fat; however, they are not severely thin. We summarize

Table 13-3
Bulimia Nervosa Diagnoses

Disorder	Bulimia Nervosa	
	DSM-5	ICD-10
Diagnostic name	Bulimia nervosa	Bulimia nervosa
Duration	Occurs at least once a week for 3 mo	

Symptom	1. Repeated binge-eating episodes
	   • Occurring within 2 hr period
	   • Loss of control during the episode
	2. Compensatory behaviors to prevent weight gain, such as
	   • Vomiting
	   • Laxatives
	   • Diuretics, other substances
	   • Excessive exercise
	   • Fasting
	3. Self-evaluation based on weight and shape
		• Binging
		• Preoccupation with weight control
		• Preoccupation with body shape and weight
		• Associated physiologic disturbances due to repeated vomiting
		• Specific compensatory behaviors:
		   • Vomiting
		   • Use of purgatives

Required number of symptom	All 3	Not specified
Exclusions	Does not occur only during episodes of anorexia nervosa	
Course specifiers	Partial remission: Full symptoms no longer met for a sustained time Full remission: No symptoms for a sustained period	
Severity specifiers	Severity is measured by the average number of compensatory behaviors in a weeks' time See DSM-5 for ranges	

the diagnostic criteria in DSM-5 and ICD-10 for the disorder in Table 13-3.

When making a diagnosis of bulimia nervosa, clinicians should explore the possibility that the patient has experienced a brief or prolonged prior bout of anorexia nervosa, which is present in approximately half of those with bulimia nervosa. The binging behavior commonly precedes vomiting by about 1 year.

Vomiting is frequent and is often induced by sticking a finger down the throat. Some patients can vomit at will. Vomiting decreases the abdominal pain and the feeling of being bloated and allows patients to continue eating without fear of gaining weight. The acid content of vomitus can damage tooth enamel, a not uncommon finding in patients with the disorder. Depression, sometimes called postbinge anguish, often follows the episode. During binges, patients eat food that is sweet, high in calories, and generally soft or smooth textured, such as cakes and pastry. Some patients prefer bulky foods without regard to taste. The food is eaten secretly and rapidly and is sometimes not even chewed.

Jean was a 25-year-old woman admitted to an inpatient unit after a superficial suicide attempt. During her initial evaluation, she revealed that she had struggled with bulimia nervosa since her early teens. She said that she has always tended "to be on the heavy side" and would respond by skipping meals during the day, only to binge on "junk food" in the evening. Her binge eating occurred almost daily, and at least two or three times a week, Jean would force herself to vomit afterward. She also used daily laxatives and ran for at least an hour a day. Despite these behaviors, she could not lose weight, which distressed her to the point that she cut her wrists, although Jean admitted she had really "only scratched myself." She drank socially and did not use

illicit drugs. On examination, she appeared somewhat overweight with a BMI of 29. Her dentition showed signs of enamel erosion, and she had calluses on her fingers from her induced vomiting. There were superficial scratches on her wrist from when she cut herself. She had normal electrolytes on laboratory evaluation.

Jean had a high school education and had been married for 2 years, and she described her marriage as "rocky" as her husband frequently traveled on business. She said she rarely saw her parents, who were "always criticizing me." She did not work and said she was bored most of the time. On several occasions, while her husband was away, she would meet up with former boyfriends and sometimes slept with them. She felt that her guilt over these affairs contributed to her depression and suicidal ideation.

During her hospital stay, she had nutritional counseling and ate regularly scheduled meals, for which she had to be observed. After meals, she could use the bathroom but was instructed not to flush the toilet. This continued for 2 days until a staff member found a plastic bag of partially digested food in a trash can, after which the staff would observe her for an hour after meals. Initially, she would use a hospital courtyard for jogging, and when that was restricted, the evening staff observed her doing calisthenics in her room. Several staff members also saw her flirting with the male patients, and her therapist reminded her of the unit rules regarding patient relationships. Her treatment consisted of a behavioral schedule and frequent observation while her therapy focused on her difficulties with self-esteem and interpersonal interactions. Her psychiatrist initiated fluoxetine, 20 mg. Her purging behaviors decreased over the next 2 weeks to the point where she was considered appropriate for outpatient treatment.

Most patients with bulimia nervosa are within their normal weight range, but some may be underweight or overweight. These patients are concerned about their body image and their appearance, worried about how others see them, and concerned about

Table 13-4
Binge-Eating Disorder

Disorder	Binge-Eating Disorder	
	DSM-5	ICD-10
Diagnostic name	Binge-eating disorder	Bulimia nervosa, nonpurging type
Duration	Occurs at least once a week for 3 mo	

Symptom	• Repeated binge-eating episodes
	  • Occurring within 2 hr period
	  • Loss of control during the episode
	• Binge-associated behaviors or reactions
	  • Eating quicker than normal
	  • Eating until uncomfortably full
	  • Eating despite not being hungry
	  • Eating alone to avoid embarrassment
	  • Feeling guilty or disgusted after eating
		Similar to ICD-10 bulimia nervosa minus the specific compensatory behaviors

Required number of symptom	Binge behaviors plus at least three of the associated behaviors or reactions	
Psychosocial consequences of symptoms	Marked distress	
Exclusions	No compensatory behavior as in bulimia nervosa	
Course specifiers	Partial remission: Occurrences are less frequent (<1 episode/wk) Full remission: No symptoms for a sustained period	
Severity specifiers	Severity is measured by the average number of compensatory behaviors in a weeks' time See DSM-5 for ranges	

their sexual attractiveness. Most are sexually active, compared with anorexia nervosa patients, who are not interested in sex. They may have a history of pica and struggles during meals.

Binge-Eating Disorder

Individuals with binge-eating disorder engage in frequent binges, often independent of feeling hungry. We summarize the diagnostic criteria in DSM-5 and ICD-10 for the disorder in Table 13-4.

Other Specified Feeding and Eating Disorder

Night-Eating Syndrome. As implied by the name, night-eating syndrome includes recurrent episodes of hyperphagia or night eating. It may be associated with insomnia and a lack of desire for food in the morning.

Patients with night-eating syndrome usually consume a large portion of their daily calorie intake after the evening meal. They may also wake up during the night and eat upon awakening. Some patients believe that they can only sleep if they eat. Depressed mood is common among these patients, especially during the evening and night hours.

PATHOLOGY AND LABORATORY EXAMINATION

Anorexia Nervosa

A patient with anorexia nervosa must have a thorough general physical and neurologic examination. If the patient is vomiting, a hypokalemic alkalosis may be present. Because most patients are dehydrated, serum electrolyte levels must be determined initially

and periodically. Hospitalization may be necessary to deal with medical complications.

A complete blood count often reveals leukopenia with a relative lymphocytosis in emaciated patients with anorexia nervosa. If binge eating and purging are present, serum electrolyte determination reveals hypokalemic alkalosis. Fasting serum glucose concentrations are often low during the emaciated phase, and serum salivary amylase concentrations may increase if the patient is vomiting.

Electrocardiographic (ECG) changes, such as T-wave flattening or inversion, ST segment depression, and lengthening of the QT interval, have been noted in the emaciated stage of anorexia nervosa. The ST segment and T-wave changes are usually secondary to electrolyte disturbances; emaciated patients have hypotension and bradycardia. ECG changes may also result from potassium loss, which can lead to death. Young girls may have a high serum cholesterol level. All these values revert to normal with nutritional rehabilitation and cessation of purging behaviors. Endocrine changes related to being underweight may occur. These can include amenorrhea, mild hypothyroidism, and hypersecretion of corticotrophin-releasing hormone, which revert to normal with weight gain (see Table 13-2).

Bulimia Nervosa

Bulimia nervosa can result in electrolyte abnormalities and various degrees of starvation, although it may not be as apparent as in low-weight patients with anorexia nervosa. Thus, even normal-weight patients with bulimia nervosa should have laboratory studies of electrolytes and metabolism. In general, thyroid function remains intact in bulimia nervosa, but patients may show nonsuppression on a dexamethasone-suppression test. Dehydration and electrolyte disturbances are likely to occur in patients with bulimia nervosa who purge regularly. These patients commonly exhibit hypomagnesemia and hyperamylasemia. Although not a core diagnostic feature, many patients with bulimia nervosa have menstrual disturbances. Hypotension and bradycardia occur in some patients.

DIFFERENTIAL DIAGNOSIS

Anorexia Nervosa

The differential diagnosis of anorexia nervosa is complicated, as patients often deny symptoms, are secretive about their eating habits, and resist seeking treatment. Thus, it may be difficult to identify the mechanism of weight loss and the patient's associated ruminative thoughts about distortions of body image.

We should differentiate the eating disorders from one another. Attention to specific criteria, including whether the patient is of average weight, is essential. However, the two conditions can coexist.

We must ascertain that a patient does not have a medical illness that can account for the weight loss (e.g., a brain tumor or cancer). Weight loss, peculiar eating behaviors, and vomiting can occur in several mental disorders. Depressive disorders and anorexia nervosa have several features in common, such as depressed feelings, crying spells, sleep disturbance, obsessive ruminations, and occasional suicidal thoughts. The two disorders, however, have several distinguishing features. In general, a patient with a depressive disorder has decreased appetite, whereas a patient with anorexia nervosa claims to have a normal appetite and to feel hungry; only in the severe stages of anorexia nervosa do patients have decreased appetite.

In contrast to depressive agitation, the hyperactivity seen in anorexia nervosa is planned and ritualistic. The preoccupation with recipes, the caloric content of foods, and the preparation of gourmet feasts is typical of patients with anorexia nervosa but is absent in patients with a depressive disorder. In depressive disorders, patients have no intense fear of obesity or disturbance of body image.

Weight fluctuations, vomiting, and peculiar food handling may occur in somatization disorder. On rare occasions, a patient may have both a somatization disorder and anorexia nervosa, in which case we should diagnose both. In general, patients with somatization disorder have less weight loss than patients with anorexia nervosa and do not fear weight gain. Amenorrhea for 3 months or longer is unusual in somatization disorder.

Patients with schizophrenia that include delusions about food rarely are concerned with caloric content. More likely, they believe someone poisoned the food. Patients with schizophrenia are rarely preoccupied with a fear of becoming obese and do not have the hyperactivity seen with anorexia nervosa. Patients with schizophrenia have bizarre eating habits but not the entire syndrome of anorexia nervosa.

There are rare conditions of unknown etiology in which a hyperactive vagus nerve causes changes in eating patterns that are associated with weight loss, sometimes severe. In such cases, we may see bradycardia, hypotension, and other parasympathomimetic signs and symptoms. Because the vagus nerve relates to the enteric nervous system, eating may be associated with gastric distress such as nausea or bloating. Patients do not generally lose their appetite. Treatment is symptomatic. Anticholinergic drugs can reverse hypotension and bradycardia, which may be life-threatening.

Bulimia Nervosa

We cannot make the diagnosis of bulimia nervosa if the binge-eating and purging behaviors occur exclusively during episodes of anorexia nervosa. In such cases, the diagnosis is anorexia nervosa, binge eating–purging type. Additionally, we should distinguish bulimia nervosa from binge-eating disorder, which typically includes binge-eating behaviors but no compensatory or purging behaviors.

We must ascertain that patients have no neurologic disease, such as epileptic-equivalent seizures, central nervous system tumors, Klüver–Bucy syndrome, or Kleine–Levin syndrome. Klüver–Bucy syndrome includes visual agnosia, compulsive licking and biting, an examination of objects by the mouth, inability to ignore any stimulus, placidity, altered sexual behavior (hypersexuality), and altered dietary habits, especially hyperphagia. The syndrome is exceedingly rare and is unlikely to cause a problem in the differential diagnosis. Kleine–Levin syndrome consists of periodic hypersomnia lasting for 2 to 3 weeks and hyperphagia. As in bulimia nervosa, the onset is usually during adolescence, but the syndrome is more common in men than in women.

Some patients with bulimia nervosa have multiple comorbid impulsive behaviors, including substance abuse, and lack of ability to control themselves in such diverse areas as money management (resulting in impulse buying and compulsive shopping) and sexual relationships (often resulting in a short, passionate attachment and promiscuity). They exhibit self-mutilation, chaotic emotions, and chaotic sleeping patterns. They usually meet the criteria for borderline personality disorder and other mixed personality disorders and, not infrequently, bipolar II disorder. When bulimia nervosa co-occurs with one of these disorders, we should note both diagnoses.

Binge-Eating Disorder

Binge-eating disorder and bulimia nervosa share the same core feature of recurrent binge eating. Binge-eating disorder is distinct from bulimia nervosa, however, in that binge-eating disorder patients do not report repetitive compensatory behaviors such as vomiting, laxative abuse, or excessive dieting. Binge-eating disorder is distinct from anorexia nervosa in that patients do not exhibit an extreme drive for thinness and are of average weight or are obese.

Other Specified Feeding and Eating Disorder

Night-Eating Syndrome.   Night-eating syndrome is common among patients with other eating disorders, particularly bulimia nervosa and binge-eating disorder. Although we can find night eating in patients with bulimia nervosa and binge-eating disorder, it is the characteristic sign of night-eating disorder. Also, the amount of food consumed during eating episodes is usually lower in night-eating disorder than in bulimia nervosa and binge-eating disorder. Unlike other eating disorders, patients with night eating syndrome are not overly concerned about body image and weight. Patients with night-eating syndrome are also at higher risk for obesity and metabolic syndrome.

Recurrent episodes of involuntary eating characterize a sleep-related eating disorder during the night. These episodes can lead to severe consequences such as the ingesting of nonedible foods or substances, dangerous behaviors while searching for or preparing food, and sleep-related injury. The eating episodes usually occur after the patient has gone to sleep and may occur while the patient is unconscious or asleep. The sleep-related eating disorder also has high comorbidity with sleepwalking, restless legs syndrome, and obstructive sleep apnea, conditions that are rarely found among night-eating syndrome patients. Episodes of sleep-related eating disorder have been reported after the use of certain medications, including zolpidem, triazolam, olanzapine, and risperidone.

COMORBIDITY

Anorexia Nervosa

Table 13-5 lists comorbid psychiatric conditions associated with anorexia nervosa. Overall, anorexia nervosa is associated with depression in 50 percent of cases, social phobia in 22 percent of cases, and obsessive-compulsive disorder (OCD) in 35 percent of cases.

The suicide rate is higher in persons with the binge eating–purging type of anorexia nervosa than in those with the restricting type.

Binge eating–purging persons are likely to be associated with substance abuse, impulse control disorders, and personality disorders. Persons with restricting anorexia nervosa often have obsessive-compulsive traits concerning food and other matters. Some persons with anorexia nervosa may purge but not binge.

Bulimia Nervosa

Bulimia nervosa occurs in individuals with high rates of mood disorders and impulse control disorders. Bulimia nervosa also co-occurs with substance use disorders, particularly alcohol. Patients with bulimia nervosa also have increased rates of anxiety disorders, bipolar I disorder, dissociative disorders, and histories of sexual abuse. Patients with bulimia nervosa who have concurrent seasonal affective disorder and patterns of atypical depression (with overeating and oversleeping in low-light months) may manifest seasonal worsening of both bulimia nervosa and depressive features. Individuals with bulimia nervosa who purge may be at risk for certain medical complications such as hypokalemia from vomiting or laxative abuse and hypochloremic alkalosis. Those who vomit repeatedly are at risk for gastric and esophageal tears, although these complications are rare.

Binge-Eating Disorder

Binge-eating disorder is associated with mood, anxiety, and substance use disorders. Also, nearly half of individuals with binge-eating disorder are obese and are at risk for medical complications associated with obesity. Patients with binge-eating disorder are also more likely to have an unstable weight history with frequent episodes of weight cycling (the gaining or losing of more than 10 kg). The disorder may be associated with insomnia, early menarche, neck or shoulder and lower back pain, chronic muscle pain, and metabolic disorders.

Table 13-5
Lifetime Comorbidities of Various Psychiatric Disorders with Eating Disorders

Diagnosis	No Eating Disorder %	Anorexia Nervosa (%) %	Anorexia Nervosa (%) AOR[a]	Bulimia Nervosa (%) %	Bulimia Nervosa (%) AOR[a]	Binge-Eating Disorder (%) %	Binge-Eating Disorder (%) AOR[a]
MDD	10	8.7	0.7	31.0	3.2[b]	35.4	3.9[b]
Dysthymia	1.7	1.1	0.6	6.7	3.6[b]	5.8	3.1[b]
Bipolar disorder type 1 or 2	2.8	2.1	0.7	18.5	7.3[b]	9.0	3[b]
Any anxiety disorder	12.8	10.9	0.7	49.9	5.7[b]	45.3	4.6[b]
Agoraphobia[c]	2.2	3.5	1.8	7.5	2.7[b]	7.1	2.6[b]
GAD	0.9	0.0	n/a[d]	4.4	4.0	2.0	1.8
Social phobia	5	9.2	1.8	20.3	3.9[b]	26.3	5.9[b]
Specific phobia	14.2	20.5	1.5	36.7	3.1[b]	32.1	2.6[b]
Panic disorder[c]	2.1	0.9	0.4	11.1	5.2[b]	8.7	4[b]
PTSD	3.4	8.7	2.0	26.5	7.6[b]	13.2	3[b]
Seasonal affective disorder	6.5	11.1	1.8	22.1	3.5[b]	16.8	2.6[b]
Any substance use or dependence	24.5	23.9	0.9	66.2	5[b]	65.2	5[b]
Alcohol use disorder	6.1	9.1	1.6	14.3	3.1[b]	13.9	2.4[b]
Substance use disorder	8.3	13.0	1.7	19.3	2.8[b]	22.5	3.2[b]
Any drug use	10.8	13.0	1.3	20.1	2.2[b]	26.8	3.1
ADHD[e]	8.6	2.3	0.2	20.0	3.6[b]	12.6	2.1[b]
Oppositional defiant disorder[e]	6.9	30.4	5.1[b]	24.4	4[b]	32.8	6.2[b]
Conduct disorder[e]	10.4	5.7	0.5	29.0	3.5[b]	28.5	3.6[b]

AOR, adjusted odds ratio.
[a]Adjusted for age, sex, and race/ethnicity.
[b]$p < 0.05$.
[c]Agoraphobia is assessed without panic disorder, while panic disorder is assessed with or without agoraphobia.
[d]No adolescents had both AN and GAD.
[e]Disorders are assessed using both parent and child report ($n = 6,483$).
Adapted from Hudson JI, Hiripi E, Pope HG Jr, Kessler RC. The prevalence and correlates of eating disorders in the National Comorbidity Survey Replication. *Biol Psychiatry.* 2007;61(3):348–358.

COURSE AND PROGNOSIS

Anorexia Nervosa

The precise course of the illness varies substantially, although specific patterns have emerged in the literature. Follow-up studies of patients with anorexia nervosa reveal that, at the time of assessment, approximately 30 to 50 percent have achieved full recovery, and 10 to 20 percent remain chronically ill. The remainder improve but continue to struggle with certain disordered behaviors. The chronically ill group often requires multiple hospitalizations. Of note, anorexia nervosa has a mortality rate as high as that associated with any psychiatric illness. Compared to the general population, individuals with the illness are up to six times more likely to die. The majority of deaths are attributable to medical complications of low weight and malnourishment, but a smaller, yet significant, proportion of deaths (approximately 1 in 5) are due to suicide.

Although additional research is needed to identify predictors of outcome in anorexia nervosa, studies have found that adolescents with a shorter duration of illness tend to have a better prognosis, emphasizing the importance of early detection and intervention. Studies examining inpatients with anorexia nervosa just before and after discharge have also identified specific predictors of posttreatment outcomes. Individuals who achieve full weight-restoration on an inpatient unit and maintain their weight in the first month after discharge are, perhaps unsurprisingly, more likely to remain at a healthy weight up to a year after treatment. Lower BMI at discharge and weight loss in the first month after treatment, on the other hand, predict more unsatisfactory long-term outcomes. Additionally, individuals who demonstrate an ability to consume a diet that is high in variety and energy density (i.e., a greater concentration of kcal/g) before discharge seem to do better after treatment.

Bulimia Nervosa

Bulimia nervosa is characterized by higher rates of partial and full recovery compared with anorexia nervosa. Those receiving treatment fare much better than those who are untreated. Untreated patients tend to remain chronic or may show small, but generally unimpressive, degrees of improvement with time. Research has yet to identify any clear predictors of outcome in bulimia nervosa. Studies have examined a variety of potential prognostic factors, including duration of illness, age of onset, illness severity, comorbid diagnoses, and personality characteristics, with mixed results. In individuals who receive treatment for bulimia nervosa, studies have found that rapid symptom reduction predicts better treatment outcomes.

Binge-Eating Disorder

We know little about the course of binge-eating disorder. Severe obesity is a long-term effect in over 3 percent of patients with the disorder. One prospective study of women in the community with binge-eating disorder suggested that by 5 years of follow-up, fewer than one-fifth of the sample still had clinically significant eating disorder symptoms.

Other Specified Feeding and Eating Disorder

Night-Eating Syndrome.   The age of onset for night-eating syndrome ranges from the late teens to the late 20s and has a long-lasting course with periods of remission with treatment. Patients who experience poor sleep quality are more likely to develop diabetes, obesity, hypertension, and cardiovascular disease.

TREATMENT APPROACH

Treatment of Anorexia Nervosa

Given the complicated psychological and medical implications of anorexia nervosa, a comprehensive treatment plan, including hospitalization when necessary and both individual and family therapy, is recommended. It is important to consider behavioral, interpersonal, and cognitive approaches. In many cases, medication may also help.

Hospitalization.   The first consideration in the treatment of anorexia nervosa is to restore patients' nutritional state; dehydration, starvation, and electrolyte imbalances can seriously compromise health and, in some cases, lead to death. When deciding whether to hospitalize a patient, we should consider the patient's medical condition and the amount of structure needed to ensure cooperation. In general, patients with anorexia nervosa who are 20 percent below the normal weight for their height require inpatient programs, and patients who are 30 percent below their expected weight require psychiatric hospitalization for 2 to 6 months.

Inpatient psychiatric programs for patients with anorexia nervosa generally use a combination of a behavioral management approach, individual psychotherapy, family education and therapy, and, in some cases, psychotropic medications. Staff members should maintain a firm yet supportive approach to patients, often through a combination of positive reinforcers (praise) and negative reinforcers (restriction of exercise). The program must have some flexibility for individualizing treatment to meet patients' needs and cognitive abilities. Patients must become willing participants for treatment to succeed in the long run.

Most patients are uninterested in psychiatric treatment and even resist it; they are brought to a doctor's office unwillingly by agonizing relatives or friends. The patients rarely accept the recommendation of hospitalization without arguing and criticizing the proposed program. Emphasizing the benefits, such as relief of insomnia and depressive signs and symptoms, may help persuade the patients to admit themselves willingly to the hospital. Relatives' support and confidence in the physicians and treatment team are essential for reinforcing the firm recommendations made on the unit. We should warn patients' families that the patients will resist admission and, for the first several weeks of treatment, will make many dramatic pleas for their families' support to obtain release from the hospital program. We should consider compulsory admission or commitment only when the risk of death from the complications of malnutrition is likely. On rare occasions, patients prove that the doctor's statements about the probable failure of outpatient treatment are wrong. They may gain a specified amount of weight by the time of each outpatient visit, but such behavior is uncommon, and a period of inpatient care is usually necessary.

HOSPITAL MANAGEMENT.   The following considerations apply to the general management of patients with anorexia nervosa during a hospitalized treatment program. Patients should be weighed daily, early in the morning after emptying the bladder. The staff should record daily fluid intake and urine output. If vomiting is occurring, hospital staff members must monitor serum electrolyte levels regularly and watch for the development of hypokalemia. Because patients often regurgitate food after meals, the staff may be able to control vomiting by making the bathroom inaccessible for at least 2 hours after meals or by having an attendant in the bathroom to prevent the opportunity for vomiting. Constipation in these patients is relieved when they begin to eat normally. We may occasionally use stool softeners, but never laxatives. If diarrhea occurs, it usually means that patients are surreptitiously taking laxatives. Because of the risk of refeeding syndrome when patients immediately start eating an enormous number of calories, the hospital staff should start patients on a low-caloric intake initially (e.g., 1,000 to 1,400 kcals/day), and increase slowly by approximately 400 kcals every few days. It is wise to give these calories in six equal feedings throughout the day so that patients need not eat a large amount of food at one sitting. Giving patients a liquid food supplement may be advisable, because they may be less apprehensive about gaining weight slowly with formula than by eating food. After discharging patients from the hospital, clinicians usually find it necessary to continue outpatient supervision of the problems identified in the patients and their families.

Psychotherapy

FAMILY-BASED THERAPY. Family-based therapy (FBT) is an effective treatment for anorexia nervosa, particularly in patients under the age of 18. FBT, also known as the Maudsley method, generally consists of three phases of treatment. In phase one, treatment focuses on the restoration of the patient's physical health, with decisions about what or when the patient will eat made by the parents. Once the patient has begun to gain weight and shown improvement in symptoms of anorexia nervosa, FBT moves on to phase two. In this phase, the patient gradually begins to take responsibility for decisions about eating. In phase three, the focus shifts to the patient's growth and development.

COGNITIVE-BEHAVIORAL THERAPY. Cognitive and behavioral therapy principles can be applied in both inpatient and outpatient settings and have been found effective for inducing weight gain. Monitoring is an essential component of cognitive-behavioral therapy (CBT). Therapists teach patients to monitor their food intake, their feelings and emotions, their binging and purging behaviors, and their problems in interpersonal relationships. They also teach the patients cognitive restructuring to identify automatic thoughts and to challenge their core beliefs. Problem-solving is a specific method whereby patients learn how to think through and devise strategies to cope with their food-related and interpersonal problems. These techniques can help address a patient's vulnerability to rely on anorectic behavior as a means of coping.

DYNAMIC PSYCHOTHERAPY. We sometimes use dynamic expressive-supportive psychotherapy in the treatment of patients with anorexia nervosa, but their resistance may make the process difficult and painstaking. Because patients view their symptoms as constituting the core of their specialness, therapists must avoid excessive investment in trying to change their eating behavior. We should gear the opening phase of the psychotherapy process toward building a therapeutic alliance. Patients may experience early interpretations as though someone else was telling them what they feel and thereby minimizing and invalidating their own experiences. Therapists who empathize with patients' points of view and take an active interest in what their patients think and feel, however, convey to patients that their autonomy is respected. Above all, psychotherapists must be flexible, persistent, and durable in the face of patients' tendencies to defeat any efforts to help them.

Pharmacotherapy. Pharmacologic studies have not yet identified any medication that yields a definitive improvement of the core symptoms of anorexia nervosa. Some reports support the use of atypical antipsychotics, particularly olanzapine, for weight gain, although larger studies or meta-analyses have not supported this. When using atypical antipsychotics, the metabolic and cardiac risks associated with these medications, particularly in a population already at risk for cardiac complications, require close monitoring. Antidepressants, including selective serotonin reuptake inhibitors (SSRIs) and tricyclic antidepressants (TCAs), have been tried by patients with anorexia nervosa with variable results, though typically antidepressants are not helpful while patients are in an undernourished state. In patients with anorexia nervosa and coexisting depressive disorders, we should treat the depressive condition. Concern exists about the use of tricyclic drugs in low-weight, depressed patients with anorexia nervosa, who may be vulnerable to hypotension, cardiac arrhythmia, and dehydration. In some patients, the depression improves with weight gain and normalized nutritional status.

Treatment of Bulimia Nervosa

Most patients with uncomplicated bulimia nervosa do not require hospitalization. In general, patients with bulimia nervosa are not as secretive about their symptoms as patients with anorexia nervosa. Therefore, outpatient treatment is usually not difficult, but psychotherapy is frequently stormy and prolonged. In some cases—when eating binges are out of control, outpatient treatment does not work, or a patient exhibits such additional psychiatric symptoms as suicidality and substance abuse—hospitalization may become necessary. Also, electrolyte and metabolic disturbances resulting from severe purging may necessitate hospitalization.

Psychotherapy

COGNITIVE-BEHAVIORAL THERAPY. CBT should be considered the benchmark, first-line treatment for bulimia nervosa. The data supporting the efficacy of CBT are based on strict adherence to rigorously implemented, highly detailed, manual-guided treatments that include about 18 to 20 sessions over 5 to 6 months. CBT implements several cognitive and behavioral procedures to (1) interrupt the self-maintaining behavioral cycle of binging and dieting and (2) alter the individual's dysfunctional cognitions; beliefs about food, weight, body image; and overall self-concept.

OTHER MODALITIES. Given its effectiveness in anorexia nervosa, clinicians have also used FBT for bulimia nervosa. Additionally, controlled trials have shown that a variety of novel ways of administering and facilitating CBT are effective for bulimia nervosa. These include "stepped-care" programs and internet-based platforms, computer-facilitated programs, email-enhanced programs, and administration of CBT via telemedicine to remote areas. Finally, emerging evidence suggests that dialectical behavior therapy may be effective.

Pharmacotherapy. Antidepressant medications help treat bulimia nervosa, particularly the SSRI fluoxetine. Fluoxetine can reduce binge eating and purging, independent of the presence of a mood disorder. Dosages of fluoxetine that are effective in decreasing binge eating, however, may be higher (60 to 80 mg a day) than those used for depressive disorders. Other antidepressants that may be helpful include other SSRIs (although concerns about prolonged QT intervals with higher doses limit the utility of citalopram in this population), TCAs (particularly amitriptyline and desipramine), trazodone, and monoamine oxidase inhibitors (MAOIs). Bupropion is contraindicated due to an increased risk of seizure in this population. In general, most of the antidepressants other than fluoxetine have been effective at dosages usually given in the treatment of depressive disorders. Medication is helpful in patients with comorbid depressive disorders and bulimia nervosa. Topiramate may have some efficacy in reducing binge episodes in bulimia nervosa, as may lisdexamfetamine. Evidence indicates that CBT and medications (particularly fluoxetine) are the most effective combination.

Treatment of Binge-Eating Disorder

Psychotherapy. CBT is the most effective psychological treatment for binge-eating disorder and should be considered a first-line treatment. CBT can lead to decreases in binge eating and associated problems (e.g., depression); however, studies have not shown marked weight loss as a result of CBT. CBT combined with psychopharmacological treatments such as SSRIs shows better results than CBT alone. Exercise has also shown a reduction in binge eating when combined with CBT. Interpersonal psychotherapy (IPT) is also effective in the treatment of binge-eating disorder; however, therapy focuses more on the interpersonal problems that contribute to the disorder rather than disturbances in eating behavior. There is also some evidence for the use of dialectical behavior therapy for binge-eating disorder.

Psychopharmacotherapy. Symptoms of binge eating may benefit from medication treatment, with strong evidence supporting the use of lisdexamfetamine for both weight loss and reduction of binge episodes. Antidepressant medications have demonstrated improvement in binge eating, but typically do not result in sustained weight loss; these include fluoxetine, fluvoxamine, citalopram, escitalopram, sertraline, duloxetine, and bupropion. The anticonvulsants topiramate and zonisamide may improve binge-eating disorder, particularly with moderate weight loss. Topiramate may also reduce binge episodes.

Most, but not all, studies show that medication added to CBT is more effective than medication alone. For example, studies indicate that CBT did better than fluvoxamine or desipramine as a monotherapy for binge-eating disorder; however, when CBT was combined with these agents, more improvement was seen in terms of weight loss compared with CBT alone.

Treating of Other Specified Feeding and Eating Disorder

Night-Eating Syndrome. Various studies have shown positive results in patients treated with SSRIs who showed improvement in nighttime awakenings, nocturnal eating, and post-evening caloric intake. Weight loss and a reduction in nocturnal eating are associated with an addition of topiramate to medication regimens.

In patients with comorbid major depression and night-eating syndrome, bright light therapy has shown to decrease depressed mood. CBT has also been helpful.

EPIDEMIOLOGY

Anorexia Nervosa

Although a substantial proportion of those diagnosed with subthreshold anorexia nervosa in DSM-IV now have a formal diagnosis in DSM-5, combined rates of subthreshold and threshold anorexia nervosa have remained relatively stable since the 1970s. Various studies have, however, documented a significant increase in incidence rates (the number of new cases in the population over a set time) in the high-risk group of 15- to 19-year-old females in recent years. It remains unclear if this increase signifies an earlier age of illness onset or more rapid recognition and intervention. Across all age groups and genders, a review of recent epidemiologic studies found that lifetime prevalence of DSM-5 anorexia nervosa is between 2.4 and 4.3 percent, approximately double the rate of cases diagnosed using DSM-IV criteria. Among girls and women, point prevalence estimates of DSM-5 anorexia nervosa is between 0.6 and 0.7 percent.

Although epidemiologic studies indicate that it may occur as many as ten times more frequently in females, anorexia nervosa does affect males. Recent research suggests that the illness, which continues to be perceived by many as a female disorder, may be even more common in men and boys than previously believed. It may go unrecognized in men for a variety of reasons. In particular, men may be reluctant to seek treatment out of shame, and clinicians may be less likely to recognize the syndrome in male versus female patients. Historically, many consider anorexia nervosa to be a disease of white, wealthy women; however, it impacts individuals of all racial and socioeconomic backgrounds.

Bulimia Nervosa

As with anorexia nervosa, rates of bulimia nervosa have increased with changes to diagnostic criteria. However, before the recent modifications appearing in DSM-5, studies suggested that the incidence of the illness had decreased in recent years. Using DSM-5 criteria, the lifetime prevalence of bulimia nervosa in women is approximately 2 percent, and point prevalence is close to 0.6 percent. The average age of onset also seems to have decreased, although this finding may be an artifact of earlier detection. Like anorexia nervosa, the disorder is more common in women than in men.

Binge-Eating Disorder

Binge-eating disorder is the most common eating disorder and the least gender-divided of the three. In the United States, the lifetime prevalence of binge-eating disorder is about 3.6 percent for women and 2.1 percent for men. Rates of binge-eating disorder are particularly high in obese and overweight individuals.

Other Specified Feeding and Eating Disorder

Night-Eating Syndrome. Night-eating syndrome occurs in approximately 2 percent of the general population; however, it has a higher prevalence among patients with insomnia, obesity (10 to 15 percent), eating disorders, and other psychiatric disorders. The disorder usually begins in early adulthood.

ETIOLOGY

Biologic, social, and psychological factors are important to the cause of feeding and eating disorders. However, the precise mechanisms of causation remain elusive. Current theories posit that individuals with eating disorders, in particular, possess a set of predisposing traits (e.g., biologic, genetic, or personality vulnerability) which, when triggered by a precipitating event (e.g., the stress of puberty, the decision to go on a diet), result in illness. Once the illness sets in, several factors work to maintain it (e.g., the social rewards of weight loss, the effects of the starvation state in anorexia nervosa). A discussion of the current understanding of the etiology of feeding and eating disorders is detailed below.

Anorexia Nervosa

Genetic and Biologic Factors. Although we have not identified a specific gene in anorexia nervosa, several lines of evidence suggest that genetic vulnerability plays an important role in the development of the illness. Family studies, in particular, have provided useful information about genetic susceptibility, demonstrating that individuals with a family history of anorexia nervosa are much more likely than those with no family history to receive a diagnosis during their lifetime. The risk of developing the illness is up to 11 times greater in individuals with a first-degree relative who has experienced the illness. A relative with a history of a different eating disorder also increases this risk. Twin studies have demonstrated that concordance rates of anorexia nervosa are substantially higher in monozygotic twins as compared to dizygotic twins, suggesting that something more than the family environment is at play in increasing the odds of illness development. Studies of the serotonin transporter offer preliminary evidence that this gene may interact with environmental stressors to play a role in the development of anorexia, further emphasizing that a convergence of elements is necessary for illness development. Finally, once the illness sets in, the biologic and psychological changes to the body that occur in the starvation state, including depression and obsessionality, may help to maintain the illness.

Developmental Factors. Anorexia nervosa tends to develop during adolescence, suggesting that factors particular to this period may put individuals at risk for the syndrome. Adolescence represents a time of increased biologic, psychological, and social change. The experience of going through puberty and experiencing changes to body shape or weight may serve as a major stressor for some, triggering or worsening body dissatisfaction and low self-esteem. Additionally, several major social and psychological transitions occur throughout adolescence, including identity and role formation, increasing independence from parents, and the initiation of romantic relationships. These stressors and others may work to catalyze the eating disorder.

Psychological Factors. Several psychological factors appear to confer added risk for developing anorexia nervosa. Certain personality traits, including high levels of perfectionism, self-discipline, harm avoidance, and self-criticism, are common in individuals with the illness. Individuals with the restricting subtype, in particular, exhibit low impulsivity and are much more likely to delay rewards than individuals without the illness. Cognitive inflexibility is usually prominent, as well. In a subset of individuals, mood and anxiety disorders or symptoms precede the development of the anorexia nervosa. OCD and obsessive-compulsive personality traits also appear to serve as vulnerability factors.

Environmental and Social Factors. Environmental and social factors, small and large, from experiences in the family or school setting to cultural ideals, may play a role in the development of anorexia nervosa. The influence of family functioning style as a potential predisposing factor remains controversial. No specific family functioning style appears to be either a necessary or sufficient requirement for developing an eating disorder. As in most psychiatric disorders, various family dysfunctional styles appear to act as nonspecific vulnerability factors and also hamper recovery.

Activities that emphasize weight may increase the probability of developing anorexia nervosa or another eating disorder. Ballet, gymnastics, modeling, and weight-restricted sports like wrestling or light-weight rowing may lead to preoccupation with body form and unhealthy attempts to control weight. As many of these activities likely select for individuals who are higher in perfectionism, another risk factor for anorexia nervosa, they may be even more likely to contribute to illness onset.

Although it is a common misperception that Western media causes eating disorders, the cultural ideal of thinness, which is certainly perpetuated by the media, may fuel the overvaluation of shape and weight that marks both anorexia nervosa and bulimia nervosa. Indeed, studies in Fiji, where Western media was not available until the 1990s, showed a significant increase in cases of eating disorders following the introduction of Western television shows to the country. Nonetheless, classic anorexia nervosa remains rare, and research has firmly established that the media alone does not cause eating disorders.

Bulimia Nervosa

Genetic and Biologic Factors. As in anorexia nervosa, genetics likely play a role in the development of bulimia nervosa, as evidenced by twin and family studies. Individuals with a family history of bulimia nervosa, mood disorder, substance use disorder, or obesity are at higher risk for developing the syndrome.

Neurobiologic disturbances are also present in individuals with bulimia nervosa and may increase the probability of binge eating. In particular, individuals with the disorder tend to display delayed gastric emptying, increased stomach capacity, and reduced secretion of cholecystokinin (CCK), a peptide hormone released by the small intestine that helps to signal satiety during food consumption. Together, disruptions to these neurobiologic processes may put individuals at elevated risk for overeating.

Developmental Factors. The same psychological and social stressors of puberty and adolescence that put individuals at risk for anorexia nervosa also confer risk for bulimia nervosa.

Psychological Factors. Unlike individuals with anorexia nervosa, those with bulimia nervosa tend to exhibit high levels of novelty seeking and impulsivity. They also tend to display elevated levels of harm avoidance, negative emotionality, and stress reactivity. Afflicted individuals are more likely than others to experience a comorbid substance use disorder and engage in self-harm, leading to speculation that a subset of individuals with bulimia nervosa may have a propensity toward impulsivity across a range of problematic behaviors. Mood and anxiety disturbances appear to serve as risk factors for bulimia nervosa, as well.

Just as the starvation state works to maintain anorexia nervosa, the cycle of binge eating and purging often becomes self-sustaining in bulimia nervosa. Individuals with bulimia nervosa tend to restrict their food intake outside of binge episodes, which puts them at increased risk for episodes of overeating. In turn, after experiencing a binge episode and the resulting compensatory behaviors, individuals often renew their commitment to restrictive eating in an attempt to avoid future overeating episodes. Thus, this cycle tends to become self-perpetuating and works to maintain the disorder.

Environmental and Social Factors.   Individuals with bulimia nervosa are likely affected by similar environmental and social stressors as those with anorexia nervosa.

Binge-Eating Disorder

We know even less about the etiology of binge-eating disorder than of anorexia or bulimia nervosa. Research thus far has suggested that a history of childhood obesity, mood disorder, and negative family dynamics may put individuals at higher risk for developing the illness. In some individuals, dietary restriction appears to play a role in precipitating episodes of binge eating, as in bulimia nervosa. Many individuals with binge-eating disorder, however, seem to experience binge eating outside of the context of dietary restriction. For these individuals, intense emotions may provoke binge episodes.

Other Specified Feeding and Eating Disorder

Night-Eating Syndrome.   We also know little about the cause of night-eating disorder. However, researchers have studied the hormones melatonin, leptin, ghrelin, and cortisol as they relate to this disorder. Night-eating syndrome also appears to run in families.

References

Allison KC, Lundgren JD, O'Reardon JP, Geliebter A, Gluck ME, Vinai P, Mitchell JE, Schenck CH, Howell MJ, Crow SJ, Engel S, Latzer Y, Tzischinsky O, Mahowald MW, Stunkard AJ. Proposed diagnostic criteria for night eating syndrome. *Int J Eat Disord*. 2010;43:241–247.

American Psychiatric Association. *Diagnostic and Statistical Manual of Mental Disorders*. 5th ed. Arlington, VA: American Psychiatric Association; 2013.

Birmingham CL, Treasure J. *Medical Management of Eating Disorders*. 2nd ed. New York: Cambridge University Press; 2010.

Brown LM, Clegg DJ. Estrogen and leptin regulation of endocrinological features of anorexia nervosa. *Neuropsychopharmacol Rev*. 2013;38:237.

Brown TA, Keel PK, Striegel RH. Feeding and eating conditions not elsewhere classified (NEC) in DSM-5. *Psych Annals*. 2012;42:421.

Call CC, Attia E, Walsh BT. Chapter 22: Feeding and eating disorders. In: Sadock BJ, Sadock VA, Ruiz P, eds. *Kaplan & Sadock's Comprehensive Textbook of Psychiatry*. 10th ed. Philadelphia, PA: Wolters Kluwer; 2017:2065–2082.

Castillo M, Weiselberg E. Bulimia nervosa/purging disorder. *Curr Probl Pediatr Adolesc Health Care*. 2017;47:85–94.

Crow SJ. Pharmacologic treatment of eating disorders. *Psychiatr Clin N Am*. 2019; 42:253–262.

De Young KP, Lavender JM, Wilson GT, Wonderlich SA. Binge eating disorder in DSM-5. *Psych Annals*. 2012;42:410.

Engel SG, Wonderlich SA, Crosby RD, Mitchell JE, Crow S, Peterson CB, Le Grange D, Simonich HK, Cao L, Lavender JM, Gordon KH. The role of affect in the maintenance of anorexia nervosa: Evidence from a naturalistic assessment of momentary behaviors and emotion. *J Abnorm Psychol*. 2013;122(3):709–719.

Fallon P, Wisniewski L. A system of evidenced-based techniques and collaborative clinical interventions with a chronically ill patient. *Int J Eat Disord*. 2013;46(5): 501–506.

Fazeli PK, Misra M, Goldstein M, Miller KK, Klibanski A. Fibroblast growth factor-21 may mediate growth hormone resistance in anorexia nervosa. *J Clin Endocrinol Metab*. 2010;95:369–374.

Fladung AK, Grön G, Grammer K, Herrnberger B, Schilly E, Grasteit S, Wolf RC, Walter H, von Wietersheim J. A neural signature of anorexia nervosa in the ventral striatal reward system. *Am J Psych*. 2009;167:206–212.

Frank GKW, Reynolds JR, Shott ME, Jappe L, Yang TT, Tregellas JR, O'Reilly RC. Anorexia nervosa and obesity are associated with opposite brain reward response. *Neuropsychopharmacology*. 2012;37:2031–2046.

Friborg O, Martinussen M, Kaiser S, Overgård KT, Martinsen EW, Schmierer P, Rosenvinge JH. Personality disorders in eating disorder not otherwise specified and binge eating disorder: A meta-analysis of comorbidity studies. *J Nerv Ment Dis*. 2014;202(2):119–125.

Friederich HC, Herzog W. Cognitive-behavioral flexibility in anorexia nervosa. In: Adan RAH, Kaye WH, eds. *Behavioral Neurobiology of Eating Disorders*. New York: Springer; 2011:111.

Germain N, Galusca B, Grouselle D, Frere D, Billard S, Epelbaum J, Estour B. Ghrelin and obestatin circadian levels differentiate bingeing-purging from restrictive anorexia nervosa. *J Clin Endocrinol Metab*. 2010;95:3057–3062.

Gianini LM, White MA, Masheb RM. Eating pathology, emotion regulation, and emotional overeating in obese adults with binge eating disorder. *Eat Behav*. 2013;14(3):309–313.

Goldschmidt AB, Grange DL, Powers P, Crow SJ, Hill LL, Peterson CB, Crosby RD, Mitchell JE. Eating disorder symptomatology in normal-weight vs. obese individuals with binge eating disorder. *Obesity*. 2011;19:1515–1518.

Guerdjikova AI, Mori N, Casuto LS, McElroy SL. Update on binge eating disorder. *Med Clin N Am*. 2019;103(4):669–680.

Hay P. A systematic review of evidence for psychological treatments in eating disorders: 2005–2012. *Int J Eat Disord*. 2013;46(5):462–469.

Hudson JI, Hiripi E, Pope HG Jr, Kessler RC. The prevalence and correlates of eating disorders in the National Comorbidity Survey replication. *Biol Psychiatry*. 2007;61:348–358.

Kaye WH, Bulik CM, Thornton L, Barbarich N, Masters K. Comorbidity of anxiety disorders in anorexia and bulimia nervosa. *Am J Psych*. 2004;161(12): 2215–2221.

Kishi T, Kafantaris V, Sunday S, Sheridan EM, Correll CU. Are antipsychotics effective for the treatment of anorexia nervosa? Results from a systematic review and meta-analysis. *J Clin Psychiatry*. 2012;73:e757–e766.

Kumar KK, Tung S, Iqbal J. Bone loss in anorexia nervosa: Leptin, serotonin, and the sympathetic nervous system. *Ann N Y Acad Sci*. 2010;1211:51–65.

Locke J, Grange DL. *Treatment Manual for Anorexia Nervosa*. 2nd ed. New York: Guilford; 2013.

Lopez C, Davies H, Tchanturia K. Neuropsychological inefficiences in anorexia nervosa targeted in clinical practice: The development of a module of cognitive remediation therapy. In: Fox J, Goss K, eds. *Eating and its Disorders*. Hoboken, NJ: Wiley; 2012:185.

Lowe MR, Witt AA, Grossman SL. Dieting in bulimia nervosa is associated with increased food restriction and psychopathology but decreased binge eating. *Eat Behav*. 2013;14(3):342–347.

Milano W, De Rosa M, Milano L, Capasso A. Night eating syndrome: An overview. *J Pharm Pharmacol*. 2012;64:2–10.

Moskowitz L, Weiselberg E. Anorexia nervosa/atypical anorexia nervosa. *Curr Probl Pediatr Adolesc Health Care*. 2017;47:70–84.

Oberndorfer TA, Frank GKW, Simmons AN, Wagner A, McCurdy D, Fudge JL, Yang TT, Paulus MP, Kaye WH. Altered insula response to sweet taste processing after recovery from anorexia and bulimia nervosa. *Am J Psychiatry*. 2013;170(10): 1143–1151.

Perez M, Warren CS. The relationship between quality of life, binge-eating disorder, and obesity status in an ethnically diverse sample. *Obesity*. 2012;20:879–885.

Pollert GA, Engel SG, Schreiber-Gregory DN, Crosby RD, Cao L, Wonderlich SA, Tanofsky-Kraff M, Mitchell JE. The role of eating and emotion in binge eating disorder and loss of control eating. *Int J Eat Disord*. 2013;46(3):233–238.

Poulsen S, Lunn S, Daniel SI, Folke S, Mathiesen BB, Katznelson H, Fairburn CG. A randomized controlled trial of psychoanalytic psychotherapy or cognitive-behavioral therapy for bulimia nervosa. *Am J Psychiatry*. 2014;171(1):109–116.

Reinecke RD. Family-based treatment of eating disorders in adolescents: Current insights. *Adolesc Health Med Ther*. 2017;8:69–79.

Sandberg K, Erford BT. Choosing assessment instruments for bulimia practice and outcome research. *J Counsel Dev*. 2013;91(3):359–366.

Schwitzer AM. Diagnosing, conceptualizing, and treating eating disorders not otherwise specified: A comprehensive practice model. *J Counsel Dev*. 2012;90: 281–289.

Tanofsky-Kraff M, Bulik CM, Marcus MD, Striegel RH, Wilfley DE, Wonderlich SA, Hudson JI. Binge eating disorder: The next generation of research. *Int J Eat Disord*. 2013;46(3):193–207.

Udo T, Grilo CM. Psychiatric and medical correlates of DSM-5 eating disorders in a nationally representative sample of adults in the United States. *Int J Eat Disord*. 2019;52:42–50.

Vander Wal JS. Night eating syndrome: A critical review of the literature. *Clin Psychol Rev*. 2012;32:49–59.

Wolfe BE, Hannon-Engel SL, Mitchell JE. Bulimia nervosa in DSM-5. *Psych Annals*. 2012;42:406–409.

Zimmerli EJ, Devlin MJ, Kissileff HR, Walsh BT. The development of satiation in bulimia nervosa. *Physiol Behav*. 2010;100:346–349.

Zipfel S, Wild B, Groß G, Friederich HC, Teufel M, Schellberg D, Giel KE, de Zwaan M, Dinkel A, Herpertz S, Burgmer M, Löwe B, Tagay S, von Wietersheim J, Zeeck A, Schade-Brittinger C, Schauenburg H, Herzog W; ANTOP study group. Focal psychodynamic therapy, cognitive behaviour therapy, and optimised treatment as usual in outpatients with anorexia nervosa (ANTOP study): Randomised controlled trial. *Lancet*. 2014;383(9912):127–137.

Zunker C, Peterson CB, Crosby RD, Cao L, Engel SG, Mitchell JE, Wonderlich SA. Ecological momentary assessment of bulimia nervosa: Does dietary restriction predict binge eating? *Behav Res Ther*. 2011;49(10):714–717.

14 ▲

Elimination Disorders

The developmental milestones of mastering control over bowel and bladder function are complex processes that involve motor and sensory functions, coordinated through frontal lobe activities, and regulated by neurons in the pons and midbrain area. Mastery of bowel and bladder function occurs over several months for the typical toddler. Infants generally void small volumes of urine approximately every hour, commonly stimulated by feeding, and may have incomplete emptying of the bladder. As the infant matures to be a toddler, bladder capacity increases, and between 1 and 3 years of age, cortical inhibitory pathways develop that allow the child to have voluntary control over reflexes that control the bladder muscles. The ability to have muscular control over the bowel occurs even before bladder control for most toddlers, and the assessment of fecal soiling includes determining whether the clinical presentation occurs with or without chronic constipation and overflow soiling. The typical sequence of developing control over bowel and bladder functions is the development of nocturnal fecal continence, diurnal fecal continence, diurnal bladder control, and nocturnal bladder control. Bowel and bladder control develops gradually over time. Toilet training is affected by many factors, such as a child's intellectual capacity and social maturity, cultural determinants, and the psychological interactions between child and parents. The ability to control bowel and bladder functions depends on the maturation of neurobiologic systems, so that children with developmental delays may also display delayed continence of bowel and bladder. When children exhibit incontinence of urine or feces regularly, it is troubling to the children and families, and often misunderstood as voluntary misbehavior.

Encopresis (repeated passage of feces into inappropriate places) and enuresis (repeated urination into bed or clothes) are the two elimination disorders described in DSM-5. ICD-10 contains the diagnoses of nonorganic encopresis and enuresis, which they list in the category of other behavioral and emotional disorders with onset usually occurring in childhood and adolescence. We should not make these diagnoses until after age 4 years, for encopresis, and after age 5 years for enuresis, the ages at which a typically developing child masters these skills. Healthy development encompasses a range of time in which a given child can devote the attention, motivation, and physiologic skills to exhibit competency in elimination processes.

We discuss each disorder separately in this chapter.

ENCOPRESIS

Clinical and Diagnostic Features

According to both DSM-5 and ICD-10, encopresis occurs when a child passes feces into inappropriate places regularly. Table 14-1 compares the diagnostic approaches for encopresis. Encopresis may be present in children who have bowel control and intentionally deposit feces in their clothes or other places for a variety of emotional reasons. Anecdotal reports have suggested that occasionally encopresis is attributable to an expression of anger or rage in a child whose parents have been punitive or of hostility at a parent. In a case such as this, once a child develops this inappropriate repetitive behavior eliciting negative attention, it is difficult to break the cycle of continuous negative attention. In other children, sporadic episodes of encopresis can occur during times of stress—for example, proximal to the birth of a new sibling—but in such cases, the behavior is usually transient and does not fulfill the diagnostic criteria for the disorder.

Encopresis can also be present on an involuntary basis in the absence of physiologic abnormalities. In these cases, a child may not exhibit adequate control over the sphincter muscles, either because the child is absorbed in another activity or because he or she is unaware of the process. The feces may be of normal, near-normal, or liquid consistency. Some involuntary soiling occurs from chronic retaining of stool, which may result in a liquid overflow. In rare cases, the involuntary overflow of stool results from psychological causes of diarrhea or anxiety disorder symptoms. DSM-5 includes specifiers to indicate whether or not the disorder includes constipation and overflow incontinence.

Studies have indicated that children with encopresis who do not have gastrointestinal illnesses have high rates of abnormal anal sphincter contractions. This finding is particularly prevalent among children with encopresis with constipation and overflow incontinence who have difficulty relaxing their anal sphincter muscles when trying to defecate. Children with constipation, who have difficulties with sphincter relaxation, are not likely to respond well to laxatives in the treatment of their encopresis. Children with encopresis without abnormal sphincter tone are likely to improve over a short period.

Jack was a 7-year-old boy with daily encopresis, enuresis, and history of hoarding behaviors, along with hiding the feces around the house. He lived with his adoptive parents, having been removed from his biologic parents at the age of 3 years because of neglect and physical abuse. He was reported to be cocaine-addicted at birth but was otherwise healthy. Jack's biologic mother was a known methamphetamine and alcohol user, and his father had spent time in jail for drug dealing. Jack had always been enuretic at night, and until this year, he had a history of daytime enuresis as well. Jack had a short attention span, was highly impulsive, and had great difficulty staying in his seat at school and remaining on task. He had reading difficulties and was in a contained special education classroom because of his disruptive behavior as well as his academic difficulties. Despite experiencing physical abuse, he has not experienced flashbacks or other symptoms that would indicate the presence of posttraumatic stress disorder. Jack was treated for attention-deficit/hyperactivity disorder (ADHD) with a good response to methylphenidate.

Table 14-1
Encopresis

	DSM-5	ICD-10
Name	**Encopresis**	**Nonorganic Encopresis**
Duration	≥1/mo for ≥3 mo	
Symptoms	Eliminating feces in clothes or floor Can be voluntary or unintentional	Eliminating feces in inappropriate places Can be voluntary or unintentional
Exclusion	Age <4 y Substance use Another medical condition (not including ones that are causing constipation)	Another medical condition
Severity specifiers	With constipation and overflow incontinence Without constipation and overflow incontinence	

Jack's adoptive family sought help at a university hospital's outpatient program that had expertise in the behavioral treatments of many psychiatric disorders, including encopresis. The treatment program combined the use of regular laxatives and a bowel training method with cognitive-behavioral therapy for Jack and his family. Jack was started on a regimen of daily polyethylene glycol (PEG) solution and was seen by a pediatrician who was able to perform a manual disimpaction under sedation. Following that, Jack was continued on daily PEG solution combined with therapy. He learned to empty his bowel while sitting on the toilet for 10 minutes after each meal, whether or not he felt like he had to go. He soon was eager to stay on this regular bathroom schedule and felt proud when he was able to have a bowel movement in the toilet. Over 3 months, Jack improved, and at 6 months, he was almost entirely better. (Courtesy of Edwin J. Mikkelsen, M.D. and Caroly Pataki, M.D.)

Pathology and Laboratory Examination

Although no specific test indicates a diagnosis of encopresis, clinicians must rule out medical illnesses, such as Hirschsprung disease, before making a diagnosis. The physician should perform an abdominal examination to help determine whether fecal retention is responsible for encopresis with constipation and overflow incontinence, and an abdominal x-ray can help determine the degree of constipation present. Tests to determine whether sphincter tone is abnormal are generally not conducted in uncomplicated cases of encopresis.

Differential Diagnosis

In encopresis with constipation and overflow incontinence, constipation can begin as early as the child's first year and can peak between the second and fourth years. Soiling usually begins by age 4. There are frequent liquid stools and hard fecal masses in the colon and the rectum on abdominal palpation and rectal examination. Complications include impaction, megacolon, and anal fissures.

The chief differential medical problem is aganglionic megacolon or Hirschsprung disease, in which a patient may have an empty rectum and no desire to defecate, but may still have an overflow of feces. The disorder occurs in 1 in 5,000 children; signs appear shortly after birth. Faulty nutrition is rarely the cause of encopresis with constipation and overflow incontinence. Other conditions are rare as well, including structural disease of the anus, rectum, and colon, adverse drug effects, or nongastrointestinal medical (endocrine or neurologic) disorders.

Course and Prognosis

The outcome of encopresis depends on the etiology, the chronicity of the symptoms, and coexisting behavioral problems. In some cases, encopresis is self-limiting, and it rarely continues beyond middle adolescence. Encopresis in children who have associated physiologic factors, such as poor gastric motility and an inability to relax the anal sphincter muscles, is more challenging to treat than that in those with constipation but normal sphincter tone.

Encopresis is a particularly objectionable disorder to family members, who may assume that the behavior is due to "laziness," and family tensions are often high. Peers are intolerant of the developmentally inappropriate behavior and typically taunt and reject a child with encopresis. Many affected children have abysmally low self-esteem and feel constant social rejection. Psychologically, a child may appear blunted toward the symptoms or less frequently may be entrenched in a pattern of encopresis as a mode of expressing anger. The outcome of encopresis is influenced by a family's willingness and ability to participate in treatment without being overly punitive and by the child's ability and motivation to engage in treatment.

Treatment

A typical treatment plan for a child with encopresis includes daily oral administration of laxatives such as PEG at 1 g/kg per day, and often a surgical disimpaction under general anesthesia before administering maintenance laxatives. Also help is a cognitive-behavioral intervention to help the child begin regular attempts to have bowel movements in the toilet, and to diminish anxiety related to bowel movement. By the time a child presents for treatment, considerable family discord and distress are common. We must reduce family tensions about the symptom and establish a nonpunitive atmosphere. Similarly, we should help to reduce the child's embarrassment at school. A treatment plan may include arranging for many changes of underwear with a minimum of embarrassment. Education of the family and correction of misperceptions that a family may have about soiling must occur before treatment. Laxatives are not necessary for children who are not constipated and do have reasonable bowel control, but regular timed intervals on the toilet may be useful with these children as well.

A report confirms the success of an interactive parent–child family guidance intervention for young children with encopresis based on psychological and behavioral interventions for children younger than age 9 years.

Supportive psychotherapy and relaxation techniques may be useful in treating the anxieties and other sequelae of children with encopresis, such as low self-esteem and social isolation. Family interventions can be helpful for children who have bowel control but who continue to deposit their feces in inappropriate locations. An optimal outcome occurs when a child achieves a feeling of control over his or her bowel function.

Epidemiology

Encopresis affects about 3 percent of 4-year-olds and 1.6 percent of 10-year-old children. Incidence rates for encopretic behavior decrease drastically with increasing age. Between the ages of 10 and 12 years, it affects about 0.75 percent of typically developing children. Globally, the community prevalence of encopresis ranges from 0.8 to 7.8 percent. In Western cultures, bowel control is established in more than 95 percent of children by their fourth birthday and 99 percent by the fifth birthday. Encopresis is virtually absent in youth with normal intellectual function by the age of 16 years. Males are from three to six times more likely to have encopresis than females. A significant relationship exists between encopresis and enuresis.

Etiology

Ninety percent of chronic childhood encopresis is likely functional. Children with this disorder typically withhold feces by contracting their gluteal muscles, holding their legs together, and tightening their external anal sphincter. In some cases, this is an entrenched behavioral response to previously painful bowel movements due to hard stool, which leads to fear of defecation and withholding behaviors. Encopresis involves an often-complicated interplay between physiologic and psychological factors leading to an avoidance of defecation. However, when children chronically hold in bowel movements, the result is often fecal impaction and eventual overflow soiling. This pattern occurs in more than 75 percent of children with encopretic behavior. This standard set of circumstances in most children with encopresis supports a behavioral intervention with a focus on ameliorating constipation while increasing appropriate toileting behavior. Inadequate training or the lack of appropriate toilet training may delay a child's attainment of continence.

Evidence indicates that some encopretic children have lifelong inefficient and ineffective sphincter control. Other children may soil involuntarily, either because of an inability to control the sphincter adequately or because of excessive fluid caused by a retentive overflow.

In about 5 to 10 percent of cases, medical conditions cause fecal incontinence, including abnormal innervation of the anorectal region, ultrashort-segment Hirschsprung disease, neuronal intestinal dysplasia, or spinal cord damage.

One study found encopresis to occur with significantly higher frequency among children with known sexual abuse and other psychiatric disorders, compared to samples of healthy children. Encopresis, however, is not a specific indicator of sexual abuse.

It is evident that once a child has developed a pattern of withholding bowel movements and attempts to defecate have become painful, the child's fear and resistance to changing the pattern are high. Battles with parents who insist that their untreated child attempts to defecate may aggravate the condition and cause secondary behavioral difficulties. Untreated children with encopresis, however, frequently end up being socially ostracized and rejected. The social consequences of soiling can lead to the development of emotional problems. On the other hand, children with encopresis who clearly can control their bowel function adequately but chronically deposit feces of relatively normal consistency in abnormal places are likely to have pre-existing neurodevelopmental problems. Occasionally, a child has a specific fear of using the toilet, leading to a phobia.

Encopresis, in some cases, can be considered secondary, that is, emerging after a period of healthy bowel habits in conjunction with a disruptive life event, such as the birth of a sibling or a move to a new home. When encopresis manifests after a long period of fecal continence, it may reflect a regressive developmental behavior based on a severe stressor, such as parental separation, loss of a best friend, or unexpected academic failure.

Megacolon. Most children with encopresis retain feces and become constipated, either voluntarily or secondary to painful defecation. In some cases, a subclinical pre-existing anorectal dysfunction exists that contributes to constipation. In either case, the resulting chronic rectal distention from large, hard fecal masses can cause loss of tone in the rectal wall and desensitization to pressure. Thus, children in this situation become even less aware of the need to defecate, and overflow encopresis occurs, usually with relatively small amounts of liquid or soft stool leaking out.

ENURESIS

Clinical and Diagnostic Features

Enuresis is the repeated voiding of urine into a child's clothes or bed; the voiding may be involuntary or intentional. The child must exhibit a developmental or chronologic age of at least 5 years. Children with enuresis are at higher risk for ADHD compared with the general population. They are also more likely to have comorbid encopresis. DSM-5 and the ICD-10 break down the disorder into three types: nocturnal only, diurnal only, and nocturnal and diurnal (Table 14-2).

Pathology and Laboratory Examination

No single laboratory finding is pathognomonic of enuresis, but clinicians must rule out organic factors, such as the presence of urinary tract infections, which may predispose a child to enuresis. Structural obstructive abnormalities may be present in up to 3 percent of children with apparent enuresis. Usually, clinicians defer sophisticated radiographic studies in uncomplicated cases of enuresis with no signs of repeated infections or other medical problems.

Table 14-2
Enuresis

Name	DSM-5 **Enuresis**	ICD-10 **Nonorganic Enuresis**
Duration	≥2/wk for ≥3 mo	
Symptoms	Urinating into bed or clothes Can be voluntary or unintentional	Involuntary voiding of urine Can be nighttime or daytime
Exclusions (not result of):	Age <5 y Substance use Another medical condition	Another medical condition (i.e., structural abnormality, epilepsy, neurologic disorder)
Symptom specifiers	Nocturnal only Diurnal only Nocturnal and Diurnal	

Differential Diagnosis

Medical causes of bladder dysfunction must be investigated and ruled out. Urinary tract infections, obstructions, or anatomical conditions are found most often in children who experience both nocturnal and diurnal enuresis combined with urinary frequency and urgency. We should consider various causes of genitourinary pathology. Depending on the signs and symptoms, these can include obstructive uropathy, spina bifida occulta, and cystitis—there are many other causes of polyuria and enuresis, such as diabetes mellitus and diabetes insipidus. Also, we should consider disturbances of consciousness and sleep, such as seizures, intoxication, and sleepwalking disorder, during which a child urinates; and adverse effects from medications.

Course and Prognosis

Enuresis is often self-limited, and a child with enuresis may have a spontaneous remission. Most children who master the task of control over their bladder gain self-esteem and improved social confidence when they become continent. About 80 percent of affected children have never achieved a year-long period of dryness. Enuresis after at least 1 dry year usually begins between the ages of 5 and 8 years; if it occurs much later, especially during adulthood, we should investigate for other causes. Some evidence indicates that the late onset of enuresis in children is more frequently associated with a concomitant psychiatric difficulty than is enuresis without at least 1 dry year. Relapses occur in children with enuresis who are becoming dry spontaneously and in those in treatment. The significant emotional and social difficulties of these children usually include poor self-image, decreased self-esteem, social embarrassment and restriction, and intrafamilial conflict. The course of children with enuresis may be influenced by whether they receive appropriate evaluation and treatment for common comorbid disorders such as ADHD.

Treatment

A relatively high rate of spontaneous remission of enuresis occurs over time in childhood; however, in many cases, interventions are necessary because enuresis is causing functional impairment. The first step in any treatment plan is to review appropriate toilet training. If the parents have not attempted toilet training with the child, we should guide the parents and the patient in this undertaking. It is helpful to keep records, to determine a baseline, and follow the child's progress; it may also be therapeutic in itself. A star chart may be particularly helpful. Other useful techniques include restricting fluids before bed and night lifting to toilet train the child. Intervention with alarm therapy, which is triggered by wet underwear, has been a mainstay of treatment for enuresis. Alarm therapy works by alerting a child to respond when voiding begins during sleep. The alarm is a battery-operated device that can be attached to a child's underwear or a mat. The alarm is triggered as soon as voiding begins by emitting a loud noise that awakens the child. The success of this method depends on the child's ability to awaken promptly and respond to the alarm by getting up and voiding in the toilet. A child who can respond optimally is at least 6 or 7 years old.

Another simple intervention for children with enuresis and bowel dysfunction is to assess whether chronic constipation is contributing to urinary dysfunction and to consider increasing dietary fiber to diminish constipation.

Behavioral Therapy.   Classical conditioning with the bell (or buzzer) and pad (alarm) apparatus is generally the most effective treatment for enuresis, with dryness resulting in more than 50 percent of cases. Bladder training—encouragement or reward for delaying micturition for increasing times during waking hours—has also been used. Although sometimes useful, this method is decidedly inferior to the bell and pad.

Pharmacotherapy.   We can consider medication when enuresis is causing social, family or functional impairment, and when dietary and behavioral interventions are not sufficient. When the problem interferes significantly with a child's functioning, we can consider several medications, although the problem often recurs when we discontinue the medications.

Desmopressin, an antidiuretic compound that is available as an intranasal spray, has shown success in reducing enuresis. The reduction of enuresis has varied from 10 to 90 percent with the use of desmopressin. In most studies, enuresis recurred shortly after discontinuation of this medication. Adverse effects that can occur with desmopressin include headache, nasal congestion, epistaxis, and stomachache. The most severe adverse effect reported with the use of desmopressin to treat enuresis was a hyponatremic seizure experienced by a child.

Antidepressants, particularly imipramine, were the first medications used for enuresis, and are still used at times. In this case, we are taking advantage of the anticholinergic side effects of the medication. However, it does have a considerable side effect profile. Reboxetine (not available in the United States), a norepinephrine reuptake inhibitor that has a noncardiotoxic side effect profile, may be a safer alternative to the classically used imipramine in the treatment of childhood enuresis.

Psychotherapy.   Psychotherapy may be useful in dealing with coexisting psychiatric problems and the emotional and family difficulties that arise secondary to chronic enuresis. However, the behavioral therapy approaches described above are the treatments of choice.

Epidemiology

The prevalence of enuresis ranges from 5 to 10 percent in 5-year-olds. It is about 1.5 to 5 percent in 9- to 10-year-olds, and about 1 percent in adolescents 15 years and older. The prevalence of enuresis decreases with increasing age. Enuretic behavior is considered developmentally appropriate among young toddlers, precluding diagnoses of enuresis; however, enuretic behavior occurs in 82 percent of 2-year-olds, 49 percent of 3-year-olds, and 26 percent of 4-year-olds regularly.

Although most children with enuresis do not have a comorbid psychiatric disorder, children with enuresis are at higher risk for the development of another psychiatric disorder.

Nocturnal enuresis is about 50 percent more common in boys and accounts for about 80 percent of children with enuresis. Diurnal enuresis is also seen more often in boys who often delay voiding until it is too late. A spontaneous resolution of nocturnal enuresis is about 15 percent per year. Nocturnal enuresis consists of an average volume of voided urine, whereas when a child voids small volumes of urine at night, other medical causes may be present.

Etiology

Enuresis involves complex neurobiologic systems that include contributions from cerebral and spinal cord centers, motor and sensory functions, and autonomic and voluntary nervous systems. Neurons regulate urination in the pons and midbrain regions. Bladder detrusor muscle contraction occurs whenever bladder capacity is reached, which can lead to enuresis in a sleeping child. Therefore, excessive volumes of urine produced at night may lead to enuresis at night in children without any physiologic abnormalities. Nighttime enuresis often occurs in the absence of a specific neurogenic cause. Daytime enuresis may develop based on behavioral habits developed over time.

Daytime enuresis may occur in the absence of neurologic abnormalities resulting from habitual, voluntary tightening of the external sphincter during urges to urinate. The pattern may become set in a young child who may start with a normal or overactive detrusor muscle in the bladder, but with repeated attempts to prevent leaking or urination when there is an urge to void. Over time, the sensation of the urge to urinate diminishes, and the bladder does not empty regularly, leading to enuresis at night when the bladder is relaxed and can empty without resistance. This immature pattern of urinating can account for some cases of enuresis, especially when the pattern has been in place since early childhood. Most children are not enuretic by intention or even with awareness until after they are wet. Physiologic factors often play a role in the development of enuresis, and behavioral patterns are likely to maintain the maladaptive urination. Healthy bladder control, which is acquired gradually, is influenced by neuromuscular and cognitive development, socioemotional factors, toilet training, and genetic factors. Difficulties in one or more of these areas can delay urinary continence.

Genetic factors play a role in the expression of enuresis, given that the emergence of enuresis is significantly higher in first-degree relatives. A longitudinal study of child development found that children with enuresis were about twice as likely to have concomitant developmental delays as those who did not have enuresis. About 75 percent of children with enuresis have a first-degree relative who has or has had enuresis. A child's risk for enuresis is more than seven times higher if the father was enuretic. The concordance rate is higher in monozygotic twins than in dizygotic twins. There is a strong genetic component, and much can be accounted for by tolerance for enuresis in some families and by other psychosocial factors.

Studies indicate that children with enuresis with a normal anatomical bladder capacity report urge to void with less urine in the bladder than children without enuresis. Other studies report that nocturnal enuresis occurs when the bladder is full because of lower than expected levels of nighttime antidiuretic hormone. This low level of the hormone could lead to higher-than-usual urine output. Enuresis does not appear to be related to a specific stage of sleep or time of night; instead, bedwetting appears randomly. In most cases, the quality of sleep is average. Little evidence indicates that children with enuresis sleep more soundly than other children.

Psychosocial stressors appear to precipitate enuresis in a subgroup of children with the disorder. In young children, the disorder may relate to the birth of a sibling, hospitalization, the start of school, separation of a family due to divorce, or a move to a new environment.

References

Baeyens D, Roeyers H, D'Haese L, Pieters F, Hoebeke P, Vande Walle J. The prevalence of ADHD in children with enuresis: Comparison between a tertiary and non-tertiary care sample. *Acta Paediatr*. 2006;95:347–352.

Benninga MA, Voskuijl WP, Akkerhius GW, Taminiau JA, Buller HA. Colonic transit times and behaviour profiles in children with defecation disorders. *Arch Dis Child*. 2004;89:13–16.

Brazzeli M, Griffiths P. Behavioural and cognitive interventions with or without other treatments for the management of faecal incontinence in children. *Cochrane Database Syst Rev*. 2006;19:CD002240.

Brown ML, Pope AW, Brown EJ. Treatment of primary nocturnal enuresis in children: A review. *Child Care Health Dev*. 2010;37:153–160.

Butler RJ, Heron J. The prevalence of infrequent bedwetting and nocturnal enuresis in childhood: A large British cohort. *Scand J Urol Nephrol*. 2008;42:257–264.

Di Lorenzo C, Benninga MA. Pathophysiology of pediatric fecal incontinence. *Gastroenterology*. 2004;126(Suppl 1):S33–S40.

Feldman AS, Bauer SB. Diagnosis and management of dysfunctional voiding. *Curr Opin Pediatr*. 2006;18:139–147.

Fitzgerald MP, Thom DH, Wassel-Fyr C, Subak L, Brubaker L, Van Den Deden SK, Brown JS; Reproductive Risks for Incontinence Study at Kaiser Research Group. Childhood urinary symptoms predict adult overactive bladder symptoms. *J Urol*. 2006;175:989–993.

Friedman FM, Weiss JP. Desmopressin in the treatment of nocturia: Clinical evidence and experience. *Ther Adv Urol*. 2013;5:310–317.

Har AF, Croffie JM. Encopresis. *Pediatr Rev*. 2010;31:368–374.

Kajiwara M, Inoue K, Kato M, Usui A, Kurihara M, Usui T. Nocturnal enuresis and overactive bladder in children: An epidemiological study. *Int J Urol*. 2006;13:36–41.

Klages T, Geller B, Tillman R, Bolhofner K, Zimerman B. Controlled study of encopresis and enuresis in children with a prepubertal and early adolescent bipolar-I disorder phenotype. *J Am Acad Child Adolesc Psychiatry*. 2005;44:1050–1057.

Landgraf JM, Abidari J, Cilento BG Jr., Cooper CS, Schulman SL, Ortenberg J. Coping, commitment, and attitude: Quantifying the everyday burden of enuresis on children and their families. *Pediatrics*. 2004;113:334–344.

Mellon MW, Whiteside SP, Friedrich WN. The relevance of fecal soiling as an indicator of child sexual abuse: A preliminary analysis. *J Dev Behav Pediatr*. 2006;27:25–32.

Mikkelsen EJ. Elimination disorders. In: Sadock BJ, Sadock VA, Ruiz P, eds. *Kaplan & Sadock's Comprehensive Textbook of Psychiatry*. 9th ed. Vol. II. Philadelphia, PA: Lippincott Williams & Wilkins; 2009:3624.

Mugie SM, Di Lorenzo C, Benninga MA. Constipation in childhood. *Nat Rev Gastroenterol Hepatol*. 2011;8:502–511.

Nevéus T. Reboxetine in therapy-resistant enuresis: Results and pathogenetic implications. *Scand J Urol Nephrol*. 2006;40:31–34.

Pennesi M, Pitter M, Borduga A, Minisini S, Peratoner L. Behavioral therapy for primary nocturnal enuresis. *J Urol*. 2004;171:408–410.

Perrin N, Sayer L, White A. The efficacy of alarm therapy versus desmopressin therapy in the treatment of primary mono-symptomatic nocturnal enuresis: A systematic review. *Prim Health Care Res Dev*. 2015;16:21–31.

Rajindrajith S, Devanarayana NM, Benninga MA. Review article: Faecal incontinence in children: Epidemiology, pathophysiology, clinical evaluation and management. *Aliment Pharmacol Ther*. 2013;37:37–48.

Reid H, Bahar RJ. Treatment of encopresis and chronic constipation in young children: Clinical results from interactive parent-child guidance. *Clin Pediatr*. 2006;45:157–164.

Reiner WG. Pharmacotherapy in the management of voiding and storage disorders, including enuresis and encopresis. *J Am Acad Child Adolesc Psychiatry*. 2008;47:5:491–498.

Rowan-Legg A; Canadian Paediatric Society, Community Paediatrics Committee. Managing functional constipation in children. *Paediatr Child Health*. 2011;16:661–670.

Rutter M, Tizard J, Yule W, Graham P, Whitmore K. Research report: Isle of Wight Studies, 1964–1974. *Psychol Med*. 1976;6:313–332.

Von Gontard A, Hollmann E. Comorbidity of functional urinary incontinence and encopresis: Somatic and behavioral associations. *J Urol*. 2004;171:2644–2647.

Yilmaz S, Bilgic A, Hergüner S. Effect of OROS methylphenidate on encopresis in children with attention-deficit/hyperactivity disorder. *J Child Adolesc Psychopharmacol*. 2014;24:158–160.

15 ▲

Sleep–Wake Disorders

To understand sleep and its disorders, it helps to begin with sleep's three essential characteristics: (1) Sleep is a process required for proper brain function. Failure to sleep impairs thought processes, mood regulation, and a host of normal physiologic functions. (2) Sleep is not a single process; there are several distinct types of sleep. These different types of sleep differ both qualitatively and quantitatively. Each type of sleep has unique characteristics, functional importance, and regulatory mechanisms. Selectively depriving one particular type of sleep produces compensatory rebound when an individual is allowed to sleep ad lib. (3) Sleep is not a passive process; during sleep, there is a high degree of brain activation and metabolism.

The science of sleep is a fascinating ever-growing topic, that is, perhaps unfortunately, beyond the repertoire of the average psychiatrist, and we refer the interested reader to the Comprehensive Textbook's discussion of the basic science of sleep, discussed about the neural sciences.

Several basic mechanisms regulate sleep, and when these systems go awry, sleep disorders occur. Sleep disorders are both dangerous and expensive. Hypersomnolence is a serious, potentially life-threatening condition affecting not only the sleepy individual but also their family, coworkers, and society in general. Sleep-related motor vehicle accidents represent a significant public safety concern, with some states enacting criminal statutes to deter sleepy driving. Investigations link many major industrial catastrophes to sleepiness. Research shows that sleep-disordered breathing contributes to hypertension, heart failure, and stroke. Sleep disorders' direct cost per annum in the United States is about $16 billion, with indirect costs ranging upward to more than $100 billion.

THE CLINICAL PRESENTATION

This chapter's disorders all describe disturbances in healthy sleep. Among them, however, there is considerable variation.

It is helpful to understand the stages of sleep and electrophysiologic criteria. Table 15-1 and Figure 15-1 illustrate some of the features of normal sleep.

Insomnia Disorder

Persons with insomnia primarily have difficulty falling asleep, difficulty staying asleep, or trouble waking early with an inability to fall back to sleep, sufficient to impair their functioning. In children, this may manifest as resistance to caregiver designation of bedtime or difficulty sleeping without some sort of intervention from the caregiver.

Hypersomnolence Disorder

Hypersomnolence broadly refers to excessive sleepiness and time sleeping. During the day, people are drowsy and have reduced

attention. Excessive sleepiness can be a serious, debilitating, potentially life-threatening condition. It affects not only the patient but their family, colleagues, and the public. Not due to disrupted sleep or circadian problems, hypersomnolence disorder likely results from some fundamental neurologic sleep regulation dysfunction.

Narcolepsy

People with narcolepsy have an overwhelming desire to sleep and may suddenly fall asleep, even if it is not appropriate to do so. Also, they may experience cataplexy, or the sudden loss of muscle tone, usually with continuing full or partial consciousness. Laughter, or other strong emotions, commonly precipitate the cataplexy. Cataplexy can range from transient weakness in the knees to total paralysis while the patient is fully conscious. Episodes may last from several seconds to minutes. Usually, the patient is unable to speak and may fall to the floor. Sleep paralysis and hypnagogic (or hypnopompic) hallucinations may occur.

Sleep-Related Breathing Disorders

People who present with sleep-related breathing disorders experience an interruption of normal respiration that impacts their sleep, often resulting in CNS arousal and, consequently, daytime sleepiness. Sleep-related breathing disorders include conditions involving large airway obstruction during sleep, breathing cessation resulting from central respiratory mechanisms, and hypoventilation without breathing cessation. Those affected may experience sleep-related breathing cessation (sleep apnea), in which the patient stops breathing for 10 seconds or more during sleep. They may instead have reduced breathing or *hypopnea*. Airway obstruction is the usual case of these impairments, however central (brainstem) pathology can also be the cause. When asleep, breathing cessations or reductions typically provoke CNS arousal, significant oxyhemoglobin desaturation, or both. Sleep apnea can *obstructive, central,* or *mixed,* depending on the cause.

The clinical presentation of the sleep-related breathing disorders varies depending on the mechanism of the disorder. Table 15-2 lists some of these symptoms.

Circadian Rhythm Sleep–Wake Disorders

Circadian rhythm sleep disorders include a wide range of conditions involving a misalignment between desired and actual sleep periods. This collection of sleep disorders shares the same primary underlying etiology—a desynchrony between an individual's internal circadian biologic clock and the desired or conventional sleep–wake cycle. The circadian pacemaker is in the suprachiasmatic nucleus (SCN). SCN firing oscillates with an almost sinusoidal pattern, the

Table 15-1
Stages of Sleep—Electrophysiologic Criteria

	Electroencephalogram	Electrooculogram	Electromyogram
Wakefulness	Low-voltage, mixed frequency activity; α (8–13 cps) activity with eyes closed	Eye movements and eye blinks	High tonic activity and voluntary movements
Non–rapid eye movement sleep			
Stage 1	Low-voltage, mixed frequency activity; θ (3–7 cps) activity, vertex sharp waves	Slow eye movements	Tonic activity slightly decreased from wakefulness
Stage 2	Low-voltage, mixed frequency background with sleep spindles (12–14 cps bursts) and K complexes (negative sharp wave followed by positive slow wave)	None	Low tonic activity
Stage 3	High-amplitude (≥75 μV) slow waves (≤2 cps) occupying 20–50% of epoch	None	Low tonic activity
Stage 4	High-amplitude slow waves occupy >50% of epoch	None	Low tonic activity
REM sleep	Low-voltage, mixed frequency activity; saw-tooth waves, θ activity, and slow α activity	REMs	Tonic atonia with phasic twitches

cps, cycles per second; REM, rapid eye movement.
Criteria from Rechtschaffen A, Kales A. *A Manual of Standardized Terminology, Techniques, and Scoring System for Sleep Stages of Human Subjects.* Los Angeles, CA: Brain Information Service/UCLA Brain Research Institute; 1968, with permission.

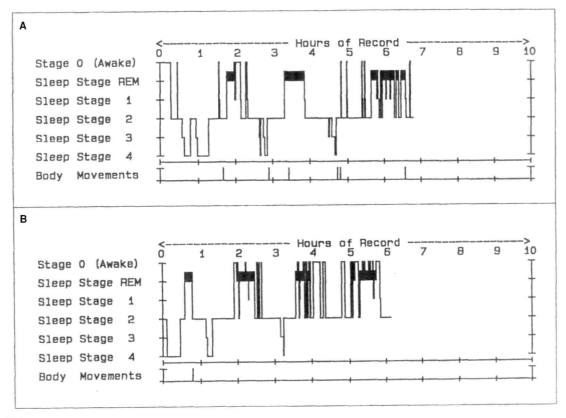

FIGURE 15-1
Sleep histograms showing normal sleep and insomnia. Sleep stage histograms comparing normal sleep (**Panel A**) with that found in a patient with major depressive disorder (**Panel B**). Difficulty maintaining sleep and early morning awakenings are common complaints in patients with depression. **Panel B** illustrates the electrophysiologic correlates of these complaints beginning, in this case, after approximately 2 hours of sleep. Sleep continuity becomes disrupted as morning approaches. Also present is a markedly reduced latency to REM sleep. This sleep feature is characteristic of this patient population and is thought by some to reflect cholinergic–aminergic imbalance.

Table 15-2
Sleep Apnea Symptoms Based on Cause

Obstructive Sleep Apnea
Excessive sleepiness
Snoring
Obesity
Restless sleep
Nocturnal awakenings with choking or gasping for breath
Morning dry mouth
Morning headaches
Heavy nocturnal sweating

Central Sleep Apnea
Breathing cessations unrelated to airway flow limitations
Insomnia
Daytime sleepiness
Morning headaches

Table 15-3
Sleep-Related Movement Disorders

Restless legs syndrome
Periodic limb movement disorder
Sleep-related leg cramps
Sleep-related bruxism
Sleep-related rhythmic movement disorder
Benign sleep myoclonus of infancy
Propriospinal myoclonus at sleep onset

Sleep-related movement disorders due to:
    Medical conditions
    Medications
    Substances

period of which is 24 hours, and the output correlates with the daily fluctuations in core body temperature. Mismatched circadian clock and desired schedules can arise from improper phase relationships between the two, travel across time zones, or dysfunctions in the basic biologic rhythm. Under normal circumstances, the internal circadian pacemaker is reset each day by bright light, social cues, stimulants, and activity. In cases in which these factors fail to reentrain the circadian rhythm, the circadian sleep disorders occur.

Parasomnias and Sleep-Related Movement Disorders

Parasomnias are disorders of partial arousal. In general, the parasomnias are a diverse collection of sleep disorders characterized by physiologic or behavioral phenomena that occur during or are potentiated by sleep. One conceptual framework views many parasomnias as overlaps or intrusions of one sleep–wake state into another. Usually, we divide sleep into three basic states: wakefulness, non–rapid eye movement (NREM) sleep, and REM. Each has a unique neurologic organization. During wakefulness, both the body and brain are active. In NREM sleep, both the body and brain are much less active. REM sleep, however, pairs an atonic body with an active brain (capable of creating elaborate dream fantasies). Regional cerebral blood flow, magnetic resonance imaging (MRI), and other imaging studies confirm increased brain activation during REM sleep. It certainly appears that in some parasomnias, there are state boundary violations. For example, arousal disorders (sleepwalking and sleep terrors) involve momentary or partial wakeful behaviors suddenly occurring in NREM sleep. Similarly, isolated sleep paralysis is the persistence of REM sleep atonia into the wakefulness transition, whereas REM sleep behavior disorder (RBD) is the failure of the mechanism creating paralytic atonia such that individuals act out their dreams.

There are many sleep-related movement disorders. These disorders typically involve relatively simple bodily movements that impact sleep. Table 15-3 lists examples of these disorders.

DIAGNOSIS

Three different nosologies provide classification systems for sleep disorders: (1) the Diagnostic and Statistical Manual of Mental Disorders, fifth edition (DSM-5), (2) the International Classification of Sleep Disorders, third edition (ICSD-3), and (3) the International Classification of Diseases, 10th edition (ICD-10). Most general psychiatrists use the DSM-5 approach. However, Sleep Medicine specialists often prefer the ICSD-3. We have included a listing of ICSD sleep–wake disorders for reference (Table 15-4).

Insomnia Disorder

The primary diagnostic criteria descriptively relate to how insomnia affects sleep. To be diagnosed with insomnia, the person must have difficulty falling asleep, staying asleep, or waking early with difficulty getting back to sleep. While there are no formal criteria for diagnostic subtypes of insomnia, the ICSD-3 does describe each subtype briefly. We describe the insomnia subtypes here to highlight possible insomnia nuances and complications. We present a comparison of the different approaches to diagnosing insomnia in Table 15-5.

Psychophysiologic Insomnia.   Psychophysiologic insomnia (PPI) involves conditioned arousal with the thought of sleeping. Objects related to sleep (e.g., the bed, the bedroom) likewise have become conditioned stimuli that evoke insomnia. Daytime adaptation is usually good; however, there can be extreme tiredness, and the affected person can become desperate. PPI often occurs in combination with stress and anxiety disorders, delayed sleep phase syndrome, and hypnotic use and withdrawal. Table 15-6 lists some typical characteristics of PPI.

DESCRIPTION

Ms. W is a 41-year-old, divorced white female presenting with a two-and one-half year complaint of sleeplessness. She has some difficulty falling asleep (30- to 45-minute sleep-onset latency) and awakens every hour or two after sleep onset. These awakenings may last 15 minutes to several hours, and she estimates approximately 4.5 hours of sleep on an average night. She rarely takes daytime naps notwithstanding feeling tired and edgy. The patient describes her sleep problem with the following words, "It seems like I never get into a deep sleep. I have never been a heavy sleeper, but now the slightest noise wakes me up. Sometimes I have a hard time getting my mind to shut down." She views the bedroom as an unpleasant place of sleeplessness and states, "I tried staying at a friend's house where it is quiet, but then I couldn't sleep because of the silence."

At times, Ms. W is unsure whether she is asleep or awake. She has a history of clock watching (to time her wakefulness) but stopped doing this when she realized it was contributing to the problem. Reportedly the insomnia is unrelated to seasonal changes, menstrual cycle, or time-zone translocation. Her basic sleep hygiene is good. Appetite and libido are unchanged. She denies mood disturbance, except that she is quite frustrated and concerned about sleeplessness and its effect on her work. Her work involves sitting at a microscope for 6 hours out of a 9-hour

Table 15-4
Outline of the International Classification of Sleep Disorders, Third Edition

I. Insomnia
  A. Chronic Insomnia Disorder
  B. Short-Term Insomnia Disorder
  C. Other Insomnia Disorder
  D. Isolated Symptoms and Normal Variants
    1. Excessive Time in Bed
    2. Short Sleeper
II. Sleep-Related Breathing Disorders
  A. Obstructive Sleep Apnea Disorders
    1. Obstructive Sleep Apnea, Adult
    2. Obstructive Sleep Apnea Disorder, Pediatric
  B. Central Sleep Apnea Syndromes
    1. Central Sleep Apnea with Cheyne–Stokes Breathing
    2. Central Apnea due to a Medical Disorder without Cheyne–Stokes Breathing
    3. Central Sleep Apnea due to High-Altitude Periodic Breathing
    4. Central Sleep Apnea due to a Medication or Substance
    5. Primary Central Sleep Apnea
    6. Primary Central Sleep Apnea of Infancy
    7. Primary Central Sleep Apnea of Prematurity
    8. Treatment-Emergent Central Sleep Apnea
  C. Sleep-Related Hypoventilation Disorders
    1. Obesity Hypoventilation Syndrome
    2. Congenital Central Alveolar Hypoventilation Syndrome
    3. Late-Onset Central Hypoventilation and Hypothalamic Dysfunction
    4. Idiopathic Central Alveolar Hypoventilation
    5. Sleep-Related Hypoventilation due to a Medication or Substance
    6. Sleep-Related Hypoventilation due to a Medical Disorder
  D. Sleep-Related Hypoxemia Disorder
    1. Sleep-Related Hypoxemia
  E. Isolated Symptoms and Normal Variants
    1. Snoring
    2. Catathrenia
III. Central Disorders of Hypersomnolence
  A. Narcolepsy type 1
  B. Narcolepsy type 2
  C. Idiopathic Hypersomnia
  D. Kleine–Levin Syndrome
  E. Hypersomnia due to a Medical Disorder
  F. Hypersomnia due to a Medication or Substance
  G. Hypersomnia Associated with a Psychiatric Disorder
  H. Insufficient Sleep Syndrome
  I. Isolated Symptoms and Normal Variants
    1. Long Sleeper

IV. Circadian Rhythm Sleep–Wake Disorders
  A. Delayed Sleep–Wake Phase Disorder
  B. Advanced Sleep–Wake Phase Disorder
  C. Irregular Sleep–Wake Rhythm Disorder
  D. Non–24-h Sleep–Wake Rhythm Disorder
  E. Shift Work Disorder
  F. Jet Lag Disorder
  G. Circadian Sleep–Wake Disorder Not Otherwise Specified
V. Parasomnias
  A. NREM-Related Parasomnias
    1. Confusional Arousals
    2. Sleepwalking
    3. Sleep Terrors
    4. Sleep-Related Eating Disorder
  B. REM-Related Parasomnias
    1. REM Sleep Behavior Disorder
    2. Recurrent Isolated Sleep Paralysis
    3. Nightmare Disorder
  C. Other Parasomnias
    1. Exploding Head Syndrome
    2. Sleep-Related Hallucinations
    3. Sleep Enuresis
    4. Parasomnia due to Medical Disorder
    5. Parasomnia due to a Medication or Substance
    6. Parasomnia, Unspecified
    7. Isolated Symptoms and Normal Variants
      a. Sleep Talking
VI. Sleep-Related Movement Disorders
  A. Restless Legs Syndrome
  B. Periodic Limb Movement Disorder
  C. Sleep-Related Leg Cramps
  D. Sleep-Related Bruxism
  E. Sleep-Related Rhythmic Movement Disorder
  F. Benign Sleep Myoclonus of Infancy
  G. Propriospinal Myoclonus at Sleep Onset
  H. Sleep-Related Movement Disorder due to Medical Disorder
  I. Sleep-Related Movement Disorder due to a Medication or Substance
  J. Sleep-Related Movement Disorder, Unspecified
  K. Isolated Symptoms and Normal Variants
    1. Excessive Fragmentary Myoclonus
    2. Hypnagogic Foot Tremor and Alternating Leg Muscle Activation
    3. Sleep Starts (Hypnic Jerks)
VII. Other Sleep Disorders

working day and meticulously documenting her findings. Her final output has not suffered, but she must now "double check" for accuracy.

She describes herself as a worrier and a Type-A personality. The patient does not know how to relax. For example, on vacation she continually worries about things that can go wrong. She will not even begin to unwind until she has arrived at the destination, checked in, and unpacked. Even then, she is unable to relax.

Medical history is unremarkable except for tonsillectomy (age 16 years), migraine headaches (current), and diet-controlled hypercholesterolemia. She takes naproxen as needed for headache. She does not currently drink caffeinated beverages, smoke tobacco, or drink alcoholic beverages. She does not use recreational drugs.

The problem with insomnia began after relocation to a new city and place of employment. She attributes her insomnia to the noisy neighborhood in which she now lives. She first sought treatment 18 months ago. Her family practice physician diagnosed depression, and she was started on fluoxetine that made her "climb the walls." Antihistamines were tried next with similar results. She was then switched to low-dose

trazodone (for sleep) and developed nausea. After these medical interventions, she sought medical care elsewhere. Zolpidem 5 mg was prescribed, but it made her feel drugged and upon discontinuation she had withdrawal effects. Another family practice physician diagnosed "nonspecific anxiety disorder" and began buspirone; an experience she describes as "having an alien try to climb out of my skin." Buspirone was discontinued. Paroxetine was tried for 8 weeks with no effect. Finally, a psychiatrist was consulted, who diagnosed adult attention-deficit disorder (without hyperactivity) and suggested treatment with methylphenidate. At this point, the patient was convinced that a stimulant would not help her insomnia and demanded referral to a sleep disorders center.

DISCUSSION

Ms. W's symptoms fall into the broad category of an insomnia, and the symptoms began after having moved from one city to another. Environmental sleep disorder (noise) and adjustment sleep disorder (new job, city, and apartment) are likely initial diagnoses. However, a more

Table 15-5
Insomnia Disorder

	DSM-5	ICSD-3	ICD-10
Name	Insomnia disorder	Insomnia disorder	Disorders of initiating and maintaining sleep (insomnias)
Duration	Symptoms occur at least 3 nights/wk, lasting at least 3 mo	Occurs at least 3×/wk	
Symptoms	Dissatisfaction with quality of sleep due to either: • Difficulty falling asleep • Difficulty maintaining sleep • Early morning awakenings	1. Problem with sleep initiation or maintenance 2. Symptoms occurring despite adequate opportunities for sleep 3. Symptoms resulting in daytime consequences due to poor sleep	Disorders characterized by difficulties with falling asleep and/or staying asleep
# Symptoms needed	Any of the above	All the above three symptoms	
Exclusion (not the result of):	Medical disorder A medication or substance Another sleep–wake disorder Insufficient opportunity for sleep		Nightmares Nonorganic sleep disorders Sleep terrors Sleepwalking
Psychosocial impact	Causes significant distress and/or impairment in functioning	Required presence of significant daytime impairment/consequences due to impaired sleep	
Symptom specifiers	• **With non-sleep disorder mental comorbidity** (including substance use disorder) • **With other medical comorbidity** • **With other sleep disorder**		
Severity specifiers			
Course specifiers	**Episodic** (lasting 1–3 mo) **Persistent** (lasting ≥3 mo) **Recurrent** (two or more episodes occurring within 1 y)	**Short-term insomnia disorder:** <3 mo **Chronic insomnia disorder:** ≥3 mo	
Comments		This is often occurring in the setting of an acute stressor	

chronic, endogenous problem has become operative. What is it? Ms. W is a "worrier" and meticulous, but she doesn't reach diagnostic criteria for personality or anxiety disorders. Dyssomnia associated with mood disorder should be considered in any patient with sleep maintenance problems and early morning awakening insomnia. However, this patient does not have other significant signs of depression. Unfortunately, many patients are misdiagnosed with depression or "masked depression" on the sole basis of an insomnia complaint and unsuccessfully treated with antidepressant medication. Ms. W's job demands long hours with focused concentration. Her job performance has been superior for many years notwithstanding insomnia. Thus, a diagnosis of attention-deficit disorder is unlikely. Idiopathic insomnia implies a childhood complaint, which Ms. W denies.

The likely working diagnosis is PPI. There may be some sleep state misperception (sometimes unclear of whether she is awake or asleep), but this cannot adequately account for the constellation of symptoms. An initial treatment plan should include further documentation of the sleep pattern using a sleep log. Behavioral treatments will likely benefit this patient. Medications with sedative effects are sometimes useful during initial treatment of PPI. However, thus far in this patient they have done more harm than good. She is likely to be a challenging patient to treat.

Idiopathic Insomnia. Idiopathic insomnia characterizes patients with a lifelong inability to obtain adequate sleep. The insomnia predates any psychiatric condition, and other etiologies must be ruled out or treated, including PPI, environmental sleep disturbances, and poor sleep hygiene.

Paradoxical Insomnia. Paradoxical insomnia, at its core, involves a dissociation between sleep and its usual attendant unconsciousness. In paradoxical insomnia, a person thinks he or she is awake and having insomnia even though the brain electrophysiologic activity pattern is consistent with the correlates of healthy sleep. We should consider this disorder when a patient complains of difficulty initiating or maintaining sleep without any objective evidence of sleep disruption. Paradoxical insomnia can occur in individuals who are free from psychopathology; however, it may represent a somatic delusion or hypochondriasis. Some patients with paradoxical insomnia have obsessional features regarding bodily functions.

Table 15-6
Some Characteristics of Psychophysiologic Insomnia

1. Excessive worry about not being able to sleep
2. Trying too hard to sleep
3. Rumination—inability to clear one's mind while trying to sleep
4. Increased muscle tension when getting into bed
5. Other somatic manifestations of anxiety
6. Ability to fall asleep when not trying (e.g., while watching television)
7. Sleeping better away from the person's own bedroom

Inadequate Sleep Hygiene.   Inadequate sleep hygiene refers to insomnia produced by behaviors that are not conducive to good sleep. Many behaviors can interfere with sleep. Some of these behaviors increase arousal, for example, consuming caffeine or nicotine at night or engaging in excessive emotional or physical stimulation within a few hours of bedtime. Other behaviors interfere with sleep architecture, including daytime naps and a significant variation of the daily sleep–wake schedule.

Behavioral Insomnia of Childhood.   Children with this subtype of insomnia depend on specific stimulation, objects, or setting for initiating or returning to sleep. Without the presence of, for example, a stuffed animal or a parent, the child has trouble falling asleep. Alternatively, without adequate limit-setting by the caregiver, bedtime stalling ("Dad, I'm thirsty—can I get some water?") or bedtime refusal ("I'm not tired! I don't want to go to sleep!") can ensue.

Insomnia Comorbid with Mental Disorder.   This type of insomnia is the most common. Sleep disorder centers report that 35 percent of patients seen with insomnia have a mental disorder. Of these, major depressive disorder (MDD) is the most common disorder. Other common disorders include bipolar disorder, schizophrenia, and generalized anxiety disorder.

Insomnia Comorbid with Medical Condition.   Insomnia accompanies many medical and neurologic conditions. Given pain's potential for disturbing sleep, all medical conditions producing pain can (and usually do) disturb sleep. Unfortunately, a synergy exists between pain and sleep, such that poor sleep lowers the pain threshold. This vicious cycle can present a difficult treatment challenge. However, reducing pain can also improve sleep, and improving sleep can reduce pain. In other medical conditions, sleep disturbance appears to be secondary. For example, patients with sleep-related gastroesophageal reflux disease (GERD) often have insomnia. Treating the reflux results in sleep improvement but insomnia treatments seldom, if ever, relieve nocturnal GERD. Patients with chronic obstructive pulmonary disease (COPD) commonly suffer from both sleep-onset and sleep-maintenance insomnia. Neurodegenerative disorders are also frequently associated with sleep disorders.

Insomnia due to Drug or Substance.   Many prescription drugs, even when taken properly, can disturb sleep. We list some common examples in Table 15-7.

Alcohol and hypnotic use initially promote sleep onset because of their sedating properties. A problem occurs when sleep quality is adversely affected, tolerance develops after chronic use, or withdrawal begins. Alcohol may relax a tense person and thereby decrease latency to sleep; however, sleep later in the night will usually be fragmented by arousals. As tolerance develops to the

Table 15-7
Medications and Drugs Causing Insomnia

Antiparkinsonian drugs
Decongestants (e.g., pseudoephedrine)
Anorectics
Stimulants
Antiepileptic medications
SSRI antidepressants
Caffeine
Alcohol (rebound insomnia)
Sedatives (rebound insomnia)

alcohol, higher amounts or more frequent dosing are needed to sustain the effects. Furthermore, during withdrawal or after tolerance develops, insomnia may rebound to a level more severe than the initial disturbance.

Caffeine (the active ingredient in coffee) and theobromine (the active ingredient in chocolate) are methylxanthines and act as psychostimulants in the central nervous system (CNS). Psychostimulants increase sleep latency, reduce sleep efficiency, and decrease total sleep time. Caffeine's half-life is 3 to 7 hours and may interfere with sleep when consumed in large quantities throughout the day or even in smaller portions closer to bedtime. Some individuals are hypersensitive to methylxanthines, and any coffee or chocolate can trigger difficulty falling asleep or awakening after a couple of hours of sleep with difficulty getting back to sleep.

Finally, abuse of illicit substances, particularly stimulants (such as cocaine and amphetamines), interfere with sleep onset and sleep maintenance. Unlike with alcohol, discontinuation of these substances will cause hypersomnolence.

Hypersomnolence Disorder

DSM-5 includes hypersomnolence disorder as a discreet diagnosis, whereas ICSD and ICD consider it more broadly. ICSD refers to it as "idiopathic hypersomnia" and questions whether it is a single disorder or rather a group of disorders with different underlying causes. Table 15-8 compares the different approaches to diagnosing hypersomnolence.

In general, we should consider this disorder when a patient complains of frequently feeling sleepy despite getting adequate sleep. They may nap during the day. Despite getting adequate sleep, they do not feel refreshed when waking.

Kleine–Levin Syndrome.   Kleine–Levin syndrome is a relatively rare condition consisting of recurrent periods of prolonged sleep (from which they are arousable) with intervening periods of healthy sleep and alert waking. During the episodes of hypersomnia, wakeful periods are usually marked by withdrawal from social contacts and return to bed at the first opportunity. Kleine–Levin syndrome is the best-recognized recurrent hypersomnia though it is uncommon. It predominantly afflicts males in early adolescence; however, it can also affect females and older people. With few exceptions, the first attack occurs between the ages of 10 and 21 years. However, there are some reports of onset in the fourth and fifth decades of life. In its classic form, the recurrent episodes include extreme sleepiness (18- to 20-hour sleep periods), voracious eating, hypersexuality, and disinhibition (e.g., aggression). Episodes typically last for a few days up to several weeks and appear once to 10 times per year. A monosymptomatic hypersomnolent form can occur. The disorder is usually sporadic but familial cases are reported.

Narcolepsy

Table 15-9 lists the criteria for narcolepsy. People with narcolepsy have irresistible sleep episodes, lapses into sleep, or nap frequently.

The discovery that narcolepsy is strongly associated with a hypocretin (orexin) deficit radically changed diagnostic practice. Cataplexy had been considered a core feature of the disorder, but we now know that there are variants that occur without cataplexy.

Sleep-Related Breathing Disorders

DSM-5 includes three disorders under the category of sleep-related breathing disorders: obstructive sleep apnea-hypopnea,

Table 15-8
Hypersomnolence Disorder

	DSM-5	ICS-3	ICD-10
Name	Hypersomnolence disorder	Idiopathic hypersomnia	Nonorganic hypersomnia
Duration	≥3×/wk for at least 3 mo		
Symptoms	Multiple episodes of sleeping within the same day Main sleep lasts >9 h, but is nonrestorative Difficult to become fully aroused when woken	Subjective sleepiness MSLT shows mean sleep latency ≤8 min <2 sleep-onset rapid eye movement periods on the MSLT and overnight polysomnogram	Excess daytime sleepiness Sleep attacks Difficult to become fully aroused when woken
# Symptoms needed	At least one of the above	All the above	
Exclusion (not the result of):	Another sleep disorder Substance use Another mental or medical disorder	Cataplexy Hypocretin-1 deficiency Sleep deprivation Other causes of hypersomnolence	Medical cause Narcolepsy
Psychosocial impact	Causes significant distress and/or impairment in functioning		
Symptom specifiers	With mental disorder With medical condition With another sleep disorder		
Severity specifiers	Mild: occurs 1–2 days a week Moderate: occurs 3–4 days a week Severe: occurs 5–7 days a week		
Course specifiers	Acute: <1 mo Subacute: 1–3 mo Persistent: >3 mo		
Comments		It is unclear whether this is a single disorder or multiple with different underlying mechanisms	This is usually associated with some other mental disorder

central sleep apnea, and sleep-related hypoventilation. Table 15-10 compares the diagnostic approaches to sleep-related breathing disorders.

Obstructive Sleep Apnea-Hypopnea. Obstructive sleep apnea/hypopnea, often called obstructive sleep apnea (OSA), occurs when the airway partially or fully collapses during sleep. Decreased oxygen saturation and increased respiratory effort leads to arousals and sleep fragmentation. Predisposing factors for OSA include being male, reaching middle age, being obese, and having micrognathia (undersized lower jaw), retrognathia (posteriorly positioned lower jaw), nasopharyngeal abnormalities, hypothyroidism, and acromegaly. Patients with OSA may also have hypertension, erectile failure in men, depression, heart failure, nocturia, polycythemia, and memory impairment as a result of obstructive sleep apnea-hypopnea. Obstructive apnea and hypopnea episodes can occur in any stage of sleep but are more typical during REM sleep, NREM stage 1, and NREM stage 2 sleep.

Mr. J is a 28-year-old single African American male with an approximately 10-year history of fatigue and sleepiness in the daytime. He began to recognize the daytime sleepiness as a problem in his freshman year of college when he would fall asleep in class or in the dormitory. He admits that his sleep–wake schedule was disrupted during college due to taking long naps and then having to stay up until 1:00 or 2:00 AM to complete his studies. His grades and social life suffered,

and he describes himself as depressed, isolated, and hopeless about his planned future as a certified public accountant.

As a child, Mr. J says he slept "normally." In high school he felt best with 10 hours of sleep per night and was able to function well in the daytime. Mr. J denies abuse of alcohol or drugs. He does not use tobacco and drinks about 8 to 10 cups of coffee per day. Family history is negative for known sleep or psychiatric disorders. Physical examination findings are noncontributory except for body mass index of 29. Routine labs were normal, including TSH.

Mr. J's excessive sleepiness has continued to the present day, notwithstanding some improved sleep hygiene. Improvements include more consistency in bedtime, trying not to nap, and a torturous month-long trial without caffeine. He remains dysphoric and discouraged about his future, blaming his chronic sleepiness as the continuing impediment to his life plans. "I'm just tired of being tired," he says.

Currently, his bedtime is between 10:00 and 10:30 PM; his wake-up alarm is set for 6:30 AM. He oversleeps at least once a week on workdays and sleeps from 10:30 PM until 10:00 AM on weekends to "catch up." He has difficulty awakening and feels unrefreshed or mildly refreshed. By drinking six to eight cups of coffee in the morning, he is usually able to avoid dozing during the morning. Luckily, he works independently and can schedule client appointments during this relatively alert time. After lunch he routinely falls asleep at the computer while working. He sleeps for 20 to 60 minutes and is usually awakened by his secretary. He then drinks another two cups of coffee and continues with his work. Unexpected napping can also occur later in the afternoon or evening, and he has "nodded off" while driving. He sleeps alone; however, he has been told that he snores loudly. He does

**Table 15-9
Narcolepsy**

	DSM-5	ICSD-3	ICD-10
Name	Narcolepsy	Narcolepsy	Narcolepsy and cataplexy
Duration	≥3×/wk for at least 3 mo		

Symptoms	Excessive daytime sleepiness with
	• Cataplexy
	• CSF hypocretin deficiency
	• REM sleep latency
	  • ≤15 min on polysomnography
	  • OR mean sleep latency ≤8 min on multiple sleep latency testing with ≥ sleep-onset REM sleep periods
		1. Excessive sleepiness
		2. Cataplexy and/or hypocretin 1 deficiency
		3. Mean sleep latency of ≤8 min and two sleep-onset rapid eye movement periods (SOREMP) within 15 min of sleep onset
			Episodes of daytime sleepiness occurring despite adequate sleep, and often associated with cataplexy, and uncontrollable lapses in consciousness

# Symptoms needed	Excessive daytime sleepiness is required, plus at least one other symptom as above.	**Type 1:** All of the above criteria met **Type 2:** Cataplexy and/or hypocretin deficiency not present	
Exclusion (not the result of):	Substance use disorder Another sleep–wake disorder	Sleep deprivation Another sleep-related disorder	Nightmares Nonorganic sleep disorders Sleep terrors Sleepwalking
Symptom specifiers	**Narcolepsy without cataplexy but with hypocretin deficiency** **Narcolepsy with cataplexy but without hypocretin deficiency** **Autosomal dominant cerebellar ataxia, deafness, and narcolepsy** (due to genetic mutation and characterized by late onset in 30s and 40s) **Autosomal dominant narcolepsy, obesity, and type 2 diabetes** (associated with mutation in myelin oligodendrocyte glycoprotein gene) **Narcolepsy secondary to another medical condition**	**Types 1 and 2** (see above)	
Severity specifiers	**Mild:** <1/wk, 1–2 naps daily mildly, or intermittently disturbed sleep. **Moderate:** cataplexy 1/day or close to that. Disturbed sleep, need for multiple naps. **Severe:** near constant. Multiple attacks/day. Disturbed sleep. Resistant to medications.		

not awaken gasping or choking. He denies hypnagogic hallucinations and sleep paralysis but thinks he may feel weak after the rare occasions when he participates in a heated argument.

DISCUSSION

Mr. J has one of the hypersomnias. Most consistent with his history are obstructive sleep apnea syndrome, idiopathic hypersomnia, sleep deprivation in a long sleeper, dyssomnia associated with mood disorder, and narcolepsy. The ancillary symptoms of narcolepsy are absent, with the possible exception of cataplexy. When cataplexy occurs clearly, the diagnosis of narcolepsy is strongly indicated. However, Mr. J's possible infrequent weakness during heated arguments is equivocal for cataplexy. His persistent desire for a 10-hour sleep period would be unusual for a patient with narcolepsy.

A long sleeper or an individual with idiopathic hypersomnia requires prolonged sleep periods and may awaken groggy as does Mr. J. The main differentiating feature is that whenever consistently given a chance to have a full nightly sleep period (usually 10 to 12 hours), the long sleeper does not experience excessive daytime sleepiness. Furthermore, there may be associated autonomic nervous

system dysfunction or polysomnographic evidence of elevated slow-wave sleep percentage in patients with idiopathic hypersomnia.

Sleepiness associated with a low-grade chronic depression may be difficult to differentiate from other causes of hypersomnolence. Polysomnography, psychiatric interview, and psychometric testing can be helpful. Mr. J relates his dysphoria to sleepiness and not vice versa; nonetheless, a dyssomnia associated with mood disorder should be considered.

Obstructive sleep apnea syndrome is a strong possibly. Mr. J is overweight (BMI = 29) and snores loudly. Many patients are unaware of gasping or choking for breath. Often, family members witness cessation of breathing during sleep and urge patients to seek treatment. However, Mr. J lives and sleeps alone.

Polysomnography is recommended in patients suspected of obstructive sleep apnea syndrome, narcolepsy, or idiopathic hypersomnia. These disorders usually require lifelong treatment and have significant morbidity and mortality if untreated.

Central Sleep Apnea. Central sleep apnea is a diminished effort to breathe. There are many possible causes, DSM defines

Table 15-10
Sleep-Related Breathing Disorders

	DSM-5	ICSD-3	ICD-10

Name	Breathing-related sleep disorders:
	• **Obstructive sleep apnea-hypopnea**
	• **Central sleep apnea**
	• **Sleep-related hypoventilation**
		Sleep-related breathing disorders:
		• **Central sleep apnea syndromes**
		  • Central sleep apnea with Cheyne–Stokes breathing
		  • Central sleep apnea due to a medical disorder without Cheyne–Stokes breathing
		  • Central sleep apnea due to high-altitude periodic breathing
		  • Primary central sleep apnea
		• **Obstructive sleep apnea disorders**
		• **Sleep-related hypoventilation disorders**
		  • Obesity hypoventilation syndrome
		  • Congenital central alveolar hypoventilation syndrome
		  • Late-onset central hypoventilation with hypothalamic dysfunction
		  • Idiopathic central alveolar hypoventilation
			Sleep apnea
			Central
			Obstructive

Symptoms	**Obstructive Sleep Apnea-Hypopnea:** Evidence on polysomnography of ≤5 obstructive apneas or hypopneas/hour of sleep with either: • Nocturnal breathing disturbance (i.e., snoring, breathing pauses) • Daytime sleepiness, fatigue Evidence on polysomnography of 15+ obstructive apneas and/or hypopneas/hour of sleep **Central Sleep Apnea:** 5+ central apneas/hour of sleep on polysomnography **Sleep-Related Hypoventilation:** Decreased respiration causing increased CO_2 levels, as correlated by polysomnography	**Obstructive Sleep Apnea-Hypopnea:** 15+ events/hour of sleep on polysomnogram OR 5 obstructive events/hour on polysomnography w/ daytime symptoms of fatigue or sleepiness **Central Sleep Apnea:** Above symptoms but they persist despite positive airway pressure relieving an obstruction **Sleep-Related Hypoventilation:** ↑ alveolar CO_2 (direct measurement or by end-tidal CO_2 measurement) *For obesity hypoventilation syndrome:* Daytime ↑ $PaCO_2$ (>45 mm Hg) in a patient with BMI of >30 kg/m^2	
# Symptoms needed	**Obstructive Sleep Apnea-Hypopnea:** One of the above criteria must be met **Central Sleep Apnea:** All criteria met **Sleep-related hypoventilation:** All criteria met	**Obstructive Sleep Apnea-Hypopnea:** One of the above criteria must be met **Central Sleep Apnea:** All criteria met **Sleep-related hypoventilation:** All criteria met	
Exclusion (not the result of):	Another sleep disorder Use of a substance or medication	Another sleep disorder Use of a substance/medication	Pickwickian syndrome Sleep apnea of newborn
Symptom specifiers	Obstructive Sleep Apnea-Hypopnea: n/a Central Sleep Apnea: • **Idiopathic central sleep apnea** • **Cheyne–Stokes breathing** • **Central sleep apnea comorbid with opioid use** Sleep-Related Hypoventilation: • **Idiopathic hypoventilation** • **Congenital central alveolar hypoventilation** • **Comorbid sleep-related hypoventilation**		

Table 15-10
Sleep-Related Breathing Disorders (*Continued*)

	DSM-5	ICSD-3	ICD-10
Severity specifiers	<u>Obstructive Sleep Apnea-Hypopnea:</u> **Mild:** apnea hypopnea index is <15 **Moderate:** apnea hypopnea index 15–30 **Severe:** apnea hypopnea index >30 <u>Central Sleep Apnea:</u> Severity based on frequency of breathing disturbance as well as severity of oxygen desaturation/sleep fragmentation <u>Sleep-Related Hypoventilation:</u> Severity based on degree of hypoxemia/hypercarbia, in addition to presence of end-organ impairment. Blood gas abnormality during wakefulness is an indicator of more severe illness.		

three of them: idiopathic CSA, Cheyne–Stokes breathing, and CSA comorbid with opioid use. Other causes include heart failure, high altitude, brainstem lesions, metabolic conditions, specific drugs or substances (CNS depressants), congenital abnormalities, and positive airway pressure (PAP) treatment. The critical characteristic linking the various CSA syndromes is the diminished breathing is not caused by airway obstruction. ICSD-3 includes several subtypes of CSA in addition to those included in DSM-5, which we discuss below, along with the DSM-5 subtypes.

IDIOPATHIC CSA. Patients with idiopathic CSA typically have low normal arterial carbon dioxide tension ($PaCO_2$) while awake and have a high ventilatory response to CO_2. They present with daytime sleepiness, insomnia, or awakening with shortness of breath. Respiratory cessations during sleep are independent of ventilatory effort. Polysomnography reveals five or more central apneas per hour of sleep.

CHEYNE–STOKES BREATHING. Cheyne–Stokes breathing is a unique breathing pattern consisting of prolonged hyperpnea during which tidal volume gradually waxes and wanes in a crescendo–decrescendo fashion. The hyperpnea alternates with apnea and hypopnea episodes that are associated with reduced ventilatory effort. This pattern is most common in older men with congestive heart failure or stroke. As with idiopathic CSA, the patient presents with daytime sleepiness, insomnia, and awakening short of breath.

CSA COMORBID WITH OPIOID USE. This syndrome is the third subtype of CSA in DSM-5, specified if opioid use disorder is present. There is an association with chronic use of long-acting opioid medications and impairment of neuromuscular respiratory control leading to CSA.

CSA DUE TO HIGH-ALTITUDE PERIODIC BREATHING. Central apnea at sleep onset is universal at elevations above 7,600 m but can occur at 1,500 m in some individuals (especially with a rapid ascent). This subtype is no longer included in DSM-5 but may still have clinical significance. Periods of central apnea alternate with periods of hyperpnea in a 12- to 34-second cycle. This response is an extension of normal respiratory control at sleep onset where medullary pH receptors raise their set-point and require lower pH to respond. At high altitudes, hyperventilation causes a hypocapnic alkalosis that reduces ventilation during sleep. Sleep architecture may suffer,

with increased duration in stages 1 and 2 and less slow-wave sleep. REM sleep may not be affected.

CSA DUE TO MEDICAL DISORDER WITHOUT CHEYNE–STOKES BREATHING. This form of CSA is usually caused by a brainstem lesion associated with a wide range of variable etiologies. Cardiac and renal disorders can also cause central apnea. Diagnostic criteria require a polysomnographically verified rate of 5 or more central apneas and hypopneas per hour of sleep.

CSA DUE TO DRUG OR SUBSTANCE USE. A variety of drugs or drug combinations can provoke central apnea episodes, most notably long-acting opiates. However, other substances or medications can also alter neuromuscular control leading to CSA. Diagnostic criteria are a central apnea index (number of episodes per hour) of 5 or more per hour.

PRIMARY SLEEP APNEA OF INFANCY. This form of CSA involves prolonged apneas or hypopneas with concomitant hypoxemia, bradycardia, or both. This condition afflicts preterm neonates, presumably because their brainstems are not fully developed. The condition may be exacerbated by other medical problems that further compromise the infant's physiologic and developmental status.

Sleep-Related Hypoventilation. DSM-5 includes three types of sleep-related hypoventilation disorders: (1) idiopathic hypoventilation, (2) congenital central alveolar hypoventilation, and (3) comorbid sleep-related hypoventilation (which results from a medical disorder, such as a cervical spinal cord injury, COPD, or a neuromuscular disorder, for example). Polysomnography must demonstrate either episodes with elevated CO_2 levels and decreased respirations or, if not monitoring the CO_2, episodes of persistently low oxyhemoglobin levels that are not provoked by apnea or hypopnea.

Circadian Rhythm Sleep–Wake Disorders

DSM-5 lists six types of circadian rhythm sleep–wake disorders: delayed sleep phase type, advanced sleep phase type, irregular sleep–wake type, non–24-hour sleep–wake type, shift work type, and unspecified type. DSM-5 does not include jet lag type, but ICSD does. Table 15-11 compares the diagnostic approaches to the circadian rhythm sleep–wake disorders.

Table 15-11
Circadian Rhythm Sleep Disorders

	DSM-5	ICSD-3	ICD-10
Name	Circadian rhythm sleep-wake disorders	Circadian rhythm sleep–wake disorders: • **Shift work disorder** • **Jet lag disorder** • **Delayed sleep–wake phase disorder** • **Advanced sleep–wake phase disorder** • **Irregular sleep–wake rhythm disorder** • **Non–24-h sleep–wake rhythm disorder**	Disorders of sleep–wake schedule **Delayed sleep phase syndrome** **Irregular sleep–wake pattern**
Duration	**Episodic** (lasting 1–3 mo) **Persistent** (lasting ≥3 mo) **Recurrent** (two or more episodes occurring within 1 y)	Symptoms ≥3 mo (exception of jet lag disorder)	
Symptoms	• Disturbed sleep due to altered circadian rhythm • Excessive daytime sleepiness and/or insomnia	Chronic pattern of sleep–wake rhythm disruption due to abnormality in circadian timing/schedule Presence of insomnia and/or excessive sleepiness	Persistent sleep disturbance (i.e., insomnia or excessive daytime sleepiness) due to altered circadian rhythm and environmental demands Disruption of normal 24-h circadian cycle
# Symptoms needed	All the above	All the above	One of the above
Exclusion (not the result of):	Substance use Another medical condition		Nightmares Nonorganic sleep disorders Sleep terrors Sleepwalking
Psychosocial impact	Marked distress and/or impairment in functioning	Distress or impairment in functioning	
Symptom specifiers	**Delayed sleep phase type** (sleep onset and awakening times are later) Specify if **familial** Specify if **overlapping with non–24-h sleep–wake type** **Advanced sleep phase type** (sleep onset and awakening times are earlier) Specify if **familial** **Irregular sleep–wake type** (disorganized cycle) **Non–24-h sleep–wake type** does not follow 24-h pattern, with daily drift of progressively later sleep onset/wake time) **Shift work type** **Unspecified type**		
Course specifiers	**Episodic** (lasting 1–3 mo) **Persistent** (lasting ≥3 mo) **Recurrent** (two or more episodes occurring within 1 y)		
Comments		Circadian rhythm disorders can be the result of underlying medical, psychiatric, or neurologic disorders	

Delayed Sleep Phase Type.   The delayed sleep phase circadian disorder occurs when the biologic clock runs slower than 24 hours or is shifted later than the desired schedule. This produces a phase delay in the sleepiness–alertness cycle. Individuals with delayed sleep phase are more alert in the evening and early nighttime, stay up later and are more tired in the morning. These individuals are sometimes called *night owls*.

Advanced Sleep Phase Type.   Advanced sleep phase occurs when the circadian rhythm cycle shifts forward. Therefore, the sleepiness cycle moves earlier. Individuals with advanced sleep phase are drowsy in the evening, want to retire to bed earlier, awaken earlier, and are more alert in the early morning. Individuals with this pattern of advanced sleep phase are sometimes called *early birds* or *larks*.

Irregular Sleep–Wake Type.   The irregular sleep–wake pattern occurs when the circadian sleep–wake rhythm is absent or pathologically diminished. The sleep–wake pattern is temporally disorganized, and the timing of sleep and wakefulness is unpredictable. Individuals with this condition have a healthy amount of sleep during 24 hours; however, it is fragmented into three or more episodes that occur irregularly. There are symptoms of insomnia at night and excessive sleepiness during the day. Long daytime naps and inappropriate nocturnal wakefulness occur. This usually impairs activities of daily life.

Non–24-Hour Sleep–Wake Type.   When the circadian sleep–wake pacemaker has a cycle length greater or less than 24 hours and is not reset each morning, a person may develop this type of circadian rhythm disorder. Under normal circumstances, resynchronization of the circadian rhythm occurs daily in response to the light–dark cycle. Problems occur incrementally when internal and environmental clocks become more and more out of phase. If the circadian clock's period is longer than 24 hours and does not reset each day, the patient experiences progressively worsening sleep-onset insomnia and daytime sleepiness. Sleep problems peak when circadian and environmental clocks are 12 hours out of phase and then begin to lessen, as the sleep phase continues to advance. Eventually, the clocks align, and the sleep–wake cycle is normal for a few days. Then, unfortunately, the problem begins again.

For this reason, non–24-hour sleep–wake disorder has been called *periodic insomnia* and *periodic excessive sleepiness.* Traumatic brain injury (TBI) can cause this, as can blindness.

Shift Work Type.   Many service industries require 24-hour operation (e.g., transportation, health care). Similarly, as cultures became more capital intensive, mining and manufacturing became around-the-clock enterprises. The number of individuals doing shift work has been increasing steadily for decades. Shift workers commonly have insomnia, excessive sleepiness, or both. Some individuals require only a short time to adjust to a shift change, whereas others have great difficulty. Frequent shift rotation adds to the problem.

Furthermore, to meet social demands, shift workers often adopt an unshifted sleep–wake schedule on weekends and holidays. Even those individuals who try to stay shifted usually retain an unshifted circadian rhythm. The result can be severe insomnia when attempting to sleep and excessive sleepiness when attempting to remain awake. The result is profound sleep deprivation as circadian rhythm continues to conflict with the sleep–wake schedule. The natural low point in the normal sleep–wake rhythm occurs at approximately 3:00 to 5:00 AM—the time frame during which transportation and industrial accidents commonly occur as a direct consequence of sleepiness.

Jet Lag Type.   Removed from DSM-5, the other classifications still recognize jet lag. With the advent of high-speed air travel, induced desynchrony between circadian and environmental clocks became possible. Thus, the term *jet lag* came into use. When an individual rapidly travels across many time zones, they either induce a circadian phase advance or a phase delay, depending on the direction of travel. Typically, traveling across one or two time zones will not cause a significant problem. However, it can be challenging to adjust to overseas travel. Individuals who frequently travel for business can find themselves quite impaired at the time they need to make crucial decisions.

Furthermore, "night owls" will experience greater difficulty adjusting to eastward travel because resynchronization requires phase advance. Similarly, "larks" theoretically will have more difficulty with westward travel. The number of time zones crossed is a critical factor. Usually, healthy individuals can quickly adapt to one or two time zone changes per day; therefore, natural adjustment to an 8-hour translocation may take 4 or more days.

Unspecified Type.   During illnesses that keep patients bedridden during hospitalizations, and in some forms of dementia, individuals often sleep erratically. The resulting chaotic sleep–wake pattern adversely affects the circadian rhythm. Medications can also exacerbate the sleep–wake cycle breakdown. Sleep in patients in the intensive care unit is disturbed by noise, light, and therapeutic and monitoring procedures. The resulting disorganized sleep–wake pattern can produce a significant sleep disorder. Also, abuse of recreational street drugs (e.g., methamphetamine, ecstasy) is associated with individuals remaining awake overnight or continuously for several days at a time. These episodes of prolonged wakefulness ultimately produce periods of profound hypersomnia.

Parasomnias and Sleep-Related Movement Disorders

DSM 5 includes only three of the 10 specific parasomnias referenced in the ICSD-3. Also, DSM-5 includes restless legs syndrome (RLS), which ICSD-3 classifies as one of the seven specific sleep-related movement disorders. We will discuss all of these disorders together.

NREM-Related Parasomnias.   Table 15-12 compares the diagnostic approaches to the NREM-related parasomnias.

SLEEPWALKING.   Sleepwalking, in its classic form, as the name implies, is a condition in which an individual arises from bed and ambulates without fully awakening. It is sometimes called somnambulism, and individuals can engage in a variety of complex behaviors while unconscious. Usually, sleepwalking occurs during slow-wave sleep, and characteristically begins toward the end of the first or second slow-wave sleep episodes. Sleep deprivation and interruption of slow-wave sleep appear to exacerbate, or even provoke, sleepwalking in susceptible individuals. Sleepwalking episodes may range from sitting up and attempting to walk to conducting an involved sequence of semipurposeful actions. The sleepwalker can often successfully interact with the environment (e.g., avoiding tripping over objects). However, the sleepwalker may interact with the environment inappropriately, which sometimes results in injury (e.g., stepping out of an upstairs window or walking into the roadway). There are cases in which sleepwalkers have committed acts of violence. An individual who is sleepwalking is difficult to awaken. Once awake, the sleepwalker will usually appear confused. It is best to gently attempt to lead sleepwalkers back to bed rather than to attempt to awaken them by grabbing, shaking, or shouting. In their confused state, sleepwalkers may think they are being attacked and may react violently to defend themselves. Sleepwalking in adults is rare, has a familial pattern, and may occur as a primary parasomnia or secondary to another sleep disorder (e.g., sleep apnea). By contrast, sleepwalking is very common in children and has a peak prevalence between the ages of 4 and 8 years. After adolescence, it usually disappears spontaneously. Nightly to weekly sleepwalking episodes associated with physical injury to the patient and others are considered severe. There are "specialized" forms of sleepwalking, most notably sleep-related eating behavior.

Table 15-12
NREM Sleep Disorders

	DSM-5	ICSD-3	ICD-10
Name	NREM sleep arousal disorders	NREM-related parasomnias	Nonorganic disorders of the sleep–wake schedule Sleepwalking (somnambulism) Sleep terrors (night terrors) Nightmares
Symptoms	Recurrent episodes of incomplete awakening from sleep, accompanied by either • Sleepwalking • Sleep terrors Little dream recall, if any Amnesia for episodes	Recurrent episodes of incomplete awakening associated with abnormal behaviors or experiences (confused arousal, sleepwalking, sleep terrors, sleep-related eating disorders) Absent or inappropriate responsiveness during episodes Limited or no cognition of dream report Partial or complete amnesia for the event	Sleepwalking: altered state of consciousness in which sleep and wakefulness are combined; episodes associated with low levels of awareness, with no recall of event on awakening Sleep terrors: nighttime episodes of terror and panic associated with motor movement and vocalization, in addition to high levels of autonomic tone; associated with little to no recall of the event Nightmares: dreams associated with fear and negative emotion, with presence of intact recall of dream content on awakening. Not associated with vocalization and body movement
# Symptoms needed	All the above criteria met		
Exclusion (not the result of):	Effects of substance or medication Other mental or medical disorders		
Psychosocial impact	Marked impairment and/or distress		
Symptom specifiers	Sleep terror type Sleepwalking type • With sleep-related eating • With sleep-related sexual behavior		DSM includes nightmare disorder as a separate category

DESCRIPTION

Ms. R is a 20-year-old white woman who was referred with symptoms of talking, mumbling, and crying out during sleep. At least twice per week she screams in her sleep. She is bothered with excessive sleepiness and falling asleep inappropriately, such as during a conversation. When inactive, she is tired and sleepy, even after a full 8-hour night of sleep. However, she has energy when motivated and leads a vigorous life. Once, she awakened outside of her apartment and her roommate had to let her back in because she had locked herself out. She does not recall the sleepwalking episode or other nocturnal wanderings but sometimes remembers yelling. From the history, crying seems to occur in light sleep but she rarely recalls any sleep-related thoughts or dreams. However, there is a history of occasional nightmares and bruxism. The patient uses an oral appliance to protect her teeth. Leg-kicking and mild snoring without gasping or choking are noted. The patient also complains of leg-kicking during sleep. Her sleep–wake schedule is irregular, and she averages between 5 and 7 hours of sleep per night. She occasionally awakens with a headache in the morning.

Previous health history includes a hospitalization for febrile convulsions during infancy, ophthalmologic surgery for strabismus during childhood, and tonsillectomy as a teenager. Health is otherwise excellent. The patient does not smoke tobacco or drink alcohol.

DISCUSSION

By history Ms. R has one or more of the parasomnias. Sleep talking alone does not require a sleep study, but this patient has nocturnal

wanderings. Polysomnography with clinical EEG is indicated to rule out unrecognized nocturnal seizure disorder or other organic factors inducing sleepwalking. Sleepwalking is common and not necessarily considered abnormal in young children; however, in the adult it is rare and merits careful evaluation. Ms. R's excessive daytime sleepiness is likely due to insufficient sleep (5 to 7 hours per night) and possibly parasomnia-related disruption. Interestingly, many parasomnias are exacerbated by sleep deprivation, as is nocturnal seizure disorder.

Sleep studies were performed using comprehensive, attended, laboratory polysomnography. Prior to the overnight study, a clinical EEG was performed. The clinical EEG study did not reveal any significant abnormal EEG activity during baseline, photic stimulation, or hyperventilation. An extended EEG montage was used during the sleep study. Overall sleep quality was within the normal range. Sleep efficiency was 96 percent and latency to sleep was 1 minute. REM sleep percentage was elevated (31 percent) and latency to REM sleep was less than normal (57 minutes). Slow-wave sleep was normal in percentage, but EEG delta activity was very high amplitude. The overall macroarchitectural sleep pattern suggested rebound from sleep deprivation.

By contrast, sleep microarchitecture contained many abnormal features. The clinicians observed high amplitude paroxysmal EEG bursts. Excessively prolonged sleep spindles were noted, and rhythmic K complexes were observed. There was one arousal out of slow-wave sleep with rhythmic EEG discharges alternating with sharp waves. Sharps and spikes occurred several times; however, the focus was difficult to localize (possibly right temporal lobe). There were frequent body movements and full body jerks, most of which occurred during NREM sleep. There were episodes of moaning during slow-wave sleep and laughing during stage 2 sleep that was followed by high amplitude theta bursts and REM sleep. The clinicians observed frequent movements and arousals from REM sleep, but no REM-related spikes or sharp waves. Seizure-like EEG activity was noted during the night and occurred predominantly during slow-wave sleep. However, the patient did not attempt to sleepwalk. Sharp wave and spike activity increased during the final 45 minutes of the sleep study.

The patient did not have any sleep-related breathing impairment and SaO_2 nadir was 90 percent. She had no periodic limb movements during sleep, and polygraphic features associated with RLS were absent.

SLEEP TERRORS. Sleep terrors involve sudden arousal with intense fearfulness. They usually begin with a piercing scream or cry and are accompanied by behavioral manifestations of intense anxiety bordering on panic. Autonomic and behavioral correlates of fear are typically present. Typically, an individual experiencing a sleep terror sits up in bed, is unresponsive to stimuli, and, if awakened, is confused or disoriented. Vocalizations may occur, but they usually are incoherent.

Notwithstanding the intensity of these events, amnesia for the episodes usually occurs. Like sleepwalking, these episodes usually arise from slow-wave sleep. Fever and CNS depressant withdrawal potentiate sleep terror episodes. Unlike nightmares, in which an elaborate dream sequence unfolds, sleep terrors may be devoid of images or contain only fragments of very brief but frighteningly vivid and sometimes static images. It is sometimes called *pavor nocturnus,* incubus, or night terror. As with other slow-wave sleep parasomnias, sleep deprivation can provoke or exacerbate sleep terrors. Psychopathology is seldom associated with sleep terrors in children; however, a history of a traumatic experience or frank psychiatric problems is often comorbid in adults with this disorder.

Severity ranges from less than once per month to almost nightly occurrence (with injury to the patient or others).

CONFUSIONAL AROUSALS. ICSD-3 defines confusional arousals as a milder form of NREM sleep parasomnias. It is common in young children. The child will typically partially awaken from sleep and sit up. The child is confused, but lies back down and resumes sleep. Confusional arousals, sleepwalking, and sleep terrors likely lie on a continuum.

SLEEP-RELATED EATING DISORDER. This diagnosis is subsumed under the DSM-5 classification NREM sleep arousal disorders and specified as "sleepwalking with sleep-related eating." In this disorder, eating may become obsessional, and the patient may eat several small meals during a night. The individual may be unaware of the activity, and weight gain can become a problem. During the recurrent sleep-related eating episodes, the individual may consume unusual foods or food combinations or may injure themselves or create a hazard while preparing food (e.g., starting a fire on the stove). They may also experience health consequences from these episodes.

REM-Related Parasomnias.

Table 15-13 compares the diagnostic approaches to the REM-related parasomnias.

NIGHTMARE DISORDER. Nightmares are frightening or terrifying dreams. Sometimes called *dream anxiety attacks,* they produce sympathetic activation and ultimately awaken the dreamer. Nightmares occur in REM sleep and usually evolve from a long, complicated dream that becomes increasingly frightening. Having aroused to wakefulness, the person typically remembers the dream (in contrast to sleep terrors). Some nightmares are recurrent, and reportedly when they occur in association with posttraumatic stress disorder, they may be recollections of actual events. Common in children ages 3 to 6 years, nightmares are rare in adults. Frequent and distressing nightmares are sometimes responsible for insomnia because the individual is afraid to sleep. Most people with nightmares are free from psychiatric conditions. Traumatic events are known to induce nightmares,

Table 15-13
REM Sleep Disorders

	DSM-5	ICSD-3	ICD-10
Name	REM sleep behavior disorder	REM-related parasomnias	REM sleep behavior disorder

Symptoms	Repeated arousal during sleep
	Vocalization or complex motor behavior
	Occurs during REM sleep
	Not confused when awakened
	Either:
	    REM sleep without atonia on polysomnography
	    OR history consistent with REM sleep behaviors with established diagnosis of a synucleinopathy (i.e., Parkinson disease)
		Sleep-related vocalizations or complex motor behaviors
		Occurs during REM sleep as documented by polysomnography (or presumed based on history)
		REM sleep without atonia on polysomnography
			Recurrent episodes of sudden, often violent behaviors during REM sleep
			May cause harm to self or others.
			Difficulty awakening
			Associated with dream enactment

# Symptoms needed	All the above	All the above	
Exclusion (not the result of):	Medication Substance use disorder Another medical condition A mental disorder	Another sleep disorder Medical or neurologic disorder Mental disorder Medication Substance use disorder Absence of epileptiform activity during REM sleep	
Psychosocial impact	Marked distress and/or impairment in functioning		

Table 15-14
Nightmare Disorder

	DSM-5	ICSD-3	ICD-10
Name	Nightmare disorder	Nightmare disorder (classified under REM-related parasomnia; see Table 15-13)	Nonorganic disorders of the sleep–wake schedule Sleep terrors Nightmares
Symptoms	Pattern of long, dysphoric, threatening, vivid dreams Dreams are recalled On awakening, quickly becomes awake and alert	Recurrent, highly dysphoric or anxiety-laden nightmares Dreams are remembered upon awakening	Sleep terrors: Nighttime episodes of terror and panic associated with motor movement and vocalization High levels of autonomic tone Little to no recall of the event Nightmares: Dreams associated with fear and negative emotion Intact recall of dream content
# Symptoms needed	All of the above		
Exclusion (not the result of):	Effects of a substance or medication Coexisting mental or medical disorder		Not associated with vocalization and body movement
Psychosocial impact	Marked distress and/or impairment in areas of functioning	Marked distress and/or impairment in areas of functioning	
Symptom specifiers	• **During sleep onset** • **With associated nonsleep disorder** (including substance use disorder) • **With associated other medical condition** • **With associated other sleep disorder**		
Severity specifiers	**Mild** (less than one episode per week) **Moderate** (one or more episodes per week, but less than nightly) **Severe** (nightly episodes)		
Course specifiers	**Acute** (duration ≤1 mo) **Subacute** (1–6 mo) **Persistent** (≥6 mo)		

sometimes immediately, but at other times delayed. The nightmares can persist for many years. Several medications can provoke nightmares, including L-DOPA and β-adrenergic blockers. Withdrawal from REM suppressant medications may induce nightmares, as well. Finally, drug or alcohol abuse is associated with nightmares.

Frequently occurring nightmares often produce a "fear of sleeping" type of insomnia. In turn, insomnia may provoke sleep deprivation, which is known to exacerbate nightmares; hence, a vicious cycle.

ICSD includes it among the REM-related sleep disorders whereas DSM-5 classifies this as a separate disorder. ICD considers this a "nonorganic disorder" of the sleep–wake schedule, along with sleep terrors. Table 15-14 compares the diagnostic approaches.

REM SLEEP BEHAVIOR DISORDER. RBD involves a failure of the patient to have atonia (sleep paralysis) during the REM stage sleep. The result is that the patient enacts his or her dreams. Under normal circumstances, the REM-related hypopolarization of α and γ motor neurons immobilizes the dreamer. Without this paralysis or with intermittent atonia, a dreamer could punch, kick, leap, while dreaming. The activity correlates with dream imagery.

Unlike sleepwalking, the individual seems unaware of the actual environment but instead is acting on the dream sensorium. Thus, a sleepwalker may calmly go to a bedroom window, open it, and step out. By contrast, a person with RBD would more likely dive through the window, thinking it is a dream-visualized lake. Patients and bed partners frequently sustain an injury, which is sometimes

severe (e.g., lacerations, fractures). A wide variety of drugs and comorbid conditions can precipitate or worsen RBD.

RECURRENT ISOLATED SLEEP PARALYSIS. Sleep paralysis is, as the name implies, an inability to make voluntary movements during sleep. It becomes a parasomnia when it occurs at sleep onset or on awakening, a time when the individual is partially conscious and aware of the surroundings. This inability to move can be extremely distressing, especially when coupled with the feeling that there is an intruder in the house or when hypnagogic hallucinations are occurring. Sleep paralysis is part of the tetrad of symptoms associated with narcolepsy; however, it can occur (with or without hypnagogia) in individuals that have neither cataplexy nor excessive daytime sleepiness. Although it is sometimes frightening, sleep paralysis is a feature of normal REM sleep, briefly intruding into wakefulness. The paralysis may last from one to several minutes.

Interestingly, the occurrence of sleep paralysis with hypnagogia may account for a variety of experiences in which the sleeper is confronted or attacked by some sort of "creature." The standard description is that the paralyzed sleeper feels a "presence" nearby, and the creature talks, attacks, or sits on the sleeper's chest and then vanishes. Whether it is called an incubus, "Old Hag," a vampire, ghost oppression (*kanashibari* in Japanese), witch riding, or an alien encounter, all these experiences have elements that are similar to descriptions of sleep paralysis. Irregular sleep, sleep deprivation, psychological stress, and shift work increase the likelihood of sleep paralysis.

Other Parasomnias

EXPLODING HEAD SYNDROME. Individuals with the parasomnia "hear" a loud imagined noise or a sense of an explosion. They experience it as inside their head as they are falling asleep or awakening. The experience can occur just once or recurrently. There is no pain associated with the noise, but the individual may be concerned that they are having a stroke or that something is very wrong. Even a single episode can trigger severe insomnia. There are no known neurologic consequences to this syndrome.

SLEEP-RELATED HALLUCINATIONS. This parasomnia typically involves visual images occurring at sleep onset (hypnagogic) or on awakening (hypnopompic) from sleep. Sometimes challenging to differentiate from dreams, they are common in patients with narcolepsy. Complex hallucinations are rare and usually happen with abrupt awakening and without remembering dreaming. Images tend to be vivid and immobile and persist for several minutes. They usually appear when turning on a light. The images can be frightening.

SLEEP ENURESIS. Sleep enuresis is a disorder in which the individual urinates during sleep while in bed. It is commonly called *bed-wetting* and has primary and secondary forms. In children, primary sleep enuresis is the continuance of bed-wetting since infancy. Secondary enuresis refers to relapse after toilet training was complete, and there was a period during which the child remained dry. Usually, after toilet training, bed-wetting spontaneously resolves before age 6 years.

Parental primary enuresis increases the likelihood that the children will also have enuresis. A single recessive gene is suspected. Secondary enuresis in children may occur with the birth of a sibling and represent a "cry for attention." Secondary enuresis can also be associated with nocturnal seizures, sleep deprivation, and urologic anomalies. In adults with sleep-disordered breathing, sleep enuresis may occur. In most cases, embarrassment, shame, and guilt are the most substantial consequences. Nonetheless, if we do not address sleep enuresis, it may leave psychosocial scars.

PARASOMNIA DUE TO DRUG OR SUBSTANCE USE AND PARASOMNIA DUE TO MEDICAL CONDITIONS. Many drugs and substances can trigger parasomnias, particularly those agents that lighten sleep; however, alcohol is notorious for producing sleepwalking (even in individuals who have taken sleeping pills). Table 15-15 lists some medications and drugs that can worsen parasomnias.

Seizure disorder should always be on the top of a differential diagnosis list for most parasomnias. The American Academy of Sleep Medicine practice guidelines concerning the indications for polysomnography includes using sleep testing to rule out seizures when diagnosing sleep terror, sleepwalking, RBD, nightmares, and other parasomnias. Sleep-related breathing disorders are also known to trigger sleepwalking, enuresis, sleep terror, confusional arousal, and nightmares. RBD is associated with a variety of neurologic conditions, including Parkinson disease, dementia, progressive supranuclear palsy, Shy–Drager syndrome (a movement disorder with autonomic arousal symptoms), narcolepsy, and others.

Restless Legs Syndrome.

RLS is an uncomfortable, subjective sensation of the limbs, usually the legs, sometimes described as a "creepy-crawly" feeling, and the irresistible urge to move the legs when at rest or while trying to fall asleep. Patients often report the sensation of ants walking on the skin and crawling feelings in their legs. It tends to be worse at night, and moving the legs or walking helps to alleviate the discomfort. Thus, as the individual is lying in bed and relaxing, he or she is disturbed by these sensations. Then he or she moves the legs and again tries to fall asleep. This cycle

Table 15-15
Medications and Drugs Causing or Worsening Certain Parasomnias

REM Sleep Behavior Disorder
Biperiden
Caffeine
Monoamine oxidase inhibitors (MAOIs)
Selegiline
Serotonin agonists
Tricyclic antidepressants
Venlafaxine
Withdrawal syndromes
  Alcohol
  Meprobamate
  Pentazocine
  Nitrazepam
Nightmares
Alcohol abuse or withdrawal
Drug-induced REM sleep rebound (e.g., withdrawal from
  REM-suppressing drugs such as methamphetamine)
L-DOPA
β-Blockers

sometimes continues for hours and results in profound insomnia. Table 15-16 compares the diagnostic approaches to RLS.

A variety of medical conditions can cause secondary RLS, and we list these in Table 15-17. A detailed history and physical examination are essential parts of the RLS workup. Also, we should check a ferritin level in every patient with symptoms consistent with RLS.

Periodic Limb Movement Disorder.

Periodic limb movement disorder (PLMD), previously called *nocturnal myoclonus*, involves brief, stereotypic, repetitive, nonepileptiform movements of the limbs, usually the legs. It occurs primarily in NREM sleep and involves an extension of the big toe. A partial flexion of the ankle, knee, and hip may also occur. These movements range from 0.5 to 5 seconds in duration and occur every 20 to 40 seconds. The leg movements are frequently associated with brief arousals from sleep and, as a result, can (but do not always) disturb sleep architecture. The prevalence of PLMD increases with aging and can occur in association with folate deficiency, renal disease, anemia, and the use of antidepressants.

Sleep-Related Leg Cramps.

Nocturnal leg cramps are much like leg cramps that occur during wakefulness. They usually affect the calf and are painful muscle contractions. The pain awakens the sleeper and thereby disrupts sleep. Metabolic disorders, mineral deficiencies, electrolytic imbalances, diabetes, and pregnancy are known precipitators. The reason that some individuals have repeated leg cramps during sleep and not during the day is not known.

Sleep-Related Bruxism.

Sleep-related bruxism occurs when an individual grinds or clenches the teeth during sleep. Formerly classified as a parasomnia, sleep bruxism can produce abnormal wear and damage to teeth, provoke tooth and jaw pain, or make loud, unpleasant sounds that disturb the bed partner. Sometimes atypical facial pain and headache also result. More than 85 percent of the population may brux at one time or another; however, it is clinically significant in only about 5 percent. Teeth grinding occurs in any sleep stage but is most common at the transition to sleep, in stage 2 sleep, and during REM sleep. Some evidence indicates that teeth grinding during REM sleep is more commonly associated with dental wear or damage. Sleep bruxism does not appear to be exacerbated by dental malocclusion. It worsens during periods of

Table 15-16
Restless Legs Syndrome

	DSM-5	ICSD-3	ICD-10
Name	Restless legs syndrome	Restless legs syndrome	Other specified extrapyramidal and movement disorders **Restless legs syndrome**
Duration	≥3×/wk for ≥3 mo		
Symptoms	Urge to move legs Worse at night Urge relieved by movement	Urge to move legs Uncomfortable sensations occurring during rest/inactivity At least partially relieved by movement Tend to have circadian pattern (occurring primarily at night)	Experiencing a strong urge to move legs to relieve discomfort often occurs while lying down or sitting and tends to be worse at night
# Symptoms needed	All the above	All the above	
Exclusion (not the result of):	Akathisia Effects of a substance or medication Another mental disorder or medical condition Behavioral condition (i.e., habitual movements)		
Psychosocial impact	Marked distress and/or impairment in areas of functioning present	Marked distress and/or impairment in areas of functioning present	

stress. Researchers studying sleep bruxism have found that many patients seem to have less frequent teeth grinding when sleeping in the laboratory; therefore, we may need repeat studies to document the disorder. By contrast, bruxism frequently appears on polysomnographic recordings made for other purposes. Sleep bruxism may occur secondary to sleep-related breathing disorders, the use of psychostimulants (e.g., amphetamine, cocaine), alcohol ingestion, and treatment with some SSRIs. Sleep bruxism can infrequently occur (monthly), regularly (weekly), or frequently (nightly). We judge the severity by considering the degree of sleep disruption, consequent pain, and dental damage.

Sleep-Related Rhythmic Movement Disorder. This sleep disorder consists of repetitive, rhythmic movements, usually involving the head and neck. Most often occurring at the transition from wakefulness to sleep, this movement disorder may also continue during light sleep. Formerly classified as a parasomnia, sleep-related rhythmic movement disorder has many names, including *jactatio capitis nocturna,* headbanging, head rolling, body rocking, and *rhythmie du sommeil.* Most infants body rock. Some clinicians believe that body rocking develops from the soothing effect of vestibular stimulation. If the rhythmic movement persists into childhood, the risk of injury increases. This is particularly true if the movement includes headbanging. The male to female ratio is 4:1. Severity

ranges from less than one episode weekly to nightly episodes producing injury.

Benign Sleep Myoclonus of Infancy. Previously called benign neonatal sleep myoclonus, this disorder is characterized by asynchronous jerking of limbs and trunk during quiet sleep in neonates. This benign, apparently rare, parasomnia usually begins within the first week of life and may last a few days or several months. It does not require any treatment and should resolve with time.

Propriospinal Myoclonus at Sleep Onset. Propriospinal myoclonus at sleep onset is a spinal cord–mediated movement disorder, sometimes associated with spinal cord lesions. Movements appear during times of wakeful relaxation and may interfere with sleep onset. They start in the abdominal and truncal muscles and then progress to the neck and proximal muscles of the limbs.

Sleep-Related Movement Disorder due to Medication or Substance Use and Sleep-Related Movement Disorder due to Medical Condition. A variety of medications, substances, and comorbid conditions can produce or exacerbate sleep-related movement disorders. Table 15-18 lists some example medications. Neurologic diseases that are associated with daytime movement disorders can also be associated with sleep-related

Table 15-17
Medical Disorders That Can Cause Secondary Restless Legs Syndrome

COPD
Diabetes
Fibromyalgia
Iron and folic acid deficiency anemias
Neuropathies
Rheumatoid arthritis
Thyroid diseases
Uremia

Table 15-18
Medications Causing Sleep-Related Movement Disorders

Antidepressants (including most tricyclics and SSRIs)
Antiemetics
Antihistamines
Antipsychotics (restless legs symptoms, periodic limb movement disorder)
Calcium channel blockers
Lithium
Stimulants (rhythmic movement disorders, bruxism)

movement disorders. Stress, anxiety, and sleep deprivation may contribute to bruxism.

Isolated Symptoms and Normal Variants

Sleep Talking. As the name implies, sleep talking in classic form involves unconscious speech during sleep. Unless it annoys the bed partner, it is seldom recognized. Fever, stress, or talking with the sleeper can all induce the behavior. Somniloquy may accompany sleep terror, sleepwalking, confusional arousals, OSAs, and RBD.

Sleep Starts (Hypnic Jerks). Sleep starts are sudden, brief muscle contractions that occur at the transition between wakefulness and sleep in 60 to 70 percent of adults. The contractions commonly involve the legs; however, sometimes there is movement in the arms and head. Sometimes called a "hypnic jerk," it is usually benign. The sleep start, however, can interfere with the ability to fall asleep and may be accompanied by sensations of falling, a hallucinated flash of light, or a loud crackling sound. In severe cases, the sleep start produces profound sleep-onset insomnia.

CLINICAL TOOLS IN SLEEP MEDICINE

Clinical Interview

A careful and thorough clinical interview is one of the most informative parts of a workup for sleep disorders. The habitual bedtime and arising times for both weekdays and weekends, the frequency, duration, and restorative nature of naps, and overall level of sleepiness are good places to begin. Specific sleep problems relating to difficulty initiating and maintaining sleep are informative, including whether there is rumination at bedtime, fear of not being able to sleep, or excessive worry when attempting to sleep. We should assess for movements, including leg movement, leg sensations, leg cramps, teeth grinding, and dream enactments (with or without injury). We should also review for morning headaches, morning dry mouth, nocturnal reflux, hyperhidrosis (excess sweating), nocturia, enuresis, nocturnal tongue biting, nightmares, sleep terrors, and other sleep-related problems. In some cases, it can be crucial to ask about the presence of family pets and whether they sleep in the bedroom (or bed). A sleep history questionnaire is often helpful in diagnosing a patient's sleep disorder (Table 15-19).

Clinical Tests

Polysomnography. Polysomnography is the continuous, attended, comprehensive recording of the physiologic changes that occur during sleep. A polysomnogram is typically recorded at night and lasts between 6 and 8 hours. Brain wave activity, eye movements, submentalis electromyography activity, nasal–oral airflow, nasal pressure, respiratory effort, oxyhemoglobin saturation, heart rhythm, and leg movements during sleep are measured. Usually, the laboratory records body position and snoring sounds. Brain wave activity, eye movements, and submentalis electromyogram are essential for identifying sleep stages and CNS arousals. Muscle tension and movements subside with deeper sleep and can also be useful in the diagnosis of PLMD and RLS. Nasal airflow, respiratory effort, and oxyhemoglobin saturation are instrumental in diagnosing sleep apnea and other sleep-related breathing disorders.

Table 15-20 lists the most common reasons for ordering polysomnography. A sleep study is not needed to diagnose RLS.

Table 15-21 lists standard polysomnographic measures.

Home Sleep Testing. Home sleep testing involves recording a limited number of cardiopulmonary parameters to assess patients for sleep-related breathing disorders. Home sleep testing is much less expensive than polysomnography. The test can record airflow, respiratory effort, heart rhythm, snoring sounds, and oximetry. Several devices are commercially available that are capable of detecting sleep apnea in patients with moderate to severe pathophysiology. Negative studies are problematic because home sleep testing is less sensitive than full laboratory polysomnography. Patients with negative tests, notwithstanding obvious symptoms or comorbidity, should be scheduled for laboratory polysomnography. Also, home sleep testing does not check for the full spectrum of sleep disorders; therefore, the presence of residual symptoms after a breathing disorder is diagnosed in this manner and treated indicates a need for careful follow-up.

Multiple Sleep Latency Test. The multiple sleep latency test (MSLT) is essential for the workup of narcolepsy. Every 2 hours, beginning 2 hours after morning awakening, the patient is provided with 20-minute nap opportunities and instructed not to resist falling asleep. During sleep, the laboratory records electroencephalographic, electrooculographic, and submentalis electromyography activity to determine the sleep stage. The latency to sleep helps assess hypersomnolence, and the appearance of REM sleep on two or more nap opportunities confirms narcolepsy (or on one nap if the previous night's polysomnography revealed REM sleep within 15 minutes of sleep onset). If the patient falls asleep on a given nap opportunity, the laboratory will wake the patient 15 minutes after initial sleep onset. If the patient does not fall asleep after 20 minutes, the laboratory will terminate the session. The laboratory gives the patient five nap opportunities during 2-hour intervals across the day.

Maintenance of Wakefulness Test. Similar to the MSLT, the maintenance of wakefulness test (MWT) provides 40-minute test sessions at 2-hour intervals across the day. However, in this test, the laboratory instructs the patient to try to remain awake. This technique is used to assess treatment outcomes and is sometimes part of "fit for duty" testing. Patients are recorded in a darkened room while sitting in a comfortable chair or a bed with a bolster pillow. The first epoch of stage 2, 3, or 4 sleep or REM or three consecutive epochs of stage 1 mark unequivocal sleep onset. Falling asleep on MWT indicates some level of sleepiness. Any sleep latency of fewer than 8 minutes is abnormal. Sleep latency ranging from 8 to 40 minutes is of unknown significance.

Actigraphy. An actigraph is a device that measures and records movement. It is usually worn on the wrist (like a watch) and is a rough measure of the sleep–wake cycle. Depending on the model and the settings, it can make continuous recordings for days or weeks. It can be especially useful for assessing insomnia, circadian rhythm disorders, movement disorders, and an assortment of rare events.

Common Test Findings in Sleep–Wake Disorders

Hypersomnolence Disorder. The EEG sleep pattern is essentially the same as that found in healthy individuals who are sleep deprived (Fig. 15-2). Unlike a sleep-deprived individual, the sleep pattern continues in this profile even after several nights of extended sleep. Also, we may see elevated slow-wave sleep.

Narcolepsy. When the diagnosis is not clinically apparent, a nighttime polysomnographic recording reveals a characteristic

Table 15-19
Example Sleep History Questionnaire

Patient name _____

Date _____

Please check the appropriate box or give short answers for the following:

	Yes	No
1. Do you feel sleepy or have sleep attacks during the day?	☐	☐
2. Do you nap during the day?	☐	☐
3. Do you have trouble concentrating during the day?	☐	☐
4. Do you have trouble falling asleep when you first go to bed?	☐	☐
5. Do you awaken during the night?	☐	☐
6. Do you awaken more than once?	☐	☐
7. Do you awaken too early in the morning?	☐	☐
8. How long have you had trouble sleeping?	☐	☐

What do you think precipitated the problem?

_____

_____

_____

9. How would you describe your usual night's sleep (hours of sleep, quality of sleep, etc.)?

_____

_____

_____

	Yes	No
10. Does your schedule for sleep and rising on the weekend differ from what it is during the week?	☐	☐
11. Do others live at home who interrupt your sleep?	☐	☐
12. Are you regularly awakened at night by pain or the need to use the bathroom?	☐	☐
13. Does your job require shift changes or travel?	☐	☐
14. Do you drink caffeinated beverages (coffee, tea, or soft drinks)?	☐	☐

15. Apart from difficulty in sleeping, what, if any, other medical problems do you have?

_____

_____

_____

16. What sleep medications, prescription or nonprescription, do you take? (Please include the dosage, how often you take it, and for how many months or years you have taken it.)

_____

_____

_____

17. What other prescription and over-the-counter medications do you regularly use? (Again, please include the dosage, the frequency, and the duration.)

_____

_____

_____

	Yes	No
18. Have you ever suffered from depression, anxiety, or similar problems?	☐	☐
19. Do you snore?	☐	☐

Questions for the Sleep Partner

	Yes	No
1. Does your sleep partner snore?	☐	☐
2. Does your sleep partner seem to stop breathing repeatedly during the night?	☐	☐
3. Does your sleep partner jerk his or her legs or kick you while he or she is sleeping?	☐	☐
4. Have you ever experienced trouble sleeping? Please explain.	☐	☐

_____

_____

_____

Table 15-20
Indications for Polysomnography

Common Reasons
Diagnosis of sleep-related breathing disorders
Positive airway pressure (PAP) titration and assessment of treatment efficacy
Evaluation of sleep-related behaviors that are violent or may potentially harm the patient or bed partner
Differentiating narcolepsy from other hypersomnolence disorders
Differentiating parasomnias from nocturnal seizures

Other Possible Uses
Diagnose atypical parasomnias
Sleep-related problems secondary to neuromuscular disorders
Periodic limb movement disorder
Arousals secondary to seizure disorder
Excessive daytime sleepiness
Waking up gasping or choking
Narcolepsy (to assess sleep quality and quantity prior to a multiple sleep latency test)

Table 15-21
Common Polysomnographic Measures

Sleep latency: Period of time from turning out the lights until the appearance of stage 2 sleep
Early morning awakening: Time of being continuously awake from the last stage of the sleep until the end of the sleep record (usually at 7 AM)
Sleep efficiency: Total sleep time or total time of the sleep record × 100
Apnea index: Number of apneas longer than 10 s/h of sleep
Nocturnal myoclonus index: Number of periodic leg movements per hour
Rapid eye movement (REM) latency: Period of time from the onset of sleep until the first REM period of the night
Sleep-onset REM period: REM sleep within the first 10 min of sleep

sleep-onset REM period (Fig. 15-3). A test of daytime MSLT shows rapid sleep onset and usually one or more sleep-onset REM periods.

Obstructive Sleep Apnea. On the polysomnogram, episodes of OSA appear as multiple periods of at least 10 seconds' duration

in which nasal and oral airflow ceases either wholly or partially. Meanwhile, the abdominal and chest expansion leads indicate the continuing efforts of the diaphragm and accessory muscles of respiration to move air through the obstruction (Fig. 15-4). The arterial oxygen saturation drops, and often we see bradycardia, along with possible arrhythmias, such as premature ventricular contractions. In the end, an arousal reflex takes place, seen as a waking signal, and possibly as a motor artifact on the EEG channels. At this

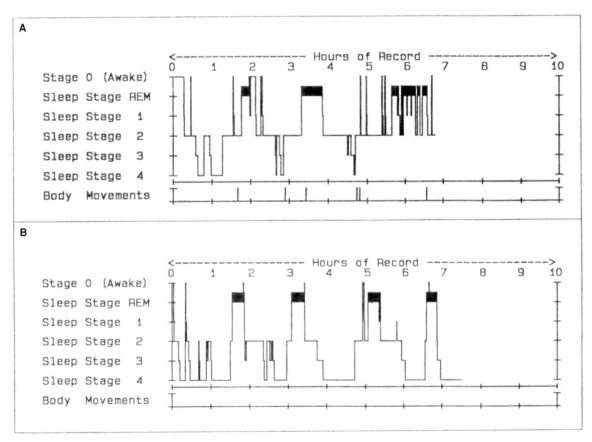

FIGURE 15-2
Sleep stage histograms comparing a normal sleep profile with that of a patient with hypersomnolence. **Panel A** illustrates the sleep pattern recorded in a healthy young adult. His sleep was interrupted several times by awakenings associated with other concurrent laboratory procedures; however, all parameters were within normal limits. **Panel B** depicts the sleep pattern of a patient with severe daytime sleepiness. The patient did not have narcolepsy or apnea. In the laboratory, sleep onset was rapid, sleep continued virtually without interruption, and he was extremely difficult to arouse. This recording was terminated after 7.5 hours to begin daytime testing; however, the patient's sleep revealed little indication of progressing toward a lighter state. In contrast to the normal sleep pattern, slow-wave sleep duration was elevated and it continued to emerge in alternation with REM sleep throughout the night. The patient awoke feeling unrefreshed and not satisfied with his sleep.

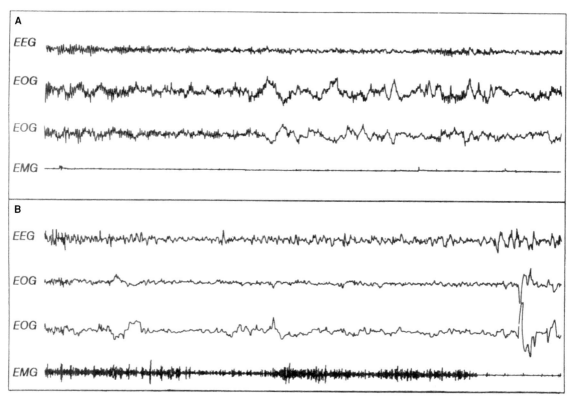

FIGURE 15-3

Polysomnographic tracing comparing normal sleep onset with that of a patient with narcolepsy. Each panel illustrates approximately 30 seconds of polysomnographic recording beginning with relaxed wakefulness. **Panel A** (normal sleep progression) shows a reduction of EEG α activity and development of slow rolling eye movements. **Panel B** shows the normally expected abatement of EEG α activity associated with increased θ activity and the appearance of a few slow eye movements. However, within 25 seconds (far right of figure) a swift loss of muscle tone occurs accompanied by rapid eye movements. This appearance of sleep-onset REM sleep (SOREM) characterizes narcolepsy and is part of the diagnostic criteria.

moment, sometimes called the *breakthrough,* the patient can make brief restless movements in bed.

Central Sleep Apnea.   The polysomnographic features of CSA are similar to those of OSA. However, during the periods of apnea, cessation of respiratory effort is seen in the abdominal and chest expansion leads. In Cheyne–Stokes breathing, polysomnography reveals five or more central apnea and hypopnea episodes per hour of sleep. In CSA, due to a medical disorder without Cheyne–Stokes breathing, diagnostic criteria require a polysomnographically verified rate of 5 or more central apneas and hypopneas per hour of sleep. Also, CSA due to medication or substance requires five or more central apneas per hour.

Sleep-Related Hypoventilation.   Polysomnography demonstrates either episodes with elevated CO_2 levels and decreased respirations or, if not monitoring CO_2, episodes of persistently low oxyhemoglobin levels that are not provoked by apnea or hypopnea.

Parasomnias.   Sleep studies help to develop a differential diagnosis and rule out that the unusual behavior is secondary to a seizure, sleep-related breathing disorder, or another sleep disorder. Figures 15-5 to 15-7 give examples of polysomnograms for sleep terrors, RLS, and sleep-related bruxism.

DIFFERENTIAL DIAGNOSIS

In general, the differential diagnosis of sleep–wake disorders should include other individual sleep–wake disorders, psychiatric disorders, medical conditions, medications and substance use, and normal variants.

Insomnia Disorder

Many psychiatric disorders can cause a person to experience insomnia. For example, MDD, bipolar disorder, and PTSD can all present with sleep disruption. Many medications and substances also affect sleep, some of which we listed in Table 15-7. Other sleep–wake disorders should also be considered, including circadian rhythm sleep–wake disorder, RLS, sleep-related breathing disorders, narcolepsy, and parasomnias. Finally, one should consider whether the sleep pattern is a normal variant in the population (e.g., a "short sleeper") or is occurring in the context of an acute stressor.

Hypersomnolence Disorder

Psychiatric disorders associated with increased sleep or fatigue, such as MDD or bipolar depression, should be considered part of the differential diagnosis. Certain medications or substances can also cause sedation, such as sedative–hypnotics and opioids. Other sleep–wake disorders should be considered, including circadian rhythm sleep–wake disorder, sleep-related breathing disorders, and parasomnias. Also, poor sleep quality can lead to excessive daytime sleepiness, and there are some persons for whom it is a normal variant to require more sleep (e.g., "long sleepers").

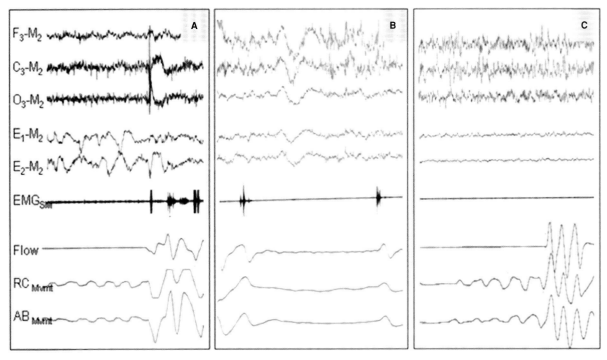

FIGURE 15-4

Polysomnographic tracings illustrating sleep apnea episodes. **Panel A** illustrates an obstructive sleep apnea, **Panel B** shows a central sleep apnea, and **Panel C** depicts a mixed sleep apnea. Note the presence of respiratory effort (rib cage and abdominal movement), notwithstanding cessation of airflow, throughout the obstructive apnea and during the latter portion of the mixed apnea. By contrast, respiratory effort is absent during the flow cessation throughout the central apnea and during the early portion of the mixed apnea. Notation: F_3 (left frontal scalp derivation); M_2 (right mastoid electrode location); C_3 (left central scalp derivation); O_3 (left occipital scalp derivation); E_1 (left outer canthus eye electrode location); E_2 (right outer canthus eye electrode location); EMG_{SM} (surface electrode electromyogram from submentalis muscle); Flow (airflow measured with nasal–nasal–oral thermistors); RC Mvmt (rib cage movement measured with inductive plethysmography); AB Mvmt (abdominal movement measured with inductive plethysmography). (From Hirshkowitz M, Sharafkhaneh A. Diagnostic assessment methods in adults. In: Kryger MH, Avidan AY, Berry RB, eds. *Atlas of Clinical Sleep Medicine*. 2nd ed. Elsevier Saunders: Philadelphia, PA; 2014:378.)

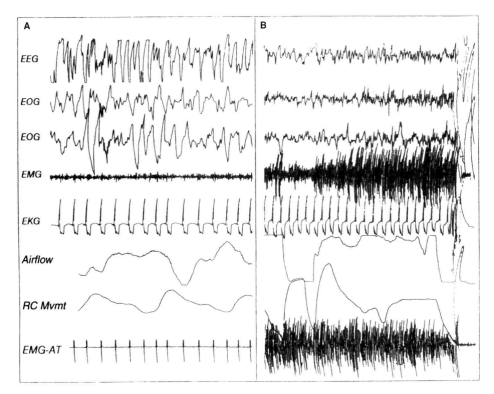

FIGURE 15-5

Polysomnographic tracing illustrating a sleep terror. **Panel A** shows approximately 14 seconds of tracing occurring immediately before the sleep terror. Prominent EEG slow-wave activity and other characteristics of stage 4 sleep are seen. **Panel B** shows the awakening, accompanied by tachycardia and movement. EEG activity is ambiguous and the patient eventually disconnected his electrodes as he thrashed about in bed (visible at far right of figure). Although the patient was screaming and greatly agitated, there was no report of dreaming. In the morning, there was little recollection of anything having occurred during the night.

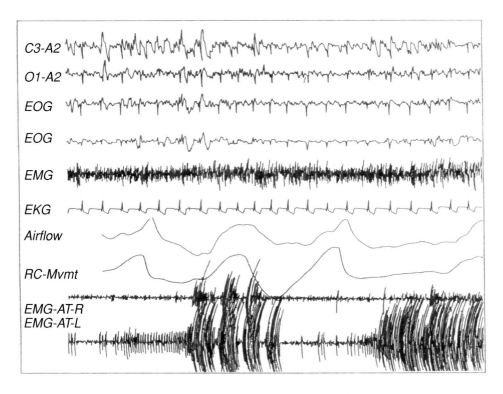

FIGURE 15-6
Restless legs syndrome. This patient presented with complaints of uncomfortable, crawling sensations in the legs when trying to fall asleep. Patients commonly report an urge to move the leg in order to dispel the sensation. This figure shows a bilateral pattern of leg EMG activity; however, the discharge is more pronounced in the left anterior tibialis (EMG-AT-L) than the right (EMG-AT-R). This pattern continued for more than an hour as the patient attempted to fall asleep; note that the sharp activity in central and occipital EEG (C3-A2 and O1-A2, respectively) and EOG is EKG artifact and not an EEG abnormality.

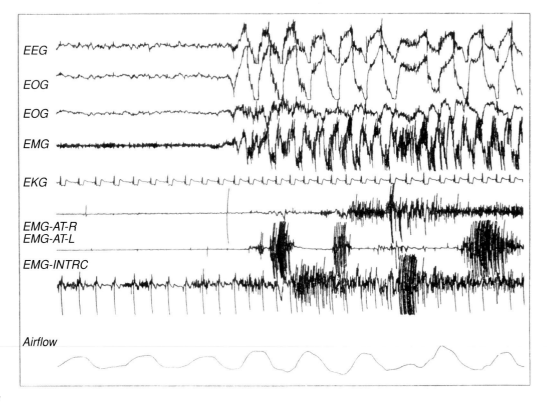

FIGURE 15-7
Polysomnographic tracing showing sleep-related bruxism. This figure showing approximately 25 seconds of tracing was obtained from a patient during an episode of bruxism. Bruxism can occur during any stage of sleep or wakefulness. The interference pattern of EEG-EOG-EMG channels is typical and reflects the rhythmic jaw movement and grinding of the teeth. This patient had many such episodes, some that caused awakening. Readily observable tooth damage and jaw pain were noted.

Table 15-22
Medical Disorders Causing Cataplexy

Disorders affecting the hypothalamus
  Tumors
  Sarcoidosis
  Multiple sclerosis plaques
Paraneoplastic syndrome
Neimann–Pick type C disease
Coffin–Lowry syndrome

Narcolepsy

The differential diagnosis of narcolepsy includes many of the same disorders as the differential diagnosis of hypersomnolence disorder. Also, cataplexy can be confused for seizures or neurologic movement disorders (e.g., chorea). Many disorders can precipitate cataplexy, and we list some of the more common in Table 15-22. All of these disorders would preclude a diagnosis of narcolepsy. Cataplexy is usually absent in narcolepsy associated with multiple sclerosis, myotonic dystrophy, Prader–Willi syndrome, Parkinson disease, and multisystem atrophy.

Sleep-Related Breathing Disorders

The differential diagnosis of sleep-related breathing disorders includes many of the same disorders as the differential diagnosis of insomnia and hypersomnolence disorders, given the clinical presentation of fatigue and daytime sleepiness. Other possible conditions include panic attacks and attention-deficit/hyperactivity disorder (as repeated apneic episodes may lead to problems with focus, attention, and school- or job-related performance).

Circadian Rhythm Sleep–Wake Disorders

The differential diagnosis of circadian rhythm sleep–wake disorders includes insomnia disorder, other sleep–wake disorders, and mood disorders. One should also consider the possibility that the sleep pattern represents a normal variant.

Parasomnias and Sleep-Related Movement Disorders

The differential diagnosis of parasomnias can be complicated and should include other individual parasomnias, sleep-related breathing disorders, nocturnal seizures, panic attacks, other sleep–wake disorders, amnestic and dissociative syndromes, and numerous medical conditions. The differential diagnosis of RLS includes multiple medical conditions, such as arthritis, neuropathy, positional ischemia, and peripheral artery disease, to name a few, while the differential diagnosis of sleep-related bruxism should include nocturnal seizures.

COMORBIDITY

Insomnia Disorder

Several psychiatric disorders are often comorbid with insomnia. We list some common ones in Table 15-23. Nearly 90 percent of patients with MDD have insomnia. Of the most significant concern, insomnia is an independent risk factor for suicide in patients with MDD. Insomnia also predicts who will develop

posttraumatic stress disorder following a trauma. For bipolar patients, lack of sleep may precipitate a manic episode. Patients with schizophrenia may deny having slept despite objective measures showing normal sleep.

Hypersomnolence Disorder

Many disorders also occur with hypersomnolence disorder, and we list some of these in Table 15-23. Medication use disorders are also common, particularly the stimulants, as the individual attempts to stay awake.

Narcolepsy

Narcolepsy is associated with psychiatric disorders in general, as well as many medical disorders. We list some of these in Table 15-23.

Sleep-Related Breathing Disorders

Table 15-23 lists several disorders associated with sleep-related breathing disorders. The section on diagnosis discusses conditions associated with central sleep apnea and sleep-related hypoventilation.

Circadian Rhythm Sleep–Wake Disorders

The circadian rhythm sleep–wake disorders can be associated with psychiatric and medical comorbidities; we list some of these in Table 15-23. The shift work type is especially associated with many psychiatric and medical disorders.

Parasomnias and Sleep-Related Movement Disorders

Each parasomnia has its own set of common comorbid diagnoses, and we list some examples in Table 15-23. Many individuals who present with RBD will go on to develop a neurodegenerative disorder.

TREATMENT APPROACH

Insomnia

Pharmacologic Treatment. For many years, benzodiazepines were the most commonly prescribed sedative–hypnotic medications for treating insomnia. Other benzodiazepine-receptor agonists (e.g., zolpidem and similar drugs) then emerged as an option to treat insomnia. The subsequent development of a low-dose antihistamine (doxepin), a melatonin receptor agonist (ramelteon), and an orexin antagonist (suvorexant) have more recently augmented the armamentarium of medications approved for treating insomnia. However, unapproved off-label (and not recommended) use of sedating antidepressants is commonplace. Additionally, a variety of over-the-counter (OTC) sleep aids is available. Nonprescription formulas include sedating antihistamines, protein precursors, and other substances. L-tryptophan was trendy and readily available at health food stores until an outbreak of eosinophilia led to pulling it off the shelves. However, the cause was a single manufacturer, and L-tryptophan subsequently became available OTC again. Melatonin is the leader among self-administered food additives believed by some to alleviate sleeplessness. Low-dose melatonin can improve sleep when

Table 15-23
Disorders That Are Commonly Comorbid with Various Sleep Disorders

Insomnia Disorder
Bipolar disorder
Generalized anxiety disorder
Major depressive disorder
Posttraumatic stress disorder
Schizophrenia
 	
Hypersomnolence Disorder
Bipolar disorder
Depressive disorders (particularly seasonal depression)
Neurodegenerative disorders
Substance use disorders (stimulants)
 	
Narcolepsy
Anxiety
Depressive disorders
Obstructive sleep apnea
Headache
Hyperlipidemia
Hypertension
Obesity
Peripheral neuropathy
Thyroid disease, other endocrinopathies
 	
Sleep-Related Breathing Disorders
Anxiety disorders
Dementia
Mood disorders
Post-traumatic stress disorder
Psychotic disorders
Cardiovascular disease
Diabetes mellitus
Heart failure
Hypertension
Obesity
	Circadian Rhythm Sleep-Wake Disorders
	Depression
	Neurodegenerative disorders
	Neurodevelopmental disorders
	Personality disorder
	Somatic symptom disorders
	Blindness
	Cardiovascular disease
	Diabetes mellitus
	Gastrointestinal disease
	Substance use disorders
	
	Parasomnias and Sleep-Related Movement Disorders
	Sleepwalking
	    Obsessive compulsive disorder
	    Major depression
	Nightmare disorder
	    Posttraumatic stress disorder
	    Acute stress disorder
	    Schizophrenia
	    Anxiety disorders
	    Personality disorders
	    Bereavement
	    Pain
	    Neurodegenerative disorders
	    Cardiovascular disease
	REM sleep behavior disorder
	    Narcolepsy
	    Neurodegenerative disorders
	Restless legs syndrome
	    Depression
	    Anxiety
	    Attentional disorders
	    Iron deficiency

used to align or reentrain the circadian rhythm with the desired sleep–wake schedule.

Drug manufacturers must rigorously test prescription medications in clinical trials; therefore, they hold an advantage over the virtually untested OTCs. Medication must be proven safe and effective to become FDA approved.

Most hypnotic medications are approved for short-, not long-term use. Exceptions include zolpidem-modified release, eszopiclone, and ramelteon, which the FDA approved for long-term therapy. When properly used, hypnotics can provide immediate and adequate relief from sleeplessness. Insomnia, however, usually returns upon discontinuation of dosing.

The clinical practice guideline from the American Academy of Sleep Medicine recommends the use of suvorexant, eszopiclone, zaleplon, zolpidem, triazolam, temazepam, ramelteon, and doxepin for the treatment of insomnia (with specific agents having different indications for sleep-onset or sleep-maintenance insomnia). They recommend against the use of trazodone, tiagabine, diphenhydramine, melatonin, tryptophan, and valerian for insomnia treatment.

Cognitive-Behavioral Therapy for Insomnia. Cognitive-behavioral therapy for insomnia (CBTi), as a treatment modality, uses a combination of behavioral and cognitive techniques to overcome dysfunctional sleep behaviors, misperceptions, and distorted, disruptive thoughts about sleep. Behavioral techniques include universal sleep hygiene, stimulus control therapy, sleep restriction therapy, relaxation therapies, and biofeedback.

Studies repeatedly show significant, sustained improvement in sleep symptoms, including number and duration of awakenings and sleep latency, from CBTi. Short-term benefits are similar to that of medication, but CBTi tends to have lasting benefits, even 36 months after treatment. With the cessation of the medication, insomnia frequently returns and is sometimes accompanied by rebound insomnia. CBTi has no apparent adverse effects. There are no established "best practice" guidelines for length or quantity of sessions. CBTi, however, is not without limitations. Most data do not compare the efficacy of the individual components of CBTi. However, sleep hygiene education alone produces an insignificant effect on sleep. Intuitively, the multicomponent approach addresses many of the variables contributing to insomnia. Other limitations of CBTi include lack of or unavailability of trained specialists, cost of sessions, and noncoverage by insurance carriers.

The effects of CBTi take longer to emerge than the effects of medications. Usually, when patients finally come for treatment of their insomnia, they are desperate. It is challenging to convince them to try a therapy that may take several weeks before it will provide relief. Furthermore, patients do not assume a passive role in this type of therapy; they must be active participants. Many individuals not only want a "quick fix," but they also want to undergo a procedure or have something administered rather than be involved in the therapeutic process. For optimal CBTi, patients must commit to come to multiple sessions and also be open to the idea that modifying thoughts and behaviors about sleep can improve the symptoms of insomnia.

Although firmly focused on cognitive and behavioral issues, it helps to extend CBT slightly into the psychodynamic sphere.

For some patients with long-standing difficulty sleeping, being an insomniac becomes an essential part of their identity. There may be primary or secondary gain to such identification. It is the negative emotional response (i.e., anger at the inability to control one's sleep, feeling like a failure because one cannot sleep) to insomnia that contributes to its chronicity. In general, these individuals tend to internalize rather than express emotion, feel a heightened need for control, experience interpersonal difficulties and have significant discontent with past events. For this subset of people, neglecting the emotional response can limit the response to treatment and cause a relapse. The clinician will be better able to intercept barriers to treatment when they attune themselves to a patient's tendency to view something as a failure rather than a challenge.

Universal Sleep Hygiene. A patient's lifestyle can lead to a sleep disturbance. We usually call this *inadequate sleep hygiene*, referring to a problem in following generally accepted practices to aid sleep. These include, for instance, keeping regular hours of bedtime and arousal, avoiding excessive caffeine, not eating heavy meals before bedtime, and getting adequate exercise. Many behaviors can interfere with sleep and may do so by increasing nervous system arousal near bedtime or by altering circadian rhythms.

The focus of universal sleep hygiene is on modifiable environmental and lifestyle components that may interfere with sleep, as well as behaviors that may improve sleep. Because some of these behaviors are difficult to change, we should concentrate on only one or two items, chosen in collaboration with the patient, to address. The patient then has the best chance at a successful intervention. We list some sleep-enhancing directives in Table 15-24. Often a few simple alterations in a patient's habits or sleep environment are useful. The clinician, however, needs to spend time reviewing both the patient's routine and its irregularity. In some respects, the essence of insomnia is its variability. The day-to-day changes in behavior and the changing severity of sleeplessness can obscure the factors responsible for the problem. A carefully explained program of sleep hygiene, with follow-up, represents a reasonably inexpensive intervention. Furthermore, improving sleep habits can enhance sleep, even when the primary cause of insomnia is physical. However, sleep hygiene education does not appear to be as effective as CBTi.

Stimulus Control Therapy. Stimulus control therapy is a deconditioning paradigm that aims to break the cycle of problems commonly associated with difficulty initiating sleep. By attempting to undo conditioning that undermines sleep, stimulus control therapy helps reduce both primary and reactive factors involved in insomnia. The rules attempt to enhance stimulus cues for sleeping and diminish associations with sleeplessness. The instructions are simple; however, the patient must consistently follow them. We list an example of these instructions in Table 15-25. Stimulus control therapy does work; however, we might not see results for weeks or even a month. If continually practiced, the bouts of insomnia lessen in both frequency and severity.

Sleep Restriction Therapy. Sleep restriction therapy is a strategy designed to increase sleep efficiency by decreasing the amount of time spent awake while lying in bed. This therapy targets explicitly those patients who lie awake in bed, unable to sleep. Restricting time in bed can help to consolidate sleep. If the patient reports sleeping only 5 hours of an 8-hour scheduled time in bed, reduce the time in bed. It is advised, however, not to reduce bedtime to less than 4 hours per night and to warn the patient about the

Table 15-24
Do's and Don'ts for Good Sleep Hygiene

	DO	DON'T
Maintain regular hours of bedtime and arising	✓	
If you are hungry, have a light snack before bedtime	✓	
Maintain a regular exercise schedule	✓	
Give yourself approximately an hour to wind down before going to bed	✓	
If you are preoccupied or worried about something at bedtime, write it down and deal with it in the morning	✓	
Keep the bedroom cool	✓	
Keep the bedroom dark	✓	
Keep the bedroom quiet	✓	
Take naps		✓
Watch the clock so you know how bad your insomnia actually is		✓
Exercise right before going to bed in order wear yourself out		✓
Watch television in bed when you cannot sleep		✓
Eat a heavy meal before bedtime to help you sleep		✓
Drink coffee in the afternoon and evening		✓
If you cannot sleep, smoke a cigarette		✓
Use alcohol to help in going to sleep		✓
Read in bed when you cannot sleep		✓
Eat in bed		✓
Exercise in bed		✓
Talk on the phone in bed		✓

hazards of daytime sleepiness. Sleep at other times during the day must be avoided, except in the elderly, who may take a 30-minute nap. The clinician then monitors sleep efficiency (time asleep as a percentage of the time in bed). When sleep efficiency reaches 85 percent (averaged over five nights), we should increase the time in bed by 15 minutes. Sleep restriction therapy produces a gradual and steady decline in nocturnal wakefulness.

Relaxation Therapy and Biofeedback. The most critical aspect of relaxation therapy is to perform it properly. Self-hypnosis,

Table 15-25
Stimulus Control Instructions

1. Go to bed only when sleepy to maximize success.
2. Use the bed only for sleeping. Do not watch television in bed, do not read, do not eat, and do not talk on the telephone while in bed.
3. Do not lie in bed and become frustrated if unable to sleep. After a few minutes (do not watch the clock), get up, go to another room, and do something nonarousing until sleepiness returns. Repeat as often as needed.
4. Awaken at the same time every morning (regardless of bedtime, total sleep time, or day of week) and totally avoid napping.

Table 15-26
Abdominal Breathing

1. In the supine position, the patient should breathe normally through his or her mouth or nose, whichever is more comfortable, and attend to his or her breathing pattern.
2. While maintaining that rhythm, the patient should begin to breathe more with his or her abdomen and less with his or her chest.
3. The patient should pause for a half second after each breath cycle (in and out) and evaluate the breath. How did it feel? Was it smooth? Eventually each breath will become uniform and smooth.
4. The patient should find a place where he or she can best feel the air move in and out. Concentrate on that spot and on the air moving in and out.
5. The patient should visualize intrusive thoughts as floating away; if there are too many thoughts, stop practicing and try again later.

progressive relaxation, guided imagery, and deep breathing exercises are all useful if they produce relaxation. The goal is to find the optimal technique for each patient, but not all patients need help in relaxing. *Progressive muscle relaxation* is especially useful for patients who experience muscle tension. The patients should purposefully tense (5 to 6 seconds) and then relax (20 to 30 seconds) muscle groups, beginning at the head and ending at the feet. The patient should appreciate the difference between tension and relaxation. *Guided imagery* has the patient visualize a pleasant, restful scene, engaging all of his or her senses.

Breathing exercises should be practiced for at least 20 min/day for 2 weeks. Once mastered, the technique should be used once at bedtime for 30 minutes. If it does not work, the patient should try a different night again. It is essential that the technique not become associated with failure to fall asleep. Table 15-26 gives example instructions for *abdominal breathing*, an important technique. The patient should become comfortable with each step before moving on to the next.

Biofeedback provides stimulus cues for physiologic markers of relaxation and can increase self-awareness. Muscle tension in the forehead or finger temperature is measured. Finger temperature rises when a person becomes more relaxed. Patients require thorough and adequate training; merely giving them an instruction tape is not especially helpful. Techniques are ideally mastered during the day for several weeks before application to the sleep problem; the patient preferably does this outside of the bed. By the time the patient uses the techniques in bed, the skill should be automatic. Relaxation techniques readily lend themselves to being combined with sleep hygiene and stimulus control therapies. Sometimes they make for good distractions from thinking about the inability to sleep. The ruminations fuel insomnia, and if the ruminator can be distracted, then the person may sleep better.

Cognitive Therapy.   This practical, validated treatment for a variety of psychiatric conditions, including major depression and generalized anxiety, has been adapted for use with insomnia. The cognitive aspect of insomnia treatment targets the negative emotional response to an appraisal of a sleep-related situation. The negative emotional response produces emotional arousal, which in turn contributes to or perpetuates insomnia. People who have maladaptive cognitions tend to exaggerate the negative consequences of insomnia: "There must be something wrong with me if I cannot fall asleep in 40 minutes." They also tend to have unrealistic expectations about their sleep requirements: "If I do not sleep 8 hours a

night, then my whole day will be ruined." The first step is to identify these cognitions, then challenge their validity, and finally, substitute them with more adaptive cognitions.

DH was a 42-year-old man with a 5-year history of insomnia. He identified losing his job and the birth of a colicky baby as precipitating factors in his inability to sleep. However, even after he found a new position with better hours and pay and with the child sleeping through the night, DH continued to experience difficulty falling and staying asleep. Perpetuating factors included low back pain and a spouse with periodic limb movement disorder. He reported spending 8 to 9 hours in bed each night and sleeping only 4 to 5 hours intermittently. He watched 1 hour of television in bed before turning out the light for bedtime. He spent hours watching the minutes tick away. He did not wake feeling rested, and when his alarm went off, he was frequently already awake and had thoughts such as, "I hardly slept at all last night. I should be able to get more sleep. There must be something wrong. Great, I'll be too tired to concentrate on anything today."

Examples of maladaptive thoughts: *"I should be able to get more sleep."* This is a faulty appraisal of sleeping ability and may relate to a need for control over sleep. This need for control interferes with having a more laissez-faire attitude about a few missed hours of rest. Such thoughts can also lead to feelings of frustration and anger. *"Great, I'll be too tired to concentrate on anything today."* This is a misattribution of daytime impairment due to poor sleep. DH was also magnifying the negative and discounting the positive with his black-and-white or all-or-nothing thinking. Could DH be too tired to concentrate on some things, but not all things? Might his inability to concentrate be due to a myriad of other factors? *"There must be something wrong with me (if I can't get enough sleep)."* This is catastrophizing and emotional reasoning: just because a person had a feeling does not mean that the thought or feeling is valid. A firmly held belief that sleeplessness negatively affects physical and mental health can set off catastrophizing. (Courtesy of Max Hirshkowitz, Ph.D., Rhoda G. Seplowitz-Hafkin, M.D., and Amir Sharafkhaneh, M.D., Ph.D.)

Paradoxical Intention.   This is a cognitive technique with conflicting evidence regarding its efficacy. In clinical practice, compliance is often a barrier, but it does work for a limited number of patients. The theory is that performance anxiety interferes with sleep onset. Thus, when the patient tries to stay awake for as long as possible rather than trying to fall asleep, performance anxiety will be reduced, and sleep latency will improve.

Hypersomnolence Disorder

We usually treat hypersomnolence disorder with medication. Although there are no medications approved for its treatment, physicians commonly use stimulants, with varying degrees of success. The wake-promoting substance modafinil or traditional psychostimulants (amphetamines and their derivatives) sometimes help manage the sleepiness. In addition to drug therapies, the overall therapeutic approach usually includes lifestyle adjustment, psychological counseling, drug holidays to reduce tolerance (if using stimulants), and careful monitoring of refills, general health, and cardiac status.

Narcolepsy

Currently, we cannot cure narcolepsy; however, the symptoms can be managed with either the wake-promoting substances modafinil or armodafinil, or traditional psychostimulants like amphetamines

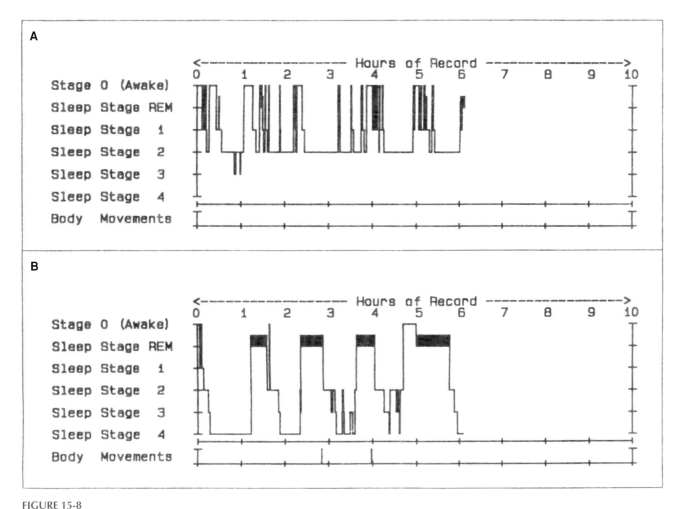

FIGURE 15-8

Sleep histogram showing CPAP-related sleep improvement. Sleep stage histogram illustrating the immediate, dramatic improvement in sleep architecture produced by treating obstructive sleep apnea with continuous positive airway pressure (CPAP) therapy. **Panel A** illustrates the abnormal sleep pattern on a night when the patient had more than 200 episodes of obstructive sleep apnea. Sleep is disturbed by frequent awakenings while REM and slow-wave (stages 3 and 4) sleep are nearly absent. **Panel B** shows data from the same patient being treated with CPAP on the next night. Normalization of sleep continuity with a massive rebound in REM and slow-wave sleep is evident.

and their derivatives. The FDA has approved two medications for the treatment of narcolepsy as wake-promoting agents: pitolisant, which is a selective H_3 receptor antagonist/inverse agonist, and solriamfetol, a selective norepinephrine–dopamine reuptake inhibitor. For managing cataplexy, clinicians often administer REM sleep–suppressing drugs (e.g., many antidepressants). This approach capitalizes on the REM sleep-suppressant properties of these drugs. Because cataplexy is presumably an intrusion of REM sleep phenomena into the awake state, the rationale is clear. Many reports indicate that imipramine and protriptyline are quite effective in reducing or eliminating cataplexy. Selective serotonin reuptake inhibitors have gained popularity because they are associated with fewer side effects than the tricyclic antidepressants. Sodium oxybate has proven extremely useful for reducing cataplexy, even in cases where clinicians thought that the cataplexy was intractable. Studies also suggest that sodium oxybate helps improve sleep and relieves some of the sleepiness associated with narcolepsy. Although drug therapy is the treatment of choice, the overall therapeutic approach should include scheduled naps, lifestyle adjustment, psychological counseling, drug holidays to reduce tolerance, and careful monitoring of drug refills, general health, and cardiac status.

Breathing-Related Sleep Disorders

Obstructive Sleep Apnea-Hypopnea.
A number of treatments are available for OSA, including PAP, oral appliances, positional therapy, surgical intervention, and weight loss. Medications have not been useful for treating OSA. Wakefulness promoting agents, such as modafinil, solriamfetol, and pitolisant, may help with the residual sleepiness that may persist despite the use of other OSA treatments such as PAP. However, these medications do not address the pathophysiology of airway occlusion.

POSITIVE AIRWAY PRESSURE. PAP is the preferred treatment for OSA (Fig. 15-8). The PAP apparatus consists of a fan-driven blower, a nasal mask or oronasal interface, and tubing connecting the two. The airflow through the interface (usually a mask or nasal pillows) provides a positive pressure that offsets oropharyngeal collapse produced by inspiratory negative thoracic pressure. In this manner, it acts as a pneumatic splint, thereby maintaining the airway. When appropriately titrating the pressure, even the most severe sleep apnea can be alleviated. Results are often dramatic. PAP devices come in several varieties. The most common are systems that provide a preset continuous positive airway pressure

(CPAP). For individuals who find it difficult to exhale against a continuous pressure, bilevel positive airway pressure (BPAP) may provide a solution. BPAP devices have different inspiratory and expiratory pressure settings. More recently, systems that sense the patient's changes in airway resistance and automatically adjust the positive airway pressure have been gaining popularity. Such automatic positive airway pressure (APAP) systems should theoretically be able to adapt to changes in pressure requirements produced by sleep deprivation, medications, weight change, sleep stage, illness, and aging. Finally, there are timed bilevel and servo-ventilation systems, but these fall into the category of noninvasive positive pressure ventilation (NIPPV) systems, which are more appropriate for treating other pulmonary diseases and breathing problems in neuromuscular diseases. The tremendous efficacy and remarkable safety of PAP therapies have made them the standard of care for patients who can tolerate sleeping with the machine. The principal therapeutic challenge is utilization. Patient education and systematic follow-up are crucial. When problems with the interface, the pressure, nasal stuffiness, and other barriers to routine, nightly use arise, we should remedy these quickly to ensure therapeutic adherence. When used properly, the success of PAP therapy has rendered surgical intervention a secondary option, resorted to mainly after PAP failure, rejection, or nonadherence.

ORAL APPLIANCE. Oral appliances represent another therapeutic option that is gaining popularity. A variety of oral appliances have also been developed to treat snoring and can provide benefit for mild to moderate OSA cases. The general approach is to manipulate the position of the mandible, lift the palate, or retain the tongue. Randomized trials indicate that some oral appliances improve airway patency sufficiently. However, in patients with severe OSA, improvement does not always reach satisfactory levels; therefore, follow-up evaluations are critically important.

POSITIONAL THERAPY. In some patients, sleep-disordered breathing occurs only in the supine position. In such situations, preventing patients from sleeping on their backs may produce beneficial results. Tennis balls sewn onto or placed into pockets on the back of the nightshirt or foam wedges may accomplish this goal. Although such interventions seem to be useful in clinical practice, large-scale systematic clinical trials are needed.

SURGICAL INTERVENTION. Aggressive surgical treatments evolved soon after OSA's pathophysiologic and potentially life-threatening consequences were recognized. The earliest surgical intervention aimed to create a patent airway; thus, in the late 1970s, tracheostomies were performed on individuals with severe apnea. Although no longer the preferred treatment, it remains a standard against which we judge newer, more refined therapies. Second-generation surgical approaches attempt to correct airway obstructions and malformations. Early studies of uvulopalatopharyngoplasty (UPPP) suggested that modification of the soft palate effectively relieved most sleep apnea. Later follow-up results were less impressive. Approximately 30 to 50 percent of patients with sleep apnea benefit from UPPP. These patients are likely those with oropharyngeal obstruction; thus, careful attention to selection criteria presumably improves outcomes. However, if obstruction occurs in the posterior airway space (PAS), maxillomandibular surgery may be appropriate. In retrognathic patients or patients with cephalometrics revealing compromised PAS, moving the jaw forward can achieve impressive normalization of breathing during sleep.

WEIGHT LOSS. Weight loss is known to help many patients. However, because losing weight and keeping it off is difficult

and unreliably achieved, the prudent clinician should recommend weight loss but also rely on other therapies.

CSA due to High-Altitude Periodic Breathing. We can treat CSA due to high-altitude periodic breathing with acetazolamide, which lowers serum pH and increases the respiratory drive. Acetazolamide side effects include metabolic acidosis, electrolyte imbalance, anaphylaxis, Stevens–Johnson syndrome, toxic epidermal necrolysis, and agranulocytosis. Common reactions include but are not limited to fatigue, anorexia, taste changes, polyuria, diarrhea, melena, tinnitus, and photosensitivity.

Circadian Rhythm Sleep–Wake Disorders

Light Therapy. Research indicates that exposing an individual to bright lights can reset the circadian pacemaker. This seems especially the case when the light is bright (higher than 10,000 lux) or in the blue spectrum. With the precise timing of bright light exposure, we can reset the biologic clock. Exposure to light modifies the set-point of the biologic clock. Using core body temperature as a physiologic marker, one can use bright lights to produce a phase delay when presented before the temperature nadir. By contrast, light exposure after the temperature nadir evokes phase advance. The closer one presents light to the point of inflection (temperature nadir), the more robust is the response in altering the cycle. Thus, we can use early-morning bright-light therapy to phase advance individuals with delayed sleep phase syndrome.

Similarly, exposure to bright light in the evening can help patients with advanced sleep phase syndrome. The blue part of the light spectrum is the crucial ingredient in phase setting and shifting. Therefore, blue light exposure (or limitation with blue-blocking eyewear) at specific times can provide therapeutic benefit. Clinicians are using light therapy to reset the circadian rhythm of shift workers, astronauts, and individuals experiencing jet lag.

Medication. Researchers posit that melatonin secretion acts as the biologic substrate for the internal circadian oscillator. Under normal circumstances, melatonin levels begin to rise at dusk and remain elevated until dawn. Bright light suppresses the release of melatonin. Melatonin, in a sense, is the signal of darkness in the brain. As such, we can use it clinically to manage sighted patients with disturbed sleep–wake cycles. Melatonin is available over the counter in the United States. A prescription synthetic melatonin agonist (ramelteon) is also available. Ramelteon is FDA approved for treating patients with sleep-onset insomnia but is used off label for the entire spectrum of circadian rhythm sleep disorders. Outside the United States, a sustained-release prescription form of melatonin is available. Of interest, the only medication approved for shift work sleep disorder is the wake-promoting compound modafinil. Modafinil treats sleepiness occurring during night shift work.

Chronotherapy. Chronotherapy is one technique used to reset the biologic clock. It involves progressively phase delaying a person until synchronizing the circadian oscillator with the desired sleep–wake schedule. Most young and middle-aged adults have a propensity to phase delay the circadian sleep–wake rhythm progressively anyhow. Thus, phase delaying each night by 2 to 3 hours is simpler than phase advancing because it capitalizes on a natural tendency. Halting the phase delay at the appropriate moment and maintaining the desired synchrony can be a challenge. The patient also has to cope with an odd sleep–wake schedule for the better part of a week during therapy (which can interfere with school or work). For these reasons, the development of light therapy and pharmacologic interventions has overshadowed chronotherapy.

Parasomnias and Sleep-Related Movement Disorders

Nightmare Disorder.
Treatment using behavioral techniques can be helpful. Desensitization and exposure therapy, image rehearsal therapy, lucid dream therapy, and cognitive therapy can help address nightmare disorder. Additionally, evidence for the use of prazosin, a CNS α-1 receptor antagonist, in the treatment of PTSD-related nightmares is growing. Nitrazepam and triazolam may also be helpful.

Recurrent Isolated Sleep Paralysis.
Improved sleep hygiene and assuring sufficient sleep are first-line therapies. Sometimes, if the individual voluntarily makes very–rapid eye movements or is touched by another person, the episode will usually terminate.

Sleep Enuresis.
Treating sleep enuresis involves medication, behavioral interventions, or both. Among medications, desmopressin acetate is the preferred choice. Other medications used to treat sleep enuresis include imipramine and oxybutynin chloride. Behavioral treatments, including bladder training, using conditioning devices (bell and pad), diet modification, and fluid restriction, have reported success when properly administered. Other treatments include psychotherapy, motivational strategies, and hypnotherapy.

Restless Legs Syndrome.
Pharmacologically, the dopaminergic agonists pramipexole, rotigotine, and ropinirole are FDA approved and represent the treatment of choice. Other agents used to treat RLS include dopamine precursors (e.g., levodopa), benzodiazepines, opiates (including prolonged-release oxycodone–naloxone), and antiepileptic drugs (e.g., gabapentin, pregabalin). When iron deficiency is present, or when ferritin levels are low, iron supplementation can also be helpful. Nonpharmacologic treatment includes avoiding alcohol or nicotine use close to bedtime, massaging the affected parts of the legs, taking hot baths, applying hot or cold to the affected areas, magnetic or electric stimulation therapy, and moderate exercise.

Periodic Limb Movement Disorder Treatment.
Pharmacotherapy for PLMD associated with RLS is the same as for RLS. Clinical trials of pharmacotherapy for other forms of PLMD are lacking. However, benzodiazepines, especially clonazepam, reportedly improve sleep in patients with PLMD.

Sleep-Related Bruxism.
The usual treatment involves having the patient wear an oral appliance to protect the teeth during sleep. There are two basic types of appliances: the soft one (mouth guard) is typically used in the short term, whereas the hard acrylic one (bite splint) is used long term and requires regular follow-up. Relaxation, biofeedback, hypnosis, physical therapy, and stress management can also treat sleep bruxism. A variety of drug therapies have been tried (benzodiazepines, muscle relaxants, dopaminergic agonists, and propranolol); however, reliable outcome data are not available. Botulinum toxin can also improve the frequency of bruxism episodes.

Benign Sleep Myoclonus of Infancy.
This benign condition typically lasts a few days to several months and does not need to be treated.

Propriospinal Myoclonus at Sleep Onset.
Treatment with clonazepam or anticonvulsants may be useful.

References

American Academy of Sleep Medicine. *International Classification of Sleep Disorders*. 3rd ed. Darien, IL: American Academy of Sleep Medicine; 2014.

American Psychiatric Association. *Diagnostic and Statistical Manual of Mental Disorders*. 5th ed. Arlington, VA: American Psychiatric Association; 2013.

Barateau L, Dauvillers Y. Recent advances in treatment for narcolepsy. *Ther Adv Neurol Disord*. 2019;12:1756286419875622.

Barclay NL, Gregory AM. Quantitative genetic research on sleep: a review of normal sleep, sleep disturbances and associated emotional, behavioural, and health-related difficulties. *Sleep Med Rev*. 2013;17(1):29–40.

Beddis H, Pemberton M, Davies S. Sleep bruxism: an overview for clinicians. *Br Dent J*. 2018;225(6):497–501.

Bianchi MT, Thomas RJ. Technical advances in the characterization of the complexity of sleep and sleep disorders. *Prog Neuropsychopharmacol Biol Psychiatry*. 2013;45:277–286.

Chung KF, Lee CT, Yeung WF, Chan MS, Chung EW, Lin WL. Sleep hygiene education as a treatment of insomnia: a systematic review and meta-analysis. *Fam Pract*. 2018;35(4):365–375.

Claassen DO, Josephs KA, Ahlskog JE, Silber MH, Tippmann-Peikert M, Boeve BF. REM sleep behavior disorder preceding other aspects of synucleinopathies by up to half a century. *Neurology*. 2010;75(6):494–499.

Costa G. Shift work and occupational medicine: an overview. *Occup Med (Lond)*. 2003;53(2):83–88.

Dauvilliers Y, Verbraecken J, Partinen M, Hedner J, Saaresranta T, Georgiev O, Tiholov R, Lecomte I, Tamisier R, Levy P, Scart-Gres C, Lecomte JM, Schwarts JC, Pepin JL; HAROSA II Study Group collaborators. Pitolisant for daytime sleepiness in patients with obstructive sleep apnea who refuse continuous positive airway pressure treatment. A randomized trial. *Am J Respir Crit Care Med*. 2020;201(9):1135–1145.

Genderson MR, Rana BK, Panizzon MS, Grant MD, Toomey R, Jacobson KC, Xian H, Cronin-Golomb A, Franz CE, Kremen WS, Lyons MJ. Genetic and environmental influences on sleep quality in middle-aged men: a twin study. *J Sleep Res*. 2013;22(5):519–526.

Gieselmann A, Aoudia MA, Carr M, Germain A, Gorzka R, Holzinger B, Kleim B, Krakow B, Kunze AE, Lancee J, Nadorff MR, Nielsen T, Riemann D, Sandahl H, Schlarb AA, Schmid C, Schredl M, Spoormaker VI, Steil R, van Schagen AM, Wittmann L, Zschoche M, Pietrowsky R. Aetiology and treatment of nightmare disorder: state of the art and future perspectives. *J Sleep Res*. 2019;28(4):e12820.

Hirshkowitz M, Sharafkhaneh A. Chapter 23: Sleep disorders. In: Sadock BJ, Sadock VA, Ruiz P, eds. *Kaplan & Sadock's Comprehensive Textbook of Psychiatry*. 10th ed. Philadelphia, PA: Wolters Kluwer; 2017:2083–2109.

Iber C, Ancoli-Israel S, Chesson A; Quan SF for the American Academy of Sleep Medicine. *The AASM Manual for the Scoring of Sleep and Associated Events: Rules, Terminology and Technical Specifications*. Westchester, IL: American Academy of Sleep Medicine; 2007.

Jenni OG. How much sleep is "normal" in children and adolescents? *JAMA Pediatr*. 2013;167(1):91–92.

Manfredini D, Winocur E, Guarda-Nardini L, Paesani D, Lobbezoo F. Epidemiology of bruxism in adults: a systematic review of the literature. *J Orofac Pain*. 2013;27(2):99–110.

Ohayon MM, Dauvilliers Y, Reynolds CF III. Operational definitions and algorithms for excessive sleepiness in the general population: implications for DSM-5 nosology. *Arch Gen Psychiatry*. 2012;69(1):71–79.

Ohayon MM, Mahowald MW, Dauvilliers Y, Krystal AD, Léger D. Prevalence and comorbidity of nocturnal wandering in the U.S. adult general population. *Neurology*. 2012;78(20):1583–1589.

Ohayon MM, Reynolds CF III, Dauvilliers Y. Excessive sleep duration and quality of life. *Ann Neurol*. 2013;73(6):785–794.

Potts KJ, Butterfield DT, Sims P, Henderson M, Shames CB. Cost savings associated with an education campaign on the diagnosis and management of sleep-disordered breathing: a retrospective, claims-based U.S. study. *Popul Health Manag*. 2013;16(1):7–13.

Qaseem A, Holty JE, Owens DK, Dallas P, Starkey M, Shekelle P; Clinical Guidelines Committee of the American College of Physicians. Management of obstructive sleep apnea in adults: a clinical practice guideline from the American College of Physicians. *Ann Intern Med*. 2013;159(7):471–483.

Richard DM, Dawes MA, Mathias CW, Acheson A, Hill-Kapturczak N, Dougherty DM. L-tryptophan: basic metabolic functions, behavioral research, and therapeutic indications. *Int J Tryptophan Res*. 2009;2:45–60.

Richardson GS. The human circadian system in normal and disordered sleep. *J Clin Psychiatry*. 2005;66(Suppl 9):3–9; quiz 42–43.

Rosipal R, Lewandowski A, Dorffner G. In search of objective components for sleep quality indexing in normal sleep. *Biol Psychol*. 2013;94(1):210–220.

Saper CB, Scammell TE. Emerging therapeutics in sleep. *Ann Neurol*. 2013;74(3):435–440.

Sateia MJ. International classification of sleep disorders-third edition: highlights and modifications. *Chest*. 2014;146(5):1387–1394.

Sateia MJ, Buysse DJ, Krystal AD, Neubauer DN, Heald JL. Clinical practice guideline for the pharmacologic treatment of chronic insomnia in adults: an American Academy of Sleep Medicine clinical practice guideline. *J Clin Sleep Med*. 2017; 13(2):307–349.

Scott AJ. Shift work and health. *Prim Care*. 2000;27(4):1057–1079.

Thomas SJ, Lichstein KL, Taylor DJ, Riedel BW, Bush AJ. Epidemiology of bedtime, arising time, and time in bed: analysis of age, gender, and ethnicity. *Behav Sleep Med*. 2014;12(3):169–182.

Trenkwalder C, Allen R, Högl B, Clemens S, Patton S, Schormair B, Winkelmann J. Comorbidities, treatment, and pathophysiology in restless legs syndrome. *Lancet Neurol*. 2018;17(11):994–1005.

Wright KP, Lowry CA, Lebourgeois MK. Circadian and wakefulness-sleep modulation of cognition in humans. *Front Mol Neurosci*. 2012;5:50.

Younes, MK, Ostrowski M, Hanly P, Raneri J. Agreement between manual and automatic scoring of polysomnograms in a broad spectrum of sleep disorders. *Am J Respir Crit Care Med*. 2014;189:A3593.

Zee PC, Vitiello MV. Circadian rhythm sleep disorder: irregular sleep wake rhythm type. *Sleep Med Clin*. 2009;4(2):213–218.

## 16

Human Sexuality and Sexual Dysfunctions

Sexuality is a broad topic, and no brief synopsis can do it justice. For the psychiatrist, it loosely divides into the subjects of normal sexuality, sexual dysfunction, paraphilias, and gender dysphoria. As with other chapters, we are focusing on the disorders that might bring a patient to a psychiatrist. There are two broad categories of disorders that we loosely group under sexual disorders: sexual dysfunction and paraphilias. By sexual dysfunctions, we are referring to disorders of normal sexual functioning. The paraphilias are unusual expressions of sexuality that are considered aberrant or even illegal. As these represent fundamentally different problems that require very different approaches, we separate these into two sections. We then discuss normal sexuality as part of our consideration of the pathology and etiology of these disorders. We will discuss gender dysphoria in the next section.

For a fuller discussion, we would refer the reader to Virginia Sadock's excellent review of the subject in the *Comprehensive Textbook*.

SEXUAL DYSFUNCTIONS

The essential features of sexual dysfunctions are an inability to respond to sexual stimulation, or the experience of pain during the sexual act. Dysfunction can be defined by a disturbance in the subjective sense of pleasure or desire usually associated with sex, or by the objective performance. According to ICD-10, sexual dysfunction refers to a person's inability "to participate in a sexual relationship as he or she would wish."

In DSM-5, the sexual dysfunctions include male hypoactive sexual desire disorder, female sexual interest/arousal disorder, erectile disorder, female orgasmic disorder, delayed ejaculation, premature (early) ejaculation, genito-pelvic pain/penetration disorder, substance/medication-induced sexual dysfunction, other specified sexual dysfunction, and unspecified sexual dysfunction. We diagnose sexual dysfunctions only when they are a significant part of the clinical picture. If more than one dysfunction exists, we should diagnose them all. Sexual dysfunctions can be lifelong or acquired, generalized or situational, and result from psychological factors, physiologic factors, combined factors, and numerous stressors, including prohibitive cultural mores, health and partner issues, and relationship conflicts. If the dysfunction is attributable entirely to a general medical condition, substance use, or adverse effects of medication, then sexual dysfunction due to a general medical condition or substance-induced sexual dysfunction is diagnosed. DSM-5 indicates the severity of the dysfunction by whether the patient's distress is mild, moderate, or severe.

Sexual dysfunctions are frequently associated with other mental disorders, such as depressive disorders, anxiety disorders, personality disorders, and schizophrenia. In many instances, sexual dysfunction is comorbid with another psychiatric disorder. If the dysfunction is mostly attributable to an underlying psychiatric disorder, we should only diagnose the underlying disorder. Sexual dysfunctions are usually self-perpetuating, with the patients increasingly subjected to ongoing performance anxiety and a concomitant inability to experience pleasure. In relationships, the sexually functional partner often reacts with distress or anger due to feelings of deprivation or a sense that he or she is an insufficiently attractive or adequate sexual partner. In such cases, the clinician must consider whether the sexual problem preceded or arose from relationship difficulties and weigh whether a diagnosis of sexual dysfunction relevant to relationship issues is appropriate.

A sex history provides essential information about patients, regardless of the presence of a sexual disorder or whether that is the patient's chief complaint. The information can be obtained gradually through open-ended questions. The outline in Table 16-1 provides a guide to the topics to be covered.

Desire, Interest, and Arousal Disorders

Male Hypoactive Sexual Desire Disorder. Male hypoactive sexual desire disorder is a deficiency or absence of sexual fantasies and desire for sexual activity for a minimum duration of approximately 6 months (Table 16-2). Men for whom this is a lifelong condition have never experienced many spontaneous erotic/sexual thoughts. Minimal spontaneous sexual thinking or minimal desire for sex ahead of sexual experiences is not a diagnosable disorder in women, primarily if the sexual encounter then triggers the desire. The reported prevalence of low desire is highest at the younger and older ends of the age spectrum, with only 2 percent of men ages 16 to 44 affected by this disorder. A reported 6 percent of men ages 18 to 24, and 40 percent of men ages 66 to 74, have problems with sexual desire. Some men may confuse decreased desire with decreased activity. Their erotic thoughts and fantasies are undiminished, but they no longer act on them due to health issues, unavailability of a partner, or another sexual dysfunction such as erectile disorder.

A variety of causative factors are associated with low sexual desire. Patients with desire problems often use inhibition of desire defensively, to protect against unconscious fears about sex.

Abstinence from sex for a prolonged period sometimes results in suppression of sexual impulses. Loss of desire may also be an expression of hostility to a partner or the sign of a deteriorating relationship. The presence of desire depends on several factors: biologic drive, adequate self-esteem, the ability to accept oneself as a sexual person, the availability of an appropriate partner, and a good relationship in nonsexual areas with a partner. Damage to, or absence of, any of these factors can diminish desire.

In making the diagnosis, clinicians must evaluate a patient's age, general health, any medication regimen, and life stresses. The

Table 16-1
Taking a Sex History

I. Identifying data
  A. Age
  B. Sex
  C. Occupation
  D. Relationship status—single, married, number of times previously married, separated, divorced, cohabiting, serious involvement, casual dating (difficulty forming or keeping relationships should be assessed throughout the interview)
  E. Sexual orientation—heterosexual, homosexual, or bisexual (this may also be ascertained later in the interview)
II. Current functioning
  A. Unsatisfactory to highly satisfactory
  B. If unsatisfactory, why?
  C. Feeling about partner satisfaction
  D. Dysfunctions?—e.g., lack of desire, erectile disorder, inhibited female interest/arousal, anorgasmia, premature ejaculation, retarded ejaculation, pain associated with intercourse (dysfunction discussed below)
    1. Onset—lifelong or acquired
      a. If acquired, when?
      b. Did onset coincide with drug use (medications or illegal recreational drugs), life stresses (e.g., loss of job, birth of child), interpersonal difficulties
    2. Generalized—occurs in most situations or with most partners
    3. Situational
      a. Only with current partner
      b. In any committed relationship
      c. Only with masturbation
      d. In socially proscribed circumstance (e.g., affair)
      e. In definable circumstance (e.g., very late at night, in parental home, when partner initiated sex play)
  E. Frequency—partnered sex (coital and noncoital sex play)
  F. Desire/libido—how often are sexual feelings, thoughts, fantasies, dreams, experienced? (per day, week, etc.)
  G. Description of typical sexual interaction
    1. Manner of initiation or invitation (e.g., verbal or physical? Does same person always initiate?)
    2. Presence, type, and extent of foreplay (e.g., kissing, caressing, manual or oral genital stimulation)
    3. Coitus? positions used?
    4. Verbalization during sex? if so, what kind?
    5. Afterplay? (whether sex act is completed or disrupted by dysfunction); typical activities (e.g., holding, talking, return to daily activities, sleeping)
    6. Feeling after sex: relaxed, tense, angry, loving
  H. Sexual compulsivity?—intrusion of sexual thoughts or participation in sexual activities to a degree that interferes with relationships or work, requires deception and may endanger the patient
III. Past sexual history
  A. Childhood sexuality
    1. Parental attitudes about sex—degree of openness or reserve (assess unusual prudery or seductiveness)
    2. Parents' attitudes about nudity and modesty
    3. Learning about sex
      a. From parents? (initiated by child's questions or parent volunteering information? which parent? what was child's age?) subjects covered (e.g., pregnancy, birth, intercourse, menstruation, nocturnal emission, masturbation)
      b. From books, magazines, or friends at school or through religious group?
      c. Significant misinformation
      d. Feeling about information
    4. Viewing or hearing primal scene—reaction?
    5. Viewing sex play or intercourse of person other than parent
    6. Viewing sex between pets or other animals
  B. Childhood sex activities
    1. Genital self-stimulation before adolescence; age? reaction if apprehended?
    2. Awareness of self as boy or girl; bathroom sensual activities? (regarding urine, feces, odor, enemas)
    3. Sexual play or exploration with another child (playing doctor)—type of activity (e.g., looking, manual touching, genital touching); reactions or consequences if apprehended (by whom?)
IV. Adolescence
  A. Age of onset of puberty—development of secondary sex characteristics, age of menarche for girl, wet dreams or first ejaculation for boy (preparation for and reaction to)
  B. Sense of self as feminine or masculine—body image, acceptance by peers (opposite sex and same sex), sense of sexual desirability, onset of coital fantasies
  C. Sex activities
    1. Masturbation—age begun; ever punished or prohibited? method used, accompanying fantasies, frequency (questions about masturbation and fantasies are among the most sensitive for patients to answer)
    2. Homosexual activities—ongoing or rare and experimental episodes, approached by others? If homosexual, has there been any heterosexual experimentation?
    3. Dating—casual or steady, description of first crush, infatuation, or first love
    4. Experiences of kissing, necking, petting ("making out" or "fooling around"), age begun, frequency, number of partners, circumstances, type(s) of activity
    5. Orgasm—when first experienced? (may not be experienced during adolescence), with masturbation, during sleep, or with partner? with intercourse or other sex play? frequency?
    6. First coitus—age, circumstances, partner, reactions (may not be experienced during adolescence); contraception and/or safe sex precautions used

Table 16-1
Taking a Sex History (*Continued*)

V. Adult sexual activities (may be experienced by some adolescents)
   A. Premarital sex
      1. Types of sex play experiences—frequency of sexual interactions, types and number of partners
      2. Contraception and/or safe sex precautions used
      3. First coitus (if not experienced in adolescence) age, circumstances, partner
      4. Cohabitation—age begun, duration, description of partner, sexual fidelity, types of sexual activity, frequency, satisfaction, number of cohabiting relationships, reasons for breakup(s)
      5. Engagement—age, activity during engagement period with fiancé(e), with others; length of engagement
   B. Marriage (if multiple marriages have occurred, explore sexual activity, reasons for marriage, and reasons for divorce in each marriage)
      1. Types and frequency of sexual interaction—describe typical sexual interaction (see above), satisfaction with sex life? view of partner's feeling
      2. First sexual experience with spouse—when? what were the circumstances? was it satisfying? disappointing?
      3. Honeymoon—setting, duration, pleasant or unpleasant, sexually active, frequency? problems? compatibility?
      4. Effect of pregnancies and children on marital sex
      5. Extramarital sex—number of incidents, partner; emotional attachment to extramarital partners? feelings about extramarital sex
      6. Postmarital masturbation—frequency? effect on marital sex?
      7. Extramarital sex by partner—effect on interviewee
      8. Ménage à trois or multiple sex (swinging)
      9. Areas of conflict in marriage (e.g., parenting, finances, division of responsibilities, priorities)
VI. Sex after widowhood, separation, divorce—celibacy, orgasms in sleep, masturbation, noncoital sex play, intercourse (number of and relationship to partners), other
VII. Special issues
   A. History of rape, incest, sexual or physical abuse
   B. Spousal abuse (current)
   C. Chronic illness (physical or psychiatric)
   D. History or presence of sexually transmitted diseases
   E. Fertility problems
   F. Abortions, miscarriages, or unwanted or illegitimate pregnancies
   G. Gender identity conflict—(e.g., transsexualism, wearing clothes of opposite sex)
   H. Paraphilias—(e.g., fetishes, voyeurism, sadomasochism)

Table 16-2
Male Hypoactive Sexual Desire Disorder

	DSM-5	ICD-10
Name	Male Hypoactive Sexual Desire Disorder	Lack or loss of sexual desire Sexual aversion and lack of sexual enjoyment
Duration	≥6 mo	
Symptoms	Decreased thoughts or interest in sex	Lack or loss of sexual desire not attributable to physiologic difficulties related to intercourse Sexual aversion due to anxiety and subsequent avoidance of sexual activity, or lack of enjoyment given that orgasm is not accompanied by appropriate pleasure
# Symptoms Needed	Symptoms should be recurrent	
Exclusions (not result of):	Sociocultural influences Age Relationship problem Substance use (including prescribed meds) Another medical condition Another psychiatric condition	
Psychosocial Impact	Marked distress	
Symptom Specifiers	Generalized vs. Situational	
Severity Specifiers	**Mild:** causes mild distress **Moderate:** causes moderate distress **Severe:** causes severe distress	
Course Specifiers	Lifelong vs. Acquired	Note: ICD-10 classifies this diagnosis as including male hypoactive sexual desire disorder as well as female sexual arousal disorder (Table 16-3)

Table 16-3
Female Sexual Interest/Arousal Disorder

	DSM-5	ICD-10
Name	Female Sexual Interest/Arousal Disorder	Lack or loss of sexual desire Sexual aversion and lack of sexual enjoyment
Duration	≥6 mo	
Symptoms	Decreased arousal or interest in sex: 　Reduced interest in sex 　Reduced sexual thoughts/fantasies 　Reduced initiation/receptiveness to sexual activity 　Absent or reduced sexual pleasure 　Absent or reduced pleasure from sexual cues 　Absent or reduced sensation during sex	Lack or loss of sexual desire not attributable to physiologic difficulties related to intercourse Sexual aversion due to anxiety and subsequent avoidance of sexual activity, or lack of enjoyment given that orgasm is not accompanied by appropriate pleasure
# Symptoms Needed	≥3 during most sexual experiences	
Exclusions (not result of):	Relationship problem Substance use (including prescribed meds) Another medical condition Another psychiatric condition	
Psychosocial Impact	Marked distress	
Symptom Specifiers	Generalized vs. Situational	
Severity Specifiers	**Mild:** causes mild distress **Moderate:** causes moderate distress **Severe:** causes severe distress	
Course Specifiers	Lifelong vs. Acquired	

clinician must attempt to establish a baseline of sexual interest before the disorder began. The need for sexual contact and satisfaction varies among persons. We should not make a diagnosis unless the lack of desire is a source of distress to a patient.

Female Sexual Interest/Arousal Disorder. The combination of interest (or desire) and arousal into one dysfunction category reflects the recognition that women do not necessarily move stepwise from desire to arousal, but often experience desire synchronously with, or even following, beginning feelings of arousal. This is particularly true for women in long-term relationships. As a corollary, women experiencing sexual dysfunction may experience either inability to feel interest or arousal, and they may also have difficulty achieving orgasm or experience pain. Some may experience dysfunction across the entire range of sexual response. Complaints in this dysfunction category present variously as a decrease or paucity of erotic feelings, thoughts, or fantasies; a decreased impulse to initiate sex; a decreased or absent receptivity to partner overtures; or an inability to respond to partner stimulation (Table 16-3).

A complicating factor in this diagnosis is that a subjective sense of arousal is often poorly correlated with genital lubrication in both normal and dysfunctional women. Therefore, complaints of lack of pleasure are sufficient for this diagnosis even when vaginal lubrication and congestion are present. A woman complaining of lack of arousal may lubricate vaginally, but may not experience a subjective sense of excitement. Alterations in testosterone, estrogen, prolactin, and thyroxin levels occur in female sexual arousal disorder. Also, medications with antihistaminic or anticholinergic properties cause a decrease in vaginal lubrication.

We should evaluate factors such as life stresses, aging, menopause, adequate sexual stimulation, and general health before making this diagnosis. Relationship problems are particularly relevant to acquired interest/arousal disorder. In one study of couples

with markedly decreased sexual interaction, the most prevalent etiology was marital discord.

Male Erectile Disorder. Male erectile disorder was historically called *impotence*. The term was dropped for a more medical designation, but also because it was considered derogatory and had negative connotations for the man with the problem. However, it describes with accuracy the feelings of powerlessness, helplessness, and resultant low self-esteem men with this dysfunction frequently suffer (Table 16-4). A man with a lifelong male erectile disorder has never been able to obtain an erection sufficient for insertion. In acquired male erectile disorder, a man has successfully achieved penetration at some time in his sexual life but is later unable to do so. In situational male erectile disorder, a man can have coitus in certain circumstances but not in others; for example, he may function effectively with a sex worker but be unable to have an erection when with his partner.

Acquired male erectile disorder occurs in 10 to 20 percent of all men. Erectile disorder is the chief complaint of more than 50 percent of all men treated for sexual disorders. Lifelong male erectile disorder is rare; it occurs in about 1 percent of men younger than age 35. The incidence of erectile disorder increases with age. It has been reported variously as 2 to 8 percent of the young adult population, and much more common in older men. Male erectile disorder, however, is not universal in aging men; having an available sex partner is related to continuing potency, as is a history of consistent sexual activity and the absence of vascular, neurologic, or endocrine disease. Twenty percent of men fear erectile dysfunction before their first coitus; the reported incidence of actual erectile dysfunction during the first coitus is 8 percent.

Male erectile disorder can be organic or psychological or a combination of both, but in young and middle-aged men, the cause is usually psychological. A good history is of primary importance in determining the cause of the dysfunction. If a man reports having

Table 16-4
Erectile Disorder or Failure of Genital Response

	DSM-5	ICD-10
Name	Erectile Disorder	Failure of genital response
Duration	≥6 mo	

Symptoms	Difficulties with erections:
	    Achieving
	    Maintaining
	    Rigidity
		Male
		Difficulty with erections:
		    developing
		    maintaining
		Female
		Difficulty with:
		    Vaginal dryness
		    Lack of adequate lubrication

# Symptoms Needed	≥1 during most sexual encounters	
Exclusions (not result of):	Relationship problem Substance use (including prescribed meds) Another medical condition Another psychiatric condition	
Psychosocial Impact	Marked distress	
Symptom Specifiers	Generalized vs. Situational	
Severity Specifiers	**Mild:** causes mild distress **Moderate:** causes moderate distress **Severe:** causes severe distress	
Course Specifiers	Lifelong vs. Acquired	
Comments		Note: ICD-10 classifies this diagnosis as including male erectile disorder as well as female sexual arousal disorder

spontaneous erections at times when he does not plan to have intercourse, having morning erections, or having good erections with masturbation or with partners other than his usual one, the physiologic causes of his erectile disorder can be considered negligible, and he can avoid costly diagnostic procedures. Male erectile disorder caused by a general medical condition or a pharmacologic substance is discussed later in this section.

A man may be unable to express a sexual impulse because of fear, anxiety, anger, or moral prohibition. In an ongoing relationship, the disorder may reflect difficulties between the partners, mainly when a man cannot communicate his needs or his anger directly and constructively. Also, episodes of erectile disorder are reinforcing, with the man becoming increasingly anxious before each sexual encounter.

Mr. Y came for therapy after his wife complained about their lack of sexual interaction. The patient avoided sex because of his frequent erectile dysfunction and the painful feelings of inadequacy he suffered after his "failures." He presented as an articulate, gentle, and self-blaming man.

He was faithful to his wife but masturbated frequently. His fantasies involved explicit sadistic components, including hanging and biting women. The contrast between his angry, aggressive fantasies and his loving, considerate behavior toward his wife symbolized his conflicts about his sexuality, his masculinity, and his mixed feelings about women. The physician diagnosed him with erectile disorder, situational type.

Orgasm Disorders

Female Orgasmic Disorder.   Female orgasmic disorder, sometimes called *inhibited female orgasm* or *anorgasmia,* is defined as the

recurrent or persistent inhibition of female orgasm, as manifested by the recurrent delay in, or absence of, orgasm after a normal sexual excitement phase that a clinician judges to be adequate in focus, intensity, and duration—in short, a woman's inability to achieve orgasm by masturbation or coitus (Table 16-5). Women who can achieve orgasm by one of these methods are not necessarily categorized as anorgasmic, although there may be some sexual inhibition. Some anorgasmic women are not distressed by the lack of climax and derive pleasure from sexual activity. However, the woman may still present for treatment as her partner is distressed by her apparent disinterest.

Research on the physiology of the female sexual response has shown that orgasms caused by clitoral stimulation and those caused by vaginal stimulation are physiologically identical. Many women achieve orgasm during coitus by a combination of manual clitoral stimulation and penile vaginal stimulation.

A woman with a lifelong female orgasmic disorder has never experienced orgasm by any kind of stimulation. A woman with an acquired orgasmic disorder has previously experienced at least one orgasm, regardless of the circumstances or means of stimulation, whether by masturbation or while dreaming during sleep. Studies have shown that women achieve orgasm more consistently with masturbation than with partnered sex. Lifelong female orgasmic disorder is more common among unmarried women than married women. Increased orgasmic potential in women older than 35 years of age may relate to less psychologic inhibition, greater sexual experience, or both.

Acquired female orgasmic disorder is a common complaint in clinical populations. One clinical treatment facility reported having about four times as many nonorgasmic women in its practice as

Table 16-5
Female Orgasmic Disorder

	DSM-5	ICD-10
Name	Female Orgasmic Disorder	Orgasmic dysfunction
Duration	≥6 mo	

Symptoms	Difficulties with orgasms
	  Delayed/reduced frequency
	  Reduced intensity
		Marked delay or absence of orgasm

# Symptoms Needed	≥1 during most sexual encounters	
Exclusions (not result of):	Relationship problem Substance use (including prescribed meds) Another medical condition Another psychiatric condition	Another medical condition
Psychosocial Impact	Marked distress	
Symptom Specifiers	Generalized vs. Situational	
Severity Specifiers	**Mild:** causes mild distress **Moderate:** causes moderate distress **Severe:** causes severe distress	
Course Specifiers	Lifelong vs. Acquired Never experienced an orgasm under any conditions	
Comments		Note: ICD 10 classifies orgasmic dysfunction as occurring in men and women, including delayed ejaculation in this category as per Table 16-6

female patients with all other sexual disorders. In another study, 46 percent of women complained of difficulty reaching orgasm. Inhibition of arousal and orgasmic problems often occur together. The overall prevalence of female orgasmic disorder from all causes is estimated to be 30 percent. Orgasmic dysfunction in some females may have a genetic basis and cannot be attributed solely to psychologic differences. That study demonstrated an estimated heritability for difficulty reaching orgasm with intercourse of 34 percent and an estimated heritability in women who could not climax with masturbation of 45 percent.

Numerous psychological factors are associated with female orgasmic disorder. They include fears of impregnation, rejection by a sex partner, and damage to the vagina; hostility toward men; poor body image; and feelings of guilt about sexual impulses. Some women equate orgasm with loss of control or with aggressive, destructive, or violent impulses; they may express their fear of these impulses through inhibition of arousal or orgasm. Cultural expectations and social restrictions on women are also relevant. Despite the sexual revolution of the 1960s, many women in the United States still grow to believe that sexual pleasure is not a natural entitlement for so-called decent women. Nonorgasmic women may be otherwise symptom-free or may experience frustration in a variety of ways; they may have such pelvic complaints as lower abdominal pain, itching, and vaginal discharge, as well as increased tension, irritability, and fatigue.

Delayed Ejaculation.   In male delayed ejaculation, sometimes called *retarded ejaculation,* a man achieves ejaculation during coitus with great difficulty, if at all (Table 16-6). The problem is rarely present with masturbation but appears as a problem during partnered sex. A man with lifelong delayed ejaculation has never been able to ejaculate during partnered sexual activity. The problem is usually most pronounced during coital activity. We would consider the disorder to be acquired if it develops after previously normal functioning. Some researchers think that orgasm and ejaculation should be differentiated, especially in the case of men who ejaculate but complain of a decreased or absent subjective sense of pleasure during the orgasmic experience (orgasmic anhedonia).

The incidence of male orgasmic disorder is much lower than the incidence of premature ejaculation or erectile disorder. The prevalence is about 5 percent. However, there may be an increase in this disorder presenting to sex therapy programs. An increase in antidepressant use may be one explanation for this. Another is the high use of Internet pornography. These sites offer a level of stimulation involving such a variety of people and acts that they may inure the man to the stimulation of more typical partnered activity. Some studies of adolescent males who use these sites frequently, before live sexual interaction, have reported that these teens do not develop neuronal synapses that will enable them to respond to usual partnered interactions with sufficient pleasure to allow them to achieve climax.

Lifelong delayed ejaculation indicates severe psychopathology. A man may come from a rigid, puritanical background; he may perceive sex as sinful and the genitals as dirty, and he may have conscious or unconscious incest wishes and guilt. He usually has difficulty with closeness in areas beyond those of sexual relations. In a few cases, an attention-deficit/hyperactivity disorder may aggravate the condition. A man's distractibility prevents sufficient arousal for climax to occur.

In an ongoing relationship, acquired male delayed ejaculation disorder frequently reflects interpersonal difficulties. The disorder may be a man's way of coping with real or fantasized changes in a relationship, such as plans for pregnancy about which the man is ambivalent, the loss of sexual attraction to the partner, or demands by the partner for greater commitment as expressed by sexual

Table 16-6
Delayed Ejaculation

	DSM-5	ICD-10
Name	Delayed Ejaculation	Orgasmic dysfunction
Duration	≥6 mo	
Symptoms	Difficulty with ejaculations: Delayed Absent or reduced frequency	Marked delay or absence of orgasm
# Symptoms Needed	≥1	
Exclusions (not result of):	Relationship problem Substance use (including prescribed meds) Another medical condition Another psychiatric condition	Another medical condition
Psychosocial Impact	Marked distress	
Symptom Specifiers	Generalized vs. Situational	
Severity Specifiers	**Mild:** causes mild distress **Moderate:** causes moderate distress **Severe:** causes severe distress	
Course Specifiers	Lifelong vs. Acquired	
Comments		Note: ICD 10 classifies orgasmic dysfunction as occurring in men and women, including delayed ejaculation in this category as per Table 16-5

performance. In some men, the inability to ejaculate reflects unexpressed hostility toward a woman. The problem is more common among men with obsessive-compulsive disorder (OCD) than among others.

> A couple presented with the man as the identified patient; he was unable to ejaculate with intercourse. He had always had difficulty reaching climax, except in rare circumstances. He ejaculated once when he was with two women at the same time and once when he was experimenting with cocaine. He currently was not using any substances except for moderate use of alcohol. This patient was committed to his marriage, although he had extramarital sexual experiences. He did not ejaculate with coitus in those situations either, although he could climax with oral sex. He stated he was more interested in "the conquest" than in the sex itself. He could climax with masturbation, although he rarely masturbated himself, but went to massage parlors. He had issues with anger at women and considered his wife to be excessively critical.
>
> He had difficulty doing any of the exercises that required him to pleasure his wife. His difficulty giving also made it hard for him to enjoy mutual pleasuring. It was easier for him to be the recipient of stimulation. Because of this patient's problems with impulsiveness, narcissism, and dependency, it was necessary to combine introspective psychotherapy with a regimen of behavioral exercises.
>
> The psychiatrist diagnosed the patient with delayed ejaculation, lifelong type.

Premature (Early) Ejaculation. In premature ejaculation, men persistently or recurrently achieve orgasm and ejaculation before they wish to. The diagnosis occurs when a man regularly ejaculates before or within approximately 1 minute after penetration. DSM-5 refers only to "vaginal penetration" in its diagnostic criteria, even though the disorder can occur in gay men or those who do not engage in vaginal penetration for other reasons. DSM-5 defines the disorder as mild if ejaculation occurs within

approximately 30 seconds to 1 minute of vaginal penetration, moderate if ejaculation occurs within approximately 15 to 30 seconds of vaginal penetration, and severe when ejaculation occurs at the start of sexual activity or within approximately 15 seconds of vaginal penetration. A difficulty with these specifiers involves time distortions, which patients make in both overestimating and underestimating time from penetration to climax. Clinicians need to consider factors that affect the duration of the excitement phase of the sexual response, such as age, the novelty of the sex partner, and the frequency of coitus (Table 16-7). As with the other sexual dysfunctions, we would not diagnose premature ejaculation when it is caused exclusively by organic factors or when it is symptomatic of another clinical psychiatric syndrome.

Premature ejaculation appears to be more common among college-educated men than among men with less education. The complaint is likely related to their concern for partner satisfaction, although data is limited, and we do not know for sure. Premature ejaculation is the chief complaint of about 35 to 40 percent of men treated for sexual disorders. In DSM-5, the writers state that the disorder, with its newly defined time parameter, would now be an accurate diagnosis for only 1 to 3 percent of men. Some researchers divide men who experience premature ejaculation into two groups: those who are physiologically predisposed to climax quickly because of shorter nerve latency time and those with a psychogenic or behaviorally conditioned cause. Difficulty in ejaculatory control can be associated with anxiety regarding the sex act, with unconscious fears about the vagina, or with negative cultural conditioning. Men whose early sexual contacts occurred mainly with sex workers who demanded that the sex act proceed quickly or whose sexual contacts took place in situations in which discovery would be embarrassing (e.g., in a shared dormitory room or the parental home) may be conditioned to orgasm rapidly. With young, inexperienced men, who have the problem, it may resolve in time. In ongoing relationships, the partner has a significant influence on a

Table 16-7
Premature (Early) Ejaculation

	DSM-5	ICD-10
Name	Premature (Early) Ejaculation	Premature ejaculation
Duration	≥6 mo	
Symptoms	Ejaculation occurs Within 1 min of penetration Before it was intended	Difficulty controlling ejaculation
# Symptoms Needed	Above occurs in most sexual encounters	
Exclusions (not result of):	Relationship problem Substance use (including prescribed meds) Another medical condition Another psychiatric condition	
Psychosocial Impact	Marked distress	Both partners do not sufficiently enjoy the sexual encounter
Symptom Specifiers	Generalized vs. Situational	
Severity Specifiers	Defined by time from penetration until ejaculation: **Mild:** 30 s–1 min **Moderate:** 15–30 s **Severe:** <15 s	
Course Specifiers	Lifelong vs. Acquired	

premature ejaculator, and a stressful marriage exacerbates the disorder. The developmental background and the psychodynamics found in premature ejaculation and erectile disorder are similar.

The focus of this diagnosis is on males, and data on premature female orgasm are lacking. There are some case reports of, for example, multiple spontaneous orgasms without sexual stimulation. In some cases, an epileptogenic focus may be the cause. There are also some rare case reports of spontaneous orgasms in women taking serotonergic antidepressants.

Orgasmic Anhedonia.

Orgasmic anhedonia is a condition in which a person has no physical sensation of orgasm, even though the physiologic component (e.g., ejaculation) remains intact. Organic causes, such as sacral and cephalic lesions that interfere with afferent pathways from the genitalia to the cortex, must be ruled out. Psychiatric causes usually relate to extreme guilt about experiencing sexual pleasure. These feelings produce a dissociative response that isolates the affective component of the orgasmic experience from consciousness. In DSM-5 this would be diagnosed as an "other specified sexual dysfunction."

Sexual Pain Disorders

Genito-Pelvic Pain/Penetration Disorder.

In DSM-5, this disorder refers to one or more of the following complaints, of which any two or more may occur together: difficulty having intercourse, genito-pelvic pain, fear of pain or penetration, and tension of the pelvic floor muscles (Table 16-8). Previously, we diagnosed these

pain disorders as *dyspareunia* or *vaginismus*. These former diagnoses could coexist, or one could lead to the other and could understandably lead to fear of pain with sex. Thus, it is reasonable to gather these diagnoses into one diagnostic category. For this clinical discussion, however, the distinct categories of dyspareunia and vaginismus remain clinically useful.

DYSPAREUNIA. Dyspareunia is recurrent or persistent genital pain occurring before, during, or after intercourse. Dyspareunia is related to and often coincides with vaginismus. Repeated episodes of vaginismus can lead to dyspareunia and vice versa; in either case, we should rule out somatic causes, or lack of lubrication. Perhaps 5 percent of women in North America report recurrent pain during intercourse.

In most cases, dynamic factors are considered causative. Chronic pelvic pain is a common complaint in women with a history of rape or childhood sexual abuse. Painful coitus can result from tension and anxiety about the sex act that causes women to contract their pelvic floor muscles involuntarily. The pain is real and makes intercourse unpleasant or unbearable. The anticipation of further pain may cause women to avoid coitus altogether. If a partner proceeds with intercourse regardless of a woman's state of readiness, this aggravates the condition. There is an increase in reported dyspareunia postmenopausally due to hormonally induced physiologic changes in the vagina; however, specific complaints of difficulty having intercourse occur more often in premenopausal women. There is some increase in dyspareunia in the immediate postpartum population, but it is usually temporary. Dyspareunia may present as any of the four complaints listed under genito-pelvic pain/penetration disorder, and we would diagnose this as a genito-pelvic pain/penetration disorder.

VAGINISMUS. Vaginismus is a constriction of the outer third of the vagina due to involuntary pelvic floor muscle tightening or spasm. It then interferes with penile insertion and intercourse. This response may occur during a gynecologic examination when involuntary vaginal constriction prevents the introduction of the speculum into the vagina. We would not make the diagnosis when the dysfunction is caused exclusively by organic factors or when it is symptomatic of another mental disorder.

Vaginismus may be complete; that is, no penetration of the vagina is possible, whether by the penis, fingers, a speculum during a gynecologic examination, or even if the woman tries to use the smallest size tampon. Many women who discover this when they become sexually active have avoided the use of tampons previously. In a less severe form of vaginismus, pelvic floor muscle tightening due to pain or fear of pain makes penetration difficult, but not impossible. Penetration may be achieved with the smallest size speculum or little fingers. In mild cases, the muscles relax after the initial difficulty with penetration, and the woman can continue with sexual play, sometimes even with coitus.

Miss B was a 27-year-old single woman who presented for therapy because of an inability to have intercourse. She described episodes with a recent boyfriend in which he had tried vaginal penetration but had been unable to enter. The boyfriend did not have erectile dysfunction. Miss B experienced desire and was able to achieve orgasm through manual or oral stimulation. For almost a year, she and her boyfriend had sex play without intercourse. However, he complained increasingly about his frustration at the lack of coitus, which he had enjoyed in previous relationships. Miss B had a conscious fear of penetration and dreaded going to the gynecologist, although she was able to use tampons when she menstruated. Her therapist diagnosed her with genito-pelvic pain/penetration disorder, lifelong type.

Table 16-8
Genito-Pelvic Pain/Penetration Disorder

	DSM-5	ICD-10
Name	**Genito-Pelvic Pain/Penetration Disorder**	**Nonorganic vaginismus** **Nonorganic dyspareunia**
Duration	≥6 mo	

Symptoms	During vaginal penetration, the woman experiences
	  Difficulties with penetration
	  Pain
	Associated symptoms during or in anticipation of penetration:
	  Fear or anxiety
	  Tension or tightening of pelvic muscles
		Vaginismus: spasm of pelvic floor muscles around the vagina, causing pain and difficulties with penetration
		Dyspareunia: pain or discomfort related to penile penetration or intercourse

# Symptoms Needed	One or more of the above	
Exclusions (not result of):	Relationship problem Substance use (including prescribed meds) Another medical condition Another psychiatric condition	Another medical condition
Psychosocial Impact	Marked distress	
Symptom Specifiers		
Severity Specifiers	**Mild:** causes mild distress **Moderate:** causes moderate distress **Severe:** causes severe distress	
Course Specifiers	Lifelong vs. Acquired	

Vaginismus is less prevalent than female orgasmic disorder. It most often afflicts highly educated women and those in high socioeconomic groups. Women with vaginismus may consciously wish to have coitus, but unconsciously wish to keep a penis from entering their bodies. Sexual trauma, such as rape, may cause vaginismus. The anticipation of pain at the first coital experience may cause vaginismus. Clinicians have noted that a strict religious upbringing in which the patient associates sex with sin is frequent in these patients. Other women have problems in dyadic relationships; if women feel emotionally abused by their partners, they may protest in this nonverbal fashion. Some women who have experienced significant pain in childhood due to surgical or dental interventions become guarded about any breach of body integrity and develop vaginismus. Vaginismus may present as any of the four complaints under genito-pelvic pain/penetration disorder, and we should diagnose this as genito-pelvic pain/penetration disorder.

Postcoital Headache. Postcoital headache, characterized by headache immediately after coitus, may last for several hours. It is usually described as throbbing and localized to the occipital or frontal area. The cause is unknown. There may be vascular, muscle contraction (tension), or psychogenic causes. Coitus may precipitate migraine or cluster headaches in predisposed persons. In DSM-5 this disorder would not be included among the above pain disorders as the pain is not directly associated with the sexual act. When it is a source of distress or dysfunction, we list it as an "other specified sexual dysfunction."

Sexual Dysfunction due to a General Medical Condition

Male Erectile Disorder due to a General Medical Condition.
The incidence of psychological male erectile disorder

has been the focus of many studies. Statistics indicate that 20 to 50 percent of men with erectile disorder have an organic basis for the disorder. A physiologic etiology is more likely in men older than 50 and the most likely cause in men older than age 60. Table 16-9 lists the medical causes of male erectile disorder. Side effects of medication can impair male sexual functioning in a variety of ways (Table 16-10). Castration (removal of the testes) does not always lead to sexual dysfunction because erection may still occur. A reflex arc, fired when stimulating the inner thigh, passes through the sacral cord erectile center to account for the phenomenon.

Several procedures, benign and invasive, are used to help differentiate the causes of erectile disorder. The procedures include monitoring nocturnal penile tumescence (erections that occur during sleep), generally associated with rapid eye movement; monitoring tumescence with a strain gauge; measuring blood pressure in the penis with a penile plethysmograph or an ultrasound (Doppler) flowmeter, both of which assess blood flow in the internal pudendal artery; and measuring pudendal nerve latency time. Other diagnostic tests that delineate physiologic bases for impotence include glucose tolerance tests, plasma hormone assays, liver and thyroid function tests, prolactin and follicle-stimulating hormone (FSH) determinations, and cystometric examinations. Invasive diagnostic studies include penile arteriography, infusion cavernosonography, and radioactive xenon penography. Invasive procedures require expert interpretation and are used only for patients who are candidates for vascular reconstructive procedures.

Dyspareunia due to a General Medical Condition.
An estimated 30 percent of all surgical procedures on the female genital area result in temporary dyspareunia. Also, 30 to 40 percent of women with the complaint seen in sex therapy clinics have pelvic

Table 16-9
Diseases and Other Medical Conditions Implicated in Male Erectile Disorder

Infectious and parasitic diseases	Neurologic disorders
Elephantiasis	Multiple sclerosis
Mumps	Transverse myelitis
Cardiovascular disease[a]	Parkinson disease
Atherosclerotic disease	Temporal lobe epilepsy
Aortic aneurysm	Traumatic and neoplastic spinal cord diseases[a]
Leriche syndrome	Central nervous system tumor
Cardiac failure	Amyotrophic lateral sclerosis
Renal and urologic disorders	Peripheral neuropathy
Peyronie disease	General paresis
Chronic renal failure	Tabes dorsalis
Hydrocele and varicocele	Pharmacologic factors
Hepatic disorders	Alcohol and other dependence-inducing substances (heroin, methadone, morphine, cocaine, amphetamines, and barbiturates)
Cirrhosis (usually associated with alcohol dependence)	Prescribed drugs (psychotropic drugs, antihypertensive drugs, estrogens, and antiandrogens)
Pulmonary disorders	Poisoning
Respiratory failure	Lead (plumbism)
Genetics	Herbicides
Klinefelter syndrome	Surgical procedures[a]
Congenital penile vascular and structural abnormalities	Perineal prostatectomy
Nutritional disorders	Abdominal–perineal colon resection
Malnutrition	Sympathectomy (frequently interferes with ejaculation)
Vitamin deficiencies	Aortoiliac surgery
Obesity	Radical cystectomy
Endocrine disorders[a]	Retroperitoneal lymphadenectomy
Diabetes mellitus	Miscellaneous
Dysfunction of the pituitary–adrenal–testis axis	Radiation therapy
Acromegaly	Pelvic fracture
Addison disease	Any severe systemic disease or debilitating condition
Chromophobe adenoma	
Adrenal neoplasia	
Myxedema	
Hyperthyroidism	

[a]In the United States an estimated 2 million men are impotent because they have diabetes mellitus; an additional 300,000 are impotent because of other endocrine diseases; 1.5 million are impotent as a result of vascular disease; 180,000 because of multiple sclerosis; 400,000 because of traumas and fractures leading to pelvic fractures or spinal cord injuries; and another 650,000 are impotent as a result of radical surgery, including prostatectomies, colostomies, and cystectomies.

pathology. Organic abnormalities leading to dyspareunia and vaginismus include irritated or infected hymenal remnants, episiotomy scars, Bartholin gland infection, various forms of vaginitis and cervicitis, endometriosis, and adenomyosis. Women with myomata, endometriosis, and adenomyosis may report postcoital pain owing to the uterine contractions during orgasm. Postmenopausal women may have dyspareunia resulting from thinning of the vaginal mucosa and reduced lubrication.

Two conditions not readily apparent on physical examination that produce dyspareunia are vulvar vestibulitis and interstitial cystitis. The former may present with chronic vulvar pain, and the latter produces pain most intensely following orgasm. Dyspareunia can also occur in men, but it is uncommon and is usually associated with an organic condition, such as Peyronie disease, which consists of sclerotic plaques on the penis that cause penile curvature.

Male Hypoactive Sexual Desire Disorder and Female Interest/Arousal Disorder due to a General Medical Condition.
Sexual desire commonly decreases after major illness or surgery, particularly when the body image is affected after such procedures as mastectomy, ileostomy, hysterectomy, and prostatectomy. Illnesses that deplete a person's energy, chronic conditions that require physical and psychological adaptation, and serious illnesses that can cause a person to become depressed can all markedly lessen sexual desire.

In some cases, biochemical correlates are associated with hypoactive sexual desire disorder (Table 16-11). A recent study found markedly lower levels of serum testosterone in men complaining of low desire than in normal controls in a sleep-laboratory situation. Drugs that depress the central nervous system (CNS) or decrease testosterone production can decrease desire.

Other Male Sexual Dysfunction due to a General Medical Condition.
Delayed ejaculation can have physiologic causes and can occur after surgery on the genitourinary tract, such as prostatectomy. It may also be associated with Parkinson disease and other neurologic disorders involving the lumbar or sacral sections of the spinal cord. The antihypertensive drug guanethidine monosulfate, methyldopa, the phenothiazines, the tricyclic drugs, and the selective serotonin reuptake inhibitors (SSRIs), among others, have been implicated in retarded ejaculation. Also, we should differentiate delayed ejaculation from retrograde ejaculation, in which ejaculation occurs but the seminal fluid passes back into the bladder. Retrograde ejaculation always has an organic cause. It can develop after genitourinary surgery, and it is also associated with medications that have anticholinergic adverse effects, such as the phenothiazines.

Other Female Sexual Dysfunction due to a General Medical Condition.
Some medical conditions—specifically, endocrine diseases such as hypothyroidism, diabetes mellitus,

Table 16-10
Some Pharmacologic Agents Implicated in Male Sexual Dysfunctions

Drug	Impairs Erection	Impairs Ejaculation
Psychiatric drugs		
Cyclic drugs[a]		
Imipramine (Tofranil)	+	+
Protriptyline (Vivactil)	+	+
Desipramine (Pertofrane)	+	+
Clomipramine (Anafranil)	+	+
Amitriptyline (Elavil)	+	+
Trazodone (Desyrel)[b]	−	−
Monoamine oxidase inhibitors		
Tranylcypromine (Parnate)	+	+
Phenelzine (Nardil)	+	+
Pargyline (Eutonyl)	−	+
Isocarboxazid (Marplan)	−	+
Other mood-active drugs		
Lithium (Eskalith)	+	+
Amphetamines	+	+
Fluoxetine (Prozac)[c]	−	+
Antipsychotics[d]		
Fluphenazine (Prolixin)	+	+
Thioridazine (Mellaril)	+	+
Chlorprothixene (Taractan)	−	+
Mesoridazine (Serentil)	−	+
Perphenazine (Trilafon)	−	+
Trifluoperazine (Stelazine)	−	+
Reserpine (Serpasil)	+	+
Haloperidol (Haldol)	−	+
Antianxiety agent[e]		
Chlordiazepoxide (Librium)	−	+
Antihypertensive drugs		
Clonidine (Catapres)	+	+
Methyldopa (Aldomet)	+	+
Spironolactone (Aldactone)	+	−
Hydrochlorothiazide	+	−
Guanethidine (Ismelin)	+	+
Commonly abused substances		
Alcohol	+	+
Barbiturates	+	+
Cannabis	+	−
Cocaine	+	+
Heroin	+	+
Methadone	+	−
Morphine	+	+
Miscellaneous drugs		
Antiparkinsonian agents	+	+
Clofibrate (Atromid-S)	+	−
Digoxin (Lanoxin)	+	−
Glutethimide (Doriden)	+	+
Indomethacin (Indocin)	+	−
Phentolamine (Regitine)	−	+
Propranolol (Inderal)	+	−

[a]The incidence of male erectile disorder associated with the use of tricyclic drugs is low.
[b]Trazodone has been causative in some cases of priapism.
[c]All SSRIs can produce sexual dysfunction, more commonly, in men.
[d]Impairment of sexual function is not a common complication of the use of antipsychotics. Priapism has occasionally occurred in association with the use of antipsychotics.
[e]Benzodiazepines have been reported to decrease libido, but in some patients the diminution of anxiety caused by those drugs enhances sexual function.

and primary hyperprolactinemia—can affect a woman's ability to have orgasms. Several drugs also affect some women's capacity to have orgasms (Table 16-12). Antihypertensive medications, CNS stimulants, tricyclic drugs, SSRIs, and, frequently, monoamine oxidase inhibitors (MAOIs) have interfered with female orgasmic capacity. One study of women taking MAOIs, however, found that after 16 to 18 weeks of pharmacotherapy, the adverse effect of the medication disappeared, and the women were able to reexperience orgasms, although they continued taking an undiminished dose of the drug.

Substance/Medication-Induced Sexual Dysfunction. We diagnose substance-induced sexual dysfunction when evidence of substance intoxication or withdrawal is apparent from the history, physical examination, or laboratory findings. The disturbance in sexual function must be predominant in the clinical picture. Distressing sexual dysfunction occurs soon after significant substance intoxication or withdrawal, or after exposure to a medication or a change in medication use. Specified substances include alcohol, amphetamines or related substances, cocaine, opioids, sedatives, hypnotics, or anxiolytics, and other or unknown substances.

Abused recreational substances affect sexual function in various ways. In small doses, many substances enhance sexual performance by decreasing inhibition or anxiety or by causing a temporary elevation of mood. With continued use, however, erectile engorgement and orgasmic and ejaculatory capacities become impaired. The abuse of sedatives, anxiolytics, hypnotics, and particularly opiates and opioids nearly always depresses desire. Alcohol may foster the initiation of sexual activity by removing inhibition, but it also impairs performance. Cocaine and amphetamines produce the similar effects. Although no direct evidence indicates that sexual drive is enhanced, users initially have feelings of increased energy and may become sexually active; ultimately, dysfunction occurs. Men usually go through two stages: an experience of prolonged erection without ejaculation, and then a gradual loss of erectile capability.

Patients recovering from substance dependency may need therapy to regain sexual function, partly because of psychological readjustment to a nondependent state. Many substance abusers have always had difficulty with intimate interactions. Others who spent their crucial developmental years under the influence of a substance have missed the experiences that would have enabled them to learn social and sexual skills.

Almost every pharmacologic agent, particularly those used in psychiatry, has been associated with an effect on sexuality. In men, these effects include decreased sex drive, erectile failure, decreased volume of ejaculate, and delayed or retrograde ejaculation. In women, decreased sex drive, decreased vaginal lubrication, inhibited or delayed orgasm, and decreased or absent vaginal contractions may occur. Drugs may also enhance sexual responses and increase the sex drive, but this is less common than adverse effects.

ANTIPSYCHOTIC DRUGS. Most antipsychotic drugs are dopamine receptor antagonists that also block adrenergic and cholinergic receptors, thus accounting for the adverse sexual effects (Table 16-13). Chlorpromazine and trifluoperazine are potent anticholinergics, and they impair erection and ejaculation. With some drugs, the seminal fluid backs up into the bladder rather than being propelled through the penile urethra. Patients still have a pleasurable sensation, but the orgasm is dry. When urinating after orgasm, the urine may be milky white because it contains the ejaculate. The condition is startling but harmless. Paradoxically, antipsychotics may rarely cause priapism.

Table 16-11
Neurophysiology of Sexual Dysfunction

	DA	5-HT	NE	ACh	Clinical Correlation
Erection	↑	°	α_1, β $\downarrow \uparrow$	M	Antipsychotics may lead to erectile dysfunction (DA block): DA agonists may lead to enhanced erection and libido; priapism with trazodone (α_1 block); β-blockers may lead to impotence
Ejaculation and orgasm	°	± $\downarrow$	α_1 $\uparrow$	M	α-Blockers (tricyclic drugs, MAOIs, thioridazine) may lead to impaired ejaculation; 5-HT agents may inhibit orgasm

↑, facilities; ↓, inhibits or decreases; ±, some; ACh, acetylcholine; DA, dopamine; 5-HT, serotonin; M, modulates; NE, norepinephrine; °, minimal.
Reprinted with permission from Segraves R. *Psychiatric Times*. 1990.

ANTIDEPRESSANT DRUGS. The tricyclic and tetracyclic antidepressants have anticholinergic effects that interfere with erection and delay ejaculation. Because the anticholinergic effects vary among the cyclic antidepressants, those with the fewest effects (e.g., desipramine) produce the fewest sexual adverse effects.

Some men report increased sensitivity of the glans that is pleasurable, and that does not interfere with erection, although it delays ejaculation. In some cases, however, the tricyclic causes painful ejaculation, perhaps as the result of interference with seminal propulsion caused by interference with, in turn, urethral, prostatic, vas, and epididymal smooth muscle contractions. Clomipramine may increase sex drive in some persons. Selegiline, a selective MAO type B (MAO_B) inhibitor, and bupropion may also increase sex drive, possibly by dopaminergic activity and increased production of norepinephrine.

Venlafaxine and the SSRIs most often have adverse effects because of the rise in serotonin levels. A lowering of the sex drive and difficulty reaching orgasm occur in both sexes. Cyproheptadine, an antihistamine with antiserotonergic effects, and methylphenidate, with adrenergic effects, may reverse those adverse effects. Trazodone is associated with the rare occurrence of priapism, the symptom of prolonged erection in the absence of sexual stimuli. That symptom appears to result from the α_1-adrenergic antagonism of trazodone.

The MAOIs affect biogenic amines broadly. Accordingly, they produce impaired erection, delayed or retrograde ejaculation, vaginal dryness, and inhibited orgasm. Tranylcypromine has a paradoxical sexually stimulating effect in some persons, possibly as a result of its amphetamine-like properties.

Mr. W presented with the complaint of inability to achieve orgasm. His problem dated from the time, 18 months previously, when he started fluoxetine. Before that time, he had been able to achieve orgasm through masturbation and coitus with his wife.

Mr. W tried several other SSRIs, as well as venlafaxine, but the side effect of delayed ejaculation persisted. None of the usual antidotes to SSRI-induced anorgasmia proved effective, and the patient then tried antidepressants of other categories. Mr. W was able to respond to bupropion and clonazepam. This combination treated his depression and anxiety, and his delayed ejaculation resolved.

His psychiatrist diagnosed pharmacologically induced delayed ejaculation.

Table 16-12
Some Pharmacologic Agents Implicated in Inhibited Female Orgasm[a]

Tricyclic antidepressants
　Imipramine (Tofranil)
　Clomipramine (Anafranil)
　Nortriptyline (Aventyl)

Monoamine oxidase inhibitors
　Tranylcypromine (Parnate)
　Phenelzine (Nardil)
　Isocarboxazid (Marplan)

Dopamine receptor antagonists
　Thioridazine (Mellaril)
　Trifluoperazine (Stelazine)

Selective serotonin reuptake inhibitors
　Fluoxetine (Prozac)
　Paroxetine (Paxil)
　Sertraline (Zoloft)
　Fluvoxamine (Luvox)
　Citalopram (Celexa)

[a]The interrelation between female sexual dysfunction and pharmacologic agents has been less extensively evaluated than male reactions. Oral contraceptives are reported to decrease libido in some women, and some drugs with anticholinergic side effects may impair arousal as well as orgasm. Prolonged use of oral contraceptives may also cause physiologic menopausal-like changes resulting in genito-pelvic pain/penetration disorder. Benzodiazepines have been reported to decrease libido, but in some patients the diminution of anxiety caused by those drugs enhances sexual function. Both increase and decrease in libido have been reported with psychoactive agents. It is difficult to separate those effects from the underlying condition or from improvement of the condition. Sexual dysfunction associated with the use of a drug disappears when use of the drug is discontinued.

Table 16-13
Diagnostic Issues with Sex and Some Antipsychotic Drugs

Differential diagnosis of drug-induced sexual dysfunction	Problem after drug therapy started or drug overdose Problem not situation or partner specific Not a lifelong or recurrent problem No obvious nonpharmacologic precipitant Dissipates with drug discontinuation
Antipsychotic drugs and ejaculatory problems	Perphenazine Chlorpromazine Trifluoperazine Haloperidol Mesoridazine Chlorprothixene
Antipsychotic drugs and priapism	Perphenazine Mesoridazine Chlorpromazine Thioridazine Fluphenazine Molindone Risperidone Clozapine

Table by R. T. Seagraves, M.D.

Because depression is associated with decreased libido, varying levels of sexual dysfunction and anhedonia are part of the disease process. Some patients report improved sexual functioning as their depression improves because of antidepressant medication. The phenomenon makes evaluating sexual side effects difficult; also, the side effects may disappear with time, perhaps because a biogenic amine homeostatic mechanism comes into play.

LITHIUM. Lithium regulates mood and, in the manic state, may reduce hypersexuality, possibly by a dopamine antagonist activity. Some patients may have impaired erections.

SYMPATHOMIMETICS. Psychostimulants, including amphetamines, methylphenidate, and pemoline, raise the plasma levels of norepinephrine and dopamine. They can increase libido. However, with prolonged use, men may experience a loss of desire and erections.

α-ADRENERGIC AND β-ADRENERGIC RECEPTOR ANTAGONISTS. α-Adrenergic and β-adrenergic receptor antagonists, used in the treatment of hypertension, angina, and certain cardiac arrhythmias, diminish tonic sympathetic nerve outflow from vasomotor centers in the brain. As a result, they can cause impotence, decrease the volume of ejaculate, and produce retrograde ejaculation. They can affect libido in both sexes.

ANTICHOLINERGICS. The anticholinergics block cholinergic receptors and include such drugs as amantadine and benztropine. They produce dryness of the mucous membranes (including those of the vagina) and erectile disorder. However, amantadine may reverse SSRI-induced orgasmic dysfunction through its dopaminergic effect.

ANTIHISTAMINES. Drugs such as diphenhydramine have anticholinergic activity and are mildly hypnotic. They may inhibit sexual function as a result. Cyproheptadine, although an antihistamine, also has potent activity as a serotonin antagonist. It can block the serotonergic sexual adverse effects produced by SSRIs, such as delayed orgasm.

ANTIANXIETY AGENTS. The dominant class of anxiolytics is the benzodiazepines. They act on the γ-aminobutyric acid (GABA) receptors, which are involved in cognition, memory, and motor control. Because benzodiazepines decrease plasma epinephrine concentrations, they diminish anxiety, and as a result, they improve sexual function in persons inhibited by anxiety.

ALCOHOL. Alcohol suppresses CNS activity generally and can produce erectile disorders in men as a result. Alcohol has a direct gonadal effect that decreases testosterone levels in men; paradoxically, it can produce a slight rise in testosterone levels in women. The latter finding may account for women who report increased libido after drinking small amounts of alcohol. The long-term use of alcohol reduces the ability of the liver to metabolize estrogenic compounds in men, which produces signs of feminization (such as gynecomastia as a result of testicular atrophy).

OPIOIDS. Opioids, such as heroin, have adverse sexual effects, such as erectile failure and decreased libido. The alteration of consciousness may enhance the sexual experience of occasional users.

HALLUCINOGENS. The hallucinogens include lysergic acid diethylamide (LSD), phencyclidine (PCP), psilocybin (from some mushrooms), and mescaline (from peyote cactus). In addition to inducing hallucinations, the drugs cause loss of contact with reality and an expanding and heightening of consciousness. Some users report that the sexual experience is similarly enhanced, but others experience anxiety, delirium, or psychosis, which interfere with sexual function.

CANNABIS. The altered state of consciousness produced by cannabis may enhance sexual pleasure for some persons. Its prolonged use depresses testosterone levels.

BARBITURATES AND SIMILARLY ACTING DRUGS. Barbiturates and similarly acting sedative-hypnotic drugs may enhance sexual responsiveness in persons who are sexually unresponsive as a result of anxiety. They have no direct effect on the sex organs; however, they do produce an alteration in consciousness that some persons find pleasurable. These drugs are subject to abuse, and use can be fatal when combined with alcohol or other CNS depressants.

Methaqualone acquired a reputation as a sexual enhancer, a reputation without basis. It is no longer legally sold in the United States.

Treatment

Before 1970, the most common treatment for sexual dysfunctions was individual psychotherapy. Classic psychodynamic theory holds that sexual inadequacy has its roots in early developmental conflicts, and the therapist treated the sexual disorder as part of a pervasive emotional disturbance. The symptoms of sexual dysfunctions, however, frequently become secondarily autonomous and continue to persist, even when other problems evolving from the patients' pathology have been resolved. The addition of behavioral techniques is often necessary to cure a sexual problem. Depending on the disorder, medications can be a first-line treatment or an adjunct to therapy.

Somatic Treatments. Biologic treatments, including pharmacotherapy, surgery, and mechanical devices, can treat specific cases of sexual disorder. Most of the recent advances involve male sexual dysfunction.

PHARMACOTHERAPY. Medications for erectile disorder include sildenafil and its congeners (Table 16–14), oral phentolamine, alprostadil, and injectable medications. Other options include papaverine, prostaglandin E1, phentolamine, or some combination of these; and transurethral alprostadil (MUSE).

Sildenafil is a nitric oxide enhancer that facilitates the inflow of blood to the penis necessary for an erection. The drug takes effect about 1 hour after ingestion, and its effect can last up to 4 hours. Sildenafil is not effective in the absence of sexual stimulation. The most common adverse events associated with its use are headaches, flushing, and dyspepsia. Persons taking organic nitrates should not take sildenafil, as the combined action of the two drugs can cause sudden, and sometimes fatal, drops in systemic blood pressure. Sildenafil is not effective in all cases of erectile dysfunction. It fails to produce an erection that is sufficiently rigid for penetration in about 50 percent of men who have had radical prostate surgery or in those with long-standing insulin-dependent diabetes. It is also ineffective in some instances of nerve damage.

A small number of patients developed nonarteritic ischemic optic neuropathy (NAION) soon after using sildenafil. This side effect may be more common in patients with cardiovascular risk factors. Although rare, sildenafil may provoke NAION in individuals with an arteriosclerotic risk profile. Exceedingly rare cases of hearing loss may also occur.

Sildenafil use in women results in vaginal lubrication, but not in increased desire. Anecdotal reports, however, describe individual women who have experienced intensified excitement with sildenafil.

Oral phentolamine and apomorphine are not FDA approved at present but have proved useful as potency enhancers in men with minimal erectile dysfunction. Phentolamine reduces sympathetic tone and relaxes corporeal smooth muscle. Adverse events include

Table 16-14
Pharmacokinetics of the PDE-5 Inhibitors

		Sildenafil (Viagra)	Vardenafil (Levitra)	Vardenafil ODT (Staxyn)	Tadalafil (Cialis)	Avanafil (Stendra)
Recommended dose (mg/day)		25–100	5–20	10	5–20	100–200
Time to peak concentration (hr)		0.5–2	0.5–2	0.75–2.5	0.5–6	0.5–0.75
Half-life (hr)		4	4–5	4–6	17.5	3–5
Usual duration of action (hr)		12		12	36	6
Delay after high fat meal (hr)		1		1	0	1–1.25
Metabolism	Major enzyme			CYP3A4		
	Additional enzymes	CYP2C9		CYP3A5, CYP2C	CYP3A5, CYP2C	CYP2C
Elimination (%)	Feces	80		91–95	61	62
	Urine	13		2–6	36	21

Sources: Prescriber's Digital Reference, https://www.pdr.net/; Huang SA, Lie JD. Phosphodiesterase-5 (PDE5) Inhibitors in the management of erectile dysfunction. *P T.* 2013;38(7):407–419; Katz EG, Tan RB, Rittenberg D, Hellstrom WJ. Avanafil for erectile dysfunction in elderly and younger adults: differential pharmacology and clinical utility. *Ther Clin Risk Manag.* 2014;10:701–711.

hypotension, tachycardia, and dizziness. Apomorphine effects are mediated by the autonomic nervous system and result in vasodilation that facilitates the inflow of blood to the penis. Adverse events include nausea and sweating.

In contrast to the oral medications, injectable and transurethral forms of alprostadil act locally on the penis and can produce erections in the absence of sexual stimulation. Alprostadil contains a naturally occurring form of prostaglandin E, a vasodilating agent. Alprostadil may be administered by direct injection into the corpora cavernosa or by intraurethral insertion of a pellet through a cannula. The firm erection produced within 2 to 3 minutes after administration of the drug may last as long as 1 hour. Infrequent and reversible adverse effects of injections include penile bruising and changes in liver function test results. Possible hazardous sequelae exist, including priapism and sclerosis of the small veins of the penis. Users of transurethral alprostadil sometimes complain of burning sensations in the penis.

Two small trials found different topical agents effective in alleviating erectile dysfunction. One cream consists of three vasoactive substances absorbed through the skin: aminophylline, isosorbide dinitrate, and co-dergocrine mesylate, which is a mixture of ergot alkaloids. The other is a gel containing alprostadil and an additional ingredient, which temporarily makes the outer layer of the skin more permeable.

Also, a cream incorporating alprostadil exists for female sexual arousal disorder. Vaginally applied phentolamine mesylate, an α-receptor antagonist, can increase vasocongestion and a subjective sense of arousal. Flibanserin is also FDA-approved to increase desire in women.

The pharmacologic treatments described in the preceding text are useful in the treatment of arousal dysfunction of various causes: neurogenic, arterial insufficiency, venous leakage, psychogenic, and mixed. When coupled with insight-oriented or behavioral sex therapy, the use of medications can reverse psychogenic arousal disorder that is resistant to psychotherapy alone, the ultimate goal being pharmacologically unassisted sexual functioning.

Other Pharmacologic Agents. Numerous other pharmacologic agents have been used to treat various sexual disorders. Intravenous methohexital sodium assists with desensitization therapy. Antianxiety agents may have some application for tense patients.

The side effects of antidepressants, in particular the SSRIs and tricyclic drugs, have been used to prolong the sexual response in patients with premature ejaculation. This approach is particularly useful in patients who are refractory to behavioral techniques. Topical anesthetic creams may help decrease the intravaginal ejaculation latency time (IELT) in cases of premature ejaculation. Antidepressants can help patients who are phobic of sex and in those with posttraumatic stress disorder following rape. Trazodone is an antidepressant that improves nocturnal erections. We should always weigh the risks of taking such medications against their possible benefits. Bromocriptine treats hyperprolactinemia, which is frequently associated with hypogonadism and any associated sexual dysfunction. In such patients, it is necessary to rule out pituitary tumors.

Several substances have popular standing as aphrodisiacs; for example, ginseng root and yohimbine. Studies, however, have not confirmed any aphrodisiac properties. Yohimbine, an α-receptor antagonist, may cause dilation of the penile artery; however, the American Urologic Association does not recommend its use to treat organic erectile dysfunction. Many recreational drugs, including cocaine, amphetamines, alcohol, and cannabis, are considered enhancers of sexual performance. Although they may provide the user with an initial benefit because of their tranquilizing, disinhibiting, or mood-elevating effects, consistent or prolonged use of any of these substances impairs sexual functioning.

Dopaminergic agents may increase libido and improve sex function. Those drugs include L-dopa, a dopamine precursor, and bromocriptine, a dopamine agonist. The antidepressant bupropion has dopaminergic effects and has increased sex drive in some patients. Selegiline, an MAOI, is selective for MAO_B and is dopaminergic. It improves sexual functioning in older persons.

Hormone Therapy. Androgens increase the sex drive in women and men with low testosterone concentrations. Women may experience virilizing effects, some of which are irreversible (e.g., deepening of the voice). In men, prolonged use of androgens produces hypertension and prostatic enlargement. Testosterone is most effective when given parenterally; however, effective oral and transdermal preparations are available.

Women who use estrogens for replacement therapy or contraception may report decreased libido; in such cases, a combined preparation of estrogen and testosterone may help. Estrogen itself prevents thinning of the vaginal mucous membrane and facilitates lubrication. Several forms of locally delivered estrogen—vaginal rings, vaginal creams, and vaginal tablets—provide alternate administration routes to treat women with arousal problems or genital atrophy. Because tablets, creams, and rings do not significantly increase circulating estrogen levels, we should consider these devices for patients with breast cancer with arousal problems.

Antiandrogens and Antiestrogens.   Estrogens and progesterone are antiandrogens that have been used to treat compulsive sexual behavior in men, usually in sex offenders. Clomiphene and tamoxifen are both antiestrogens, and both stimulate gonadotropin-releasing hormone (GnRH) secretion and increase testosterone concentrations, thereby increasing libido. Women treated for breast cancer with tamoxifen report an increased libido. However, tamoxifen may cause uterine cancer.

Mechanical Treatment Approaches.   Male patients with arteriosclerosis (especially of the distal aorta, known as Leriche syndrome), may lose their erection during active pelvic thrusting. The need for increased blood in the gluteal muscles and others served by the ilial or hypogastric arteries takes blood away (steals) from the pudendal artery and, thus, interferes with penile blood flow. They can obtain relief by decreasing pelvic thrusting, which is also aided by the woman's superior coital position.

Vacuum Pump.   Vacuum pumps are mechanical devices that patients without a vascular disease can use to obtain erections. The vacuum draws blood to the penis and kept there by a ring at the base of the penis. This device has no adverse effects, but it is cumbersome, and partners must be willing to accept its use. Some women complain that the penis is redder and cooler than a natural erection or find the process objectionable.

A similar device, called EROS, has been developed to create clitoral erections in women. EROS is a small suction cup that fits over the clitoral region and draws blood into the clitoris. Studies have reported its success in treating female sexual arousal disorder. Vibrators used to stimulate the clitoral area have been successful in treating anorgasmic women.

OTHER SOMATIC TREATMENTS

Male Prostheses.   Surgical treatment is rarely indicated, but penile prosthetic devices are available for men with inadequate erectile responses who are resistant to other treatment methods or who have medically caused deficiencies. The two main types of prostheses are (1) a semi-rigid rod prosthesis that produces a permanent erection that can be positioned close to the body for concealment and (2) an inflatable type that is implanted with its reservoir and pump for inflation and deflation. The latter type can mimic normal physiologic functioning.

Vascular Surgery.   When vascular insufficiency is present due to atherosclerosis or other blockages, bypass surgery of penile arteries may help in selected cases.

Psychosocial Treatments

DUAL-SEX THERAPY.   The theoretical basis of dual-sex therapy is the concept of the marital unit or dyad as the object of therapy; the approach represented the significant advance in the diagnosis and treatment of sexual disorders in the 20th century. The methodology was originated and developed by Masters and Johnson. In dual-sex therapy, when a dysfunctional person is in a relationship, the couple must be treated. Because both are involved in a sexually distressing situation, both must participate in the therapy program. The sexual problem often reflects other areas of disharmony or

misunderstanding in the relationship so that the entire relationship is treated, with emphasis on the sexual functioning of the partners.

The keystone of the program is the roundtable session in which a male and female therapy team clarifies, discusses, and works through problems with the couple. The four-way sessions require active participation by the patients. Therapists and patients discuss the psychological and physiologic aspects of sexual functioning, and therapists have an educative attitude. Therapists suggest specific sexual activities for the couple to follow in the privacy of their home. The therapy aims to establish or reestablish communication within the partner unit. Sex is emphasized as a natural function that flourishes in the appropriate domestic climate, and improved communication is encouraged toward that end. In a variation of this therapy that has proved useful, one therapist may treat the couple. Treatment is short term and is behaviorally oriented. The therapists attempt to reflect the situation as they see it, rather than interpret underlying dynamics. An undistorted picture of the relationship presented by the therapists often corrects the myopic, narrow view held by each partner. This new perspective can interrupt the couple's destructive pattern of relating and can encourage improved, more effective communication. Specific exercises are prescribed for the couple to treat their particular problems. Sexual inadequacy often involves a lack of information, misinformation, and performance fear. Therefore, the therapist prohibits any sexual play other than what was prescribed. Beginning exercises usually focus on heightening sensory awareness to touch, sight, sound, and smell. Initially, the therapist also prohibits intercourse, and the couple learns to give and receive bodily pleasure without the pressure of performance or penetration. At the same time, they learn how to communicate nonverbally in a mutually satisfactory way, and they learn that sexual foreplay is an enjoyable alternative to intercourse and orgasm.

During the sensate focus exercises, the couple receives much reinforcement to reduce anxiety. They can use fantasies to distract them from obsessive concerns about performance (spectatoring). They should consider the needs of both the dysfunctional partner and the nondysfunctional partner. If either partner becomes sexually excited by the exercises, the other is encouraged to bring them to orgasm by manual or oral means. Open communication and the expression of mutual needs are encouraged. Resistances, such as claims of fatigue or not enough time to complete the exercises, are common and must be dealt with by the therapists. Issues of body image, fear of being touched, and difficulty touching oneself arise frequently. Eventually, the therapy allows genital stimulation in addition to general body stimulation. The couple should sequentially to try various positions for intercourse, without necessarily completing the act, and to use varieties of stimulating techniques before they proceed with intercourse.

Psychotherapy sessions follow each new exercise period, and problems and satisfactions, both sexual and in other areas of the couple's lives, are discussed. The therapist reviews specific instructions and introduces new exercises geared to the individual couple's progress. Gradually, the couple gains confidence and learns to communicate, verbally and sexually. Dual-sex therapy is most effective when sexual dysfunction exists apart from other psychopathology. The more difficult treatment cases involve couples with severe marital discord. Desire disorders are particularly challenging to treat. They require more extended and intensive therapy than some other disorders, and their outcomes vary greatly.

SPECIFIC TECHNIQUES AND EXERCISES.   Various techniques can treat various sexual dysfunctions. In cases of vaginismus, a woman is advised to dilate her vaginal opening with her fingers or with size-graduated dilators. Dilators can also treat cases of dyspareunia.

Sometimes, specially trained physiotherapists can assist the treatment by helping the patients to relax their perineal muscles.

In cases of premature ejaculation, an exercise known as the squeeze technique can raise the threshold of penile excitability. In this exercise, the man or the woman stimulates the erect penis until feeling the earliest sensations of impending ejaculation. At this point, the partner forcefully squeezes the coronal ridge of the glans, diminishing the erection and inhibiting ejaculation. The exercise program eventually raises the threshold of the sensation of ejaculatory inevitability and allows the man to focus on the sensations of arousal without anxiety and develop confidence in his sexual performance. A variant of the exercise is the stop-start technique developed by James H. Semans, in which the woman stops all stimulation of the penis when the man first senses an impending ejaculation without squeezing. Research has shown that the presence or absence of circumcision has no bearing on a man's ejaculatory control; the glans is equally sensitive in the two states. Sex therapy has been most successful in the treatment of premature ejaculation.

A man with a sexual desire disorder or male erectile disorder can masturbate to prove that full erection and ejaculation are possible. Delayed ejaculation is managed initially by extravaginal ejaculation and then by gradual vaginal entry after stimulation to a point near ejaculation. Most importantly, the early exercises forbid ejaculation to remove the pressure to climax and allow the man to immerse himself in sexual pleasuring.

In cases of lifelong female orgasmic disorder, the woman is directed to masturbate, sometimes using a vibrator. The shaft of the clitoris is the masturbatory site most preferred by women, and orgasm depends on adequate clitoral stimulation. An area on the anterior wall of the vagina exists in some women as a site of sexual excitation, known as the *G-spot*, but reports of an ejaculatory phenomenon at orgasm in women following the stimulation of the G-spot is only anecdotal.

BEHAVIOR THERAPY. Behavioral approaches were initially designed for the treatment of phobias but are now used to treat other problems as well. Behavior therapists assume that the patient learns sexual dysfunction as maladaptive behavior, which causes them to fear sexual interaction. Using traditional techniques, therapists set up a hierarchy of anxiety-provoking situations, ranging from least threatening (e.g., the thought of kissing) to most threatening (e.g., the thought of penile penetration). The behavior therapist enables the patient to master the anxiety through a standard program of systematic desensitization, which inhibits the learned anxious response by encouraging behaviors antithetical to anxiety. The patient first deals with the least anxiety-producing situation in fantasy and progresses by steps to the most anxiety-producing situation. Medication, hypnosis, and specialized training in deep muscle relaxation can help with the initial mastery of anxiety.

Assertiveness training can help teach patients to express sexual needs openly and without fear. The patient receives exercises in assertiveness, given in conjunction with sex therapy, and they are encouraged to make sexual requests and to refuse to comply with requests perceived as unreasonable. Sexual exercises may be prescribed for patients to perform at home, and the therapist helps the patient to establish a hierarchy, starting with those activities that have proved most pleasurable and successful in the past.

One treatment variation involves the participation of the patient's sexual partner in the desensitization program. The partner, rather than the therapist, presents items of increasing stimulation value to the patient. A cooperative partner is necessary to help the patient carry gains made during treatment sessions to sexual activity at home.

Couples who regularly practice assigned exercises appear to have a much higher likelihood of success than do more resistant couples or those whose interaction involves sadomasochistic or depressive features or mechanisms of blame and projection. Attitude flexibility is also a favorable prognostic factor. Overall, younger couples tend to complete sex therapy more often than older couples. Couples whose interactional difficulties center on their sex problems, such as inhibition, frustration, or fear of performance failure, are also likely to respond well to therapy.

MINDFULNESS. Mindfulness is a cognitive technique that has been helpful in the treatment of sexual dysfunction. The patient focuses on the moment and maintains an awareness of sensations—visual, tactile, auditory, and olfactory—that he or she experiences in the moment. The aim is to distract the patient from "spectatoring" (watching him or herself) and center the person on the sensations that lead to arousal or orgasm. Hopefully, this shift in focus allows patients to become immersed in the pleasure of the experience and remove themselves from self-judgment and performance anxiety.

GROUP THERAPY. Group therapy helps to examine both intrapsychic and interpersonal problems in patients with sexual disorders. A therapy group provides a strong support system for a patient who feels ashamed, anxious, or guilty about a particular sexual problem. It is a useful forum in which to counteract sexual myths, correct misconceptions, and provide accurate information about sexual anatomy, physiology, and varieties of behavior.

One can organize the groups in several ways. Members may all share the same problem, such as premature ejaculation; members may all be of the same sex with different sexual problems, or groups may be composed of both men and women who are experiencing a variety of sexual problems. Group therapy can be an adjunct to other forms of therapy or the prime mode of treatment. Groups organized to treat a particular dysfunction are usually behavioral in approach.

Groups composed of married couples with sexual dysfunctions are also useful. A group provides the opportunity to gather accurate information, offers consensual validation of individual preferences, and enhances self-esteem and self-acceptance. Techniques, such as role-playing and psychodrama, may be used in treatment. Such groups are not indicated for couples when one partner is uncooperative, when a patient has a severe depressive disorder or psychosis, when a patient finds explicit sexual audiovisual material repugnant, or when a patient fears or dislikes groups.

HYPNOTHERAPY. Hypnotherapists focus specifically on the anxiety-producing situation—that is, the sexual interaction that results in dysfunction. The successful use of hypnosis enables patients to gain control over the symptom that has been lowering self-esteem and disrupting psychological homeostasis. The patient's cooperation is first obtained and encouraged during a series of nonhypnotic sessions with the therapist. Those discussions permit the development of a secure doctor–patient relationship, a sense of physical and psychological comfort on the part of the patient, and the establishment of mutually desired treatment goals. During this time, the therapist assesses the patient's capacity for the trance experience. The nonhypnotic sessions also permit the clinician to take a psychiatric history and perform a mental status examination before beginning hypnotherapy. The focus of treatment is on symptom removal and attitude alteration. The patient develops alternative means of dealing with the anxiety-provoking situation, the sexual encounter.

Also, the therapist teaches relaxation techniques for use before sexual relations. With these methods to alleviate anxiety, the physiologic responses to sexual stimulation can more readily result in pleasurable excitation and discharge. The therapy helps to remove psychological impediments to vaginal lubrication, erection, and orgasms so that normal sexual functioning ensues. Hypnosis may be added to a basic individual psychotherapy program to accelerate the effects of psychotherapeutic intervention.

ANALYTICALLY ORIENTED SEX THERAPY.   Some therapists combine sex therapy with psychodynamic psychotherapy. The therapy occurs over a more extended period than usual, which allows learning or relearning of sexual satisfaction under the realities of patients' day-to-day lives. The addition of psychodynamic conceptualizations to behavioral techniques used to treat sexual dysfunctions allows the treatment of patients with sexual disorders associated with other psychopathology.

The material and dynamics that emerge in patients in analytically oriented sex therapy are the same as those in psychoanalytic therapy, such as dreams, fear of punishment, aggressive feelings, difficulty trusting a partner, fear of intimacy, oedipal feelings, and fear of genital mutilation. The combined approach of analytically oriented sex therapy is used by the general psychiatrist, who carefully judges the optimal timing of sex therapy and the ability of patients to tolerate the directive approach that focuses on their sexual difficulties.

PARAPHILIC DISORDERS

Paraphilias or perversions are sexual stimuli or acts that are deviations from normal sexual behaviors but are necessary for some persons to experience arousal and orgasm. DSM-5 only considers this a disorder when a person has acted on the fantasy or impulse, or if the fantasies or impulses lead to significant distress. Individuals with paraphilic interests can experience sexual pleasure, but they do not respond to stimuli that are typically considered erotic. The paraphiliac person's sexuality is mainly restricted to specific deviant stimuli or acts. Persons who occasionally experiment with paraphilic behavior (e.g., infrequent episode of bondage or dressing in costumes), but can respond to more typical erotic stimuli, do not have paraphilic disorders.

Paraphilic disorders can range from nearly normal behavior to behavior that is destructive or hurtful only to a person's self or to a person's self and partner, and finally to behavior that is deemed destructive or threatening to the community at large. DSM-5 lists pedophilia, frotteurism, voyeurism, exhibitionism, sexual sadism, sexual masochism, fetishism, and transvestism with explicit diagnostic criteria because of their threat to others or because they are relatively common paraphilias. Many other paraphilias exist.

A particular fantasy with its unconscious and conscious components is the pathognomonic element of the paraphilia, with sexual arousal and orgasm being associated phenomena that *reinforce the fantasy or impulse.* The influence of these fantasies and their behavioral manifestations often extend beyond the sexual sphere to pervade people's lives.

The primary functions of human sexual behavior are to assist in bonding, to create mutual pleasure in cooperation with a partner, to express and enhance love between two persons, and to procreate.

Paraphilic disorders entail divergent behaviors in that those acts involve aggression, victimization, and extreme one-sidedness. The behaviors exclude or harm others and disrupt the potential for bonding between persons. Moreover, paraphilic sexual scripts often serve other vital psychic functions. They may assuage anxiety, bind aggression, or stabilize identity.

The Clinical Presentation and Diagnosis

In DSM-5, the criteria for paraphilic disorder require the patient to experience intense and recurrent arousal from their deviant fantasy for at least 6 months and to either act on the paraphilic impulse or experience significant distress as a result of the impulse. The fantasy distressing the patient contains unusual sexual material that is relatively fixed and shows only minor variations. Arousal and orgasm depend on the mental elaboration, if not the behavioral playing out of the fantasy. Sexual activity is ritualized or stereotyped and makes use of degraded, reduced, or dehumanized objects.

Exhibitionism

Exhibitionism is the recurrent urge to expose the genitals to a stranger or an unsuspecting person. Sexual excitement occurs in anticipation of the exposure, and orgasm is brought about by masturbation during or after the event. In almost 100 percent of cases, those with exhibitionism are men exposing themselves to women. The dynamic of men with exhibitionism is to assert their masculinity by showing their penises and by watching the victims' reactions—fright, surprise, and disgust. In other related paraphilias, the central themes involve derivatives of looking or showing.

A substance-abusing professional was finally able to attain sobriety at age 33 years. With this accomplishment, he met a woman and got married, began to work steadily for the first time in his life, and was able to impregnate his new wife. His preferred sexual activity had been masturbation in semi-public places. The patient had a strong sense that his mother had always thought him to be inadequate, did not like to spend time with him, and constantly made negative comparisons between him and his "all-boy" younger brother. He recalled several times when his father had tried to explain his mother's antipathy: "It is just one of those things, son: your mother does not seem to like you." Without substance abuse, he gave up his exhibitionism, but he quickly developed sexual incapacity with his wife and became "addicted" to phone sex. (Courtesy of Stephen B. Levine, M.D.)

Specifiers added to exhibitionistic disorder by DSM-5 differentiate between arousal from exposing genitals to prepubertal children, to physically mature individuals, or both (Table 16-15).

Fetishism

In fetishism, the sexual focus is on objects (e.g., shoes, gloves, pantyhose, and stockings) that are intimately associated with the human body, or on nongenital body parts. The latter focus is sometimes called *partialism.* DSM-5 applies the diagnosis of fetishistic disorder to partialism and attaches the following specifiers to fetishistic disorder: body part(s); nonliving parts; other (Table 16-16). The particular fetish used is linked to someone closely involved with a patient during childhood and has a quality associated with

Table 16-15
Exhibitionism

	DSM-5	ICD-10
Name	Exhibitionistic Disorder	Exhibitionism
Duration	≥6 mo	
Symptoms	Sexual arousal/fantasies/ urges/behaviors that result from exposing one's genitals to unsuspecting individuals	Exposing genitals to strangers or in public, often of the opposite sex sexual excitement/ arousal/ masturbation associated
Psychosocial Impact	Marked distress and/ or psychosocial impairment	
Symptom Specifiers	Sexually aroused by: exposing genitals to prepubertal children exposing genitals to physically mature individuals both	
Severity Specifiers	**In a controlled environment** lives in institution/ other controlled environment	
Course Specifiers	**In full remission:** no symptoms or distress for ≥5 yr	

Table 16-16
Fetishism

	DSM-5	ICD-10
Name	Fetishistic Disorder	F65.0 Fetishism
Duration	≥6 mo	
Symptoms	Sexual arousal/fantasies/ urges/behaviors that result from objects/ nongenital body parts	Sexual arousal/ gratification from nonliving objects
Psychosocial Impact	Marked distress and/ or psychosocial impairment	
Exclusions (not result of):	Transvestic disorder Using genital stimulation devices	
Symptom Specifiers	Body Part(s) Nonliving object(s) Other	
Severity Specifiers	**In a controlled environment** (lives in institution/ other controlled environment)	
Course Specifiers	**In full remission:** no symptoms or distress for ≥5 yr	

this loved, needed, or even traumatizing person. Usually, the disorder begins by adolescence, although the fetish may begin in childhood. Once established, the disorder tends to be chronic.

The patient may direct sexual activity at the fetish itself (e.g., masturbation with or into a shoe), or may incorporate the fetish into sexual intercourse (e.g., the demand that high-heeled shoes be worn). The disorder is almost exclusively found in men. Learning theorists believe that the object was associated with sexual stimulation at an early age.

A 50-year-old man entered treatment with a chief complaint of erectile disorder experienced primarily with his wife. He was suffering from a moderate depression that related to both his marital issues and business problems. He had no erectile problems with women he picked up in bars or knew and arranged to meet in bars, partly because where he lived, smoking was allowed in bars. The woman's act of smoking a cigarette was necessary to his sexual arousal. His family history included an alcoholic mother and an emotionally abusive father who was a chain smoker. On family car trips, the father would smoke, with all the car windows up. If the patient complained of feeling nauseous, the father would tell him to "shut up." He recalled being very attracted to a Sunday school teacher who smoked when he was six years old. He first smoked when he was 13, sneaking and hiding behind his house. His first cigarette was one he stole from a pack on his mother's night table.

Frotteurism

Frotteurism is usually characterized by a man's rubbing his penis against the buttocks or other body parts of a fully clothed woman to achieve orgasm (Table 16-17). At other times, he may use his hands to rub an unsuspecting victim. The acts usually occur in crowded places, particularly in subways and buses. Those with frotteurism are passive and isolated, and frottage is often their only source of sexual gratification. The expression of aggression in this paraphilia is readily apparent.

Pedophilia

Pedophilia involves recurrent intense sexual urges toward, or arousal by, children. Per DSM-5, the child must be under 14 years old, and the patient must be at least 16 years old and at least five years older than the victims.

Most child molestations involve genital fondling or oral sex. Vaginal or anal penetration of children infrequently occurs, except in cases of incest. Although most child victims coming to public attention are girls, this finding may be a product of the referral process. Offenders report that when they touch a child, most (60 percent) of the victims are boys. This figure is in sharp contrast to the figure for nontouching victimization of children, such as window peeping and exhibitionism; 99 percent of all such cases occur against girls. DSM-5 includes criteria to specify the genders of the patient's target, and Table 16-18 compares the criteria for this disorder.

Of persons with pedophilia, 95 percent are heterosexual, and 50 percent have consumed alcohol to excess at the time of the incident. Many perpetrators concomitantly or have previously committed exhibitionism, voyeurism, or rape.

Incest is related to pedophilia by the frequent selection of an immature child as a sex object, the subtle or overt element of coercion, and occasionally the preferential nature of the adult–child liaison.

Table 16-17
Frotteurism

	DSM-5	ICD-10
Name	Frotteuristic Disorder	Other disorders of sexual preference *Frotteurism*
Duration	≥6 mo	
Symptoms	Sexual arousal/fantasies/urges/behaviors that result from touching/rubbing against a nonconsenting individual	Sexual arousal from rubbing against people in public spaces
Psychosocial Impact	Marked distress and/or psychosocial impairment	
Severity Specifiers	**In a controlled environment** (lives in institution/other controlled environment)	
Course Specifiers	**In full remission:** no symptoms or distress for ≥5 yr	
Comments		This category also includes *Necrophilia,* in addition to behaviors such as making obscene phone calls, engaging in sexual activity with animals, and use of strangulation for sexual excitement

A 62-year-old married janitor had worked as a fourth-grade school teacher for 26 years before he transferred school districts, and several years later mysteriously lost his second job. He was referred for help after his family discovered that he had repeatedly fondled the genitals of his 4- and 6-year-old granddaughters. A father of five who had not had sex with his wife for 30 years after strenuously objecting to her cigarette smoking, he was generous, helpful, and cooperative with his children and grandchildren. Intellectually slow, he preferred comic books and had a charming manner of playing with young children "like he was one himself." By his estimate, he had touched the buttocks and genitals of at least 300 girl students, thinking only of how they did not know what he was doing because he was affectionate, and they were too young to realize what was happening. He loved the anticipation and excitement of this behavior. His teaching career ended when parents complained to a principal. The principal discovered that the man had lost his last job for the same reason. (Courtesy of Stephen B. Levine, M.D.)

Sexual Masochism

Masochism takes its name from the 19th-century novelist Sacher-Masoch, whose characters derived sexual pleasure from being abused and dominated by women. According to the DSM-5, persons with sexual masochism have a recurrent preoccupation with sexual urges and fantasies involving the act of being humiliated, beaten, bound, or otherwise made to suffer (Table 16-19). The diagnosis includes asphyxiophilia or autoerotic asphyxiation as a subtype. It is the practice of achieving or heightening sexual arousal with restriction of breathing. Sexual masochistic practices are more common among men than among women. Persons with sexual masochism may have had childhood experiences that convinced them that pain is a prerequisite for sexual pleasure. About 30 percent of those with sexual masochism also have sadistic fantasies. Moral masochism involves a need to suffer but does not include sexual fantasies.

Table 16-18
Pedophilia

	DSM-5	ICD-10
Name	Pedophilic Disorder	Pedophilia
Duration	≥6 mo	
Symptoms	Sexual arousal/fantasies/urges/behaviors that result from sexual activity with prepubescent children Individual must be 16 yr or older at time of diagnosis, and must also be a minimum of 5 yr older than the child of sexual interest	Sexually preferring young boys and girls Often preferring prepubertal or early pubertal age
# Symptoms Needed	Both of the above	
Exclusion	≤16 yr old Adolescent in relationship with child aged 12 or 13	
Psychosocial Impact	Marked distress and/or psychosocial impairment	
Symptom Specifiers	**Exclusive type** (attracted only to children) **Nonexclusive type** **Sexually attracted to males** **Sexually attracted to females** **Sexually attracted to both males and females** **Limited to incest**	

Table 16-19
Sexual Masochism

	DSM-5	ICD-10
Name	Sexual Masochism Disorder	Sadomasochism
Duration	≥6 mo	
Symptoms	Sexual arousal/fantasies/urges/behaviors that result from being humiliated/hit/bound/made to suffer	Preference for sexual activity to include: Bondage Infliction of pain or humiliation (as the recipient)
Psychosocial Impact	Marked distress and/or psychosocial impairment	
Symptom Specifiers	**With asphyxiophilia:** arousal from restriction of breathing	
Severity Specifiers	**In a controlled environment:** lives in institution/other controlled environment	
Course Specifiers	**In full remission:** no symptoms or distress for ≥5 yr	
Comments		ICD combined masochism and sadism into one diagnosis

A 27-year-old woman presented for a job interview. She was accompanied by a man whom she introduced, saying, "This is my lover." When asked about this, the woman said that her companion had ordered her to bring him and introduce him in that way. She further explained that she was part of a group that utilized sadomasochistic techniques in their sexual play.

Sexual Sadism

Sexual sadism is recurrent and intense sexual arousal from the physical and psychological suffering of another person. The name is from the Marquis de Sade, an 18th-century French author who wrote novels detailing violent sexual acts against women, and was himself imprisoned for such acts. A person must have experienced these feelings for at least 6 months and must have either acted on sadistic fantasies or experienced significant distress as a result of these fantasies to receive a diagnosis of sexual sadism disorder (Table 16-20).

The onset of the disorder is usually before the age of 18 years, and most persons with sexual sadism are male. Sexual sadism likely derives from early abusive life experiences. However, there is little data about how the disorder develops. Sexual sadism is related

to rape, although rape is more aptly considered an expression of power. Some sadistic rapists, however, kill their victims after having sex (so-called lust murders). In many cases, these persons have underlying schizophrenia, and they may also suffer from a dissociative disorder or have a history of head trauma.

Voyeurism

Voyeurism, also known as *scopophilia,* is the recurrent preoccupation with fantasies and acts that involve observing unsuspecting persons who are naked or engaged in grooming or sexual activity (Table 16-21). Masturbation to orgasm usually accompanies or follows the event. The first voyeuristic act usually occurs during childhood, and the paraphilia is most common in men. When persons with voyeurism are apprehended, the charge is usually loitering.

Transvestism

Transvestism, formerly called transvestic fetishism, is described as fantasies and sexual urges to dress in opposite gender clothing as a means of arousal and as an adjunct to masturbation or coitus. DSM also has various specifiers depending on the exact nature of the fantasy, and Table 16-22 compares the criteria for this disorder.

Table 16-20
Sexual Sadism

	DSM-5	ICD-10
Name	Sexual Sadism Disorder	Sadomasochism
Duration	≥6 mo	
Symptoms	Sexual arousal/fantasies/urges/behaviors that result from inflicting physical or psychological suffering/humiliation on others	Preference for sexual activity to include: Bondage Infliction of pain or humiliation (as the provider)
Psychosocial Impact	Marked distress and/or psychosocial impairment or engaging with nonconsenting person	
Severity Specifiers	**In a controlled environment:** lives in institution/other controlled environment	
Course Specifiers	**In full remission:** no symptoms or distress for ≥5 yr	
Comments		ICD combined masochism and sadism into one diagnosis

Table 16-21
Voyeurism

	DSM-5	ICD-10
Name	Voyeuristic Disorder	Voyeurism
Duration	≥6 mo	
Symptoms	Sexual arousal/fantasies/urges/behaviors that result from observing an unaware person as they undress/have sex	Experiencing sexual pleasure from watching unaware people engage in: sex other intimate activities (undressing)
# Symptoms Needed		
Exclusion	≤18 yr old	
Psychosocial Impact	Marked distress and or impairment	
Symptom Specifiers		
Severity Specifiers	**In a controlled environment:** lives in institution/other controlled environment	
Course Specifiers	**In full remission:** no symptoms or distress for ≥5 yr	

Transvestism typically begins in childhood or early adolescence. With time, some men want to dress and live permanently as women. Very rarely, women want to dress and live as men. DSM-5 considers this to be a combination of transvestic disorder and gender dysphoria. Usually, a person wears more than one article of opposite sex clothing; frequently, this involves an entire wardrobe. When a man with transvestism cross-dresses, the appearance of femininity may be striking, although not usually to the degree found in transsexualism. When not dressed in women's clothes, men with transvestism may be hypermasculine in appearance and occupation. Cross-dressing can range from solitary, guilt-ridden behaviors to ego-syntonic, social membership in a subculture.

The overt clinical syndrome of transvestism may begin in latency but is more often seen around pubescence or in adolescence. Frank dressing in opposite-sex clothing usually does not begin until the person is relatively independent of their parents.

Other Specified Paraphilic Disorder

DSM-5 includes a generalized category for paraphilias that cause distress but do not fit into one of the previous categories. We describe some examples of these next.

In some cases, we may not wish to specify the exact paraphilia, such as when we do not yet have enough information; in these cases, we would diagnose an unspecified paraphilic disorder.

Telephone and Computer Scatologia. Telephone scatologia involves obscene phone calling to an unsuspecting recipient. Tension and arousal begin in anticipation of phoning; the recipient of the call listens while the telephoner (usually male) verbally exposes his preoccupations or induces her to talk about her sexual activity. The conversation is accompanied by masturbation.

Persons also use interactive computer networks, sometimes compulsively, to send obscene messages by electronic mail and to transmit sexually explicit messages and video images. Because of the anonymity of the users in chat rooms who use aliases, on-line or computer sex (cybersex) allows some persons to play the role of the opposite sex ("genderbending"), which represents an alternative method of expressing transvestic or other fantasies. A danger of on-line cybersex is that pedophiles often make contact with children or adolescents who lure children into meeting and then molest them. Many on-line contacts develop into off-line liaisons. Although some persons report that the off-line encounters develop into meaningful relationships, most such

Table 16-22
Transvestism

	DSM-5	ICD-10
Name	Transvestic Disorder	Fetishistic transvestism
Duration	≥6 mo	
Symptoms	Sexual arousal/fantasies/urges/behaviors that result from cross-dressing	Sexual excitement from wearing opposite sex clothes Desire to remove after arousal declines
Psychosocial Impact	Marked distress and/or impairment	
Symptom Specifiers	**With fetishism** (sexually aroused by specific fabrics or garments) **With autogynephilia** (sexually aroused by imagining self as female)	
Severity Specifiers	**In a controlled environment:** lives in institution/other controlled environment	
Course Specifiers	**In full remission:** no symptoms or distress for ≥5 yr	

meetings are filled with disappointment and disillusionment, as the fantasized person fails to meet the unconscious expectations of the ideal partner. In other situations, when adults meet, rape or even homicide may occur.

Necrophilia. Necrophilia is an obsession with obtaining sexual gratification from cadavers. Most persons with this disorder find corpses in morgues, but some may rob graves or even murder to satisfy their sexual urges. In the few cases studied, those with necrophilia believed that they were inflicting the greatest conceivable humiliation on their lifeless victims. Some experts consider this a type of psychosis.

Partialism. Persons with the disorder of partialism concentrate their sexual activity on one part of the body to the exclusion of all others. Mouth–genital contacts—such as cunnilingus (oral contact with a woman's external genitals), fellatio (oral contact with the penis), and anilingus (oral contact with the anus)—is typically associated with foreplay. However, when a person uses these activities as the sole source of sexual gratification and cannot have or refuses to have coitus, a paraphilia exists. It is also known as *oralism.* As described earlier, transvestism is a type of partialism but differs in that the focus is not on a sexual organ.

Zoophilia. In zoophilia, persons incorporate animals into arousal fantasies or sexual activities, including intercourse, masturbation, and oral–genital contact. Zoophilia, as an organized paraphilia, is rare. For many persons, animals are the primary source of relatedness, so it is not surprising that some may use a broad variety of domestic animals sensually or sexually.

Sexual relations with animals may occasionally be an outgrowth of availability or convenience, especially in parts of the world where rigid convention precludes premarital sexuality and in situations of enforced isolation. Because masturbation is also available in such situations, however, a predilection for animal contact is probably present in opportunistic zoophilia.

Coprophilia, Urophilia, and Klismaphilia. Coprophilia is sexual pleasure associated with the desire to defecate on a partner, to be defecated on, or to eat feces (coprophagia). A variant is the compulsive utterance of obscene words (coprolalia). Urophilia, a form of urethral eroticism, is an interest in sexual pleasure associated with the desire to urinate on a partner or to be urinated on. The disorder may be associated with masturbatory techniques involving the insertion of foreign objects into the urethra for sexual stimulation. Similarly, klismaphilia is the use of enemas for sexual stimulation.

Hypoxyphilia. Hypoxyphilia is the desire to achieve an altered state of consciousness secondary to hypoxia while experiencing orgasm. Persons may use a drug (e.g., a volatile nitrite or nitrous oxide) to produce hypoxia. Autoerotic asphyxiation is related and is a form of sexual masochism.

Differential Diagnosis

Clinicians must differentiate a paraphilia from an experimental act that is not recurrent or compulsive and done for its novelty. Paraphilic activity most likely begins during adolescence. Some paraphilias (especially the bizarre types) are associated with other mental disorders, such as schizophrenia. Brain diseases can also release perverse impulses.

Course and Prognosis

The difficulty in controlling or curing paraphilic disorders rests in the fact that it is hard for people to give up sexual pleasure with no assurance that alternative approaches will be as sexually gratifying. The prognosis is poor when it begins at an early age, and when it occurs frequently. Also, a lack of guilt is a bad predictor of outcome, as is a substance use disorder. The course and the prognosis are better when patients also engage in regular sexual activity. It may also be better when patients self-refer than are forced to present for legal reasons.

Treatment

There are five types of psychiatric interventions used to treat persons with paraphilic disorder: external control, reduction of sexual drives, treatment of comorbid conditions (e.g., depression or anxiety), cognitive-behavioral therapy, and dynamic psychotherapy.

Prison is an external control mechanism for sexual crimes that usually does not contain a treatment element. When victimization occurs in a family or work setting, the external control comes from informing supervisors, peers, or other adult family members of the problem and advising them about eliminating opportunities for the perpetrator to act on urges.

Drug therapy, including antipsychotic or antidepressant medication, is indicated for the treatment of schizophrenia or depressive disorders if the paraphilia is associated with these disorders. Antiandrogens, such as cyproterone acetate in Europe and medroxyprogesterone acetate (Depo-Provera) in the United States, may reduce the drive to behave sexually by decreasing serum testosterone levels to subnormal concentrations. Serotonergic agents, such as fluoxetine, have been used with limited success in some patients with paraphilia.

Cognitive-behavioral therapy can disrupt learned paraphilic patterns and modify behavior to make it socially acceptable. The interventions include social skills training, sex education, cognitive restructuring (confronting and destroying the rationalizations used to support the victimization of others), and development of victim empathy. The therapist can also teach the patient imaginal desensitization and relaxation technique. The patient can also learn what triggers the paraphilic impulse so that they can avoid these stimuli. In modified aversive behavior rehearsal, the therapist videotapes the perpetrators acting out their paraphilia with a mannequin. Then the therapist or a peer group may confront the patient with questions about feelings, thoughts, motives associated with the act and repeatedly try to correct cognitive distortions and point out the lack of victim empathy to the patient.

Insight-oriented psychotherapy is a long-standing treatment approach. Patients have the opportunity to understand their dynamics and the events that caused the paraphilia to develop. In particular, they become aware of the daily events that cause them to act on their impulses (e.g., a real or fantasized rejection). Treatment helps them deal more effectively with life stresses and enhances their capacity to relate to a life partner. Also, psychotherapy allows patients to regain self-esteem, which in turn allows them to approach a partner in a more normal sexual manner. Sex therapy is an appropriate adjunct to the treatment of patients with specific sexual dysfunctions when they attempt nondeviant sexual activities.

Good treatment predictors include the presence of a single paraphilia, normal intelligence, the absence of substance abuse, the absence of nonsexual antisocial personality traits, and the presence of a successful adult attachment. Paraphilic disorders, however, remain significant treatment challenges even under these circumstances.

Epidemiology

Paraphilias are rare, but the insistent, repetitive nature of the disorders results in a high frequency of such acts. Thus, many people are victims of persons with paraphilic disorders. It may be that the prevalence of paraphilias is much higher than that found in clinical care, given the large commercial market in paraphilic pornography and paraphernalia. We do not know how many consumers of these materials act on their fantasies or cannot respond to typical erotic stimuli.

Among legally identified cases of paraphilic disorders, pedophilia is most common. Of all children, 10 to 20 percent have been molested by age 18. Because the act involves a child, it has gotten more attention than some other paraphilic disorders. Persons with exhibitionism who publicly display themselves to young children are also commonly apprehended. Those with voyeurism may be apprehended, but their risk is not considerable. Of adult females, 20 percent have been the targets of persons with exhibitionism and voyeurism. Sexual masochism and sexual sadism are underrepresented in any prevalence estimates. Sexual sadism usually comes to attention only in sensational cases of rape, brutality, and lust murder. The excretory paraphilic disorders rarely come to clinical attention, as it usually takes place between consenting adults or between a sex worker and client. Persons with fetishism rarely become entangled in the legal system. Those with transvestism may be arrested occasionally for disturbing the peace or on other misdemeanor charges if they are men dressed in women's clothes, but an arrest is more common among those with gender identity disorders. Zoophilia, as an actual paraphilic disorder, is rare (Table 16-23).

As usually defined, the paraphilias seem to be mostly male conditions. Fetishism almost always occurs in men. More than 50 percent of all paraphilias have their onset before age 18. Patients with paraphilia frequently have three to five paraphilias, either concurrently or at different times in their lives. This pattern of occurrence is especially the case with exhibitionism, fetishism, sexual

Table 16-23
Frequency of Paraphilic Acts Committed by Patients with Paraphilia Seeking Outpatient Treatment

Diagnostic Category	Patients with Paraphilia Seeking Outpatient Treatment (%)	Paraphilic Acts per Patient with Paraphilia
Pedophilia	45	5
Exhibitionism	25	50
Voyeurism	12	17
Frotteurism	6	30
Sexual masochism	3	36
Transvestic fetishism	3	25
Sexual sadism	3	3
Fetishism	2	3
Zoophilia	1	2

[a]Median number.
Courtesy of Gene G. Abel, M.D.

masochism, sexual sadism, transvestic fetishism, voyeurism, and zoophilia (see Table 16-23). The occurrence of paraphilic behavior peaks between ages 15 and 25 and gradually declines. DSM-5 suggests the paraphilia designation be reserved for those ages 18 and older to avoid pathologizing healthy sexual curiosity and occasional experimentation in adolescence. In men older than 50, criminal paraphilic acts are rare. Those that occur are practiced in isolation or with a cooperative partner.

Etiology

Psychosocial Factors. Many paraphilias can be traced back to childhood experiences that condition or socialize children into committing a paraphilic act. The first shared sexual experience can be significant in that regard. Molestation as a child can predispose a person to accept continued abuse as an adult or, conversely, to become an abuser of others. Also, early experiences of abuse that are not explicitly sexual, such as spanking, enemas, or verbal humiliation, can be sexualized by a child and can form the basis for a paraphilia. Such experiences can result in the development of an *eroticized child.*

> A 34-year-old man presented for the treatment of an erectile disorder. He was frequently unable to obtain an erection sufficient for coitus with his wife. The problem disappeared whenever she was willing to act out his bondage fantasy and tie him up with ropes, a scenario he intensely desired. He explained that he felt free to be sexual when tied up because it reassured him that he could move vigorously and not hurt the woman. Also, he gave a history of being tied up "in fun" when he was a child by a babysitter who would then tickle him until he begged her to stop.

The onset of paraphilic acts can result from persons' modeling their behavior on the behavior of others who have carried out paraphilic acts, mimicking sexual behavior depicted in the media, or recalling emotionally laden events from the past, such as their molestation. Learning theory indicates that because the fantasizing of paraphilic interests begins at an early age and because children are likely to hide their fantasies from others (who might discourage them), the use and misuse of paraphilic fantasies and urges continue uninhibited until late in life. Only then do persons begin to realize that such paraphilic interests and urges are inconsistent with societal norms. By that time, however, the repetitive use of such fantasies has become ingrained, and sexual thoughts and behaviors have become associated with or conditioned to paraphilic fantasies.

In the classic psychoanalytic model, persons with a paraphilia have failed to complete the normal developmental process toward sexual adjustment, but new psychoanalytic approaches have modified the model. What distinguishes one paraphilia from another is the method chosen by a person (usually male) to cope with the anxiety caused by the threat of castration by the father and separation from the mother. However bizarre its manifestation, the resulting behavior provides an outlet for the sexual and aggressive drives that would otherwise channel into normal sexual behavior.

Biologic Factors. Several studies have identified abnormal biologic findings in persons with paraphilias. None has used random samples of such persons; instead, they have extensively investigated patients with paraphilia at large medical centers. Among these patients, those with positive physical findings included 74 percent with abnormal hormone levels, 27 percent with hard or soft neurologic signs, 24 percent with chromosomal abnormalities, 9 percent with seizures, 9 percent with dyslexia, 4 percent with abnormal electroencephalography (EEG) studies, 4 percent with major mental disorders, and 4 percent with an intellectual disorder. It is not clear whether these abnormalities are causally related or incidental to the paraphilia.

Psychophysiological tests can measure the penile volumetric size in response to paraphilic and nonparaphilic stimuli. The procedures may be of use in diagnosis and treatment but are of questionable diagnostic validity because some men can suppress their erectile responses.

SEX ADDICTION AND COMPULSIVITY

The concept of sex addiction developed over the last two decades to refer to persons who compulsively seek out sexual experiences and whose behavior becomes impaired if they are unable to gratify their sexual impulses. This concept derives from the model of substance addiction or such addictive behaviors as gambling. Addiction implies psychological dependence, physical dependence, and the presence of a withdrawal syndrome if the substance or behavior is not available.

DSM-5 does not contain the diagnosis of sex addiction or compulsive sexuality, and the concept remains controversial. Nevertheless, the phenomenon of a person whose life revolves around sex-seeking behavior and activities, who spends an excessive amount of time in such behavior, and who often tries to stop such behavior but is unable to do so is well known to clinicians. Such persons show repeated and increasingly frequent attempts to have a sexual experience, deprivation of which gives rise to symptoms of distress. When encountering such a story, this should alert the clinician to find an underlying cause for the behavior.

Sex addicts cannot control their sexual impulses, which can involve the entire spectrum of sexual fantasy or behavior. Eventually, the need for sexual activity increases, and the person's behavior is mainly motivated by the persistent desire to experience the sex act. The history usually reveals a long-standing pattern of such behavior, which the person repeatedly has tried to stop, but without success. Although a patient may have feelings of guilt and remorse after the act, these feelings do not suffice to prevent its recurrence. The patient may report that their need to act out is most severe during stressful periods or when angry, depressed, anxious, or otherwise dysphoric. Most acts culminate in sexual orgasm. Eventually, the sexual activity interferes with the person's social, vocational, or marital life, which begins to deteriorate. Table 16-24 lists the signs of sexual addiction.

Table 16-24
Signs of Sexual Addiction

1. Out-of-control behavior
2. Severe adverse consequences (medical, legal, interpersonal) due to sexual behavior
3. Persistent pursuit of self-destructive or high-risk sexual behavior
4. Repeated attempts to limit or stop sexual behavior
5. Sexual obsession and fantasy as a primary coping mechanism
6. The need for increasing amounts of sexual activity
7. Severe mood changes related to sexual activity (e.g., depression, euphoria)
8. Inordinate amount of time spent in obtaining sex, being sexual, or recovering from sexual experience
9. Interference of sexual behavior in social, occupational, or recreational activities

Some men who appear to be hypersexual, as manifested by their need to have many sexual encounters or conquests, use their sexual activities to mask deep feelings of inferiority, this is sometimes called *Don Juanism*. Some are unconsciously attracted to other men, which they deny by compulsive sexual contact with women. After having sex, most Don Juans are no longer interested in the woman. The condition is also called *satyriasis*.

In a woman, a similar condition is called nymphomania. Of the few scientific studies of the condition, those patients who were studied usually have had one or more sexual disorders, often including female orgasmic disorder. The woman often has an intense fear of losing love and, through her actions, attempts to satisfy her dependence needs rather than gratify her sexual impulses.

Comorbidity

Many sex addicts have an associated psychiatric disorder. The comorbid diagnosis may be challenging to recognize, given that the addictive disorder produces considerable stress and anxiety on its own. Most common are substance use disorders (up to 80 percent in some studies), which not only complicates the task of diagnosis, but also complicates treatment.

Treatment

Self-help groups based on the 12-step concept used in Alcoholics Anonymous (AA) have been used successfully with many sex addicts. They include such groups as Sexaholics Anonymous (SA), Sex and Love Addicts Anonymous (SLAA), and Sex Addicts Anonymous (SAA). The groups differ in that some are for men or women, or married persons or couples. All advocate some abstinence from either the addictive behavior or sex in general. Should a substance use disorder also be present, the patient often requires referral to AA or Narcotics Anonymous (NA) as well. Patients may enter an inpatient treatment unit when they lack sufficient motivation to control their behavior on an outpatient basis or pose a danger to themselves or others. Also, severe medical or psychiatric symptoms may require careful supervision and treatment best carried out in a hospital.

A 42-year-old married businessman with two children was considered a model of virtue in his community. He was active in his church and on the boards of several charitable organizations. He was living a secret life, however, and would lie to his wife, telling her that he was at a board meeting when he was visiting massage parlors for paid sex. He eventually was engaging in the behavior four to five times a day, and although he tried to quit many times, he was unable to do so. He knew that he was harming himself by putting his reputation and marriage at risk.

The patient presented himself to the psychiatric emergency room, stating that he would prefer to be dead rather than continue the behavior described. He was admitted with a diagnosis of major depressive disorder and started on a daily dose of 20 mg of fluoxetine. He also received 100 mg of medroxyprogesterone intramuscularly once a day. His need to masturbate diminished markedly and ceased entirely on the third hospital day, as did his mental preoccupation with sex. His clinicians discontinued the medroxyprogesterone on the sixth day and discharged him. He continued to take fluoxetine, enrolled in a local SA group, and entered individual and couples psychotherapy. His addictive behavior eventually stopped, he was having satisfactory sexual relations with his wife, and he was no longer suicidal or depressed.

Pharmacotherapy. Certain medications may be of use in treating sex addiction, however, because of their specific effects on reducing the sex drive. SSRIs reduce libido in some persons. Compulsive masturbation is an example of a behavioral pattern that may benefit from such medication. Medroxyprogesterone acetate diminishes libido in men and, thus, makes it easier to control sexually addictive behavior.

There is little information on the use of antiandrogens in women to control hypersexuality; however, they might be of benefit. Antiandrogenic agents (e.g., cyproterone acetate) are not available in the United States, but in Europe, they have had varying success. Antiandrogenic medications remain controversial, and some clinicians see it as chemical castration.

Psychotherapy. Insight-oriented psychotherapy may help patients understand the dynamics of their behavioral patterns. Supportive psychotherapy can help repair the interpersonal, social, or occupational damage that occurs. Cognitive behavioral therapy helps the patient recognize dysphoric states that precipitate sexual acting out. Marital therapy or couples therapy can help the patient regain self-esteem. It is also helpful to the partners who need assistance in understanding the disease and dealing with their complex reactions to the situation. Finally, psychotherapy may help in the treatment of any associated psychiatric disorder.

NORMAL SEXUALITY

Sexuality is determined by anatomy, physiology, the culture in which a person lives, relationships with others, and developmental experiences throughout the life cycle. It includes the perception of being male or female and private thoughts and fantasies as well as behavior. To the average person, sexual attraction to another person and the passion and love that follow are deeply associated with feelings of intimate happiness.

Healthy sexual behavior brings pleasure to oneself and one's partner and involves stimulation of the primary sex organs, including coitus; it is devoid of inappropriate feelings of guilt or anxiety and is not compulsive. Societal understanding of what defines normal sexual behavior is inconstant and varies from era to era, reflecting the cultural mores of the time.

Terms

Sexuality and personality cannot be separated as they are related; hence the term *psychosexual,* to describe personality development and functioning as affected by sexuality. The term *psychosexual* applies to more than sexual feelings and behavior, and it is not synonymous with *libido* in the Freudian sense.

Childhood Sexuality

Before Freud described the effects of childhood experiences on the personalities of adults, the universality of sexual activity and sexual learning in children was unrecognized. Most sexual learning experiences in childhood occur without the parents' knowledge, but awareness of a child's sex does influence parental behavior. Male infants, for instance, tend to be handled more vigorously, and female infants cuddled more. Fathers spend more time with their infant sons than with their daughters, and they also tend to be more aware of their sons' adolescent concerns than of their daughters' anxieties. Boys are more likely than girls to be physically disciplined. A child's sex affects parental tolerance for aggression and reinforcement or extinction of activity and intellectual, aesthetic, and athletic interests.

Observation of children reveals that genital play in infants is part of healthy development. According to Harry Harlow, interaction with mothers and peers is necessary for the development of active adult sexual behavior in monkeys, a finding that has relevance to the socialization of children. During a critical period in development, infants are especially susceptible to certain stimuli; later, they may be immune to these stimuli. We do not entirely understand the detailed relation of critical periods to psychosexual development; Freud's stages of psychosexual development—oral, anal, phallic, latent, and genital—presumably provide a broad framework.

Psychosexual Factors

Sexuality depends on four interrelated psychosexual factors: sexual identity, gender identity, sexual orientation, and sexual behavior. These factors affect personality, growth, development, and functioning. Sexuality is something more than physical sex, coital or noncoital, and something less than all behaviors directed toward attaining pleasure.

Sexual Identity, Gender Identity, and Sexual Orientation

Sexual identity is the pattern of a person's biologic sexual characteristics: chromosomes, external genitalia, internal genitalia, hormonal composition, gonads, and secondary sex characteristics. In healthy development, these characteristics form a cohesive pattern that leaves a person in no doubt about his or her sex. Gender identity is a person's sense of maleness or femaleness. Sexual identity and gender identity are interactive. Genetic influences and hormones affect behavior, and the environment affects hormonal production and gene expression (Table 16-25).

Sexual Identity. Modern embryologic studies have shown that all mammalian embryos, whether genetically male (XY genotype) or genetically female (XX genotype), are anatomically female during the early stages of fetal life. Differentiation of the male from the female results from the action of fetal androgens; the action begins about the sixth week of embryonic life and finishes by the end of the third month. Recent research has focused on the possible roles of critical genes in fetal sexual development. A testis develops because of SRY and SOX9 action, and an ovary develops in the absence of such action. DAX1 plays a part in the fetal development of both sexes, and WNT4 action is needed for the development of the müllerian ducts in the female fetus. Other studies have explained the effects of fetal hormones on the masculinization or feminization of the brain. In animals, prenatal hormonal stimulation of the brain is necessary for male and female reproductive and copulatory behavior. The fetus is also vulnerable to exogenously administered androgens during that period. For instance, if a pregnant woman receives sufficient exogenous androgens, her female fetus that possesses ovaries can develop external genitalia resembling those of a male fetus.

In the past, newborns with ambiguous genitalia were assigned their sexual identity at birth. The theory underlying this action was that parents and child would feel less confusion and that the child would accept the assigned sex and more easily develop a stable sense of being male or female. Although this worked for some children, others developed a gender identity at odds with their assigned sex.

Table 16-25
Classification of Intersexual Disorders[a]

Syndrome	Description
Virilizing adrenal hyperplasia (adrenogenital syndrome)	Results from excess androgens in fetus with XX genotype; most common female intersex disorder; associated with enlarged clitoris, fused labia, hirsutism in adolescence
Turner syndrome	Results from absence of second female sex chromosome (XO); associated with web neck, dwarfism, cubitus valgus; no sex hormones produced; infertile
Klinefelter syndrome	Genotype is XXY; male habitus present with small penis and rudimentary testes because of low androgen production; weak libido; usually assigned as male
Androgen insensitivity syndrome (testicular-feminizing syndrome)	Congenital X-linked recessive disorder that results in inability of tissues to respond to androgens; external genitals look female and cryptorchid testes present; in extreme form patient has breasts, normal external genitals, short blind vagina, and absence of pubic and axillary hair
Enzymatic defects in XY genotype (e.g., 5-α-reductase deficiency, 17-hydroxy-steroid deficiency)	Congenital interruption in production of testosterone that produces ambiguous genitals and female habitus
Hermaphroditism	True hermaphrodite is rare and characterized by both testes and ovaries in same person (may be 46 XX or 46 XY)
Pseudohermaphroditism	Usually the result of endocrine or enzymatic defect (e.g., adrenal hyperplasia) in persons with normal chromosomes; female pseudohermaphrodites have masculine-looking genitals but are XX; male pseudohermaphrodites have rudimentary testes and external genitals and are XY

[a]Intersexual disorders include a variety of syndromes that produce persons with gross anatomical or physiologic aspects of the opposite sex.

For example, an infant designated female at birth could instead feel male throughout childhood, and more emphatically at puberty. In some cases, this conflict led to depression and even suicide. Current practice usually allows the child to develop with the ambiguity, which permits a sense of gender identity to evolve as the child grows. The gender identity is then more congruent with the child's emotional sense of maleness or femaleness. Ideally, the family receives support from a medical team composed of a pediatrician, an endocrinologist, and a psychiatrist throughout this developmental process.

Gender Identity.   In infants with an unambiguous sexual identity, almost everyone has a firm conviction that "I am male" or "I am female" by 2 to 3 years of age. However, even if maleness and femaleness develop typically, persons must still develop a sense of masculinity or femininity.

Gender identity, according to Robert Stoller, "connotes psychological aspects of behavior related to masculinity and femininity." Stoller considers gender social and sex biologic: "Most often, the two are relatively congruent, that is, males tend to be manly and females womanly." Nevertheless, sex and gender can develop in conflicting or even opposite ways. Gender identity results from an almost infinite series of cues derived from experiences with family members, teachers, friends, and coworkers, and from cultural phenomena. Physical characteristics derived from a person's biologic sex—such as physique, body shape, and physical dimensions—interrelate with an intricate system of stimuli, including rewards and punishment and parental gender labels, to establish gender identity.

Thus, the formation of gender identity arises from parental and cultural attitudes, the infant's external genitalia, and genetic influence, which is physiologically active by the sixth week of fetal life. Although family, cultural, and biological influences may complicate the establishment of a sense of masculinity or femininity, persons usually develop a relatively secure sense of identification with their biologic sex—a stable gender identity.

GENDER ROLE.   Related to, and in part derived from, gender identity is gender role behavior. John Money and Anke Ehrhardt described gender role behavior as all those things that a person says or does to disclose himself or herself as having the status of boy or man, girl or woman, respectively. A gender role is not established at birth, but builds gradually through (1) experiences encountered and transacted through casual and unplanned learning, (2) explicit instruction and inculcation, and (3) spontaneously putting two and two together to sometimes make four and sometimes five. The usual outcome is a congruence of gender identity and gender roles. Although biologic attributes are significant, the primary factor in achieving the role appropriate to a person's sex is learning.

Research on sex differences in children's behavior reveals more psychological similarities than differences. Girls, however, are found to be less susceptible to tantrums after the age of 18 months than are boys, and boys generally are more physically and verbally aggressive than are girls from age two onward. Little girls and little boys are similarly active, but boys are more easily stimulated to sudden bursts of activity when they are in groups. Some researchers speculate that, although aggression is a learned behavior, male hormones may have sensitized boys' neural organizations to absorb these lessons more readily than do girls.

Persons' gender roles can seem to be opposed to their gender identities. They may identify with their sex and yet adopt the dress, hairstyle, or other characteristics of the opposite sex. Alternatively, they may identify with the opposite sex and yet for expediency adopt many behavioral characteristics of their sex. A further discussion of gender issues appears in Chapter 17.

Sexual Orientation.   Sexual orientation describes the object of a person's sexual impulses: opposite sex, same-sex, or both sexes. A group of people have defined themselves as "asexual" and assert this as a positive identity. Some researchers believe this lack of attraction to any object is a manifestation of a desire disorder. Other people wish not to define their sexual orientation at all and avoid labels. Still, others describe themselves as polysexual or pansexual.

The Biology of Sexual Behavior

The Brain

CORTEX.   The cortex is involved both in controlling sexual impulses and in processing sexual stimuli that may lead to sexual activity. In studies of young men, some areas of the brain are more active during sexual stimulation than others. These include the orbitofrontal cortex, which is involved in emotions; the left anterior cingulate cortex, which is involved in hormone control and sexual arousal; and the right caudate nucleus, whose activity is a factor in whether sexual activity follows arousal.

LIMBIC SYSTEM.   In all mammals, the limbic system is directly involved with elements of sexual functioning. Chemical or electrical stimulation of the lower part of the septum and the contiguous preoptic area, the fimbria of the hippocampus, the mammillary bodies, and the anterior thalamic nuclei have all elicited penile erections.

Studies of the brain in women have revealed that those areas activated by emotions of fear or anxiety are notably quiescent when the woman experiences an orgasm.

BRAINSTEM.   Brainstem sites exert inhibitory and excitatory control over spinal sexual reflexes. The nucleus paragigantocellularis projects directly to pelvic efferent neurons in the lumbosacral spinal cord, apparently causing them to secrete serotonin, which is known to inhibit orgasms. The lumbosacral cord also receives projections from other serotonergic nuclei in the brainstem.

BRAIN NEUROTRANSMITTERS.   Many neurotransmitters, including dopamine, epinephrine, norepinephrine, and serotonin, are produced in the brain and affect sexual function. For example, an increase in dopamine likely increases libido. Serotonin, produced in the upper pons and midbrain, exerts an inhibitory effect on sexual function. Oxytocin is released with orgasm and may reinforce pleasurable activities.

Spinal Cord.

Ultimately, sexual arousal and climax are organized at the spinal level. Afferents from the pudendal, pelvic, and hypogastric nerves convey the sensory stimuli related to sexual function. Several separate experiments suggest that spinal neurons mediate sexual reflexes in the central gray region of the lumbosacral segments.

Physiologic Responses.

Sexual response is a psychophysiological experience. Both psychological and physical stimuli trigger arousal and an aroused person experiences both physiologic and emotional tension. With orgasm, usually, subjective perception of a peak of physical reaction and release occurs along with a feeling of well-being. Psychosexual development, psychological attitudes toward sexuality, and attitudes toward one's sexual partner are directly involved with, and affect, the physiology of human sexual response.

Usually, men and women experience a sequence of physiologic responses to sexual stimulation. In the first detailed description of these responses, Masters and Johnson observed that the physiologic process involves increasing levels of vasocongestion and myotonia (tumescence) and the subsequent release of the vascular activity and muscle tone as a result of orgasm (detumescence). Tables 16-26 and 16-27 describe the physiologic male and female sexual response cycles. It is important to remember that the sequence of responses can overlap and fluctuate. A sexual fantasy or the desire to have sex frequently precedes the physiologic responses of excitement, orgasm, and resolution, particularly in the male. Also, a person's subjective experiences are as relevant to sexual satisfaction as the objective physiologic response. Figures 16-1 and 16-2 illustrate several possible patterns in the phases of the male sexual response and female sexual response, respectively.

Hormones and Sexual Behavior.

In general, substances that increase dopamine levels in the brain increase desire, whereas substances that augment serotonin decrease desire. Testosterone increases libido in both men and women, although estrogen is a crucial factor in the lubrication involved in female arousal and may increase sensitivity in the woman to stimulation. Recent studies indicate that estrogen is also a factor in the male sexual response and that a decrease in estrogen in the middle-aged male results in higher fat accumulation just as it does in women. Progesterone mildly depresses desire in men and women as do excessive prolactin and cortisol. Oxytocin is involved in pleasurable sensations during sex and increases in men and women after orgasm.

Gender Differences in Desire and Erotic Stimuli

Sexual impulses and desire exist in men and women. In measuring desire by the frequency of spontaneous sexual thoughts, interest in participating in sexual activity, and alertness to sexual cues, males generally possess a higher baseline level of desire than do women, which may be biologically determined. Motivations for having sex, other than desire, exist in both men and women but seem to be more varied and prevalent in women. In women, they may include a wish to reinforce the pair bond, the need for a feeling of closeness, a way of preventing the man from straying, or a desire to please the partner.

Although explicit sexual fantasies are common to both sexes, the external stimuli for the fantasies frequently differ for men and women. Many men respond sexually to visual stimuli of nude or barely dressed women. Women report responding sexually to romantic stories such as a demonstrative hero whose passion for the heroine impels him toward a lifetime commitment to her. A complicating factor is that a woman's subjective sense of arousal is not always congruent with her physiologic state of arousal. Her sense of excitement may reflect a readiness to be aroused rather than physiologic lubrication. Conversely, she may experience signs of arousal, including vaginal lubrication, without being aware of them. This situation rarely occurs in men.

Masturbation

Masturbation is usually a standard precursor of object-related sexual behavior. To paraphrase MS Patton, no other form of sexual activity is more discussed, more condemned, and more universally practiced. Research by Kinsey into the prevalence of masturbation indicated that nearly all men and three-fourths of all women masturbate sometime during their lives.

Longitudinal studies of development show that sexual self-stimulation is common in infancy and childhood. Just as infants learn to explore the functions of their fingers and mouths, they learn to do the same with their genitalia. At about 15 to 19 months of age, both sexes begin genital self-stimulation. Pleasurable sensations result from any gentle touch to the genital region. Those sensations, coupled with the ordinary desire for exploration of the body, produce a healthy interest in masturbatory pleasure at that time. Children also develop an increased interest in the genitalia of others—parents, children, and even animals. As youngsters acquire playmates, the curiosity about their own and others' genitalia motivates episodes of exhibitionism or genital exploration. Such experiences, unless blocked by guilty fear, contribute to continued pleasure from sexual stimulation.

With the approach of puberty, the upsurge of sex hormones, and the development of secondary sex characteristics, sexual curiosity

Table 16-26
Male Sexual Response Cycle[a]

Organ	Excitement Phase	Orgasmic Phase	Resolution Phase
	Lasts several minutes to several hours; heightened excitement before orgasm, 30 s to 3 min	3–5 s	10–15 min; if no orgasm, ½–1 day
Skin	Just before orgasm: sexual flush inconsistently appears; maculopapular rash originates on abdomen and spreads to anterior chest wall, face, and neck and can include shoulders and forearms	Well-developed flush	Flush disappears in reverse order of appearance; inconsistently appearing film of perspiration on soles of feet and palms of hands
Penis	Erection in 10–30 s caused by vasocongestion of erectile bodies of corpus cavernosa of shaft; loss of erection may occur with introduction of asexual stimulus, loud noise; with heightened excitement, size of glands and diameter of penile shaft increase further	Ejaculation; emission phase marked by three to four 0.8-s contractions of vas, seminal vesicles, prostate; ejaculation proper marked by 0.8-s contractions of urethra and ejaculatory spurt of 12–20 in at age 18, decreasing with age to seepage at 70	Erection: partial involution in 5–10 s with variable refractory period; full detumescence in 5–30 min
Scrotum and testes	Tightening and lifting of scrotal sac and elevation of testes; with heightened excitement, 50% increase in size of testes over unstimulated state and flattening against perineum, signaling impending ejaculation	No change	Decrease to baseline size because of loss of vasocongestion; testicular and scrotal descent within 5–30 min after orgasm; involution may take several hours if no orgasmic release takes place
Cowper glands	2–3 drops of mucoid fluid that contain viable sperm are secreted during heightened excitement	No change	No change
Other	Breasts: inconsistent nipple erection with heightened excitement before orgasm Myotonia: semispastic contractions of facial, abdominal, and intercostal muscles Tachycardia: up to 175 beats a minute Blood pressure: rise in systolic 20–80 mm; in diastolic 10–40 mm Respiration: increased	Loss of voluntary muscular control Rectum: rhythmical contractions of sphincter Heart rate: up to 180 beats a minute Blood pressure: up to 40–100 mm systolic; 20–50 mm diastolic Respiration: up to 40 respirations a minute	Return to baseline state in 5–10 min A refractory period follows orgasm, during which time the male cannot be rearoused to erection and is unresponsive to stimulation. The length of the refractory period is age and situation dependent

[a]A desire phase consisting of sex fantasies and desire to have sex precedes excitement phase.
Table by Virginia Sadock, M.D.

intensifies, and masturbation increases. Adolescents are physically capable of coitus and orgasm but are usually inhibited by social restraints. The dual and often conflicting pressures of establishing their sexual identities and controlling their sexual impulses produce a strong physiologic sexual tension in teenagers that demands release, and masturbation is a healthy way to reduce sexual tensions. In general, males learn to masturbate to orgasm earlier than females and masturbate more frequently. An important emotional difference between the adolescent and the youngster of earlier years is the presence of coital fantasies during masturbation in the adolescent. These fantasies are an essential adjunct to the development of sexual identity; in the comparative safety of the imagination, the adolescent learns to perform the adult sex role. This autoerotic activity continues into the young adult years when coitus becomes more common.

Couples in a sexual relationship do not abandon masturbation entirely. When coitus is unsatisfactory or is unavailable because of illness or the absence of the partner, self-stimulation often serves an adaptive purpose, combining sensual pleasure and tension release.

Kinsey reported that when women masturbate, most prefer clitoral stimulation. Masters and Johnson stated that women prefer the shaft of the clitoris to the glans because the glans is hypersensitive to intense stimulation. Most men masturbate by vigorously stroking the penile shaft and glans.

Several studies found that in men, orgasm from masturbation raised the serum prostate-specific antigen (PSA) significantly. Male patients scheduled for PSA tests should be advised not to masturbate (or have coitus) for at least seven days before the examination.

Moral taboos against masturbation have generated myths that masturbation causes mental illness or decreased sexual potency. No scientific evidence supports such claims. Masturbation is a psychopathological symptom only when it becomes a compulsion beyond a person's willful control. Then, it is a symptom of emotional disturbance, not because it is sexual, but because it is compulsive. Masturbation is probably a universal aspect of psychosexual development, and, in most cases, it is adaptive.

Coitus

The first coitus is a rite of passage for both men and women. In the United States, most people have experienced coitus by young

Table 16-27
Female Sexual Response Cycle[a]

Organ	Excitement Phase	Orgasmic Phase	Resolution Phase
	Lasts several minutes to several hours; heightened excitement before orgam, 30 s to 3 min	3–15 seconds	10–15 minutes; if no orgasm, $\frac{1}{2}$–1 day
Skin	Just before orgam: sexual flush inconsistently appears; maculopapular rash originates on abdomen and spreads to anterior chest wall, face, and neck; can include shoulders and forearms	Well-developed flush	Flush disappears in reverse order of appearance; inconsistently appearing film of perspiration on soles of feet and palms of hands
Breasts	Nipple erection in two-thirds of women, venous congestion and areolar enlargement; size increases to one-fourth over normal	Breasts may become tremulous	Return to normal in about 30 min
Clitoris	Enlargement in diameter of glans and shaft; just before orgasm, shaft retracts into prepuce	No change	Shaft returns to normal position in 5–10 s; detumescence in 5–30 min; if no orgasm, detumescence takes several hours
Labia majora	Nullipara: elevate and flatten against perineum	No change	Nullipara: decrease to normal size in 1–2 min
	Multipara: congestion and edema		Multipara: decrease to normal size in 10–15 min
Labia minora	Size increased two to three times over normal; change to pink, red, deep red before orgasm	Contractions of proximal labia minora	Return to normal within 5 min
Vagina	Color change to dark purple; vaginal transudate appears 10–30 s after arousal; elongation and ballooning of vagina; lower third of vagina constricts before orgasm	3–15 contractions of lower third of vagina at intervals of 0.8 s	Ejaculate forms seminal pool in upper two-thirds of vagina; congestion disappears in seconds or, if no orgasm, in 20–30 min
Uterus	Ascends into false pelvis; labor-like contractions begin in heightened excitement just before orgasm	Contractions throughout orgasm	Contractions cease, and uterus descends to normal position
Other	Myotonia A few drops of mucoid secretion from Bartholin glands during heightened excitement Cervix swells slightly and is passively elevated with uterus	Loss of voluntary muscular control Rectum: rhythmical contractions of sphincter Hyperventilation and tachycardia	Return to baseline status in seconds to minutes Cervix color and size return to normal, and cervix descends into seminal pool

[a]A desire phase consisting of sex fantasies and desire to have sex may precede or overlap with the excitement phase.
Table by Virginia Sadock, M.D.

adulthood. In a study of people ages 18 to 59, over 95 percent had included coitus in their last sexual interaction.

The young man experiencing intercourse for the first time is vulnerable in his pride and self-esteem. Cultural myths still perpetuate the idea that he should be able to have an erection with no, or little, stimulation, and that he should have an effortless mastery over the situation, even though it is an act that he has never before experienced. Cultural pressure on the woman with her first coitus reflects remaining cultural ambivalence about her loss of virginity, despite the current era of sexual liberality. This reality is illustrated

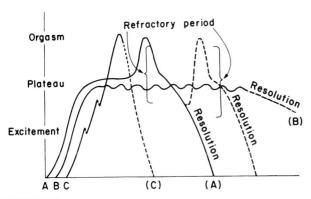

FIGURE 16-1
Male sexual response. An individual man may experience any of these three patterns (**A, B,** or **C**) during a particular sexual experience. (From Walker JI, ed. *Essentials of Clinical Psychiatry*. Philadelphia, PA: JB Lippincott; 1985:276, with permission.)

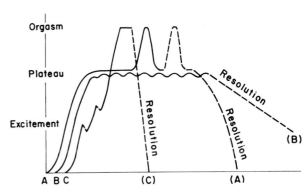

FIGURE 16-2
Female sexual response. An individual woman may experience any of these three patterns (**A, B,** or **C**) during a particular sexual experience. (From Walker JI, ed. *Essentials of Clinical Psychiatry*, Philadelphia, PA: JB Lippincott; 1985:276. with permission.)

by a survey that found only 50 percent of young women use contraception during their first coitus, and of that 50 percent, an even smaller number use it consistently after that. Young women with a history of masturbation are more likely to approach intercourse with positive anticipation and confidence.

In the last decade, coitus has also been part of the sexual repertoire of elderly adults, due to the development of sildenafil type drugs, which facilitate erections in men, and hormonally enhanced creams or hormonal pills, which counteract vaginal atrophy in postmenopausal women. Before the development of these drugs, many elderly adults enjoyed gratifying sex play, exclusive of coitus.

References

Arnold P, Agate RJ, Carruth LL. Hormonal and nonhormonal mechanisms of sexual differentiation of the brain. In: Legato M, ed. *Principles of Gender Specific Medicine*. San Diego: Elsevier Science; 2004:84.

Bancroft J. Alfred C. Kinsey and the politics of sex research. *Ann Rev Sex Res*. 2004;15:1–39.

Basson R. Clinical practice. Sexual desire and arousal disorders in women. *N Engl J Med*. 2006;354(15):1497–1506.

Brotto LA. "Efficacy of psychological interventions for sexual dysfunction: A systematic review and meta-analysis": Comment. *J Sex Med*. 2013;10:1904–1906.

Carnes PJ, Murray R, Charpantier L. Addiction interaction disorder. In: Combs RH, ed. *Handbook of Addictive Disorders: A Practical Guide to Diagnosis and Treatment*. Hoboken, NJ: John Wiley & Sons; 2004:31.

Ceccarelli P. Perversion on the other side of the couch. *Int Forum Psychoanalysis*. 2005;14:176–182.

Charnigo R, Noar SM, Garnett C, Crosby R, Palmgreen P, Zimmerman RS. Sensation seeking and impulsivity: Combined associations with risky sexual behavior in a large sample of young adults. *J Sex Res*. 2013;50(5):480–488.

Chirban JT. Integrative strategies for treating internet sexuality: A case study of paraphilias. *Clin Case Stud*. 2006;5:126–141.

Dimen M. Perversion is us? Eight notes. In: *Sexuality, Intimacy, Power*. Hillsdale, NJ: The Analytic Press; 2003:257–291.

Drescher J, Stein TS, Byne WM. Homosexuality, gay and lesbian identities and homosexual behavior. In: Sadock BJ, Sadock VA, eds. *Kaplan & Sadock's Comprehensive Textbook of Psychiatry*. 9th ed. Vol. 1. Philadelphia, PA: Lippincott Williams & Wilkins; 2009:2060.

Egan V, Parmar R. Dirty habits? Online pornography use, personality, obsessionality, and compulsivity. *J Sex Marital Ther*. 2013;39(5):394–409.

Federman DD. Current concepts: The biology of human sex differences. *N Engl J Med*. 2006;354(14):1507.

Fisher WA, Rosen RC, Mollen M, Brock G, Karlin G, Pommerville P, Goldstein I, Bangerter K, Bandel TJ, Derogatis LR, Sand M. Improving the sexual quality of life of couples affected by erectile dysfunction: A double-blind, randomized, placebo-controlled trial of vardenafil. *J Sex Med*. 2005;2(5):699–708.

Freud S. General theory of the neuroses. In: Strachey J, Freud A, eds. *Standard Edition of the Complete Psychological Works of Sigmund Freud*. Vol. 16. London: Hogarth Press; 1966:241.

Freud S. Letter to an American mother. *Am J Psychiatry*. 1951;102:786.

Frohman EM. Sexual dysfunction in neurological disease. *Clin Neuropharmacol*. 2002;25(3):126–132.

Fugl-Meyer KS, Oberg K, Lundberg PO, Lewin B, Fugl-Meyer A. On orgasm, sexual techniques, and erotic perceptions in 18- to 74-year-old Swedish women. *J Sex Med*. 2006;3(1):56–68.

Gopalakrishnan R, Jacob KS, Kuruvilla A, Vasantharaj B, John JK. Sildenafil in the treatment of antipsychotic-induced erectile dysfunction: A randomized, double-blind, placebo-controlled, flexible-dose, two-way crossover trial. *Am J Psychiatry*. 2006;163(3):494–499.

Gross G, Blundo R. Viagra: Medical technology constructing aging masculinity. *J Sociol Soc Welf*. 2005;32(1):85–97.

Hines M. *Brain Gender*. New York: Oxford University Press; 2004.

Humphreys TP. Cognitive frameworks of virginity and first intercourse. *J Sex Res*. 2013;50(7):664–675.

Jacobson L. On the use of "sexual addiction": The case for "perversion." *Contemp Psychoanal*. 2003;39:107–113.

Kafka MP, Hennen J. Hypersexual desire in males: Are males with paraphilias different from males with paraphilia-related disorders? *Sex Abuse*. 2003;15(4):307–321.

Kafka MP. The monoamine hypothesis for the pathophysiology of paraphilic disorders: An update. *Ann N Y Acad Sci*. 2003;989:86–94.

Kristen PN, Kristen NJ. The mediating role of sexual and nonsexual communication between relationship and sexual satisfaction in a sample of college-age heterosexual couples. *J Sex Marital Ther*. 2013;39(5):410–427

Gutmann P. About confusions of the mind due to abnormal conditions of the sexual organs. In: Löwenstein HJ, ed. *History of Psychiatry*. SAGE Publications; 2006;17(1):107–133. ff10.1177/0957154X06061724ff.ffhal-00570853f.

Lowenstein L, Mustafa S, Burke Y. Pregnancy and normal sexual function. Are they compatible? *J Sex Med*. 2013;10(3):621–622.

Melby T. Asexuality: Is it a sexual orientation? *Contemporary Sexuality*. 2005;39(11):1.

Nestler EJ, Malenka RC. The addicted brain. *Sci Am*. 2004;290(3):78–85.

Oliviera C, Nobre PJ. The role of trait-affect, depression, and anxiety in women with sexual dysfunction: A pilot study. *J Sex Marital Ther*. 2013;39(5):436–452.

Patrick K, Heywood W, Simpson JM, Pitts MK, Richters J, Shelley JM, Smith AM. Demographic predictors of consistency and change in heterosexuals' attitudes toward homosexual behavior over a two-year period. *J Sex Res*. 2013;50(6):611–619.

Patton MS. Twentieth-century attitudes toward masturbation. *J Relig Health*. 1986;25:291–302.

Pauls RN, Kleeman SD, Karram MM. Female sexual dysfunction: Principles of diagnosis and therapy. *Obstet Gynecol Surv*. 2005;60(3):196–205.

Person ES. As the wheel turns: A centennial reflection on Freud's three essays on the theory of sexuality. *J Am Psychoanal Assoc*. 2005;53(4):1257–1282.

Person ES. Paraphilias. In: Sadock BJ, Sadock VA, eds. *Kaplan & Sadock's Comprehensive Textbook of Psychiatry*. 9th ed. Vol. 1. Philadelphia, PA: Lippincott Williams & Wilkins; 2009:1965.

Puppo V. Comment on 'New findings and concepts about the G-spot in normal and absent vagina: Precautions possibly needed for preservation of the G-spot and sexuality during surgery'. *J Obstet Gynaecol Res*. 2014; 40(2):639–640.

Raymond NC, Coleman E, Miner MH. Psychiatric comorbidity and compulsive/impulsive traits in compulsive sexual behavior. *Compr Psychiatry*. 2003;44(5):370–380.

Reichenpfader U, Gartlehner G, Morgan LC, Greenblatt A, Nussbaumer B, Hansen RA, Van Noord N, Lux L, Gaynes BN. Sexual dysfunction associated with second-generation antidepressants in patients with major depressive disorder: Results from a systematic review with network meta-analysis. *Drug Saf*. 2014;37(1):19–31.

Rhoden EL, Morgentaler A. Risks of testosterone-replacement therapy and recommendations deficiency. *N Engl J Med*. 2004;350(5):482–492.

Richards AK. A fresh look at perversion. *J Am Psychoanal Assoc*. 2003;51(4):1199–1218.

Rosen R, Shabsigh R, Berber M, Assalian P, Menza M, Rodriguez-Vela L, Porto R, Bangerter K, Seger M, Montorsi F; Vardenafil Study Site Investigators. The Vardenafil Study Site Investigators. Efficacy and tolerability of vardenafil in men with mild depression and erectile dysfunction: The depression-related improvement with vardenafil for erectile response study. *Am J Psychiatry*. 2006;163(1):79–87.

Sadock VA. Group psychotherapy of psychosexual dysfunctions. In: Kaplan HI, Sadock BJ, eds. *Comprehensive Group Psychotherapy*. Baltimore, MD: Williams & Wilkins; 1983:286.

Sadock VA. Normal human sexuality and sexual dysfunction. In: Sadock BJ, Sadock VA, eds. *Kaplan & Sadock's Comprehensive Textbook of Psychiatry*. 10th ed. Vol. 1. Philadelphia, PA: Lippincott Williams & Wilkins; 2017.

Sadock VA. Sexual addiction. In: Ruiz P, Strain E, eds. *Lowinson and Ruiz's Substance Abuse: A Comprehensive Textbook*. 5th ed. Lippincott William & Wilkins; 2011.

Serretti A, Chiesa A. Sexual dysfunction and antidepressants: Identification, epidemiology, and treatment. *Directions in Psychiatry*. 2013;33:1–11.

Simkovic M, Stulhofer A, Bozic J. Revisiting the association between pornography use and risky sexual behaviors: The role of early exposure to pornography and sexual sensation seeking. *J Sex Res*. 2013;50(7):633–641.

van Lankveld J. Does "normal" sexual functioning exist? *J Sex Res*. 2013;50(3–4):205–206.

Woodward TL, Nowak NT, Balon R, Tancer M, Diamond MP. Brain activation patterns in women with acquired hypoactive desire disorder and women with normal function: A cross-sectional pilot study. *Fertil Steril*. 2013;100(4):1068–1076.

Yakeley J, Wood H. Paraphilias and paraphilic disorders: Diagnosis, assessment and management. *Adv Psychiatr Treat*. 2014;20:202–213.

17

Gender Dysphoria, Gender Identity, and Related Conditions

INTRODUCTION

In this chapter, we discuss gender identity and associated disorders. We start with gender identity and related conditions.

Gender identity refers to the sense one has of being male or female, which corresponds most often to the person's anatomical sex. Persons with gender dysphoria express their discontent with their assigned sex as a desire to have the body of the other sex or to be regarded socially as a person of the other sex.

The term gender dysphoria appears as a diagnosis for the first time in DSM-5 to refer to those persons with a marked incongruence between their experienced or expressed gender and the one assigned at birth. It was known as gender identity disorder in the previous edition of DSM.

In ICD-10, gender identity issues appear under Disorders of Adult Behavior and Personality in the category Gender Identity Disorders and include five diagnoses: transsexualism, dual-role transvestic, gender identity disorder of childhood, other gender identity disorders, and gender identity disorder, unspecified.

The ICD Working Group on the Classification of Sexual Disorders and Sexual Health is recommending that for ICD-11, gender identity concerns be moved from the psychological sections and is considering options that would list these concerns in a separate chapter, as medical diagnoses, or as part of a new chapter on sexual health and sexual disorders.

The term *transgender* is a general term used to refer to those who identify with a gender different from the one they were born with (sometimes referred to as their assigned gender). Transgender people are a diverse group: those who want to have the body of another sex known as transsexuals; those who feel they are between genders, of both genders, or neither gender known as genderqueer; and those who wear clothing traditionally associated with another gender, but who maintain a gender identity that is the same as their birth-assigned gender known as cross-dressers. Contrary to popular belief, most transgender people do not have genital surgery. Some do not desire it, and others who do may be unable to afford it. Transgender people may be of any sexual orientation. For example, a transgender man, assigned female at birth, may identify as gay (attracted to other men), straight (attracted to women), or bisexual (attracted to both men and women).

DIAGNOSIS AND CLINICAL FEATURES

Children

The DSM-5 defines gender dysphoria in children as incongruence between expressed and assigned gender, with the most critical criterion being a desire to be another gender or insistence that one is another gender. By emphasizing the importance of the child's self-perception, the creators of the diagnosis attempt to limit its use to those children who clearly state their wishes to be another gender, rather than encompassing a broader group of children who might be considered by adults to be gender nonconforming. However, a child's behavior may also lead to this diagnosis. Table 17-1 compares the approaches to diagnosing gender dysphoria or gender identity disorder.

Many children with gender dysphoria prefer clothing typical of another gender, preferentially choose playmates of another gender, enjoy games and toys associated with another gender, and take on the roles of another gender during play. In gender dysphoria, these social characteristics accompany other traits that are less likely to be socially influenced, such as a strong desire to be the other gender, dislike of one's sexual anatomy, or desire for primary or secondary sexual characteristics of the desired gender. Children may express a desire to have different genitals, state that their genitals are going to change, or urinate in the position (standing or sitting) typical of another gender. Also, although the caregivers may be distressed, it is the child who must feel clinically significant distress or impairment because of the condition for there to be a diagnosis.

Adolescents and Adults

Adolescents and adults diagnosed with gender dysphoria must also show an incongruence between expressed and assigned gender. Also, they must meet at least two of six criteria, half of which are related to their current (or in the cases of early adolescents, future) secondary sex characteristics or desired secondary sex characteristics. Other criteria include a strong desire to be another gender, be treated as another gender, or the belief that one has the typical feelings and reactions of another gender (see Table 17-1).

In practice, most adults who present to mental health practitioners with reports of gender-related concerns are aware of the concept of transgender identity. They may be interested in therapy to explore gender issues. They may also make contact to request a letter recommending hormone treatment or surgery. The cultural trope of being "trapped in the wrong body" does not apply to all, or even most, people who identify as transgender, so clinicians should be aware of using open and affirming approaches, taking language cues from their patients.

The DSM-5 criteria are noticeably open to the idea that some people do not fit into the traditional gender binary and might desire to be alternative genders, such as genderqueer. As with children, adolescents and adults should be personally distressed or impaired by their feelings. The adolescent and adult criteria also contain a

Table 17-1
Gender Dysphoria

	DSM-5	ICD-10
Name	Gender Dysphoria	Gender Identity Disorder (Several Disorders)
Duration	≥6 mo	
Symptoms	Conflict between experienced and assigned gender: **Children** • Desire or insistence of being another gender • Dressing like the other gender • Preference for other gender roles during play • Preference for other gender toys, games, or stereotypes • Rejection of same gender toys, games, or stereotypes • Preferences for other gender playmates • Dislike of one's anatomy • Desire for physical characteristics of other gender **Adults** • Conflict between experienced gender and primary/secondary sex characteristics • Desire to remove one's primary/secondary sex characteristics • Desire for other another gender's primary/secondary sex characteristics • Desire to be another gender • Feeling one has the psychological characteristics of another gender	**Transsexualism:** desire to live as member of the opposite sex **Dual-role transvestism:** temporarily wearing clothes of opposite sex to experience the other gender, but not desiring sex change. **Gender identity disorder of childhood:** • Distress about assigned sex • Desire to be other sex • Dressing like other sex • Disliking one's assigned sex
# Symptoms needed	Children: ≥6 Adults: ≥2	

Exclusions (not result of):		Not motivated by sexual excitement
		In children:
		  Normal variants ("tomboyishness" or effeminate behavior)
		  Ego-dystonic sexual orientation
		  Sexual maturation disorder

Psychosocial impact	Distress or functional impairment	Distress
Symptom specifiers	With a disorder of sex development	
Course specifiers	Post transition: ≥1 procedure/treatment for gender change and is living as the other gender	

posttransition specifier, which is for people living in their affirmed genders. For this specifier, they have to have had at least one medical or surgical procedure or be preparing for one.

Other Specified

The category *other specified gender dysphoria* is for cases where the presentation causes clinically significant distress or impairment but does not meet the full criteria for gender dysphoria. When using this diagnosis, the clinician should specify why the full criteria were not met.

Unspecified

The category *unspecified gender dysphoria* can be applied when full criteria are not met, and the clinician chooses not to specify the reason.

A 27-year-old assigned female at birth was referred to a gender identity clinic reporting having felt different as a child from other girls, although unable then to identify the source. As a young girl, she enjoyed playing sports with girls and boys but generally preferred the companionship of boys. She preferred wearing unisex or boyish clothes and resisted wearing a skirt or dress. Everyone referred to her as a tomboy. She tried to hide her breast development by wearing loose-fitting tops and stooping forward. Menses were embarrassing and poignantly reminded her of her femaleness, which was becoming increasingly alienating. As sexual attractions evolved, they were directed exclusively to female partners. In her late teens, she had one sexual experience with a man, and it was aversive. She began socializing in lesbian circles, but did not feel comfortable there and did not consider herself lesbian, but more a man. For sexual partners, she wanted heterosexual women and wanted to be considered by the partner as a man. As gender dysphoric feelings became increasingly pronounced, she consulted transsexual sites on the Internet and contacted a female-to-male transsexual community support group. She then set into motion the process of clinical referral. She transitioned to living as a man, had a name change, and received androgen injections. The patient's voice deepened, facial and body hair grew, menses stopped, and sex drive increased, along with clitoral hypertrophy. After 2 years, the patient underwent a bilateral mastectomy and was on the waitlist for phalloplasty and hysterectomy–oophorectomy. Employment as a man continues, as does a 3-year relationship with a female partner. The partner has a child from a previous marriage. (Adapted from a case of Richard Green, M.D.)

DIFFERENTIAL DIAGNOSIS

Differential Diagnosis of Children

Children diagnosed with gender dysphoria predicted to be more likely than others to identify as transgender as adults are differentiated from other gender-nonconforming children by statements about desired anatomical changes, as well as the persistence of the diagnosis over time. Children whose gender dysphoria persists over time may make repeated statements about a desire to be or believe that they are another gender. Other gender-nonconforming children may make these statements for short periods but not repeatedly, or may not make these types of statements, and may instead prefer clothing and behaviors associated with another gender but show contentment with their birth-assigned gender.

The diagnosis of gender dysphoria no longer excludes intersex people and instead is coded with a specifier in the cases where intersex people are gender dysphoric about their birth-assigned gender. Medical history is important to distinguish between children with or without intersex conditions. The standards of care for intersex children have changed dramatically over the last few decades due to activism by intersex adults and supportive medical and mental health professionals. Historically, intersex babies were often subjected to early surgical procedures to create a more standard male or female appearance. These procedures had the potential to cause sexual dysfunction, such as inability to orgasm, and permanent sterility. Recently, these practices have changed considerably so that more intersex people can make decisions about their bodies later in life.

Differential Diagnosis of Adolescents and Adults

Those who meet the criteria for a diagnosis of gender dysphoria must experience clinical distress or impairment related to their gender identity. This requirement excludes the diagnosis of transgender or gender-nonconforming people who are not clinically distressed by their gender identities. There are certain mental illnesses in which transgender identity may be a component of delusional thinking, such as in schizophrenia. However, this is extremely rare and is different from transgender identity or gender dysphoria as the gender identity issues diminish with the treatment of the psychosis. Body dysmorphic disorder may be a differential diagnosis for some patients who present with a desire to change gendered body parts. However, with body dysmorphic disorder, the focus is on the body part looking abnormal, not on gender. Transvestic disorder, discussed in the previous chapter, is a recurrent and intense sexual arousal from cross-dressing that causes clinically significant distress or impairment. This diagnosis is differentiated from gender dysphoria by the patient's gender identity being consistent with their gender assigned at birth, and by sexual excitement linked to cross-dressing coming to interfere with the person's life.

COURSE AND PROGNOSIS

Children

Children typically begin to develop a sense of their gender identity around age 3. At this point, they may develop gendered behaviors and interests, and some may begin to express a desire to be another gender. It is often around school age that children are first brought for clinical consultations, as this is when they begin to interact with classmates closely and to be scrutinized by adults other than their caregivers. Some adults who identify as transgender recall that as children, they did not show behaviors consistent with another gender then. Some say later that they worked hard to appear stereotypical to their assigned gender, whereas others deny being able to recall gender identity concerns. Approaching puberty, many children diagnosed with gender dysphoria begin to show increased levels of anxiety related to anticipated changes to their bodies.

Children diagnosed with gender dysphoria do not necessarily grow up to identify as transgender adults. Several studies have demonstrated that more than half of those diagnosed with gender identity disorder, based on the DSM-IV, later identify with their birth-assigned gender once they reach adulthood. Those children who do identify as transgender as adults tend to have more extreme gender dysphoria as children. Many studies show increased rates of gay and bisexual identity among those who were gender nonconforming as children.

COMORBIDITY

Comorbidity in Children

Children diagnosed with gender dysphoria show higher rates than other children of depressive disorders, anxiety disorders, and impulse control disorders. This high rate is likely related to the stigma faced by these children related to their gendered behaviors and identities. There are also reports that those diagnosed with gender dysphoria are more likely than others to fall on the autism spectrum. Some researchers posit that this may be related to intrauterine hormone exposure.

Comorbidity in Adults

Adults diagnosed with gender dysphoria show higher rates than other adults of depressive disorders, anxiety disorders, suicidality, self-harming behaviors, and substance abuse. The lifetime rate of suicidal thoughts in transgender people is about 40 percent. The minority stress model predicts increases in mental illness in groups that are stigmatized, discriminated against, harassed, and abused at higher rates than others. DSM-5 reports that persons with late-onset gender dysphoria may have more significant fluctuations in the extent of their distress and more ambivalence about and less satisfaction after sex reassignment surgery.

TREATMENT

Children

Treatment of gender identity issues in children typically consists of individual, family, and group therapy that guides children in exploring their gendered interests and identities. Some providers practice reparative, or conversion therapy, which attempts to change a person's gender identity or sexual orientation. This type of therapy is contrary to position statements by the American Psychiatric Association and practice guidelines of the American Academy of Child and Adolescent Psychiatry, and we consider this to treatment to be unethical.

Adolescents

As gender-nonconforming children approach puberty, some show intense fear and preoccupation related to the physical changes they anticipate or are beginning to experience. In addition to providing psychotherapy, many clinicians use these adolescents' reactions to the first signs of puberty as a compass to determine if puberty-blocking medications should be a consideration.

Puberty-blocking medications are gonadotropin-releasing hormone (GnRH) agonists that can temporarily block the release of hormones that lead to secondary sex characteristics, giving adolescents and their families time to reflect on the best options moving forward. GnRH agonists are used in other populations (e.g., children with precocious puberty) and thought safe. However, we should consider such steps carefully.

Adults

Treatment of adults who identify as transgender may include psychotherapy to explore gender issues, hormonal treatment, and surgical treatment. Hormonal and surgical interventions may decrease depression and improve the quality of life for such persons.

Mental Health Treatment

The history of poor treatment and medicalization of transgender people by mental health providers has led to a decreased interest on the part of trans-identified people in engaging in mental health care. Many surgeons, and some physicians who prescribe transition-related hormones, require a letter from a mental health provider, so for many transgender people, the mental health worker is a gatekeeper. Many community clinics are now using informed consent models for hormone treatment, thereby decreasing the need for mental health providers to play the role of gatekeepers. The World Professional Association for Transgender Health (WPATH) Standards of Care (SOC) for the health of transsexual, transgender, and gender-nonconforming people have recently become more flexible and open to informed consent models. Some mental health providers are specializing in working with transgender populations, and this is increasing the rate at which transgender people engage in psychotherapy.

Hormones

Hormone treatment of transgender men most often involves testosterone, usually taken by injection every week or every other week. Initial changes with testosterone therapy include increased acne, muscle mass, and libido, as well as a cessation of menses, usually within the first few months. Subsequent and more permanent changes include deepening of the voice, increased body hair, and enlargement of the clitoris. Monitoring includes hemoglobin/hematocrit levels, as testosterone can rarely cause an increase in red blood cell counts that can lead to stroke. Like all steroid hormones, the liver metabolizes testosterone, so we should obtain routine liver function tests. Clinicians also want to monitor cholesterol and screen for diabetes, as testosterone treatment may increase the likelihood of lipid abnormalities and diabetes. Those beginning hormone treatments are routinely counseled on fertility, as future fertility may be affected by testosterone.

Transgender women may take estrogen, testosterone-blockers, or progesterone, often in combination. These hormones can cause softening of the skin and redistribution of fat, as well as breast growth. Breast development varies between people but does not generally exceed bra cup size B. Experts recommend for patients to be on hormones for 18 to 24 months before having breast augmentation, allowing the breasts to develop to their final size. Sex drive can decrease, as well as erections and ejaculation. Body hair can decrease somewhat, but often not as much as desired, prompting many women to obtain electrolysis. There is no change in voice, as testosterone has permanently altered the vocal cords, and many women seek out voice coaching. Those on estrogen should avoid cigarette smoking, as the combination can lead to an increased risk of blood clots. We should monitor blood pressure, as well as liver function and cholesterol. Also, providers routinely test prolactin as this hormone can increase with estrogen therapy, and in rare cases, transgender women may develop prolactinomas. Reproductive counseling is essential before beginning estrogen treatment because permanent sterility is almost always the outcome.

Surgery

Many fewer people undergo gender-related surgeries than take hormones. Some people do not desire gender-related surgeries. Others cannot afford them or are not convinced that they will be satisfied with the currently available results.

The most common type of surgery for both trans men and trans women is "top surgery," or chest surgery. Transgender men may have surgery to construct a male-contoured chest. Trans-women may have breast augmentation.

"Bottom surgery" is less common. Transgender men may have a metoidioplasty, in which the surgeon frees the clitoris from the ligament, attaching it to the body, and adds tissue increasing its length and girth. Scrotoplasty, the placement of testicular implants, is another way to create male-appearing genitalia. Phalloplasty, the creation of a penis, is less commonly performed because it is expensive, involves multiple procedures, requires donor skin from another part of the body, and has limited functionality. Bottom surgery for women is typically vaginoplasty, also commonly known as Sex Reassignment Surgery (SRS). Here, the surgeon removes the testicles, reconstructs the penis to form a clitoris, and creates a vagina. Techniques for vaginoplasty are becoming very good, but the procedure remains expensive. Because of this, some women, especially those with less money, may have orchiectomies, where the surgeon removes the testicles. These can be in-office procedures with a local anesthetic. The procedure is useful for substantially decreasing the body's production of androgens like testosterone. Less widely discussed, but essential to many women, are facial feminization surgeries that alter the cheeks, forehead, nose, and lips to create a more feminine facial appearance. The face is often used by persons to recognize gender in another person, and having facial features that match the affirmed gender can facilitate social interaction and provide safety from harassment and violence. Transgender men rarely undergo facial surgeries, as testosterone typically causes the face to appear more masculine.

Because surgery is inaccessible to many, there are rare cases of self-surgery, and some people have surgeries performed under unsafe conditions. Women may inject industrial-grade silicone to produce body curves. Silicone injection done without the supervision of a medical professional can result in body mutilation, infection, and even silicone blood clots that can lead to embolism and death.

EPIDEMIOLOGY

Children

Most children with gender dysphoria come to clinical attention in early grade school years. Parents, however, typically report that the cross-gender behaviors were apparent before 3 years of age. Among a sample of boys younger than age 12 referred for a range of clinical problems, the reported desire to be the other sex was 10 percent. For clinically referred girls younger than age 12, the reported desire to be the other sex was 5 percent. The sex ratio of children referred for gender dysphoria is 4 to 5 boys for each girl, which is likely due in part to societal stigma directed toward feminine boys. The sex ratio is equal in adolescents referred for gender dysphoria. Researchers have observed that many children considered to have shown gender-nonconforming behavior do not grow up to be transgender adults; conversely, many people who later come out as transgender adults report that they were not identified as gender nonconforming during childhood.

Adults

The estimates of gender dysphoria in adults emanate from European hormonal/surgical clinics with a prevalence of 1 in 11,000 male- and 1 in 30,000 female-assigned people. DSM-5 reports a prevalence rate ranging from 0.005 to 0.014 percent for male- and 0.002 to 0.003 percent for female-assigned people. Most clinical centers report a sex ratio of three to five male patients for each female patient. Most adults with gender dysphoria report having felt different from other children of their same sex, although, in retrospect, many could not identify the source of that difference. Many report feeling extensively cross-gender identified from the earliest years, with the cross-gender identification becoming more profound in adolescence and young adulthood. Overall the prevalence of male to female dysphoria is higher than female to male dysphoria. An important factor in diagnosis is that there is greater social acceptance of birth-assigned females dressing and behaving as boys (so-called tomboys) than there is of birth-assigned males acting as females (so-called sissies). Some researchers speculate that 1 in 500 adults may fall somewhere on a transgender spectrum, based on population data rather than clinical data.

ETIOLOGY

Biologic Factors

For mammals, the resting state of tissue is initially female. Males only develop if the body introduces androgen, which is set off by the Y chromosome. The result is testicular development. Without testes and androgen, female external genitalia develop. Thus, maleness and masculinity depend on fetal and perinatal androgens. Sex steroids govern sexual behavior in lower animals, but this effect diminishes as the evolutionary tree is scaled. Sex steroids influence the expression of sexual behavior in mature men or women; that is, testosterone can increase libido and aggressiveness in women, and estrogen can decrease libido and aggressiveness in men. However, masculinity, femininity, and gender identity are more a product of postnatal life events than the prenatal hormonal organization.

Brain organization theory refers to the masculinization or feminization of the brain in utero. Testosterone affects brain neurons that contribute to the masculinization of the brain in such areas as the hypothalamus. Whether testosterone contributes to so-called masculine or feminine behavioral patterns remains a controversial issue.

Genetic causes of gender dysphoria are under study, but we have not identified candidate genes, and chromosomal variations are uncommon in transgender populations. Case reports of identical twins have shown some pairs that are concordant for transgender issues and others that are not.

A variety of other approaches to understanding gender dysphoria are underway. These include imaging studies that have shown changes in white matter tracts, cerebral blood flow, and cerebral activation patterns in patients with gender dysphoria, but this is preliminary work. An incidental finding is that transgender persons are likely to be left-handed, the significance of which is unknown.

Psychosocial Factors

Children usually develop a gender identity consonant with their assigned sex. Many factors influence the formation of gender identity, including children's temperament and the interaction of that with parents' qualities and attitudes. Culturally acceptable gender roles exist: Society does not expect boys to be effeminate, or girls to be masculine. There are boys' games (e.g., cops and robbers) and girls' toys (e.g., dolls and dollhouses). Children learn these roles, although some investigators believe that some boys are temperamentally delicate and sensitive and that some girls are aggressive and energized—traits that are stereotypically known in today's culture as feminine and masculine, respectively. However, in Western society, we have a higher tolerance for "nontraditional" gender role behaviors than we once did.

Sigmund Freud believed that gender identity problems resulted from conflicts experienced by children within the oedipal triangle. In his view, both real family events and children's fantasies fuel these conflicts. Whatever interferes with a child loving the opposite-sex parent and identifying with the same-sex parent interferes with healthy gender identity development.

Since Freud, psychoanalysts have postulated that the quality of the mother–child relationship in the first years of life is paramount in establishing gender identity. During this period, mothers usually facilitate their children's awareness of, and pride in, their gender: they value their children as little boys and girls. Analysts argue that devaluing, hostile mothering can result in gender problems. At the same time, the separation–individuation process is unfolding. When gender problems become associated with separation–individuation problems, the result can be the use of sexuality to remain in relationships characterized by shifts between a desperate infantile closeness and a hostile, devaluing distance.

Some children receive the message that they would be more valued if they adopted the gender identity of the opposite sex. Rejected or abused children may act on such a belief. A mother's death, extended absence, or depression can influence the process, and a young boy may react by totally identifying with her—that is, by becoming a mother to replace her.

The father's role is also vital in the early years, and his presence can help the separation–individuation process. Without a father, the mother and child may remain overly close. For a girl, the father usually is the prototype of future love objects; for a boy, the father is a model for male identification.

Learning theory postulates that children may be rewarded or punished by parents and teachers based on gendered behavior, thus influencing the way children express their gender identities. Children also learn how to label people according to gender. Eventually, they also learn that we should not dictate gender based on surface appearances such as clothing or hairstyle.

References

Adelson SL; American Academy of Child and Adolescent Psychiatry (AACAP) Committee on Quality Issues (CQI). Practice parameter on gay, lesbian, or bisexual sexual orientation, gender nonconformity, and gender discordance in children and adolescents. *J Am Acad Child Adolesc Psychiatry*. 2011;51(9):957–974.

Carmel T, Hopwood R, Dickey L. Mental health concerns. In: Erickson-Schroth L, ed. *Trans Bodies, Trans Selves*. New York: Oxford University Press; 2014.

Devor AH. Witnessing and mirroring: a fourteen stage model of transsexual identity formation. *JGLP*. 2004;8(1/2):41–67.

Drescher J. Queer diagnoses: parallels and contrasts in the history of homosexuality, gender variance, and the Diagnostic and Statistical Manual. *Arch Sex Behav*. 2009;39:427–460.

Drescher J, Cohen-Kettenis P, Winter S. Minding the body: situating gender identity diagnoses in the ICD-11. *Int Rev Psychiatry*. 2012;24(6):568–577.

Erickson-Schroth L. Update on the biology of transgender identity. *J Gay Lesbian Ment Health*. 2013;17(2):150–174.

Erickson-Schroth L, Gilbert MA, Smith TE. Sex and gender development. In: Erickson-Schroth L, ed. *Trans Bodies, Trans Selves*. New York: Oxford University Press; 2014.

Grant JM, Mottet LA, Tanis J, Harrison J, Herman JL, Keisling M. Injustice at every turn: a report of the national transgender discrimination survey. Washington, DC: National Center for Transgender Equality and National Gay and Lesbian Task Force; 2011. Retrieved from http://www.thetaskforce.org/reports_and_research/ntds

Green R. Gender identity disorders. In: Sadock BJ, Sadock VA, Ruiz P, eds. *Kaplan & Sadock's Comprehensive Textbook of Psychiatry*. 9th ed. Philadelphia, PA: Lippincott Williams & Wilkins; 2009.

Lev AI. Transgender emergence: therapeutic guidelines for working with gender variant people and their families. Binghamton, New York: The Haworth Press; 2004.

Meier SC, Labuski CM. The demographics of the transgender population. In: Baumle AK, ed. *International Handbook on the Demography of Sexuality*. New York: Springer; 2013.

Spack NP, Edwards-Leeper L, Feldman HA, Leibowitz S, Mandel F, Diamond DA, Vance SR. Children and adolescents with gender identity disorder referred to a pediatric medical center. *Pediatrics*. 2012;129(3):418–425.

Wallien MSC, Cohen-Kettenis P. Psychosexual outcome of gender dysphoric children. *J Am Acad Child Adolesc Psychiatry*. 2008;47(12):1413–1423.

Wylie K, Barrett J, Besser M, Bouman WP, Bridgman M, Clayton A, Green R, et al. Good practice guidelines for the assessment and treatment of adults with gender dysphoria. *Sex Relatsh Ther*. 2014;29(2):154–214.

18 ▲

Disruptive, Impulse-Control, and Conduct Disorders

Six conditions comprise the category of *disruptive, impulse-control, and conduct disorders.* They include two that are associated with childhood: (1) oppositional defiant disorder and (2) conduct disorder; we discuss both in Chapter 2. DSM-5 includes antisocial personality disorder in both this section and in the personality disorders section; we will consider that with the personality disorders (Chapter 19). The remaining three disorders are intermittent explosive disorder, kleptomania, and pyromania, which are discussed here as well as other specified and unspecified disorders that relate to this category.

THE CLINICAL PRESENTATION

Persons suffering from one of these disorders have either an inability to resist an intense impulse or drive or are tempted to perform a particular act that is clearly harmful to themselves or others, or both. Before the event, the individual usually experiences mounting tension and arousal, sometimes—but not consistently—mingled with conscious anticipatory pleasure. Completing the action brings immediate gratification and relief. Within a variable time afterward, the individual experiences a conflation of remorse, guilt, self-reproach, and dread. Shameful secretiveness about the repeated impulsive activity frequently expands to permeate the individual's entire life, often delaying treatment.

Intermittent Explosive Disorder

Patients with intermittent explosive disorder have discrete episodes of losing control of their aggressive impulses; these episodes can result in severe assault or the destruction of property. The aggressiveness expressed is grossly out of proportion to any stressors that may have helped elicit the events. The episodes appear within minutes or hours and, regardless of duration, remit spontaneously and quickly. After each episode, patients usually show genuine regret or guilt, and signs of generalized impulsivity or aggressiveness are absent between events. Clinicians should not diagnose intermittent explosive disorder if they can better explain the symptoms with another disorder: one can imagine a long list of possible disorders, and we discuss some differentials in that section.

A 36-year-old real estate agent sought assistance for difficulty with his anger. He was quite competent at his job, although he frequently lost clients when he became enraged over their indecisiveness. On several occasions, he became verbally abusive, leading clients to find ways out of escrow closings. The impulsive aggression also led to the termination of multiple relationships because sudden angry outbursts contained demeaning accusations toward his girlfriends. These outbursts frequently occurred in the absence of any apparent conflict. On numerous occasions, the patient became so uncontrollably enraged that he threw things across the room, including books, his desk, and the contents of the refrigerator. Between episodes, he was a kind and likable individual with many friends. He enjoyed drinking on the weekends and had a history of two arrests for driving while intoxicated. On one of these occasions, he became involved in a verbal altercation with a police officer. He had a history of drug experimentation in college that included cocaine and marijuana.

A mental status examination revealed a generally cooperative patient. However, he became quite defensive when questioned about his anger and quickly felt accused and blamed by the interviewer for his past behaviors. He had no significant medical history and no signs of neurologic problems. He had never been in psychiatric treatment before this evaluation. He was on no medications. He denied any symptoms of a mood disorder or any other antisocial activity.

Treatment included the use of carbamazepine and a combination of supportive and cognitive-behavioral psychotherapy. The patient's angry outbursts improved as he became aware of the early signs that he was about to lose control. He learned techniques to avoid confrontation when such warning signs occurred. (Courtesy of Vivien K. Burt, M.D., Ph.D. and Jeffrey William Katzman, M.D.)

Kleptomania

Patients with kleptomania (from the Greek *kleptēs,* "thief") describe a recurrent failure to resist the impulse to steal objects, even though they have no need for the objects—often it has no value to the person, monetary or otherwise, and the patient could have easily afforded it. For patients with this disorder, the goal is not to obtain a specific item, it is the act of stealing itself. After taking the objects, the patient often gives them away, returns them secretly, or hides them.

As with other impulse-control disorders, patients with kleptomania experience mounting tension before the act, followed by gratification and lessening of tension after the action. They may or may not feel guilt or remorse and might feel depressed about their behavior. The theft is not planned and does not involve others. Although patients are unlikely to take something when immediate arrest is probable (e.g., in front of a security guard at a store), they may not rationally consider the risks involved even though repeated arrests lead to pain and humiliation. Patients may feel guilt and anxiety after the theft, but they do not feel anger or vengeance.

Jane was a 42-year-old, highly successful, single executive from a wealthy background. She called herself a "shop-'til-you-drop type" and had always been able to afford the expensive designer clothing that she loved. Since college, her "legit" shopping had been paralleled by "boosting" cheap panties and brassieres from discount stores. She did not wear the stolen items; indeed, she considered them "sleazy." She could never bring herself to get rid of them either and kept boxes filled with stolen lingerie in a storage facility.

Jane talked or bought her way out of trouble until her 30s when she was arrested while stealing pantyhose from the same K-Mart for the third time in as many months. As a condition of probation, she was ordered to see a psychiatrist. Her attendance was sporadic, and several more thefts occurred over the next 2 years. She also experienced substantial depression, which she tried to alleviate by heavy drinking.

Jane finally began taking her problem seriously after yet another arrest precipitated a suicidal gesture. She started keeping appointments regularly and consented to take citalopram and naltrexone. She believes that her participation in an Alcoholics Anonymous (AA) group for high-pressured executives has been at least as effective—if not more so—in controlling her stealing. (Courtesy of Harvey Roy Greenberg, M.D.)

Pyromania

Patients with pyromania repeatedly and deliberately set fires. They feel an urge to do this and relief or pleasure after they do. They typically are fascinated with all aspects of fires and may set off false alarms. They often are attracted to firefighting, may spend time at their local fire department, volunteer, or even become professional firefighters. Their curiosity is evident, but they show no remorse and may be indifferent to the consequences for life or property. Firesetters may gain satisfaction from the resulting destruction; frequently, they leave apparent clues.

DIAGNOSIS

Intermittent Explosive Disorder

Table 18-1 lists the diagnostic approaches to intermittent explosive disorder in DSM-5 and ICD-10. The key feature of this disorder is an aggressive outburst that has a rapid onset, typically without warning, lasting for less than 30 minutes. There is usually some provocation, although the response is disproportionate to that provocation. A less severe episode may occur in between the more severe ones.

As with most psychiatric disorders, the disorders cause significant distress or impairment in psychosocial functioning and are not better accounted for by another psychiatric, substance use, or other medical disorder. Relatively unique to this disorder is an age requirement, in which the individual has to be above the age of 6 years (or of comparable developmental level).

The diagnosis of intermittent explosive disorder should be the result of history-taking that reveals several episodes of loss of control associated with aggressive outbursts. One discrete episode does not justify the diagnosis. The histories typically describe a childhood in an atmosphere of an alcohol use disorder, violence, and emotional instability. Patients' work histories are poor; they report job losses, marital difficulties, and trouble with the law. Most patients have sought psychiatric help in the past but to no avail. Anxiety, guilt, and depression usually follow an outburst, but this is not a constant finding.

Kleptomania

Table 18-2 lists the diagnostic approaches to kleptomania in DSM-5 and ICD-10. The essential feature of kleptomania is recurrent, intrusive, and irresistible urges or impulses to steal unneeded objects. The act is accompanied by tension before the action and pleasure, gratification, or relief after it. It is not associated with anger or vengeance and is not better explained by some other disorder, as discussed in the Differential section.

Table 18-1
Intermittent Explosive Disorder

	Intermittent Explosive Disorder	
Disorder	DSM-5	ICD-10
Diagnostic name	Intermittent explosive disorder	Other habit and impulse disorders (intermittent explosive disorder)
Duration	If symptom 1, average of 2×/wk for 3 mo If symptom 2, occurs for at least 1 y	
Symptoms	Nonpremeditated, unmotivated verbal or physical aggression, out of proportion to the provocation 1. Not causing damage 2. Causing damage	Persistently repeated maladaptive behavior Failure to resist the impulse Preceded by a period of tension Followed by a period of release
Required number of symptoms	Either 1 or 2 above If symptom 2, has to occur at least 3 times within the year	All of above
Psychosocial consequences of symptoms	Distress or impaired functioning (social, occupational, or other significant areas) Or, financial or legal consequences	
Exclusions (not result of):	Medical illness Substance Other psychiatric disorder Age <6	Not secondary to another psychiatric syndrome
Comments		This is diagnosed as a habit and impulse disorder, "other," and not specifically defined

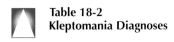

Table 18-2
Kleptomania Diagnoses

| Disorder | Kleptomania | |
	DSM-5	ICD-10
Diagnostic name	Kleptomania	Kleptomania
Symptoms	Recurrent stealing • Failure to resist the impulse to steal • Items stolen are not needed • Preceded by a period of tension • Followed by a period of gratification or release	Persistently repeated maladaptive behavior • Failure to resist the impulse • Preceded by a period of tension • Followed by a period of release
Required number of symptoms	All of above	All of above
Exclusions (not result of):	Anger Vengeance Psychosis Conduct disorder Mania Antisocial personality disorder	Not secondary to another psychiatric syndrome
Comments		Included among the habit and impulse disorders

Pyromania

Table 18-3 lists the diagnostic approaches to kleptomania in DSM-5 and ICD-10. To be diagnosed with pyromania, patients must set fires, not just desire or imagine them. This action is repetitive, deliberate, and purposeful. They feel tension or arousal before setting the fires as well as a fascination and attraction to fires. They may make considerable preparations before starting the fire. After setting the fire, they feel pleasure, gratification or relief when witnessing or participating in the aftermath of the fire. Perhaps related to that gratification, they also feel a similar attraction and interest with firefighting, including the activities and equipment associated with that profession. Like the discussion of kleptomania, they do not personally benefit, financially or otherwise, from the fire, hence the distinction between pyromania and arson, and the disorder is not better explained by another cause (see the Differential section).

Other Specified or Unspecified Disorders

DSM includes "other specified or unspecified disorders" for most of the diagnostic categories. This is usually a residual category for disorders that do not meet the criteria for the major disorders in the class. In this case, this group includes some unique disorders, some of which stand at the border between impulsive and compulsive disorders (see the section on Differential Diagnosis for a discussion of the difference). Many of these, such as Internet gaming disorder and related, are better considered as addictive disorders and included in our substance use disorders chapter. This is because even though not due to substances, the phenomenology, pathology, course, and treatment approach of disorders such as Internet gaming disorder appears to be very similar.

OBJECTIVE TESTS FOR THE DISORDERS

Physical Findings and Laboratory Examination

Blood chemistry (liver and thyroid function tests, fasting blood glucose, electrolytes), urinalysis (including drug toxicology), and syphilis serology may help rule out other causes of aggression or impulsive behavior. Magnetic resonance imaging (MRI) may reveal changes in the prefrontal cortex, which is associated with loss of impulse control.

DIFFERENTIAL DIAGNOSIS FOR THE DISRUPTIVE AND IMPULSE-CONTROL DISORDERS

It can be challenging to distinguish between impulse disorders and compulsive disorders, and the terms in practice are sometimes vague and overlapping. Technically, an *impulse* is a tension state that can exist without an action; a *compulsion* is a tension state that always has an action component. In the case of compulsive disorders (such as obsessive-compulsive disorder [OCD] or trichotillomania), the patients feel "compelled" to act out their pathologic behavior; they cannot resist the impulse to do so. Impulses and compulsions also differ by their expected result: people acting on an impulse expect to receive some pleasure, whereas compulsions are often ego-dystonic, meaning that a person does not desire or enjoy the act despite feeling compelled to do it. Even this is complicated, as in some cases impulse-control disorders also elicit guilt, which disturbs the sense of pleasure. Similarly, not all compulsions are ego-dystonic; for example, compulsive video game playing may have a pleasurable component. Both impulsive and compulsive behaviors are repetitive; however, the repeated acting out of impulses leads to psychosocial impairment, whereas compulsive behavior does not always carry that risk.

Intermittent Explosive Disorder

One should only diagnose an intermittent explosive disorder after other disorders associated with the occasional loss of control of aggressive impulses have been ruled out as the primary cause. These other disorders include psychotic disorders, personality change because of a general medical condition, antisocial or borderline personality disorder, substance intoxication (e.g., alcohol, barbiturates, hallucinogens, amphetamines), epilepsy, brain tumors, degenerative diseases, and endocrine disorders.

Table 18-3
Pyromania

| | Pyromania | |
Disorder	DSM-5	ICD-10
Diagnostic name	Pyromania	Pyromania
Symptoms	Fire setting • 1+ incidents • Deliberate and purposeful • Preoccupied by fire, burning, and related phenomena • Followed by a period of gratification or release	Fire setting • Multiple acts or attempts • No apparent motive • Preoccupied by fire, burning, and related phenomena • Preceded by a period of tension • Followed by a period of excitement
Required number of symptoms	All of above	All of above
Exclusions (not result of):	• Conduct disorder • Mania • Antisocial personality disorder • Psychosis • Impaired cognition or judgment Motivated by: • Desire for a perceived financial or social benefit • Sociopolitical ideology • Need to conceal criminal activity • Anger • Vengeance	• Dissocial personality disorder • Alcohol or substance disorder • Feigned illness • Conduct disorder • Organic mental disorder • Schizophrenia
Comments		Included among the habit and impulse disorders

The episodic and discrete nature of intermittent explosive disorder differentiates it from conduct disorder and antisocial personality disorder, which are more pervasive patterns of behavior in which aggression is a consistent feature, and not just associated with discrete outbursts.

In schizophrenia, patients may display violent behavior in response to delusions and hallucinations, and they show gross impairments in reality testing. Hostile patients with mania may be impulsively aggressive, but the underlying diagnosis is generally apparent from their mental status examinations and clinical presentations.

Amok is a culture-bound syndrome usually associated with southeastern Asia (but also seen elsewhere), which consists of episodes of acute violent behavior for which the person claims amnesia. It is distinguished from intermittent explosive disorder by a single episode and prominent dissociative features.

Among medical disorders, certain neurologic disorders can resemble impulse-control disorders. The best-documented examples are with Parkinson disease, which can resemble both impulse-control disorders and addictive disorder.

Kleptomania

Shoplifting has become a national epidemic. Few shoplifters have true kleptomania; most are teenagers and young adults who steal in pairs or small groups for "kicks" as well as goods and do not have a psychiatric disorder.

Individuals with an antisocial personality disorder steal for personal gain, with some degree of premeditation and planning. Often they convince others to rob for them. Antisocial stealing regularly involves the threat of harm or actual violence, mainly to elude capture. Guilt and remorse are distinctively lacking, or patients are patently insincere.

Episodes of theft occasionally occur during psychotic illness, for example, acute mania, major depression with psychotic features, or schizophrenia. Psychotic stealing is a product of pathologic elevation or depression of mood or command hallucinations or delusions.

Acute intoxication with drugs or alcohol may precipitate theft in an individual with another psychiatric disorder or without significant psychopathology. Patients with Alzheimer disease or other dementing organic illness may leave a store without paying, owing to forgetfulness rather than larcenous intent.

Some individuals with an antisocial personality disorder or no disorder may steal and then claim to suffer from kleptomania. This would be an example of malingering, not kleptomania, although with sufficiently intelligent perpetrators it may be challenging to tell the difference.

Pyromania

Clinicians should have little trouble distinguishing between pyromania and the fascination of many young children with matches, lighters, and fire as part of the normal investigation of their environments. One should also separate pyromania from incendiary acts of sabotage carried out by dissident political extremists or by arsonists.

When a fire setting occurs in conduct disorder and antisocial personality disorder, it is a deliberate act, not a failure to resist an impulse. Such individuals may set fires for profit, sabotage, or retaliation. Patients with schizophrenia or mania may set fires in response to delusions or hallucinations. Patients with brain dysfunction (e.g., dementia), mental retardation, or substance intoxication may set fires because of a failure to appreciate the consequences of the act.

COMORBIDITY

Intermittent Explosive Disorder

More than 80 percent of individuals with intermittent explosive disorder meet the criteria for another psychiatric disorder. These include other disorders of impulse-control and substance use, and mood, anxiety, personality (antisocial and borderline), posttraumatic stress, and eating disorders. Also, individuals with intermittent explosive disorder have been reported to be at increased risk of self-harm.

Kleptomania

Patients with kleptomania are said to have high lifetime comorbidity of major mood disorders (usually, but not exclusively, depressive) and various anxiety disorders. Associated conditions also include other disorders such as pathologic gambling and compulsive shopping, eating disorders (especially bulimia nervosa), personality disorders, OCD, and substance use disorders, especially alcohol use disorder. Individuals with kleptomania are also reported to have higher rates of suicide.

Pyromania

Pyromania is significantly associated with substance use disorders (especially alcohol and marijuana use disorders), affective disorders, depressive or bipolar, and other impulse-control disorders. They are also reported to have increased suicidal thoughts.

COURSE AND PROGNOSIS

Intermittent Explosive Disorder

Intermittent explosive disorder may begin at any stage of life but usually appears between late adolescence and early adulthood. The onset can be sudden or insidious, and the course can be episodic or chronic. In most cases, the disorder decreases in severity with the start of middle age, but heightened organic impairment can lead to frequent and severe episodes. Intermittent explosive disorder is more common in men than women.

Kleptomania

Kleptomania may begin in childhood, although most children and adolescents who steal do not become kleptomaniac adults. The onset of the disorder generally is adolescence. In quiescent cases, loss or disappointment may precipitate new bouts of the disorder.

The course of the disorder waxes and wanes but tends to be chronic—the frequency of stealing ranges from less than one to multiple episodes per month. Most patients with kleptomania steal from retail stores, but they may also take from family members in their households. People with the disorder sometimes have bouts of being unable to resist the impulse to steal, followed by free periods that last for weeks or months. The spontaneous recovery rate of kleptomania is unknown.

Severe impairment and complications are usually secondary to being caught, particularly to being arrested. Many persons seem never to have consciously considered the possibility of facing the consequences of their acts. Often, the disorder in no way impairs a person's social or work functioning.

The prognosis with treatment can be good, but few patients come for help of their own accord.

Pyromania

It should not be too surprising that we know very little about the development and course of pyromania. Most individuals with pyromania start setting fires in adolescence or young adulthood. The frequency and intensity of fire setting may increase over time or may wax and wane. The course of pyromania is unknown, but smaller studies suggest it may be chronic. Pyromania occurs more frequently in males with weaker social skills and learning difficulties.

TREATMENT APPROACH

Intermittent Explosive Disorder

A combined pharmacologic and psychotherapeutic approach has the best chance of success. Psychotherapy with patients who have an intermittent explosive disorder is difficult, however, because of their angry outbursts. Therapists may have problems with countertransference and limit-setting. Group psychotherapy may be helpful, and family therapy is useful, especially when the explosive patient is an adolescent or a young adult. A goal of treatment is to have the patient recognize and verbalize the thoughts or feelings that precede the explosive outbursts instead of acting them out. Cognitive-behavioral therapy and contingency management may be helpful.

Anticonvulsants have long been used, with mixed results, in treating explosive patients. Lithium has been reported useful in generally lessening aggressive behavior, and carbamazepine, valproate, and phenytoin have been reported helpful. Some clinicians have also used other anticonvulsants (e.g., topiramate). Clinicians occasionally use benzodiazepines but the meds can cause disinhibition, thus worsening the behaviors.

Antipsychotics and tricyclic drugs have been effective in some cases, but clinicians must then question whether schizophrenia or a mood disorder is the correct diagnosis. With a likelihood of subcortical seizure-like activity, medications that lower the seizure threshold can aggravate the situation. Selective serotonin reuptake inhibitors (SSRIs), trazodone, and buspirone are useful in reducing impulsivity and aggression. Propranolol and other β-adrenergic receptor antagonists and calcium channel inhibitors have also been effective in some cases.

Some neurosurgeons have performed operative treatments for intractable violence and aggression. No evidence indicates that such treatment is effective.

Kleptomania

Because true kleptomania is rare, reports of treatment tend to be individual case descriptions or a short series of cases. Insight-oriented psychotherapy and psychoanalysis have been successful but depend on patients' motivations. Those who feel guilt and shame may be helped by insight-oriented psychotherapy because of their increased motivation to change their behavior.

Case reports and case series suggest that cognitive-behavioral therapy may be helpful. Specific behavior therapies, including systematic desensitization, aversive conditioning, and a combination of aversive conditioning and altered social contingencies, have been reported successful, even when motivation was lacking.

SSRIs, such as fluoxetine and fluvoxamine, appear to be effective in some patients with kleptomania; however, there are also reports of fluoxetine having no benefit in kleptomania. Case reports indicated successful treatment with tricyclic drugs, trazodone, lithium, valproate, topiramate, naltrexone, methylphenidate, and electroconvulsive therapy. In a controlled trial of antidepressants, escitalopram was found to have no benefit in treating kleptomania. Though limited by small sample size and open-label design, high-dose naltrexone was reported to be effective in reducing the urge to steal in patients with kleptomania.

Pyromania

Little has been written about the treatment of pyromania, and treating firesetters has been difficult because of their lack of motivation. No single treatment has been proved effective; as a result, most therapists try various modalities, including behavioral approaches. Among the treatments attempted, CBT appears to be the most promising.

Because of the recurrent nature of pyromania, any treatment program should include the supervision of patients to prevent a repeated episode of fire setting. Incarceration may be the only method of avoiding a recurrence while their therapy can commence.

We should treat firesetting by children with the utmost seriousness. When possible we should consider intensive interventions, but as therapeutic and preventive measures, not as punishment. In the case of children and adolescents, treatment of pyromania or fire setting should include family therapy.

Several case reports have been published using SSRIs, lithium, naltrexone, stimulants, topiramate, valproate, carbamazepine, antiandrogen agents, clonazepam, and olanzapine. Unfortunately, many have reported no benefit from pharmacotherapy.

EPIDEMIOLOGY

For all these disorders, we do not know much about their epidemiology, as they are all underreported. This is understandable given the potential ramifications of self-reporting what is usually illegal behavior.

The lifetime prevalence rate for intermittent explosive disorder is estimated to be around 5 to 8 percent, and it appears to be more common in men than in women. The men are likely to be found in correctional institutions and the women in psychiatric facilities. In one study, about 2 percent of all persons admitted to a university hospital psychiatric service had an intermittent explosive disorder; 80 percent were men.

The prevalence of kleptomania is not known, but it is estimated to be about 0.6 percent. The range varies from 4 to 24 percent of those arrested for shoplifting. The male-to-female ratio is 1:3 in clinical samples.

No information is available on the prevalence of pyromania, but only a small percentage of adults who set fires have pyromania. The disorder is found far more often in men than in women. In the United States, 60 percent of individuals who set fires are adolescents; most, however, would not meet the criteria for pyromania.

ETIOLOGY

For all of these disorders, the cause is not known. Psychodynamic, psychosocial, and biologic factors all undoubtedly play an essential role. Some disruptive and impulse-control disorders may have common underlying neurobiologic mechanisms. Fatigue, constant stimulation, and psychic trauma can lower a person's resistance to control impulses.

Intermittent Explosive Disorder

Other factors associated with impulsive aggression include childhood exposure to violence, maltreatment, and neglect. One study found that there was significant association between intermittent explosive disorder and aversive childhood parenting environment comparable to other psychopathologies. Another study found that physical abuse in childhood was independently associated with intermittent explosive disorder, with impulsivity and aggression as the mediators of the relationship between physical abuse and intermittent explosive disorder. Others have shown that intermittent explosive disorder is associated with childhood exposure to interpersonal traumatic events.

Prefrontal cortical dysfunction has been associated with impulsive aggression. Some investigators suggest that disordered brain physiology, particularly in the limbic system, is involved in most cases of episodic violence. Compelling evidence indicates that serotonergic neurons mediate behavioral inhibition. Decreased serotonergic transmission, which can be induced by inhibiting serotonin synthesis or by antagonizing its effects, reduces the impact of punishment as a deterrent to behavior. The restoration of serotonin activity (e.g., by administering L-tryptophan, a serotonin precursor) restores the behavioral effect of punishment and may aid the control of violent tendencies. Low levels of CSF 5-hydroxyindoleacetic acid (5-HIAA) correlate with violent suicide attempts and impulsive aggression in some studies. High CSF testosterone concentrations are associated with aggressiveness and interpersonal violence in men. Antiandrogenic agents have been shown to decrease aggression.

Evidence indicates that intermittent explosive disorder is more common in first-degree biologic relatives of persons with the disorder than in the general population. This association does not imply a genetic etiology, as many other familial and social factors are surely influential. A gene–environment interaction may exist where individuals who have specific serotonin gene polymorphisms may be more prone to impulsive aggression behavior after exposure to childhood maltreatment.

Kleptomania

We know little about the etiology of kleptomania. There have been case reports of kleptomania associated with head trauma, frontal lobe lesions, cortical atrophy, dementia, and hypoglycemia secondary to insulinoma. There are implications for subtle white matter pathology based on diffusion tensor imaging results. Another study found that although, as a group, patients with kleptomania did not show deficits on neuropsychological testing, the severity of illness was associated with impairment in executive functioning.

Data are lacking and limited regarding the genetics of kleptomania. A study found that individuals with kleptomania had more first-degree relatives with alcohol use disorders compared to controls. Serotonin and dopamine, as well as the opioid and glutamatergic neurotransmitter systems, may play a role in kleptomania. Additionally, there are higher rates of OCD in relatives of individuals with kleptomania compared to the general population.

Pyromania

The etiology of pyromania is also poorly understood. The literature on the origins of pyromania has suggested factors ranging from temperament to environmental factors and parental psychopathology. Other authors have suggested pyromania, and the other impulse-control disorders, may share a neurobiologic link with substance use disorders. Limited studies suggest that pyromania may be associated with lower concentration of norepinephrine and serotonin metabolites 3-methoxy-4-hydroxyphenylglycol (MHPG) and 5-hydroxyindoleacetic acid (5-HIAA).

References

American Psychiatric Association. *Diagnostic and Statistical Manual of Mental Disorders*. 5th ed. Arlington, VA: American Psychiatric Association; 2013.

Dannon PN. Topiramate for the treatment of kleptomania: a case series and review of the literature. *Clin Neuropharmacol*. 2003;26:1.

Grant JE, Kim SW. An open-label study of naltrexone in the treatment of kleptomania. *J Clin Psychiatry*. 2002;63:349–356.

Grant JE, Potenza MN. Impulse control disorders: clinical characteristics and pharmacological management. *Ann Clin Psychiatry*. 2004;16:27–34.

Greenberg HR. Impulse-control disorders not elsewhere classified. In: Sadock BJ, Sadock VA, eds. *Kaplan & Sadock's Comprehensive Textbook of Psychiatry*. 8th ed. Vol. 1. Philadelphia, PA: Lippincott Williams & Wilkins; 2005:2035.

Hassamal S, Ramesh D, Moeller FG. Chapter 24: Impulse control disorders: pyromania. In: Sadock BJ, Sadock VA, Ruiz P, eds. *Kaplan & Sadock's Comprehensive Textbook of Psychiatry*. 10th ed. Philadelphia, PA: Wolters Kluwer; 2017: 2113–2114.

Hassamal S, Ramesh D, Moeller FG. Chapter 24: Impulse control disorders: kleptomania. In: Sadock BJ, Sadock VA, Ruiz P, eds. *Kaplan & Sadock's Comprehensive Textbook of Psychiatry*. 10th ed. Philadelphia, PA: Wolters Kluwer; 2017: 2114–2115.

Hollander E, Baker BR, Kahn J, Stein DJ. Conceptualizing and assessing impulse-control disorders. In: Hollander E, Stein DJ, eds. *Clinical Manual of Impulse-Control Disorders*. Washington, DC: American Psychiatric Publishing; 2006:1–18.

Koran LM, Aboujaoude EN, Gamel NN. Escitalopram treatment of kleptomania: an open-label trial followed by double-blind discontinuation. *J Clin Psychiatry*. 2007;68:422–427.

Kuzma JM, Black DW. Disorders characterized by poor impulse control. *Ann Clin Psychiatry*. 2005;17:219–226.

Lyke J. A psychiatric perspective on the variety of impulsive behaviors. *PsycCRITIQUES*. 2006;51(12).

Mandy W, Skuse D, Steer C, St Pourcain B, Oliver BR. Oppositionality and socioemotional competence: interacting risk factors in the development of childhood conduct disorder symptoms. *J Am Acad Child Adolesc Psychiatry*. 2013;52(7):718–727.

Olson SL, Sameroff AJ, Lansford JE, Sexton H, Davis-Kean P, Bates JE, Pettit GS, Dodge KA. Deconstructing the externalizing spectrum: growth patterns of overt aggression, covert aggression, oppositional behavior, impulsivity/inattention, and emotion dysregulation between school entry and early adolescence. *Dev Psychopathol*. 2013;25(3):817–842.

Ramesh D, Hassamal S, Moeller FG. Chapter 24: Impulse control disorders: intermittent explosive disorder. In: Sadock BJ, Sadock VA, Ruiz P, eds. *Kaplan & Sadock's Comprehensive Textbook of Psychiatry*. 10th ed. Philadelphia, PA: Wolters Kluwer; 2017:2110–2113.

Reimherr FW, Marchant BK, Olsen JL, Wender PH, Robison RJ. Oppositional defiant disorder in adults with ADHD. *J Attent Dis*. 2013;17(2):102–113.

Reist C, Nakamura K, Sagart E, Sokolski KN, Fujimoto KA. Impulsive aggressive behavior: open-label treatment with citalopram. *J Clin Psychiatry*. 2003;64:81.

Stein DJ, Harvey B, Seedat S, Hollander E. Treatment of impulse-control disorders. In: Hollander E, Stein DJ, eds. *Clinical Manual of Impulse-Control Disorders*. Washington, DC: American Psychiatric Publishing; 2006:309–325.

Voon V, Rizos A, Chakravartty R, Mulholland N, Robinson S, Howell NA, Harrison N, Vivian G, Chaudhuri KR. Impulse control disorders in Parkinson's disease: decreased striatal dopamine transporter levels. *J Neurol Neurosurg Psychiatry*. 2014;85(2):148–152.

Zhang Z, Huang F, Liu D. Kleptomania: recent advances in symptoms, etiology and treatment. *Curr Med Sci*. 2018;38:937–940.

The person-centered approach to understanding personality and its disorders distinguish psychiatry fundamentally from all other branches of medicine. A person is a self-aware human being, as C. Robert Cloninger said, not "a machine-like object that lacks self-awareness." Personality refers to all of the characteristics that distinguish a continually developing, self-organizing human being from a predictable machine-like object. In other words, personality refers to all the ways someone shapes and adapts in a unique way to an ever-changing internal and external environment.

Persons with personality disorders are far more likely to refuse psychiatric help and to deny their problems than persons with anxiety disorders, depressive disorders, or obsessive-compulsive disorder. In general, personality disorder symptoms are ego-syntonic (i.e., acceptable to the ego, as opposed to ego-dystonic) and alloplastic (i.e., adapt by trying to alter the external environment rather than themselves). Persons with personality disorders do not feel anxiety about their maladaptive behavior. Because they do not routinely acknowledge pain from what others perceive as their symptoms, they often seem disinterested in treatment and impervious to recovery.

THE CLINICAL PRESENTATION

Persons suffering from one of these disorders have long-standing, maladaptive behavior traits that are pervasive and apparent in a wide range of personal and social contexts.

Paranoid Personality Disorder

Persons with paranoid personality disorder have long-standing suspiciousness and mistrust of persons in general. They refuse responsibility for their feelings and assign responsibility to others. They are often hostile, irritable, and angry.

Schizoid Personality Disorder

Schizoid personality disorder is characterized by a lifelong pattern of social withdrawal. Others often see persons with schizoid personality disorder as eccentric, isolated, or lonely. Their discomfort with human interaction, their introversion, and their bland, constricted affect are noteworthy.

Schizotypal Personality Disorder

Persons with schizotypal personality disorder are strikingly odd or strange, even to laypersons. Magical thinking, peculiar notions, ideas of reference, illusions, and derealization are commonplace.

Antisocial Personality Disorder

Antisocial personality disorder is an inability to conform to the social norms that ordinarily govern many aspects of a person's adolescent and adult behavior. Although often characterized by continual antisocial or criminal acts, the disorder is not synonymous with criminality.

Borderline Personality Disorder

Patients with borderline personality disorder stand on the border between neurosis and psychosis, and they have extraordinarily unstable affect, mood, behavior, object relations, and self-image.

Histrionic Personality Disorder

Persons with histrionic personality disorder are excitable and emotional and behave in a colorful, dramatic, extroverted fashion. Accompanying their flamboyant aspects, however, is often an inability to maintain sincere, long-lasting attachments.

Narcissistic Personality Disorder

Individuals with narcissistic personality disorder have a heightened sense of self-importance, lack of empathy, and grandiose feelings of uniqueness. Underneath, however, their self-esteem is fragile and vulnerable to even minor criticism.

Avoidant Personality Disorder

Persons with avoidant personality disorder show extreme sensitivity to rejection and may lead socially withdrawn lives. Although shy, they are not asocial and show a great desire for companionship, but they need unusually strong guarantees of uncritical acceptance. We often describe this group as having an inferiority complex.

Dependent Personality Disorder

Patients with dependent personality disorder subordinate their own needs to those of others, get others to assume responsibility for significant areas of their lives, lack self-confidence, and may experience intense discomfort when alone for more than a brief period.

Obsessive-Compulsive Personality Disorder

Persons with obsessive-compulsive personality disorder typically are emotionally constricted, orderly, perseverative, stubborn, and indecisive. The essential feature of the disorder is a pervasive pattern of perfectionism and inflexibility.

Personality Change due to a General Medical Condition

Personality change due to a general medical condition is a significant occurrence. ICD-10 includes the category personality and behavioral disorders due to brain disease, damage, and dysfunction, which includes organic personality disorder, postencephalitic syndrome, and postconcussional syndrome. Persons with this disorder have a marked change in personality style and traits from their previous level of functioning. Patients must show evidence of a causative medical factor antedating the onset of personality change.

DIAGNOSIS

DSM-5's categorical approach to personality disorders is problematic. It seems counterintuitive to think that we can boil down disturbed personality into a few symptoms. Experts in the field have argued for a more dimensional approach that is grounded in research on temperament and personality, some of which we later describe. The DSM-5 Personality Disorders Workgroup did work on such a change, in which the clinician would focus on the impairments in a person's personality functioning, using an approach based on a widely accepted model of personality. Although the authors of DSM-5 did consider such a change, they felt it too radical a leap for clinical use. Instead, they included the approach that the workgroup recommended in a later section of the book, "Emerging Measures and Models." For now, the categorical approach remains. However, this remains a controversial area of psychiatry, and many rightly question the validity of this approach.

ICD-10, with its more descriptive approach, is a little less controversial. However, despite some wording differences, its approach is similar to DSM-5's, although it lists more disorders than does DSM-5.

Table 19-1 compares the general approaches to diagnosing personality disorders.

DSM-5 divides the disorders into three categories, or clusters: A, B, and C. Cluster A includes three personality disorders with odd, aloof features (paranoid, schizoid, and schizotypal). Cluster B includes four personality disorders with dramatic, impulsive, exploitative, and erratic features (borderline, antisocial, narcissistic, and histrionic). Cluster C includes three personality disorders sharing anxious and fearful features (avoidant, dependent, and obsessive-compulsive). Individuals frequently exhibit traits that are not limited to a single personality disorder. When a patient meets the criteria for more than one personality disorder, clinicians should diagnose each.

Many of the features of various personality disorders can occur during an episode of another mental disorder. We should only use a diagnosis of personality disorder when the features are typical of long-term functioning and are not limited to a discrete episode of another mental disorder. Likewise, when maladaptive behavior features are due to the direct psychological effects of another mental disorder, including substance use, a diagnosis of personality disorder is not warranted. However, it is possible to diagnose personality change due to another medical condition such as temporal lobe epilepsy; in this case, we must specify the medical condition along with the associated diagnosis of personality change.

Table 19-1
Personality Disorders

Name	DSM-5 **General Personality Disorder**	ICD-10 **Disorders of Adult Personality and Behavior**
Duration	Persistent, long duration, usually since teens or early adulthood	Persistent
Symptoms	The symptoms comprise a fixed pattern of behavior. The domains include: • Cognitive and perceptual • Mood and affect • Interpersonal • Behavioral	Consistent, fixed, and inflexible pattern of behaviors, involving • Dysfunctional relationships • Distorted view of oneself
# Symptoms Needed	2/4 of the domains above	
Exclusions (not result of):	Another mental disorder Substance use Another medical illness	
Psychosocial Impact	Distress, functional impairment	Usually causes distress Difficulties with social performance
Specific Disorders	• **Cluster A:** paranoid personality disorder, schizoid personality disorder, schizotypal personality disorder • **Cluster B:** antisocial personality disorder, borderline personality disorder, histrionic personality disorder, narcissistic personality disorder • **Cluster C:** avoidant personality disorder, dependent personality disorder, obsessive-compulsive personality disorder	• **Specific personality disorder:** Paranoid personality disorder, schizoid personality disorder, dissocial personality disorder, emotionally unstable personality disorder, histrionic personality disorder, anankastic personality disorder, anxious [avoidant] personality disorder, dependent personality disorder, other specific personality disorder (eccentric, haltlose, immature, narcissistic, passive-aggressive, psychoneurotic), personality disorder unspecified • **Mixed and other personality disorders** • **Enduring personality changes:** due to brain damage and disease, after catastrophic experience, after psychiatric illness, chronic pain personality syndrome, enduring personality change unspecified

This compares the general criteria for all the disorders. Please see additional tables for specific personality disorders.

Table 19-2
Paranoid Personality Disorder: Specific Symptoms

DSM-5		ICD-10	
Paranoid Personality Disorder		**Paranoid Personality Disorder**	
Suspiciousness, evident from the following (≥4): • Suspicion/persecutory thoughts • Doubting others' loyalty • Distrust, inability to confide in others • Interpreting experiences as threatening or hostile • Holds grudges • Feeling attacked by others • Distrusting partner's faithfulness	Exclusions (not result of): • Schizophrenia • Depression with psychotic features • Other psychoses • Substance use • A medical condition	• Excessive sensitivity to setbacks or insults • Suspiciousness • Interpreting experiences as threatening or hostile • Distrusting partner's faithfulness • May also be self-important or overall self-referential	Exclusions (not result of): • Psychosis • Schizophrenia • Paranoid state

Cluster A: Odd and Eccentric

Paranoid Personality Disorder. The hallmarks of paranoid personality disorder are excessive suspiciousness and distrust of others expressed as a pervasive tendency to interpret the actions of others as deliberately demeaning, malevolent, threatening, exploiting, or deceiving. This tendency begins in early adulthood and appears in a variety of contexts. Almost invariably, those with the disorder expect to be exploited or harmed by others in some way. They frequently dispute, without any justification, friends' or associates' loyalty or trustworthiness. Such persons are often pathologically jealous and, for no reason, question the fidelity of their spouses or sexual partners. Persons with this disorder externalize their own emotions and use the defense of projection; they attribute to others the impulses and thoughts that they cannot accept in themselves. Ideas of reference and logically defended illusions are common. Table 19-2 compares the different approaches to diagnosing paranoid personality disorder.

On psychiatric examination, patients with paranoid personality disorder may be formal in their style and act baffled about having to seek psychiatric help. Muscular tension, an inability to relax, and a need to scan the environment for clues may be evident, and the patient's manner is often severe and humorless. Although some premises of their arguments may be false, their speech is goal-directed and logical. Their thought content shows evidence of projection, prejudice, and occasional ideas of reference.

Schizoid Personality Disorder. Persons with schizoid personality disorder seem to be cold and aloof; they display a remote reserve and show no involvement with everyday events and the concerns of others. They appear quiet, distant, seclusive, and unsociable. They may pursue their own lives with remarkably little need or longing for emotional ties, and they are the last to be aware of changes in popular fashion. Table 19-3 compares the different approaches to diagnosing schizoid personality disorder.

The life histories of such persons reflect solitary interests and success at noncompetitive, lonely jobs that others find difficult to tolerate. Their sexual lives may exist exclusively in fantasy, and they may postpone mature sexuality indefinitely. Persons with schizoid personality disorder usually reveal a lifelong inability to express anger directly. They often lack close friends or confidants and are indifferent to praise and criticism. Although persons with schizoid personality disorder appear self-absorbed and lost in daydreams, they have an average capacity to recognize reality.

On an initial psychiatric examination, patients with schizoid personality disorder may appear ill at ease. They rarely tolerate eye contact, and interviewers may surmise that such patients are eager for the interview to end. Their affect may be constricted, aloof, or inappropriately severe, but underneath the aloofness, sensitive clinicians can recognize fear. These patients find it challenging to be lighthearted: their efforts at humor may seem adolescent and off the mark. Their speech is goal-directed, but they are likely to

Table 19-3
Schizoid Personality Disorder: Specific Symptoms

DSM-5		ICD-10	
Schizoid Personality Disorder		**Schizoid Personality Disorder**	
Detachment from interpersonal relationships (≥4): • Doesn't enjoy relationships • Prefers doing things alone • Not interested in sexual relations • Doesn't enjoy activities • Few if any friends or acquaintances • Doesn't care what others think of them • Emotionally constricted	Exclusions (not result of): • Schizophrenia • Depression with psychotic features • Bipolar disorder with psychotic features • Autism spectrum disorder • Another psychotic disorder • Another medical condition	• Retreats from close contact or emotional encounters • Prefers fantasy, isolation, and introspection • Difficulty expressing emotions • Difficulty experiencing pleasure	Exclusions (not result of): • Asperger syndrome • Delusional disorder • Schizophrenia • Schizotypal disorder

Table 19-4
Schizotypal Personality Disorder: Specific Symptoms

DSM-5		ICD-10	
Schizotypal Personality Disorder		**Schizotypal Disorder (classified under the psychotic disorders in ICD-10, not personality disorders)**	
Social difficulties and perceptual disturbances (≥5): • Ideas of reference • Magical/strange thinking • Odd perceptions • Odd speech/thoughts • Odd affect • Odd behavior • Suspicious or persecutory thoughts • Few if any friends or acquaintances • Socially anxious (because of thoughts)	Exclusions (not result of): • Schizophrenia • Depression with psychotic features • Bipolar disorder with psychotic features • Autism spectrum disorder • Another psychotic disorder	• Eccentric behavior • Abnormal thinking • Cold affect • Odd behavior • Social isolation • Perceptual disturbances: Quasi-psychotic episodes Illusions Delusional-like ideas Hallucinations • Starts suddenly, course is more like that for personality disorders	Exclusions (not result of): • Schizophrenia, other psychiatric disorders • Asperger syndrome • Schizoid personality disorder

give short answers to questions and to avoid spontaneous conversation. They may occasionally use unusual figures of speech, such as an odd metaphor, and may be fascinated with inanimate objects or metaphysical constructs. Their sensorium is intact, their memory functions well, and their proverb interpretations are abstract.

Schizotypal Personality Disorder. Schizotypal personality disorder is characterized by pervasive discomfort with and inability to maintain close relationships, as well as eccentric behavior. These individuals demonstrate peculiarities of thinking, behavior, and appearance. Taking a history may be difficult because of the patients' unusual way of communicating.

Patients with schizotypal personality disorder exhibit disturbed thinking and communicating. Although frank thought disorder is absent, their speech may be distinctive or peculiar, may have meaning only to them, and often needs interpretation. These patients may be superstitious or claim powers of clairvoyance and may believe that they have other special powers of thought and insight. Their inner world may contain vivid imaginary relationships and child-like fears and fantasies, and they may experience perceptual illusions, as well. Table 19-4 compares the different approaches to diagnosing schizotypal personality disorder.

Because persons with schizotypal personality disorder have poor interpersonal relationships and may act inappropriately, they are isolated and have few, if any, friends. Under stress, patients with schizotypal personality disorder may decompensate and have psychotic symptoms, but these are usually brief. Patients with severe cases of the disorder may exhibit anhedonia and severe depression.

Cluster B: Dramatic

Antisocial Personality Disorder. The hallmarks of antisocial personality disorder are pervasive disrespect for and infringement on the rights of others. A person has to be 18 years of age or older, has to have demonstrated this pattern of behavior since age 15, and must have demonstrated evidence of conduct disorder before the age of 15 years (conduct disorder involves a repetitive and persistent pattern of behavior in which they violate the fundamental rights of others or major age-appropriate social rules). Table 19-5 compares the different approaches to diagnosing antisocial personality disorder.

Patients with antisocial personality disorder can often seem to be normal and even charming and ingratiating. Their histories, however, reveal many areas of disordered life functioning. Lying,

Table 19-5
Antisocial Personality Disorder: Specific Symptoms

DSM-5		ICD-10	
Antisocial Personality Disorder		**Dissocial Personality Disorder**	
≥age 18 Began by age 15 Conduct disorder before age 15 (diagnosed or evidence for) (≥3): • Disregards legal and social rules/norms • Lies • Impulsive • Irritable or aggressive • Neglects safety (self/others) • Irresponsible • No remorse	Exclusions (not result of): • Schizophrenia • Bipolar disorder	• Disregards social norms • Unconcerned by others' feelings • Easily frustrated/distressed • Easily becomes aggressive • Blames others	Exclusions (not result of): • Conduct disorders • Emotionally unstable personality disorder

truancy, running away from home, thefts, fights, substance abuse, and illegal activities are typical experiences that patients report as beginning in childhood. These patients often impress clinicians with the colorful, seductive aspects of their personalities, but the clinician may also regard them as manipulative and demanding. They frequently have a heightened sense of reality testing and often impress observers as having excellent verbal intelligence.

Persons with antisocial personality disorder are highly representative of the so-called con men. They are incredibly manipulative and can frequently talk others into participating in schemes for easy ways to make money or to achieve fame or notoriety. These schemes may eventually lead the unwary to financial ruin, social embarrassment, or both. Those with this disorder do not tell the truth and cannot be trusted to carry out any task or adhere to any conventional standard of morality. Promiscuity, spousal abuse, child abuse, and drunk driving are frequent events in their lives. A notable finding is a lack of remorse for these actions; that is, they appear to lack a conscience.

Patients with antisocial personality disorder can fool even the most experienced clinicians. In an interview, patients can appear composed and credible, but beneath the veneer lurks tension, hostility, irritability, and rage. A stress interview, in which the clinician vigorously confronts the patient with inconsistencies in their histories, may be necessary to reveal the pathology. A diagnostic workup should include a thorough neurologic examination. Because patients often show abnormal EEG results and soft neurologic signs suggesting minimal brain damage in childhood, these findings may support the clinical impression.

Borderline Personality Disorder. Persons with borderline personality disorder almost always appear to be in a state of crisis. Mood swings are frequent. Patients can be argumentative at one moment, depressed the next, and later complain of having no feelings. Patients can have short-lived psychotic episodes rather than full-blown psychotic breaks, and the symptoms are circumscribed, fleeting, or questionable. The behavior of patients with borderline personality disorder is highly unpredictable, and their achievements are rarely at the level of their abilities. The painful nature of their lives reflects in their repetitive self-destructive acts. Such patients may slash their wrists and perform other self-mutilation to elicit help from others, to express anger, or to numb themselves to overwhelming affect. Table 19-6 compares the different approaches to diagnosing borderline personality disorder.

Because they feel both dependent and hostile, persons with this disorder have tumultuous interpersonal relationships. They can be dependent on those with whom they are close and, when frustrated, can express enormous anger toward their intimate friends. Patients with borderline personality disorder cannot tolerate being alone, and they prefer a frantic search for companionship, no matter how unsatisfactory, to their own company. To assuage loneliness, if only for brief periods, they accept a stranger as a friend or behave promiscuously. They often complain about chronic feelings of emptiness and boredom and the lack of a consistent sense of identity (identity diffusion); when pressed, they may complain about how depressed they usually feel, despite the flurry of other affects.

Functionally, patients with borderline personality disorder distort their relationships by considering each person to be either all good or all bad. They see persons as either nurturing attachment figures or as hateful, sadistic figures who deprive them of security needs and threaten them with abandonment whenever they feel dependent. As a result of this splitting, the good person is idealized, and the bad person devalued. Shifts of allegiance from one person or group to another are frequent. Some clinicians use the concepts of panphobia, pananxiety, panambivalence, and chaotic sexuality to delineate these patients' characteristics.

Projective identification is a defense mechanism that often occurs in patients with borderline personality disorder. In this primitive defense mechanism, the patient projects intolerable aspects of themselves onto another person, inducing them to play the projected role, and the two persons act in unison. Therapists must be aware of this process so they can act neutrally toward such patients.

Histrionic Personality Disorder. Persons with histrionic personality disorder show a high degree of attention-seeking behavior. They tend to exaggerate their thoughts and feelings and make everything sound more vital than it is. They display temper tantrums, tears, and accusations when they are not the center of attention or are not receiving praise or approval. Table 19-7 compares the different approaches to diagnosing histrionic personality disorder.

Seductive behavior is typical in both sexes. Sexual fantasies about persons with whom patients are involved are common, but patients are inconsistent about verbalizing these fantasies and may be coy or flirtatious rather than sexually aggressive. Despite these behaviors, they may have a psychosexual dysfunction, such as anorgasmia. They may act on their sexual impulses to reassure themselves that they are attractive to the other sex. Their relationships tend to be superficial, however, and they can be vain, self-absorbed, and fickle. Their deep dependence needs make them overly trusting and gullible.

**Table 19-6
Borderline Personality Disorder: Specific Symptoms**

DSM-5	ICD-10	
Borderline Personality Disorder	**Emotionally Unstable Personality Disorder**	
Conflict/impulsivity (≥5): • Avoids abandonment • Intense, unstable relations marked by splitting • Unstable self-image • Self-harm, other impulsive behaviors • Suicidal ideation or behavior • Labile affect • Feeling empty inside • Poor anger management • Paranoia/dissociation, usually due to stress	• Impulsiveness • Labile mood • Outbursts • Interpersonal conflict Two subtypes: (1) Impulsive type (emotional lability and lack of impulse control) (2) Borderline type (poor self-image, self-worth, relationships, with associated self-harm)	Exclusions (not result of): • Dissocial personality disorder

Table 19-7
Histrionic Personality Disorder: Specific Symptoms

DSM-5	ICD-10
Histrionic Personality Disorder	**Histrionic Personality Disorder**
Needing attention, very emotional (≥5): • Uncomfortable when not the center of attention • Flirtatious, provocatively sexual • Emotionally labile • Physically provocative or flamboyant • Speech is vague • Speech is exaggerated/ dramatic • Suggestible • Overestimates the intimacy of relationships	• Affect is shallow/labile • Self-dramatization • Speech and emotions are exaggerated • Suggestible • Egocentric • Not concerned with others • Attention seeking • Easily offended or hurt

Table 19-8
Narcissistic Personality Disorder: Specific Symptoms

DSM-5	ICD-10
Narcissistic Personality Disorder	**Narcissistic Personality**
Self-important, lacking empathy for others (≥5): • Grandiose • Preoccupied with fantasies about success • Feeling special/unique • Needing others to admire them for validation • Expecting special treatment • Exploiting others • Lacking empathy • Jealous of others' success, assuming others are jealous of them • Arrogance	Not described. Listed as an "other specific personality disorder"

The major defenses of patients with histrionic personality disorder are repression and dissociation. Accordingly, such patients are unaware of their true feelings and cannot explain their motivations. Under stress, reality testing quickly becomes impaired.

In interviews, patients with histrionic personality disorder are generally cooperative and eager to give a detailed history. Gestures and dramatic punctuation in their conversations are commonplace; they may make frequent slips of the tongue, and their language is colorful. Affective display is typical, but when pressed to acknowledge certain feelings (e.g., anger, sadness, and sexual wishes), they may respond with surprise, indignation, or denial. The results of the cognitive examination are usually normal, although they may show a lack of perseveration on arithmetic or concentration tasks, and the patients' forgetfulness of affect-laden material may be astonishing.

Narcissistic Personality Disorder.   Persons with narcissistic personality disorder have a grandiose sense of self-importance; they consider themselves special and expect special treatment. Their sense of entitlement is striking. They handle criticism poorly and may become enraged when someone dares to criticize them, or they may appear utterly indifferent to criticism. Persons with this disorder want their way and are frequently ambitious to achieve fame and fortune. Their relationships are tenuous, and they can make others furious by their refusal to obey conventional rules of behavior. Interpersonal exploitativeness is commonplace. They cannot show empathy, and they feign sympathy only to achieve their selfish ends. Because of their fragile self-esteem, they are susceptible to depression. Interpersonal difficulties, occupational problems, rejection, and loss are among the stresses that narcissists commonly produce by their behavior—stresses they are least able to handle. Table 19-8 compares the different approaches to diagnosing narcissistic personality disorder.

Cluster C: Anxious

Avoidant Personality Disorder.   Hypersensitivity to rejection by others is the central feature of avoidant personality disorder, and timidity is the primary personality trait that is displayed. These persons desire the warmth and security of human companionship but justify their avoidance of relationships by their fear of rejection. When talking with someone, they express uncertainty, show

a lack of self-confidence, and may speak in a self-effacing manner. Because they are hypervigilant about rejection, they are afraid to speak up in public or to make requests of others. They are apt to misinterpret others' comments as derogatory or ridiculing. The refusal of any request leads them to withdraw from others and to feel hurt. Table 19-9 compares the different approaches to diagnosing avoidant personality disorder.

In the vocational sphere, patients with avoidant personality disorder often take jobs on the sidelines. They rarely attain much personal advancement or exercise much authority but seem shy and eager to please. These persons are generally unwilling to enter relationships unless they have an unusually strong guarantee of uncritical acceptance. Consequently, they often have no close friends or confidants.

In clinical interviews, patients' most striking aspect is anxiety about talking with an interviewer. Their nervous and tense manner may wax and wane depending on whether they think the interviewer likes them. They may also seem vulnerable to the interviewer's comments and suggestions and may regard a clarification or interpretation as criticism.

Dependent Personality Disorder.   Dependent personality disorder is a pervasive pattern of dependent and submissive behavior.

Table 19-9
Avoidant Personality Disorder: Specific Symptoms

DSM-5	ICD-10
Avoidant Personality Disorder	**Anxious [Avoidant] Personality Disorder**
Hypersensitive, lacking confidence (≥4): • Avoids others • Fears being disliked • Avoids relationships for fear of shame • Fears rejection/criticism • Inhibited in relationships • Avoids novelty for fear of embarrassment	• Fearful, insecure, feels inferior to others • Craves acceptance • Fears or is sensitive to rejection • Relationships are superficial • Avoids activities/situations perceived as risky

Table 19-10
Dependent Personality Disorder: Specific Symptoms

DSM-5	ICD-10
Dependent Personality Disorder	**Dependent Personality Disorder**
Fears separation, needs others to care for them (≥5): • Cannot make decisions alone • Avoids taking on responsibility for important things • Cannot disagree with others for fear they will disapprove of them • Lacks confidence, cannot initiate new things • Seeks acceptance of others • Fears being alone/independence • When relationship ends, quickly seeks new one • Fears having to take care of self	• Relies on others and needs them for validation • Cannot make decisions without another's approval • Fears abandonment • Fears helplessness/incompetence • Passive, lets another make decisions • Avoids responsibility

Persons with the disorder cannot make decisions without significant and unwarranted advice and encouragement from others. They avoid positions of responsibility and become anxious if asked to assume a leadership role. They prefer to be submissive. When on their own, they find it difficult to persevere at tasks but may find it easy to perform these tasks for someone else. Table 19-10 compares the different approaches to diagnosing dependent personality disorder.

Because persons with the disorder do not like to be alone, they seek out others on whom they can depend; their relationships, thus, are distorted by their need to be attached to another person. In a shared psychotic disorder (folie à deux), one member of the pair usually has dependent personality disorder; the submissive partner takes on the delusional system of the more aggressive, assertive partner on whom he or she depends.

Pessimism, self-doubt, passivity, and fears of expressing sexual and aggressive feelings all typify the behavior of persons with a dependent personality disorder. An abusive, unfaithful, or alcoholic spouse may be tolerated for long periods to avoid disturbing the sense of attachment.

In interviews, patients appear compliant. They try to cooperate, welcome specific questions and look for guidance.

Obsessive-Compulsive Personality Disorder.   Persons with obsessive-compulsive personality disorder are preoccupied with rules, regulations, orderliness, neatness, details, and the achievement of perfection. These traits account for the general constriction of the entire personality. They insist that rules be followed rigidly and cannot tolerate what they consider infractions. Accordingly, they lack flexibility and are intolerant. They are capable of prolonged work, provided it is routinized and does not require changes to which they cannot adapt. Table 19-11 compares the different approaches to diagnosing obsessive-compulsive personality disorder.

Persons with obsessive-compulsive personality disorder have limited interpersonal skills. They are formal and severe and often lack a sense of humor. They alienate those around them, are unable to compromise, and insist that others submit to their needs. They are eager to please those whom they see as more powerful, however, and they carry out these persons' wishes in an authoritarian manner. Because they fear to make mistakes, they are indecisive and ruminate about making decisions. Although a stable marriage and occupational adequacy are common, persons with obsessive-compulsive personality disorder have few friends. Anything that threatens to upset their perceived stability or the routine of their lives can precipitate much anxiety otherwise bound up in the rituals that they impose on their lives and try to impose on others.

In interviews, patients with an obsessive-compulsive personality disorder may have a stiff, formal, and rigid demeanor. Their affect is not blunted or flat but often constricted. They lack spontaneity, and their mood is usually serious. Such patients may be anxious about not being in control of the interview. Their answers to questions are unusually detailed. The defense mechanisms they use are rationalization, isolation, intellectualization, reaction formation, and undoing.

Other Personality Disorders

Personality Change due to Another Medical Condition. This diagnosis involves a change in personality from previous patterns of behavior or an exacerbation of previous personality characteristics. Impaired control of the expression of emotions and impulses is a cardinal feature. Emotions are characteristically labile and shallow, although euphoria or apathy may be prominent. The euphoria may mimic hypomania, but genuine elation is absent, and patients may admit to not feeling happy. There is a hollow and silly ring to their excitement and facile jocularity, particularly when the frontal lobes are involved. Also associated with damage to the frontal lobes, the so-called frontal lobe syndrome, consists of prominent indifference and apathy, characterized by a lack of concern for events in the immediate environment. Temper outbursts, which can occur with little or no provocation, especially after alcohol ingestion, can result in violent behavior. The expression of impulses may include inappropriate jokes, a coarse manner, improper sexual advances, and antisocial conduct resulting in conflicts with the law, such as assaults on others, sexual misdemeanors, and shoplifting.

Table 19-11
Obsessive-Compulsive Personality Disorder: Specific Symptoms

Obsessive-Compulsive Personality Disorder		Anankastic Personality Disorder	
Orderliness, perfectionism, self-control (≥4): • Attention to rules/details/order • Cannot complete things because of needing it to be perfect • Relationships neglected because of devotion to work • Inflexible thinking • Cannot part with things	• Cannot delegate • Stingy • Stubborn/rigid	• Plagued by doubt • Perfectionism, checking, attention to detail • Stubborn/rigid • Overly cautious • Unwanted thoughts or impulses, but not to the point of obsessions or compulsions	Exclusions (not result of): • Obsessive-compulsive disorder

They typically have diminished foresight, and cannot anticipate the social or legal consequences of actions. Persons with temporal lobe epilepsy characteristically show humorlessness, hypergraphia, hyperreligiosity, and marked aggressiveness during seizures.

Persons with personality change due to a general medical condition have a clear sensorium. Mild disorders of cognitive function often coexist but do not amount to intellectual deterioration. Patients may be inattentive, which may account for disorders of recent memory. With some prodding, however, patients are likely to recall what they claim to have forgotten. We should suspect the diagnosis in patients who show marked changes in behavior or personality involving emotional lability and impaired impulse control, who have no history of mental disorder, and whose personality changes occur abruptly or over a relatively brief time.

Other Specified Personality Disorder.   DSM-5 reserves the category of other specified personality disorder for situations that meet the general criteria for a personality disorder, but the presentation does not fit into any of the personality disorder categories described above. Passive-aggressive personality and depressive personality are examples. A narrow spectrum of behavior or a particular trait—such as oppositionalism, sadism, or masochism—can also be classified in this category. A patient with features of more than one personality disorder but without the complete criteria of any one disorder can be assigned this classification.

Unspecified Personality Disorder.   This diagnosis is like the above Other Specified Personality Disorder but is used in situations when we may choose not to indicate why the patient does not meet the criteria for a specific personality disorder. A typical example is a case in which there is not enough information to make a specific personality disorder diagnosis.

DIFFERENTIAL DIAGNOSIS

Many of the features of various personality disorders may occur during an episode of another mental disorder. Some of the personality disorders, particularly within a given cluster, may also share common features.

Paranoid Personality Disorder

Paranoid personality disorder can usually be differentiated from delusional disorder by the absence of fixed delusions. Unlike persons with schizophrenia, those with personality disorders typically lack hallucinations or formal thought disorder. However, when a brief reactive psychosis with delusions complicates the clinical picture of paranoid personality disorder, this distinction is far more complicated. Paranoid personality disorder can be distinguished from a borderline personality disorder because patients who are paranoid are rarely capable of overly involved, tumultuous relationships with others. Patients with paranoia lack the long history of antisocial behavior of persons with antisocial character. Persons with schizoid personality disorder are withdrawn and aloof and do not have paranoid ideation.

Schizoid Personality Disorder

Schizoid personality disorder differs from schizophrenia, delusional disorder, and affective disorder with psychotic features based on periods with positive psychotic symptoms, such as delusions and hallucinations, in the latter. Although patients with paranoid personality disorder share many traits with those with schizoid personality disorder, the former exhibit more social engagement, a history of aggressive verbal behavior, and a greater tendency to project their feelings onto others. If just as emotionally constricted, patients with obsessive-compulsive and avoidant personality disorders experience loneliness as dysphoric, possess a more abundant history of past object relations, and do not engage as much in autistic reverie. The chief distinction between a patient with schizotypal personality disorder and one with schizoid personality disorder is that the patient who is schizotypal is more similar to a patient with schizophrenia in oddities of perception, thought, behavior, and communication. Patients with avoidant personality disorder are isolated but do wish to participate in activities, a characteristic absent in those with schizoid personality disorder. Schizoid personality disorder is distinguished from autism spectrum disorder by more severely impaired social interactions and stereotypical behaviors and interests with autism.

Schizotypal Personality Disorder

Persons with schizotypal personality disorder can be distinguished from those with schizoid and avoidant personality disorders by the presence of oddities in their behavior, thinking, perception, and communication. Schizotypal personality disorder is difficult to distinguish from the heterogeneous group of solitary, odd children whose behavior is characterized by social isolation, eccentricity, and peculiarities in language seen in autism spectrum disorder and communication disorders. We distinguish the latter by the primacy and severity of the language disorder and accompanying compensatory efforts by the patient. Also, individuals with autism often have more severely impaired social interactions and restricted behaviors and interests than those with schizotypal disorder. Patients with schizotypal personality disorder can be distinguished from those with schizophrenia by the absence of psychosis. If psychotic symptoms do appear, they are brief and fragmentary. Patients with paranoid personality disorder are suspicious but lack the odd behavior of patients with schizotypal personality disorder.

Antisocial Personality Disorder

Antisocial personality disorder differs from mere illegal behavior in that antisocial personality disorder involves many areas of a person's life. When illegal behavior is only for gain and does not include rigid, maladaptive, and persistent personality traits, we classify it as criminal behavior not associated with a personality disorder in DSM-5.

Many of these persons have a neurologic or mental disorder that has been either overlooked or undiagnosed. More difficult is the differentiation of antisocial personality disorder from substance use disorders. When both substance use disorders and antisocial behavior begin in childhood and continue into adult life, we should diagnose both disorders. When, however, the antisocial behavior is secondary to premorbid alcohol use disorder or another substance use disorder, the diagnosis of antisocial personality disorder is not warranted.

In diagnosing antisocial personality disorder, clinicians must adjust for the distorting effects of socioeconomic status, cultural background, and sex. Furthermore, the diagnosis of antisocial personality disorder is not warranted when intellectual disability, schizophrenia, or mania can explain the symptoms. Other personality disorders, such as narcissistic, histrionic, and paranoid, can be differentiated from antisocial personality disorder as the former personality disorders rarely include serious criminality and aggressiveness. Borderline personality disorder can sometimes be associated with criminality. However, individuals with borderline personality who commit crimes tend to display high novelty seeking and high harm avoidance behaviors, whereas those with antisocial personality tend to display high novelty seeking and low harm avoidance behaviors.

Borderline Personality Disorder

Borderline personality disorder differs from major depressive disorder, bipolar disorder, dysthymic disorder, and cyclothymia based on the presence of core borderline personality symptoms that are not typically present in mood disorders (e.g., fear of abandonment, highly unpredictable behavior, tumultuous interpersonal relationships, seeing others as either all good or all bad, complaints of being numb or empty, and the lack of a consistent sense of identity). It differs from identity problems, which are typically limited to a developmental stage.

Borderline personality disorder differs from schizophrenia on the basis that the patient with borderline personality lacks prolonged psychotic episodes, thought disorder, and other classic schizophrenic signs. Patients with schizotypal personality disorder show marked peculiarities of thinking, strange ideation, and recurrent ideas of reference. Those with paranoid personality disorder have extreme suspiciousness. In contrast, patients with borderline personality disorder generally have short-lived psychotic episodes, when present.

Histrionic Personality Disorder

Distinguishing between histrionic personality disorder and borderline personality disorder is challenging, but in borderline personality disorder, suicide attempts, identity diffusion, and brief psychotic episodes are more likely. Although both conditions can exist in the same patient, clinicians should separate the two. Somatic symptom disorder may occur in conjunction with histrionic personality disorder, and we should diagnose both as well. Patients with brief psychotic disorder and dissociative disorders may warrant a coexisting diagnosis of histrionic personality disorder.

Narcissistic Personality Disorder

Borderline, histrionic, and antisocial personality disorders often accompany narcissistic personality disorder, so differential diagnosis is difficult. Patients with narcissistic personality disorder have less anxiety than those with borderline personality disorder; their lives tend to be less chaotic, and they are less likely to attempt suicide. Patients with antisocial personality disorder have a history of impulsive behavior, often associated with alcohol or other substance use, which frequently gets them into trouble with the law. Patients with histrionic personality disorder show features of exhibitionism and interpersonal manipulativeness that resemble those of patients with narcissistic personality disorder. Narcissistic personality disorder can be distinguished from the grandiosity of mania by the episodic course, associated euphoria, and functional impairment in a manic or hypomanic episode.

Avoidant Personality Disorder

Avoidant personality disorder is complicated to distinguish from social anxiety disorder. In social anxiety disorder, specific situations, rather than interpersonal contact in general, are avoided.

They may co-occur. Panic disorder with agoraphobia also manifests avoidance, but usually after the onset of panic attacks.

Patients with schizoid and schizotypal personality disorders may be indistinguishable from those with avoidant personality disorder. However, patients with avoidant personality disorder desire social interaction, unlike patients with schizoid personality disorder, who want to be alone. Patients with avoidant personality disorder are not as demanding, irritable, or unpredictable as those with borderline and histrionic personality disorders. Avoidant personality disorder and dependent personality disorder are similar. Patients with dependent personality disorder are presumed to have a greater fear of being abandoned or unloved than those with avoidant personality disorder, but the clinical picture may be indistinguishable.

Dependent Personality Disorder

The traits of dependence occur in many psychiatric disorders, so the differential diagnosis is difficult. Dependence is a prominent factor in patients with histrionic and borderline personality disorders. However, those with dependent personality disorder usually have a long-term relationship with one person rather than a series of persons on whom they are dependent, and they do not tend to be overly manipulative. Dependent behavior can also occur in patients with agoraphobia, panic disorder, and depressive disorders, but these patients tend to have a high level of overt anxiety, panic, or depression, respectively.

Obsessive-Compulsive Personality Disorder

When recurrent obsessions or compulsions are present, we should diagnose an obsessive-compulsive disorder. Perhaps the most challenging distinction is between outpatients with some obsessive-compulsive traits and those with an obsessive-compulsive personality disorder. We should reserve the personality disorder diagnosis for those with significant impairments in their occupational or social effectiveness. In some cases, delusional disorder coexists with personality disorders, and we should diagnose both.

Personality Change due to Another Medical Condition

Dementia involves global deterioration in intellectual and behavioral capacities, of which personality change is just one category. A personality change may herald a cognitive disorder that eventually will deteriorate into dementia. In these cases, as deterioration begins to encompass significant memory and cognitive deficits, the diagnosis of the disorder changes from personality change caused by a general medical condition to dementia. In differentiating the specific syndrome from other disorders in which personality change may occur—such as schizophrenia, delusional disorder, mood disorders, and impulse control disorders—physicians must consider the most critical factor, the presence of a personality change due to a specific organic causative factor.

COMORBIDITY

Personality disorders occur in 10 to 20 percent of the general population and about half of psychiatric inpatients or outpatients. Personality disorders are frequently comorbid with other clinical syndromes and are predisposing factors for other psychiatric disorders and symptoms (e.g., substance use, suicide, affective disorders, impulse-control disorders, eating disorders, and anxiety disorders).

Paranoid Personality Disorder

These individuals are at increased risk for major depression, obsessive-compulsive disorder, agoraphobia, and substance use disorders. The most common co-occurring personality disorders are schizotypal, schizoid, narcissistic, avoidant, and borderline. Paranoid personality disorder may be a premorbid antecedent of delusional disorder, persecutory type.

Schizoid Personality Disorder

This personality disorder sometimes appears as the premorbid antecedent of delusional disorder, schizophrenia, or rarely major depression. Paranoid, schizotypal, and avoidant are the most common co-occurring personality disorders.

Schizotypal Personality Disorder

More than half of these patients have had at least one episode of major depression, and 30 to 50 percent have major depression concurrent with this personality disorder. The most common co-occurring personality disorders are schizoid, paranoid, avoidant, and borderline.

Antisocial Personality Disorder

These patients are at increased risk for impulse control disorders, major depression, substance use disorders, pathologic gambling, anxiety disorders, and somatic symptom disorder. Narcissistic, borderline, and histrionic are the most common co-occurring personality disorders.

Borderline Personality Disorder

These individuals are at increased risk for major depression, substance use disorders, eating disorders (notably bulimia), posttraumatic stress disorder, attention-deficit hyperactivity disorder, and somatic symptom disorder. Borderline personality disorder can co-occur with most other personality disorders.

Histrionic Personality Disorder

Patients with histrionic personality disorder are at increased risk for major depression, somatic symptom disorder, and conversion disorder. Narcissistic, borderline, antisocial, and dependent are the most common co-occurring personality disorders.

Narcissistic Personality Disorder

These patients are at increased risk for major depression and substance use disorders (especially cocaine use). The most common co-occurring personality disorders are borderline, antisocial, histrionic, and paranoid.

Avoidant Personality Disorder

Patients with avoidant personality disorder are at increased risk for mood and anxiety disorders (especially social anxiety disorder). The most common co-occurring personality disorders are schizotypal, schizoid, paranoid, dependent, and borderline. Somatic symptom disorder may be comorbid.

Dependent Personality Disorder

These patients are at increased risk for major depression, anxiety disorders, and adjustment disorder. Somatic symptom disorder may be comorbid. The personality disorders that co-occur most commonly are histrionic, avoidant, and borderline.

Obsessive-Compulsive Personality Disorder

These individuals are at increased risk for major depression and anxiety disorder. Equivocal evidence exists for an increased risk of obsessive-compulsive disorder.

COURSE AND PROGNOSIS

Personality disorders are chronic, and they last over decades. They often interfere with the treatment outcomes of comorbid psychiatric disorders and lead to personal incapacitation, morbidity, and mortality in these patients. People with personality disorders have chronic impairments in their ability to work and love, tend to be less educated, drug dependent, single, unemployed, and to have marital difficulties. They consume a large portion of community services, social welfare benefits, public health, and prison resources.

Paranoid Personality Disorder

There are no adequate, systematic long-term studies of paranoid personality disorder. In some, paranoid personality disorder is lifelong; in others, it is a harbinger of schizophrenia. In still others, paranoid traits give way to reaction formation, appropriate concern with morality, and altruistic concerns as they mature or as stress diminishes. In general, however, those with paranoid personality disorder have lifelong problems working and living with others.

Occupational and marital problems are common. Complications may include brief reactive psychosis, particularly in response to stress.

Schizoid Personality Disorder

The onset of schizoid personality disorder usually occurs in early childhood or adolescence. As with all personality disorders, schizoid personality disorder is long-lasting but not necessarily lifelong. The proportion of patients who incur schizophrenia is unknown. These individuals frequently have severe problems in social relations, and occupational problems develop when interpersonal involvement is required. Solitary work sometimes favorably affects overall performance. Complications may include very brief reactive psychosis, particularly in response to stress.

Schizotypal Personality Disorder

This disorder can be the premorbid personality of the patient with schizophrenia. Some, however, maintain a stable schizotypal personality throughout their lives and marry and work, despite their oddities. Complications may include transient psychotic episodes, particularly in response to stress. Symptoms sometimes become so significant that individuals meet the criteria for schizophreniform disorder, delusional disorder, and brief psychotic disorder. One long-term study reported that 10 percent of those with schizotypal personality disorder eventually committed suicide.

Antisocial Personality Disorder

When an antisocial personality disorder develops, it runs an unremitting course, with the height of antisocial behavior usually occurring in late adolescence. The prognosis varies. Some reports indicate that symptoms decrease as a person ages. Even after the severe antisocial behavior "burns out," people diagnosed with antisocial personality disorder usually continue to be irritable, impulsive, and detached. Complications may include dysphoria, tension, low tolerance for boredom, depressed mood, and premature, violent death.

Borderline Personality Disorder

The course of borderline personality disorder is variable and most commonly follows a pattern of chronic instability in early adulthood, with episodes of severe affective and impulsive dyscontrol. The impairment and the risk of suicide are highest in the young adult years and gradually wane with advancing age. In the fourth and fifth decades, these individuals tend to attain greater stability in their relationships and functioning. Impairment typically involves frequent job losses, interrupted education, and broken marriages. Complications may include psychotic-like symptoms (hallucinations, body image distortions, hypnagogic phenomena, ideas of reference) in response to stress, as well as premature death or physical handicaps from suicide and suicidal gestures, failed suicide, and self-injurious behavior.

Histrionic Personality Disorder

With age, persons with histrionic personality disorder show fewer symptoms, but because they lack the energy of earlier years, the difference in the number of symptoms may be more apparent than real. Persons with this disorder are sensation seekers, and they may get into trouble with the law, abuse substances, and act promiscuously. Complications may include frequent suicidal gestures and threats to coerce better caregiving; interpersonal relations that are unstable, shallow, and generally ungratifying; and frequent marital problems secondary to the tendency to neglect long-term relationships for the excitement of new relationships.

Narcissistic Personality Disorder

Narcissistic personality disorder is chronic and difficult to treat. Patients with the disorder must continuously deal with blows to their narcissism resulting from their behavior or life experience. Patients handle aging poorly; they value beauty, strength, and youthful attributes, to which they cling inappropriately. They may be more vulnerable, therefore, to midlife crises than are other groups. However, narcissistic symptoms tend to diminish after the age of 40 years, when pessimism usually develops. Impairment is frequently severe and includes marital problems and interpersonal relationships in general. Complications may include social withdrawal, depressed mood, and dysthymic or major depressive disorder in reaction to criticism or failure.

Avoidant Personality Disorder

Avoidant personality disorder frequently begins in childhood with shyness and fear of strangers and new situations. Impairment can be severe and typically includes occupational and social difficulties. However, many persons with avoidant personality disorder can function in a protected environment. Some marry, have children, and live their lives surrounded only by family members. If their support system fails, however, they are subject to depression, anxiety, and anger. Phobic avoidance is common, and patients with the disorder may give histories of social anxiety disorder or incur social anxiety disorder in the course of their illness.

Dependent Personality Disorder

We know little about the course of dependent personality disorder. Occupational functioning tends to be impaired because persons with the disorder cannot act independently and without close supervision. Social relationships are limited to those on whom they can depend, and many suffer physical or mental abuse because they cannot assert themselves. They risk major depressive disorder if they lose the person on whom they depend, but with treatment, the prognosis is favorable. Complications may include low socioeconomic status and inadequate family and marital functioning, as well as mood disorders, anxiety disorders, adjustment disorder, and social anxiety disorder.

Obsessive-Compulsive Personality Disorder

The course of obsessive-compulsive personality disorder is variable and unpredictable. Occupational and social difficulties are typical. From time to time, persons may develop obsessions or compulsions in the course of their disorder. Some adolescents with obsessive-compulsive personality disorder evolve into warm, open, and loving adults; in others, the disorder can be either the harbinger of schizophrenia or—decades later and exacerbated by the aging process—major depressive disorder.

Persons with obsessive-compulsive personality disorder may flourish in positions demanding methodical, deductive, or detailed work, but they are vulnerable to unexpected changes, and their personal lives may remain barren. Depressive disorders, especially those of late-onset, are common. Complications may include distress and difficulties when confronted with new situations that require flexibility and compromise, as well as myocardial infarction secondary to features typical of type A personalities, such as time urgency, hostility, and competitiveness.

Personality Change due to Another Medical Condition

Both the course and the prognosis of personality change due to a general medical condition depend on its cause. If the disorder results from structural damage to the brain, the disorder tends to persist. In cases of head trauma or vascular accident, the disorder may follow a period of coma and delirium, and it may be permanent. The personality change can evolve into dementia in cases of brain tumors, multiple sclerosis, and Huntington disease. Personality changes produced by chronic intoxication, medical illness, or drug therapy (such as levodopa for parkinsonism) may reverse with appropriate treatment of the cause. Some patients require custodial care or at least close supervision to meet their basic needs, avoid repeated conflicts with the law, and protect themselves and their families from the hostility of others and destitution resulting from impulsive and ill-considered actions.

TREATMENT APPROACH

Individuals with personality disorders do not recognize that they are ill and seldom seek help unless others (such as a spouse or parents) are insistent. This usually happens when maladaptive behaviors create marital, family, and career problems, or when other disorders (e.g., anxiety, depression, substance use) or somatic symptoms (e.g., obesity, heart disease, COPD) complicate their clinical picture. In general, patients with personality disorders require a multifaceted treatment plan that often combines psychotherapy and pharmacotherapy.

Combining Psychotherapy and Pharmacotherapy

Most patients with a personality disorder will require a combination of psychotherapy and pharmacotherapy. Psychotherapy is the primary treatment, as it promotes the maturation of character and, ultimately, the encouragement of the patient's capacity to develop better adaptive solutions. However, psychotherapy is very hard to implement in the setting of unstable affect and risky or self-destructive behaviors, all very common in the initial stages of treatment. During these early stages, pharmacotherapy achieves a relatively prompt control of affect and behavior. Most importantly, this nonspecific improvement sets a more suitable platform for the work in psychotherapy.

Pharmacotherapy. In the treatment of patients with personality disorders, medications can target specific symptoms of their disorders with the goals of relieving subjective distress, risky or self-destructive behaviors, or conflict with others, thereby preparing them for or allowing them to participate in psychotherapeutic approaches. We should identify target symptoms, in order to choose agents that effect those symptoms. Table 19-12 summarizes drug choices for various target symptoms of personality disorders.

Paranoid Personality Disorder

Psychotherapy. Psychotherapy is the treatment of choice for those with paranoid personality disorder. Therapists should be straightforward in all their dealings with these patients. If the patient accuses the therapist of an inconsistency or a fault, such as lateness for an appointment, honesty and an apology are preferable to a defensive explanation. Therapists must remember that trust and tolerance of intimacy are troubled areas for patients with this disorder. Individual psychotherapy thus requires a professional and not overly warm style from therapists. Clinicians' overzealous use of interpretation—especially interpretation about deep feelings of dependence, sexual concerns, and wishes for intimacy—increases patients' mistrust significantly. Generally, patients who are paranoid do not do well in group psychotherapy, although it can be useful for improving social skills and diminishing suspiciousness through role-playing. Many cannot tolerate the intrusiveness of behavior therapy, also used for social skills training.

At times, patients with paranoid personality disorder behave so threateningly that therapists must control or set limits on their actions. Delusional accusations should be realistically handled, but gently and without humiliating patients. Patients who are paranoid are profoundly frightened when they feel that those trying to help them are weak and helpless; therefore, therapists should never offer to take control unless they are willing and able to do so.

Pharmacotherapy. There is little evidence to guide the use of pharmacotherapy in paranoid personality disorder. Treatment selection should be tailored to the individual patient and guided by target symptoms, such as the use of low-dose novel antipsychotics for psychotic symptoms or the use of anticonvulsants for irritability.

Schizoid Personality Disorder

Psychotherapy. The treatment of patients with schizoid personality disorder is similar to that of those with paranoid personality disorder. Patients who are schizoid tend toward introspection; however, these tendencies are consistent with psychotherapists' expectations, and such patients may become devoted if distant patients. As trust develops, patients who are schizoid may, with great trepidation, reveal a plethora of fantasies, imaginary friends, and fears of unbearable dependence—even of merging with the therapist.

In group therapy settings, patients with schizoid personality disorder may be silent for long periods; nonetheless, they do become involved. The patients should be protected against aggressive attack by group members for their proclivity to be silent. With time, the group members become important to patients who are schizoid and may provide the only social contact in their otherwise isolated existence.

Pharmacotherapy. Limited evidence exists to guide the psychopharmacologic treatment of patients with schizoid personality disorder. The use of psychotropics to target specific symptoms, such as social and emotional detachment, may be appropriate.

Schizotypal Personality Disorder

Psychotherapy. The principles of treatment of schizotypal personality disorder do not differ from those of schizoid personality disorder, but clinicians must deal sensitively with the former, mainly using care to avoid ridiculing or judging patients' odd beliefs. Schizotypal patients have peculiar patterns of thinking, and some are involved in cults, strange religious practices, or the occult.

Pharmacotherapy. Antipsychotic medication may be useful for dealing with ideas of reference, illusions, and other symptoms of the disorder and can be an adjunct to psychotherapy. Antidepressants are useful when a depressive component of the personality is present.

Antisocial Personality Disorder

Psychotherapy. There is limited evidence to guide the use of psychotherapeutic approaches in antisocial personality disorder. Overall, the limited evidence suggests that these individuals seem to respond better to contingency management and other reward-based interventions than they do to cognitive behavioral therapy.

Pharmacotherapy. Pharmacotherapy can deal with incapacitating symptoms such as anxiety, rage, and depression, but because patients often misuse substances, we should use medications judiciously. One might use anticonvulsants to treat aggressive behaviors, especially if there are abnormal waveforms on an EEG. β-Adrenergic receptor antagonists, lithium, and antipsychotics may also reduce aggression.

Borderline Personality Disorder

Psychotherapy. Psychotherapy for patients with borderline personality disorder is an area of intensive investigation and has been the treatment of choice. It seems to be most successful in combination with pharmacotherapy.

Psychotherapy is difficult for the patient and therapist alike. Patients regress quickly, act out their impulses, and show labile or

Table 19-12
Pharmacotherapy of Target Symptom Domains of Personality Disorders

Choice of Drugs According to Target Symptoms of Personality Disorders

Target Symptom	Drug/Treatment of Choice	Not Recommended
I. Mood Dysregulation and Anxiety		
Anxiety		
Chronic cognitive	Psychotherapy, SSRIs, SNRIs, MAOIs, Low-Dose Novel Psychotropics (aripiprazole, quetiapine) Valproate and other GABA analogs (clonazepam and buspirone)	Benzodiazepines
Chronic somatic	MAOIs, SNRIs (duloxetine, milnacipran) Pregabalin and other GABA analogs, TCAs, beta-blockers	If used—benzodiazepines with long half-life and short trials preferred
Obsessions	SSRIs, Antipsychotics (quetiapine), TCAs (clomipramine), Mild NMDA antagonists (riluzole, memantine)	
Acute and severe	Mirtazapine, Novel Psychotropics (quetiapine, aripiprazole, clozapine), TCAs, clonazepam, valproates, lithium	
Depression		
Atypical depression/dysphoria Classical depression	MAOIs, SSRIs, SNRIs, Aripiprazole, Lurasidone, ziprasidone, quetiapine, Atypical antipsychotics (as monotherapy or augmentation)	TCAs
Emotional lability/rapid cycling	Lithium, Lamotrigine, Valproate, Lower-dose antipsychotics (olanzapine, aripiprazole, clozapine, ziprasidone)	TCAs ("catecholamine stress"), Standard antidepressants (risk of switching to mania)
II. Behavior Dyscontrol		
Aggression/impulsivity		
Affective aggression "Hot temper" with normal EEG	Lithium, SSRIs, Anticonvulsants, Low-dose antipsychotics	Benzodiazepines (disinhibition)
Predatory aggression (cold blooded revenge/cruelty)	No Effective Pharmacologic Tx	Benzodiazepines (disinhibition)
Organic-like aggression (traumatic brain injury)	Beta-Blockers, Valproates, Quetiapine, Carbamazepine (CBMZ), TCAs, cholinesterase inhibitors (donepezil)	Benzodiazepines (disinhibition, delirium)
Ictal aggression (abnormal EEG)	CBMZ, Diphenylhydantoin, Valproate Benzodiazepines (clonazepam)	TCAs, Low-potency typical antipsychotics (both increase risk of seizures)
III. Social and Emotional Detachment		
Chronic asociality and disinterest		
Blunted affect	Low-Dose Antipsychotics (aripiprazole, olanzapine, low-dose clozapine, sulpiride)	
IV. Cognitive-Perceptual Distortions/ Psychotic Symptoms		
Acute and brief psychotic episodes	Novel Antipsychotics (Risperdal, olanzapine) Typical neuroleptics (for the duration of psychosis)	
Chronic and low-level psychotic-like symptoms	Novel Antipsychotics	

Adapted with permission of the Center for Well-Being at Washington University.

fixed negative or positive transferences, which are difficult to analyze. Projective identification may also cause countertransference problems when therapists are unaware that patients are unconsciously trying to coerce them to act out a particular behavior. The splitting defense mechanism causes patients to love and hate therapists and others in the environment alternately. A reality-oriented approach is more effective than in-depth interpretations of the unconscious.

Therapists have used behavior therapy to help patients manage their impulses and angry outbursts and to reduce their sensitivity to criticism and rejection. Social skills training, especially with videotape playback, helps patients to see how their actions affect others and thereby improve their interpersonal behavior.

Patients with borderline personality disorder often do well in a hospital setting in which they receive intensive psychotherapy on both an individual and a group basis. In a hospital, they can also interact with trained staff members from a variety of disciplines and receive occupational, recreational, and vocational therapy. Such programs are especially helpful when the home environment is detrimental to a patient's rehabilitation because of intrafamilial conflicts or other stresses, such as abuse. Within the protected environment of the hospital, we can give limits to patients who are excessively impulsive, self-destructive, or self-mutilating, and observe their actions. Under ideal circumstances, patients remain in the hospital until they show marked improvement, up to 1 year in some cases. We can then discharge patients to specialized support systems, such as day hospitals, night hospitals, and halfway houses.

DIALECTICAL BEHAVIOR THERAPY. Dialectical behavior therapy (DBT) is the psychosocial treatment that has received the most empirical support for patients with borderline personality disorder. The method is eclectic, drawing on concepts derived from supportive, cognitive, and behavioral therapies. There are four primary modes of treatment in DBT: group skill training, individual therapy, phone consultation, and consultation team. Patients are seen weekly, with the goal of improving interpersonal skills and decreasing self-destructive behavior. Patients with borderline personality disorder receive help in dealing with the ambivalent feelings that are characteristic of the disorder. As with other behavioral approaches, DBT assumes all behavior (including thoughts and feelings) is learned and that patients with borderline personality disorder behave in ways that reinforce or even reward their behavior, regardless of how maladaptive it is. See Chapter 23 for a more detailed discussion of DBT.

MENTALIZATION-BASED TREATMENT. Another type of psychotherapy for borderline personality disorder is called mentalization-based therapy (MBT). Mentalization is a social construct that allows a person to be attentive to the mental states of oneself and of others; it comes from a person's awareness of mental processes and subjective states that arise in interpersonal interactions. MBT is based on a theory that borderline personality symptoms, such as difficulty regulating emotions and managing impulsivity, are a result of patients' reduced capacities to mentalize. Thus, recovery of mentalization should help patients build relationship skills as they learn to regulate their thoughts and feelings better. MBT was effective for borderline personality disorder in several randomized, controlled research trials.

TRANSFERENCE-FOCUSED PSYCHOTHERAPY. Transference-focused psychotherapy (TFP) is a modified form of psychodynamic psychotherapy used for the treatment of borderline personality disorder grounded in object relations theory. The therapist relies on two major processes in working with the patient: the first is clarification, in which the transference is analyzed more directly than in traditional psychotherapy so that the patient becomes quickly aware of his or her distortions about the therapist, and the second is confrontation, whereby the therapist points out how these transferential distortions interfere with interpersonal relations toward others (objects). The mechanism of splitting used by borderline patients is characterized by their having a good object and a bad object, and they use this as a defense against anxiety. If therapy is successful, then the need for splitting diminishes, object relations are improved, and the patient achieves a more normal level of functioning. Studies comparing TFP, DBT, psychodynamic psychotherapy, and supportive psychotherapy show that all are useful and all show varying degrees of success.

Pharmacotherapy. Pharmacotherapy is useful to deal with specific personality features that interfere with patients' overall functioning. Antipsychotics may help control anger, hostility, and brief psychotic episodes. Antidepressants improve the depressed mood common in patients with borderline personality disorder. Benzodiazepines should be avoided not only due to the risk of abuse, but also because patients may become disinhibited with this class of drugs. Anticonvulsants, such as carbamazepine, may improve functioning for some patients. Serotonergic agents, such as selective serotonin reuptake inhibitors (SSRIs), have been helpful in some cases.

Histrionic Personality Disorder

Psychotherapy. Patients with histrionic personality disorder are often unaware of their real feelings; clarification of their inner feelings is a necessary therapeutic process. Psychoanalytically oriented psychotherapy is probably the treatment of choice for histrionic personality disorder.

Pharmacotherapy. Pharmacotherapy can be adjunctive to target symptoms (e.g., the use of antidepressants for depression and somatic complaints, antianxiety agents for anxiety, and antipsychotics for derealization and illusions).

Narcissistic Personality Disorder

Psychotherapy. Because patients must renounce their narcissism to make progress, the treatment of narcissistic personality disorder is challenging. Some experts have advocated using psychoanalytic approaches to effect change, but much research is required to validate the diagnosis and to determine the best treatment. Some clinicians advocate group therapy for their patients so they can learn how to share with others and, under ideal circumstances, can develop an empathic response to others.

Pharmacotherapy. Lithium can help patients whose clinical picture includes mood swings. Because patients with narcissistic personality disorder tolerate rejection poorly and are susceptible to depression, antidepressants, especially serotonergic drugs, may also be of use.

Avoidant Personality Disorder

Psychotherapy. Psychotherapeutic treatment depends on solidifying an alliance with patients. As trust develops, a therapist must convey an accepting attitude toward the patient's fears, especially the fear of rejection. The therapist eventually encourages a patient to move out into the world to take what they perceive as significant risks of humiliation, rejection, and failure. However, therapists should be cautious when giving assignments to exercise new social skills outside therapy; failure can reinforce the patient's already weak self-esteem. Group therapy may help patients understand how their sensitivity to rejection affects them and others. Assertiveness training is a form of behavior therapy that may teach patients to express their needs openly and to enlarge their self-esteem.

Pharmacotherapy. Pharmacotherapy can help manage anxiety and depression when they are associated with the disorder. Some patients are helped by β-adrenergic receptor antagonists, such as atenolol, to manage autonomic nervous system hyperactivity, which tends to be high in patients with avoidant personality disorder, especially when they approach feared situations. Serotonergic agents may help with rejection sensitivity. Theoretically, dopaminergic drugs might engender novelty-seeking behavior in these patients; however, the patient must be psychologically prepared for any new experience that might result.

Dependent Personality Disorder

Psychotherapy. The treatment of dependent personality disorder is often successful. Insight-oriented therapies enable patients to understand the antecedents of their behavior, and with the support of a therapist, patients can become more independent, assertive, and self-reliant. Behavioral therapy, assertiveness training, family therapy, and group therapy have all been used, with successful outcomes in many cases.

A pitfall may arise in treatment when a therapist encourages a patient to change the dynamics of a pathologic relationship (e.g., supports a physically abused wife in seeking help from the police). At this point, patients may become anxious and unable to cooperate in therapy; they may feel torn between complying with the therapist and losing an external pathologic relationship. Therapists must show great respect for these patients' feelings of attachment, no matter how pathologic these feelings may seem.

Pharmacotherapy.   Pharmacotherapy can help deal with specific symptoms, such as anxiety and depression, which are commonly associated features of dependent personality disorder. Patients who experience panic attacks or who have high levels of separation anxiety may benefit from symptom-targeted pharmacotherapy, such as antidepressant agents.

Obsessive-Compulsive Personality Disorder

Psychotherapy.   Unlike patients with other personality disorders, some individuals with obsessive-compulsive personality disorder are often aware of their suffering and seek treatment on their own. Though limited evidence exists to guide treatment, there have been several studies that support cognitive therapy or cognitive behavioral therapy as an effective treatment for individuals with this disorder, delivered either individually or in a group. Additionally, interpersonal psychotherapy may improve depressive symptoms in individuals with obsessive-compulsive personality disorder.

Pharmacotherapy.   There is limited evidence for the pharmacologic treatment of obsessive-compulsive personality disorder. Some studies have suggested benefits from fluvoxamine and carbamazepine, and in those patients with comorbid depression, citalopram may be helpful. In one study comparing citalopram and sertraline, both medications reduced the number of obsessive-compulsive personality disorder traits, though citalopram performed better than sertraline.

Personality Change due to Another Medical Condition

Management of personality change disorder involves the treatment of the underlying medical condition when possible. Psychopharmacological treatment of specific symptoms may help in some cases, such as antidepressants for depression or anticonvulsants for irritability, aggression, or impulsivity.

Patients with severe cognitive impairment or weakened behavioral controls may need counseling to help avoid difficulties at work or to prevent social embarrassment. As a rule, patients' families need emotional support and concrete advice on how to help minimize patients' undesirable conduct. Patients should avoid alcohol, and we should curtail social engagements when patients tend to act in a grossly offensive manner.

EPIDEMIOLOGY

Personality disorders are common. They occur in 10 to 20 percent of the general population, and approximately 50 percent of all psychiatric patients.

Paranoid Personality Disorder

Data suggest that the prevalence of paranoid personality disorder is 0.5 to 4.4 percent of the general population. Those with the disorder rarely seek treatment themselves; when referred to treatment by a spouse or an employer, they can often pull themselves together and appear undistressed. Relatives of patients with schizophrenia show a higher incidence of paranoid personality disorder than control participants. Some evidence suggests a more specific familial relationship with delusional disorder, persecutory type. The diagnosis is more common in men.

Schizoid Personality Disorder

The prevalence of schizoid personality disorder is estimated to be 3.1 to 4.9 percent of the general population, according to DSM-5. This diagnosis is more common in men. Persons with the disorder tend to gravitate toward solitary jobs that involve little or no contact with others. Many prefer night work to day work so that they need not deal with many persons. There appears to be an increased prevalence among the relatives of individuals with schizophrenia or schizotypal personality disorder.

Schizotypal Personality Disorder

Schizotypal personality disorder occurs in 3.9 to 4.6 percent of the population, according to DSM-5. The sex ratio is unknown; however, it is frequent in females with fragile X syndrome. A higher association of cases exists among the biologic relatives of patients with schizophrenia than among control participants and a higher incidence among monozygotic twins than among dizygotic twins (33 percent vs. 4 percent in one study).

Antisocial Personality Disorder

According to DSM-5, prevalence rates for antisocial personality disorder are 3 percent for males and 1 percent for females in the general population. It is frequent among the first-degree biologic relatives of individuals with this disorder. Biologic relatives of females with antisocial personality disorder are at increased risk for the same disorder compared to biologic relatives of males with antisocial personality disorder. Genetic studies have suggested familial transmission of antisocial personality disorder, substance use, and somatic symptom disorder (most studies used the previous criteria for the related somatization disorder), the former two being characteristic of males, and the latter of females in the same family. Adoption studies have shown that both genetic and environmental factors contribute to the risk of this disorder. Both adopted and biologic children of parents with antisocial personality disorder are at increased risk for this disorder. Conduct disorder (before the age of 10 years) and accompanying attention-deficit hyperactivity disorder increases the likelihood of developing antisocial personality in adult life. Conduct disorder is more likely to develop into antisocial personality disorder with erratic parenting, neglect, or inconsistent parental discipline.

Borderline Personality Disorder

Borderline personality disorder is thought to be present in about 2 percent of the general population and is more common in women than in men. The disorder is more common in younger than in older samples, suggesting a natural tendency toward maturation and remission. Physical and sexual abuse, neglect, hostile conduct, and early parental loss or separation are common in the childhood histories of patients with this disorder. Borderline personality disorder is five times more common among relatives of individuals with the same disorder than the general population. An increased prevalence of mood disorders, antisocial personality disorder, and substance use disorder is common in first-degree relatives of persons with borderline personality disorder.

Histrionic Personality Disorder

Limited data from general population studies suggest a prevalence of histrionic personality disorder of about 2 percent. Although traditionally thought to occur more frequently in women, there is some evidence to suggest that this disorder might be equally frequent among men and women. Histrionic personality disorder tends to run in families. Some experts suggest that there is a genetic link between histrionic and antisocial personality disorder and alcohol use disorder.

Narcissistic Personality Disorder

According to DSM-5, estimates of the prevalence of narcissistic personality disorder range from less than 1 percent in the general population to 2 to 16 percent in the clinical population; this disorder is more common in men.

Avoidant Personality Disorder

The prevalence of the disorder is about 0.5 to 2 percent of the general population, according to DSM-5. It occurs in men and women equally.

Dependent Personality Disorder

Dependent personality disorder is equally common in women and men. DSM-5 reports an estimated prevalence of 0.5 to 0.6 percent. Persons with chronic physical illness in childhood or separation anxiety disorder may be most susceptible to dependent personality disorder.

Obsessive-Compulsive Personality Disorder

DSM-5 reports an estimated prevalence ranging from 2 to 8 percent of the general population. It is more common in men than in women. Some studies have demonstrated a familial aggregation of this disorder.

ETIOLOGY

Genetic Factors

The best evidence that genetic factors contribute to personality disorders comes from investigations of more than 15,000 pairs of twins in the United States. The concordance for personality disorders among monozygotic twins was several times that among dizygotic twins. Moreover, according to one study, monozygotic twins reared apart are about as similar as monozygotic twins reared together. Similarities include multiple measures of personality and temperament, occupational and leisure-time interests, and social attitudes.

Cluster A personality disorders are more common in the biologic relatives of patients with schizophrenia than in control groups. Adoption, family, and twin studies demonstrate an increased prevalence of schizotypal features in the families of schizophrenic patients, mainly when schizotypal features were not associated with comorbid affective symptoms. Less correlation exists between paranoid or schizoid personality disorder and schizophrenia.

Cluster B personality disorders have a genetic basis. Antisocial personality disorder is associated with alcohol use disorders. Depression is common in the family backgrounds of patients with borderline personality disorder. These patients have more relatives with mood disorders than do control groups, and persons with borderline personality disorder often have a mood disorder as well. There is a strong association between histrionic personality disorder and somatic symptom disorder; patients with each disorder show an overlap of symptoms.

Cluster C personality disorders may also have a genetic base. Patients with avoidant personality disorder often have high anxiety levels. Obsessive-compulsive traits are more common in monozygotic twins than in dizygotic twins, and patients with obsessive-compulsive personality disorder show some signs associated with depression—for example, shortened rapid eye movement (REM) latency period and abnormal dexamethasone-suppression test (DST) results.

Biologic Factors

Hormones. Persons who exhibit impulsive traits also often show high levels of testosterone, 17-estradiol, and estrone. In nonhuman primates, androgens increase the likelihood of aggression and sexual behavior, but the role of testosterone in human aggression is unclear. DST results are abnormal in some patients with borderline personality disorder who also have depressive symptoms.

Platelet Monoamine Oxidase. Low platelet monoamine oxidase (MAO) levels are associated with activity and sociability in monkeys. College students with low platelet MAO levels report spending more time in social activities than students with high platelet MAO levels. Low platelet MAO levels occur in some patients with schizotypal disorders.

Smooth Pursuit Eye Movements. Smooth pursuit eye movements are saccadic (i.e., jumpy) in persons who are introverted, who have low self-esteem and tend to withdraw, and who have schizotypal personality disorder. These findings have no clinical application, but they do indicate the role of inheritance.

Neurotransmitters. Studies of personality traits and the dopaminergic and serotonergic systems indicate an arousal-activating function for these neurotransmitters. Levels of 5-hydroxyindoleacetic acid (5-HIAA), a metabolite of serotonin, are low in persons who attempt suicide and in patients who are impulsive and aggressive. Raising serotonin levels with serotonergic agents such as fluoxetine can produce dramatic changes in some character traits of personality. In many persons, serotonin reduces depression, impulsiveness, and rumination and can produce a sense of general well-being. Increased dopamine concentrations in the central nervous system produced by certain psychostimulants (e.g., amphetamines) can induce euphoria. The effects of neurotransmitters on personality traits have generated much interest and controversy about whether personality traits are inborn or acquired.

Table 19-13
Medical Conditions Associated with Personality Change

Head trauma
Cerebrovascular diseases
Cerebral tumors
Epilepsy (particularly, complex partial epilepsy)
Huntington disease
Multiple sclerosis
Endocrine disorders
Heavy metal poisoning (manganese, mercury)
Neurosyphilis
Acquired immune deficiency syndrome (AIDS)

Electrophysiology.   Changes in electrical conductance on the electroencephalogram (EEG) occur in some patients with personality disorders, most commonly antisocial and borderline types; these changes appear as slow-wave activity on EEGs.

Other Biologic Factors.   In the case of personality change due to another medical condition, structural damage to the brain is usually the cause, and head trauma is probably the most common cause. Cerebral neoplasms and vascular accidents, particularly of the temporal and frontal lobes, are also common causes. The conditions most often associated with personality change are listed in Table 19-13.

Psychoanalytic Factors

Sigmund Freud suggested that personality traits are related to a fixation at one psychosexual stage of development. For example, those with an oral character are passive and dependent because they are fixated at the oral stage when the dependence on others for food is prominent. Those with an anal character are stubborn, parsimonious, and highly conscientious because of struggles over toilet training during the anal period.

Wilhelm Reich subsequently coined the term *character armor* to describe individuals' characteristic defensive styles for protecting themselves from internal impulses and interpersonal anxiety in significant relationships. Reich's theory has had a broad influence on contemporary concepts of personality and personality disorders. For example, each human being's unique stamp of personality depends on their characteristic defense mechanisms. Each personality disorder has a cluster of defenses that help psychodynamic clinicians recognize the type of character pathology present. Persons with paranoid personality disorder, for instance, use projection, whereas schizoid personality disorder is associated with withdrawal.

When defenses work effectively, persons with personality disorders master feelings of anxiety, depression, anger, shame, guilt, and other affects. Their behavior is ego-syntonic; that is, it creates no distress for them even though it may adversely affect others. They may also be reluctant to engage in a treatment process; because their defenses are essential to controlling unpleasant affects, they are not interested in surrendering them.

In addition to characteristic defenses in personality disorders, another central feature is internal object relations. During development, a person develops particular patterns of the self in relation to others. Through introjection, children internalize a parent or another significant person as an internal presence that continues to feel like an object rather than a self. Through identification, children internalize parents and others in such a way that they

incorporate the traits of the external object into the self, and the child "owns" the traits. These internal self-representations and object representations are crucial in developing the personality and, through externalization and projective identification, are played out in interpersonal scenarios in which they coerce others into playing a role in the person's internal life. Hence, persons with personality disorders are also identified by particular patterns of interpersonal relatedness that stem from these internal object relations patterns.

Defense Mechanisms.   To help those with personality disorders, psychiatrists must appreciate patients' underlying defenses, the unconscious mental processes that the ego uses to resolve conflicts among the four lodestars of the inner life: instinct (wish or need), reality, important persons, and conscience. When defenses are most effective, especially in those with personality disorders, they can abolish anxiety and depression at the conscious level. Thus, abandoning a defense increases conscious awareness of anxiety and depression—a primary reason that those with personality disorders are reluctant to alter their behavior.

Although we tend to characterize patients with personality disorders by their most dominant or rigid mechanism, each patient uses several defenses. Therefore, the management of defense mechanisms used by patients with personality disorders is discussed here as a general topic and not as an aspect of the specific disorders. While many formulations are presented here in the language of psychoanalytic psychiatry, it is possible to translate them into principles consistent with cognitive and behavioral approaches.

FANTASY.   Many people who are labeled schizoid—those who are eccentric, lonely, or frightened—seek solace and satisfaction within themselves by creating imaginary lives, especially imaginary friends. In their extensive dependence on fantasy, these persons often seem to be strikingly aloof. Therapists must understand that the unsociableness of these patients rests on a fear of intimacy. Rather than criticizing them or feeling rebuffed by their rejection, therapists should maintain a quiet, reassuring, and considerate interest without insisting on reciprocal responses. Recognition of patients' fear of closeness and respect for their eccentric ways are both therapeutic and useful.

DISSOCIATION.   Dissociation is an unconscious defense mechanism that involves separating a mental or behavioral process (e.g., thought, feeling) from the rest of the person's psychic activity. Patients with borderline personality disorder may demonstrate dissociation during times of increased stress, including derealization or depersonalization.

ISOLATION.   Isolation involves the separation of an idea or memory from its attached emotion. It is characteristic of controlled, orderly persons who are often labeled obsessive-compulsive personalities. These individuals remember the truth in fine detail but without affect. In a crisis, patients may show intensified self-restraint, overly formal social behavior, and obstinacy. Patients' quests for control may annoy clinicians or make them anxious. Often, such patients respond well to precise, systematic, and rational explanations and value efficiency, cleanliness, and punctuality as much as they do clinicians' effective responsiveness. Whenever possible, therapists should allow such patients to control their own care and should not engage in a battle of wills.

PROJECTION.   In projection, patients attribute their unacknowledged feelings to others. Patients' excessive faultfinding and sensitivity to criticism may appear to therapists as prejudiced, hypervigilant, and injustice-collecting, but the therapist should not respond with defensiveness and argument. Instead, clinicians should frankly acknowledge even minor mistakes on their part and should discuss the possibility of future difficulties. Strict honesty, concern for patients' rights, and maintaining the same formal, concerning distance as used with patients who use fantasy defenses are all helpful. Confrontation guarantees a lasting enemy and early termination of the interview. Therapists need not agree with patients' injustice-collecting, but they should ask whether both can agree to disagree.

The technique of counterprojection is especially helpful. Clinicians acknowledge and give paranoid patients full credit for their feelings and perceptions; they neither dispute patients' complaints nor reinforce them but agree that the world described by patients is conceivable. Interviewers can then talk about real motives and feelings, misattributed to someone else, and begin to cement an alliance with patients.

SPLITTING. In splitting, the patient divides persons toward whom they are, or have been, ambivalent into good and bad. For example, in an inpatient setting, a patient may idealize some staff members and uniformly disparage others. This defense behavior can be highly disruptive in a hospital ward and can ultimately provoke the staff to turn against the patient. When staff members anticipate the process, discuss it at staff meetings, and gently confront the patient with the fact that no one is all good or all bad, the phenomenon of splitting can be dealt with effectively.

ACTING OUT. In acting out, patients directly express unconscious wishes or conflicts through action to avoid being conscious of either the accompanying idea or the affect. Tantrums, apparently motiveless assaults and pleasureless promiscuity are typical examples. Because the behavior occurs outside reflective awareness, acting out appears to observers to be unaccompanied by guilt, but when acting out is impossible, the conflict behind the defense may be accessible. The clinician faced with acting out, either aggressive or sexual, in an interview situation, must recognize that the patient has lost control, that the patient will mishear anything the interviewer says, and that getting the patient's attention is of paramount importance. Depending on the circumstances, a clinician's response may be, "How can I help you if you keep screaming?" Alternatively, if the patient's loss of control seems to be escalating, say, "If you continue screaming, I will leave." An interviewer who feels genuinely frightened of the patient can simply leave and, if necessary, ask for help from ward attendants or the police.

PROJECTIVE IDENTIFICATION. The defense mechanism of projective identification appears mainly in borderline personality disorder and consists of three steps. First, the patient projects an aspect of the self onto someone else. The projector then tries to coerce the other person into identifying what they projected. Finally, the recipient of the projection and the projector feel a sense of oneness or union.

Temperament

Temperament refers to the body's biases in the modulation of conditioned behavioral responses to prescriptive physical stimuli. Behavioral conditioning (i.e., procedural learning) involves presemantic sensations that elicit basic emotions, such as fear or anger, independent of conscious recognition, descriptive observation, reflection, or reasoning. Pioneering work by A. Thomas and S. Chess conceptualized temperament as the stylistic component ("how") of behavior, as differentiated from the motivation ("why") and the content ("what") of behavior. Modern concepts of temperament emphasize its emotional, motivational, and adaptive aspects.

Specifically, four major temperament traits have been identified and subjected to extensive neurobiologic, psychosocial, and clinical investigation: harm avoidance, novelty seeking, reward dependence, and persistence. These four temperaments are now understood to be genetically independent dimensions that occur in all possible combinations within the same individual rather than as mutually exclusive categories.

Psychobiology of Temperament. Temperament traits of harm avoidance, novelty seeking, reward dependence, and persistence are heritable differences underlying one's automatic response to danger, novelty, social approval, and intermittent reward, respectively. These four temperaments are closely associated with the four basic emotions of fear (harm avoidance), anger (novelty seeking), attachment (reward dependence), and ambition (persistence).

Individual differences in temperament and basic emotions modify the processing of sensory information and shape early learning characteristics, especially associative conditioning of unconscious behavior responses and preattentive components of perception. Temperament occurs in terms of heritable biases in emotionality and learning that underlie the acquisition of emotion-based, automatic behavioral traits and habits observable early in life and relatively stable over one's lifespan.

Each of the four major dimensions is a normally distributed quantitative trait, moderately heritable, observable early in childhood, relatively stable in time, and moderately predictive of adolescent and adult behavior. The four dimensions are genetically homogeneous and independently inherited from one another, as per several extensive international twin studies. Temperamental differences, which are not very stable initially, tend to stabilize during the second and third years of life. Accordingly, ratings of these four temperament traits at ages 10 to 11 years were moderately predictive of personality traits at ages 15, 18, and 27 years in a large sample of Swedish children.

The four dimensions are universal across different cultures, ethnic groups, and political systems on every inhabited continent. We call these aspects of personality temperaments because they are heritable, manifest early in life, are developmentally stable, and are consistent in different cultures. Temperament traits are similar to crystallized intelligence in that they do not show the rapid changes with increasing age or across birth cohorts found for fluid intelligence and character traits. Table 19-14 summarizes contrasting sets of behaviors that distinguish extreme scorers on the four dimensions of temperament. Note that each extreme of these dimensions has specific adaptive advantages and disadvantages so that neither high nor low scores inherently mean better adaptation.

Each of the four temperament dimensions has unique genetic determinants according to family and twin studies, as well as studies of genetic associations with specific DNA markers.

HARM AVOIDANCE. Harm avoidance involves a heritable bias in the inhibition of behavior in response to signals of punishment and frustrative non-reward. High harm avoidance is a fear of uncertainty, social inhibition, shyness, passive avoidance of problems/danger, rapid fatigability, and pessimistic worry in anticipation of problems even in situations that do not worry others. Those low in harm avoidance are carefree, courageous, energetic, outgoing, and optimistic, even in situations that worry most people.

The psychobiology of harm avoidance is complex. Benzodiazepines disinhibit avoidance by γ-aminobutyric acid (GABA)-ergic inhibition of serotonergic neurons originating in the dorsal raphe nuclei. The anterior serotonergic cells in the dorsal raphe nucleus

Table 19-14
Descriptors of Individuals Who Score High or Low on the Four Temperament Dimensions

Temperament Dimension	Descriptors of Extreme Variants	
	High	Low
Harm avoidance	Pessimistic	Optimistic
	Fearful	Daring
	Shy	Outgoing
	Fatigable	Energetic
Novelty seeking	Exploratory	Reserved
	Impulsive	Deliberate
	Extravagant	Thrifty
	Disorderly	Orderly
Reward dependence	Sentimental	Detached
	Open	Aloof
	Warm	Cold
	Affectionate	Independent
Persistence	Industrious	Lazy
	Determined	Spoiled
	Ambitious	Underachiever
	Perfectionist	Pragmatist

intermingle with the dopaminergic cells of the ventral tegmental area, and both groups innervate the same structures (e.g., basal ganglia, accumbens, amygdala), providing opposing dopaminergic-serotonergic influences in the modulation of approach and avoidance behavior. Persons given serotonin drugs show decreased harm avoidance behavior.

NOVELTY SEEKING. Novelty seeking reflects a heritable bias in the initiation or activation of appetitive approach in response to novelty, approach to signals of reward, active avoidance of conditioned signals of punishment, and escape from unconditioned punishment.

Novelty seeking is an exploratory activity in response to novelty, impulsiveness, extravagance in approach to cues of reward, and active avoidance of frustration. Individuals high in novelty seeking are quick-tempered, curious, easily bored, impulsive, extravagant, and disorderly. Those low in novelty seeking are slow tempered, uninquiring, stoical, reflective, frugal, reserved, tolerant of monotony, and orderly.

Dopaminergic projections have a crucial role in novelty seeking. Novelty seeking seems to involve increased reuptake of dopamine at presynaptic terminals, thereby requiring frequent stimulation to maintain optimal levels of postsynaptic dopaminergic stimulation. Studies of candidate genes involved in dopamine neurotransmission, have provided evidence of association with novelty seeking and no other dimension of temperament.

REWARD DEPENDENCE. Reward dependence reflects the maintenance of behavior in response to cues of social reward. Individuals high in reward dependence are tender-hearted, sensitive, dedicated, dependent, and warmly sociable. Those low in reward dependence are practical, tough-minded, cold, socially insensitive, irresolute, and indifferent if alone.

Noradrenergic projections from the locus coeruleus and serotonergic projections from the median raphe likely influence such reward conditioning. The "love hormone" oxytocin's plasma level is positively correlated ($r = 0.5$) with individual differences in reward dependence but not other dimensions of personality.

PERSISTENCE. Persistence reflects the maintenance of behavior despite frustration, fatigue, and intermittent reinforcement. It manifests as industriousness, determination, ambitiousness, and perfectionism. Highly persistent individuals are hard-working, perseverant, and ambitious overachievers who tend to intensify their effort in response to anticipated rewards and view frustration and fatigue as personal challenges. Those low in persistence are indolent, inactive, unstable, and erratic; they tend to give up easily when faced with frustration, rarely strive for higher accomplishments,

FIGURE 19-1

Correlations between individual personality disorder subtypes and temperament traits of harm avoidance (HA), novelty seeking (NS), and reward dependence (RD). A, antisocial; Ac, antisocial children; B, borderline; D, dependent; F, self-defeating; G, passive aggressive; H, histrionic; N, narcissistic; O, obsessive; P, paranoid; S, sadistic; GT, schizotypal; V, avoidant; Z, schizoid.

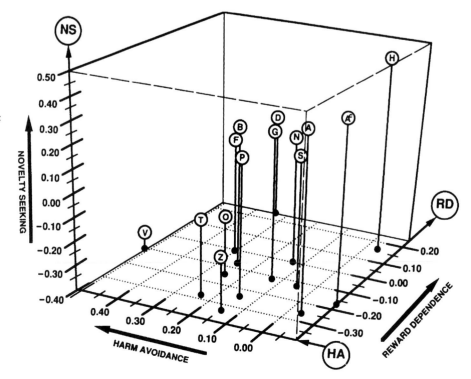

and manifest little perseverance even in response to intermittent reward.

Individual differences in persistence have been strongly correlated ($r = 0.8$) with responses measured by fMRI in a circuit involving the ventral striatum, orbitofrontal cortex/rostral insula, and dorsal anterior cingulate cortex.

Figure 19-1 illustrates the interrelationships between the personality disorders and the temperament traits of harm avoidance, novelty seeking, and reward dependence.

References

American Psychiatric Association. *Diagnostic and Statistical Manual of Mental Disorders*. 5th ed. Arlington, VA: American Psychiatric Association; 2013.

Apt C, Hurlbert DF. The sexual attitudes, behavior, and relationships of women with histrionic personality disorder. *J Sex Marital Ther*. 1994;20(2):125–133.

Bateman A, Fonagy P. 8-year follow-up of patients treated for borderline personality disorder: mentalization-based treatment versus treatment as usual. *Focus*. 2013;11(2):261–268.

Bornstein RF, Gold SH. Comorbidity of personality disorders and somatization disorder: a meta-analytic review. *J Psychopathol Behav Assess*. 2008;30:154–161.

Boudreaux MJ. "Personality-related problems and the five-factor model of personality." *Personality Disord*. 2016;7(4):372–383.

Brazil IA, van Dongen JDM, Maes JHR, Mars RB, Baskin-Sommers AR. Classification and treatment of antisocial individuals: from behavior to biocognition. *Neurosci Biobehav Rev*. 2018;91:259–277.

Cloninger CR. *Feeling Good: The Science of Well Being*. New York: Oxford University Press; 2004.

Cloninger CR, Svrakic DM. Chapter 26: Personality disorders. In: Sadock BJ, Sadock VA, Ruiz P, eds. *Kaplan & Sadock's Comprehensive Textbook of Psychiatry*. 10th ed. Philadelphia, PA: Wolters Kluwer; 2017:2126–2176.

Crawford TN, Cohen P, Johnson JG, Sneed Joel R, Brook JS. The course and psychosocial correlates of personality disorder symptoms in adolescence: Erikson's developmental theory revisited. *J Youth Adolesc*. 2004;33:373–387.

Diedrich A, Voderholzer U. Obsessive-compulsive personality disorder: a current review. *Curr Psychiatry Rep*. 2015;17:2–10.

Forster C, Berthollier N, Rawlinson D. A systematic review of potential mechanisms of change in psychotherapeutic interventions for personality disorder. *J Psychol Psychother*. 2014;4(133):2161–0487.

Helgeland MI, Kjelsberg E, Torgersen S. Continuities between emotional and disruptive behavior disorders in adolescence and personality disorders in adulthood. *Am J Psychiatry*. 2005;162:1941–1947.

Johnson JG, First MB, Cohen P, Skodol AE, Kasen S, Brook JS. Adverse outcomes associated with personality disorder not otherwise specified in a community sample. *Am J Psychiatry*. 2005;162:1926–1932.

Koch J, Modesitt T, Palmer M, Ward S, Martin B, Wyatt R, Thomas C. Review of pharmacologic treatment in cluster a personality disorders. *Ment Health Clin*. 2016;6(2):75–81.

Linehan MM, Comtois KA, Murray AM, Brown MZ, Gallop RJ, Heard HL, Korslund KE, Tutek DA, Reynolds SK, Lindenboim N. Two-year randomized controlled trial and follow-up of dialectical behavior therapy vs therapy by experts for suicidal behaviors and borderline personality disorder. *Arch Gen Psychiatry*. 2006;63(7):757–766.

Nickel MK, Muehlbacher M, Nickel C, Kettler C, Pedrosa Gil F, Bachler E, Buschmann W, Rother N, Fartacek R, Egger C, Anvar J, Rother WK, Loew TH, Kaplan P. Aripiprazole in the treatment of patients with borderline personality disorder: a double-blind, placebo-controlled study. *Am J Psychiatry*. 2006;163(5):833–838.

Ozkan M, Altindag A. Comorbid personality disorders in subjects with panic disorder: do personality disorders increase clinical severity? *Compr Psychiatry*. 2005;46:20–26.

Pagan JL, Oltmanns TF, Whitmore MJ, Turkheimer E. Personality disorder not otherwise specified: searching for an empirically based diagnostic threshold. *J Pers Disord*. 2005;19:674–689.

Papaioannou D, Brazier J, Parry G. How to measure quality of life for cost effectiveness analyses of personality disorders: a systematic review. *J Pers Disord*. 2013;27(3):383–401.

Rosenthal MZ, Rodriguez MA. Chapter 33.9: Dialectical behavior therapy. In: Sadock BJ, Sadock VA, Ruiz P, eds. *Kaplan & Sadock's Comprehensive Textbook of Psychiatry*. 10th ed. Philadelphia, PA: Wolters Kluwer; 2017:2784–2795.

Schwarze C, Mobascher A, Pallasch B, Hoppe G, Kurz M, Hellhammer DH, Lieb K. Prenatal adversity: a risk factor in borderline personality disorder? *Psychol Med*. 2013;43(6):1279–1291.

Silk KR. "Caught in an unconscious split: commentary on 'the ironic fate of the personality disorders in DSM-5.'" *Personality Disord*. 2013;4(4): 350–351.

Skodol AE, Morey LC, Bender DS, Oldham JM. "The ironic fate of the personality disorders in DSM-5." *Personality Disord*. 2013;4(4): 342–349.

Sussman N. Borderline personality and bipolar disorders: Is there a connection? *Primary Psychiatry*. 2004;11:13.

Witkiewitz K, King K, McMahon RJ, Wu J, Luk J, Bierman KL, Coie JD, Dodge KA, Greenberg MT, Lochman JE, Pinderhughes EE, Conduct Problems Prevention Research Group. Evidence for a multi-dimensional latent structural model of externalizing disorders. *J Abnorm Child Psychol*. 2013;41(2):223–237.

Zimmerman M, Rothschild L, Chelminski I. The prevalence of DSM-IV personality disorders in psychiatric outpatients. *Am J Psychiatry*. 2005;162:1911–1918.

20 ◢

Other Conditions that May be a Focus of Clinical Attention

INTRODUCTION

DSM-5 includes a section called Other Conditions that May be a Focus of Clinical Attention. ICD-10 has a similar section called Factors Influencing Health Status and Contact with Health Services. These sections are for conditions that are not mental disorders but that have led to contact with the mental health care system. In some instances, one of these conditions will be noted during a psychiatric evaluation (e.g., divorce), although there is no mental disorder. In other instances, the diagnostic evaluation reveals no mental disorder, but there is a need to note the primary reason for contact with the mental health care system (e.g., homelessness).

In some cases, we may eventually find a mental disorder, but the focus of attention or treatment is on a condition that is not caused by a mental disorder. For example, a patient with an anxiety disorder may receive treatment for a marital problem that is unrelated to the anxiety disorder itself.

Table 20-1 includes the many conditions DSM-5 lists that may be a focus of clinical attention, or that may influence the diagnosis, treatment, or course of a mental disorder contained in DSM-5. The list of conditions that make up this category covers the entire life cycle from infancy through childhood, adolescence, adulthood, and old age. The list of conditions covers almost every conceivable life circumstance, from divorce to problems related to being in military service. Each of these conditions or circumstances is capable of having a profound input on a particular mental illness or the human experience in general.

MALINGERING

Malingering is the deliberate falsification of physical or psychological symptoms in an attempt to achieve a secondary gain such as avoiding military duty, avoiding work, obtaining financial compensation, evading criminal prosecution, or obtaining drugs. Under some circumstances, malingering may represent adaptive behavior—for example, as mentioned below, feigning illness while a captive of the enemy during wartime.

The clinician should consider possible malingering when encountering any combination of the following: (1) medicolegal context of presentation (e.g., the person is referred by an attorney to the clinician for examination), (2) evident discrepancy between the individual's claimed stress or disability and the objective findings, (3) lack of cooperation during the diagnostic evaluation and in complying with the prescribed treatment regimen, and (4) the presence of antisocial personality disorder.

Diagnosis and Clinical Features

Avoidance of Criminal Responsibility, Trial, and Punishment. Criminals may pretend to be incompetent to avoid standing trial; they may feign insanity at the time of the perpetration of the crime, malinger symptoms to receive a less harsh penalty, or attempt to act too incapacitated (incompetent) for punishment.

Avoidance of Military Service or Particularly Hazardous Duties. Persons may malinger to avoid conscription into the armed forces, and, after being conscripted, they may feign illness to escape from particularly onerous or hazardous duties.

Financial Gain. Malingerers may seek financial gain in the form of undeserved disability insurance, veterans' benefits, workers' compensation, or tort damages for purported psychological injury.

Avoidance of Work, Social Responsibility, and Social Consequences. Individuals may malinger to escape from unpleasant vocational or social circumstances or to avoid the social and litigation-related consequences of vocational or social improprieties.

An owner of a previously successful photographic equipment supplier declared bankruptcy in a way that the government maintained was illegal. Subsequently, the government indicted the defendant on various counts of fraud. The defendant's counsel maintained that the defendant was too depressed to cooperate with him and that, because of that depression, he experienced memory loss that made it impossible to understand what had occurred and, therefore, impossible to provide a meaningful defense. The government's forensic psychiatrist evaluated the defendant to ascertain the nature of his depression and to determine whether it was causing cognitive problems.

When asked early in his evaluation when his birthday was, he responded, "Oh, what does it matter? It was in the 40s or 50s." Similarly, when queried about where he was born, he said, "Somewhere in Hungary." Even when pressed for more specifics, he refused to elaborate. Nevertheless, at many points later in his evaluation, he responded with complete, often detailed information about transactions not related to those for which he was under indictment. It was the impression of the evaluator that the defendant was malingering grossly and inconsistently, incompatible with the kinds of decreases in cognitive skills that occasionally attend major depression. (Adapted from a case of Mark J. Mills, J.D., M.D. and Mark S. Lipian, M.D., Ph.D.)

Table 20-1
Conditions that May be a Focus of Clinical Attention

Relational Problems
- Problems Related to Family Upbringing
  - Parent–Child Problem
  - Sibling Problem
  - Upbringing Away from Parents
  - Parental Relationship Distress
- Other Problems Related to Primary Support System
  - Relationship Distress with Spouse or Partner
  - Separation or Divorce
  - Emotional Distress within Family
  - Uncomplicated Bereavement

Abuse and Neglect
- Problems of Child Maltreatment and Neglect
  - Child Physical Abuse
  - Child Sexual Abuse
  - Child Neglect
  - Child Psychological Abuse
- Problems of Adult Maltreatment and Neglect
  - Physical Violence of Spouse or Partner
  - Sexual Violence of Spouse or Partner
  - Spouse or Partner Neglect
  - Psychological Spouse or Partner Abuse
  - Adult Abuse by Nonspouse or Nonpartner (e.g., Physical, Sexual, Psychological)

Educational and Occupational Problems
- Educational Problems
- Occupational Problems
  - Related to Current Military Deployment Status
  - Other (e.g., Job change, Loss of job, Stress)

Housing and Economic Problems
- Housing Problems
  - Homelessness
  - Inadequate Housing (e.g., Lack of Heat or Electricity, Insect or Rodent Infestation)
  - Neighbor, Lodger, or Landlord Discord
  - Residential Institution (Does Not Include Psychological Reaction to Change in Living Situation; see Adjustment Disorders, Chapter 10)
- Economic Problems
  - Lack of Adequate Food or Safe Drinking Water
  - Extreme Poverty
  - Low Income

Other Problems Related to the Social Environment
- Phase of Life Problem
- Acculturation Difficulty
- Social Exclusion or Rejection
- Discrimination or Persecution

Problems Related to Crime or Interaction with the Legal System (e.g., Victim of Crime, Imprisonment, Release from Prison)

Other Health Service Encounters for Counseling and Medical Advice (e.g., Sexual Counseling)

Problems Related to Other Psychological, Personal, and Environmental Circumstances
- Religious or Spiritual Problem
- Victim of Terrorism or Torture
- Exposure to Disaster or War

Other Circumstances of Personal History
- Adult Antisocial Behavior
- Child or Adolescent Antisocial Behavior
- Problems Related to Access to Medical and Other Health Care
- Nonadherence to Medical Treatment (e.g., Overweight or Obesity, Malingering, Wandering Associated with a Mental Disorder)
- Borderline Intellectual Functioning

Adapted from *Diagnostic and Statistical Manual of Mental Disorders*. 5th ed., American Psychiatric Association; 2013.

Facilitation of Transfer from Prison to Hospital. Prisoners may malinger (fake bad) to obtain a transfer to a psychiatric hospital from which they may hope to escape or in which they expect to do "easier time." The prison context may also give rise to dissimulation (faking good). However, the prospect of an indeterminate number of days on a mental health ward may prompt an inmate with actual psychiatric symptoms to make every effort to conceal them.

Admission to a Hospital. In this era of deinstitutionalization and homelessness, individuals may malinger to gain admission to a psychiatric hospital. The individual may see such institutions as providing free room and board, a haven from the police, or refuge from rival gang members or disgruntled drug cronies who have made street life even more unbearable and hazardous than it usually is.

A robust, neatly attired man presented to the psychiatric emergency department in the early-morning hours. He stated that "the voices" were worse than before and that he wished readmission to the hospital. When the psychiatrist challenged him, observing that his discharge was just that afternoon, that he routinely left the hospital in the morning and demanded rehospitalization at night, and that, despite multiple hospitalizations, clinicians increasingly doubted his reported history of hallucinations, the man became belligerent. When the psychiatrist still refused to admit him, the patient grabbed the psychiatrist's clothes, threatening him but inflicting no harm. The psychiatrist asked the hospital police to escort him off the grounds. The treatment team told the patient that he could seek readmission to his regular ward during the day. Subsequent contact with the patient's ward revealed that their diagnoses were substance abuse and homelessness; his apparent schizophrenia appeared never to have been an actual issue in his treatment. (Courtesy of Mark J. Mills, J.D., M.D. and Mark S. Lipian, M.D., Ph.D.)

Drug Seeking. Malingerers may feign illness to obtain favored medications, either for personal use or, in a prison setting, as currency to barter for cigarettes, protection, or other inmate-provided favors.

The plaintiff, a woman in her late 20s, was injured while dancing at a club. Although her claim initially appeared bona fide, subsequent investigation cast doubt on the mechanism of injury that she claimed—namely, that a misplaced electrical cord under a carpet caused her to slip. This was true, she claimed, even though she had been dancing in a particularly jerky manner that could have easily caused problems without tripping.

Subsequently, she sought medical and surgical treatment for torn cartilage in her injured knee. Even though the initial surgery went well, she kept reinjuring the knee with various "slips." As a result, she requested narcotic analgesics. A careful medical record review revealed that she was obtaining such medications from multiple practitioners and that she had forged at least one prescription.

In reviewing the case before binding arbitration, it was the opinion of the orthopedic and psychiatric consultants that, although the initial injury and reported pain were real, the plaintiff consciously elaborated her injuries to obtain the desired narcotic analgesics. (Courtesy of Mark J. Mills, J.D., M.D. and Mark S. Lipian, M.D., Ph.D.)

Child Custody. Minimizing difficulties or faking good for the sake of obtaining child custody can occur when one party accurately accuses the other of being an unfit parent because of psychological conditions. The accused party may feel compelled to minimize symptoms or to portray him- or herself in a positive light to reduce the chances of being deemed unfit and losing custody.

Differential Diagnosis

The challenge is to differentiate malingering from an actual physical or psychiatric illness. Furthermore, the possibility of partial malingering, which is an exaggeration of existing symptoms, must be entertained. Also, the possibility exists of unintentional, dynamically driven misattribution of genuine symptoms (e.g., of depression) to an incorrect environmental cause (e.g., to sexual harassment rather than to narcissistic injury).

We should also remember that a real psychiatric disorder and malingering are not mutually exclusive.

Factitious disorder is distinguished from malingering by motivation (sick role vs. tangible pain), whereas the somatoform disorders involve no conscious volition. In conversion disorder, as in malingering, objective signs cannot account for subjective experience, and differentiation between the two disorders can be difficult. Table 20-2 lists some variables that may aid in distinguishing between these two conditions.

Epidemiology

There is perhaps a 1 percent prevalence of malingering among mental health patients in civilian clinical practice, with the estimate rising to 5 percent in the military. In a litigious context, during interviews of criminal defendants, the estimated prevalence of malingering is much higher—between 10 and 20 percent. Approximately 50 percent of children presenting with conduct disorders have reported lying-related issues.

Although there is no apparent familial or genetic patterns, and no clear-cut sex or age bias at onset, malingering does appear to be highly prevalent in some military, prison, and litigious populations and, in Western society, in men from youth through middle age. Associated disorders include conduct and anxiety disorders in children and antisocial, borderline, and narcissistic personality disorders in adults.

Etiology

Although there do not seem to be any biologic factors causally related to malingering, its frequent association with antisocial

Table 20-2
Factors Aiding in the Differentiation between Malingering and Conversion Disorder

1. Malingerers are more likely to be suspicious, uncooperative, aloof, and unfriendly; patients with conversion disorder are likely to be friendly, cooperative, appealing, dependent, and clinging.
2. Malingerers may try to avoid diagnostic evaluations and refuse recommended treatment; patients with conversion disorder likely welcome evaluation and treatment, "searching for an answer."
3. Malingerers likely refuse employment opportunities designed to circumvent their disability; patients with conversion disorder likely accept such opportunities.
4. Malingerers are more likely to provide extremely detailed and exacting descriptions of events precipitating their "illness"; patients with conversion disorder are more likely to report historical gaps, inaccuracies, and vagaries.

personality disorder raises the possibility that hypoarousability may be an underlying metabolic factor. Still, no predisposing genetic, neurophysiologic, neurochemical, or neuroendocrinologic forces are presently known.

Course and Prognosis

Malingering persists as long as the malingerer believes it will likely produce the desired rewards. In the absence of concurrent diagnoses, after the individual has attained the goal, the feigned symptoms disappear. In some structured settings, such as the military or prison units, ignoring the malingered behavior may result in its disappearance, mainly if an expectation of continued productive performance, despite complaints, is made clear. In children, malingering is most likely associated with a predisposing anxiety or conduct disorder; proper attention to this developing problem may alleviate the child's propensity to malinger.

Treatment

The appropriate stance for the psychiatrist is clinical neutrality. If malingering is suspected, a careful differential investigation should ensue. If, after the diagnostic evaluation, malingering seems most likely, the clinician should tactfully but firmly confront the patient with the apparent outcome. The clinician should also try to understand the underlying reasons for the ruse, and explore alternative, more acceptable pathways to the desired outcome. Coexisting psychiatric disorders should be thoroughly assessed. Only if the patient is utterly unwilling to interact with the physician under any terms other than manipulation should the physician abandon the interaction.

BEREAVEMENT

Normal bereavement begins immediately after or within a few months of the loss of a loved one. Typical signs and symptoms include feelings of sadness, preoccupation with thoughts about the deceased, tearfulness, irritability, insomnia, and difficulties concentrating and carrying out daily activities. Based on the cultural group, bereavement is limited to a varying time, usually 6 months, but it can be longer. Normal bereavement, however, can lead to a full depressive disorder that requires treatment. Some grieving individuals present with symptoms characteristic of a major depressive episode such as depressed mood, insomnia, anorexia, and weight loss. The duration of grief and bereavement varies considerably among different cultural groups and within the same cultural group. The diagnosis of depressive disorder is generally not given unless the symptoms are still present 2 months after the loss. However, the presence of specific symptoms that are not characteristic of a "normal" grief reaction may help differentiate bereavement from depression. These include (1) guilt about things other than actions taken or not taken by the survivor at the time of the death, (2) thoughts of death other than the survivor feeling that he or she would be better off dead or should have died with the deceased person, (3) morbid preoccupation with worthlessness, (4) marked psychomotor retardation, (5) prolonged and marked functional impairment, and (6) hallucinatory experiences other than thinking that he or she hears the voice of or transiently sees the image of the deceased person.

OCCUPATIONAL PROBLEMS

Occupational problems often arise during stressful changes in work, namely, at initial entry into the workforce or when making job changes within the same organization to a higher position because of excellent quality performance or to a parallel position because of corporate need. Distress often occurs when not choosing these changes or if the person feels unprepared for the change. It is also true during layoffs and at retirement, especially if retirement is mandatory, and the person is unprepared for this event. Work distress can result if one's work situation changes to work overload, or conversely, a lack of challenge. Also, an individual may feel unable to fulfill work expectations, perhaps because they lack sufficient authority to enact any change or meet with conflicting expectations. Working with harsh or unreasonable superiors can be another common source of work distress.

Work Choices and Changes

Young adults without role models or guidance from families, mentors, or others in their communities too often underestimate their potential lifetime abilities to learn a trade or earn a college or postgraduate degree. Also, women and members of minority groups often feel less prepared to accept work challenges, fear rejection, and do not apply for jobs for which they are qualified. On the other hand, men, in fields in which they are underrepresented, often and confidently move up the career ladder faster (glass elevator). As part of initial interviews for evaluation of occupational problems, patients should be encouraged to consider their heretofore unrecognized, unadmitted talents; long-held, yet unexpressed, dreams and goals regarding work; actual successes in work and school; and motivation to risk learning what they would find satisfying.

Minorities and those in low-paying and low-skilled jobs too often have less job security. Business and institutional reorganization and consequent downsizing, factory closings, and moves affect many, often leaving these workers feeling hopeless and helpless about future employment, on welfare, angry, and depressed.

With ongoing and often sudden downsizing of corporations and businesses, men and women continue to struggle with unexpected job loss and premature retirement even when finances are not an issue. Also, men, in particular, define themselves by their work roles and thus experience more occupational distress from these changes. Women may adjust faster to retirement, but they often have less financial security than men. Even today, white women earn approximately 80 cents on the dollar, and African American and Hispanic women earn even less for comparable work. In addition to lower pay, women may have lower status, find themselves widowed more often than men, and are more likely to be caring for children, grandchildren, and elderly relatives. Women represent more of the single working parent group and the working poor.

Stress and the Workplace

More than 30 percent of workers report that they are under stress at work. At least 15 percent of occupational disability claims involve workplace distress. Expected distress follows recognized and uncontrollable work changes—downsizing, mergers and acquisitions; work overload; and chronic physical strains, including work noise, temperature, bodily injuries, and strain from performing computer work.

Work frustration can also arise from an individual worker's unrecognized (and therefore unresolved) psychodynamic issues, such as working appropriately with superiors and not relating to one's supervisor as a parent figure. Other developmental issues include unresolved problems with competition, assertiveness, envy,

fear of success, and the inability to communicate verbally in a constructive manner.

> After the September 11, 2001, World Trade Center tragedy, a 32-year-old married male firefighter, who had been away on vacation that day with his wife and children, began to exhibit changed behaviors at home and work. At home, he appeared not to listen to his two children and, instead, focused his attention on television sporting events. At work, he also appeared to be more focused on cooking the same dinners for his peers and watching television than on interacting verbally with his remaining peers and the new chief. In several months, a chaplain visited the station several times and talked to the firefighters about survivor guilt and the 9/11 tragedy, and the firefighter began to return somewhat to his former healthier behaviors. (Courtesy of Leah J. Dickstein, M.D.)

Often, work conflicts reflect similar conflicts in the worker's personal life, and referral for treatment, unless there is insight, is in order. Some studies have found that massage therapy, meditation, and yoga at intervals during the workday relieve stress when used regularly. Approaches using cognitive therapy have also helped people reduce work pressure.

Suicide Risk

Some occupations—health professionals, financial service workers, and police, the first and latter groups because of more access to lethal drugs and weapons—both attract persons with high suicide risk and involve increased chronic distress that may lead to higher suicide rates.

Career and Job Problems of Women

Most women work outside the home out of necessity to support themselves or their dependents (whether children or adults) or as part of a working couple. With the divorce rate remaining at the 50 percent level, many women find themselves economically more impoverished after a divorce than when married, although divorced men usually find their economic status improved. Despite more than four decades of increasing knowledge about and concern for women's status in the workplace, unique gender issues, bias, and lack of accommodation to their unique needs at certain life stages (i.e., pregnancy and postpartum, the primary responsibility for young healthy and ill children) continue. However, women were the largest group establishing new small businesses in the 1990s. Many have left large corporations where they felt undervalued because of their gender. Women experience problems when they are the sole woman in a man's field. Despite increasing recognition of the need for men in relationships with women to assume home and family responsibilities, fewer than 25 percent of men do so equitably.

Women of childbearing and child-rearing ages continue to find themselves in conflict with job expectations, opportunities, and personal responsibilities. High-quality, on-site, dependent-care facilities with extended hours are rare and often out of range financially. Major unresolved work issues that are unique to women at certain life stages include flextime and paid and unpaid dependent leave options. Beyond dependent care issues, women in the workforce continue to experience distress after chronic and repeated sexual harassment, despite its illegality and media attention. Increasingly, more women have travel responsibilities, work long hours, work shifts beyond daylight hours, and experience personal workplace violence.

Among dual-career families and partners, the woman is more likely to move when the man chooses to move for a work opportunity than vice versa. Consequently, a woman's career is interrupted more often. There is now less hesitation to have the two members of a relationship work for the same organization than previously, albeit usually in different departments. Work distress may also stem from continuous miscommunication, especially that based on gender.

Working Teenagers

With unemployment increasing, many teenagers work part time while attending high school. Consequently, stress can arise because of less parent–teenager interaction and constructive parental control issues about teens' use of earnings, time spent away from home, and consequent behaviors both in and outside the home. When both parents or a single parent, as well as the teenager, work outside the home, often on different schedules, parent–teen verbal communication must be proactive, transparent, and ongoing.

Working within the Home

Although most women with children of all ages must work outside the home, at times, they may be home full time or part time or may work at home. When their husbands or partners work full time outside the home, problems may develop from each one's perceived expectations of the other. Women who care for children and their home exclusively may be seen by their partners as not only economically dependent and inferior but also not as competent and not understanding of the man's stressors and needs. Ongoing respectful listening and verbal communication must be encouraged.

People in organizations are increasingly taking work home as their work expectations increase. This work-at-home experience can and does interfere with personal lives and satisfaction, which can then have further repercussions at work.

Chronic Illness

As general and other medical and psychiatric treatments for chronic diseases improve, employers have been increasingly concerned about accommodating patients with acquired immunodeficiency syndrome (AIDS), diabetes mellitus, and other disorders. The issue of mandatory testing for AIDS and substance abuse (alcohol and other illegal substances) continues to be of concern. Employee assistance programs offering education about general and mental health topics have proved timely and cost-effective.

Domestic Violence

Although occurring in the home, signs and symptoms that interfere with work may help identify victims of domestic violence. Trained professionals must question all employees experiencing work distress about domestic violence and, when indicated, refer individuals for assistance, which includes safety in the workplace.

Job Loss

Regardless of the reason for job loss, most people experience distress, at least temporarily, including symptoms of normal grief, loss of self-esteem, anger, and reactive depressive and anxiety symptoms, as well as somatic symptoms and possibly the onset of or increase in substance abuse or domestic violence. Timely education,

support programs, and vocational guidance can be helpful, as is access to treatment.

Vocational Rehabilitation

Rehabilitation is often necessary for those traumatized by stresses in the workplace, those who had to take a leave for medical or psychiatric reasons, and those who lose their jobs. Individual or group counseling enables persons to improve personal relationships, raise self-esteem, or learn new work skills. Patients with schizophrenia may benefit from sheltered workshops in which they perform work geared to their level of function. Some patients with schizophrenia or autism do well in tasks that are repetitive or require obsessive concern with details.

ADULT ANTISOCIAL BEHAVIOR

Characterized by activities that are illegal, immoral, or both, antisocial behavior usually begins in childhood and often persists throughout life. The term *antisocial behavior* somewhat confusingly applies both to persons' actions that are not due to a mental disorder and to actions by those who never received a neuropsychiatric workup to determine the presence or absence of a mental disorder. As Dorothy Lewis noted, the term can apply to behavior by otherwise normal persons who "struggle to make a dishonest living."

Diagnosis and Clinical Features

The diagnosis of adult antisocial behavior is one of exclusion. Substance dependence in such behavior often makes it difficult to separate the antisocial behavior related primarily to substance dependence from disordered behaviors that occurred either before substance use or during episodes unrelated to substance dependence.

It is also essential that we differentiate this from an antisocial personality disorder, and when a patient meets the criteria for the personality disorder, that diagnosis would supersede this one.

During the manic phases of bipolar I disorder, certain aspects of behavior, such as wanderlust, sexual promiscuity, and financial difficulties can be similar to adult antisocial behavior. Patients with schizophrenia may have episodes of adult antisocial behavior, but the symptom picture is usually clear, especially regarding thought disorder, delusions, and hallucinations on the mental status examination.

Neurologic conditions can be associated with adult antisocial behavior, and, when indicated, a full workup, including neuroimaging, can help identify a cause of the behavior. We should consider complex partial seizures in the differential diagnosis. When making a clear-cut diagnosis of epilepsy or encephalitis, we should then consider whether the disorder is contributing to antisocial behavior. Abnormal EEG findings are prevalent among violent offenders: an estimated 50 percent of aggressive criminals have abnormal EEG findings.

Persons with adult antisocial behavior have difficulties in work, marriage, and money matters and conflicts with various authorities. Table 20-3 summarizes the symptoms of adult antisocial behavior.

Epidemiology

Depending on the specifics of the case finding, adult antisocial behavior may range from 5 to 15 percent of the population. Within

Table 20-3
Symptoms of Adult Antisocial Behavior

Life Area	Antisocial Patients with Significant Problems in Area (%)
Work problems	85
Marital problems	81
Financial dependence	79
Arrests	75
Alcohol abuse	72
School problems	71
Impulsiveness	67
Sexual behavior	64
Wild adolescence	62
Vagrancy	60
Belligerence	58
Social isolation	56
Military record (of those serving)	53
Lack of guilt	40
Somatic complaints	31
Use of aliases	29
Pathologic lying	16
Drug abuse	15
Suicide attempts	11

Data from Robins L. *Deviant Children Grown Up: A Sociological and Psychiatric Study of Sociopathic Personality*. Baltimore, MD: Williams & Wilkins; 1966.

prison populations, investigators report prevalence figures between 20 and 80 percent. Men account for more adult antisocial behavior than do women.

Etiology

Antisocial behaviors in adulthood are characteristic of a variety of persons, ranging from those with no demonstrable psychopathology to those who are severely impaired and have psychotic disorders, cognitive disorders, and retardation, among other conditions. A comprehensive neuropsychiatric assessment of antisocial adults is indicated and may reveal potentially treatable psychiatric and neurologic impairments. Only in the absence of mental disorders can patients be categorized as displaying adult antisocial behavior. Genetic and social factors may influence adult antisocial behavior.

Genetic Factors.   Some studies found a 60 percent concordance rate in monozygotic twins and about a 30 percent concordance rate in dizygotic twins. Adoption studies show a high rate of antisocial behavior in the biologic relatives of adoptees identified with antisocial behavior and a high incidence of antisocial behavior in the adopted-away offspring of those with antisocial behavior. The prenatal and perinatal periods of those who subsequently display antisocial behavior often are associated with low birth weight, mental retardation, and prenatal exposure to alcohol and other drugs of abuse.

Social Factors.   Studies have shown that in neighborhoods in which families with low socioeconomic status (SES) predominate, the sons of unskilled workers are more likely to commit more offenses and more serious criminal offenses than do the sons of middle-class and skilled workers, at least during adolescence and early adulthood. These data are not as precise for women, but the findings are generally similar in studies from many countries. Areas of family training differ by SES group. Middle-SES parents use love-oriented techniques in discipline. They withdraw affection rather than impose physical punishment, as is done in low-SES groups. Negative parental attitudes toward aggressive behavior attempt to curb that behavior, and the ability to communicate parental values are more characteristic of middle- and high-SES groups than of low ones. Adult antisocial behavior is associated with the use and abuse of alcohol and other substances and with the easy availability of handguns.

Treatment

In general, therapists are pessimistic about treating adult antisocial behavior. They have little hope of changing a pattern that has been present almost continuously throughout a person's life. Psychotherapy has not been effective, and no breakthroughs with biologic treatments, including medications, have occurred.

Therapists show more enthusiasm for the use of therapeutic communities and other forms of group treatment, although the data provide little basis for optimism. Many adult criminals, incarcerated in institutional settings, have shown some response to group therapy approaches. The history of violence, criminality, and antisocial behavior has shown that such behaviors seem to decrease after age 40 years. Recidivism in criminals, which can reach 90 percent in some studies, also decreases in middle age.

Prevention.   Because antisocial behavior often begins during childhood, the primary focus must be on delinquency prevention. Any measures that improve the physical and mental health of socioeconomically disadvantaged children and their families are likely to reduce delinquency and violent crime. Often, recurrently violent persons have sustained many insults to the central nervous system (CNS) prenatally and throughout childhood and adolescence. Consequently, we need to develop programs to educate parents about the dangers to their children of CNS injury from maltreatment, including the effects of psychoactive substances on the brains of growing fetuses. Public education about the releasing effect of alcohol on violent behaviors (as well as its contribution to vehicular homicide) may also reduce crime.

In a Surgeon General's Workshop on Violence and Public Health (1985), the work group on preventing assault and homicide emphasized the importance of discouraging corporal punishment in the home, forbidding it in the schools, and even abolishing capital punishment by the state, saying that all are models and sanctions for violence. No evidence indicates that capital punishment reduces crime in the states that have it. Opponents of capital punishment see it as "vengeance," not punishment.

Although persons disagree about the contribution of violence in the media to violent crime, the propaganda potential of the media is universally recognized. We have not fully realized the extent to which the media, such as television, can be used to transmit positive social values. The guidelines issued by the television industry to indicate the amount of sex and violence in programs is an attempt to deal with the issue; however, program content that espouses traditional societal values would be beneficial.

The most successful preventive measures within the field of medicine have come from community-wide public health programs (e.g., campaigns against smoking) and from programs that detect individual vulnerabilities (e.g., individual monitoring of blood pressure). Studies of adult antisocial behavior reveal the contribution of broad cultural factors and constellations of individual biopsychosocial vulnerabilities. Prevention programs must recognize and address both kinds of factors.

RELIGIOUS OR SPIRITUAL PROBLEM

A religious or spiritual problem can bring the person to the psychiatrist under one of several circumstances. For example, a person may begin to question his or her faith and choose not to discuss the problem with a spiritual advisor. Alternatively, a person may wish to convert to a new faith, to marry or improve a marriage when the partner is of a different faith.

Psychiatrists must enable and assist patients in distinguishing religious thought or experience from psychopathology and, if this is a problem, encourage patients to work through the issues independently or with assistance. Religious imagery may be recognized in mental illness when persons state they believe that they have been commanded by God to take a dangerous or grandiose action.

Religious experiences may factor into a person's life in unexpected ways, as in the following case. A midcareer male surgeon who was very successful but long overcommitted to his private practice and his academic responsibilities revealed to his often-neglected wife that, at age 9 years, he was approached by his religious leader to get close physically and ultimately engaged in sexual acts over several years. Believing it was his fault, he never told anyone and decided never to have children. After telling his wife about the experience, they engaged in family therapy to work through the stresses the confession produced in their marriage.

Cults

Recently, cults have appeared to be less popular and less attractive to naïve late adolescents and young adults seeking assistance in discovering who they are as they struggle to develop more mature relationships with their parents. Cults are led by charismatic leaders, often out of control themselves, with inappropriate and often unethical values but purporting to offer acceptance and guidance to troubled followers. Cult members are actively controlled and forced to dissolve allegiance to family and others to serve the cult leader's directives and personal needs. These young members often come from educated families who then seek professional help in persuading their children to leave the cult and enter deprogramming therapy to restore psychological stability to the former cult members. Deprogramming and adjustment back into the family, society, and an independent life are time-intensive and long term with resultant posttraumatic stress disorder (PTSD), which must be recognized and treated.

ACCULTURATION PROBLEM

Acculturation is the process whereby a person from one culture changes in their manner, custom, and dress to adapt to a different culture. It leads to assimilation in which the person has identified with the new culture, usually without conflict or ambivalence. In some cases, however, significant cultural change can evoke severe distress, termed *culture shock.* This condition arises when individuals suddenly find themselves in a new culture in which they feel entirely alien. They may also feel conflict over which lifestyles to maintain, change, or adopt. Children and young adult immigrants often adapt more quickly than do middle-aged and elderly immigrants. Younger immigrants often learn the new language more efficiently and continue to mature in the new culture, but those who are more senior, having had more stability and unchanging routines in their former culture, struggle more to adapt. Culture shock from immigration differs from the restless and continuous moving of psychiatric patients secondary to their illness.

Culture shock can occur within a person's own country with geographic, school, and work changes, such as joining the military, experiencing school busing, moving across the country, or moving to a vastly different neighborhood or from a rural area to a metropolis. Reactive symptoms, which are understandable, include anxiety, depression, isolation, fear, and a sense of loss of identity as the person adjusts. If the person is part of a family or group making this transition and the move is positive and planned, stress can be lower. Furthermore, if one can maintain selected cultural mores safely as they integrate into the new culture, it may be less stressful.

Constant geographic moves because of chosen work opportunities or necessity involve a large proportion of workers in the United States. Joining activities in the new community and actively trying to meet neighbors and coworkers can lessen the culture shock.

An 18-year-old, first-year female college student offered an academic scholarship by a small Southern college with a major in her field of interest, realized on her return home to the Midwest for winter break that she felt like a misfit among her dorm peers. They were friendly yet generally kept their distance from her after class. At home, she discussed her experiences with high school friends, who replied that they had heard about such cultural dissonance from peers at their Midwestern colleges. The student returned to college feeling that it was not her fault or imagination and slowly began to reach out more assertively to her peers so they could get to know her beyond stereotypical beliefs and so she could do the same.

Brainwashing

First practiced by the Chinese Communists on American prisoners during the Korean War, *brainwashing* is the deliberate creation of culture shock. Individuals are isolated, intimidated, and made to feel different and out of place to break their spirits and destroy their coping skills. When a person appears mentally weak and helpless, the aggressors impose new ideas on them that they would never have accepted in their normal state. As with those involved in cults, on release and return to their homes, brainwashed individuals with PTSD require deprogramming treatment, including re-education and ongoing supportive psychotherapy, both on an individual and group basis. Treatment is usually long-term to rebuild healthy self-esteem and coping skills.

Prisoners of War and Torture Victims

Prisoners who survive war or torture experiences do so because of personal inner strengths developed in their earlier lives, beginning within their emotionally healthy and caring families; if they come from troubled families, they are more likely to commit suicide during imprisonment and torture. Prisoners must continuously cope with ongoing anxiety, fear, isolation from known lives, and complete loss of all control over their lives. Those who appear to cope best believe they must survive for a reason (e.g., to tell others what they experienced or to find and return to loved ones). Prisoners who cope best describe living simultaneously on two levels—coping in the here and now to survive the situation while maintaining constant mental connections to their past values and experiences and those important to them.

Beyond the surviving prisoner's personal difficulties, including PTSD, if and when his or her survival behavior continues, his or her family may be affected by the surviving prisoner's inordinate fear of police and strangers, overprotection and overburdening of children to replace those significant others lost, lack of sharing of the past, continued isolation from current communities, or inappropriately expressed anger. Thus, another generation (i.e., children of survivors) can be affected in their personal development and psychological functioning and may require psychiatric evaluation and treatment. (See also Chapter 10, Trauma and Stressor-Related Disorders, for further discussion of these topics.)

A 75-year-old Catholic female survivor of the Pawiak prison in Warsaw, Poland, and then of a concentration camp after her capture as a member of the underground in World War II stated that she had wanted to become a painter. In camp, she carved the Madonna and Child on her toothbrush and sent it home to her mother. She made other clandestine carvings for several women in her barracks to send home to their families, which pleased everyone. After the war, she became a well-known sculptress with exhibits throughout Europe. Many of her art pieces taught people about suffering and respect for others who are of different religions and cultures.

PHASE OF LIFE PROBLEM

Phase of life problems may occur at any point along the life cycle: the first day of school as a child, the divorce of a parent during adolescence, starting college as a young adult, marriage, having children, illness, caring for aged parents, and many others. Although, on some level, adults recognize that life events will intrude on expected plans in the course of a lifetime, unexpected, multiple, significant negative occurrences, especially if they are chronic, overwhelm a person's ability to recover and function constructively. The typical phase of life problems include relationship changes, such as a changed significant personal relationship or loss, job crises, and parenthood.

Because of sex-role socialization and consequent cultural expectations, where men appear externally better able to handle these phases of life problems, women, people with lower SES, and minority group members appear more vulnerable to negative experiences, perhaps because they feel less empowered psychologically. Significant life changes precipitate distress in the form of anxiety and depressive symptoms, an inability to express reactive emotions directly, and often difficulties in coping with ongoing or changed life responsibilities.

Individuals with positive attitudes, healthy family and personal relationships, and mature defense mechanisms and coping styles, including essential trust in self and others, good verbal communication skills, a capacity for creative and positive thinking, and the ability to be flexible, reliable, and energetic, appear to be best able to cope with phase of life problems. Furthermore, a capacity for sublimation; adequate financial and work status; solid values; and healthy, feasible goals can enable people to face, accept, and deal realistically with expected and unexpected life problems and changes.

NONCOMPLIANCE WITH TREATMENT

Compliance is the degree to which a patient carries out the recommendations of the treating physician. A positive doctor–patient relationship can help foster compliance, but even in those circumstances, the patient may be reluctant to comply with a physician's advice. In psychiatry, a significant concern is medication noncompliance, which may result from discomforting side effects, expense, personal value judgments, and denial of illness, among many others. We should only use this category when the problem is sufficiently severe to warrant independent clinical attention.

RELATIONAL PROBLEMS

An adult's psychological health and sense of well-being depend, to a significant degree, on the quality of his or her critical relationships—that is, on patterns of interaction with a partner and children, parents and siblings, and friends and colleagues. Problems in the interaction between any of these significant others can lead to clinical symptoms and impaired functioning among one or more members of the relational unit. Relational problems may be a focus of clinical attention (1) when a relational unit is distressed and dysfunctional or threatened with dissolution and (2) when the relational problems precede, accompany, or follow other psychiatric or medical disorders. Indeed, the relational context of the patient influences other medical or psychiatric symptoms. Conversely, the functioning of a relational unit is affected by a member's general and other medical or psychiatric illness. Relational disorders require a different clinical approach than other disorders. Instead of focusing primarily on the link between symptoms, signs, and the workings of the individual mind, the clinician must also focus on interactions between the individuals involved. Also, the clinician should consider how these interactions are related to the general and other medical or psychiatric symptoms in a meaningful way.

Definition

Relational problems are patterns of interaction between members of a relational unit that are associated with significantly impaired functioning in one or more individual members. Thus one may have parent–child problems, sibling-related problems, or other dyad or triad impairments. At times the entire unit, such as the family itself, may be dysfunctional.

Epidemiology

No reliable figures are available on the prevalence of relational problems. They can be assumed to be ubiquitous; however, most relational problems resolve without professional intervention. We should consider the nature, frequency, and effects of the problem on those involved before using this diagnosis. For example, divorce, which occurs in just under 50 percent of marriages, is a problem that partners resolve through the remedy of divorce. We do not need to use this diagnosis for most divorces. If the persons cannot resolve their disputation and continue to live together in a sadomasochistic or pathologically depressed relationship with unhappiness and abuse, then they should be so labeled. Relationship problems between involved persons that cannot be resolved by friends, family, or clergy require professional intervention by psychiatrists, clinical psychologists, social workers, and other mental health professionals.

Relational Problem Related to a Mental Disorder or General Medical Condition

When a family member is ill either from a psychiatric or medical illness, there are reverberations throughout the family unit. Studies indicate that whereas satisfying relationships may have a health-protective influence, relationship distress tends to be associated with an increased incidence of illness. Psychophysiologic mechanisms help to explain how relational systems affect physical or mental health—for example, the intense emotions generated in human attachment systems can affect vascular reactivity and immune processes. Thus, stress-related psychological or physical symptoms can be an expression of family dysfunction.

Adults must often assume responsibility for caring for aging parents while they are still caring for their children, and this dual obligation can create stress. When adults take care of their parents, both parties must adapt to a reversal of their former roles, and the caretakers not only face the potential loss of their parents but also must cope with evidence of their mortality.

Some caretakers abuse their aging parents, a problem that is now receiving attention. Abuse is most likely to occur when the caretaking offspring have substance abuse problems, are under economic stress, and have no relief from their caretaking duties or when the parent is bedridden or has a chronic illness requiring constant nursing attention. Women suffer abuse more often than men, and most abuse occurs in persons older than age 75 years.

The development of chronic illness in a family member stresses the family system and requires adaptation by both the sick person and the other family members. The person who has become sick must frequently face a loss of autonomy, an increased sense of vulnerability, and sometimes a taxing medical regimen. The other family members must experience the loss of the person as he or she was before the illness, and they usually have substantial caretaking responsibility—for example, in debilitating neurologic diseases, including dementia of the Alzheimer's type, and diseases such as AIDS and cancer. In these cases, the whole family must deal with the stress of prospective death as well as the current illness. Some families use the anger engendered by such situations to create support organizations, increase public awareness of the disease, and rally around the sick member. However, chronic illness frequently produces depression in family members and can cause them to withdraw from or attack one another. The burden of caring for ill family members falls disproportionately on the women in a family—mothers, daughters, and daughters-in-law.

Chronic emotional illness also requires major adaptations by families. For instance, family members may react with chaos or fear of the psychotic productions of a family member with schizophrenia. The regression, exaggerated emotions, frequent hospitalizations, and economic and social dependence of a person with schizophrenia can stress the family system. Family members may react with hostile feelings (referred to as expressed emotion) that are associated with a poor prognosis for the person who is sick. Similarly, a family member with bipolar I disorder can disrupt a family, particularly during manic episodes.

Family devastation can occur when illness (1) suddenly strikes a previously healthy person, (2) occurs earlier than expected in the life cycle (some impairment of physical capacities is expected in old age, although many older persons are healthy), (3) affects the economic stability of the family, and (4) when there are few options for improving the condition of the sick family member.

Parent–Child Relational Problem

Parents differ widely in sensing the needs of their infants. Some quickly note their child's moods and needs; others are slow to respond. Parental responsiveness interacts with the children's temperament to affect the quality of the attachment between child and parent. The diagnosis of the parent–child relational problem applies when the focus of clinical attention is a pattern of interaction between parent and child that is associated with clinically significant impairment in individual or family functioning or with clinically significant symptoms. Examples include impaired communication, overprotection, and inadequate discipline.

Research on parenting skills has isolated two primary dimensions: (1) a permissive–restrictive dimension and (2) a warm and accepting versus a cold and hostile dimension. A typology that separates parents on these dimensions distinguishes among *authoritarian* (restrictive and cold), *permissive* (minimally restrictive and accepting), and *authoritative* (restrictive as needed but also warm and accepting) parenting styles. Children of authoritarian parents tend to be withdrawn or conflicted; those of permissive parents are likely to be more aggressive, impulsive, and low achievers; and children of authoritative parents seem to function at the highest level, socially and cognitively. However, switching from an authoritarian to a permissive mode may create a negative reinforcement pattern.

Difficulties in many situations stress the usual parent–child interaction. Substantial evidence indicates that marital discord leads to problems in children, from depression and withdrawal to conduct disorder and poor performance at school. Parents may resort to *triangulation*, where they recruit a child as an ally in the struggle with the partner. Divorces and remarriages stress the parent–child relationship and may create painful loyalty conflicts. Stepparents often find it challenging to assume a parental role and may resent the special relationship that exists between their new marital partner and the children from that partner's previous marriages. The resentment of a stepparent by a stepchild and the favoring of a natural child are usual reactions in a new family's initial phases of adjustment. When a second child is born, both familial stress and happiness may result, although happiness is the dominant emotion in most families. The birth of a child can also be troublesome when parents had adopted a child in the belief that they were infertile. Single-parent families usually consist of a mother and children, and their relationship is often affected by financial and emotional problems.

Other situations that can produce a parent–child problem are the development of fatal, disabling, or chronic illness, such as leukemia, epilepsy, sickle-cell anemia, or spinal cord injury, in either the parent or child. The birth of a child with congenital disabilities, such as cerebral palsy, blindness, or deafness, may also produce parent–child problems. These situations, which are not rare, challenge the emotional resources of those involved. Parents and the child must face present and potential loss and must adjust their day-to-day lives physically, economically, and emotionally. These situations can strain the healthiest families and produce parent–child problems not only with the sick person but also with the unaffected family members. In a family with a severely sick child, parents may resent, prefer, or neglect the other children because the ill child requires much time and attention.

Parents with children who have emotional disorders face particular problems, depending on the child's illness. In families with a child with schizophrenia, family treatment is beneficial and improves the social adjustment of the patient. Similarly, family therapy is useful when a child has a mood disorder. In families with a substance-abusing child or adolescent, family involvement is crucial to help control the drug-seeking behavior and to allow family members to verbalize the feelings of frustration and anger that are invariably present.

Normal developmental crises can also be related to parent–child problems. For instance, adolescence is a time of frequent conflict as the adolescent resists rules and demands, increasing autonomy and, at the same time, elicits protective control by displaying immature and dangerous behavior.

The parents of sons ages 18, 15, and 11 years presented with distress about the behavior of their middle child. The family had been cohesive with satisfactory relationships among all members until 6 months before this consultation. At that time, the 15-year-old son began seeing a girl from a comparatively unsupervised household. Frequent arguments had developed between parents and son regarding going out on school nights, curfews, and neglect of schoolwork. The son's combativeness and lowered academic achievement upset his parents to a great deal. They had not experienced similar conflicts with their oldest child. The adolescent, however, maintained a good relationship with his siblings and friends, did not have behavior problems at school, continued to participate in the school basketball team, and was not a substance user.

Daycare Centers. Quality of care during the first 3 years of life is crucial to neuropsychologic development. The National Institute of Child Health and Human Development does not consider daycare harmful to children, especially when the caregivers and daycare teachers provide consistent, empathetic, nurturing care. Not all daycare centers can meet that level of care, however, especially those located in impoverished urban areas. Children receiving less than optimal caring exhibit decreased intellectual and verbal skills that indicate delayed neurocognitive development. They may also become irritable, anxious, or depressed, which interferes with the parent–child bonding experience, and they are less assertive and less effectively toilet trained by the age of 5 years.

Currently, more than 55 percent of women are in the workforce, many of whom have no choice but to place their children in daycare centers. Close to 50 percent of entering medical students are women; few medical centers, however, make adequate provisions for on-site daycare centers for their students or staff. Similarly, corporations need to provide on-site, high-quality care for the children of their employees. Not only will that approach benefit the children, but also corporate economic benefits will accrue as a result of reduced absenteeism, increased productivity, and happier working mothers. Such programs have the added benefit of decreasing stresses on marriages.

Partner Relational Problem

Partner relational problems may include negative communication (e.g., criticisms), distorted communication (e.g., unrealistic expectations), or noncommunication (e.g., withdrawal) associated with clinically significant impairment in individual or family functioning or symptoms in one or both partners.

When persons have partner relational problems, psychiatrists must assess whether a patient's distress arises from the relationship or a mental disorder. Mental disorders are more common in single persons—those who never married or who are widowed, separated,

or divorced—than among married persons. Clinicians should evaluate developmental, sexual, and occupational and relationship histories, for purposes of diagnosis.

Marriage demands a sustained level of adaptation from both partners. In a troubled marriage, a therapist can encourage the partners to explore areas such as the extent of communication between the partners, their ways of solving disputes, their attitudes toward childbearing and child-rearing, their relationships with their in-laws, their attitudes toward social life, their handling of finances, and their sexual interaction. The birth of a child, abortion or miscarriage, economic stresses, moves to new areas, episodes of illness, significant career changes, and any situations that involve a significant change in marital roles can precipitate stressful periods in a relationship. Illness in a child exerts the most significant strain on a marriage, and marriages in which a child has died through illness or accident more often than not end in divorce. Complaints of lifelong anorgasmia or impotence by marital partners usually indicate intrapsychic problems, although sexual dissatisfaction is involved in many cases of marital maladjustment.

Adjustment to marital roles can be a problem when partners are from different backgrounds and have grown up with different value systems. For example, members of low SES groups perceive a wife as making most of the decisions in the family, and they accept physical punishment as a way to discipline children. Middle-class persons perceive family decision-making processes as shared, with the husband often being the final arbiter, and they prefer to discipline children verbally. Therapists and partners can handle the problems involving conflicts in values, adjustment to new roles, and poor communication by examining the couple's relationship, as in marital therapy.

Epidemiologic surveys show that unhappy marriages are a risk factor for major depressive disorders. Marital discord also affects physical health. For example, in a study of women age 30 to 65 years with coronary artery disease, marital stress worsened the prognosis 2.9 times for recurrent coronary events. Marital conflict was also associated with a 46 percent higher relative death risk among female patients having hemodialysis and with elevations in serum epinephrine, norepinephrine, and corticotrophin levels in both men and women. In one study, patients with high levels of hostile marital behavior had slower healing wounds, lower production of proinflammatory cytokines, and higher cytokine production in peripheral blood. Overall, women show better psychological and physiologic responsiveness to conflict than men.

Physician Marriages. Physicians have a higher risk of divorce than other occupational groups. The incidence of divorce among physicians is about 25 to 30 percent. Specialty choice influenced divorce. The highest rate of divorce occurred in psychiatrists (50 percent) followed by surgeons (33 percent) and internists, pediatricians, and pathologists (31 percent). The average age at first marriage was 26 years among all groups.

It is not clear why physicians are at high risk for divorce. Factors implicated include the stresses of dealing with dying patients, making life-and-death decisions, working long hours, and the constant risk of malpractice litigation. Such stressors may predispose physicians to a variety of emotional ills, with the most common being depression and substance abuse, including alcoholism. Such persons generally cannot deal with the complex interactions required to maintain successful long-term relationships of any kind, and marriage requires the most interpersonal skills of all.

Sibling Relational Problem

Sibling relationships tend to be characterized by competition, comparison, and cooperation. Intense sibling rivalry can occur with the birth of a child and can persist as the children grow up, compete for parental approval, and measure their accomplishments against one another. Alliances between siblings are equally common. Siblings may learn to protect one another against parental control or aggression. In households with three children, one pair tends to become tightly involved with one another, leaving the extra child in the position of an outsider.

Relational problems can arise when a family treats siblings unequally; for instance, idealizing one child while casting another in the role of the family scapegoat. Differences in gender roles and expectations expressed by the parents can underlie sibling rivalry. Parent–child relationships also are dependent on personality interactions. A child's resentment directed at a parental figure or a child's own disavowed dark emotions can be projected onto a sibling and can fuel an intense hate relationship.

An ill child creates stress for the child's siblings. Parental concern and attention to the sick child can elicit envy in the siblings. Also, chronic disability can leave the sick child feeling devalued and rejected by siblings, and the latter may develop a sense of superiority and may feel embarrassed about having a disabled sister or brother. Twin relationships have become an area of increasing study. Preliminary data show that twins are more likely to be cooperative than competitive. Whether or not identical twins should be dressed differently during their toddler years to ensure a separate identity is open to question as is the issue of whether or not they should be in separate classrooms when they begin school.

Other Relational Problems

People, across the life cycle, may become involved in relational problems with leaders and others in their communities at large. In such relationships, conflicts are frequent and can bring about stress-related symptoms. Many relational problems of children occur in the school setting and involve peers. Impaired peer relationships can be the chief complaint in attention-deficit or conduct disorders, as well as in depressive and other psychiatric disorders of childhood, adolescence, and adulthood.

Racial, ethnic, and religious prejudices and ignorance cause problems in interpersonal relationships. In the workplace and communities at large, sexual harassment is often a combination of inappropriate sexual interactions, inappropriate displays of abuse of power and dominance, and expressions of negative gender stereotypes. This harassment most often victimizes women and gay men. However, it can also affect children and adolescents of both sexes.

References

Barzilai-Pesach V, Sheiner EK, Sheiner E, Potashnik G, Shoham-Vardi I. The effect of women's occupational psychologic stress on outcome of fertility treatments. *J Occup Environ Med*. 2006;48(1):56–62.

Bhugra D. Migration and depression. *Acta Psychiatr Scand Suppl*. 2003;418:67–72.

Bogduk N. Diagnostic blocks: A truth serum for malingering. *Clin J Pain*. 2004;20(6):409–414.

Bosco SM, Harvey D. Effects of terror attacks on employment plans and anxiety levels of college students. *College Student J*. 2003;37:438–446.

Campagna AF. Sexual abuse of males: The SAM model of theory and practice. *J Am Acad Child Adolesc Psychiatry*. 2005;44(10):1064–1065.

Costigan CL, Cox MJ, Cauce AM. Work-parenting linkage among dual-earner couples at the transition to parenthood. *J Fam Psychol*. 2003;17:397–408.

Dagan E, Gil S. BRCA1/2 mutation carriers: Psychological distress and ways of coping. *J Psychol Oncol*. 2004;22(3):93–106.

Guriel J, Fremouw W. Assessing malingered posttraumatic disorder: A critical review. *Clin Psychol Rev*. 2003;23(7):881–904.

Johnston D. What makes a difference to patients? *Int Rev Psychiatry*. 2013;25(3):319–328.

Langan J, Mercer SW, Smith DJ. Multimorbidity and mental health: Can psychiatry rise to the challenge? *Br J Psychiatry*. 2013;202(6):391–393.

Larrabee GJ. Detection of malingering using atypical performance patterns on standard neuropsychological tests. *Clin Neuropsychol*. 2003;17(3):410–425.

Mason AM, Cardell R, Armstrong M. Malingering psychosis: Guidelines for assessment and management. *Perspect Psychiatr Care*. 2014;50(1):51–57.

Mills MJ, Lipian MS. Malingering. In: Sadock BJ, Sadock VA, eds. *Kaplan & Sadock's Comprehensive Textbook of Psychiatry*. 8th ed. Vol. 2. Philadelphia, PA: Lippincott Williams & Wilkins; 2005:2247.

Ninivaggi FJ. Malingering. In: Sadock BJ, Sadock VA, Ruiz P, eds. *Kaplan & Sadock's Comprehensive Textbook of Psychiatry*. 10th ed. Philadelphia, PA. Wolters Kluwer; 2017.

O'Bryant SE, Hilsabeck RC, Fisher JM, McCaffrey RJ. Utility of the trail making test in the assessment of malingering in a sample of mild traumatic brain injury litigants. *Clin Neuropsychol*. 2003;17(1):69–74.

Stansfeld SA, Pike C, McManus S, Harris J, Bebbington P, Brugha T, Hassiotis A, Jenkins R, Meltzer H, Moran P, Clark C. Occupations, work characteristics and common mental disorder. *Psychol Med*. 2013;43(5):961–973.

Zierold KM, Anderson H. The relationship between work permits, injury, and safety training among working teenagers. *Am J Ind Med*. 2006;49(5):360–366.

21 ▲

Psychopharmacology

Psychopharmacologic advances continue to expand the parameters of psychiatric treatments dramatically. Our increasing understanding of the brain has led to more effective, less toxic, better-tolerated, and more specific therapeutic agents. With the ever-increasing sophistication and array of treatment options, clinicians, however, must remain aware of potential adverse effects, drug–drug (and drug–food or drug–supplement) interactions, and how to manage the emergence of unwanted or unintended consequences. Newer drugs often cause side effects that are not recognized initially. Keeping up with the latest research findings is important as these findings proliferate. A thorough understanding of the management of medication-induced side effects (either through treating the effect with another agent or substituting another primary agent) is necessary.

Medications used to treat psychiatric disorders are sometimes referred to as *psychotropic drugs.* These drugs are commonly described by their primary clinical application, for example, *antidepressants, antipsychotics, mood stabilizers, anxiolytics, hypnotics, cognitive enhancers,* and *stimulants.* A problem with this approach is that, in many instances, drugs have multiple indications. For example, drugs such as the selective serotonin reuptake inhibitors (SSRIs) are both antidepressants and anxiolytics, and the serotonin-dopamine antagonists (SDAs) are both antipsychotics and mood stabilizers. The term is largely synonymous with simply "psychiatric drugs" and we use both terms synonymously in this book.

Psychotropic drugs have also been organized according to structure (e.g., tricyclic), mechanism (e.g., monoamine oxidase inhibitor [MAOI]), history (e.g., first-generation, traditional), uniqueness (e.g., atypical), or indication (e.g., antidepressant). A further source of confusion is that many drugs used to treat medical and neurologic conditions are routinely used to treat psychiatric disorders.

Also, psychotropic drug terminology can be confusing. The first pharmaceutical agents used to treat schizophrenia were termed *tranquilizers.* When newer drugs emerged as therapies for anxiety, a distinction was drawn between *major* and *minor tranquilizers.* At first, antidepressants were tricyclic antidepressants (TCAs) or MAOIs. In the 1970s and 1980s, as newer antidepressant drugs emerged, they were labeled as *second-* or *third-generation antidepressants.* More recently, older agents used as treatments for psychosis became known as *typical, conventional,* or first-generation *traditional* neuroleptics. Newer ones became *atypical neuroleptics* or second-generation antipsychotics.

In this chapter, we still start with a general review of psychopharmacology, as it applies to psychotropic medications. We will then review the major classes of drugs. For the purposes here, we will use the first system of organization described above; that is, we will classify them by their primary application. Also, we will divert from our usual practice of mainly using generic names of the drugs to, in many cases, include brand names as well. However, in practice, most psychotropic medications are now available through generic preparations, and few patients receive the brand version of a medication. Also, the brand names here reflect US brands. Drug companies in other countries may produce medications under a different brand name.

DRUG SELECTION

Although all U.S. Food and Drug Administration (FDA)-approved psychotropics are similar in overall effectiveness for their indicated disorder, they differ considerably in their pharmacology and their efficacy and adverse effects on individual patients. The ability of a drug to prove effective, thus, is only partially predictable and is dependent on poorly understood patient variables. Nevertheless, some drugs may have a niche in which they can be uniquely helpful for a subgroup of patients, without demonstrating any overall superiority in efficacy. No drug is universally effective, and no evidence indicates the unambiguous superiority of any single agent as a treatment for any major psychiatric disorders. The only exception, clozapine (Clozaril), has been approved by the FDA as a treatment for cases of treatment-refractory schizophrenia.

Decisions about drug selection and use are made on a case-by-case basis, relying on individual judgment by the physician. Other factors in drug selection are the characteristics of the drug and the nature of the patient's illness. Each of these components affects the probability of a successful outcome.

DRUG FACTORS

Pharmacodynamics

Both genetic and environmental factors influence individual response to and tolerability of psychotropic agents. Thus, a drug that may not prove effective in many patients with a disorder can dramatically improve symptoms in others. In these cases, identification of characteristics that might predict potential candidates for that drug becomes important but often remains elusive.

Drugs, even within the same class, are distinguished from one another by often subtle differences in molecular structure, types of interactions with neurotransmitter systems, differences in pharmacokinetics, the presence or absence of active metabolites, and protein binding. These differences, along with patient biochemical variations, account for the profile of efficacy, tolerability, and safety and the risk-to-benefit ratio for the individual. These multiple variables, some poorly understood, make it difficult to predict a drug's effect with certainty. Nevertheless, knowledge of the nature of each property increases the likelihood of successful treatment. The clinical effects of drugs are best understood in terms of *pharmacokinetics* and *pharmacodynamics.* Pharmacokinetics describes *what the body does to a drug*, whereas pharmacodynamics is *what the drug does to the body.*

Pharmacokinetics and pharmacodynamics need to be seen in the context of the underlying variability among patients for how drug effects are expressed clinically. Patients differ in their therapeutic response to a drug, and the experience of side effects. It is increasingly clear that these differences have a strong genetic basis. Pharmacogenetics research is attempting to identify the role of genetics in drug response.

Primary pharmacodynamic considerations include receptor mechanisms, the dose–response curve, the therapeutic index, and the development of tolerance, dependence, and withdrawal phenomena. The drug's mechanism of action is subsumed under pharmacodynamics. The clinical response to a drug, including adverse reactions, results from an interaction between that drug and a patient's susceptibility to those actions. Pharmacogenetic studies are beginning to identify genetic polymorphisms linked to individual differences in treatment response and sensitivity to side effects.

Mechanisms

The mechanisms through which most psychotropic drugs produce their therapeutic effects remain poorly understood. Standard explanations focus on ways that drugs alter synaptic concentrations of dopamine, serotonin, norepinephrine, histamine, γ-aminobutyric acid (GABA), or acetylcholine. These changes are said to result from receptor antagonists or agonists, interference with neurotransmitter reuptake, enhancement of neurotransmitter release, or inhibition of enzymes. Specific drugs are associated with permutations or combinations of these actions. For example, a drug can be an agonist for a receptor, thus stimulating the specific biologic activity of the receptor, or an antagonist, thus inhibiting the biologic activity. Some drugs are partial agonists because they are not capable of fully activating a specific receptor. Some psychotropic drugs also produce clinical effects through mechanisms other than receptor interactions. For example, lithium (Eskalith) can act by directly inhibiting the enzyme inositol-1-phosphatase. Some effects are closely linked to a specific synaptic effect. For example, most medications that treat psychosis share the ability to block the dopamine type 2 (D_2) receptor. Similarly, benzodiazepine agonists bind a receptor complex that contains benzodiazepine and GABA receptors.

Additionally, illustrating the fact that the mechanisms of action of psychotropic drugs remain only partially understood are observations that medications that do not directly target monoamine neurotransmitters can be remarkably effective in treating some psychiatric disorders. For example, ketamine (Ketalar), an anesthetic agent that targets glutamate, can rapidly and dramatically alleviate symptoms of depression when given as a slow infusion. Another example involves the antibiotic minocycline (Solodyn), which has been shown to have antidepressant effects. Along with other findings, this suggests that the immune system and inflammatory responses may underlie some mood disorders.

Accounts of the so-called mechanisms of action should nevertheless be kept in perspective. Explanations of how psychotropic drugs work that focus on synaptic elements represent an oversimplification of a complex series of events. If merely raising or lowering levels of neurotransmitter activity is associated with the clinical effects of a drug, then all drugs that cause these changes should produce equivalent benefits. This predictability is not the case. Multiple obscure actions, several steps removed from events

at neuronal receptor sites, are probably responsible for the therapeutic effects of psychotropic drugs. These *downstream* elements are postulated to represent the actual reasons that these drugs produce clinical improvement. A glossary of terms related to receptor drug interactions is given in Table 21-1.

SIDE EFFECTS

Side effects are an unavoidable risk of medication treatment. Although it is impossible to have an encyclopedic knowledge of all possible adverse drug effects, prescribing clinicians should be familiar with the more common adverse effects, as well as those with serious medical consequences. No single text or document, including the product information, contains a complete list of possible treatment-emergent events.

Side effect considerations include the probability of its occurrence, its impact on a patient's quality of life, its time course, and its cause. Just as no one drug is sure to produce clinical improvement in all patients, no side effect, no matter how common, occurs in every patient. When concurrent medical disorders or a history of a similar adverse reaction puts a patient at increased risk for a side effect, it is logical to consider prescribing a compound not typically associated with that adverse reaction.

Side effects can result from the same pharmacologic action that is responsible for a drug's therapeutic activity or from an unrelated property. In examples of the latter, some of the most common adverse effects of the TCAs are caused by blockade of muscarinic acetylcholine receptors or histamine receptors. If a patient is sensitive to these effects, alternative agents without these properties should be prescribed. When side effects are manifestations of the drug's presumed mechanism of action, side effects may be unavoidable. Thus, blockade of serotonin reuptake by SSRIs can cause nausea and sexual dysfunction. The D_2 blockade of drugs used to treat psychosis can cause extrapyramidal side effects. Agonist action of benzodiazepine receptors can cause ataxia and daytime sleepiness. In these cases, additional medications are frequently used to make the primary agent better tolerated.

Time Course

Adverse effects differ in terms of their onset and duration. Some side effects appear at the outset of treatment and then rapidly diminish. Nausea occurring with SSRIs or venlafaxine (Effexor) and sedation occurring with mirtazapine (Remeron) are good examples of early, time-limited side effects. Early-onset, but persistent, side effects include a dry mouth that is associated with noradrenergic reuptake inhibition or antimuscarinic activity. Some side effects appear later in treatment (*late-appearing side effects*) and, sometimes may be just the opposite of adverse events early in treatment. For example, patients may typically lose weight during early treatment with SSRIs, only to find, over time, a reversal occurs, so that they gain weight.

Similarly, early activation or agitation may be followed by constant fatigue or apathy. Because most data about new drugs come from short-term studies, generally 8 weeks in duration, early-onset side effects are overrepresented in product information and descriptions of newly marketed information. Clinicians must follow the letters to the editor sections of journals and other sources of information to update their understanding of the real side effect profile of a drug.

Adverse effects differ in their impact on compliance and the potential to cause harm. Depending on a patient's threshold

Table 21-1
Glossary of Receptor Drug Interactions

Receptor Interaction	Definition	Examples and Comments
Agonist (full agonist)	A drug or medication that binds to a specific receptor producing an effect identical to that usually produced by the neurotransmitter affecting that receptor. Drugs are often designed as receptor agonists to treat a variety of diseases and disorders in which the original neurotransmitter is missing or diminished.	Full agonists include opioids such as morphine, methadone, oxycodone, hydrocodone, heroin, codeine, meperidine, propoxyphene, and fentanyl. Benzodiazepines act as agonists at the GABA receptor complex.
Antagonist	A compound that binds to a receptor that blocks or reduces the action of another substance (agonist) at the receptor site involved. Antagonists that compete with an agonist for a receptor are *competitive antagonists*. Those that antagonize by other means are *noncompetitive antagonists*.	Flumazenil is a competitive benzodiazepine receptor antagonist. It competitively inhibits the activity at the benzodiazepine recognition site on the GABA/benzodiazepine receptor complex. It is the purest antagonist synthesized. Drugs used in the treatment of schizophrenia block dopamine 2 receptors. Examples of opioid antagonists include naltrexone and naloxone.
Partial agonist (mixed agonist)	A compound that (even when fully occupying a receptor) possesses affinity for a receptor, but elicits a partial pharmacologic response at the receptor involved. Partial agonists are often structural analogs of agonist molecules. If neurotransmitter concentrations are low, partial agonists may behave as an agonist. This is why these medications are sometimes called mixed agonists.	Buprenorphine is a partial agonist that produces typical opioid agonist effects and side effects, such as euphoria and respiratory depression, but its maximal effects are less than those of full agonists like heroin and methadone. When used at low doses buprenorphine produces sufficient agonist effect to enable opioid-addicted individuals to discontinue the drugs with fewer withdrawal symptoms.
Inverse agonist	An inverse agonist is an agent that binds to the same receptor as an agonist for that receptor but produces the opposite pharmacologic effect.	Several inverse agonists are currently in clinical development. One particular example is RO15-4513, which is the inverse agonist of the benzodiazepine class of drugs. RO15-4513 and the benzodiazepines both utilize the same GABA binding site on neurons, yet RO15-4513 has the opposite effect, producing severe anxiety rather than the sedative and anxiolytic effects associated with benzodiazepines. Cannabinoid inverse agonists have been found to reduce appetite, the opposite of the craving effect associated with cannabis.

GABA, γ-aminobutyric acid.
Table by Norman Sussman, M.D.

of tolerance for a side effect and the impact on the quality of life, side effects can lead to drug discontinuation. Examples of serious side effects include agranulocytosis (clozapine), Stevens–Johnson syndrome (lamotrigine [Lamictal]), hepatic failure (nefazodone [Serzone]), stroke (phenelzine [Nardil]), and heart block (thioridazine [Mellaril]). Overall, the risk of life-threatening side effects with psychotropics is low. Drugs that carry such a risk should be monitored more closely, and the prescribing physician should take into account whether the potential clinical benefits justify the additional risk. Any drug with a serious risk, as reflected in a black box warning, is generally used less extensively than would otherwise be the case.

In the case of haloperidol (Haldol) and other dopamine receptor antagonists (DRAs), long-term complications, such as tardive dyskinesia, have been well documented. Emerging evidence also suggests that the use of dopamine antagonists is associated with a small increase in the risk of breast cancer and that this is related to larger cumulative doses. In cases in which serious risk is associated with a drug, closer medical monitoring of medication treatment is warranted. Because the most widely used psychotropics, such as the SSRIs and SDAs, have only been in use since the 1980s or 1990s, there is less certainty about long-term effects, but no evidence indicates that side effects are not merely extensions of those

already evident during initial therapy. It should also be kept in mind that most drugs used in the treatment of chronic medical disorders have not been in use sufficiently long to provide assurances about unintended long-term adverse effects.

Suicidal Ideation and Antidepressant Treatment

The issue of antidepressant-associated suicide has become front-page news, the result of an analysis suggesting a link between medication use and suicidal ideation among children, adolescents, and adults up to age 24 in short-term (4 to 16 weeks), placebo-controlled trials of nine newer antidepressant drugs. The data from trials involving more than 4,400 patients suggested that the average risk of suicidal thinking or behavior (suicidality) during the first few months of treatment in those receiving antidepressants was 4 percent, twice the placebo risk of 2 percent. No suicides occurred in these trials. The analysis also showed no increase in suicide risk among the 25- to 65-age group. Antidepressants reduced suicidality among those over age 65.

Following public hearings on the subject, in October 2004, the FDA requested the addition of black box warnings—the most severe warning placed on the labeling of prescription medication—to all antidepressant drugs, old and new. This action raised the alarm among parents and physicians and prompted an explosion of advertisements by malpractice attorneys. Most important, antidepressant prescriptions written for adolescents declined, whereas those for adults flattened, after years of growth.

A large study of real-world patients published in the January 2006 issue of the *American Journal of Psychiatry* raised severe doubt about antidepressants and actual suicidality and about the wisdom of the FDA's decision to change the labeling. The study examined suicides and hospitalizations for suicide attempts in the medical records of 65,103 members of a nonprofit insurer in the Pacific Northwest that covers about 500,000 people who received antidepressants from 1992 to 2003. It found that (1) newer antidepressants were associated with a more rapid and more significant reduction in risk than older types of antidepressants, and (2) patients were significantly more likely to attempt or commit suicide in the month before they began drug therapy than in the 6 months after starting it.

This controversy is not the first time credible evidence has contradicted a significant link between antidepressant use and increased risk of suicide. At the hearings that led to the black box warning, John Mann of Columbia University presented population data showing that since 1987, the year before fluoxetine (Prozac) became the first marketed SSRI, suicide rates in the United States began dropping and that areas in the United States with the highest SSRI prescription rates had the most significant decline in suicides. For every 10 percent increase in prescription rates, the US suicide rate declined 3 percent.

Another study, a review of 588 case files of patients aged 10 to 19, found that a 1 percent increase in antidepressant use was associated with a decrease of 0.23 suicides per 100,000 adolescents per year.

A more critical question, given how slight the risk may be, if indeed it exists, is whether as a result of the FDA's ill-considered actions, some depressed patients are not getting potentially lifesaving treatment. Epidemiologic findings from several countries, including the United States, have shown that decreased prescribing of antidepressants for depressed children and adolescents resulted in an increase in suicide rates in those populations.

Medication-Induced Movement Disorders

Medication-induced movement disorders are commonly associated with the use of psychotropic drugs. Although most frequently associated with drugs that block dopamine type 2 (D_2) receptors, abnormal motor activity may occur with other types of medications as well. Sometimes it can be challenging to determine if abnormal motor movements are an adverse event or a symptom of an underlying disorder. For example, anxiety can resemble akathisia, and alcohol or benzodiazepine withdrawal can cause tremors. The American Psychiatric Association has decided to retain the term *neuroleptic* when discussing side effects associated with drugs used to treat psychosis—the DRAs and second-generation antipsychotics (SGAs). The rationale for continued use of the term is that it was initially used to describe the tendency of these drugs to cause abnormal movements. Note that SGA and SDA are often used interchangeably when referring to the second-generation antipsychotics.

The most common neuroleptic-related movement disorders are parkinsonism, acute dystonia, and acute akathisia. The neuroleptic malignant syndrome is a life-threatening and often misdiagnosed condition. Neuroleptic-induced tardive dyskinesia is a late-appearing adverse effect of neuroleptic drugs and can be irreversible; recent data, however, indicate that the syndrome, although still severe and potentially disabling, is less pernicious than was previously thought in patients taking DRAs. The newer antipsychotics, the SDAs, block binding to dopamine receptors to a much lesser degree and thereby are presumed to be less likely to produce such movement disorders. Nevertheless, this risk remains, and vigilance is still required when these drugs are prescribed.

Table 21-2 lists the selected medications associated with movement disorders and their impact on relevant neuroreceptors.

Neuroleptic-Induced Parkinsonism and Other Medication-Induced Parkinsonism

DIAGNOSIS, SIGNS, AND SYMPTOMS. Symptoms of neuroleptic-induced parkinsonism and other medication-induced parkinsonism include muscle stiffness (lead pipe rigidity), cogwheel rigidity, shuffling gait, stooped posture, and drooling. The pill-rolling tremor of idiopathic parkinsonism is rare, but a regular, coarse tremor similar to essential tremor may be present. The so-called *rabbit syndrome,* a tremor affecting the lips and perioral muscles, is another parkinsonian effect seen with antipsychotics, although perioral tremor is more likely than other tremors to occur late in the course of treatment.

EPIDEMIOLOGY. Parkinsonian adverse effects typically occur within 5 to 90 days of the initiation of treatment. Patients who are elderly and female are at the highest risk for neuroleptic-induced parkinsonism, although the disorder can occur at all ages.

ETIOLOGY. The blockade of D_2 receptors causes neuroleptic-induced parkinsonism in the caudate at the termination of the nigrostriatal dopamine neurons. All antipsychotics can cause the symptoms, especially high-potency drugs with low levels of anticholinergic activity, most notably haloperidol (Haldol).

DIFFERENTIAL DIAGNOSIS. Included in the differential diagnosis are idiopathic parkinsonism, other organic causes of parkinsonism, and depression, which can also be associated with parkinsonian symptoms. Decreased psychomotor activity and blunted facial expression are symptoms of depression and idiopathic parkinsonism.

TREATMENT. Parkinsonism can be treated with anticholinergic agents, benztropine (Cogentin), amantadine (Symmetrel), or diphenhydramine (Benadryl) (Table 21-3). Anticholinergics should be withdrawn after 4 to 6 weeks to assess whether tolerance to the parkinsonian effects has developed; about half of patients with neuroleptic-induced parkinsonism require continued treatment. Even after the antipsychotics are withdrawn, parkinsonian symptoms can last up to 2 weeks. In elderly patients, this may last as long as 3 months. With such patients, the clinician may continue the anticholinergic drug after the antipsychotic has been stopped until the parkinsonian symptoms resolve completely.

Neuroleptic Malignant Syndrome

DIAGNOSIS, SIGNS, AND SYMPTOMS. *Neuroleptic malignant syndrome* is a life-threatening complication that can occur anytime during antipsychotic treatment. The motor and behavioral symptoms include muscular rigidity and dystonia, akinesia, mutism, obtundation, and agitation. The autonomic symptoms include hyperthermia, diaphoresis, and increased pulse and blood pressure (BP). Laboratory findings include an increased white blood cell (WBC) count and increased levels of creatinine phosphokinase, liver enzymes, plasma myoglobin, and myoglobinuria, occasionally associated with renal failure.

Table 21-2
Selected Medications Associated with Movement Disorders: Impact on Relevant Neuroreceptors

Type (Subtype)	Name (Brand)	D₂ Blockade	5-HT₂ Blockade	mACh Blockade
Antipsychotics				
Phenothiazine (Aliphatic)	Chlorpromazine (Thorazine)	Low	High	High
Phenothiazine (Piperidines)	Thioridazine (Mellaril)	Low	Med	High
	Mesoridazine (Serentil)	Low	Med	High
Phenothiazine (Piperazines)	Trifluoperazine (Stelazine)	Med	Med	Med
	Fluphenazine (Prolixin)	High	Low	Low
	Perphenazine (Trilafon)	High	Med	Low
Thioxanthenes	Thiothixene (Navane)	High	Med	Low
	Chlorprothivene (Taractan)	Med	High	Med
Dibenzoxazepines	Loxapine (Loxitane)	Med	High	Low
Butyrophenones	Haloperidol (Haldol)	High	Low	Low
	Droperidol (Inapsine)	High	Med	—
Diphenyl-butylpiperidines	Pimozide (Orap)	High	Med	Low
Dihydroindolones	Molindone (Moban)	Med	Low	Low
Dibenzodiazepines	Clozapine (Clozaril)	Low	High	High
Benzisoxazole	Risperidone (Risperdal)	High	High	Low
Thienobenzodiazepines	Olanzapine (Zyprexa)	Low	High	High
Dibenzothiazepines	Quetiapine (Seroquel)	Low/med	Low/med	Low
Benzisothiazolvils	Ziprasidone (Geodon)	Med	High	Low
Quinolones	Aripiprazole (Abilify)	High (as partial agonist)	High	Low
Nonantipsychotic psychotropics	Lithium (Eskalith)	N/A	N/A	N/A
Anticonvulsants		Low	Low	Low
Antidepressants		Low (except amoxapine)	(Varies)	(Varies)
Nonpsychotropics	Prochlorperazine (Compazine)	High	Med	Low
	Metoclopramide (Reglan)	High	High	—

D₂, dopamine type 2; 5-HT₂, 5-hydroxytryptomine type 2; mACh, muscarinic acetylcholine; N/A, not applicable.
Adapted from Janicak PG, Davis JM, Preskorn SH, Ayd Fj Jr. *Principles and Practice of Psychopharmacotherapy*. 3rd ed. Philadelphia, PA: Lippincott Williams & Wilkins; 2001, with permission.

EPIDEMIOLOGY. About 0.01 to 0.02 percent of patients treated with antipsychotics develop neuroleptic malignant syndrome. Men are affected more frequently than women, and young patients are affected more commonly than elderly patients. The mortality rate can reach 10 to 20 percent or even higher when depot antipsychotic medications are involved.

COURSE AND PROGNOSIS. The symptoms usually evolve over 24 to 72 hours, and the untreated syndrome lasts 10 to 14 days. The diagnosis is often missed in the early stages, and the withdrawal or agitation may mistakenly be considered to reflect an exacerbation of the psychosis.

TREATMENT. In addition to supportive medical treatment, the most commonly used medications for the condition are dantrolene (Dantrium) and bromocriptine (Parlodel), although amantadine (Symmetrel) is sometimes used (Table 21-4). Bromocriptine and amantadine pose direct DRA effects and may overcome the antipsychotic-induced dopamine receptor blockade. We should reduce the antipsychotic dose to the lowest effective dose possible. High-potency drugs, such as haloperidol, pose the greatest risk. Antipsychotic drugs with anticholinergic effects seem less likely to cause neuroleptic malignant syndrome. Electroconvulsive therapy (ECT) has been used.

Medication-Induced Acute Dystonia

DIAGNOSIS, SIGNS, AND SYMPTOMS. *Dystonias* are brief or prolonged contractions of muscles that result in obviously abnormal movements or postures, including oculogyric crises, tongue protrusion, trismus, torticollis, laryngeal–pharyngeal dystonias, and dystonic postures of the limbs and trunk. Other dystonias include blepharospasm and glossopharyngeal dystonia; the latter results in dysarthria, dysphagia, and even difficulty in breathing, which can cause cyanosis. Children are particularly likely to evidence opisthotonos, scoliosis, lordosis, and writhing movements. Dystonia can be painful and frightening and often results in noncompliance with future drug treatment regimens.

EPIDEMIOLOGY. Their early-onset characterizes the development of acute dystonic symptoms during treatment with neuroleptics. There is a higher incidence of acute dystonia in men, in patients younger than age 30 years, and patients who were given high dosages of high-potency medications.

ETIOLOGY. Although it is most frequent with intramuscular doses of high-potency antipsychotics, dystonia can occur with any antipsychotic. The mechanism of action is thought to be dopaminergic hyperactivity in the basal ganglia that occurs when the central nervous system (CNS) levels of the antipsychotic drug begin to fall between doses.

Table 21-3
Drug Treatment of Extrapyramidal Disorders

Generic Name	Trade Name	Usual Daily Dosage	Indications
Anticholinergics			
Benztropine	Cogentin	PO 0.5–2 mg tid; IM or IV 1–2 mg	Acute dystonia, parkinsonism, akinesia, akathisia
Biperiden	Akineton	PO 2–6 mg tid; IM or IV 2 mg	
Procyclidine	Kemadrin	PO 2.5–5 mg bid-qid	
Trihexyphenidyl	Artane, Tremin	PO 2–5 mg tid	
Orphenadrine	Norflex, Disipal	PO 50–100 mg bid-qid; IV 60 mg	Rabbit syndrome
Antihistamine			
Diphenhydramine	Benadryl	PO 25 mg qid; IM or IV 25 mg	Acute dystonia, parkinsonism, akinesia, rabbit syndrome
Amantadine	Symmetrel	PO 100–200 mg bid	Parkinsonism, akinesia, rabbit syndrome
β-Adrenergic Antagonist			
Propranolol	Inderal	PO 20–40 mg tid	Akathisia, tremor
α-Adrenergic Antagonist			
Clonidine	Catapres	PO 0.1 mg tid	Akathisia
Benzodiazepines			
Clonazepam	Klonopin	PO 1 mg bid	Akathisia, acute dystonia
Lorazepam	Ativan	PO 1 mg tid	
Buspirone	BuSpar	PO 20–40 mg qid	Tardive dyskinesia
Vitamin E	—	PO 1,200–1,600 IU/day	Tardive dyskinesia

PO, orally; IM, intramuscularly; IV, intravenously; bid, twice a day; tid, three times a day; qid; four times a day.

DIFFERENTIAL DIAGNOSIS. The differential diagnosis includes seizures and tardive dyskinesia.

COURSE AND PROGNOSIS. Dystonia can fluctuate spontaneously and respond to reassurance, so the clinician gets the false impression that the movement is hysterical or entirely under conscious control.

TREATMENT. Prophylaxis with anticholinergics or related drugs (outlined in Table 21-3) usually prevents dystonia, although the risks of prophylactic treatment weigh against that benefit. Treatment with intramuscular anticholinergics or intravenous or intramuscular diphenhydramine (Benadryl) (50 mg) almost always relieves the symptoms. Diazepam (Valium) (10 mg intravenously), amobarbital (Amytal), caffeine sodium benzoate, and hypnosis have also been

Table 21-4
Treatment of Neuroleptic Malignant Syndrome

Intervention	Dosing	Effectiveness
Amantadine	200–400 mg PO/day in divided doses	Beneficial as monotherapy or in combination; decrease in death rate
Bromocriptine	2.5 mg PO bid or tid, may increase to a total of 45 mg/day	Mortality reduced as a single or combined agent
Levodopa/carbidopa	Levodopa 50–100 mg/day IV as continuous infusion	Case reports of dramatic improvement
Electroconvulsive therapy	Reports of good outcome with both unilateral and bilateral treatments; response may occur in as few as three treatments	Effective when medications have failed; also may treat underlying psychiatric disorder
Dantrolene	1 mg/kg/day for 8 days, then continue as PO for 7 additional days	Benefits may occur in minutes or hours as a single agent or in combination
Benzodiazepines	1–2 mg IM as test dose; if effective, switch to PO; consider use if underlying disorder has catatonic symptoms	Has been reported effective when other agents have failed
Supportive measures	IV hydration, cooling blankets, ice packs, ice-water enema, oxygenation, antipyretics	Often effective as initial approach early in the episode

PO, orally; bid, twice a day; tid, three times a day; IV, intravenously; IM, intramuscularly.
Adapted from Davis JM, Caroif SN, Mann SC. Treatment of neuroleptic malignant syndrome. *Psychiatr Ann.* 2000;30:325–331, with permission.

reported to be effective. Although tolerance for the adverse effects usually develops, it is prudent to change the antipsychotic if the patient is particularly concerned that the reaction may recur.

Medication-Induced Acute Akathisia

DIAGNOSIS, SIGNS, AND SYMPTOMS.   *Akathisia* is subjective feelings of restlessness, objective signs of restlessness, or both. Examples include a sense of anxiety, inability to relax, jitteriness, pacing, rocking motions while sitting, and rapid alternation of sitting and standing. Akathisia has been associated with the use of a wide range of psychiatric drugs, including antipsychotics, antidepressants, and sympathomimetics. Once akathisia is recognized and diagnosed, the antipsychotic dose should be reduced to a minimally adequate level. Akathisia may be associated with a poor treatment outcome.

EPIDEMIOLOGY.   Middle-aged women are at increased risk of akathisia, and the time course is similar to that for neuroleptic-induced parkinsonism.

TREATMENT.   Three necessary steps in the treatment of akathisia are reducing medication dosage, attempting treatment with appropriate drugs, and considering changing the neuroleptic. The most efficacious drugs are β-adrenergic receptor antagonists, although anticholinergic drugs, benzodiazepines, and cyproheptadine (Periactin) may benefit some patients. In some cases of akathisia, no treatment seems to be effective.

Tardive Dyskinesia

DIAGNOSIS, SIGNS, AND SYMPTOMS.   *Tardive dyskinesia* is a delayed effect of antipsychotics; it rarely occurs until after 6 months of treatment. The disorder consists of abnormal, involuntary, irregular choreoathetoid movements of the muscles of the head, limbs, and trunk. The severity of the movements ranges from minimal—often missed by patients and their families—to grossly incapacitating. Perioral movements are the most common and include darting, twisting, and protruding movements of the tongue; chewing and lateral jaw movements; lip-puckering; and facial grimacing. Finger movements and hand clenching are also typical. Torticollis, retrocollis, trunk twisting, and pelvic thrusting occur in severe cases. In the most severe cases, patients may have breathing and swallowing irregularities that result in aerophagia, belching, and grunting. Respiratory dyskinesia has also been reported. Dyskinesia is exacerbated by stress and disappears during sleep.

EPIDEMIOLOGY.   Tardive dyskinesia develops in about 10 to 20 percent of patients who are treated for more than a year. About 20 to 40 percent of patients who require long-term hospitalization have tardive dyskinesia. Women are more likely to be affected than men. Children, patients who are more than 50 years of age, and patients with brain damage or mood disorders are also at high risk.

COURSE AND PROGNOSIS.   Between 5 and 40 percent of all cases of tardive dyskinesia eventually remit, and between 50 and 90 percent of all mild cases remit. Tardive dyskinesia is less likely to remit in elderly patients than in young patients, however.

TREATMENT.   The three basic approaches to tardive dyskinesia are prevention, diagnosis, and management. Prevention is best achieved by using antipsychotic medications only when indicated and in the lowest effective doses. The atypical antipsychotics are associated with less tardive dyskinesia than the older antipsychotics. Clozapine (Clozaril) is the only antipsychotic to have minimal risk of tardive dyskinesia and can even help improve preexisting symptoms of tardive dyskinesia. This quality of the drug may be due to its low affinity for D_2 receptors and high affinity for 5-hydroxytryptamine (5-HT) receptor antagonism. Patients who are receiving antipsychotics should be examined regularly for the appearance of abnormal movements, preferably with the use of a standardized rating scale (Table 21-5). Patients frequently

Table 21-5
Abnormal Involuntary Movement Scale (AIMS) Examination Procedure

Patient Identification	**Date**

Rated by

Either before or after completing the examination procedure, observe the patient unobtrusively at rest (e.g., in waiting room).

The chair to be used in this examination should be a hard, firm one without arms.

After observing the patient, rate him or her on a scale of 0 (none), 1 (minimal), 2 (mild), 3 (moderate), and 4 (severe), according to the severity of the symptoms.

Ask patient whether there is anything in his or her mouth (e.g., gum, candy) and, if so, to remove it.

Ask patient about the current condition of his or her teeth. Ask patient if he or she wears dentures. Do teeth or dentures bother patient now?

Ask patient whether he or she notices movement in mouth, face, hands, or feet. If yes, ask patient to describe and indicate to what extent movements currently bother patient or interfere with his or her activities.

0 1 2 3 4 Have patient sit in chair with hands on knees, legs slightly apart, and feet flat on floor. (Look at entire body for movement while in this position.)

0 1 2 3 4 Ask patient to sit with hands hanging unsupported—If male, between legs; if female and wearing a dress, hanging over knees. (Observe hands and other body areas.)

0 1 2 3 4 Ask patient to open mouth. (Observe tongue at rest within mouth.) Do this twice.

0 1 2 3 4 Ask patient to protrude tongue. (Observe abnormalities of tongue movement.) Do this twice.

0 1 2 3 4 Ask patient to tap thumb, with each finger, as rapidly as possible for 10–15 seconds; separately with right hand, then with left hand. (Observe facial and leg movements.)

0 1 2 3 4 Flex and extend patient's left and right arms. (One at a time.)

0 1 2 3 4 Ask patient to stand up. (Observe in profile. Observe all body areas again, hips included.)

0 1 2 3 4 ᵃAsk patient to extend both arms outstretched in front with palms down. (Observe trunk, legs, and mouth.)

0 1 2 3 4 ᵃHave patient walk a few paces, turn, and walk back to chair. (Observe hands and gait.)

Do this twice.

ᵃActivated movements.

experience an exacerbation of their symptoms when the DRA is withheld, whereas substitution of an SDA may limit the abnormal movements without worsening the progression of the dyskinesia.

Once tardive dyskinesia is recognized, the clinician should consider reducing the dose of the antipsychotic or even stopping the medication altogether. Alternatively, the clinician may switch the patient to clozapine or one of the new SDAs. In patients who cannot continue taking any antipsychotic medication, lithium (Eskalith), carbamazepine (Tegretol), or benzodiazepines may effectively reduce the symptoms of both the movement disorder and the psychosis. In 2017, the FDA-approved valbenazine (Ingrezza) for the treatment of adults with tardive dyskinesia, making this the first approved medication for tardive dyskinesia.

Tardive Dystonia and Tardive Akathisia.
On occasion, dystonia and akathisia emerge late in the course of treatment. These symptoms may persist for months or years despite drug discontinuation or dose reduction.

Medication-Induced Postural Tremor

DIAGNOSIS, SIGNS, AND SYMPTOMS. *Tremor* is a rhythmic alteration in a movement that is usually faster than one beat per second. Fine tremor (8 to 12 Hz) is most common.

EPIDEMIOLOGY. Typically, tremors decrease during periods of relaxation and sleep and increase with stress or anxiety.

ETIOLOGY. Whereas all the above diagnoses specifically include an association with a neuroleptic, a range of psychiatric medications can produce tremors—most notably, lithium, stimulants, antidepressants, caffeine, and valproate (Depakene).

TREATMENT. The treatment involves four principles:

1. The lowest possible dose of the psychiatric drug should be taken.
2. Patients should minimize caffeine consumption.
3. The psychiatric drug should be taken at bedtime to minimize the amount of daytime tremor.
4. β-Adrenergic receptor antagonists (e.g., propranolol [Inderal]) can be given to treat drug-induced tremors.

Other Medication-Induced Movement Disorders

NOCTURNAL MYOCLONUS. *Nocturnal myoclonus* consists of highly stereotyped, abrupt contractions of specific leg muscles during sleep. Patients lack any subjective awareness of the leg jerks. The condition may be present in about 40 percent of persons over 65 years of age. The cause is unknown, but it is a rare side effect of SSRIs.

The repetitive leg movements occur every 20 to 60 seconds, with extensions of the large toe and flexion of the ankle, the knee, and the hips. Frequent awakenings, unrefreshing sleep, and daytime sleepiness are significant symptoms. No treatment for nocturnal myoclonus is universally effective. Benzodiazepines, levodopa (Larodopa), quinine, and, in rare cases, opioids may be useful.

RESTLESS LEG SYNDROME. In *restless leg syndrome,* persons feel deep sensations of creeping inside the calves whenever sitting or lying down. The dysesthesias are rarely painful but are agonizingly relentless and cause an almost irresistible urge to move the legs; thus, this syndrome interferes with sleep and with falling asleep. It peaks in middle age and occurs in 5 percent of the population. The cause is unknown, but it is a rare side effect of SSRIs.

Symptoms are relieved by movement and by leg massage. The dopamine receptor agonists ropinirole (Requip) and pramipexole (Mirapex) are effective in treating this syndrome. Other treatments include the benzodiazepines, levodopa, quinine, opioids, propranolol, valproate, and carbamazepine.

Hyperthermic Syndromes.
All the medication-induced movement disorders may be associated with hyperthermia. Table 21-6 lists the various conditions associated with hyperthermia.

Side Effects Associated with Newer Medications

All medications are associated with side effects. The clinician should be aware of these, be able to recognize them, and take appropriate measures to treat them.

Somnolence.
Sedation is often an intended effect of many psychotropic drugs, mainly when used to treat insomnia, anxiety, or agitation. Daytime sleepiness, or somnolence, is also an unwanted adverse event, however. It is essential for the clinician to alert patients to the possibility of sedation and to document that the person was advised to exercise caution when operating any type of vehicle or mechanical equipment. Some somnolence results from a carryover of nighttime use of drugs as hypnotics. Even with drugs such as the SSRIs, which are activating for many patients, somnolence can be problematic. In some instances, it results from impairment of sleep quality. Chronic use of SSRIs can cause some patients to experience a subjective sense of fatigue, exhaustion, or yawning, even with adequate amounts of sleep. Management of unwanted somnolence includes adjustment of dose or timing of administration, switching to alternative medications, the addition of small doses of stimulants, or the addition of modafinil (Provigil).

Gastrointestinal Disturbances.
The significant gastrointestinal (GI) side effects of the older antidepressant and antipsychotic drugs consisted primarily of constipation and dry mouth, a consequence of their antimuscarinic activity. Most of the newer drugs have little antimuscarinic activity but do have effects on the serotonin system. Most of the body's serotonin is in the GI tract, and serotonergic drugs often cause varying degrees of stomach pain, nausea, flatulence, and diarrhea. In most cases, these side effects are transient, but some persons never accommodate and must switch to another class of drugs. The initial use of lower doses or the use of delayed-release preparations are the most effective strategies for minimizing GI side effects.

Movement Disorders.
The introduction of SDAs has dramatically reduced the incidence of medication-induced movement disorders, but varying degrees of dose-related parkinsonism, akathisia, and dystonia still occur. Risperidone (Risperdal) most closely resembles the older agents in terms of these side effects. Olanzapine (Zyprexa) also causes more extrapyramidal effects than clinical trials suggested. Aripiprazole (Abilify) causes severe akathisia. There have been rare reports of SSRI-induced movement disorders, ranging from akathisia to tardive dyskinesia.

Sexual Dysfunction.
The use of psychiatric drugs can be associated with sexual dysfunction—decreased libido, impaired ejaculation and erection, and inhibition of female orgasm. In clinical trials with the SSRIs, the extent of sexual side effects was grossly underestimated because data were based on spontaneous reports by patients. The rate of sexual dysfunction in the original fluoxetine product information, for example, was less than 5 percent. In subsequent studies in which specific questions elicited information about sexual side effects, the rate of SSRI-associated sexual

Table 21-6
Drug-Induced Central Hyperthermic Syndromes[a]

Condition (and Mechanism)	Common Drug Causes	Frequent Symptoms	Possible Treatment[b]	Clinical Course
Hyperthermia (↓ heat dissipation, ↑ heat production)	Atropine, lidocaine, meperidine NSAID toxicity, pheochromocytoma, thyrotoxicosis	Hyperthermia, diaphoresis, malaise	Acetaminophen per rectum (325 mg every 4 hr), diazepam oral or per rectum (5 mg every 8 hr) for febrile seizures	Benign, febrile seizures in children
Malignant hyperthermia (↑ heat production)	NMJ blockers (succinylcholine), halothane	Hyperthermia, muscle rigidity, arrhythmias, ischemia,[c] hypotension, rhabdomyolysis; disseminated intravascular coagulation	Dantrolene sodium (1–2 mg/kg/min IV infusion)[d]	Familial, 10% mortality if untreated
Tricyclic overdose (↑ heat production)	Tricyclic antidepressants, cocaine	Hyperthermia, confusion, visual hallucinations, agitation, hyperreflexia, muscle relaxation, anticholinergic effects (dry skin, pupil dilation), arrhythmias	Sodium bicarbonate (1 mEq/kg IV bolus) if arrhythmia is present, physostigmine (1–3 mg IV) with cardiac monitoring	Fatalities have occurred if untreated
Autonomic hyperreflexia (↑ heat production)	CNS stimulants (amphetamines)	Hyperthermia, excitement, hyperreflexia	Trimethaphan (0.3–7 mg/min IV infusion)	Reversible
Lethal catatonia (↓ heat dissipation)	Lead poisoning	Hyperthermia, intense anxiety, destructive behavior, psychosis	Lorazepam (1–2 mg IV every 4 hr), antipsychotics may be contraindicated	High mortality if untreated
Neuroleptic malignant syndrome (mixed; hypothalamic, ↓ heat dissipation, ↑ heat production)	Antipsychotics (neuroleptics), methyldopa, reserpine	Hyperthermia, muscle rigidity, diaphoresis (60%), leukocytosis, delirium, rhabdomyolysis, elevated CPK, autonomic deregulation, extrapyramidal symptoms	Bromocriptine (2–10 mg every 8 hr orally or nasogastric tube), lysuride (0.02–0.1 mg/hr IV infusion), carbidopa-levodopa (Sinemet) (25/100 PO every 8 hr), dantrolene sodium (0.3–1 mg/kg IV every 6 hr)	Rapid onset, 20% mortality if untreated

NSAID, nonsteroidal anti-inflammatory drug; MAOI, monoamine oxidase inhibitor; NMJ, neuromuscular junction; CNS, central nervous system; CPK, creatine phosphokinase; PO, orally; IV, intravenously.
[a]Boldface indicates features that may be used to distinguish one syndrome from another.
[b]Gastric lavage and supportive measures, including cooling, are required in most cases.
[c]Oxygen consumption increases by 7% for every 1°F increase in body temperature.
[d]Has been associated with idiosyncratic hepatocellular injury, as well as severe hypotension in one case.
From Theoharides TC, Harris RS, Weckstein D. Neuroleptic malignant-like syndrome due to cyclobenzaprine? [letter]. *J Clin Psychopharmacol.* 1995;15:80, with permission.

dysfunction was found to be between 35 and 75 percent. In clinical practice, patients are not likely to report sexual dysfunction spontaneously to the physician, so it is essential to ask about this side effect. Also, some sexual dysfunctions may be related to the primary psychiatric disorder.

Nevertheless, if sexual dysfunction emerges after pharmacotherapy has begun and the primary response to treatment has been positive, it may be worthwhile to attempt to treat the symptoms. Long lists of possible antidotes to these side effects have evolved, but few interventions are consistently effective, and few have more than anecdotal evidence to support their use. The clinician and patient should consider the possibility of sexual side effects when selecting a drug and switching treatment to another drug that is less or not at all associated with sexual dysfunction if this adverse effect is not acceptable to the patient.

Weight Gain. Weight gain accompanies the use of many psychotropic drugs as a result of retained fluid, increased caloric intake, decreased exercise, or altered metabolism. Weight gain can also occur as a symptom of a disorder, as in bulimia or atypical depression. In these cases, it may be a sign of recovery. Treatment-emergent increase in body weight is a common reason for noncompliance with a drug regimen. No specific mechanisms have been identified as causing weight gain, and it appears that the histamine and serotonin systems mediate changes in weight associated with many drugs used to treat depression and psychosis. Metformin (Glucophage) has been reported to facilitate weight loss among patients whose weight gain is attributed to the use of serotonin-dopamine reuptake inhibitors and valproic acid (Depakene). Valproate (Depacon), as well as olanzapine, has been linked to the development of insulin resistance, which could induce appetite increase, with the subsequent weight increase. Weight gain is a noteworthy side effect of clozapine (Clozaril) and olanzapine. Genetic factors that regulate body weight, as well as the related problem of diabetes mellitus, seem to involve the 5-HT_{2C} receptor. There is a genetic polymorphism of the promoter region of this receptor, and patients with a variant allele have less weight gain. Drugs with a strong 5-HT_{2C} affinity would be expected to have a more significant impact on body weight of patients with a polymorphism of the 5-HT_{2C} receptor promoter region.

Weight Loss. Initial weight loss is associated with SSRI treatment but is usually transient, with most weight being regained within the first few months. Bupropion (Wellbutrin) has been shown to cause modest weight loss that is sustained. When combined with diet and lifestyle changes, bupropion can facilitate more significant weight loss. Topiramate (Topamax) and zonisamide (Zonegran), marketed as treatments for epilepsy, sometimes produce substantial, sustained loss of weight.

Glucose Changes. Increased risk of glucose abnormalities, including diabetes mellitus, is associated with weight increase during psychotropic drug therapy. Clozapine and olanzapine are associated with a greater risk than other SDAs of abnormalities in fasting glucose levels, as well as hyperosmolar diabetes and keto-acidosis. This dysregulation of glucose homeostasis appears to be drug-induced and increases glucagon.

Hyponatremia. Hyponatremia is associated with oxcarbaze-pine (Trileptal) and SSRI treatment, especially in elderly patients. Confusion, agitation, and lethargy are common symptoms.

Cognitive Impairment. Cognitive impairment means a disturbance in the capacity to think. Some agents, such as the benzodiazepine agonists, are recognized as causes of cognitive impairment. Other widely used psychotropics, such as the SSRIs, lamotrigine (Lamictal), topiramate (Topamax), gabapentin (Neurontin), lithium, TCAs, and bupropion, however, are also associated with varying degrees of memory impairment and word-finding difficulties. In contrast to the benzodiazepine-induced anterograde amnesia, these agents cause a more subtle type of absent-mindedness. Drugs with anticholinergic properties are likely to worsen memory performance.

Sweating. Severe perspiration unrelated to ambient temperature is associated with TCAs, SSRIs, and venlafaxine. This side effect is often socially disabling. Attempts can be made to treat this side effect with alpha agents, such as terazosin (Hytrin) and oxybutynin (Ditropan).

Cardiovascular Disturbances. Newer agents are less likely to have direct cardiac effects. Many older agents, such as TCAs and phenothiazines, affected BP and cardiac conduction. Thioridazine (Mellaril), which has been in use for decades, has been shown to prolong the QTc interval in a dose-related manner and may increase the risk of sudden death by delaying ventricular repolarization and causing torsades de pointes. Newer drugs are now routinely scrutinized for evidence of cardiac effects. A promising treatment for psychosis, sertindole (Serlect), was not marketed because the FDA would have required a black box warning. Slight QTc effects noted with ziprasidone (Geodon) delayed the marketing of that drug. Clozapine can cause myocarditis in rare cases.

Rash. Any medication is a potential source of a drug rash. Some psychotropics, such as carbamazepine (Equetro, Tegretol) and lamotrigine, have been linked to an increased risk of severe exfoliative dermatitis. Commonly referred to as Stevens–Johnson syndrome, this condition is a systemic, immune-mediated reaction that can prove fatal or result in permanent scarring or blindness. All patients should be informed about the potential seriousness of widespread lesions that occur above the neck, that involve the mucous membranes, and that may be associated with fever and lymphadenopathy. If such symptoms manifest, a patient should be instructed at the time that the medication is prescribed to go immediately to an emergency department.

Idiosyncratic and Paradoxical Drug Responses

Idiosyncratic reactions occur in a tiny percentage of patients taking a drug. The reactions are not related to the known pharmacologic properties, and most likely represent a genetically based abnormal sensitivity to a drug. A paradoxical response represents the manifestation of a clinical effect the opposite of what is expected. In March 2007, the FDA reported dissociative-like states associated with certain sedative-hypnotics. These included behaviors such as sleepwalking, binge eating, aggressive outbursts, and night driving, of which the patient was unaware. Table 21-7 lists the drugs required to have warning labels for that effect.

Therapeutic Index

The therapeutic index is a relative measure of the toxicity or safety of a drug and is defined as the ratio of the median toxic dose to the median effective dose. The median toxic dose is the dose at which 50 percent of patients experience a specific toxic effect, and the median effective dose is the dose at which 50 percent of patients have a specified therapeutic effect. When the therapeutic index is high, as it is for haloperidol, it is reflected by the wide range of dosages in which that drug is prescribed. Conversely, the therapeutic index for lithium is relatively low, thus requiring careful monitoring of serum lithium levels in patients for whom the drug is prescribed.

Overdose

Safety in overdose is always a consideration in drug selection. Almost all of the newer agents, however, have a wide margin of safety when taken in overdose. By contrast, a 1-month supply of TCAs could be fatal. The depressed patients they were used to treat are the group most at risk of attempting suicide. Because even the safest drugs can sometimes produce severe medical complications, especially when combined with other agents, clinicians must recognize that the prescribed medication can be used in an

**Table 21-7
Sedative-Hypnotics Cited by the U.S. Food and Drug Administration**

Drug	Manufacturer
Zolpidem (Ambien/Ambien CR)	Sanofi Aventis
Butabarbital (Butisol Sodium)	MedPointe Pharmaceuticals
Pentobarbital and carbromal (Carbrital)	Parke-Davis
Flurazepam (Dalmane)	Valeant Pharmaceuticals
Quazepam (Doral)	Questcor Pharmaceuticals
Triazolam (Halcion)	Pfizer
Eszopiclone (Lunesta)	Sepracor
Ethchlorvynol (Placidyl)	Abbott
Estazolam (Prosom)	Abbott
Temazepam (Restoril)	Tyco Healthcare
Ramelteon (Rozerem)	Takeda
Secobarbital (Seconal)	Lilly
Zaleplon (Sonata)	King Pharmaceuticals

attempt to commit suicide. Although it is prudent to write nonre-fillable prescriptions for small quantities, this practice passes along increased copay costs to the patient. Many pharmacy benefit management programs encourage the prescribing of a 3-month supply of medication.

In cases in which suicide is a significant concern, an attempt should be made to verify that the medication is not being hoarded for a later overdose attempt. Random pill counts or asking a family member to dispense daily doses may be helpful. Some patients attempt suicide just as they are beginning to recover. Large quantities of medications with a low therapeutic index should be prescribed judiciously. Another reason to limit the number of pills prescribed is the possibility of accidental ingestion of medications by children in the household. Psychotherapeutic medications should be kept in a safe place.

Physicians who work in emergency departments should know which drugs can be hemodialyzed. The issues involved are complex and are not based on any single chemical property of the drug. For example, it is generally presumed that drugs with low protein binding are good candidates for dialysis. Venlafaxine, however, is only 27 percent protein-bound and is too large as a molecule dialyzed. Hemodialysis is useful for treating overdose of lithium and valproic acid.

Pharmacokinetics

Pharmacokinetic drug interactions are the effects of drugs on the plasma concentrations of each other, and *pharmacodynamic drug interactions* are the effects of drugs on the biologic activities of each other. Pharmacokinetic concepts are used to describe and predict the time course of drug concentrations in different parts of the body, such as plasma, adipose tissue, and the CNS. From a clinical perspective, pharmacokinetic methods help explain or predict the onset and duration of drug activity and interactions between drugs that alter their metabolism or excretion.

Pharmacogenetic research focuses on finding variant alleles that alter drug pharmacokinetics and pharmacodynamics. Researchers are attempting to identify genetic differences in how enzymes metabolize psychotropics, as well as CNS proteins directly involved in drug action. Likely, identification of patient genotypes will facilitate the prediction of clinical response to different types of drugs.

Most clinicians need to consult charts or computer programs to determine when potential interactions may occur and, if so, how clinically relevant they may be. Whenever possible, it is preferable to use a medication that produces the minimal risk of drug interactions. Also, it is recommended that prescribers know the interaction profiles of the drugs they most commonly prescribe.

Examples of pharmacokinetic interactions include one drug increasing or decreasing the concentrations of a coadministered compound. These types of interactions can also lead to altered concentrations of metabolites. In some cases, there may also be interference with the conversion of a drug to its active metabolite. Enormous variability exists among patients concerning pharmacokinetic parameters, such as drug absorption and metabolism. Another type of interaction is represented by interactions involving the kidney. Commonly used medications, such as angiotensin-converting enzyme inhibitors (ACEIs), nonsteroidal anti-inflammatory drugs (NSAIDs), and thiazides, decrease the renal clearance of lithium, increasing the likelihood of severe elevations of lithium. Drug interactions can occur pharmacokinetically or pharmacodynamically.

Pharmacogenetics is being used to study why patients differ in the way they metabolize drugs. In patients who are ultrarapid or extensive metabolizers, the concentrations of a drug may be lower than expected.

PATIENT-RELATED FACTORS

Response to medication and sensitivity to side effects are influenced by factors related to the patient. This response is why there is no one-size-fits-all approach to pharmacologic treatment. Patient-related variables include diagnosis, genetic factors, lifestyle, overall medical status, concurrent disorders, and history of drug response. A patient's attitude toward medication in general, aversion to certain types of side effects, and preference for a specific agent also need to be considered.

Diagnosis

Failure to correctly diagnose a disorder diminishes the likelihood of optimal drug selection. Misdiagnosis not only can result in a missed opportunity, but it also can, at times, produce worsening of symptoms. Inadvertently diagnosing a patient in the depressed phase of bipolar disorder as having unipolar depression can induce mania or rapid cycling. Treatment failure or exacerbation of symptoms should prompt a reassessment of the working diagnosis.

Past Treatment Response

A specific drug should be selected according to the patient's history of drug response (compliance, therapeutic response, adverse effects), the patient's family history of drug response, the profile of adverse effects for that drug concerning the particular patient, and the prescribing clinician's usual practice. If a drug has previously been effective in treating a patient or a family member, the same drug should be used again. For reasons that are not understood, however, some patients fail to respond to a previously effective agent when it is resumed. A history of severe adverse effects from a specific drug is a strong indicator that the patient would not be compliant with that particular drug.

It is helpful if patients can recall the details of past psychotropic drug treatment: the drugs prescribed, in what dosages, for how long, and in what combinations. Because of their psychiatric disorders, many patients, however, are poor historians. If possible, patients' medical records should be obtained to confirm their reports. Family members are a good source of collateral information.

Response in Family Members

It is widely held that drug responses cluster in families. Response to a drug in a relative may predict a patient's response. Although no conclusive evidence supports this as a consideration in drug selection, existing studies do confirm that a history of positive response to treatment with a drug should be considered in making treatment decisions. Of course, certain drugs may not have been available to a family member depending on the era in which they were treated.

Concurrent Medical or Psychiatric Disorders

The initial assessment should elicit information about coexisting medical disorders. In some cases, a medical disorder may be responsible for the symptoms. Patients with thyroid disease who are not adequately treated may appear depressed. Sleep apnea produces depression and cognitive impairment. Rare conditions, such as Kleine–Levin syndrome, can mimic bipolar disorder. A drug should be selected that minimally exacerbates any preexisting medical problems that a particular patient may have.

Recreational drug use, excessive consumption of alcohol, and frequent ingestion of caffeine-containing beverages can complicate and even undermine psychotropic drug treatment. These compounds possess significant psychoactive properties and, in some cases, may represent the source of the patient's symptoms. It is reasonable to ask patients to abstain from the use of these substances, at least until the benefits of psychotropic drug treatment have been unequivocally established. Gradual reintroduction of moderate amounts of alcohol, tea, and coffee can then take place. Patients can then observe for themselves whether there are any untoward effects on their clinical status.

INFORMED CONSENT AND PATIENT EDUCATION

Establishing trust and motivating the patient to comply with the medication regimen are essential components of successful treatment. Patients should be informed about treatment options and the probable side effects and unique benefits of each treatment. Patient preference should be respected unless a compelling advantage exists involving efficacy, tolerability, or safety with an alternative agent. If a particular medication is being recommended, the reasons for this recommendation should be explained. Patients are more likely to continue taking their medication if they fully understand the reasons why it is being prescribed.

A strong therapeutic alliance between a clinician and a patient is always helpful. Given the unpredictability of medication response, the frequent occurrence of side effects, and underlying ambivalence about, or fear of taking, medication, a constructive, trusting relationship serves to improve patient compliance. Repeated failed trials may be needed before a response is seen. A patient's confidence in the physician's knowledge and judgment enables medication trials and more complex regimens, such as the use of multiple medications.

Discussions about drug selection should be documented in notes, but a signed informed consent is not needed. Surprisingly, patients who are informed of potential adverse effects report a higher incidence of side effects but do not have higher rates of premature discontinuation.

How the patient and family are engaged in the treatment plan can determine the success of treatment. The psychodynamic meaning of pharmacotherapy to the patient and family and environmental influences, psychosocial stressors, and support should be explored. Some patients may view drug treatment as a panacea, and others may view it as the enemy. With the patient's consent, relatives and other clinicians should be instructed about the reasons for the drug treatment, as well as the expected benefits and potential risks.

DOSING, DURATION, AND MONITORING

Dosing

The clinically effective dose for treatment depends on the characteristics of the drug and patient factors, such as inherited sensitivity and ability to metabolize a drug, concurrent medical disorders, use of concurrent medications, and history of exposure to previous medications.

Plasma concentrations of many psychotropics can vary up to 10-fold. Thus, to some extent, the optimal dose for an individual is ultimately determined by trial and error, guided by the empirical evidence of the usual dose range for that drug. In some cases, it may prove helpful to test patients for genetic polymorphisms involving hepatic enzymes. Patients who are ultrarapid metabolizers of certain drugs may require higher than standard dosing. Slow metabolizers might demonstrate side effects and even toxicity at very low doses.

Some drugs demonstrate a clear relationship between increases in the dose and clinical response. This dose–response curve plots the drug concentration against the effects of the drug.

The *potency* of a drug refers to the relative dose required to achieve specific effects, not to its efficacy. Haloperidol, for example, is more potent than chlorpromazine (Thorazine) because approximately 5 mg of haloperidol is required to achieve the same therapeutic effect as 100 mg of chlorpromazine. These drugs, however, are equal in their clinical efficacy—that is, the maximal clinical response achievable by the administration of a drug.

Drugs must be used in effective dosages for sufficient periods. Although drug tolerability and safety are always considerations, subtherapeutic doses and incomplete therapeutic trials should be avoided. The use of inadequate doses merely exposes the patient to the risk of side effects without providing the probability of therapeutic benefit. Because of the wide margin of safety associated with most currently prescribed medications, more risk exists in underdosing than in overshooting the recommended dose range.

The time of dosing is usually based on the plasma half-life of a drug and its side effect profile. Sedating drugs are given all at night or with disproportionate daily doses at night. The opposite is true with activating drugs. The frequency of dosing is not as straightforward as with sedating drugs. Most dosing regimens of psychotropic drugs, such as once-a-day versus divided doses, are based on measurements of plasma concentrations rather than receptor occupancy in the brain. Evidence suggests a significant dissociation exists between the brain and plasma kinetics. Reliance on plasma kinetics as the basis for dosing regimens leads to a misunderstanding of necessary schedules.

As a rule, psychotropic drugs should be used continuously. There are some possible exceptions, such as when treating insomnia, agitation, or situational anxiety. A common mistake is the use of high-potency benzodiazepines, such as alprazolam (Xanax) and clonazepam (Klonopin), only after an attack has begun. These drugs should be used as part of a regular schedule to prevent attacks.

Some patients who experience sexual dysfunction while being treated with SSRIs take a drug holiday; that is, they skip a daily dose from time to time to facilitate sexual performance.

Intermittent dosing regimens of SSRIs are effective as a treatment for premenstrual dysphoric disorder (PMDD). The drugs are taken daily during the 2-week luteal phase of the menstrual cycle.

Duration of Treatment

A common question from a patient is, "How long do I need to take the medication?" The answer depends on multiple variables. These include the specific disorder, the symptom duration, and family history. We should also consider the patient's tolerance of and benefit from the medication. Patients can be given a reasonable explanation of the probabilities but should be told that it is first best to see if the medication works for them and whether any side effects are acceptable. Any more definitive discussion of treatment duration can be held once we can assess the degree of success. Even patients with a philosophical aversion to the use of psychotropic drugs may elect to stay on the medication indefinitely if the magnitude of improvement is excellent. Most psychiatric disorders have high rates of chronicity and relapse. Because of this, long-term treatment is often needed to prevent a recurrence. Nevertheless, the fact remains that psychotropic drugs are not said to cure the disorders they treat but rather to help control the symptoms.

Treatment is conceptually broken down into three phases: the initial therapeutic trial, the continuation, and the maintenance phase. The initial period of treatment should last at least several weeks because of the delay in therapeutic effects that characterize most classes of psychotropic drugs. The required duration of a *therapeutic trial* of a drug should be discussed at the outset of treatment so that the patient does not have unrealistic expectations of an immediate improvement in symptoms. Patients are more likely to experience side effects early in the course of pharmacotherapy than any relief from their disorder. In some cases, medication may even exacerbate some symptoms. Patients should be counseled that a meager initial reaction to medication is not an indicator of the outcome of treatment. For instance, many patients with panic disorder develop jitteriness or an increase in panic attacks after starting on tricyclic or SSRI treatment. Benzodiazepine agonists are an exception to the rule that clinical onset is delayed. In most cases, their hypnotic and antianxiety effects are evident immediately.

Ongoing use of medication, however, does not provide absolute protection against relapse. Continuation therapy provides clinically and statistically significant protective effects against relapse. The optimal duration of continuation or maintenance therapy is variable and dependent on the clinical history of the patient. Early-onset chronic major depression, for example, has a more severe course and more significant comorbidity than late-onset chronic major depression. In addition to early-onset, a history of multiple past episodes and the severity and length of a current episode would suggest that longer, even indefinite, treatment is appropriate.

Frequency of Visits

Until an unequivocal response to treatment occurs, patients should be seen as frequently as circumstances warrant. The frequency of follow-up or monitoring visits is determined by clinical judgment. In severely ill patients, this might mean several times a week. Patients on maintenance therapy, even when stable, need monitoring, but no consensus exists on the frequency of follow-up therapy. Three months is a reasonable interval between visits, but 6 months may be adequate after long-standing treatment.

LABORATORY TESTS AND THERAPEUTIC BLOOD MONITORING

Laboratory testing and therapeutic blood monitoring should be based on clinical circumstances and the drugs being used. For most commonly used psychotropic drugs, routine testing is not required.

Pretreatment tests are routine as part of a workup to establish baseline values and to rule out underlying medical problems that may be causing the psychiatric symptoms or that might complicate treatment with drugs. Results of recently performed tests should be obtained. With agents known to cause cardiac conduction changes, a pretreatment electrocardiogram (ECG) should be obtained before initiating treatment. With lithium and clozapine, the possibility of severe changes in thyroid, renal, hepatic, or hematologic functions requires pretreatment and ongoing monitoring with appropriate laboratory tests.

As a result of both anecdotal and research findings of sometimes severe glucose dysregulation during treatment primarily

with SDAs, the FDA has suggested that patients being treated with any atypical antipsychotic be monitored for the emergence of diabetes.

Certain circumstances present in which it is necessary or useful to use plasma concentrations to monitor a patient's condition. The most common is the monitoring of drugs with narrow therapeutic indexes, such as lithium. Also, we may monitor drugs with a therapeutic window, which is the optimal dose range for a therapeutic response; drug combinations that can lead to interactions that raise drug concentrations of medications or their metabolites, which can cause toxicity; unexplained toxicity at average therapeutic doses; and failure to respond in a patient who may be noncompliant. A clinician should have no reservations about requesting random urine toxicologic tests in a patient who abuses substances.

TREATMENT OUTCOMES

The goal of psychotropic treatment is to eliminate all manifestations of a disorder, thus enabling the patient to regain the ability to function as well and to enjoy life as fully as before they became ill. This degree of improvement to below the syndromal threshold is defined as *remission.*

Response and Remission

Remission is the preferred outcome of treatment, not only because of the immediate impact on functioning and state of mind but also because emerging evidence suggests that patients in remission are less likely to experience relapse and recurrence of their disorder.

Patients who improve but do not experience a full resolution are considered to be responders. They may exhibit significant improvement but continue to experience symptoms. In depression studies, the *response* is usually defined as a 50 percent or more significant decrease from baseline on a standard rating scale, such as the Hamilton Depression (HAM-D) Scale or the Montgomery-Asberg Depression Rating Scale (MADRS). The scales define r*emission* as an absolute score of 7 or less on the HAM-D or 10 or less on the MADRS.

Our expectations around improvement derive from what we know about the disorder and its response to treatment. Obsessive-compulsive disorder (OCD) and schizophrenia, for example, are more likely to be associated with residual manifestations of illness than major depression or panic disorder. The probability of full remission from OCD with SSRI treatment alone over 2 years is less than 12 percent, and the probability of partial remission is approximately 47 percent.

Treatment Failure

The initial treatment plan should anticipate that the medication may be ineffective. A next-step strategy should be in place at the initiation of treatment. Repeated drug failures should prompt a reassessment of the patient. First, was the original diagnosis correct? In answering this question, the clinician should include the possibility of an undiagnosed medical condition or recreational drug use as the cause of the psychiatric symptoms.

Second, are the observed symptoms related to the original disorder, or are they adverse effects of the drug treatment? Some antipsychotic drugs, for example, can produce akinesia, which resembles psychotic withdrawal, or akathisia and neuroleptic malignant syndrome, which resemble increased psychotic agitation. Long-term use of SSRIs can produce emotional blunting, which can mimic depression. Intolerance of side effects may be the most common reason for treatment failure.

Third, was the drug administered at an appropriate dosage for a sufficient length of time? Because absorption and metabolism of drugs can vary significantly in patients, the clinician may need to measure plasma levels of a drug to ensure a sufficient dose of the drug.

Fourth, did a pharmacokinetic or pharmacodynamic interaction with another drug that the patient was taking reduce the efficacy of the newly prescribed drug?

Fifth, did the patient take the drug as directed? Drug noncompliance is a common clinical problem that arises as a result of complicated drug regimens (more than one drug in more than one daily dosage), adverse effects (mainly if unnoticed by the clinician), and poor patient education about the drug treatment plan. Patients may discontinue medication when they recover, thinking that they are cured and no longer benefiting from the medication.

Treatment Resistance

Some patients fail to respond to repeated trials of medication. No single factor can explain the ineffectiveness of the various interventions in these cases. Strategies in these cases include the use of drug combinations, high-dose therapy, and the use of unconventional drugs. Limited evidence is available on the comparative success rates associated with any given strategy.

Tolerance

The development of tolerance is marked by a need, over time, to use increased doses of a drug for it to maintain a clinical effect. This decreased responsiveness to a drug occurs after repeated doses. Tolerance also describes decreased sensitivity to adverse effects of the drug, such as nausea. This phenomenon is used as the basis for starting some drugs at subtherapeutic doses, with the plan to adjust the schedule once the patient can tolerate higher doses. Clinical tolerance appears to represent changes in the CNS, such as altered receptor configuration or density. Drugs with similar pharmacologic actions often exhibit cross-tolerance.

Sensitization

Clinically manifested as the reverse of tolerance, sensitization is said to occur when sensitivity to a drug effect increases over time. In these cases, the same dose typically produces more pronounced effects as treatment progresses.

Withdrawal

The development of physiologic adaptation to a drug, with a subsequent risk of withdrawal symptoms, has been reported for many classes of psychotropic drugs. Technically, withdrawal should be considered a side effect. The probability and severity of these reactions are remote with most drugs and more frequent with others. As a general rule, the more abruptly a drug is stopped and the shorter its elimination half-life, the more likely it is that clinically significant withdrawal symptoms will occur. When using some short-acting drugs, withdrawal reactions can result from missed doses and during daily intervals between doses. Gradual tapering of medications after prolonged use is recommended whenever possible. Although this reduces the risk of withdrawal reactions, it does not ensure they will not occur. The so-called sedative-hypnotics

and opiates are the agents most often associated with mentally and physically distressing discontinuation reactions. In some cases, such as barbiturate use, withdrawal can be fatal.

Marked differences are found among agents, even within a given class, concerning the probability and severity of discontinuation effects. For example, the benzodiazepines alprazolam and triazolam (Halcion) commonly produce more immediate and intense withdrawal symptoms than other compounds. Among the SSRIs, there is a well-described withdrawal syndrome that appears to be more frequent and severe with paroxetine (Paxil). It can, however, occur with any SSRI. Even fluoxetine can be associated with discontinuation symptoms, but the symptoms may be delayed and attenuated because of the long elimination half-life of its active metabolite. These manifestations are subtle and are delayed for weeks after the last dose. Venlafaxine also produces severe SSRI-like withdrawal syndrome.

In addition to half-life, many variables can influence the likelihood and degree of discontinuation symptoms. Changes in the rate of drug metabolism, as an example, can play a role. Paroxetine is primarily metabolized by the cytochrome P450 (CYP) 2D6 isoenzyme. However, it is also a potent inhibitor of CYP 2D6. This results in *autoinhibition,* dose-dependent inhibition of its metabolism, with a subsequent increase in plasma concentrations of paroxetine. If the dose of paroxetine is decreased or the drug is stopped, the decline in its plasma concentrations can be steep, causing withdrawal to occur. Withdrawal can occur in rare cases in which the dose of a drug is not decreased, but a second agent, which had been inhibiting its metabolism, was stopped. For example, alprazolam is metabolized via the CYP 3A3/4 enzyme system. Nefazodone inhibits that enzyme. If a patient taking both agents for several weeks discontinues the nefazodone, it could result in a rapid increase in the rate of alprazolam metabolism and a consequent drop in plasma concentrations.

The development of sustained-release versions of drugs, such as alprazolam, paroxetine, and venlafaxine, has not reduced the severity of their withdrawal reactions. The prolonged half-life of those agents results from delayed absorption rather than prolongation of the elimination phase. The frequency of drug dosing is reduced but not the rate of the falloff in plasma concentrations.

Low bioavailability with a generic agent may account for the unexpected loss of clinical effect in the emergence of withdrawal symptoms. The occurrence of these events soon after refilling a prescription should prompt examination of the new medication. It should be confirmed whether the dispensed medication and dose are both correct. It is difficult to ascertain whether generic medications are genuinely equivalent, so the possibility exists that differences in potency may underlie adverse changes in clinical status.

Withdrawal symptoms invariably occur hours or days after dose reduction or discontinuation. Symptoms resolve within a few weeks, so the persistence of symptoms argues against withdrawal. Although depletion studies have been shown to provoke the rapid return of symptoms, in clinical practice, psychotic and mood symptoms do not usually reappear abruptly after long-term treatment.

COMBINATION OF DRUGS

According to the American Psychiatric Association Practice Guidelines for the Treatment of Psychiatric Disorders, "the use of multiple agents should be avoided if possible" in the treatment of psychiatric disorders. Although *monotherapy* represents the ideal, *polypharmacy,* the simultaneous use of psychotropic medications,

Table 21-8
Selected Combination Drugs Used in Psychiatry

Ingredients	Preparation	Amount of Each	Recommended Dosage	Indications
Perphenazine and amitriptyline	—	Tablet: 2:25, 4:25, 4:50, 2:10, 4:10	Initial therapy: tablet of 2:25 or 4:25 qid Maintenance therapy: tablet 2:25 or 4:25 bid or qid.	Depression and associated anxiety
Dextroamphetamine and amphetamine	Adderall	Tablet: 5, 7.5, 10.0, 12.5, 15.0, 20.0, 30.0 mg	3–5 yr: 2.5 mg/day; 6 yr and older: 5 mg/day	Attention-deficit/hyperactivity disorder
	Adderall XR	Capsule: 5, 10, 15, 20, 25, 30 mg	—	—
Chlordiazepoxide and clidinium bromide	—	Capsule: 5:25	One or two capsules tid or qid before meals and at bedtime	Peptic ulcer, gastritis, duodenitis, irritable bowel syndrome, spastic colitis, and mild ulcerative colitis
Chlordiazepoxide and amitriptyline	—	Tablet: 5.0:12.5, 10:25	Tablet of 5:12.5 tid or qid; tablet of 10:25 tid or qid, initially, then may increase to six tablets daily as required	Depression and associated anxiety
Olanzapine and fluoxetine	Symbyax	Capsule: 6:25, 6:50, 12:25, 12:50	Once daily in the evening in a dose range of olanzapine 6–12 mg and fluoxetine 25–50 mg	Depressive episodes associated with bipolar I disorder

qid, four times daily; bid, twice daily; tid, three times daily.

has been commonplace since chlorpromazine was combined with reserpine (Diupres) in the early 1950s. The practice of combining drugs and the merits of various *augmentation* or *combination* strategies are routinely discussed in the literature and at scientific meetings. The mean number of simultaneously prescribed medications has increased in recent decades. Among psychiatric inpatients, the mean number of psychotropics prescribed is approximately three. Fixed combinations—drugs that contain more than one active ingredient—have been successfully marketed in the past, and research on new combinations is ongoing. A fluoxetine-olanzapine fixed combination has been approved as a treatment for bipolar disorder. The use of such drugs may increase the patients' compliance by simplifying the drug regimen. A problem with combination drugs, however, is that the clinician has less flexibility in adjusting the dosage of one of the components; that is, the use of combination drugs can cause two drugs to be administered when only one drug continues to be necessary for therapeutic efficacy (Table 21-8).

Sometimes distinctions are made between augmentation and combination therapy. When two psychotropics with the same approved indications are used concurrently, this is termed *combination therapy*. Adding a drug with another indication is termed *augmentation*. Augmentation often entails the use of a drug that is not primarily considered a psychotropic. For example, in treating depression, it is not common to add thyroid hormone to an approved antidepressant.

Almost all patients with bipolar disorder are taking more than one psychotropic agent. Combination treatment with drugs that treat depression and DRA or SDA has long been held as preferable in patients with psychotic depression. Similarly, SSRIs typically produce partial improvement in patients with OCD, so the addition of an SDA may be helpful.

Medications also can be combined to counteract side effects, to treat specific symptoms, and as a temporary measure to transition from one drug to another. It is common practice to add a new medication without the discontinuation of a prior drug, mainly when the first drug has provided partial benefit. This addition can be part of a plan to transition from an agent that is not producing a satisfactory response or an attempt to maintain the patient on combined therapy.

The advantages of combining drugs include building on the existing response, which may be less demoralizing, and the possibility that combinations produce new mechanisms that no single agent can provide. One limitation is that noncompliance and adverse effects increase, and the clinician may not be able to determine whether it was the second drug alone or the combination of drugs that resulted in a therapeutic success or a particular adverse effect. Combining drugs can create a broad spectrum effect and also changes the ratio of metabolites.

COMBINED PSYCHOTHERAPY AND PHARMACOTHERAPY

Many psychiatrists believe that patients are best treated with a combination of medication and psychotherapy. Studies have demonstrated that the results of combined therapy are superior to those of either type of therapy alone. When pharmacotherapy and psychotherapy are used together, the approach should be coordinated, integrated, and synergistic. If two separate clinicians direct psychotherapy and pharmacotherapy, the clinicians must communicate with each other clearly and often.

SPECIAL POPULATIONS

Although every patient brings a unique combination of demographic and clinical variables to the clinical setting, specific patient populations require special consideration. When treating the young, the elderly, those with medical disorders, and women who want to conceive or are pregnant or nursing, awareness of risks associated with medication assumes increased importance. Data derived from clinical trials are of limited value in guiding many decisions because populations in these studies consisted of healthy young adults and, until recently, excluded many women of child-bearing age. Studies of children and adolescents have become more common, so understanding of treatment effects in this population has grown.

Children

Understanding of the safety and efficacy of most psychotropic drugs, when used to treat children, is based more on clinical experience than on evidence from extensive clinical trial data. Often, so results from adult studies are extrapolated to children. This extrapolation is not necessarily appropriate because of developmental differences in pharmacokinetics and pharmacodynamics. Dosing is another special consideration in drug use with children. Although the small volume of distribution suggests the use of lower doses than those used in adults, a child's higher rate of metabolism suggests that a higher ratio of milligrams of a drug to kilograms of body weight should be used. In practice, beginning with a small dose is best, then increasing it until clinical effects are observed. The clinician should not hesitate, however, to use adult dosages in children if these dosages are effective and the adverse effects are acceptable.

The paucity of research data is a legacy of many years in which manufacturers avoided conducting trials in children because of liability concerns, small market share, and, hence, limited profit potential represented by this population. To correct this problem, the FDA Modernization Act (FDAMA) of 1997 provided for special encouragement and incentives to study drugs for pediatric use.

Pregnant and Nursing Women

No definitive assurances exist that any drug is entirely without risk during pregnancy and lactation. No psychotropic medication is absolutely contraindicated during pregnancy, although drugs with known risks of congenital disabilities, premature birth, or neonatal complications should be avoided if acceptable alternatives are available.

Women who are pregnant or lactating are excluded from clinical trials, and it is only recently that women of child-bearing age have been able to participate in these studies. As a result, there are large gaps in knowledge of the effects of psychotropic agents on the developing fetus and the neonate. Most of what is known are the result of anecdotal reports or data from registries. The basic rule is to avoid administering any drug to a woman who is pregnant (particularly during the first trimester) or who is breastfeeding a child unless the mother's psychiatric disorder is severe, and the therapeutic value of the drug outweighs the theoretical adverse effects on the fetus or newborn. A woman may elect to continue on medication because she does not want to chance a possible recurrence of painful or disabling symptoms.

Among the newer antidepressants, paroxetine is the only one to carry a warning from the FDA, the result of an increased risk of cardiac malformation. The agents with the most well-documented risk of specific congenital disabilities are lithium, carbamazepine, and valproate. Lithium administration during pregnancy is associated with Ebstein anomaly, a severe abnormality of cardiac development, although recent evidence suggests that the risk is not as significant as previously believed. Carbamazepine and valproic acid are associated with neural tube defects, which can be prevented by the use of folate during pregnancy. Lamotrigine may cause oral clefts when used during the first trimester. Some experts advise that

all women of child-bearing age who are treated with psychotropics take supplemental folate.

The administration of psychotherapeutic drugs at or near delivery can cause the baby to be overly sedated at delivery and require a respirator. They may also be physically dependent on the drug, requiring detoxification and the treatment of a withdrawal syndrome. Reports exist of a neonatal withdrawal syndrome associated with third-trimester use of SSRIs in pregnant women. They have also been implicated in producing pulmonary hypertension in newborns.

Virtually all psychiatric drugs are secreted in the milk of a nursing mother; therefore, mothers on those agents should be advised not to breastfeed their infants.

Elderly Patients

The two major concerns when treating geriatric patients with psychotherapeutic drugs are that elderly persons may be more susceptible to adverse effects (particularly cardiac effects) and may metabolize and excrete drugs more slowly, thus requiring lower dosages of medication. In practice, clinicians should begin treating geriatric patients with a small dose, usually approximately half of the usual starting dose. The dose should be raised in small increments, more slowly than for middle-aged adults, until a clinical benefit is achieved or unacceptable adverse effects appear. Although many geriatric patients require a small dose of medication, many others require a full therapeutic dose.

Elderly patients account for approximately one-third of all prescription drug use and a substantial percentage of over-the-counter preparations as well. Even more significant is the incidence of polypharmacy. Recent surveys have found that elderly patients in the community are taking between three and five medications, and that hospitalized elderly patients are treated with an average of ten drugs. Nearly half of all patients in long-term care facilities are prescribed one or more psychotropic agents. Because of these statistics, clinicians need to consider potential types and likelihood of drug interactions when selecting medications.

Psychotropic drugs are causally related to falls in the elderly. Discontinuation of psychotropic drugs results in an estimated 40 percent risk reduction for falls. This association between psychotropics and falls and hip fractures may weaken as newer agents become widely used. As a rule, new-generation compounds produce less unwanted sedation, dizziness, parkinsonism, and postural hypotension.

Age-related changes in renal clearance and hepatic metabolism make it more important to be conservative with the starting doses of medication as well as the rate of dose titration. Within any class of psychotropic agents, those with potentially serious consequences, such as hypotension, cardiac conduction abnormalities, anticholinergic activity, and respiratory depression, are not suitable choices. Drugs that cause cognitive impairment, such as benzodiazepines and anticholinergics, can mimic or exacerbate symptoms of dementia. Similarly, DRAs can worsen or induce Parkinson disease, another age-related disorder. Some side effects, such as SSRI-associated syndrome of inappropriate secretion of antidiuretic hormone (SIADH) and oxcarbazepine-associated hyponatremia, occur more commonly in older patients.

A common ethical dilemma with the medically ill elderly or those with dementia is the question of their capacity to give informed consent before treatment with psychotropic drugs or ECT.

Medically Ill Patients

There are special considerations, diagnostic and therapeutic, when administering psychiatric drugs to medically ill patients. The medical disorder should be ruled out as a cause of psychiatric symptoms. For example, patients with neurologic or endocrine disorders or those infected with human immunodeficiency virus (HIV) may experience disturbances of mood and cognition. Common medications, such as corticosteroids and L-dopa, are associated with the induction of mania.

A patient with diabetes mellitus is better treated with an agent without the risk of weight gain or glucose dysregulation. Depending on the diagnosis, drugs that might treat the primary psychiatric disorder and also cause weight loss, drugs such as bupropion, topiramate, and zonisamide, should be prescribed for these patients. Patients with obstructive pulmonary disease should not be given sedating drugs, which raise the arousal threshold and suppress respiration. Patients with medical disorders are also taking other medications, which can result in pharmacodynamic and pharmacokinetic interactions. Combined treatment with an inducer of multiple CYP enzymes and a drug that is a substrate for those enzymes could result in subtherapeutic levels, leading to inadequate symptom control. The use of the tuberculosis treatment rifampicin (Rifadin) with carbamazepine is an example of this. The use of drugs that inhibit CYP 2D6, agents such as paroxetine and fluoxetine, can prevent the conversion of hydrocodone (Robidone) and other opiates into an active analgesic form. NSAIDs are also a rare cause of perceptual disturbances and psychotic symptoms.

Other issues include a potentially increased sensitivity to adverse effects, including increased or decreased metabolism and excretion of the drug, and interactions with other medications. Drug interactions are an obvious concern when drugs with a narrow therapeutic range are being used. Any change in the rate of metabolism or interference with the formation and elimination of metabolites can profoundly influence the activity of that drug. Similarly, interactions that interfere with drug metabolism can produce an increase in side effects and toxicity.

As with children and geriatric patients, the most reasonable clinical practice is to begin with a small dosage, to increase it slowly, and to watch for clinical benefit and adverse effects. Determining the plasma drug concentrations may be helpful for such patients, but therapeutic blood concentrations for most psychotropic drugs are neither necessary nor routinely available.

Substance Abuse

Many patients who seek or need treatment for a psychiatric disorder chronically use illicit substances or drink excessive amounts of alcohol. Discontinuation of chronic drug or alcohol use can result not only in craving but also in clinically significant psychiatric and physiologic withdrawal symptoms. For many patients, successful treatment of their underlying psychiatric disorder may not be possible in the presence of ongoing marijuana, cocaine, and alcohol use. If several trials of medications fail, hospitalization for detoxification may be necessary. Little research and no consensus exist about how to use psychotropic agents in patients who are regular users of cocaine, marijuana, or other recreational drugs.

REGULATORY ISSUES

The FDA has the authority to approve a drug for clinical use and to ensure that product labeling is truthful and contains all information pertinent to the safe and effective use of that drug.

Product information that is FDA approved for marketed drugs appears as a package insert that lists potential side effects, drug interactions, the need for special monitoring, and restrictions for use. In some cases, these adverse reactions and potential safety hazards warrant a warning label called a *black box label*. The FDA typically negotiates final labeling language with the company; however, in cases where a company refuses to satisfy the FDA, the agency may initiate proceedings to remove the drug from clinical use. In recent years, warning labels have been applied to entire classes of psychotropic drugs, including the SDAs and antidepressants such as the SSRIs.

The product information may also contain a "Contraindications" heading. This section describes instances in which the drug should not be used because the risk of using it outweighs the benefit. If no contraindications are known, this section of the labeling will state "None known."

A Precautions section may contain precautions for most individuals taking the drug, as well as for specific groups, such as pregnant women, nursing mothers, or children. In this section, one will find recommendations for patients to ensure the safe and effective use of the drug. For example, there may be precautions about driving when taking the medication or using substances such as other drugs, food, or alcohol that may have harmful effects if taken while using the medication. The precautions section also provides information about laboratory tests needed to track responses or to identify adverse reactions to the drug or about known interactions with other drugs, foods, or ingredients.

Every product label has an Adverse Reaction section that lists the frequency of undesirable effects that may be associated with the use of a drug. Causes of adverse reactions can include medication errors, such as overdosage, or interactions between different drugs or between drugs and certain foods.

NONAPPROVED DOSAGES AND USES

It is now common practice to treat psychiatric disorders with drugs that are approved for nonpsychiatric conditions. Some examples include propranolol (Inderal) for social anxiety and treatment of lithium-induced tremor; verapamil (Calan, Isoptin) for mania and treatment of MAOI-induced hypertensive crisis; levothyroxine (Levoxyl) for antidepressant augmentation; clonidine (Catapres) and guanfacine (Tenex) for posttraumatic stress disorder (PTSD); dextroamphetamine (Dexedrine) for antidepressant augmentation; and riluzole (Rilutek) for self-injurious behavior. Off-label use of a drug is not a violation of law or a departure from good medical practice. The FDA does not limit how a physician may use an approved drug. Medications can be prescribed for any reason shown to be medically indicated for the welfare of the patient. Once a drug is approved for commercial use, a physician can, as part of the practice of medicine, lawfully prescribe a different dosage for a patient or may otherwise vary the conditions of use from what is approved in the package labeling without notifying the FDA or obtaining its approval.

Failure to follow the information on the drug label does not in itself impose liability and should not preclude a physician from using sound clinical judgment in the service of the patient. Physicians are permitted to use a drug for indications not included on the drug's official labeling without violating the FDA rules. This fact, however, does not absolve the physician of responsibility for an untoward result from treatment. Patients can still sue for possible medical malpractice with the reasoning that the failure to follow the FDA-approved label can be interpreted as deviating from the prevailing standard of care.

When using a drug off-label or in doses outside the usual range, we should explain to the patient the reasons for this approach. We should also document it in the chart. When doubting the plan to use a drug off label, a consultation with a colleague should be obtained.

In some cases, a drug has obtained limited approval for an indication. Divalproex (Depakote) and risperidone, for example, are approved by the FDA for the acute, but not long-term, treatment of mania. Nevertheless, these drugs are routinely used for long-term prevention of recurrences of mania and bipolar disorder. In the case of lamotrigine, it was accepted as a first-choice agent for the treatment of bipolar disorder long before the FDA approved that indication.

PLACEBOS

Pharmacologically inactive substances have long been known sometimes to produce significant clinical benefits. A patient who believes that a compound is helpful may often derive considerable benefit from taking that substance, whether it is known to be pharmacologically active or not. For many psychiatric disorders, including mild to moderate depression and some anxiety disorders, well over 30 percent of patients can exhibit significant improvement or remission of symptoms on a placebo. For other conditions, such as schizophrenia, manic episodes, and psychotic depression, the placebo response rate is meager. Whereas suggestion is undoubtedly crucial in the efficacy of placebos (and active drugs), placebos can produce biologic effects. For example, placebo-induced analgesia may sometimes be blocked by naloxone (Narcan), which suggests that endorphins may mediate the analgesia derived from taking a placebo. It is conceivable that placebos may also stimulate endogenous anxiolytic and antidepressant factors, resulting in clinical improvement in patients with depression and anxiety disorders.

Just as placebos can produce benefits, they can also have adverse effects. In many studies, some adverse effects are likely to be more frequent with placebos than with the active drug. Some patients will not tolerate placebos, although they are supposedly inert, and they exhibit adverse effects (called the *nocebo phenomenon*). It is easy to discount such patients as overly suggestible; however, if placebos can stimulate beneficial endogenous factors, perhaps toxic endogenous factors can also be produced.

Prudence is needed in contemplating the use of a placebo in clinical practice. Treating a patient with a placebo without consent can seriously undermine a patient's confidence in the physician if, and when, it is discovered.

▲ 21.1 Antipsychotics

SEROTONIN–DOPAMINE ANTAGONISTS AND SIMILARLY ACTING DRUGS (SECOND-GENERATION OR ATYPICAL ANTIPSYCHOTICS)

The SGAs, also known as second-generation or atypical antipsychotic drugs, are a group of pharmacologically diverse drugs that have largely supplanted the older DRAs. The term *atypical* is used because these drugs differ in their side effect profiles, most notably lower risk of extrapyramidal side effects (EPS), and have spectra of action that are broader than those of the DRAs. However, this term is becoming something of a misnomer, as the drugs are now more commonly used than the "typical" antipsychotics. In contrast

to the earlier antipsychotic drugs, the SGAs have significant effects on both the dopamine and serotonin systems. Their pharmacology is complex, with individual drugs in this group having multiple neurotransmitter effects. All SGAs are indicated for the treatment of schizophrenia. Most of these SGA drugs have also received approval as monotherapy or adjunctive therapy in the treatment of bipolar disorder. Some have also been approved as adjuncts for the treatment of major depression.

As of 2020, 13 SGA drugs were approved by the FDA. These include the following:

Aripiprazole (marketed as Abilify)
Asenapine Maleate (marketed as Saphris)
Brexpiprazole (marketed as Rexulti)
Cariprazine (marketed as Vraylar)
Clozapine (marketed as Clozaril)
Iloperidone (marketed as Fanapt)
Lumateperone (marketed as Caplyta)
Lurasidone (marketed as Latuda)
Olanzapine (marketed as Zyprexa, and as Symbyax in combination with fluoxetine)
Paliperidone (marketed as Invega)
Quetiapine (marketed as Seroquel)
Risperidone (marketed as Risperdal)
Ziprasidone (marketed as Geodon)

It is arguable whether the SGAs represent an improvement in overall tolerability than the DRAs. Although there is an improvement concerning a lowered, not absent, risk of EPS, most of the drugs in this group often produce substantial weight gain, which in turn increases the potential for the development of diabetes mellitus. Olanzapine and clozapine appear to account for most cases of weight gain and drug-induced diabetes mellitus. The other agents pose a smaller risk of these side effects; nevertheless, the FDA has requested that all SGAs carry a warning label that patients taking the drugs need to be monitored closely, and has recommended the following factors be considered for all patients prescribed SGAs:

1. Personal and family history of obesity, diabetes, dyslipidemia, hypertension, and cardiovascular disease
2. Weight and height (so that body mass index can be calculated)
3. Waist circumference (at the level of the umbilicus)
4. BP
5. Fasting plasma glucose level
6. Fasting lipid profile

Patients with preexisting diabetes should have regular monitoring, including hemoglobin A1C (HbA1C) and, in some cases, insulin levels. Among these drugs, clozapine sits apart. It is not considered a first-line agent because of side effects (hematologic) and the need for weekly blood tests. Although highly effective in treating both mania and depression, clozapine does not have an FDA indication for these conditions.

Mechanisms of Action

The presumed antipsychotic effects of the SDAs are blockade of D_2 dopamine receptors. Where the SDAs differ from older antipsychotic drugs is their higher ratio interactions with serotonin receptor subtypes, most notably the 5-HT_{2A} subtype, as well as with other neurotransmitter systems. It is hypothesized that these properties account for the distinct tolerability profiles associated with each of the SDAs. All SDAs have different chemical structures, receptor affinities, and side effect profiles. No SDA is identical in its combination of receptor affinities, and the relative contribution of each receptor interaction to the clinical effects is unknown.

Therapeutic Indications

Although initially approved for the treatment of schizophrenia and acute mania, some of these drugs have also been approved as adjunctive therapy in treatment-resistant depression and as adjunctive therapy in major depressive disorder (MDD). They are also useful in PTSD and anxiety disorders. Although clinicians tend to use them in behavioral disturbances associated with dementia, all SDAs carry an FDA boxed warning regarding adverse effects when used in elderly persons with dementia-related psychoses, because elderly patients with dementia-related psychoses are at an increased risk (1.6 to 1.7 times) of death compared with placebo. All of these agents are considered first-line drugs for schizophrenia except clozapine, which may cause adverse hematologic effects that require weekly blood sampling.

Schizophrenia and Schizoaffective Disorder.
The SDAs are useful for treating acute and chronic psychoses such as schizophrenia and schizoaffective disorder, in both adults and adolescents. SDAs are as good as or better than typical antipsychotics (DRAs) for the treatment of positive symptoms in schizophrenia and superior to DRAs for the treatment of negative symptoms. Compared with persons treated with DRAs, persons treated with SDAs have fewer relapses and require less frequent hospitalization, fewer emergency department visits, less phone contact with mental health professionals, and less treatment in day programs.

Because clozapine has potentially life-threatening adverse effects, it is appropriate only for patients with schizophrenia who are resistant to all other antipsychotics. Other indications for clozapine include treatment of persons with severe tardive dyskinesia—which can be reversed with high dosages in some cases—and those with a low threshold for EPS. Persons who tolerate clozapine have done well on long-term therapy. The effectiveness of clozapine may be increased by augmentation with risperidone, which raises clozapine concentrations and sometimes results in dramatic clinical improvement.

Mood Disorders.
Most of the SDAs (clozapine being a notable exception) are FDA approved for the treatment of acute mania. Some of these agents, including aripiprazole, olanzapine, quetiapine, and quetiapine XR, are also approved for the maintenance treatment in bipolar disorder as monotherapy or adjunctive therapy. The SDAs improve depressive symptoms in schizophrenia, and both clinical experience and clinical trials show that all of the SDAs augment antidepressants in the acute management of major depression. At this time, olanzapine, in combination with fluoxetine, has been approved for treatment-resistant depression, and aripiprazole and quetiapine XR are indicated for adjunctive therapy to antidepressants in MDDs. Quetiapine and quetiapine XR are also approved in bipolar depression. A fixed combination of olanzapine and fluoxetine (Symbyax) is approved as a treatment for acute bipolar depression.

Other Indications.
About 10 percent of patients with schizophrenia exhibit outwardly aggressive or violent behavior, and the SDAs are effective for the treatment of such aggression. Other off-label indications include acquired immunodeficiency syndrome (AIDS) dementia, autism spectrum disorders, Tourette disorder, Huntington disease, and Lesch–Nyhan syndrome. Risperidone and olanzapine have been used to control aggression and self-injury in children. These drugs are sometimes coadministered with stimulants to children with ADHD who are comorbid for either oppositional–defiant disorder or conduct disorder. SDAs—especially olanzapine, quetiapine, and clozapine—are useful in persons who have severe tardive dyskinesia. The SDAs are also effective for treating psychotic depression and for psychosis secondary to head trauma, dementia, or treatment drugs.

Treatment with SDAs decreases the risk of suicide and water intoxication in patients with schizophrenia. Patients with treatment-resistant OCD have responded to the SDAs; however, a few persons treated with the SDAs have been noted to develop treatment-emergent symptoms of OCD. Some patients with borderline personality disorder may improve with the SDAs.

Some data suggest that treatment with conventional DRAs has protective effects against the progression of schizophrenia when used during the first episode of psychosis. Ongoing studies are looking at whether the use of SDAs in at-risk patients with early evidence of disease prevents deterioration, thus improving long-term outcomes.

Adverse Effects

The SDAs share a similar spectrum of adverse reactions but differ considerably in terms of frequency or severity of their occurrence. Specific side effects that are more common with an individual SDA are emphasized in the discussion of each drug in subsequent text.

Risperidone (Risperdal)

Indications. Risperidone is indicated for the acute and maintenance treatment of schizophrenia in adults and the treatment of schizophrenia in adolescents ages 13 to 17 years. Risperidone is also indicated for the short-term treatment of acute manic or mixed episodes associated with bipolar I disorder in adults and children and adolescents ages 10 to 17 years. The combination of risperidone with lithium or valproate is indicated for the short-term treatment of acute manic or mixed episodes associated with bipolar I disorder.

Risperidone is also indicated for the treatment of irritability associated with an autistic spectrum disorder in children and adolescents ages 5 to 16 years, including symptoms of aggression toward others, deliberate self-injuriousness, temper tantrums, and quickly changing moods.

Pharmacology. Risperidone is a benzisoxazole. It undergoes extensive first-pass hepatic metabolism to 9-hydroxy risperidone, a metabolite with equivalent antipsychotic activity. Peak plasma levels of the parent compound occur within 1 hour for the parent compound and 3 hours for the metabolite. Risperidone has bioactivity of 70 percent. The combined half-life of risperidone and 9-hydroxy risperidone averages 20 hours, so it is useful in once-daily dosing. Risperidone is an antagonist of the serotonin 5-HT$_{2A}$, dopamine D$_2$, α_1-adrenergic and α_2-adrenergic, and histamine H$_1$ receptors. It has a low affinity for α-adrenergic and muscarinic cholinergic receptors. Risperidone is a potent antagonist of D$_2$ receptors, as potent as haloperidol, however unlike haloperidol it causes less EPS.

Dosages. The recommended dose range and frequency of risperidone dosing have changed since the drug first came into clinical use. Risperidone is available in 0.25-, 0.5-, 1-, 2-, 3-, and 4-mg tablets and a 1-mg/mL oral solution. The initial dosage is usually 1 to 2 mg at night, which can then be increased to 4 mg/day. Positron emission tomography (PET) studies have shown that dosages of 1 to 4 mg/day provide the required D_2 blockade for a therapeutic effect. At first, it was believed that because of its short elimination half-life, risperidone should be given twice a day, but studies have shown equal efficacy with once-a-day dosing. Dosages above 6 mg a day are associated with a higher incidence of adverse effects, particularly EPS. There is no correlation between plasma concentrations and therapeutic effects. Dosing guidelines for adolescents and children are different from those for adults, requiring lower starting dosages; higher dosages are associated with more adverse effects.

Side Effects.   The EPS of risperidone is largely dosage dependent, and there has been a trend to using lower doses than initially recommended. Weight gain, anxiety, nausea and vomiting, rhinitis, erectile dysfunction, orgasmic dysfunction, and increased pigmentation are associated with risperidone use. The most common drug-related reasons for discontinuation of risperidone use are EPS, dizziness, hyperkinesias, somnolence, and nausea. Marked elevation of prolactin may occur. Weight gain occurs more commonly with risperidone use in children than in adults.

Risperidone is also available as an orally disintegrating tablet (Risperdal M-Tab), which is available in 0.5, 1, and 2 mg strengths, and in a depot formulation (Risperdal Consta), which is given as an intramuscular (IM) injection formulation every 2 weeks. The dose may be 25, 50, or 75 mg. Oral risperidone should be coadministered with Risperdal Consta for the first 3 weeks before being discontinued.

Drug Interactions.   Inhibition of CYP2D6 by drugs such as paroxetine and fluoxetine can block the formation of risperidone's active metabolite. Risperidone is a weak inhibitor of CYP2D6 and has little effect on other drugs. Combined use of risperidone and SSRIs may result in significant elevation of prolactin, with associated galactorrhea and breast enlargement.

Paliperidone (Invega)

Indications.   Paliperidone is indicated for the acute and maintenance treatment of schizophrenia. Paliperidone is also indicated for the acute treatment of schizoaffective disorder as monotherapy or as an adjunct to mood stabilizers or antidepressants.

Pharmacology.   Paliperidone is a benzisoxazole derivative and is the primary active metabolite of risperidone. Peak plasma concentrations (C_{max}) are achieved approximately 24 hours after dosing, and steady-state concentrations of paliperidone are attained within 4 or 5 days. The hepatic isoenzymes CYP2D6 and CYP3A4 play a limited role in the metabolism and elimination of paliperidone, so no dose adjustment is required in patients with mild or moderate hepatic impairment.

Dosage.   Paliperidone is available in 3-, 6-, and 9-mg tablets. The recommended dosage is 6 mg once daily administered in the morning. It can be taken with or without food. It is also available as extended-release tablets, which are also available in 3-, 6-, and 9-mg tablets administered once daily. It is recommended that no more than 12 mg should be administered per day. A long-acting formulation of paliperidone (Invega Sustenna) is given by injection once a month. Invega Sustenna is available as a white to off-white sterile aqueous extended-release suspension for intramuscular

injection in dose strengths of 39-, 78-, 117-, 156-, and 234-mg paliperidone palmitate. The drug product hydrolyzes to the active moiety, paliperidone, resulting in dose strengths of 25, 50, 75, 100, and 150 mg of paliperidone, respectively.

Invega Sustenna is provided in a prefilled syringe with a plunger stopper and tip cap. The kit also contains two safety needles (a 1½-in 22-gauge safety needle and a 1-in 23-gauge safety needle). It has a half-life of 25 to 49 days. Monthly injections of 117 mg are recommended, although higher or lower dosages can be used depending on the clinical situation. The first two injections should be in the deltoid muscle because plasma concentrations are 28 percent higher with deltoid versus gluteal administration. Subsequent injections can alternate between gluteal and deltoid sites.

Side Effects.   The dose of paliperidone should be reduced in patients with renal impairment. It may cause more sensitivity to temperature extremes, such as very hot or cold conditions. Paliperidone may cause an increase in QT (QTc) interval and should be avoided in combination with other drugs that cause prolongation of QT interval. It may cause orthostatic hypotension, tachycardia, somnolence, akathisia, dystonia, EPS, and parkinsonism.

Olanzapine (Zyprexa)

Indications.   Olanzapine is indicated for the treatment of schizophrenia. Oral olanzapine is indicated for use as monotherapy for the acute treatment of manic or mixed episodes associated with bipolar I disorder and maintenance treatment of bipolar I disorder. Oral olanzapine is also indicated for the treatment of manic or mixed episodes associated with bipolar I disorder as an adjunct to lithium or valproate, and olanzapine can also be used in combination with fluoxetine (Symbyax) for the treatment of depressive episodes associated with bipolar I disorder.

Oral olanzapine and fluoxetine in combination (Symbyax) is indicated for the treatment of treatment-resistant depression. Olanzapine monotherapy is not indicated for the treatment of treatment-resistant depression.

Pharmacology.   Approximately 85 percent of olanzapine is absorbed from the GI tract, and about 40 percent of the dosage is inactivated by first-pass hepatic metabolism. Peak concentrations are reached in 5 hours, and the half-life averages 31 hours (range 21 to 54 hours). It is given in once-daily dosing. In addition to $5\text{-}HT_{2A}$ and D_2 antagonism, olanzapine is an antagonist of the D_1, D_4, α_1, $5\text{-}HT_{1A}$, muscarinic M_1 to M_5, and H_1 receptors.

Dosages.   Olanzapine is available in 2.5-, 5-, 7.5-, 10-, 15-, and 20-mg oral and Zydis form (orally disintegrating) tablets. The initial dosage for the treatment of psychosis is usually 5 or 10 mg. For acute mania, it is usually 10 or 15 mg given once daily. It is also available as 5-, 10-, 15-, and 20-mg orally disintegrating tablets that might be useful for patients who have difficulty swallowing pills or who "cheek" their medication.

A starting daily dose of 5 to 10 mg is recommended. After 1 week, the dosage can be raised to 10 mg a day. Given the long half-life, 1 week must be allowed to achieve each new steady-state blood level. Dosages in clinical use ranges vary, with 5 to 20 mg a day is most commonly used, but 30 to 40 mg a day is needed in treatment-resistant patients. A word of caution, however, is that the higher dosages are associated with increased EPS and other adverse effects, and dosages above 20 mg a day were not studied in the pivotal trials that led to the approval of olanzapine. The parenteral form of olanzapine is indicated for the treatment of acute agitation associated with schizophrenia and bipolar disorder, and the IM dosage is 10 mg. Coadministration with benzodiazepines is not approved.

Other Formulations. Olanzapine is available as an extended-release injectable suspension (Relprevv), which is a long-acting atypical IM injection indicated for the treatment of schizophrenia. It is injected deep in the gluteal region and should not be administered intravenously or subcutaneously, nor is it approved for deltoid administration. Before administering the injection, the administrator should aspirate the syringe for several seconds to ensure that no blood is visible. It carries a boxed warning for postinjection delirium sedation syndrome (PDSS). Patients are at risk for severe sedation (including coma) and must be observed for 3 hours after each injection in a registered facility. In controlled studies, all patients with PDSS recovered, and there were no deaths reported. It is postulated that PDSS is secondary to increased levels of olanzapine secondary to accidental rupture of a blood vessel, causing extreme sedation or delirium. Patients should be managed as clinically appropriate and, if necessary, monitored in a facility capable of resuscitation. The injection can be given every 2 or 4 weeks, depending on the dosing guidelines.

Drug Interactions. Fluvoxamine (Luvox) and cimetidine (Tagamet) increase, and carbamazepine and phenytoin decrease, serum concentrations of olanzapine. Ethanol increases olanzapine absorption by more than 25 percent, leading to increased sedation. Olanzapine has little effect on the metabolism of other drugs.

Side Effects. Other than clozapine, olanzapine consistently causes a more significant amount and more frequent weight gain than other atypicals. This effect is not dose-related and continues over time. Clinical trial data suggest it peaks after 9 months, after which it may continue to increase more slowly. Somnolence, dry mouth, dizziness, constipation, dyspepsia, increased appetite, akathisia, and tremor are associated with olanzapine use. A small number of patients (2 percent) may need to discontinue the use of the drug because of transaminase elevation. There is a dose-related risk of EPS. The manufacturer recommends a "periodic" assessment of blood sugar and transaminases during treatment with olanzapine. There is an FDA-mandated warning about an increased risk of stroke among patients with dementia treated with SDAs, but this risk is small and is outweighed by improved behavioral control that treatment may produce.

Quetiapine (Seroquel)

Indications. Quetiapine is indicated for the treatment of schizophrenia. It is also indicated for the acute treatment of manic episodes associated with bipolar I disorder, both as monotherapy and as an adjunct to lithium or sodium valproate. It is also indicated as monotherapy for the acute treatment of depressive episodes associated with bipolar disorder and maintenance treatment of bipolar I disorder as an adjunct to lithium or divalproex. It also is indicated as adjunctive therapy to antidepressants for the treatment of MDD.

Pharmacology. Quetiapine is a dibenzothiazepine structurally related to clozapine, but it differs markedly from that agent in biochemical effects. It is rapidly absorbed from the GI tract, with peak plasma concentrations reached in 1 to 2 hours. The steady-state half-life is about 7 hours, and optimal dosing is two or three times per day. Quetiapine, in addition to being an antagonist of D_2 and 5-HT_2, also blocks 5-HT_6, D_1 and H_1, and α_1 and α_2 receptors. It does not block muscarinic or benzodiazepine receptors. The receptor antagonism for quetiapine is generally lower than that for other antipsychotic drugs, and it is not associated with EPS.

Dosages. Quetiapine is available in 25-, 50-, 100-, 200-, 300-, and 400-mg tablets. Quetiapine dosing should begin at 25 mg twice daily, with doses then increased by 25 to 50 mg/dose every 2 to 3 days, up to a target of 300 to 400 mg a day. Studies have shown efficacy in the range of 300 to 800 mg a day. In reality, more aggressive dosing is both tolerated and more effective. It has become evident that the target dose can be achieved more rapidly and that some patients benefit from dosages of as much as 1,200 to 1,600 mg a day. When used at higher doses, serial ECG studies are required. Despite its short elimination half-life, quetiapine can be given to many patients once a day. This dosing is consistent with the observation that quetiapine receptor occupancy remains even when concentrations in the blood have markedly declined. Quetiapine in doses of 25 to 300 mg at night has been used for insomnia.

Other Formulations. Quetiapine XR has comparable bioavailability to an equivalent dose of quetiapine administered two or three times daily. Quetiapine XR is given once daily, preferably in the evening, 3 to 4 hours before bedtime without food or a light meal to prevent an increase in C_{max}. The usual starting dose is 300 mg, and it may be increased to 400 to 800 mg.

Drug Interactions. The potential interactions between quetiapine and other drugs have been well studied. Phenytoin increases quetiapine clearance fivefold; no significant pharmacokinetic interactions have been noted. Avoid the use of quetiapine with drugs that increase the QT interval and in patients with risk factors for prolonged QT interval. The FDA has added a new warning about quetiapine, cautioning prescribers about potential prolongation of the QT interval when above-recommended amounts of quetiapine are combined with specific drugs. Quetiapine should not be combined with other drugs that are known to prolong QTc. This includes class 1A antiarrhythmics (e.g., quinidine, procainamide) or class III antiarrhythmics (e.g., amiodarone, sotalol), antipsychotic medications (e.g., ziprasidone, chlorpromazine, thioridazine), antibiotics (e.g., gatifloxacin, moxifloxacin), or any other class of medications known to prolong the QTc interval (e.g., pentamidine, levomethadyl acetate, methadone). Quetiapine should also be avoided in circumstances that may increase the risk of occurrence of torsade de pointes or sudden death, including (1) a history of cardiac arrhythmias such as bradycardia; (2) hypokalemia or hypomagnesemia; (3) concomitant use of other drugs that prolong the QTc interval; and (4) presence of congenital prolongation of the QT interval. Postmarketing cases also show increases in QT interval in patients who overdose on quetiapine.

Side Effects. Somnolence, postural hypotension, and dizziness are the most common adverse effects of quetiapine. These are usually transient and are best managed with initial gradual upward titration of the dosage. Quetiapine is the SDA least likely to cause EPS, regardless of dose. This makes it particularly useful in treating patients with Parkinson disease who develop dopamine agonist-induced psychosis. Prolactin elevation is rare and both transient and mild when it occurs. Quetiapine is associated with modest transient weight gain in some persons, but some patients occasionally gain a considerable amount of weight. The relationship between quetiapine and the development of diabetes is not as clearly established as are the cases involving the use of olanzapine. Small increases in heart rate, constipation, and a transient increase in liver transaminases may also occur. Initial concerns about cataract formation, based on animal studies, have not been borne out since the drug has been in clinical use. Nevertheless, it might be prudent to test for lens abnormalities early in treatment and periodically after that.

Ziprasidone (Geodon)

Indications.   Ziprasidone is indicated for the treatment of schizophrenia. Ziprasidone is also indicated as monotherapy for the acute treatment of manic or mixed episodes associated with bipolar I disorder and as an adjunct to lithium or valproate for the maintenance treatment of bipolar I disorder.

Pharmacology.   Ziprasidone is a benzisothiazole piperazine. Peak plasma concentrations of ziprasidone are reached in 2 to 6 hours. Steady-state levels ranging from 5 to 10 hours are reached between the first and the third days of treatment. The mean terminal half-life at steady state ranges from 5 to 10 hours, which accounts for the recommendation that twice-daily dosing is necessary. Bioavailability doubles when ziprasidone is taken with food, and therefore it should be taken with food.

Peak serum concentrations of IM ziprasidone occur after approximately 1 hour, with a half-life of 2 to 5 hours.

Ziprasidone, similar to the other SDAs, blocks $5-HT_{2A}$ and D_2 receptors. It is also an antagonist of $5-HT_{1D}$, $5-HT_{2C}$, D_3, D_4, α_1, and H_1 receptors. It has a very low affinity for D_1, M_1, and α_2 receptors. Also, ziprasidone has agonist activity at the serotonin $5-HT_{1A}$ receptors and is an SSRI and a norepinephrine reuptake inhibitor. This action is consistent with clinical reports that ziprasidone has antidepressant-like effects in nonschizophrenic patients.

Dosages.   Ziprasidone is available in 20-, 40-, 60-, and 80-mg capsules. Ziprasidone for IM use comes as a single-use 20 mg/mL vial. Oral ziprasidone dosing should be initiated at 40 mg a day, divided into two daily doses. Studies have shown efficacy in the range of 80 to 160 mg a day, divided twice daily. In clinical practice, doses as high as 240 mg a day are being used. The recommended IM dosage is 10 to 20 mg every 2 hours for the 10-mg dose and every 4 hours for the 20-mg dose. The maximum total daily dose of IM ziprasidone is 40 mg.

Other than interactions with other drugs that prolong the QTc complex, ziprasidone appears to have a low potential for clinically significant drug interactions.

Side Effects.   Somnolence, headache, dizziness, nausea, and lightheadedness are the most common adverse effects in patients taking ziprasidone. The drug has almost no significant effects outside the CNS, is associated with almost no weight gain, and does not cause sustained prolactin elevation. Concerns about prolongation of the QTc complex have deterred some clinicians from using ziprasidone as a first choice. The QTc interval has been shown to increase in patients treated with 40 and 120 mg/day. Ziprasidone is contraindicated in combination with other drugs known to prolong the QTc interval. These include, but are not limited to, dofetilide, sotalol, quinidine, other class IA and III antiarrhythmics, mesoridazine, thioridazine, chlorpromazine, droperidol, pimozide, sparfloxacin, gatifloxacin, moxifloxacin, halofantrine, mefloquine, pentamidine, arsenic trioxide, levomethadyl acetate, dolasetron mesylate, probucol, and tacrolimus. Ziprasidone should be avoided

in patients with congenital long QT syndrome and patients with a history of cardiac arrhythmias.

Aripiprazole (Abilify)

Aripiprazole is a potent $5-HT_{2A}$ antagonist and is indicated for the treatment of both schizophrenia and acute mania. It is also approved for the augmentation of antidepressant agents in MDD. Aripiprazole is a D_2 antagonist, but can also act as a partial D_2 agonist. Partial D_2 agonists compete at D_2 receptors for endogenous dopamine, thereby producing a functional reduction of dopamine activity.

Indications.   Aripiprazole is indicated for the treatment of schizophrenia. Short-term, 4- to 6-week studies comparing aripiprazole with haloperidol and risperidone in patients with schizophrenia and schizoaffective disorder have shown comparable efficacy. Dosages of 15, 20, and 30 mg a day were found to be effective. Long-term studies suggest that aripiprazole is effective as a maintenance treatment at a daily dose of 15 to 30 mg.

Aripiprazole is also indicated for the acute and maintenance treatment of manic and mixed episodes associated with bipolar I disorder. It is also used as adjunctive therapy to either lithium or valproate for the acute treatment of manic and mixed episodes associated with bipolar I disorder.

Aripiprazole is indicated for use as adjunctive therapy to antidepressants for the treatment of MDD. Aripiprazole is also indicated for the treatment of irritability associated with autistic disorder.

Pharmacology.   Aripiprazole is well absorbed, reaching peak plasma concentrations after 3 to 5 hours. Absorption is not affected by food. The mean elimination half-life of aripiprazole is about 75 hours. It has a weakly active metabolite with a half-life of 96 hours. These relatively long half-lives make aripiprazole suitable for once-daily dosing. Clearance is reduced in elderly persons. Aripiprazole exhibits linear pharmacokinetics and is primarily metabolized by CYP3A4 and CYP2D6 enzymes. It is 99 percent protein-bound. Aripiprazole is excreted in breast milk in lactating rats.

Mechanistically, aripiprazole acts as a modulator, rather than a blocker, and acts on both postsynaptic D_2 receptors and presynaptic autoreceptors. In theory, this mechanism addresses excessive limbic dopamine (hyperdopaminergic) activity and decreased dopamine (hypodopaminergic) activity in frontal and prefrontal areas—abnormalities that are thought to be present in schizophrenia. The absence of a complete D_2 blockade in the striatal areas would be expected to minimize EPS. Aripiprazole is an α_1-adrenergic receptor antagonist, which may cause some patients to experience orthostatic hypotension. Similar to the so-called atypical antipsychotic agents, aripiprazole is a $5-HT_{2A}$ antagonist.

Other Uses.   A study of aggressive children and adolescents with oppositional defiant disorder or conduct disorder found that there was a positive response in about 60 percent of the subjects. In this study, vomiting and somnolence led to a reduction in initial aripiprazole dosage.

Drug Interactions.   Whereas carbamazepine and valproate reduce serum concentrations, ketoconazole, fluoxetine, paroxetine, and quinidine increase aripiprazole serum concentrations. Lithium and valproic acid, two drugs likely to be combined with aripiprazole when treating bipolar disorder, do not affect the steady-state concentrations of aripiprazole. Combined use with antihypertensives may cause hypotension. Drugs that inhibit CYP2D6 activity reduce aripiprazole elimination.

Dosage and Clinical Guidelines.   Aripiprazole is available as 5-, 10-, 15-, 20-, and 30-mg tablets. The effective dosage range is 10 to 30 mg/day. Although the starting dosage is 10 to 15 mg/day, problems with nausea, insomnia, and akathisia have led to the use of lower than recommended starting dosages of aripiprazole. Many clinicians find that an initial dose of 5 mg increases tolerability.

Side Effects.   The most commonly reported side effects of aripiprazole are headache, somnolence, agitation, dyspepsia, anxiety, and nausea. Although it is not a frequent cause of EPS, aripiprazole does cause akathisia-like activation. Described as restlessness or agitation, it can be highly distressing and often leads to discontinuation of the medication. Insomnia is another common complaint. Data so far do not indicate that weight gain or diabetes mellitus have an increased incidence with aripiprazole. Prolactin elevation does not typically occur. Aripiprazole does not cause significant QTc interval changes. There have been reports of seizures.

Asenapine (Saphris)

Indications.   Asenapine is approved for the acute treatment of adults with schizophrenia and acute treatment of manic or mixed episodes associated with bipolar I disorder with or without psychotic features in adults.

Pharmacology.   Asenapine has an affinity for several receptors, including serotonin (5-HT$_{2A}$ and 5-HT$_{2C}$), noradrenergic (α_2, and α_1), dopaminergic (D$_3$ and D$_4$ receptors is higher than its affinity for D$_2$ receptors), and histamine (H$_1$). It has a negligible affinity for muscarinic-1 cholinergic receptors and hence less incidence of dry mouth, blurred vision, constipation, and urinary retention. The bioavailability is 35 percent via the sublingual (preferred) route, and it achieves peak plasma concentration in 1 hour. Asenapine is metabolized through glucuronidation and oxidative metabolism by CYP1A2, so coadministration with fluvoxamine and other CYP1A2 inhibitors should be done cautiously.

Dosage.   Asenapine is available as 5- and 10-mg sublingual tablets and should be placed under the tongue. This method is because the bioavailability of asenapine is less than 2 percent when swallowed, but is 35 percent when absorbed sublingually. The agent dissolves in saliva within seconds and is absorbed through the oral mucosa. Sublingual administration avoids first-pass hepatic metabolism. Patients should be advised to avoid drinking or eating for 10 minutes after taking asenapine because this may lower the blood levels. The recommended starting and target dose for schizophrenia is 5 mg twice a day. In bipolar disorder, the patient may be started on 10 mg twice a day, and if necessary, the dosage may be lowered to 5 mg twice a day, depending on the tolerability issues. In acute schizophrenia treatment, there is no evidence of added benefit with a 10 mg twice-daily dose, but there is an apparent increase in specific adverse reactions. In both bipolar I disorder and schizophrenia, the maximum dose should not exceed 10 mg two times a day. The safety of doses above 10 mg twice a day has not been evaluated in clinical studies.

Side Effects.   The most common side effects observed in schizophrenic and bipolar disorders are somnolence, dizziness, EPS other than akathisia, and increased weight. In clinical trials, the mean weight gain after 52 weeks is 0.9 kg, and there were no clinically relevant differences in lipid profile and blood glucose after 52 weeks. In clinical trials, asenapine was found to increase the QTc interval in a range of 2 to 5 milliseconds compared to placebo. No patients treated with asenapine experienced QTc increases 60 milliseconds or greater from baseline measurements, nor did any experience a QTc of 500 milliseconds or more. Nevertheless, asenapine should be avoided in combination with other drugs known to prolong QTc interval in patients with congenital prolongation of QT interval or a history of cardiac arrhythmias, and in circumstances that may increase the occurrence of torsades de pointes. Asenapine can elevate prolactin levels, and the elevation can persist during chronic administration. Galactorrhea, amenorrhea, gynecomastia, and impotence may occur.

Clozapine (Clozaril)

Indications.   In addition to being the most effective drug treatment for patients who have failed to respond to standard therapies, clozapine has been shown to benefit patients with severe tardive dyskinesia. Clozapine suppresses these dyskinesias, but the abnormal movements return when clozapine is discontinued. This suppression is true even though clozapine, on rare occasions, may cause tardive dyskinesia. Other clinical situations in which clozapine may be used include the treatment of psychotic patients intolerant of EPS caused by other agents, treatment-resistant mania, severe psychotic depression, idiopathic Parkinson disease, Huntington disease, and suicidal patients with schizophrenia or schizoaffective disorder. Other treatment-resistant disorders that have demonstrated response to clozapine include pervasive developmental disorder, autism of childhood, and OCD (either alone or in combination with an SSRI). Used by itself, clozapine may very rarely induce obsessive-compulsive symptoms.

Pharmacology.   Clozapine is a dibenzothiazepine. It is rapidly absorbed, with peak plasma levels reached in about 2 hours. Steady state is achieved in less than 1 week if twice-daily dosing is used. The elimination half-life is about 12 hours. Clozapine has two significant metabolites, one of which, *N*-dimethyl clozapine, may have some pharmacologic activities. Clozapine is an antagonist of 5-HT$_{2A}$, D$_1$, D$_3$, D$_4$, and α (especially α_1) receptors. It has relatively low potency as a D$_2$ receptor antagonist. Data from PET scanning show that whereas 10 mg of haloperidol produces 80 percent occupancy of striatal D$_2$ receptors, clinically significant dosages of clozapine occupy only 40 to 50 percent of striatal D$_2$ receptors. This difference in D$_2$ receptor occupancy is probably why clozapine does not cause EPS. It has also been postulated that clozapine and other SDAs bind more loosely to the D$_2$ receptor, and because of this "fast dissociation," more normal dopamine neurotransmission is possible.

Dosages.   Clozapine is available in 25- and 100-mg tablets. The initial dosage is usually 25 mg one or two times daily, although a conservative initial dosage is 12.5 mg twice daily. The dosage can then be increased gradually (25 mg a day every 2 or 3 days) to 300 mg a day in divided doses, usually two or three times a day. Dosages up to 900 mg a day can be used. Testing for blood concentrations of clozapine may be helpful in patients who fail to respond. Studies have found that plasma concentrations greater than 350 μg/mL are associated with a better likelihood of response.

Drug Interactions.   Clozapine should not be used with any other drug that is associated with the development of agranulocytosis or bone marrow suppression. Such drugs include carbamazepine, phenytoin, propylthiouracil, sulfonamides, and captopril (Capoten). Lithium combined with clozapine may increase the risk of seizures, confusion, and movement disorders. Lithium should not be used in combination with clozapine by persons who have experienced an episode of neuroleptic malignant syndrome. Clomipramine (Anafranil) can increase the risk of seizure by lowering the seizure threshold and by increasing clozapine plasma concentrations. Risperidone, fluoxetine, paroxetine, and fluvoxamine increase serum concentrations of clozapine. The addition of paroxetine may precipitate clozapine-associated neutropenia.

Side Effects.   The most common drug-related adverse effects are sedation, dizziness, syncope, tachycardia, hypotension, electrocardiography (ECG) changes, nausea, and vomiting. Other common adverse effects include fatigue, weight gain, various GI symptoms (most commonly constipation), anticholinergic effects, and subjective muscle weakness. Sialorrhea, or hypersalivation, is a side effect that begins early in treatment and is most evident at night. Patients report that their pillows are drenched with saliva. This side effect is most likely the result of impairment of swallowing. Although there are reports that clonidine or amitriptyline may help reduce hypersalivation, the most practical solution is to put a towel over the pillow.

The risk of seizures is about 4 percent in patients taking dosages greater than 600 mg a day. Leukopenia, granulocytopenia, agranulocytosis, and fever occur in about 1 percent of patients. During the first year of treatment, there is a 0.73 percent risk of clozapine-induced agranulocytosis. The risk during the second year is 0.07 percent. For neutropenia, the risk is 2.32 percent and 0.69 percent, respectively, during the first and second years of treatment. The only contraindications to the use of clozapine are a WBC count below 3,500 cells/mm^3; a previous bone marrow disorder; a history of agranulocytosis during clozapine treatment; or the use of another drug that is known to suppress the bone marrow, such as carbamazepine (Tegretol).

During the first 6 months of treatment, weekly WBC counts are indicated to monitor the patient for the development of agranulocytosis. If the WBC count remains normal, the frequency of testing can be decreased to every 2 weeks. Although monitoring is expensive, an early indication of agranulocytosis can prevent a fatal outcome. Clozapine should be discontinued if the WBC count is below 3,000 cells/mm^3 or the granulocyte count is below 1,500/mm^3. Also, a hematologic consultation should be obtained, and obtaining a bone marrow sample should be considered. Persons with agranulocytosis should not be reexposed to the drug. Clozapine cannot be dispensed without proof of monitoring.

Patients exhibiting symptoms of chest pain, shortness of breath, fever, or tachypnea should be immediately evaluated for myocarditis or cardiomyopathy, an infrequent but serious adverse effect ending in death. Serial CPK-MB (creatine phosphokinase with myocardial band fractions), troponin levels, and ECG studies are recommended, with immediate discontinuation of clozapine.

Iloperidone (Fanapt)

Indications.   Iloperidone (Fanapt) is indicated for the acute treatment of schizophrenia in adults. The safety and efficacy of iloperidone in children and adolescents has not been established.

Pharmacology.   Iloperidone is not a derivative of another antipsychotic agent. It has complex multiple antagonist effects on several neurotransmitter systems. Iloperidone has a strong affinity for dopamine D_3 receptors, followed by decreasing affinities of α_{2c}-noradrenergic, $5\text{-}HT_{1a}$, D_{2a}, and $5\text{-}HT_6$ receptors. Iloperidone has a low affinity for histaminergic receptors. As with other antipsychotics, the clinical significance of this receptor binding affinity is unknown.

Iloperidone has a peak concentration of 2 to 4 hours and a half-life that is dependent on hepatic isoenzyme metabolism. It is metabolized primarily through CYP2D6 and CYP3A4, and the dosage should be reduced by half when administered concomitantly with potent inhibitors of these two isoenzymes. The half-life is 18 to 26 hours in CYP2D6 extensive metabolizers and is 31 to 37 hours in CYP2D6 poor metabolizers. Of note, approximately 7 to 10 percent of whites and 3 to 8 percent of African Americans cannot metabolize CYP2D6 substrates; hence, dosing should be determined with this caveat in mind. Iloperidone should be used with caution in persons with severe hepatic impairment.

Side Effects.   Iloperidone prolongs the QT interval and may be associated with arrhythmia and sudden death. Iloperidone prolongs the QTc interval by 9 milliseconds at dosages of 12 mg twice daily. Concurrent use with other agents that prolong the QTc interval may result in additive effects on the QTc interval. The concurrent use of iloperidone with agents that prolong the QTc interval may result in potentially life-threatening cardiac arrhythmias, including torsades de pointes. Concurrent administration of other drugs that are known to prolong the QTc interval should be avoided. Cardiovascular disease, hypokalemia, hypomagnesemia, bradycardia, congenital prolongation of the QT interval, and concurrent use of inhibitors of CYP3A4 or CYP2D6, which metabolize iloperidone, may increase the risk of QT prolongation.

The most common adverse effects reported are dizziness, dry mouth, fatigue, sedation, tachycardia, and orthostatic hypotension (depending on dosing and titration). Despite being a robust D_2 antagonist, the rates of EPS and akathisia are similar to those of placebo. The mean weight gain in short- and long-term trials is 2.1 kg. Due to its relatively limited use, there is no accurate understanding of iloperidone's effects on weight and lipids. Some patients exhibit elevated prolactin levels. Three cases of priapism have been reported in the premarketing phase.

Dosing.   Iloperidone must be titrated slowly to avoid orthostatic hypotension. It is available in a titration pack, and the effective dose (12 mg) should be reached in approximately 4 days based on a twice-a-day dosing schedule. It is usually started on day 1 at 1 mg twice a day and increased daily on a twice-a-day schedule to reach 12 mg by day 4. The maximum recommended dose is 12 mg twice a day (24 mg a day), and it can be administered without regard to food.

Lurasidone HCL (Latuda)

Indications.   Lurasidone hydrochloride is an oral, once-daily atypical antipsychotic indicated for the treatment of patients with schizophrenia. To date, there has not been extensive clinical experience with lurasidone.

Side Effects.   The most commonly observed adverse reactions associated with the use of lurasidone are similar to those seen with other new-generation antipsychotics. These include, but are not limited to, somnolence, akathisia, nausea, parkinsonism, and agitation. Based on clinical trial data, lurasidone appears to cause less weight gain and metabolic changes than the two other most recently approved SDAs, asenapine and iloperidone. More extensive clinical experience with the drug is required to determine whether this is, in fact, the case.

Drug Interactions.   When coadministration of lurasidone with a moderate CYP3A4 inhibitor such as diltiazem is considered, the dose should not exceed 40 mg/day. Lurasidone should not be used in combination with a potent CYP3A4 inhibitor (e.g., ketoconazole). Lurasidone also should not be used in combination with a potent CYP3A4 inducer (e.g., rifampin).

Dosages.   Lurasidone is available as 20-, 40-, 80-, and 120-mg tablets. Initial dose titration is not required. The recommended starting dose is 40 mg once daily, and the medication should be taken with food. It is effective in a dose range of 40 to 120 mg/day. Although there is no proven added benefit with the 120 mg/day dose, there may be a dose-related increase in adverse reactions. Still, some patients may benefit from the maximum recommended dose of 160 mg/day. Dose adjustment is recommended in patients with renal impairment. The dose in moderate to severe renal impairment should not exceed 80 mg/day. The dose in severe hepatic impairment patients should not exceed 40 mg/day.

Lumateperone (Caplyta)

Lumateperone was approved by the FDA for the treatment of schizophrenia in adults in December 2019 and became available in February 2020. It antagonizes several receptors, including 5-HT$_{2A}$ receptor, D$_1$, D$_2$, and D$_4$. Although effective for schizophrenia, several studies of its effectiveness in bipolar depression had disappointing results. It is available in several doses, although the highest FDA-approved dose is 42 mg. As this is a new drug, experience with it in post study clinical samples is very limited.

Clinical Guidelines for SDAs

All SDAs are appropriate for the management of an initial psychotic episode, but clozapine is reserved for persons who are refractory to all other antipsychotic drugs. If a person does not respond to the first SDA, other SDAs should be tried. The choice of drug should be based on the patient's clinical status and history of response to medication. Recent studies have challenged the notion that SDAs require 4 to 6 weeks to reach full effectiveness, and it may take up to 8 weeks for the full clinical effects of an SDA to become apparent. The newer meta-analyses suggest that the apparent benefits may be seen as early as 2 to 3 weeks, and early response or failure is an indicator of subsequent response or failure.

Nevertheless, it is acceptable practice to augment an SDA with a high-potency DRA or benzodiazepine in the first few weeks of use. Lorazepam (Ativan) 1 to 2 mg orally or IM can be used as needed for acute agitation. Once effective, dosages can be lowered as tolerated. Clinical improvement may take 6 months of treatment with SDAs in some, particularly treatment-refractory persons.

The use of all SDAs must be initiated at low dosages and gradually tapered upward to therapeutic dosages. The potential development of adverse effects necessitates the gradual increase in dosage. If a person stops taking an SDA for more than 36 hours, drug use should be resumed at the initial titration schedule. After the decision to terminate olanzapine or clozapine use, dosages should be tapered whenever possible to avoid cholinergic rebound symptoms such as diaphoresis, flushing, diarrhea, and hyperactivity.

After assuring themselves of the appropriateness of SDA treatment, the clinician should explain the risks and benefits of SDA treatment to the person and the family. In the case of clozapine, an informed consent procedure should be documented in the person's chart. The patient's history should include information about blood disorders, epilepsy, cardiovascular disease, hepatic and renal diseases, and drug abuse. The presence of a hepatic or renal disease necessitates using low starting dosages of the drug. The physical examination should include supine and standing BP measurements to screen for orthostatic hypotension. The laboratory examination should include an ECG and several complete blood counts (CBCs) with WBC counts, which can then be averaged; and liver and renal function tests. Periodic monitoring of blood glucose, lipids, and body weight is recommended.

Although the transition from a DRA to an SDA may be made abruptly, it is wiser to taper off the DRA slowly while titrating up the SDA. Clozapine and olanzapine both have anticholinergic effects, and the transition from one to the other can usually be accomplished with little risk of cholinergic rebound. The transition from risperidone to olanzapine is best accomplished by tapering the risperidone off over 3 weeks while simultaneously beginning olanzapine at 10 mg a day. Risperidone, quetiapine, and ziprasidone lack anticholinergic effects, and the abrupt transition from a DRA, olanzapine, or clozapine to one of these agents may cause cholinergic rebound, which consists of excessive salivation, nausea, vomiting, and diarrhea. The risk of cholinergic rebound can be mitigated by initially augmenting risperidone, quetiapine, or ziprasidone with an anticholinergic drug, which is then tapered off slowly. Any initiation and termination of SDA use should be accomplished gradually.

It is wise to overlap the administration of the new drug with the old drug. Of interest, some people have a more robust clinical response while taking the two agents during the transition and then regressing on monotherapy with the newer drug. We know little about the safety of combination antipsychotic treatment.

Persons receiving regular injections of depot formulations of a DRA who are to switch to SDA use are given the first dose of the SDA on the day the next injection is due.

Persons who developed agranulocytosis while taking clozapine can safely switch to olanzapine use, although initiation of olanzapine use amid clozapine-induced agranulocytosis can prolong the time of recovery from the usual 3 to 4 days up to 11 to 12 days. It is prudent to wait for the resolution of agranulocytosis before initiating olanzapine use. Emergence or recurrence of agranulocytosis has not been reported with olanzapine, even in persons who developed it while taking clozapine.

SDA use by pregnant women has not been studied, but consideration should be given to the potential of risperidone to raise prolactin concentrations, sometimes up to three to four times the upper limit of the normal range. Because the drugs can be excreted in breast milk, they should not be taken by nursing mothers. The dosages for selected SDAs are given in Table 21-9.

DOPAMINE RECEPTOR ANTAGONISTS (FIRST-GENERATION ANTIPSYCHOTICS)

The DRAs represent the first group of effective agents for schizophrenia and other psychotic illnesses. The first of these drugs, the phenothiazine chlorpromazine (Thorazine), was introduced in the early 1950s. Other DRAs include all of the antipsychotics in the following groups: phenothiazines, butyrophenones, thioxanthenes, dibenzoxazepines, dihydroindoles, and diphenylbutylpiperidines. Because these agents are associated with extrapyramidal side effects (EPS)

Table 21-9
Comparison of Usual Dosing[a] for Some Available Second-Generation Antipsychotics in Schizophrenia

Antipsychotic	Typical Starting Dosage	Maintenance Therapy Dose Range	Titration	Maximum Recommended Dosage
Aripiprazole (Abilify)	10–15 mg tablets once a day	10–30 mg/day	Dosage increases should not be made before 2 wk	30 mg/day
Asenapine (Saphris)	5 mg twice a day	10 mg twice a day	Titration not necessary	20 mg/day
Clozapine (Clozaril)	12.5-mg tablets once or twice a day	150–300 mg/day in divided doses or 200 mg as a single dose in the evening	The dosage should be increased to 25–50 mg on the second day. Further increases may be made in daily increments of 25–50 mg to a target dosage of 300–450 mg/day. Subsequent dosage increases should be made no more than once or twice weekly in increments of no more than 100 mg	900 mg/day
Iloperidone (Fanapt)	1 mg twice a day	12–24 mg a day in divided dose	Start at 1 mg twice a day then move to 2, 4, 6, 8 and 12 mg twice a day. Do this over the course of 7 days	24 mg/day
Lurasidone (Latuda)	40 mg/day	40–80 mg/day	Titration not necessary	120 mg/day
Olanzapine (Zyprexa)	5–10 mg/day tablets or orally disintegrating tablets	10–20 mg/day	Dosage increments of 5 mg once a day are recommended when required at intervals of not less than 1 wk	20 mg/day
Paliperidone (Invega)	3–9 mg extended-release tablets once a day	3–6 mg/day	Plasma concentration rises to a peak approximately 24 hr after dosing	12 mg/day
Quetiapine (Seroquel)	25-mg tablets twice a day	Lowest dose needed to maintain remission	Increase in increments of 25–50 mg two or three times a day on the second and the third day, as tolerated, to a target dosage of 500 mg daily by the fourth day (given in two or three doses/day). Further dosage adjustments, if required, should be of 25–50 mg twice a day and occur at intervals of not fewer than 2 days	800 mg/day
Risperidone (Risperdal)	1-mg tablet and oral solution once a day	2–6 mg once a day	Increase to 2 mg once a day on the second day and 4 mg once a day on the third day. In some patients, a slower titration may be appropriate. When dosage adjustments are necessary, further dosage increments of 1–2 mg/day at intervals of not less than 1 wk are recommended	1–6 mg/day
Risperidone IM long-acting (Consta)	25–50 mg IM injection every 2 wk	Start with oral risperidone for 3 wk	Starting dose: 25 mg every 2 wk	50 mg for 2 wk
Ziprasidone (Geodon)	20-mg capsules twice a day with food	20–80 mg twice a day	Dosage adjustments based on individual clinical status may be made at intervals of not fewer than 2 days	80 mg twice a day
Ziprasidone (IM)	For acute agitation: 10–20 mg, as required, up to a maximum of 40 mg/day	Not applicable	For acute agitation: Doses of 10 mg may be administered every 2 hr, and doses of 20 mg may be administered every 4 hr up to a maximum of 40 mg/day	For acute agitation: 40 mg/day, for not more than 3 consecutive days

Note: Information taken from U.S. Prescribing Information for individual agents.
[a]Dosage adjustments may be required in special populations.
IM, intramuscular.

at clinically effective dosages, newer antipsychotic drugs—the SDAs—have gradually replaced the older agents in the United States. The SDAs are differentiated from earlier drugs by their lower liability to cause extrapyramidal side effects. These newer drugs have other liabilities, most notably a propensity to cause weight gain, lipid elevations, and diabetes. Therefore, a reason to still consider the use of the DRAs is their lower risk of causing significant metabolic abnormalities. Intermediate-potency DRAs, such as perphenazine (Trilafon), are as effective and well tolerated as the SDAs. Manufacturing of molindone (Moban), the DRA with

the lowest risk of weight gain and metabolic side effects, was discontinued in the United States.

Pharmacologic Actions

All of the DRAs are well absorbed after oral administration, with liquid preparations being absorbed more efficiently than tablets or capsules. Peak plasma concentrations are usually reached 1 to 4 hours after oral administration and 30 to 60 minutes after parenteral administration. Smoking, coffee, antacids, and food interfere

Table 21-10
Factors Influencing the Pharmacokinetics of Antipsychotics

Age	Elderly patients may demonstrate reduced clearance rates.
Medical condition	Decreased hepatic blood flow can reduce clearance. Hepatic disease can decrease clearance.
Enzyme inducers	Carbamazepine, phenytoin, ethambutol, barbiturates.
Clearance inhibitors	Include SSRIs, TCAs, cimetidine, β-blockers, isoniazid, methylphenidate, erythromycin, triazolobenzodiazepines, ciprofloxacin, and ketoconazole.
Changes in binding protein	Hypoalbuminemia can occur with malnutrition or hepatic failure.

SSRI, selective serotonin reuptake inhibitor; TCA, tricyclic antidepressant.
Adapted from Ereshefsky L. Pharmacokinetics and drug interactions: update for new antipsychotics. *J Clin Psychiatry*. 1996;57(Suppl 11):12–25.

with the absorption of these drugs. Steady-state levels are reached in approximately 3 to 5 days. The half-lives of these drugs are approximately 24 hours. All can be given in one daily oral dose if tolerated after the patient is in a stable condition. Most DRAs are highly protein-bound. Parenteral formulation of the DRAs results in a more rapid and more reliable onset of action. Bioavailability is also up to 10-fold higher with parenteral administration. Most DRAs are metabolized by cytochrome P450 (CYP) CYP2D6 and 3A isozymes. However, there are differences among the specific agents.

Long-acting depot parenteral formulations of haloperidol (Haldol Decanoate) and fluphenazine are available in the United States. These agents are usually administered once every 1 to 4 weeks, depending on the dose and the patient. It can take up to 6 months of treatment with depot formulations to reach steady-state plasma levels, indicating that oral therapy should be continued during the first month or so of depot antipsychotic treatment.

Antipsychotic activity derives from the inhibition of dopaminergic neurotransmission. The DRAs are effective when approximately 72 percent of dopamine D_2 receptors in the brain are occupied. The DRAs also block noradrenergic, cholinergic, and histaminergic receptors, with different drugs having different effects on these receptor systems.

Some generalizations can be made about the DRAs based on their potency. Potency refers to the amount of drug that is required to achieve therapeutic effects. Low-potency drugs such as chlorpromazine and thioridazine (Mellaril), given in doses of several 100 mg/day, typically produce more weight gain and sedation than high-potency agents such as haloperidol and fluphenazine, usually given in doses of less than 10 mg/day. High-potency agents are also more likely to cause EPS. Some factors influencing the pharmacologic actions of DRAs are listed in Table 21-10.

Therapeutic Indications

Many types of psychiatric and neurologic disorders may benefit from treatment with DRAs. Some of these indications are shown in Table 21-11.

Schizophrenia and Schizoaffective Disorder.
The DRAs are useful in both the short- and long-term management of schizophrenia and schizoaffective disorder. They both reduce acute

Table 21-11
Indications for Dopamine Receptor Antagonists

Acute psychotic episodes in schizophrenia and schizoaffective disorder
Maintenance treatment in schizophrenia and schizoaffective disorders
Mania
Depression with psychotic symptoms
Delusional disorder
Borderline personality disorder
Substance-induced psychotic disorder
Delirium and dementia
Mental disorders caused by a medical condition
Childhood schizophrenia
Autism spectrum disorder
Tourette disorder
Huntington disease

symptoms and prevent future exacerbations. These agents produce their most dramatic effects on the positive symptoms of schizophrenia (e.g., hallucinations, delusions, and agitation). Negative symptoms (e.g., emotional withdrawal and ambivalence) are less likely to improve significantly, and they may appear to worsen because these drugs produce constriction of facial expression and akinesia, side effects that mimic negative symptoms.

Schizophrenia and schizoaffective disorder are characterized by remission and relapse. DRAs decrease the risk of reemergence of psychosis in patients who have recovered while on medication. After the first episode of psychosis, patients should be maintained on medication for 1 to 2 years; after multiple episodes, for 2 to 5 years.

Mania.
DRAs are useful for treating psychotic symptoms of acute mania. Because antimanic agents (e.g., lithium) generally have a slower onset of action than do antipsychotics in the treatment of acute symptoms, it is standard practice to initially combine either a DRA or an SDA with lithium (Eskalith), sodium valproate (Depakote), lamotrigine (Lamictal), or carbamazepine (Tegretol) and then to withdraw the antipsychotic gradually.

Depression with Psychotic Symptoms.
Combination treatment with an antipsychotic and an antidepressant is one of the treatments of choice for MDD with psychotic features; the other is ECT.

Delusional Disorder.
Patients with delusional disorder often respond favorably to treatment with these drugs. Some persons with borderline personality disorder who develop paranoid thinking may respond to antipsychotic drugs.

Severe Agitation and Violent Behavior.
Severely agitated and violent patients, regardless of diagnosis, may be treated with DRAs. Symptoms such as extreme irritability, lack of impulse control, severe hostility, gross hyperactivity, and agitation respond to short-term treatment with these drugs. Children with mental disabilities, especially those with profound intellectual disabilities and autistic disorder, often have associated episodes of violence, aggression, and agitation that respond to treatment with antipsychotic drugs; however, the repeated administration of antipsychotics to control disruptive behavior in children is controversial.

Tourette Disorder.
DRAs are used to treat Tourette's disorder, a neurobehavioral disorder marked by motor and vocal tics. Haloperidol and pimozide (Orap) are the drugs most frequently used, but other DRAs are also useful. Some clinicians prefer to use clonidine (Catapres) for this disorder because of its lower risk of neurologic side effects.

Borderline Personality Disorder.   Patients with borderline personality disorder who experience transient psychotic symptoms, such as perceptual disturbances, suspiciousness, ideas of reference, and aggression, may need to be treated with a DRA. This disorder is also associated with mood instability, so patients should be evaluated for possible treatment with mood-stabilizing agents.

Dementia and Delirium.   About two-thirds of agitated, elderly patients with various forms of dementia improve when given a DRA. Low doses of high-potency drugs (e.g., 0.5 to 1 mg a day of haloperidol) are recommended. DRAs are also used to treat psychotic symptoms and agitation associated with delirium. The cause of the delirium needs to be determined because toxic deliriums caused by anticholinergic agents can be exacerbated by low-potency DRAs, which often have significant antimuscarinic activity. Orthostasis, parkinsonism, and worsened cognition are the most problematic side effects in this elderly population.

Substance-Induced Psychotic Disorder.   Intoxication with cocaine, amphetamines, alcohol, phencyclidine, or other drugs can cause psychotic symptoms. Because these symptoms tend to be time-limited, it is preferable to avoid the use of a DRA unless the patient is severely agitated and aggressive. Usually, benzodiazepines can be used to calm the patient. Benzodiazepines should be used instead of DRAs in cases of phencyclidine intoxication. When a patient is experiencing hallucinations or delusions as a result of alcohol withdrawal, DRAs may increase the risk of seizure.

Childhood Schizophrenia.   Children with schizophrenia benefit from treatment with antipsychotic medication, although considerably less research has been devoted to this population. Studies are underway to determine if intervention with medication at the very earliest signs of disturbance in children genetically at risk for schizophrenia can prevent the emergence of more florid symptoms. Careful consideration needs to be given to side effects, especially those involving cognition and alertness.

Other Psychiatric and Nonpsychiatric Indications.   The DRAs reduce the chorea in the early stages of Huntington disease. Patients with this disease may develop hallucinations, delusions, mania, or hypomania. These and other psychiatric symptoms respond to DRAs. High-potency DRAs should be used. However, clinicians should be aware that patients with a rigid form of this disorder may experience acute EPS. The use of DRAs to treat impulse control disorders should be reserved for patients in whom other interventions have failed. Patients with autism spectrum disorder may exhibit hyperactivity, screaming, and agitation with combativeness. Some of these symptoms respond to high-potency DRAs, but there is little research evidence supporting benefits in these patients.

The rare neurologic disorders ballismus and hemiballismus (which affect only one side of the body), characterized by propulsive movements of the limbs away from the body, also respond to treatment with antipsychotic agents. Other miscellaneous indications for the use of DRAs include the treatment of nausea, emesis, intractable hiccups, and pruritus. Endocrine disorders and temporal lobe epilepsy may be associated with psychosis that responds to antipsychotic treatment.

The most common side effects of DRAs are neurologic. As a rule, low-potency drugs cause the most nonneurologic adverse effects, and high-potency drugs cause the most neurologic adverse effects.

Table 21-12
Dopamine Receptor Antagonists: Potency and Adverse Effects

Drug Name	Chemical Classification	Therapeutically Equivalent Oral	Side Effects		
			Sedation	Autonomic[a]	Extrapyramidal Reactions[b]
Pimozide[c]	Diphenylbutyl-piperidine	1.5	+	+	+++
Fluphenazine	Phenothiazine: piperazine compound	2	+	+	+++
Haloperidol	Butyrophenone	2	+	+	+++
Thiothixene	Thioxanthene	4	+	+	+++
Trifluoperazine	Phenothiazine: piperazine compound	5	++	+	+++
Perphenazine	Phenothiazine: piperazine compound	8	++	+	++/+++
Molindone	Dihydroindolone	10	++	+	+
Loxapine	Dibenzoxazepine	10	++	+/++	++/+++
Prochlor-perazine[c]	Phenothiazine: piperazine compound	15	++	+	+++
Aceto-phenazine	Phenothiazine: piperazine compound	20	++	+	++/+++
Triflupromazine	Phenothiazine: aliphatic compound	25	+++	++/+++	++
Mesoridazine	Phenothiazine: piperidine compound	50	+++	++	+
Chlorpromazine	Phenothiazine: aliphatic compound	100	+++	+++	++
Chlorprothixene	Thioxanthene	100	+++	+++	+/++
Thioridazine	Phenothiazine: piperidine compound	100	+++	+++	+

[a]Anti–α-adrenergic and anticholinergic effects.
[b]Excluding tardive dyskinesia, which appears to be produced to the same degree and frequency by all agents with equieffective antipsychotic dosages.
[c]Pimozide is used principally in the treatment of Tourette disorder; prochlorperazine is used rarely, if ever, as an antipsychotic agent.
Adapted from American Medical Association. *AMA Drug Evaluations: Annual 1992.* Chicago: American Medical Association, 1992.

Precautions and Adverse Reactions

Table 21-12 summarizes the most common adverse events associated with the use of DRAs.

Neuroleptic Malignant Syndrome. A potentially fatal side effect of DRA treatment, neuroleptic malignant syndrome, can occur at any time during DRA treatment. Symptoms include extreme hyperthermia, severe muscular rigidity and dystonia, akinesia, mutism, confusion, agitation, and increased pulse rate and BP. Laboratory findings include increased WBC count and levels of creatinine phosphokinase, liver enzymes, plasma myoglobin, and myoglobinuria, occasionally associated with renal failure. The symptoms usually evolve over 24 to 72 hours, and the untreated syndrome lasts 10 to 14 days. The diagnosis is often missed in the early stages, and the withdrawal or agitation may mistakenly be considered to reflect increased psychosis. Men are affected more frequently than are women, and young persons are affected more commonly than are elderly persons. The mortality rate can reach 20 to 30 percent, or even higher, when depot medications are involved. Rates are also increased when high doses of high-potency agents are used.

If the neuroleptic malignant syndrome is suspected, the DRA should be stopped immediately, and the following done: medical support to cool the person; monitoring of vital signs, electrolytes, fluid balance, and renal output; and symptomatic treatment of fever. Antiparkinsonian medications may reduce some of the muscle rigidity. Dantrolene (Dantrium), a skeletal muscle relaxant (0.8 to 2.5 mg/kg every 6 hours, up to a total dosage of 10 mg a day), may be useful in the treatment of this disorder. When the person can take oral medications, dantrolene can be given in doses of 100 to 200 mg a day. Bromocriptine (20 to 30 mg a day in four divided doses) or amantadine can be added to the regimen. Treatment should usually be continued for 5 to 10 days. When drug treatment is restarted, the clinician should consider switching to a low-potency drug or an SDA, although these agents—including clozapine—may also cause the neuroleptic malignant syndrome.

Seizure Threshold. DRAs may lower the seizure threshold. Chlorpromazine, thioridazine, and other low-potency drugs are thought to be more epileptogenic than are high-potency drugs. The risk of inducing a seizure by drug administration warrants consideration when the person already has a seizure disorder or brain lesion.

Sedation. The blockade of histamine H_1 receptors is the usual cause of sedation associated with DRAs. Chlorpromazine is the most sedating typical antipsychotic. The relative sedative properties of the drugs are summarized in Table 21-12. Giving the entire daily dose at bedtime usually eliminates any problems from sedation, and tolerance for this adverse effect often develops.

Central Anticholinergic Effects. The symptoms of central anticholinergic activity include severe agitation; disorientation to time, person, and place; hallucinations; seizures; high fever; and dilated pupils. Stupor and coma may ensue. The treatment of anticholinergic toxicity consists of discontinuing the causal agent or agents, close medical supervision, and physostigmine (Antilirium, Eserine), 2 mg by slow intravenous (IV) infusion, repeated within 1 hour as necessary. Too much physostigmine is dangerous, and symptoms of physostigmine toxicity include hypersalivation and sweating. Atropine sulfate (0.5 mg) can reverse the effects of physostigmine toxicity.

Cardiac Effects. The DRAs decrease cardiac contractility, disrupt enzyme contractility in cardiac cells, increase circulating levels of catecholamines, and prolong atrial and ventricular conduction time and refractory periods. Low-potency DRAs, particularly the phenothiazines, are usually more cardiotoxic than are high-potency drugs. One exception is haloperidol, which has been linked to abnormal heart rhythm, ventricular arrhythmias, torsades de pointes, and sudden death when injected IV. Pimozide, sulpiride, and droperidol (a butyrophenone) also prolong the QTc interval and have been associated with torsades de pointes and sudden death. In one study, thioridazine was responsible for 28 (61 percent) of the 46 sudden antipsychotic deaths. In 15 of these cases, it was the only drug ingested. Chlorpromazine also causes prolongation of the QT and PR intervals, blunting of the T waves, and depression of the ST segment. These drugs are thus indicated only when other agents have been ineffective.

Sudden Death. Occasional reports of sudden cardiac death during treatment with DRAs may be the result of cardiac arrhythmias. Other causes may include seizure, asphyxiation, malignant hyperthermia, heatstroke, and neuroleptic malignant syndrome. However, there does seem to be an overall increased incidence of sudden death with antipsychotics.

Orthostatic (Postural) Hypotension. Orthostatic (postural) hypotension is most frequent with low-potency drugs, particularly chlorpromazine, thioridazine, and chlorprothixene. When using intramuscular (IM) low-potency DRAs, the clinician should measure the patient's BP (lying and standing) before and after the first dose and during the first few days of treatment.

Orthostatic hypotension is mediated by adrenergic blockade and occurs most frequently during the first few days of treatment. Tolerance often develops for this side effect, which is why the initial dosing of these drugs is lower than the usual therapeutic dose. Fainting or falls, although uncommon, may lead to injury. Patients should be warned of this side effect and instructed to rise slowly after sitting and reclining. Patients should avoid all caffeine and alcohol; should drink at least 2 L of fluid a day; and if not under treatment for hypertension, should add liberal amounts of salt to their diet. Support hose may help some persons.

Hypotension can usually be managed by having patients lie down with their feet higher than their heads and pump their legs as if bicycling. Volume expansion or vasopressor agents, such as norepinephrine (Levophed), may be indicated in severe cases. Because hypotension is produced by α-adrenergic blockade, the drugs also block the α-adrenergic stimulating properties of epinephrine, leaving the β-adrenergic stimulating effects untouched. Therefore, the administration of epinephrine results in a paradoxical worsening of hypotension and is contraindicated in cases of antipsychotic-induced hypotension. Pure α-adrenergic pressor agents, such as metaraminol (Aramine) and norepinephrine, are the drugs of choice in the treatment of the disorder.

Hematologic Effects. Temporary leukopenia with a WBC count of about 3,500 is a common but not a serious problem. Agranulocytosis, a life-threatening hematologic problem, occurs in about 1 in 10,000 persons treated with DRAs. Thrombocytopenic or nonthrombocytopenic purpura, hemolytic anemias, and pancytopenia may rarely occur in persons treated with DRAs. Although routine CBCs are not indicated, if a person reports a sore throat and fever, a CBC should be done immediately to check for the possibility of a severe blood dyscrasia. If blood index values are low, the administration of DRAs should be stopped, and the patient should be transferred to a medical facility. The mortality rate for the complication may be as high as 30 percent.

Peripheral Anticholinergic Effects.   Peripheral anticholinergic effects, such as dry mouth and nose, blurred vision, constipation, urinary retention, and mydriasis, are common. This is especially true with low-potency DRAs, for example, chlorpromazine, thioridazine, mesoridazine (Serentil). Some persons may also have nausea and vomiting.

Constipation should be treated with the usual laxative preparations, but severe constipation can progress to paralytic ileus. A decrease in the DRA dosage is warranted in such cases. Pilocarpine (Salagen) may be used to treat paralytic ileus, although the relief is only transitory. Bethanechol (Urecholine) (20 to 40 mg a day) may be useful in some persons with urinary retention.

Weight gain is associated with increased mortality and morbidity and with medication noncompliance. Low-potency DRAs may cause significant weight gain but not as much as is seen with the SDAs olanzapine (Zyprexa) and clozapine (Clozaril). Molindone and perhaps loxapine (Loxitane) appear to be least likely to cause weight gain.

Endocrine Effects.   Blockade of the dopamine receptors in the tuberoinfundibular tract results in the increased secretion of prolactin, which can result in breast enlargement, galactorrhea, amenorrhea, and inhibited orgasm in women and impotence in men. The SDAs, except risperidone (Risperdal), are not significantly associated with an increase in prolactin levels and may be the drugs of choice for persons experiencing disturbing side effects from increased prolactin release.

Sexual Adverse Effects.   Both men and women taking DRAs can experience anorgasmia and decreased libido. Up to 50 percent of men who take antipsychotics report ejaculatory and erectile disturbances. Sildenafil (Viagra), vardenafil (Levitra), and tadalafil (Cialis) are often used to treat psychotropic-induced orgasmic dysfunction, but they have not been studied in combination with the DRAs. Thioridazine is mainly associated with decreased libido and retrograde ejaculation in men. Priapism and reports of painful orgasms have also been described, both possibly resulting from α_1-adrenergic antagonist activity.

Skin and Eye Effects.   Allergic dermatitis and photosensitivity may occur, especially with low-potency agents. Urticarial, maculopapular, petechial, and edematous eruptions may occur early in treatment, generally in the first few weeks, and remit spontaneously. A photosensitivity reaction that resembles a severe sunburn also occurs in some persons taking chlorpromazine. Persons should be warned of this adverse effect, should spend no more than 30 to 60 minutes in the sun, and should use sunscreens. Long-term chlorpromazine use is associated with blue-gray discoloration of skin areas exposed to sunlight. The skin changes often begin with a tan or golden brown color and progress to such colors as slate gray, metallic blue, and purple. These discolorations resolve when the patient is switched to another medication.

Irreversible retinal pigmentation is associated with the use of thioridazine at dosages above 1,000 mg a day. An early symptom of the side effect can sometimes be nocturnal confusion related to difficulty with night vision. The pigmentation can progress even after thioridazine administration is stopped, finally resulting in blindness. It is for this reason that the maximum recommended dosage of thioridazine is 800 mg/day.

Patients taking chlorpromazine may develop a relatively benign pigmentation of the eyes, characterized by whitish brown granular deposits concentrated in the anterior lens and posterior cornea and visible only by slit-lens examination. The deposits can progress to opaque white and yellow-brown granules, often stellate. Occasionally, the conjunctiva is discolored by a brown pigment. No retinal damage is seen, and vision is rarely impaired. This condition gradually resolves when chlorpromazine is discontinued.

Jaundice.   Elevations of liver enzymes during treatment with a DRA tend to be transient and not clinically significant. When chlorpromazine first came into use, cases of obstructive or cholestatic jaundice were reported, usually in the first month of treatment and heralded by symptoms of upper abdominal pain, nausea, and vomiting. This adverse effect was followed by fever, rash, eosinophilia, bilirubin in the urine, and increases in levels of serum bilirubin, alkaline phosphatase, and hepatic transaminases. Reported cases are now sporadic, but if jaundice occurs, the medication should be discontinued.

Overdoses.   Overdoses typically consist of exaggerated DRA side effects. Symptoms and signs include CNS depression, EPS, mydriasis, rigidity, restlessness, decreased deep tendon reflexes, tachycardia, and hypotension. The severe symptoms of overdose include delirium, coma, respiratory depression, and seizures. Haloperidol may be among the safest typical antipsychotics in overdose. After an overdose, electroencephalography (EEG) shows diffuse slowing and low voltage. An extreme overdose may lead to delirium and coma, with respiratory depression and hypotension. Life-threatening overdose usually involves the ingestion of other CNS depressants, such as alcohol or benzodiazepines.

Activated charcoal, if possible, and gastric lavage should be administered if the overdose is recent. Emetics are not indicated because the antiemetic actions of the DRAs inhibit their efficacy. Seizures can be treated with IV diazepam or phenytoin. Hypotension can be treated with either norepinephrine or dopamine but not epinephrine.

Pregnancy and Lactation.   There is a low correlation between the use of antipsychotics during pregnancy and congenital malformations. Nevertheless, antipsychotics should be avoided during pregnancy, particularly in the first trimester, unless the benefit outweighs the risk. High-potency drugs are preferable to low-potency drugs because low-potency drugs are associated with hypotension.

DRAs are secreted in the breast milk, although concentrations are low. Women taking these agents should be advised against breastfeeding.

Drug Interactions

Many pharmacokinetic and pharmacodynamic drug interactions are associated with these drugs (Table 21-13). CYP2D6 is the most common hepatic isozyme involved in DRA pharmacokinetic interactions. Other common drug interactions affect the absorption of the DRAs.

Antacids, activated charcoal, cholestyramine (Questran), kaolin, pectin, and cimetidine (Tagamet) taken within 2 hours of antipsychotic administration can reduce the absorption of these drugs. Anticholinergics may decrease the absorption of the DRAs.

Table 21-13
Antipsychotic Drug Interactions

Interacting Medication	Mechanism	Clinical Effect
Drug Interactions Assessed to Have Major Severity		
β-Adrenergic receptor antagonists	Synergistic pharmacologic effect; antipsychotic inhibits metabolism of propranolol; antipsychotic increases plasma concentrations	Severe hypotension
Anticholinergics	Pharmacodynamic effects Additive anticholinergic effect	Decreased antipsychotic effect Anticholinergic toxicity
Barbiturates	Phenobarbital induces antipsychotic metabolism	Decreased antipsychotic concentrations
Carbamazepine	Induces antipsychotic metabolism	Up to 50% reduction in antipsychotic concentrations
Charcoal	Reduces GI absorption of antipsychotic and adsorbs drug during enterohepatic circulation	May reduce antipsychotic effect or cause toxicity when used to treat overdose or for GI disturbances
Cigarette smoking	Induction of microsomal enzymes	Reduced plasma concentrations of antipsychotic agents
Epinephrine, norepinephrine	Antipsychotic antagonizes pressor effect	Hypotension
Ethanol	Additive CNS depression	Impaired psychomotor status
Fluvoxamine	Fluvoxamine inhibits metabolism of haloperidol and clozapine	Increased concentrations of haloperidol and clozapine
Guanethidine	Antipsychotic antagonizes guanethidine reuptake	Impaired antihypertensive effect
Lithium	Unknown	Rare reports of neurotoxicity
Meperidine	Additive CNS depression	Hypotension and sedation
Drug Interactions Assessed to Have Minor or Moderate Severity		
Amphetamines, anorexiants	Decreased pharmacologic effect of amphetamine	Diminished weight loss effect; amphetamines may exacerbate psychosis
ACEIs	Additive hypotensive crisis	Hypotension, postural intolerance
Antacids containing aluminum	Insoluble complex formed in GI tract	Possible reduced antipsychotic effect
AD nonspecific	Decreased metabolism of AD through competitive inhibition	Increased AD concentration
Benzodiazepines	Increased pharmacologic effect of the benzodiazepine	Respiratory depression, stupor, hypotension
Bromocriptine	Antipsychotic antagonizes dopamine receptor stimulation	Increased prolactin
Caffeinated beverages	Form precipitate with antipsychotic solutions	Possible diminished antipsychotic effect
Cimetidine	Reduced antipsychotic absorption and clearance	Decreased antipsychotic effect
Clonidine	Antipsychotic potentiates α-adrenergic hypotensive effect	Hypotension or hypertension
Disulfiram	Impairs antipsychotic metabolism	Increased antipsychotic concentrations
Methyldopa	Unknown	BP elevations
Phenytoin	Induction of antipsychotic metabolism; decreased phenytoin metabolism	Decreased antipsychotic concentrations: increased phenytoin levels
SSRIs	Impair antipsychotic metabolism; pharmacodynamic interaction	Sudden onset of extrapyramidal symptoms
Valproic acid	Antipsychotic inhibits valproic acid metabolism	Increased valproic acid half-life and levels

ACEI, angiotensin-converting enzyme inhibitor; AD, antidepressant; BP, blood pressure; CNS, central nervous system; GI, gastrointestinal; SSRI, selective serotonin reuptake inhibitor.
From Ereshosky L, Overman GP, Karp JK. Current psychotropic dosing and monitoring guidelines. *Prim Psychiatry.* 1996;3:21, with permission.

The additive anticholinergic activity of the DRAs, anticholinergics, and tricyclic drugs may result in anticholinergic toxicity. Digoxin (Lanoxin) and steroids, both of which decrease gastric motility, can increase DRA absorption.

Phenothiazines, especially thioridazine, may decrease the metabolism of and cause toxic concentrations of phenytoin. Barbiturates may increase the metabolism of DRAs.

Tricyclic drugs and SSRIs that inhibit CYP2D6—paroxetine (Paxil), fluoxetine (Prozac), and fluvoxamine (Luvox)—interact with DRAs, resulting in increased plasma concentrations of both drugs. The anticholinergic, sedative, and hypotensive effects of the drugs may also be cumulative.

Typical antipsychotics may inhibit the hypotensive effects of α-methyldopa (Aldomet). Conversely, typical antipsychotics may have an additive effect on some hypotensive drugs. Antipsychotic drugs have a variable effect on the hypotensive effects of clonidine. Propranolol (Inderal) coadministration increases the blood concentrations of both drugs.

The DRAs potentiate the CNS-depressant effects of the sedatives, antihistamines, opiates, opioids, and alcohol, particularly in persons with impaired respiratory status. When these agents are taken with alcohol, the risk for heatstroke may be increased.

Cigarette smoking may decrease the plasma levels of the typical antipsychotic drugs. Epinephrine has a paradoxical hypotensive effect in persons taking typical antipsychotics. These drugs may decrease the blood concentration of warfarin (Coumadin), resulting in decreased bleeding time. The phenothiazines, thioridazine, and pimozide should not be coadministered with other agents that prolong the QT interval. Thioridazine is contraindicated in patients taking drugs that inhibit the CYP2D6 isoenzyme or in patients with reduced levels of CYP2D6.

Laboratory Interferences

Chlorpromazine and perphenazine (Trilafon) may cause both false-positive and false-negative results in immunologic pregnancy tests and falsely elevated bilirubin (with reagent test strips) and urobilinogen (with Ehrlich reagent test) values. These drugs are associated with an abnormal shift in the results of the glucose tolerance test. However, that shift may reflect the effects of the drugs on the glucose-regulating system. Phenothiazines have been reported to interfere with the measurement of 17-ketosteroids and 17-hydroxycorticosteroids and produce false-positive results in tests for phenylketonuria.

Dosage and Clinical Guidelines

Contraindications to the use of DRAs include the following: (1) a history of a severe allergic response; (2) the possible ingestion of a substance that will interact with the antipsychotic to induce CNS depression (e.g., alcohol, opioids, barbiturates, and benzodiazepines) or anticholinergic delirium (e.g., scopolamine and possibly phencyclidine [PCP]); (3) the presence of a severe cardiac abnormality; (4) a high risk for seizures; (5) the presence of narrow-angle glaucoma or prostatic hypertrophy if a drug with high anticholinergic activity is to be used; and (6) the presence or a history of tardive dyskinesia. Antipsychotics should be administered with caution in persons with hepatic disease because impaired hepatic metabolism may result in high plasma concentrations. The usual assessment should include a CBC with WBC indexes, liver function tests, and electrocardiography (ECG), especially in women older than 40 years of age and men older than 30 years of age. Elderly persons and children are more sensitive to side effects than are young adults, so the dosage of the drug should be adjusted accordingly.

Various patients may respond to widely different dosages of antipsychotics; therefore, there is no set dosage for any given antipsychotic drug. Because of side effects, it is a reasonable clinical practice to begin at a low dosage and increase as necessary. It is important to remember that the maximal effects of a particular dosage may not be evident for 4 to 6 weeks. Available preparations and dosages of the DRAs are given in Table 21-14.

Short-Term Treatment.   The equivalent of 5 to 20 mg of haloperidol is a reasonable dose for an adult in an acute state. An older adult may benefit from as little as 1 mg of haloperidol. The administration of more than 25 mg of chlorpromazine in one injection

may result in profound hypotension. IM administration results in peak plasma levels in about 30 minutes versus 90 minutes using the oral route. Doses of drugs for IM administration are about half those given by the oral route. In a short-term treatment setting, the person should be observed for 1 hour after the first dose of medication. After that time, most clinicians administer a second dose or a sedative agent (e.g., a benzodiazepine) to achieve effective behavioral control. Possible sedatives include lorazepam (Ativan) (2 mg IM) and amobarbital (50 to 250 mg IM).

Rapid Neuroleptization.   Rapid neuroleptization (also called psychotolysis) is the practice of administering hourly IM doses of antipsychotic medications until marked sedation is achieved. However, several research studies have shown that merely waiting several more hours after one dose yields the same clinical improvement as is seen with repeated doses. Nevertheless, clinicians must be careful to keep patients from becoming violent while they are psychotic. Clinicians can help prevent violent episodes by using adjuvant sedatives or by temporarily using physical restraints until the persons can control their behavior.

Early Treatment.   A full 6 weeks may be necessary to evaluate the extent of the improvement in psychotic symptoms. However, agitation and excitement usually improve quickly with antipsychotic treatment. About 75 percent of persons with a short history of illness show significant improvement in their psychosis. Psychotic symptoms, both positive and negative, usually continue to improve 3 to 12 months after the initiation of treatment.

About 5 mg of haloperidol or 300 mg of chlorpromazine is a usual effective daily dose. In the past, much higher doses were used, but evidence suggests that it resulted in more side effects without additional benefits. A single daily dose is usually given at bedtime to help induce sleep and to reduce the incidence of adverse effects. However, bedtime dosing for elderly persons may increase their risk of falling if they get out of bed during the night. The sedative effects of typical antipsychotics last only a few hours, in contrast to the antipsychotic effects, which last for 1 to 3 days.

Intermittent Medications.   It is a common clinical practice to order medications to be given intermittently as needed (PRN). Although this practice may be reasonable during the first few days that a person is hospitalized, the amount of time the person takes antipsychotic drugs, rather than an increase in dosage, is what produces therapeutic improvement. Clinicians on inpatient services may feel pressured by staff members to write PRN antipsychotic orders; such orders should include specific symptoms, how often the drugs should be given, and how many doses can be given each day. Clinicians may choose to use small doses for the PRN doses (e.g., 2 mg of haloperidol) or use a benzodiazepine instead (e.g., 2 mg of lorazepam IM). If PRN doses of an antipsychotic are necessary after the first week of treatment, the clinician may want to consider increasing the standing daily dose of the drug.

Maintenance Treatment.   The first 3 to 6 months after a psychotic episode are usually considered a period of stabilization. After that time, the dosage can be decreased by about 20 percent every 6 months until the minimum effective dosage is found. A person is usually maintained on antipsychotic medications for 1 to 2 years after the first psychotic episode. Antipsychotic treatment is often continued for 5 years after a second psychotic episode, and lifetime maintenance is considered after the third psychotic episode, although attempts to reduce the daily dosage can be made every 6 to 12 months.

Table 21-14
Dopamine Receptor Antagonists

Name		Tablets (mg)	Capsules (mg)	Solution	Parenteral	Rectal Suppositories (mg)	Adult Dose Range (mg/day)	
Generic or Chemical	Trade						Acute	Maintenance
Chlorpromazine	Thorazine	10, 25, 50, 100, 200	30, 75, 150, 200, 300	10 mg/5 mL, 30 mg/mL, 100 mg/mL	25 mg/mL	25, 100	100–1,600 PO, 25–400 IM	50–400 PO
Prochlorperazine	Compazine	5, 10, 25	10, 15, 30	5 mg/5 mL	5 mg/mL	2.5, 5, 25	15–200 PO, 40–80 IM	15–60 PO
Perphenazine	Trilafon	2, 4, 8, 16	—	16 mg/5 mL	5 mg/mL	—	12–64 PO, 15–30 IM	8–24 PO
Trifluoperazine	Stelazine	1, 2, 5, 10	—	10 mg/mL	2 mg/mL	—	4–40 PO, 4–10 IM	5–20 PO
Fluphenazine	Prolixin	1, 2.5, 5, 10	—	2.5 mg/5 mL, 5 mg/mL	2.5 mg/mL (IM only)	—	2.5–40.0 PO, 5–20 IM	1.0–15.0 PO, 12.5–50.0 IM (decanoate or enanthate, weekly or biweekly)
Fluphenazine decanoate	—	—	—	—	2.5 mg/mL	—	—	—
Fluphenazine enanthate	—	—	—	2.5 mg/mL	—	—	—	—
Thioridazine	Mellaril	10, 15, 25, 50, 100, 150, 200	—	25 mg/5 mL, 100 mg/5 mL, 30 mg/mL, 100 mg/mL	—	—	200–800 PO	100–300 PO
Mesoridazine	Serentil	10, 25, 50, 100	—	25 mg/mL	25 mg/mL	—	100–400 PO, 25–200 IM	30–150 PO
Haloperidol	Haldol	0.5, 1, 2, 5, 10, 20	—	2 mg/5 mL	5 mg/mL (IM only)	—	5–20 PO, 12.5–25 IM	1–10 PO
Haloperidol decanoate	—	—	—	—	50 mg/mL, 100 mg/mL (IM only)	—	—	25–200 IM (decanoate, monthly)
Chlorprothixene	Taractan	10, 25, 50, 100	—	100 mg/5 mL (suspension)	12.5 mg/mL	—	75–600 PO, 75–200 IM	50–400 PO
Thiothixene	Navane	—	1, 2, 5, 10, 20	5 mg/mL	5 mg/mL (IM only), 20 mg/mL (IM only)	—	60–100 PO, 8–30 IM	6–30 PO
Loxapine	Loxitane	—	5, 10, 25, 50	25 mg/5 mL	50 mg/mL	—	20–250 PO, 20–75 IM	20–100 PO
Molindone	Moban	5, 10, 25, 50, 100	—	20 mg/mL	—	—	50–225 PO	5–150 PO
Pimozide	Orap	2	—	—	—	—	0.5–20 PO	0.5–5.0 PO

IM, intramuscular; PO, oral.

Antipsychotic drugs are effective in controlling psychotic symptoms, but persons may report that they prefer being off the drugs because they feel better without them. The clinician must discuss maintenance medication with patients and take into account their wishes, the severity of their illnesses, and the quality of their support systems. The clinician needs to know enough about the patient's life to try to predict upcoming stressors that might require increasing the dosage or closely monitoring compliance.

Long-Acting Depot Medications.   Long-acting depot preparations may be needed to overcome problems with compliance. IM preparations are typically given once every 1 to 4 weeks.

Two depot preparations, a decanoate and an enanthate of fluphenazine, and a decanoate preparation of haloperidol, are available in the United States. The preparations are injected IM into an area of extensive muscle tissue, from which they are absorbed slowly into the blood. Decanoate preparations can be given less frequently than enanthate preparations because they are absorbed more slowly. Although stabilizing a person on the oral preparation of the specific drugs is not necessary before initiating the depot form, it is good practice to give at least one oral dose of the drug to assess the possibility of an adverse effect, such as severe EPS or an allergic reaction.

It is reasonable to begin with either 12.5 mg (0.5 mL) of fluphenazine preparation or 25 mg (0.5 mL) of haloperidol decanoate. If symptoms emerge in the next 2 to 4 weeks, the person can be treated temporarily with additional oral medications or with additional small depot injections. After 3 to 4 weeks, the depot injection can be increased to a single dose equal to the total of the doses given during the initial period.

A good reason to initiate depot treatment with low doses is that the absorption of the preparations may be faster than usual at the onset of treatment, resulting in frightening episodes of dystonia that eventually discourage compliance with the medication. Some clinicians keep patients drug free for 3 to 7 days before initiating depot treatment and give small doses of the depot preparations (3.125 mg of fluphenazine or 6.25 mg of haloperidol) every few days to avoid those initial problems.

Plasma Concentrations

Genetic differences among persons and pharmacokinetic interactions with other drugs influence the metabolism of the antipsychotics. If a person has not improved after 4 to 6 weeks of treatment, the plasma concentration of the drug should be determined if feasible. After a patient has been on a particular dosage for at least five times the half-life of the drug and thus approaches steady-state concentrations, blood levels may be helpful. It is standard practice to obtain plasma samples at trough levels—just before the daily dose is given, usually at least 12 hours after the previous dose, and most commonly 20 to 24 hours after the previous dose. Most antipsychotics have no well-defined dose–response curve. The best-studied drug is haloperidol, which may have a therapeutic window ranging from 2 to 15 ng/mL. Other therapeutic ranges that have been reasonably well documented are 30 to 100 ng/mL for chlorpromazine and 0.8 to 2.4 ng/mL for perphenazine.

Treatment-Resistant Persons.   Unfortunately, 10 to 35 percent of persons with schizophrenia do not obtain significant benefit from the antipsychotic drugs. Treatment resistance is a failure on at least two adequate trials of antipsychotics from two pharmacologic classes. It is useful to determine plasma concentrations for such

persons because it is possible that they are slow or rapid metabolizers or are not taking their medication. Clozapine has been conclusively shown to be effective when given to patients who have failed multiple trials of DRAs.

Adjunctive Medications.   It is common practice to use DRAs in conjunction with other psychotropic agents, either to treat side effects or to improve symptoms further. Most commonly, this involves the use of lithium or other mood-stabilizing agents, SSRIs, or benzodiazepines. It was once held that antidepressant drugs exacerbated psychosis in patients with schizophrenia. In all likelihood, this observation involved patients with bipolar disorder who were misdiagnosed as having schizophrenia. Abundant evidence suggests that antidepressants improve symptoms of depression in patients with schizophrenia. In some cases, amphetamines can be added to DRAs if patients remain withdrawn and apathetic.

Choice of Drug

Given their proven efficacy in managing acute psychotic symptoms and the fact that prophylactic administration of antiparkinsonian medication prevents or minimizes acute motor abnormalities, DRAs are still valuable, especially for short-term therapy. There is a considerable cost advantage to a DRA antiparkinsonian regimen compared with monotherapy with a newer antipsychotic agent. Concern about the development of DRA-induced tardive dyskinesia is the primary deterrent to long-term use of these drugs, yet it is not clear that SDAs are entirely free of this complication. Thus, DRAs still occupy an important role in psychiatric treatment. DRAs are not predictably interchangeable. For reasons that cannot be explained, some patients do better on one drug than another. The choice of a particular DRA should be based on the known adverse effect profile of the drugs. Other than a significant advantage in terms of medication cost, the choice currently would be an SDA. If a DRA is thought to be preferable, a high-potency antipsychotic is favored, even though it may be associated with more neurologic adverse effects, mainly because there is a higher incidence of other adverse effects (e.g., cardiac, hypotensive, epileptogenic, sexual, and allergic) with the low-potency drugs. If sedation is the desired goal, either a low-potency antipsychotic can be given in divided doses, or a benzodiazepine can be coadministered.

An unpleasant or dysphoric reaction (a subjective sense of restlessness, oversedation, and acute dystonia) to the first dose of an antipsychotic predicts future inadequate response and noncompliance. Prophylactic use of antiparkinsonian medications may prevent this reaction. In general, clinicians should be vigilant about serious side effects and adverse events (described above) regardless of which drug is used.

▲ 21.2 Antidepressants

SELECTIVE SEROTONIN REUPTAKE INHIBITORS

Fluoxetine (Prozac), the first SSRI marketed in the United States, rapidly captured the favor of both clinicians and the general public as reports emerged of dramatic patient responses to treatment of depression. Patients no longer experienced such side effects as dry mouth, constipation, sedation, orthostatic hypotension, and tachycardia, typical side effects associated with the earlier antidepressant drugs—the TCAs and MAOIs. It was also significantly safer when

Table 21-15
Currently Approved Indications of the Selective Serotonin Reuptake Inhibitors in the United States for Adult and Pediatric Populations

	Citalopram (Celexa)	Escitalopram (Lexapro)	Fluoxetine (Prozac)	Fluvoxamine (Luvox)	Paroxetine (Paxil)	Sertraline (Zoloft)	Vilazodone (Viibryd)
Major depressive disorder	Adult	Adult	Adult[a] and pediatric	—	Adult[b]	Adult	Adult
Generalized anxiety disorder	—	Adult	—	—	Adult	—	—
OCD	—	—	Adult and pediatric	Adult and pediatric	Adult	Adult and pediatric	—
Panic disorder	—	—	Adult	—	Adult[b]	Adult	—
PTSD	—	—	—	—	Adult	Adult	—
Social anxiety disorder	—	—	—	—	Adult[b]	Adult	—
Bulimia nervosa	—	—	Adult	—	—	—	—
Premenstrual dysphoric disorder	—	—	Adult[c]	—	Adult[d]	Adult	—

OCD, obsessive-compulsive disorder; PTSD, posttraumatic stress disorder.
[a]Weekly fluoxetine is approved for continuation and maintenance therapy in adults.
[b]Paroxetine and paroxetine controlled-release.
[c]Marketed as Sarafem.
[d]Paroxetine-controlled release is approved for premenstrual dysphoric disorder.

taken in overdose than any previously available antidepressant. A significant effect of fluoxetine's popularity was that it helped ameliorate the long-standing stigma of depression and its treatment.

Other SSRIs followed fluoxetine. These include sertraline (Zoloft), paroxetine (Paxil), fluvoxamine (Luvox), citalopram (Celexa), escitalopram (Lexapro), and vilazodone (Viibryd). These drugs are all equally effective in treating depression. However, some are approved by the U.S. FDA for multiple indications, such as major depression, OCD, PTSD, PMDD, panic disorder, and social phobia (social anxiety disorder) (Table 21-15). Note that fluvoxamine is not FDA approved as an antidepressant, a fact that is due to a marketing decision. It is considered an antidepressant in other countries.

Although all SSRIs are equally effective, there are meaningful differences in pharmacodynamics, pharmacokinetics, and side effects, differences that might affect clinical responses among individual patients. This would explain why some patients have better clinical responses to a particular SSRI than another. The SSRIs have proven more problematic in terms of some side effects than the original clinical trials suggested. Quality-of-life–associated adverse effects such as nausea, sexual dysfunction, and weight gain sometimes mitigate the therapeutic benefits of the SSRIs. There can also be distressing withdrawal symptoms when SSRIs are stopped abruptly. This withdrawal is especially true with paroxetine but also occurs when other SSRIs with short half-lives are stopped.

Pharmacologic Actions

Pharmacokinetics.   A significant difference among the SSRIs is their broad range of serum half-lives. Fluoxetine has the most prolonged half-life: 4 to 6 days; its active metabolite has a half-life of 7 to 9 days. The half-life of sertraline is 26 hours, and its less active metabolite has a half-life of 3 to 5 days. The half-lives of the other three, which do not have metabolites with significant pharmacologic activity, are 35 hours for citalopram, 27 to 32 hours for escitalopram, 21 hours for paroxetine, and 15 hours for fluvoxamine. As a rule, the SSRIs are well absorbed after oral administration and

have their peak effects in the range of 3 to 8 hours. Absorption of sertraline may be slightly enhanced by food.

There are also differences in plasma protein–binding percentages among the SSRIs, with sertraline, fluoxetine, and paroxetine being the most highly bound and escitalopram being the least bound.

All SSRIs are metabolized in the liver by the CYP450 enzymes. Because the SSRIs have such a broad therapeutic index, other drugs rarely produce problematic increases in SSRI concentrations. The most critical drug–drug interactions involving the SSRIs occur as a result of the SSRIs inhibiting the metabolism of the coadministered medication. Each of the SSRIs possesses a potential for slowing or blocking the metabolism of many drugs (Table 21-16). Fluvoxamine is the most problematic of the drugs in this respect. It has a marked effect on several of the CYP enzymes. Examples of clinically significant interactions include fluvoxamine and theophylline (Slo-Bid, Theo-Dur) through CYP1A2 interaction, fluvoxamine and clozapine (Clozaril) through CYP1A2 inhibition; and fluvoxamine with alprazolam (Xanax) or clonazepam (Klonopin) through CYP3A4 inhibition. Fluoxetine and paroxetine also possess significant effects on the CYP2D6 isozyme, which may interfere with the efficacy of opiate analogs, such as codeine and hydrocodone, by blocking the conversion of these agents to their active form. Thus, coadministration of fluoxetine and paroxetine with an opiate interferes with its analgesic effects. Sertraline, citalopram, and escitalopram are least likely to complicate treatment because of interactions.

The pharmacokinetics of vilazodone (5 to 80 mg) is dose-proportional. Steady-state plasma levels are achieved in about 3 days. The elimination of vilazodone is primarily by hepatic metabolism with a terminal half-life of approximately 25 hours.

Pharmacodynamics.   The SSRIs are believed to exert their therapeutic effects through serotonin reuptake inhibition. They derive their name because they have little effect on the reuptake of norepinephrine or dopamine. Often, adequate clinical activity and saturation of the 5-HT transporters are achieved at starting dosages.

Table 21-16
CYP450 Inhibitory Potential of Commonly Prescribed Antidepressants

Relative Rank	CYP1A2	CYP2C	CYP2D6	CYP3A
Higher	Fluvoxamine (Luvox)	Fluoxetine Fluvoxamine	Bupropion Fluoxetine Paroxetine	Fluvoxamine Nefazodone Tricyclics
Moderate	Tertiary amine tricyclics Fluoxetine (Prozac)	Sertraline	Secondary amine tricyclics Citalopram (Celexa) Escitalopram (Lexapro) Sertraline	Fluoxetine Sertraline
Low or minimal	Bupropion (Wellbutrin) Mirtazapine (Remeron) Nefazodone (Serzone) Paroxetine (Paxil) Sertraline (Zoloft) Venlafaxine (Effexor)	Paroxetine Venlafaxine	Fluvoxamine Mirtazapine Nefazodone Venlafaxine	Citalopram Escitalopram Mirtazapine Paroxetine Venlafaxine

CYP, cytochrome P450.

As a rule, higher dosages do not increase antidepressant efficacy but may increase the risk of adverse effects.

Citalopram and escitalopram are the most selective inhibitors of serotonin reuptake, with very little inhibition of norepinephrine or dopamine reuptake and very low affinities for histamine H_1, GABA, or benzodiazepine receptors. The other SSRIs have a similar profile except that fluoxetine weakly inhibits norepinephrine reuptake and binds to 5-HT_{2C} receptors, sertraline weakly inhibits norepinephrine and dopamine reuptake, and paroxetine has significant anticholinergic activity at higher dosages and binds to nitric oxide synthase. The SSRI vilazodone has 5-HT_{1A} receptor agonist properties. The clinical implications of the 5-HT_{1A} receptor agonist effects are not yet evident.

A pharmacodynamic interaction appears to underlie the antidepressant effects of combined fluoxetine–olanzapine. When taken together, these drugs increase brain concentrations of norepinephrine. Concomitant use of SSRIs and drugs in the triptan class (sumatriptan [Imitrex], naratriptan [Amerge], rizatriptan [Maxalt], and zolmitriptan [Zomig]) may result in a severe pharmacodynamic interaction—the development of serotonin syndrome (see "Precautions and Adverse Reactions"). However, many people use triptans while taking low doses of an SSRI for headache prophylaxis without adverse reaction. A similar reaction may occur when SSRIs are combined with tramadol (Ultram).

Therapeutic Indications

Depression. In the United States, all SSRIs other than fluvoxamine have been approved by the FDA for the treatment of depression. Several studies have found that antidepressants with serotonin-norepinephrine activity—drugs such as the MAOIs, TCAs, venlafaxine (Effexor), and mirtazapine (Remeron)—may produce higher rates of remission than SSRIs in head-to-head studies. The continued role of SSRIs as first-line treatment thus reflects their simplicity of use, safety, and a broad spectrum of action.

Direct comparisons of individual SSRIs have not revealed any to be consistently superior to another. There nevertheless can be considerable diversity in response to the various SSRIs among individuals. For example, more than 50 percent of people who respond poorly to one SSRI will respond favorably to another. Thus, before shifting to non-SSRI antidepressants, it is most reasonable to try other agents in the SSRI class for persons who did not respond to the first SSRI.

Some clinicians have attempted to select a particular SSRI for a specific person based on the drug's unique adverse effect profile. For example, thinking that fluoxetine is an activating and stimulating SSRI, they may assume it is a better choice for an abulic person than paroxetine, which is presumed to be a sedating SSRI. These differences, however, usually vary from person to person. Analyses of clinical trial data show that SSRIs are more effective in patients with more severe symptoms of major depression than those with milder symptoms.

SUICIDE. The FDA has issued a black box warning for antidepressants and suicidal thoughts and behavior in children and young adults. This warning is based on a decade-old analysis of clinical trial data. More recent, comprehensive reanalysis of data has shown that suicidal thoughts and behavior decreased over time for adult and geriatric patients treated with antidepressants as compared with placebo. No differences were found for youths. In adults, reduction in suicide ideation and attempts occurred through a reduction in depressive symptoms. In all age groups, the severity of depression improved with medication and was significantly related to suicide ideation or behavior. It appears that SSRIs, as well as serotonin-norepinephrine reuptake inhibitors (SNRIs), have a protective effect against suicide that is mediated by decreases in depressive symptoms with treatment. For youths, no significant effects of treatment on suicidal thoughts and behavior were found, although depression responded to treatment. No evidence of increased suicide risk was observed in youths receiving active medication. It is crucial to keep in mind that SSRIs, like all antidepressants, prevent potential suicides as a result of their primary action, the shortening and prevention of depressive episodes. In clinical practice, a few patients become anxious and agitated when started on an SSRI. The appearance of these symptoms could conceivably provoke or aggravate suicidal ideation. Thus, all depressed patients should be closely monitored during the period of maximum risk, the first few days and weeks they are taking SSRIs.

DEPRESSION DURING PREGNANCY AND POSTPARTUM. Rates of relapse of major depression during pregnancy among women who discontinue, attempt to discontinue, or modify their antidepressant regimens are very high. Rates range from 68 to 100 percent of patients. Thus, many women need to continue taking their medication during pregnancy and postpartum. The impact of maternal depression on infant development is unknown. There is no significantly increased risk for major congenital malformations after exposure to SSRIs during pregnancy (with the exception of paroxetine, discussed below). Thus, the risk of relapse into depression when a newly pregnant mother is taken off SSRIs is severalfold higher than the risk to the fetus of exposure to SSRIs.

There is some evidence suggesting increased rates of special care nursery admissions after delivery for children of mothers taking SSRIs. There is also a potential for a discontinuation syndrome with paroxetine. However, there is an absence of clinically significant neonatal complications associated with SSRI use.

Studies that have followed children into their early school years have failed to find any perinatal complications, congenital fetal anomalies, decreases in global intelligence quotient (IQ), language delays, or specific behavioral problems attributable to the use of fluoxetine during pregnancy.

Postpartum depression (with or without psychotic features) affects a small percentage of mothers. Some clinicians start administering SSRIs if the postpartum blues extend beyond a few weeks or if a woman becomes depressed during pregnancy. The head start afforded by starting SSRI administration during pregnancy if a woman is at risk for postpartum depression also protects the newborn, toward whom the woman may have harmful thoughts after parturition.

Babies whose mothers are taking an SSRI in the latter part of pregnancy may be at a slight risk of developing pulmonary hypertension. Data about the risk of this side effect are inconclusive, but it is estimated to involve 1 to 2 babies for 1,000 births. Paroxetine should be avoided during pregnancy.

The FDA classified paroxetine as a pregnancy Category D medication in the former FDA classification system. In 2005, the FDA issued an alert that paroxetine increases the risk of congenital disabilities, particularly heart defects, when women take it during the first 3 months of pregnancy. Paroxetine should usually not be taken during pregnancy, but for some women who have already been taking paroxetine, the benefits of continuing paroxetine may be greater than the potential risk to the baby. Women taking paroxetine who are pregnant, think they may be pregnant, or plan to become pregnant should talk to their physicians about the potential risks of taking paroxetine during pregnancy.

The FDA alert was based on the findings of studies that showed that women who took paroxetine during the first 3 months of pregnancy were about one-and-a-half to two times as likely to have a baby with a heart defect as women who received other antidepressants or women in the general population. Most of the heart defects in these studies were not life-threatening and happened mainly in the inside walls of the heart muscle, where repairs can be made if needed (atrial and ventricular septal defects). Sometimes these septal defects resolve without treatment. In one of the studies, the risk of heart defects in babies whose mothers had taken paroxetine early in pregnancy was 2 percent, compared with a 1 percent risk in the whole population. In the other study, the risk of heart defects in babies whose mothers had taken paroxetine in the first 3 months of pregnancy was 1.5 percent, compared with 1 percent in babies whose mothers had taken other antidepressants in the first 3 months of pregnancy. This study also showed that women who took paroxetine in the first 3 months of pregnancy were about twice as likely to have a baby with any congenital disability as women who took other antidepressants.

Minimal amounts of SSRIs are found in breast milk, and no harmful effects have been found in breastfed babies. Concentrations of sertraline and escitalopram are exceptionally low in breast milk. However, in some cases, reported concentrations might be higher than average. No decision regarding the use of an SSRI is risk-free. It is thus essential to document that communication of potential risks to the patient has taken place.

DEPRESSION IN ELDERLY AND MEDICALLY ILL PERSONS. The SSRIs are safe and well tolerated when used to treat elderly and medically ill persons. As a class, they have little or no cardiotoxic, anticholinergic, antihistaminergic, or α-adrenergic adverse effects. Paroxetine does have some anticholinergic activity, which may lead to constipation and worsening of cognition. The SSRIs can produce subtle cognitive deficits, prolonged bleeding time, and hyponatremia, all of which may impact the health of this population. The SSRIs are effective in poststroke depression and dramatically reduce the symptom of crying.

DEPRESSION IN CHILDREN. The use of SSRI antidepressants in children and adolescents has been controversial. Few studies have shown clear-cut benefits from the use of these drugs, and studies show that there may be an increase in suicidal or aggressive impulses. However, some children and adolescents do exhibit dramatic responses to these drugs in terms of depression and anxiety. Fluoxetine has most consistently demonstrated effectiveness in reducing symptoms of depressive disorder in both children and adolescents. This fact may be a function of the quality of the clinical trials involved. Sertraline is effective in treating social anxiety disorder in this population, especially when combined with cognitive-behavioral therapy. Given the potential adverse effect of untreated depression and anxiety in a young population and the uncertainty about many aspects of how children and adolescents might react to medication, any use of SSRIs should be undertaken only within the context of comprehensive management of the patient.

Anxiety Disorders

OBSESSIVE-COMPULSIVE DISORDER. Fluvoxamine, paroxetine, sertraline, and fluoxetine are indicated for the treatment of OCD in persons older than the age of 18 years. Fluvoxamine, fluoxetine, and sertraline have also been approved for the treatment of children with OCD (ages 6 to 17 years). About 50 percent of persons with OCD begin to show symptoms in childhood or adolescence, and more than half of these respond favorably to medication. Beneficial responses can be dramatic. Long-term data support the model of OCD as a genetically determined, lifelong condition that is best treated continuously with drugs and cognitive-behavioral therapy from the onset of symptoms in childhood throughout the lifespan.

SSRI dosages for OCD may need to be higher than those required to treat depression. Although some responses can be seen in the first few weeks of treatment, it may take several months for the maximum effects to become evident. Patients who fail to obtain adequate relief of their OCD symptoms with an SSRI will usually benefit from the addition of a small dose of risperidone (Risperdal). Apart from the extrapyramidal side effects of risperidone, patients should be monitored for increases in prolactin levels when this combination is used. Clinically, hyperprolactinemia may manifest as gynecomastia and galactorrhea (in both men and women) and loss of menses.

Several disorders are now considered to be within the OCD spectrum. This spectrum includes several conditions and symptoms characterized by nonsuicidal self-mutilation, such as trichotillomania, eyebrow picking, nose picking, nail-biting, compulsive picking of skin blemishes, and cutting. Patients with these behaviors benefit from treatment with SSRIs. Other spectrum disorders include compulsive gambling, compulsive shopping, hypochondriasis, and body dysmorphic disorder.

PANIC DISORDER. Paroxetine, fluoxetine, and sertraline are indicated for the treatment of panic disorder, with or without agoraphobia. These agents work less rapidly than do benzodiazepines but are far superior to them for the treatment of panic disorder with comorbid depression. Citalopram and fluvoxamine also may reduce spontaneous or induced panic attacks. Because fluoxetine can initially heighten anxiety symptoms, persons with panic disorder must begin taking small dosages (5 mg a day) and increase the dosage slowly. Low doses of benzodiazepines may be given to manage this side effect.

SOCIAL ANXIETY DISORDER. SSRIs are effective agents in the treatment of social phobia. They reduce both symptoms and disability. The response rate is comparable to that seen with the MAOI phenelzine (Nardil), the previous standard treatment. The SSRIs are safer to use than MAOIs or benzodiazepines.

POSTTRAUMATIC STRESS DISORDER. Pharmacotherapy for PTSD must target specific symptoms in four clusters: reexperiencing, avoidance, negative changes in mood and thinking, and arousal. For long-term treatment, SSRIs appear to have a broader spectrum of therapeutic effects on specific PTSD symptom clusters than do TCAs and MAOIs. Benzodiazepine augmentation is useful in the acute symptomatic state. The SSRIs are associated with marked improvement of both intrusive and avoidant symptoms.

GENERALIZED ANXIETY DISORDER. The SSRIs may be useful for the treatment of specific phobias, generalized anxiety disorder (GAD), and separation anxiety disorder. A thorough, individualized evaluation is the first approach, with particular attention to identifying conditions amenable to drug therapy. Also, cognitive-behavioral or other psychotherapies can be added for greater efficacy.

Bulimia Nervosa and Other Eating Disorders.

Fluoxetine is indicated for the treatment of bulimia, which is best done in the context of psychotherapy. Dosages of 60 mg a day are significantly more effective than 20 mg a day. In several well-controlled studies, fluoxetine in dosages of 60 mg a day was superior to placebo in reducing binge eating and induced vomiting. Some experts recommend an initial course of cognitive-behavioral therapy alone. If there is no response in 3 to 6 weeks, then fluoxetine administration is added. The appropriate duration of treatment with fluoxetine and psychotherapy has not been determined.

Fluvoxamine was not effective at a statistically significant level in one double-blind, placebo-controlled trial for inpatients with bulimia.

ANOREXIA NERVOSA. Fluoxetine has been used in inpatient treatment of anorexia nervosa to attempt to control comorbid mood disturbances and obsessive-compulsive symptoms. However, at least two careful studies, one of 7 months' and one of 24 months' duration, failed to find that fluoxetine affected the overall outcome and the maintenance of weight. Effective treatments for anorexia include cognitive-behavioral, interpersonal, psychodynamic, and family therapies in addition to a trial with SSRIs.

OBESITY. Fluoxetine, in combination with a behavioral program, is only modestly beneficial for weight loss. A significant percentage of all persons who take SSRIs, including fluoxetine, lose weight initially but later may gain weight. However, all SSRIs may cause initial weight gain.

PREMENSTRUAL DYSPHORIC DISORDER. PMDD is characterized by debilitating mood and behavioral changes in the week preceding menstruation that interferes with normal functioning. Sertraline,

paroxetine, fluoxetine, and fluvoxamine have been reported to reduce the symptoms of PMDD. Controlled trials of fluoxetine and sertraline administered either throughout the cycle or only during the luteal phase (the 2 weeks between ovulation and menstruation) showed both schedules to be equally effective.

An additional observation of unclear significance was that fluoxetine was associated with changing the duration of the menstrual period by more than 4 days, either lengthening or shortening it. The effects of SSRIs on menstrual cycle length are mostly unknown and may warrant careful monitoring in women of reproductive age.

Off-Label Uses

PREMATURE EJACULATION. The anorgasmic effects of SSRIs make them useful as a treatment for men with premature ejaculation. The SSRIs permit intercourse for a significantly more extended period and are reported to improve sexual satisfaction in couples in which the man has premature ejaculation. Fluoxetine and sertraline are useful for this purpose.

PARAPHILIAS. The SSRIs may reduce obsessive-compulsive behavior in people with paraphilias. The SSRIs diminish the average time per day spent in unconventional sexual fantasies, urges, and activities. Evidence suggests a more significant response to sexual obsessions than for paraphilic behavior.

AUTISM. Obsessive-compulsive behavior, poor social relatedness, and aggression are prominent autistic features that may respond to serotonergic agents such as SSRIs and clomipramine (Anafranil). Sertraline and fluvoxamine have been shown in controlled and open-label trials to mitigate aggressiveness, self-injurious behavior, repetitive behaviors, some degree of language delay, and (rarely) lack of social relatedness in adults with autistic spectrum disorders. Fluoxetine has been reported to be useful for features of autism in children, adolescents, and adults.

Precautions and Adverse Reactions. SSRI side effects need to be considered in terms of their onset, duration, and severity. For example, nausea and jitteriness are early, generally mild, and time-limited side effects. Although SSRIs share similar side effect profiles, individual drugs in this class may cause a higher rate or carry a more severe risk of specific side effects depending on the patient.

Sexual Dysfunction. All SSRIs cause sexual dysfunction, and it is the most common adverse effect of SSRIs associated with long-term treatment. It has an estimated incidence of between 50 and 80 percent. The most common complaints are anorgasmia, inhibited orgasm, and decreased libido. Some studies suggest that sexual dysfunction is dose-related, but this has not been established. Unlike most of the other adverse effects of SSRIs, sexual inhibition rarely resolves in the first few weeks of use but usually continues as long as the drug is taken. In some cases, there may be an improvement over time.

Strategies to counteract SSRI-induced sexual dysfunction are numerous, and none has been proven to be very useful. Some reports suggest decreasing the dosage or adding bupropion (Wellbutrin) or amphetamine. Reports have described successful treatment of SSRI-induced sexual dysfunction with agents such as sildenafil (Viagra), which are used to treat erectile dysfunction. Ultimately, patients may need to be switched to antidepressants that do not interfere with sexual functioning, drugs such as mirtazapine or bupropion.

Gastrointestinal Adverse Effects. GI side effects are widespread and are mediated mainly through effects on the serotonin

5-HT$_3$ receptor. The most frequent GI complaints are nausea, diarrhea, anorexia, vomiting, flatulence, and dyspepsia. Sertraline and fluvoxamine produce the most intense GI symptoms. Delayed-release paroxetine, compared with the immediate-release preparation of paroxetine, has less intense GI side effects during the first week of treatment. However, paroxetine, because of its anticholinergic activity, frequently causes constipation. Nausea and loose stools are usually dose-related and transient, usually resolving within a few weeks. Sometimes flatulence and diarrhea persist, especially during sertraline treatment. Initial anorexia may also occur and is most frequent with fluoxetine. SSRI-induced appetite and weight loss begin as soon as the drug is taken and peak at 20 weeks, after which weight often returns to baseline. Up to one-third of persons taking SSRIs will gain weight, sometimes more than 20 lb. This effect is mediated through a metabolic mechanism, an increase in appetite, or both. It happens gradually and is usually resistant to diet and exercise regimens. Paroxetine is associated with more frequent, rapid, and pronounced weight gain than the other SSRIs, especially among young women.

Cardiovascular Effects. All SSRIs can lengthen the QT interval in otherwise healthy people and cause drug-induced long QT syndrome, especially when taken in overdose. The risk of QTc prolongation increases when an antidepressant and an antipsychotic are used in combination, an increasingly common practice. Citalopram stands out as the SSRI with the most pronounced effect on QT intervals. A QT study to assess the effects of 20- and 60-mg doses of citalopram on the QT interval in adults, compared with placebo, found a maximum mean prolongation in the individually corrected QT intervals were 8.5 milliseconds for 20-mg citalopram and 18.5 milliseconds for 60 mg. For 40 mg, prolongation of the corrected QT interval was estimated to be 12.6 milliseconds. Based on these findings, the FDA has issued the following recommendation regarding citalopram use:

▶ 20 mg a day is the maximum recommended dose for patients with hepatic impairment, who are older than 60 years of age, who are CYP2C19 poor metabolizers, or who are taking concomitant cimetidine (Tagamet).
▶ No longer prescribe at doses greater than 40 mg a day.
▶ Do not use in patients with congenital long QT syndrome.
▶ Correct hypokalemia and hypomagnesemia before administering citalopram.
▶ Monitor electrolytes as clinically indicated.

Consider more frequent electrocardiograms in patients with congestive heart failure, bradyarrhythmias, or patients on concomitant medications that prolong the QT interval.

The fact that citalopram carries a greater risk of causing fatal rhythm abnormalities was confirmed in a review of 469 SSRI poisoning admissions. Accordingly, patients should be advised to contact their prescriber immediately if they experience signs and symptoms of an abnormal heart rate or rhythm while taking citalopram.

The effect of vilazodone (20, 40, 60, and 80 mg) on the QT interval was evaluated, and a small effect was observed. The upper bound of the 90 percent confidence interval for the largest placebo-adjusted, baseline-corrected QTc interval was below 10 milliseconds, based on the individual correction method (QTcI). This interval is below the threshold for clinical concern. However, it is unknown whether 80 mg is adequate to represent a high clinical exposure condition.

Physicians should consider whether the benefits of androgen deprivation therapy outweigh the potential risks in SSRI treated patients with prostate cancer, as reductions in androgen levels can cause QTc interval prolongation.

Dextromethorphan/Quinidine (Nuedexta) is available as a treatment for pseudobulbar affect, which is defined by involuntary, sudden, and frequent episodes of laughing or crying that are generally out of proportion or inappropriate to the situation. Quinidine can prolong the QT interval and is a potent inhibitor of CYP2D6. It should not be used with other medications that prolong the QT interval and are metabolized by CYP2D6. This drug should be used with caution with any medications that can prolong the QT interval and inhibit CYP3A4, particularly in patients with cardiac disease.

Antepartum use of SSRIs is sometimes associated with QTc interval prolongation in exposed neonates. In a review of 52 newborns exposed to SSRIs in the immediate antepartum period and 52 matched control subjects, the mean QTc was significantly longer in the group of newborns exposed to antidepressants as compared with control subjects. Five (10 percent) newborns exposed to SSRIs had a markedly prolonged QTc interval (greater than 460 milliseconds) compared with none of the unexposed newborns. The most extended QTc interval observed among exposed newborns was 543 milliseconds. All of the drug-associated repolarization abnormalities normalized in subsequent electrocardiographic tracings.

Headaches. The incidence of headache in SSRI trials was 18 to 20 percent, only one percentage point higher than the placebo rate. Fluoxetine is the most likely to cause headaches. On the other hand, all SSRIs are effective prophylaxis against both migraine and tension-type headaches in many persons.

Central Nervous System Adverse Effects

ANXIETY.   Fluoxetine may cause anxiety, particularly in the first few weeks of treatment. However, these initial effects usually give way to an overall reduction in anxiety after a few weeks. Increased anxiety is caused considerably less frequently by paroxetine and escitalopram, which may be better choices if sedation is desired, as in mixed anxiety and depressive disorders.

INSOMNIA AND SEDATION.   The primary effect SSRIs exert in the area of insomnia and sedation is improved sleep resulting from the treatment of depression and anxiety. However, as many as 25 percent of persons taking SSRIs note trouble sleeping, excessive somnolence, or overwhelming fatigue. Fluoxetine is the most likely to cause insomnia, for which reason it is often taken in the morning. Sertraline and fluvoxamine are about equally likely to cause insomnia as somnolence, and citalopram and especially paroxetine often cause somnolence. Escitalopram is more likely to interfere with sleep than its isomer, citalopram. Some persons benefit from taking their SSRI dose before going to bed, but others prefer to take it the morning. SSRI-induced insomnia can be treated with benzodiazepines, trazodone (Desyrel) (clinicians must explain the risk of priapism), or other sedating medicines. Significant SSRI-induced somnolence often requires switching to the use of another SSRI or bupropion.

OTHER SLEEP EFFECTS.   Many persons taking SSRIs report recalling extremely vivid dreams or nightmares. They describe sleep as "busy." Other sleep effects of the SSRIs include bruxism, restless legs, nocturnal myoclonus, and sweating.

EMOTIONAL BLUNTING.   Emotional blunting is a largely overlooked but frequent side effect associated with chronic SSRI use. Patients report an inability to cry in response to emotional situations, a feeling of apathy or indifference, or a restriction in the intensity of emotional experiences. This side effect often leads to treatment discontinuation, even when the drugs provide relief from depression or anxiety.

YAWNING.   Close clinical observation of patients taking SSRIs reveals an increase in yawning. This side effect is not a reflection of fatigue or poor nocturnal sleep but is the result of SSRI effects on the hypothalamus.

SEIZURES.   Seizures have been reported in 0.1 to 0.2 percent of all patients treated with SSRIs, an incidence comparable to that reported with other antidepressants and not significantly different from that with placebo. Seizures are more frequent at the highest doses of SSRIs (e.g., fluoxetine 100 mg a day or higher) than at standard doses.

EXTRAPYRAMIDAL SYMPTOMS.   The SSRIs may rarely cause aka-thisia, dystonia, tremor, cogwheel rigidity, torticollis, opisthotonos, gait disorders, and bradykinesia. Rare cases of tardive dyskinesia have been reported. Some people with well-controlled Parkinson disease may experience acute worsening of their motor symptoms when they take SSRIs.

Anticholinergic Effects.

Paroxetine has a mild anticholin-ergic activity that causes dry mouth, constipation, and sedation in a dose-dependent fashion. Nevertheless, most persons taking paroxetine do not experience cholinergic adverse effects. Other SSRIs are associated with dry mouth, but this effect is not mediated by muscarinic activity.

Hematologic Adverse Effects.

The SSRIs can cause functional impairment of platelet aggregation but not a reduction in platelet number. This pharmacologic effect can manifest through easy bruising and excessive or prolonged bleeding. When patients exhibit these signs, a test for bleeding time should be performed. Special monitoring is suggested when patients use SSRIs in conjunction with anticoagulants or aspirin. Concurrent use of SSRIs and NSAIDs is associated with a significantly increased risk of gastric bleeding. In cases where this combination is necessary, we should consider using proton pump inhibitors.

Electrolyte and Glucose Disturbances.

The SSRIs may acutely decrease glucose concentrations; therefore, diabetic patients should be carefully monitored. Long-term use may be associated with increased glucose levels, although it remains to be proven whether this is the result of a pharmacologic effect. Antide-pressant users may have other characteristics that raise their odds of developing diabetes, or may be more likely to be diagnosed with diabetes or other medical conditions as a result of being in treatment for depression.

Cases of SSRI-associated hyponatremia and the syndrome of inappropriate antidiuretic hormone have been seen in some patients, especially those who are older or treated with diuretics.

Endocrine and Allergic Reactions.

The SSRIs can increase prolactin levels and cause mammoplasia and galactorrhea in both men and women. Breast changes are reversible upon discontinuation of the drug, but this may take several months to occur.

Various types of rashes appear in about 4 percent of all patients; in a small subset of these patients, the allergic reaction may generalize and involve the pulmonary system, rarely resulting in fibrotic damage and dyspnea. SSRI treatment may have to be discontinued in patients with drug-related rashes.

Serotonin Syndrome.

Concurrent administration of an SSRI with an MAOI, L-tryptophan, or lithium (Eskalith) can raise plasma serotonin concentrations to toxic levels, producing a constellation of symptoms called *serotonin syndrome*. This severe and possibly fatal syndrome of serotonin overstimulation comprises, in order of appearance as the condition worsens, (1) diarrhea; (2) restless-ness; (3) extreme agitation, hyperreflexia, and autonomic insta-bility with possible rapid fluctuations in vital signs; (4) myoclonus, seizures, hyperthermia, uncontrollable shivering, and rigidity; and (5) delirium, coma, status epilepticus, cardiovascular collapse, and death.

Treatment of serotonin syndrome consists of removing the offending agents and promptly instituting comprehensive sup-portive care. Supportive care and treatment may include nitroglyc-erine, cyproheptadine (Periactin), methysergide (Sansert), cooling blankets, chlorpromazine (Thorazine), dantrolene (Dantrium), benzodiazepines, anticonvulsants, mechanical ventilation, and paralyzing agents.

Sweating.

Some patients experience sweating while being treated with SSRIs. This sweating is independent of the tempera-ture in the environment. Nocturnal sweating may drench bed sheets and require a change of nightclothes. Terazosin (Hytrin), 1 or 2 mg/day, is often dramatically effective in counteracting sweating.

Overdose.

The adverse reactions associated with overdose of vilazodone at doses of 200 to 280 mg, as observed in clinical trials, included serotonin syndrome, lethargy, restlessness, hallucinations, and disorientation.

Selective Serotonin Reuptake Inhibitor Withdrawal.

The abrupt discontinuance of SSRI use, especially one with a shorter half-life such as paroxetine or fluvoxamine, has been associated with a withdrawal syndrome that may include dizziness, weak-ness, nausea, headache, rebound depression, anxiety, insomnia, poor concentration, upper respiratory symptoms, paresthesias, and migraine-like symptoms. It usually does not appear until after at least 6 weeks of treatment and usually resolves spontaneously in 3 weeks. Persons who experienced transient adverse effects in the first weeks of taking an SSRI are more likely to experience discon-tinuation symptoms.

Fluoxetine is the SSRI least likely to be associated with this syn-drome because the half-life of its metabolite is more than 1 week, and it effectively tapers itself. Fluoxetine has therefore been used in some cases to treat the discontinuation syndrome caused by the termination of other SSRIs. Nevertheless, a delayed and attenuated withdrawal syndrome occurs with fluoxetine as well.

Drug Interactions

The SSRIs do not interfere with most other drugs. A serotonin syn-drome (Table 21-17) can develop with concurrent administration of

Table 21-17
Serotonin Syndrome Symptoms

Diarrhea	Myoclonus
Diaphoresis	Hyperactive reflexes
Tremor	Disorientation
Ataxia	Lability of mood

MAOIs, L-tryptophan, lithium, or other antidepressants that inhibit the reuptake of serotonin. Fluoxetine, sertraline, and paroxetine can raise plasma concentrations of TCAs, which can cause clinical toxicity. Several potential pharmacokinetic interactions have been described based on in vitro analyses of the CYP enzymes, but clinically relevant interactions are rare. SSRIs that inhibit CYP2D6 may interfere with the analgesic effects of hydrocodone and oxycodone. These drugs can also reduce the effectiveness of tamoxifen (Nolvadex, Soltamox). The combined use of SSRIs and NSAIDs increases the risk of gastric bleeding.

The SSRIs, particularly fluvoxamine, should not be used with clozapine because it raises clozapine concentrations, increasing the risk of seizure. The SSRIs may increase the duration and severity of zolpidem (Ambien)-induced side effects, including hallucinations.

Fluoxetine. Fluoxetine can be administered with tricyclic drugs, but the clinician should use low dosages of the tricyclic drug. Because the hepatic enzyme CYP2D6 metabolizes it, fluoxetine may interfere with the metabolism of other drugs in the 7 percent of the population who have an inefficient isoform of this enzyme, the so-called poor metabolizers. Fluoxetine may slow down the metabolism of carbamazepine (Tegretol), antineoplastic agents, diazepam (Valium), and phenytoin (Dilantin). Drug interactions have been described for fluoxetine that may affect the plasma levels of benzodiazepines, antipsychotics, and lithium. Fluoxetine and other SSRIs may interact with warfarin (Coumadin), increasing the risk of bleeding and bruising.

Sertraline. Sertraline may displace warfarin from plasma proteins and may increase the prothrombin time. The drug interaction data on sertraline support a generally similar profile to that of fluoxetine, although sertraline does not interact as strongly with the CYP2D6 enzyme.

Paroxetine. Paroxetine has a higher risk for drug interactions than does either fluoxetine or sertraline because it is a more potent inhibitor of the CYP2D6 enzyme. Cimetidine can increase the concentration of sertraline and paroxetine, and phenobarbital (Luminal) and phenytoin can decrease the concentration of paroxetine. Because of the potential for interference with the CYP2D6 enzyme, the coadministration of paroxetine with other antidepressants, phenothiazines, and antiarrhythmic drugs should be undertaken with caution. Paroxetine may increase the anticoagulant effect of warfarin. Coadministration of paroxetine and tramadol may precipitate serotonin syndrome in elderly persons.

Fluvoxamine. Among the SSRIs, fluvoxamine appears to present the most risk for drug–drug interactions. Fluvoxamine is metabolized by the enzyme CYP3A4, which may be inhibited by ketoconazole (Nizoral). Fluvoxamine may increase the half-life of alprazolam, triazolam (Halcion), and diazepam, and it should not be coadministered with these agents. Fluvoxamine may increase theophylline levels threefold and warfarin levels twofold, with significant clinical consequences; thus, the serum levels of the latter drugs should be closely monitored, and the doses adjusted accordingly. Fluvoxamine raises concentrations and may increase the activity of clozapine, carbamazepine, methadone (Dolophine, Methadose), propranolol (Inderal), and diltiazem (Cardizem). Fluvoxamine has no significant interactions with lorazepam (Ativan) or digoxin (Lanoxin).

Citalopram. Citalopram is not a potent inhibitor of any CYP enzymes. Concurrent administration of cimetidine increases concentrations of citalopram by about 40 percent. Citalopram does not significantly affect the metabolism of, nor is its metabolism significantly affected by, digoxin, lithium, warfarin, carbamazepine, or imipramine (Tofranil). Citalopram increases the plasma concentrations of metoprolol (Lopressor) twofold, but this usually does not affect BP or heart rate. Data on coadministration of citalopram and potent inhibitors of CYP3A4 or CYP2D6 are not available.

Escitalopram. Escitalopram is a moderate inhibitor of CYP2D6 and has been shown to raise desipramine (Norpramin) and metoprolol concentrations significantly.

Vilazodone. Vilazodone dose should be reduced to 20 mg when coadministered with CYP3A4 potent inhibitors. Concomitant use with inducers of CYP3A4 can result in inadequate drug concentrations and may diminish effectiveness. The effect of CYP3A4 inducers on the systemic exposure of vilazodone has not been evaluated.

Laboratory Interferences

In general, the SSRIs do not interfere with any laboratory tests. There have been some reports of false-positive urine toxicology for benzodiazepines in patients taking sertraline; if this is suspected, additional confirmation can be sought via gas chromatography-mass spectrometry.

Dosage and Clinical Guidelines

Fluoxetine. Fluoxetine is available in 10- and 20-mg capsules, in a scored 10-mg tablet, as a 90-mg enteric-coated capsule for once-weekly administration, and as an oral concentrate (20 mg/5 mL). Fluoxetine is also marketed as Sarafem for PMDD. For depression, the initial dosage is usually 10 or 20 mg orally each day, usually given in the morning, because insomnia is a potential adverse effect of the drug. Fluoxetine should be taken with food to minimize possible nausea. The long half-lives of the drug and its metabolite contribute to 4 weeks to reach steady-state concentrations. Twenty milligrams is often as effective as higher doses for treating depression. The maximum dosage recommended by the manufacturer is 80 mg a day. To minimize the early side effects of anxiety and restlessness, some clinicians initiate fluoxetine use at 5 to 10 mg a day, either with the scored 10-mg tablet or by using the liquid preparation. Alternatively, because of the long half-life of fluoxetine, its use can be initiated with an every-other-day administration schedule. The dosage of fluoxetine (and other SSRIs) that is effective in other indications may differ from the dosage generally used for depression.

Sertraline. Sertraline is available in scored 25-, 50-, and 100-mg tablets. For the initial treatment of depression, sertraline use should be initiated with a dosage of 50 mg once daily. To limit the GI effects, some clinicians begin at 25 mg a day and increase to 50 mg a day after 3 weeks. Patients who do not respond after 1 to 3 weeks may benefit from dosage increases of 50 mg every week up to a maximum of 200 mg given once daily. Sertraline can be administered in the morning or in the evening. Administration after eating may reduce the GI adverse effects. Sertraline oral concentrate (1 mL = 20 mg) has 12 percent alcohol content and must be diluted before use. When used to treat panic disorder, sertraline should be initiated at 25 mg to reduce the risk of provoking a panic attack.

Paroxetine. Immediate-release paroxetine is available in scored 20-mg tablets; in unscored 10-, 30-, and 40-mg tablets; and as an orange-flavored 10-mg/5-mL oral suspension. Paroxetine use for the treatment of depression is usually initiated at a dosage of 10 or 20 mg a day. An increase in the dosage should be considered when an adequate response is not seen in 1 to 3 weeks. At that point, the clinician can initiate upward dose titration in 10-mg increments at weekly intervals to a maximum of 50 mg a day. Persons who experience GI upset may benefit from taking the drug with food. Paroxetine can be taken initially as a single daily dose in the evening; higher dosages may be divided into two doses per day.

A delayed-release formulation of paroxetine, paroxetine CR, is available in 12.5-, 25-, and 37.5-mg tablets. The starting dosages of paroxetine CR are 25 mg/day for depression and 12.5 mg/day for panic disorder.

Paroxetine is the SSRI most likely to produce a discontinuation syndrome, because plasma concentrations decrease rapidly in the absence of continuous dosing. Paroxetine use should be tapered gradually to limit the symptoms of abrupt discontinuation, with dosage reductions every 2 to 3 weeks.

Fluvoxamine. Fluvoxamine is the only SSRI not approved by the FDA as an antidepressant. It is indicated for OCD. It is available in unscored 25-mg tablets and scored 50- and 100-mg tablets. The effective daily dosage range is 50 to 300 mg a day. A usual starting dosage is 50 mg once a day at bedtime for the first week, after which the dosage can be adjusted according to the adverse effects and clinical response. Dosages above 100 mg a day may be divided into twice-daily dosing. A temporary dosage reduction or slower upward titration may be necessary if nausea develops over the first 2 weeks of therapy. Although fluvoxamine can also be administered as a single evening dose to minimize its adverse effects, its short half-life may lead to interdose withdrawal. An extended-release formulation is available in 100- and 150-mg dose strengths. All fluvoxamine formulations should be swallowed with food without chewing the tablet. Abrupt discontinuation of fluvoxamine may cause a discontinuation syndrome owing to its short half-life.

Citalopram. Citalopram is available in 20- and 40-mg scored tablets and as a liquid (10 mg/5 mL). The usual starting dosage is 20 mg a day for the first week, after which it usually is increased to 40 mg a day. For elderly persons or persons with hepatic impairment, 20 mg a day is recommended. Tablets should be taken once daily in either the morning or the evening with or without food.

Escitalopram. Escitalopram is available as 10- and 20-mg scored tablets, as well as an oral solution at a concentration of 5 mg/5 mL. The recommended dosage of escitalopram is 10 mg/day. In clinical trials, no additional benefit was noted when 20 mg/day was used.

Vilazodone. Vilazodone is available as 10-, 20-, and 40-mg tablets. The recommended therapeutic dose of vilazodone is 40 mg once daily. Treatment should be titrated, starting with an initial dose of 10 mg once daily for 7 days, followed by 20 mg once daily for an additional 7 days, and then an increase to 40 mg once daily. Vilazodone should be taken with food. If vilazodone is taken without food, inadequate drug concentrations may result, and the drug's effectiveness may be diminished. Vilazodone is not approved for use in children. The safety and efficacy of vilazodone in pediatric patients have not been studied. The patient's age should not influence the dose, nor does mild or moderate hepatic impairment. Vilazodone has not been studied in patients with severe hepatic impairment. No dose adjustment is recommended in patients with mild, moderate, or severe renal impairment.

Pregnancy and Breastfeeding. Except for paroxetine, the SSRIs are safe to take during pregnancy when deemed necessary for the treatment of the mother. There are no controlled human data regarding vilazodone use during pregnancy, nor are there human data regarding drug concentrations in breast milk. Transient QTc prolongation has been noted in newborns whose mother was being treated with an SSRI during pregnancy.

Loss of Efficacy. Some patients report a diminished response or total loss of response to SSRIs with recurrence of depressive symptoms while remaining on a full dose of medication. The exact mechanism of this so-called "poop-out" is unknown, but the phenomenon is genuine. Potential remedies for the attenuation of the response to SSRIs include increasing or decreasing the dosage, tapering drug use, and then rechallenging with the same medication, switching to another SSRI or non-SSRI antidepressant, and augmenting with bupropion or another augmentation agent.

Vortioxetine (Trintellix). Vortioxetine works mainly as an inhibitor of serotonin (5-HT) reuptake, but it has a more complex pharmacologic profile than other SSRIs. It also acts as an agonist at 5-HT$_{1A}$ receptors, a partial agonist at 5-HT$_{1B}$ receptors, and an antagonist at 5-HT$_3$, 5-HT$_{1D}$, and 5-HT$_7$ receptors. The contribution of each of these activities to the drug's antidepressant effect has not been established, but it is the only compound with this combination of pharmacodynamic actions.

Side effects seen during the trials include, but are not limited to, nausea, constipation, and vomiting.

The recommended starting dose is 10 mg administered orally once daily without regard to meals. The dose should then be increased to 20 mg/day, as tolerated. A dose of 5 mg/day should be considered for patients who do not tolerate higher doses.

The maximum recommended dose of vortioxetine is 10 mg/day in known CYP2D6 poor metabolizers. Reduction of the dose of vortioxetine by one-half is suggested when patients are receiving a CYP2D6 potent inhibitor (e.g., bupropion, fluoxetine, paroxetine, or quinidine) concomitantly. The dose should be increased to the original dose of vortioxetine in patients who stop taking CYP inducers (e.g., rifampin, carbamazepine, or phenytoin). This adjustment is especially essential when a potent CYP inducer is coadministered for greater than 14 days. The maximum recommended dose should not exceed three times the original dose. The dose of vortioxetine should be reduced to the original level within 14 days when the inducer is discontinued.

Although vortioxetine can be abruptly discontinued, in placebo-controlled trials, patients experienced transient adverse reactions such as headache and muscle tension following abrupt discontinuation of vortioxetine 15 or 20 mg/day. It is recommended that the dose be decreased to 10 mg/day for 1 week before full discontinuation of vortioxetine 15 or 20 mg/day.

Vortioxetine is available in 5-, 10-, 15-, and 20-mg tablets.

SELECTIVE SEROTONIN–NOREPINEPHRINE REUPTAKE INHIBITORS

There are currently four SNRIs approved for use in the United States: venlafaxine (Effexor and Effexor XR), desvenlafaxine succinate (DVS; Pristiq), duloxetine (Cymbalta), and levomilnacipran (Fetzima). A fifth SNRI, milnacipran (Savella), available in other countries as an antidepressant, has U.S. FDA approval in the United States as a treatment for fibromyalgia. The term SNRI reflects the belief that the therapeutic effects of these medications are mediated by concomitant blockade of neuronal serotonin (5-HT) and norepinephrine uptake transporters. The SNRIs are also sometimes referred to as dual reuptake inhibitors, a broader functional class of antidepressant medications that include TCAs such as clomipramine (Anafranil) and, to a lesser extent, imipramine (Tofranil) and amitriptyline (Elavil). What distinguishes the SNRIs from TCAs is their relative lack of affinity for other receptors, especially muscarinic, histaminergic, and the families of α- and β-adrenergic receptors. This distinction is an important one because the SNRIs have a more favorable tolerability profile than the older dual reuptake inhibitors.

Venlafaxine and Desvenlafaxine

Therapeutic Indications. Venlafaxine is approved for the treatment of four disorders: MDD, GAD, social anxiety disorder, and panic disorder. MDD is currently the only FDA-approved indication for DVS.

DEPRESSION. The FDA does not recognize any class of antidepressants as being more effective than any other. This does not mean that differences do not exist, but no study to date has sufficiently demonstrated such superiority. It has been argued that direct modulation of serotonin and norepinephrine may convey more significant antidepressant effects than are exerted by medications that selectively enhance only noradrenergic or serotoninergic neurotransmission. This more significant therapeutic benefit could result from an acceleration of postsynaptic adaptation to increased neuronal signaling, simultaneous activation of two pathways for intracellular signal transduction, additive effects on the activity of relevant genes such as brain-derived neurotrophic factor, or, quite simply, broader coverage of depressive symptoms. Clinical evidence supporting this hypothesis first emerged in a pair of studies conducted by the Danish University Antidepressant Group, which found an advantage for the dual reuptake inhibitor clomipramine compared with SSRIs citalopram (Celexa) and paroxetine (Paxil). Another report, which compared the results of a group of patients prospectively treated with the combination of desipramine (Norpramin) and fluoxetine (Prozac) with a historical comparison group treated with desipramine alone, provided additional support. A meta-analysis of 25 inpatient studies comparing the efficacy of TCAs and SSRIs yielded the most substantial evidence. Specifically, although the TCAs were found to have a modest overall advantage, superiority versus SSRIs was almost entirely explained by the studies that used the TCAs that are considered to be dual reuptake inhibitors—clomipramine, amitriptyline, and imipramine. Meta-analyses of head-to-head studies suggest that venlafaxine has the potential to induce higher rates of remission in depressed patients than do the SSRIs. This difference in the venlafaxine advantage is about 6 percent. DVS has not been extensively compared with other classes of antidepressants concerning efficacy.

GENERALIZED ANXIETY DISORDER. The extended-release formulation of venlafaxine is approved for the treatment of GAD. In clinical trials lasting 6 months, dosages of 75 to 225 mg a day were effective in treating insomnia, poor concentration, restlessness, irritability, and excessive muscle tension related to GAD.

SOCIAL ANXIETY DISORDER. The extended-release formulation of venlafaxine is approved for the treatment of social anxiety disorder. Its efficacy was established in 12-week studies.

OTHER INDICATIONS. Case reports and uncontrolled studies have indicated that venlafaxine may be beneficial in the treatment of obsessive-compulsive disorder, panic disorder, agoraphobia, social phobia, ADHD, and patients with a dual diagnosis of depression and cocaine dependence. It has also been used in chronic pain syndromes with good effect.

Precautions and Adverse Reactions. Venlafaxine has a safety and tolerability profile similar to that of the more widely prescribed SSRI class. Nausea is the most frequently reported treatment-emergent adverse effect associated with venlafaxine and DVS therapy. Initiating therapy at lower dosages may also attenuate nausea. When extremely problematic, treatment-induced nausea can be controlled by prescribing a selective 5-HT$_3$ antagonist or mirtazapine (Remeron).

Venlafaxine and DVS therapy is associated with sexual side effects, predominantly decreased libido and a delay to orgasm or ejaculation. The incidence of these side effects may exceed 30 to 40 percent when there is a direct, detailed assessment of sexual function.

Other common side effects include headache, insomnia, somnolence, dry mouth, dizziness, constipation, asthenia, sweating, and nervousness. Although several side effects are suggestive of anticholinergic effects, these drugs have no affinity for muscarinic or nicotinic receptors. Thus, noradrenergic agonism is likely to be the culprit.

Higher-dose venlafaxine therapy is associated with an increased risk of sustained elevations of BP. Experience with the instant-release (IR) formulation in studies of depressed patients indicated that sustained hypertension was dose-related, increasing from 3 to 7 percent at doses of 100 to 300 mg/day and 13 percent at doses greater than 300 mg/day. In this dataset, venlafaxine therapy did not adversely affect BP control of patients taking antihypertensives and lowered the mean values of patients with elevated BP readings before therapy. In controlled studies of the extended-release formulation, venlafaxine therapy resulted in only approximately 1 percent greater risk of high BP when compared with the placebo. Arbitrarily capping the upper dose of venlafaxine used in these studies, thus, significantly attenuated concerns about elevated BP. When higher doses of the extended-release formulation are used, however, monitoring of BP is recommended.

Venlafaxine and DVS are commonly associated with discontinuation syndrome. This syndrome is characterized by the appearance of a constellation of adverse effects during a rapid taper or abrupt cessation, including dizziness, dry mouth, insomnia, nausea, nervousness, sweating, anorexia, diarrhea, somnolence, and sensory disturbances. It is recommended that, whenever possible, a slow taper schedule should be used when longer-term treatment must be stopped. On occasion, substituting a few doses of the sustained-release formulation of fluoxetine may help to bridge this transition.

There were no overdose fatalities in premarketing trials of venlafaxine, although electrocardiographic changes (e.g., prolongation of QT interval, bundle branch block, QRS interval prolongation), tachycardia, bradycardia, hypotension, hypertension, coma, serotonin syndrome, and seizures were reported. Fatal overdoses have been documented subsequently, typically involving venlafaxine ingestion in combination with other drugs, alcohol, or both.

Information concerning the use of venlafaxine and DVS by pregnant and nursing women is not available at this time. Venlafaxine and DVS are excreted in breast milk. Clinicians should carefully weigh the risks and benefits of venlafaxine use by pregnant and nursing women.

Drug Interactions. Venlafaxine is metabolized in the liver primarily by the CYP2D6 isoenzyme. Because the parent drug and principal metabolite are essentially equipotent, medications that inhibit this isoenzyme usually do not adversely affect therapy. Venlafaxine is itself a relatively weak inhibitor of CYP2D6, although it can increase levels of substrates, such as desipramine or risperidone (Risperdal). In vitro and in vivo studies have shown venlafaxine to cause little or no inhibition of CYP1A2, CYP2C9, CYP2C19, and CYP3A4.

Venlafaxine is contraindicated in patients taking MAOIs because of the risk of a pharmacodynamic interaction (i.e., serotonin syndrome). An MAOI should not be started for at least 7 days after stopping venlafaxine. Few data are available regarding the combination of venlafaxine with atypical neuroleptics, benzodiazepines, lithium (Eskalith), and anticonvulsants; therefore, clinical judgment should be exercised when combining medications.

Laboratory Interferences. Data are not currently available on laboratory interferences with venlafaxine. There have been some reports of patients taking venlafaxine who have false-positive results on liquid chromatography testing for tramadol.

Dosage and Administration. Venlafaxine is available in 25-, 37.5-, 50-, 75-, and 100-mg tablets and 37.5-, 75-, and 150-mg extended-release capsules. The tablets and the extended-release capsules are equally potent, and persons stabilized with one can switch to an equivalent dosage of the other. Because the immediate-release tablets are rarely used due to their tendency to cause nausea and the need for multiple-daily doses, the dosage recommendations that follow refer to the use of the extended-release capsules.

In depressed persons, venlafaxine demonstrates a dose–response curve. The initial therapeutic dosage is 75 mg a day, given once a day. However, most persons are started at a dosage of 37.5 mg for 4 to 7 days to minimize adverse effects, particularly nausea. A convenient starter kit for the drug contains a 1-week supply of both the 37.5- and 75-mg strengths. If a rapid titration is preferred, the dosage can be raised to 150 mg/day after day 4. As a rule, the dosage can be raised in increments of 75 mg a day every 4 or more days. Although the recommended upper dosage of the extended-release preparation (venlafaxine XR) is 225 mg/day, it is approved by the FDA for use at dosages up to 375 mg a day. The dosage of venlafaxine should be halved in persons with significantly diminished hepatic or renal function. If discontinued, venlafaxine use should be gradually tapered over 2 to 4 weeks to avoid withdrawal symptoms.

There are minor differences in the doses used for major depression, GAD, and social anxiety disorder. In the treatment of these disorders, for example, a dose–response effect has not been found. Also, lower mean dosages are typically used, with most patients taking 75 to 150 mg/day.

DVS is available as 50- and 100-mg extended-release tablets. The therapeutic dose for most patients is 50 mg a day. Although some patients may need higher doses, in clinical trials, no more significant therapeutic benefit was noted when the dose was increased. At higher doses, adverse events and discontinuation rates were increased.

Duloxetine

Pharmacologic Actions. Duloxetine is formulated as a delayed-release capsule to reduce the risk of severe nausea associated with the drug. It is well absorbed, but there is a 2-hour delay before absorption begins. Peak plasma concentrations occur 6 hours after ingestion. Food delays the time to achieve maximum concentrations from 6 to 10 hours and reduces the extent of absorption by about 10 percent. Duloxetine has an elimination half-life of about 12 hours (range, 8 to 17 hours). Steady-state plasma concentrations occur after 3 days. Duloxetine's elimination is mainly through the isozymes CYP2D6 and CYP1A2. Duloxetine undergoes extensive hepatic metabolism to numerous metabolites. About 70 percent of the drug appears in the urine as metabolites, and about 20 percent is excreted in the feces. Duloxetine is 90 percent protein-bound.

Therapeutic Indications

DEPRESSION. In contrast to venlafaxine, a small number of studies have compared duloxetine with the SSRIs. Although these studies are suggestive of some advantage in efficacy, their findings are limited by the use of fixed, low starting doses of paroxetine and fluoxetine, but dosages of duloxetine in some studies were as high as 120 mg/day. Any inferences on whether duloxetine is superior to the SSRIs in any aspect of treatment for depression thus await more evidence from adequately designed trials.

NEUROPATHIC PAIN ASSOCIATED WITH DIABETES AND STRESS URINARY INCONTINENCE. Duloxetine is the first drug to be approved by the FDA as a treatment for neuropathic pain associated with diabetes. Its pain effects have not been compared with other agents, such as venlafaxine and the TCAs. Duloxetine is currently awaiting approval as a treatment for stress urinary incontinence, the inability to voluntarily control bladder voiding, which is the most frequent type of incontinence in women. The action of duloxetine in the treatment of stress urinary incontinence is associated with its effects in the sacral spinal cord, which in turn increases the activity of the striated urethral sphincter. Duloxetine is marketed under the name Yentreve for this indication which has not been approved for this indication in the United States but is available in the European Union and other countries.

PRECAUTIONS AND ADVERSE REACTIONS. The most common adverse reactions are nausea, dry mouth, dizziness, constipation, fatigue, decreased appetite, anorexia, somnolence, and increased sweating. Nausea was the most common side effect that led to treatment discontinuation in clinical trials. The true incidence of sexual dysfunction is unknown; the long-term effects on body weight are also unknown. In clinical trials, treatment with duloxetine was associated with mean increases in BP averaging 2 mm Hg systolic and 0.5 mm Hg diastolic versus placebo. No studies have compared the BP effects of venlafaxine and duloxetine at equivalent therapeutic doses.

Close monitoring is suggested when using duloxetine in patients who have or are at risk for diabetes. Duloxetine has been shown to increase blood sugar and hemoglobin A1C levels during long-term treatment.

Patients with substantial alcohol use should not be treated with duloxetine because of possible hepatic effects. It also should not be prescribed for patients with hepatic insufficiency and end-stage renal disease or patients with uncontrolled narrow-angle glaucoma.

Abrupt discontinuation of duloxetine should be avoided because it may produce a discontinuation syndrome similar to that of venlafaxine. A gradual dose reduction is recommended.

Clinicians should avoid the use of duloxetine by pregnant and nursing women unless the potential benefits justify the potential risks.

Drug Interactions. Duloxetine is a moderate inhibitor of CYP450 enzymes.

Laboratory Interferences.   Data are not currently available on laboratory interferences with duloxetine.

Dosage and Administration.   Duloxetine is available in 20-, 30-, and 60-mg tablets. The recommended therapeutic and maximum dosage is 60 mg/day. The 20- and 30-mg doses are useful for either initial therapy or for twice-daily use as strategies to reduce side effects. In clinical trials, dosages of up to 120 mg/day were studied, but no consistent advantage in efficacy was noted at doses higher than 60 mg/day. Duloxetine thus does not appear to demonstrate a dosage–response curve. However, there were difficulties in tolerability with single doses above 60 mg. Accordingly, when dosages of 80 and 120 mg/day were used, they were administered as 40 or 60 mg twice daily. It remains to be seen to what extent dosages above 60 mg/day will be necessary and whether this will require divided doses to make the drug tolerable.

Milnacipran and Levomilnacipran

Milnacipran is only FDA approved for the treatment of fibromyalgia. Although some countries have approved milnacipran for general use as an antidepressant, efficacy is not as well established. Compared with venlafaxine, milnacipran is approximately five times more potent for inhibition of norepinephrine uptake than for 5-HT reuptake inhibition. Milnacipran has a half-life of approximately 8 hours and shows linear pharmacokinetics between doses of 50 and 250 mg/day. Milnacipran has no active metabolites, and it is directly metabolized in the liver. The kidneys primarily excrete milnacipran.

Milnacipran is available as 12.5-, 25-, 50-, and 100-mg tablets. The standard recommended milnacipran dose is as follows: day 1, 12.5 mg once daily; days 2 and 3, 12.5 mg twice daily; days 4 to 7, 25 mg twice daily; and day 7 and beyond, 50 mg twice daily.

Levomilnacipran was approved in 2013 by the FDA as a treatment for MDD in adults. Levomilnacipran is an active enantiomer of the racemic drug milnacipran. In vitro studies have shown that it has greater potency for norepinephrine reuptake inhibition than for serotonin reuptake inhibition and does not directly affect the uptake of dopamine or other neurotransmitters. It is taken once daily as a sustained-release formulation. In clinical trials, doses of 40, 80, or 120 mg improved symptoms compared with placebo.

The most common adverse reactions in the placebo-controlled trials were nausea, constipation, hyperhidrosis, increased heart rate, erectile dysfunction, tachycardia, vomiting, and palpitations. Rates of adverse events were generally consistent across the 40- to 120-mg dose range. The only dose-related adverse events were urinary hesitation and erectile dysfunction.

BUPROPION

Bupropion (Wellbutrin, Wellbutrin SR, Wellbutrin XL) is an antidepressant drug that inhibits the reuptake of norepinephrine and, possibly, dopamine. Most significantly, it does not act on the serotonin system like SSRI antidepressants. This novel action results in a side effect profile characterized by a low risk of sexual dysfunction and sedation and with modest weight loss during acute and long-term treatment. No withdrawal syndrome has been linked to discontinuation of bupropion. Although increasingly used as first-line monotherapy, a significant percentage of bupropion use occurs as add-on therapy to other antidepressants, usually SSRIs. Bupropion was marketed under the name Zyban for use in smoking cessation regimens. However, the manufacturer has discontinued that brand in the United States.

Pharmacologic Actions

Three formulations of bupropion are available: immediate-release (taken three times daily), sustained-release (taken twice daily), and extended-release (taken once daily). The different versions of the drug contain the same active ingredient but differ in their pharmacokinetics and dosing. There have been reports of inconsistencies in bioequivalence between various branded and generic versions of bupropion. If a patient experiences changes in adverse effects or efficacy, the clinician should inquire whether there has been a change of formulation.

Immediate-release bupropion is well absorbed from the GI tract. Peak plasma concentrations of bupropion are usually reached within 2 hours of oral administration, and peak levels of the sustained-release version are seen after 3 hours. The mean half-life of the compound is 12 hours, ranging from 8 to 40 hours. Peak levels of extended-release bupropion occur 5 hours after ingestion. This pharmacokinetic profile provides a longer time to maximum plasma concentration (t_{max}) but comparable peak and trough plasma concentrations. The 24-hour exposure occurring after administration of the extended-release version of 300 mg once daily is equivalent to that provided by sustained release of 150 mg twice daily. Clinically, this permits the drug to be taken once a day in the morning. Plasma levels are also reduced in the evening, making it less likely for some patients to experience treatment-related insomnia.

The mechanism of action for the antidepressant effects of bupropion is presumed to involve the inhibition of dopamine and norepinephrine reuptake. Bupropion binds to the dopamine transporter in the brain. The effects of bupropion on smoking cessation may be related to its effects on dopamine reward pathways or inhibition of nicotinic acetylcholine receptors.

Therapeutic Indications

Depression.   Although overshadowed by the SSRIs as first-line treatment for major depression, the therapeutic efficacy of bupropion in depression is well established in both outpatient and inpatient settings. Observed rates of response and remission are comparable to those seen with the SSRIs. Bupropion has been found to prevent seasonal major depressive episodes in patients with a history of seasonal patterns or affective disorder.

Smoking Cessation.   Bupropion is indicated for use in combination with behavioral modification programs for smoking cessation. It is intended to be used in patients who are highly motivated and who receive some form of structured behavioral support. Bupropion is most effective when combined with nicotine substitutes (Nico-Derm, Nicotrol).

Bipolar Disorders.   Bupropion is less likely than TCAs to precipitate mania in persons with bipolar I disorder and less likely than other antidepressants to exacerbate or induce rapid-cycling bipolar II disorder; however, the evidence about the use of bupropion in the treatment of patients with bipolar disorder is limited.

Attention-Deficit/Hyperactivity   Disorder.   Bupropion is used as a second-line agent, after the sympathomimetics, for treatment of ADHD. It has not been compared with proven ADHD medications such as methylphenidate (Ritalin) or atomoxetine (Strattera) for childhood and adult ADHD. Bupropion is an appropriate choice for persons with comorbid ADHD and depression or persons with comorbid ADHD, conduct disorder, or substance use disorder. It may also be considered for use in patients who develop tics when treated with psychostimulants.

Cocaine Detoxification.   Bupropion may be associated with a euphoric feeling; thus, it may be contraindicated in persons with histories of substance abuse. However, because of its dopaminergic effects, bupropion has been explored as a treatment for cocaine cravings. Results have been inconclusive, with some patients showing a reduction in drug craving and others finding their cravings increased.

Hypoactive Sexual Desire Disorder.   Bupropion is often added to drugs such as SSRIs to counteract sexual side effects and may be helpful as a treatment for nondepressed individuals with a disorder of sexual desire. Bupropion may improve sexual arousal, orgasm completion, and sexual satisfaction.

Precautions and Adverse Reactions

Headache, insomnia, dry mouth, tremor, and nausea are the most common side effects. Restlessness, agitation, and irritability may also occur. Patients with severe anxiety or panic disorder should not be prescribed bupropion. Most likely, because of its potentiating effects on dopaminergic neurotransmission, bupropion can cause psychotic symptoms, including hallucinations, delusions, and catatonia, as well as delirium. Most notable about bupropion is the absence of significant drug-induced orthostatic hypotension, weight gain, daytime drowsiness, and anticholinergic effects. Some persons, however, may experience dry mouth or constipation and weight loss. Hypertension may occur in some patients, but bupropion causes no other significant cardiovascular or clinical laboratory changes. Bupropion exerts indirect sympathomimetic activity, producing positive inotropic effects in the human myocardium, an effect that may reflect catecholamine release. Some patients experience cognitive impairment, most notably word-finding difficulties.

Concern about seizure has deterred some physicians from prescribing bupropion. The risk of seizure is dose-dependent. Studies show that at dosages of 300 mg a day or less of sustained-release bupropion, the incidence of seizures is 0.05 percent, which is no worse than the incidence of seizures with other antidepressants. The risk of seizures increases to about 0.1 percent with dosages of 400 mg a day.

Changes in electroencephalographic (EEG) waveforms have been reported to be associated with bupropion use. About 20 percent of individuals treated with bupropion exhibit spike waves, sharp waves, and focal slowing. The likelihood of women having sharp waves is higher than for men. The presence of these waveforms in individuals taking a medication known to lower the seizure threshold may be a risk factor for developing seizures. Other risk factors for seizures include a history of seizures, use of alcohol, recent benzodiazepine withdrawal, organic brain disease, head trauma, or pretreatment epileptiform discharges on EEG.

The use of bupropion by pregnant women is not associated with a specific risk of an increased rate of congenital disabilities. Bupropion is secreted in breast milk, so the use of bupropion in nursing women should be based on the clinical circumstances of the patient and the judgment of the clinician.

Few deaths have been reported after overdoses of bupropion. Poor outcomes are associated with cases of massive doses and mixed-drug overdoses. Seizures occur in about one-third of all overdoses and are dose-dependent, with those having seizures ingesting a significantly higher median dose. Fatalities can involve uncontrollable seizures, sinus bradycardia, and cardiac arrest. Symptoms of poisoning most often involve seizures, sinus tachycardia, hypertension, GI symptoms, hallucinations, and agitation. All seizures are typically brief and self-limited. In general, however, bupropion is safer in overdose cases than are other antidepressants except for perhaps SSRIs.

Drug Interactions

Given the fact that bupropion is frequently combined with SSRIs or venlafaxine, potential interactions are significant. Bupropion has been found to affect the pharmacokinetics of venlafaxine. One study noted a significant increase in venlafaxine levels and a consequent decrease in its main metabolite O-desmethylvenlafaxine during combined treatment with sustained-release bupropion. Bupropion hydroxylation is weakly inhibited by venlafaxine. No significant changes in plasma levels of the SSRIs paroxetine and fluoxetine have been reported. However, few case reports indicate that the combination of bupropion and fluoxetine (Prozac) may be associated with panic, delirium, or seizures. Bupropion, in combination with lithium (Eskalith), may rarely cause CNS toxicity, including seizures.

Because of the possibility of inducing a hypertensive crisis, bupropion should not be used concurrently with MAOIs. At least 14 days should pass after the discontinuation of an MAOI before initiating treatment with bupropion. In some cases, the addition of bupropion may permit persons taking antiparkinsonian medications to lower the doses of their dopaminergic drugs. However, delirium, psychotic symptoms, and dyskinetic movements may occur with the coadministration of bupropion and dopaminergic agents, such as antiparkinsonian meds. Sinus bradycardia may occur when bupropion is combined with metoprolol.

Carbamazepine (Tegretol) may decrease plasma concentrations of bupropion, and bupropion may increase plasma concentrations of valproic acid (Depakene).

In vitro biotransformation studies of bupropion have found that the formation of a major active metabolite, hydroxybupropion, is mediated by CYP2B6. Bupropion has a significant inhibitory effect on CYP2D6.

Laboratory Interferences

A report has appeared indicating that bupropion may give a false-positive result on urinary amphetamine screens. No other reports have appeared of laboratory interferences associated with bupropion treatment. Clinically nonsignificant changes in the electrocardiogram (premature beats and nonspecific ST-T changes) and decreases in the WBC count (by about 10 percent) have been reported in a small number of persons.

Dosage and Clinical Guidelines

Immediate-release bupropion is available in 75-, 100-, and 150-mg tablets. Sustained-release bupropion is available in 100-, 150-, 200-, and 300-mg tablets. Extended-release bupropion comes in 150- and 300-mg strengths.

There have been problems associated with one of the extended-release generic versions called Budeprion XL 300-mg tablets, which was found not to be therapeutically equivalent to Wellbutrin XL 300 mg and was removed from the market.

The initiation of immediate-release bupropion in the average adult person should be 75 mg orally twice a day. On the fourth day of treatment, the dosage can be increased to 100 mg three times a day. Because 300 mg is the recommended dose, the person should be maintained on this dose for several weeks before increasing it further. The maximum dosage, 450 mg a day, should be given as 150 mg three times a day. Because of the risk of seizures, increases in dose should never exceed 100 mg in 3 days; a single dose of immediate-release bupropion should never exceed 150 mg, and the total daily dosage should not exceed 450 mg. The maximum of 400 mg of the sustained-release version should be used as a twice-a-day regimen of either 200 mg twice daily or 300 mg in the morning and 100 mg in the afternoon. A starting dosage of the sustained-release version, 100 mg once a day, can be increased to 100 mg twice a day after 4 days. Then 150 mg twice a day may be used. A single dose of sustained-release bupropion should never exceed 300 mg. The maximum dosage is 200 mg twice a day of the immediate-release or extended-release formulations. An advantage of the extended-release preparation is that the patient can take a single daily dose of 450 mg after proper titration.

For smoking cessation, the patient should start taking 150 mg a day of sustained-release bupropion 10 to 14 days before quitting smoking. On the fourth day, the dosage should be increased to 150 mg twice daily. Treatment generally lasts 7 to 12 weeks.

MIRTAZAPINE

Mirtazapine (Remeron) is unique among drugs used to treat major depression in that it increases both norepinephrine and serotonin through a mechanism other than reuptake blockade (as in the case of tricyclic agents or SSRIs) or monoamine oxidase inhibition (as in the case of phenelzine or tranylcypromine). Mirtazapine is also more likely to reduce rather than cause nausea and diarrhea, the result of its effects on serotonin 5-HT$_3$ receptors. Characteristic side effects include increased appetite and sedation.

Pharmacologic Actions

Mirtazapine is administered orally and is rapidly and completely absorbed. It has a half-life of about 30 hours. Peak concentration is achieved within 2 hours of ingestion, and steady state is reached after 6 days. Plasma clearance may be slowed up to 30 percent in persons with impaired hepatic function, up to 50 percent in those with impaired renal function, up to 40 percent slower in older men, and up to 10 percent slower in older women.

The mechanism of action of mirtazapine is the antagonism of central presynaptic α_2-adrenergic receptors and blockade of post-synaptic serotonin 5-HT$_2$ and 5-HT$_3$ receptors. The α_2-adrenergic receptor antagonism causes the increased firing of norepinephrine and serotonin neurons. The potent antagonist of serotonin 5-HT$_2$ and 5-HT$_3$ receptors serves to decrease anxiety, relieve insomnia, and stimulate the appetite. Mirtazapine is a potent antagonist of histamine H$_1$ receptors and is a moderately potent antagonist at α_1-adrenergic and muscarinic-cholinergic receptors.

Therapeutic Indications

Mirtazapine is effective for the treatment of depression. It is highly sedating, making it a reasonable choice for use in depressed patients with severe or long-standing insomnia. Some patients find the residual daytime sedation associated with the initiation of treatment to be quite pronounced. However, the more extreme sedating properties of the drug generally lessen over the first week of treatment. Combined with the tendency to sometimes cause a ravenous appetite, mirtazapine is well suited for depressed patients with melancholic features such as insomnia, weight loss, and agitation. Elderly depressed patients, in particular, are good candidates for mirtazapine; young adults are more likely to object to this side effect profile.

Mirtazapine's blockade of 5-HT$_3$ receptors, a mechanism associated with medications used to combat the severe GI side effects of cancer chemotherapy agents, has led to the use of the drug in a similar role. In this population, sedation and stimulation of appetite clearly could be seen as being beneficial instead of unwelcome side effects.

Mirtazapine is often combined with SSRIs or venlafaxine to augment antidepressant response or counteract serotonergic side effects of those drugs, particularly nausea, agitation, and insomnia. Mirtazapine has no significant pharmacokinetic interactions with other antidepressants.

Precautions and Adverse Reactions

Somnolence, the most common adverse effect of mirtazapine, occurs in more than 50 percent of persons (Table 21-18). Persons starting mirtazapine should thus exercise caution when driving or operating dangerous machinery and even when getting out of bed at night. This adverse effect is why mirtazapine is almost always given before sleep. Mirtazapine potentiates the sedative effects of other CNS depressants, so potentially sedating prescription or over-the-counter drugs and alcohol should be avoided during the use of mirtazapine. Mirtazapine also causes dizziness in 7 percent of persons. It does not appear to increase the risk of seizures. Mania or hypomania occurred in clinical trials at a rate similar to that of other antidepressant drugs.

Mirtazapine increases appetite in about one-third of patients. Mirtazapine may also increase serum cholesterol concentration to 20 percent or more above the upper limit of normal in 15 percent of persons and increase triglycerides to 500 mg/dL or more in 6 percent of persons. Elevations of alanine transaminase levels to more than three times the upper limit of normal were seen in 2 percent of mirtazapine-treated persons as opposed to 0.3 percent of placebo control subjects.

In limited premarketing experience, the absolute neutrophil count dropped to 500/mm^3 or less within 2 months of the onset of

Table 21-18
Adverse Reactions Reported with Mirtazapine

Event	Patients (%)
Somnolence	54
Dry mouth	25
Increased appetite	17
Constipation	13
Weight gain	12
Dizziness	7
Myalgias	5
Disturbing dreams	4

use in 0.3 percent of persons, some of whom developed symptomatic infections. This hematologic condition was reversible in all cases and was more likely to occur when other risk factors for neutropenia were present. Increases in the frequency of neutropenia have not, however, been reported during the extensive postmarketing period. Persons who develop fever, chills, sore throat, mucous membrane ulceration, or other signs of infection should nevertheless be evaluated medically. If a low WBC count is found, mirtazapine should be immediately discontinued, and the infectious disease status should be followed closely.

A small number of persons experience orthostatic hypotension while taking mirtazapine. Although no data exist regarding the effects on fetal development, mirtazapine should be used with caution during pregnancy.

Mirtazapine use by pregnant women has not been studied, but because the drug may be excreted in breast milk, it should not be taken by nursing mothers. Because of the risk of agranulocytosis associated with mirtazapine use, persons should be attuned to signs of infection. Because of the sedating effects of mirtazapine, persons should determine the degree to which they are affected before engaging in driving or other potentially dangerous activities.

Drug Interactions

Mirtazapine can potentiate the sedation of alcohol and benzodiazepines. Mirtazapine should not be used within 14 days of use of an MAOI.

Laboratory Interferences

No laboratory interferences have yet been described for mirtazapine.

Dosage and Administration

Mirtazapine is available in 15-, 30-, and 45-mg scored tablets. Mirtazapine is also available in 15-, 30-, and 45-mg orally disintegrating tablets for persons who have difficulty swallowing pills. If persons fail to respond to the initial dose of 15 mg of mirtazapine before sleep, the dose may be increased in 15-mg increments every 5 days to a maximum of 45 mg before sleep. Lower dosages may be necessary for elderly persons or persons with renal or hepatic insufficiency.

NEFAZODONE AND TRAZODONE

Nefazodone (Serzone) and Trazodone (Desyrel) are mechanistically and structurally related drugs approved as treatments for depression. Nefazodone (Serzone) is an analog of trazodone. When nefazodone was introduced in 1995, there were expectations that it would become widely used because it did not cause the sexual side effects and sleep disruption associated with the selective SSRIs. Although it was devoid of these side effects, it was nevertheless found to produce problematic sedation, nausea, dizziness, and visual disturbances. Consequently, nefazodone was never extensively adopted in clinical practice. This fact, as well as reports of rare cases of sometimes fatal hepatotoxicity, led the original manufacturer to discontinue the production of branded nefazodone in 2004. Generic nefazodone remains available in the United States.

Trazodone received FDA approval in 1981 as a treatment for MDD. Its novel triazolopyridine chemical structure distinguished it from the TCAs, and clinical trials suggested improved safety and

tolerability compared with TCAs. There were high expectations that it would replace the older drugs as a mainstay of treatment for depression. However, the extreme sedation associated with trazodone, even at subtherapeutic doses, limited the clinical effectiveness of the drug. However, its soporific properties made trazodone a favorite alternative to standard hypnotics as a sleep-inducing agent. Unlike conventional sleeping pills, trazodone is not a controlled substance.

Nefazodone

Pharmacologic Actions.   Nefazodone is rapidly and completely absorbed but is then extensively metabolized so that the bioavailability of active compounds is about 20 percent of the oral dose. Its half-life is 2 to 4 hours. Steady-state concentrations of nefazodone and its principal active metabolite, hydroxynefazodone, are achieved within 4 to 5 days. Metabolism of nefazodone in elderly persons, especially women, is about half of that seen in younger persons, so lowered doses are recommended for elderly persons. An important metabolite of nefazodone is meta-chlorophenylpiperazine (mCPP), which has some serotonergic effects and may cause migraine, anxiety, and weight loss.

Although nefazodone is an inhibitor of serotonin uptake and, more weakly, of norepinephrine reuptake, its antagonism of serotonin 5-HT$_A$ receptors is thought to produce its antianxiety and antidepressant effects. Nefazodone is also a mild antagonist of the α_1-adrenergic receptors, which predisposes some persons to orthostatic hypotension but is not sufficiently potent to produce priapism.

Therapeutic Indications.   Nefazodone is effective for the treatment of major depression. The usual effective dosage is 300 to 600 mg a day. In direct comparison with SSRIs, nefazodone is less likely to cause inhibition of orgasm or decreased sexual desire. Nefazodone is also effective for the treatment of panic disorder and panic with comorbid depression or depressive symptoms, GAD, and PMDD and management of chronic pain. It is not useful for the treatment of OCD. Nefazodone increases rapid eye movement (REM) sleep and increases sleep continuity. Nefazodone is also of use in patients with PTSD and chronic fatigue syndrome. It may also be effective in patients who have been treatment-resistant to other antidepressant drugs.

Precautions and Adverse Reactions.   The most common reasons for discontinuing nefazodone use are sedation, nausea, dizziness, insomnia, weakness, and agitation (Table 21-19). Many patients report no specific side effects but describe a vague sense of feeling medicated. Nefazodone also causes visual trails, in which patients see an afterimage when looking at moving objects or when moving their heads quickly.

A significant safety concern with the use of nefazodone is a severe elevation of hepatic enzymes, and, in some instances, liver failure. Accordingly, serial hepatic function tests need to be done when patients are treated with nefazodone. Hepatic effects can be seen early in treatment and are more likely to develop when nefazodone is combined with other drugs metabolized in the liver.

Some patients taking nefazodone may experience a decrease in BP that can cause episodes of postural hypotension. Nefazodone should therefore be used with caution by persons with underlying cardiac conditions or history of stroke or heart attack, dehydration, or hypovolemia or by persons being treated with antihypertensive medications. Patients switched from SSRIs to nefazodone may experience an increase in side effects, possibly because nefazodone

Table 21-19
Adverse Reactions Reported with Nefazodone
(300–600 mg a day)

Reaction	Patients (%)
Headache	36
Dry mouth	25
Somnolence	25
Nausea	22
Dizziness	17
Constipation	14
Insomnia	11
Weakness	11
Lightheadedness	10
Blurred vision	9
Dyspepsia	9
Infection	8
Confusion	7
Scotomata	7

does not protect against SSRI withdrawal symptoms. One of its metabolites, mCPP, may intensify these discontinuation symptoms. Patients have survived nefazodone overdoses above 10 g, but deaths have been reported when it has been combined with alcohol. Nausea, vomiting, and somnolence are the most common signs of toxicity.

There are few studies or clinical reports of nefazodone during pregnancy. Nefazodone should, therefore, be used during pregnancy only if the potential benefit to the mother outweighs the potential risks to the fetus. It is not known whether nefazodone is excreted in human breast milk. Therefore, it should be used with caution by lactating mothers. The nefazodone dosage should be lowered in persons with severe hepatic disease, but no adjustment is necessary for persons with renal disease.

Drug Interactions and Laboratory Interferences. Nefazodone should not be given concomitantly with MAOIs. Also, nefazodone has particular drug–drug interactions with the triazolobenzodiazepines triazolam (Halcion) and alprazolam (Xanax) because of the inhibition of CYP3A4 by nefazodone. Potentially elevated levels of each of these drugs can develop after administration of nefazodone, but the levels of nefazodone are generally not affected. The dose of triazolam should be lowered by 75 percent, and the dose of alprazolam should be lowered by 50 percent, when given concomitantly with nefazodone.

Nefazodone may slow the metabolism of digoxin; therefore, digoxin levels should be monitored carefully in persons taking both medications. Nefazodone also slows the metabolism of haloperidol (Haldol) so that the dosage of haloperidol should be reduced in persons taking both medications. The addition of nefazodone may also exacerbate the adverse effects of lithium carbonate (Eskalith).

There are no known laboratory interferences associated with nefazodone.

Dosage and Clinical Guidelines. Nefazodone is available in 50-, 200-, and 250-mg unscored tablets and 100- and 150-mg scored tablets. The recommended starting dosage of nefazodone is 100 mg twice a day, but 50 mg twice a day may be better tolerated, especially by elderly persons. The dosage should be slowly raised in increments of 100 to 200 mg a day at intervals of no less than 1 week per increase to limit the development of adverse effects. The optimal dosage is 300 to 600 mg daily in two divided doses. However, some studies report that nefazodone is effective when taken once a day, especially at bedtime. Geriatric persons should receive dosages about two-thirds of the usual nongeriatric dosages, with a maximum of 400 mg a day. Similar to other antidepressants, the clinical benefit of nefazodone usually appears after 2 to 4 weeks of treatment. Patients with the premenstrual syndrome are treated with a flexible dosage that averages about 250 mg a day.

Trazodone

Pharmacologic Actions.   Trazodone is readily absorbed from the GI tract and reaches peak plasma levels in about 1 hour. It has a half-life of 5 to 9 hours. Trazodone is metabolized in the liver, and 75 percent of its metabolites are excreted in the urine.

Trazodone is a weak inhibitor of serotonin reuptake and a potent antagonist of serotonin 5-HT_{2A} and 5-HT_{2C} receptors. The active metabolite of trazodone is mCPP, which is an agonist at 5-HT_{2C} receptors and has a half-life of 14 hours. mCPP has been associated with migraine, anxiety, and weight loss. The adverse effects of trazodone are partially mediated by α_1-adrenergic receptor antagonism.

Therapeutic Indications

DEPRESSIVE DISORDERS.   The main indication for the use of trazodone is MDD. There is a dose–response relationship, with dosages of 250 to 600 mg a day being necessary for trazodone to have therapeutic benefit. Trazodone increases total sleep time, decreases the number and the duration of nighttime awakenings, and decreases the amount of REM sleep. Unlike tricyclic drugs, trazodone does not decrease stage 4 sleep. Trazodone is thus useful for depressed persons with anxiety and insomnia.

INSOMNIA.   Trazodone is a first-line agent for the treatment of insomnia because of its marked sedative qualities and favorable effects on sleep architecture (see above) combined with its lack of anticholinergic effects. Trazodone is effective for insomnia caused by depression or the use of drugs. When used as a hypnotic, the usual initial dosage is 25 to 100 mg at bedtime.

ERECTILE DISORDER.   Trazodone is associated with an increased risk of priapism. Trazodone can potentiate erections resulting from sexual stimulation. It has thus been used to prolong erectile time and turgidity in some men with erectile disorder. The dosage for this indication is 150 to 200 mg a day. Trazodone-triggered priapism (an erection lasting more than 3 hours with pain) is a medical emergency. The use of trazodone for the treatment of male erectile dysfunction has diminished considerably since the introduction of phosphodiesterase (PDE)-5 agents (see Chapter 16).

OTHER INDICATIONS.   Trazodone may be useful in low dosages (50 mg a day) for controlling severe agitation in children with developmental disabilities and elderly persons with dementia. At dosages above 250 mg a day, trazodone reduces the tension and apprehension associated with GAD. It has been used to treat depression in patients with schizophrenia. Trazodone may have a beneficial effect on insomnia and nightmares in persons with PTSD.

Precautions and Adverse Reactions. The most common adverse effects associated with trazodone are sedation, orthostatic hypotension, dizziness, headache, and nausea. Some persons experience dry mouth or gastric irritation. The drug is not associated with anticholinergic adverse effects, such as urinary retention, weight gain, and constipation. A few case reports have noted an association between trazodone and arrhythmias in persons with preexisting premature ventricular contractions or mitral valve prolapse. Neutropenia, usually not of clinical significance, may develop, which should be considered if persons have a fever or sore throat.

Trazodone may cause significant orthostatic hypotension 4 to 6 hours after a dose is taken, especially if taken concurrently with antihypertensive agents or if a large dose is taken without food. Administration of trazodone with food slows absorption and reduces the peak plasma concentration, thus reducing the risk of orthostatic hypotension.

Because suicide attempts often involve the ingestion of sleeping pills, it is essential to be familiar with the symptoms and treatment of trazodone overdose. Patients have survived trazodone overdoses of more than 9 g. Symptoms of overdose include lethargy, vomiting, drowsiness, headache, orthostasis, dizziness, dyspnea, tinnitus, myalgias, tachycardia, incontinence, shivering, and coma. Treatment consists of emesis or lavage and supportive care. Forced diuresis may enhance elimination. Treat hypotension and sedation as appropriate.

Trazodone causes priapism, prolonged erection in the absence of sexual stimuli, in one of every 10,000 men. Trazodone-induced priapism usually appears in the first 4 weeks of treatment but may occur as late as 18 months into treatment. It can appear at any dose. In such cases, trazodone use should be discontinued, and another antidepressant should be used. Painful erections or erections lasting more than 1 hour are warning signs that warrant immediate discontinuation of the drug and medical evaluation. The first step in the emergency management of priapism is an intracavernosal injection of an α_1-adrenergic agonist pressor agent, such as metaraminol (Aramine) or epinephrine. In about one-third of reported cases, surgical intervention was required. In some cases, permanent impairment of erectile function or impotence resulted.

The use of trazodone is contraindicated in pregnant and nursing women. Trazodone should be used with caution in persons with hepatic and renal diseases.

Drug Interactions. Trazodone potentiates the CNS depressant effects of other centrally acting drugs and alcohol. Concurrent use of trazodone and antihypertensives may cause hypotension. No cases of hypertensive crisis have been reported when trazodone has been used to treat MAOI-associated insomnia. Trazodone can increase levels of digoxin and phenytoin. Trazodone should be used with caution in combination with warfarin. Drugs that inhibit CYP3A4 can increase levels of trazodone's primary metabolite, mCPP, leading to an increase in side effects.

Laboratory Interferences. No known laboratory interferences are associated with the administration of trazodone.

Dosage and Clinical Guidelines. Trazodone is available in 50-, 100-, 150-, and 300-mg tablets. Once-a-day dosing is as effective as divided dosing and reduces daytime sedation. The usual starting dose is 50 mg before sleep. The dosage can be increased in increments of 50 mg every 3 days if sedation or orthostatic hypotension does not become a problem. The therapeutic range for trazodone is 200 to 600 mg a day in divided doses. Some reports indicate that dosages of 400 to 600 mg a day are required for maximal therapeutic effects; other reports indicate that 250 to 400 mg a day is sufficient. The dosage may be titrated up to 300 mg a day; then, the person can be evaluated for the need for further dosage increases based on the presence or the absence of signs of clinical improvement.

TRICYCLICS AND TETRACYCLICS

The observation in 1957 that imipramine (Tofranil) had antidepressant effects led to the development of a new class of antidepressant compounds, the tricyclics (TCAs). In turn, the finding that imipramine blocked reuptake of norepinephrine led to research into the role of catecholamines in depression. After the introduction of imipramine, several other antidepressant compounds were developed that shared a basic tricyclic structure and had relatively similar effects. Later, other heterocyclic compounds were also marketed that were somewhat similar in structure and that had relatively comparable secondary properties. At one time, amitriptyline (Elavil, Endep) and imipramine were the two most commonly prescribed antidepressants in the United States. However, because of their anticholinergic and antihistaminic side effects, they are rarely used for depression. Nortriptyline (Aventyl, Pamelor) and desipramine (Norpramin, Pertofrane) became preferred. Nortriptyline has the least effect on orthostatic hypotension, and desipramine is the least anticholinergic. Although introduced as antidepressants, the therapeutic indications for these agents have grown to include panic disorder, GAD, PTSD, OCD, and pain syndromes. The introduction of newer antidepressant agents with more selective actions on neurotransmitters or with unique mechanisms of action has sharply reduced the prescribing of TCAs and tetracyclics. The improved safety profiles of the newer drugs, especially when taken in overdose, also contributed to the decline in the use of older drugs. Nevertheless, the TCAs and tetracyclics remain unsurpassed in terms of their antidepressant efficacy. Table 21-20 lists TCA and tetracyclic drugs and their available preparations.

Pharmacologic Actions

The absorption of most TCAs is complete after oral administration, and there is significant metabolism from the first-pass effect. Peak plasma concentrations occur within 2 to 8 hours, and the half-lives of the TCAs vary from 10 to 70 hours; nortriptyline, maprotiline (Ludiomil), and particularly protriptyline (Vivactil) can have longer half-lives. The long half-lives allow all the compounds to be given once daily; 5 to 7 days is needed to reach steady-state plasma concentrations. Imipramine pamoate (Tofranil) is a depot form of the drug for intramuscular (IM) administration; indications for the use of this preparation are limited.

The TCAs undergo hepatic metabolism by the CYP450 enzyme system. Clinically relevant drug interactions may result from competition for enzyme CYP2D6 among TCAs and quinidine, cimetidine (Tagamet), fluoxetine (Prozac), sertraline (Zoloft), paroxetine (Paxil), phenothiazines, carbamazepine (Tegretol), and the type IC antiarrhythmics propafenone (Rythmol) and flecainide (Tambocor). Concomitant administration of TCAs and these inhibitors may slow down the metabolism and raise the plasma concentrations of TCAs. Additionally, genetic variations in the activity of CYP2D6 may account for up to a 40-fold difference in plasma TCA

Table 21-20
Tricyclic and Tetracyclic Drug Preparations

Drug	Tablets (mg)	Capsules (mg)	Parenteral (mg/mL)	Solution
Imipramine (Tofranil)	10, 25, and 50	75, 100, 125, and 150	12.5	—
Desipramine (Norpramin, Pertofrane)	10, 25, 50, 75, 100, and 150	—	—	—
Trimipramine (Surmontil)	—	25, 50, and 100	—	—
Amitriptyline (Elavil)	10, 25, 50, 75, 100, and 150	—	10	—
Nortriptyline (Aventyl, Pamelor)	—	10, 25, 50, and 75	—	10 mg/5 mL
Protriptyline (Vivactil)	5 and 10	—	—	—
Amoxapine (Asendin)	25, 50, 100, and 150	—	—	—
Doxepin (Sinequan)	—	10, 25, 50, 75, 100, and 150	—	10 mg/mL
Maprotiline (Ludiomil)	25, 50, and 75	—	—	—
Clomipramine (Anafranil)	—	25, 50, and 75	—	—

concentrations in different persons. The dosage of the TCA may need to be adjusted to correct changes in the rate of hepatic TCA metabolism.

The TCAs block the transporter site for norepinephrine and serotonin, thus increasing synaptic concentrations of these neurotransmitters. Each drug differs in its affinity for each of these transporters, with clomipramine (Anafranil) being the most serotonin selective and desipramine the most norepinephrine selective of the TCAs. Secondary effects of the TCAs include antagonism at the muscarinic acetylcholine, histamine H_1, and α_1- and α_2-adrenergic receptors. The potency of these effects on other receptors largely determines the side effect profile of each drug. Amoxapine, nortriptyline, desipramine, and maprotiline have the least anticholinergic activity; doxepin has the most antihistaminergic activity. Although they are more likely to cause constipation, sedation, dry mouth, or lightheadedness than the SSRIs, the TCAs are less prone to cause sexual dysfunction, significant long-term weight gain, and sleep disturbances than the SSRIs. The half-lives and plasma clearance for most TCAs are very similar.

Therapeutic Indications

The indications are similar to those for the SSRIs, which have widely replaced the TCAs. However, the TCAs represent a reasonable alternative for persons who cannot tolerate the adverse effects of the SSRIs.

Major Depressive Disorder. The treatment of a major depressive episode and the prophylactic treatment of MDD are the principal indications for using TCAs. Although the TCAs are effective in the treatment of depression in persons with bipolar I disorder, they are more likely to induce mania, hypomania, or cycling than the newer antidepressants, most notably the SSRIs and bupropion. It is thus not advised that TCAs be routinely used to treat depression associated with bipolar I or bipolar II disorder.

Melancholic features, prior major depressive episodes, and a family history of depressive disorders increase the likelihood of therapeutic response. All of the available TCAs are equally effective in the treatment of depressive disorders. In the case of a person, however, one tricyclic or tetracyclic may be useful, and another one may be ineffective. The treatment of a major depressive episode

with psychotic features almost always requires the coadministration of an antipsychotic drug and an antidepressant.

Although it is used worldwide as an antidepressant, clomipramine is only approved in the United States for the treatment of OCD.

Panic Disorder with Agoraphobia. Imipramine is the TCA most studied for panic disorder with agoraphobia, but other TCAs are also useful when taken at the usual antidepressant dosages. Because of the potential initial anxiogenic effects of the TCAs, starting dosages should be small, and the dosage should be titrated upward slowly. Small doses of benzodiazepines may be used initially to deal with this side effect.

Generalized Anxiety Disorder. The FDA approves the use of doxepin for the treatment of anxiety disorders. Some research data show that imipramine may also be useful. Although rarely used anymore, a chlordiazepoxide–amitriptyline combination (Limbitrol) is available for mixed anxiety and depressive disorders.

Obsessive-Compulsive Disorder. Patients with OCD appear to respond specifically to clomipramine, as well as the SSRIs. Some improvement is usually seen in 2 to 4 weeks, but a further reduction in symptoms may continue for the first 4 to 5 months of treatment. None of the other TCAs appears to be nearly as effective as clomipramine for the treatment of this disorder. Clomipramine may also be a drug of choice for depressed persons with marked obsessive features.

Pain. The TCAs are widely used to treat chronic neuropathic pain and in the prophylaxis of migraine headache. Amitriptyline is the TCA most often used in this role. During the treatment of pain, doses are generally lower than those used in depression; for example, 75 mg of amitriptyline may be sufficient. These effects also appear more rapidly.

Other Disorders. Childhood enuresis is often treated with imipramine. Peptic ulcer disease can be treated with doxepin, which has marked antihistaminergic effects. Other indications for the TCAs are narcolepsy, nightmare disorder, and PTSD. The drugs are sometimes used for the treatment of children and adolescents with ADHD, sleepwalking disorder, separation anxiety disorder, and sleep terror disorder. Clomipramine has also been used to treat premature ejaculation, movement disorders, and compulsive behavior in children with autistic disorders; however, because the TCAs have caused sudden death in several children and adolescents, they should not be used in children.

Precautions and Adverse Reactions

The TCAs are associated with a wide range of problematic side effects and can be lethal when taken in overdose.

Psychiatric Effects.   The TCAs can induce a switch to mania or hypomania in susceptible individuals. The TCAs may also exacerbate psychotic disorders in susceptible persons. At high plasma concentrations (levels above 300 ng/mL), the anticholinergic effects of the TCAs can cause confusion or delirium. Patients with dementia are particularly vulnerable to this development.

Anticholinergic Effects.   Anticholinergic effects often limit the tolerable dosage to relatively low ranges. Some persons may develop a tolerance for the anticholinergic effects with continued treatment. Anticholinergic effects include dry mouth, constipation, blurred vision, delirium, and urinary retention. Sugarless gum, candy, or fluoride lozenges can alleviate dry mouth. Bethanechol (Urecholine), 25 to 50 mg three or four times a day, may reduce urinary hesitancy and may be helpful in erectile dysfunction when the drug is taken 30 minutes before sexual intercourse. Anticholinergic drugs can also aggravate narrow-angle glaucoma, and the precipitation of glaucoma requires emergency treatment with a miotic agent. The TCAs should be avoided in persons with narrow-angle glaucoma, and an SSRI should be substituted. Severe anticholinergic effects can lead to CNS anticholinergic syndrome. This syndrome includes symptoms of confusion and delirium, especially if the TCAs are administered with DRAs or anticholinergic drugs. IM or IV physostigmine (Antilirium, Eserine) is used to diagnose and treat anticholinergic delirium.

Cardiac Effects.   When administered in their usual therapeutic dosages, the TCAs may cause tachycardia, flattened T waves, prolonged QT intervals, and depressed ST segments in the electrocardiographic (ECG) recording. Imipramine has a quinidine-like effect at therapeutic plasma concentrations and may reduce the number of premature ventricular contractions. Because the drugs prolong conduction time, their use in persons with preexisting conduction defects is contraindicated. In persons with a history of any type of heart disease, the TCAs should be used only after SSRIs or other newer antidepressants have been found ineffective, and if used, they should be introduced at low dosages, with gradual increases in dosage and monitoring of cardiac functions. All of the TCAs can cause tachycardia, which may persist for months and is one of the most common reasons for drug discontinuation, especially in younger persons. At high plasma concentrations, as seen in overdoses, the drugs become arrhythmogenic.

Other Autonomic Effects.   Orthostatic hypotension is the most common cardiovascular autonomic adverse effect, and the most common reason TCAs are discontinued. It can result in falls and injuries in affected persons. Nortriptyline may be the drug least likely to cause this problem. Orthostatic hypotension is treated with avoidance of caffeine, intake of at least 2 L of fluid per day, and addition of salt to the diet unless the person is being treated for

hypertension. In persons taking antihypertensive agents, reduction of the dosage may reduce the risk of orthostatic hypotension. Other possible autonomic effects are profuse sweating, palpitations, and increased BP. Although some persons respond to fludrocortisone (Florinef), 0.02 to 0.05 mg twice a day, the drug has potential toxicities. It is preferable to substitute an SSRI than to use a mineralocorticoid such as fludrocortisone. The TCAs' use should be discontinued several days before elective surgery because of the occurrence of hypertensive episodes during surgery in persons receiving TCAs.

Sedation.   Sedation is a common effect of the TCAs and may be welcomed if sleeplessness has been a problem. The sedative effect of the TCAs is a result of anticholinergic and antihistaminergic activities. Amitriptyline, trimipramine, and doxepin are the most sedating agents; imipramine, amoxapine, nortriptyline, and maprotiline are less sedating; and desipramine and protriptyline are the least sedating agents.

Neurologic Effects.   A fine, rapid tremor may occur. Myoclonic twitches and tremors of the tongue and the upper extremities are common. Rare effects include speech blockage, paresthesia, peroneal palsies, and ataxia.

Amoxapine is unique in causing parkinsonian symptoms, akathisia, and even dyskinesia because of the dopaminergic blocking activity of one of its metabolites. Amoxapine may also cause neuroleptic malignant syndrome in rare cases. Maprotiline may cause seizures when the dosage is increased too quickly or is kept at high levels for too long. Clomipramine and amoxapine may lower the seizure threshold more than other drugs in the class. As a class, however, the TCAs have a relatively low risk for inducing seizures except in persons who are at risk for seizures (e.g., persons with epilepsy and those with brain lesions). Although such persons can still use the TCAs, the initial dosages should be lower than usual, and subsequent dosage increases should be gradual.

Allergic and Hematologic Effects.   Exanthematous rashes are seen in 4 to 5 percent of all persons treated with maprotiline. Jaundice is rare. Agranulocytosis, leukocytosis, leukopenia, and eosinophilia are rare complications of TCA treatment. However, a person who has a sore throat or a fever during the first few months of TCA treatment should have a CBC done immediately.

Hepatic Effects.   Mild and self-limited increases in serum transaminase concentrations may occur and should be monitored. The TCAs can also produce a fulminant acute hepatitis in 0.1 to 1 percent of persons. This side effect can be life-threatening, and the antidepressant should be discontinued.

Other Adverse Effects.   Modest weight gain is typical. Amoxapine exerts a DRA effect and may cause hyperprolactinemia, impotence, galactorrhea, anorgasmia, and ejaculatory disturbances. Other TCAs have also been associated with gynecomastia and amenorrhea. The syndrome of inappropriate secretion of antidiuretic hormone has also been reported with TCAs. Other effects include nausea, vomiting, and hepatitis.

TERATOGENICITY AND PREGNANCY-RELATED RISKS.   A definitive link between the tricyclic compounds and tetracyclic compounds and teratogenic effects has not been established, but isolated reports of morphogenesis have been reported. TCAs cross the placenta, and neonatal drug withdrawal can occur. This syndrome includes tachypnea, cyanosis, irritability, and poor sucking reflex. If possible, tricyclic and tetracyclic medications should be discontinued 1 week before delivery. Recently, norepinephrine and serotonin transporters have been identified in the placenta. They appear to play an essential role in the clearance of these amines in the fetus. The understanding of the effects of reuptake inhibitors on these transporters during pregnancy is limited. However, one study compared intelligence and language development in 80 children exposed to TCAs during pregnancy with 84 children exposed to other nonteratogenic agents and found no deleterious effects of the TCAs. The TCAs are excreted in breast milk at concentrations similar to plasma. The actual quantity delivered, however, is small, so drug levels in the infant are usually undetectable or very low. Because the risk of relapse is a serious concern in patients with recurrent depression, and these risks may be increased during pregnancy or the postpartum period, the risks and benefits of continuing or withdrawing treatment need to be discussed with the patient and weighed carefully.

Precautions. The TCAs may cause a withdrawal syndrome in newborns consisting of tachypnea, cyanosis, irritability, and poor sucking reflex. The drugs do pass into breast milk but at concentrations that are usually undetectable in the infant's plasma. We should use these drugs cautiously in patients with hepatic or renal diseases. The TCAs should not be administered during a course of ECT, primarily because of the risk of serious adverse cardiac effects.

Drug Interactions

Monoamine Oxidase Inhibitors. The TCAs should not be taken within 14 days of administration of an MAOI.

Antihypertensives. The TCAs block the therapeutic effects of antihypertensive medication. The TCAs may block the antihypertensive effects of the β-adrenergic receptor antagonists (e.g., propranolol [Inderal] and clonidine [Catapres]). The coadministration of a TCA and α-methyldopa (Aldomet) may cause behavioral agitation.

Antiarrhythmic Drugs. The antiarrhythmic properties of TCAs can be additive to those of quinidine, an effect that is further exacerbated by the inhibition of TCA metabolism by quinidine.

Dopamine Receptor Antagonists. Concurrent administration of TCAs and DRAs increases the plasma concentrations of both drugs. Desipramine plasma concentrations may increase twofold during concurrent administration with perphenazine (Trilafon). The DRAs also add to the anticholinergic and sedative effects of the TCAs. Concomitant use of SDAs also increases those effects.

Central Nervous System Depressants. Opioids, alcohol, anxiolytics, hypnotics, and over-the-counter cold medications have additive effects by causing CNS depression when coadministered with TCAs. Persons should be advised to avoid driving or using dangerous equipment if sedated by TCAs.

Sympathomimetics. Tricyclic drug use with sympathomimetic drugs may cause serious cardiovascular effects.

Oral Contraceptives. Birth control pills may decrease TCA plasma concentrations through the induction of hepatic enzymes.

Other Drug Interactions. Nicotine may reduce TCA concentrations. Plasma concentrations may also be lowered by ascorbic

acid, ammonium chloride, barbiturates, cigarette smoking, carbamazepine, chloral hydrate, lithium (Eskalith), and primidone (Mysoline). TCA plasma concentrations may be increased by concurrent use of acetazolamide (Diamox), sodium bicarbonate, acetylsalicylic acid, cimetidine, thiazide diuretics, fluoxetine, paroxetine, and fluvoxamine (Luvox). Plasma concentrations of the TCAs may rise three- to fourfold when administered concurrently with fluoxetine, fluvoxamine, and paroxetine.

Laboratory Interferences

The tricyclic compounds are present at low concentrations and are not likely to interfere with other laboratory assays. They may interfere with the determination of conventional neuroleptic blood concentrations because of their structural similarity and the low concentrations of some neuroleptics.

Dosage and Clinical Guidelines

Persons who intend to take TCAs should undergo routine physical and laboratory examinations, including a CBC, a WBC count with differential, and serum electrolytes with liver function tests. An ECG should be obtained for all persons, especially women older than 40 years of age and men older than 30 years of age. The TCAs are contraindicated in persons with a QT_c greater than 450 milliseconds. The initial dose should be small and should be raised gradually. Because of the availability of highly effective alternatives to TCAs, a newer agent should be used if there is any medical condition that may interact adversely with the TCAs.

Elderly persons and children are more sensitive to TCA adverse effects than are young adults. In children, the ECG should be regularly monitored during the use of a TCA.

The available preparations of TCAs are presented in Table 21-20. The dosages and therapeutic blood levels for the TCAs vary among the drugs (Table 21-21). Except for protriptyline, all of the TCAs should be started at 25 mg a day and increased as tolerated. Divided doses at first reduce the severity of the adverse effects, although most of the dosage should be given at night to help induce sleep if a sedating drug such as amitriptyline is used. Eventually, the entire daily dose can be given at bedtime. A common clinical mistake is to stop increasing the dosage when the person is tolerating the drug but taking less than the maximum therapeutic dose and does not show clinical improvement. The clinician should routinely assess the person's pulse and orthostatic changes in BP while the dosage is being increased.

Nortriptyline use should be started at 25 mg a day. Most patients need only 75 mg a day to achieve a blood level of 100 mg/nL. However, the dosage may be raised to 150 mg a day if needed. Amoxapine use should be started at 150 mg a day and raised to 400 mg a day. Protriptyline use should be started at 15 mg a day and raised to 60 mg a day. Maprotiline has been associated with an increased incidence of seizures. This risk is most significant if the dosage is raised too quickly or is maintained at too high a level. Maprotiline use should be started at 25 mg a day and increased over 4 weeks to 225 mg a day. It should be kept at that level for only 6 weeks and then be reduced to 175 to 200 mg a day.

Persons with chronic pain may be particularly sensitive to adverse effects when TCA use is started. Therefore, treatment should begin with low dosages that are raised in small increments. However, persons with chronic pain may experience relief on long-term low-dosage therapy, such as amitriptyline or nortriptyline at 10 to 75 mg a day.

Table 21-21
General Information for the Tricyclic and Tetracyclic Antidepressants

Generic Name	Trade Name	Usual Adult Dosage Range (mg/day)	Therapeutic Plasma Concentrations (µg/mL)
Imipramine	Tofranil	150–300	150–300[a]
Desipramine	Norpramin, Pertofrane	150–300	150–300[a]
Trimipramine	Surmontil	150–300	150–300
Amitriptyline	Elavil, Endep	150–300	100–250[b]
Nortriptyline	Pamelor, Aventyl	50–150	50–150[a] (maximum)
Protriptyline	Vivactil	15–60	75–250
Amoxapine	Asendin	150–400	200–500[c]
Doxepin	Adapin, Sinequan	150–300	100–250[a]
Maprotiline	Ludiomil	150–230	150–300[a]
Clomipramine	Anafranil	130–250	50 to 250[c]

[a]Exact range may vary among laboratories.
[b]Includes parent compound and desmethyl metabolite.
[c]Estimated from limited studies.

The TCAs should be avoided in children except as a last resort. Dosing guidelines in children for imipramine include initiation at 1.5 mg/kg a day. The dosage can be titrated to no more than 5 mg/kg a day. In enuresis, the dosage is usually 50 to 100 mg a day, taken at bedtime. Clomipramine use can be initiated at 50 mg a day and increased to no more than 3 mg/kg per day or 200 mg a day.

When TCA treatment is discontinued, the dosage should first be decreased to three-fourths the maximal dosage for a month. At that time, if no symptoms are present, drug use can be tapered by 25 mg (5 mg for protriptyline) every 4 to 7 days. Slow tapering avoids a cholinergic rebound syndrome consisting of nausea, upset stomach, sweating, headache, neck pain, and vomiting. This syndrome can be treated by reinstituting a small dosage of the drug and tapering more slowly than before. Several case reports note the appearance of rebound mania or hypomania after the abrupt discontinuation of TCA use.

Plasma Concentrations and Therapeutic Drug Monitoring.
Clinical determinations of plasma concentrations should be conducted after 5 to 7 days on the same dosage of medication and 8 to 12 hours after the last dose. Because of variations in absorption and metabolism, there may be a 30- to 50-fold difference in the plasma concentrations in persons given the same dosage of a TCA. Nortriptyline is unique in its association with a therapeutic window—that is, plasma concentrations below 50 ng/mL or above 150 ng/mL may reduce its efficacy.

Plasma concentrations may be useful in confirming compliance, assessing reasons for drug failures, and documenting effective plasma concentrations for future treatment. Clinicians should always treat the person and not the plasma concentration. Some persons have adequate clinical responses with seemingly subtherapeutic plasma concentrations, and other persons only respond at supratherapeutic plasma concentrations without experiencing adverse effects. The latter situation, however, should alert the clinician to monitor the person's condition with, for example, serial ECG recordings.

Overdose Attempts. Overdose attempts with TCAs are severe and can often be fatal. Prescriptions for these drugs should be non-refillable and for no longer than 1 week at a time for patients at risk for suicide. Amoxapine may be more likely than the other TCAs to result in death when taken in overdose. The newer antidepressants are safer in overdose.

Symptoms of overdose include agitation, delirium, convulsions, hyperactive deep tendon reflexes, bowel and bladder paralysis, dysregulation of BP and temperature, and mydriasis. The patient then progresses to coma and perhaps respiratory depression. Cardiac arrhythmias may not respond to treatment. Because of the long half-lives of TCAs, the patients are at risk of cardiac arrhythmias for 3 to 4 days after the overdose, so they should be monitored in intensive care medical settings.

MONOAMINE OXIDASE INHIBITORS

Introduced in the late 1950s, MAOIs were the first class of approved antidepressant drugs. The first of these drugs, isoniazid, was intended to be used as a treatment for tuberculosis, but its antidepressant properties were discovered by chance when some treated patients experienced elevation of mood during treatment. Despite their effectiveness, prescription of MAOIs as first-line agents has always been limited by concern about the development of potentially lethal hypertension and the consequent need for a restrictive diet. The use of MAOIs declined further after the introduction of the SSRIs and other new agents. They are now mainly relegated to use in treatment-resistant cases. Thus, the second-line status of MAOIs has less to do with considerations of efficacy than with safety concerns. The currently available MAOIs include phenelzine (Nardil), isocarboxazid (Marplan), tranylcypromine (Parnate), rasagiline (Azilect), moclobemide (Manerix), and selegiline (Eldepryl).

Two subsequent advances in the field of antidepressant MAOIs involve the introduction of a selective reversible inhibitor of MAO_A (RIMA), moclobemide (Manerix), in the early 1990s into most countries except the United States, and in 2005, the introduction of a transdermal delivery form of selegiline (Emsam) in the United States that is used for the treatment of parkinsonism. Other RIMA agents, including brofaromine (Consonar) and befloxatone, have not been submitted for registration despite favorable outcomes in clinical trials.

Pharmacologic Actions

Phenelzine, tranylcypromine, and isocarboxazid are readily absorbed after oral administration and reach peak plasma concentrations within 2 hours. Whereas their plasma half-lives are in the range of 2 to 3 hours, their tissue half-lives are considerably longer. Because they irreversibly inactivate MAOs, the therapeutic effect of a single dose of irreversible MAOIs may persist for as long as 2 weeks. The RIMA moclobemide is rapidly absorbed and has a half-life of 0.5 to 3.5 hours. Because it is a reversible inhibitor, moclobemide has a much briefer clinical effect after a single dose than do irreversible MAOIs.

The MAO enzymes are found on the outer membranes of mitochondria, where they degrade cytoplasmic and extraneuronal monoamine neurotransmitters such as norepinephrine, serotonin, dopamine, epinephrine, and tyramine. MAOIs act in the CNS, the sympathetic nervous system, the liver, and the GI tract. There are two types of MAOs, MAO_A and MAO_B. MAO_A primarily metabolizes norepinephrine, serotonin, and epinephrine; both MAO_A and MAO_B metabolize dopamine and tyramine.

The structures of phenelzine and tranylcypromine are similar to those of amphetamine and have similar pharmacologic effects in that they increase the release of dopamine and norepinephrine with attendant stimulant effects on the brain.

Therapeutic Indications

MAOIs are used for the treatment of depression. Some research indicates that phenelzine is more effective than TCAs in depressed patients with mood reactivity, extreme sensitivity to interpersonal loss or rejection, prominent anergia, hyperphagia, and hypersomnia—a constellation of symptoms conceptualized as atypical depression. Evidence also suggests that MAOIs are more effective than TCAs as a treatment for bipolar depression.

Patients with panic disorder and social phobia respond well to MAOIs. MAOIs have also been used to treat bulimia nervosa, PTSD, anginal pain, atypical facial pain, migraine, ADHD, idiopathic orthostatic hypotension, and depression associated with traumatic brain injury.

Precautions and Adverse Reactions

The most frequent adverse effects of MAOIs are orthostatic hypotension, insomnia, weight gain, edema, and sexual dysfunction. Orthostatic hypotension can lead to dizziness and falls. Thus, cautious upward tapering of the dosage should be used to determine the maximum tolerable dosage. Treatment for orthostatic hypotension includes avoidance of caffeine; intake of 2 L of fluid per day; addition of dietary salt or adjustment of antihypertensive drugs (if applicable); support stockings; and in severe cases, treatment with fludrocortisone (Florinef), a mineralocorticoid, 0.1 to 0.2 mg a day. Orthostatic hypotension associated with tranylcypromine use can usually be relieved by dividing the daily dosage.

Insomnia can be treated by dividing the dose, not giving the medication after dinner, and using a benzodiazepine hypnotic if necessary. Weight gain, edema, and sexual dysfunction often do not respond to any treatment and may warrant switching to another agent. When switching from one MAOI to another, the clinician should taper and stop the use of the first drug for 10 to 14 days before beginning the use of the second drug.

Paresthesias, myoclonus, and muscle pains are occasionally seen in persons treated with MAOIs. Paresthesias may be secondary to MAOI-induced pyridoxine deficiency, which may respond to supplementation with pyridoxine, 50 to 150 mg orally each day. Occasionally, persons complain of feeling drunk or confused, perhaps indicating that the dosage should be reduced and then increased gradually. Reports that the hydrazine MAOIs are associated with hepatotoxic effects are relatively uncommon. MAOIs are less cardiotoxic and less epileptogenic than are the tricyclic and tetracyclic drugs.

The most common adverse effects of the RIMA moclobemide are dizziness, nausea, and insomnia or sleep disturbance. RIMAs cause fewer GI adverse effects than do SSRIs. Moclobemide does not have adverse anticholinergic or cardiovascular effects, and it has not been reported to interfere with sexual function.

MAOIs should be used with caution by persons with renal disease, cardiovascular disease, or hyperthyroidism. MAOIs may alter the dosage of a hypoglycemic agent required by persons with diabetes. MAOIs have been significantly associated with the induction of mania in persons in the depressed phase of bipolar I disorder and triggering a psychotic decompensation in persons with schizophrenia. MAOIs are contraindicated during pregnancy, although data on their teratogenic risk are minimal. Nursing women should not take MAOIs because the drugs can pass into breast milk.

Tyramine-Induced Hypertensive Crisis. The most worrisome side effect of MAOIs is the tyramine-induced hypertensive crisis. The amino acid tyramine is usually transformed via GI metabolism. However, MAOIs inactivate GI metabolism of dietary tyramine, thus allowing intact tyramine to enter the circulation. A hypertensive crisis may subsequently occur as a result of a powerful pressor effect of the amino acid. Tyramine-containing foods should be avoided for 2 weeks after the last dose of an irreversible MAOI to allow the resynthesis of adequate concentrations of MAO enzymes.

Accordingly, foods rich in tyramine (Table 21-22) or other sympathomimetic amines, such as ephedrine, pseudoephedrine

Table 21-22
Tyramine-Rich Foods to Be Avoided in Planning Monoamine Oxidase Inhibitor Diets

---

High Tyramine Content[a] (≥2 mg of tyramine a serving)
  Cheese: English Stilton, blue cheese, white (3 yr old), extra old, old cheddar, Danish blue, mozzarella, cheese snack spreads
  Fish, cured meats, sausage; pâtés and organs, salami, mortadella, air-dried sausage
  Alcoholic beverages[b]: Liqueurs and concentrated after-dinner drinks
  Marmite (concentrated yeast extract)
  Sauerkraut (Krakus)
Moderate Tyramine Content[a] (0.5–1.99 mg of tyramine a serving)
  Cheese: Swiss Gruyere, muenster, feta, parmesan, gorgonzola, blue cheese dressing, Black Diamond
  Fish, cured meats, sausage, pâtés and organs: Chicken liver (5 days old); bologna; aged sausage, smoked meat; salmon mousse
  Alcoholic beverages: Beer and ale (12 oz per bottle)—Amstel, Export Draft, Blue Light, Guinness Extra Stout, Old Vienna, Canadian, Miller Light, Export, Heineken, Blue Wines (per 4-oz glass)—Rioja (red wine)
Low Tyramine Content[a] (0.01 to >0.49 mg of tyramine a serving)
  Cheese: Brie, Camembert, Cambozola with or without rind
  Fish, cured meat, sausage, organs, and pâtés; pickled herring; smoked fish; kielbasa sausage; chicken liver; liverwurst (<2 days old)
  Alcoholic beverages: Red wines, sherry, scotch[c]
  Others: Banana or avocado (ripe or not), banana peel

---

[a]Any food left out to age or spoil can spontaneously develop tyramine through fermentation.
[b]Alcohol can produce profound orthostasis interacting with monoamine oxidase inhibitors (MAOIs) but cannot produce direct hypotensive reactions.
[c]White wines, gin, and vodka have no tyramine content.
Table by Jonathan M. Himmelhoch, M.D.

(Sudafed), or dextromethorphan (Trocal), should be avoided by persons who are taking irreversible MAOIs. Patients should be advised to continue the dietary restrictions for 2 weeks after they stop MAOI treatment to allow the body to resynthesize the enzyme. Bee stings may cause a hypertensive crisis. In addition to severe hypertension, other symptoms may include headache, stiff neck, diaphoresis, nausea, and vomiting. A patient with these symptoms should seek immediate medical treatment.

An MAOI-induced hypertensive crisis should be treated with α-adrenergic antagonists—for example, phentolamine (Regitine) or chlorpromazine (Thorazine). These drugs lower BP within 5 minutes. IV furosemide (Lasix) can be used to reduce fluid load, and a β-adrenergic receptor antagonist can control tachycardia. A sublingual 10-mg dose of nifedipine (Procardia) can be given and repeated after 20 minutes. Persons with thyrotoxicosis or pheochromocytoma should not use MAOIs.

The risk of tyramine-induced hypertensive crises is relatively low for persons who are taking RIMAs, such as moclobemide and befloxatone. These drugs have relatively little inhibitory activity for MAO$_B$, and because they are reversible, regular activity of existing MAO$_A$ returns within 16 to 48 hours of the last dose of a RIMA. Therefore, the dietary restrictions are less stringent for RIMAs, applying only to foods containing high concentrations of tyramine, which need to be avoided for 3 days after the last dose of a RIMA. A reasonable dietary recommendation for persons taking RIMAs is to avoid eating tyramine-containing foods 1 hour before and 2 hours after taking a RIMA.

Spontaneous, nontyramine-induced hypertensive crisis is a rare occurrence, usually shortly after the first exposure of an MAOI. Persons experiencing such a crisis should avoid MAOIs altogether.

Withdrawal.   Abrupt cessation of regular doses of MAOIs may cause a self-limited discontinuation syndrome consisting of arousal, mood disturbances, and somatic symptoms. Dosages should be gradually tapered over several weeks to avoid these symptoms.

Overdose.   It often takes 1 to 6 hours after an overdose for the toxic symptoms to occur. MAOI overdose is characterized by agitation that can progress to coma with hyperthermia, hypertension, tachypnea, tachycardia, dilated pupils, and hyperactive deep tendon reflexes. Involuntary movements may be present, particularly in the face and the jaw. Acidification of the urine markedly hastens the excretion of MAOIs, and dialysis can be of some use. Phentolamine or chlorpromazine may be useful if hypertension is a problem. Moclobemide alone in overdosage causes relatively mild and reversible symptoms.

Drug Interactions

The significant drug–drug interactions involving MAOIs are listed in Table 21-23. Most antidepressants, as well as precursor agents, should be avoided. Persons should be instructed to tell any other physicians or dentists who are treating them that they are taking an MAOI. MAOIs may potentiate the action of CNS depressants, including alcohol and barbiturates. MAOIs should not be coadministered with serotonergic drugs, such as SSRIs and clomipramine (Anafranil), because this combination can trigger serotonin syndrome. The use of lithium or tryptophan with an irreversible MAOI may also induce serotonin syndrome. Initial symptoms of serotonin syndrome can include tremor, hypertonicity, myoclonus, and autonomic signs, which can then progress to hallucinosis, hyperthermia, and even death. Fatal reactions had occurred when MAOIs were combined with meperidine (Demerol) or fentanyl (Sublimaze).

Table 21-23
Drugs to Be Avoided during Monoamine Oxidase Inhibitor Treatment (Partial Listing)

Never Use
  Antiasthmatics
  Antihypertensives (methyldopa, guanethidine, reserpine)
  Buspirone
  Levodopa
  Opioids (especially meperidine, dextromethorphan, propoxyphene, tramadol; morphine or codeine may be less dangerous)
  Cold, allergy, or sinus medications containing dextromethorphan or sympathomimetics
  SSRIs, clomipramine, venlafaxine, sibutramine
  Sympathomimetics (amphetamines, cocaine, methylphenidate, dopamine, epinephrine, norepinephrine, isoproterenol, ephedrine, pseudoephedrine, phenylpropanolamine)
  L-Tryptophan

Use Carefully
  Anticholinergics
  Antihistamines
  Disulfiram
  Bromocriptine
  Hydralazine
  Sedative-hypnotics
  Terpin hydrate with codeine
  Tricyclics and tetracyclics (avoid clomipramine)

SSRI, selective serotonin reuptake inhibitor.

When switching from an irreversible MAOI to any other type of antidepressant drug, persons should wait at least 14 days after the last dose of the MAOI before beginning the use of the next drug to allow replenishment of the body's MAOs. When switching from an antidepressant to an irreversible MAOI, persons should wait 10 to 14 days (or 5 weeks for fluoxetine [Prozac]) before starting the use of the MAOI to avoid drug–drug interactions. In contrast, MAO activity recovers completely 24 to 48 hours after the last dose of a RIMA.

The effects of the MAOIs on hepatic enzymes are poorly studied. Tranylcypromine inhibits CYP2C19. Moclobemide inhibits CYP2D6, CYP2C19, and CYP1A2 and is a substrate for 2C19.

Cimetidine (Tagamet) and fluoxetine significantly reduce the elimination of moclobemide. Modest doses of fluoxetine and moclobemide administered concurrently may be well tolerated, with no significant pharmacodynamic or pharmacokinetic interactions.

Laboratory Interferences

MAOIs may lower blood glucose concentrations. MAOIs artificially raise urinary metanephrine concentrations and may cause a false-positive test result for pheochromocytoma or neuroblastoma. MAOIs have been reported to be associated with a minimal false elevation in thyroid function test results.

Dosage and Clinical Guidelines

There is no definitive rationale for choosing one irreversible MAOI over another. Table 21-24 lists MAOI preparations and typical dosages. Phenelzine use should begin with a test dose of 15 mg on the first day. The dosage can be increased to 15 mg three times daily during the first week and increased by 15 mg a day each week after that until the dosage of 90 mg a day, in divided doses, is reached by the end of the fourth week. Tranylcypromine and isocarboxazid use should begin with a test dosage of 10 mg and may be increased to 10 mg three times daily by the end of the first week. Many clinicians

Table 21-24
Typical Dosage Forms and Recommended Dosages for Currently Available Monoamine Oxidase Inhibitors

Drug	Usual Dose (mg/day)	Maximum Dose (mg/day)	Dosage (Oral) Formulation
Isocarboxazid (Marplan)	20–40	60	10-mg tablets
Phenelzine (Nardil)	30–60	90	15-mg tablets
Tranylcypromine (Parnate)	20–60	60	10-mg tablets
Rasagiline	0.5–1.0	1.0	0.5- or 1.0-mg tablets
Selegiline (Eldepryl)	10	30	5-mg tablets
Moclobemide (Manerix)	300–600	600	100- or 150-mg tablets

and researchers have recommended upper limits of 50 mg a day for isocarboxazid and 40 mg a day for tranylcypromine. Administration of tranylcypromine in multiple small daily doses may reduce its hypotensive effects.

Even though coadministration of MAOIs with TCAs, SSRIs, or lithium is generally contraindicated, these combinations have been used successfully and safely to treat patients with refractory depression. However, they should be used with extreme caution.

Hepatic transaminase serum concentrations should be monitored periodically because of the potential for hepatotoxicity, especially with phenelzine and isocarboxazid. Elderly persons may be more sensitive to MAOI adverse effects than are younger adults. MAO activity increases with age, so MAOI dosages for elderly persons are the same as those required for younger adults. We know little about using MAOIs in children.

Studies have suggested that transdermal selegiline has antidepressant properties. Although selegiline is a type B inhibitor at low doses, it becomes less selective as the dose is increased.

THYROID HORMONES

Thyroid hormones—levothyroxine (Synthroid, Levothroid, Levoxine) and liothyronine (Cytomel)—are used in psychiatry either alone or as an augmentation to treat persons with depression or rapid-cycling bipolar I disorder. They can convert an antidepressant-nonresponsive person into an antidepressant-responsive person. Thyroid hormones are also used as replacement therapy for persons treated with lithium (Eskalith) who have developed a hypothyroid state. Successful use of thyroid hormone as an intervention for treatment-resistant patients was first reported in the early 1970s. Study results since then have been mixed; however, most show that patients taking triiodothyronine (T_3) are twice as likely to respond to antidepressant treatment versus placebo. These studies have found that augmentation with T_3 is significant with TCAs and SSRIs. Nevertheless, many endocrinologists object to the use of thyroid hormones as antidepressant augmentation agents, citing such risks as osteoporosis and cardiac arrhythmias.

Pharmacologic Actions

Thyroid hormones are administered orally, and their absorption from the GI tract is variable. Absorption is increased if the drug is administered on an empty stomach. Thyroxine (T_4) crosses the blood–brain barrier and diffuses into neurons, where it is converted into T_3, which is the physiologically active form. The half-life of T_4 is 6 to 7 days, and that of T_3 is 1 to 2 days.

The mechanism of action for thyroid hormone effects on antidepressant efficacy is unknown. Thyroid hormone binds to intracellular receptors that regulate the transcription of a wide range of genes, including several receptors for neurotransmitters.

Therapeutic Indications

The primary indication for thyroid hormones in psychiatry is as an adjuvant to antidepressants. There is no clear correlation between the laboratory measures of thyroid function and the response to thyroid hormone supplementation of antidepressants. If a patient has not responded to a 6-week course of antidepressants at appropriate dosages, adjuvant therapy with either lithium or a thyroid hormone is an alternative. Most clinicians use adjuvant lithium before trying a thyroid hormone. Several controlled trials have indicated that liothyronine use converts about 50 percent of antidepressant nonresponders to responders.

The dosage of liothyronine is 25 or 50 µg a day added to the patient's antidepressant regimen. Liothyronine has been used primarily as an adjuvant for tricyclic drugs; however, evidence suggests that liothyronine augments the effects of all of the antidepressant drugs.

Thyroid hormones have not been shown to cause particular problems in pediatric or geriatric patients; however, the hormones should be used with caution in elderly persons who may have occult heart disease.

Precautions and Adverse Reactions

At the dosages usually used for augmentation—25 to 50 µg a day—adverse effects occur infrequently. The most common adverse effects associated with thyroid hormones are transient headache, weight loss, palpitations, nervousness, diarrhea, abdominal cramps, sweating, tachycardia, increased BP, tremors, and insomnia. Osteoporosis may also occur with long-term treatment, but this has not been found in studies involving liothyronine augmentation. Overdoses of thyroid hormones can lead to cardiac failure and death.

Patients with cardiac disease, angina, or hypertension should not take thyroid hormones. The hormones are contraindicated in thyrotoxicosis and uncorrected adrenal insufficiency and persons with acute myocardial infarctions. Thyroid hormones can be administered safely to pregnant women, provided that laboratory thyroid indexes are monitored. Thyroid hormones are minimally excreted in breast milk and have not been shown to cause problems in nursing babies.

Drug Interactions

Thyroid hormones can potentiate the effects of warfarin (Coumadin) and other anticoagulants by increasing the catabolism of clotting factors. They may increase the insulin requirement for diabetic persons and the digitalis requirement for persons with cardiac disease. We should not coadminister with sympathomimetics, ketamine (Ketalar), or maprotiline (Ludiomil) because of the risk of cardiac decompensation. Administration of SSRIs, tricyclic and tetracyclic drugs, lithium, or carbamazepine (Tegretol) can mildly lower serum T_4 and raise serum thyrotropin concentrations in euthyroid persons or persons taking thyroid replacements. This interaction warrants close serum monitoring and may require an increase in the dosage or initiation of thyroid hormone supplementation.

Laboratory Interferences

Levothyroxine has not been reported to interfere with any laboratory test other than thyroid function indexes. Liothyronine, however, suppresses the release of endogenous T_4, thereby lowering the result of any thyroid function test that depends on the measure of T_4.

Thyroid Function Tests

Several thyroid function tests are available, including tests for T_4 by competitive protein binding (T_4 [D]) and by radioimmunoassay (T_4 RIA) involving a specific antigen–antibody reaction. More than 90 percent of T_4 is bound to serum protein and is responsible for thyroid-stimulating hormone (TSH) secretion and cellular metabolism. Other thyroid measures include the free T_4 index (FT_4I), T_3 uptake, and total serum T_3 measured by radioimmunoassay (T_3 RIA). Those tests are used to rule out hypothyroidism, which can be associated with symptoms of depression. In some studies, up to 10 percent of patients complaining of depression and associated fatigue had an incipient hypothyroid disease. Lithium can cause hypothyroidism and, more rarely, hyperthyroidism. Neonatal hypothyroidism results in intellectual disability and is preventable if the diagnosis is made at birth.

Thyrotropin-Releasing Hormone Stimulation Test. The thyrotropin-releasing hormone (TRH) stimulation test is indicated for patients who have marginally abnormal thyroid test results with suspected subclinical hypothyroidism, which may account for clinical depression. It is also used in patients with possible lithium-induced hypothyroidism. The procedure entails an intravenous injection of 500 mg of protirelin (TRH), which produces a sharp increase in serum TSH levels are measured at 15, 30, 60, and 90 minutes. An increase in serum TSH of 5 to 25 mIU/mL above the baseline is normal. An increase of less than 7 mIU/mL is considered a blunted response, which may correlate with a diagnosis of depression. Eight percent of all patients with depression have some thyroid illness.

Dosage and Clinical Guidelines

Liothyronine is available in 5-, 25-, and 50-µg tablets. Levothyroxine is available in 12.5-, 25-, 50-, 75-, 88-, 100-, 112-, 125-, 150-, 175-, 200-, and 300-µg tablets; it is also available in a 200 and 500 µg parenteral form. The dosage of liothyronine is 25 or 50 µg a day added to the person's antidepressant regimen. Liothyronine has been used as an adjuvant for all of the available antidepressant drugs. An adequate trial of liothyronine supplementation should last 2 to 3 weeks. If liothyronine supplementation is successful, it should be continued for 2 months and then tapered off at a rate of 12.5 µg a day every 3 to 7 days.

NOVEL AGENTS

Several agents with novel mechanisms are currently approved for use. They are usually given in specialized centers, and clinicians should only administer after special training to manage their significant safety profile.

NMDA Receptor Antagonists

Ketamine, an anesthetic agent, is used in specialized centers for depression. It has a unique action, as after a single low dose, much lower than the usual anesthetic dose, it can produce rapid relief from depression. This effect often occurs within 4 hours of IV administration. The effects persist for several weeks, but then without additional intervention, the depression often relapses. The drug has several significant side effects, including its general anesthetic effect as well as its psychotomimetic effect. Most experts consider it safe at lower doses; however, the clinical team should be ready to provide medical treatment should the drug have a profound effect on a patient's breathing or cause significant bradycardia.

Ketamine's enantiomer, esketamine (Ketanest), was approved by the FDA for the treatment of depression in adults in 2019. It has the advantage over ketamine, in that in addition to an injectable form, it is available as a nasal spray. Esketamine's mechanism of action is similar to ketamine's, although not identical; for example, both are noncompetitive NMDA receptor antagonist and inhibit dopamine transporters. However, esketamine does not act on the sigma receptors, which may account for part of ketamine's antidepressant effect. This lack of effect on sigma receptors is thought to reduce the psychotomimetic properties of the drug. It must be provided in a clinical setting that has the staff and facilities to observe the patient for at least 2 hours following administration. The main side effects are sedation, difficulties with vision and speaking, and cognitive effects, including confusion, dissociation, and potentially delirium. It may also cause anxiety and increased BP in some patients.

GABA$_A$ Allosteric Modulators

Brexanolone, also called allopregnanolone, was approved in the United States in 2019 under the priority review process as a breakthrough therapy for the treatment of postpartum depression. It is a neurosteroid which positively modulates the GABA$_A$ receptor. It is also a negative allosteric modulator of the nicotinic acetylcholine receptor and may have action on serotonin HT_3 as well. The mechanism of its antidepressant effect is not clear, as other positive allosteric modulators of GABA$_A$, such as benzodiazepines, do not have a significant antidepressant effect. However, like ketamine, it provides a rapid response in patients who respond to the drug, usually within 2 to 3 days. We know little about the long term efficacy of the drug.

The drug is marketed under the brand name Zulresso and is a Schedule IV controlled substance. It is only available through a national registry and has several other drawbacks limiting its widespread acceptance. One is its long administration time, as the drug must be given by continuous IV infusion over 60 hours, during which the dose is slowly increased. This extended hospitalization is to prevent excess sedation or syncope.

Perhaps the most significant drawback of the medication is its cost. Currently, the drug costs about $34,000 for a single dose, as well as the price of remaining in a medical facility for 60 hours, and is not currently covered by most insurance companies.

▲ 21.3 Mood Stabilizers

LITHIUM

The effectiveness of lithium for mania and the prophylactic treatment of manic–depressive disorder was established in the early 1950s as a result of research done by John F.J. Cade, an Australian psychiatrist. Concerns about toxicity limited initial acceptance of lithium use in the United States, but its use increased gradually in the late 1960s. It was not until 1970 that the FDA approved its labeling for the treatment of mania. The only other approved FDA indication came in 1974 when it was accepted as maintenance therapy in patients with a history of mania. For several decades, lithium was the only drug approved for both acute and maintenance treatment. It is also used as an adjunctive medication in the treatment of MDD.

Lithium (Li), a monovalent ion, is a member of the group IA alkali metals on the periodic table, a group that also includes sodium, potassium, rubidium, cesium, and francium. Lithium exists in nature as both ^{6}Li (7.42 percent) and ^{7}Li (92.58 percent). The latter isotope allows the imaging of lithium by magnetic resonance spectroscopy. Some 300 mg of lithium is contained in 1,597 mg of lithium carbonate (Li_2CO_3). Most lithium used in the United States is obtained from dry lake mining in Chile and Argentina.

Pharmacologic Actions

Lithium is rapidly and completely absorbed after oral administration, with peak serum concentrations occurring in 1 to 1.5 hours with standard preparations and in 4 to 4.5 hours with slow-release and controlled-release preparations. Lithium does not bind to plasma proteins, is not metabolized, and is excreted through the kidneys. The plasma half-life is initially 1.3 days and is 2.4 days after administration for more than 1 year. The blood–brain barrier permits only the slow passage of lithium, which is why a single overdose does not necessarily cause toxicity and why long-term lithium intoxication is slow to resolve. The elimination half-life of lithium is 18 to 24 hours in young adults but is shorter in children and more prolonged in elderly persons. Renal clearance of lithium is decreased with renal insufficiency. Equilibrium is reached after 5 to 7 days of regular intake. Obesity is associated with higher rates of lithium clearance. The excretion of lithium is complex during pregnancy; excretion increases during pregnancy but decreases after delivery. Lithium is excreted in breast milk and insignificant amounts in the feces and sweat. Thyroid and renal concentrations of lithium are higher than serum levels.

An explanation for the mood-stabilizing effects of lithium remains elusive. Theories include alterations of ion transport and effects on neurotransmitters and neuropeptides, signal transduction pathways, and second messenger systems.

Therapeutic Indications

Bipolar I Disorder

MANIC EPISODES. Lithium controls acute mania and prevents relapse in about 80 percent of persons with bipolar I disorder and in a somewhat smaller percentage of persons with mixed (mania and depression) episodes, rapid-cycling bipolar disorder, or mood changes in encephalopathy. Lithium has a relatively slow onset of action when used and exerts its antimanic effects over 1 to 3 weeks. Thus, a benzodiazepine, DRA, SDA, or valproic acid is usually administered for the first few weeks. Patients with mixed or dysphoric mania, rapid cycling, comorbid substance abuse, or organicity respond less well to lithium than those with classic mania.

BIPOLAR DEPRESSION. Lithium is effective in the treatment of depression associated with bipolar I disorder, as well as in the role of add-on therapy for patients with severe MDD. Augmentation of lithium therapy with valproic acid (Depakene) or carbamazepine (Tegretol) is usually well tolerated, with little risk of precipitation of mania.

When a depressive episode occurs in a person taking maintenance lithium, the differential diagnosis should include lithium-induced hypothyroidism, substance abuse, and lack of compliance with lithium therapy. One approach is to increase the lithium concentration (up to 1 to 1.2 mEq/L). Alternately we may augment with valproate or carbamazepine. It may also help to add supplemental thyroid hormone (e.g., 25 µg a day of liothyronine [Cytomel]), even in the presence of normal findings on thyroid function tests. Antidepressants or ECT are sometimes added judiciously. After the acute depressive episode resolves, other therapies should be tapered in favor of lithium monotherapy, if clinically tolerated.

MAINTENANCE. Maintenance treatment with lithium markedly decreases the frequency, severity, and duration of manic and depressive episodes in persons with bipolar I disorder. Lithium provides relatively more effective prophylaxis for mania than for depression, and supplemental antidepressant strategies may be necessary either intermittently or continuously. Lithium maintenance is almost always indicated after the first episode of bipolar I disorder, depression or mania, and should be considered after the first episode for adolescents or for persons who have a family history of bipolar I disorder. Others who benefit from lithium maintenance are those who have poor support systems, had no precipitating factors for the first episode, have a high suicide risk, had a sudden onset of the first episode, or had a first episode of mania. Clinical studies have shown that lithium reduces the incidence of suicide in bipolar I disorder patients six- or sevenfold. Lithium is also an effective treatment for persons with severe cyclothymic disorder.

It is wise to initiate maintenance therapy after the first manic episode, based on several observations. First, each episode of mania increases the risk of subsequent episodes. Second, among people responsive to lithium, relapses are 28 times more likely after lithium use is discontinued. Third, case reports describe persons who initially responded to lithium, discontinued taking it, and then had a relapse but no longer responded to lithium in subsequent episodes. Continued maintenance treatment with lithium is often associated with increased efficacy and reduced mortality. Therefore, an episode of depression or mania that occurs after a relatively short time on lithium maintenance does not necessarily represent treatment failure. However, lithium treatment alone may begin to lose its effectiveness after several years of successful use. If this occurs, then supplemental treatment with carbamazepine or valproate may be useful.

Maintenance lithium dosages can often be adjusted to achieve plasma concentration somewhat lower than that needed for the treatment of acute mania. If lithium use is to be discontinued, then the dosage should be slowly tapered. Abrupt discontinuation of lithium therapy is associated with an increased risk of recurrence of manic and depressive episodes.

Major Depressive Disorder.

Lithium is effective in the long-term treatment of major depression, but it is not more effective than antidepressant drugs. The most common role for lithium in MDD is as an adjuvant to antidepressant use in persons who have failed to respond to the antidepressants alone. About 50 to 60 percent of antidepressant nonresponders do respond when lithium, 300 mg three times daily, is added to the antidepressant regimen. In some cases, a response may be seen within days, but most often, several weeks are required to see the efficacy of the regimen. Lithium alone may effectively treat depressed persons who have bipolar I disorder but have not yet had their first manic episode. Lithium has been reported to be effective in persons with MDD whose disorder has marked cyclicity.

Schizoaffective Disorder and Schizophrenia. Persons with prominent mood symptoms—either bipolar type or depressive type—with schizoaffective disorder are more likely to respond to lithium than those with predominant psychotic symptoms. Although SDAs and DRAs are the treatments of choice for persons with schizoaffective disorder, lithium is a useful augmentation agent. This approach is particularly true for persons whose symptoms are resistant to treatment with SDAs and DRAs. Lithium augmentation of an SDA or DRA medication may be an effective treatment for persons with schizoaffective disorder even in the absence of a prominent mood disorder component. Some persons with schizophrenia who cannot take antipsychotic drugs may benefit from lithium treatment alone.

Other Indications. Over the years, reports have appeared about the use of lithium to treat a wide range of other psychiatric and nonpsychiatric conditions (Tables 21-25 and 21-26). The

Table 21-25
Psychiatric Uses of Lithium

Well established (FDA approved)
  Bipolar disorder
    Manic episode
    Maintenance therapy

Reasonably well established
  Bipolar I disorder, depressive episode
  Bipolar II disorder
  Rapid-cycling bipolar I disorder
  Cyclothymic disorder
  Major depressive disorder
    Acute depression (as an augmenting agent)
    Maintenance therapy
  Schizoaffective disorder

Evidence of benefit in particular groups
  Schizophrenia
  Aggression (episodic), explosive behavior, and self-mutilation
  Conduct disorder in children and adolescents
  Intellectual disability
  Cognitive disorders
  Aggressive prisoners

Anecdotal, controversial, unresolved, or doubtful
  Alcohol and other substance-related disorders
  Cocaine abuse
  Substance-induced mood disorder with manic features
  Obsessive-compulsive disorder
  Phobias
  Posttraumatic stress disorder
  ADHD
  Eating disorders
    Anorexia nervosa
    Bulimia nervosa
  Impulse-control disorders
  Kleine–Levin syndrome
  Mental disorders caused by a general medical condition (e.g., mood disorder caused by a general medical condition with manic features)
  Periodic catatonia
  Periodic hypersomnia
  Personality disorders (e.g., antisocial, borderline, emotionally unstable, schizotypal)
  Premenstrual dysphoric disorder
  Sexual disorders
    Transvestism
    Exhibitionism
    Pathologic hypersexuality

FDA, Food and Drug Administration; ADHD, attention-deficit/hyperactivity disorder.

Table 21-26
Nonpsychiatric Uses of Lithium[a]

Neurologic
  Epilepsy
  Headache (chronic cluster, hypnic, migraine, particularly cyclic)
  Ménière disease (not supported by controlled studies)
  Movement disorders
  Huntington disease
  L-Dopa–induced hyperkinesias
  On–off phenomenon in Parkinson disease (controlled study found decreased akinesia but development of dyskinesia in a few cases)
  Spasmodic torticollis
  Tardive dyskinesia (not supported by controlled studies, and pseudoparkinsonism has been reported)
  Tourette disorder
  Pain (facial pain syndrome, painful shoulder syndrome, fibromyalgia)
  Periodic paralysis (hypokalemic and hypermagnesic but not hyperkalemic)
Hematologic
  Aplastic anemia
  Cancer—chemotherapy-induced, radiotherapy-induced
  Neutropenia (one study found increased risk of sudden death in patients with preexisting cardiovascular disorder)
  Drug-induced neutropenia (e.g., from carbamazepine, antipsychotics, immunosuppressives, and zidovudine)
  Felty syndrome
  Leukemia
Endocrine
  Thyroid cancer as an adjunct to radioactive iodine
  Thyrotoxicosis
  Syndrome of inappropriate antidiuretic hormone secretion
Cardiovascular
  Antiarrhythmic agent (animal data only)
Dermatologic
  Genital herpes (controlled studies support topical and oral use)
  Eczematoid dermatitis
  Seborrheic dermatitis (controlled study supports)
Gastrointestinal
  Cyclic vomiting
  Gastric ulcers
  Pancreatic cholera
  Ulcerative colitis
Respiratory
  Asthma (controlled study did not support)
  Cystic fibrosis
Other
  Bovine spastic paresis

[a]All the uses listed here do not have Food and Drug Administration(FDA)–approved labeling. There are conflicting reports about many of these uses—some have negative findings in controlled studies, and a few involve reports of possible adverse effects.
L-Dopa, levodopa.

effectiveness and safety of lithium for most of these disorders have not been confirmed. Lithium has an anti-aggressive activity that is separate from its effects on mood. Aggressive outbursts in persons with schizophrenia, violent prison inmates, and children with conduct disorder and aggression, or self-mutilation in persons with intellectual disability, can sometimes be controlled with lithium.

Precautions and Adverse Effects

More than 80 percent of patients taking lithium experience side effects. It is crucial to minimize the risk of adverse events through monitoring of lithium blood levels and to use appropriate pharmacologic interventions to counteract unwanted effects when they occur. The most common adverse effects are summarized

Table 21-27
Adverse Effects of Lithium

Neurologic
- Benign, nontoxic: dysphoria, lack of spontaneity, slowed reaction time, memory difficulties
- Tremor: postural, occasional extrapyramidal
- Toxic: coarse tremor, dysarthria, ataxia, neuromuscular irritability, seizures, coma, death
- Miscellaneous: peripheral neuropathy, benign intracranial hypertension, myasthenia gravis–like syndrome, altered creativity, lowered seizure threshold

Endocrine
- Thyroid: goiter, hypothyroidism, exophthalmos, hyperthyroidism (rare)
- Parathyroid: hyperparathyroidism, adenoma

Cardiovascular
- Benign T-wave changes, sinus node dysfunction

Renal
- Concentrating defect, morphologic changes, polyuria (nephrogenic diabetes insipidus), reduced GFR, nephrotic syndrome, renal tubular acidosis

Dermatologic
- Acne, hair loss, psoriasis, rash

Gastrointestinal
- Appetite loss, nausea, vomiting, diarrhea

Miscellaneous
- Altered carbohydrate metabolism, weight gain, fluid retention

GFR, glomerular filtration rate.

in Table 21-27. Patient education can play an essential role in reducing the incidence and severity of side effects. Patients taking lithium should be advised that changes in the body's water and salt content can affect the amount of lithium excreted, resulting in either increases or decreases in lithium concentrations. Excessive sodium intake (e.g., a dramatic dietary change) lowers lithium concentrations.

Conversely, too little sodium (e.g., fad diets) can lead to potentially toxic concentrations of lithium. Decreases in body fluid (e.g., excessive perspiration) can lead to dehydration and lithium intoxication. Patients should report whenever another clinician prescribes medications, because many commonly used agents can affect lithium concentrations.

Cardiac Effects. Lithium can cause diffuse slowing, widening of the frequency spectrum, and potentiation and disorganization of background rhythm on electrocardiography (ECG). Bradycardia and cardiac arrhythmias may occur, especially in people with cardiovascular disease. Lithium infrequently reveals Brugada syndrome, an inherited, life-threatening heart problem that some people may have without knowing it. It can cause a severe abnormal heartbeat and other symptoms (such as severe dizziness, fainting, shortness of breath) that need medical attention right away. Before starting lithium treatment, clinicians should ask about known heart conditions, unexplained fainting, and family history of problems or sudden unexplained death before age 45.

Gastrointestinal Effects. GI symptoms—which include nausea, decreased appetite, vomiting, and diarrhea—can be diminished by dividing the dosage, administering the lithium with food, or switching to another lithium preparation. The lithium preparation least likely to cause diarrhea is lithium citrate. Some lithium preparations contain lactose, which can cause diarrhea in lactose-intolerant persons. Persons taking slow-release formulations of lithium who experience diarrhea caused by unabsorbed medication in the lower part of the GI tract may experience less diarrhea than

with standard-release preparations. Diarrhea may also respond to antidiarrheal preparations such as loperamide (Imodium, Kaopectate), bismuth subsalicylate (Pepto-Bismol), or diphenoxylate with atropine (Lomotil).

Weight Gain. Weight gain results from a poorly understood effect of lithium on carbohydrate metabolism. Weight gain can also result from lithium-induced hypothyroidism, lithium-induced edema, or excessive consumption of soft drinks and juices to quench lithium-induced thirst.

Neurologic Effects

TREMOR. A lithium-induced postural tremor may occur that is usually 8 to 12 Hz and is most notable in outstretched hands, especially in the fingers, and during tasks involving fine manipulations. The tremor can be reduced by dividing the daily dosage, using a sustained-release formulation, reducing caffeine intake, reassessing the concomitant use of other medicines, and treating comorbid anxiety. β-Adrenergic receptor antagonists, such as propranolol, 30 to 120 mg a day in divided doses, and primidone (Mysoline), 50 to 250 mg a day, are usually effective in reducing the tremor. In persons with hypokalemia, potassium supplementation may improve the tremor. When a person taking lithium has a severe tremor, the possibility of lithium toxicity should be suspected and evaluated.

COGNITIVE EFFECTS. Lithium use has been associated with dysphoria, lack of spontaneity, slowed reaction times, and impaired memory. We should note these symptoms carefully because they are a frequent cause of noncompliance. The differential diagnosis for such symptoms should include depressive disorders, hypothyroidism, hypercalcemia, other illnesses, and other drugs. Some, but not all, persons have reported that fatigue and mild cognitive impairment decrease with time.

OTHER NEUROLOGIC EFFECTS. Uncommon neurologic adverse effects include symptoms of mild parkinsonism, ataxia, and dysarthria, although the last two symptoms may also be attributable to lithium intoxication. Lithium is rarely associated with the development of peripheral neuropathy, benign intracranial hypertension (pseudotumor cerebri), findings resembling myasthenia gravis, and increased risk of seizures.

Renal Effect. The most common adverse renal effect of lithium is polyuria with secondary polydipsia. The symptom is particularly a problem in 25 to 35 percent of persons taking lithium who may have a urine output of more than 3 L a day (reference range: 1 to 2 L a day). The polyuria primarily results from lithium antagonism to the effects of antidiuretic hormone, which thus causes diuresis. When polyuria is a significant problem, the person's renal function should be evaluated and followed up with 24-hour urine collections for creatinine clearance determinations. Treatment consists of fluid replacement, the use of the lowest effective dosage of lithium, and single daily dosing of lithium. Treatment can also involve the use of a thiazide or potassium-sparing diuretic. For example, amiloride (Midamor), spironolactone (Aldactone), triamterene (Dyrenium), or amiloride–hydrochlorothiazide (Moduretic) may help. If treatment with a diuretic is initiated, the lithium dosage should be halved, and the diuretic should not be started for 5 days, because the diuretic is likely to increase lithium retention.

The most severe renal adverse effects, which are rare and associated with continuous lithium administration for 10 years or more, involve the appearance of nonspecific interstitial fibrosis, associated with gradual decreases in glomerular filtration rate and increases in serum creatinine concentrations, and rarely with renal failure. Lithium is occasionally associated with nephrotic syndrome and features of distal renal tubular acidosis. Another pathologic finding in patients with lithium nephropathy is the presence of micro-cysts. Magnetic resonance imaging (MRI) can be used to demon-strate renal microcysts secondary to chronic lithium nephropathy and therefore avoid renal biopsy. It is prudent for persons taking lithium to check their serum creatinine concentration, urine chem-istries, and 24-hour urine volume at 6-month intervals. If creati-nine levels do rise, then more frequent monitoring and MRI might be considered.

Thyroid Effects. Lithium causes a generally benign and often transient diminution in the concentrations of circulating thyroid hormones. Reports have attributed goiter (5 percent of persons), benign reversible exophthalmos, hyperthyroidism, and hypothy-roidism (7 to 10 percent of persons) to lithium treatment. Lithium-induced hypothyroidism is more common in women (14 percent) than in men (4.5 percent). Women are at the highest risk during the first 2 years of treatment. Persons taking lithium to treat bipolar disorder are twice as likely to develop hypothyroidism if they develop rapid cycling. About 50 percent of persons receiving long-term lithium treatment have laboratory abnormalities, such as an abnormal TRH response, and about 30 percent have elevated concentrations of TSH. If symptoms of hypothyroidism are present, replacement with levothyroxine (Synthroid) is indicated. Even in the absence of hypothyroid symptoms, some clinicians treat per-sons with significantly elevated TSH concentrations with levothy-roxine. In lithium-treated persons, TSH concentrations should be measured every 6 to 12 months. Lithium-induced hypothyroidism should be considered when evaluating depressive episodes that emerge during lithium therapy.

Cardiac Effects. The cardiac effects of lithium resemble those of hypokalemia on ECG. The displacement of intracellular potas-sium by the lithium ion causes this. The most common changes on the ECG are T-wave flattening or inversion. The changes are benign and disappear after lithium is excreted from the body.

Lithium depresses the pacemaking activity of the sinus node, sometimes resulting in sinus dysrhythmias, heart block, and episodes of syncope. Lithium treatment, therefore, is contraindi-cated in persons with sick sinus syndrome. In rare cases, ventricular arrhythmias and congestive heart failure have been associated with lithium therapy. Lithium cardiotoxicity is prevalent in persons on a low-salt diet, those taking certain diuretics or ACEIs, and those with fluid–electrolyte imbalances or any renal insufficiency.

Dermatologic Effects. Dermatologic effects may be dose-dependent. They include acneiform, follicular, and maculopapular eruptions; pretibial ulcerations; and worsening of psoriasis. Occa-sionally, aggravated psoriasis or acneiform eruptions may force the discontinuation of lithium treatment. Alopecia has also been reported. Persons with many of those conditions respond favorably to changing to another lithium preparation and the usual dermato-logic measures. Lithium concentrations should be monitored if tet-racycline is used for the treatment of acne because it can increase the retention of lithium.

Lithium Toxicity and Overdoses. The early signs and symp-toms of lithium toxicity include neurologic symptoms, such as coarse tremor, dysarthria, and ataxia; GI symptoms; cardiovascular changes; and renal dysfunction. The later signs and symptoms

Table 21-28
Signs and Symptoms of Lithium Toxicity

1. Mild to moderate intoxication (lithium level, 1.5–2.0 mEq/L)

GI	Vomiting
	Abdominal pain
	Dryness of mouth
Neurologic	Ataxia
	Dizziness
	Slurred speech
	Nystagmus
	Lethargy or excitement
	Muscle weakness

2. Moderate to severe intoxication (lithium level: 2.0–2.5 mEq/L)

GI	Anorexia
	Persistent nausea and vomiting
Neurologic	Blurred vision
	Muscle fasciculations
	Clonic limb movements
	Hyperactive deep tendon reflexes
	Choreoathetoid movements
	Convulsions
	Delirium
	Syncope
	Electroencephalographic changes
	Stupor
	Coma
	Circulatory failure (lowered BP, cardiac arrhythmias, and conduction abnormalities)

3. Severe lithium intoxication (lithium level >2.5 mEq/L)

	Generalized convulsions
	Oliguria and renal failure
	Death

include impaired consciousness, muscular fasciculations, myoc-lonus, seizures, and coma. Signs and symptoms of lithium tox-icity are outlined in Table 21-28. Risk factors include exceeding the recommended dosage, renal impairment, low-sodium diet, drug interaction, and dehydration. Elderly persons are more vulner-able to the effects of increased serum lithium concentrations. The greater the degree and duration of elevated lithium concentrations, the worse are the symptoms of lithium toxicity.

Lithium toxicity is a medical emergency, potentially causing per-manent neuronal damage and death. In cases of toxicity (Table 21-29), lithium should be stopped and dehydration treated. Unabsorbed lithium can be removed from the GI tract by ingestion of sodium polystyrene sulfonate (Kayexalate) or polyethylene glycol solu-tion (GoLYTELY), but not activated charcoal. Ingestion of a single

Table 21-29
Management of Lithium Toxicity

1. Contact personal physician or go to a hospital emergency department
2. Lithium should be discontinued
3. Vital signs and a neurologic examination with complete formal mental status examination
4. Lithium level, serum electrolytes, renal function tests, and ECG
5. Emesis, gastric lavage, and absorption with Kayexalate or GoLYTELY
6. For any patient with a serum lithium level greater than 4.0 mEq/L, hemodialysis

ECG, electrocardiography.

large dose may create clumps of medication in the stomach, which can be removed by gastric lavage with a wide-bore tube. The value of forced diuresis is still debated. In severe cases, hemodialysis rapidly removes excessive amounts of serum lithium. Postdialysis serum lithium concentrations may increase as lithium is redistributed from tissues to the blood, so repeat dialysis may be needed. Neurologic improvement may lag behind the clearance of serum lithium by several days because lithium crosses the blood–brain barrier slowly.

Adolescents.   The serum lithium concentrations for adolescents are similar to those for adults. Weight gain and acne associated with lithium use can be particularly troublesome to adolescents.

Elderly Persons.   Lithium is a safe and effective drug for elderly persons. However, the treatment of elderly persons taking lithium may be complicated by the presence of other medical illnesses, decreased renal function, special diets that affect lithium clearance, and generally increased sensitivity to lithium. Elderly persons should initially be given low dosages, their dosages should be switched less frequently than those of younger persons, and a longer time must be allowed for renal excretion to equilibrate with absorption before lithium can be assumed to have reached its steady-state concentrations.

Pregnant Women.   Lithium should not be administered to pregnant women in the first trimester because of the risk of congenital disabilities. The most common malformations involve the cardiovascular system, most commonly Ebstein anomaly of the tricuspid valves. The risk of Ebstein malformation in lithium-exposed fetuses is 1 in 1,000, which is 20 times the risk in the general population. The possibility of fetal cardiac anomalies can be evaluated with fetal echocardiography. The teratogenic risk of lithium (4 to 12 percent) is higher than that for the general population (2 to 3 percent) but appears to be lower than that associated with the use of valproate or carbamazepine. A woman who continues to take lithium during pregnancy should use the lowest effective dosage. The maternal lithium concentration must be monitored closely during pregnancy, and especially after pregnancy, because of the significant decrease in renal lithium excretion as the renal function returns to normal in the first few days after delivery. Adequate hydration can reduce the risk of lithium toxicity during labor. Lithium prophylaxis is recommended for all women with bipolar disorder as they enter the postpartum period. Lithium is excreted into breast milk and should be taken by a nursing mother only after careful evaluation of potential risks and benefits. Signs of lithium toxicity in infants include lethargy, cyanosis, abnormal reflexes, and sometimes hepatomegaly.

Miscellaneous Effects.   Lithium should be used with caution in diabetic persons, who should monitor their blood glucose concentrations carefully to avoid diabetic ketoacidosis. Benign, reversible leukocytosis is commonly associated with lithium treatment. Dehydrated, debilitated, and medically ill persons are most susceptible to adverse effects and toxicity.

Drug Interactions

Lithium drug interactions are summarized in Table 21-30.

Lithium is commonly used in conjunction with DRAs. This combination is typically sufficient and safe. However, coadministration of higher dosages of a DRA and lithium may result in a

synergistic increase in the symptoms of lithium-induced neurologic side effects and neuroleptic extrapyramidal symptoms. In rare instances, encephalopathy has been reported with this combination.

The coadministration of lithium and carbamazepine, lamotrigine, valproate, and clonazepam may increase lithium concentrations and aggravate lithium-induced neurologic adverse effects. Treatment with the combination should be initiated at slightly lower dosages than usual, and the dosages should be increased gradually. Changes from one to another treatment for mania should be made carefully, with as little temporal overlap between the drugs as possible.

Most diuretics (e.g., thiazide and potassium-sparing) can increase lithium concentrations; when treatment with such a diuretic is stopped, the clinician may need to increase the person's daily lithium dosage. Osmotic and loop diuretics, carbonic anhydrase inhibitors, and xanthines (including caffeine) may reduce lithium concentrations to below therapeutic concentrations. Whereas ACEIs may cause an increase in lithium concentrations, the AT_1 angiotensin II receptor inhibitors losartan (Cozaar) and irbesartan (Avapro) do not alter lithium concentrations. A wide range of NSAIDs can decrease lithium clearance, thereby increasing lithium concentrations. These drugs include indomethacin (Indocin), phenylbutazone (Azolid), diclofenac (Voltaren), ketoprofen (Orudis), oxyphenbutazone (Oxalid), ibuprofen (Motrin, Advil), piroxicam (Feldene), and naproxen (Naprosyn). Aspirin and sulindac (Clinoril) do not affect lithium concentrations.

The coadministration of lithium and quetiapine (Seroquel) may cause somnolence but is otherwise well tolerated. The coadministration of lithium and ziprasidone (Geodon) may modestly increase the incidence of tremors. The coadministration of lithium and calcium channel inhibitors should be avoided because of potentially fatal neurotoxicity.

A person taking lithium who is about to undergo ECT should discontinue taking lithium 2 days before beginning ECT to reduce the risk of delirium.

Laboratory Interferences

Lithium does not interfere with any laboratory tests, but lithium-induced alterations include an increased WBC count, decreased serum thyroxine, and increased serum calcium. Blood collected in a lithium–heparin anticoagulant tube will produce falsely elevated lithium concentrations.

Dosage and Clinical Guidelines

Initial Medical Workup.   All patients should have a routine laboratory workup and physical examination before being started on lithium. The laboratory tests should include serum creatinine concentration (or a 24-hour urine creatinine if the clinician has any reason to be concerned about renal function), electrolytes, thyroid function (TSH, T_3 [triiodothyronine], and T_4 [thyroxine]), a CBC, ECG, and a pregnancy test in women of childbearing age.

Dosage Recommendations.   Lithium formulations include immediate-release 150-, 300-, and 600-mg lithium carbonate capsules (Eskalith and generic), 300 mg lithium carbonate tablets (Lithotabs), 450-mg controlled-release lithium carbonate capsules (Eskalith CR and Lithonate), and 8 mEq/5 mL of lithium citrate syrup.

The starting dosage for most adults is 300 mg of the regular-release formulation three times daily. The starting dosage for

Table 21-30
Drug Interactions with Lithium

Drug Class	Reaction
Antipsychotics	Case reports of encephalopathy, worsening of extrapyramidal adverse effects, and neuroleptic malignant syndrome; inconsistent reports of altered red blood cell and plasma concentrations of lithium, antipsychotic drug, or both
Antidepressants	Occasional reports of a serotonin-like syndrome with potent serotonin reuptake inhibitors
Anticonvulsants	No significant pharmacokinetic interactions with carbamazepine or valproate; reports of neurotoxicity with carbamazepine; combinations helpful for treatment resistance
NSAIDs	May reduce renal lithium clearance and increase serum concentration; toxicity reported (exception is aspirin)
Diuretics	
Thiazides	Well-documented reduced renal lithium clearance and increased serum concentration; toxicity reported
Potassium sparing	Limited data; may increase lithium concentration
Loop	Lithium clearance unchanged (some case reports of increased lithium concentration)
Osmotic (mannitol, urea)	Increase renal lithium clearance and decrease lithium concentration
Xanthine (aminophylline, caffeine, theophylline)	Increase renal lithium clearance and decrease lithium concentration
Carbonic anhydrase inhibitors (acetazolamide)	Increase renal lithium clearance
ACEIs	Reports of reduced lithium clearance, increased concentrations, and toxicity
Calcium channel inhibitors	Case reports of neurotoxicity; no consistent pharmacokinetic interactions
Miscellaneous	
Succinylcholine, pancuronium	Reports of prolonged neuromuscular blockade
Metronidazole	Increased lithium concentration
Methyldopa	Few reports of neurotoxicity
Sodium bicarbonate	Increased renal lithium clearance
Iodides	Additive antithyroid effects
Propranolol	Used for lithium tremor; possible slight increase in lithium concentration

NSAID, nonsteroidal anti-inflammatory drug; ACEI, angiotensin-converting enzyme inhibitor.

elderly persons or persons with renal impairment should be 300 mg once or twice daily. After stabilization, dosages between 900 and 1,200 mg a day usually produce a therapeutic plasma concentration of 0.6 to 1 mEq/L, and a daily dose of 1,200 to 1,800 mg usually produces a therapeutic concentration of 0.8 to 1.2 mEq/L. Maintenance dosing can be given either in two or three divided doses of the regular-release formulation or in a single dosage of the sustained-release formulation equivalent to the combined daily dosage of the regular-release formulation. The use of divided doses reduces gastric upset and avoids single high-peak lithium concentrations. Discontinuation of lithium should be gradual to minimize the risk of early recurrence of mania and to permit recognition of early signs of recurrence.

Laboratory Monitoring. The periodic measurement of serum lithium concentration is an essential aspect of patient care, but it should always be combined with sound clinical judgment. A laboratory report listing the therapeutic range as 0.5 to 1.2 mEq/L may lull a clinician into disregarding early signs of lithium intoxication in patients whose levels are around 1.2 mEq/L. Clinical toxicity, especially in elderly persons, has been well documented at or slightly above the upper limit of the therapeutic range.

Regular monitoring of serum lithium concentrations is essential. Lithium levels should be obtained every 2 to 6 months except when there are signs of toxicity, during dosage adjustments, and in persons suspected to be noncompliant with the prescribed dosages. Under these circumstances, levels may be done weekly. Baseline ECG studies are essential and should be repeated annually.

When obtaining blood for lithium levels, patients should be at steady-state lithium dosing (usually after 5 days of constant dosing), preferably using a twice-daily or thrice-daily dosing regimen, and the blood sample must be drawn 12 hours (±30 minutes) after a given dose. Lithium concentrations 12 hours postdose in persons treated with sustained-release preparations are generally about 30 percent higher than the corresponding concentrations obtained from those taking the regular-release preparations. Because available data are based on a sample population following a multiple-dosage regimen, regular-release formulations given at least twice daily should be used for the initial determination of the appropriate dosages. Factors that may cause fluctuations in lithium measurements include dietary sodium intake, mood state, activity level, body position, and use of an improper blood sample tube.

Laboratory values that do not seem to correspond to clinical status may result from the collection of blood in a tube with a lithium–heparin anticoagulant (which can give results falsely elevated by as much as 1 mEq/L) or aging of the lithium ion-selective electrode (which can cause inaccuracies of up to 0.5 mEq/L). After the daily dose has been set, it is reasonable to change to the sustained-release formulation given once daily.

Effective serum concentrations for mania are 1.0 to 1.2 mEq/L, a level associated with 1,800 mg a day. The recommended range for maintenance treatment is 0.4 to 0.8 mEq/L, which is usually achieved with a daily dose of 900 to 1,200 mg. A small number of persons will not achieve therapeutic benefit with a lithium concentration of 1.2 mEq/L, yet will have no signs of toxicity. For such persons, titration of the lithium dosage to achieve a concentration above 1.2 mEq/L may be warranted. Some patients can be maintained at concentrations below 0.4 mEq/L. There may be considerable variation from patient to patient, so it is best to follow the maxim, "treat the patient, not the laboratory results." The only way to establish an optimal dose for a patient may be through trial and error.

Package inserts (US) for lithium products list effective serum concentrations for mania between 1.0 and 1.2 mEq/L (usually achieved with 1,800 mg of lithium carbonate daily) and for long-term maintenance between 0.6 and 1.2 mEq/L (usually achieved with 900 to 1,200 mg of lithium carbonate daily). The dose–blood level relationship may vary considerably from patient to patient. The likelihood of achieving a response at levels above 1.2 mEq/L is usually significantly outweighed by the increased risk of toxicity, although rarely a patient may both require and tolerate a higher-than-usual blood concentration.

What constitutes the lower end of the therapeutic range remains a matter of debate. A prospective 3-year study found patients who maintained a concentration between 0.4 and 0.6 mEq/L (mean 0.54) were 2.6 times more likely to relapse than those who maintained between 0.8 and 1.0 mEq/L (mean 0.83). However, higher blood concentrations produced more adverse effects and were less well tolerated.

If there is no response after 2 weeks at a concentration that is beginning to cause adverse effects, then the person should taper off lithium over 1 to 2 weeks, and other mood-stabilizing drugs should be tried.

Patient Education. Lithium has a narrow therapeutic index, and many factors can upset the balance between lithium concentrations that are well tolerated and therapeutic, and those that produce side effects or toxicity. It is thus imperative that persons taking lithium be educated about signs and symptoms of toxicity, factors that affect lithium levels, how and when to obtain laboratory testing, and the importance of regular communication with the prescribing physician. Lithium concentrations can be disrupted by common factors such as excessive sweating from ambient heat or exercise or the use of widely prescribed agents such as ACEIs or NSAIDs. Patients may stop taking their lithium because they are feeling well or because they are experiencing side effects. They should be advised against discontinuing or modifying their lithium regimen. Table 21-31 lists some essential instructions for patients.

VALPROATE

Valproate (Depakene, Depakote), or valproic acid, is approved for the treatment of manic episodes associated with bipolar I disorder and is one of the most widely prescribed mood stabilizers in psychiatry. It has a rapid onset of action and is well-tolerated, and numerous studies suggest that it reduces the frequency and intensity of recurrent manic episodes over extended periods.

Table 21-31
Instructions to Patients Taking Lithium

Lithium can be remarkably effective in treating your disorder. If not used appropriately and not monitored closely, it can be ineffective and potentially harmful. It is important to keep the following instructions in mind.

Dosing

Take lithium exactly as directed by your doctor—never take more or less than the prescribed dose.

Do not stop taking without speaking to your doctor.

If you miss a dose, take it as soon as possible. If it is within 4 hr of the next dose, skip the missed dose (about 6 hr in the case of extended-release or slow-release preparations). Never double up doses.

Blood Tests

Comply with the schedule of recommended regular blood tests.

Despite their inconvenience and discomfort, your lithium blood levels, thyroid function, and kidney status need to be monitored as long as you take lithium.

When going to have lithium levels checked, you should have taken your last lithium dose 12 hr earlier.

Use of Other Medications

Do not start any prescription or over-the-counter medications without telling your doctor.

Even drugs such as ibuprofen (Advil, Motrin) and naproxen (Aleve) can significantly increase lithium levels.

Diet and Fluid Intake

Avoid sudden changes in your diet or fluid intake. If you do go on a diet, your doctor may need to increase the frequency of blood tests.

Caffeine and alcohol act as diuretics and can lower your lithium concentrations.

During treatment with lithium, it is recommended that you drink about 2 or 3 quarts of fluid daily and use normal amounts of salt.

Inform your doctor if you start or stop a low-salt diet.

Recognizing Potential Problems

If you engage in vigorous exercise or have an illness that causes sweating, vomiting, or diarrhea, consult your doctor because these might affect lithium levels.

Nausea, constipation, shakiness, increased thirst, frequency of urination, weight gain, or swelling of the extremities should be reported to your doctor.

Blurred vision, confusion, loss of appetite, diarrhea, vomiting, muscle weakness, lethargy, shakiness, slurred speech, dizziness, loss of balance, inability to urinate, or seizures could indicate severe toxicity and should prompt immediate medical attention.

Chemistry

Valproate is a simple-chain branch carboxylic acid. It is called valproic acid because it is rapidly converted to the acid form in the stomach. Multiple formulations of valproic acid are marketed. These include valproic acid (Depakene), divalproex sodium (Depakote), an enteric-coated delayed-release 1:1 mixture of valproic acid and sodium valproate available in tablet and sprinkle formulation (can be opened and spread on food); and sodium valproate injection (Depacon). Extended-release preparation is also available. Each of these is therapeutically equivalent because, at physiologic pH, valproic acid dissociates into valproate ion.

Pharmacologic Actions

Regardless of how it is formulated, valproate is rapidly and completely absorbed 1 to 2 hours after oral administration, with peak concentrations occurring 4 to 5 hours after oral administration. The plasma half-life of valproate is 10 to 16 hours. Valproate is highly protein-bound. Protein binding becomes saturated at higher dosages, and concentrations of therapeutically effective free valproate increase at serum concentrations above 50 to 100 μg/mL. The unbound portion of valproate is considered to be pharmacologically active and can cross the blood–brain barrier. The extended-release preparation produces lower peak concentrations and higher minimum concentrations and can be given once a day. Valproate is metabolized primarily by hepatic glucuronidation and mitochondrial β oxidation.

The biochemical basis of valproate's therapeutic effects remains poorly understood. Postulated mechanisms include enhancement of GABA activity, modulation of voltage-sensitive sodium channels, and action on extrahypothalamic neuropeptides.

Therapeutic Indications

Valproate is currently approved as monotherapy or adjunctive therapy of complex partial seizures, monotherapy and adjunctive therapy of simple and complex absence seizures, and adjunctive therapy for patients with multiple seizures that include absence seizures. Divalproex has additional indications for prophylaxis of migraine.

Bipolar I Disorder

ACUTE MANIA.   About two-thirds of persons with acute mania respond to valproate. The majority of patients with mania usually respond within 1 to 4 days after achieving valproate serum concentrations above 50 μg/mL. The antimanic response is generally associated with levels greater than 50 μg/mL, in a range of 50 to 125 μg/mL. This serum concentration may be gradually achieved within 1 week of initiation of dosing, but rapid oral loading strategies achieve therapeutic serum concentrations in 1 day and can control manic symptoms within 5 days. The short-term antimanic effects of valproate can be augmented with the addition of lithium, carbamazepine (Tegretol), SDAs, or DRAs. Numerous studies have suggested that the irritable manic subtype responds significantly better to sodium valproate than lithium or placebo. Because of its more favorable profile of cognitive, dermatologic, thyroid, and renal adverse effects, valproate is preferred to lithium for the treatment of acute mania in children and elderly persons.

ACUTE BIPOLAR DEPRESSION.   Valproate possesses some activity as a short-term treatment of depressive episodes in bipolar I disorder, but this effect is far less pronounced than for the treatment of manic episodes. Among depressive symptoms, valproate is more useful for the treatment of agitation than dysphoria. In clinical practice, valproate is most often used as add-on therapy to an antidepressant to prevent the development of mania or rapid cycling.

PROPHYLAXIS.   Studies suggest that valproate is useful in the prophylactic treatment of bipolar I disorder, resulting in fewer, less severe, and shorter manic episodes. In direct comparison, valproate is at least as effective as lithium and is better tolerated than lithium. It may be particularly useful in persons with rapid-cycling and ultrarapid-cycling bipolar disorders, dysphoric or mixed mania, and mania caused by a general medical condition as well as in persons who have comorbid substance use disorders or panic attacks and in persons who have not had complete favorable responses to lithium treatment.

Schizophrenia and Schizoaffective Disorder.   Valproate may accelerate response to antipsychotic therapy in patients with schizophrenia or schizoaffective disorder. Valproate alone is generally less effective in schizoaffective disorder than in bipolar I disorder. Valproate alone is ineffective for the treatment of psychotic symptoms and is typically used in combination with other drugs in patients with these symptoms.

Other Mental Disorders.   Valproate has been studied for possible efficacy in a broad range of psychiatric disorders. These include alcohol withdrawal and relapse prevention, panic disorder, PTSD, impulse control disorder, borderline personality disorder, and behavioral agitation and dementia. Evidence supporting use in these cases is weak, and any observed therapeutic effects may be related to the treatment of a comorbid bipolar disorder.

Precautions and Adverse Reactions

Although valproate treatment is generally well tolerated and safe, it carries quite a few black box warnings and other warnings (Table 21-32). The two most serious adverse effects of valproate treatment affect the pancreas and liver. Risk factors for potentially fatal hepatotoxicity include young age (younger than 3 years); concurrent use of phenobarbital; and the presence of neurologic disorders, especially inborn errors of metabolism. The rate of fatal

Table 21-32
Black Box Warnings and Other Warnings for Valproate

More Serious Side Effect	Management Considerations
Hepatotoxicity	Rare, idiosyncratic event Estimated risk, 1:118,000 (adults) Greatest risk profile (polypharmacy, younger than 2 yr of age, intellectual disability): 1:800
Pancreatitis	Rare, similar pattern to hepatotoxicity Incidence in clinical trial data is 2 in 2,416 (0.0008%) Postmarketing surveillance shows no increased incidence Relapse with rechallenge Asymptomatic amylase not predictive
Hyperammonemia	Rare; more common in combination with carbamazepine (Tegretol) Associated with coarse tremor and may respond to L-carnitine administration
Associated with urea cycle disorders	Discontinue valproate and protein intake Assess underlying urea cycle disorder Divalproex is contraindicated in patients with urea cycle disorders
Teratogenicity	Neural tube defect: 1–4% with valproate Preconceptual education and folate–vitamin B complex supplementation for all young women of childbearing potential
Somnolence in elderly persons	Slower titration than conventional doses Regular monitoring of fluid and nutritional intake
Thrombocytopenia	Decrease dose if clinically symptomatic (i.e., bruising, bleeding gums) Thrombocytopenia more likely with valproate levels ≥110 μg/mL (women) and ≥135 μg/mL (men)

hepatotoxicity in persons who have been treated with valproate alone is 0.85 per 100,000 persons; no persons older than the age of 10 years have been reported to have died from hepatotoxicity. Therefore, the risk of this adverse reaction in adult psychiatric patients is low.

Nevertheless, if symptoms of lethargy, malaise, anorexia, nausea and vomiting, edema, and abdominal pain occur in a person treated with valproate, the clinician must consider the possibility of severe hepatotoxicity. A modest increase in liver function test results does not correlate with the development of severe hepatotoxicity. Rare cases of pancreatitis have been reported; they occur most often in the first 6 months of treatment, and the condition occasionally results in death. The pancreatic function can be assessed and followed by serum amylase concentrations. Other potentially severe consequences of treatment include hyperammonemia-induced encephalopathy and thrombocytopenia. Thrombocytopenia and platelet dysfunction occur most commonly at high dosages and result in the prolongation of bleeding times.

There are multiple concerns regarding the use of valproate during pregnancy. Women who require valproate therapy should, therefore, inform their physicians if they intend to become pregnant. First-trimester use of valproate has been associated with a 3 to 5 percent risk of neural tube defects, as well as an increased risk of other malformations affecting the heart and other organ systems. Multiple reports have also indicated that in utero exposure to valproate may negatively affect cognitive development in children of mothers who take valproate during pregnancy. They have lower IQ scores at age 6 years compared with those exposed to other antiepileptic drugs. Fetal valproate exposure has dose-dependent associations with reduced cognitive abilities across a range of domains at 6 years of age. Valproate exposure may also increase the risk of autistic spectrum disorder.

Valproate is also associated with teratogenicity, most notably neural tube defects (e.g., spina bifida). The risk is about 1 to 4 percent of all women who take valproate during the first trimester of pregnancy. The risk of valproate-induced neural tube defects can be reduced with daily folic acid supplements (1 to 4 mg a day). All women with childbearing potential who take the drug should be given folic acid supplements. Infants breastfed by mothers taking valproate develop serum valproate concentrations 1 to 10 percent of maternal serum concentrations, but no data suggest that this poses a risk to the infant. Valproate is not contraindicated in nursing mothers. We should avoid this drug in patients with hepatic diseases. Valproate may be especially problematic for adolescents and young women. Cases of polycystic ovarian disease have been reported in women using valproate. Even when the full syndromal criteria for this syndrome are not met, many of these women develop menstrual irregularities, hair loss, and hirsutism. These effects are thought to result from a metabolic syndrome that is driven by insulin resistance and hyperinsulinemia.

The common adverse effects associated with valproate (Table 21-33) are those affecting the GI system, such as nausea, vomiting, dyspepsia, and diarrhea. The GI effects are generally most common in the first month of treatment, significantly if the dosage is increased rapidly. Unbuffered valproic acid (Depakene) is more likely to cause GI symptoms than the enteric-coated "sprinkle" or the delayed-release divalproex sodium formulations. Other common adverse effects involve the nervous system, such as sedation, ataxia, dysarthria, and tremor. Valproate-induced tremor may respond well to treatment with β-adrenergic receptor antagonists or gabapentin. Treatment of the other neurologic adverse effects usually requires lowering the valproate dosage.

Table 21-33
Adverse Effects of Valproate

Common
    GI irritation
    Nausea
    Sedation
    Tremor
    Weight gain
    Hair loss

Uncommon
    Vomiting
    Diarrhea
    Ataxia
    Dysarthria
    Persistent elevation of hepatic transaminases

Rare
    Fatal hepatotoxicity (primarily in pediatric patients)
    Reversible thrombocytopenia
    Platelet dysfunction
    Coagulation disturbances
    Edema
    Hemorrhagic pancreatitis
    Agranulocytosis
    Encephalopathy and coma
    Respiratory muscle weakness and respiratory failure

GI, gastrointestinal.

Weight gain is a common adverse effect, especially in long-term treatment, and can best be treated by strict limitation of caloric intake. Hair loss may occur in 5 to 10 percent of all persons treated, and rare cases of complete loss of body hair have been reported. Some clinicians have recommended treatment of valproate-associated hair loss with vitamin supplements that contain zinc and selenium. About 5 to 40 percent of persons experience a persistent but clinically insignificant elevation in liver transaminases up to three times the upper limit of normal, which is usually asymptomatic and resolves after discontinuation of the drug. High dosages of valproate (above 1,000 mg a day) may rarely produce mild to moderate hyponatremia, most likely because of some degree of the syndrome of secretion of inappropriate antidiuretic hormone, which is reversible upon lowering of the dosage. Overdoses of valproate can lead to coma and death.

Drug Interactions

Valproate is commonly prescribed as part of a regimen involving other psychotropic agents. The only consistent drug interaction with lithium, if both drugs are maintained in their respective therapeutic ranges, is the exacerbation of drug-induced tremors, which can usually be treated with β-receptor antagonists. The combination of valproate and DRAs may result in increased sedation, as can be seen when valproate is added to any CNS depressant (e.g., alcohol), and increased severity of extrapyramidal symptoms, which usually responds to treatment with antiparkinsonian drugs. Valproate can usually be safely combined with carbamazepine or SDAs. Perhaps the most worrisome interaction of valproate and a psychotropic drug involves lamotrigine. Since the approval of lamotrigine for the treatment of bipolar disorder, it is more likely that patients will be treated with both agents. Valproate more than doubles lamotrigine concentrations, increasing the risk of a severe rash (Stevens–Johnson syndrome and toxic epidermal necrolysis).

The plasma concentrations of carbamazepine, diazepam (Valium), amitriptyline (Elavil), nortriptyline (Pamelor), and phenobarbital (Luminal) may also be increased when these drugs are coadministered with valproate. Also, the plasma concentrations

Table 21-34
Interactions of Valproate with Other Drugs

Drug	Interactions Reported with Valproate
Lithium	Increased tremor
Antipsychotics	Increased sedation; increased extrapyramidal effects; delirium and stupor (single report)
Clozapine	Increased sedation; confusional syndrome (single report)
Carbamazepine	Acute psychosis (single report); ataxia, nausea, lethargy (single report); may decrease valproate serum concentrations
Antidepressants	Amitriptyline and fluoxetine may increase valproate serum concentrations
Diazepam	Serum concentration increased by valproate
Clonazepam	Absence status (rare; reported only in patients with preexisting epilepsy)
Phenytoin	Serum concentration decreased by valproate
Phenobarbital	Serum concentration increased by valproate; increased sedation
Other CNS depressants	Increased sedation
Anticoagulants	Possible potentiation of effect

CNS, central nervous system.

of phenytoin (Dilantin) and desipramine (Norpramin) may be decreased when they are combined with valproate. The plasma concentrations of valproate may be decreased when the drug is coadministered with carbamazepine and may be increased when coadministered with guanfacine (Tenex), amitriptyline, or fluoxetine (Prozac). Valproate can be displaced from plasma proteins by carbamazepine, diazepam, and aspirin. Persons who are treated with anticoagulants (e.g., aspirin and warfarin [Coumadin]) should also be monitored when valproate use is initiated to assess the development of any undesired augmentation of the anticoagulation effects. Interactions of valproate with other drugs are listed in Table 21-34.

Laboratory Interferences

Valproate may cause a laboratory increase of serum-free fatty acids. Valproate metabolites may produce a false-positive test result

Table 21-35
Recommended Laboratory Tests during Valproate Therapy

Before Treatment
Standard chemistry screen with special attention to liver function tests
CBC, including WBC and platelet count

During Treatment
Liver function tests at 1 mo; then every 6–24 mo if no abnormalities are found.
Complete blood count with platelet count at 1 mo; then every 6–24 mo if findings are normal.

If Liver Function Test Results Become Abnormal
Mild transaminase elevation (less than three times normal): monitoring every 1–2 wk; if stable and patient is responding to valproate, results are monitored monthly to every 3 mo.
Pronounced transaminase elevation (more than three times normal): dosage reduction or discontinuation of valproate; increase dose or rechallenge if transaminases normalize and if the patient is a valproate responder.

CBC, complete blood count; WBC, white blood cell.

for urinary ketones as well as falsely abnormal thyroid function test results.

Dosage and Clinical Guidelines

When starting valproate therapy, a baseline hepatic panel, CBC and platelet counts, and pregnancy testing should be ordered. Additional testing should include amylase and coagulation studies if baseline pancreatic disease or coagulopathy is suspected. In addition to baseline laboratory tests, hepatic transaminase concentrations should be obtained 1 month after initiation of therapy and every 6 to 24 months after that. However, because even frequent monitoring may not predict severe organ toxicity, it is more prudent to reinforce the need for prompt evaluation of any illnesses when reviewing the instructions with patients. Asymptomatic elevation of transaminase concentrations up to three times the upper limit of normal are typical and do not require any change in dosage. Table 21-35 lists the recommended laboratory tests for valproate treatment.

Valproate is available in several formulations (Table 21-36). For the treatment of acute mania, an oral loading strategy of initiation with 20 to 30 mg/kg a day can be used to accelerate the control of symptoms. This strategy is usually well tolerated but can cause excessive sedation and tremor in elderly persons. Agitated behavior can be rapidly stabilized with IV infusion of valproate.

Table 21-36
Valproate Preparations Available in the United States

Generic Name	Trade Name, Form (Doses)	Time to Peak
Valproate sodium injection	Depacon injection (100-mg valproic acid/mL)	1 hr
Valproic acid	Depakene, syrup (250 mg/5 mL)	1–2 hr
	Depakene, capsules (250 mg)	1–2 hr
Divalproex sodium	Depakote, delayed-released tablets (125, 250, 500 mg)	3–8 hr
Divalproex sodium-coated particles in capsules	Depakote, sprinkle capsules (125 mg)	Compared with divalproex tablets, divalproex sprinkle has earlier onset and slower absorption, with slightly lower peak plasma concentration
Divalproex sodium extended-release	Depakote ER (250, 500 mg)	4–17 hr

If acute mania is absent, it is best to initiate drug treatment gradually to minimize the common adverse effects of nausea, vomiting, and sedation. The dose on the first day should be 250 mg administered with a meal. The dosage can be raised to 250 mg orally three times daily for over 3 to 6 days. The plasma concentrations can be assessed in the morning before the first daily dose is administered. Therapeutic plasma concentrations for the control of seizures range between 50 and 100 µg/mL. It is reasonable to use the same range for the treatment of mental disorders; most of the controlled studies have used 50 to 125 µg/mL. Most persons attain therapeutic plasma concentrations on a dosage between 1,200 and 1,500 mg a day in divided doses. After a person's symptoms are well controlled, the full daily dose can be taken all at once before sleep.

LAMOTRIGINE

Lamotrigine (Lamictal) was developed as a result of screening folate antagonists as anticonvulsants. Lamotrigine proved effective in several animal models of epilepsy, was developed as an anti-epileptic drug, and was marketed for the adjunctive treatment of partial seizures in the United States in 1995. Initial, postmarketing, open, clinical experience suggested efficacy in a variety of neurologic and psychiatric conditions, coupled with good tolerability (aside from the risk of rash). Later, double-blind, placebo-controlled studies revealed that lamotrigine was useful for some, but not all, of the neurologic and psychiatric conditions reported in open studies. Therefore, lamotrigine appeared effective as a maintenance treatment for bipolar disorder and was approved for the maintenance treatment of bipolar I disorder in 2003. Lamotrigine also appeared to have potential utility in acute bipolar depression. However, the magnitude of the effect was too modest to yield consistently superior performance compared with placebo, and hence lamotrigine did not receive approval for the treatment of acute bipolar depression.

Similarly, limited data suggested that lamotrigine had potential utility in rapid-cycling bipolar disorder. Lamotrigine did not appear to be as effective as the primary intervention in acute mania. Thus, lamotrigine has emerged as an agent that appears to "stabilize mood from below" in the sense that it may maximally impact the depressive component of bipolar disorders.

Pharmacologic Actions

Lamotrigine is wholly absorbed, has a bioavailability of 98 percent, and has a steady-state plasma half-life of 25 hours. However, the rate of metabolism of lamotrigine varies over a sixfold range, depending on which other drugs are administered concomitantly. Dosing is escalated slowly to twice-a-day maintenance dosing. Food does not affect its absorption, and it is 55 percent protein-bound in the plasma; 94 percent of lamotrigine and its inactive metabolites are excreted in the urine. Among the better-delineated biochemical actions of lamotrigine is the blockade of voltage-sensitive sodium channels, which in turn modulates the release of glutamate and aspartate and has a slight effect on calcium channels. Lamotrigine modestly increases plasma serotonin concentrations, possibly through inhibition of serotonin reuptake, and is a weak inhibitor of serotonin 5-HT$_3$ receptors.

Therapeutic Indications

Bipolar Disorder. Lamotrigine is indicated in the treatment of bipolar disorder and may prolong the time between episodes of depression and mania. It is more effective in lengthening the intervals between depressive episodes than manic episodes. It is also useful as a treatment for rapid-cycling bipolar disorder.

Other Indications. There have been reports of therapeutic benefit in the treatment of borderline personality disorder and the treatment for various pain syndromes.

Precautions and Adverse Reactions

Lamotrigine is remarkably well tolerated. The absence of sedation, weight gain, and other metabolic effects are noteworthy. The most common adverse effects—dizziness, ataxia, somnolence, headache, diplopia, blurred vision, and nausea—are typically mild. Anecdotal reports of cognitive impairment and joint or back pain are standard.

The appearance of a rash, which is common and occasionally very severe, is a source of concern. About 8 percent of patients started on lamotrigine develop a benign maculopapular rash during the first 4 months of treatment, and the drug should be discontinued if a rash develops. Even though these rashes are benign, there is concern that, in some cases, they may represent early manifestations of Stevens–Johnson syndrome or toxic epidermal necrolysis. Nevertheless, even if lamotrigine is discontinued immediately upon the development of a rash or other signs of hypersensitivity reaction, such as fever and lymphadenopathy, this may not prevent subsequent development of a life-threatening rash or permanent disfiguration.

Estimates of the rate of severe rash vary, depending on the source of the data. In some studies, the incidence of severe rashes was 0.08 percent in adult patients receiving lamotrigine as initial monotherapy and 0.13 percent in adult patients receiving lamotrigine as adjunctive therapy. German registry data, based on clinical practice, suggest that the risk of rash may be as low as 1 in 5,000 patients. The appearance of any rash necessitates immediate discontinuation of drug administration.

It is known that the likelihood of a rash increases if the recommended starting dose and speed of dose increase exceed what is recommended. Concomitant administration of valproic acid also increases risk and should be avoided if possible. If valproate is used, a more conservative dosing regimen is followed. Children and adolescents younger than age 16 years appear to be more susceptible to rash with lamotrigine. If patients miss more than 4 consecutive days of lamotrigine treatment, they need to restart therapy at the initial starting dose and titrate upward as if they had not already been on the medication.

Laboratory Testing

There is no proven correlation between lamotrigine blood concentrations and either antiseizure effects or efficacy in bipolar disorders. Laboratory tests are not useful in predicting the occurrence of adverse events.

Drug Interactions

Lamotrigine has significant, well-characterized drug interactions involving other anticonvulsants. The most potentially serious lamotrigine drug interaction involves concurrent use of valproic acid, which doubles serum lamotrigine concentrations. Lamotrigine decreases the plasma concentration of valproic acid by 25 percent. Sertraline (Zoloft) also increases plasma lamotrigine concentrations, but to a lesser extent than does valproic acid. Lamotrigine concentrations are decreased by 40 to 50 percent with concomitant administration of carbamazepine, phenytoin, or phenobarbital. Combinations of lamotrigine and other anticonvulsants have complex effects on the time of peak plasma concentration and the plasma half-life of lamotrigine.

Laboratory Interferences

Lamotrigine does not interfere with any laboratory tests.

Dosage and Administration

In the clinical trials leading to the approval of lamotrigine as a treatment for bipolar disorder, no consistent increase in efficacy was associated with doses above 200 mg/day. Most patients should take between 100 and 200 mg a day. In epilepsy, the drug is administered twice daily, but in bipolar disorder, the total dose can be taken once a day, either in the morning or night, depending on whether the patient finds the drug activating or sedating.

Lamotrigine is available as unscored 25-, 100-, 150-, and 200-mg tablets. The primary determinant of lamotrigine dosing is the minimization of the risk of rash. Lamotrigine should not be taken by anyone younger than 16 years of age. Because valproic acid markedly slows the elimination of lamotrigine, concomitant administration of these two drugs necessitates a much slower titration (Table 21-37). People with renal insufficiency should aim for a lower maintenance dosage. The appearance of any rash necessitates immediate discontinuation of lamotrigine administration. Lamotrigine should usually be discontinued gradually over 2 weeks unless a rash emerges, in which case it should be discontinued over 1 to 2 days.

Lamotrigine orally disintegrating tablets (Lamictal ODT) are available for patients who have difficulty swallowing. It is the only antiepileptic treatment that is available in an orally disintegrating formulation. It is available in 25, 50, 100, and 200 mg strengths and matches the dose of lamotrigine tablets. Chewable dispersible tablets of 2, 5, and 25 mg are also available.

CARBAMAZEPINE AND OXCARBAZEPINE

Carbamazepine (Tegretol) possesses some structural similarity to the TCA imipramine (Tofranil). It was approved for use in the United States for the treatment of trigeminal neuralgia in 1968 and temporal lobe epilepsy (complex partial seizures) in 1974. Interestingly, carbamazepine was first synthesized as a potential antidepressant, but because of its atypical profile in several animal models, it was initially developed for use in pain and seizure disorders. It is now recognized in most guidelines as a second-line mood

stabilizer useful in the treatment and prevention of both phases of bipolar affective disorder. A long-acting sustained release formulation (Equetro) was approved by the U.S. FDA for the treatment of acute mania in 2002.

An analog of carbamazepine, oxcarbazepine (Trileptal), was marketed as an antiseizure medication in the United States in 2000. Previously it was used as a treatment for pediatric epilepsy in Europe since 1990. Because of its similarity to carbamazepine, many clinicians began to use it as a treatment for patients with bipolar disorder. Despite some reports that oxcarbazepine has mood-stabilizing properties, this has not been confirmed in large, placebo-controlled trials.

Carbamazepine

Pharmacologic Actions.   The absorption of carbamazepine is slow and unpredictable. Food enhances absorption. Peak plasma concentrations are reached 2 to 8 hours after a single dose, and steady-state levels are reached after 2 to 4 days on a steady dosage. It is 70 to 80 percent protein-bound. The half-life of carbamazepine ranges from 18 to 54 hours, with an average of 26 hours. However, with chronic administration, the half-life of carbamazepine decreases to an average of 12 hours. This results from the induction of hepatic CYP450 enzymes by carbamazepine, specifically the autoinduction of carbamazepine metabolism. The induction of hepatic enzymes reaches its maximum level after about 3 to 5 weeks of therapy.

The pharmacokinetics of carbamazepine are different for two long-acting preparations of carbamazepine, each of which uses slightly different technology. One formulation, Tegretol XR, requires food to ensure standard GI transit time. The other preparation, Carbatrol, relies on a combination of intermediate, extended-release, and very slow release beads, making it suitable for bedtime administration.

Carbamazepine is metabolized in the liver, and the 10,11-epoxide metabolite is active as an anticonvulsant. Its activity in the treatment of bipolar disorders is unknown. Long-term use of carbamazepine is associated with an increased ratio of the epoxide to the parent molecule.

The anticonvulsant effects of carbamazepine are thought to be mediated mainly by binding to voltage-dependent sodium channels in the inactive state and prolonging their inactivation. This action secondarily reduces voltage-dependent calcium channel activation and, thus, synaptic transmission. Additional effects include reduction of currents through N-methyl-D-aspartate (NMDA) glutamate-receptor channels, competitive antagonism of adenosine a_1-receptors, and potentiation of CNS catecholamine neurotransmission. Whether any or all of these mechanisms also result in mood stabilization is not known.

Therapeutic Indications

Bipolar Disorder

ACUTE MANIA.   The acute antimanic effects of carbamazepine are typically evident within the first several days of treatment. About 50 to 70 percent of all persons respond within 2 to 3 weeks of initiation. Studies suggest that carbamazepine may be especially useful in persons who are not responsive to lithium (Eskalith), such as persons with dysphoric mania, rapid cycling, or an adverse family history of mood disorders. The antimanic effects of carbamazepine can be, and often are, augmented by concomitant administration of lithium, valproic acid (Depakene), thyroid hormones, DRAs,

Table 21-37
Lamotrigine Dosing (mg/day)

Treatment	Weeks 1–2	Weeks 3–4	Weeks 4–5
Lamotrigine monotherapy	25	50	100–200 (200 maximum)
Lamotrigine + carbamazepine	50	100	200–400 (400 maximum)
Lamotrigine + valproate	25 every other day	25	50–100 (100 maximum)

or SDAs. Some persons may respond to carbamazepine but not lithium or valproic acid and vice versa.

PROPHYLAXIS. Carbamazepine is effective in preventing relapses, particularly among patients with bipolar II disorder and schizoaffective disorder, and dysphoric mania.

ACUTE DEPRESSION. A subgroup of treatment-refractory patients with acute depression responds well to carbamazepine. Patients with more severe episodic and less chronic depression seem to be better responders to carbamazepine. Nevertheless, carbamazepine remains an alternative drug for depressed persons who have not responded to conventional treatments, including ECT.

OTHER DISORDERS. Carbamazepine helps to control symptoms associated with acute alcohol withdrawal, although benzodiazepines are more effective in this population. Carbamazepine has been suggested as a treatment for the recurrent paroxysmal component of PTSD. Uncontrolled studies suggest that carbamazepine is effective in controlling impulsive, aggressive behavior in nonpsychotic persons of all ages, including children and elderly persons. Carbamazepine is also effective in controlling nonacute agitation and aggressive behavior in patients with schizophrenia and schizoaffective disorder. Persons with prominent positive symptoms (e.g., hallucinations) may be likely to respond, as are persons who display impulsive aggressive outbursts.

Precautions and Adverse Reactions.
Carbamazepine is relatively well tolerated. Mild GI (nausea, vomiting, gastric distress, constipation, diarrhea, and anorexia) and CNS (ataxia, drowsiness) side effects are the most common. The severity of these adverse effects is reduced if the dosage of carbamazepine is increased slowly and kept at the minimal effective plasma concentration. In contrast to lithium and valproate (other drugs used to manage bipolar disorder), carbamazepine does not appear to cause weight gain. Because of the phenomena of autoinduction, with consequent reductions in carbamazepine concentrations, side effect tolerability may improve over time. Most of the adverse effects of carbamazepine are correlated with plasma concentrations above 9 µg/mL. The rarest but most serious adverse effects of carbamazepine are blood dyscrasias, hepatitis, and severe skin reactions (Table 21-38).

BLOOD DYSCRASIAS. The drug's hematologic effects are not dose-related. Severe blood dyscrasias (aplastic anemia, agranulocytosis) occur in about 1 in 125,000 persons treated with carbamazepine. There does not appear to be a correlation between the degree of benign WBC suppression (leukopenia), which is seen in 1 to 2 percent of persons, and the emergence of life-threatening blood dyscrasias. Persons should be warned that the emergence of such symptoms as fever, sore throat, rash, petechiae, bruising, and easy

bleeding can potentially herald a serious dyscrasia, and they should seek medical evaluation immediately. Routine hematologic monitoring in carbamazepine-treated persons is recommended at 3, 6, 9, and 12 months. If there is no significant evidence of bone marrow suppression by that time, many experts will reduce the interval of monitoring. However, even assiduous monitoring may fail to detect severe blood dyscrasias before they cause symptoms.

HEPATITIS. Within the first few weeks of therapy, carbamazepine can cause both hepatitis associated with increases in liver enzymes, particularly transaminases, and cholestasis associated with elevated bilirubin and alkaline phosphatase. Mild transaminase elevations warrant observation only, but persistent elevations more than three times the upper limit of normal indicate the need to discontinue the drug. Hepatitis can recur if the drug is reintroduced to the person and can result in death.

DERMATOLOGIC EFFECTS. About 10 to 15 percent of those treated with carbamazepine develop a benign maculopapular rash within the first 3 weeks of treatment. Stopping the medication usually leads to resolution of the rash. Some patients may experience life-threatening dermatologic syndromes, including exfoliative dermatitis, erythema multiforme, Stevens–Johnson syndrome, and toxic epidermal necrolysis. The possible emergence of these serious dermatologic problems causes most clinicians to discontinue carbamazepine use in people who develop any rash. The risk of drug rash is about equal between valproic acid and carbamazepine in the first 2 months of use but is subsequently much higher for carbamazepine. If carbamazepine seems to be the only effective drug for a person who has a benign rash with carbamazepine treatment, a retrial of the drug can be undertaken. Many patients can be rechallenged without reemergence of the rash. Pretreatment with prednisone (Deltasone; 40 mg a day) may suppress the rash, although other symptoms of an allergic reaction (e.g., fever and pneumonitis) may develop even with steroid pretreatment.

RENAL EFFECTS. Carbamazepine is occasionally used to treat diabetes insipidus not associated with lithium use. This activity results from direct or indirect effects at the vasopressin receptor. It may also lead to the development of hyponatremia and water intoxication in some patients, mainly elderly persons, or when used in high doses.

OTHER ADVERSE EFFECTS. Carbamazepine decreases cardiac conduction (although less than the tricyclic drugs do) and can thus exacerbate preexisting cardiac disease. Carbamazepine should be used with caution in persons with glaucoma, prostatic hypertrophy, diabetes, or a history of alcohol abuse. Carbamazepine occasionally activates vasopressin receptor function, which results in a condition resembling the syndrome of secretion of inappropriate antidiuretic hormone, characterized by hyponatremia and, rarely, water intoxication. This effect is the opposite of the renal effects of lithium (i.e., nephrogenic diabetes insipidus). Augmentation of lithium with carbamazepine does not reverse the lithium effect, however. The emergence of confusion, severe weakness, or headache in a person taking carbamazepine should prompt the measurement of serum electrolytes.

Carbamazepine use rarely elicits an immune hypersensitivity response consisting of fever, rash, eosinophilia, and possibly fatal myocarditis.

Cleft palate, fingernail hypoplasia, microcephaly, and spina bifida in infants may be associated with the maternal use of carbamazepine during pregnancy. Pregnant women should not use

Table 21-38
Adverse Events Associated with Carbamazepine

Dosage-Related Adverse Effects	Idiosyncratic Adverse Effects
Double or blurred vision	Agranulocytosis
Vertigo	Stevens–Johnson syndrome
Gastrointestinal disturbances	Aplastic anemia
Task performance impairment	Hepatic failure
Hematologic effects	Rash
	Pancreatitis

carbamazepine unless necessary. All women with childbearing potential should take 1 to 4 mg of folic acid daily, even if they are not trying to conceive. Carbamazepine is secreted in breast milk.

Drug Interactions.   Carbamazepine decreases serum concentrations of numerous drugs as a result of the prominent induction of hepatic CYP3A4 (Table 21-39). Monitoring for a decrease in clinical effects is frequently indicated. Carbamazepine can decrease the blood concentrations of oral contraceptives, resulting in breakthrough bleeding and uncertain prophylaxis against pregnancy. Carbamazepine should not be administered with MAOIs, which should be discontinued at least 2 weeks before initiating treatment with carbamazepine. Grapefruit juice inhibits the hepatic metabolism of carbamazepine. When carbamazepine and valproate are used in combination, the dosage of carbamazepine should be decreased because valproate displaces carbamazepine binding on proteins, and the dosage of valproate may need to be increased.

**Table 21-39
Carbamazepine: Drug Interactions**

Effect of Carbamazepine on Plasma Concentrations of Concomitant Agents	Agents that May Affect Carbamazepine Plasma Concentrations
Carbamazepine may decrease drug plasma concentration of:	*Agents that may increase carbamazepine plasma concentration:*
Acetaminophen	Allopurinol
Alprazolam	Cimetidine
Amitriptyline	Clarithromycin
Bupropion	Danazol
Clomipramine	Diltiazem
Clonazepam	Erythromycin
Clozapine	Fluoxetine
Cyclosporine	Fluvoxamine
Desipramine	Gemfibrozil
Dicumarol	Itraconazole
Doxepin	Ketoconazole
Doxycycline	Isoniazid[a]
Ethosuximide	Itraconazole
Felbamate	Lamotrigine
Fentanyl	Loratadine
Fluphenazine	Macrolides
Haloperidol	Nefazodone
Hormonal contraceptives	Nicotinamide
Imipramine	Propoxyphene
Lamotrigine	Terfenadine
Methadone	Troleandomycin
Methsuximide	Valproate[a]
Methylprednisolone	Verapamil
Nimodipine	Viloxazine
Pancuronium	
Phensuximide	*Drugs that may decrease carbamazepine plasma concentrations*
Phenytoin	
Primidone	Carbamazepine (autoinduction)
Theophylline	Cisplatin
Valproate	Doxorubicin HCl
Warfarin	Felbamate
Carbamazepine may increase drug plasma concentrations of	Phenobarbital
Clomipramine	Phenytoin
Phenytoin	Primidone
Primidone	Rifampin[b]
	Theophylline
	Valproate

[a]Increased concentrations of the active 10,11-epoxide.
[b]Decreased concentrations of carbamazepine and increased concentrations of the 10,11-epoxide.
Table by Carlos A. Zarate, Jr., M.D. and Mauricio Tohen, M.D.

Laboratory Interferences.   Circulating levels of thyroxine and triiodothyronine are associated with a decrease in TSH and may be associated with treatment. Carbamazepine is also associated with an increase in total serum cholesterol, primarily by increasing high-density lipoproteins. The thyroid and cholesterol effects are not clinically significant. Carbamazepine may interfere with the dexamethasone (Decadron) suppression test and may also cause false-positive pregnancy test results.

Dosing and Administration.   The target dose for antimanic activity is 1,200 mg a day, although this varies considerably. Immediate-release carbamazepine needs to be taken three or four times a day, which leads to lapses in compliance. Extended-release formulations are thus preferred because they can be taken once or twice a day. One form of extended-release carbamazepine, Carbatrol, comes as 100-, 200-, and 300-mg capsules. Another form, Equetro, is identical to Carbatrol and is marketed as a treatment for bipolar disorder. These capsules contain tiny beads with three different types of coatings, so they dissolve at different times. Capsules should not be crushed or chewed. However, the contents can be sprinkled over food without affecting the extended-release qualities. This formulation can be taken either with or without meals. The entire daily dose can be given at bedtime. The rate of absorption is faster when it is given with a high-fat meal. Another extended-release form of carbamazepine, Tegretol XR, uses a different drug-delivery system than Carbatrol. It is available in 100-, 200-, and 300-mg tablets.

Preexisting hematologic, hepatic, and cardiac diseases can be relative contraindications for carbamazepine treatment. Persons with hepatic disease require only one-third to one-half the usual dosage; the clinician should be cautious about raising the dosage in such persons and should do so only slowly and gradually. The laboratory examination should include a CBC with platelet count, liver function tests, serum electrolytes, and an electrocardiogram in persons older than 40 years of age or with preexisting cardiac disease. An electroencephalogram is not necessary before the initiation of treatment, but it may be helpful in some cases for the documentation of objective changes correlated with clinical improvement. Table 21-40 presents a brief user's guide to carbamazepine in bipolar disorder.

Routine Laboratory Monitoring.   Serum levels for antimanic efficacy have not been established. The anticonvulsant blood concentration range for carbamazepine is 4 to 12 μg/mL, and this range should be reached before determining that carbamazepine is not effective in the treatment of a mood disorder. A clinically insignificant suppression of the WBC count commonly occurs during carbamazepine treatment. This benign decrease can be reversed by adding lithium, which enhances colony-stimulating factor. Potential serious hematologic effects of carbamazepine, such as pancytopenia, agranulocytosis, and aplastic anemia, occur in about 1 in 125,000 patients. Complete laboratory blood assessments may be performed every 2 weeks for the first 2 months of treatment and quarterly after that, but the FDA has revised the package insert for carbamazepine to suggest that blood monitoring be performed at the discretion of the physician. Patients should be informed that fever, sore throat, rash, petechiae, bruising, or unusual bleeding may indicate a hematologic problem and should prompt immediate notification of a physician. This approach is probably more useful than is frequent blood monitoring during long-term treatment. It has also been suggested that liver and renal function tests be conducted quarterly, although the benefit of conducting tests

Table 21-40
Carbamazepine in Bipolar Illness: A Brief User's Guide

1. Start with low (200 mg) bedtime dose in depression or euthymia; higher doses (600–800 mg/day in divided doses) in manic inpatients.
2. All bedtime dosing is reasonable with carbamazepine extended-release preparation.
3. Titrate slowly to the individual's response or side effects threshold.
4. Hepatic enzyme CYP450 (3A4) induction and autoinduction occur in 2–3 wk; slightly higher doses may be needed or tolerated at that time.
5. Warn regarding benign rash, which occurs in 5–10% of those taking the drug; progression to rare, severe rash is unpredictable, so the drug should be discontinued if any rash develops.
6. Benign white blood cell count decreases occur regularly (usually inconsequential).
7. Rarely, agranulocytosis and aplastic anemia may develop (several per million new exposures); warn regarding appearance of fever, sore throat, petechiae, and bleeding gums and to check with physician to obtain an immediate complete blood cell count.
8. Use adequate birth control methods, including higher dosage forms of estrogen (as carbamazepine lowers estrogen levels).
9. Avoid carbamazepine in pregnancy (spina bifida occurs in 0.5%; other severe adverse outcomes occur in about 8%).
10. Some people will respond well to carbamazepine and not other mood stabilizers (lithium) or anticonvulsants (valproic acid).
11. Combination treatment often required to maintain remission and prevent loss of effect via tolerance.
12. Major drug interactions associated with increases in carbamazepine and potential toxicity from 3A4 enzyme inhibition include calcium channel blockers (isradipine and verapamil); erythromycin and related macrolide antibiotics; and valproate.

this frequently has been questioned. It seems reasonable, however, to assess hematologic status, along with liver and renal functions, whenever a routine examination of the person is being conducted. A monitoring protocol is listed in Table 21-41.

Carbamazepine treatment should be discontinued, and a consult with a hematologist should be obtained, if the following laboratory values are found: total WBC count below 3,000/mm³, erythrocytes below 4.0×10^6/mm³, neutrophils below 1,500/mm³, hematocrit less than 32 percent, hemoglobin less than 11 g/100 mL, platelet

Table 21-41
Laboratory Monitoring of Carbamazepine for Adult Psychiatric Disorders

	Baseline	Weekly to Stability	Monthly for 6 Months	6–12 Months
CBC	+	+	+	+
Bilirubin	+		+	+
Alanine aminotransferase	+		+	+
Aspartate aminotransferase	+		+	+
Alkaline phosphatase	+		+	+
Carbamazepine level	+	+		+

CBC, complete blood count.

count below 100,000/mm³, reticulocyte count below 0.3 percent, and a serum iron concentration below 150 mg/100 mL.

Oxcarbazepine

Although structurally related to carbamazepine, the usefulness of oxcarbazepine as a treatment for mania has not been established in controlled trials.

Pharmacokinetics. Absorption is rapid and unaffected by food. Peak concentrations occur after about 45 minutes. The elimination half-life of the parent compound is 2 hours, which remains stable over long-term treatment. The monohydroxide has a half-life of 9 hours. Most of the drug's anticonvulsant activity is presumed to result from this monohydroxy derivative.

Side Effects. The most common side effects are sedation and nausea. Less frequent side effects are cognitive impairment, ataxia, diplopia, nystagmus, dizziness, and tremor. In contrast to carbamazepine, oxcarbazepine does not have an increased risk of severe blood dyscrasias, so hematologic monitoring is not necessary. The frequency of benign rash is lower than observed with carbamazepine, and severe rashes are extremely rare. However, about 25 to 30 percent of patients who develop an allergic rash while taking carbamazepine also develop a rash with oxcarbazepine. Oxcarbazepine is more likely to cause hyponatremia than carbamazepine. Approximately 3 to 5 percent of patients taking oxcarbazepine develop this side effect. It is advisable to obtain serum sodium concentrations early in the course of treatment because hyponatremia may be clinically silent. In severe cases, confusion and seizure may occur.

Dosing and Administration. Oxcarbazepine dosing for bipolar disorder has not been established. It is available in 150-, 300-, and 600-mg tablets. The dose range may vary from 150 to 2,400 mg/day, given in divided doses twice a day. In clinical trials for mania, the doses typically used were from 900 to 1,200 mg/day with a starting dose of 150 or 300 mg at night.

Drug Interactions. Drugs such as phenobarbital and alcohol, which induce CYP34A, increase clearance and reduce oxcarbazepine concentrations. Oxcarbazepine induces CYP3A4/5 and inhibits CYP2C19, which may affect the metabolism of drugs that use that pathway. Women taking oral contraceptives should be told to consult with their gynecologists, because oxcarbazepine may reduce concentrations of their contraceptive and thus decrease its efficacy.

OTHER ANTICONVULSANTS

The anticonvulsants described in this section were developed for the treatment of epilepsy but were also found to have beneficial effects in psychiatric disorders. Also, these agents are used as skeletal muscle relaxants and in neurogenic pain. These drugs have a variety of mechanisms, including increasing GABAergic function or decreasing glutamatergic function. This section includes seven anticonvulsants: gabapentin (Neurontin), levetiracetam (Keppra), pregabalin (Lyrica), tiagabine (Gabitril), topiramate (Topamax), and zonisamide (Zonegran), as well as one of the first used anticonvulsants, phenytoin (Dilantin). Carbamazepine (Tegretol), valproate (Depakene, Depakote), lamotrigine (Lamictal), and oxcarbazepine (Trileptal) are discussed in separate sections.

In 2008, the FDA issued a warning that these drugs may increase the risk of suicidal ideation or act in some persons compared with placebo; however, the relative risk for suicidality was higher in patients with epilepsy compared with those with psychiatric disorders. However, some published data contradict this warning. These studies suggest that anticonvulsants may have a protective effect on suicidal thoughts in bipolar disorder. Considering the inherently increased risk of suicide in persons with bipolar disorder, clinicians should be aware of these warnings.

Gabapentin

Gabapentin was first introduced as an antiepileptic drug and was found to have sedative effects that were useful in some psychiatric disorders, especially insomnia. It was also found to be beneficial in reducing neuropathic pain, including postherpetic neuralgia. It is used in anxiety disorders (social phobia and panic disorder), but not as the primary intervention in mania or treatment-resistant mood disorders.

Pharmacologic Actions. Gabapentin circulates in the blood primarily unbound and is not appreciably metabolized in humans. It is eliminated unchanged by renal excretion and can be removed by hemodialysis. Food only moderately affects the rate and extent of absorption. Clearance is decreased in elderly persons, requiring dosage adjustments. Gabapentin appears to increase cerebral GABA and may inhibit glutamate synthesis as well. It increases human whole blood serotonin concentrations and modulates calcium channels to reduce monoamine release. It has antiseizure as well as antispastic activity and antinociceptive effects in pain.

Therapeutic Indications. In neurology, gabapentin is used for the treatment of both general and partial seizures. It is useful in reducing the pain of postherpetic neuralgia and other pain syndromes associated with diabetic neuropathy, neuropathic cancer pain, fibromyalgia, meralgia paresthetica, amputation, and headache. It is useful in some cases of chronic pruritus.

In psychiatry, gabapentin is used as a hypnotic agent because of its sedating effects. It has anxiolytic properties and benefits patients with social anxiety and panic disorder. It may decrease the craving for alcohol in some patients and improve mood as well; hence, it may have some use in depressed patients. Some bipolar patients have benefited when gabapentin is used adjunctively with mood stabilizers.

Precautions and Adverse Reactions. Adverse effects are mild, with the most common being daytime somnolence, ataxia, and fatigue, which are usually dose-related. Overdose (over 45 g) has been associated with diplopia, slurred screech, lethargy, and diarrhea, but all patients recovered. The drug was classified as pregnancy category C in the former FDA classification system and is excreted in breast milk, so it is best to avoid it in pregnant women and nursing mothers.

Drug Interactions. Gabapentin bioavailability may decrease as much as 20 percent when administered with antacids. In general, there are no drug interactions. Chronic use does not interfere with lithium administration.

Laboratory Interferences. Gabapentin does not interfere with any laboratory tests, although spontaneous reports of false-positive drug toxicology screenings for amphetamines, barbiturates, benzodiazepines, and marijuana have been reported.

Dosages and Clinical Guidelines. Gabapentin is well tolerated, and the dosage can be increased to the maintenance range within a few days. A general approach is to start with 300 mg on day 1, increase to 600 mg on day 2, 900 mg on day 3, and subsequently increase up to 1,800 mg/day in divided doses as needed to relieve symptoms. Final total daily doses tend to be between 1,200 and 2,400 mg/day, but occasionally results may be achieved with dosages as low as 200 to 300 mg/day, especially in elderly persons. Sedation is usually the limiting factor in determining the dosage. Some patients have taken dosages as high as 4,800 mg/day.

Gabapentin is available as 100-, 300-, and 400-mg capsules and as 600- and 800-mg tablets. A 250-mg/5-mL oral solution is also available. Although abrupt discontinuation of gabapentin does not cause withdrawal effects, the use of all anticonvulsant drugs should be gradually tapered.

Topiramate

Topiramate (Topamax) was developed as an anticonvulsant and was found useful in a variety of psychiatric and neurologic conditions, including migraine prevention, treatment of obesity, bulimia, binge eating, and alcohol dependence.

Pharmacologic Actions. Topiramate has GABAergic effects and increases cerebral GABA in humans. It has 80 percent oral bioavailability and is not significantly altered by food. It is 15 percent protein-bound, and about 70 percent of the drug is eliminated by renal excretion. With renal insufficiency, topiramate clearance decreases by about 50 percent, so the dosage needs to be decreased. It has a half-life of around 24 hours.

Therapeutic Indications. Topiramate is used mainly as an antiepileptic medication and has been found superior to placebo as monotherapy in patients with seizure disorders. It is also used in the prevention of migraine, smoking cessation, pain syndromes (e.g., low back pain), PTSD, and essential tremor. The drug has been associated with weight loss, and that fact has been used to counteract the weight gain caused by many psychotropic drugs. It has also been used in general obesity and the treatment of bulimia and binge-eating disorder. Self-mutilating behavior may be decreased in borderline personality disorder. It is of little or no benefit in the treatment of psychotic disorders. In one study, the combination of topiramate with bupropion (Wellbutrin) showed some efficacy in bipolar depression, but double-blind, placebo-controlled trials failed to demonstrate topiramate monotherapy efficacy in acute mania in adults.

Precautions and Adverse Reactions. The most common adverse effects of topiramate include paresthesias, weight loss, somnolence, anorexia, dizziness, and memory problems. Sometimes disturbances in the sense of taste occur. In many cases, the adverse effects are mild to moderate and can be attenuated by decreasing the dose. No deaths have been reported during an overdose. The drug affects acid–base balance (low serum bicarbonate), which can be associated with cardiac arrhythmias and the formation of renal calculi in about 1.5 percent of cases. Patients taking the drug should be encouraged to drink plenty of fluids. It is not known if the drug passes through the placenta or is present in breast milk, and pregnant women or nursing mothers should avoid it.

Drug Interactions. Topiramate has few drug interactions with other anticonvulsant drugs. Topiramate may increase phenytoin concentrations up to 25 percent and valproic acid 11 percent; it does not affect the concentration of carbamazepine, phenobarbital

(Luminal), or primidone. Topiramate concentrations are decreased by 40 to 48 percent with concomitant administration of carbamazepine or phenytoin. We should not combine topiramate with other carbonic anhydrase inhibitors, as it increases the risk of nephrolithiasis or heat-related problems (oligohidrosis and hyperthermia). These include acetazolamide (Diamox) or dichlorphenamide (Daranide).

Laboratory Interferences.   Topiramate does not interfere with any laboratory tests.

Dosages and Clinical Guidelines.   Topiramate is available as unscored 25-, 100-, and 200-mg tablets. Topiramate dosage is titrated gradually over 8 weeks to a maximum of 200 mg twice a day to reduce the risk of adverse cognitive and sedative effects. Off-label topiramate is typically used adjunctively, starting with 25 mg at bedtime and increasing weekly by 25 mg as necessary and tolerated. Final doses in efforts to promote weight loss are often between 75 and 150 mg/day at bedtime. Doses higher than 400 mg are not associated with increased efficacy. All of the doses can be given at bedtime to take advantage of the sedative effects. Persons with renal insufficiency should reduce doses by half.

Tiagabine

Tiagabine was introduced as a treatment for epilepsy in 1997 and was found to have efficacy in some psychiatric conditions, including acute mania. However, safety concerns (see later), along with a lack of controlled data, have limited the use of tiagabine in disorders other than epilepsy.

Pharmacologic Actions.   Tiagabine is well absorbed with a bioavailability of about 90 percent and is extensively (96 percent) bound to plasma proteins. Tiagabine is a cytochrome P450 CYP3A substrate and is extensively transformed into inactive 5-oxo-tiagabine and glucuronide metabolites, with only 2 percent being excreted unchanged in the urine. The remainder is excreted as metabolites in the feces (65 percent) and the urine (25 percent). Tiagabine blocks the uptake of the inhibitory amino acid neurotransmitter GABA into neurons and glia, enhancing the inhibitory action of GABA at both $GABA_A$ and $GABA_B$ receptors, putatively yielding anticonvulsant and antinociceptive effects, respectively. It has mild blocking effects on histamine 1 (H_1), serotonin type 1B ($5-HT_{1B}$), benzodiazepine, and chloride channel receptors.

Therapeutic Indications.   Tiagabine is rarely used for psychiatric disorders, and then it is used only for GAD and insomnia. Its main indication is in generalized epilepsy.

Precautions and Adverse Reactions.   Tiagabine may cause withdrawal seizures, cognitive or neuropsychiatric problems (impaired concentration, speech or language problems, somnolence, and fatigue), status epilepticus, and sudden unexpected death in epilepsy (SUDEP). Acute oral overdoses of tiagabine have been associated with seizures, status epilepticus, coma, ataxia, confusion, somnolence, drowsiness, impaired speech, agitation, lethargy, myoclonus, stupor, tremors, disorientation, vomiting, hostility, temporary paralysis, and respiratory depression. Deaths have been reported in polydrug overdoses involving tiagabine. Cases of severe rash may occur, including Stevens–Johnson syndrome.

Tiagabine was classified as pregnancy category C in the former FDA classification system because fetal loss and teratogenicity have been demonstrated in animals. It is not known if the drug is excreted in breast milk. Pregnant women and nursing mothers should not be given the drug.

Laboratory Tests.   Tiagabine does not interfere with any laboratory tests.

Dosage and Administration.   Tiagabine should not be rapidly loaded or rapidly initiated because of the risk of severe adverse effects. In adults and adolescents 12 years of age or older with epilepsy who are also taking enzyme inducers, tiagabine should be initiated at 4 mg/day and increased weekly by 4 mg/day during the first month. The dose should then be increased weekly by 4 to 8 mg/day for weeks 5 and 6, yielding 24 to 32 mg/day administered in two to four divided doses by week 6. In adults (but not adolescents), tiagabine doses may be further increased weekly by 4 to 8 mg/day to as high as 56 mg/day. Plasma concentrations in patients with epilepsy commonly range between 20 and 100 ng/mL but do not appear to be systematically related to antiseizure effects and thus are not routinely monitored.

Levetiracetam

Initially developed as a nootropic (memory enhancing) drug, levetiracetam proved to be a potent anticonvulsant and marketed as a treatment for partial seizures. It has been used to treat acute mania and anxiety and to augment antidepressant drug therapy.

Pharmacologic Actions.   The CNS effects are not well understood, but it appears to enhance GABA inhibition indirectly. It is wholly and rapidly absorbed, and peak concentrations are reached in 1 hour. Food delays the rate of absorption and decreases the amount of absorption. Levetiracetam is not significantly plasma protein-bound and is not metabolized through the hepatic CYP system. Its metabolism involves the hydrolysis of the acetamide group. Serum concentrations are not correlated with therapeutic effects.

Therapeutic Indications.   The primary indication is for the treatment of convulsive disorders, including partial-onset seizures, myoclonic seizures, and idiopathic generalized epilepsy. In psychiatry, levetiracetam has been used off label to treat acute mania, as an add-on treatment for major depression, and as an anxiolytic agent.

Precautions and Adverse Reactions.   The most common side effects of levetiracetam include drowsiness, dizziness, ataxia, diplopia, memory impairment, apathy, and paresthesias. Some patients develop behavioral disturbances during treatment, and hallucinations may occur. Suicidal patients may become agitated. It should not be used in pregnant or lactating women.

Drug Interactions.   There are few if any interactions with other drugs, including other anticonvulsants. There is no interaction with lithium.

Laboratory Interferences.   No laboratory interferences have been reported.

Dosages and Clinical Guidelines.   The drug is available as 250-, 500-, 750-, and 1,000-mg tablets; 500-mg extended-release tablets; a 100-mg/mL oral solution; and a 100-mg/mL intravenous solution. In epilepsy, the typical adult daily dose is 1,000 mg.

Because of its renal clearance, dosages should be reduced in patients with impaired renal function.

Zonisamide

Zonisamide, another anticonvulsant, was also found to be useful in bipolar disorder, obesity, and binge-eating disorder.

Pharmacologic Actions.   Zonisamide blocks sodium channels and may weakly potentiate dopamine and serotonin activity. It also inhibits carbonic anhydrase. Some evidence suggests that it may block calcium channels. The hepatic CYP3A system metabolizes zonisamide, so enzyme-inducing agents such as carbamazepine, alcohol, and phenobarbital increase the clearance and reduce the availability of the drug. Zonisamide does not affect the metabolism of other drugs. It has a long half-life of 60 hours, so it is efficiently dosed once daily, preferably at nighttime.

Therapeutic Indications.   Its primary use is in the treatment of generalized seizure disorders and refractory partial seizures. In psychiatry, controlled studies found it to be of use in obesity and binge-eating disorder. Uncontrolled trials have found it useful in bipolar disorder, particularly mania; however, further studies are warranted for this indication.

Precautions and Adverse Reactions.   Zonisamide is a sulfonamide and thus may cause a fatal rash and blood dyscrasias, although these events are rare. About 4 percent of patients develop kidney stones. The most common side effects are drowsiness, cognitive impairment, insomnia, ataxia, nystagmus, paresthesia, speech abnormalities, constipation, diarrhea, nausea, and dry mouth. Weight loss is also a common side effect, which has been exploited as a therapy for patients who have gained weight during treatment with psychotropics or, as mentioned above, have ongoing difficulty controlling their eating. Zonisamide should not be used in pregnant women or breastfeeding mothers.

Drug Interactions.   Zonisamide does not inhibit CYP isoenzymes and does not instigate drug interactions. It is important not to combine carbonic anhydrase inhibitors with zonisamide because of an increased risk of nephrolithiasis related to increased blood levels of urea.

Laboratory Interferences.   Zonisamide can elevate hepatic alkaline phosphatase and increase blood urea nitrogen and creatinine.

Dosages and Clinical Guidelines.   Zonisamide is available in 100- and 200-mg capsules. In epilepsy, the dosage range is 100 to 400 mg/day, with side effects becoming more pronounced at doses above 300 mg. Because of its long half-life, zonisamide can be given once a day.

Pregabalin

Pregabalin is pharmacologically similar to gabapentin. It is believed to work by inhibiting the release of excess excitatory neurotransmitters. It increases neuronal GABA levels, its binding affinity is six times greater than that of gabapentin, and it has a longer half-life.

Pharmacologic Actions.   Pregabalin exhibits linear pharmacokinetics. It is rapidly absorbed in proportion to its dose. The time to maximal plasma concentration is about 1 hour, and to steady state is within 24 to 48 hours. Pregabalin demonstrates high bioavailability, and it has a mean elimination half-life of about 6.5 hours. Food does not affect absorption. Pregabalin does not bind to plasma proteins and is excreted virtually unchanged (<2 percent metabolism) by the kidneys. It is not subject to hepatic metabolism and does not induce or inhibit liver enzymes. Dose reduction may be necessary for patients with creatinine clearance (CLcr) less than 60 mL/min. Daily doses should be further reduced by approximately 50 percent for each additional 50 percent decrease in CLcr. Pregabalin is highly cleared by hemodialysis so that additional doses may be needed for patients on chronic hemodialysis treatment after each hemodialysis treatment.

Therapeutic Indications.   Pregabalin is approved for the management of diabetic peripheral neuropathy and postherpetic neuralgia and adjunctive treatment of partial-onset seizures. It is of benefit to some patients with GAD. In studies, no consistent dose–response relationship was found, although 300 mg of pregabalin per day was more effective than 150 or 450 mg. Some patients with panic disorder or social anxiety disorder may benefit from pregabalin, but little evidence supports its routine use in treating persons with these disorders. It was most recently approved for the treatment of fibromyalgia.

Precautions and Adverse Reactions.   The most common adverse events associated with pregabalin use are dizziness, somnolence, blurred vision, peripheral edema, amnesia or loss of memory, and tremors. Pregabalin potentiates the sedating effects of alcohol, antihistamines, benzodiazepines, and other CNS depressants. It remains to be seen if pregabalin is associated with benzodiazepine-type withdrawal symptoms. There are scant data about its use in pregnant women or nursing mothers, and it is best avoided in these patients.

Drug Interactions.   Given the absence of hepatic metabolism, pregabalin lacks metabolic drug interactions.

Laboratory Interferences.   There are no effects on laboratory tests.

Dosage and Clinical Guidelines.   The recommended dose for postherpetic neuralgia is 50 or 100 mg orally three times a day. The recommended dose for diabetic peripheral neuropathy is 100 to 200 mg orally three times a day. Patients with fibromyalgia may require up to 450 to 600 mg/day given in divided doses. Pregabalin is available as 25-, 50-, 75-, 100-, 150-, 200-, 225-, and 300-mg capsules.

Phenytoin

Phenytoin sodium (Dilantin) is an antiepileptic drug and is related to the barbiturates in chemical structure. It is indicated for the control of generalized tonic–clonic (grand mal) and complex partial (psychomotor, temporal lobe) seizures and prevention and treatment of seizures occurring during or after neurosurgery. Studies have shown comparable efficacy of phenytoin to other anticonvulsants in bipolar disorder, but clinicians should take into account the danger of gingival hyperplasia, leukopenia, or anemia and the danger of toxicity caused by nonlinear pharmacokinetics.

Pharmacologic Action.   Similar to other anticonvulsants, phenytoin causes blockade of voltage-activated sodium channels and hence is efficacious as an antimanic agent. The plasma half-life after oral administration averages 22 hours, with a range of 7 to

42 hours. Steady-state therapeutic levels are achieved at least 7 to 10 days (5 to 7 half-lives) after initiation of therapy, with recommended doses of 300 mg/day. Serum level should be obtained at least 5 to 7 half-lives after treatment initiation. Phenytoin is excreted in the bile, which is then reabsorbed from the intestinal tract and excreted in the urine. Urinary excretion of phenytoin occurs partly with glomerular filtration and by tubular secretion. Small incremental doses of phenytoin may increase the half-life and produce very substantial increases in serum levels. Patients should adhere strictly to the prescribed dosage, and serial monitoring of phenytoin levels is recommended.

Therapeutic Indications. Apart from its indication in generalized tonic–clonic (grand mal) and complex partial (psychomotor, temporal lobe) seizures, phenytoin is also used for the treatment of acute mania in bipolar disorder.

Precautions and Adverse Reactions. The most common adverse reactions reported with phenytoin therapy are usually dose-related and include nystagmus, ataxia, slurred speech, decreased coordination, and mental confusion. Other side effects include dizziness, insomnia, transient nervousness, motor twitching, and headaches. There have been rare reports of phenytoin induced dyskinesias, similar to those induced by phenothiazine and other neuroleptic drugs. More severe side effects include thrombocytopenia, leukopenia, agranulocytosis, and pancytopenia, with or without bone marrow suppression.

Several reports have suggested the development of lymphadenopathy (local or generalized), including benign lymph node hyperplasia, pseudolymphoma, lymphoma, and Hodgkin's disease. Prenatal exposure to phenytoin may increase the risks for congenital malformations, and a potentially life-threatening bleeding disorder related to decreased levels of vitamin K–dependent clotting factors may occur in newborns exposed to phenytoin in utero. Hyperglycemia has been reported with phenytoin use; also, the agent may increase the serum glucose level in patients with diabetes.

Drug Interactions. Acute alcohol intake, amiodarone, chlordiazepoxide, cimetidine, diazepam, disulfiram, estrogens, fluoxetine, H2-antagonists, isoniazid, methylphenidate, phenothiazines, salicylates, and trazodone may increase phenytoin serum levels. Drugs that may lower phenytoin levels include carbamazepine, chronic alcohol abuse, and reserpine.

Laboratory Interferences. Phenytoin may decrease serum concentrations of thyroxine. It may cause increased serum levels of glucose, alkaline phosphatase, and γ-glutamyl transpeptidase.

Dosage and Clinical Guidelines. Patients may be started on one 100-mg extended oral capsule three times daily, and the dosage then adjusted to suit individual requirements. Patients may then be switched to once-a-day dosing, which is more convenient. In this case, extended-release capsules may be used. Serial monitoring of phenytoin levels is recommended, and the normal range is usually 10 to 20 µg/mL.

CALCIUM CHANNEL BLOCKERS

The intracellular calcium ion regulates the activity of multiple neurotransmitters such as serotonin and dopamine, and that action may account for its role as a treatment in mood disorders. Calcium channel inhibitors are used in psychiatry as antimanic agents for persons who are refractory to or cannot tolerate treatment with first-line mood-stabilizing agents such as lithium (Eskalith), carbamazepine (Tegretol), and sodium valproate (Depakote). Calcium channel inhibitors include nifedipine (Procardia, Adalat), nimodipine (Nimotop), isradipine (DynaCirc), amlodipine (Norvasc, Lotrel), nicardipine (Cardene), nisoldipine (Sular), nitrendipine, and verapamil (Calan). They are used for control of mania and ultradian bipolar disorder (mood cycling in less than 24 hours).

The results of a large genetic study have rekindled interest in the potential clinical uses of calcium channel blockers (CCBs). Two genome-wide findings implicated genes encoding L-type voltage-gated calcium channel subunits as susceptibility genes for bipolar disorder, schizophrenia, MDD, ADHD, and autism.

Pharmacologic Actions

The calcium channel inhibitors are nearly completely absorbed after oral use, with significant first-pass hepatic metabolism. Considerable intraindividual and interindividual variations are seen in the plasma concentrations of the drugs after a single dose. Peak plasma levels of most of these agents are achieved within 30 minutes. Amlodipine does not reach peak plasma levels for about 6 hours. The half-life of verapamil after the first dose is 2 to 8 hours; the half-life increases to 5 to 12 hours after the first few days of therapy. The half-lives of the other CCBs range from 1 to 2 hours for nimodipine and isradipine to 30 to 50 hours for amlodipine (Table 21-42).

Table 21-42
Half-Lives, Dosages, and Effectiveness of Selected Calcium Channel Inhibitors in Psychiatric Disorders

	Verapamil (Calan, Isoptin)	Nimodipine (Nimotop)	Isradipine (DynaCirc)	Amlodipine (Norvasc)
Half-Life	Short (5–12 hr)	Short (1–2 hr)	Short (1–2 hr)	Long (30–50 hr)
Starting Dosage	30 mg TID	30 mg TID	2.5 mg BID	5 mg HS
Peak Daily Dosage	480 mg	240–450 mg	20 mg	10–15 mg
Antimanic	++	++	++	[a]
Antidepressant	±	+	+	[a]
Antiultradian[b]	±	++	(++)	[a]

BID, twice a day; HS, bedtime; TID, three times a day.
[a]No systematic studies, only case reports.
[b]Rapid-cycling bipolar disorder.
Adapted from Robert M. Post, M.D.

The primary mechanism of action of CCBs in bipolar illness is not known. The calcium channel inhibitors discussed in this section inhibit the influx of calcium into neurons through L-type (long-acting) voltage-dependent calcium channels.

Therapeutic Indications

Bipolar Disorder. Nimodipine and verapamil have been demonstrated to be effective as maintenance therapy in persons with bipolar illness. Patients who respond to lithium appear to also respond to treatment with verapamil. Nimodipine may be useful for ultradian cycling and recurrent brief depression. The clinician should begin treatment with a short-acting drug such as nimodipine or isradipine, beginning with a low dosage and increasing the dosage every 4 to 5 days until clinical response is seen or adverse effects appear. When symptoms are controlled, a longer-acting drug, such as amlodipine, can be substituted as maintenance therapy. Failure to respond to verapamil does not exclude a favorable response to one of the other drugs. Verapamil has been shown to prevent antidepressant-induced mania. The CCBs can be combined with other agents, such as carbamazepine, in patients who are partial responders to monotherapy.

Depression. None of the CCBs is effective as a treatment for depression and may prevent response to antidepressants.

Other Psychiatric Indications. Nifedipine is used to treat hypertensive crises associated with the use of MAOIs. Isradipine may reduce the subjective response to methamphetamine. Calcium channel inhibitors may be beneficial in Tourette disorder, Huntington disease, panic disorder, intermittent explosive disorder, and tardive dyskinesia.

Other Medical Uses. These drugs have been used to treat medical conditions such as angina, hypertension, migraine headaches, Raynaud phenomenon, esophageal spasm, premature labor, and headache. Verapamil has antiarrhythmic activity and has been used to treat superventricular arrhythmias.

Precautions and Adverse Reactions

The most common adverse effects associated with calcium channel inhibitors are those attributable to vasodilation: dizziness, headache, tachycardia, nausea, dysesthesias, and peripheral edema. Verapamil and diltiazem (Cardizem), in particular, can cause hypotension, bradycardia, and atrioventricular (AV) heart block, which necessitate close monitoring and sometimes discontinuation of the drugs. In all patients with cardiovascular disease, the drugs should be used with caution. Other common adverse effects include constipation, fatigue, rash, coughing, and wheezing. Adverse effects noted with diltiazem include hyperactivity, akathisia, and parkinsonism; with verapamil, delirium, hyperprolactinemia, and galactorrhea; with nimodipine, subjective sense of chest tightness and skin flushing; and with nifedipine, depression. The drugs have not been evaluated for safety in pregnant women and are best avoided. Because the drugs are secreted in breast milk, nursing mothers should also avoid the drugs.

Drug Interactions

All CCBs have the potential for drug–drug interactions. The types and risks of these interactions vary by the compound. Verapamil raises serum levels of carbamazepine, digoxin, and other CYP3A4 substrates. Verapamil and diltiazem but not nifedipine have been reported to precipitate carbamazepine-induced neurotoxicity. Calcium channel inhibitors should not be used by persons taking β-adrenergic receptor antagonists, hypotensives (e.g., diuretics, vasodilators, and ACEIs), or antiarrhythmic drugs (e.g., quinidine and digoxin) without consultation with an internist or cardiologist. Cimetidine (Tagamet) has been reported to increase plasma concentrations of nifedipine and diltiazem. Some patients who are treated with lithium and calcium channel inhibitors concurrently may be at increased risk for the signs and symptoms of neurotoxicity, and deaths have occurred.

Laboratory Interferences

No known laboratory interferences are associated with the use of calcium channel inhibitors.

Dosage and Clinical Guidelines

Verapamil is available in 40-, 80-, and 120-mg tablets; 120-, 180-, and 240-mg sustained-release tablets; and 100-, 120-, 180-, 200-, 240-, 300-, and 360-mg sustained-release capsules. The starting dosage is 40 mg orally three times a day and can be increased in increments every 4 to 5 days up to 80 to 120 mg three times a day. The patient's BP, pulse, and electrocardiogram (in patients older than 40 years old or with a history of cardiac illness) should be routinely monitored.

Nifedipine is available in 10- and 20-mg capsules and 30-, 60-, and 90-mg extended-release tablets. The administration should be started at 10 mg orally three or four times a day and can be increased up to a maximum dosage of 120 mg a day.

Nimodipine is available in 30-mg capsules. It has been used at 60 mg every 4 hours for ultra–rapid-cycling bipolar disorder and sometimes briefly at up to 360 mg/day.

Isradipine is available in 2.5- and 5-mg capsules, with a maximum of 20 mg/day. An extended-release formulation of isradipine has been discontinued.

Amlodipine is available in 2.5-, 5-, and 10-mg tablets. The administration should start at 5 mg once at night and can be increased to a maximum dosage of 10 to 15 mg a day.

Diltiazem is available in 30-, 60-, 90-, and 120-mg tablets; 60-, 90-, 120-, 180-, 240-, 300-, and 360-mg extended-release capsules; and 60-, 90-, 120-, 180-, 240-, 300-, and 360-mg extended-release tablets. The administration should start with 30 mg orally four times a day and can be increased up to a maximum of 360 mg a day.

Elderly persons are more sensitive to calcium channel inhibitors than are younger adults. No specific information is available regarding the use of the agents for children.

▲ 21.4 Anxiolytics

BENZODIAZEPINES AND DRUGS ACTING ON GABA RECEPTORS

The first benzodiazepine to be introduced was chlordiazepoxide (Librium), in 1959. In 1963, diazepam (Valium) became available. Over the next three decades, superior safety and tolerability helped the benzodiazepines replace the older antianxiety and hypnotic medications, such as the barbiturates and meprobamate (Miltown).

Dozens of benzodiazepines and drugs acting on benzodiazepine receptors have been synthesized and marketed worldwide. Many of these agents are not available in the United States. Also, some benzodiazepines have been discontinued because of a lack of use. Table 21-43 lists agents currently available in the United States.

The benzodiazepines derive their name from their molecular structure. They share a common effect on receptors that have been termed benzodiazepine receptors, which in turn modulate GABA activity. Nonbenzodiazepine agonists, such as zolpidem (Ambien), zaleplon (Sonata), and eszopiclone (Lunesta), are similar to these drugs as they bind at a location close to the benzodiazepine receptor. However, we discuss these with the medications for insomnia. Flumazenil (Romazicon), a benzodiazepine receptor antagonist used to reverse benzodiazepine-induced sedation and in emergency care of benzodiazepine overdosage, is also covered here.

Because benzodiazepines have a rapid anxiolytic sedative effect, they are most commonly used for acute treatment of insomnia, anxiety, agitation, or anxiety associated with any psychiatric disorder. Also, the benzodiazepines are used as anesthetics, anticonvulsants, and muscle relaxants and as the preferred treatment for catatonia. Because of the risk of psychological and physical dependence associated with long-term use of benzodiazepines, ongoing assessment should be made as to the continued clinical need for these drugs in treating patients. In most patients, given the nature of their disorders, it is often best if benzodiazepine agents are used in conjunction with psychotherapy and when alternative agents have been tried and proven ineffective or poorly tolerated. In many forms of chronic anxiety disorders, antidepressant drugs such as SSRIs and SNRIs are now used as primary treatments, with benzodiazepines used as adjuncts. Benzodiazepine abuse is rare, usually found in patients who abuse multiple prescription and recreational drugs.

Pharmacologic Actions

All benzodiazepines except clorazepate (Tranxene) are completely absorbed after oral administration and reach peak serum levels within 30 minutes to 2 hours. Metabolism of clorazepate in the stomach converts it to desmethyldiazepam, which is then completely absorbed.

The absorption, the attainment of peak concentrations, and the onset of action are quickest for diazepam (Valium), lorazepam (Ativan), alprazolam (Xanax), triazolam (Halcion), and estazolam (ProSom). The rapid onset of effects is vital to persons who take a single dose of a benzodiazepine to calm an episodic burst of anxiety or to fall asleep rapidly. Several benzodiazepines are effective after intravenous (IV) injection, but only lorazepam and midazolam (Versed) have rapid and reliable absorption after intramuscular (IM) administration.

Diazepam, chlordiazepoxide, clonazepam (Klonopin), clorazepate, flurazepam (Dalmane), and quazepam (Doral) have plasma

Table 21-43
Preparations and Doses of Medications Acting on the Benzodiazepine Receptor Available in the United States

Medication	Brand Name	Dose Equivalent	Usual Adult Dose (mg)	How Supplied
Diazepam	Valium	5	2.5–40.0	2-, 5-, and 10-mg tablets 15-mg slow-release tablets
Clonazepam	Klonopin	0.25	0.5–4.0	0.5-, 1.0-, and 2.0-mg tablets
Alprazolam	Xanax	0.5	0.5–6.0	0.25-, 0.5-, 1.0-, and 2.0-mg tablets 1.5-mg sustained-release tablet
Lorazepam	Ativan	1	0.5–6.0	0.5-, 1.0-, and 2.0-mg tablets 4 mg/mL parenteral
Oxazepam	Serax	15	15–120	7.5-, 10.0-, 15.0-, and 30.0-mg capsules 15-mg tablets
Chlordiazepoxide	Librium	25	10–100	5-, 10-, and 25-mg capsules and tablets
Clorazepate	Tranxene	7.5	15–60	3.75-, 7.50-, and 15.00-mg tablets 11.25- and 22.50-mg slow-release tablets
Midazolam	Versed	0.25	1–50	5 mg/mL parenteral 1-, 2-, 5-, and 10-mL vials
Flurazepam	Dalmane	15	15–30	15- and 30-mg capsules
Temazepam	Restoril	15	7.5–30.0	7.5-, 15.0-, and 30.0-mg capsules
Triazolam	Halcion	0.125	0.125–0.250	0.125- and 0.250-mg tablets
Estazolam	ProSom	1	1–2	1- and 2-mg tablets
Quazepam	Doral	5	7.5–15.0	7.5- and 15.0-mg tablets
Zolpidem	Ambien Ambien CR	10 5	5–10 6.25–12.5	5- and 10-mg tablets 6.25- and 12.5-mg tablets
Zaleplon	Sonata	10	5–20	5- and 10-mg capsules
Eszopiclone	Lunesta	1	1–3	1-, 2- and 3-mg tablets
Flumazenil	Romazicon	0.05	0.2–0.5/min	0.1 mg/mL 5- and 10-mL vials

half-lives of 30 hours to more than 100 hours and are technically described as long-acting benzodiazepines. The plasma half-lives of these compounds can be as high as 200 hours in persons whose metabolism is genetically slow. Because the attainment of steady-state plasma concentrations of the drugs can take up to 2 weeks, persons may experience symptoms and signs of toxicity after only 7 to 10 days of treatment with a dosage that seemed initially to be in the therapeutic range.

Clinically, half-life alone does not necessarily determine the duration of therapeutic action for most benzodiazepines. The fact that all benzodiazepines are lipid-soluble to varying degrees means that benzodiazepines and their active metabolites bind to plasma proteins. The extent of this binding is proportional to their lipid solubility. The amount of protein binding varies from 70 to 99 percent. Distribution, onset, and termination of action after a single dose are thus determined mainly by benzodiazepine lipid solubility, not elimination half-life. Preparations with high lipid solubility, such as diazepam and alprazolam, are absorbed rapidly from the GI tract and distribute rapidly to the brain by passive diffusion along a concentration gradient, resulting in a rapid onset of action. However, as the concentration of the medication increases in the brain and decreases in the bloodstream, the concentration gradient reverses itself, and these medications leave the brain rapidly, resulting in fast cessation of drug effect. Drugs with longer elimination half-lives, such as diazepam, may remain in the bloodstream for a substantially more extended time than their actual pharmacologic action at benzodiazepine receptors because the concentration in the brain decreases rapidly below the level necessary for a noticeable effect.

In contrast, lorazepam, which has a shorter elimination half-life than diazepam but is less lipid-soluble, has a slower onset of action after a single dose because the drug is absorbed and enters the brain more slowly. However, the duration of action after a single dose is longer because it takes longer for lorazepam to leave the brain and for brain levels to decrease below the concentration that produces an effect. In chronic dosing, some of these differences are not as apparent because brain levels are in equilibrium with higher and more consistent steady-state blood levels, but additional doses still produce a more rapid but briefer action with diazepam than with lorazepam. Benzodiazepines are distributed widely in adipose tissue. As a result, medications may persist in the body after discontinuation longer than would be predicted from their elimination half-lives. Also, the dynamic half-life (i.e., duration of action on the receptor) may be longer than the elimination half-life.

The advantages of long–half-life drugs over short–half-life drugs include less frequent dosing, less variation in plasma concentration, and less severe withdrawal phenomena. The disadvantages include drug accumulation, increased risk of daytime psychomotor impairment, and increased daytime sedation.

The half-lives of lorazepam, oxazepam (Serax), temazepam (Restoril), and estazolam are between 8 and 30 hours. Alprazolam has a half-life of 10 to 15 hours, and triazolam has the shortest half-life (2 to 3 hours) of all the orally administered benzodiazepines. Rebound insomnia and anterograde amnesia are thought to be more of a problem with the short–half-life drugs than with the long–half-life drugs.

Because the administration of medications more frequently than the elimination half-life leads to drug accumulation, medications such as diazepam and flurazepam accumulate with daily dosing, eventually resulting in increased daytime sedation.

Some benzodiazepines (e.g., oxazepam) are conjugated directly by glucuronidation and are excreted. Most benzodiazepines are oxidized first by CYP3A4 and CYP2C19, often to active metabolites. These metabolites may then be hydroxylated to another active metabolite. For example, diazepam is oxidized to desmethyldiazepam, which, in turn, is hydroxylated to produce oxazepam. These products undergo glucuronidation to inactive metabolites. Several benzodiazepines (e.g., diazepam, chlordiazepoxide) have the same active metabolite (desmethyldiazepam), which has an elimination half-life of more than 120 hours. Flurazepam (Dalmane), a lipid-soluble benzodiazepine used as a hypnotic that has a short elimination half-life, has an active metabolite (desalkylflurazepam) with a half-life greater than 100 hours. This is another reason that the duration of action of a benzodiazepine may not correspond to the half-life of the parent drug.

Therapeutic Indications

Insomnia. Because insomnia may be a symptom of a physical or psychiatric disorder, hypnotics should not be used for more than 7 to 10 consecutive days without a thorough investigation of the cause of insomnia. However, many patients have long-standing sleep difficulties and benefit significantly from the long-term use of hypnotic agents. Temazepam, flurazepam, and triazolam are benzodiazepines with a sole indication for insomnia.

Flurazepam, temazepam, quazepam, estazolam, and triazolam are the benzodiazepines approved for use as hypnotics. The benzodiazepine hypnotics differ principally in their half-lives; flurazepam has the most prolonged half-life, and triazolam has the shortest. Flurazepam may be associated with minor cognitive impairment on the day after its administration, and triazolam may be associated with mild rebound anxiety and anterograde amnesia. Quazepam may be associated with daytime impairment when used for a long time. Temazepam or estazolam may be a reasonable compromise for most adults. Estazolam produces rapid onset of sleep and a hypnotic effect for 6 to 8 hours.

Anxiety Disorders

GENERALIZED ANXIETY DISORDER. Benzodiazepines are highly effective for the relief of anxiety associated with GAD. Most persons should be treated for a predetermined, specific, and relatively brief period. However, because GAD is a chronic disorder with a high rate of recurrence, some persons with GAD may warrant long-term maintenance treatment with benzodiazepines.

PANIC DISORDER. Alprazolam and clonazepam, both high-potency benzodiazepines, are commonly used medications for panic disorder with or without agoraphobia. Although the SSRIs are also indicated for the treatment of panic disorder, benzodiazepines have the advantage of working quickly and not causing significant sexual dysfunction and weight gain. However, the SSRIs are still often preferred because they target common comorbid conditions, such as depression or OCD. Benzodiazepines and SSRIs can be initiated together to treat acute panic symptoms; use of the benzodiazepine can be tapered after 3 to 4 weeks once the therapeutic benefits of the SSRI have emerged.

SOCIAL ANXIETY DISORDER. Clonazepam is an effective treatment for social anxiety disorder. Also, several other benzodiazepines (e.g., diazepam) have been used as adjunctive medications for the treatment of social anxiety disorder.

OTHER ANXIETY DISORDERS. Benzodiazepines are used adjunctively for treatment of adjustment disorder with anxiety, pathologic anxiety associated with life events (e.g., after an accident), OCD, and PTSD.

ANXIETY ASSOCIATED WITH DEPRESSION. Depressed patients often experience significant anxiety, and antidepressant drugs may cause initial exacerbation of these symptoms. Accordingly, benzodiazepines are indicated for the treatment of anxiety associated with depression.

Bipolar I and II Disorders

Clonazepam, lorazepam, and alprazolam are useful in the management of acute manic episodes and as an adjuvant to maintenance therapy instead of antipsychotics. As an adjuvant to lithium (Eskalith) or lamotrigine (Lamictal), clonazepam may result in an increased time between cycles and fewer depressive episodes. Benzodiazepines may help patients with bipolar disorder sleep better.

Catatonia. Lorazepam, sometimes in low doses (less than 5 mg/day) and sometimes in very high doses (12 mg/day or more), is regularly used to treat acute catatonia, which is more frequently associated with bipolar disorder than with schizophrenia. Other benzodiazepines have also been said to be helpful. However, there are no valid controlled trials of benzodiazepines in catatonia. Chronic catatonia does not respond as well to benzodiazepines. The definitive treatment for catatonia is ECT.

Akathisia. The first-line drug for akathisia is most commonly a β-adrenergic receptor antagonist. However, benzodiazepines are also useful in treating some patients with akathisia.

Other Psychiatric Indications. Chlordiazepoxide (Librium) and clorazepate (Tranxene) are used to manage the symptoms of alcohol withdrawal. The benzodiazepines (especially IM lorazepam) are used to manage substance-induced and psychotic agitation in the emergency department. Benzodiazepines have been used instead of amobarbital (Amytal) for drug-assisted interviewing.

Flumazenil for Benzodiazepine Overdosage. Flumazenil is used to reverse the adverse psychomotor, amnestic, and sedative effects of benzodiazepine receptor agonists. Flumazenil is administered IV and has a half-life of 7 to 15 minutes. The most common adverse effects of flumazenil are nausea, vomiting, dizziness, agitation, emotional lability, cutaneous vasodilation, injection-site pain, fatigue, impaired vision, and headache. The most common serious adverse effect associated with the use of flumazenil is the precipitation of seizures, which is most likely to occur in persons with seizure disorders, those who are physically dependent on benzodiazepines, and those who have ingested large quantities of benzodiazepines. Flumazenil alone may impair memory retrieval.

In mixed-drug overdosage, the toxic effects (e.g., seizures and cardiac arrhythmias) of other drugs (e.g., TCAs) may emerge with the reversal of the benzodiazepine effects of flumazenil. For example, seizures caused by an overdosage of TCAs may have been partially treated in a person who had also taken an overdosage of benzodiazepines. With flumazenil treatment, the tricyclic-induced seizures or cardiac arrhythmias may appear and result in a fatal outcome. Flumazenil does not reverse the effects of ethanol, barbiturates, or opioids.

For the initial management of a known or suspected benzodiazepine overdosage, the recommended initial dosage of flumazenil is 0.2 mg (2 mL) administered IV over 30 seconds. If the desired consciousness is not obtained after 30 seconds, a further dose of 0.3 mg (3 mL) can be administered over 30 seconds. Further doses of 0.5 mg (5 mL) can be administered over 30 seconds at 1-minute intervals up to a cumulative dose of 3.0 mg. The clinician should not rush the administration of flumazenil. A secure airway and IV access should be established before the administration of the drug. Persons should be awakened gradually.

Most persons with a benzodiazepine overdosage respond to a cumulative dose of 1 to 3 mg of flumazenil; doses above 3 mg of flumazenil do not reliably produce additional effects. If a person has not responded 5 minutes after receiving a cumulative dose of 5 mg of flumazenil, the primary cause of sedation is probably not benzodiazepine receptor agonists, and additional flumazenil is unlikely to help.

Sedation can return in 1 to 3 percent of persons treated with flumazenil. It can be prevented or treated by giving repeated dosages of flumazenil at 20-minute intervals. For repeat treatment, no more than 1 mg (given as 0.5 mg a minute) should be given at any one time, and no more than 3 mg should be given in any 1 hour.

Precautions and Adverse Reactions

The most common adverse effect of benzodiazepines is drowsiness, which occurs in about 10 percent of all persons. Because of this adverse effect, persons should be advised to be careful while driving or using dangerous machinery when taking drugs. Drowsiness can be present during the day after the use of a benzodiazepine for insomnia the previous night, the so-called residual daytime sedation. Some persons also experience ataxia (fewer than 2 percent) and dizziness (less than 1 percent). These symptoms can result in falls and hip fractures, especially in elderly persons. The most severe adverse effects of the benzodiazepines occur when other sedative substances, such as alcohol, are taken concurrently. These combinations can result in marked drowsiness, disinhibition, or even respiratory depression. Infrequently, benzodiazepine receptor agonists cause mild cognitive deficits that may impair job performance. Persons taking benzodiazepine receptor agonists should be advised to exercise additional caution when driving or operating dangerous machinery.

High-potency benzodiazepines, especially triazolam, can cause anterograde amnesia. A paradoxical increase in aggression has been reported in persons with preexisting brain damage. Allergic reactions to the drugs are rare, but a few studies report maculopapular rashes and generalized itching. The symptoms of benzodiazepine intoxication include confusion, slurred speech, ataxia, drowsiness, dyspnea, and hyporeflexia.

Triazolam has received significant attention in the media because of an alleged association with aggression. Therefore, the manufacturer recommends that the drug be used for no more than 10 days for the treatment of insomnia and that physicians carefully evaluate the emergence of any abnormal thinking or behavioral changes in persons treated with triazolam, giving appropriate consideration to all potential causes. Triazolam was banned in Great Britain in 1991.

Persons with hepatic disease and elderly persons are particularly likely to have adverse effects and toxicity from the benzodiazepines, including hepatic coma, especially when the drugs are administered repeatedly or in high dosages. Benzodiazepines can produce clinically significant impairment of respiration in persons with chronic obstructive pulmonary disease and sleep apnea. Alprazolam may exert a direct appetite stimulant effect and may cause weight gain. The benzodiazepines should be used with caution by persons with a history of substance abuse, cognitive disorders, renal disease, hepatic disease, porphyria, CNS depression, or myasthenia gravis.

Some data indicate that benzodiazepines are teratogenic; therefore, their use during pregnancy is not advised. Moreover, the use of benzodiazepines in the third trimester can precipitate a withdrawal syndrome in newborns. The drugs are secreted in the breast milk in sufficient concentrations to affect newborns. Benzodiazepines may cause dyspnea, bradycardia, and drowsiness in nursing babies.

Tolerance, Dependence, and Withdrawal.   When benzodiazepines are used for short periods (1 to 2 weeks) in moderate dosages, they usually cause no significant tolerance, dependence, or withdrawal effects. The short-acting benzodiazepines (e.g., triazolam) may be an exception to this rule because some persons have reported increased anxiety the day after taking a single dose of the drug and then stopping its use. Some persons also report a tolerance for the anxiolytic effects of benzodiazepines and require increased doses to maintain the clinical remission of symptoms.

The appearance of a withdrawal syndrome, also called discontinuation syndrome, depends on how long a person takes the drug, what dose, how quickly they taper it, and the half-life of the compound. Benzodiazepine withdrawal syndrome consists of anxiety, nervousness, diaphoresis, restlessness, irritability, fatigue, lightheadedness, tremor, insomnia, and weakness (Table 21-44). Abrupt discontinuation of benzodiazepines, particularly those with short half-lives, is associated with severe withdrawal symptoms, which may include depression, paranoia, delirium, and seizures. These severe symptoms are more likely to occur if flumazenil is used for the rapid reversal of the benzodiazepine receptor agonist effects. Some features of the syndrome may occur in as many as 90 percent of persons treated with the drugs. The development of severe withdrawal syndrome is seen only in persons who have taken high dosages for long periods. The syndrome may be delayed for 1 or 2 weeks in persons who had been taking benzodiazepines with long half-lives. Alprazolam seems to be significantly associated with an immediate and severe withdrawal syndrome and should be tapered gradually.

When the medication is to be discontinued, the drug must be tapered slowly (25 percent a week); otherwise, recurrence or rebound of symptoms is likely. Monitoring of any withdrawal symptoms (possibly with a standardized rating scale) and psychological support of the person are helpful in the successful accomplishment of benzodiazepine discontinuation. Concurrent use of carbamazepine (Tegretol) during benzodiazepine discontinuation has been reported to permit a more rapid and better-tolerated withdrawal than does a gradual taper alone. The dosage range of carbamazepine used to facilitate withdrawal is 400 to 500 mg a day. Some clinicians report particular difficulty in tapering and discontinuing alprazolam, especially in persons who have been receiving high dosages for long periods. There have been reports of successful discontinuation of alprazolam by switching to clonazepam, which is then gradually withdrawn.

Table 21-44
Signs and Symptoms of Benzodiazepine Withdrawal

Anxiety	Tremor
Irritability	Depersonalization
Insomnia	Hyperesthesia
Hyperacusis	Myoclonus
Nausea	Delirium
Difficulty concentrating	Seizures

Drug Interactions

The most common and potentially severe benzodiazepine receptor agonist interaction is excessive sedation and respiratory depression occurring when benzodiazepines are administered concomitantly with other CNS depressants, such as alcohol, barbiturates, tricyclic and tetracyclic drugs, DRAs, opioids, and antihistamines. Ataxia and dysarthria may be likely to occur when lithium, antipsychotics, and clonazepam are combined. The combination of benzodiazepines and clozapine (Clozaril) has been reported to cause delirium and should be avoided. Cimetidine (Tagamet), disulfiram (Antabuse), isoniazid, estrogen, and oral contraceptives increase the plasma concentration of diazepam, chlordiazepoxide, clorazepate, and flurazepam. However, antacids may reduce the GI absorption of benzodiazepines. The plasma concentrations of triazolam and alprazolam are increased to potentially toxic concentrations by nefazodone (Serzone) and fluvoxamine (Luvox).

The manufacturer of nefazodone recommends that the dosage of triazolam be lowered by 75 percent, and the dosage of alprazolam be lowered by 50 percent, when given concomitantly with nefazodone. Over-the-counter preparations of the kava plant, advertised as a "natural tranquilizer," can potentiate the action of benzodiazepine receptor agonists through synergistic overactivation of GABA receptors. Carbamazepine can lower the plasma concentration of alprazolam. Antacids and food may decrease the plasma concentrations of benzodiazepines, and smoking may increase the metabolism of benzodiazepines. The benzodiazepines may increase the plasma concentrations of phenytoin and digoxin (Lanoxin). The SSRIs may prolong and exacerbate the severity of zolpidem-induced hallucinations. Deaths have been reported when parental lorazepam is given with parental olanzapine.

Dosage and Clinical Guidelines

The clinical decision to treat an anxious person with a benzodiazepine should be carefully considered. Medical causes of anxiety (e.g., thyroid dysfunction, caffeinism, and prescription medications) should be ruled out. Benzodiazepine use should be started at a low dosage, and the person should be instructed regarding the drug's sedative properties and abuse potential. An estimated length of therapy should be decided at the beginning of therapy, and the need for continued therapy should be reevaluated at least monthly because of the problems associated with long-term use. However, certain persons with anxiety disorders are unresponsive to treatments other than benzodiazepines in long-term use.

Benzodiazepines are available in a wide range of formulations. Clonazepam is available in a wafer formulation that facilitates its use in patients who have trouble swallowing pills. Alprazolam is available in an extended-release form, which reduces the frequency of dosing. Some benzodiazepines are more potent than others in that one compound requires a relatively smaller dosage than another compound to achieve the same effect. For example, clonazepam requires 0.25 mg to achieve the same effect as 5 mg of diazepam; thus, clonazepam is considered a high-potency benzodiazepine. Conversely, oxazepam has an approximate dosage equivalence of 15 mg and is a low-potency drug.

Table 21-43 lists preparations and doses of medications discussed in this chapter.

BUSPIRONE

Buspirone hydrochloride (BuSpar) is classified as an azapirone and is chemically distinct from other psychotropic agents. It acts on two types of receptors, serotonin (5-HT) and dopamine (D). It has a high affinity for the 5-HT_{1A} serotonin receptor, acting as an agonist or partial agonist, and moderate affinity for the D_2 dopamine receptor, acting as both an agonist and an antagonist. The approved indication for this psychotropic drug is for the treatment of GAD. It was initially believed to be a better alternative to the benzodiazepine drug group because buspirone does not possess anticonvulsant and muscle relaxant effects. Reports continue to appear that some patients benefit from the addition of buspirone to their antidepressant regimen. Its use in this role is more common than its use as an anxiolytic. Interestingly, the antidepressant drug vilazodone (Viibryd) inhibits 5-HT reuptake and acts as a 5-HT_{1A} receptor partial agonist.

Pharmacologic Actions

Buspirone is well absorbed from the GI tract, but absorption is delayed by food ingestion. Peak plasma levels are achieved 40 to 90 minutes after oral administration. At doses of 10 to 40 mg, single-dose linear pharmacokinetics are observed. Nonlinear pharmacokinetics are observed after multiple doses. Because of its short half-life (2 to 11 hours), buspirone is dosed three times daily. An active metabolite of buspirone, 1-pyrimidinylpiperazine (1-PP), is about 20 percent less potent than buspirone but is up to 30 percent more concentrated in the brain than the parent compound. The elimination half-life of 1-PP is 6 hours.

Buspirone does not affect the GABA-associated chloride ion channel or the serotonin reuptake transporter, targets of other drugs that are effective in GAD. Buspirone also has activity at 5-HT_2 and dopamine type 2 (D_2) receptors, although the significance of the effects at these receptors is unknown. At D_2 receptors, it has properties of both an agonist and an antagonist.

Therapeutic Indications

Generalized Anxiety Disorder. Buspirone is a narrow-spectrum antianxiety agent with demonstrated efficacy only in the treatment of GAD. In contrast to the SSRIs or venlafaxine, buspirone is not effective in the treatment of panic disorder, OCD, or social phobia. Buspirone, however, has an advantage over these agents in that it does not typically cause sexual dysfunction or weight gain.

Some evidence suggests that, compared with benzodiazepines, buspirone is generally more useful for symptoms of anger and hostility, equally effective for psychic symptoms of anxiety, and less effective for somatic symptoms of anxiety. The full benefit of buspirone is evident only at dosages above 30 mg a day. Compared with the benzodiazepines, buspirone has a delayed onset of action and lacks any euphoric effect. Unlike benzodiazepines, buspirone has no immediate effects, and patients should be told that a full clinical response may take 2 to 4 weeks. If an immediate response is needed, patients can be started on a benzodiazepine and then withdrawn from the drug after buspirone's effects begin. Sometimes the sedative effects of benzodiazepines, which are not found with buspirone, are desirable; however, these sedative effects may cause impaired motor performance and cognitive deficits.

Other Disorders. Many other clinical uses of buspirone have been reported, but most have not been confirmed in controlled trials. Evidence of the efficacy of high-dosage buspirone (30 to 90 mg a day) for depressive disorders is mixed. Buspirone appears to have weak antidepressant activity, which has led to its use as an augmenting agent in patients who have failed standard antidepressant

therapy. In a large study, buspirone augmentation of SSRIs worked as well as other commonly used strategies. Buspirone is sometimes used to augment SSRIs in the treatment of OCD. There are reports that buspirone may be beneficial against the increased arousal and flashbacks associated with PTSD.

Because buspirone does not act on the GABA–chloride ion channel complex, the drug is not recommended for the treatment of withdrawal from benzodiazepines, alcohol, or sedative-hypnotic drugs, except as treatment of comorbid anxiety symptoms.

Scattered trials suggest that buspirone reduces aggression and anxiety in persons with organic brain disease or traumatic brain injury. It is also used for SSRI-induced bruxism and sexual dysfunction, nicotine craving, and ADHD.

Precautions and Adverse Reactions

Buspirone does not cause weight gain, sexual dysfunction, discontinuation symptoms, or significant sleep disturbance. It does not produce sedation or cognitive and psychomotor impairment. The most common adverse effects of buspirone are headache, nausea, dizziness, and (rarely) insomnia. No sedation is associated with buspirone. Some persons may report a minor feeling of restlessness, although that symptom may reflect an incompletely treated anxiety disorder. No deaths have been reported from overdoses of buspirone, and the median lethal dose is estimated to be 160 to 550 times the recommended daily dose. Buspirone should be used with caution by persons with hepatic and renal impairment, pregnant women, and nursing mothers. Buspirone can be used safely by the elderly.

Drug Interactions

The coadministration of buspirone and haloperidol (Haldol) results in increased blood concentrations of haloperidol. Buspirone should not be used with MAOIs to avoid hypertensive episodes, and a 2-week washout period should pass between the discontinuation of MAOI use and the initiation of treatment with buspirone. Drugs or foods that inhibit CYP3A4, for example, erythromycin, itraconazole (Sporanox), nefazodone (Serzone), and grapefruit juice, increase buspirone plasma concentrations.

Laboratory Interferences

Single doses of buspirone can cause transient elevations in growth hormone, prolactin, and cortisol concentrations, although the effects are not clinically significant.

Dosage and Clinical Guidelines

Buspirone is available in single-scored 5- and 10-mg tablets and triple-scored 15- and 30-mg tablets; treatment is usually initiated with either 5 mg orally three times daily or 7.5 mg orally twice daily. The dosage can be raised 5 mg every 2 to 4 days to the usual dosage range of 15 to 60 mg a day.

Buspirone should not be used in patients with past hypersensitivity to buspirone, in cases of diabetes-associated metabolic acidosis, or patients with severely compromised liver or renal function.

Switching from a Benzodiazepine to Buspirone. Buspirone is not cross-tolerant with benzodiazepines, barbiturates, or alcohol. A common clinical problem, therefore, is how to initiate buspirone therapy in a person who is currently taking benzodiazepines. There are two alternatives. First, the clinician can start buspirone treatment gradually while the benzodiazepine is being withdrawn. Second, the clinician can start buspirone treatment and bring the person up to a therapeutic dosage for 2 to 3 weeks while the person is still receiving the regular dosage of the benzodiazepine and then slowly taper the benzodiazepine dosage. Patients who have received benzodiazepines in the past, especially in recent months, may find that buspirone is not as effective as the benzodiazepines in the treatment of their anxiety. This difference might be explained by the absence of the immediate mildly euphoric and sedative effects of benzodiazepines. The coadministration of buspirone and benzodiazepines may be useful in the treatment of persons with anxiety disorders who have not responded to treatment with either drug alone.

β-ADRENERGIC RECEPTOR ANTAGONISTS

Because of the innervations of many, if not most, peripheral organs and vasculature by the sympathetic division of the autonomic nervous system, their functions are ultimately controlled, in part, by one of the two major classes of adrenergic receptors: α-receptors (see Table 33-2) and β-receptors. These receptors are further subdivided based on their action and location, and they are located both peripherally and in the CNS. Shortly after being introduced for cardiac indications, propranolol (Inderal) was reported to be useful for agitation, and its use in psychiatry spread rapidly. The five most commonly used β-receptor antagonists in psychiatry are propranolol, nadolol (Corgard), metoprolol (Lopressor, Toprol), pindolol (Visken), and atenolol (Tenormin) (Table 21-45).

Pharmacologic Actions

The β-receptor antagonists differ concerning lipophilicities, metabolic routes, β-receptor selectivity, and half-lives. The absorption of the β-receptor antagonists from the GI tract is variable. The agents that are most soluble in lipids (i.e., are lipophilic) are likely to cross the blood–brain barrier and enter the brain; those agents that are least lipophilic are less likely to enter the brain. When CNS effects are desired, a lipophilic drug may be preferred; when only peripheral effects are desired, a less lipophilic drug may be indicated.

Whereas propranolol, nadolol, pindolol, and labetalol (Normodyne, Trandate) have nearly equal potency at both the β_1- and β_2-receptors, metoprolol and atenolol have a greater affinity for the β_1-receptor than for the β_2-receptor. Relative β_1-selectivity confers few pulmonary and vascular effects of these drugs, although they must be used with caution in persons with asthma because the drugs retain some activity at the β_2-receptors.

Pindolol has sympathomimetic effects in addition to its β-antagonist effects, which has allowed its use for augmentation of antidepressant drugs. Pindolol, propranolol, and nadolol possess some antagonist activity at the serotonin 5-HT$_{1A}$ receptors.

Therapeutic Indications

Anxiety Disorders. Propranolol is useful for the treatment of social anxiety disorder, primarily of the performance type (e.g., disabling anxiety before a musical performance). Data are also available for its use in the treatment of panic disorder, PTSD, and GAD. In social anxiety disorder, the standard treatment approach is to take 10 to 40 mg of propranolol 20 to 30 minutes before the anxiety-provoking situation. The β-receptor antagonists are less useful for the treatment of panic disorder than are benzodiazepines or SSRIs.

Lithium-Induced Postural Tremor. The β-receptor antagonists are beneficial for lithium-induced postural tremor and other medication-induced postural tremors—for example, those induced by TCAs and valproate (Depakene). The initial approach to this movement disorder includes lowering the dose of lithium (Eskalith), eliminating aggravating factors, such as caffeine, and administering lithium at bedtime. If these interventions are inadequate, however, propranolol in the range of 20 to 160 mg a day taken two or three times daily is generally sufficient for the treatment of lithium-induced postural tremor.

Neuroleptic-Induced Acute Akathisia. Many studies have shown that β-receptor antagonists can be effective in the treatment of neuroleptic-induced acute akathisia. They are generally more effective for this indication than are anticholinergics and

Table 21-45
β-Adrenergic Drugs Used in Psychiatry

Drug	Pregnancy Category (former FDA classification system)	Protein Binding (%)	Lipophilic	ISA	Metabolism	Receptor Selectivity	Half-Life (hr)	Usual Starting Dosage (mg)	Usual Maximal Dosage (mg)
Atenolol (Tenormin)	D	6–16	No		Renal	$\beta_1 > \beta_2$	6–9	50 OD	50–100 OD
Metoprolol (Lopressor)	C	5–10	Yes		Hepatic	$\beta_1 > \beta_2$	3–4	50 bid	75–150 bid
Nadolol (Corgard)	C	30	No		Renal	$\beta_1 = \beta_2$	14–24	40 OD	80–240 OD
Propranolol (Inderal)	C	>90	Yes		Hepatic	$\beta_1 = \beta_2$	3–6	10–20 bid/tid	80–140 tid
Pindolol (Visken)	B	40	Yes	Minimal	Hepatic	$\beta_1 > \beta_2$	3–4	5 tid/qid	60 bid/tid

Note: In 2015, the FDA changed the pregnancy classification system from a letter-based system to a descriptive system. We refer here to the letter-based system in order to simplify the summary of data into a table.
ISA, intrinsic sympathomimetic activity; OD, once daily; bid, twice a day; tid, three times a day; qid, four times a day.

benzodiazepines. The β-receptor antagonists are not effective in the treatment of such neuroleptic-induced movement disorders as acute dystonia and parkinsonism.

Aggression and Violent Behavior. The β-receptor antagonists may be useful in reducing the number of aggressive and violent outbursts in persons with impulse disorders, schizophrenia, and aggression associated with brain injuries such as trauma, tumors, anoxic injury, encephalitis, alcohol use disorders, and degenerative disorders (e.g., Huntington disease).

Alcohol Withdrawal. Propranolol is reported to be useful as an adjuvant to benzodiazepines but not as a sole agent in the treatment of alcohol withdrawal. The following dose schedule is suggested: no propranolol for a pulse rate below 50 beats/min; 50-mg propranolol for a pulse rate between 50 and 79 beats/min; and 100-mg propranolol for a pulse rate of 80 beats/min or above.

Antidepressant Augmentation. Pindolol has been used to augment and hasten the antidepressant effects of SSRIs, tricyclic drugs, and ECT. Small studies have shown that pindolol administered at the onset of antidepressant therapy may shorten the usual 2- to 4-week latency of antidepressant response by several days. Because the β-receptor antagonists may induce depression in some persons, augmentation strategies with these drugs need to be further clarified in controlled trials.

Other Disorders. Several case reports and controlled studies have reported data indicating that β-receptor antagonists may be of modest benefit for persons with schizophrenia and manic symptoms. They have also been used in some cases of stuttering (see Table 21-46).

Precautions and Adverse Reactions

The β-receptor antagonists are contraindicated for use in people with asthma, insulin-dependent diabetes, congestive heart failure, significant vascular disease, persistent angina, and hyperthyroidism. The contraindication in diabetic persons is because the drugs antagonize the normal physiologic response to hypoglycemia. The β-receptor antagonists can worsen AV conduction defects and lead to complete AV heart block and death. If the clinician decides that the risk-to-benefit ratio warrants a trial of a β-receptor antagonist in a person with one of these coexisting medical conditions, a β₁-selective agent should be the first choice, and the patient should

Table 21-46
Psychiatric Uses for β-Adrenergic Receptor Antagonists

Definitely effective
Performance anxiety
Lithium-induced tremor
Neuroleptic-induced akathisia

Probably effective
Adjunctive therapy for alcohol withdrawal and other substance-related disorders
Adjunctive therapy for aggressive or violent behavior

Possibly effective
Antipsychotic augmentation
Antidepressant augmentation

Table 21-47
Adverse Effects and Toxicity of β-Adrenergic Receptor Antagonists

Cardiovascular
   Hypotension
   Bradycardia
   Congestive heart failure (in patients with compromised myocardial function)
Respiratory
   Asthma (less risk with β₁-selective drugs)
Metabolic
   Worsened hypoglycemia in diabetic patients on insulin or oral agents
Gastrointestinal
   Nausea
   Diarrhea
   Abdominal pain
Sexual function
   Impotence
Neuropsychiatric
   Lassitude
   Fatigue
   Dysphoria
   Insomnia
   Vivid nightmares
   Depression (rare)
   Psychosis (rare)
Other (rare)
   Raynaud phenomenon
   Peyronie disease
Withdrawal syndrome
   Rebound worsening of preexisting angina pectoris when β-adrenergic receptor antagonists are discontinued

be monitored. All currently available β-receptor antagonists are excreted in breast milk and should be administered with caution to nursing women.

The most common adverse effects of β-receptor antagonists are hypotension and bradycardia. In persons at risk for these adverse effects, a test dosage of 20 mg a day of propranolol can be given to assess the reaction to the drug. Depression has been associated with lipophilic β-receptor antagonists, such as propranolol, but it is probably rare. Nausea, vomiting, diarrhea, and constipation can also be caused by treatment with these agents. The β-receptor antagonists may blunt cognition in some people. Other more severe CNS adverse effects (e.g., agitation, confusion, and hallucinations) are rare. Table 21-47 lists the possible adverse effects of β-receptor antagonists.

Drug Interactions

Antipsychotics, anticonvulsants, theophylline (Theo-Dur, Slo-bid), and levothyroxine (Synthroid) have increased plasma concentrations when given with propranolol. Other β-receptor antagonists may have similar effects. The β-receptor antagonists that are eliminated by the kidneys may have similar effects on drugs that are also eliminated by the renal route. Barbiturates, phenytoin (Dilantin), and cigarette smoking increase the elimination of β-receptor antagonists that are metabolized by the liver. Several reports have associated hypertensive crises and bradycardia with the coadministration of β-receptor antagonists and MAOIs. Depressed myocardial contractility and AV nodal conduction can occur from concomitant administration of a β-receptor antagonist and calcium channel inhibitors.

Laboratory Interferences

The β-receptor antagonists do not interfere with standard laboratory tests.

Dosage and Clinical Guidelines

Propranolol is available in 10-, 20-, 40-, 60-, 80-, and 90-mg tablets; 4-, 8-, and 80-mg/mL solutions; and 60-, 80-, 120-, and 160-mg sustained-release capsules. Nadolol is available in 20-, 40-, 80-, 120-, and 160-mg tablets. Pindolol is available in 5- and 10-mg tablets. Metoprolol is available in 50- and 100-mg tablets and 50-, 100-, and 200-mg sustained-release tablets. Atenolol is available in 25-, 50-, and 100-mg tablets. Acebutolol is available in 200- and 400-mg capsules.

For the treatment of chronic disorders, propranolol administration is usually initiated at 10 mg by mouth three times a day or 20 mg by mouth twice daily. The dosage can be raised by 20 to 30 mg a day until a therapeutic effect emerges. The dosage should be leveled off at the appropriate range for the disorder under treatment. The treatment of aggressive behavior sometimes requires dosages up to 80 mg a day, and therapeutic effects may not be seen until the person has been receiving the maximal dosage for 4 to 8 weeks. For the treatment of social phobia, primarily the performance type, the patient should take 10 to 40 mg of propranolol 20 to 30 minutes before the performance.

Pulse and BP readings should be taken regularly, and the drug should be withheld if the pulse rate is below 50 beats/min or the systolic BP is below 90 mm Hg. The drug should be temporarily discontinued if it produces severe dizziness, ataxia, or wheezing. Treatment with β-receptor antagonists should never be discontinued abruptly. Propranolol should be tapered by 60 mg a day until a dosage of 60 mg a day is reached. After that, the drug should be tapered by 10 to 20 mg a day every 3 or 4 days.

The clinical guidelines for the other drugs listed in this chapter are similar to propranolol, taking into consideration the different doses used. For example, if propranolol is prescribed initially at the lowest available dose (e.g., 10 mg), then metoprolol should be prescribed at its lowest available dose (e.g., 50 mg).

BARBITURATES AND SIMILARLY ACTING DRUGS

The first barbiturate to be used in medicine was barbital (Veronal), which was introduced in 1903. It was followed by phenobarbital (Luminal), amobarbital (Amytal), pentobarbital (Nembutal), secobarbital (Seconal), and thiopental (Pentothal). Many others have been synthesized, but only a handful have been used clinically (Table 21-48). Many problems are associated with these drugs, including high abuse and addiction potential, a narrow therapeutic range with low therapeutic index, and unfavorable side effects. The use of barbiturates and similar compounds such as meprobamate (Miltown) has practically been eliminated by the benzodiazepines and hypnotics, such as zolpidem (Ambien), eszopiclone (Lunesta), and zaleplon (Sonata), which have a lower abuse potential and a higher therapeutic index than the barbiturates. Nevertheless, barbiturates still have a role in the treatment of certain mental and convulsive disorders.

Pharmacologic Actions

The barbiturates are well absorbed after oral administration. The binding of barbiturates to plasma proteins is high, but lipid solubility varies. The individual barbiturates are metabolized by the liver and excreted by the kidneys. The half-lives of specific barbiturates range from 1 to 120 hours. The barbiturates may also induce hepatic enzymes (cytochrome P450, CYP), thereby reducing the levels of both the barbiturate and any other concurrently administered drugs metabolized by the liver. The mechanism of action of barbiturates involves the GABA receptor–benzodiazepine receptor–chloride ion channel complex.

Therapeutic Indications

Electroconvulsive Therapy. Methohexital (Brevital) is commonly used as an anesthetic agent for ECT. It has lower cardiac risks than other barbiturate anesthetics. Used intravenously (IV),

Table 21-48
Barbiturate Dosages (Adult)

Drug	Trade Name	Available Preparations	Hypnotic Dose Range	Anticonvulsant Dose Range
Amobarbital	Amytal	200 mg	50–300 mg	65–500 mg IV
Aprobarbital	Alurate	40 mg/5 mL elixir	40–120 mg	Not established
Butabarbital	Butisol	15-, 30-, and 50-mg tablets 30 mg/5 mL elixir	45–120 mg	Not established
Mephobarbital	Mebaral	32, 50, and 100 mg tablets	100–200 mg	200–600 mg
Methohexital	Brevital	500 mg/50 mL	1 mg/kg for electroconvulsive therapy	Not established
Pentobarbital	Nembutal	50- and 100-mg capsules 50 mg/mL injection or elixir 30, 60, 120, and 200 mg suppository	100–200 mg	100 mg IV, each minute up to 500 mg
Phenobarbital	Luminal	Tablets range from 15–100 mg 20 mg/5 mL elixir 30–130 mg/mL injection	30–150 mg	100–300 mg IV, up to 600 mg/day
Secobarbital	Seconal	100-mg capsule, 50 mg/mL injection	100 mg	5.5 mg/kg IV

IV, intravenous.

methohexital produces rapid unconsciousness, and because of its rapid redistribution, it has a brief duration of action (5 to 7 minutes). Typical dosing for ECT is 0.7 to 1.2 mg/kg. Methohexital can also be used to abort prolonged seizures in ECT or to limit postictal agitation.

Seizures. Phenobarbital (Solfoton, Luminal), the most commonly used barbiturate for treatment of seizures, has indications for the treatment of generalized tonic–clonic and simple partial seizures. Parenteral barbiturates are used in the emergency management of seizures independent of cause. Intravenous phenobarbital should be administered slowly at 10 to 20 mg/kg for status epilepticus.

Narcoanalysis. Amobarbital (Amytal) has been used historically as a diagnostic aid in several clinical conditions, including conversion reactions, catatonia, hysterical stupor, and unexplained muteness, and to differentiate stupor of depression, schizophrenia, and structural brain lesions.

The *Amytal interview* is performed by placing the patient in a reclining position and administering amobarbital IV at 50 mg a minute. Infusion is continued until lateral nystagmus is sustained or drowsiness is noted, usually at 75 to 150 mg. After this, 25 to 50 mg can be administered every 5 minutes to maintain narcosis. The patient should be allowed to rest for 15 to 30 minutes after the interview before attempting to walk.

Because of the risk of laryngospasm with IV amobarbital, diazepam has become the drug of choice for narcoanalysis.

Sleep. The barbiturates reduce sleep latency and the number of awakenings during sleep, although tolerance to these effects generally develops within 2 weeks. Discontinuation of barbiturates often leads to rebound increases in electroencephalographic measures of sleep and a worsening of insomnia.

Withdrawal from Sedative-Hypnotics

Barbiturates are sometimes used to determine the extent of tolerance to barbiturates or other hypnotics to guide detoxification. After intoxication has been resolved, a test dose of pentobarbital (200 mg) is given orally. One hour later, the patient is examined. Tolerance and dose requirements are determined by the degree to which the patient is affected. If the patient is not sedated, another 100 mg of pentobarbital can be administered every 2 hours, up to three times (maximum, 500 mg over 6 hours). The amount needed for mild intoxication corresponds to the approximate daily dose of barbiturate used. Phenobarbital (30 mg) may then be substituted for each 100 mg of pentobarbital. This daily dose requirement can be administered in divided doses and gradually tapered by 10 percent a day, with adjustments made according to withdrawal signs.

Precautions and Adverse Reactions

Some adverse effects of barbiturates are similar to those of benzodiazepines, including paradoxical dysphoria, hyperactivity, and cognitive disorganization. Rare adverse effects associated with barbiturate use include the development of Stevens–Johnson syndrome, megaloblastic anemia, and neutropenia.

Before the advent of benzodiazepines, the widespread use of barbiturates as hypnotics and anxiolytics made them the most common cause of acute porphyria reactions. Severe attacks of porphyria have decreased, mainly because barbiturates are now seldom used and are contraindicated in patients with the disease.

A significant difference between the barbiturates and the benzodiazepines is the low therapeutic index of the barbiturates. An overdose of barbiturates can easily prove fatal. In addition to narrow therapeutic indexes, the barbiturates are associated with a significant risk of abuse potential and the development of tolerance and dependence. Barbiturate intoxication is manifested by confusion, drowsiness, irritability, hyporeflexia or areflexia, ataxia, and nystagmus. The symptoms of barbiturate withdrawal are similar to but more marked than those of benzodiazepine withdrawal.

Ten times the daily dose or 1 g of most barbiturates causes severe toxicity; 2 to 10 g generally proves fatal. Manifestations of barbiturate intoxication may include delirium, confusion, excitement, headache, and CNS and respiratory depression, ranging from somnolence to coma. Other adverse reactions include Cheyne–Stokes respiration, shock, miosis, oliguria, tachycardia, hypotension, hypothermia, irritability, hyporeflexia or areflexia, ataxia, and nystagmus. Treatment of overdose includes induction of emesis or lavage, activated charcoal, and saline cathartics; supportive treatment, including maintaining airway and respiration and treating shock as needed; maintaining vital signs and fluid balance; alkalinizing the urine, which increases excretion; forced diuresis if renal function is typical, or hemodialysis in severe cases.

Because of some evidence of teratogenicity, barbiturates should not be used by pregnant women or women who are breastfeeding. Barbiturates should be used with caution by patients with a history of substance abuse, depression, diabetes, hepatic impairment, renal disease, severe anemia, pain, hyperthyroidism, or hypoadrenalism. Barbiturates are also contraindicated in patients with acute intermittent porphyria, impaired respiratory drive, or limited respiratory reserve.

Drug Interactions

The primary area for concern about drug interactions is the potentially dangerous effects of respiratory depression. Barbiturates should be used with great caution with other prescribed CNS drugs (including antipsychotic and antidepressant drugs) and nonprescribed CNS agents (e.g., alcohol). Also, caution must be exercised when prescribing barbiturates to patients who are taking other drugs that are metabolized in the liver, especially cardiac drugs and anticonvulsants. Because individual patients have a wide range of sensitivities to barbiturate-induced enzyme induction, it is not possible to predict the degree to which the metabolism of concurrently administered medications may be affected. Drugs that have their metabolism enhanced by barbiturate administration include opioids, antiarrhythmic agents, antibiotics, anticoagulants, anticonvulsants, antidepressants, β-adrenergic receptor antagonists, DRAs, contraceptives, and immunosuppressants.

Laboratory Interferences

No known laboratory interferences are associated with the administration of barbiturates.

Dose and Clinical Guidelines

Barbiturates and other drugs described later begin to act within 1 to 2 hours of administration. The doses of barbiturates vary, and treatment should begin with low doses that are increased to achieve a clinical effect. Children and older people are more sensitive to the effects of barbiturates than are young adults. The most commonly used barbiturates are available in a variety of dose forms. Barbiturates with half-lives in the 15- to 40-hour range are preferable, because long-acting drugs tend to accumulate in the body. Clinicians should instruct patients clearly about the adverse effects and the potential for dependence associated with barbiturates.

Although determining plasma concentrations of barbiturates is rarely necessary for psychiatry, monitoring of phenobarbital concentrations is standard practice when the drug is used as an anticonvulsant. The therapeutic blood concentrations for phenobarbital in this indication range from 15 to 40 mg/L, although some patients may experience significant adverse effects in that range.

Barbiturates are contained in combination products with which the clinician should be familiar.

Other Similarly Acting Drugs

Several agents that act similarly to the barbiturates have been used in the treatment of anxiety and insomnia. Three such available drugs are paraldehyde (Paral), meprobamate, and chloral hydrate (Noctec). These drugs are rarely used because of their abuse potential and potential toxic effects and some of them are now banned in other countries such as the European Union and Canada.

Paraldehyde. Paraldehyde is a cyclic ether and was first used in 1882 as a hypnotic. It has also been used to treat epilepsy, alcohol withdrawal symptoms, and delirium tremens. Because of its low therapeutic index, it has been supplanted by the benzodiazepines and other anticonvulsants.

PHARMACOLOGIC ACTIONS. Paraldehyde is rapidly absorbed from the GI tract and intramuscular (IM) injections. It is primarily metabolized to acetaldehyde by the liver, and the lungs expire the unmetabolized drug. Reported half-lives range from 3.4 to 9.8 hours. The onset of action is 15 to 30 minutes.

THERAPEUTIC INDICATIONS. Paraldehyde is not indicated as an anxiolytic or a hypnotic and has little place in current psychopharmacology.

PRECAUTIONS AND ADVERSE REACTIONS. Paraldehyde frequently causes foul breath because of the expired unmetabolized drug. It can inflame pulmonary capillaries and cause coughing. It can also cause local thrombophlebitis with IV use. Patients may experience nausea and vomiting with oral use. Overdose leads to metabolic acidosis and decreased renal output. There is a risk of abuse among drug addicts.

DRUG INTERACTIONS. Disulfiram (Antabuse) inhibits acetaldehyde dehydrogenase and reduces the metabolism of paraldehyde, leading to a possible toxic concentration of paraldehyde. Paraldehyde has additive sedating effects in combination with other CNS depressants such as alcohol or benzodiazepines.

LABORATORY INTERFERENCES. Paraldehyde can interfere with the metyrapone, phentolamine, and urinary 17-hydroxycorticosteroid tests.

DOSING AND CLINICAL GUIDELINES. Paraldehyde is available in 30-mL vials for oral, IV, or rectal use. For seizures in adults, up to 12 mL (diluted to a 10 percent solution) can be administered by gastric tube every 4 hours. For children, the oral dose is 0.3 mg/kg.

Meprobamate. Meprobamate, a carbamate, was introduced shortly before the benzodiazepines, specifically to treat anxiety. It is also used for muscle relaxant effects.

PHARMACOLOGIC ACTIONS. Meprobamate is rapidly absorbed from the GI tract and IM injections. It is metabolized primarily by the liver, and a small portion is excreted unchanged in the urine. The plasma half-life is approximately 10 hours.

THERAPEUTIC INDICATIONS. Meprobamate is indicated for the short-term treatment of anxiety disorders. It has also been used as a hypnotic and is prescribed as a muscle relaxant.

PRECAUTIONS AND ADVERSE REACTIONS. Meprobamate can cause CNS depression and death in overdose and carries the risk of abuse by patients with drug or alcohol use disorders. Abrupt cessation after long-term use can lead to withdrawal syndrome, including seizures and hallucinations. Meprobamate can exacerbate acute intermittent porphyria. Other rare side effects include hypersensitivity reactions, wheezing, hives, paradoxical excitement, and leukopenia. It should not be used in patients with hepatic compromise.

DRUG INTERACTIONS. Meprobamate has additive sedating effects in combination with other CNS depressants, such as alcohol, barbiturates, or benzodiazepines.

LABORATORY INTERFERENCES. Meprobamate can interfere with the metyrapone, phentolamine, and urinary 17-hydroxycorticosteroid tests.

DOSING AND CLINICAL GUIDELINES. Meprobamate is available in 200-, 400-, and 600-mg tablets; 200- and 400-mg extended-release capsules; and various combinations, for example, aspirin 325 mg and 200 mg of meprobamate (Equagesic) for oral use. For adults, the usual dose is 400 to 800 mg twice daily. Elderly patients and children aged 6 to 12 years require half the adult dose.

Chloral Hydrate. Chloral hydrate is a hypnotic agent rarely used in psychiatry because numerous safer options, such as benzodiazepines, are available.

PHARMACOLOGIC ACTIONS. Chloral hydrate is well absorbed from the GI tract. The parent compound is metabolized within minutes by the liver to the active metabolite trichloroethanol, which has a half-life of 8 to 11 hours. A dose of chloral hydrate induces sleep in about 30 to 60 minutes and maintains sleep for 4 to 8 hours. It probably potentiates GABAergic neurotransmission, which suppresses neuronal excitability.

THERAPEUTIC INDICATIONS. The FDA lists chloral hydrate as an unapproved drug that is still prescribed by clinicians, however it has no FDA-approved indication. The primary use in clinical practice for chloral hydrate is to induce sleep. It should be used for no more than 2 or 3 days because longer-term treatment is associated with an increased incidence and severity of adverse effects. Tolerance develops to the hypnotic effects of chloral hydrate after 2 weeks of treatment. The benzodiazepines are superior to chloral hydrate for all psychiatric uses.

PRECAUTIONS AND ADVERSE REACTIONS. Chloral hydrate has adverse effects on the CNS, GI system, and skin. High doses (>4 g) may be associated with stupor, confusion, ataxia, falls, or coma. The GI effects include nonspecific irritation, nausea, vomiting, flatulence, and an unpleasant taste. With long-term use and overdose, gastritis and gastric ulceration can develop. Along with tolerance, dependence on chloral hydrate can occur. The symptoms are similar to those of alcohol dependence. With a lethal dose between 5,000 and 10,000 mg, chloral hydrate is a particularly poor choice for potentially suicidal persons.

DRUG INTERACTIONS. Because of metabolic interference, chloral hydrate should be strictly avoided with alcohol, a notorious concoction known as a *Mickey Finn*. Chloral hydrate may displace warfarin (Coumadin) from plasma proteins and enhance anticoagulant activity; this combination should be avoided.

LABORATORY INTERFERENCES.   Chloral hydrate administration can lead to false-positive results for urine glucose determinations that use cupric sulfate (e.g., Clinitest) but not in tests that use glucose oxidase (e.g., Clinistix and Tes-Tape). Chloral hydrate can also interfere with the determination of urinary catecholamines and 17-hydroxycorticosteroids.

DOSING AND CLINICAL GUIDELINES.   Chloral hydrate is available in 500-mg capsules; 500-mg/5-mL solution; and 324-, 500-, and 648-mg rectal suppositories. The standard dose of chloral hydrate is 500 to 2,000 mg at bedtime. Because the drug is a GI irritant, it should be administered with excess water, milk, other liquids, or antacids to decrease gastric irritation.

Propofol.   Propofol (Diprivan) is a $GABA_A$ agonist that is used as an anesthetic. It induces the presynaptic release of GABA and dopamine (the latter possibly through action on $GABA_B$ receptors) and is a partial agonist at dopamine D_2 and NMDA receptors. Because it is very lipid-soluble, it crosses the blood–brain barrier readily and induces anesthesia in less than 1 minute. Rapid redistribution from the CNS results in an offset of action within 3 to 8 minutes after the infusion is discontinued. It is well tolerated when used for conscious sedation, but it has a potential for acute adverse effects, including respiratory depression, apnea, and bradyarrhythmias, and the prolonged infusion can cause acidosis and mitochondrial myopathies. The carrier used for the infusion is a soybean emulsion that can be a culture medium for various organisms. Also, the carrier can impair macrophage function and cause hematologic and lipid abnormalities and anaphylactic reactions.

Etomidate.   Etomidate is a carboxylated imidazole that acts at the β_2 and β_3 subunits of the $GABA_A$ receptor. It has a rapid onset (1 minute) and short duration (less than 5 minutes) of action. The propylene glycol vehicle has been linked to hyperosmolar metabolic acidosis. It has both proconvulsant and anticonvulsant properties, and it inhibits cortisol release, with possible adverse consequences after long-term use. It has been used in anesthesia as it is unlikely to affect blood pressure, however it has largely been replaced by newer medications.

▲ 21.5 Drugs Used to Treat Sleep Disorders

NONBENZODIAZEPINE GABA AGONISTS

Several of the benzodiazepines are commonly used for sleep, such as flurazepam, temazepam, quazepam, estazolam, and triazolam. Temazepam, flurazepam, and triazolam are benzodiazepines used for insomnia; these are discussed with the other benzodiazepines under the anxiolytic section. Nonbenzodiazepine agonists, such as zolpidem (Ambien), zaleplon (Sonata), and eszopiclone (Lunesta)—the so-called "Z drugs"—are similar to these drugs as they bind at a location close to the benzodiazepine receptor

Pharmacologic Action

Zaleplon, zolpidem, and eszopiclone are structurally distinct and vary in their binding to the GABA receptor subunits.

Benzodiazepines activate all three specific GABA–benzodiazepine (GABA–BZ) binding sites of the $GABA_A$-receptor, which opens chloride channels and reduces the rate of neuronal and muscle firing. Zolpidem, zaleplon, and eszopiclone have selectivity for specific subunits of the GABA receptor. This specificity may account for their selective sedative effects and relative lack of muscle relaxant and anticonvulsant effects.

Zolpidem, zaleplon, and eszopiclone are rapidly and well absorbed after oral administration, although absorption can be delayed by as long as 1 hour if they are taken with food. Zolpidem reaches peak plasma concentrations in 1.6 hours and has a half-life of 2.6 hours. Zaleplon reaches peak plasma concentrations in 1 hour and has a half-life of 1 hour. Eszopiclone reaches peak plasma concentrations in 1 hour. If taken immediately after a high-fat or heavy meal, the peak is delayed by approximately 1 hour, reducing the effects of eszopiclone on sleep onset. The terminal-phase elimination half-life is approximately 6 hours in healthy adults. Eszopiclone is weakly bound to plasma protein (52 to 59 percent).

The rapid metabolism and lack of active metabolites of zolpidem, zaleplon, and eszopiclone avoid the accumulation of plasma concentrations compared with the long-term use of benzodiazepines such as flurazepam or diazepam.

Flumazenil for Benzodiazepine Overdosage.   Similar to the benzodiazepines, flumazenil can reverse the adverse psychomotor, amnestic, and sedative effects of zolpidem and zaleplon.

Therapeutic Indications

Insomnia.   Zolpidem, zaleplon, and eszopiclone are also indicated only for insomnia. Although these "Z drugs" are not usually associated with rebound insomnia after the discontinuation of their use for short periods, some patients experience increased sleep difficulties the first few nights after discontinuing their use. The use of zolpidem, zaleplon, and eszopiclone for periods more extended than 1 month is not associated with the delayed emergence of adverse effects. No development of tolerance to any parameter of sleep measurement was observed over 6 months in clinical trials of eszopiclone.

γ-Hydroxybutyrate (GHB, Xyrem), which is approved for the treatment of narcolepsy and improves slow-wave sleep, is also an agonist at the $GABA_A$ receptor, where it binds to specific GHB receptors. GHB has the capacity both to reduce drug craving and to induce dependence, abuse, and absence seizures as a result of complex actions on tegmental dopaminergic systems.

Parkinson Disease.   A small number of persons with idiopathic Parkinson disease respond to long-term use of zolpidem with reduced bradykinesia and rigidity. Zolpidem dosages of 10 mg four times daily may be tolerated without sedation for several years.

Precautions and Adverse Reactions

Zolpidem and zaleplon are generally well tolerated. At zolpidem dosages of 10 mg/day and zaleplon dosages above 10 mg/day, a small number of persons will experience dizziness, drowsiness, dyspepsia, or diarrhea. Zolpidem and zaleplon are secreted in breast milk and are therefore contraindicated for use by nursing mothers. The dosage of zolpidem and zaleplon should be reduced in elderly persons and persons with hepatic impairment.

Zolpidem (Ambien) has been associated with automatic behavior and amnesia. In rare cases, zolpidem may cause hallucinations and behavioral changes. The coadministration of zolpidem and SSRIs may extend the duration of hallucinations in susceptible patients. Eszopiclone exhibits a dose–response relationship in elderly adults for the side effects of pain, dry mouth, and unpleasant taste.

Zolpidem and zaleplon can produce a mild withdrawal syndrome lasting 1 day after prolonged use at higher therapeutic dosages. Rarely, a person taking zolpidem has self-titrated up the daily dosage to 30 to 40 mg a day. Abrupt discontinuation of such a high dosage of zolpidem may cause withdrawal symptoms for 4 or more days. Tolerance does not develop to the sedative effects of zolpidem and zaleplon.

Drug Interactions

These agents are most dangerous when used with other CNS depressants, such as alcohol, barbituates, opioids, and similar drugs. Cimetidine increases the plasma concentrations of zaleplon.

Rifampin (Rifadin), phenytoin (Dilantin), carbamazepine, and phenobarbital (Solfoton, Luminal) significantly increase the metabolism of zaleplon.

The CYP3A4 and CYP2E1 enzymes are involved in the metabolism of eszopiclone. Eszopiclone did not show any inhibitory potential on CYP450 1A2, 2A6, 2C9, 2C19, 2D6, 2E1, and 3A4 in cryopreserved human hepatocytes.

Laboratory Interferences

No known laboratory interferences are associated with the use of zolpidem and zaleplon.

Dosage and Clinical Guidelines

Zaleplon is available in 5- and 10-mg capsules. A single 10-mg dose is the usual adult dose. The dose can be increased to a maximum of 20 mg as tolerated. A single dose of zaleplon can be expected to provide 4 hours of sleep with minimal residual impairment. For persons older than age 65 years or persons with hepatic impairment, an initial dose of 5 mg is advised.

Eszopiclone is available in 1-, 2-, and 3-mg tablets. The starting dose should not exceed 1 mg in patients with severe hepatic impairment or those taking potent CYP3A4 inhibitors. The recommended dosing to improve sleep onset or maintenance is 2 or 3 mg for adult patients (ages 18 to 64 years) and 2 mg for older adult patients (ages 65 years and older). The 1-mg dose is for sleep onset in older adult patients whose primary complaint is difficulty falling asleep.

Zolpidem is available in 5- and 10-mg capsules, and 6.25- and 12.5-mg capsules for the controlled-release capsules. There is also a sublingual tablet and an oropharyngeal spray. The controlled-release form is usually for problems with sleep maintenance. The sublingual and oropharyngeal forms are for difficulties with taking the pill, or in particular circumstances. For example, the sublingual can be used for middle of the night awakening. With the oral capsule, the starting dose is 5 mg for females and 5 to 10 mg for males before bedtime. A single 10-mg dose is the usual adult dose (6.25- or 12.5-mg of the controlled release). The capsule should only be taken at the beginning of the night, as the drug can impair a person if they attempt activity within 7 to 8 hours of using the drug. For persons older than age 65 years or persons who are medically frail, 5 mg is the recommended dose.

MELATONIN AGONISTS: RAMELTEON AND MELATONIN

There are two melatonin receptor agonists commercially available in the United States: (1) melatonin, a dietary supplement available in various preparations in health food stores, and not under FDA regulations; (2) and ramelteon (Rozerem), an FDA-approved drug for the treatment of insomnia characterized by difficulties with sleep onset. Both exogenous melatonin and ramelteon are thought to exert their effects by interaction with central melatonin receptors.

Ramelteon

Ramelteon (Rozerem) is a melatonin receptor agonist used to treat sleep-onset insomnia. Unlike the benzodiazepines, ramelteon has no appreciable affinity for the GABA receptor complex.

Pharmacologic Actions. Ramelteon essentially mimics melatonin's sleep-promoting properties and has a high affinity for melatonin MT_1 and MT_2 receptors in the brain. These receptors are thought to be critical in the regulation of the body's sleep–wake cycle.

Ramelteon is rapidly absorbed and eliminated over a dose range of 4 to 64 mg. Maximum plasma concentration (C_{max}) is reached approximately 45 minutes after administration, and the elimination half-life is 1 to 2.6 hours. The total absorption of ramelteon is at least 84 percent, but extensive first-pass metabolism results in a bioavailability of approximately 2 percent. Ramelteon is metabolized primarily through the CYP1A2 pathway and eliminated principally in urine. Repeated once-daily dosing does not appear to result in accumulation, likely because of the compound's short half-life.

Therapeutic Indications. The FDA-approved ramelteon for the treatment of insomnia characterized by difficulty with sleep onset. Potential off-label use is centered on the application in circadian rhythm disorders, predominantly jet lag, delayed sleep phase syndrome, and shift work sleep disorder.

Clinical trials and animal studies have failed to demonstrate evidence of rebound insomnia or withdrawal effects.

Precautions and Adverse Events. Headache is the most common side effect of ramelteon. Other adverse effects may include somnolence, fatigue, dizziness, worsening insomnia, depression, nausea, and diarrhea. We should not use the drug in patients with severe hepatic impairment. It is also not recommended in patients with severe sleep apnea or severe chronic obstructive pulmonary disease. Prolactin levels may be increased in women. The drug should be used with caution, if at all, in nursing mothers and pregnant women.

Ramelteon has been found sometimes to decrease blood cortisol and testosterone and to increase prolactin. Female patients should be monitored for the cessation of menses and galactorrhea, decreased libido, and fertility problems. The safety and effectiveness of ramelteon in children has not been established.

Drug Interactions. CYP1A2 is the major isozyme involved in the hepatic metabolism of ramelteon. Accordingly, fluvoxamine (Luvox) and other CYP1A2 inhibitors may increase the side effects of ramelteon.

Ramelteon should be administered with caution in patients taking CYP1A2 inhibitors, potent CYP3A4 inhibitors such as ketoconazole, and strong CYP2C inhibitors such as fluconazole (Diflucan). No clinically meaningful interactions were found when ramelteon was coadministered with omeprazole, theophylline, dextromethorphan, midazolam, digoxin, and warfarin.

Dosing and Clinical Guidelines. The usual dose of ramelteon is 8 mg within 30 minutes of going to bed. It should not be taken with or immediately after high-fat meals.

Melatonin

Melatonin (*N*-acetyl-5-methoxytryptamine) is a hormone produced mainly at night in the pineal gland. Ingested melatonin can reach and bind to melatonin-binding sites in the brains of mammals and produce somnolence when used at high doses. Melatonin is available as a dietary supplement and is not a medication. Few well-controlled clinical trials have been conducted to determine its effectiveness in treating such conditions as insomnia, jet lag, and sleep disturbances related to shift work.

Pharmacologic Actions. Melatonin's secretion is stimulated by the dark and inhibited by the light. It is naturally synthesized from the amino acid tryptophan, which is converted to serotonin and finally converted to melatonin. The suprachiasmatic nuclei (SCN) of the hypothalamus have melatonin receptors, and melatonin may have a direct action on SCN to influence circadian rhythms, which are relevant for jet lag and sleep disturbances. In addition to the pineal gland, melatonin is also produced in the retina and GI tract.

Melatonin has a very short half-life of 0.5 to 6 minutes. Plasma concentrations are a function of the dose administered and the endogenous rhythm. Approximately 90 percent of melatonin is cleared through the first-pass metabolism by way of the CYP1A1 and CYP1A2 pathways. Elimination occurs principally in urine.

Exogenous melatonin interacts with the melatonin receptors that suppress neuronal firing and promote sleep. There does not appear to be a dose–response relationship between exogenous melatonin administrations and sleep effects.

Therapeutic Indications. Melatonin is approved for insomnia in the European Union and several other countries, however, it is not approved by the FDA for any medical use. It is sold over the counter in the United States and Canada but requires a prescription in some other countries such as the United Kingdom. Individuals have used exogenous melatonin to address sleep difficulties (insomnia, circadian rhythm disorders), cancer (breast, prostate, colorectal), seizures, depression, anxiety, and seasonal affective disorder. Some studies suggest that exogenous melatonin may have some antioxidant effects and antiaging properties.

Precautions and Adverse Reactions. Adverse events associated with melatonin include fatigue, dizziness, headache, irritability, and somnolence. Disorientation, confusion, sleepwalking, vivid dreams, and nightmares have also been observed, often with effects resolving after melatonin administration was suspended.

Melatonin may reduce fertility in both men and women. In men, exogenous melatonin reduces sperm motility, and long-term administration has been shown to inhibit testicular aromatase levels. In women, exogenous melatonin may inhibit ovarian function, and for that reason, it has been evaluated as a contraceptive, but with inconclusive results.

Drug Interactions. As a dietary supplement preparation, exogenous melatonin is not regulated by the FDA and has not been subjected to the same type of drug interaction studies that were performed for ramelteon. Caution is suggested in coadministering melatonin with blood thinners (e.g., warfarin [Coumadin], aspirin, and heparin), antiseizure medications, and medications that lower BP.

Laboratory Interference. Melatonin is not known to interfere with any commonly used clinical laboratory tests.

Dosage and Administration. Over-the-counter melatonin is available in the following formulations: 1-, 2.5-, 3-, and 5-mg capsules; 1-mg/4-mL liquid; 0.5- and 3-mg lozenges; 2.5-mg sublingual tablets; and 1-, 2-, and 3-mg timed-release tablets.

Standard recommendations are to take the desired melatonin dose at bedtime, but some evidence from clinical trials suggests that dosing up to 2 hours before habitual bedtime may produce a more significant improvement in sleep onset.

Agomelatine (Valdoxan). Agomelatine is structurally related to melatonin and is used in Europe as a treatment for MDD. It acts as an agonist at melatonin (MT_1 and MT_2) receptors. It also acts as a serotonin antagonist. Analysis of agomelatine clinical trial data raised serious questions about the efficacy and safety of the drug. The drug is not being marketed in the United States.

PRAZOSIN

Prazosin (Minipress) is a quinazoline derivative and one of a new chemical class of antihypertensives. It is an α_1-adrenergic receptor antagonist as opposed to the drugs mentioned above, which are α_2-blockers.

Pharmacologic Actions

The exact mechanism of the hypotensive action of prazosin, and how it suppresses nightmares, is unknown. Prazosin causes a decrease in total peripheral resistance that is related to its action as an α_1-adrenergic receptor antagonist. BP is lowered in both the supine and standing positions. This effect is most pronounced on the diastolic BP. After oral administration, human plasma concentrations reach a peak at about 3 hours with a plasma half-life of 2 to 3 hours. The drug is highly bound to plasma protein. Tolerance has not been observed to develop with long-term therapy.

Therapeutic Action

Prazosin is used in psychiatry to suppress nightmares, particularly those associated with PTSD.

Precautions and Adverse Reactions

During clinical trials and subsequent marketing experience, the most frequent reactions were dizziness (10.3 percent); headache (7.8 percent); drowsiness (7.6 percent); lack of energy (6.9 percent); weakness (6.5 percent); palpitations (5.3 percent); and nausea (4.9 percent). In most instances, side effects disappeared with continued therapy or have been tolerated with no decrease in the dose of the drug. Prazosin should not be used in nursing mothers or during pregnancy.

Drug Interactions

No adverse drug interactions have been reported.

Laboratory Interferences

No laboratory interferences have been reported.

Dosage and Clinical Guidelines

The drug is supplied in 1-, 2-, and 5-mg capsules and a nasal spray. The therapeutic dosages most commonly used have ranged from 6 to 15 mg daily given in divided doses. Doses higher than 20 mg do not increase efficacy. When adding a diuretic or other antihypertensive agent, the dose should be reduced to 1 or 2 mg three times a day, and retitration then carried out. Concomitant use with a PDE-5 inhibitor can result in additive BP-lowering effects and symptomatic hypotension; therefore, PDE-5 inhibitor therapy should be initiated at the lowest dose in patients taking prazosin.

▲ 21.6 Stimulants

STIMULANT DRUGS AND ATOMOXETINE

Stimulant drugs increase motivation, mood, energy, and wakefulness. They are also called sympathomimetics because they mimic the physiologic effects of the neurotransmitter epinephrine. Several chemical classes are included in this group.

Currently, these drugs are most commonly used to treat symptoms of poor concentration and hyperactivity in children and adults with ADHD. Paradoxically, many patients with ADHD find that these drugs can have a calming effect. Sympathomimetics are also approved for use in increasing alertness in narcolepsy.

Amphetamines were the first stimulants to be synthesized. They were created in the late 19th century and were used by Bavarian soldiers in the mid-1880s to maintain wakefulness, alertness, energy, and confidence in combat. They have been used similarly in most wars since then. They were not widely used clinically until the 1930s when they were marketed as Benzedrine inhalers for relief of nasal congestion. When their psychostimulant effects were noted, these drugs were used to treat sleepiness associated with narcolepsy. They have been classified as controlled drugs because of their rapid onset, immediate behavioral effects, and propensity to develop tolerance, which leads to the risk of abuse and dependence in vulnerable individuals. State and federal agencies regulate their manufacture, distribution, and use. In 2005, pemoline was withdrawn from the market because of significant risks of treatment-emergent hepatotoxicity.

Sympathomimetics have been widely used in persons with ADHD and narcolepsy because no equally effective agents have been available. They have also been found useful in treating certain cognitive disorders that result in secondary depression or profound apathy (e.g., AIDS, multiple sclerosis, poststroke depression, dementia, closed head injury) as well as in the augmentation of antidepressant medications in specific treatment-resistant depressions.

Atomoxetine is included in this section because it is used to treat ADHD, even though it is not a psychostimulant.

Pharmacologic Actions

All of these drugs are well absorbed from the GI tract. Amphetamine (Adderall) and dextroamphetamine (Dexedrine, Dextrostat) reach peak plasma concentrations in 2 to 3 hours and have a half-life of about 6 hours, thereby necessitating once- or twice-daily dosing. Methylphenidate is available in immediate-release (Ritalin), sustained-release (Ritalin SR), and extended-release (Concerta) formulations. Immediate-release methylphenidate reaches peak plasma concentrations in 1 to 2 hours and has a short half-life of 2 to 3 hours, thereby necessitating multiple-daily dosing. The sustained-release formulation reaches peak plasma concentrations in 4 to 5 hours and doubles the effective half-life of methylphenidate. The extended-release formulation reaches peak plasma concentrations in 6 to 8 hours and is designed to be effective for 12 hours in once-daily dosing. Dexmethylphenidate (Focalin) reaches peak plasma concentration in about 3 hours and is prescribed twice daily.

Lisdexamfetamine dimesylate, also known as L-lysine D-amphetamine (Vyvanse), is an amphetamine prodrug. In this formulation, dextroamphetamine is coupled with the amino acid L-lysine. Lisdexamfetamine becomes active upon cleavage of the lysine portion of the molecule by enzymes in the red blood cells. This results in the gradual release of dextroamphetamine into the bloodstream. Apart from having an extended duration of action, this formulation reduces its abuse potential. It is the only prodrug of its kind. Lisdexamfetamine is indicated for the treatment of ADHD in children 6 years and up and in adults as an integral part of a total treatment program that may include other measures (i.e., psychological, educational, social). The safety and efficacy of lisdexamfetamine dimesylate in patients 3 to 5 years old has not been established. In contrast to Adderall, which contains approximately 75 percent dextroamphetamine and 25 percent levoamphetamine, lisdexamfetamine is a single, dextro-enantiomer amphetamine molecule. In most cases, this makes the drug better tolerated, but some patients experience a more significant benefit from the mixed isomer preparation.

Methylphenidate, dextroamphetamine, and amphetamine are indirectly acting sympathomimetics, with the primary effect causing the release of catecholamines from presynaptic neurons. Their clinical effectiveness is associated with increased release of both dopamine and norepinephrine. Dextroamphetamine and methylphenidate are also weak inhibitors of catecholamine reuptake and inhibitors of monoamine oxidase.

In recent years, there has been an explosion of new brand name stimulants. Most of these are variations of the generic methylphenidate or mixed amphetamine salts that provide additional options to customize treatment in terms of dosing and duration of effect.

For modafinil, the specific mechanism of action is unknown. Narcolepsy–cataplexy results from a deficiency of hypocretin, a hypothalamic neuropeptide. Hypocretin-producing neurons are activated after modafinil administration. Modafinil does not appear to work through a dopaminergic mechanism. It does have α_1-adrenergic agonist properties, which may account for its alerting effects, because the wakefulness induced by modafinil can be attenuated by prazosin, an α_1-adrenergic antagonist. Some evidence suggests that modafinil has some norepinephrine reuptake blocking effects. Armodafinil (Nuvigil) is the R-enantiomer of modafinil. Both drugs have similar clinical effects and side effects.

Therapeutic Indications

Attention-Deficit/Hyperactivity Disorder (ADHD). Sympathomimetics are the first-line drugs for the treatment of ADHD in children and are effective about 75 percent of the time. Methylphenidate and dextroamphetamine are equally effective and work within 15 to 30 minutes. Sympathomimetic drugs decrease hyperactivity, increase attentiveness, and reduce impulsivity. They may also reduce comorbid oppositional behaviors associated with ADHD. Many persons take these drugs throughout their schooling and beyond. In responsive persons, the use of a sympathomimetic may be a critical determinant of scholastic success.

Sympathomimetics improve the core ADHD symptoms of hyperactivity, impulsivity, and inattentiveness and permit improved social interactions with teachers, family, other adults, and peers. The success of long-term treatment of ADHD with sympathomimetics, which are efficacious for most of the various constellations of ADHD symptoms present from childhood to adulthood, supports a model in which ADHD results from a genetically determined neurochemical imbalance that requires lifelong pharmacologic management.

Methylphenidate is the most commonly used initial agent at a dosage of 5 to 10 mg every 3 to 4 hours. Dosages may be increased to a maximum of 20 mg four times daily or 1 mg/kg a day. Use of the 20-mg sustained-release formulation to achieve 6 hours of benefit and eliminate the need for dosing at school is supported by many experts, although other authorities believe it is less effective than the immediate-release formulation. Dextroamphetamine is about twice as potent as methylphenidate on a per milligram basis and provides 6 to 8 hours of benefit. Some 70 percent of nonresponders to one sympathomimetic may benefit from another. All of the sympathomimetic drugs should be tried before switching to drugs of a different class. The previous dictum that sympathomimetics worsen tics and, therefore, should be avoided by persons with comorbid ADHD and tic disorders has been questioned. Small dosages of sympathomimetics do not appear to cause an increase in the frequency and severity of tics. Alternatives to sympathomimetics for ADHD include bupropion (Wellbutrin), venlafaxine (Effexor), guanfacine (Tenex), clonidine (Catapres), and tricyclic drugs. Further studies are needed to determine whether modafinil improves the symptoms of ADHD.

Short-term use of sympathomimetics induces a euphoric feeling; however, tolerance develops for both the euphoric feeling and the sympathomimetic activity.

Narcolepsy and Hypersomnolence.
Narcolepsy consists of sudden sleep attacks (*narcolepsy*), sudden loss of postural tone (*cataplexy*), loss of voluntary motor control going into (hypnagogic) or coming out of (hypnopompic) sleep (*sleep paralysis*), and hypnagogic or hypnopompic *hallucinations.* Sympathomimetics reduce narcoleptic sleep attacks and improve wakefulness in other types of hypersomnolent states. Modafinil is approved as an antisomnolence agent for the treatment of narcolepsy, for people who cannot adjust to night shift work, and for those who do not sleep well because of obstructive sleep apnea.

Other sympathomimetics are also used to maintain wakefulness and accuracy of motor performance in persons subject to sleep deprivation, such as pilots and military personnel. Persons with narcolepsy, unlike persons with ADHD, may develop a tolerance for the therapeutic effects of sympathomimetics.

In direct comparison with amphetamine-like drugs, modafinil is equally useful at maintaining wakefulness, with a lower risk of excessive activation.

Depressive Disorders.
Sympathomimetics may be used for treatment-resistant depressive disorders, usually as augmentation of standard antidepressant drug therapy. Possible indications for the use of sympathomimetics as monotherapy include depression in elderly persons, who are at increased risk for adverse effects from standard antidepressant drugs; depression in medically ill persons, especially persons with AIDS; obtundation caused by chronic use of opioids; and clinical situations in which a rapid response is necessary but for which ECT is contraindicated. Depressed patients with abulia and anergia may also benefit.

Dextroamphetamine may be useful in differentiating pseudodementia of depression from dementia. A depressed person generally responds to a 5-mg dose with increased alertness and improved cognition. Sympathomimetics are thought to provide only short-term benefit (2 to 4 weeks) for depression because most persons rapidly develop a tolerance for the antidepressant effects of the drugs. However, some clinicians report that long-term treatment with sympathomimetics can benefit some persons.

Encephalopathy Caused by Brain Injury.
Sympathomimetics increase alertness, cognition, motivation, and motor performance in persons with neurologic deficits caused by strokes, trauma, tumors, or chronic infections. Treatment with sympathomimetics may permit earlier and more robust participation in rehabilitative programs. Poststroke lethargy and apathy may respond to long-term use of sympathomimetics.

Obesity.
Sympathomimetics are used in the treatment of obesity because of their anorexia-inducing effects. Because tolerance develops for the anorectic effects and because of the drugs' high abuse potential, their use for this indication is limited. Of the sympathomimetic drugs, phentermine (Adipex-P, Fastin) is the most widely used for appetite suppression. Phentermine was the second half of "fen-phen," an off-label combination of fenfluramine and phentermine, widely used to promote weight loss. Fenfluramine and dexfenfluramine were withdrawn from the market because of their adverse effect, including cardiac valvular insufficiency, primary pulmonary hypertension, and irreversible loss of cerebral serotoninergic nerve fibers. The toxicity of fenfluramine is attributed to the fact that it stimulates the release of massive amounts of serotonin from nerve endings, a mechanism of action not shared by phentermine. The use of phentermine alone has not been reported to cause the same adverse effects like those caused by fenfluramine or dexfenfluramine.

Careful limitations of caloric intake and judicious exercise are at the core of any successful weight loss program. Sympathomimetic drugs facilitate the loss of, at most, an additional fraction of a pound per week. Sympathomimetic drugs are effective appetite suppressants only for the first few weeks of use; then, the anorexigenic effects tend to decrease.

Fatigue.
Between 70 and 90 percent of individuals with multiple sclerosis experience fatigue. Modafinil, armodafinil, amphetamines, methylphenidate, and the dopamine receptor agonist amantadine (Symmetrel) are sometimes useful in combating this symptom. Other causes of fatigue, such as chronic fatigue syndrome, respond to stimulants in many cases.

Precautions and Adverse Reactions

The most common adverse effects associated with amphetamine-like drugs are stomach pain, anxiety, irritability, insomnia, tachycardia, cardiac arrhythmias, and dysphoria. Sympathomimetics cause a decreased appetite, although tolerance usually develops for this effect. The treatment of common adverse effects in children with ADHD is usually straightforward (Table 21-49). The drugs can also cause increases in heart rate and BP and may cause palpitations. Less common adverse effects include the possible induction of movement disorders, such as tics, Tourette disorder–like symptoms, and dyskinesias, all of which are often self-limited over 7 to 10 days. If a person taking a sympathomimetic develops one of these movement disorders, a correlation between the dose of the medication and the severity of the disorder must be firmly established before adjustments are made in the medication dosage. In severe cases, augmentation with risperidone (Risperdal), clonidine (Catapres), or guanfacine (Tenex) is necessary. Methylphenidate may worsen tics in one-third of persons; these persons fall into two groups: those whose methylphenidate-induced tics resolve immediately upon the metabolism of the dosage, and a smaller group in whom methylphenidate appears to trigger tics that persist for several months but eventually resolve spontaneously.

Table 21-49
Management of Common Stimulant-Induced Adverse Effects in Attention-Deficit/Hyperactivity Disorder

Adverse Effect	Management
Anorexia, nausea, weight loss	• Administer stimulant with meals. • Use caloric-enhanced supplements. Discourage forcing meals.
Insomnia, nightmares	• Administer stimulants earlier in day. • Change to short-acting preparations. • Discontinue afternoon or evening dosing. • Consider adjunctive treatment (e.g., antihistamines, clonidine, antidepressants).
Dizziness	• Monitor BP. • Encourage fluid intake. • Change to long-acting form.
Rebound phenomena	• Overlap stimulant dosing. • Change to long-acting preparation or combine long- and short-acting preparations. • Consider adjunctive or alternative treatment (e.g., clonidine, antidepressants).
Irritability	• Assess timing of phenomena (during peak or withdrawal phase). • Evaluate comorbid symptoms. • Reduce dose. • Consider adjunctive or alternative treatment (e.g., lithium, antidepressants, anticonvulsants).
Dysphoria, moodiness, agitation	• Consider comorbid diagnosis (e.g., mood disorder). • Reduce dosage or change to long-acting preparation. • Consider adjunctive or alternative treatment (e.g., lithium, anticonvulsants, antidepressants).

BP, blood pressure.
From Wilens TE, Blederman J. The stimulants. In: Shaffer D, ed. *The Psychiatric Clinics of North America: Pediatric Psychopharmacology*. Philadelphia, PA: Saunders; 1992, with permission.

Longitudinal studies do not indicate that sympathomimetics cause growth suppression. Sympathomimetics may exacerbate glaucoma, hypertension, cardiovascular disorders, hyperthyroidism, anxiety disorders, psychotic disorders, and seizure disorders.

High dosages of sympathomimetics can cause dry mouth, pupillary dilation, bruxism, formication, excessive ebullience, restlessness, emotional lability, and occasionally seizures. Long-term use of high dosages can cause a delusional disorder that resembles paranoid schizophrenia. Seizures can be treated with benzodiazepines, cardiac effects with β-adrenergic receptor antagonists, fever with cooling blankets, and delirium with DRAs. Overdosages of sympathomimetics result in hypertension, tachycardia, hyperthermia, toxic psychosis, delirium, hyperpyrexia, convulsions, coma, chest pain, arrhythmia, heart block, hypertension or hypotension, shock, and nausea. Toxic effects of amphetamines can be seen at 30 mg, but idiosyncratic toxicity can occur at doses as low as 2 mg. Conversely, survival has been reported up to 500 mg.

The most limiting adverse effect of sympathomimetics is their association with psychological and physical dependence. At the doses used for the treatment of ADHD, the development of psychological dependence virtually never occurs. The more considerable concern is the presence of adolescent or adult cohabitants who might confiscate the supply of sympathomimetics for abuse or sale.

The use of sympathomimetics should be avoided during pregnancy, especially during the first trimester. Dextroamphetamine and methylphenidate pass into the breast milk, and it is not known whether modafinil or armodafinil do.

Drug Interactions

Sympathomimetics decrease the metabolism of several drugs, thus increasing their plasma levels. These drugs include tricyclic or tetracyclic antidepressants, warfarin (Coumadin), primidone (Mysoline), phenobarbital (Luminal), phenytoin (Dilantin), or phenylbutazone (Butazolidin). Sympathomimetics decrease the therapeutic efficacy of many antihypertensive drugs, especially guanethidine (Esimil, Ismelin). The sympathomimetics should be used with extreme caution with MAOIs.

Laboratory Interferences

Dextroamphetamine may elevate plasma corticosteroid levels and interfere with some assay methods for urinary corticosteroids.

Dosage and Administration

Many psychiatrists believe that governmental authorities have overly regulated amphetamine use. Amphetamines are listed as schedule II drugs by the Drug Enforcement Agency. Some states keep a registry of patients who receive amphetamines. Such mandates worry both patients and physicians about breaches in confidentiality, and physicians are concerned that official agencies may misinterpret their prescribing practices. Consequently, some physicians may withhold prescription of sympathomimetics, even from persons who may benefit from the medications.

The dosage ranges and the available preparations for sympathomimetics are presented in Table 21-50. Vyvanse dosing is a particular case because many patients are switched to this formulation after being treated with other stimulants. A conversion table is shown in Table 21-51. It is available in 20-, 30-, 40-, 50-, 60-, and 70-mg capsules. Dosage should be individualized according to the therapeutic needs and response of the patient. Lisdexamfetamine (Vyvanse) should be administered at the lowest effective dosage. In patients who are either starting treatment for the first time or switching from another medication, 30 mg once daily in the morning is the recommended dose. Dosages may go up or down in 10 or 20 mg increments in intervals of approximately 1 week. Patients should avoid taking the drug in the afternoon, as this may cause insomnia. The drug may be taken with or without food.

Dextroamphetamine, methylphenidate, amphetamine, benzphetamine, and methamphetamine are schedule II drugs and, in some states, require triplicate prescriptions. Phendimetrazine (Adipost, Bontril) and phenmetrazine (Prelude) are schedule III drugs, and modafinil, armodafinil, phentermine, diethylpropion (Tenuate), and mazindol (Mazanor, Sanorex) are schedule IV drugs.

Pretreatment evaluation should include an evaluation of the patient's cardiac function, with particular attention to the presence of hypertension or tachyarrhythmias. The clinician should also examine the patient for the presence of movement disorders, such as tics and dyskinesia, because the administration of sympathomimetics can exacerbate these conditions. If tics are present, many experts will not prescribe sympathomimetics but will instead choose clonidine or antidepressants. However, recent data indicate that sympathomimetics may cause only a mild increase in motor tics and may suppress vocal tics. Liver function and renal function

Table 21-50
Selected Sympathomimetics Commonly Used in Psychiatry

Generic Name	Trade Name	Preparations	Initial Daily Dose	Usual Daily Dose for ADHD[a]	Usual Daily Dose for Disorders Associated with Excessive Daytime Somnolence	Maximum Daily Dose
Amphetamine–dextroamphetamine	Adderall	5-, 10-, 20-, and 30-mg tablets	5–10 mg	20–30 mg	5–60 mg	Children: 40 mg Adults: 60 mg
Armodafinil	Nuvigil	50-, 150-, and 250-mg tablets	50–150 mg	150–250 mg	250 mg	
Atomoxetine	Strattera	10-, 18-, 25-, 40-, and 60-mg tablets	20 mg	40–80 mg	Not used	Children: 80 mg Adults: 100 mg
Dexmethylphenidate	Focalin	2.5-, 5-, and 10-mg capsules	5 mg	5–20 mg	Not used	20 mg
Dextroamphetamine	Dexedrine, Dextrostat	5-, 10-, and 15-mg ER capsules; 5- and 10-mg tablets	5–10 mg	20–30 mg	5–60 mg	Children: 40 mg Adults: 60 mg
Lisdexamfetamine	Vyvanse	20-, 30-, 40-, 50-, 60-, and 70-mg capsules	20–30 mg			70 mg
Methamphetamine	Desoxyn	5-mg tablets; 5-, 10-, and 15-mg ER tablets	5–10 mg	20–25 mg	Not generally used	45 mg
Methylphenidate	Ritalin, Methidate, Methylin, Attenade	5-, 10-, and 20-mg tablets; 10- and 20-mg SR tablets	5–10 mg	5–60 mg	20–30 mg	Children: 80 mg Adults: 90 mg
	Concerta	18- and 36-mg ER tablets	18 mg	18–54 mg	Not yet established	54 mg
Modafinil*	Provigil	100- and 200-mg tablets	100 mg	Not used	400 mg	400 mg

*Obstructive sleep apnea, narcolepsy, and shift work disorder
[a]For children 6 years of age and older.
ER, extended release; SR, sustained release.

Table 21-51
Lisdexamfetamine (Vyvanse) Dosage Equivalency Conversions

Vyvanse and Adderall XR	
Vyvanse	**Adderall XR**
20 mg	5 mg
30 mg	10 mg
40 mg	15 mg
50 mg	20 mg
60 mg	25 mg
70 mg	30 mg

Vyvanse, Adderall IR, and Dexedrine		
Vyvanse	**Adderall IR**	**Dexedrine**
70 mg	30 mg	22.5 mg
50 mg	20 mg	15 mg
30 mg	10 mg	7.5 mg

XR, extended release; IR, immediate-release.

should be assessed, and dosages of sympathomimetics should be reduced for persons with impaired metabolism.

Persons with ADHD can take immediate-release methylphenidate at 8 AM, 12 noon, and 4 PM. Dextroamphetamine, Adderall, sustained-release methylphenidate, or 18 mg of extended-release methylphenidate may be taken once at 8 AM. The starting dose of methylphenidate ranges from 2.5 mg of regular to 20 mg of the sustained-release formulation. If this is inadequate, it may be increased to a maximum dose of 80 mg in children and 90 mg daily in adults. The dosage of dextroamphetamine is 2.5 to 40 mg a day up to 0.5 mg/kg a day.

The starting dosage of modafinil is 200 mg in the morning in medically healthy individuals and 100 mg in the morning in persons with hepatic impairment. Some persons take a second 100- or 200-mg dose in the afternoon. The maximum recommended daily dosage is 400 mg, although dosages of 600 to 1,200 mg a day have been used safely. Adverse effects become prominent at dosages greater than 400 mg a day. Compared with amphetamine-like drugs, modafinil promotes wakefulness but produces less attentiveness and less irritability. Some persons with excessive daytime sleepiness extend the activity of the morning modafinil dose with an afternoon dose of methylphenidate. Armodafinil is virtually identical to modafinil but is dosed differently, the dosing range being 50 to 250 mg daily.

ATOMOXETINE (STRATTERA)

Atomoxetine is the first nonstimulant drug to be approved by the FDA as a treatment of ADHD in children, adolescents, and adults.

It is included in this chapter because it shares this indication with the stimulants described earlier.

Pharmacologic Actions

Atomoxetine is believed to produce a therapeutic effect through selective inhibition of the presynaptic norepinephrine transporter. It is well absorbed after oral administration and is minimally affected by food. High-fat meals may decrease the rate but not the extent of absorption. Maximum plasma concentrations are reached after approximately 1 to 2 hours. At therapeutic concentrations, 98 percent of atomoxetine in plasma is bound to protein, mainly albumin. Atomoxetine has a half-life of approximately 5 hours and is metabolized principally by the CYP2D6 pathway. Poor metabolizers of this compound reach a fivefold higher area under the curve and fivefold higher peak plasma concentration than normal or extensive metabolizers. This variation is critical to consider in patients receiving medications that inhibit the CYP2D6 enzyme. For example, the antidepressant-like pharmacology of atomoxetine has led to its use as an add-on to SSRIs or other antidepressants. Drugs such as fluoxetine (Prozac), paroxetine (Paxil), and bupropion (Wellbutrin) are CYP2D6 inhibitors and may raise atomoxetine levels.

Therapeutic Indications

Atomoxetine is used for the treatment of ADHD. It should be considered for use in patients who find stimulants too activating or who experience other intolerable side effects. Because atomoxetine has no abuse potential, it is a reasonable choice in the treatment of patients with both ADHD and substance abuse, patients who complain of ADHD symptoms but are suspected of seeking stimulant drugs, and patients who are in recovery.

Atomoxetine may enhance cognition when used to treat patients with schizophrenia. It may also be used as an alternative or add-on to antidepressants in patients who fail to respond to standard therapies.

Precautions and Adverse Reactions

Common side effects of atomoxetine include abdominal discomfort, decreased appetite with resulting weight loss, sexual dysfunction, dizziness, vertigo, irritability, and mood swings. Minor increases in BP and heart rate have also been observed. There have been cases of severe liver injury in a small number of patients taking atomoxetine. The drug should be discontinued in patients with jaundice (yellowing of the skin or whites of the eyes, itching) or laboratory evidence of liver injury. Atomoxetine should not be taken at the same time as, or within 2 weeks of taking, an MAOI or by patients with narrow-angle glaucoma.

The effects of overdose greater than twice the maximum recommended daily dose in humans are unknown. No specific information is available on the treatment of overdose with atomoxetine.

Dosage and Clinical Guidelines

Atomoxetine is available as 10-, 18-, 25-, 40-, and 60-mg capsules. In children and adolescents who weigh up to 70 kg, atomoxetine should be initiated at a total daily dose of approximately 0.5 mg/kg and increased after a minimum of 3 days to a target total daily dose of approximately 1.2 mg/kg, administered either as a single daily dose in the morning or as evenly divided doses in the morning and late afternoon or early evening. The total daily dose in smaller children and adolescents should not exceed 1.4 mg/kg or 100 mg,

whichever is less. Dosing of children and adolescents who weigh more than 70 kg and adults should start at a total daily dose of 40 mg and then be increased after a minimum of 3 days to a target total daily dose of approximately 80 mg. The doses can be administered either as a single daily dose in the morning or as evenly divided doses in the morning and late afternoon or early evening. After 2 to 4 additional weeks, the dose may be increased to a maximum of 100 mg in patients who have not achieved an optimal response. The maximum recommended total daily dose in children and adolescents over 70 kg and adults is 100 mg.

▲ 21.7 Drugs Used to Treat Substance Use Disorders

OPIOID RECEPTOR AGONISTS

Opioid receptor agonists are a structurally diverse group of compounds that are used for pain management. These drugs are also called narcotics. Although highly effective as analgesics, they often cause dependence and are frequently diverted for recreational use. Commonly used opioid agonists for pain relief include morphine, hydromorphone (Dilaudid), codeine, meperidine (Demerol), oxycodone (OxyContin), buprenorphine (Buprenex), hydrocodone (Robidone), tramadol (Ultram), and fentanyl (Durogesic). Heroin is used as a street drug. Methadone is used both for pain management and for the treatment of opiate addiction. This chapter focuses on the μ-opioid receptor agonists that are most likely to be used in the treatment of psychiatric disorders instead of pain management.

It is now recognized that the pharmacology of the opioid system is complex. There are multiple types of opioid receptors, with μ- and κ-opioid receptors representing functionally opposing endogenous systems (Table 21-52). All of the compounds above, which represent the most extensively used narcotic analgesics, are agonists at μ-opioid receptors. However, analgesic effects also result from agonist effects on the κ-opioid receptor. Buprenorphine has mixed receptor effects, being primarily a μ-opioid receptor agonist as well as a κ-opioid antagonist.

There is growing interest in the use of some drugs that act on opioid receptors as alternative treatments for a subpopulation of patients with refractory depression, as well as treatment for cutting behavior in patients with borderline personality disorder.

Ongoing, regular use of opioids produces dependence and tolerance and may lead to maladaptive use, functional impairment, and withdrawal symptoms. This well-known fact tempers consideration of such off-label use. The prevalence of opioid use, abuse,

Table 21-52
μ- and κ-Opiate Receptors

Receptor	Agonist Effects	Antagonist Effects
Mu (μ)	Analgesia Euphoria Antidepressant Anxiety	Anxiety Hostility
Kappa (κ)	Analgesia Dysphoria Depression Stress-induced anxiety	Antidepressant

and dependence, particularly with prescription opioids, has risen in recent years.

Before using opioid receptor agonists with patients who have failed on multiple conventional therapeutic agents, screen carefully for a history of drug use disorders, document the rationale for off-label use, establish treatment ground rules, obtain written consent, consult with primary care physician, and monitor closely. Avoid replacing "lost" prescriptions and providing early prescription renewals.

Pharmacologic Actions

Methadone and buprenorphine are absorbed rapidly from the GI tract. Hepatic first-pass metabolism significantly affects the bioavailability of each of the drugs but in markedly different ways. For methadone, hepatic enzymes reduce the bioavailability of an oral dosage by about half, an effect that is easily managed with dosage adjustments.

For buprenorphine, first-pass intestinal and hepatic metabolism eliminates oral bioavailability almost wholly. When used in opioid detoxification, buprenorphine is given sublingually in either a liquid or a tablet formulation.

The peak plasma concentrations of oral methadone are reached within 2 to 6 hours, and the plasma half-life initially is 4 to 6 hours in opioid-naive persons and 24 to 36 hours after steady dosing of any type of opioid. Methadone is highly protein-bound and equilibrates widely throughout the body, which ensures little post dosage variation in steady-state plasma concentrations.

Elimination of a sublingual dosage of buprenorphine occurs in two phases: an initial phase with a half-life of 3 to 5 hours and a terminal phase with a half-life of more than 24 hours. Buprenorphine dissociates from its receptor binding site slowly, which permits an every-other-day dosing schedule.

Methadone acts as a pure agonist at μ-opioid receptors and has negligible agonist or antagonist activity at κ- or δ-opioid receptors. Buprenorphine is a partial agonist at μ-receptors, a potent antagonist at κ-receptors, and neither an agonist nor an antagonist at δ-receptors.

Therapeutic Indications

Methadone. Methadone is used for short-term detoxification (7 to 30 days), long-term detoxification (up to 180 days), and maintenance (treatment beyond 180 days) of opioid-dependent individuals. For these purposes, it is only available through designated clinics called methadone maintenance treatment programs (MMTPs) and in hospitals and prisons. Methadone is a schedule II drug, which means that specific federal laws and regulations tightly govern its administration.

Enrollment in a methadone program reduces the risk of death by 70 percent; reduces illicit use of opioids and other substances of abuse; reduces criminal activity; reduces the risk of infectious diseases of all types, most importantly HIV and hepatitis B and C infection; and in pregnant women, reduces the risk of fetal and neonatal morbidity and mortality. The use of methadone maintenance frequently requires lifelong treatment.

Some opioid-dependence treatment programs use a stepwise detoxification protocol in which a person addicted to heroin switches first to the potent agonist methadone; then to the weaker agonist buprenorphine; and finally to maintenance on an opioid receptor antagonist, such as naltrexone (ReVia). This approach minimizes the appearance of opioid withdrawal effects, which,

if they occur, are mitigated with clonidine (Catapres). However, compliance with opioid receptor antagonist treatment is low outside of settings using intensive cognitive-behavioral techniques. In contrast, noncompliance with methadone maintenance precipitates opioid withdrawal symptoms, which serve to reinforce the use of methadone and make cognitive-behavioral therapy less than essential. Thus, some well-motivated, socially integrated former heroin addicts can use methadone for years without participation in a psychosocial support program.

Data pooled from many reports indicate that methadone is more effective when taken at dosages above 60 mg a day. The analgesic effects of methadone are sometimes used in the management of chronic pain when less addictive agents are ineffective.

PREGNANCY. Methadone maintenance, combined with effective psychosocial services and regular obstetric monitoring, significantly improves obstetric and neonatal outcomes for women addicted to heroin. Enrollment of a heroin-addicted pregnant woman in such a maintenance program reduces the risk of malnutrition, infection, preterm labor, spontaneous abortion, preeclampsia, eclampsia, abruptio placenta, and septic thrombophlebitis.

The dosage of methadone during pregnancy should be the lowest effective dosage, and no withdrawal to abstinence should be attempted during pregnancy. Methadone is metabolized more rapidly in the third trimester, which may necessitate higher dosages. The daily dose can be administered in two divided doses during the third trimester to avoid potentially sedating postdose peak plasma concentrations. Methadone treatment has no known teratogenic effects.

NEONATAL METHADONE WITHDRAWAL SYMPTOMS. Withdrawal symptoms in newborns frequently include tremor, a high-pitched cry, increased muscle tone and activity, poor sleep and eating, mottling, yawning, perspiration, and skin excoriation. Convulsions that require aggressive anticonvulsant therapy may also occur. Withdrawal symptoms may be delayed in onset and prolonged in neonates because of their immature hepatic metabolism. Women taking methadone are sometimes counseled to initiate breastfeeding as a means of gently weaning their infants from methadone dependence, but they should not breastfeed their babies while still taking methadone.

Buprenorphine. The analgesic effects of buprenorphine are sometimes used in the management of chronic pain when less addictive agents are ineffective. Because buprenorphine is a partial agonist rather than a full agonist at the μ-receptor and is a weak antagonist at the κ-receptor, this agent produces a milder withdrawal syndrome and has a wider margin of safety than the full μ-agonist compounds generally used in treatment. Buprenorphine has a ceiling effect beyond which dose increases prolong the duration of action of the drug without further increasing the agonist effects. Because of this, buprenorphine has a high clinical safety profile, with limited respiratory depression, therefore decreasing the likelihood of lethal overdose. Buprenorphine does have the capacity to cause typical side effects associated with opioids, including sedation, nausea and vomiting, constipation, dizziness, headache, and sweating. A relevant pharmacokinetic consideration when using buprenorphine is the fact that it requires hepatic conversion to become analgesic (*N*-dealkylation catalyzed by CYP3A4). This may explain why some patients do not benefit from buprenorphine. Genetics, grapefruit juice, and many medications (including fluoxetine and fluvoxamine) can reduce a person's ability to metabolize buprenorphine into its bioactive form.

Buprenorphine has been combined with the narcotic antagonist naloxone for sublingual administration (Suboxone). This combination reduces the likelihood of abusing buprenorphine via the IV route. Because the sublingual route poorly absorbs naloxone, when the combination drug is taken sublingually, there is no effect of the naloxone on the efficacy of buprenorphine. If an opioid-dependent individual injects the combination medication, the naloxone precipitates a withdrawal reaction, therefore reducing the likelihood of illicit injection use of the sublingual preparation.

Inducting and stabilizing a patient on buprenorphine is analogous to inducting and stabilizing a patient on methadone except that, as a partial agonist, buprenorphine has the potential to cause precipitated withdrawal in patients who have recently taken full agonist opioids. Thus, a patient must avoid short-acting opioids for 12 to 24 hours before starting buprenorphine. Similarly, they should abstain from longer-acting opioids such as methadone for 24 to 48 hours or longer. The physician must assess the patient clinically and determine that the patient is in mild to moderate opioid withdrawal with objectively observable withdrawal signs before initiating buprenorphine.

In most instances, a relatively low dose of buprenorphine (2 to 4 mg) can then be administered, with additional doses given in 1 to 2 hours if withdrawal signs persist. The goal for the first 24 hours is to suppress withdrawal signs and symptoms, and the total 24-hour dose to do so can range from 2 to 16 mg on the first day. In subsequent days, the dose can be adjusted upward or downward to resolve withdrawal fully and, as with methadone, to achieve an absence of craving, adequate tolerance to prevent reinforcement from the use of other opioids, and ultimately abstinence from other opioids while minimizing side effects. Dose-ranging studies have demonstrated that dosages of 6 to 16 mg/day are associated with improved treatment outcomes compared with lower doses of buprenorphine (1 to 4 mg). Sometimes patients seem to need dosages higher than 16 mg/day, although there is no evidence for any benefit of dosages beyond 32 mg/day. For the treatment of opioid dependence, a dose of approximately 4 mg of sublingual buprenorphine is the equivalent of a daily dose of 40 mg of oral methadone. It has also been demonstrated that daily, alternate-day or three-times-per-week administration has equivalent effects in suppressing the symptoms of opioid withdrawal for dependent individuals. The combination tablet is recommended for most clinical purposes, including induction and maintenance. The buprenorphine mono (Subutex) should be used only for pregnant patients (although recent studies are investigating whether the combination of buprenorphine/naloxone is safe in pregnancy) or for patients who have a documented anaphylactic reaction to naloxone.

Newer forms of buprenorphine delivery, including a transdermal skin patch, a long-acting depot intramuscular injection that provides therapeutic plasma levels for several weeks (Sublocade), and subcutaneous buprenorphine implants that may provide therapeutic plasma levels for 6 months (Probuphine), are also FDA approved, although the latter treatment requires special training to administer.

Tramadol.   There are multiple reports of tramadol's antidepressant effects, both as monotherapy and augmentation agent in treatment-resistant depression. Clinical and experimental data suggest that tramadol has an inherent antidepressant-like activity. Tramadol has complex pharmacology. It is a weak μ-opioid receptor agonist, a 5-HT releasing agent, a DA-releasing agent, a 5-HT$_{2C}$ receptor antagonist, a norepinephrine reuptake inhibitor, an NMDA receptor antagonist, a nicotinic acetylcholine receptor antagonist, a TRPV$_1$ receptor agonist, and an M$_1$ and M$_3$ muscarinic acetylcholine receptor antagonist. Consistent with the evidence of

its antidepressant effects is the fact that tramadol has a close structural similarity to the antidepressant venlafaxine.

Both venlafaxine and tramadol inhibit norepinephrine/serotonin reuptake and inhibit the reserpine-induced syndrome completely. Both compounds also have an analgesic effect on chronic pain. Venlafaxine may have an opioid component, and naloxone reverses the antipain effect of venlafaxine. Nonopioid activity is demonstrated by the fact that the μ-opioid receptor antagonist naloxone does not fully antagonize its analgesic effect. Indicative of their structural similarities, venlafaxine may cause false-positive results on liquid chromatography tests to detect urinary tramadol levels.

Another relevant property of tramadol is its relatively long half-life, which reduces the potential for misuse. Its habituating effects are found to be much less than other opiate agonists, but abuse, withdrawal, and dependence are risks. Tramadol requires metabolism to become analgesic: individuals who are CYP2D6 "poor metabolizers" or use drugs that are CYP2D6 inhibitors reduce the efficacy of tramadol (the same is true of codeine).

Precautions and Adverse Reactions

The most common adverse effects of opioid receptor agonists are lightheadedness, dizziness, sedation, nausea, constipation, vomiting, perspiration, weight gain, decreased libido, inhibition of orgasm, and insomnia or sleep irregularities. Opioid receptor agonists are capable of inducing tolerance as well as producing physiologic and psychological dependence. Other CNS adverse effects include depression, sedation, euphoria, dysphoria, agitation, and seizures. Delirium has been reported in rare cases. Occasional non-CNS adverse effects include peripheral edema, urinary retention, rash, arthralgia, dry mouth, anorexia, biliary tract spasm, bradycardia, hypotension, hypoventilation, syncope, antidiuretic hormone-like activity, pruritus, urticaria, and visual disturbances. Menstrual irregularities are frequent in women, especially in the first 6 months of use. Various abnormal endocrine laboratory indexes of little clinical significance may also be seen.

Most persons develop tolerance to the pharmacologic adverse effects of opioid agonists during long-term maintenance, and relatively few adverse effects are experienced after the induction period.

Overdosage.   The acute effects of opioid receptor agonist overdosage include sedation, hypotension, bradycardia, hypothermia, respiratory suppression, miosis, and decreased GI motility. Severe effects include coma, cardiac arrest, shock, and death. The risk of overdosage is most significant in the induction stage of treatment and in persons with slow drug metabolism caused by preexisting hepatic insufficiency. Deaths have been caused during the first week of induction by methadone dosages of only 50 to 60 mg a day.

The risk of overdosage with buprenorphine appears to be lower than with methadone. However, deaths have been caused by the use of buprenorphine in combination with benzodiazepines.

Withdrawal Symptoms.   Abrupt cessation of methadone use triggers withdrawal symptoms within 3 to 4 days, which usually reaches peak intensity on the sixth day. Withdrawal symptoms include weakness, anxiety, anorexia, insomnia, gastric distress, headache, sweating, and hot and cold flashes. The withdrawal symptoms usually resolve after 2 weeks. However, a protracted methadone abstinence syndrome is possible that may include restlessness and insomnia.

The withdrawal symptoms associated with buprenorphine are similar to but less marked than those caused by methadone. In particular, buprenorphine is sometimes used to ease the transition from methadone to opioid receptor antagonists or abstinence because of the relatively mild withdrawal reaction associated with discontinuation of buprenorphine.

Drug–Drug Interactions

Opioid receptor agonists can potentiate the CNS-depressant effects of alcohol, barbiturates, benzodiazepines, other opioids, low-potency DRAs, tricyclic and tetracyclic drugs, and MAOIs. Carbamazepine (Tegretol), phenytoin (Dilantin), barbiturates, rifampin (Rimactane, Rifadin), and heavy long-term consumption of alcohol may induce hepatic enzymes, which may lower the plasma concentration of methadone or buprenorphine and thereby precipitate withdrawal symptoms. In contrast, however, hepatic enzyme induction may increase the plasma concentration of active levomethadyl metabolites and cause toxicity.

Acute opioid withdrawal symptoms may be precipitated in persons on methadone maintenance therapy who take pure opioid receptor antagonists such as naltrexone, nalmefene (Revex, Selincro), and naloxone (Narcan); partial agonists such as buprenorphine; or mixed agonist–antagonists such as pentazocine (Talwin). These symptoms may be mitigated by the use of clonidine, a benzodiazepine, or both.

Competitive inhibition of methadone or buprenorphine metabolism after short-term use of alcohol or administration of cimetidine (Tagamet), erythromycin, ketoconazole (Nizoral), fluoxetine (Prozac), fluvoxamine (Luvox), loratadine (Claritin), quinidine (Quinidex), and alprazolam (Xanax) may lead to higher plasma concentrations or a prolonged duration of action of methadone or buprenorphine. Medications that alkalinize the urine may reduce methadone excretion.

Methadone maintenance may also increase plasma concentrations of desipramine (Norpramin, Pertofrane) and fluvoxamine. The use of methadone may increase zidovudine (Retrovir) concentrations, which increases the possibility of zidovudine toxicity at otherwise standard dosages. Moreover, in vitro human liver microsome studies demonstrate competitive inhibition of methadone demethylation by several protease inhibitors, including ritonavir (Norvir), indinavir (Crixivan), and saquinavir (Invirase). The clinical relevance of this finding is unknown.

Fatal drug–drug interactions with the MAOIs are associated with the use of the opioids fentanyl (Sublimaze) and meperidine (Demerol) but not with the use of methadone, levomethadyl, or buprenorphine.

Tramadol may interact with drugs that inhibit serotonin reuptake. Such combinations can trigger seizures and serotonin syndrome. These events may also develop during tramadol monotherapy, either at routine or excessive doses. The risk of interactions is increased when tramadol is combined with virtually all classes of antidepressants and with drugs that lower the seizure threshold, especially the antidepressant bupropion.

Laboratory Interferences

Methadone and buprenorphine can be tested separately in urine toxicology to distinguish them from other opioids. No known laboratory interferences are associated with the use of methadone or buprenorphine.

Dosage and Clinical Guidelines

Methadone. Methadone is supplied in 5-, 10-, and 40-mg dispersible scored tablets; 40-mg scored wafers; 5-mg/5-mL,

10-mg/5-mL, and 10-mg/mL solutions; and a 10-mg/mL parenteral form. In maintenance programs, methadone is usually dissolved in water or juice, and dose administration is directly observed to ensure compliance. For induction of opioid detoxification, an initial methadone dose of 15 to 20 mg will usually suppress craving and withdrawal symptoms. However, some individuals may require up to 40 mg a day in single or divided doses. Higher dosages should be avoided during induction of treatment to reduce the risk of acute toxicity from overdosage.

Over several weeks, the dosage should be raised to at least 70 mg a day. The maximum dosage is usually 120 mg a day, and higher dosages require prior approval from regulatory agencies. Dosages above 60 mg a day are associated with much more complete abstinence from the use of illicit opioids than are dosages less than 60 mg a day.

The duration of treatment should not be predetermined but should be based on response to treatment and assessment of psychosocial factors. All studies of methadone maintenance programs endorse long-term treatment (i.e., several years) as more effective than short-term programs (i.e., less than 1 year) for the prevention of relapse into opioid abuse. In actual practice, however, a minority of programs are permitted by policy or approved by insurers to provide even 6 months of continuous maintenance treatment. Moreover, some programs encourage withdrawal from methadone in less than 6 months after induction. This practice is quite ill-conceived, because more than 80 percent of persons who terminate methadone maintenance treatment eventually return to illicit drug use within 2 years. In programs that offer both maintenance and withdrawal treatments, the overwhelming majority of participants enroll in the maintenance treatment.

Buprenorphine. Buprenorphine is supplied as a 0.3-mg/mL solution in 1-mL ampules. Sublingual tablet formulations of buprenorphine containing buprenorphine only or buprenorphine combined with naloxone in a 4:1 ratio are used for opioid maintenance treatment. Physicians must be trained and certified to carry out this therapy in their private offices. There are several approved training programs in the United States. As noted above, an extended release and subcutaneous extended formulation are also available but require some special skill and training.

Tramadol. No controlled trials exist that establish the appropriate dosing schedule for tramadol when used for conditions other than pain. Tramadol is available in many formulations. These range from capsules (regular and extended-release) to tablets (regular, extended-release, chewable tablets) that can be taken sublingually, suppositories, and injectable ampules. It also comes as tablets and capsules containing acetaminophen or aspirin. Doses in case reports of treatment for depression or OCD range from 50 to 200 mg a day and involve short-term use. The long-term use of tramadol in the treatment of psychiatric disorders has not been studied.

OPIOID RECEPTOR ANTAGONISTS: NALTREXONE, NALMEFENE, AND NALOXONE

Naltrexone (Revia, Depade) and naloxone (Narcan) are competitive opioid antagonists. They bind to opioid receptors without causing their activation. Because these drugs induce opioid withdrawal effects in people using full opioid agonists, these drugs are classified as opioid antagonists.

Naltrexone is the most widely used of these drugs. It has a relatively long half-life, is orally effective, is not associated with dysphoria, and is administered once daily. Naloxone, which predated naltrexone to treat narcotic overdose, became less widely used for preventing relapse to opiate use in detoxified opiate addicts. Since its introduction, naltrexone has been tried for the treatment of a wide range of psychiatric disorders, including, among others, eating disorders, autism, self-injurious behavior, cocaine dependence, gambling, and alcoholism. Naltrexone was approved for the treatment of alcohol dependence in 1994. Several generic formulations are also available. An extended-release, once-a-month injectable suspension (Vivitrol) was also approved in 2006. Nalmefene (Revex) is indicated for the complete or partial reversal of opioid drug effects and in the management of known or suspected opioid overdose. An oral formulation of nalmefene is available in some countries but not in the United States. Nalmefene (Revex, Selincro) is an opioid receptor antagonist that is sometimes used in the management of alcohol dependence.

Pharmacologic Actions

The GI tract rapidly absorbs oral opioid receptor antagonists. However, because of first-pass hepatic metabolism, only 60 percent of a dose of naltrexone and 40 to 50 percent of a dose of nalmefene reach the systemic circulation unchanged. Peak concentrations of naltrexone and its active metabolite, 6-β-naltrexol, are achieved within 1 hour of ingestion. The half-life of naltrexone is 1 to 3 hours, and the half-life of 6-β-naltrexol is 13 hours. Peak concentrations of nalmefene are achieved in about 1 to 2 hours, and the half-life is 8 to 10 hours. Clinically, a single dose of naltrexone effectively blocks the rewarding effects of opioids for 72 hours. Traces of 6-β-naltrexol may linger for up to 125 hours after a single dose.

Naltrexone and nalmefene are competitive antagonists of opioid receptors. Understanding the pharmacology of opioid receptors can explain the difference in adverse effects caused by naltrexone and nalmefene. Opioid receptors in the body are typed pharmacologically as μ, κ, or δ. Whereas activation of the κ- and δ-receptors is thought to reinforce opioid and alcohol consumption centrally, activation of μ-receptors is more closely associated with central and peripheral antiemetic effects. Because naltrexone is a relatively weak antagonist of κ- and δ-receptors and a potent μ-receptor antagonist, dosages of naltrexone that effectively reduce opioid and alcohol consumption also strongly block μ-receptors and, therefore, may cause nausea. Nalmefene, in contrast, is an equally potent antagonist of all three opioid receptor types, and dosages of nalmefene that effectively reduce opioid and alcohol consumption have no significantly increased effect on μ-receptors. Thus, nalmefene is associated clinically with few GI adverse effects.

Naloxone has the highest affinity for the μ-receptor but is a competitive antagonist at the μ-, κ-, and δ-receptors.

Whereas the effects of opioid receptor antagonists on opioid use are easily understood in terms of competitive inhibition of opioid receptors, the effects of opioid receptor antagonists on alcohol dependence are less straightforward. That likely relates to the fact that the desire for and the effects of alcohol consumption appear to be regulated by several neurotransmitter systems, both opioid and nonopioid.

Therapeutic Indications

The combination of a cognitive-behavioral program plus the use of opioid receptor antagonists is more successful than either the cognitive-behavioral program or the use of opioid receptor antagonists alone. Naloxone is used as a screening test to ensure that

Table 21-53
Naloxone (Narcan) Challenge Test

The naloxone challenge test should not be performed in a patient showing clinical signs or symptoms of opioid withdrawal or in a patient whose urine contains opioids. The naloxone challenge test may be administered by either the intravenous (IV) or the subcutaneous route.

IV challenge: After appropriate screening of the patient, 0.8 mg of naloxone should be drawn into a sterile syringe. If the IV route of administration is selected, 0.2 mg of naloxone should be injected, and while the needle is still in the patient's vein, the patient should be observed for 30 s for evidence of withdrawal signs or symptoms. If there is no evidence of withdrawal, the remaining 0.6 mg of naloxone should be injected and the patient observed for an additional 20 min for signs and symptoms of withdrawal.

Subcutaneous challenge: If the subcutaneous route is selected, 0.8 mg should be administered subcutaneously and the patient observed for signs and symptoms of withdrawal for 20 min.

Conditions and technique for observation of patient: During the appropriate period of observation, the patient's vital signs should be monitored, and the patient should be monitored for signs of withdrawal. It is also important to question the patient carefully. The signs and symptoms of opioid withdrawal include, but are not limited to, the following:

Withdrawal signs: Stuffiness or running nose, tearing, yawning, sweating, tremor, vomiting, or piloerection

Withdrawal symptoms: Feeling of temperature change, joint or bone and muscle pain, abdominal cramps, and formication (feeling of bugs crawling under skin)

Interpretation of the challenge: Warning—the elicitation of the enumerated signs or symptoms indicates a potential risk for the subject, and naltrexone should not be administered. If no signs or symptoms of withdrawal are observed, elicited, or reported, naltrexone may be administered. If there is any doubt in the observer's mind that the patient is not in an opioid-free state or is in continuing withdrawal, naltrexone should be withheld for 24 hr and the challenge repeated.

the patient is opioid-free before the induction of therapy with naltrexone (see "Naloxone Challenge Test" in Table 21-53).

Opioid Dependence. Patients in detoxification programs are usually weaned from potent opioid agonists such as heroin over days to weeks, during which emergent adrenergic withdrawal effects are treated as needed with clonidine (Catapres). A serial protocol is sometimes used in which potent agonists are gradually replaced by weaker agonists followed by mixed agonist–antagonists and then finally by pure antagonists. For example, an abuser of the potent agonist heroin would switch first to the weaker agonist methadone (Dolophine), then to the partial agonist buprenorphine (Buprenex) or levomethadyl acetate (ORLAAM)—commonly called LAAM—and finally, after a 7- to 10-day washout period, to a pure antagonist, such as naltrexone or nalmefene. However, even with gradual detoxification, some persons continue to experience mild adverse effects or opioid withdrawal symptoms for the first several weeks of treatment with naltrexone.

As the opioid receptor agonist potency diminishes, so do the adverse consequences of discontinuing the drug. Thus, because there are no pharmacologic barriers to discontinuation of pure opioid receptor antagonists, the social environment and frequent cognitive-behavioral intervention become significant factors supporting continued opioid abstinence. Because of poorly tolerated adverse symptoms, most persons not simultaneously enrolled in a cognitive-behavioral program stop taking opioid receptor antagonists within 3 months. Compliance with the administration of an opioid receptor antagonist regimen can also be increased with participation in a well-conceived voucher program.

Issues of medication compliance should be a central focus of treatment. If a person with a history of opioid addiction stops taking a pure opioid receptor antagonist, the person's risk of relapse into opioid abuse is exceedingly high, because the reintroduction of a potent opioid agonist would yield a very rewarding subjective "high." In contrast, compliant persons do not develop tolerance to the therapeutic benefits of naltrexone even if it is administered continuously for 1 year or longer. Individuals may undergo several relapses and remissions before achieving long-term abstinence.

Persons taking opioid receptor antagonists should also be warned that sufficiently high dosages of opioid agonists can overcome the receptor antagonism of naltrexone or nalmefene, which may lead to hazardous and unpredictable levels of receptor activation (see "Precautions and Adverse Reactions").

Rapid Detoxification. The recommended period of opioid abstinence before starting opioid receptor antagonists is 7 to 10 days. However, to avoid this, rapid detoxification protocols have been developed. Continuous administration of adjunct clonidine—to reduce the adrenergic withdrawal symptoms—and adjunct benzodiazepines, such as oxazepam (Serax)—to reduce muscle spasms and insomnia—can permit the use of oral opioid receptor antagonists on the first day of opioid cessation. Detoxification can thus be completed within 48 to 72 hours, at which point opioid receptor antagonist maintenance is initiated. Moderately severe withdrawal symptoms may be experienced on the first day, but they taper off rapidly after that.

Because of the potential hypotensive effects of clonidine, the BP of persons undergoing rapid detoxification must be closely monitored for the first 8 hours. Outpatient rapid detoxification settings must therefore be adequately prepared to administer emergency care.

The main advantage of rapid detoxification is that the transition from opioid abuse to maintenance treatment occurs over just 2 or 3 days. The completion of detoxification in as little time as possible minimizes the risk that the person will relapse into opioid abuse during the detoxification protocol.

Alcohol Use Disorder. Opioid receptor antagonists are also used as adjuncts to cognitive-behavioral programs for the treatment of alcohol use disorder. Opioid receptor antagonists reduce alcohol craving and alcohol consumption, and they ameliorate the severity of relapses. Concomitant opioid receptor antagonist treatment added to an effective cognitive-behavioral program may halve the risk of relapse into heavy alcohol consumption.

The newer agent, nalmefene, has several potential pharmacologic and clinical advantages over its predecessor, naltrexone, for the treatment of alcohol use disorder. Whereas naltrexone may cause reversible transaminase elevations in persons who take dosages of 300 mg a day (which is six times the recommended dosage for treatment of alcohol and opioid dependence [50 mg a day]), nalmefene has not been associated with any hepatotoxicity. Clinically effective dosages of naltrexone are discontinued by 10 to 15 percent of persons because of adverse effects, most commonly nausea. In contrast, discontinuation of nalmefene because of an adverse event is rare at the clinically effective dosage of 20 mg a day and in the range of 10 percent at excessive dosages—that is, 80 mg a day. Because of its pharmacokinetic profile, a given dosage of nalmefene may also produce a more sustained opioid antagonist effect than does naltrexone.

The efficacy of opioid receptor antagonists in reducing alcohol craving may be augmented with an SSRI, although data from large trials are needed to assess this potential synergistic effect more fully.

Precautions and Adverse Reactions

Because opioid receptor antagonists are used for sustaining a drug-free state after opioid detoxification, great care must be taken to ensure that an adequate washout period elapses. This detox requires at least 5 days for a short-acting opioid such as heroin and at least 10 days for longer-acting opioids such as methadone—after the last dose of opioids and before the first dose of an opioid receptor antagonist is taken. Self-report and urine toxicology screens should determine the opioid-free state. If any question persists of whether opioids are in the body despite a negative urine screen result, then a *naloxone challenge test* should be performed. Naloxone challenge is used because its opioid antagonism lasts less than 1 hour, but those of naltrexone and nalmefene may persist for more than 24 hours. Thus, any withdrawal effects elicited by naloxone will be relatively short-lived (see "Dosage and Clinical Guidelines"). Symptoms of acute opioid withdrawal include drug craving, a feeling of temperature change, musculoskeletal pain, and GI distress. Signs of opioid withdrawal include confusion, drowsiness, vomiting, and diarrhea. Naltrexone and nalmefene should not be taken if naloxone infusion causes any signs of opioid withdrawal except as part of a supervised rapid detoxification protocol.

A set of adverse effects resembling a vestigial withdrawal syndrome tends to affect up to 10 percent of persons who take opioid receptor antagonists. Up to 15 percent of persons taking naltrexone may experience abdominal pain, cramps, nausea, and vomiting, which may be limited by transiently halving the dosage or altering the time of administration. Adverse CNS effects of naltrexone, experienced by up to 10 percent of persons, include headache, low energy, insomnia, anxiety, and nervousness. Joint and muscle pains may occur in up to 10 percent of persons taking naltrexone, as may rash.

Naltrexone may cause dosage-related hepatic toxicity at dosages well above 50 mg a day; 20 percent of persons taking 300 mg a day of naltrexone may experience serum aminotransferase concentrations 3 to 19 times the upper limit of normal. The hepatocellular injury of naltrexone appears to be a dose-related toxic effect rather than an idiosyncratic reaction. At the lowest dosages of naltrexone required for significant opioid antagonism, hepatocellular injury is not typically observed. However, naltrexone dosages as low as 50 mg a day may be hepatotoxic in persons with underlying liver disease, such as persons with cirrhosis of the liver caused by chronic alcohol abuse. Serum aminotransferase concentrations should be monitored monthly for the first 6 months of naltrexone therapy and after that based on clinical suspicion. Hepatic enzyme concentrations usually return to normal after discontinuation of naltrexone therapy.

If analgesia is required while a dose of an opioid receptor antagonist is pharmacologically active, opioid agonists should be avoided in favor of benzodiazepines or other nonopioid analgesics. Persons taking opioid receptor antagonists should be instructed that low dosages of opioids will not affect them. However, larger dosages could overcome the receptor blockade and suddenly produce symptoms of profound opioid overdosage, with sedation possibly progressing to coma or death. Use of opioid receptor antagonists is contraindicated in persons who are taking opioid agonists, small amounts of which may be present in over-the-counter antiemetic and antitussive preparations; in persons with acute hepatitis or hepatic failure; and in persons who are hypersensitive to the drugs.

Because naltrexone is transported across the placenta, opioid receptor antagonists should only be taken by pregnant women if a compelling need outweighs the potential risks to the fetus. It is not known whether opioid receptor antagonists are distributed into breast milk.

Opioid receptor antagonists are relatively safe drugs, and the ingestion of high doses of opioid receptor antagonists should be treated with supportive measures combined with efforts to decrease GI absorption.

Because buprenorphine has a high affinity and slow displacement from the opioid receptors, nalmefene may not wholly reverse buprenorphine-induced respiratory depression.

Drug Interactions

Many drug interactions involving opioid receptor antagonists have been discussed earlier, including those with opioid agonists associated with drug abuse as well as those involving antiemetics and antitussives. Because of its extensive hepatic metabolism, naltrexone may affect or be affected by other drugs that influence hepatic enzyme levels. However, the clinical importance of these potential interactions is not known.

One potentially hepatotoxic drug that has been used in some cases with opioid receptor antagonists is disulfiram (Antabuse). Although no adverse effects were observed, frequent laboratory monitoring is indicated when such combination therapy is contemplated. Opioid receptor antagonists have been reported to potentiate the sedation associated with the use of thioridazine (Mellaril), an interaction that probably applies equally to all low-potency DRAs.

Intravenous nalmefene has been administered after benzodiazepines, inhalational anesthetics, muscle relaxants, and muscle relaxant antagonists were administered in conjunction with general anesthetics without any adverse reactions. Care should be taken when using flumazenil (Romazicon) and nalmefene together because both of these agents have been shown to induce seizures in preclinical studies.

Laboratory Interferences

The potential for false-positive urine for opiates using less specific urine screens such as enzyme-multiplied immunoassay technique (EMIT) may exist, given that naltrexone and nalmefene are derivatives of oxymorphone. Naltrexone does not interefere with thin-layer, gas-liquid, and high-pressure liquid chromatographic methods used for the detection of opiates in the urine.

Dosage and Clinical Guidelines

We should take several steps to ensure that the person is opioid-free. These steps are meant to avoid the possibility of precipitating an acute opioid withdrawal syndrome. Within a supervised detoxification setting, at least 5 days should elapse after the last dose of short-acting opioids, such as heroin, hydromorphone (Dilaudid), meperidine (Demerol), or morphine, and at least 10 days should elapse after the last dose of longer-acting opioids, such as methadone, before opioid antagonists are initiated. Some rapid detoxification protocols use shorter abstinence periods, however these require special expertise to do safely. Urine toxicologic screens should demonstrate no opioid metabolites, and detoxification should be complete. However, an individual may have a negative urine opioid screen result, yet still be physically dependent on opioids and thus susceptible to antagonist-induced withdrawal effects. Therefore, after the urine screen result is negative, a naloxone challenge test is recommended unless an adequate period of opioid abstinence can be reliably confirmed by observers (Table 21-53).

The initial dosage of naltrexone for the treatment of opioid or alcohol dependence is 50 mg a day, which should be achieved through a gradual introduction, even when the naloxone challenge test result is negative. Various authorities begin with 5, 10, 12.5, or 25 mg and titrate up to the 50-mg dosage over a period ranging from 1 hour to 2 weeks while continually monitoring for evidence of opioid withdrawal. When a daily dose of 50 mg is well tolerated, it may be averaged over a week by giving 100 mg on alternate days or 150 mg every third day. Such schedules may increase compliance. The corresponding therapeutic dosage of nalmefene is 20 mg a day, divided into two equal doses. Gradual titration of nalmefene to this daily dose is probably a wise strategy, although clinical data on dosage strategies for nalmefene are not yet available.

It is recommended that family members directly observe the ingestion of each dose. This strategy helps to maximize compliance. Random urine tests for opioid receptor antagonists and their metabolites, as well as for ethanol or opioid metabolites, should also be taken. Opioid receptor antagonists should be continued until the person is no longer considered psychologically at risk for relapse into opioid or alcohol abuse. This treatment generally requires at least 6 months but may take longer, mainly if there are external stresses.

Nalmefene is available as a sterile solution for intravenous, intramuscular, and subcutaneous administration in two concentrations, containing 100 µg or 1.0 mg of nalmefene free base per milliliter. The 100 µg/mL concentration contains 110.8 µg of nalmefene hydrochloride, and the 1.0 mg/mL concentration contains 1.108 mg of nalmefene hydrochloride per milliliter. Both concentrations contain 9.0 mg of sodium chloride per milliliter, and the pH is adjusted to 3.9 with hydrochloric acid. Pharmacodynamic studies have shown that nalmefene has a longer duration of action than naloxone at fully reversing opiate activity.

Rapid Detoxification.   Rapid detoxification has been standardized using naltrexone, although nalmefene would be expected to be equally effective with fewer adverse effects. In rapid detoxification protocols, the addicted person stops opioid use abruptly and begins the first opioid-free day by taking clonidine 0.2 mg orally every 2 hours for nine doses, to a maximum dose of 1.8 mg, during which time the BP is monitored every 30 to 60 minutes for the first 8 hours. Naltrexone 12.5 mg is administered 1 to 3 hours after the first dose of clonidine. To reduce muscle cramps and later insomnia, a short-acting benzodiazepine, such as oxazepam 30 to 60 mg, is administered simultaneously with the first dose of clonidine, and half of the initial dose is readministered every 4 to 6 hours as needed. The maximum daily dosage of oxazepam should not exceed 180 mg. The person undergoing rapid detoxification should be accompanied home by a reliable escort. On the second day, similar doses of clonidine and the benzodiazepine are administered but with a single dose of naltrexone 25 mg taken in the morning. Relatively asymptomatic persons may return home after 3 to 4 hours. Administration of the daily maintenance dose of 50 mg of naltrexone is begun on the third day, and the dosages of clonidine and the benzodiazepine are gradually tapered off over 5 to 10 days.

DISULFIRAM AND ACAMPROSATE

Disulfiram (Antabuse) and acamprosate (Campral) are drugs used to treat alcohol use disorder. Disulfiram has suffered from a reputation as a dangerous medication only suitable for highly motivated and strictly supervised drinkers because of the severe physical reactions the drug causes after drinking. Experience has shown, however, that at recommended doses, it is an acceptable and safe medication for dependent drinkers seeking to sustain abstinence. The properties that constitute disulfiram's main therapeutic effect (i.e., the ability to produce unpleasant symptoms after alcohol intake, also known as disulfiram–alcohol reaction) have created that perception of dangerousness.

In the most severe cases, when disulfiram is combined with alcohol, severe clinical conditions can occur. These include respiratory depression, cardiovascular collapse, acute heart failure, convulsions, loss of consciousness, and death in rare cases. These potential complications, as well as the development of alternative antialcohol medications, have been the limiting factors for the broader use of disulfiram. Unlike disulfiram, acamprosate, the other drug discussed in this section, does not produce aversive side effects. Acamprosate is now prescribed more commonly than disulfiram in outpatient settings, but disulfiram is prescribed more often in inpatient settings because it helps facilitate initial abstinence.

Other drugs that are useful in reducing alcohol consumption include naltrexone (ReVia, Trexan), nalmefene (Revex), topiramate (Topamax), and gabapentin (Neurontin). These agents are discussed in their respective sections.

Disulfiram

Pharmacologic Actions.   Disulfiram is almost completely absorbed from the GI tract after oral administration. Its half-life is estimated to be 60 to 120 hours. Therefore, it may take 1 or 2 weeks to eliminate disulfiram from the body after taking the last dose.

The metabolism of ethanol proceeds through oxidation via alcohol dehydrogenase to the formation of acetaldehyde, which is further metabolized to acetyl-coenzyme A (acetyl-CoA) by aldehyde dehydrogenase. Disulfiram is an aldehyde dehydrogenase inhibitor that interferes with the metabolism of alcohol by producing a marked increase in blood acetaldehyde concentration. The accumulation of acetaldehyde (to a level up to 10 times higher than occurs in the normal metabolism of alcohol) produces a wide array of unpleasant reactions, called the *disulfiram–alcohol reaction,* characterized by nausea, throbbing headache, vomiting, hypertension, flushing, sweating, thirst, dyspnea, tachycardia, chest pain, vertigo, and blurred vision. The reaction occurs almost immediately after the ingestion of one alcoholic drink and may last from 30 minutes to 2 hours.

BLOOD CONCENTRATIONS IN RELATION TO ACTION.   Plasma concentrations of disulfiram vary among individuals because of several factors, most notably age and hepatic function. In general, the severity of disulfiram–alcohol reaction is proportional to the amount of the ingested disulfiram and alcohol. Nevertheless, disulfiram plasma levels are rarely obtained in clinical practice. The positive correlation between plasma concentrations of alcohol and the intensity of the reaction is described as follows: in sensitive individuals, as little as a 5 to 10 mg/100 mL increase of the plasma alcohol level may produce mild symptoms; fully developed symptoms occur at alcohol levels of 50 mg/100 mL, and levels as high as 125 to 150 mg/100 mL result in loss of consciousness and coma.

Therapeutic Indications.   The primary indication for disulfiram use is as an aversive conditioning treatment for alcohol use disorder. Either the fear of having a disulfiram–alcohol reaction or the memory of having had one is meant to condition the person not to use alcohol. Usually, describing the severity and the unpleasantness of the disulfiram–alcohol reaction graphically enough discourages the person from imbibing alcohol. Disulfiram treatment should be combined with such treatments as psychotherapy, group therapy, and support groups such as Alcoholics Anonymous (AA). Treatment with disulfiram requires careful monitoring because a person can decide not to take the medication.

Precautions and Adverse Reactions

WITH ALCOHOL CONSUMPTION.   The intensity of the disulfiram–alcohol reaction varies with each person. In extreme cases, it is marked by respiratory depression, cardiovascular collapse, myocardial infarction, convulsions, and death. Therefore, disulfiram is contraindicated for persons with significant pulmonary or cardiovascular disease. Also, disulfiram should be used with caution, if at all, by persons with nephritis, brain damage, hypothyroidism, diabetes, hepatic disease, seizures, polydrug dependence, or an abnormal electroencephalogram. Most fatal reactions occur in persons who take more than 500 mg a day of disulfiram and who consume more than 3 oz of alcohol. The treatment of a severe disulfiram–alcohol reaction is primarily supportive to prevent shock. The use of oxygen, intravenous vitamin C, ephedrine, and antihistamines have been reported to aid in recovery.

WITHOUT ALCOHOL CONSUMPTION.   The adverse effects of disulfiram in the absence of alcohol consumption include fatigue, dermatitis, impotence, optic neuritis, a variety of mental changes, and hepatic damage. A metabolite of disulfiram inhibits dopamine-β-hydroxylase, the enzyme that metabolizes dopamine into norepinephrine and epinephrine, and thus may exacerbate psychosis in persons with psychotic disorders. Catatonic reactions may also occur.

Drug Interactions.   Disulfiram increases the blood concentration of diazepam (Valium), paraldehyde, phenytoin (Dilantin), caffeine, tetrahydrocannabinol (the active ingredient in marijuana), barbiturates, anticoagulants, isoniazid (Nydrazid), and tricyclic drugs. Disulfiram should not be administered concomitantly with paraldehyde because paraldehyde is metabolized to acetaldehyde in the liver.

Laboratory Interferences.   In rare instances, disulfiram has been reported to interfere with the incorporation of iodine-131 into protein-bound iodine. Disulfiram may reduce urinary concentrations of homovanillic acid, the major metabolite of dopamine, because it inhibits dopamine hydroxylase.

Dosage and Clinical Guidelines.   Disulfiram is supplied in 250- and 500-mg tablets. The usual initial dosage is 500 mg a day, taken by mouth for the first 1 or 2 weeks, followed by a maintenance dosage of 250 mg a day. The dosage should not exceed 500 mg a day. The maintenance dosage range is 125 to 500 mg a day.

Persons taking disulfiram must be instructed that the ingestion of even the smallest amount of alcohol will bring on a disulfiram–alcohol reaction, with all of its unpleasant effects. Also, persons should be warned against ingesting any alcohol-containing preparations, such as cough drops, tonics of any kind, and alcohol-containing foods and sauces. Some reactions have occurred in patients who used alcohol-based lotions, toilet water, colognes, or perfumes and inhaled the fumes; therefore, precautions must be explicit and should include any topically applied preparations containing alcohol, such as perfume.

Disulfiram should not be administered until the person has abstained from alcohol for at least 12 hours. Persons should be warned that the disulfiram–alcohol reaction may occur as long as 1 or 2 weeks after the last dose of disulfiram. Persons taking disulfiram should carry identification cards describing the disulfiram–alcohol reaction and listing the name and telephone number of the physician to be called.

Acamprosate

Pharmacologic Actions. Acamprosate's mechanism of action is not fully understood, but it is thought to antagonize neuronal overactivity related to the actions of the excitatory neurotransmitter glutamate. In part, this may result from antagonism of NMDA receptors.

Indications. Acamprosate is used for treating alcohol-dependent individuals seeking to continue to remain alcohol-free after they have stopped drinking. Its efficacy in promoting abstinence has not been demonstrated in persons who have not undergone detoxification and who have not achieved alcohol abstinence before beginning treatment.

Precautions and Adverse Effects. Side effects are mostly seen early in treatment and are usually mild and transient. The most common side effects are headache, diarrhea, flatulence, abdominal pain, paresthesias, and various skin reactions. No adverse events occur after abrupt withdrawal of acamprosate, even after long-term use. There is no evidence of addiction to the drug. Patients with severe renal impairment (creatinine clearance of less than 30 mL/min) should not be given acamprosate.

Drug Interactions. Alcohol and acamprosate do not affect each other's pharmacokinetics. The same is true when adding disulfiram or diazepam to acamprosate. Coadministration of naltrexone with acamprosate produces an increase in concentrations of acamprosate. No adjustment of dosage is recommended in such patients. The pharmacokinetics of naltrexone and its major metabolite 6-β-naltrexol were unaffected after coadministration with acamprosate. During clinical trials, patients taking acamprosate concomitantly with antidepressants more commonly reported both weight gain and weight loss compared with patients taking either medication alone.

Laboratory Interferences. Acamprosate has not been shown to interfere with commonly performed laboratory tests.

Dosage and Clinical Guidelines. It is important to remember that acamprosate should not be used to treat alcohol withdrawal symptoms. It should only be started after the individual has been successfully weaned off alcohol. Patients should show a commitment to remaining abstinent, and treatment should be part of a comprehensive management program that includes counseling or support group attendance.

Each tablet contains acamprosate calcium 333 mg, which is equivalent to 300 mg of acamprosate. The dose of acamprosate is different for different patients. The recommended dosage is two 333-mg tablets (each dose should total 666 mg) taken three times daily. Although dosing may be done without regard to meals, dosing with meals was used during clinical trials and is suggested as an aid to compliance in patients who regularly eat three meals daily. A

lower dose may be useful in some patients. A missed dose should be taken as soon as possible. However, if it is almost time for the next dose, the missed dose should be skipped, and then the regular dosing schedule should be resumed. Doses should not be doubled up. For patients with moderate renal impairment (creatinine clearance of 30 to 50 mL/min), a starting dosage of one 333-mg tablet taken three times daily is recommended. People with severe renal insufficiency should not take acamprosate.

CLONIDINE AND GUANFACINE

Clonidine and guanfacine are marketed as hypertension treatments. Guanfacine is more selective and less potent than clonidine, but clonidine is the most widely used α_2-agonist.

Pharmacologic Actions

Clonidine and guanfacine are presynaptic α_2-receptor agonists. They inhibit sympathetic outflow and cause vasodilation of blood vessels. Clonidine and guanfacine are well absorbed from the GI tract and reach peak plasma levels 1 to 3 hours after oral administration. The half-life of clonidine is 6 to 20 hours, and that of guanfacine is 10 to 30 hours.

The agonist effects of clonidine and guanfacine on presynaptic α_2-adrenergic receptors in the sympathetic nuclei of the brain result in a decrease in the amount of norepinephrine released from the presynaptic nerve terminals. This decrease serves to reset the body's sympathetic tone at a lower level and decrease arousal. Table 21-54 provides a summary of α_2-adrenergic receptor agonists used in psychiatry.

Therapeutic Indications

There is considerably more experience in clinical psychiatry with clonidine than with guanfacine. There is recent interest in the use of guanfacine for the same indications that respond to clonidine due to guanfacine's longer half-life and relative lack of sedative effects.

Withdrawal from Opioids, Alcohol, Benzodiazepines, or Nicotine. Clonidine and guanfacine are effective in reducing the autonomic symptoms of rapid opioid withdrawal (e.g., hypertension, tachycardia, dilated pupils, sweating, lacrimation, and rhinorrhea) but not the associated subjective sensations. Clonidine administration (0.1 to 0.2 mg two to four times a day) is initiated before detoxification and is then tapered off over 1 to 2 weeks (Table 21-55).

Clonidine and guanfacine can reduce symptoms of alcohol and benzodiazepine withdrawal, including anxiety, diarrhea, and tachycardia. They can reduce craving, anxiety, and irritability symptoms of nicotine withdrawal. The transdermal patch formulation of clonidine is associated with better long-term compliance for purposes of detoxification than is the tablet formulation.

Tourette Disorder. Clonidine and guanfacine are effective drugs for the treatment of Tourette disorder. Most clinicians begin treatment for Tourette disorder with the standard DRAs haloperidol (Haldol) and pimozide (Orap) and the SDAs risperidone (Risperdal) and olanzapine (Zyprexa). However, if concerned about the adverse effects of these drugs, the clinician may begin treatment with clonidine or guanfacine. The starting dose of clonidine for children is 0.05 mg a day; it can be increased to 0.3 mg a day in divided doses. Clonidine may take long periods (e.g., 4 to 6 months) to positively effect the symptoms of the disorder. The response rate has been reported to be up to 70 percent.

Table 21-54
α_2-Adrenergic Receptor Agonists Used in Psychiatry[a]

Drug	Preparations	Usual Child Starting Dosage	Usual Child Dosage Range	Usual Adult Starting Dosage	Usual Adult Dosage
Clonidine tablets (Catapres)	0.1, 0.2, 0.3 mg	0.05 mg/day	Up to 0.3 mg/day tablets in divided doses	0.1–0.2 mg, two to four times a day (0.2–0.8 mg/day)	0.3–1.2 mg/day, two to three times a day (1.2 mg/day maximal dosage)
Clonidine transdermal system (Catapres-TTS)	0.1, 0.2, 0.3 mg/day	0.05 mg/day	Up to 0.3 mg/day patch every 5 days (0.5 mg/day every 5 days maximal dosage)	0.1 mg/day every 7 days	0.1 mg/day patch per week (0.6 mg/day every 7 days)
Guanfacine (Tenex)	1- and 2-mg tablets	1 mg/day at bedtime	1–2 mg/day at bedtime (3 mg/day maximal dosage)	1 mg/day at bedtime	1–2 mg at bedtime (3 mg/day maximal dosage)

[a]Dosages for medical indications, such as hypertension, vary.

Other Tic Disorders. Clonidine and guanfacine reduce the frequency and severity of tics in persons with tic disorder with or without comorbid ADHD.

Hyperactivity and Aggression in Children. Clonidine and guanfacine can be useful alternatives for the treatment of ADHD. They are used in place of sympathomimetics and antidepressants, which may produce a paradoxical worsening of hyperactivity in some children with intellectual disability, aggression, or features on the spectrum of autism. Clonidine and guanfacine can improve mood, reduce activity level, and improve social adaptation. Some impaired children may respond favorably to clonidine, but others may become sedated. The starting dose is 0.05 mg a day; it can be raised to 0.3 mg a day in divided doses. The efficacy of clonidine and guanfacine for control of hyperactivity and aggression often diminishes over several months of use.

Clonidine and guanfacine can be combined with methylphenidate (Ritalin) or dextroamphetamine (Dexedrine) to treat hyperactivity and inattentiveness, respectively. A small number of cases have been reported of the sudden death of children taking clonidine together with methylphenidate; however, it has not been conclusively demonstrated that these medications contributed to these deaths. The clinician should explain to the family that the efficacy and safety of this combination have not been investigated in controlled trials. Periodic cardiovascular assessments, including vital signs and electrocardiograms, are warranted if this combination is used.

Posttraumatic Stress Disorder. Acute exacerbations of PTSD may be associated with hyperadrenergic symptoms such as hyperarousal, exaggerated startle response, insomnia, vivid nightmares, tachycardia, agitation, hypertension, and perspiration. Preliminary reports suggested that these symptoms may respond to the use of clonidine or, especially for an overnight benefit, to the use of guanfacine. More recent studies have failed to demonstrate that guanfacine produces an improvement in PTSD symptoms.

Other Disorders. Other potential indications for clonidine include other anxiety disorders (panic disorder, phobias, obsessive-compulsive disorder, and GAD) and mania, in which it may be synergistic with lithium (Eskalith) or carbamazepine (Tegretol). There are anecdotal accounts suggesting the efficacy of clonidine in schizophrenia and tardive dyskinesia. A clonidine patch can reduce the hypersalivation and dysphagia caused by clozapine. Low-dose use has been reported effective in hallucinogen-persisting perceptive disorders.

Precautions and Adverse Reactions

The most common adverse effects associated with clonidine are dry mouth and eyes, fatigue, sedation, dizziness, nausea, hypotension,

Table 21-55
Oral Clonidine Protocols for Opioid Detoxification

Clonidine 0.1–0.2 mg PO four times a day; hold for systolic BP <90 mm Hg or bradycardia; stabilize for 2–3 days, then taper over 5–10 days
OR
Clonidine 0.1–0.2 mg PO q4–6h as needed for withdrawal signs or symptoms; stabilize for 2–3 days, then taper over 5–10 days
OR
Test dose with clonidine 0.1–0.2 mg PO or SL (for patients weighing over 200 lb); check BP after 1 hr. If diastolic BP >70 mm Hg and no symptoms of hypotension, begin treatment as follows:

Weight (lb)	Number of Clonidine Patches
<110	1 patch
110–160	2 patches
160–200	2 patches
>200	2 patches

OR
Test dose of oral clonidine 0.1 mg; check BP after 1 hr (if systolic BP <90 mm Hg, do not give patch)
Place two TTS-2 clonidine patches (or three patches if patient weighs >150 lb) on hairless area of upper body; then
For first 23 hr after patch application, give oral clonidine 0.2 mg q6h; then
For next 24 hr, give oral clonidine 0.1 mg q6h
Change patches weekly
After 2 wk of two patches, switch to one patch (or two patches if patient weighs >150 lb)
After 1 wk of one patch, discontinue patches

BP, blood pressure; PO, oral; q, every; SL, sublingual; TTS, through the skin.
From American Society of Addiction Medicine. Detoxification: principle and protocols. In: *The Principles Update Series: Topics in Addiction Medicine*, Section 11. American Society of Addiction; 1997, with permission.

and constipation, which result in discontinuation of therapy by about 10 percent of all persons taking the drug. Some persons also experience sexual dysfunction. Tolerance may develop to these adverse effects. A similar but milder adverse profile is seen with guanfacine, especially in doses of 3 mg or more per day. Adults should not take clonidine and guanfacine if their BP is below 90/60 mm Hg or if they have cardiac arrhythmias, especially bradycardia. Development of bradycardia warrants gradual, tapered discontinuation of the drug. Clonidine, in particular, is associated with sedation, and tolerance does not usually develop to this adverse effect. Uncommon CNS adverse effects of clonidine include insomnia, anxiety, and depression; rare CNS adverse effects include vivid dreams, nightmares, and hallucinations. Fluid retention associated with clonidine treatment can be treated with diuretics.

The transdermal patch formulation of clonidine may cause local skin irritation, which can be minimized by rotating the sites of application.

Overdose. Persons who take an overdose of clonidine may present with coma and constricted pupils, symptoms similar to those of an opioid overdose. Other symptoms of overdose are decreased BP, pulse, and respiratory rate. Guanfacine overdose produces a milder version of these symptoms. Clonidine and guanfacine should be avoided during pregnancy and by nursing mothers. Elderly persons are more sensitive to the drug than are younger adults. Children are susceptible to the same adverse effects as are adults.

Withdrawal. Abrupt discontinuation of clonidine can cause anxiety, restlessness, perspiration, tremor, abdominal pain, palpitations, headache, and a dramatic increase in BP. These symptoms may appear about 20 hours after the last dose of clonidine, and these may also be seen if one or two doses are skipped. A similar set of symptoms occasionally occurs 2 to 4 days after discontinuation of guanfacine, but the usual course is a gradual return to baseline BP over 2 to 4 days. Because of the possibility of discontinuation symptoms, doses of clonidine and guanfacine should be tapered slowly.

Drug Interactions

Clonidine and guanfacine cause sedation, especially early in therapy, and when administered with other centrally active depressants, such as barbiturates, alcohol, and benzodiazepines, the potential for additive sedative effects should be considered. Dose reduction may be required in patients receiving agents that interfere with AV node and sinus node conduction such as β-blockers, CCBs, and digitalis. This combination increases the risk of AV block and bradycardia. Clonidine should not be given with TCAs, which can inhibit the hypotensive effects of clonidine.

Laboratory Interferences

No known laboratory interferences are associated with the use of clonidine or guanfacine.

Dosage and Clinical Guidelines

Clonidine is available in 0.1-, 0.2-, and 0.3-mg tablets. The usual starting dosage is 0.1 mg orally twice a day; the dosage can be raised by 0.1 mg a day to an appropriate level (up to 1.2 mg/day). Clonidine must always be tapered when it is discontinued to avoid rebound hypertension, which may occur about 20 hours after the last clonidine dose. A weekly transdermal formulation of clonidine

is available at doses of 0.1, 0.2, and 0.3 mg/day. The usual starting dosage is the 0.1-mg-a-day patch, which is changed each week for adults and every 5 days for children; the dose can be increased, as needed, every 1 to 2 weeks. The transition from the oral to the transdermal formulations should be accomplished gradually by overlapping them for 3 to 4 days.

Guanfacine is available in 1- and 2-mg tablets. The usual starting dosage is 1 mg before sleep, and this can be increased to 2 mg before sleep after 3 to 4 weeks, if necessary. Regardless of the indication for which clonidine or guanfacine is being used, the drug should be withheld if a person becomes hypotensive (BP below 90/60 mm Hg).

An extended-release preparation of guanfacine (Intuniv) is also available. Extended-release guanfacine should be dosed once daily. Tablets should not be crushed, chewed, or broken before swallowing because this will increase the rate of guanfacine release. It should not be administered with high-fat meals due to increased exposure. The extended-release formulation should not be substituted for immediate-release guanfacine tablets on a milligram-per-milligram basis because of differing pharmacokinetic profiles. If switching from immediate-release guanfacine, discontinue that treatment, and titrate with extended-release guanfacine according to the following recommended schedule:

1. Begin at a dose of 1 mg/day, and adjust in increments of no more than 1 mg/wk for both monotherapy and adjunctive therapy to a psychostimulant.
2. For both monotherapy and adjunctive therapy (with a stimulant), maintain the dose within the range of 1 to 4 mg once daily, depending on clinical response and tolerability. In clinical trials, patients were randomized or dose optimized to doses of 1, 2, 3, or 4 mg and received extended-release guanfacine once daily in the morning in monotherapy trials and once daily in the morning or the evening in the adjunctive therapy trial.
3. In monotherapy trials, clinically relevant improvements were observed beginning at doses in the range 0.05 to 0.08 mg/kg once daily. Efficacy increased with increasing weight-adjusted dose (mg/kg). If well tolerated, doses up to 0.12 mg/kg once daily may provide additional benefit. Doses above 4 mg/day have not been systematically studied in controlled clinical trials.
4. In the adjunctive trial, the majority of subjects reached optimal doses in the 0.05 to 0.12 mg/kg/day range.

In clinical trials, there were dose-related and exposure-related risks for several clinically significant adverse reactions (e.g., hypotension, bradycardia, sedative events). Thus, consideration should be given to dosing an extended-release preparation of guanfacine on a milligram-per-kilogram basis in order to balance the exposure-related potential benefits and risks of treatment.

▲ 21.8 Drugs Used for Cognitive Enhancement

CHOLINESTERASE INHIBITORS

Donepezil (Aricept), rivastigmine (Exelon), and galantamine (Reminyl) are cholinesterase inhibitors used to treat mild to moderate cognitive impairment in dementia of the Alzheimer type. They reduce the inactivation of the neurotransmitter acetylcholine and, thus, potentiate cholinergic neurotransmission, which in turn produces a modest improvement in memory and goal-directed thought. Memantine (Namenda) is not a cholinesterase inhibitor, producing its effects through blockade of NMDA receptors. Unlike the cholinesterase inhibitors, which are indicated for the mild to moderate stages of Alzheimer disease, memantine is indicated for the moderate to severe stages of the disease. Tacrine (Cognex), the first cholinesterase inhibitor to be introduced, is no longer used because of its multiple-daily dosing regimens, its potential for hepatotoxicity, and the consequent need for frequent laboratory monitoring. Clinicians often combine a cholinesterase inhibitor with memantine, as this combination may provide a beneficial response compared with only cholinesterase inhibitor pharmacotherapy.

Pharmacologic Actions

Donepezil is entirely absorbed from the GI tract. Peak plasma concentrations are reached about 3 to 4 hours after oral dosing. The half-life of donepezil is 70 hours in elderly persons, and it is taken only once daily. Steady-state levels are achieved within about 2 weeks. The presence of stable alcoholic cirrhosis reduces the clearance of donepezil by 20 percent. Rivastigmine (Exelon) is rapidly and completely absorbed from the GI tract and reaches peak plasma concentrations in 1 hour, but this is delayed by up to 90 minutes if rivastigmine is taken with food. The half-life of rivastigmine is 1 hour, but because it remains bound to cholinesterases, a single dose is therapeutically active for 10 hours, and it is taken twice daily. Galantamine (Reminyl) is an alkaloid similar to codeine and is extracted from daffodils of the plant *Galanthus nivalis*. It is readily absorbed, with maximum concentrations reached after 30 minutes to 2 hours. Food decreases the maximum concentration by 25 percent. The elimination half-life of galantamine is approximately 6 hours.

Tacrine (Cognex) is absorbed rapidly from the GI tract. Peak plasma concentrations are reached about 90 minutes after oral dosing. The half-life of tacrine is about 2 to 4 hours, thereby necessitating four-times-daily dosing.

Cholinesterase inhibitors are reversible, nonacylating inhibitors of either acetylcholinesterase or butyrylcholinesterase, the enzymes that catabolize choline-based esthers in the CNS. The enzyme inhibition increases synaptic concentrations of acetylcholine, especially in the hippocampus and cerebral cortex. Unlike tacrine, which is nonselective for all forms of acetylcholinesterase, donepezil appears to be selectively active within the CNS and has little activity in the periphery. Donepezil's favorable side effect profile appears to correlate with its lack of inhibition of cholinesterases in the GI tract. Rivastigmine appears to have somewhat more peripheral activity than donepezil and is thus more likely to cause GI adverse effects than is donepezil.

Therapeutic Indications

Cholinesterase inhibitors are effective for the treatment of mild to moderate cognitive impairment in dementia of the Alzheimer type. In long-term use, they slow the progression of memory loss and diminish apathy, depression, hallucinations, anxiety, euphoria, and purposeless motor behaviors. Functional autonomy is less well preserved. Some persons note an immediate improvement in memory, mood, psychotic symptoms, and interpersonal skills. Others note little initial benefit but can retain their cognitive and adaptive faculties at a relatively stable level for many months. A practical benefit of cholinesterase inhibitor use is a delay or reduction of the need for nursing home placement.

Donepezil and rivastigmine may be beneficial for patients with Parkinson disease and Lewy body disease and treatment of cognitive deficits caused by traumatic brain injury. Donepezil is under study for the treatment of mild cognitive impairment that is less severe than that caused by Alzheimer disease. People with vascular dementia may respond to acetylcholinesterase inhibitors. Occasionally, cholinesterase inhibitors elicit an idiosyncratic catastrophic reaction, with signs of grief and agitation, which is self-limited after the drug is discontinued. The use of cholinesterase inhibitors to improve cognition by nondemented individuals should be discouraged.

Precautions and Adverse Reactions

Donepezil.   Donepezil is generally well tolerated at recommended dosages. Fewer than 3 percent of those taking donepezil experience nausea, diarrhea, and vomiting. These mild symptoms are more frequent with a 10-mg dose than with a 5-mg dose, and when present, they tend to resolve after 3 weeks of continued use. Donepezil may cause weight loss. Donepezil treatment has been infrequently associated with bradyarrhythmias, especially in those with underlying cardiac disease. A small number of persons experience syncope.

Rivastigmine.   Rivastigmine is generally well tolerated but recommended dosages may need to be scaled back in the initial period of treatment to limit GI and CNS adverse effects. These mild symptoms are more common at dosages above 6 mg a day, and when present, they tend to resolve after the dosage is lowered. The most common adverse effects associated with rivastigmine are nausea, vomiting, dizziness, headache, diarrhea, abdominal pain, anorexia, fatigue, and somnolence. Rivastigmine may cause weight loss, but it does not appear to cause hepatic, renal, hematologic, or electrolyte abnormalities.

Galantamine.   The most common side effects of galantamine are dizziness, headache, nausea, vomiting, diarrhea, and anorexia. These side effects tend to be mild and transient.

Tacrine.   Tacrine is the least used of the cholinesterase inhibitors but requires more discussion than the others because it is cumbersome to titrate and use, and it poses the risk of potentially significant elevations in hepatic transaminase levels. These increases occur in 25 to 30 percent of persons. Aside from elevated transaminase levels, the most common specific adverse effects associated with tacrine treatment are nausea, vomiting, myalgia, anorexia, and rash, but only nausea, vomiting, and anorexia have been found to have a clear relation to the dosage. Transaminase elevations characteristically develop during the first 6 to 12 weeks of treatment, and cholinergically mediated events are dosage related.

HEPATOTOXICITY.   Tacrine is associated with increases in the plasma activities of alanine aminotransferase (ALT) and aspartate aminotransferase (AST). The ALT measurement is the more sensitive indicator of the hepatic effects of tacrine. About 95 percent of patients who develop elevated ALT serum levels do so in the first 18 weeks of treatment. The average length of time for elevated ALT concentrations to return to normal after stopping tacrine treatment is 4 weeks.

For routine monitoring of hepatic enzymes, AST and ALT activities should be measured weekly for the first 18 weeks, every month for the second 4 months, and every 3 months after that. Weekly assessments of AST and ALT should be performed for at least 6 weeks after an increase in dosage. Patients with mildly elevated ALT activity should be monitored weekly and not be rechallenged

Table 21-56
Incidence of Major Adverse Side Effects with Cholinesterase Inhibitors (%)

Drug	Dose (mg/day)	Nausea	Vomiting	Diarrhea	Dizziness	Muscle Cramps	Insomnia
Donepezil	5	4	3	9	15	9	7
Donepezil	10	17	10	17	13	12	8
Rivastigmine	1–4	14	7	10	15	NR	NR
Rivastigmine	6–12	48	27	17	24	NR	NR
Galantamine	8	5.7	3.6	5	NR	NR	NR
Galantamine	16	13.3	6.1	12.2	NR	NR	NR
Galantamine	24	16.5	9.9	5.5	NR	NR	NR

NR, not reported from clinical trial data; incidence less than 5%.

with tacrine until the ALT activity returns to the normal range. For any patient with elevated ALT activity and jaundice, tacrine treatment should be stopped, and the patient should not be given the drug again.

Table 21-56 summarizes the incidence of significant adverse side effects associated with each of the cholinesterase inhibitors.

Drug Interactions. All cholinesterase inhibitors should be used cautiously with drugs that also possess cholinomimetic activity. Such drugs include succinylcholine (Anectine) and bethanechol (Urecholine). The coadministration of cholinesterase inhibitors and drugs that have cholinergic antagonist activity (e.g., tricyclic drugs) is probably counterproductive. Paroxetine is the most anticholinergic of the SSRIs, and we avoid it in patients taking cholinesterase inhibitors.

Donepezil undergoes extensive metabolism via both CYP2D6 and 3A4 isozymes. The metabolism of donepezil may be increased by phenytoin (Dilantin), carbamazepine (Tegretol), dexamethasone (Decadron), rifampin (Rifadin), and phenobarbital (Solfoton). Commonly used agents such as paroxetine, ketoconazole (Nizoral), and erythromycin can significantly increase donepezil concentrations. Donepezil is highly protein-bound, but it does not displace other protein-bound drugs, such as furosemide (Lasix), digoxin (Lanoxin), or warfarin (Coumadin). Rivastigmine circulates mostly unbound to serum proteins and has no significant drug interactions.

Similar to donepezil, galantamine is metabolized by both CYP2D6 and 3A4 isozymes and thus may interact with drugs that inhibit these pathways. Paroxetine and ketoconazole should be used with great caution.

Laboratory Interferences. No laboratory interferences have been associated with the use of cholinesterase inhibitors.

Dosage and Clinical Guidelines. Before initiation of cholinesterase inhibitor therapy, potentially treatable causes of dementia should be ruled out, and the diagnosis of dementia of the Alzheimer type established.

Donepezil is available in 5- and 10-mg tablets. Treatment should be initiated at 5 mg each night. If well tolerated and of some discernible benefit after 4 weeks, the dosage should be increased to a maintenance dosage of 10-mg each night. Donepezil absorption is unaffected by meals.

Rivastigmine is available in 1.5-, 3-, 4.5-, and 6-mg capsules. The recommended initial dosage is 1.5 mg twice daily for a minimum of 2 weeks, after which increases of 1.5 mg a day can be made at intervals of at least 2 weeks to a target dosage of 6 mg a day, taken in two equal dosages. If tolerated, the dosage may be further titrated upward to a maximum of 6 mg twice daily. The administration of rivastigmine with food can reduce the risk of adverse GI events.

Galantamine is available in 4-, 8-, and 16-mg tablets. The suggested dose range is 16 to 32 mg/day given twice a day. The higher dose is better tolerated than lower doses. The initial dosage is 8 mg/day, and after a minimum of 4 weeks, the dose can be raised. All subsequent dosage increases should occur at 4-week intervals and should be based on tolerability.

Tacrine is available in 10-, 20-, 30-, and 40-mg capsules. Before the initiation of tacrine treatment, a complete physical and laboratory examination should be conducted, with particular attention to liver function tests and baseline hematologic indexes. Treatment should be initiated at 10 mg four times a day and then raised by increments of 10 mg a dose every 6 weeks up to 160 mg a day; the person's tolerance of each dosage is indicated by the absence of unacceptable side effects and lack of elevation of ALT activity. Tacrine should be given four times daily—ideally 1 hour before meals because the absorption of tacrine is reduced by about 25 percent when it is taken during the first 2 hours after meals. If tacrine is used, the specific guidelines for tacrine-induced ALT listed above should be followed.

MEMANTINE

Pharmacologic Actions

Memantine is well absorbed after oral administration. It reaches peak concentrations in about 3 to 7 hours. Food does not affect the absorption of memantine. Memantine has linear pharmacokinetics over the therapeutic dosage range and has a terminal elimination half-life of about 60 to 80 hours. Plasma protein binding is 45 percent.

Memantine undergoes little metabolism, with the majority (57 to 82 percent) of an administered dose excreted unchanged in the urine; the remainder is converted primarily to three polar metabolites: the N-gludantan conjugate, 6-hydroxy memantine, and 1-nitroso-deaminated memantine. These metabolites possess minimal NMDA receptor antagonist activity. Memantine is a low- to moderate-affinity NMDA receptor antagonist. It is thought that the overexcitation of NMDA receptors by the neurotransmitter glutamate may play a role in Alzheimer disease because glutamate plays an integral role in the neural pathways associated with learning and memory. Excess glutamate overstimulates NMDA receptors to allow too much calcium into nerve cells, leading to the eventual cell death observed in Alzheimer disease. Memantine may protect cells against excess glutamate by partially blocking NMDA receptors associated with the abnormal transmission of glutamate while allowing for physiologic transmission associated with normal cell functioning.

Therapeutic Indications

Memantine is the only approved therapy in the United States for moderate to severe Alzheimer disease.

Precautions and Adverse Reactions

Memantine is safe and well tolerated. The most common adverse effects are dizziness, headache, constipation, and confusion. The use of memantine in patients with severe renal impairment is not recommended. In a documented case of an overdose with up to 400 mg of memantine, the patient experienced restlessness, psychosis, visual hallucinations, somnolence, stupor, and loss of consciousness. The patient recovered without permanent sequelae.

Drug Interactions

In vitro studies conducted with marker substrates of CYP450 enzymes (CYP1A2, 2A6, 2C9, 2D6, 2E1, and 3A4) showed minimal inhibition of these enzymes by memantine. No pharmacokinetic interactions with drugs metabolized by these enzymes are expected.

Because memantine is eliminated in part by tubular secretion, coadministration of drugs that use the same renal cationic system, including hydrochlorothiazide triamterene (Dyrenium), cimetidine (Tagamet), ranitidine (Zantac), quinidine, and nicotine, could potentially result in altered plasma levels of both agents. Coadministration of memantine with a combination of hydrochlorothiazide and triamterene did not affect the bioavailability of either memantine or triamterene, and the bioavailability of hydrochlorothiazide decreased by 20 percent.

Urine pH is altered by diet, drugs (e.g., carbonic anhydrase inhibitors, topiramate [Topamax], sodium bicarbonate), and the clinical state of the patient (e.g., renal tubular acidosis or severe infections of the urinary tract). The clearance of memantine is reduced by about 80 percent under alkaline urine conditions at pH 8. Therefore, alterations of urine pH toward the alkaline condition may lead to an accumulation of the drug with a possible increase in adverse effects. Hence, memantine should be used with caution under these conditions.

Laboratory Interferences

No laboratory interferences have been associated with the use of memantine.

Dosage and Clinical Guidelines

Memantine is available in 5- and 10-mg tablets, with a recommended starting dose of 5 mg daily. The recommended target dose is 20 mg/day. The drug is administered twice daily in separate doses with 5-mg increment increases weekly depending on tolerability.

Patients with mild to moderate disease receiving memantine in combination with a cholinesterase inhibitor have not been found to experience significantly greater benefit in cognition or overall function than those who receive a cholinesterase inhibitor alone.

▲ 21.9 Drugs Used to Treat Sexual Disorders

PHOSPHODIESTERASE-5 INHIBITORS

Phosphodiesterase (PDE)-5 inhibitors, such as sildenafil (Viagra), which was developed in 1998, revolutionized the treatment of erectile disorder. Two congeners have since come on the market—vardenafil (Levitra) and tadalafil (Cialis). All have a similar method of action and have changed people's expectations of sexual functioning. Although indicated only for the treatment of male erectile dysfunction, there is anecdotal evidence of these drugs being effective in women. They are also being misused as recreational drugs to enhance sexual performance. These drugs have been used by more than 20 million men around the world.

The development of sildenafil provided important information about the physiology of erection. Sexual stimulation causes the release of the neurotransmitter nitric oxide (NO), which increases the synthesis of cyclic guanosine monophosphate (cGMP), causing smooth muscle relaxation in the corpus cavernosum that allows blood to flow into the penis and results in turgidity and tumescence. The concentration of cGMP is regulated by the enzyme PDE-5, which, when inhibited, allows cGMP to increase and enhance erectile function. Because sexual stimulation is required to cause the release of NO, PDE-5 inhibitors do not affect in the absence of such stimulation, an important point to understand when providing information to patients about their use. The congeners vardenafil and tadalafil work in the same way, by inhibiting PDE-5, thus allowing an increase in cGMP and enhancing the vasodilatory effects of NO. For this reason, these drugs are sometimes referred to as NO enhancers.

Pharmacologic Actions

All three substances are relatively rapidly absorbed from the GI tract, with maximum plasma concentrations reached in 30 to 120 minutes (median, 60 minutes) in the fasting state. Because it is lipophilic, concomitant ingestion of a high-fat meal delays the rate of absorption by up to 60 minutes and reduces the peak concentration by one-quarter. These drugs are principally metabolized by the CYP3A4 system, which may lead to clinically significant drug–drug interactions, not all of which have been documented. Excretion of 80 percent of the dose is via feces, and another 13 percent is eliminated in the urine. Elimination is reduced in persons older than age 65 years, which results in plasma concentrations 40 percent higher than in persons ages 18 to 45 years. Elimination is also reduced in the presence of severe renal or hepatic insufficiency.

The mean half-lives of sildenafil and vardenafil are 3 to 4 hours, and that of tadalafil is about 18 hours. Tadalafil can be detected in the bloodstream 5 days after ingestion, and because of its long half-life, it has been marketed as effective for up to 36 hours—the so-called weekend pill. The onset of sildenafil occurs about 30 minutes after ingestion on an empty stomach; tadalafil and vardenafil act somewhat more quickly.

Clinicians need to be aware of the crucial clinical observation that these drugs do not by themselves create an erection. Instead, the mental state of sexual arousal brought on by erotic stimulation must first lead to activity in the penile nerves, which then release NO into the cavernosum, triggering the erectile cascade, the resulting erection being prolonged by the NO enhancers. Thus, a full advantage may be taken of a sexually exciting stimulus, but the drug is not a substitute for foreplay and emotional arousal.

Therapeutic Indications

Erectile dysfunctions have traditionally been classified as organic, psychogenic, or mixed. Over the past 20 years, the prevailing view of the cause of erectile dysfunction has shifted away from psychological causes toward organic causes. The latter include diabetes mellitus, hypertension, hypercholesterolemia, cigarette smoking, peripheral vascular disease, pelvic or spinal cord injury, pelvic or abdominal surgery (especially prostate surgery), multiple sclerosis, peripheral neuropathy, and Parkinson disease. Erectile dysfunction is often induced by alcohol, nicotine, and other substances of abuse and prescription drugs.

These drugs are effective regardless of the baseline severity of erectile dysfunction, race, or age. Among those responding to sildenafil are men with coronary artery disease, hypertension, other cardiac diseases, peripheral vascular disease, diabetes mellitus, depression, coronary artery bypass graft surgery, radical prostatectomy, transurethral resection of the prostate, spina bifida, and spinal cord injury, as well as persons taking antidepressants, antipsychotics, antihypertensives, and diuretics. However, the response rate is variable.

Sildenafil has been reported to reverse SSRI-induced anorgasmia in men. There are anecdotal reports of sildenafil having a therapeutic effect on sexual inhibition in women as well.

Precautions and Adverse Reactions

A significant potential adverse effect associated with the use of these drugs is myocardial infarction (MI). The U.S. FDA distinguished the risk of MI caused directly by these drugs from that caused by underlying conditions such as hypertension, atherosclerotic heart disease, diabetes mellitus, and other atherogenic conditions. The FDA concluded that when used according to the approved labeling, the drugs do not by themselves confer an increased risk of death. However, there is increased oxygen demand and stress placed on the cardiac muscle by sexual intercourse. Thus, coronary perfusion may be severely compromised, and cardiac failure may occur as a result. For that reason, any person with a history of MI, stroke, renal failure, hypertension, or diabetes mellitus and any person older than the age of 70 years should discuss plans to use these drugs with an internist or a cardiologist. The cardiac evaluation should specifically address exercise tolerance and the use of nitrates.

The use of PDE-5 inhibitors is contraindicated in persons who are taking organic nitrates in any form. Also, amyl nitrate (poppers), a popular substance of abuse used by gay men to enhance the intensity of orgasm, should not be used with any of the erection-enhancing drugs. The combination of organic nitrates and PDE inhibitors can cause a precipitous lowering of BP and can reduce coronary perfusion to the point of causing MI and death.

Adverse effects are dose-dependent, occurring at higher rates with higher dosages. The most common adverse effects are headache, flushing, and stomach pain. Other less common adverse effects include nasal congestion, urinary tract infection, abnormal vision (colored tinge [usually blue], increased sensitivity to light, or blurred vision), diarrhea, dizziness, and rash. No cases of priapism were reported in premarketing trials. Supportive management is indicated in cases of overdosage. Tadalafil has been associated with back and muscle pain in about 10 percent of patients.

Recently, there have been 50 reports and 14 verified cases of a severe condition in men taking sildenafil called nonarteritic anterior ischemic optic neuropathy. This condition is an eye ailment that causes restriction of blood flow to the optic nerve and can result in permanent vision loss. The first symptoms appear within 24 hours after the use of sildenafil and include blurred vision and some degree of vision loss. The incidence of this effect is infrequent—1 in 1 million. In the reported cases, many patients had preexisting eye problems that may have increased their risk, and many had a history of heart disease and diabetes, which may indicate vulnerability in these men to endothelial damage.

In 2010, possible hearing loss was reported based on 29 incidents of the problem since the introduction of these drugs. Hearing loss usually occurs within hours or days of using the drug. In some cases, the loss is both unilateral and temporary.

No data are available on the effects on human fetal growth and development or testicular morphologic or functional changes. However, because these drugs are not considered an essential treatment, they should not be used during pregnancy.

Treatment of Priapism

Phenylephrine (Neo-Synephrine) is the drug of choice and first-line treatment of priapism, because the drug has almost pure α-agonist effects and minimal β activity. In short-term priapism (less than 6 hours), especially for drug-induced priapism, intracavernosal injection of phenylephrine can be used to cause detumescence. A mixture of 1 ampule of phenylephrine (1 mL/1,000 μg) should be diluted with an additional 9 mL of normal saline. 0.3 to 0.5 mL should be injected into the corpora cavernosa, using a 29-gauge needle with 10 to 15 minutes between injections. Vital signs should be monitored, and compression should be applied to the area of injection to help prevent hematoma formation.

Phenylephrine can also be used orally, 10 to 20 mg every 4 hours as needed, but it may not be as effective or act as rapidly as the injectable route.

Drug Interactions

The primary route of PDE-5 metabolism is through CYP3A4, and the minor route is through CYP2C9. Inducers or inhibitors of these enzymes will therefore affect the plasma concentration and half-life of sildenafil. For example, 800 mg of cimetidine (Tagamet), a nonspecific CYP inhibitor, increases plasma sildenafil concentrations by 56 percent, and erythromycin (E-mycin) increases plasma sildenafil concentrations by 182 percent. Other, more potent inhibitors of CYP3A4 include ketoconazole (Nizoral), itraconazole (Sporanox), and mibefradil (Posicor). In contrast, rifampicin, a CYP3A4 inducer, decreases plasma concentrations of sildenafil.

Laboratory Interferences

No laboratory interferences have been described.

Dosage and Clinical Guidelines

Sildenafil is available as 25-, 50-, and 100-mg tablets. The recommended dose of sildenafil is 50 mg taken by mouth 1 hour before intercourse. However, sildenafil may take effect within 30 minutes. The duration of the effect is usually 4 hours, but in healthy young men, the effect may persist for 8 to 12 hours. Based on effectiveness and adverse effects, the dose should be titrated between 25 and 100 mg. Sildenafil is recommended for use no more than once a day. The dosing guidelines for use by women as off-label use are the same as those for men.

Increased plasma concentrations of sildenafil may occur in persons older than 65 years of age and those with cirrhosis or severe renal impairment or using CYP3A4 inhibitors. A starting dose of 25 mg should be used in these circumstances.

An investigational nasal spray formulation of sildenafil has been developed that acts within 5 to 15 minutes of administration. This formulation is highly water-soluble, and it is rapidly absorbed directly into the bloodstream. Such a formulation would permit more ease of use.

Vardenafil is supplied in 2.5-, 5-, 10-, and 20-mg tablets. The initial dose is usually 10 mg taken with or without food about 1 hour before sexual activity. The dose can be increased to a maximum of 20 mg or decreased to 5 mg based on efficacy and side effects. The maximum dosing frequency is once per day. As with sildenafil, dosages may have to be adjusted in patients with hepatic impairment or patients using specific CYP3A4 inhibitors. A 10 mg orally disintegrating form of vardenafil (Staxyn) is available. It is placed on the tongue approximately 60 minutes before sexual activity and should not be used more than once a day.

Tadalafil is available in 2.5-, 5-, or 20-mg tablets for oral administration. The recommended dose of tadalafil is 10 mg before sexual activity, which may be increased to 20 mg or decreased to 5 mg depending on efficacy and side effects. Once-a-day use of the 2.5- or 5-mg pill is acceptable for most patients. Similar cautions apply as mentioned earlier in patients with hepatic impairment and those taking concomitant potent inhibitors of CYP3A4. As with other PDE-5 inhibitors, concomitant use of nitrates in any form is contraindicated.

YOHIMBINE

Yohimbine (Yocon) is an α_2-adrenergic receptor antagonist that is used as a treatment for both idiopathic and medication-induced erectile disorder. Currently, sildenafil (Viagra) and its congeners and alprostadil (Impulse, Edex) are considered more efficacious for this indication than yohimbine. Yohimbine is derived from an alkaloid found in *Rubiaceae* and related trees and the *Rauwolfia serpentina* plant.

Pharmacologic Actions

Yohimbine is erratically absorbed after oral administration, with bioavailability ranging from 7 to 87 percent. There is extensive hepatic first-pass metabolism. Yohimbine affects the sympathomimetic autonomic nervous system by increasing plasma concentrations of norepinephrine. The half-life of yohimbine is 0.5 to 2 hours. Clinically, yohimbine produces increased parasympathetic (cholinergic) tone.

Therapeutic Indications

Yohimbine has been used to treat erectile dysfunction. Penile erection has been linked to cholinergic activity and to the α_2-adrenergic blockade, which theoretically results in an increased penile inflow of blood, decreased penile outflow of blood, or both. Yohimbine is reported to help counteract the loss of sexual desire and the orgasmic inhibition caused by some serotonergic antidepressants (e.g., SSRIs). It has not been found useful in women for these indications.

Precautions

The side effects of yohimbine include anxiety, elevated BP and heart rate, increased psychomotor activity, irritability, tremor, headache, skin flushing, dizziness, urinary frequency, nausea, vomiting, and sweating. Patients with panic disorder show heightened sensitivity to yohimbine and experience increased anxiety, increased BP, and increased plasma 3-methoxy-4-hydroxyphenylglycol (MHPG).

Yohimbine should be used with caution in female patients and should not be used in patients with renal disease, cardiac disease, glaucoma, or a history of gastric or duodenal ulcers.

Drug Interactions

Yohimbine blocks the effects of clonidine, guanfacine, and other α_2-receptor agonists.

Laboratory Interferences

No known laboratory interferences are associated with yohimbine use.

Dosage and Clinical Guidelines

Yohimbine is available in 5.4-mg tablets. The dosage of yohimbine in the treatment of erectile disorder is approximately 16 mg a day, given in doses that range from 2.7 to 5.4 mg three times a day. In the event of significant adverse effects, the dose should first be reduced and then gradually increased again. Yohimbine should be used judiciously in psychiatric patients because it may worsen their mental status. Because yohimbine has no consistent effect on erectile dysfunction, its use remains controversial. Phosphodiesterase-5 (PDE-5) inhibitors are the preferred medication for this disorder.

▲ 21.10 Drugs Used to Treat the Side Effects of Psychotropic Drugs

ANTICHOLINERGIC AGENTS

Anticholinergic drugs block the actions of atropine. In the clinical practice of psychiatry, the anticholinergic drugs are primarily used to treat medication-induced movement disorders, particularly neuroleptic-induced parkinsonism, neuroleptic-induced acute dystonia, and medication-induced postural tremor.

Anticholinergics

Pharmacologic Actions. All anticholinergic drugs are well absorbed from the GI tract after oral administration, and all are sufficiently lipophilic to enter the CNS. Trihexyphenidyl (Artane) and benztropine (Cogentin) reach peak plasma concentrations in 2 to 3 hours after oral administration, and their duration of action is 1 to 12 hours. Benztropine is absorbed equally rapidly by intramuscular (IM) and intravenous (IV) administration; IM administration is preferred because of its low risk for adverse effects.

All six anticholinergic drugs listed in this section (Table 21-57) block muscarinic acetylcholine receptors, and benztropine has some antihistaminergic effects. None of the available anticholinergic drugs has any effect on the nicotinic acetylcholine receptors. Of these drugs, trihexyphenidyl is the most stimulating agent, perhaps acting through dopaminergic neurons, and

Table 21-57
Anticholinergic Drugs

Generic Name	Brand Name	Tablet Size	Injectable	Usual Daily Oral Dosage	Short-Term Intramuscular or Intravenous Dosage
Benztropine	Cogentin	0.5, 1, 2 mg	1 mg/mL	1–4 mg one to three times	1–2 mg
Biperiden	Akineton	2 mg	5 mg/mL	2 mg one to three times	2 mg
Ethopropazine	Parsidol	10, 50 mg	—	50–100 mg one to three times	—
Orphenadrine	Norflex, Disipal	100 mg	30 mg/mL	50–100 mg three times	60 mg IV given over 5 min
Procyclidine	Kemadrin	5 mg	—	2.5–5 mg three times	—
Trihexyphenidyl	Artane, Trihexane, Trihexy-5	2, 5 mg elixir 2 mg/5 mL	—	2–5 mg two to four times	—

IV, intravenous.

benztropine is the least stimulating and thus is least associated with abuse potential.

Therapeutic Indications. The primary indication for the use of anticholinergics in psychiatric practice is for the treatment of *neuroleptic-induced parkinsonism,* characterized by tremor, rigidity, cogwheeling, bradykinesia, sialorrhea, stooped posture, and festination. All of the available anticholinergics are equally effective in the treatment of parkinsonian symptoms. Neuroleptic-induced parkinsonism is most common in elderly persons and is most frequently seen with high-potency DRAs, for example, haloperidol (Haldol). The onset of symptoms usually occurs after 2 or 3 weeks of treatment. The incidence of neuroleptic-induced parkinsonism is lower with the newer antipsychotic drugs of the SDA class.

Another indication for the use of anticholinergics is for the treatment of *neuroleptic-induced acute dystonia,* which is most common in young men. The syndrome often occurs early in the course of treatment; it is commonly associated with high-potency DRAs (e.g., haloperidol); and most commonly affects the muscles of the neck, tongue, face, and back. Anticholinergic drugs are useful both in the short-term treatment of dystonias and in prophylaxis against neuroleptic-induced acute dystonias.

Akathisia is characterized by a subjective and objective sense of restlessness, anxiety, and agitation. Although a trial of anticholinergics for the treatment of neuroleptic-induced acute akathisia is reasonable, these drugs are not generally considered as effective as the β-adrenergic receptor antagonists, the benzodiazepines, and clonidine (Catapres).

Precautions and Adverse Reactions. The adverse effects of the anticholinergic drugs result from the blockade of muscarinic acetylcholine receptors. Anticholinergic drugs should be used cautiously, if at all, by persons with prostatic hypertrophy, urinary retention, and narrow-angle glaucoma. The anticholinergics are occasionally used as drugs of abuse because of their mild mood-elevating properties, most notably, trihexyphenidyl.

The most severe adverse effect associated with anticholinergic toxicity is anticholinergic intoxication. The intoxication includes symptoms of delirium, coma, seizures, agitation, hallucinations, severe hypotension, supraventricular tachycardia, and peripheral manifestations (flushing, mydriasis, dry skin, hyperthermia, and decreased bowel sounds). Treatment should begin with the immediate discontinuation of all anticholinergic drugs. We can both diagnose and treat anticholinergic intoxication with physostigmine (Antilirium, Eserine), an inhibitor of anticholinesterase, 1 to 2 mg

IV (1 mg every 2 minutes) or IM every 30 or 60 minutes. Because physostigmine can lead to severe hypotension and bronchial constriction, it should be used only in severe cases, and only when emergency cardiac monitoring and life-support services are available.

Drug Interactions. The most common drug–drug interactions with the anticholinergics occur when they are coadministered with psychotropics that also have high anticholinergic activity, such as DRAs, tricyclic and tetracyclic drugs, and MAOIs. Many other prescription drugs and over-the-counter cold preparations also induce significant anticholinergic activity. The coadministration of those drugs can result in a life-threatening anticholinergic intoxication syndrome. Also, anticholinergic drugs can delay gastric emptying, thereby decreasing the absorption of drugs that are broken down in the stomach and usually absorbed in the duodenum (e.g., levodopa [Larodopa] and DRAs).

Laboratory Interferences. No known laboratory interferences have been associated with anticholinergics.

Dosage and Clinical Guidelines. The six anticholinergic drugs discussed in this chapter are available in a range of preparations (see Table 21-57).

NEUROLEPTIC-INDUCED PARKINSONISM. For the treatment of neuroleptic-induced parkinsonism, the equivalent of 1 to 3 mg of benztropine should be given one to two times daily. The anticholinergic drug should be administered for 4 to 8 weeks, and then it should be discontinued to assess whether the person still requires the drug. Anticholinergic drugs should be tapered over 1 to 2 weeks.

Treatment with anticholinergics as prophylaxis against the development of neuroleptic-induced parkinsonism is usually not indicated because the onset of its symptoms is usually sufficiently mild and gradual to allow the clinician to initiate treatment only after it is indicated. In young men, prophylaxis may be indicated, however, mainly if a high-potency DRA is being used. The clinician should attempt to discontinue the antiparkinsonian agent in 4 to 6 weeks to assess whether its continued use is necessary.

NEUROLEPTIC-INDUCED ACUTE DYSTONIA. For the short-term treatment and prophylaxis of neuroleptic-induced acute dystonia, 1 to 2 mg of benztropine or its equivalent in another drug should be given IM. The dose can be repeated in 20 to 30 minutes, as needed. If the person still does not improve in another 20 to 30 minutes, a benzodiazepine (e.g., 1 mg IM or IV lorazepam

[Ativan]) should be given. Laryngeal dystonia is a medical emergency and should be treated with benztropine, up to 4 mg in 10 minutes, followed by 1 to 2 mg of lorazepam, administered slowly by the IV route.

Prophylaxis against dystonias is indicated in persons who have had one episode or in persons at high risk (young men taking high-potency DRAs). Prophylactic treatment is given for 4 to 8 weeks and then gradually tapered over 1 to 2 weeks to allow assessment of its continued need. The prophylactic use of anticholinergics in persons requiring antipsychotic drugs has mostly become a moot issue because of the availability of SDAs, which are relatively free of parkinsonian effects.

AKATHISIA.   As mentioned, anticholinergics are not the drugs of choice for this syndrome. The β-adrenergic receptor antagonists and perhaps the benzodiazepines and clonidine are preferable drugs to try initially.

ANTIHISTAMINES

Antihistamines are frequently used in the treatment of a variety of psychiatric disorders because of their sedative and anticholinergic activities. Certain antihistamines (antagonists of histamine H_1 receptors) are used to treat neuroleptic-induced parkinsonism and neuroleptic-induced acute dystonia and as hypnotics and anxiolytics. Diphenhydramine (Benadryl) is used to treat neuroleptic-induced parkinsonism and neuroleptic-induced acute dystonia and sometimes as a hypnotic. Hydroxyzine hydrochloride (Atarax) and hydroxyzine pamoate (Vistaril) are used as anxiolytics. Promethazine (Phenergan) is used for its sedative and anxiolytic effects. Cyproheptadine (Periactin) has been used for the treatment of anorexia nervosa and inhibited male and female orgasms caused by serotonergic agents. The antihistamines most commonly used in psychiatry are listed in Table 21-58. Second-generation, "nonsedating" H_1 blockers, such as fexofenadine (Allegra), loratadine (Claritin), and cetirizine (Zyrtec) are less commonly used in psychiatric practice. The H_2-receptor antagonists, such as cimetidine, work primarily on gastric mucosa, inhibiting gastric secretion.

Table 21-59 lists antihistaminic drugs not used in psychiatry, but that may have psychiatric adverse effects or drug–drug interactions.

Pharmacologic Actions

The H_1 antagonists used in psychiatry are well absorbed from the GI tract. The antiparkinsonian effects of intramuscular (IM) diphenhydramine have their onset in 15 to 30 minutes and the sedative effects of diphenhydramine peak in 1 to 3 hours. The sedative effects of hydroxyzine and promethazine begin after 20 to 60 minutes and last for 4 to 6 hours. Because all three drugs are metabolized in the liver, persons with hepatic disease, such as cirrhosis, may attain

Table 21-58
Histamine Antagonists Commonly Used in Psychiatry

Generic Name	Trade Name	Duration of Action (hr)
Diphenhydramine	Benadryl	4–6
Hydroxyzine	Atarax, Vistaril	6–24
Promethazine	Phenergan	4–6
Cyproheptadine	Periactin	4–6

Table 21-59
Other Histamine Antagonists often Prescribed

Class	Generic Name	Trade Name
Second-generation histamine 1 receptor antagonists	Cetirizine	Zyrtec
	Loratadine	Claritin
	Fexofenadine	Allegra
Histamine 2 receptor antagonists	Nizatidine	Axid
	Famotidine	Pepcid
	Ranitidine	Zantac
	Cimetidine	Tagamet

high plasma concentrations with long-term administration. Cyproheptadine is well absorbed after oral administration, and its metabolites are excreted in the urine.

Activation of H_1 receptors stimulates wakefulness; therefore, receptor antagonism causes sedation. All four agents also possess some antimuscarinic cholinergic activity. Cyproheptadine is unique among the drugs because it has both potent antihistamine and serotonin $5-HT_2$-receptor antagonist properties.

Therapeutic Indications

Antihistamines are useful as a treatment for neuroleptic-induced parkinsonism, neuroleptic-induced acute dystonia, and neuroleptic-induced akathisia. They are an alternative to anticholinergics and amantadine for these purposes. The antihistamines are relatively safe hypnotics, but they are not superior to the benzodiazepines, which have been much better studied in terms of efficacy and safety. The antihistamines have not been proven effective for long-term anxiolytic therapy; therefore, the benzodiazepines, buspirone (BuSpar), or SSRIs are preferable for such treatment. Cyproheptadine is sometimes used to treat impaired orgasms, especially delayed orgasm resulting from treatment with serotonergic drugs.

Because it promotes weight gain, cyproheptadine may be of some use in the treatment of eating disorders, such as anorexia nervosa. Cyproheptadine can reduce recurrent nightmares with posttraumatic themes. The antiserotonergic activity of cyproheptadine may counteract the serotonin syndrome caused by concomitant use of multiple serotonin-activating drugs, such as SSRIs and MAOIs.

Precautions and Adverse Reactions

Antihistamines are commonly associated with sedation, dizziness, and hypotension, all of which can be severe in elderly persons, who are also likely to experience the anticholinergic effects of those drugs. Paradoxical excitement and agitation is an adverse effect seen in a small number of persons. Poor motor coordination can result in accidents; therefore, persons should be warned about driving and operating dangerous machinery. Other common adverse effects include epigastric distress, nausea, vomiting, diarrhea, and constipation. Because of mild anticholinergic activity, some people experience dry mouth, urinary retention, blurred vision, and constipation.

For this reason, also, antihistamines should be used only at very low doses, if at all, by persons with narrow-angle glaucoma or obstructive GI, prostate, or bladder conditions. Either cyproheptadine or diphenhydramine may induce a central anticholinergic syndrome with psychosis. The use of cyproheptadine in some persons has been associated with weight gain, which may contribute to its reported efficacy in some persons with anorexia nervosa.

In addition to the above adverse effects, antihistamines have some potential for abuse. The coadministration of antihistamines and opioids can increase the euphoria experienced by persons with substance use disorders. Overdoses of antihistamines can be fatal. Antihistamines are excreted in breast milk, so nursing mothers should avoid their use. Because of some potential for teratogenicity, pregnant women should avoid the use of antihistamines.

Drug Interactions

The sedative property of antihistamines can be additive with other CNS depressants, such as alcohol, other sedative-hypnotic drugs, and many psychotropic drugs, including tricyclic drugs and DRAs. Anticholinergic activity can be cumulative when using other anticholinergic drugs and may sometimes result in severe anticholinergic symptoms or intoxication.

Laboratory Interferences

H_1 antagonists may eliminate the wheal and induration that form the basis of allergy skin tests. Promethazine may interfere with pregnancy tests and may increase blood glucose concentrations. Diphenhydramine may yield a false-positive urine test result for phencyclidine (PCP). Hydroxyzine use can falsely elevate the results of specific tests for urinary 17-hydroxycorticosteroids.

Dosage and Clinical Guidelines

The antihistamines are available in a variety of preparations (Table 21-60). IM injections should be deep because superficial administration can cause local irritation.

Intravenous (IV) administration of 25 to 50 mg of diphenhydramine is an effective treatment for neuroleptic-induced acute dystonia, which may immediately disappear. Treatment with 25 mg three times a day—up to 50 mg four times a day, if necessary—can be used to treat neuroleptic-induced parkinsonism, akinesia, and buccal movements. Diphenhydramine can be used as a hypnotic at a 50-mg dose for mild transient insomnia. Doses of 100 mg are not superior to doses of 50 mg, but they produce more anticholinergic effects than doses of 50 mg.

Hydroxyzine is most commonly used as a short-term anxiolytic. Hydroxyzine should not be given IV because it is irritating to the blood vessels. Dosages of 50 to 100 mg given orally four times a day for long-term treatment or 50 to 100 mg IM every 4 to 6 hours for short-term treatment are usually effective.

SSRI-induced anorgasmia may sometimes be reversed with 4 to 16 mg a day of cyproheptadine taken by mouth 1 or 2 hours before anticipated sexual activity. Several case reports and small studies have also reported that cyproheptadine may be of some use in the treatment of eating disorders, such as anorexia nervosa. Cyproheptadine is available in 4-mg tablets and a 2-mg/5-mL solution. Children and elderly patients are more sensitive to the effects of antihistamines than are young adults.

DOPAMINE RECEPTOR AGONISTS AND PRECURSORS

Dopamine agonists activate dopamine receptors in the absence of endogenous dopamine and have been widely used to treat idiopathic Parkinson disease, hyperprolactinemia, and certain pituitary tumors (prolactinoma). Because dopamine stimulates the heart and increases blood flow to the liver, kidneys, and other organs, low levels of dopamine are associated with low BP and low cardiac

Table 21-60
Dosage and Administration of Common Histamine Antagonists

Medication	Route	Preparation	Common Dosage
Diphenhydramine (Benadryl)	PO	Capsules and tablets: 25 mg, 50 mg Liquid: 12.5 mg/5.0 mL	Adults: 25–50 mg three to four times per day Children: 5 mg/kg three to four times per day, not to exceed 300 mg/day
	Deep IM or IV	Solution: 10 or 50 mg/mL	Same as oral
Hydroxyzine Hydrochloride (Atarax)	PO	Tablets: 10, 25, 50, and 100 mg Syrup: 10 mg/5 mL	Adults: 50–100 mg three to four times daily Children younger than 6 yr of age: 2 mg/kg/day in divided doses Children older than 6 yr of age: 12.5–25.0 mg three to four times daily
	IM	Solution: 25 or 50 mg/mL	Same as oral
Hydroxyzine Pamoate (Vistaril)	PO	Suspension: 25 mg/mL Capsules: 25, 50, and 100 mg	Same as dosages for hydroxyzine hydrochloride
Promethazine (Phenergan)	PO	Tablets: 15.2, 25.0, and 50.0 mg Syrup: 3.25 mg/5 mL	Adults: 50–100 mg three to four times daily for sedation Children: 12.5–25.0 mg at night for sedation
	Rectal	Suppositories: 12.5, 25.0, and 50.0 mg	
	IM	Solution: 25 and 50 mg/mL	
Cyproheptadine (Periactin)	PO	Tablets: 4 mg Syrup: 2 mg/5 mL	Adults: 4–20 mg/day Children 2–7 yr of age: 2 mg two to three times daily (maximum, 12 mg/day) Children 7–14 yr of age: 4 mg two to three times daily (maximum of 16 mg/day)

IM, intramuscular; IV, intravenous; PO, oral.

input. Dopamine agonist drugs are also administered to treat shock and congestive heart failure.

Their use in psychiatry has been limited to treat such adverse effects of antipsychotic drugs as parkinsonism, extrapyramidal symptoms, akinesia, focal perioral tremors, hyperprolactinemia, galactorrhea, and neuroleptic malignant syndrome. The drugs in this class most commonly prescribed are bromocriptine (Parlodel), levodopa (also called L-Dopa; Larodopa), carbidopa-levodopa (Sinemet), and amantadine (Symmetrel). Amantadine is used primarily for the treatment of medication-induced movement disorders, such as neuroleptic-induced parkinsonism. It is also used as an antiviral agent for the prophylaxis and treatment of influenza A infection and Cotard syndrome, a rare neuropsychiatric disorder in which a person holds a delusional belief that he or she is dead. There are also a few reports of amantadine's role in augmenting antidepressant medications in patients with treatment-resistant depression.

New dopamine receptor agonists include ropinirole (Requip), pramipexole (Mirapex), apomorphine (Apokyn), and pergolide (Permax). Of these drugs, pramipexole is the most widely prescribed in psychiatry as an augmenter of antidepressants. In 2007, pergolide was removed from the market because of the risk of severe damage to patients' heart valves. In 2012, the U.S. FDA notified health care professionals about a possible increased risk of heart failure with pramipexole. This warning was based on studies that suggested a potential risk of heart failure; however, further review is required because of study limitations.

Pharmacologic Actions

L-Dopa is rapidly absorbed after oral administration, and peak plasma levels are reached after 30 to 120 minutes. The half-life of L-Dopa is 90 minutes. Absorption of L-Dopa can be significantly reduced by changes in gastric pH and by ingestion with meals. Bromocriptine and ropinirole are rapidly absorbed but undergo first-pass metabolism such that only about 30 to 55 percent of the dose is bioavailable. Peak concentrations are achieved 1.5 to 3 hours after oral administration. The half-life of ropinirole is 6 hours. Pramipexole is rapidly absorbed with little first-pass metabolism and reaches peak concentrations in 2 hours. Its half-life is 8 hours. Oral forms of apomorphine have been studied, but this form is not available in the United States. Subcutaneous apomorphine injection results in rapid and controlled systemic delivery, with linear pharmacokinetics over a dose ranging from 2 to 8 mg.

After L-Dopa enters the dopaminergic neurons of the CNS, it is converted into the neurotransmitter dopamine. Apomorphine, bromocriptine, ropinirole, and pramipexole act directly on dopamine receptors. L-Dopa, pramipexole, and ropinirole bind about 20 times more selectively to dopamine D_3 than D_2 receptors; the corresponding ratio for bromocriptine is less than 2 to 1. Apomorphine binds selectively to D_1 and D_2 receptors, with little affinity for D_3 and D_4 receptors. L-Dopa, pramipexole, and ropinirole have no significant activity at nondopaminergic receptors. However, bromocriptine binds to serotonin 5-HT$_1$ and 5-HT$_2$ and α_1-, α_2-, and β-adrenergic receptors.

Therapeutic Indications

Medication-Induced Movement Disorders.
In present-day clinical psychiatry, dopamine receptor agonists are used for the treatment of medication-induced parkinsonism, extrapyramidal symptoms, akinesia, and focal perioral tremors. Their use has

diminished sharply, however, because the incidence of medication-induced movement disorders is much lower with the use of the newer, atypical antipsychotics (SDAs). Dopamine receptor agonists are effective in treating idiopathic restless legs syndrome and may also be helpful when this is a medication side effect. Ropinirole can treat restless legs syndrome.

For the treatment of medication-induced movement disorders, most clinicians rely on anticholinergics, amantadine, and antihistamines because they are equally effective and have few adverse effects. Bromocriptine remains in use in the treatment of neuroleptic malignant syndrome; however, the incidence of this disorder is diminishing with the decreased use of DRAs.

Dopamine receptor agonists are also used to counteract the hyperprolactinemic effects of DRAs, which result in the side effects of amenorrhea and galactorrhea.

Mood Disorders.
Bromocriptine has long been used to enhance response to antidepressant drugs in refractory patients. Ropinirole has been reported to be useful as an augmentation of antidepressant therapy and as a treatment for medication-resistant bipolar II depression. Ropinirole may also be helpful in the treatment of antidepressant-induced sexual dysfunction. Pramipexole is often used in the augmentation of antidepressants in treatment-resistant depression. Some studies have found pramipexole to be superior to sertraline (Zoloft) in the treatment of depression in Parkinson disease, as well as in reducing anhedonia in Parkinson patients.

Sexual Dysfunction.
Dopamine receptor agonists improve erectile dysfunction in some patients. However, they are rarely used because they frequently cause adverse effects at therapeutic dosages. Phosphodiesterase-5 inhibitor agents are better tolerated and more effective (see Chapter 16).

Precautions and Adverse Reactions

Adverse effects are common with dopamine receptor agonists, thus limiting the usefulness of these drugs. Adverse effects are dosage-dependent and include nausea, vomiting, orthostatic hypotension, headache, dizziness, and cardiac arrhythmias. To reduce the risk of orthostatic hypotension, the initial dosage of all dopamine receptor agonists should be relatively low, with incremental increases at intervals of at least 1 week. These drugs should be used with caution in persons with hypertension, cardiovascular disease, and hepatic disease. After long-term use, persons, particularly elderly persons, may experience choreiform and dystonic movements and psychiatric disturbances—including hallucinations, delusions, confusion, depression, and mania—and other behavioral changes.

Long-term use of bromocriptine can produce retroperitoneal and pulmonary fibrosis, pleural effusions, and pleural thickening.

In general, ropinirole and pramipexole have a similar but milder adverse effect profile than L-Dopa and bromocriptine. Pramipexole and ropinirole may cause irresistible sleep attacks that occur suddenly without warning and have caused motor vehicle accidents.

The most common adverse effects of apomorphine are yawning, dizziness, nausea, vomiting, drowsiness, bradycardia, syncope, and perspiration. Hallucinations have also been reported. Apomorphine's sedative effects are exacerbated with concurrent use of alcohol or other CNS depressants.

Dopamine receptor agonists are contraindicated during pregnancy, especially for nursing mothers, because they inhibit lactation.

Drug Interactions

DRAs are capable of reversing the effects of dopamine receptor agonists, but this is not usually clinically significant. The concurrent use of tricyclic drugs and dopamine receptor agonists has been reported to cause symptoms of neurotoxicity, such as rigidity, agitation, and tremor. They may also potentiate the hypotensive effects of diuretics and other antihypertensive medications. Dopamine receptor agonists should not be used in conjunction with MAOIs, including selegiline (Eldepryl), and MAOIs should be discontinued at least 2 weeks before the initiation of dopamine receptor agonist therapy.

Benzodiazepines, phenytoin (Dilantin), and pyridoxine may interfere with the therapeutic effects of dopamine receptor agonists. We should not combine ergot alkaloids and bromocriptine because they may cause hypertension and myocardial infarction. Progestins, estrogens, and oral contraceptives may interfere with the effects of bromocriptine and may raise plasma concentrations of ropinirole. Ciprofloxacin (Cipro) can raise plasma concentrations of ropinirole, and cimetidine (Tagamet) can raise plasma concentrations of pramipexole.

Laboratory Interferences

L-Dopa administration has been associated with false reports of elevated serum and urinary uric acid concentrations, urinary glucose test results, urinary ketone test results, and urinary catecholamine concentrations. No laboratory interferences have been associated with the administration of the other dopamine receptor agonists.

Dosage and Clinical Guidelines

Table 21-61 lists the various dopamine receptor agonists and their formulations. For the treatment of antipsychotic-induced parkinsonism, the clinician should start with a 100-mg dose of levodopa three times a day, which may be increased until the person is functionally improved. The maximum dosage of L-Dopa is 2,000 mg a day, but most persons respond to dosages below 1,000 mg/day. The dosage of the carbidopa component of the L-Dopa-carbidopa formulation should total at least 75 mg a day.

The dosage of bromocriptine for mental disorders is uncertain, although it seems prudent to begin with low dosages (1.25 mg twice daily) and to increase the dosage gradually. Bromocriptine is usually taken with meals to help reduce the likelihood of nausea.

The starting dosage of pramipexole is 0.125 mg three times daily, which is increased to 0.25 mg three times daily in the second week and is increased by 0.25 mg/dose each week until therapeutic benefit or adverse effects emerge. Persons with idiopathic Parkinson disease usually experience benefits at total daily doses of 1.5 mg, and the maximum daily dose is 4.5 mg.

For ropinirole, the starting dosage is 0.25 mg three times daily and is increased by 0.25 mg/dose each week to a total daily dose of 3 mg, then by 0.5 mg/dose each week to a total daily dose of 9 mg, and then by 1 mg/dose each week to a maximum dosage of 24 mg a day until therapeutic benefit or adverse effects emerge. The average daily dose for persons with idiopathic Parkinson disease is about 16 mg.

The recommended subcutaneous dose of apomorphine in Parkinson disease is 0.2 to 0.6 mL subcutaneously during acute hypomobility episodes delivered via metered injector pen. Apomorphine can be administered three times daily, with a maximum dose of 0.6 mL five times daily.

Table 21-61
Available Preparations of Dopamine Receptor Agonists and Carbidopa

Generic Name	Trade Name	Preparations
Amantadine	Symmetrel	100-mg capsule, 50-mg/5-mL syrup (teaspoon)
Bromocriptine	Parlodel	2.5-, 5-mg tablets
Carbidopa	Lodosyn	25 mg[a]
Levodopa (L-Dopa)	Larodopa	100-, 250-, 500-mg tablets
Levodopa-carbidopa (co-careldopa)	Sinemet, Atamet	100/10-mg, 100/25-mg, 250/25-mg tablets; 100/25-, 200/50-mg extended-release tablets
Pramipexole	Mirapex	0.125-, 0.375-, 0.75-, 1.5-, 3-, 4-mg extended-release tablets
Ropinirole	Requip	0.25-, 0.5-, 1-, 2-, 5-mg tablets

[a]Drug only available directly through the manufacturer.

Amantadine

Amantadine is an antiviral drug used for the prophylaxis and treatment of influenza. It was found to have antiparkinsonian properties and is now used to treat that disorder as well as akinesias and other extrapyramidal signs, including focal perioral tremors (rabbit syndrome).

Pharmacologic Actions. Amantadine is well absorbed from the GI tract after oral administration, reaches peak plasma concentrations in approximately 2 to 3 hours, has a half-life of about 12 to 18 hours, and attains steady-state concentrations after approximately 4 to 5 days of therapy. Amantadine is excreted unmetabolized in the urine. Amantadine plasma concentrations can be twice as high in elderly persons as in younger adults. Patients with renal failure accumulate amantadine in their bodies.

Amantadine augments dopaminergic neurotransmission in the CNS; however, the precise mechanism is unknown. The mechanism may involve dopamine release from presynaptic vesicles, blocking the reuptake of dopamine into presynaptic nerve terminals, or an agonist effect on postsynaptic dopamine receptors.

Therapeutic Indications. The primary indication for amantadine use in psychiatry is to treat extrapyramidal signs and symptoms, such as parkinsonism, akinesia, and rabbit syndrome (focal perioral tremor of the choreoathetoid type) caused by the administration of DRA or SDA drugs. Amantadine is as effective as the anticholinergics (e.g., benztropine [Cogentin]) for these indications and results in an improvement in approximately half of all persons who take it. Amantadine, however, is not generally considered as effective as the anticholinergics for the treatment of acute dystonic reactions and is not effective in treating tardive dyskinesia and akathisia.

Amantadine is a reasonable compromise for persons with extrapyramidal symptoms who would be sensitive to additional anticholinergic effects, particularly those taking a low-potency DRA or the elderly. Elderly persons are susceptible to anticholinergic adverse effects, both in the CNS, such as anticholinergic delirium, and in the peripheral nervous system, such as urinary retention. Amantadine is associated with less memory impairment than are the anticholinergics.

Amantadine has been reported to be of benefit in treating some SSRI-associated side effects, such as lethargy, fatigue, anorgasmia, and ejaculatory inhibition.

Amantadine is used in general medical practice for the treatment of parkinsonism of all causes, including idiopathic parkinsonism.

Precautions and Adverse Effects. The most common CNS effects of amantadine are mild dizziness, insomnia, and impaired concentration (dosage related), which occur in 5 to 10 percent of all persons. Irritability, depression, anxiety, dysarthria, and ataxia occur in 1 to 5 percent of all persons. More severe CNS adverse effects, including seizures and psychotic symptoms, have been reported. Nausea is the most common peripheral adverse effect of amantadine. Headache, loss of appetite, and blotchy spots on the skin have also been reported.

Livedo reticularis of the legs (a purple discoloration of the skin caused by dilation of blood vessels) has been reported in up to 5 percent of persons who take the drug for longer than 1 month. It usually diminishes with the elevation of the legs and resolves in almost all cases when drug use is terminated.

Amantadine is relatively contraindicated in persons with renal disease or a seizure disorder. Amantadine should be used with caution in persons with edema or cardiovascular disease. Some evidence indicates that amantadine is teratogenic and, therefore, should not be taken by pregnant women. Because amantadine is excreted in breast milk, breastfeeding women should not take the drug.

Suicide attempts with amantadine overdosages are life-threatening. Symptoms can include toxic psychoses (confusion, hallucinations, aggressiveness) and cardiopulmonary arrest. Emergency treatment beginning with gastric lavage is indicated.

Drug Interactions. Coadministration of amantadine with phenelzine (Nardil) or other MAOIs can result in a significant increase in resting BP. The coadministration of amantadine with CNS stimulants can result in insomnia, irritability, nervousness, and possibly seizures or irregular heartbeat. Amantadine should not be coadministered with anticholinergics because unwanted side effects—such as confusion, hallucinations, nightmares, dry mouth, and blurred vision—may be exacerbated.

Dosage and Clinical Guidelines. Amantadine is available in 100-mg capsules and as a 50-mg/5-mL syrup. The usual starting dosage of amantadine is 100 mg given twice a day orally, although the dosage can be cautiously increased up to 200 mg given twice a day orally if indicated. Amantadine should be used in persons with renal impairment *only* in consultation with the physician treating the renal condition. If amantadine is successful in the treatment of the drug-induced extrapyramidal symptoms, it should be continued for 4 to 6 weeks and then discontinued to see whether the person has become tolerant to the neurologic adverse effects of the antipsychotic medication. Amantadine should be tapered over 1 to 2 weeks after a decision has been made to discontinue the drug. Persons taking amantadine should not drink alcoholic beverages.

DRUGS TO TREAT PSYCHOTROPIC-INDUCED WEIGHT GAIN

Weight management is a critical element of psychotropic drug treatment because obesity is common among persons with mental disorders. Thus, medical conditions such as hypertension, diabetes mellitus, and hyperlipidemia need to be taken into account when selecting medications. With few exceptions, most psychotropic drugs used to manage mood disorders, anxiety disorders, and psychosis are associated with a significant risk of weight gain as a side effect. Many patients may refuse or discontinue treatment if weight gain occurs, even if the drug is effective in treating their symptoms. For this and other reasons, clinicians need to be well informed about treatment strategies for mitigating drug-induced weight gain and obesity in general.

The standard recommendation for weight loss regimens consists of attempting to manage body weight through consistent dietary modifications and regular physical activity. This behavioral approach may be difficult for patients struggling with psychiatric symptoms, because their mental disorder can compromise their ability to be disciplined in this effort. Also, the physiologic effects of some psychotropic drugs on the regulation of satiety and body metabolism are difficult, if not impossible, to overcome through diet and exercise alone. For these reasons, it may be necessary to use prescription medications to facilitate weight loss.

In this section, drugs used to manage obesity are categorized in two ways: (1) drugs approved by the U.S. FDA as diet pills; and (2) drugs with primary indications other than weight loss but produce weight loss as a side effect.

Drugs with U.S. Food and Drug Administration Approval for Weight Loss

All of the drugs approved by the FDA as weight loss agents are specifically indicated as an adjunct to a reduced-calorie diet and increased physical activity for chronic weight management in adult patients with an initial body mass index (BMI) of 30 kg/m^2 or greater (obese) or 27 kg/m^2 or greater (overweight) in the presence of at least one weight-related comorbidity such as hypertension, type 2 diabetes mellitus, or dyslipidemia.

Phentermine. Phentermine hydrochloride (Adipex-P) is a sympathomimetic amine with pharmacologic activity similar to the amphetamines. It is indicated as a short-term adjunct in a regimen of weight reduction, but in fact, many patients use the drug for extended periods. As with all sympathomimetics, contraindications include advanced arteriosclerosis, cardiovascular disease, moderate to severe hypertension, hyperthyroidism, known hypersensitivity or idiosyncrasy to the sympathomimetic amines, agitated states, and glaucoma.

The drug should be prescribed with caution to patients with a history of drug abuse. Hypertensive crises may result if phentermine is used during or within 14 days following the administration of MAOIs. Insulin requirements in diabetes mellitus may be altered in association with the use of phentermine hydrochloride and the concomitant dietary regimen. Phentermine hydrochloride may decrease the hypotensive effect of guanethidine. Phentermine was pregnancy Category X in the former FDA classification system and thus contraindicated during pregnancy. Studies have not been performed with phentermine hydrochloride to determine the potential for carcinogenesis, mutagenesis, or impairment of fertility.

Phentermine should be taken on an empty stomach once daily, before breakfast. Tablets may be broken or cut in half but should not be crushed. It should be dosed early in the day to avoid disrupting normal sleep patterns. If taking more than one dose a day, the last dose should be taken approximately 4 to 6 hours before going to bed. The recommended dose of phentermine may be different for different patients. Adults under age 60 taking phentermine using 15- to

37.5-mg capsules should take them once per day before breakfast or 1 to 2 hours after breakfast. Those using 15- to 37.5-mg tablets should take them once per day before breakfast or 1 to 2 hours after breakfast. Instead of taking it once a day, some patients may take 15 to 37.5 mg in divided doses a half hour before meals. An oral resin formulation is available in 15- and 30-mg capsules, which should be taken once per day before breakfast.

Phentermine/Topiramate Extended Release (Qsymia).

This drug is a combination of phentermine and topiramate (Topamax). The FDA approved the phentermine/topiramate combination in 2012 as an extended-release formulation. Both active agents in this formulation are associated with weight loss through separate mechanisms.

Adverse events associated with the use of this drug may include, but are not limited to, paresthesia, dizziness, dysgeusia, insomnia, constipation, dry mouth, kidney stones, metabolic acidosis, and secondary angle-closure glaucoma. The use of this drug is associated with a fivefold increased risk of infants with cleft palate and was classified as pregnancy Category X in the former FDA classification system. It can only be prescribed by clinicians who have been certified in the use of this drug.

It is available as a tablet and should be administered once daily in the morning with or without food. Avoid dosing with the drug in the evening due to the possibility of insomnia. The recommended dose is as follows: Start treatment with 3.75 mg/ 23 mg (phentermine/topiramate extended-release) daily for 14 days; after 14 days, increase the dose to 7.5 mg/46 mg once daily. Evaluate for weight loss after 12 weeks of treatment at the 7.5 mg/ 46 mg dose. If at least 3 percent of baseline body weight has not been lost on 7.5 mg/46 mg, discontinue the drug or escalate the dose. To escalate the dose, increase to 11.25 mg/69 mg daily for 14 days, followed by dosing 15 mg/92 mg daily. Evaluate weight loss following dose escalation to 15 mg/92 mg after an additional 12 weeks of treatment. If at least 5 percent of baseline body weight has not been lost on 15 mg/92 mg, discontinue the medication gradually.

Phendimetrazine (Bontril PDM, Adipost, Phendiet, Statobex).

Phendimetrazine is a sympathomimetic amine that is closely related to the amphetamines. It is classified by the Drug Enforcement Agency (DEA) as a Schedule III controlled substance.

The overall prescribing of this agent is limited. The most commonly used formulation is the 105-mg extended-release capsule, which approximates the action of three 35-mg immediate-release doses taken at 4-hour intervals. The average half-life of elimination, when studied under controlled conditions, is about 3.7 hours for both the extended-release and immediate-release forms. The absorption half-life of the drug from the immediate-release 35-mg phendimetrazine tablets is appreciably more rapid than the absorption rate of the drug from the extended-release formulation. The primary route of elimination is via the kidneys, where most of the drug and metabolites are excreted.

Phendimetrazine contraindications are similar to those of phentermine. They include a history of cardiovascular disease (e.g., coronary artery disease, stroke, arrhythmias, congestive heart failure, uncontrolled hypertension, pulmonary hypertension); use during or within 14 days following the administration of MAOIs; hyperthyroidism; glaucoma; agitated states; a history of drug abuse; pregnancy; nursing; use in combination with other anorectic agents or CNS stimulants; and known hypersensitivity or idiosyncratic reactions to sympathomimetics. Given the lack of systematic research, phendimetrazine should not be used in combination with over-the-counter preparations and herbal products that claim to promote weight loss.

Phendimetrazine tartrate was considered pregnancy Category X in the former FDA classification system and is contraindicated during pregnancy because weight loss offers no potential benefit to a pregnant woman and may result in fetal harm. Studies with phendimetrazine tartrate sustained release have not been performed to evaluate carcinogenic potential, mutagenic potential, or effects on fertility.

Interactions may occur with MAOIs, alcohol, insulin, and oral hypoglycemic agents. Phendimetrazine may decrease the hypotensive effect of adrenergic neuron blocking drugs. The effectiveness and safety of phendimetrazine in pediatric patients have not been established. It is not recommended in patients less than 17 years of age.

Adverse reactions reported with phendimetrazine include sweating, flushing, tremor, insomnia, agitation, dizziness, headache, psychosis, and blurred vision. Elevated BP, palpitations, and tachycardia are frequent. GI side effects include dry mouth, nausea, stomach pain, diarrhea, and constipation. Genitourinary side effects include frequency, dysuria, and changes in libido.

Phendimetrazine tartrate is related chemically and pharmacologically to the amphetamines. Amphetamines and related stimulant drugs have been extensively abused, and the possibility of abuse of phendimetrazine should be kept in mind when evaluating the desirability of including a drug as part of a weight reduction program.

Acute overdose with phendimetrazine may manifest itself by restlessness, confusion, belligerence, hallucinations, and panic states. Fatigue and depression usually follow central stimulation. Cardiovascular effects include tachycardia, arrhythmias, hypertension or hypotension, and circulatory collapse. GI symptoms include nausea, vomiting, diarrhea, and abdominal cramps. Poisoning may result in convulsions, coma, and death. The management of acute overdose is mainly symptomatic. It includes lavage and sedation with a barbiturate. If hypertension is marked, the use of a nitrate or rapid-acting α-receptor–blocking agent should be considered.

Diethylpropion (Tenuate).

Diethylpropion preceded its analog, the antidepressant drug bupropion (Wellbutrin). Diethylpropion comes in two formulations: a 25-mg tablet and a 75-mg extended-release tablet (Tenuate Dospan). It is usually taken three times a day, 1 hour before meals (regular tablets), or once a day in midmorning (extended-release tablets). The extended-release tablets should be swallowed whole, never crushed, chewed, or cut. The maximum daily dose is 75 mg.

Side effects include dry mouth, unpleasant taste, restlessness, anxiety, dizziness, depression, tremors, upset stomach, vomiting, and increased urination. Side effects that warrant medical attention include tachycardia, palpitations, blurred vision, skin rash, itching, difficulty breathing, chest pain, fainting, swelling of the ankles or feet, fever, sore throat, chills, and painful urination. Diethylpropion was classified as pregnancy Category B in the former FDA classification system and has low abuse potential. It is listed as a Schedule IV drug by the DEA.

Orlistat (Xenical, Alli).

Orlistat interferes with the absorption of dietary fats, causing reduced caloric intake. It works by inhibiting gastric and pancreatic lipases, the enzymes that break down triglycerides in the intestine. When lipase activity is blocked, triglycerides from the diet are not hydrolyzed into absorbable free fatty acids and are excreted undigested instead. Only trace amounts of orlistat are absorbed systemically; it is almost entirely eliminated through the feces.

The effectiveness of orlistat in promoting weight loss is definite, though modest. When used as part of a weight loss program, between 30 and 50 percent of patients can expect a 5 percent or more significant decrease in body mass. About 20 percent achieve at least a 10 percent decrease in body mass. After orlistat is stopped, up to a third of people gain the weight they lose.

Among the benefits of orlistat treatment is a decrease in BP and a reduced risk of developing type 2 diabetes.

The most common subjective side effects of orlistat are GI related and include steatorrhea, flatulence, fecal incontinence, and frequent or urgent bowel movements. Patients should avoid foods with high-fat content to minimize these effects. Also, they should eat a reduced-calorie diet. Because of this side effect, orlistat can be used with high-fat content diets to treat constipation that results from treatment with some psychotropic drugs, such as the TCAs. Side effects are most severe when beginning therapy and may decrease in frequency with time. Hepatic and renal injuries are potentially severe side effects of orlistat use. In 2010, new safety information about rare cases of severe liver injury was added to the product label of orlistat. The rate of acute kidney injury is more common among orlistat users than nonusers. It should be used with caution in patients with impaired liver function and renal function, as well as those with an obstructed bile duct and pancreatic disease. Orlistat is contraindicated in malabsorption syndromes, hypersensitivity to orlistat, reduced gallbladder function, and in pregnancy and breastfeeding. Orlistat was rated pregnancy Category X in the former FDA classification system.

The use of orlistat inhibits the absorption of fat-soluble vitamins and other fat-soluble nutrients. Multivitamin supplements that contain vitamins A, D, E, K, as well as β-carotene, should be taken once a day, preferably at bedtime.

Orlistat can reduce plasma levels of the immunosuppressant cyclosporine (Sandimmune), so the two drugs should, therefore, not be administered concomitantly. Orlistat can also impair the absorption of the antiarrhythmic amiodarone (Nexterone).

At the standard prescription dose of 120 mg three times daily before meals, orlistat prevents approximately 30 percent of dietary fat from being absorbed. Higher doses have not been shown to produce more pronounced effects.

An over-the-counter formulation of orlistat (Alli) is available as 60-mg capsules—half the dosage of prescription orlistat.

Drugs without U.S. Food and Drug Administration Approval for Weight Loss

Topiramate. Topiramate and zonisamide (Zonegran) are discussed more fully among the mood stabilizers earlier in this chapter, but are mentioned here because both agents can have a substantial effect on weight loss.

Topiramate is approved as an antiepileptic drug and for prevention of migraine headaches in adults. The degree of weight loss associated with topiramate may be comparable to the weight loss that other FDA-approved antiobesity drugs induce. Small studies and extensive anecdotal reports indicate that topiramate can help to offset weight gain associated with SSRIs and SGA drugs. Its impact on body weight may be due to its effects on both appetite suppression and satiety enhancement. These may be the result of a combination of pharmacologic effects including augmenting GABA activity, modulation of voltage-gated ion channels, inhibition of excitatory glutamate receptors, or inhibition of carbonic anhydrase.

The duration and dosage of treatment affect the weight loss benefits of topiramate. Weight loss is higher when the drug is prescribed at doses of 100 to 200 mg/day for more than a month compared with less than a month. In a large study, it was shown that compared to those who took a placebo, topiramate-treated patients were seven times more likely to lose more than 10 percent of their body weight. In clinical practice, many patients experience weight loss at a starting dose of 25 mg/day.

The most common side effects of topiramate are paresthesias, typically around the mouth, impaired taste (taste perversion), and psychomotor disturbances, including slowed cognition and reduced physical movements. Concentration and memory impairment, often characterized by word finding and name recall problems, is often reported. Some patients may experience emotional lability and mood changes. Medical side effects include increased risk of kidney stones and acute-angle closure glaucoma. Patients should report any change in visual acuity. Those with a history of kidney stones should be instructed to drink adequate amounts of fluid.

Topiramate is available as 25-, 50- 100-, and 200-mg tablets and as 15-, 25-, and 50-mg capsules.

Zonisamide. Zonisamide is a sulfonamide-related drug, similar in many ways to topiramate. Its exact mechanism of action is not known. Like topiramate, it can cause cognitive problems, but the incidence is lower than that with topiramate.

Zonisamide was assigned to pregnancy Category C in the former FDA classification system. Animal studies have revealed evidence of teratogenicity. Fetal abnormalities or embryo-fetal deaths have been reported in animal tests at zonisamide dosage and maternal plasma levels similar to, or lower than, human therapeutic levels. Therefore, the use of this drug in human pregnancy may expose the fetus to significant risk.

The most common side effects include drowsiness, loss of appetite, dizziness, headache, nausea, and agitation or irritability. Zonisamide has also been associated with hypohidrosis. There is a 2 to 4 percent risk of kidney stones. Other drugs known to provoke stones, such as topiramate or acetazolamide (Diamox), should not be combined with zonisamide. Severe, but rare, adverse drug reactions include Stevens–Johnson syndrome, toxic epidermal necrolysis, and metabolic acidosis.

Typical dosing for weight loss has not been established. Generally, zonisamide is started at 100 mg at night for 2 weeks, and increased by 100 mg daily every 2 weeks to a target dose of 200 to 600 mg/day in one or two daily doses.

Metformin (Glucophage). Metformin is a medication for type 2 diabetes mellitus. Its actions include reduction of hepatic glucose production, reduced intestinal glucose absorption, increased insulin sensitivity, and improved peripheral glucose uptake and regulation. It does not increase insulin secretion.

When used as an adjunct to SGAs, it has consistently been shown to reduce body weight and waist circumference. Metformin probably has the best evidence of therapeutic benefit for the treatment of antipsychotic drug-induced metabolic syndrome. In several studies, metformin has been shown to attenuate or reverse some of the weight gain induced by antipsychotics. The degree of effect on body weight compares favorably with the effect of other treatment options that are approved for weight reduction. The weight loss effect of adjunctive metformin appears to be stronger in drug-naive patients treated with SGA medications. This effect is most evident for those being treated with clozapine (Clozaril) and olanzapine (Zyprexa). Based on the existing evidence, if weight gain occurs after SGA initiation, despite lifestyle intervention, metformin should be considered.

Common side effects include nausea, vomiting, abdominal pain, and loss of appetite. GI side effects can be mitigated by dividing the dose, taking the drug after meals, or using delayed-release formulations.

One serious treatment risk is that of lactic acidosis. This side effect is more common in those with reduced renal function than other patients. Although very rare (approximately 9 in 100,000 persons/yr), it has a 50 percent mortality rate. Alcohol use, along with metformin, can increase the risk of acidosis. Renal function monitoring and alcohol avoidance are essential.

The weight loss effects of metformin are also evident in chronically ill patients with schizophrenia. Long-term use of metformin appears to be safe and effective.

There is no established dose range for metformin when used as an adjunct for weight loss. In most reports, the usual dose ranged from 500 to 2,000 mg/day. The maximum dose used in treating diabetes is 850 mg three times daily. Patients usually start with a low dose to see how the drug affects them.

Metformin is available in 500-, 850-, and 1,000-mg tablets, all now generic. Metformin SR (slow release) or XR (extended-release) is available in 500- and 750-mg strengths. These formulations are intended to reduce GI side effects and to increase patient compliance by reducing the pill burden.

Amphetamine.   Amphetamine is a psychostimulant approved for the treatment of ADHD and narcolepsy. It has the effect of reducing appetite and has been used off label for that purpose for many years. Some of the drugs discussed above have amphetamine-like properties, which account for their effectiveness. Amphetamines and other psychostimulants are discussed earlier in the stimulant section of this chapter.

▲ 21.11 Nutritional Supplements and Related

NUTRITIONAL SUPPLEMENTS AND MEDICAL FOODS

Thousands of herbal and dietary supplements are being marketed today. Some are purported to have psychoactive properties. A number have even shown promise in the treatment of specific psychiatric symptoms. Although certain compounds may be beneficial, in many cases, the quantity and quality of data have been insufficient to make definitive conclusions. Nevertheless, some patients prefer to use these substances in place of, or in conjunction with, standard pharmaceutical treatments. If electing to use herbal drugs or nutritional supplements, bear in mind that their use may come at the expense of proven interventions and that adverse effects are possible. Though more research is needed, information published to date is still of clinical interest in diagnosing and treating patients who may be taking dietary supplements.

Additionally, herbal and nonherbal supplements may augment or antagonize the actions of prescription and nonprescription drugs. Thus, clinicians need to remain informed on the latest research involving these substances. Because of the paucity of clinical trials, the clinician must be extraordinarily alert to the possibility of adverse effects as a result of drug–drug interactions, mainly if psychotropic agents are prescribed, because many phytomedicines have ingredients that produce physiologic changes in the body.

Nutritional Supplements

In the United States, the term *nutritional supplement* is used interchangeably with the term *dietary supplement.* The Dietary Supplement Health and Education Act (DHSEA) of 1994 defined nutritional supplements as items taken by mouth that contain a "dietary ingredient" meant to supplement the diet. These ingredients may include vitamins, minerals, herbs, botanicals, amino acids, and substances such as enzymes, tissues, glandulars, and metabolites. By law, such products must be labeled as supplements and may not be marketed as conventional food.

The DSHEA places dietary supplements in a select category, and therefore the regulations governing them are laxer than those for prescription and over-the-counter drugs. Unlike pharmaceutical drugs, nutritional supplements do not need the approval of the U.S. FDA, and the FDA does not evaluate their effectiveness. Because the FDA does not regulate dietary supplements, the contents and quality on store shelves vary dramatically. Contamination, mislabeling, and misidentification of herbs and supplements are problems. Table 21-62 provides a list of dietary supplements used in psychiatry.

Medical Foods

In recent years the FDA has introduced a new category of nutritional supplement called *medical foods.* According to the FDA, medical food, as defined in the Orphan Drug Act, is "a food which is formulated to be consumed or administered enterally under the supervision of a physician and which is intended for the specific dietary management of a disease or condition for which distinctive nutritional requirements, based on recognized scientific principles, are established by medical evaluation."

A clear distinction can be made between the regulatory classifications of medical foods and dietary supplements. Medical foods must be shown, by medical evaluation, to meet the distinctive nutritional needs of a specific population of patients with a specific disease being targeted. Dietary supplements, on the other hand, are intended for normal, healthy adults and may not require proof of the efficacy of the finished product. Medical foods are distinguished from the broader category of foods for special dietary use and from foods that make health claims by the requirement that medical foods are to be used under medical supervision.

Medical foods do not have to undergo premarket approval by the FDA. However, medical food firms must comply with other requirements, such as acceptable manufacturing practices and registration of food facilities. Medical foods do have some additional regulations that dietary supplements do not because medical foods are intended to treat illnesses. For example, a compliance program requires annual inspections of all medical food manufacturers.

In summary, to be considered a medical food, a product must, at a minimum, meet the following criteria: (1) The product must be a

Table 21-62
Dietary Supplements Used in Psychiatry

Name	Ingredients/What Is It?	Uses	Adverse Effects	Interactions	Dosage	Comments
Docosahexaenoic acid (DHA)	Omega-3 polyunsaturated fatty acid	ADD, dyslexia, cognitive impairment, dementia	Anticoagulant properties, mild GI distress	Warfarin	Varies with indication	Stop using prior to surgery
Choline	Choline	Fetal brain development, manic conditions, cognitive disorders, tardive dyskinesia, cancers	Restrict in patients with primary genetic trimethyluria, sweating, hypotension, depression	Methotrexate, works with B_6, B_{12}, and folic acid in metabolism of homocysteine	300–1,200 mg, doses >3 g associated with fishy body odor	Needed for structure and function of all cells
L-α-Glyceryl-phosphorylcholine (α-GPC)	Derived from soy lecithin	To increase growth hormone secretion, cognitive disorders	None known	None known	500 mg–1 g daily	Remains poorly understood
Phosphatidylcholine	Phospholipid that is part of cell membranes	Manic conditions, Alzheimer disease, and cognitive disorders, tardive dyskinesia	Diarrhea, steatorrhea in those with malabsorption, avoid with antiphospholipid antibody syndrome	None known	3–9 g/day in divided doses	Soybeans, sunflower, and rapeseed are major sources
Phosphatidylserine	Phospholipid isolated from soya and egg yolks	Cognitive impairment including Alzheimer disease, may reverse memory problems	Avoid with antiphospholipid antibody syndrome, GI side effects	None known	For soya-derived variety, 100 mg tid	Type derived from bovine brain carries hypothetical risk of bovine spongiform encephalopathy
Zinc	Metallic element	Immune impairment, wound healing, cognitive disorders, prevention of neural tube defects	GI distress, high doses can cause copper deficiency, immunosuppression	Bisphosphonates, quinolones, tetracycline, penicillamine, copper, cysteine-containing foods, caffeine, iron	Typical dose 15 mg/day, adverse effects >30 mg	Claims that zinc can prevent and treat the common cold are supported in some studies but not in others; more research needed
Acetyl-L-carnitine	Acetyl ester of L-carnitine	Neuroprotection, Alzheimer disease, Down syndrome, strokes, antiaging, depression in geriatric patients	Mild GI distress, seizures, increased agitation in some with Alzheimer disease	Nucleoside analogs, valproic acid, and pivalic acid–containing antibiotics	500 mg–2 g daily in divided doses	Found in small amounts in milk and meat
Huperzine A	Plant alkaloid derived from Chinese club moss	Alzheimer disease, age-related memory loss, inflammatory disorders	Seizures, arrhythmias, asthma, irritable bowel disease	Acetylcholinesterase inhibitors and cholinergic drugs	60 μg–200 μg/day	*Huperzia serrata* has been used in Chinese folk medicine for the treatment of fevers and inflammation
NADH (nicotinamide adenine dinucleotide)	Dinucleotide located in mitochondria and cytosol of cells	Parkinson disease, Alzheimer disease, chronic fatigue, CV disease	GI distress	None known	5 mg/day or 5 mg bid	Precursor of NADH is nicotinic acid

(continued)

711

Table 21-62
Dietary Supplements Used in Psychiatry (*Continued*)

Name	Ingredients/What Is It?	Uses	Adverse Effects	Interactions	Dosage	Comments
S-Adenosyl-L-methionine (SAMe)	Metabolite of essential amino acid L-methionine	Mood elevation, osteoarthritis	Hypomania, hyperactive muscle movement, caution in patients with cancer	None known	200–1,600 mg daily in divided doses	Several trials demonstrate some efficacy in the treatment of depression
5-Hydroxytryptophan (5-HTP)	Immediate precursor of serotonin	Depression, obesity, insomnia, fibromyalgia, headaches	Possible risk of serotonin syndrome in those with carcinoid tumors or taking MAOIs	SSRIs, MAOIs, methyl-dopa, St. John's wort, phenoxybenzamine, 5-HT antagonists, 5-HT receptor agonists	100 mg–2 g daily, safer with carbidopa	5-HTP along with carbidopa is used in Europe for the treatment of depression
Phenylalanine	Essential amino acid	Depression, analgesia, vitiligo	Contraindicated in patients with PKU, may exacerbate tardive dyskinesia or hypertension	MAOIs and neuroleptic drugs	Comes in 2 forms: 500 mg–1.5 g daily for DL-phenylalanine, 375 mg–2.25 g for DL-phenylalanine	Found in vegetables, juices, yogurt, and miso
Myoinositol	Major nutritionally active form of inositol	Depression, panic attacks, OCD	Caution in patients with bipolar disorder, GI distress	Possible additive effects with SSRIs and 5-HT receptor agonists (sumatriptan)	12 g in divided doses for depression and panic attacks	Studies have *not* shown effectiveness in treating Alzheimer disease, autism, or schizophrenia
Vinpocetine	Semisynthetic derivative of vincamine (plant derivative)	Cerebral ischemic stroke, dementias	GI distress, dizziness, insomnia, dry mouth, tachycardia, hypotension, flushing	Warfarin	5–10 mg daily with food, no more than 20 mg/day	Used in Europe, Mexico, and Japan as pharmaceutical agent for treatment of cerebrovascular and cognitive disorders
Vitamin E family	Essential fat-soluble vitamin, family made of tocopherols and tocotrienols	Immune-enhancing, antioxidant, some cancers, protection in CV disease, neurologic disorders, diabetes, premenstrual syndrome	May increase bleeding in those with propensity to bleed, possible increased risk of hemorrhagic stroke, thrombophlebitis	Warfarin, antiplatelet drugs, neomycin, may be additive with statins	Depends on form: tocotrienols, 200–300 mg daily with food; tocopherols, 200 mg/day	Stop members of vitamin E family 1 mo prior to surgical procedures
Glycine	Amino acid	Schizophrenia, alleviating spasticity, and seizures	Avoid in those who are anuric or have hepatic failure	Additive with antispasmodics	1 g/day in divided doses for supplement; 40–90 g/day for schizophrenia	
Melatonin	Hormone of pineal gland	Insomnia, sleep disturbances, jet lag, cancer	May inhibit ovulation in 1-g doses, seizures, grogginess, depression, headache, amnesia	Aspirin, NSAIDs, β-blockers, INH, sedating drugs, corticosteroids, valerian, kava kava, 5-HTP, alcohol	0.3–3 mg hs for short periods of time	Melatonin sets the timing of circadian rhythms and regulates seasonal responses
Fish oil	Lipids found in fish	Bipolar disorder, lowering triglycerides, hypertension, decrease blood clotting	Caution in hemophiliacs, mild GI upset, "fishy"-smelling excretions	Coumadin, aspirin, NSAIDs, garlic, ginkgo	Varies depending on form and indication—usually about 3–5 g daily	Stop prior to any surgical procedure

ADD, attention-deficit disorder; CV, cardiovascular; OCD, obsessive-compulsive disorder; GI, gastrointestinal; hs, at night; MAOIs; monamine oxidase inhibitors; PKU, phenylketonuria; SSRIs, serotonin reuptake inhibitors; NSAIDs, nonsteroidal anti-inflammatory drugs; INH, isoniazid; 5-HTP, 5-hydroxytryptophan; tid, three times a day; bid, twice a day.
Table by Mercedes Blackstone, M.D.

Table 21-63
Some Common Medical Foods

Medical Food	Indication	Mechanism of Action
Caprylic-triglyceride (Axona)	Alzheimer disease	Increases plasma concentration of ketones as an alternative energy source in the brain; metabolized in the liver
L-methylfolate (Deplin)	Depression	Regulates synthesis of serotonin, norepinephrine, and dopamine; adjunctive to selective serotonin reuptake inhibitors (SSRIs); 15 mg/day
S-adenosyl-L-methionine (SAMe)	Depression	Naturally occurring molecule involved in synthesis of hormones and neurotransmitters including serotonin and norepinephrine
L-Tryptophan	Sleep disturbance Depression	Essential amino acid; precursor of serotonin; reduces sleep latency; usual dose 4–5 g/day
Omega-3 fatty acid	Depression Cognition	Eicosapentaenoic (EPA) and docosahexaenoic (DHA) acids; direct effect on lipid metabolism; used for augmentation of antidepressant drugs
Theramine (Sentra)	Sleep disturbances Cognitive enhancer	Cholinergic modulator; increases acetylcholine and glutamate
N-Acetylcysteine	Depression Obsessive-compulsive disorder	Amino acid that attenuates glutamatergic neurotransmission; used to augment SSRIs
L-Tyrosine	Depression	Amino acid precursor to biogenic amines epinephrine and norepinephrine
Glycine	Depression	Amino acid that activates N-methyl-D-aspartate (NMDA) receptors; may facilitate excitatory transmission in the brain
Citicoline	Alzheimer disease Ischemic brain injury	Choline donor involved in synthesis of brain phosopholipids and acetylcholine; 300–1,000 mg/day; may improve memory
Acetyl L-carnitine (Alcar)	Alzheimer disease Memory loss	Antioxidant that may prevent oxidative damage in the brain

food for oral or tube feeding; (2) the product must be labeled for the dietary management of a specific medical disorder, disease, or condition for which there are distinctive nutritional requirements; and (3) the product must be intended to be used under medical supervision. The most common medical foods with psychoactive claims are listed in Table 21-63.

PHYTOMEDICINES

The term *phytomedicines* (from the Greek *phyto,* meaning "plant") refers to herb and plant preparations that are used or have been used for centuries for the treatment of a variety of medical conditions. Phytomedicines are categorized as dietary supplements, not drug products, and are therefore exempt from the regulations that govern prescription and over-the-counter medications. Manufacturers of phytomedicines are not required to provide the FDA with safety information before marketing a product or give the FDA postmarketing safety reports. Thousands of herbal drugs are being marketed today; the most common with psychoactive properties are listed in Table 21-64. Ingredients, when identified, are listed, as are indications, adverse events, dosages, and comments, particularly on interactions with commonly prescribed drugs used in psychiatry. For example, St. John's wort (*wort* is an old English word meaning "root or herb" and a familiar term for home brewers), which is used to treat depression, decreases the effectiveness of certain psychotropic drugs such as amitriptyline (Elavil), alprazolam (Xanax), paroxetine (Paxil), and sertraline (Zoloft), among others. Kava kava, which is used to treat anxiety states, has been associated with liver toxicity.

Adverse Effects

Adverse effects are possible, and toxic interactions with other drugs may occur with all phytomedicines, dietary supplements, and medicinal foods. Adulteration is possible, especially with phytomedicines. There are few or no consistent standard preparations available for most herbs. The FDA does not test medical foods; however, strict voluntary compliance is required. Safety profiles and knowledge of adverse effects of most of these substances have not been studied rigorously, however. Because of the paucity of clinical trials, all of these agents should be avoided during pregnancy; some herbs may act as abortifacients, for example. Because most of these substances or their metabolites are secreted in breast milk, they are contraindicated during lactation.

Clinicians should always attempt to obtain a history of herbal use or the use of medical foods or nutritional supplements during the psychiatric evaluation.

It is important to be nonjudgmental in dealing with patients who use these substances. Many do so for various reasons: (1) as part of their cultural tradition, (2) because they mistrust physicians or are dissatisfied with conventional medicine, or (3) because they experience relief of symptoms with the particular substance. Because patients will be more cooperative with traditional psychiatric treatments if they are allowed to continue using their preparations, psychiatrists should keep an open mind and not attribute all effects to suggestion. If psychotropic agents are prescribed, the clinician must be extraordinarily alert to the possibility of adverse effects as a result of drug–drug interactions, because many of these compounds have ingredients that produce physiologic changes in the body.

Table 21-64
Phytomedicinals with Psychoactive Effects

Name	Ingredients	Use	Adverse Effects[a]	Interactions	Dosage[a]	Comments
Arctic weed, golden root	MAOI and β endorphin	Anxiolytic, mood enhancer, antidepressant	No side effect yet documented in trials		100 mg bid to 200 mg tid	Use caution with drugs that mimic MAOIs
Areca, areca nut, betel nut, L. Areca catechu	Arecoline, guvacoline	For alteration of consciousness to reduce pain and elevate mood	Parasympathomimetic overload: increased salivation, tremors, bradycardia, spasms, GI disturbances, ulcers of the mouth	Avoid with parasympathomimetic drugs; atropine-like compounds reduce effect	Undetermined: 8–10 g is toxic dose for humans	Used by chewing the nut; used in the past as a chewing balm for gum disease and as a vermifuge; long-term use may result in malignant tumors of the oral cavity
Ashwaganda	Also called Indian Winter Cherry or Indian Ginseng, native to India Flavonoids	Antioxidant, may decrease anxiety levels Improved libido in men and women May lower levels of the stress hormone cortisol	Drowsiness and sleepiness	None	Dosage is 1 tablet twice daily before meals with a gradual increase to 4 tablets per day	None
Belladonna, L. Atropa belladonna, deadly nightshade	Atropine, scopolamine, flavonoids[b]	Anxiolytic	Tachycardia, arrhythmias, xerostomia, mydriasis, difficulties with micturition and constipation	Synergistic with anticholinergic drugs; avoid with TCAs, amantadine, and quinidine	0.05–0.10 mg a day; maximum single dose is 0.20 mg	Has a strong smell, tastes sharp and bitter, and is poisonous
Biota, Platycladus orientalis	Plant derivative	Used as a sedative. Other uses are to treat heart palpitations, panic, night sweats, and constipation. May be useful in ADHD	No known adverse effects	None	No clear established doses exist	None
Bitter orange flower, citrus aurantium	Flavonoids, limonene	Sedative, anxiolytic, hypnotic	Photosensitization	Undetermined	Tincture, 2–3 g/day; drug, 4–6 g/day; extract, 1–2 g/day	Contradictory evidence; some refer to it as a gastric stimulant
Black cohosh, L. Cimicifuga racemosa	Triterpenes, isoferulic acid	For PMS, menopausal symptoms, dysmenorrhea	Weight gain, GI disturbances	Possible adverse interaction with male or female hormones	1–2 g/day; over 5 g can cause vomiting, headache, dizziness, cardiovascular collapse	Estrogen-like effects questionable because root may act as an estrogen-receptor blocker
Black haw, cramp bark, L. Viburnum prunifolium	Scopoletin, flavonoids, caffeic acids, triterpenes	Sedative, antispasmodic action on uterus; for dysmenorrhea	Undetermined	Anticoagulant-enhanced effects	1–3 g/day	Insufficient data
California poppy, L. Eschscholtzia californica	Isoquinoline alkaloids, cyanogenic glycosides	Sedative, hypnotic, anxiolytic; for depression	Lethargy	Combination of California poppy, valerian, St. John's wort, and passion flowers can result in agitation	2 g/day	Clinical or experimental documentation of effects is unavailable

Name	Active constituents	Uses	Adverse effects	Drug interactions	Dosage	Comments
Casein	Casein peptides	Used as antistress agent; May improve sleep	Usually consumed though milk products. May interact with antihypertensive medicine and lower the blood pressure. May cause drowsiness and should be avoided when taking alcohol or benzodiazepines	None	One to two tablets once or twice daily	
Catnip, L. Nepeta cataria	Valeric acid	Sedative, antispasmodic; for migraine	Headache, malaise, nausea, hallucinogenic effects	Undetermined	Undetermined	Delirium produced in children
Chamomile, L. Matricaria chamomilla	Flavonoids	Sedative, anxiolytic	Allergic reaction	Undetermined	2–4 g/day	May be GABAergic
Coastal water hyssop		Anxiolytic, sedative, epilepsy, asthma	Mild GI discomfort	May stimulate	300–450 mg qid	Insufficient data
Cordyceps sinensis	A genus of fungi that includes about 400 described species, found primarily in the high altitudes of the Tibetan plateau in China; Antioxidant	Has been used for weakness, fatigue, to improve sexual drive in the elderly	GI discomfort, dry mouth, and nausea	None	Dosage in ranges of 3–6 g daily	None
Corydalis, L. Corydalis cava	Isoquinoline alkaloids	Sedative, antidepressant; for mild depression	Hallucination, lethargy	Undetermined	Undetermined	Clonic spasms and muscular tremor with overdose
Cyclamen, L. Cyclamen europaeum	Triterpene	Anxiolytic; for menstrual complaints	Small doses (e.g., 300 mg) can lead to nausea, vomiting, and diarrhea	Undetermined	Undetermined	High doses can lead to respiratory collapse
Echinacea, L. Echinacea purpurea	Flavonoids, polysaccharides, caffeic acid derivatives, alkamides	Stimulates immune system; for lethargy, malaise, respiratory infections and lower UTIs	Allergic reaction, fever, nausea, vomiting	Undetermined	1–3 g/day	Use in HIV and AIDS patients is controversial; may not be effective in coryza
Ephedra, ma-huang L. Ephedra sinica	Ephedrine, pseudoephedrine	Stimulant; for lethargy, malaise, diseases of respiratory tract	Sympathomimetic overload: arrhythmias, increased BP, headache, irritability, nausea, vomiting	Synergistic with sympathomimetics, serotonergic agents; avoid with MAOIs	1–2 g/day	Tachyphylaxis and dependence can occur (taken off market)
Ginkgo, L. Ginkgo biloba	Flavonoids, ginkgolide A, B	Symptomatic relief of delirium, dementia; improves concentration and memory deficits; possible antidote to SSRI-induced sexual dysfunction	Allergic skin reactions, GI upset, muscle spasms, headache	Anticoagulant: use with caution because of its inhibitory effect on PAF; increased bleeding possible	120–240 mg/day	Studies indicate improved cognition in persons with Alzheimer disease after 4–5 wk of use, possibly because of increased blood flow

(continued)

Table 21-64
Phytomedicinals with Psychoactive Effects (*Continued*)

Name	Ingredients	Use	Adverse Effects[a]	Interactions	Dosage[a]	Comments
Ginseng, *L. Panax ginseng*	Triterpenes, ginsenosides	Stimulant; for fatigue, elevation of mood, immune system	Insomnia, hypertonia, and edema (called ginseng abuse syndrome)	Not to be used with sedatives, hypnotic agents, MAOIs, antidiabetic agents, or steroids	1–2 g/day	Several varieties exist; Korean (most highly valued), Chinese, Japanese, American (*Panax quinquefolius*)
Heather, *L. Calluna vulgaris*	Flavonoids, triterpenes	Anxiolytic, hypnotic	Undetermined	Undetermined	Undetermined	Efficacy for claimed uses is not documented
Holy Basil formula, *Ocimum tenuiflorum*	*Ocimum tenuiflorum,* an aromatic plant native to the tropics, part of the *Lamiaceae* family Flavonoids	Used to combat stress, also used for common colds, headaches, stomach disorders, inflammation, heart disease	No data exist regarding the long-term effects. May prolong clotting time, increase the risk of bleeding during surgery, and lower blood sugar	None	Dosage depends on the formulation type, recommended dose is 2 softgel capsules taken with 8 oz water daily	None
Hops, *L. Humulus lupulus*	Humulone, lupulone, flavonoids	Sedative, anxiolytic, hypnotic; for mood disturbances, restlessness	Contraindicated in patients with estrogen-dependent tumors (breast, uterine, cervical)	Hyperthermia effects with phenothiazine antipsychotics and with CNS depressants	0.5 g/day	May decrease plasma levels of drugs metabolized by CYP450 system
Horehound, *L. Ballota nigra*	Diterpenes, tannins	Sedative	Arrhythmias, diarrhea, hypoglycemia, possible spontaneous abortions	May enhance serotonergic drug effects, may augment hypoglycemic effects of drugs	1–4 g/day	May cause abortion
Jambolan, *L. Syzygium cumini*	Oleic acid, myristic acid, palmitic and linoleic acids, tannins	Anxiolytic, antidepressant	Undetermined	Undetermined	1–2 g/day	In folk medicine, a single dose is 30 seeds (1.9 g) of powder
Kanna, *Sceletium tortuosum*	Alkaloid, mesembrine	Anxiolytic, mood enhancer, empathogen, COPD treatment	Sedation, vivid dreams, headache	Potentiates cannabis, PDE inhibitor	50–100 mg	Insufficient data
Kava kava, *L. Piperis methysticum*	Kava lactones, kava pyrone	Sedative, hypnotic, antispasmodic	Lethargy, impaired cognition, dermatitis with long-term usage, liver toxicity	Synergistic with anxiolytics, alcohol; avoid with levodopa and dopaminergic agents	600–800 mg/day	May be GABAergic; contraindicated in patients with endogenous depression; may increase the danger of suicide
Kratom, *Mitragyna speciosa*	Alkaloid	Stimulant and depressant	Priapism, testicular enlargement, withdrawal, depression, fatigue, insomnia	Structurally similar to yohimbine	Undetermined	Chewed, extracted into water, tar formulations

716

Name	Constituents	Uses	Adverse effects	Interactions/Contraindications	Dose	Comments
Lavender, L. *Lavandula angustifolia*	Hydroxycoumarin, tannins, caffeic acid	Sedative, hypnotic	Headache, nausea, confusion	Synergistic with other sedatives	3–5 g/day	May cause death in overdose
Lemon balm, sweet Mary, *L. Melissa officinalis*	Flavonoids, caffeic acid, triterpenes	Hypnotic, anxiolytic, sedative	Undetermined	Potentiates CNS depressant; adverse reaction with thyroid hormone	8–10 g/day	Insufficient data
L-methylfolate	Folate is a B vitamin found in some foods, needed to form healthy red blood cells. L-methylfolate and levomefolate are names for the active form of folic acid	Adjunctive L is used for major depression, not an antidepressant when used alone. Folate and L-methylfolate are also used to treat folic acid deficiency in pregnancy, to prevent spinal cord birth defects	GI side effects reported	None	15 mg once a day by mouth with or without food	Considered a "medical food" by the FDA and only available by prescription. Safe to take during pregnancy when used as directed
Mistletoe, *L. Viscum album*	Flavonoids, triterpenes, lectins, polypeptides	Anxiolytic; for mental and physical exhaustion	Berries said to have emetic and laxative effects	Contraindicated in patients with chronic infections (e.g., tuberculosis)	10 per day	Berries have caused death in children
Mugwort, *L. Artemisia vulgaris*	Sesquiterpene lactones, flavonoids	Sedative, antidepressant, anxiolytic	Anaphylaxis, contact dermatitis, may cause hallucinations	Potentiates anticoagulants	5–15 g/day	May stimulate uterine contractions, can induce abortion
N-acetylcysteine (NAC)	Amino acid	Used as an antidote for acetaminophen overdose, treatment of trichotillomania	Rash, cramps, and angioedema may occur	Activated charcoal, ampicillin, carbamazepine, cloxacillin, oxacillin, nitroglycerin, and penicillin G	1,200–2,400 mg/day	Acts as an antioxidant and a glutamate modulating agent. When used as an antidote for acetaminophen overdose, the dose is 20–40 times higher than those used in OCD trials. It has not been shown to be effective in treating schizophrenia
Nux vomica, *L. Strychnos nux vomica*, poison nut	Indole alkaloids: strychnine and brucine, polysaccharides	Antidepressant; for migraine, menopausal symptoms	Convulsions, liver damage, death; severely toxic because of strychnine	Undetermined	0.02–0.05 g/day	Symptoms of poisoning can occur after ingestion of one bean; lethal dose is 1–2 g
Oats, *L. Avena sativa*	Flavonoids, oligo and polysaccharides	Anxiolytic, hypnotic; for stress, insomnia, opium, and tobacco withdrawal	Bowel obstruction or other bowel dysmotility syndromes, flatulence	Undetermined	3 g/day	Oats have sometimes been contaminated with aflatoxin, a fungal toxin linked with some cancers

(continued)

Table 21-64
Phytomedicinals with Psychoactive Effects (*Continued*)

Name	Ingredients	Use	Adverse Effects[a]	Interactions	Dosage[a]	Comments
Omega-3 fatty acid	Comes in three forms, eicosapentaenoic acid (EPA), docosahexaenoic acid (DHA), and alpha-linolenic acid (LNA)	Used as a supplement in the treatment of heart disease, high cholesterol, high blood pressure. May also be helpful in treatment of depression, bipolar disorder, schizophrenia, and ADHD. May reduce the risk of ulcers when used in conjunction with NSAID pain relievers	Can cause gas, bloating, belching, and diarrhea	May increase effectiveness of blood thinners, may increase fasting blood sugar levels when used with diabetes medications such as insulin and metformin	Doses vary from 1 to 4 g/day	Can be contaminated with mercury and PCBs
Passion flower, *L. Passiflora incarnata*	Flavonoids, cyanogenic glycosides	Anxiolytic, sedative, hypnotic	Cognitive impairment	Undetermined	4–8 g/day	Overdose causes depression
Phosphatidylserine and Phosphatidylcholine	Phospholipids	Used for Alzheimer disease, age-related decline in mental function, improving thinking skills in young people, ADHD, depression, preventing exercise-induced stress, and improving athletic performance	Insomnia and stomach upset	None	100 mg three times daily	None
Polygala	Polygala is a genus of about 500 species of flowering plants belonging to the family *Polygalaceae*, commonly known as milkwort or snakeroot	Used for insomnia, forgetfulness, mental confusion, palpitation, seizures, anxiety, and listlessness	Contraindicated in patients who have ulcers or gastritis, should not be used long term	None	Dosage of polygala is 1.5–3 g of dried root, 1.5–3 g of a fluid extract, or 2.5–7.5 g of a tincture. A polygala tea can also be made, with a maximum of three cups per day	None
Rehmannia	Iridoid glycosides	Stimulates the release of cortisol. Used in lupus, rheumatoid arthritis (RA), fibromyalgia, and multiple sclerosis. May improve asthma and urticaria. Used to treat menopause, hair loss, and impotence	Loose bowel movements, bloating, nausea, and abdominal cramps	None	Exact dosage unknown	None
Rhodiola rosea	Potentiator, monoterpene alcohols, flavonoids					

Herb	Active components	Uses	Side effects/Toxicity	Interactions	Dose	Comments
S-adenosyl-L-methionine (SAMe)	S-adenosyl-L-methionine	Used for arthritis and fibromyalgia, may be effective as an augmentation strategy for SSRI in depression	GI symptoms, anxiety, nightmares, insomnia, and worsening of Parkinson symptoms	Use with SSRIs or SNRIs may result in serotonin syndrome. Interacts with levodopa, meperidine, pentazocine, and tramadol	400–1,600 mg/day	A naturally occurring molecule made from the amino acid methionine and ATP, serves as a methyl donor in human cellular metabolism
Scarlet Pimpernel, L. Anagallis arvensis	Flavonoids, triterpenes, cucurbitacins, caffeic acids	Antidepressant	Overdose or long-term doses may lead to gastroenteritis and nephritis	Undetermined	1.8 g of powder four times a day	Flowers are poisonous
Skullcap, L. Scutellaria lateriflora	Flavonoid, monoterpenes	Anxiolytic, sedative, hypnotic	Cognitive impairment, hepatotoxicity	Disulfiram-like reaction may occur if used with alcohol	1–2 g/day	Little information exists to support the use of this herb in humans
St. John's wort, L. Hypericum perforatum	Hypericin, flavonoids, xanthones	Antidepressant, sedative, anxiolytic	Headaches, photosensitivity (may be severe), constipation	Report of manic reaction when used with sertraline (Zoloft); do not combine with SSRIs or MAOs; possible serotonin syndrome; do not use with alcohol, opioids	100–950 mg/day	Mixed results on effectiveness for depression; may act as MAOI or SSRI; 4- to 6-wk trial for mild depressive moods; if no apparent improvement, another therapy should be tried
Strawberry leaf, L. Fragaria vesca	Flavonoids, tannins	Anxiolytic	Contraindicated with strawberry allergy	Undetermined	1 g/day	Little information exists to support the use of this herb in humans
Tarragon, L. Artemisia dracunculus	Flavonoids, hydroxycoumarins	Hypnotic, appetite stimulant	Undetermined	Undetermined	Undetermined	Little information exists to support the use of this herb in humans
Valerian, L. Valeriana officinalis	Valepotriates, valerenic acid, caffeic acid	Sedative, muscle relaxant, hypnotic	Cognitive and motor impairment, GI upset, hepatotoxicity; long-term use: contact allergy, headache, restlessness, insomnia, mydriasis, cardiac dysfunction	Avoid concomitant use with alcohol or CNS depressants	1–2 g/day	May be chemically unstable
Wild lettuce, Lactuca, Virosa	Flavonoids, coumarins, lactones	Sedative, anesthetic, galactagogue	Tachycardia, tachypnea, visual disturbance, diaphoresis	Undetermined	Undetermined	Bitter taste, added to salad or drinks, active compound closely resembles opium
Winter cherry, withania, somnifera	Alkaloids, steroidal lactones	Sedative, treatment for arthritis, possible anticarcinogenic	Thyrotoxicosis, unfavorable effects on heart and adrenal gland	Undetermined	Undetermined	Smoke inhaled

ADHD, attention-deficit/hyperactivity disorder; AIDS, acquired immunodeficiency syndrome; ATP, adenosine triphosphate; bid, twice a day; BP, blood pressure; CNS, central nervous system; COPD, chronic obstructive pulmonary disease; FDA, U.S. Food and Drug Administration; GABA, γ-aminobutyric acid; GI, gastrointestinal; MAOI, monoamine oxidase inhibitor; PAF, platelet-activating factor; PCB, polychlorinated biphenyl; PDE, phosphodiesterase; PMS, premenstrual syndrome; NSAID, nonsteroidal anti-inflammatory drug; OCD, obsessive-compulsive disorder; qid, four times a day; SNRI, serotonin and norepinephrine reuptake inhibitor; SSRI, selective serotonin reuptake inhibitor; TCA, tricyclic antidepressant; tid, three times a day; UTI, urinary tract infection.

[a] There are no reliable, consistent, or valid data exist on dosages or adverse effects of most phytomedicinals.

[b] Flavonoids are common to many herbs. They are plant byproducts that prevent the deterioration of material such as deoxyribonucleic acid (DNA) via oxidation).

References

Introduction

Ananth J, Parameswaran S, Gunatilake S, Burgoyne K, Sidhom T. Neuroleptic malignant syndrome and atypical antipsychotic drugs. *J Clin Psychiatry.* 2004;65(4):464–470.

Bai YM, Yu SC, Chen JY, Lin CY, Chou P. Risperidone for pre-existing severe tardive dyskinesia: a 48-week prospective follow-up study. *Int Clin Psychopharmacol.* 2005;20:79–85.

Balk EM, Bonis PA, Moskowitz H, Schmid CH, Ioannidis JP. Correlation of quality measures with estimates of treatment effect in meta-analyses of randomized controlled trials. *JAMA.* 2002;287:2973.

Bratti IM, Kane JM, Marder SR. Chronic restlessness with antipsychotics. *Am J Psychiatry.* 2007;164(11):1648–1654.

Caroff SN, Mann SC, Campbell EC, Sullivan KA. Movement disorders associated with atypical antipsychotic drugs. *J Clin Psychiatry.* 2002;63(Suppl 4):12–19.

Chuang DM. The antiapoptotic actions of mood stabilizers: molecular mechanisms and therapeutic potentials. *Ann N Y Acad Sci.* 2005;1053:195–204.

Damier P, Thobois S, Witjas T, Cuny E, Derost P. Bilateral deep brain stimulation of the globus pallidus to treat tardive dyskinesia. *Arch Gen Psychiatry.* 2007;64:170–176.

Dayalu P, Chou KL. Antipsychotic-induced extrapyramidal symptoms and their management. *Expert Opin Pharmacother.* 2008;9:1451–1462.

DeVeaugh-Geiss J, March J, Shapiro M, Andreason PJ, Emslie G, Ford LM, Greenhill L, Murphy D, Prentice E, Roberts R, Silva S, Swanson JM, van Zwieten-Boot B, Vitiello B, Wagner KD, Mangum B. Child and adolescent psychopharmacology in the new millennium: A workshop for academia, industry, and government. *J Am Acad Child Adolesc Psychiatry.* 2006;45(3):261–270.

Factor SA, Lang AE, Weiner WJ, eds. *Drug Induced Movement Disorders.* 2nd ed. Malden, MA: Blackwell Futura; 2005.

Fava GA, Tomba E, Tossani E. Innovative trends in the design of therapeutic trials in psychopharmacology and psychotherapy. *Prog Neuropsychopharmacol Biol Psychiatry.* 2013;40:306–311.

Gunes A, Dahl ML, Spina E, Scordo MG. Further evidence for the association between 5-HT2C receptor gene polymorphisms and extrapyramidal side effects in male schizophrenic patients. *Eur J Clin Pharmacol.* 2008;64:477–482.

Gunes A, Scordo MG, Jaanson P, Dahl ML. Serotonin and dopamine receptor gene polymorphisms and the risk of extrapyramidal side effects in perphenazine-treated schizophrenic patients. *Psychopharmacology.* 2007;190:479–484.

Guzey C, Scordo MG, Spina E, Landsem VM, Spigset O. Antipsychotic-induced extrapyramidal symptoms in patients with schizophrenia: associations with dopamine and serotonin receptor and transporter polymorphisms. *Eur J Clin Pharmacol.* 2007;63:233–241.

Janicak PG, Beedle D. Medication-induced movement disorders. In: Sadock BJ, Sadock VA, Ruiz P, eds. *Kaplan & Sadock's Comprehensive Textbook of Psychiatry.* 9th ed. Vol. 2. Philadelphia, PA: Lippincott Williams & Wilkins; 2009:2996.

Janno S, Holi M, Tuisku K, Wahlbeck K. Prevalence of neuroleptic-induced movement disorders in chronic schizophrenic inpatients. *Am J Psychiatry.* 2004;161:160–163.

Koning JP, Tenback DE, van Os J, Aleman A, Kahn RS, van Harten PN. Dyskinesia and parkinsonism in antipsychotic-naive patients with schizophrenia, first-degree relatives and healthy controls: a meta-analysis. *Schizophr Bull.* 2010;36(4):723–731.

Kosky N. A possible association between high normal and high dose olanzapine and prolongation of the PR interval. *J Psychopharmacol.* 2002;16:181–182.

Lam RW, Wan DDC, Cohen NL, Kennedy SH. Combining antidepressants for treatment-resistant depression: a review. *J Clin Psychiatry.* 2002;63:685–693.

Lee PE, Sykora K, Gill SS, Mamdani M, Marras C, Anderson G, Shulman KI, Stukel T, Normand SL, Rochon PA. Antipsychotic medications and drug-induced movement disorders other than parkinsonism: a population-based cohort study in older adults. *J Am Geriatr Soc.* 2005;53(8):1374–1379.

Lencer R, Eismann G, Kasten M, Kabakci K, Geithe V. Family history of movement disorders as a predictor for neuroleptic-induced extrapyramidal symptoms. *Br J Psychiatry.* 2004;185:465–471.

Lieberman JA, Stroup TS, McEvoy JP, Swartz MS, Rosenheck RA. Clinical Antipsychotic Trials of Intervention Effectiveness (CATIE) investigators. *N Engl J Med.* 2005;353:1209–1223.

Liguori A. Psychopharmacology of attention: the impact of drugs in an age of increased distractions. *Exp Clin Psychopharmacol.* 2013;21(5):343–344.

Lyons KE, Pahwa R. Efficacy and tolerability of levetiracetam in Parkinson disease patients with levodopa-induced dyskinesia. *Clin Neuropharmacol.* 2006;29(3):148–153.

Malizia AL. The role of emission tomography in pharmacokinetic and pharmacodynamic studies in clinical psychopharmacology. *J Psychopharmacol.* 2006;20(Suppl 4):100–107.

McGrath PJ, Stewart JW, Quitkin FM, Chen Y, Alpert JE. Predictors of relapse in a prospective study of fluoxetine treatment of major depression. *Am J Psychiatry.* 2006;163(9):1542–1548.

Meco G, Fabrizio E, Epifanio A, Morgante F, Valente M. Levetiracetam in tardive dyskinesia. *Clin Neuropharmacol.* 2006;29:265.

Meyer JH, Ginovart N, Boovariwala A, Sagrati S, Hussey D. Elevated monoamine oxidase a levels in the brain: an explanation for the monoamine imbalance of major depression. *Arch Gen Psychiatry.* 2006;63:1209–1216.

Miller del D, Caroff SN, Davis SM, Rosenheck RA, McEvoy JP. Clinical Antipsychotic Trials of Intervention Effectiveness (CATIE) investigators: extrapyramidal side-effects of antipsychotics in a randomised trial. *Br J Psychiatry.* 2008;193:279.

Moncrieff J. Magic bullets for mental disorders: the emergence of the concept of an "antipsychotic" drug. *J Hist Neurosci.* 2013;22(1):30–46.

Pappa S, Dazzan P. Spontaneous movement disorders in antipsychotic-naive patients with first-episode psychoses: a systematic review. *Psychol Med.* 2009;39:1065–1076.

Poyurovsky M, Pashinian A, Weizman R, Fuchs C, Weizman A. Low-dose mirtazapine: a new option in the treatment of antipsychotic-induced akathisia. A randomized, double-blind, placebo- and propranolol-controlled trial. *Biol Psychiatry.* 2006;59:1071–1077.

Preskorn SH. Pharmacogenomics, informatics, and individual drug therapy in psychiatry: past, present and future. *J Psychopharmacol.* 2006;20(Suppl 4):85–94.

Soares-Weiser K, Fernandez HH. Tardive dyskinesia. *Semin Neurol.* 2007;27:159–169.

Strous RD, Stryjer R, Maayan R, Gal G, Viglin D. Analysis of clinical symptomatology, extrapyramidal symptoms and neurocognitive dysfunction following dehydroepiandrosterone (DHEA) administration in olanzapine treated schizophrenia patients: a randomized, double-blind placebo controlled trial. *Psychoneuroendocrinology.* 2007;32:96–105.

Sussman N. General principles of psychopharmacology. In: Sadock BJ, Sadock VA, Ruiz P, eds. *Kaplan & Sadock's Comprehensive Textbook of Psychiatry.* 9th ed. Vol. 2. Philadelphia, PA: Lippincott Williams & Wilkins; 2009:2965.

Wadsworth EJK, Moss SC, Simpson SA, Smith AP. Psychotropic medication use and accidents, injuries, and cognitive failures. *Hum Psychopharmacol.* 2005;20(6):391–400.

Zajecka J, Goldstein C. Combining and augmenting: choosing the right therapies for treatment-resistant depression. *Psychiatr Ann.* 2005;35(12):994–1000.

Zarrouf FA, Bhanot V. Neuroleptic malignant syndrome: don't let your guard down yet. *Curr Psychiatry.* 2007;6(8):89.

Antipsychotics

Cameron K, Kolanos R, Vekariya R, De Felice L, Glennon RA. "Mephedrone and methylenedioxypyrovalerone (MDPV), major constituents of "bath salts," produce opposite effects at the human dopamine transporter": erratum. *Psychopharmacology.* 2013;227(3):501.

Davidson M, Emsley R, Kramer M, Ford L, Pan G, Lim P, Eerdekens M. Efficacy, safety and early response of paliperidone extended-release tablets (paliperidone ER): Results of a 6-week, randomized, placebo-controlled study. *Schizophr Res.* 2007;93(1–3):117–130.

Dean AC, Groman SM, Morales AM, London ED. An evaluation of the evidence that methamphetamine abuse causes cognitive decline in humans. *Neuropsychopharmacology.* 2013;38(2):259–274.

Frieling H, Hillemacher T, Ziegenbein M, Neundorfer B, Bleich S. Treating dopamimetic psychosis in Parkinson's disease: structured review and meta-analysis. *Eur Neuropsychopharmacol.* 2007;17(3):165–171.

Isom AM, Gudelsky GA, Benoit SC, Richtand NM. Antipsychotic medications, glutamate, and cell death: a hidden, but common medication side effect? *Med Hypotheses.* 2013;80(3):252–258.

Jones PB, Barnes TR, Davies L, Dunn G; Lloyd H. Randomized controlled trial of the effect on quality of life of second- vs first-generation antipsychotic drugs in schizophrenia: Cost Utility of the Latest Antipsychotic Drugs in Schizophrenia Study (CUtLASS 1). *Arch Gen Psychiatry.* 2006;63:1079–1087.

Kahn RS, Fleischhacker WW, Boter H, Davidson M, Vergouwe Y, Keet IP, Gheorghe MD, Rybakowski JK, Galderisi S, Libiger J, Hummer M, Dollfus S, Lopez-Ibor JJ, Hranov LG, Gaebel W, Peuskens J, Lindefors N, Riecher-Rossler A, Grobbee DE. Effectiveness of antipsychotic drugs in first-episode schizophrenia and schizophreniform disorder: an open randomised clinical trial. *Lancet.* 2008;371(9618):1085–1097.

Kane J, Canas F, Kramer M, Ford L, Gassmann-Mayer C, Lim P, Eerdekens M. Treatment of schizophrenia with paliperidone extended-release tablets: a 6-week placebo-controlled trial. *Schizophr Res.* 2007;90(1–3):147–161.

Kane JM, Meltzer HY, Carson WH Jr, McQuade RD, Marcus RN. Aripiprazole for treatment-resistant schizophrenia: results of a multicenter, randomized, double-blind, comparison study versus perphenazine. *J Clin Psychiatry.* 2007;68(2):213–223.

Keefe RS, Bilder RM, Davis SM. Neurocognitive effects of antipsychotic medications in patients with chronic schizophrenia in the CATIE Trial. *Arch Gen Psychiatry.* 2007;64(6):633–647.

Kumra S, Kranzler H, Gerbino-Rosen G, Kester HM, De Thomas C, Kafantaris V, Correll CU, Kane JM. Clozapine and "high-dose" olanzapine in refractory early-onset schizophrenia: a 12-week randomized and double-blind comparison. *Biol Psychiatry.* 2008;63(5):524–529.

Kumra S, Oberstar JV, Sikich L, Findling RL, McClellan JM. Efficacy and tolerability of second-generation antipsychotics in children and adolescents with schizophrenia. *Schizophr Bull.* 2008;34(1):60–71.

Leucht S, Cores C, Arbter D, Engel R, Li C, Davis J. Second-generation versus first-generation antipsychotic drugs for schizophrenia: a meta-analysis. *Lancet.* 2009;373:31–41.

Leucht S, Komossa K, Rummel-Kluge C, Corves C, Hunger H, Schmid F, Lobos CA, Schwartz S, Davis JM. A meta-analysis of head-to-head comparisons of second-generation antipsychotics in the treatment of schizophrenia. *Am J Psychiatry.* 2009;166(2):152–163.

Leucht S, Pitschel-Walz G, Abraham D, Kissling W. Efficacy and extrapyramidal side-effects of the new antipsychotics olanzapine, quetiapine, risperidone, and sertindole compared to conventional antipsychotics and placebo. A meta-analysis of randomized controlled trials. *Schizophr Res.* 1999;35(1):51–68.

Lieberman JA, Stroup TS, McEvoy JP, Swartz MS, Rosenheck RA. Clinical Antipsychotic Trials of Intervention Effectiveness (CATIE) investigators. *N Engl J Med.* 2005;353:1209.

Mamo D, Graff A, Mizrahi R, Shammi CM, Romeyer F. Differential effects of aripiprazole on D(2), 5-HT(2), and 5-HT(1A) receptor occupancy in patients with schizophrenia: a triple tracer PET study. *Am J Psychiatry.* 2007;164(9):1411–1417.

Marder SR, Essock SM, Miller AL, Buchanan RW, Davis JM. The Mount Sinai conference on the pharmacotherapy of schizophrenia. *Schizophr Bull.* 2002;28(1):5.

Marder SR, Hurford IM, van Kammen DP. Second-generation antipsychotics. In: Sadock BJ, Sadock VA, Ruiz P, eds. *Kaplan & Sadock's Comprehensive Textbook of Psychiatry.* 9th ed. Vol. 2. Philadelphia, PA: Lippincott Williams & Wilkins; 2009:3206.

McEvoy JP, Lieberman JA, Perkins DO, Hamer RM, Gu H. Efficacy and tolerability of olanzapine, quetiapine, and risperidone in the treatment of early psychosis: a randomized, double-blind 52-week comparison. *Am J Psychiatry.* 2007;164(7):1050–1060.

McEvoy JP, Lieberman JA, Stroup TS. Effectiveness of clozapine versus olanzapine, quetiapine, and risperidone in patients with chronic schizophrenia who did not respond to prior atypical antipsychotic treatment. *Am J Psychiatry.* 2006;163(4):600–610.

Novick D, Haro JM, Suarez D, Vieta E, Naber D. Recovery in the outpatient setting: 36-month results from the Schizophrenia Outpatients Health Outcomes (SOHO) study. *Schizophr Res.* 2009;108(1–3):223–230.

Owen RT. Inhaled loxapine: a new treatment for agitation in schizophrenia or bipolar disorder. *Drugs Today.* 2013;49(3):195–201.

Pacciardi B, Mauri M, Cargioli C, Belli S, Cotugno B, Di Paolo L, Pini S. Issues in the management of acute agitation: how much current guidelines consider safety? *Front Psychiatry.* 2013;4:26.

Patil ST, Zhang L, Martenyi F, Lowe SL, Jackson KA. Activation of mGlu2/3 receptors as a new approach to treat schizophrenia: a randomized phase 2 clinical trial. *Nat Med.* 2007;13(9):1102–1107.

Ray WA, Chung CP, Murray KT, Hall K, Stein CM. Atypical antipsychotic drugs and the risk of sudden cardiac death. *N Engl J Med.* 2009;360(3):225–235.

Sikich L, Frazier JA, McClellan J, Findling RL, Vitiello B, Ritz L, Ambler D, Puglia M, Maloney AE, Michael E, De Jong S, Slifka K, Noyes N, Hlastala S, Pierson L, McNamara NK, Delporto-Bedoya D, Anderson R, Hamer RM, Lieberman JA. Double-blind comparison of first- and second-generation antipsychotics in early-onset schizophrenia and schizoaffective disorder: findings from the treatment of early-onset schizophrenia spectrum disorders (TEOSS) study. *Am J Psychiatry.* 2008;165(11):1420.

Smith RC, Segman RH, Golcer-Dubner T, Pavlov V, Lerer B. Allelic variation in ApoC3, ApoA5 and LPL genes and first and second generation antipsychotic effects on serum lipids in patients with schizophrenia. *Pharmacogenomics J.* 2008;8:228–236.

Stroup TS, Lieberman JA, McEvoy JP. Results of phase 3 of the CATIE schizophrenia trial. *Schizophr Res.* 2009;107(1):1–12.

Suzuki H, Gen K, Inoue Y. Comparison of the anti-dopamine D(2) and anti-serotonin 5-HT(2A) activities of chlorpromazine, bromperidol, haloperidol and second-generation antipsychotics parent compounds and metabolites thereof. *J Psychopharmacol.* 2013;27(4):396–400.

Tandon R, Belmaker RH, Gattaz WF, Lopez-Ibor JJ Jr, Okasha A, Singh B, Stein DJ, Olie JP, Fleischhacker WW, Moeller HJ. World Psychiatric Association Pharmacopsychiatry Section statement on comparative effectiveness of antipsychotics in the treatment of schizophrenia. *Schizophr Res.* 2008;100(1–3):20–38.

van Kammen DP, Hurford I, Marder SR. First-generation antipsychotics. In: Sadock BJ, Sadock VA, Ruiz P, eds. *Kaplan & Sadock's Comprehensive Textbook of Psychiatry.* 9th ed. Vol. 2. Philadelphia, PA: Lippincott Williams & Wilkins; 2009:3105.

Wu B-J, Chen H-K, Lee S-M. Do atypical antipsychotics really enhance smoking reduction more than typical ones? The effects of antipsychotics on smoking reduction in patients with schizophrenia. *J Clin Psychopharmacol.* 2013;33(3):319–328.

Antidepressants

Adli M, Pilhatsch M, Bauer M, Köberle U, Ricken R, Janssen G, Ulrich S, Bschor T. Safety of high-intensity treatment with the irreversible monoamine oxidase inhibitor tranylcypromine in patients with treatment-resistant depression. *Pharmacopsychiatry.* 2008;41:252–257.

Altshuler LL, Bauer M, Frye MA, Gitlin MJ, Mintz J. Does thyroid supplementation accelerate tricyclic antidepressant response? A review in meta-analysis of the literature. *Am J Psychiatry.* 2001;158:1617–1622.

Amsterdam JD, Bodkin JA. Selegiline transdermal system in the prevention of relapse of major depressive disorder: a 52-week, double-blind, placebo-substitution, parallel-group clinical trial. *J Clin Psychopharmacol.* 2006;26:579–586.

Amsterdam JD, Wang CH, Shwarz M, Shults J. Venlafaxine versus lithium monotherapy of rapid and non-rapid cycling patients with bipolar II major depressive episode: a randomized, parallel group, open-label trial. *J Affect Disord.* 2009;112(1–3):219–230.

Anderson I. Selective serotonin reuptake inhibitors versus tricyclics antidepressant: a meta-analysis of efficacy and tolerability. *J Affect Disord.* 2000;58:19.

Andrisano C, Chiesa A, Serretti A. Newer antidepressants and panic disorder: a meta-analysis. *Int Clin Psychopharmacol.* 2013;28(1):33–45.

Anton RF, Burch EA. Amoxapine versus amitriptyline combined with perphenazine in the treatment of psychotic depression. *Am J Psychiatry.* 1990;147:1203–1208.

Appelhof BC, Brouwer JP, van Dyck R, Fliers E, Hoogendijk WJ. Triiodothyronine addition to paroxetine in the treatment of major depressive disorder. *J Clin Endocrinol Metab.* 2004;89:6271–6276.

Aronson R, Offman HJ, Joffe RT, Naylor CD. Triiodothyronine augmentation and the treatment of refractory depression: a meta-analysis. *Arch Gen Psychiatry.* 1996;53:842–848.

Ashton AK, Longdon MC. SSNRI-induced, dose dependent, nonmenstrual, vaginal spotting and galactorrhea accompanied by prolactin elevation (Letter). *Am J Psychiatry.* 2007;164:1121.

Baker GB, Sowa S, Todd KG. Amine oxidases and their inhibitors: what can they tell us about neuroprotection and the development of drugs for neuropsychiatric disorders? *J Psychiatr Neurosci.* 2007;32:313–315.

Baldessarini RJ, Pompili M, Tondo L. Suicidal risk in antidepressant drug trials. *Arch Gen Psychiatry.* 2006;63:246–248.

Balu DT, Hoshaw BA, Malberg JE. Differential regulation of central BDNF protein levels by antidepressant and non-antidepressant drug treatments. *Brain Res.* 2008;1211:37–43.

Banerjee S, Hellier J, Romeo R, Dewey M, Knapp M, Ballard C, Baldwin R, Bentham P, Fox C, Holmes C, Katona C, Lawton C, Lindesay J, Livingston G, McCrae N, Moniz-Cook E, Murray J, Nurock S, Orrell M, O'Brien J, Poppe M, Thomas A, Walwyn R, Wilson K, Burns A. Study of the use of antidepressants for depression in dementia: the HTA-SADD trial—a multicentre, randomised, double-blind, placebo-controlled trial of the clinical effectiveness and cost-effectiveness of sertraline and mirtazapine. *Health Technol Assess.* 2013;17(7):1–166.

Barbui C, Esposito E, Cipriani A. Selective serotonin reuptake inhibitors and risk of suicide: a systematic review of observational studies. *CMAJ.* 2009;180:291–297.

Bauer M, Baur H, Bergebifer A, Strohle A, Hellweg R. Effects of supraphysiological thyroxine administration in healthy controls in patients with depressive disorders. *J Affect Dis.* 2002;68:285–294.

Baungartner A. Thyroxine and the treatment of affective disorders: an overview of the results of basic and clinical research. *Int J Neuropsychopharmacol.* 2000;3:149–165.

Bech P, Allerup P, Larsen E, Csillag C, Licht R. Escitalopram versus nortriptyline: how to let the clinical GENDEP data tell us what they contained. *Acta Psychiatr Scand.* 2013;127(4):328–329.

Cettomai D, McArthur JC. Mirtazapine use in human immunodeficiency virus-infected patients with progressive multifocal leukoencephalopathy. *Arch Neurol.* 2009;66(2):255–258.

Chambers CD, Hernandez-Diaz S, Van Marter LJ, Werler MM, Louik C. Selective serotonin-reuptake inhibitors and risk of persistent pulmonary hypertension of the newborn. *N Engl J Med.* 2006;354:579–587.

Charney DS, Delgado PL, Price LH, Heninger GR. The receptor sensitivity hypothesis of antidepressant action: a review of antidepressant effects on serotonin function. In: Brown SL, van Praag HM, eds. *The Role of Serotonin in Psychiatric Disorders.* New York: Brunner/Mazel; 1991:29.

Choung RS, Cremonini F, Thapa P, Zinsmeister AR, Talley NJ. The effect of short-term, low-dose tricyclic and tetracyclic antidepressant treatment on satiation, postnutrient load gastrointestinal symptoms and gastric emptying: a double-blind, randomized, placebo-controlled trial. *Neurogastroenterol Motil.* 2008;20:220–227.

Cipriani A, Barbui C, Brambilla P, Furukawa TA, Hotopf M. Are all antidepressants really the same? The case of fluoxetine: a systematic review. *J Clin Psychiatry.* 2006;67:850–864.

Cipriani A, Furukawa TA, Salanti G, Geddes JR, Higgins JPT. Comparative efficacy and acceptability of 12 new-generation antidepressants: a multiple-treatments meta-analysis. *Lancet.* 2009;373:746–758.

Ciraulo DA, Knapp C, Rotrosen J, Sarid-Segal O, Seliger C. Nefazodone treatment of cocaine dependence with comorbid depressive symptoms. *Addiction.* 2005; 100(Suppl 1):23–31.

Clayton A, Kornstein S, Prakash A, Mallinckrodt C, Wohlreich M. Changes in sexual functioning associated with duloxetine, escitalopram, and placebo in the treatment of patients with major depressive disorder. *J Sex Med.* 2007;4:917–929.

Clayton AH, Montejo AL. Major depressive disorder, antidepressants, and sexual dysfunction. *J Clin Psychiatry.* 2006;67(Suppl 6):33.

Cohen LS, Altshuler LL, Harlow BL, Nonacs R, Newport DJ. Relapse of major depression during pregnancy in women who maintain or discontinue antidepressant treatment. *JAMA.* 2006;295:499.

Cooper-Kazaz A, Apter JT, Cohen R, Karapichev L, Mohammed-Moussa S. Combined treatment with sertraline and liothyronine in major depression: a randomized, double-blind, placebo-controlled trial. *Arch Gen Psychiatry.* 2007;64:679–688.

Couturier J, Sy A, Johnson N, Findlay S. Bone mineral density in adolescents with eating disorders exposed to selective serotonin reuptake inhibitors. *Eat Disord.* 2013;21(3):238–248.

Cowen P, Sherwood AC. The role of serotonin in cognitive function: evidence from recent studies and implications for understanding depression. *J Psychopharmacol.* 2013;27(7):575–583.

Danish University Antidepressant Group. Paroxetine: a selective serotonin reuptake inhibitor showing better tolerance, but weaker antidepressant effect than clomipramine in a controlled multicenter study. *J Affect Dis.* 1990;18:289.

DeBattista C, Schatzberg AF. Bupropion. In: Sadock BJ, Sadock VA, Ruiz P, eds. *Kaplan & Sadock's Comprehensive Textbook of Psychiatry.* 9th ed. Vol. 2. Philadelphia, PA: Lippincott Williams & Wilkins; 2009:3056.

DeBattista C, Solvason B, Poirier J, Kendrick E, Loraas E. A placebo-controlled, randomized, double-blind study of adjunctive bupropion sustained release in the treatment of SSRI-induced sexual dysfunction. *J Clin Psychiatry.* 2005; 66(7):844–848.

DeBattista C, Solvason HB, Poirier J, Kendrick E, Schatzberg AF. A prospective trial of bupropion SR augmentation of partial and non-responders to serotonergic antidepressants. *J Clin Psychopharmacol*. 2003;23(1):27–30.

DeBattista C. Augmentation and combination strategies for depression. *J Psychopharmacol*. 2006;20(3 Suppl):11–18.

DellaGioia N, Devine L, Pittman B, Hannestad J. Bupropion pretreatment of endotoxin-induced depressive symptoms. *Brain Behav Immun*. 2013;31:197–204.

DeSanty KP, Amabile CM. Antidepressant-induced liver injury. *Ann Pharmacother*. 2007;41(7):1201.

Diem SJ, Blackwell TL, Stone KL, Yaffe K, Haney EM. Use of antidepressants and rates of hip bone loss in older women: the study of osteoporotic fractures. *Arch Intern Med*. 2007;167:1240–1245.

Duman RS, Heninger GR, Nestler EJ. A molecular and cellular theory of depression. *Arch Gen Psychiatry*. 1997;54:597–606.

Dykens JA, Jamieson JD, Marroquin LD, Nadanaciva S, Xu JJ, Dunn MC, Smith AR, Will Y. In vitro assessment of mitochondrial dysfunction and cytotoxicity of nefazodone, trazodone, and buspirone. *Toxicol Sci*. 2008;103(2):335–345.

Elkin I, Shea T, Watkins JT. NIMH treatment of depression collaborative research program: general effectiveness of treatments. *Arch Gen Psychiatry*. 1989;46:971.

Elmer LW, Bertoni JM. The increasing role of monoamine oxidase type B inhibitors in Parkinson's disease therapy. *Expert Opin Pharmacother*. 2008;9:2759–2772.

Fava M, Rush AJ, Wisniewski SR, Nierenberg AA, Alpert JE. A comparison of mirtazapine and nortriptyline following two consecutive failed medication treatments for depressed outpatients: a STAR*D report. *Am J Psychiatry*. 2006;163(7):1161–1172.

Foley KF, DeSanty KP, Kast RE. Bupropion: pharmacology and therapeutic applications. *Expert Rev Neurother*. 2006;6(9):1249–1265.

Frampton JE, Plosker GL. Duloxetine: a review of its use in the treatment of major depressive disorder. *CNS Drugs*. 2007;21:581–609.

Frampton JE, Plosker GL, Masand PS. Selegiline transdermal system in the treatment of major depressive disorder. *Drugs*. 2007;67:257.

Frank E, Kupfer DJ, Perel JM. Three-year outcomes for maintenance therapies in recurrent depression. *Arch Gen Psychiatry*. 1990;47:1093.

Glassman AH, O'Connor CM, Califf RM, Swedberg K, Schwartz P. Association of low bone mineral density with selective serotonin reuptake inhibitor use by older men. *Arch Intern Med*. 2007;167(12):1246–1251.

Goldberg JF. A preliminary open trial of nefazodone added to mood stabilizers for bipolar depression. *J Affect Disord*. 2013;144(1–2):176–178.

Goldberg JF, Thase ME. Monoamine oxidase inhibitors revisited: what you should know. *J Clin Psychiatry*. 2013;74(2):189–191.

Hettema JM, Kornstein SG. Trazodone. In: Sadock BJ, Sadock VA, Ruiz P, eds. *Kaplan & Sadock's Comprehensive Textbook of Psychiatry*. 9th ed. Vol. 2. Philadelphia, PA: Lippincott Williams & Wilkins; 2009:3253.

Holt A, Berry MD, Boulton AA. On the binding of monoamine oxidase inhibitors to some sites distinct from the MAO active site, and effects thereby elicited. *Neurotoxicology*. 2004;25:251–266.

Hu X-Z, Rush AJ, Charney D, Wilson AF, Sorant AJM. Association between a functional serotonin transporter promoter polymorphism and citalopram treatment in adult outpatients with major depression. *Arch Gen Psychiatry*. 2007;64:783–792.

Joffe RT. Thyroid hormones. In: Sadock BJ, Sadock VA, Ruiz P, eds. *Kaplan & Sadock's Comprehensive Textbook of Psychiatry*. 9th ed. Vol. 2. Philadelphia, PA: Lippincott Williams & Wilkins; 2009:3248.

Joffe RT, Sokolov ST, Levitt AJ. Lithium and triiodothyronine augmentation of antidepressants. *Can J Psychiatry*. 2006;51:791–793.

Johansson P, Almqvist EG, Johansson J-O, Mattsson N, Hansson O, Wallin A, Blennow K, Zetterberg H, Svensson J. Reduced cerebrospinal fluid level of thyroxine in patients with Alzheimer's disease. *Psychoneuroendocrinology*. 2013;38(7):1058–1066.

Kasper S, Corruble E, Hale A, Lemoine P, Montgomery SA, Quera-Salva M-A. Antidepressant efficacy of agomelatine versus SSRI/SNRI: results from a pooled analysis of head-to-head studies without a placebo control. *Int Clin Psychopharmacol*. 2013;28(1):12–19.

Keller MB, Trivedi MH, Thase ME, Shelton RC, Kornstein SG, Nemeroff CB, Friedman ES, Gelenberg AJ, Kocsis JH, Dunner DL, Hirschfeld RMA, Rothschild AJ, Ferguson JM, Schatzberg AF, Zajecka JM, Pedersen RD, Yan B, Ahmed S, Musgnung J, Ninan PT. The Prevention of Recurrent Episodes of Depression with Venlafaxine for Two Years (PREVENT) Study: outcomes from the 2-year and combined maintenance phases. *J Clin Psychiatry*. 2007;68:1246–1256.

Kennedy SH, Holt A, Baker GB. Monoamine oxidase inhibitors. In: Sadock BJ, Sadock VA, Ruiz P, eds. *Kaplan & Sadock's Comprehensive Textbook of Psychiatry*. 9th ed. Vol. 2. Philadelphia, PA: Lippincott Williams & Wilkins; 2009:3154.

Khan AA, Kornstein SG. Nefazodone. In: Sadock BJ, Sadock VA, Ruiz P, eds. *Kaplan & Sadock's Comprehensive Textbook of Psychiatry*. 9th ed. Vol. 2. Philadelphia, PA: Lippincott Williams & Wilkins; 2009:3164.

Kim SW, Shin IS, Kim JM, Park KH, Youn T, Yoon JS. Factors potentiating the risk of mirtazapine-associated restless legs syndrome. *Hum Psychopharmacol*. 2008;(7):615–620.

Kocsis JH, Leon AC, Markowitz JC, Manber R, Arnow B, Klein DN, Thase ME. Patient preference as a moderator of outcome for chronic forms of major depressive disorder treated with nefazodone, cognitive behavioral analysis system of psychotherapy, or their combination. *J Clin Psychiatry*. 2009;70(3):354–361.

Koibuchi N. The role of thyroid hormone on functional organization in the cerebellum. *Cerebellum*. 2013;12(3):304–306.

Kostrubsky SE, Strom SC, Kalgutkar AS, Kulkarni S, Atherton J. Inhibition of hepatobiliary transport as a predictive method for clinical hepatotoxicity of nefazodone. *Toxicol Sci*. 2006;90(2):451–459.

Lai MW, Klein-Schwartz W, Rodgers GC, Abrams JY, Haber DA. 2005 Annual report of the American Association of Poison Control Centers' national poisoning and exposure database. *Clin Toxicol*. 2006;44:803–932.

Lam RW, Andersen HF, Wade AG. Escitalopram and duloxetine in the treatment of major depressive disorder: a pooled analysis of two trials. *Int Clin Psychopharmacol*. 2008;23(4):181.

Lapierre YD. A review of trimipramine: 30 years of clinical use. *Drugs*. 1989;38(Suppl 1):17–24.

Lieberman DZ, Montgomery SA, Tourian KA, Brisard C, Rosas G. A pooled analysis of two placebo-controlled trials of desvenlafaxine in major depressive disorder. *Int Clin Psychopharmacol*. 2008;23:188–197.

Liebowitz MR, Manley AL, Padmanabhan SK, Ganguly R, Tummala R. Efficacy, safety, and tolerability of desvenlafaxine 50 mg/day and 100 mg/day in outpatients with major depressive disorder. *Curr Med Res Opin*. 2008;24:1877–1890.

Liebowitz MR, Quitkin FM, Stewart JW. Antidepressant specificity in atypical depression. *Arch Gen Psychiatry*. 1988;45:129–137.

Lojko D, Rybakowski JK. L-Thyroxine augmentation of serotonergic antidepressants in female patients with refractory depression. *J Affect Disord*. 2007;103(1–3):253–256.

Looper KL. Potential medical and surgical complications of serotonergic antidepressant medications. *Psychosomatics*. 2007;48:1–9.

Maruyama W, Naoi M. "70th birthday professor riederer" induction of glial cell line-derived and brain-derived neurotrophic factors by rasagiline and (-)deprenyl: a way to a disease-modifying therapy? *J Neural Transm*. 2013;120(1):83–89.

McGrath PJ, Stewart JW, Fava M, Trivedi MH, Wisniewski SR. Tranylcypromine versus venlafaxine plus mirtazapine following three failed antidepressant medication trials for depression: a STAR*D report. *Am J Psychiatry*. 2006;163(9):1531–1541.

McIntyre RS, Panjwani ZD, Nguyen HT, Woldeyohannes HO, Alsuwaidan M. The hepatic safety profile of duloxetine: a review. *Expert Opin Drug Metab Toxicol*. 2008;4:281–285.

Montgomery SA, Baldwin DS, Blier P, Fineberg NA, Kasper S. Which antidepressants have demonstrated superior efficacy? A review of the evidence. *Int Clin Psychopharmacol*. 2007;22:323–329.

Nasky KM, Cowan GL, Knittel DR. False-positive urine screening for benzodiazepines: an association with sertraline? A two-year retrospective analysis. *Psychiatry (Edgemont)*. 2009;6(7):36–39.

Nelson JC. Tricyclics and tetracyclics. In: Sadock BJ, Sadock VA, Ruiz P, eds. *Kaplan & Sadock's Comprehensive Textbook of Psychiatry*. 9th ed. Vol. 2. Philadelphia, PA: Lippincott Williams & Wilkins; 2009:3259.

Nelson JC, Mazure G, Jatlow PI. Antidepressant activity of 2-hydroxy-desipramine. *Clin Pharmacol Ther*. 1988;44:283.

Nemeroff CB, Entsuah R, Benattia I, Demitrack M, Sloan DM. Comprehensive analysis of remission (COMPARE) with venlafaxine versus SSRIs. *Biol Psychiatry*. 2008;63:424–434.

Nierenberg AA, Fava M, Trivedi MH, Wisniewski SR, Thase ME, McGrath PJ, Alpert JE, Warden D, Luther JF, Niederehe G, Lebowitz B, Shores-Wilson K, Rush AJ. A comparison of lithium and T(3) augmentation following two failed medication treatments for depression: a STAR*D report. *Am J Psychiatry*. 2006;163:1519–1530.

Nolen WA, Kupka RW, Hellemann G, Frye MA, Altshuler LL. Tranylcypromine vs. lamotrigine in the treatment of refractory bipolar depression: a failed but clinically useful study. *Acta Psychiatr Scand*. 2007;115:360–365.

Nurnberg GH, Hensley PL, Heiman JR, Croft HA, Debattista C. Sildenafil treatment of women with antidepressant-associated sexual dysfunction: a randomized controlled trial. *JAMA*. 2008;300:395–404.

O'Malley PG, Jackson JL, Santoro J, Tomkins G, Balden E. Antidepressant therapy for unexplained symptoms and symptom syndromes. *J Fam Pract*. 1999;48:980.

Owens MJ, Dole KC, Knight DL, Nemeroff CB. Preclinical evaluation of the putative antidepressant nefazodone. *Depression*. 2008;1(6):315.

Owens MJ, Krulewicz S, Simon JS, Sheehan DV, Thase ME. Estimates of serotonin and norepinephrine transporter inhibition in depressed patients treated with paroxetine or venlafaxine. *Neuropsychopharmacology*. 2008;33:3201–3212.

Pae CU, Lim HK, Ajwani N, Lee C, Patkar AA. Extended-release formulation of venlafaxine in the treatment of posttraumatic stress disorder. *Expert Rev Neurother*. 2007;7:603–615.

Papakostas GI, Fava M. A meta-analysis of clinical trials comparing milnacipran, a serotonin–norepinephrine reuptake inhibitor, with a selective serotonin reuptake inhibitor for the treatment of major depressive disorder. *Eur Neuropsychopharmacol*. 2007;17:32.

Papakostas GI, Fava M. A meta-analysis of clinical trials comparing the serotonin (5HT)-2 receptor antagonists trazodone and nefazodone with selective serotonin reuptake inhibitors for the treatment of major depressive disorder. *Eur Psychiatry*. 2007;22(7):444–447.

Papakostas GI, Homberger CH, Fava M. A meta-analysis of clinical trials comparing mirtazapine with selective serotonin reuptake inhibitors for the treatment of major depressive disorder. *J Psychopharmacol*. 2008;22(8):843–848.

Papakostas GI, Thase ME, Fava M, Nelson JC, Shelton RC. Are antidepressant drugs that combine serotonergic and noradrenergic mechanisms of action more effective than the selective serotonin reuptake inhibitors in treating major depressive disorder? A meta-analysis of studies of newer agents. *Biol Psychiatry*. 2007;62:1217–1227.

Passos SR, Camacho LA, Lopes CS, dos Santos MAB. Nefazodone in out-patient treatment of inhaled cocaine dependence: a randomized double-blind placebo-controlled trial. *Addiction*. 2005;100(4):489–494.

Perahia DG, Pritchett YL, Kajdasz DK, Bauer M, Jain R. A randomized, double-blind comparison of duloxetine and venlafaxine in the treatment of patients with major depressive disorder. *J Psychiatr Res*. 2008;42:22–34.

Perkins KA, Karelitz JL, Jao NC, Stratton E. Possible reinforcement enhancing effects of bupropion during initial smoking abstinence. *Nicotine Tob Res.* 2013;15(6): 1141–1145.

Posternak M, Novak S, Stern A, Hennessey J, Joffe A. A pilot effectiveness study: placebo-controlled trial of adjunctive L-triiodothyronine (T₃) used to accelerate and potentiate the antidepressant response. *Int J Neuropsychopharmacol.* 2008;11(1):15–25.

Reeves RR, Ladner ME. Additional evidence of the abuse potential of bupropion. *J Clin Pharmacol.* 2013;33(4):584–585.

Roose S, Laghrissi-Thode F, Kennedy JS, Nelson JC, Bigger JT. A comparison of paroxetine and nortriptyline in depressed patients with ischemic heart disease. *JAMA.* 1998;279:287–91.

Rynn M, Russell J, Erickson J, Detke MJ, Ball S. Efficacy and safety of duloxetine in the treatment of generalized anxiety disorder: a flexible-dose, progressive-titration, placebo-controlled trial. *Depress Anxiety.* 2008;25:182–189.

Salahudeen MS, Wright C M, Peterson GM. "Esketamine: new hope for the treatment of treatment-resistant depression? A narrative review." *Ther Adv Drug Saf.* 2020;11: 2042098620937899. https://doi.org/10.1177/2042098620937899.

Salsali M, Holt A, Baker GB. Inhibitory effects of the monoamine oxidase inhibitor tranylcypromine on the cytochrome P450 enzymes CYP2C19, CYP2C6, and CYP2D6. *Cell Mol Neurobiol.* 2004;24:63–76.

Sasada K, Iwamoto K, Kawano N, Kohmura K, Yamamoto M, Aleksic B, Ebe K, Noda Y, Ozaki N. Effects of repeated dosing with mirtazapine, trazodone, or placebo on driving performance and cognitive function in healthy volunteers. *Hum Psychopharmacol.* 2013;28(3):281–286.

Scarff JR. "Use of Brexanolone for Postpartum Depression." *Innov Clin Neurosci.* 2019;16(11–12):32–35.

Schatzberg AF, Kremer C, Rodrigues HE, Murphy GM Jr. Double-blind, randomized comparison of mirtazapine and paroxetine in elderly depressed patients. *Am J Geriatr Psychiatry.* 2002;10:541–550.

Schatzberg AF, Prather MR, Keller MB, Rush AJ, Laird LK. Clinical use of nefazodone in major depression: a 6-year perspective. *J Clin Psychiatry.* 2002;63(1):18–31.

Schatzberg AF, Rush AJ, Arnow BA, Banks PL, Blalock JA. Chronic depression: medication (nefazodone) or psychotherapy (CBASP) is effective when the other is not. *Arch Gen Psychiatry.* 2005;62(5):513–520.

Schittecatte M, Dumont F, Machowski R, Fontaine E, Cornil C, Mendlewicz J, Wilmotte J. Mirtazapine, but not fluvoxamine, normalizes the blunted REM sleep response to clonidine in depressed patients: implications for subsensitivity of alpha(2)-adrenergic receptors in depression. *Psychiatry Res.* 2002;109:1–8.

Shenouda R, Desan PH. Abuse of tricyclic antidepressant drugs: a case series. *J Clin Psychopharmcol.* 2013;33(3):440–442.

Smith T, Nicholson RA. Review of duloxetine in the management of diabetic peripheral neuropathic pain. *Vasc Health Risk Manag.* 2007;3:833–844.

Stahl SM, Felker A. Monoamine oxidase inhibitors: a modern guide to an unrequited class of antidepressants. *CNS Spectr.* 2008;13:855–870.

Stenberg JH, Terevnikov V, Joffe M, Tiihonen J, Chukhin E, Burkin M, Joffe G. Predictors and mediators of add-on mirtazapine-induced cognitive enhancement in schizophrenia—a path model investigation. *Neuropharmacology.* 2013;64:248–253.

Sussman N. Selective serotonin reuptake inhibitors. In: Sadock BJ, Sadock VA, Ruiz P, eds. *Kaplan & Sadock's Comprehensive Textbook of Psychiatry.* 9th ed. Vol. 2. Philadelphia, PA: Lippincott Williams & Wilkins; 2009:3190.

Sylven SM, Elenis E, Michelakos T, Larsson A, Olovsson M, Poromaa IS, Skalkidou A. Thyroid function tests at delivery and risk for postpartum depressive symptoms. *Psychoneuroendocrinology.* 2013;38(7):1007–1013.

Tanimukai H, Murai T, Okazaki N, Matsuda Y, Okamoto Y, Kabeshita Y, Ohno Y, Tsuneto S. An observational study of insomnia and nightmare treated with trazodone in patients with advanced cancer. *Am J Hosp Palliat Care.* 2013;30(3):359–362.

Thase ME. Mirtazapine. In: Sadock BJ, Sadock VA, Ruiz P, eds. *Kaplan & Sadock's Comprehensive Textbook of Psychiatry.* 9th ed. Vol. 2. Philadelphia, PA: Lippincott Williams & Wilkins: 2009:3152.

Thase ME. Selective serotonin-norepinephrine reuptake inhibitors. In: Sadock BJ, Sadock VA, Ruiz P, eds. *Kaplan & Sadock's Comprehensive Textbook of Psychiatry.* 9th ed. Vol. 2. Philadelphia, PA: Lippincott Williams & Wilkins; 2009:3184.

Thase ME, Haight BR, Richard N, Rockett CB, Mitton M. Remission rates following antidepressant therapy with bupropion or selective reuptake inhibitors: a meta-analysis of original data from 7 randomized controlled trials. *J Clin Psychiatry.* 2005;66:974–981.

Thase ME, Pritchett YL, Ossanna MJ, Swindle RW, Xu J. Efficacy of duloxetine and selective serotonin reuptake inhibitors: comparisons as assessed by remission rates in patients with major depressive disorder. *J Clin Psychopharmacol.* 2007;27:672–676.

Tremblay P, Blier P. Catecholaminergic strategies for the treatment of major depression. *Curr Drug Targets.* 2006;7:149.

Trivedi MH, Rush AJ, Wisniewski SR, Nierenberg AA, Warden D, Ritz L, Norquist G, Howland RH, Lebowitz B, McGrath PJ, Shores-Wilson K, Biggs MM, Balasubramani GK, Fava M, STAR*D Study Team. Evaluation of outcomes with citalopram for depression using measurement-based care in STAR*D: implications for clinical practice. *Am J Psychiatry.* 2006;163:28–40.

Tulen JH, Volkers AC, van den Broek WW, Bruijn JA. Sustained effects of phenelzine and tranylcypromine on orthostatic challenge in antidepressant-refractory depression. *J Clin Psychopharmacol.* 2006;26:542–544.

Van Ameringen M, Mancini C, Oakman J. Nefazodone in the treatment of generalized social phobia: a randomized, placebo-controlled trial. *J Clin Psychiatry.* 2007; 68(2):288–295.

Verena H, Mergl R, Allgaier AK, Kohnen R, Möller HJ. Treatment of depression with atypical features: a meta-analytic approach. *Psychiatry Res.* 2006;141:89–101.

Weissman AM, Levy BT, Hartz, AJ, Bentler S, Donohue M. Pooled analysis of antidepressant levels in lactating mothers, breast milk, and nursing infants. *Am J Psychiatry.* 2004;161:1066.

Whitmyer VG, Dunner DL, Kornstein SG, Meyers AL, Mallinckrodt CH. A comparison of initial duloxetine dosing strategies in patients with major depressive disorder. *J Clin Psychiatry.* 2007;68:1921.

Wilens TE, Spencer TJ, Biederman J, Girard K, Doyle R. A controlled clinical trial of bupropion for attention deficit hyperactivity disorder in adults. *Am J Psychiatry.* 2001;158(2):282.

Wood PL, Khan MA, Moskal JR, Todd KG, Tanay VAMI. Aldehyde load in ischemia-reperfusion injury: neuroprotection by neutralization of reactive aldehydes with phenelzine. *Brain Res.* 2006;184–190.

Xu JJ, Henstock PV, Dunn MC, Smith AR, Chabot JR, de Graaf D. Cellular imaging predictions of clinical drug-induced liver injury. *Toxicol Sci.* 2008;105(1):97–105.

Yoshimura M, Furue H. Mechanisms for the anti-nociceptive actions of the descending noradrenergic and serotonergic systems in the spinal cord. *J Pharmacol Sci.* 2006;101:107–117.

Zanos P, Gould T D. "Mechanisms of ketamine action as an antidepressant." *Mol Psychiatry.* 2018;23(4): 801–811. https://doi.org/10.1038/mp.2017.255.

Zisook S, Rush AJ, Haight BR, Clines DC, Rockett CB. Use of bupropion in combination with serotonin reuptake inhibitors. *Biol Psychiatry.* 2006;59(3):203–210.

Mood Stabilizers

Alvarez G, Marsh W, Camacho IA, Gracia SL. Effectiveness and tolerability of carbamazepine vs. oxcarbazepine as mood stabilizers. *Clin Res Reg Affairs.* 2003;20:365.

Atmaca M, Ozdemir H, Cetinkaya S, Parmaksiz S, Poyraz AK. Cingulate gyrus volumetry in drug free bipolar patients and patients treated with valproate or valproate and quetiapine. *J Psychiatr Res.* 2007;41:821–827.

Atmaca M, Yildirim H, Ozdemir H, Ogur E, Tezcan E. Hippocampal 1H MRS in patients with bipolar disorder taking valproate versus valproate plus quetiapine. *Psychol Med.* 2007;37:121–129.

Bachmann RF, Schloesser RJ, Gould TD, Manji HK. Mood stabilizers target cellular plasticity and resilience cascades. *Mol Neurobiol.* 2005;32:173–202.

Bauer M, Grof P, Müller-Oerlinghausen B. *Lithium in Neuropsychiatry: The Comprehensive Guide.* Oxon, UK: Informa UK; 2006.

Bearden CE, Thompson PM, Dalwani M, Hayashi KM, Lee AD. Greater cortical gray matter density in lithium-treated patients with bipolar disorder. *Biol Psychiatry.* 2007;62:7–16.

Benedetti A, Lattanzi L, Pini S, Musetti L, Dell'Osso L. Oxcarbazepine as add-on treatment in patients with bipolar manic, mixed, or depressive episode. *J Affect Disord.* 2004;79:273–277.

Bialer M. Extended-release formulations for the treatment of epilepsy. *CNS Drugs.* 2007;21:765–774.

Bowden CL, Swann AC, Calabrese JR, Rubenfaer LM, Wozniak PJ. Depakote ER Mania Study Group. A randomized, placebo-controlled, multicenter study of divalproex sodium extended release in the treatment of acute mania. *J Clin Psychiatry.* 2006;67:1501.

Bray GA, Hollander P, Klein S, Kushner R, Levy B. A 6-month randomized, placebo-controlled, dose-ranging trial of topiramate for weight loss in obesity. *Obes Res.* 2003;11(6):722–733.

Calabrese JR, Huffman RF, White RL. Lamotrigine in the acute treatment of bipolar depression: results of five double-blind, placebo-controlled clinical trials. *Bipolar Disord.* 2008;10:323–333.

Chen PS, Wang CC, Bortner CD, Peng GS, Wu X, Pang H. Valproic acid and other histone deacetylase inhibitors induce microglial apoptosis and attenuate lipopolysaccharide-induced dopaminergic neurotoxicity. *Neuroscience.* 2007;149:203–212.

Chustecka Z. Hydralazine and valproate appear to overcome resistance to chemotherapy. *Ann Oncol.* 2007;18:1529.

Cipriani A, Hawton K, Stockton S, Geddes JR. Lithium in the prevention of suicide in mood disorders: updated systematic review and meta-analysis. *BMJ.* 2013;346: f3646.

Cohen LS, Friedman JM, Jefferson JW, Johnson EM, Weiner ML. A reevaluation of risk of in utero exposure to lithium. *JAMA.* 1994;271:146–150.

Collins J, McFarland B. Divalproex, lithium and suicide among medicaid patients with bipolar disorder. *J Affect Dis.* 2008;107:23–28.

Cousins DA, Aribisala B, Ferrier I, Blamire AM. Lithium, gray matter, and magnetic resonance imaging signal. *Biol Psychiatry.* 2013;73(7):652–657.

Crofford LJ, Rowbotham MC, Mease PJ, Russell IJ, Dworkin RH. Pregabalin for the treatment of fibromyalgia syndrome: results of a randomized, double-blind, placebo-controlled trial. *Arthritis Rheum.* 2005;52(4):1264.

Delvendahl I, Lindemann H, Heidegger T, Normann C, Ziemann U, Mall V. Effects of lamotrigine on human motor cortex plasticity. *Clin Neurophysiol.* 2013;124(1): 148–153.

Du J, Suzuki K, Wei Y, Wang Y, Blumenthal R. The anticonvulsants lamotrigine, riluzole, and valproate differentially regulate AMPA receptor membrane localization: Relationship to clinical effects in mood disorders. *Neuropsychopharmacology.* 2007;32:793–802.

Dubovsky SL. Calcium channel inhibitors. In: Sadock BJ, Sadock VA, Ruiz P, eds. *Kaplan & Sadock's Comprehensive Textbook of Psychiatry.* 9th ed. Vol. 2. Philadelphia, PA: Lippincott Williams & Wilkins; 2009:3065.

Dubovsky SL, Buzan RD, Thomas M, Kassner C, Cullum CM. Nicardipine improves the antidepressant action of ECT but does not improve cognition. *J ECT.* 2001;17: 3–10.

Einat H, Manji HK. Cellular plasticity cascades: genes-to-behavior pathways in animal models of bipolar disorder. *Biol Psychiatry*. 2006;59:1160–1171.

Findling RL, Frazier TW, Youngstrom EA, McNamara NK, Stansbrey RJ. Double-blind, placebo-controlled trial of divalproex monotherapy in the treatment of symptomatic youth at high risk for developing bipolar disorder. *J Clin Psychiatry*. 2007;68:781–788.

Freeman R, Durso-Decruz E, Emir B. Efficacy, safety, and tolerability of pregabalin treatment for painful diabetic peripheral neuropathy: findings from seven randomized, controlled trials across a range of doses. *Diabetes Care*. 2008;31:1448–1454.

Frye MA, Ketter TA, Kimbrell TA, Dunn RT, Speer AM. A placebo-controlled study of lamotrigine and gabapentin monotherapy in refractory mood disorders. *J Clin Psychopharmacol*. 2000;20(6):607–614.

Gadde KM, Franciscy DM, Wagner HR 2nd, Krishnan KR. Zonisamide for weight loss in obese adults: a randomized controlled trial. *JAMA*. 2003;289(14):1820–1825.

Geddes JR, Burgess S, Hawton K, Jamison K, Goodwin GM. Long-term lithium therapy for bipolar disorder: systematic review and meta-analysis of randomized controlled trials. *Am J Psychiatry*. 2004;161:217–222.

Geddes JR, Calabrese JR, Goodwin GM. Lamotrigine for treatment of bipolar depression: Independent meta-analysis and meta-regression of individual patient data from five randomised trials. *Br J Psychiatry*. 2009;194:4.

Ghaemi NS, Ko JY, Katzow JJ. Oxcarbazepine treatment of refractory bipolar disorder: a retrospective chart review. *Bipolar Disord*. 2002;4(1):70–74.

Goldberg JF, Bowden CL, Calabrese JR. Six-month prospective life charting of mood symptoms with lamotrigine monotherapy versus placebo in rapid cycling bipolar disorder. *Biol Psychiatry*. 2008;63:125.

Goodwin FK, Jamison KR. *Manic-Depressive Illness*. 2nd ed. New York: Oxford University Press; 2007.

Goodwin GM, Bowden CL, Calabrese JR, Grunze H, Kasper S. A pooled analysis of 2 placebo-controlled 18-month trials of lamotrigine and lithium maintenance in bipolar I disorder. *J Clin Psychiatry*. 2004;65:432–441.

Grunze H, Erfurth A, Marcuse A, Amann B, Normann C. Tiagabine appears not to be efficacious in the treatment of acute mania. *J Clin Psychiatry*. 1999;60(11):759–762.

Hartong EG, Moleman P, Hoogduin CA, Broekman TG, Nolen WA. Prophylactic efficacy of lithium versus carbamazepine in treatment-naive bipolar patients. *J Clin Psychiatry*. 2003;64:144–151.

Harwood AJ. Lithium and bipolar mood disorder: the inositol-depletion hypothesis revisited. *Mol Psychiatry*. 2005;10:117.

Hasan M, Pulman J, Marson AG. Calcium antagonists as an add-on therapy for drug-resistant epilepsy. *Cochrane Database Syst Rev*. 2013;3:CD002750.

Hoopes SP, Reimherr FW, Hedges DW, Rosenthal NR, Kamin M. Treatment of bulimia nervosa with topiramate in a randomized, double-blind, placebo-controlled trial, part 1: improvement in binge and purge measures. *J Clin Psychiatry*. 2003;64(11):1335–1341.

Ikeda A, Kato T. Biological predictors of lithium response in bipolar disorder. *Psychiatry Clin Neurosci*. 2003;57:243–250.

Ishioka M, Yasui-Furukori N, Hashimoto K, Sugawara N. Neuroleptic malignant syndrome induced by lamotrigine. *Clin Neuropharmacol*. 2013;36(4):131–132.

Isojarvi JI, Huuskonen UE, Pakarinen AJ, Vuolteenaho O, Myllyla VV. The regulation of serum sodium after replacing carbamazepine with oxcarbazepine. *Epilepsia*. 2001;42(6):741–745.

Jefferson JW, Greist JH. Lithium. In: Sadock BJ, Sadock VA, Ruiz P, eds. *Kaplan & Sadock's Comprehensive Textbook of Psychiatry*. 9th ed. Vol. 2. Philadelphia, PA: Lippincott Williams & Wilkins; 2009:3132

Johnson BA, Rosenthal N, Capece JA. Improvement of physical health and quality of life of alcohol-dependent individuals with topiramate treatment: US multisite randomized controlled trial. *Arch Intern Med*. 2008;168:1188–1199.

Johnson BA, Rosenthal N, Capece JA, Wiegand F, Mao L. Topiramate for treating alcohol dependence: a randomized controlled trial. *JAMA*. 2007;298(14):1641.

Kamalinia G, Brand S, Ghaeli P, Abedi N, Bajoghli H, Sharifi V, Zahiroddin A, Amini M, Rouini MR, Holsboer-Trachsler E, Mohammadpoor AH. Serum levels of sodium valproate in patients suffering from bipolar disorders: comparing acute and maintenance phases of mania. *Pharmacopsychiatry*. 2013;46(3):83–87.

Kato T, Ishiwata M, Mori K, Washizuka S, Tajima O. Mechanisms of altered Ca^{2+} signaling in transformed lymphoblastoid cells from patients with bipolar disorder. *Int J Neuropsychopharmacol*. 2003;6:379–389.

Ketter TA, Brooks JO, Hoblyn JC. Effectiveness of lamotrigine in bipolar disorder in a clinical setting. *J Psychiatr Res*. 2008;43:13–23.

Ketter TA, Greist JH, Graham JA, Roberts JN, Thompson TR. The effect of dermatologic precautions on the incidence of rash with addition of lamotrigine in the treatment of bipolar I disorder: a randomized trial. *J Clin Psychiatry*. 2006;67(3):400–406.

Ketter TA, Wang PW. Anticonvulsants: Gabapentin, levetiracetam, pregabalin, tiagabine, topiramate, zonisamide. In: Sadock BJ, Sadock VA, Ruiz P, eds. *Kaplan & Sadock's Comprehensive Textbook of Psychiatry*. 9th ed. Vol. 2. Philadelphia, PA: Lippincott Williams & Wilkins; 2009:3021.

Ketter TA, Wang PW. Lamotrigine. In: Sadock BJ, Sadock VA, Ruiz P, eds. *Kaplan & Sadock's Comprehensive Textbook of Psychiatry*. 9th ed. Vol. 2. Philadelphia, PA: Lippincott Williams & Wilkins; 2009:3127.

Ketter TA, Wang PW, Becker OV, Nowakowska C, Yang YS. The diverse roles of anticonvulsants in bipolar disorders. *Ann Clin Psychiatry*. 2003;15:95–108.

Klitgaard H. Epilepsy therapy: anticonvulsants, lessons learned and unmet medical needs. *Expert Rev Neurother*. 2013;13(1):13–14.

Kozaric-Kovacic D, Eterovic M. Lamotrigine abolished aggression in a patient with treatment-resistant posttraumatic stress disorder. *Clin Neuropharmacol*. 2013;36(3):94–95.

Kremer I, Vass A, Gorelik I, Bar G, Blanaru M, Javitt DC. Placebo-controlled trial of lamotrigine added to conventional and atypical antipsychotics in schizophrenia. *Biol Psychiatry*. 2004;56(6):441–446.

Kushner SF, Khan A, Lane R, Olson WH. Topiramate monotherapy in the management of acute mania: results of four double-blind placebo-controlled trials. *Bipolar Disord*. 2006;8(1):15–27.

Livingston C, Rampes H. Lithium: a review of its metabolic adverse effects. *J Psychopharmacol*. 2006;20:347–355.

McClellan J, Kowatch R, Findling RL, Work Group on Quality Issues. Practice parameter for the assessment and treatment of children and adolescents with bipolar disorder. *J Am Acad Child Adolesc Psychiatry*. 2007;46:107–125.

McElroy SL, Hudson JI, Capece JA, Beyers K, Fisher AC. Topiramate for the treatment of binge eating disorder associated with obesity: a placebo-controlled study. *Biol Psychiatry*. 2007;61(9):1039–1048.

McElroy SL, Kotwal R, Guerdjikova AI, Welge JA, Nelson EB. Zonisamide in the treatment of binge eating disorder with obesity: a randomized controlled trial. *J Clin Psychiatry*. 2006;67(12):1897–906.

Mease PJ, Russell IJ, Arnold LM. A randomized, double-blind, placebo-controlled, phase III trial of pregabalin in the treatment of patients with fibromyalgia. *J Rheumatol*. 2008;35:502–514.

Merideth CH. A single-center, double-blind, placebo-controlled evaluation of lamotrigine in the treatment of obesity in adults. *J Clin Psychiatry*. 2006;67(2):258–262.

Nahorski SR. Pharmacology of intracellular signaling pathways. *Br J Pharmacol*. 2006;147:S38.

Perucca P, Mula M. Antiepileptic drug effects on mood and behavior: molecular targets. *Epilepsy Behav*. 2013;26(3):440–449.

Post RM, Frye MA. Carbamazepine. In: Sadock BJ, Sadock VA, Ruiz P, eds. *Kaplan & Sadock's Comprehensive Textbook of Psychiatry*. 9th ed. Vol. 2. Philadelphia, PA: Lippincott Williams & Wilkins; 2009:3073.

Post RM, Frye MA. Valproate. In: Sadock BJ, Sadock VA, Ruiz P, eds. *Kaplan & Sadock's Comprehensive Textbook of Psychiatry*. 9th ed. Vol. 2. Philadelphia, PA: Lippincott Williams & Wilkins; 2009:3271.

Raedler TJ, Wiedemann K. Lithium-induced nephropathies. *Psychopharmacol Bull*. 2007;40:134.

Rao JS, Bazinet RP, Rapoport SL, Lee HJ. Chronic treatment of rats with sodium valproate downregulates frontal cortex NF-kappaB DNA binding activity and COX-2 mRNA Bipolar Disord. 2007;9:513–520.

Redmond JR, Jamison KL, Bowden CL. Lamotrigine combined with divalproex or lithium for bipolar disorder: a case series. *CNS Spectr*. 2006;11:12.

Rosenberg G. The mechanisms of action of valproate in neuropsychiatric disorders: can we see the forest for the trees? *Cell Mol Life Sci*. 2007;64:2090.

Rowe MK, Wiest C, Chuang D-M. GSK-3 is a viable potential target for therapeutic intervention in bipolar disorder. *Neurosci Biobehav Rev*. 2007;31:920.

Shaltiel G, Chen G, Manji HK. Neurotrophic signaling cascades in the pathophysiology and treatment of bipolar disorder. *Curr Opin Pharmacol*. 2007;7:22.

Sienaert P, Geeraerts I, Wyckaert S. How to initiate lithium therapy: a systematic review of dose estimation and level prediction methods. *J Affect Dis*. 2013;146(1):15–33.

Simeon D, Baker B, Chaplin W, Braun A, Hollander E. An open-label trial of divalproex extended-release in the treatment of borderline personality disorder. *CNS Spectr*. 2007;12:6.

Suppes T, Marangell LB, Bernstein IH. A single blind comparison of lithium and lamotrigine for the treatment of bipolar II depression. *J Affect Disord*. 2008;111:334–343.

Suzuki K, Kusumi I, Sasaki A, Koyama T. Serotonin-induced platelet intracellular calcium mobilization in various psychiatric disorders: is it specific to bipolar disorder? *J Affect Disord*. 2001;64:291–296.

Thomas SV, Ajaykumar B, Sindhu K, Nair MK, George B, Sarma PS. Motor and mental development of infants exposed to antiepileptic drugs in utero. *Epilepsy Behav*. 2008;13:229.

Tiihonen J, Hallikainen T, Ryynanen OP, Repo-Tiihonen E, Kotilainen I. Lamotrigine in treatment-resistant schizophrenia: a randomized placebo-controlled crossover trial. *Biol Psychiatry*. 2003;54(11):1241–1248.

Trankner A, Sander C, Schonknecht P. A critical review of the recent literature and selected therapy guidelines since 2006 on the use of lamotrigine in bipolar disorder. *Neuropsychiatr Dis Treat*. 2013;9:101–111.

Triggle DJ. Calcium channel antagonists: clinical uses—past, present and future. *Biochem Pharmacol*. 2007;74:1–9.

Trinka E, Marson AG, Paesschen WV, Kälviäinen R, Marovac J, Duncan B, Buyle S, Hallström Y, Hon P, Muscas GC, Newton M, Meencke HJ, Smith PE, Pohlmann-Eden B, KOMET Study Group. KOMET: an unblinded, randomised, two parallel group, stratified trial comparing the effectiveness of levetiracetam with controlled-release carbamazepine and extended-release sodium valproate as monotherapy in patients with newly diagnosed epilepsy. *J Neurol Neurosurg Psychiatry*. 2013;84(10):1138–1147.

Tritt K, Nickel C, Lahmann C, Leiberich PK, Rother WK. Lamotrigine treatment of aggression in female borderline-patients: a randomized, double-blind, placebo-controlled study. *J Psychopharmacol*. 2005;19(3):287–291.

Viguera AC, Newport DJ, Ritchie J, Stowe Z, Whitfield T. Lithium in breast milk and nursing infants: clinical implications. *Am J Psychiatry*. 2007;164:342–345.

Vrielynck P. Current and emerging treatments for absence seizures in young patients. *Neuropsychiatr Dis Treat*. 2013;9:963–975.

Wagner KD, Kowatch RA, Emslie GJ, Findling RL, Wilens TE, McCague K. A double-blind, randomized, placebo-controlled trial of oxcarbazepine in the treatment of bipolar disorder in children and adolescents. *Am J Psychiatry*. 2006;163(7):1179–1186.

Walz JC, Frey BN, Andreazza AC, Cereser KM, Cacilhas AA. Effects of lithium and valproate on serum and hippocampal neurotrophin-3 levels in an animal model of mania. *J Psychiatr Res*. 2008;42(5):416–421.

Wang HY, Friedman E. Increased association of brain protein kinase C with the receptor for activated C kinase-1 (RACK1) in bipolar affective disorder. *Biol Psychiatry*. 2001;50:364.

Waring WS. Management of lithium toxicity. *Toxicol Rev*. 2006;25:221.

Weisler RH, Kalali AK, Ketter TA. A multicenter, randomized, placebo-controlled trial of extended-release carbamazepine capsules as monotherapy for bipolar disorder patients with manic or mixed episodes. *J Clin Psychiatry*. 2004;65(4):478–484.

Wisner KL, Peindl KS, Perel JM, Hanusa BH, Piontek CM. Verapamil treatment for women with bipolar disorder. *Biol Psychiatry*. 2002;51:745–752.

Yatham LN, Kennedy SH, O'Donovan C, Parikh S, MacQueen G. Canadian network for mood and anxiety treatments (CANMAT) guidelines for the management of patients with bipolar disorder; consensus and controversies. *Bipolar Disord*. 2005;7(Suppl 3):5–69.

Yatham LN, Vieta E, Young AH, Moller HJ, Paulsson B. A double-blind, randomized, placebo-controlled trial of quetiapine as an add-on therapy to lithium or divalproex for the treatment of bipolar mania. *Int Clin Psychopharmacol*. 2007;22:212–220.

Yingling DR, Utter G, Vengalil S, Mason B. Calcium channel blocker, nimodipine, for the treatment of bipolar disorder during pregnancy. *Am J Obstet Gynecol*. 2002;187:1711–1712.

Zhang ZJ, Kang WH, Tan QR, Li Q, Gao CG, Zhang FG. Adjunctive herbal medicine with carbamazepine for bipolar disorders: a double-blind, randomized, placebo-controlled study. *J Psychiatr Res*. 2007;41(3–4):360–369.

Zoccali R, Muscatello MR, Bruno A, Cambria R, Mico U. The effect of lamotrigine augmentation of clozapine in a sample of treatment-resistant schizophrenic patients: a double-blind, placebo-controlled study. *Schizophr Res*. 2007;93(1–3):109–116.

Anxiolytics

Antonelli-Incalzi R, Pedone C. Respiratory effects of beta-adrenergic receptor blockers. *Curr Med Chem*. 2007;14(10):1121–1128.

Appelberg BG, Syvalahti EK, Koskinen TE, Mehtonen OP, Muhonen TT, Naukkarinen HH. Patients with severe depression may benefit from buspirone augmentation of selective serotonin reuptake inhibitors: results from a placebo-controlled, randomized, double-blind, placebo wash-in study. *J Clin Psychiatry*. 2001;62:448.

Bahmad FM Jr, Venosa AR, Oliveira CA. Benzodiazepines and GABAergics in treating severe disabling tinnitus of predominantly cochlear origin. *Int Tinnitus J*. 2006;12:140–144.

Baker JG. The selectivity of beta-adrenoceptor antagonists at the human beta1, beta2 and beta3 adrenoceptors. *Br J Pharmacol*. 2005;144(3):317–322.

Ballesteros J, Callado LF. Effectiveness of pindolol plus serotonin uptake inhibitors in depression: a meta-analysis of early and late outcomes from randomised controlled trials. *J Affect Disord*. 2004;79(1–3):137.

Benyamina A, Lecacheux M, Blecha L, Reynaud M, Lukasiewcz M. Pharmacotherapy and psychotherapy in cannabis withdrawal and dependence. *Expert Rev Neurother*. 2008;8:479–491.

Bigal ME, Lipton RB. Excessive acute migraine medication use and migraine progression. *Neurology*. 2008;71:1821.

Brands B, Blake J, Marsh DC, Sproule B, Jeypalan R, Li S. The impact of benzodiazepine use on methadone maintenance treatment outcomes. *J Addictive Disease*. 2008; 27:37–48.

Chen HI, Malhotra NR, Oddo M, Heuer GG, Levine JM, Le Roux PD. Barbiturate infusion for intractable intracranial hypertension and its effect on brain oxygenation. *Neurosurgery*. 2008;63:880–886.

Das RK, Freeman TP, Kamboj SK. The effects of N-methyl D-aspartate and β-adrenergic receptor antagonists on the reconsolidation of reward memory: a meta-analysis. *Neurosci Biobehav Rev*. 2013;37(3):240–255.

de Quervain DJ, Aerni A, Roozendaal B. Preventive effect of beta-adrenoceptor blockade on glucocorticoid-induced memory retrieval deficits. *Am J Psychiatry*. 2007;164(6):967–969.

Dell' osso B, Lader M. Do benzodiazepines still deserve a major role in the treatment of psychiatric disorders? A critical reappraisal. *Eur Psychiatry*. 2013;28(1):7–20.

Dubovsky SL. Barbiturates and similarly acting substances. In: Sadock BJ, Sadock VA, Ruiz P, eds. *Kaplan & Sadock's Comprehensive Textbook of Psychiatry*. 9th ed. Vol. 2. Philadelphia, PA: Lippincott Williams & Wilkins; 2009:3038.

Dubovsky SL. Benzodiazepine receptor agonists and antagonists. In: Sadock BJ, Sadock VA, Ruiz P, eds. *Kaplan & Sadock's Comprehensive Textbook of Psychiatry*. 9th ed. Vol. 2. Philadelphia, PA: Lippincott Williams & Wilkins; 2009:3044.

Faber J, Sansone RA. Buspirone: a possible cause of alopecia. *Innov Clin Neurosci*. 2013;10(1):12–13.

Flomenbaum NE, Goldfrank LR, Hoffman RS, Howland MA, Lewin NA. *Goldfrank's Toxicologic Emergencies*. 8th ed. New York: McGraw-Hill; 2006.

Hutto B, Fairchild A, Bright R. γ-Hydroxybutyrate withdrawal and chloral hydrate. *Am J Psychiatry*. 2000;157:1706.

Jovaisas B; and Canadian Pharmacists Association. *CPS 2020: Compendium of Pharmaceuticals and Specialities: Canada's Trusted Drug Reference*. Canadian Pharmacists Association, 2020.

Kaplan GB, Greenblatt DJ, Ehrenberg BL, Goddard JE, Harmatz JS. Differences in pharmacodynamics but not pharmacokinetics between subjects with panic disorder and healthy subjects after treatment with a single dose of alprazolam. *J Clin Psychopharmacol*. 2000;20:338–346.

Katsura M. Functional involvement of cerebral diazepam binding inhibitor (DBI) in the establishment of drug dependence. *Nippon Yakurigaku Zasshi*. 2001;117:159–168.

Koerner IK, Brambrink AM. Brain protection by anesthetic agents. *Curr Opin Anaesthesiol*. 2006;19:481.

Korpi ER, Matila MJ, Wisden W, Luddens H. GABA(A)-receptor subtypes: clinical efficacy and selectivity of benzodiazepine site ligands. *Ann Med*. 1997;29:275–282.

Le Foll B, Boileau I. Repurposing buspirone for drug addiction treatment. *Int J Neuropsychopharmacol*. 2013;16(2):251–253.

Levitt AJ, Schaffer A, Lanctôt KL. Buspirone. In: Sadock BJ, Sadock VA, Ruiz P, eds. *Kaplan & Sadock's Comprehensive Textbook of Psychiatry*. 9th ed. Vol. 2. Philadelphia, PA: Lippincott Williams & Wilkins: 2009:3060.

McAinsh J, Cruickshank JM. Beta-blockers and central nervous system side effects. *Pharmacol Ther*. 1990;46(2):163–197.

McCarron MM, Schulze BW, Walberg CB, Thompson GA, Ansari A. Short acting barbiturate overdosage: correlation of intoxication score with serum barbiturate concentration. *JAMA*. 1982;248:55.

McIntyre RS. β-Adrenergic receptor antagonists. In: Sadock BJ, Sadock VA, Ruiz P, eds. *Kaplan & Sadock's Comprehensive Textbook of Psychiatry*. 9th ed. Vol. 2. Philadelphia, PA: Lippincott Williams & Wilkins; 2009:3009.

Myers RA, Plym MJ, Signor LJ, Lodge NJ. 1-(2-pyrimidinyl)-piperazine, a buspirone metabolite, modulates bladder function in the anesthetized rat. *Neurourol Urodyn*. 2004;23(7):709–115.

Navines R, Martin-Santos R, Gomez-Gil E, Martinez De Osaba MJ, Gasto C. Interaction between serotonin 5-Htla receptors and beta-endorphins modulates antidepressant response. *Prog Neuropsychopharmacol Biol Psychiatry*. 2008;32:1804–1809.

Peskind ER, Tsuang DW, Bonner LT, Pascualy M, Riekse RG. Propranolol for disruptive behaviors in nursing home residents with probable or possible Alzheimer disease: a placebo-controlled study. *Alzheimer Dis Assoc Disord*. 2005;19(1):23–28.

Rosa MA, Rosa MO, Marcolin MA, Fregni F. Cardiovascular effects of anesthesia in ECT: a randomized, double-blind comparison of etomidate, propofol and thiopental. *J ECT*. 2007;23:6–8.

Sempere T, Urbina M, Lima L. 5-HT1A and beta-adrenergic receptors regulate proliferation of rat blood lymphocytes. *Neuroimmunomodulation*. 2004;11(5):307.

Silberstein SD, McCrory DC. Butalbital in the treatment of headache: history, pharmacology, and efficacy. *Headache*. 2001;41:953–967.

Smith MC, Riskin BJ. The clinical use of barbiturates in neurological disorders. *Drugs*. 1991;42:365–378.

Syvalahti E, Penttila J, Majasuo H, Palvimaki EP, Laakso A. Combined treatment with citalopram and buspirone: effects on serotonin 5-HT$_{2A}$ and 5-HT$_{2C}$ receptors in the rat brain. *Pharmacopsychiatry*. 2006;39(1):1–8.

Van Oudenhove L, Kindt S, Vos R, Coulie B, Tack J. Influence of buspirone on gastric sensorimotor function in man. *Aliment Pharmacol Ther*. 2008;28:1326–1333.

Wheeler DS, Jensen RA, Poss WB. A randomized, blinded comparison of chloral hydrate and midazolam sedation in children undergoing echocardiography. *Clin Pediatr*. 2001;40:381–387.

Wong H, Dockens RC, Pajor L, Yeola S, Grace JE Jr. 6-Hydroxybuspirone is a major active metabolite of buspirone: assessment of pharmacokinetics and 5-hydroxytryptamine 1A receptor occupancy in rats. *Drug Metab Dispos*. 2007;35(8):1387–1392.

Drugs Used to Treat Sleep Disorders

Bannan N, Rooney S, O'Connor J. Zopiclone misuse: an update from Dublin. *Drug Alcohol Rev*. 2007;26:83–85.

Boehlein JK, Kinzie JD. Pharmacologic reduction of CNS noradrenergic activity in PTSD: the case for clonidine and prazosin. *J Psychiatr Pract*. 2007;13:72–78.

Calvo JR, Gonzalez-Yanes C, Maldonado M. The role of melatonin in the cells of the innate immunity: a review. *J Pineal Res*. 2013;55(2):103–120.

DeMicco M, Wang-Weigand S, Zhang J. Long-term therapeutic effects of ramelteon treatment in adults with chronic insomnia: a 1-year study. *Sleep*. 2006; 29(Suppl):A234.

Doghramji K. Melatonin and its receptors: a new class of sleep-promoting agents. *J Clin Sleep Med*. 2007;3(5 Suppl):S17.

Erman M, Seiden D, Zammit G, Sainati S, Zhang J. An efficacy, safety, and dose-response study of ramelteon in patients with chronic primary insomnia. *Sleep Med*. 2006;7(1):17–24.

Johnson MW, Suess PE, Griffiths RR. Ramelteon: a novel hypnotic lacking abuse liability and sedative adverse effects. *Arch Gen Psychiatry*. 2006;63(10):1149–1157.

Karim A, Bradford D, Siebert F, Zhao Z. Pharmacokinetic effect of multiple oral doses of donepezil on ramelteon, and vice versa, in healthy adults. *Sleep*. 2007; 30(Suppl):A244.

Kato K, Hirai K, Nishiyama K, Uchikawa O, Fukatsu K. Neurochemical properties of ramelteon (TAK-375), a selective MT$_1$/MT$_2$ receptor agonist. *Neuropharmacology*. 2005;48(2):301–310.

Lemmer B. The sleep–wake cycle and sleeping pills. *Physiol Behav*. 2009;90:285.

Lieberman JA. Update on the safety considerations in the management of insomnia with hypnotics: incorporating modified-release formulations into primary care. *Prim Care Companion J Clin Psychiatry*. 2007;9(1):25–31.

Mahajan B, Kaushal S, Chopra SC. Ramelteon: a new melatonin receptor agonist. *J Anaesth Clin Pharmacol*. 2008;24(4):463.

Mundey K, Benloucif S, Harsanyi K, Dubocovich ML, Zee PC. Phase-dependent treatment of delayed sleep phase syndrome with melatonin. *Sleep*. 2005;28(10):1271–1278.

Najib J. Eszopiclone, a nonbenzodiazepine sedative-hypnotic agent for the treatment of transient and chronic insomnia. *Clin Ther*. 2006;28:490–516.

Natural Standard Research Collaboration. Melatonin. *Medline Plus—Herbs and Supplements*. 2007. Available at http://www.nlm.nih.gov/medlineplus/druginfo/natural/patient-melatonin.html.

Norris ER, Karen B, Correll JR, Zemanek KJ, Lerman J, Primelo RA, Kaufmann MW. A double-blind, randomized, placebo-controlled trial of adjunctive ramelteon for the treatment of insomnia and mood stability in patients with euthymic bipolar disorder. *J Affect Disord*.2013;144(1–2):141–147.

Roth T, Seiden D, Sainati S, Wang-Weigand S, Zhang J. Effects of ramelteon on patient-reported sleep latency in older adults with chronic insomnia. *Sleep Med*. 2006;7(4):312–318.

Roth T, Stubbs C, Walsh JK. Ramelteon (TAK-375), a selective MT$_1$/MT$_2$-receptor agonist, reduces latency to persistent sleep in a model of transient insomnia related to a novel sleep environment. *Sleep*. 2005;28(3):303–307.

Scharf MB, Lankford A. Melatonin receptor agonists: ramelteon and melatonin. In: Sadock BJ, Sadock VA, Ruiz P, eds. *Kaplan & Sadock's Comprehensive Textbook of Psychiatry*. 9th ed. Vol. 2. Philadelphia, PA: Lippincott Williams & Wilkins; 2009:3145.

Srinivasan V, Ohta Y, Espino J, Pariente JA, Rodriguez AB, Mohamed M, Zakaria R. Metabolic syndrome, its pathophysiology and the role of melatonin. *Recent Pat Endocr Metab Immune Drug Discov*. 2013;7(1):11–25.

Turek FW, Gillette MU. Melatonin, sleep, and circadian rhythms: rationale for development of specific melatonin agonists. *Sleep Med*. 2004;5(6):523.

Zammit G, Erman M, Wang-Weigand S, Sainati S, Zhang J. Evaluation of the efficacy and safety of ramelteon in subjects with chronic insomnia. *J Clin Sleep Med*. 2007;3(5):495.

Stimulants

Adler LA, Sutton VK, Moore RJ, Dietrich AP, Reimherr FW. Quality of life assessment in adult patients with attention-deficit/hyperactivity disorder treated with atomoxetine. *J Clin Psychopharmacol*. 2006;26(6):648–652.

Aiken CB. Pramipexole in psychiatry: a systematic review of the literature. *J Clin Psychiatry*. 2007;68(8):1230–1236.

Amiri S, Mohammadi MR, Mohammadi M, Nouroozinejad GH, Kahbazi M. Modafinil as a treatment for attention-deficit/hyperactivity disorder in children and adolescents: a double-blind, randomized clinical trial. *Prog Neuropsychopharmacol Biol Psychiatry*. 2008;32(1):145–149.

Bangs ME, Emsile GJ, Spencer TJ, Ramsey JL, Carlson C. Efficacy and safety of atomoxetine in adolescents with attention-deficit/hyperactivity disorder and major depression. *J Child Adolesc Psychopharmacol*. 2007;17(4):407–420.

Barone P, Scazella L, Marconi R, Antonini A, Morgante L. Pramipexole versus sertraline in the treatment of depression in Parkinson's disease: a national multicenter parallel-group randomized study. *J Neuro*. 2006;253(5):601–607.

Cheng JY, Chen RY, Ko JS, Ng EM. Efficacy and safety of atomoxetine for attention-deficit/hyperactivity disorder in children and adolescents-meta-analysis and meta-regression analysis. *Psychopharmacology (Berl)*. 2007;194(2):197.

Eliyahu U, Berlin S, Hadad E, Heled Y, Moran DS. Psychostimulants and military operations. *Mil Med*. 2007;172(4):383.

Fava M, Thase ME, DeBattista C, Doghramji K, Arora S. Modafinil augmentation of selective serotonin reuptake inhibitor therapy in MDD partial responders with persistent fatigue and sleepiness. *Ann Clin Psychiatry*. 2007;19(3):153.

Fawcett J. Sympathomimetics and dopamine receptor agonists. In: Sadock BJ, Sadock VA, Ruiz P, eds. *Kaplan & Sadock's Comprehensive Textbook of Psychiatry*. 9th ed. Vol. 2. Philadelphia, PA: Lippincott Williams & Wilkins; 2009:3241.

Fleckenstein AE, Volz TJ, Riddle EL, Gibb JW, Hanson GR. New insights into the mechanism of action of amphetamines. *Annu Rev Pharmacol Toxicol*. 2007;47:681–698.

Frye MA, Grunze H, Suppes T, McElroy SL, Keck PE Jr. A placebo-controlled evaluation of adjunctive modafinil in the treatment of bipolar depression. *Am J Psychiatry*. 2007;164(8):1242–1249.

Geller D, Donnelly C, Lopez F, Rubin R, Newcorn J. Atomoxetine treatment for pediatric patients with attention-deficit/hyperactivity disorder with comorbid anxiety disorder. *J Am Acad Child Adolesc Psychiatry*. 2007;46(9):1119–1127.

Hirshkowitz M, Black J. Effect of adjunctive modafinil on wakefulness and quality of life in patients with excessive sleepiness-associated obstructive sleep apnoea/hypopnoea syndrome: a 12-month, open-label extensions study. *CNS Drugs*. 2007;21(5):407–416.

Makris AP, Rush CR, Frederich RC, Taylor AC, Kelly TH. Behavioral and subjective effects of d-amphetamine and modafinil in healthy adults. *Exp Clin Psychopharmacol*. 2007;15(2):123–133.

McElroy SL, Guerdjikova A, Kotwal R, Weige JA, Nelson EB. Atomoxetine in the treatment of binge-eating disorder: a randomized placebo-controlled trial. *J Clin Psychiatry*. 2007;68(3):390–398.

Minzenberg MJ, Carter CS. Modafinil: a review of neurochemical actions and effects on cognition. *Neuropsychopharmacology*. 2008;97(7):1477.

Pivonello R, De Martino MC, Cappabianca P, De Leo M, Faggiano A, Lombardi G, Hofland LJ, Lamberts SWJ, Colao A. The medical treatment of Cushing's disease: effectiveness of chronic treatment with the dopamine agonist cabergoline in patients unsuccessfully treated by surgery. *J Clin Endocrinology Metabolism*. 2009;94(1):223–230.

Pizzagalli DA, Evins AE, Schetter EC, Frank MJ, Pajtas PE, Santesso DL, Culhane M. Single dose of a dopamine agonist impairs reinforcement learning in humans:

behavioral evidence from a laboratory-based measure of reward responsiveness. *Psychopharmacology*. 2008;196(2):221–232.

Quintana H, Cherlin EA, Duesenberg DA, Bangs ME, Ramsey JL. Transition from methylphenidate or amphetamine to atomoxetine in children and adolescents with attention-deficit/hyperactivity disorder: a preliminary tolerability and efficacy study. *Clin Ther*. 2007;29(6):1168–1177.

Rothenhausler HB, Ehrentraut S, von Degenfeld G, Weis M, Tichy M. Treatment of depression with methylphenidate in patients difficult to wean from mechanical ventilation in the intensive care unit. *J Clin Psychiatry*. 2007;61(10):750.

Scott JC, Woods SP, Matt GE, Meyer RA, Heaton RK. Neurocognitive effects of methamphetamine: a critical review with meta-analysis. *Neuropsychol Rev*. 2007;17(3):275–297.

Weisler RH. Review of long-acting stimulants in the treatment of attention deficit hyperactivity disorder. *Exper Opin Pharmacother*. 2007;8(6):745–758.

Wernicke JF, Holdridge KC, Jin L, Edison T, Zhang S. Seizure risk in patients with attention-deficit-hyperactivity disorder treated with atomoxetine. *Dev Med Child Neurol*. 2007;49(7):498–502.

Drugs Used to Treat Substance Use Disorders

Anton RF, O'Malley SS, Ciraulo DA, Cisler RA, Couper D. Combined pharmacotherapies and behavioral interventions for alcohol dependence:the COMBINE study: a randomized controlled trial. *JAMA*. 2006;295(17):2003–2017.

Arnsten AFT, Li B. Neurobiology of executive functions: catecholamine influences on prefrontal cortical functions. *Biol Psychiatry*. 2005;57:1377.

Biederman J, Melmed RD, Patel A, McBurnett K, Konow J, Lyne A, Scherer N. A randomized, double blind, placebo-controlled study of guanfacine extended release in children and adolescents with attention-deficit/hyperactivity disorder. *Pediatrics*. 2008;121(1):e73–e84.

Carroll KM, Ball SA, Nich C, O'Connor PG, Eagan D. Targeting behavioral therapies to enhance naltrexone treatment of opioid dependence: efficacy of contingency management and significant other involvement. *Arch Gen Psychiatry*. 2001;58:755–761.

Center for Substance Abuse Treatment. Medication-Assisted Treatment for Opioid Addiction in Opioid Treatment Programs. *Treatment Improvement Protocol (TIP) Series 43*. DHHS Publication No. (SMA) 05–4048. Rockville, MD: Substance Abuse and Mental Health Services Administration; 2005.

Collins ED, Kleber HD, Whittington RA, Heitler NE. Anesthesia-assisted vs. buprenorphine- or clonidine-assisted heroin detoxification and naltrexone induction: a randomized trial. *JAMA*. 2005;294(8):903–913.

Ducharme LJ, Knudsen HK, Roman PM. Trends in the adoption of medications for alcohol dependence. *J Clin Psychopharmacol*. 2006;26(Suppl 1):S13.

Ehret GB, Voide C, Gex-Fabry M, Chabert J, Shah D. Drug-induced long QT syndrome in injection drug users receiving methadone: high frequency in hospitalized patients and risk factors. *Arch Intern Med*. 2006;166(12):1280–1287.

Fiellin DA, Moore BA, Sullivan LE, Becker WC, Pantalon MV, Chawarski MC, Barry DT, O'Connor PG, Schottenfeld RS. Long-term treatment with buprenorphine/naloxone in primary care: results at 2–5 years. *Am J Addict*. 2008;17:116.

Fuehrlein BS, Gold MS. Medication-assisted recovery in alcohol and opioid dependence. *Dir Psychiatry*. 2013;33(1):15–27.

Gibson A, Degenhardt L, Mattick RP, Ali R, White J, O'Brien S. Exposure to opioid maintenance treatment reduces long-term mortality. *Addiction*. 2008;103:462.

Grant JE, Kim SW, Potenza MN. Advances in the pharmacological treatment of pathological gambling. *J Gambling Stud*. 2003;19:85.

Grant JE, Kim SW. An open-label study of naltrexone in the treatment of kleptomania. *J Clin Psychiatry*. 2002;63(4):349.

Gryczynski J, Jaffe JH, Schwartz RP, Dušek KA, Gugsa N, Monroe CL, O'Grady KE, Olsen YK, Mitchell SG. Patient perspectives on choosing buprenorphine over methadone in an urban, equal-access system. *Am J Addict*. 2013;22(3):285–291.

Gueorguieva R, Wu R, Pittman B, O'Malley S, Krystal JH. New insights into the efficacy of naltrexone for alcohol dependence from the trajectory-based analyses. *Biol Psychiatry*. 2007;61(11):1290–1295.

Heit HA, Gourlay DL. Buprenorphine: new tricks with an old molecule for pain management. *Clin J Pain*. 2008;24:93–97.

Helm SI, Trescot AM, Colson J, Sehgal N, Silverman S. Opioid antagonists, partial agonists, and agonists/antagonists: the role of office-based detoxification. *Pain Physician* 2008;11:225.

Hollander E, Petras JN. α_2-Adrenergic receptor agonists: clonidine and guanfacine. In: Sadock BJ, Sadock VA, Ruiz P, eds. *Kaplan & Sadock's Comprehensive Textbook of Psychiatry*. 9th ed. Vol. 2. Philadelphia, PA: Lippincott Williams & Wilkins; 2009:3004.

Hser YI, Hoffman V, Grella CE, Anglin MD. A 33-year follow-up of narcotics addicts. *Arch Gen Psychiatry*. 2001;58:503–508.

Ivanov I. Disulfiram and acamprosate. In: Sadock BJ, Sadock VA, Ruiz P, eds. *Kaplan & Sadock's Comprehensive Textbook of Psychiatry*. 9th ed. Vol. 2. Philadelphia, PA: Lippincott Williams & Wilkins; 2009:3099.

Johnson BA. Update on neuropharmacological treatments for alcoholism: scientific basis and clinical findings. *Biochem Pharmacol*. 2008;75(1):34.

Johnson BA, Ait-Daoud N, Prihoda TJ. Combining ondansetron and naltrexone effectively treats biologically predisposed alcoholics: from hypotheses to preliminary clinical evidence. *Alcoholism Clin Exp Res*. 2000;24(5):737–742.

Karachalios GN, Charalabopoulos A, Papalimneou V, Kiortsis D, Dimicco P. Withdrawal syndrome following cessation of antihypertensive drug therapy. *Int J Clin Pract*. 2005;5:562.

King A, De Wit H, Riley RC, Cao D, Niaura R. Efficacy of naltrexone in smoking cessation: a preliminary study and an examination of sex differences. *Nicotine Tobacco Res.* 2006;8(5):671–682.

Kleber HD. Methadone maintenance 4 decades later: thousands of lives saved but still controversial. *JAMA.* 2008;300:2303.

Kornfield R, Watson S, Higashi AS, Conti RM, Dusetzina SB, Garfield CF, Dorsey ER, Huskamp HA, Alexander GC. Effects of FDA advisories on the pharmacologic treatment of ADHD, 2004–2008. *Psychiatr Serv.* 2013;64(4):339–346.

Krishnan-Sarin S, Rounsaville BJ, O'Malley SS. Opioid receptor antagonists: naltrexone and nalmefene. In: Sadock BJ, Sadock VA, Ruiz P, eds. *Kaplan & Sadock's Comprehensive Textbook of Psychiatry.* 9th ed. Vol. 2. Philadelphia, PA: Lippincott Williams & Wilkins; 2009:3171.

Krystal JH, Cramer JA, Kroll WF, Kirk GF, Rosenheck RA. Naltrexone in the treatment of alcohol dependence. *N Engl J Med.* 2001;345(24):1734.

Laaksonen E, Koski-Jännes A, Salaspuro M, Ahtinen H, Alho H. A randomized, multicentre, open-label, comparative trial of disulfiram, naltrexone and acamprosate in the treatment of alcohol dependence. *Alcohol.* 2008;43(1):53–61.

Likar R, Kayser H, Sittl R. Long-term management of chronic pain with transdermal buprenorphine: a multicenter, open-label, follow-up study in patients from three short-term clinical trials. *Clin Ther.* 2006;28(6):943–952.

Mann K, Kiefer F, Spanagel R, Littleton J. Acamprosate: recent findings and future research directions. *Alcohol Clin Exp Res.* 2008;32(7):1105–1110.

Marsch LA, Bickel WK, Badger GJ, Stothart ME, Quesnel KJ. Comparison on pharmacological treatments for opioid-dependent adolescents: a randomized controlled trial. *Arch Gen Psychiatry.* 2005;62:1157.

Mattick RP, Kimber J. Breen C, Davoli M. Buprenorphine maintenance versus placebo or methadone maintenance for opioid dependence. *Cochrane Database Syst Rev.* 2008:CD002207.

Ming X, Gordon E, Kang N, Wagner GC. Use of clonidine in children with autism spectrum disorders. *Brain Dev.* 2008;30(7):454–760.

Monterosso JR, Flannery BA, Pettinati HM, Oslin DW, Rukstalis M. Predicting treatment response to naltrexone: the influence of craving and family history. *Am J Addict.* 2001;10(3):258–268.

Myers SM. The status of pharmacotherapy for autism spectrum disorders. *Expert Opin Pharmacother.* 2007;8(11):1579.

Neumann AM, Blondell RD, Jaanimagi U, Giambrone AK, Homish GG, Lozano JR, Kowalik U, Azadfard M. A preliminary study comparing methadone and buprenorphine in patients with chronic pain and coexistent opioid addiction. *J Addict Dis.* 2013;32(1):68–78.

Niederhofer H, Staffen W. Naltrexone and disulfiram in patients with alcohol dependence and comorbid psychiatric disorders. *Biol Psychiatry.* 2005;57(10):1128.

Oliva EM, Trafton JA, Harris AH, Gordon AJ. Trends in opioid agonist therapy in the Veterans Health Administration: is supply keeping up with demand? *Am J Drug Alcohol Abuse.* 2013;39(2):103–107.

O'Malley SS, Cooney JL, Krishnan-Sarin S, Dubin J, McKee SA. A controlled trial of naltrexone augmentation of nicotine replacement for smoking cessation. *Arch Intern Med.* 2006;166:667.

Raymond NC, Grant JE, Kim SW, Coleman E. Treatment of compulsive sexual behavior with naltrexone and serotonin reuptake inhibitors: two case studies. *Int Clin Psychopharmacol.* 2002;17(4):201.

Ritvo JI, Park C. The psychiatric management of patients with alcohol dependence. *Curr Treat Options Neurol.* 2007;9(5):381.

Sallee F, Connor DF, Newcorn JH. A review of the rationale and clinical utilization of 2-adrenoceptor agonists for the treatment of attention-deficit/hyperactivity and related disorders. *J Child Adolesc Psychopharmacol.* 2013;23(5):308–319.

Savage SR. Principles of pain treatment in the addicted patient. In: Graham AW, Schultz TK, eds. *Principles of Addiction Medicine.* 2nd ed. Chevy Chase, MD: American Society of Addiction Medicine; 1998:919.

Saxon AJ, McRae-Clark AL, Brady KT. Opioid receptor agonists: methadone and buprenorphine. In: Sadock BJ, Sadock VA, Ruiz P, eds. *Kaplan & Sadock's Comprehensive Textbook of Psychiatry.* 9th ed. Vol. 2. Philadelphia, PA: Lippincott Williams & Wilkins; 2009:3171.

Schmitz JM, Stotts AL, Rhoades HM, Grabowski J. Naltrexone and relapse prevention treatment for cocaine-dependent patients. *Addict Behav.* 2001;26(2):167.

Sigmon SC, Moody DE, Nuwayser ES, Bigelow GE. An injection depot formulation of buprenorphine: extended bio-delivery and effects. *Addiction.* 2006;101(3):420.

Srisurapanont M, Jarusuraisin N. Opioid antagonists for alcohol dependence. *Cochrane Database Syst Rev.* 2002(2):CD001867.

Strain EC, Moody DE, Stoller KB, Walsh SL, Bigelow GE. Relative bioavailability of different buprenorphine formulations under chronic dosing conditions. *Drug Alcohol Depend.* 2004;74:37.

Substance Abuse and Mental Health Services Administration. Results from the 2005 National Survey on Drug Use and Health: National Findings (Office of Applied Studies, NSDUH Series H-30, DHHS Publication No. SMA 06–4194). Rockville, MD: Department of Health and Human Services; 2006.

Swift RM. Naltrexone and nalmefene: any meaningful difference? *Biol Psychiatry.* 2013;73(8):700–701.

Tetrault JM, Kozal MJ, Chiarella J, Sullivan LE, Dinh AT, Fiellin DA. Association between risk behaviors and antiretroviral resistance in HIV-infected patients receiving opioid agonist treatment. *J Addict Med.* 2013;7(2):102–107.

Vaglini F, Viaggi C, Piro V, Pardini C, Gerace C, Scarselli M. Acetaldehyde and parkinsonism: role of CYP450 2E1. *Front Behav Neurosci.* 2013;7:71.

Weiss RD, Kueppenbender KD. Combining psychosocial treatment with pharmacotherapy for alcohol dependence. *J Clin Psychopharmacol.* 2006;26(Suppl 1):S37.

Weiss RD, O'malley SS, Hosking JD, Locastro JS, Swift R, COMBINE Study Research Group. Do patients with alcohol dependence respond to placebo? Results from the COMBINE Study. *J Stud Alcohol Drugs.* 2008;69(6):878.

Zarkin GA, Bray JW, Aldridge A, Mitra D, Mills MJ, Couper DJ, Cisler RA, COMBINE Cost-Effectiveness Research Group. Cost and cost-effectiveness of the COMBINE study in alcohol-dependent patients. *Arch Gen Psychiatry.* 2008;65(10):1214–1221.

Drugs Used for Cognitive Enhancement

Auchus AP, Brasher HR, Salloway S, Korczyn AD, DeDeyn PP. Galantamine treatment of vascular dementia: a randomized trial. *Neurology.* 2007;69:448.

Black SE, Doody R, Li H, McRae T, Jambor KM. Donepezil preserves cognition and global function in patients with severe Alzheimer's disease. *Neurology.* 2007; 69:459.

Cummings J, Lefevre G, Small G, Appel-Dingemanse S. Pharmacokinetic rationale for rivastigmine patch. *Neurology.* 2007;69(4 Suppl 1):S10.

Droogsma E, Veeger N, van Walderveen P, Niemarkt S, van Asselt D. Effect of treatment gaps in elderly patients with dementia treated with cholinesterase inhibitors. *Neurology.* 2013;80(17):1622.

Edwards K, Royall D, Hershey L, Lichter D, Ake A. Efficacy and safety of galantamine in patients with dementia with Lewy body: a 24-week open-label study. *Dement Geriatr Cogn Disord.* 2007;23:401.

Jann MW, Small GW. Cholinesterase inhibitors. In: Sadock BJ, Sadock VA, Ruiz P, eds. *Kaplan & Sadock's Comprehensive Textbook of Psychiatry.* 9th ed. Vol. 2. Philadelphia, PA: Lippincott Williams & Wilkins; 2009:3089.

Porsteinsson AP, Grossberg GT, Mintzer J, Memantine MEM MD 12 Study Group. Memantine treatment in patients with mild to moderate Alzheimer's disease already receiving a cholinesterase inhibitor: a randomized, double-blind, placebo-controlled trial. *Curr Alzheimer Res.* 2008;5:83–89.

Qassem A, Snow V, Cross JT Jr, Forciea MA, Hopkins R Jr, Shekelle P, Adelman A, Mehr D, Schellhase K, Campos-Outcalt D, Santagoida P, Owens DK. Current pharmacologic treatment of dementia: a clinical practice guideline from the American College of Physicians and the American Academy of Family Physicians. *Ann Intern Med.* 2008;148:370–378.

Reisberg B, Doody R, Stoffer A, Schmidt F, Ferris S. A 24-week open label extension study on memantine in moderate to severe Alzheimer's disease. *Arch Neurol.* 2006;63:49.

Ritchie C, Zhinchin G. Low dose, high dose, or no dose: better prescribing of cholinesterase inhibitors for Alzheimer's disease. *Int Psychogeriatr.* 2013;25(4):511–515.

Seltzer B. Donepezil: an update. *Expert Opin Pharmacother.* 2007;8:1011–1023.

Wagle KC, Rowan PJ, Poon O-YI, Kunik ME, Taffet GE, Braun UK. Initiation of cholinesterase inhibitors in an inpatient setting. *Am J Alzheimer Dis Other Demen.* 2013;28(4):377–383.

Drugs Used to Treat Sexual Disorders

Chivers ML, Rosen RC. Phosphodiesterase type 5 inhibitors and female sexual response: faulty protocols or paradigms? *J Sex Med.* 2010;7(2 Pt 2):858–872.

Claes HI, Goldstein I, Althof SE, Berner MM, Cappelleri JC, Bushmakin AG, Symonds T, Schnetzler G. Understanding the effects of sildenafil treatment on erection maintenance and erection hardness. *J Sex Med.* 2010;7(6):2184–2191.

Hatzimouratidis K, Burnett AL, Hatzichristou D, McCullough AR, Montorsi F, Mulhall JP. Phosphodiesterase type 5 inhibitors in postprostatectomy erectile dysfunction: a critical analysis of the basic science rationale and clinical application. *Eur Urol.* 2009;55(2):334–347.

Hosain G, Latini DM, Kauth M, Goltz HH, Helmer DA. Sexual dysfunction among male veterans returning from Iraq and Afghanistan: prevalence and correlates. *J Sex Med.* 2013;10(2):516–523.

Khan AS, Sheikh Z, Khan S, Dwivedi R, Benjamin E. Viagra deafness—Sensorineural hearing loss and phosphodiesterase-5 inhibitors. *Laryngoscope.* 2011;121(5): 1049–1054.

Kotera J, Mochida H, Inoue H, Noto T, Fujishige K, Sasaki T, Kobayashi T, Kojima K, Yee S, Yamada Y, Kikkawa K, Omori K. Avanafil, a potent and highly selective phosphodiesterase-5 inhibitor for erectile dysfunction. *J Urol.* 2012;188(2): 668–674.

McCullough AR, Hellstrom WG, Wang R, Lepor H, Wagner KR, Engel JD. Recovery of erectile function after nerve sparing radical prostatectomy and penile rehabilitation with nightly intraurethral alprostadil versus sildenafil citrate. *J Urol.* 2010;183(6):2451–2456.

Reffelmann T, Kloner RA. Phosphodiesterase 5 inhibitors: are they cardioprotective? *Cardiovasc Res.* 2009;83(2):204–212.

Roberson DW, Kosko DA. Men living with HIV and experiencing sexual dysfunction: an analysis of treatment options. *J Assoc Nurses AIDS Care.* 2013;24(1 Suppl): S135–S145.

Roustit M, Blaise S, Allanore Y, Carpentier PH, Caglayan E, Cracowski JL. Phosphodiesterase-5 inhibitors for the treatment of secondary Raynaud's phenomenon: systematic review and meta-analysis of randomised trials. *Ann Rheum Dis.* 2013; 72(10):1696–1699.

Schwartz BG, Kloner RA. Drug interactions with phosphodiesterase-5 inhibitors used for the treatment of erectile dysfunction or pulmonary hypertension. *Circulation.* 2010;122(1):88–95.

Tuncel A, Nalcacioglu V, Ener K, Aslan Y, Aydin O, Atan A. Sildenafil citrate and tamsulosin combination is not superior to monotherapy in treating lower urinary tract symptoms and erectile dysfunction. *World J Urol.* 2010;28(1):17–22.

Drugs Used to Treat the Side Effects of Psychotropic Drugs

Adan RA. Mechanisms underlying current and future antiobesity drugs. *Trend Neurosci.* 2013;36(2):133–140.

Ahmad S. Anticholinergics and amantadine. In: Sadock BJ, Sadock VA, Ruiz P, eds. *Kaplan & Sadock's Comprehensive Textbook of Psychiatry.* 9th ed. Vol. 2. Philadelphia, PA: Lippincott Williams & Wilkins; 2009:3009.

Armstrong SC, Cozza KL. Antihistamines. *Psychosomatics.* 2003;44(5):430.

Astrup A, Carraro R, Finer N, Harper A, Kunesova M, Lean MEJ, Niskanen L, Rasmussen MF, Rissanen A, Rössner S, Savolainen MJ, Van Gaal L, NN8022-1807 Investigators. Safety, tolerability and sustained weight loss over 2 years with the once-daily human GLP-1 analog, liraglutide. *Int J Obes.* 2012;36(6):843–854.

Brown RE, Stevens DR, Haas HL. The physiology of brain histamine. *Prog Neurobiol.* 2001;63(6):637.

Buhrich N, Weller A, Kevans P. Misuse of anticholinergic drugs by people with serious mental illness. *Psychiatr Serv.* 2000;51:928.

Caligiuri MR, Jeste DV, Lacro JP. Antipsychotic-induced movement disorders in the elderly: epidemiology and treatment recommendations. *Drugs Aging.* 2000; 17:363.

Camelo-Nunes IC. New antihistamines: a critical view. *J Pediatr (Rio J).* 2006;82(5 Suppl):S173.

Colman E, Golden J, Roberts M, Egan A, Weaver J, Rosebraugh C. The FDA's assessment of two drugs for chronic weight management. *N Engl J Med.* 2012; 367(17):1577–1579.

Davies AJ, Harindra V, McEwan A. Cardiotoxic effect with convulsions in terfenadine overdose. *BMJ.* 1989;298(6669):325.

Dose M. Tempel HD: abuse potential of anticholinergics. *Pharmacopsychiatry.* 2000;33:43.

Drimer T, Shahal B, Barak Y. Effects of discontinuation of long-term anticholinergic treatment in elderly schizophrenia patients. *Int Clin Pharmacol.* 2004;19(1):27.

Finnema SJ, Bang-Andersen B, Jørgensen M, Christoffersen CT, Gulyás B, Wikström HV, Farde L, Halldin C. The dopamine D_1 receptor agonist (S)-[11C] N-methyl-NNC 01-0259 is not sensitive to changes in dopamine concentration—a positron emission tomography examination in the monkey brain. *Synapse.* 2013;67(9): 586–595.

Garvey WT. New tools for weight-loss therapy enable a more robust medical model for obesity treatment: rationale for a complications-centric approach. *Endocr Pract.* 2013;19(5):864–874.

Haas H, Panula P. The role of histamine and the tuberomammillary nucleus in the nervous system. *Nat Rev Neurosci.* 2003;4(2):121.

Hampl JS, Lehmann J, Fielder EG. How United States newspapers framed weight-loss drugs. *J Acad Nutr Diet.* 2013;113(9):A20.

Javitt DC, Zukin SR, Heresco-Levy U, Umbricht D. Has an angel shown the way? Etiological and therapeutic implications of the PCP/NMDA model of schizophrenia. *Schizophr Bull.* 2012;38(5):958–966.

Kelly AS, Metzig AM, Rudser KD, Fitch AK, Fox CK, Nathan BM, Deering MM, Schwartz BL, Abuzzahab MJ, Gandrud LM, Moran A, Billington CJ, Schwarzenberg SJ. Exenatide as a weight-loss therapy in extreme pediatric obesity: a randomized, controlled pilot study. *Obesity.* 2012;20(2):364–370.

Linnet K, Ejsing TB. A review on the impact of P-glycoprotein on the penetration of drugs into the brain. Focus on psychotropic drugs. *Eur Neuropsychopharmacol.* 2008;18(3):157.

McIntyre RS. Antihistamines. In: Sadock BJ, Sadock VA, Ruiz P, eds. *Kaplan & Sadock's Comprehensive Textbook of Psychiatry.* 9th ed. Vol. 2. Philadelphia, PA: Lippincott Williams & Wilkins; 2009:3033.

Melis M, Scheggi S, Carta G, Madeddu C, Lecca S, Luchicchi A, Cadeddu F, Frau R, Fattore L, Fadda P, Ennas MG, Castelli MP, Fratta W, Schilstrom B, Banni S, De Montis MG, Pistis M. PPARα regulates cholinergic-driven activity of midbrain dopamine neurons via a novel mechanism involving α7 nicotinic acetylcholine receptors. *J Neurosci.* 2013;33(14):6203–6211.

Miller CH, Fleischhacker WW. Managing antipsychotic-induced acute and chronic akathisia. *Drug Saf.* 2000;22:73.

Monn JA, Valli MJ, Massey SM, Hao J, Reinhard MR, Bures MG, Heinz BA, Wang X, Carter JH, Getman BG, Stephenson GA, Herin M, Catlow JT, Swanson S, Johnson BG, McKinzie DL, Henry SS. Synthesis and pharmacological characterization of 4-substituted-2-aminobicyclo [3.1. 0] hexane-2, 6-dicarboxylates: Identification of new potent and selective metabotropic glutamate 2/3 receptor agonists. *J Med Chem.* 2013;56(11):4442–4555.

Montoro J, Sastre J, Bartra J, del Cuvillo A, Davila I. Effect of H_1 antihistamines upon the central nervous system. *J Investig Allergol Clin Immunol.* 2006;16(Suppl 1):24.

Naicker P, Anoopkumar-Dukie S, Grant GD, Kavanagh JJ. The effects of antihistamines with varying anticholinergic properties on voluntary and involuntary movement. *Clin Neurophysiol.* 2013;124(9):1840–1845.

O'Neil PM, Smith SR, Weissman NJ, Fidler MC, Sanchez M, Zhang J, Brian Raether, Anderson CM, Shanahan WR. Randomized placebo-controlled clinical trial of lorcaserin for weight loss in type 2 diabetes mellitus: the BLOOM-DM study. *Obesity.* 2012;20(7):1426–1436.

Papanastasiou E, Stone JM, Shergill S. When the drugs don't work: the potential of glutamatergic antipsychotics in schizophrenia. *Br J Psychiatry.* 2013;202(2):91–93.

Shapiro BJ, Lynch KL, Toochinda T, Lutnick A, Cheng HY, Kral AH. Promethazine misuse among methadone maintenance patients and community-based injection drug users. *J Addict Med.* 2013;7(2):96–101.

Simons FE. Advances in H_1-antihistamines. *N Engl J Med.* 2004;351(21):2203.

Suplicy H, Boguszewski CL, dos Santos CMC, de Figueiredo MD, Cunha DR, Radominski R. A comparative study of five centrally acting drugs on the pharmacological treatment of obesity. *Int J Obes.* 2014:1–7.

Tejeda HA, Shippenberg TS, Henriksson R. The dynorphin/κ-opioid receptor system and its role in psychiatric disorders. *Cell Mol Life Sci.* 2012;69(6):857–896.

Theunissen EL, Vermeeren A, Vuurman EF, Ramaekers JG. Stimulating effects of H_1-antagonists. *Curr Pharm Des.* 2006;12(20):2501.

Vilsbøll T, Christensen M, Junker AE, Knop FK, Gluud LL. Effects of glucagon-like peptide-1 receptor agonists on weight loss: systematic review and meta-analyses of randomised controlled trials. *BMJ.* 2012;344.

Welch MJ, Meltzer EO, Simons FE. H_1-antihistamines and the central nervous system. *Clin Allergy Immunol.* 2002;17:337.

Wright JM, Dobosiewicz MR, Clarke PB. The role of dopaminergic transmission through D1-like and D2-like receptors in amphetamine-induced rat ultrasonic vocalizations. *Psychopharmacology.* 2013;225(4):853–868.

Yanai K, Tashiro M. The physiological and pathophysiological roles of neuronal histamine: an insight from human positron emission tomography studies. *Pharmacol Ther.* 2007;113(1):1.

Nutritional Supplements and Related

Camp KM, Lloyd-Puryear MA, Huntington KL. Nutritional treatment for inborn errors of metabolism: Indications, regulations, and availability of medical foods and dietary supplements using phenylketonuria as an example. *Mol Gen Metab.* 2012;107(1–2):3–9.

Long SJ, Benton D. Effects of vitamin and mineral supplementation on stress, mild psychiatric symptoms, and mood in nonclinical samples: a meta-analysis. *Psychosom Med.* 2013;75(2):144–153.

Nelson JC. The evolving story of folate in depression and the therapeutic potential of l-methylfolate. *Am J Psychiatry.* 2012;169(12):1223–1225.

Reichenbach S, Jüni P. Medical food and food supplements: not always as safe as generally assumed. *Ann Intern Med.* 2012;156(12):894–895.

Shah R. The role of nutrition and diet in Alzheimer disease: a systematic review. *J Am Med Dir Assoc.* 2013;14(6):398–402.

Sonuga-Barke EJS, Brandeis D, Cortese S, Daley D, Ferrin M, Holtmann M, Stevenson S, Danckaerts M, van der Oord S, Döpfner M, Dittmann RW, Simonoff E, Zuddas A, Banaschewski T, Buitelaar J, Coghill D, Hollis C, Konofal E, Lecendreux M, Wong IC, Sergeant J, European ADHD Guidelines Group. Nonpharmacological interventions for ADHD: systematic review and meta-analyses of randomized controlled trials of dietary and psychological treatments. *Am J Psychiatry.* 2013;170(3):275–289.

Thaipisuttikul P, Galvin JE. Use of medical foods and nutritional approaches in the treatment of Alzheimer's disease. *Clin Pract.* 2012;9(2):199–209.

Umhau JC, Garg K, Woodward AM. Dietary supplements and their future in health care: commentary on draft guidelines proposed by the Food and Drug Administration. *Antioxid Redox Signal.* 2012;16(5):461–462.

22 ▲

Other Somatic Therapies

ELECTROCONVULSIVE THERAPY

Convulsive therapies for major psychiatric illnesses predate the modern therapeutic era, with the use of camphor reported as early as the 16th century and the existence of several accounts of camphor convulsive therapies from the late 1700s to the mid-1800s.

Unaware of the history of camphor convulsive therapy, the Hungarian neuropsychiatrist Ladislas von Meduna observed that the brains of people with epilepsy had more glial cells than other brains. In contrast, the brains of patients with schizophrenia had fewer glial cells, and von Meduna hypothesized that there might be a biologic antagonism between convulsions and schizophrenia. Following animal experimentation, camphor was (again) selected as the appropriate agent to use for the therapeutic induction of seizures. In 1934, the first catatonic psychotic patient was successfully treated using intramuscular injections of camphor in oil to produce therapeutic seizures. Later, other chemicals were used, including pentylenetetrazol. Insulin coma was also used in the 1940s and 1950s, which also sometimes induced seizures. Lucio Bini and Ugo Cerletti were interested in the use of electricity to induce seizures, and, after a series of animal experiments and observation of the use of electricity commercially, they were able to safely apply current across the heads of animals for this purpose. In 1938, the first electroconvulsive treatment was administered to a delusional and incoherent patient, who improved with one treatment and remitted after 11 treatments. Electrical induction of convulsive therapy could be made more reliable and shorter-acting than chemically induced convulsive therapies, and, by the early 1940s, it had replaced them. In 1940, the first use of electroconvulsive therapy (ECT) occurred in the United States.

Explorations of nondominant electrode placement and alternative, more efficient waveforms were then undertaken to reduce the retrograde memory problems that persisted for some patients after the initial recovery period post-ECT. The practice of ECT also benefited from the introduction of controlled trials methodology, which demonstrated its safety and efficacy, and from refinements made in diagnostic systems and the process of informed consent. In the 1980s and 1990s, efforts to ensure uniformly high standards of practice were underway with the publication of recommendations for treatment delivery, education, and training by professional organizations in the United States, England, Scandinavia, and Canada, among others.

With the widespread use of pharmacologic agents as first-line treatments for major psychiatric disorders, ECT is now more commonly used for patients with resistance to those treatments, except in the case of life-threatening illness due to inanition, severe suicidal symptoms, or catatonia. Although subconvulsive stimulation was ineffective and a seizure is necessary, it is now known that there is a dose–response relationship with right unilateral ECT and bilateral ECT is likely to be ineffective with ultrabrief pulse widths.

Work continues to explore the underlying mechanisms and biologic characteristics of effective ECT treatments, with interest in having the treatment focus on appropriate neural networks with a more efficient stimulus as a method of reducing cognitive side effects. With the growing understanding that depression is a chronic disease for many patients, more emphasis has been placed on continuation and maintenance treatments following an acute course of ECT. Utilization of ECT has diminished since the middle of the 20th century, but because ECT remains the most effective treatment for major depression and is a rapidly effective treatment for life-threatening psychiatric conditions, ECT, unlike its contemporaneous somatic therapies, such as insulin coma, remains in the active treatment portfolio of modern therapeutics. Its use has shifted from public to private institutions, and it is estimated that approximately 100,000 patients have received ECT annually over the past few decades in the United States (Table 22-1).

The Nobel Laureate Paul Greengard has suggested that the term *electrocortical therapy* might be used to replace the current term electroconvulsive therapy (ECT). Greengard has acknowledged that if the mechanism of action of ECT, as yet unknown, turns out to be subcortical, then the term might have limited use. Until that time, however, the authors of this text think Greengard's suggestion deserves consideration. It would help diminish the fear associated with the word convulsion and help destigmatize a very effective treatment method.

Electrophysiology in Electroconvulsive Therapy

Neurons maintain a resting potential across the plasma membrane and may propagate an action potential, which is a transient reversal of the membrane potential. Regular brain activity is desynchronized; that is, neurons fire action potentials asynchronously. A convulsion, or seizure, occurs when a large percentage of neurons fire in unison. Such rhythmical changes in the extracellular potential entrain neighboring neurons, propagate the seizure activity across the cortex and into deeper structures, and eventually engulf the entire brain in high-voltage synchronous neuronal firing. Cellular mechanisms work to contain the seizure activity and to maintain cellular homeostasis, and the seizure eventually ends. In epilepsy, any of possibly several hundred genetic defects can alter the balance in favor of unrestrained activity. In ECT, seizures are triggered in normal neurons by application through the scalp of pulses of current, under conditions that are carefully controlled to create a seizure of a particular duration over the entire brain.

Ohm's law can describe the qualities of the electricity used in ECT: $E = IR$, or $I = E/R$, in which E is voltage, I is current, and R is resistance. The intensity or dose of electricity in ECT is measured in terms of charge (milliampere-seconds or millicoulombs) or energy (watt-seconds or joules). Resistance is synonymous with impedance, and, in the case of ECT, both the electrode's

Table 22-1
Milestones in the History of Convulsive Therapy

1500s	Paracelsus induces seizures by administering camphor (by mouth) to treat psychiatric illness.
1785	First published report of the use of seizure induction to treat mania, again using camphor.
1934	Ladislas von Meduna begins the modern era of convulsive therapy using intramuscular injection of camphor for catatonic schizophrenia. Camphor is soon replaced with pentylenetetrazol.
1938	Ugo Cerletti and Lucio Bini conduct the first electrical induction of a series of seizures in a catatonic patient and produce a successful treatment response
1940s	ECT is introduced to the United States.
	Curare developed for use as a muscle relaxant at ECT.
1951	Introduction of succinylcholine.
1958	First controlled study of unilateral ECT.
1960	Attenuation of seizure expression with an anticonvulsant agent (lidocaine) reduces the efficacy of ECT. Subconvulsive treatment produces only weak clinical responses; the hypothesis that seizure activity is necessary and sufficient for efficacy is upheld.
1960s	Randomized clinical trials of the efficacy of ECT versus medications in the treatment of depression yield response rates that are significantly higher with ECT.
	Comparisons of neuroleptics and ECT show that neuroleptic medication is superior for acute treatment, although ECT may be more effective in the long term.
1970	The most common electrode positioning for right unilateral ECT developed.
1976	A constant current, brief pulse ECT device, the prototype for modern devices, is developed.
1978	The American Psychiatric Association publishes the first Task Force Report on ECT with the aim of establishing standards for consent and the technical and clinical aspects of the conduct of ECT.
Late 1970s–early 1980s	Randomized, controlled trials demonstrate that ECT is more effective than sham treatment for major depression.
1985	The National Institutes of Health and National Institute of Mental Health Consensus Conference on ECT endorse a role for the use of ECT and advocate research and national standards of practice.
1987	The belief that the seizure in itself is sufficient for clinical response is challenged by H. A. Sackheim and collaborators, who report that the combination of dosage just above seizure threshold and right unilateral electrode placement, while producing a seizure of sufficient duration, is ineffective.
1988	Randomized, controlled clinical trials of ECT versus lithium demonstrate them to be equally effective in mania.
2000	In controlled trials, the dose–response relationship for right unilateral ECT is validated; high-dose right unilateral and bilateral ECT show equal response rates in major depression, but right unilateral electrode placement is associated with fewer adverse cognitive effects.
	Convulsive treatment is induced with magnetic stimulation by S. H. Lisanby and colleagues.
2001	The largest modern controlled trial of relapse prevention post-ECT with continuation pharmacotherapy demonstrates a significantly better outcome for combined treatment with a tricyclic antidepressant (nortriptyline) plus lithium compared with nortriptyline alone or placebo during the first 6 months post-ECT.

ECT, electroconvulsive therapy.

contact with the body and the nature of the bodily tissues are the significant determinants of resistance. The skull has a high impedance; the brain has a low impedance. Because scalp tissues are much better conductors of electricity than bone, only about 20 percent of the applied charge enters the skull to excite neurons. The ECT machines that are now widely used can be adjusted to administer the electricity under conditions of constant current, voltage, or energy.

Mechanism of Action

The induction of a bilateral generalized seizure is necessary for both the beneficial and adverse effects of ECT. Although a seizure superficially seems as though it is an all-or-none event, some data indicate that not all generalized seizures involve all the neurons in deep brain structures (e.g., the basal ganglia and

the thalamus); recruitment of these deep neurons may be necessary for full therapeutic benefit. After the generalized seizure, the electroencephalogram (EEG) shows about 60 to 90 seconds of postictal suppression. This period is followed by high-voltage delta and theta waves, with a return to preseizure activity in about 30 minutes. During a series of ECT treatments, the interictal EEG is generally slower and of greater amplitude than usual, but the EEG returns to pretreatment appearance 1 month to 1 year after the end of the course of treatment.

Positron emission tomography (PET) studies of both cerebral blood flow and glucose use have shown that during seizures, cerebral blood flow, use of glucose and oxygen, and permeability of the blood–brain barrier increase. After the seizure, blood flow and glucose metabolism are decreased, perhaps most markedly in the frontal lobes. Some research indicates that the degree of decrease in cerebral metabolism is correlated with therapeutic response.

Seizure foci in idiopathic epilepsy are hypometabolic during interictal periods; ECT itself acts as an anticonvulsant because its administration is associated with an increase in the seizure threshold as treatment progresses. Recent data suggest that for 1 to 2 months following a session of ECT, EEGs record a massive increase in slow-wave activity located over the prefrontal cortex in patients who responded well to the ECT. High-intensity, bilateral stimulation produced the best response; low-intensity, unilateral stimulation, the weakest. These data are of unclear significance, however, because the specific EEG correlate disappears 2 months after ECT, whereas the clinical benefit persists.

ECT affects the cellular mechanisms of memory and mood regulation and raises the seizure threshold. The latter effect may be blocked by the opioid antagonist naloxone.

Neurochemical research into the mechanisms of action of ECT has focused on changes in neurotransmitter receptors and, recently, changes in second-messenger systems. Virtually every neurotransmitter system is affected by ECT, but a series of ECT sessions results in the downregulation of postsynaptic β-adrenergic receptors, the same receptor change observed with virtually all antidepressant treatments. The effects of ECT on serotonergic neurons remain controversial. Various research studies have reported an increase in postsynaptic serotonin receptors, no change in serotonin receptors, and a change in the presynaptic regulation of serotonin release. ECT has also been reported to effect changes in the muscarinic, cholinergic, and dopaminergic neuronal systems. In second-messenger systems, ECT has been reported to affect the coupling of G-proteins to receptors, the activity of adenylyl cyclase and phospholipase C, and the regulation of calcium entry into neurons.

Recently, there has been increased interest in structural changes in the brain associated with psychiatric syndromes and response to treatment. This interest has been particularly so for microscopic changes associated with electroconvulsive stimulation, as well as antidepressants and other medications. In animals, mostly rodents, synaptic plasticity in the hippocampus, including mossy fiber sprouting, alterations in cytoskeletal structure, increased connectivity in perforant pathways, promotion of neurogenesis, and suppression of apoptosis have been observed. We also see many of these structural events, although less often, with antidepressant medications such as fluoxetine. These reports have also galvanized controversy over various aspects of the technical validity of the observations. It is unknown whether such changes occur clinically and, if they do, what significance to efficacy and cognitive side effects might be discovered.

Indications

Major Depressive Disorder. The most common indication for ECT is major depressive disorder, for which ECT is the fastest and most effective available therapy. ECT should be considered for use in patients who have failed medication trials, have not tolerated medications, have severe or psychotic symptoms, are acutely suicidal or homicidal, or have marked symptoms of agitation or stupor. Controlled studies have shown that up to 70 percent of patients who fail to respond to antidepressant medications may respond positively to ECT. Table 22-2 presents the indications for the use of ECT.

ECT is effective for depression in both major depressive disorder and bipolar I disorder. Delusional or psychotic depression has long been considered exceptionally responsive to ECT, but recent studies have indicated that major depressive episodes with psychotic features are no more responsive to ECT than nonpsychotic

Table 22-2
Indications for the Use of Electroconvulsive Therapy

Major diagnostic indications
Major depressive disorder
Mania, including mixed episodes
Schizophrenia with acute exacerbation or catatonic subtype
Schizoaffective disorder

Other diagnostic indications
Parkinson disease
Neuroleptic malignant disorder

Clinical indications
Primary use
Rapid definitive response required on medical or psychiatric grounds
Risks of alternative treatments outweigh benefits
Past history of poor response to medications or good response to ECT
Patient preference

Secondary use
Failure to respond to pharmacotherapy in the current episode
Intolerance of pharmacotherapy in the current episode
Rapid definitive response necessitated by deterioration of the patient's condition

ECT, electroconvulsive therapy.

depressive disorders. Nevertheless, because major depressive episodes with psychotic features respond poorly to antidepressant pharmacotherapy alone, ECT should be considered much more often as the first-line treatment for patients with the disorder. Major depressive disorder with melancholic features (e.g., markedly severe symptoms, psychomotor retardation, early morning awakening, diurnal variation, decreased appetite and weight, and agitation) is considered likely to respond to ECT. ECT is particularly indicated for persons who are severely depressed, who have psychotic symptoms, who show suicidal intent, or who refuse to eat. Depressed patients less likely to respond to ECT include those with somatic symptom disorder. Elderly patients tend to respond to ECT more slowly than do young patients. ECT is a treatment for major depressive episode and does not provide prophylaxis unless it is administered on a long-term maintenance basis.

Manic Episodes. ECT is at least equal to lithium for the treatment of acute manic episodes. The pharmacologic treatment of manic episodes, however, is so effective in the short term and for prophylaxis that the use of ECT to treat manic episodes is generally limited to situations with specific contraindications to all available pharmacologic approaches. The relative rapidity of the ECT response indicates its usefulness for patients whose manic behavior has produced dangerous levels of exhaustion. ECT should not be used for a patient who is receiving lithium because lithium can lower the seizure threshold and may be more likely to predispose the patient to delirium.

Schizophrenia. Although an effective treatment for the symptoms of acute schizophrenia, ECT is not for those of chronic schizophrenia. Patients with schizophrenia who have marked positive symptoms, catatonia, or affective symptoms are considered most likely to respond to ECT. In such patients, the efficacy of ECT is about equal to that of antipsychotics, but improvement may occur faster.

Other Indications.   Small studies have found ECT effective in the treatment of catatonia, a symptom associated with mood disorders, schizophrenia, and medical and neurologic disorders. ECT is also reportedly useful to treat episodic psychoses, atypical psychoses, obsessive-compulsive disorder (OCD), and delirium and such medical conditions as a neuroleptic malignant syndrome, hypopituitarism, intractable seizure disorders, and the on–off phenomenon of Parkinson disease. ECT may also be the treatment of choice for depressed, suicidal pregnant women who cannot take medication. It also may be the treatment of choice for geriatric and medically ill patients who cannot take antidepressant drugs safely. It may also be appropriate for severely depressed and suicidal children and adolescents who may be less likely to respond to antidepressant drugs compared with adults. ECT is not effective in somatic symptom disorder (unless accompanied by depression), personality disorders, or anxiety disorders.

Clinical Guidelines

Patients and their families are often apprehensive about ECT; therefore, clinicians must explain both beneficial and adverse effects and alternative treatment approaches. The informed-consent process should be documented in the patients' medical records and should include a discussion of the disorder, its natural course, and the option of receiving no treatment. Printed literature and videotapes about ECT may be useful in attempting to obtain genuinely informed consent. The use of involuntary ECT is rare today and should be reserved for patients who urgently need treatment and who have a legally appointed guardian who has agreed to its use. Clinicians must know local, state, and federal laws about the use of ECT.

Pretreatment Evaluation.   Pretreatment evaluation should include standard physical, neurologic, and preanesthesia examinations and complete medical history. Laboratory evaluations should include blood and urine chemistries, a chest x-ray, and an electrocardiogram (ECG). A dental examination to assess the state of patients' dentition is advisable for elderly patients and patients who have had inadequate dental care. An x-ray of the spine is needed if other evidence of a spinal disorder is seen. Computed tomography (CT) or magnetic resonance imaging (MRI) should be performed if a clinician suspects the presence of a seizure disorder or a space-occupying lesion. Practitioners of ECT no longer consider even a space-occupying lesion to be an absolute contraindication to ECT, but with such patients, the procedure should be performed only by experts.

CONCOMITANT MEDICATIONS.   Patients' ongoing medications should be assessed for possible interactions with the induction of a seizure, for effects (both positive and negative) on the seizure threshold, and drug interactions with the medications used during ECT. Most antidepressants except bupropion, monoamine oxidase inhibitors, and antipsychotics are generally acceptable. Benzodiazepines should be withdrawn because of their anticonvulsant activity; lithium should be withdrawn because it can result in increased postictal delirium and can prolong seizure activity; clozapine and bupropion should be withdrawn because they are associated with the development of late-appearing seizures. Lidocaine should not be administered during ECT because it markedly increases the seizure threshold; theophylline is contraindicated because it increases the duration of seizures. Reserpine is also contraindicated because it is associated with the further compromise of the respiratory and cardiovascular systems during ECT.

Premedications, Anesthetics, and Muscle Relaxants.
Patients should not be given anything orally for 6 hours before treatment. Just before the procedure, the patient's mouth should be checked for dentures and other foreign objects, and an intravenous (IV) line should be established. A bite block is inserted in the mouth just before the treatment is administered to protect the patient's teeth and tongue during the seizure. Except for the brief interval of electrical stimulation, 100 percent oxygen is administered at a rate of 5 L a minute during the procedure until spontaneous respiration returns. Emergency equipment for establishing an airway should be immediately available in case it is needed.

MUSCARINIC ANTICHOLINERGIC DRUGS.   Muscarinic anticholinergic drugs are administered before ECT to minimize oral and respiratory secretions and to block bradycardias and asystoles unless the resting heart rate is above 90 beats a minute. Some ECT centers have stopped the routine use of anticholinergics as premedications, although their use is still indicated for patients taking β-adrenergic receptor antagonists and those with ventricular ectopic beats. The most commonly used drug is atropine, which can be administered 0.3 to 0.6 mg intramuscularly (IM) or subcutaneously (SC) 30 to 60 minutes before the anesthetic or 0.4 to 1.0 mg IV 2 or 3 minutes before the anesthetic. An option is to use glycopyrrolate (0.2 to 0.4 mg IM, IV, or SC), which is less likely to cross the blood–brain barrier and less likely to cause cognitive dysfunction and nausea, although it is thought to have less cardiovascular protective activity than does atropine.

ANESTHESIA.   The administration of ECT requires general anesthesia and oxygenation. The depth of anesthesia should be as light as possible, not only to minimize adverse effects but also to avoid elevating the seizure threshold associated with many anesthetics. Methohexital (0.75 to 1.0 mg/kg IV bolus) is the most commonly used anesthetic because of its shorter duration of action and lower association with postictal arrhythmias than thiopental (usual dose 2 to 3 mg/kg IV). However, this difference in cardiac effects is not universally accepted. Four other anesthetic alternatives are etomidate, ketamine, alfentanil, and propofol. Etomidate (0.15 to 0.3 mg/kg IV) is sometimes used because it does not increase the seizure threshold; this effect is particularly useful for elderly patients because the seizure threshold increases with age. Ketamine (6 to 10 mg/kg IM) is sometimes used because it does not increase the seizure threshold, although its use is limited by the association of psychotic symptoms with emergence from anesthesia with this drug. Alfentanil (2 to 9 mg/kg IV) is sometimes coadministered with barbiturates to allow the use of low doses of the barbiturate anesthetics and, thus, reduce the seizure threshold less than usual, although its use can be associated with an increased incidence of nausea. Propofol (0.5 to 3.5 mg/kg IV) has anticonvulsant properties.

MUSCLE RELAXANTS.   After the onset of the anesthetic effect, usually within a minute, a muscle relaxant is administered to minimize the risk of bone fractures and other injuries resulting from motor activity during the seizure. The goal is to produce profound relaxation of the muscles, not necessarily to paralyze them, unless the patient has a history of osteoporosis or spinal injury or has a pacemaker and, therefore, is at risk for injury related to motor activity during the seizure. Succinylcholine, an ultrafast-acting depolarizing blocking agent, has gained virtually universal acceptance for the purpose. Succinylcholine is usually administered in a dose of 0.5 to 1 mg/kg as an IV bolus or drip. Because succinylcholine is a depolarizing agent, its action is marked by the presence of muscle fasciculations, which move in a rostrocaudal progression. The disappearance of these movements in the feet or the absence of muscle contractions after peripheral nerve stimulation indicates maximal muscle relaxation. In some patients, tubocurarine (3 mg IV) is administered to prevent myoclonus and increases in potassium and muscle enzymes; these reactions can be a problem in patients with musculoskeletal or cardiac disease. A blood pressure cuff may be inflated at the ankle to apply pressure over the systolic pressure before infusion of the muscle relaxant to allow observation of relatively innocuous seizure activity in the foot muscles to monitor the duration of the convulsion.

If a patient has a known history of pseudocholinesterase deficiency, atracurium (0.5 to 1 mg/kg IV) or curare can be used instead of succinylcholine. In such a patient, the metabolism of succinylcholine is disrupted, and prolonged apnea may necessitate emergency airway management. In general, however, because of the short half-life of succinylcholine, the duration of apnea after its administration is generally shorter than the delay in regaining consciousness caused by the anesthetic and the postictal state.

ELECTRODE PLACEMENT.   Historically, most practitioners have used bifrontotemporal electrode placement because of its reliability in producing efficacy and its ease of use. This electrode placement is also associated with more short- and long-term adverse cognitive effects and is more likely to produce delirium, which may require interrupting a course of ECT and perhaps even terminating it before optimal therapeutic effects have been obtained. Hence, when bifrontotemporal ECT is used, attention should be paid to restricting the dose to a moderately suprathreshold level to attenuate adverse cognitive effects as much as possible. It should be emphasized that the combination of ultrabrief pulse and bifrontotemporal electrode placement has not been demonstrated to be effective. Treatment with bilateral electrode placements, particularly a bifrontal configuration, is more likely to manifest EEG seizure without a motor seizure, and EEG monitoring can be particularly useful in detecting its occurrence.

Newer electrode placements include bifrontal configuration and asymmetrical placements. There are limitations to these strategies, imposed by the fact that the high impedance of the skull and scalp causes the spreading of the electrical stimulus and restricts possibilities for localization of the stimulus. Bifrontal electrode placement, located sufficiently lateral to minimize interference with impedance relations, has been investigated. There have been several demonstrations that bifrontal electrode placements are equally effective as bifrontotemporal and adequately dosed right unilateral electrode configurations. Evidence of advantages in sparing of cognitive effects is quite preliminary, and adequately powered investigations with more extensive and sensitive cognitive batteries are needed. The seizure threshold is likely to be relatively higher with bifrontal ECT.

The relatively better cognitive side effect profile of right unilateral ECT (also called the d'Elia placement) should encourage wider use now that the efficacy of this electrode placement can be ensured with adequate dosing strategies. In contrast to bilateral ECT, a dose closer to 500 percent above the seizure threshold is more likely to ensure efficacy. ECT devices in the United States are restricted to an output in the range of 504 to 576 mCi. Approximately 90 percent of patients have seizure thresholds that can accommodate optimal dosing with brief pulse right unilateral ECT, and the combination of right unilateral electrode placement with ultrabrief pulse width extends the range of US devices, so that most patients can be treated within these constraints. Individuals with an exceptionally high seizure threshold may require bilateral electrode placements

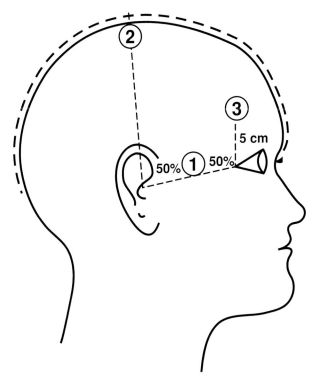

FIGURE 22-1
Electrode placements. Position 1 represents the frontotemporal position, used for both electrodes, one on each side of the head, in conducting bilateral electroconvulsive therapy (ECT). For right unilateral ECT, one electrode is in the right frontotemporal position, and the other is just to the right of the vertex at position 2. (Courtesy of American Psychiatric Association, with permission.)

to remain within the device restrictions. Maximizing interelectrode distance by using the d'Elia placement may also be optimal. Many other right unilateral placements have been described, but there is little work to support their use (Fig. 22-1).

There has been some concern that left-handed patients may require different electrode placement than right-handed patients, especially if a unilateral placement is desired. Even when handedness is lateralized to the left, the anatomic localization of language function in 70 percent of left-handed individuals is the same as in those who are right-handed. Furthermore, there is evidence for independent lateralization of affect, with the right hemisphere involved in sustaining depressed mood regardless of handedness. Because of limited indications that affective function and efficacy of ECT are associated with handedness, handedness is not generally used to guide the choice of electrode placement.

Electrical Stimulus.   The electrical stimulus must be sufficiently strong to reach the seizure threshold (the level of intensity needed to produce a seizure). The electrical stimulus is given in cycles, and each cycle contains a positive and a negative wave. Old machines use a sine wave; however, this type of machine is now considered obsolete because of the inefficiency of that wave shape. When a sine wave is delivered, the electrical stimulus in the sine wave before the seizure threshold is reached and after the seizure is activated is unnecessary and excessive. Modern ECT machines use a brief pulse waveform that administers the electrical stimulus, usually in 1 to 2 milliseconds, at a rate of 30 to 100 pulses a second. Machines that use an ultrabrief pulse (0.5 milliseconds) are not as effective as brief pulse machines.

Establishing a patient's seizure threshold is not straightforward. A 40 times variability in seizure thresholds occurs among patients. Also, during ECT treatment, a patient's seizure threshold may increase 25 to 200 percent. The seizure threshold is also higher in men than in women and higher in older than in younger adults. A common technique is to initiate treatment at an electrical stimulus that is thought to be below the seizure threshold for a particular patient and then to increase this intensity by 100 percent for unilateral placement and by 50 percent for bilateral placement until the seizure threshold is reached. A debate in the literature concerns whether a minimally suprathreshold dose, a moderately suprathreshold dose (one and a half times the threshold), or a high suprathreshold dose (three times the threshold) is preferable. The debate about stimulus intensity resembles the debate about electrode placement. Essentially, the data support the conclusion that doses of three times the threshold are the most rapidly effective and that minimal suprathreshold doses are associated with the fewest and least severe cognitive adverse effects.

Induced Seizures. A brief muscular contraction, usually strongest in a patient's jaw and facial muscles, is seen concurrently with the flow of stimulus current, regardless of whether a seizure occurs. The first behavioral sign of the seizure is often a plantar extension, which lasts 10 to 20 seconds and marks the tonic phase. This phase is followed by rhythmic (i.e., clonic) contractions that decrease in frequency and finally disappear. The tonic phase is marked by high-frequency, sharp EEG activity on which a higher-frequency muscle artifact may be superimposed. During the clonic phase, bursts of polyspike activity coincide with the muscular contractions but usually persist for at least a few seconds after the clonic movements stop.

MONITORING SEIZURES. A physician must have an objective measure that a bilateral generalized seizure has occurred after the stimulation. The physician should be able to observe either some evidence of tonic–clonic movements or electrophysiologic evidence of seizure activity from the EEG or electromyogram (EMG). Seizures with unilateral ECT are asymmetrical, with higher ictal EEG amplitudes over the stimulated hemisphere than over the nonstimulated hemisphere. Occasionally, unilateral seizures are induced; for this reason, at least a single pair of EEG electrodes should be placed over the contralateral hemisphere when using unilateral ECT. For a seizure to be effective in the course of ECT, it should last at least 25 seconds.

FAILURE TO INDUCE SEIZURES. If a particular stimulus fails to cause a seizure of sufficient duration, up to four attempts at seizure induction can be tried during a course of treatment. The onset of seizure activity is sometimes delayed as long as 20 to 40 seconds after the stimulus administration. If a stimulus fails to result in a seizure, the contact between the electrodes and the skin should be checked, and the intensity of the stimulus should be increased by 25 to 100 percent. The clinician can also change the anesthetic agent to minimize increases in the seizure threshold caused by the anesthetic. Additional procedures to lower the seizure threshold include hyperventilation and administration of 500 to 2,000 mg IV of caffeine sodium benzoate 5 to 10 minutes before the stimulus.

PROLONGED AND TARDIVE SEIZURES. Prolonged seizures (seizures lasting more than 180 seconds) and status epilepticus can be terminated either with additional doses of the barbiturate anesthetic agent or with IV diazepam (5 to 10 mg). Management of such complications should be accompanied by intubation because

the oral airway is insufficient to maintain adequate ventilation over an extended apneic period. Tardive seizures—that is, additional seizures appearing sometime after the ECT treatment—may develop in patients with preexisting seizure disorders. Rarely, ECT precipitates the development of an epileptic disorder in patients. Such situations should be clinically managed as if they were pure epileptic disorders.

Number and Spacing of Treatments. ECT treatments are usually administered two to three times a week; twice-weekly treatments are associated with less memory impairment than thrice-weekly treatments. In general, the course of treatment of major depressive disorder can take 6 to 12 treatments (although up to 20 sessions are possible); the treatment of manic episodes can take 8 to 20 treatments; the treatment of schizophrenia can take more than 15 treatments, and the treatment of catatonia and delirium can take as few as 1 to 4 treatments. Treatment should continue until the patient achieves what is considered the maximal therapeutic response. Further treatment does not yield any therapeutic benefit but increases the severity and duration of the adverse effects. The point of maximal improvement is usually thought to occur when a patient fails to continue to improve after two consecutive treatments. If a patient is not improving after 6 to 10 sessions, bilateral placement and high-density treatment (three times the seizure threshold) should be attempted before ECT is abandoned.

MULTIPLE-MONITORED ELECTROCONVULSIVE THERAPY. Multiple-monitored ECT (MMECT) involves giving multiple ECT stimuli during a single session, most commonly two bilateral stimuli within 2 minutes. This approach may be warranted in severely ill patients and those at exceptionally high risk from the anesthetic procedures. MMECT is associated with the most frequent occurrences of serious cognitive adverse effects.

Maintenance Treatment. A short-term course of ECT induces remission in symptoms but does not, of itself, prevent a relapse. Post-ECT maintenance treatment should always be considered. Maintenance therapy is generally pharmacologic, but maintenance ECT treatments (weekly, biweekly, or monthly) have been reported to be effective relapse prevention treatments, although data from extensive studies are lacking. Indications for maintenance ECT treatments can include rapid relapse after initial ECT, severe symptoms, psychotic symptoms, and the inability to tolerate medications. If ECT was used because a patient was unresponsive to a specific medication, then, following ECT, the patient should be given a trial of different medications.

Failure of Electroconvulsive Therapy Trial. Patients who fail to improve after a trial of ECT should have another medication trial, even if that agent previously failed. Although the data are primarily anecdotal, many reports indicate that patients who had previously failed to improve while taking an antidepressant drug do improve while taking the same drug after receiving a course of ECT treatments, even if the ECT seemed to be a therapeutic failure. Nonetheless, with the increased availability of drugs that act at diverse receptor sites, it is less often necessary to return to a drug that has failed than it was formerly.

Adverse Effects

Contraindications. ECT has no absolute contraindications, only situations in which a patient is at increased risk and has an increased need for close monitoring. Pregnancy is not a contra-indication for ECT, and fetal monitoring is generally considered unnecessary unless the pregnancy is high risk or complicated. Patients with space-occupying central nervous system lesions are at increased risk for edema and brain herniation after ECT. If the lesion is small, however, pretreatment with dexamethasone is given, and hypertension is controlled during the seizure, and the risk of serious complications minimized for these patients. Patients who have increased intracerebral pressure or are at risk for cerebral bleeding (e.g., those with cerebrovascular diseases and aneurysms) are at risk during ECT because of the increased cerebral blood flow during the seizure. This risk can be lessened, although not eliminated, by control of the patient's blood pressure during the treatment. Patients with recent myocardial infarctions are another high-risk group, although the risk is greatly diminished 2 weeks after the myocardial infarction and is even further reduced 3 months after the infarction. Patients with hypertension should be stabilized on their antihypertensive medications before ECT is administered. Propranolol and sublingual nitroglycerin can also be used to protect such patients during treatment.

Mortality.   The mortality rate with ECT is about 0.002 percent per treatment and 0.01 percent for each patient. These numbers compare favorably with the risks associated with general anesthesia and childbirth. ECT death is usually from cardiovascular complications and is most likely to occur in patients whose cardiac status is already compromised.

Central Nervous System Effects.   Common adverse effects associated with ECT are headache, confusion, and delirium shortly after the seizure while the patient is coming out of anesthesia. Marked confusion may occur in up to 10 percent of patients within 30 minutes of the seizure and can be treated with barbiturates and benzodiazepines. Delirium is usually most pronounced after the first few treatments and in patients who receive bilateral ECT or who have coexisting neurologic disorders. The delirium characteristically clears within days or a few weeks at the longest.

MEMORY.   The most significant concern about ECT is the association between ECT and memory loss. About 75 percent of all patients given ECT say that memory impairment is the worst adverse effect. Although memory impairment during a course of treatment is almost the rule, follow-up data indicate that almost all patients are back to their cognitive baselines after 6 months. Some patients, however, complain of persistent memory difficulties. For example, a patient may not remember the events leading up to the hospitalization and ECT, and such autobiographical memories may never be recalled. The degree of cognitive impairment during treatment and the time it takes to return to baseline are related, in part, to the amount of electrical stimulation used during treatment. Memory impairment is most often reported by patients who have experienced little improvement with ECT. Despite the memory impairment, which usually resolves, no evidence indicates brain damage caused by ECT. This subject has been the focus of several brain-imaging studies, using a variety of modalities; virtually all concluded that permanent brain damage is not an adverse effect of ECT. Neurologists and epileptologists generally agree that seizures that last less than 30 minutes do not cause permanent neuronal damage.

Other Adverse Effects of Electroconvulsive Therapy.   Fractures often accompanied treatments in the early days of ECT. With routine use of muscle relaxants, fractures of long bones or

vertebrae should not occur. Some patients, however, may break teeth or experience back pain because of contractions during the procedure. Muscle soreness can occur in some individuals, but it often results from the effects of muscle depolarization by succinylcholine and is most likely to be particularly troublesome after the first session in a series. This soreness can be treated with mild analgesics, including nonsteroidal anti-inflammatory drugs (NSAIDs). A significant minority of patients experience nausea, vomiting, and headaches following an ECT treatment. Nausea and vomiting can be prevented by treatment with antiemetics at the time of ECT (e.g., metoclopramide, 10 mg IV, or prochlorperazine, 10 mg IV; ondansetron is an acceptable alternative if adverse effects preclude the use of dopamine receptor antagonists).

ECT can be associated with headaches, although this effect is usually readily manageable. Headaches often respond to NSAIDs given in the ECT recovery period. In patients with severe headaches, pretreatment with ketorolac (30 to 60 mg IV), an NSAID approved for brief parenteral use, can be helpful. Acetaminophen, tramadol, and more potent analgesia provided by opioids can be used individually or in various combinations to manage more intractable headache. ECT can induce migrainous headache and related symptoms; sumatriptan (6 mg SC or 25 mg orally) may be a useful addition to the agents described above. Ergot compounds can exacerbate cardiovascular changes observed during ECT and probably should not be a component of ECT pretreatment.

Investigations in Electrical Brain Stimulation Treatment

There is interest in continued refinements of ECT techniques. Common themes in these approaches are focusing the treatment spatially to optimize dosing in brain areas associated with putative neural networks involved in depression and other psychopathologies that are indications for ECT, diminishing dosing in areas associated with adverse cognitive effects, and improving the efficiency of a noninvasive electrical stimulus in direction and amplitude, even to a subconvulsive level. This research is parallel to investigations in magnetic stimulation (e.g., repetitive transcranial magnetic stimulation [TMS]) and the renaissance of invasive electrical techniques (e.g., vagal nerve stimulation and deep brain stimulation [DBS]).

OTHER BRAIN STIMULATION METHODS

Brain stimulation in psychiatric practice and research uses electrical currents or magnetic fields to alter neuronal firing. There is a growing list of tools capable of eliciting such neuromodulation, each with a different spectrum of action. These tools either apply electrical or magnetic fields transcranially or involve the surgical implantation of electrodes to deliver electrical currents to a cranial nerve or the brain directly. The transcranial techniques include cranial electrical stimulation (CES), ECT, transcranial direct current stimulation (tDCS, also called direct current polarization), TMS, and magnetic seizure therapy (MST). The surgical techniques include cortical brain stimulation (CBS), DBS, and vagus nerve stimulation (VNS).

In 1985, nearly 50 years after the first use of ECT, Anthony Barker and colleagues published on the first use of pulsed magnetic fields to stimulate the brain with a procedure called *transcranial magnetic stimulation.* TMS was initially used in neurology for studies of nerve conduction, but it quickly caught the attention of psychiatrists eager to explore other, less invasive alternatives to ECT. This nonconvulsive stimulation method through TMS is under active study, with some promising results in the treatment of various psychiatric disorders, including depression, anxiety, and schizophrenia. A convulsive treatment derived from the application of more powerful magnetic stimulation has been under investigation in nonhuman primates and human studies in both the United States and Europe. The first MST procedure was performed in an animal in 1998 and a human in 2000. MST is under development as a more focal means of inducing seizures in an attempt to retain the thus-far-unparalleled efficacy of ECT with fewer cognitive side effects.

Two more additions to brain stimulation methods, DBS and VNS, were introduced about a decade following the first trials of TMS. Both were first approved by the U.S. Food and Drug Administration (FDA) in 1997 in the realm of treating sequelae of neurologic syndromes. DBS was initially approved for the treatment of essential tremor and Parkinson tremors, whereas VNS was approved for the treatment of epilepsy. Five years later, in 2002, indications for DBS were expanded to include treatment of all symptoms of Parkinson disease, including tremor, slowness, and stiffness, as well as involuntary movements induced by medications. TMS, DBS, and VNS originated in the field of neurology. Psychiatrists quickly saw the potential for those tools in the treatment of psychiatric conditions, however, and as a result of clinical trials in depression, VNS subsequently received FDA approval for the long-term adjunctive treatment of chronic or recurrent depression in adults. Also, human studies are underway to validate the efficacy of DBS in the treatment of depression and OCD.

Therapeutic Neuromodulation: Treating Psychiatric Disorders Through Brain Stimulation

Mechanism of Action

ELECTRICAL STIMULATION—COMMON PATHWAY. The brain stimulation modalities just reviewed generate either electrical or magnetic pulses. However, both of these share a common final pathway—they affect the neurons electrically. That electrical effect may either be through the direct application of electricity or the indirect induction of electricity via magnetic stimulation. The direct forms of electrical stimulation are exemplified in either *transcranial* delivery, as with ECT, CES, and tDCS, or *intracerebral* delivery, as in the case of DBS or direct cortical stimulation (epidural or subdural). The indirect forms of electrical stimulation include TMS and MST, which induce electrical fields in the brain through the application of alternating magnetic fields. Of note, both the epidural and intracerebral modalities are more focal than the transcranial application of electricity because electrodes are placed directly in the neuronal tissue, bypassing the impedance of the scalp and skull. The relatively more contemporary magnetic stimulation methods (TMS and MST) also bypass the impedance of the scalp and skull and are thus likewise more focal. However, magnetic stimulation is, in fact, an example of an indirect method of electrical brain stimulation, in that the changing magnetic fields from these devices induce electricity in the brain, the latter acting as a conductor, according to the principle first described by Michael Faraday in a law that bears his name and later incorporated into James Clerk Maxwell's equations, which unify all of electromagnetism. The magnetic modalities achieve their enhanced focality noninvasively, in contrast to the intracerebral and epidural methods, and are thus at the center of intensive research in that they offer the promise of an unparalleled degree of spatial specificity without the need for surgery.

All but one of the brain stimulation modalities described here act by stimulating neurons. The one exception is tDCS, which does not stimulate but instead polarizes. In this sense, the "S" of tDCS is a misnomer. It is more accurate to conceptualize tDCS as exerting a polarizing effect that may alter the likelihood of neuronal firing.

The action of the subconvulsive modalities of stimulation relies on the effects of the repeated stimulation of the targeted neural circuitry. However, in the case of the convulsive modalities (ECT and MST), the action depends on the seizure induced by the stimulation and the effects of repeated seizure induction on brain processes. This is not to say that the form of stimulation that triggers the seizure does not affect the outcome. Indeed, it is well replicated that electrode placement and electrical stimulus parameters have a profound effect on the efficacy and side effects of ECT. Whether the same will be valid for MST is under active investigation.

ACUTE VERSUS PROLONGED EFFECTS. Brain stimulation can have immediate or lasting effects. A single electrical pulse delivered at sufficient intensity can induce depolarization, trigger an action potential, release neurotransmitters at the synapse, and result in transsynaptic propagation with subsequent activation of a functional circuit. For example, brain stimulation applied to the hand area of the primary motor cortex may activate the corticospinal tract and induce a muscle twitch in the contralateral hand. Such stimulation can result acutely in the induction of either a positive effect, as in the case of a muscle twitch or visualization of phosphenes, or a disruptive effect, as in the case of visual masking.

Repetitive pulses delivered at fixed frequencies can exert even more powerful effects. Epstein and colleagues described in 1999 how repetitive TMS (rTMS) applied to the language-dominant hemisphere induced an arrest of speech. After termination of the stimulation, speech returned to normal.

Some more invasive brain stimulation modalities, such as DBS or VNS, are programmed to operate chronically, thus extending the acute action for as long as the stimulation is turned on. In the case of DBS, the pulses are typically given continuously at a high frequency, whereas in the case of VNS, the pulses are given in trains lasting up to 30 seconds and typically repeated every 5 minutes. The less invasive modalities, such as rTMS, tDCS, CES, and even ECT, presumably require the induction of some form of neuroplasticity for their effect to become lasting.

Transcranial Magnetic Stimulation

Definition. TMS is the application of a rapidly changing magnetic field to the superficial layers of the cerebral cortex, which locally induces small electric currents, also referred to as *eddy* currents. This induction was initially discovered by Faraday through his experiments in 1831 and later quantified in Maxwell's equations of electromagnetism. Thus, TMS may be referred to as electrical stimulation without an electrode, in that it uses magnetic fields to induce electrical pulses indirectly. TMS devices deliver intense magnetic pulses via a coil that is held on the scalp. Because magnetic fields are unaffected by the electrical impedance of the scalp and skull, this method of stimulation enables the focal stimulation of smaller areas of the brain than is possible with other noninvasive devices that use either alternating (ECT, CES) or direct (tDCS) electrical current for primary stimulation. TMS is an example of noninvasive stimulation of focal regions of the brain and, as such, can be used for research or therapeutically without the need for anesthesia.

Mechanisms of Action. At sufficient intensity, electrical currents will stimulate neuronal depolarization, which can result in an action potential. For example, when the TMS coil is positioned over the hand area of the cerebral cortex's motor strip, the changing magnetic field generated by the repetitive pulses induces local currents immediately below the site of stimulation that cause the neurons in area M1 to fire. In turn, this action potential propagates through the polysynaptic corticospinal tract and results in a twitch in the contralateral hand muscle. In essence, TMS uses magnetic fields to indirectly induce focal electrical currents in the brain, thereby triggering the firing of functional neuronal circuits that can lead to observable behavioral effects. This effect can be easily demonstrated by single TMS pulses that can be used to map the homunculus by merely moving the TMS coil across the cortical representation of neighboring muscle groups and simultaneously to study the excitability of the corticospinal system.

Single TMS pulses can exert other effects when moved to different cortical areas. When positioned over the primary visual cortex (V1), scotomas, or "blind spots," are often elicited. This illustrates that TMS can transiently disrupt functions.

Activation of motor neurons resulting in a muscle twitch and disruption of visual perception with a single-pulse TMS represent examples of the acute effects of TMS-induced neuronal depolarization, as shown in Table 22-3. The effects of single TMS pulses are believed to be immediate and short-lived. The muscle twitch, as induced by TMS to area M1, is nearly instantaneous, with the hand movement occurring approximately 20 milliseconds after the TMS pulse is applied. The visual masking likewise operates on a similar time scale measured in milliseconds. TMS can, however, exert longer-lasting effects when the pulses are repeated at regular intervals in the process of rTMS. It also occurs when they are paired with other forms of stimulation in which TMS pulses are coupled with electrical stimulation of a peripheral nerve (as in paired associative stimulation [PAS]) or when TMS is paired with audiovisual stimuli, as in the example of classical conditioning of the brain response to TMS. The mechanisms underlying these lasting effects of TMS have been described by various researchers and are thought to be related to neuroplasticity and alterations in synaptic efficacy.

Treatment of psychiatric disorders with rTMS has been informed by attempts to focally alter pathologic cortical excitability, believed to be linked to a specific illness. Reduced activity in the left dorsolateral prefrontal cortex has been implicated in several studies as a physiologic correlate of affective disorders. Numerous studies have applied high frequencies of rTMS, which have been reported to increase excitability to the left dorsolateral prefrontal cortex (DLPFC) in an attempt to normalize activity in this region. In a related approach, some investigators who implicated abnormal interhemispheric balance in activation between the right and left DLPFC applied low-frequency rTMS, which has been reported to be inhibitory, to the right DLPFC in an attempt to normalize this balance.

Side Effects, Interactions with Medications, and Other Risks. Administration of TMS is a noninvasive, relatively benign procedure when applied by a knowledgeable professional to a subject who has been appropriately evaluated. However, it is not entirely without risk. The most severe known risk of TMS is an unintended seizure. Several factors may contribute to seizure risk. Primarily, these include the form of TMS, with single-pulse stimulation less likely to result in a seizure than rTMS, and, in an equally important manner, the dose, which is the combination of treatment parameters including frequency, power, train duration, and inter-train interval. Also, subject factors can be significant, such as the presence of a neurologic disorder (epilepsy or a focal brain lesion) or the use of seizure-lowering medications.

Single-pulse TMS is generally considered to be of minimal risk when administered to appropriately screened adults without seizure risk factors. On the other hand, rTMS can induce seizures in individuals without predisposing conditions when given at sufficiently high doses.

Patient Selection. Patients who have failed a trial of one or more antidepressant medications or have untoward side effects to medications may be good candidates for TMS. However, given the lower effect size of TMS, for urgent or severely refractory cases, ECT would remain the gold standard treatment.

Future Directions and Controllable Pulse Shape TMS. TMS and other forms of magnetic stimulation hold a tremendous promise in psychiatric treatment due to their focality and noninvasiveness. However, much research is needed to replicate preliminary findings, improve optimal dosing, establish the patient characteristics that predict response, and examine the influence of concomitant medications on the TMS effect. Posttreatment relapse prevention is one of many areas that have to be adequately explored. Other vigorously pursued directions are attempts to develop stimulation coils that will allow deeper brain penetration and work on pulse shapes that may be more physiologically optimal for human stimulation.

Transcranial Direct Current Stimulation

Definition. tDCS is a noninvasive form of treatment that uses very weak (1 to 3 mA) direct electrical current applied to the scalp. Because direct current (DC) polarizes rather than stimulates with discrete pulses, its action does not appear directly to result in action potential firing in cortical neurons. It is also this DC form of electrical stimulation that distinguishes it from devices that use alternating currents (AC) as found in CES, ECT, VNS, and DBS, which produce discrete pulse stimulation. Also, because tDCS works via polarization and does not affect action potential firing in cortical neurons, the term *transcranial direct current polarization* is favored by some modern investigators, and both terms appear interchangeably in the literature today. The small device is very portable and usually operated by readily available DC batteries.

Side Effects. There are no known severe adverse effects of tDCS. It is well tolerated, with reported common side effects in the

Table 22-3
Acute and Prolonged Mechanisms of Action

Acute Effects
Phasic activation of neural circuits
Observable motor responses (e.g., twitch)
Temporary disruption (e.g., speech arrest) or facilitation of ongoing
    processing (e.g., speeds reaction time)

Prolonged Effects
Neuroplasticity
- Change in synaptic efficacy, akin to long-term potentiation or
    depression
- Alterations in neurotrophic factors
- Modulation of cortical excitability
- Modulation of functional connectivity

literature listing mostly minimal tingling at the site of stimulation, with a few reported cases of skin irritation.

Mechanism of Action. tDCS is believed to act via the alteration of neuronal membrane polarization, but little is known about the actual mechanism of action of tDCS. Polarization may affect the firing and conductance of neurons by either lowering or raising the threshold of activation. Because tDCS involves the application of low currents to the scalp via cathodal and anodal electrodes, depending on the direction of current flow, polarization can either inhibit (cathodal) or facilitate (anodal) function.

Clinical Studies. Preliminary research suggests that tDCS may enhance certain brain functions independent of mood; however, tDCS technology and its use in psychiatry are in the early stages of exploration. Research is focusing on its potential effectiveness in facilitating recovery from stroke and certain forms of dementia.

Future Directions. Most of the current tDCS devices use large, saline solution–soaked electrodes. Future device development will most likely investigate electrode shape and contact material to optimize the intended clinical effects and further improve ease of use. However, fundamental questions of efficacy, indications, and dose–response relationships, as well as predictors of response, will need to be explored first.

Cranial Electrical Stimulation

Definition. CES, like tDCS, uses a weak (1- to 4-mA) current. However, with CES, the current is alternating. It is traditionally applied via saline-soaked, felt-covered electrodes clipped onto the earlobes. Other placement strategies are also being investigated.

Mechanism of Action. The exact mechanism of action has not been elicited, and there is no agreement among researchers on the predominant mode of action. Previous hypotheses proposed that the stimulation with the alternating microcurrent affects the thalamic and hypothalamic brain tissue and facilitates the release of neurotransmitters. Claims have been made that through interaction with cell membranes, the stimulation produces changes in signal transduction associated with classic second-messenger pathways, including calcium channels and cyclic adenosine monophosphate (AMP). There are summary reports that CES causes increases in plasma serotonin, norepinephrine, dopamine, and monoamine oxidase type B (MAO_B) in blood platelets and cerebrospinal fluid (CSF), as well as the release of 5-hydroxyindoleacetic acid, dehydroepiandrosterone (DHEA), and enkephalins and reduction of cortisol and tryptophan. However, most of these reports have not been validated through modern research.

Side Effects. It is believed that the CES stimulation is not harmful, primarily due to its low-voltage power supply (9-V battery) and lack of any reported adverse event by the FDA. Local skin effects, as well as a general feeling of dizziness, have been reported, however, and device manufacturers do not advise the use of the device during pregnancy, in those with low blood pressure, or in people who have arrhythmias or pacemakers.

Clinical Studies. In a meta-analysis by the Harvard School of Public Health, 18 human clinical trials were examined that used CES to treat depression, anxiety, drug addiction, insomnia, headache, and pain. The overall pooled result showed CES to be better than sham treatment for anxiety at a statistically significant level.

Current Status in Treatment Algorithms, Patient Selection, and Dosing. The use of CES has not been studied sufficiently in the United States, and it does not have a specific place in any algorithm of standard US psychiatric practice.

Future Directions. As with tDCS, fundamental issues of indications, patient selection, dose–response relationship, and efficacy are under active research and remain to be optimized.

Magnetic Seizure Therapy

Definition. MST is a novel form of convulsive treatment that is under development in several research institutions in the United States and Europe. The treatment uses an alternating magnetic field that crosses the scalp and the calvarium bone unaffected by their high electrical impedance, to in turn induce a more-localized electrical current in the targeted regions of the cerebral cortex than is possible with ECT. The aim is to produce a seizure whose focus and patterns of spread may be controlled.

MST is a convulsive treatment that is similar to ECT. It is performed under general anesthesia. It requires approximately the same preparation and infrastructure as ECT. However, MST is given using a modified TMS device, one that can administer higher output than the conventional TMS devices and thus relies on magnetic stimulation, unlike electric stimulation in ECT. The MST procedure is performed under general anesthesia with a muscle relaxant. MST is under investigation and is not FDA approved.

Mechanism of Action. Induction of a seizure is hypothesized to be the underlying event responsible for the likely multiple specific mechanisms of action of MST treatment. As in ECT, these are not fully understood. However, due to its focality, MST appears to represent a tool better suited than ECT to study the mechanisms of action of convulsive therapy through its potential of inducing seizures initiated in different regions of the brain.

Side Effects. Adverse effects from MST, like those of ECT, are primarily connected to the risks associated with anesthesia and generalized seizure. Also, the MST magnetic coil produces a clicking noise that may potentially affect hearing. Earplugs should be worn by both the patient and members of the treating team to mitigate that risk and prevent any cumulative damage. Studies suggest that MST results in less retrograde and anterograde amnesia than ECT, although this result should be replicated in a larger trial.

Current Status in Treatment Algorithms. No clinical algorithms exist for MST, given that it is still an investigational protocol, and treatments outside of research are not FDA approved. Assuming the hypothesis that MST can approach the efficacy of ECT (but with fewer side effects) is correct, this magnetically induced convulsive treatment will play an essential role before referral for ECT.

Future Directions. MST is a novel treatment in the early phases of clinical testing. Clinical treatment variables, including dosing, optimal coil placement, patient selection, and mechanisms of action, are the topics of ongoing and future studies.

Vagus Nerve Stimulation

Definition.   VNS is the direct, intermittent electrical stimulation of the left cervical vagus nerve via an implanted pulse generator, usually in the left chest wall. The electrode is wrapped around the left vagus nerve in the neck and is connected to the generator subcutaneously.

Mechanisms of Action.   The majority of the fibers contained in the left vagus are afferents. It is estimated that as many as 80 percent of these fibers are up-going afferents. Thus chronic stimulation of these nerve fibers predominantly changes activity in the brainstem nuclei such as the nucleus of the tractus solitarius and other neighboring nuclei (e.g., raphe) that alter serotonergic activity in cortical and limbic structures. Also, persistent stimulation of the vagal afferents is anticonvulsant, an effect that appears to depend on the norepinephrine-producing locus ceruleus.

Side Effects and Contraindications.   To date, reasonably comprehensive literature confirms that VNS is generally well tolerated. The adverse events that are most frequently reported are voice alteration, dyspnea, and neck pain. Besides of the risk of perioperative infection, the surgical implantation carries a small risk of vocal cord paralysis, bradycardia, or asystole.

Current Status in Treatment Algorithms.   The FDA indicated VNS for the long-term adjunctive treatment of chronic or recurrent depression in patients 18 years or older experiencing a major depressive episode in the setting of unipolar or bipolar disease who have not had an adequate response to four or more adequate antidepressant treatments. Consultation with another clinician experienced with treatment-resistant depression and VNS is recommended.

VNS treatment success rates are lower than those with ECT. Its onset of action is also comparatively slow—typically, an approximately 30 percent response rate is observed after 1 year. VNS may be worth considering, therefore, when patients have failed to respond to less invasive treatments, ECT was ineffective, or post-ECT relapse cannot be prevented with less invasive means. VNS might be helpful with longer-term relapse prevention, but results of controlled trials would be useful to guide practice.

Patient Selection.   VNS is approved as a long-term adjunctive treatment for chronic or recurrent depressive episodes in adults with a major depressive episode who have not had a satisfactory response to four or more adequate antidepressant trials. The efficacy of VNS in other disorders is unknown.

ECT can be safely used in patients with an implant as long as the VNS generator is turned off during the convulsive treatment. This precaution is needed because of the anticonvulsant effects of VNS. It remains to be studied whether VNS could be useful in relapse prevention post-ECT.

Dosing.   The optimal dosing for psychiatric applications of VNS is still mostly an area of investigation. The published studies do not identify optimal dosing parameters like time on, time off, frequency, current, or pulse width. However, the epilepsy literature suggests that there is a threshold current for efficacy. Given current knowledge of VNS dosing, electrical current is typically increased up to greater than 1 mA, and clinical benefit is assessed over several months. Because the adverse effects of VNS are known to be dose-dependent, treatment parameters are often chosen to mitigate specific side effects. For example, lowering the pulse width reduces neck pain, allowing patients to tolerate higher currents.

Future Directions.   More research is required to establish dose–response relationships for VNS. Future studies may explore optimal medication strategies to augment responses, test the potential role of VNS for long-term relapse prevention (e.g., after ECT), and study its mechanism of action.

Implanted Cortical Stimulation

Definition.   CBS is a novel neurosurgical approach in which electrodes are implanted over the surface of the cortex to provide electrical brain stimulation in a targeted superficial region. This approach is being studied for the treatment of conditions like stroke, tinnitus, and treatment-resistant depression.

NEUROSURGICAL TREATMENTS AND DEEP BRAIN STIMULATION

After a long and checkered history, neurosurgical treatments for psychiatric illness have reemerged as a focus of great interest. Many still associate psychiatric neurosurgery with the bygone era of crude freehand "psychosurgery" when prefrontal lobotomy saw broad and indiscriminate use. Those primitive operations, which predated modern psychopharmacology, yielded modest reductions in symptoms but were accompanied by unacceptable adverse effects. Over nearly five decades, techniques, and significantly, procedures and practices have evolved tremendously. First, ablative lesions are now accurately, precisely, and reproducibly placed in specific brain targets stereotactically guided by MRI and specialized software. Alternative methods include radiosurgery, which allows stereotactic lesion placement without craniotomy. DBS, while requiring craniotomy to implant stimulating electrodes in specific brain targets, is intentionally nonablative and allows flexible and reversible modulation of brain function. Second, strict criteria for patient selection are observed, and the process of determining appropriate candidacy has been formalized.

Currently, surgical intervention is predominantly reserved for patients with severe, incapacitating major depression or OCD who have failed an exhaustive array of standard treatments. Surgery is not approved unless a multidisciplinary committee reaches consensus regarding its appropriateness for a given candidate, and the patient renders informed consent. Although a large body of clinical data has already been collected that indicates the effectiveness and safety of modern neurosurgical interventions, major centers providing these treatments continue to gather information prospectively, and controlled trials are underway or planned. With these advances in neurosurgical techniques and better-established selection criteria and long-term follow-up procedures, available data suggest that psychiatric neurosurgery yields a substantial improvement in symptoms and functioning in approximately 40 to 70 percent of cases, with morbidity and mortality drastically lower than for earlier procedures.

Although lesion procedures have been influenced by theories implicating corticolimbic systems in disordered behavior, they were initially mainly developed empirically. Although psychiatric neurosurgery is sometimes criticized for this reason, as for any clinical therapy, the relevant issues are safety and efficacy, not a correction of pathophysiologic processes that are not yet fully understood. However, psychiatric neurosurgery is now developing in a scientific context where the translation of data between clinical results to cross-species anatomical, neuroimaging, and physiologic studies of neural networks involved a promise to illuminate mechanisms of therapeutic action.

History

Trephination performed by ancient civilizations probably represents the earliest form of surgical intervention for psychopathology. In 1891, the first formal report of neurosurgical treatment in psychiatry was published, describing bilateral cortical excisions in demented and depressed patients, which yielded mixed results. After four decades in which little progress was made, in 1935, John Fulton and Charles Jacobsen presented their research on primate behavior following frontal cortical ablation. They observed that lobectomized chimpanzees showed a reduction in "experimental neurosis" and were less fearful while retaining an ability to perform complex tasks. António Egaz Moniz, a renowned Portuguese neurologist, pioneered prefrontal leukotomy in collaboration with his neurosurgical colleague, Almeida Lima. First, by using absolute alcohol injections and subsequently by mechanical means with a leucotome, Moniz and Lima performed "psychosurgery" on 20 severely ill institutionalized patients; 14 were said to have exhibited worthwhile improvement. In an era of overflowing asylums and few effective treatments for chronic debilitating psychiatric illness, this mode of therapy was initially enthusiastically embraced, and Moniz won the 1949 Nobel Prize in Physiology or Medicine for this contribution.

From the mid-1930s until the emergence of the phenothiazines in the mid-1950s, these techniques proliferated globally. Walter Freeman, a neuropsychiatrist, was perhaps the most zealous promoter of psychosurgery in the United States. Pioneering a series of freehand procedures to achieve prefrontal lobotomy (i.e., severing the white matter connections between the prefrontal cortex and the rest of the brain), Freeman, together with neurosurgeon James Watts, reported on their first 200 cases by 1942. Although the benefits of the surgery were highlighted, others acknowledged a significant complication rate, including frontal lobe syndrome, seizures, and even deaths. At its peak, lobotomy was being performed on approximately 5,000 patients per year in the United States alone. A review of the results of 10,365 prefrontal lobotomies performed from 1942 to 1954 in Britain concluded that, while 70 percent showed an improvement, adverse effects included 6 percent mortality, seizures in 1 percent, and disinhibition syndromes in 1.5 percent. There were widespread reports of blunted personality and socially inappropriate behavior. In the late 1940s and early 1950s, recognition of these risks prompted attempts to develop modified stereotactic surgical procedures that might yield better results. For example, Ernest Spiegel and Henry Wycis, who began stereotactic neurosurgery in humans, reported in the 1940s that dorsomedial thalamotomies improved obsessive-compulsive symptoms. However, with the introduction of chlorpromazine in 1954, medical management of psychiatric illness became possible. Following this, psychiatric neurosurgery was all but abandoned in favor of nonsurgical therapies.

Patient Selection: Indications and Contraindications

Although limited reports have suggested efficacy across a broad range of psychiatric conditions and research is expanding rapidly, as of this writing, the best-established indications for psychiatric neurosurgery remain major depression and OCD. In evaluating candidates, several factors are considered:

1. *Primary diagnosis:* The patient must meet clinical criteria for the diagnostic indication, and this disorder should be a primary cause of the patient's debility and suffering.
2. *Severity:* The patient must have a chronic, severe, and debilitating illness; the duration of the primary illness must exceed 1 year and typically exceeds 5 years. Severity is gauged on standardized instruments (e.g., patients with OCD typically have Yale-Brown Obsessive-Compulsive Scale scores of 25 to 30; patients with major depression typically have Beck Depression Inventory scores of 30 or higher), while a low level of functioning should indicate debility (e.g., a Global Assessment of Functioning score of 50 or less) and a low quality of life.
3. *Adequacy of previous treatment:* Patients must have already undergone an exhaustive array of other available established treatments, which are documented in detail.
4. *Psychiatric comorbidity:* Appropriate treatment must have been rendered for any comorbid psychiatric disorder; the presence of psychoactive substance use or severe personality disorders are considered strong relative contraindications.
5. *Medical comorbidity and surgical fitness:* Structural brain lesions or significant central nervous system injuries are strong contraindications. Medical conditions that increase neurosurgical risks (e.g., cardiopulmonary disease) and age greater than 65 years are relative contraindications for lesion procedures, while for DBS, the relative age restriction might be older. A history of past seizures is a risk factor for perioperative seizures after lesion procedures and must be weighed in the overall risk–benefit assessment (again, data are currently less clear in this regard for psychiatric DBS).
6. *Access to postoperative care:* The psychiatric neurosurgery procedures themselves represent the beginning of a new episode of care. Patients must have access to adequate postoperative treatment, including a psychiatrist (typically the referring physician) who will accept responsibility for managing the case after discharge. Arrangements for postoperative care (e.g., intensive behavior therapy) should be confirmed ahead of time. Notably, after lesion procedures, care can generally be delivered in standard treatment settings without the need for highly specialized psychiatric neurosurgery teams. For DBS, access to such teams is essential over the long term. Once implanted, patients require clinical monitoring and device adjustment, which can be intensive and time-consuming, especially early in treatment. Device monitoring and replacements may need to occur on a relatively urgent basis. The continuing costs incurred can be substantial, and adequacy of third-party reimbursement needs to be ensured in advance to the extent possible. After either lesion procedures or DBS, family or significant others may be needed to support and accompany patients to follow-up care, similar to the level of support that is usually necessary during the intensive evaluation process.
7. *Informed consent:* Under no circumstances should psychiatric neurosurgery be performed on patients against their will. The patient must be able and willing to render informed consent. Formal consent monitoring may be used to ensure that the consent process is adequate. In rare instances, these procedures are performed with the assent of the patient and formal consent from a legal guardian. In this context, age less than 18 years also represents a relative contraindication.

Postoperative Care

Immediate postoperative care includes the standard medical and surgical considerations following any stereotactic neurosurgical procedure. Special attention is paid to signs or symptoms of potential surgical complications, including infection, hemorrhage, seizures, or altered mental status. A postoperative MRI should be obtained to document the placement and extent of lesions. Intensive postoperative psychiatric treatment is recommended since the efficacy of the surgery may rely on some synergy between the neurosurgical intervention itself and enhanced response to pharmacologic or behavioral therapies. Although dosages of psychotropic medications may be reduced during the immediate perioperative period, the medication regimen should be readjusted as tolerated postoperatively. Moreover, in the case of OCD, intensive behavior therapy should be initiated as soon as possible, preferably within the first month postoperatively.

For DBS, electrode implantation is usually followed by a several-week delay to enable resolution of local edema and stabilization of other factors that might influence the response to stimulation. Then, systematic outpatient adjustment of stimulation parameters is performed before initial settings are determined. This adjustment is often a time-consuming process, lasting hours over one or more days. Ongoing protocols for DBS entail frequent follow-up, especially during the approximate 6 months after implantation, to enable optimization of stimulation parameters, monitoring of the patient, and coordination of other pharmacologic and behavioral therapies.

Lesion Procedures

Although numerous approaches have been tried, four lesion procedures have evolved as the safest and most effective for treating psychiatric disorders. All four entail bilateral lesions and are performed using modern stereotactic methods.

Subcaudate Tractotomy. Subcaudate tractotomy was introduced by Geoffrey Knight in Great Britain in 1964 as one of the first attempts to limit adverse effects by restricting lesion size. By targeting the substantia innominata (just inferior to the head of the caudate nucleus), the goal was to interrupt white matter tracts connecting the orbitofrontal cortex and subcortical structures. The surgery involved the placement of radioactive yttrium-90 seeds at the desired centroid, yielding lesion volumes of approximately 2 cc on each side. Indications for subcaudate tractotomy are major depression, OCD, and other severe anxiety disorders.

Anterior Cingulotomy. Anterior cingulotomy remains the most commonly employed neurosurgical treatment for psychiatric disease in North America. The surgery is conducted under local anesthesia, and two or three approximately 1-cc lesions are made on each side by thermocoagulation through bilateral burr holes. The target is within the anterior cingulate cortex (Brodmann areas 24 and 32), at the margin of the white matter bundle known as the cingulum. Initially, the placement of lesions was determined by ventriculography; however, since 1991, anterior cingulotomy has been conducted via MRI guidance. Approximately 40 percent of patients return several months following the first operation for a second procedure to extend the first set of lesions. The indications for anterior cingulotomy include major depression and OCD.

Limbic Leukotomy. Desmond Kelly and colleagues introduced limbic leukotomy in England in 1973. The procedure combines the targets of subcaudate tractotomy and anterior cingulotomy. The lesions have typically been made via thermocoagulation or with a cryoprobe. Historically, the precise placement of the lesions was guided by intraoperative stimulation;

pronounced autonomic responses were believed to designate the optimal lesion site. The indications for limbic leukotomy include major depression, OCD, and other severe anxiety disorders. More recently, there is also some evidence that this procedure might be beneficial for repetitive self-injurious behaviors or in the context of severe tic disorders.

Anterior Capsulotomy. Anterior capsulotomy or its newer variant, Gamma Knife (Elekta, Stockholm) capsulotomy, are used in Scandinavia, the United States, Belgium, Brazil, and elsewhere. The procedure places lesions within the anterior limb of the internal capsule, which impinges on the adjacent ventral striatum, thereby interrupting fibers of passage between the prefrontal cortex and subcortical nuclei, including the dorsomedial thalamus. Although the original anterior capsulotomy procedure is performed using thermocoagulation via burr holes in the skull, for the past 15 years, capsulotomy has used the Gamma Knife as an alternative. This radiosurgical instrument makes craniotomy unnecessary. Typically, gamma capsulotomy lesions are smaller than those induced by thermocapsulotomy, remaining within the ventral portion of the anterior capsule. Hence, the term *gamma ventral capsulotomy* is coming into use to describe this procedure.

In contrast to thermocapsulotomy, gamma ventral capsulotomy may be performed as an outpatient procedure, and at most, the patient might require one night of hospitalization. The relative advantages and disadvantages of this radiosurgical approach are the focus of ongoing research. Some data suggest, unsurprisingly, that the rates of neuropsychiatric adverse effects may be considerably lower for gamma ventral capsulotomy than for earlier procedures in which much larger tissue volumes were lesioned. Indications for anterior capsulotomy include major depression, OCD, and other severe anxiety disorders.

Deep Brain Stimulation

DBS for psychiatric illness is not a new idea, although the devices, surgical techniques, and theoretical models of relevant neurocircuitry have all advanced. The procedure involves the placement of small-diameter brain "leads" (e.g., approximately 1.3 mm) with multiple electrode contacts into subcortical nuclei or specific white matter tracts. The surgeon drills burr holes in skull bone under local anesthesia and then places the leads, guided by multimodal imaging and precise stereotactic landmarking. Usually, this is done bilaterally. The patient is typically sedated but awake during surgery. Later, the "pacemaker" (also known as an implantable neurostimulator or pulse generator) is implanted subdermally (e.g., in the upper chest wall) and connects via extension wires tunneled under the skin to the brain leads. The goals of DBS are to achieve improved efficacy and more favorable adverse effect profiles in comparison with ablation. Because various combinations of electrodes can be activated, at adjustable polarity, intensity, and frequency, DBS allows more flexible modulation of brain function, referred to as *neuromodulation*. Thus, parameters can be optimized for individual patients, but the process, typically performed by a specially trained psychiatrist in the outpatient setting, can be quite time-consuming and requires attentive long-term follow-up. In cases where no beneficial settings can be identified despite extensive efforts, the electrodes can be inactivated, and devices may be removed. In that event, devices are usually only partly explanted, with the brain electrodes left in place given the small risk of hemorrhage upon removal. The relative advantages and disadvantages of DBS are the focus of very active research.

Treatment Outcome

For all four contemporary ablative procedures, outcomes cannot be fairly assessed for a considerable period postoperatively, which could extend from 6 months to 2 years. In the first two or three decades of this work, clinical reports usually employed measures of global improvements, such as the Pippard Postoperative Rating Scale, which rates outcomes as follows: (1) symptom-free, (2) much improved, (3) slightly improved, (4) unchanged, and (5) worse. Most studies have operationalized significant improvement as categories 1 and 2. Also, many of the reports employ a measure of symptom severity that is specific to the indication for the procedure (e.g., the Yale-Brown Obsessive-Compulsive Scale for OCD and the Beck Depression Inventory for major depression). Most studies focus on one or another of the procedures and are best reviewed according to the surgical approach.

Outcome with Subcaudate Tractotomy.

Significant improvement was seen in 68 percent of patients with major depression, 50 percent of patients with OCD, and 62.5 percent of patients with other anxiety disorders. Patients with schizophrenia, substance abuse, or personality disorders did poorly. Short-term side effects include transient headache and confusion or somnolence, which typically resolve in less than 1 week. Patients are usually ambulatory by the third postoperative day. Transient disinhibition syndromes were common. In 1994, a large-scale review of 1,300 cases was conducted and concluded that the procedure enables 40 to 60 percent of patients to lead normal or near-normal lives, with a reduction in suicide rate to 1 percent versus 15 percent in a similarly affected control group with major affective disorders.

Outcome with Anterior Cingulotomy.

Significant improvement occurred in 62 percent of patients with affective disorders, 56 percent with OCD, and 79 percent with other anxiety disorders. Among patients with unipolar depression, 60 percent responded favorably; among patients with bipolar disorder, 40 percent responded favorably; and among patients with OCD, 27 percent were classified as responders with another 27 percent categorized as possible responders. Short-term side effects include headache, nausea, or difficulty with urination; however, these typically resolve within a few days. Patients are usually ambulatory within 12 hours following the operation and discharged on the third to fifth postoperative day. Over the past 10 years, the practice of treating patients who experience perioperative seizures with chronic anticonvulsant therapy has been discontinued, and no cases of new-onset recurrent seizures have been seen. Although patients have occasionally (5 percent or less) noted transient problems with memory, an independent analysis of 34 patients was performed. It demonstrated no significant intellectual or behavioral impairments attributable to anterior cingulotomy; a subsequent study of 57 patients likewise found no evidence for lasting neurologic or behavioral adverse effects.

Outcome with Limbic Leukotomy.

Significant improvement occurred in 89 percent of patients with OCD, 78 percent with major depression, and 66 percent with other anxiety conditions. Short-term side effects include headache, lethargy or apathy, confusion, and lack of sphincter control, which may last from a few days to a few weeks. In particular, it is common for postoperative confusion to last at least several days, and patients are often not discharged in less than 1 week. There were no seizures and no deaths; however, one patient suffered severe memory loss due to improper lesion placement, and enduring lethargy was present in 12 percent of cases.

Outcome with Anterior Capsulotomy

THERMOCAPSULOTOMY. A favorable response occurred in 50 percent of those with OCD and 48 percent of those with major depression. Short-term side effects can include transient headache or incontinence. Postoperative confusion often lasts for up to 1 week. Recovery from gamma capsulotomy is swifter and characterized by less discomfort and virtually no confusion, but side effects from radiation exposure, principally cerebral edema, may be delayed for up to 8 to 12 months. For the open capsulotomy, patients are typically ambulatory in a matter of hours to days following the operation, although the duration of confusion may influence the length of hospital stay. Weight gain has been noted to be a common enduring side effect with a mean increase in the mass of 10 percent.

GAMMA VENTRAL CAPSULOTOMY. Gamma capsulotomy was generally well tolerated and effective for patients with otherwise intractable OCD. Adverse events included cerebral edema and headache, small asymptomatic caudate infarctions, and possible exacerbation of preexisting bipolar mania. A therapeutic response, defined conservatively, was seen in 60 percent of over 50 patients receiving a gamma capsulotomy procedure, in which pairs of lesions in the ventral capsule are made bilaterally, impinging on the ventral striatum. The therapeutic benefit was achieved over 1 to 2 years and was essentially stable by 3 years. Adverse effects of gamma ventral capsulotomy include significant radiation-induced edema, appearing months after the procedure, apparently due to differential sensitivity to radiation that remains poorly understood. Long-term follow-up will be necessary to clarify the risks and benefits of gamma ventral capsulotomy. The same applies to any neurosurgery, including lesion procedures and DBS.

Outcomes with DBS

OBSESSIVE-COMPULSIVE DISORDER. Long-term outcomes of open stimulation in 26 patients showed clinically significant symptom reductions and functional improvement in about two-thirds of patients overall. Conservatively defined responses (35 percent or more significant reductions on the Yale-Brown Obsessive-Compulsive Scale) were seen in one-third of patients in the initial group, irrespective of the study center, while the response rate was over 70 percent in the second and third patient cohorts treated. The development of psychiatric DBS is following the path of stimulation for movement disorders, where several targets have been pursued with therapeutic benefit. As in movement disorders, overlapping or converging effects of DBS at different anatomical sites on the neurocircuitry involved are likely and are a focus of active research. The same reasoning applies to DBS for depression.

MAJOR DEPRESSION. A body of functional neuroimaging research implicates the subgenual cingulate cortex as a node in circuits involved in the normal experience of sadness, symptoms of depressive illness, and responses to depression treatments. Chronic DBS for up to 6 months was associated with sustained remission of depression in four of the six patients studied. Another line of research on DBS for depression was prompted by the OCD research discussed above and also by the reported antidepressant effects of anterior capsulotomy on which the VC/VS (ventral capsule/ventral striatum) stimulation target was initially based. The OCD patients, who had very high rates of comorbid depression, characteristically responded to stimulation onset with mood enhancement and reductions in nonspecific as well as OCD-related anxiety. Such effects were accompanied, or even preceded by, improvements in social interaction and daily functioning. Worsening in these same clinical domains was noted in some patients with the cessation of VC/VS stimulation. Moreover, DBS-induced changes in mood and non-specific anxiety often seemed to precede reductions in core OCD symptoms.

Outcome Across Contemporary Neurosurgical Procedures.

Although the field is developing rapidly, the conclusion reached is that 40 to 70 percent of carefully selected psychiatric patients should meaningfully benefit from contemporary neurosurgical treatment. Twenty-five percent or more might be expected to show outstanding improvement. Responses to ablative procedures have appeared marginally superior for major depression than for OCD generally. The adverse effect profiles of this group of procedures are influenced by lesion size, the surgical approach, and whether radio-surgical methods (in which the tempo of lesion development is very slow vs. thermocoagulation) are used. However, adverse effects are greatly minimized in comparison with the procedures of the past. Although minor short-term side effects may be expected after some modern ablative procedures, severe or enduring adverse consequences are relatively rare. These can include seizures in about 1 to 5 percent of cases. Although frontal syndromes, confusion, or subtle cognitive deficits can still be seen, overall cognitive function, as indicated by the standard intelligence quotient, is generally enhanced, a finding that has been attributed to the overriding beneficial effects of symptomatic improvement. Psychiatric neurosurgery likely reduces mortality, as evidenced by data on comparative suicide rates. Nonetheless, patients who undergo and fail to benefit from these procedures are at exceptionally high risk for completed suicide. Therefore, as with any therapy, the potential risks and benefits of psychiatric neurosurgery must be weighed against the potential risks and benefits of undergoing this brand of treatment.

The advent of DBS in psychiatry has created tremendous interest and considerable research activity. This therapy is intentionally nonablative, can be optimized for individual patients, is reversible, and is based on devices that are (to varying degrees) removable. DBS may therefore be accepted by patients who would not choose to undergo lesion procedures (although the reverse is also true). With all of its advantages, DBS requires that patients be treated by highly specialized teams willing and able to provide long-term care. The logistics and expenses involved can represent significant barriers.

In contrast, psychiatric care can be delivered in standard treatment settings after lesion procedures. However, although the relative risks of enduring adverse effects after psychiatric DBS remain to be established, at this stage, ablative methods appear to carry a more significant risk. Because rates of adverse outcomes are low when modern lesion procedures are performed at highly experienced centers, there may be a particularly strong rationale for referral of appropriate patients to such expert centers.

References

Belmaker R, Agam G. Deep brain drug delivery. *Brain Stimulation.* 2012;6(3):455–456.

Boggio PS, Rigonatti SP, Ribeiro RB, Myczkowski ML, Nitsche MA, Pascual-Leone A, Fregni F. A randomized, double-blind clinical trial on the efficacy of cortical direct current stimulation for the treatment of major depression. *Int J Neuropsychopharmacol.* 2008;11(2):249–254.

Byrne P, Cassidy B, Higgins P. Knowledge and attitudes towards electroconvulsive therapy among health care professionals and students. *J ECT.* 2006;22(2):133–138.

Cristancho MA, Alici Y, Augoustides JG, O'Reardon JP. Uncommon but serious complications associated with electroconvulsive therapy: Recognition and management for the clinician. *Curr Psychiatry Rep.* 2008;10(6):474–480.

deSouza RM, Moro E, Lang AE, Schapira AH. Timing of deep brain stimulation in Parkinson disease: a need for reappraisal. *Ann Neurol.* 2013;73(5):565–575.

Dougherty DD, Baer L, Cosgrove GR, Cassem EH, Price BH, Nierenberg AA, Jenike MA, Rauch SL. Prospective long-term follow-up of 44 patients who received cingulotomy for treatment-refractory obsessive-compulsive disorder. *Am J Psychiatry.* 2002;159(2):269–275.

Englot DJ. Vagus nerve stimulation versus "best drug therapy" in epilepsy patients who have failed best drug therapy. *Seizure.* 2013;22(5):409–410.

Esser SK, Huber R, Massimini M, Peterson MJ, Ferrarelli F, Tononi G. A direct demonstration of cortical LTP in humans: a combined TMS/EEG study. *Brain Res Bull.* 2006;69(1):86–94.

Fins JJ, Rezai AR, Greenberg BD. Psychosurgery: Avoiding an ethical redux while advancing a therapeutic future. *Neurosurgery.* 2006;59(4):713–716.

Fitzgerald PB, Brown TL, Marston NAU, Oxley T, de Castella A, Daskalakis ZJ, Kulkarni J. Reduced plastic brain responses in schizophrenia: a transcranial magnetic stimulation study. *Schizophren Res.* 2004;71(1):17–26.

Fregni F, Boggio PS, Nitsche M, Pascual-Leone A. Transcranial direct current stimulation. *Br J Psychiatry.* 2005;186(5):446–467.

Gabriels L, Nuttin B, Cosyns P. Applicants for stereotactic neurosurgery for psychiatric disorders: the role of the Flemish advisory board. *Acta Psychiatr Scand.* 2008;17(5):381–389.

Greenberg BD, Gabriels LA, Malone DA Jr, Rezai AR, Friehs GM, Okun MS, Shapira NA, Foote KD, Cosyns PR, Kubu CS, Malloy PF, Salloway SP, Giftakis JE, Rise MT, Machado AG, Baker KB, Stypulkowski PH, Goodman WK, Rasmussen SA, Nuttin BJ. Deep brain stimulation of the ventral internal capsule/ventral striatum for obsessive-compulsive disorder: worldwide experience. *Mol Psychiatry.* 2010;15(1):64–79.

Greenberg BD, Price LH, Rauch SL, Friehs G, Noren G, Malone D, Carpenter LL, Rezai AR, Rasmussen SA. Neurosurgery for intractable obsessive-compulsive disorder and depression: critical issues. *Neurosurg Clin North Am.* 2003;14(2):199–212.

Heeramun-Aubeeluck A, Lu Z. Neurosurgery for mental disorders: a review. *Afr J Psychiatry.* 2013;16(3):177–181.

Hooten WM, Rasmussen KG Jr. Effects of general anesthetic agents in adults receiving electroconvulsive therapy: a systematic review. *J ECT.* 2008;24(3):208–223.

Ingram A, Saling MM, Schweitzer I. Cognitive side effects of brief pulse electroconvulsive therapy: a review. *J ECT.* 2008;24(1):3–9.

Kellner CH, Knapp RG, Petrides G, Rummans TA, Husain MM, Rasmussen K, Mueller M, Bernstein HJ, O'Connor K, Smith G, Biggs M, Bailine SH, Malur C, Yim E, McClintock S, Sampson S, Fink M. Continuation electroconvulsive therapy vs pharmacotherapy for relapse prevention in major depression: a multisite study from the Consortium for Research in Electroconvulsive Therapy (CORE). *Arch Gen Psychiatry.* 2006;63(12):1337–1344.

Lapidus KA, Shin JS, Pasculli RM, Briggs MC, Popeo DM, Kellner CH. Low-dose right unilateral electroconvulsive therapy (ECT): effectiveness of the first treatment. *J ECT.* 2013;29(2):83–85.

Lisanby SH, Kinnunen LH, Crupain MJ. Applications of TMS to therapy in psychiatry. *J Clin Neurophysiol.* 2002;19(4):344–360.

Lisanby SH, Luber B, Schlaepfer TE, Sackeim HA. Safety and feasibility of magnetic seizure therapy (MST) in major depression: randomized within-subject comparison with electroconvulsive therapy. *Neuropsychopharmacology.* 2003;28(10):1852–1865.

Luber B, Kinnunen LH, Rakitin BC, Ellsasser R, Stern Y, Lisanby SH. Facilitation of performance in a working memory task with rTMS stimulation of the precuneus: frequency- and time-dependent effects. *Brain Res.* 2007;1128(1):120–129.

Luber B, Stanford AD, Malaspina D, Lisanby SH. Revisiting the backward masking deficit in schizophrenia: individual differences in performance and modeling with transcranial magnetic stimulation. *Biol Psychiatry.* 2007;62(7):793–799.

Mall V, Berweck S, Fietzek UM, Glocker FX, Oberhuber U, Walther M, Schessl J, Schulte-Mönting J, Korinthenberg R, Heinen F. Low level of intracortical inhibition in children shown by transcranial magnetic stimulation. *Neuropediatrics.* 2004;35(2):120–125.

Mayberg HS, Lozano AM, Voon V, McNeely HE, Seminowicz D, Hamani C, Schwalb JM, Kennedy SH. Deep brain stimulation for treatment-resistant depression. *Neuron.* 2005;45(5):651–650.

Montoya A, Weiss AP, Price BH, Cassem EH, Dougherty DD, Nierenberg AA, Rauch SL, Cosgrove GR. Magnetic resonance imaging-guided stereotactic limbic leukotomy for treatment of intractable psychiatric disease. *Neurosurgery.* 2002;50(5):1043–1049; discussion 1049–1052.

Munk-Olsen T, Laursen TM, Videbech P, Rosenberg R, Mortensen PB. Electroconvulsive therapy: predictors and trends in utilization from 1976 to 2000. *J ECT.* 2006;22(2):127–132.

OCD-DBS Collaborative Group. Deep brain stimulation for psychiatric disorders. *Neurosurgery.* 2002;51(2):519.

Painuly N, Chakrabarti S. Combined use of electroconvulsive therapy and antipsychotics in schizophrenia: the Indian evidence. a review and a meta-analysis. *J ECT.* 2006;22(1):59–66.

Peterchev AV, Kirov G, Ebmeier K, Scott A, Husain M, Lisanby SH. Frontiers in TMS technology development: controllable pulse shape TMS (cTMS) and magnetic seizure therapy (MST) at 100 Hz. *Biol Psychiatry.* 2007;61(8):107S.

Prudic J. Electroconvulsive therapy. In: Sadock BJ, Sadock VA, Ruiz P, eds. *Kaplan & Sadock's Comprehensive Textbook of Psychiatry.* 9th ed. Vol. 2. Philadelphia, PA: Lippincott Williams & Wilkins; 2009:3285.

Prudic J. Strategies to minimize cognitive side effects with ECT: aspects of ECT technique. *J ECT.* 2008;24(1):46–51.

Rapinesi C, Serata D, Casale AD, Carbonetti P, Fensore C, Scatena P, Caccia F, Di Pietro S, Angeletti G, Tatarelli R, Kotzalidis GD, Giradi P. Effectiveness of electroconvulsive therapy in a patient with a treatment-resistant major depressive episode and comorbid body dysmorphic disorder. *J ECT.* 2013;29(2):145–146.

Rauch SL, Dougherty DD, Malone D, Rezai A, Friehs G, Fischman AJ, Alpert NM, Haber SN, Stypulkowski PH, Rise MT, Rasmussen SA, Greenberg BD. A functional neuroimaging investigation of deep brain stimulation in patients with obsessive-compulsive disorder. *J Neurosurg.* 2006;104(4):558–565.

Rauch SL. Neuroimaging and neurocircuitry models pertaining to the neurosurgical treatment of psychiatric disorders. *Neurosurg Clin N Am.* 2003;14(2):213–223, vii–viii.

Rush AJ, Marangell LB, Sackeim HA, George MS, Brannan SK, Davis SM, Howland R, Kling MA, Rittberg BR, Burke WJ, Rapaport MH, Zajecka J, Nierenberg AA, Husain MM, Ginsberg D, Cooke RG. Vagus nerve stimulation for treatment-resistant depression: A randomized, controlled acute phase trial. *Biol Psychiatry.* 2005;58(5):347–354.

Sackeim HA, Prudic J, Nobler MS, Fitzsimons L, Lisanby SH, Payne N, Berman RM, Brakemeier EL, Perera T, Devanand DP. Effects of pulse width and electrode placement on the efficacy and cognitive effects of electroconvulsive therapy. *Brain Stimul.* 2008;1(2):71–83.

Schestatsky P, Simis M, Freeman R, Pascual-Leone A, Fregni F. Non-invasive brain stimulation and the autonomic nervous system. *Clin Neurophysiol.* 2013;124(9):1716–1728.

Schlaepfer TE, Lancaster E, Heidbreder R, Strain EC, Kosel M, Fisch HU, Pearlson GD. Decreased frontal white-matter volume in chronic substance abuse. *Int J Neuropsychopharmacol.* 2006;9(2):147–153.

Schmidt EZ, Reininghaus B, Enzinger C, Ebner C, Hofmann P, Kapfhammer HP. Changes in brain metabolism after ECT-positron emission tomography in the assessment of changes in glucose metabolism subsequent to electroconvulsive therapy–lessons, limitations and future applications. *J Affect Disord.* 2008;106(1–2):203–208.

Shorter E, Healy D. *Shock Therapy: The History of Electroconvulsive Therapy in Mental Illness.* Piscataway, NJ: Rutgers University Press; 2007.

Tomlinson SP, Davis NJ, Bracewell R. Brain stimulation studies of non-motor cerebellar function: a systematic review. *Neurosci Biobehav Rev.* 2013;37(5):766–789.

Van Laere K, Nuttin B, Gabriels L, Dupont P, Rasmussen S, Greenberg BD, Cosyns P. Metabolic imaging of anterior capsular stimulation in refractory obsessive-compulsive disorder: a key role for the subgenual anterior cingulate and ventral striatum. *J Nucl Med.* 2006;47(5):740–747.

Weiner R, Lisanby SH, Husain MM, Morales OG, Maixner DF, Hall SE, Beeghly J, Greden JF, National Network of Depression Centers. Electroconvulsive therapy device classification: response to FDA advisory panel hearing and recommendations. *J Clin Psychiatry.* 2013;74(1):38–42.

23 △

Psychotherapy

This chapter provides an overview of common psychotherapeutic approaches, covering a broad spectrum of therapy modalities.

PSYCHOANALYSIS AND PSYCHOANALYTIC PSYCHOTHERAPY

As broadly practiced today, psychoanalytic treatment encompasses a wide range of uncovering strategies used in varying degrees and blends. Despite the inevitable blurring of boundaries in actual application, we describe the original modality of classic psychoanalysis and major modes of psychoanalytic psychotherapy (expressive and supportive) separately here (Table 23-1). Analytical practice, in all its complexity, resides on a continuum. The individual technique is always a matter of emphasis, as the therapist titrates the treatment according to the needs and capacities of the patient at every moment.

Psychoanalysis is virtually synonymous with the renowned name of its founding father, Sigmund Freud. It is also referred to as "classic" or "orthodox" psychoanalysis to distinguish it from more recent variations known as *psychoanalytic psychotherapy.*

Psychoanalysis is based on the theory of sexual repression and traces the unfulfilled infantile libidinal wishes in the individual's unconscious memories. It remains unsurpassed as a method to discover the meaning and motivation of behavior, especially the unconscious elements that inform thoughts and feelings.

Psychoanalysis

Psychoanalytic Process. The psychoanalytic process involves bringing to the surface repressed memories and feelings through a scrupulous unraveling of hidden meanings of verbalized material and of the unwitting ways in which the patient wards off underlying conflicts through defensive forgetting and repetition of the past.

The overall process of analysis is one in which unconscious neurotic conflicts are recovered from memory and verbally expressed, reexperienced in the transference, reconstructed by the analyst, and, ultimately, resolved through understanding. Freud referred to these processes as *recollection, repetition,* and *working through,* which make up the totality of remembering, reliving, and gaining insight. *Recollection* entails the extension of memory back to early childhood events, a time in the distant past when the core of neurosis developed. The actual reconstruction of these events comes through reminiscence, associations, and autobiographical linking of developmental events. *Repetition* involves more than mere mental recall; it is an emotional replay of former interactions with significant individuals in the patient's life. The replay occurs within

the unique context of the analyst as a projected parent, a fantasized object from the patient's past with whom the latter unwittingly reproduces forgotten, unresolved feelings and experiences from childhood. Finally, *working through* is both an affective and cognitive integration of previously repressed memories that are brought into consciousness and through which the patient is gradually set free (cured of neurosis). The analytical course includes three major stages (Table 23-2).

Indications and Contraindications. In general, all of the so-called *psychoneuroses* are suitable for psychoanalysis. These include anxiety disorders, obsessional thinking, compulsive behavior, conversion disorder, sexual dysfunction, depressive states, and many other nonpsychotic conditions, such as personality disorders. Significant suffering must be present so that patients are motivated to make the sacrifices of time and financial resources required for psychoanalysis. Patients who enter analysis must have a genuine wish to understand themselves, not a desperate hunger for symptomatic relief. They must be able to withstand frustration, anxiety, and other strong affects that emerge in the analysis without fleeing or acting out their feelings in a self-destructive manner. They must also have a reasonable, mature superego that allows them to be honest with the analyst. Intelligence must be at least average, and above all, they must be psychologically minded in the sense that they can think abstractly and symbolically about the unconscious meanings of their behavior.

Many contraindications for psychoanalysis are the flip side of the indications. The absence of suffering, poor impulse control, inability to tolerate frustration and anxiety, and low motivation to understand are all contraindications. The presence of extreme dishonesty or antisocial personality disorder contraindicates analytic treatment. Concrete thinking or the absence of psychological mindedness is another contraindication. Some patients who might ordinarily be psychologically minded are not suitable for analysis because they are in the midst of a major upheaval or life crisis, such as a job loss or a divorce. Serious physical illness can also interfere with a person's ability to invest in a long-term treatment process. Patients of low intelligence generally do not understand the procedure or cooperate in the process. An age older than 40 years was once considered a contraindication, but today analysts recognize that patients are malleable and analyzable in their 60s or 70s. One final contraindication is a close relationship with the analyst. Analysts should avoid analyzing friends, relatives, or persons with whom they have other involvements.

Patient Requisites. Table 23-3 lists the most important patient requisites for psychoanalysis.

Table 23-1
Scope of Psychoanalytic Practice: A Clinical Continuum

Features	"Classic" Analytic	Expressive Mode (Exploratory)	Supportive Mode
Frequency	Regular 4–5 times/wk; "50-minute hour"	Regular 1–3 times/wk; 1/2 to full hour	Flexible 1 time/wk or less; or as needed 1/2 to full hour
Duration	Long term; usually 3–5+ yr; maybe considerably longer	Short or long term; several sessions to months or years	Short or intermittent long term; single session to lifetime
Setting	Patient primarily on couch with analyst out of view	Patient and therapist face to face; occasional use of couch	Patient and therapist face-to-face; couch contraindicated
Modus operandi	Systematic analysis of all positive and negative transference and resistance; primary focus on analyst and intrasession events; transference neurosis facilitated; regression encouraged	Partial analysis of dynamics and defenses; focus on current interpersonal events and transference to others outside of sessions; analysis of negative transference; positive transference left unexplored unless it impedes progress; limited regression encouraged	Formation of therapeutic alliance and real object relationship; analysis of transference contraindicated with rare exceptions; focus on conscious external events; regression discouraged
Analyst/therapist role	Absolute neutrality; frustration of patient; reflector/mirror role	Modified neutrality; implicit gratification of patient and greater activity of therapist	Neutrality suspended; limited explicit gratification, direction, and disclosure
Mutative change agents	Insight predominates within relatively deprived environment	Insight within more empathic environment; identification with benevolent object	Auxiliary or surrogate ego as a temporary substitute; holding environment; insight to the degree possible
Patient population	Neuroses; mild character psychopathology	Neuroses; mild to moderate character psychopathology, especially narcissistic and borderline disorders	Severe character disorders, latent or manifest psychoses, acute crises, physical illness
Patient requisites	High motivation, psychological mindedness, good previous object relationships, ability to maintain transference neuroses, good frustration tolerance	High moderate motivation and psychological-mindedness, ability to form therapeutic alliance, some frustration tolerance	Some degree of motivation and ability to form therapeutic alliance
Basic goals	Structural reorganization of personality; resolution of unconscious conflicts; insight into intrapsychic events; symptom relief an indirect result	Partial reorganization of personality and defenses; resolution of preconscious and conscious derivatives of conflicts; insight into current interpersonal events; improved object relations; symptom relief a goal or prelude to further exploration	Reintegration of self and ability to cope; stabilization or restoration of preexisting equilibrium; strengthening of defenses; better adjustment or acceptance of pathology; symptom relief and environmental restructuring as primary goals
Major techniques	Free association method predominates; full dynamic interpretation (including confrontation, clarification, and working through), with emphasis on genetic reconstruction	Limited free association; confrontation, clarification, and partial interpretation predominate, with emphasis on here-and-now interpretation and limited genetic interpretation	Free association method contraindicated; suggestion (advice) predominates; abreaction useful; confrontation, clarification, and interpretation in the here-and-now are secondary; genetic interpretation is contraindicated
Adjunct treatment	Primarily avoided; if applied, all negative and positive meanings and implications thoroughly analyzed more recently, medication adjunct	May be necessary, e.g., psychotropic drugs as temporary measure; if applied, negative implications are explored and diffused	Often necessary, e.g., psychotropic drugs, family rehabilitative therapy, or hospitalization; if applied, positive implications are emphasized

This division is not categorical; all practice resides on a clinical continuum.

Ms. M, a 29-year-old unmarried woman who worked in a low-level capacity for a magazine, presented for consultation with the chief complaints of considerable sadness and distress over her parent's reaction when they found that she had had a homosexual relationship. She also realized that she had been working far below her potential. She had never sought any treatment before. She was clearly intelligent, sensitive, self-reflective, and insightful. When she learned about the possibility of psychoanalysis as a treatment option, she worried that meant she was "sicker." Ms. M, however, began reading Freud, realized that analysis was actually recommended for those who are higher functioning, and became intrigued by the idea. She agreed to come 4 days a week for 50-minute sessions.

She was the oldest of three children and the only girl. Ms. M's father, a successful professional, was described as very demanding and intrusive; someone who never thought anything was good enough. He had always expected his children to do the "extra credit" assignments as part of their regular work. Ms. M, however, was very proud of her father's accomplishments. She spoke of her mother in conflicting terms as well: she was a homemaker, weak, and sometimes acquiescent to the powerful father but also an individual in her own right who was involved in community volunteer work and could be a powerful public speaker.

Just before beginning her analysis, Ms. M had had her wallet stolen. In her first analytic session, she spoke of losing all of her identification cards, and to her, it seemed as if she were starting analysis "with a completely new identity." Initially, she was somewhat hesitant to use the couch because she wanted to see her analyst's reactions, but Ms. M quickly appreciated that she could associate more easily without seeing the analyst.

As her analysis proceeded, through dreams and free associations, Ms. M became quite focused on the analyst. She became extremely curious about the analyst's life. What emerged from her associations to seeing the analyst's appointment book on the desk was that she felt "slotted in." Whenever Ms. M saw other patients, she felt the office was "like an assembly line." Further associations led to her feeling slotted in by her parents as they ran from one activity to another. Her resistance manifested itself in Ms. M, often coming as much or more than 15 minutes late to her sessions. Her associations led to her admitting that she did not want her analyst to think that she was "too eager." Ms. M was able to see that she needed to devalue her analyst and her importance to Ms. M as a defense against an overwhelmingly positive and even erotic transference toward her.

For example, Ms. M wanted to improve her appearance so that the therapist, whom she called a "role model," would find her more attractive. Her negative transference, however, was never far from the surface, and she denigrated the analyst by wondering if the analyst were a "clothes-horse" who was financing her wardrobe with the patient's payments.

Her conflicts about her sexual orientation were a central preoccupation in the course of her analysis, particularly because her father was homophobic. Early on, Ms. M felt awkward and uncomfortable when she went to a lesbian bar, and when asked if she qualified for the "lesbian discount," she said she did not. At one point, she began seeing several men, including a male psychologist. The analyst made the transference interpretation, which Ms. M accepted, that a date with this man seemed as if it were a date with the analyst, and sleeping with him would be equivalent to sleeping with the analyst. Ms. M was also able to see that her transient choice of dating a male therapist was a defensive compromise. Although her homosexual object choice was multidetermined, Ms. M came to appreciate, through her work in analysis, that at least a part of her conflicts about homosexuality stemmed from her relationship with her father. It was a means of securing his attention as well as infuriating him.

Over 4 years, Ms. M performed considerably better at work and earned a promotion to a job commensurate with her potential. She was also able to deal better with both her parents and particularly her father, regarding her sexual orientation. She became much more comfortable with her "new identity" and became involved in a relationship with a professional woman. At the end of therapy, Ms. M and this woman were committed to each other and considering adopting a child. (Courtesy of T. Byram Karasu, M.D. and S. R. Karasu, M.D.)

Goals. In developmental terms, psychoanalysis aims at the gradual removal of amnesias rooted in early childhood based on the assumption that filling all gaps in memory will lead to cessation of the morbid condition because the patient no longer needs to repeat or remain fixated to the past. The patient should be better able to relinquish former regressive patterns and to develop new, more adaptive ones, particularly as he or she learns the reasons for his or her behavior. A related goal of psychoanalysis is for the patient to achieve some measure of self-understanding or insight.

Table 23-2
Stages of Psychoanalysis

Stage one: Patient becomes familiar with the methods, routines, and requirements of analysis, and a realistic therapeutic alliance is formed between patient and analyst. Basic rules are established; the patient describes his or her problems; there is some review of history, and the patient gains initial relief through catharsis and a sense of security before delving more deeply into the source of the illness. The patient is primarily motivated by the wish to get well.

Stage two: Transference neurosis emerges that substitutes for the actual neurosis of the patient and in which the wish for health comes into direct conflict with the simultaneous wish to receive emotional gratification from the analyst. There is a gradual surfacing of unconscious conflicts; an increased irrational attachment to the analyst, with regressive and dependent concomitants of that bond; a developmental return to earlier forms of relating (sometimes compared with that of mother and infant); and a repetition of childhood patterns and recall of traumatic memories through transfer to the analyst of unresolved libidinal wishes.

Stage three: The termination phase is marked by the dissolution of the analytical bond as the patient prepares for leave-taking. The irrational attachment to the analyst in the transference neurosis has subsided because it has been worked through, and more rational aspects of the psyche preside, providing greater mastery and more mature adaptation to the patient's problems. Termination is not a hard-and-fast event, and the patient invariably has to continue to work through any problems outside of the therapy situation without the analyst or may need intermittent assistance after analysis has technically terminated.

Courtesy of T. Byram Karasu, M.D.

Table 23-3
Patient Prerequisites for Psychoanalysis

High motivation. The patient needs a strong motivation to persevere, in light of the rigors of intense and lengthy treatment. The desire for health and self-understanding must surpass the neurotic need for unhappiness. The patient must be willing to face issues of time and money and to endure the pain and frustration associated with sacrificing rapid relief in favor of future cure and with foregoing the secondary gains of illness.

Ability to form a relationship. The capacity to form and maintain, as well as to detach from, a trusting object relationship is essential. The patient also has to withstand a frustrating and regressive transference without decompensating or becoming excessively attached. Patients with a history of impaired or transient interpersonal relations who cannot establish a viable connection to another human make poor candidates for psychoanalysis.

Psychological mindedness and capacity for insight. As an introspective process, psychoanalysis requires curiosity about oneself and the capacity for self-scrutiny. Those who are unable to articulate and comprehend their inner thoughts and feelings cannot negotiate with the fundamental analytical coin words and their meanings. The inability to examine one's own motivations and behaviors precludes benefits from the analytical method.

Ego strength. Ego strength is the integrative capacity to oscillate appropriately between two antithetical types of ego functioning: On the one hand, the patient must be able to reflect temporarily, to relinquish reality for fantasy, and to be dependent and passive. On the other hand, the patient has to be able to accept analytical rules, to integrate interpretations, to defer important decisions, to shift perspectives to become an observer of his or her intrapsychic processes, and to function in a sustained interpersonal relationship as a responsible adult.

Courtesy of T. Byram Karasu, M.D.

Psychoanalytic goals often seem formidable (e.g., a total personality change), involving the radical reorganization of old developmental patterns based on earlier affects and the entrenched defenses built up against them. Goals may also be elusive, framed as they are in theoretical intrapsychic terms (e.g., greater ego strength) or conceptually ambiguous ones (resolution of the transference neurosis). Criteria for successful psychoanalysis may be largely intangible and subjective, and it is best to view them as conceptual endpoints of treatment that the therapist must translate into more realistic and practical terms.

In practice, the goals of psychoanalysis for any patient naturally vary, as do the many manifestations of neuroses. The form that the neurosis takes—unsatisfactory sexual or object relationships, inability to enjoy life, underachievement, and fear of work or academic success, or excessive anxiety, guilt, or depressive ideation—determines the focus of attention and the general direction of treatment, as well as the specific goals. Such goals may change at any time during analysis, especially as many years of treatment may be involved.

Major Approach and Techniques. Structurally, *psychoanalysis* usually refers to individual (dyadic) treatment that is frequent (four or five times per week) and long term (several years). All three features take their precedent from Freud himself.

The dyadic arrangement is a direct function of the Freudian theory of neurosis as an intrapsychic phenomenon, which takes place within the person as instinctual impulses continually seek discharge. Because it is crucial to resolve dynamic conflicts internally if structural personality reorganization is to take place, the individual's memory and perceptions of the repressed past are pivotal.

Freud initially saw patients 6 days a week for 1 hour each day, a routine now reduced to four or five sessions per week of the classic 50-minute hour, which leaves time for the analyst to take notes and organize relevant thoughts before the next patient. Therapists should avoid long intervals between sessions so that the momentum gained in uncovering conflictual material is not lost, and confronted defenses do not have time to restrengthen.

Freud's belief that successful psychoanalysis always takes a long time because profound changes in the mind occur slowly still holds. The process is similar to the fluid sense of time that is characteristic of our unconscious processes. Moreover, because psychoanalysis involves a detailed recapitulation of present and past events, any compromise in time presents the risk of losing pace with the patient's mental life.

PSYCHOANALYTIC SETTING. As with other forms of psychotherapy, psychoanalysis takes place in a professional setting, apart from the realities of everyday life, in which the therapist offers the patient a temporary sanctuary in which to ease psychic pain and reveal intimate thoughts to an accepting expert. The design of the psychoanalytic environment promotes relaxation and regression. The setting is usually spartan and sensorially neutral and minimizes external stimuli.

Use of the Couch. The couch has several clinical advantages that are both real and symbolic: (1) the reclining position is relaxing because it is associated with sleep and so eases the patient's conscious control of thoughts; (2) it minimizes the intrusive influence of the analyst, thus curbing unnecessary cues; (3) it permits the analyst to make observations of the patient without interruption; and (4) it holds a symbolic value for both parties, a tangible reminder of the Freudian legacy that gives credibility to the analyst's professional identity, allegiance, and expertise. The reclining position of the patient with analyst nearby can also generate threat and discomfort, however, as it recalls anxieties derived from the earlier parent–child configuration that it physically resembles. It may also have personal meanings—for some, a portent of dangerous impulses or submission to an authority figure; for others, relief from confrontation by the analyst (e.g., fear of the use of the couch and over-eagerness to lie down may reflect resistance and, thus, need to be analyzed). Although the use of the couch is requisite to the analytical technique, it is not applied automatically; the therapist introduces it gradually and may suspend its use whenever additional regression is unnecessary or countertherapeutic.

Fundamental Rule. The fundamental rule of free association requires patients to tell the analyst everything that comes into their heads—however disagreeable, unimportant, or nonsensical—and to let themselves go as they would in a conversation that leads from "cabbages to kings." It differs decidedly from ordinary conversation—instead of connecting personal remarks with a rational thread, the therapist asks the patient to reveal those very thoughts and events that are objectionable precisely because of being averse to doing so.

This directive represents an ideal because free association does not arise freely but is guided and inhibited by a variety of conscious and unconscious forces. The analyst must not only encourage free association through the physical setting and a nonjudgmental attitude toward the patient's verbalizations but also examine those very instances when the flow of associations is diminished or comes to a halt—they are as important analytically as the content of the associations. The analyst should also be alert to how individual patients use or misuse the fundamental rule.

Aside from its primary purpose of eliciting recall of deeply hidden early memories, the fundamental rule reflects the analytical priority placed on verbalization, which translates the patient's thoughts into words, so the patient does not channel them physically or behaviorally. As a direct concomitant of the fundamental rule, which prohibits action in favor of verbal expression, patients should postpone making significant alterations in their lives, such as marrying or changing careers, until they discuss and analyze them within the context of treatment.

Principle of Evenly Suspended Attention. As a reciprocal corollary to the rule that patients communicate everything that occurs to them without criticism or selection, the principle of evenly suspended attention requires the analyst to suspend judgment and to give impartial attention to every detail equally. The method consists simply of making no effort to concentrate on anything specific while maintaining a neutral, quiet attentiveness to all that the patient says.

Analyst as Mirror. A second principle is the recommendation that the analyst is impenetrable to the patient and, like a mirror, only reflect what the patient shows. Analysts should be neutral blank screens and not bring their personalities into treatment. They are not to bring their values or attitudes into the discussion or to share personal reactions or mutual conflicts with their patients, although they may sometimes feel the temptation to do so. The bringing in of reality and external influences can interrupt or bias the patient's unconscious projections. Neutrality also allows the analyst to accept without censure all forbidden or objectionable responses.

Rule of Abstinence. The fundamental rule of abstinence does not mean corporal or sexual abstinence but refers to the frustration of emotional needs and wishes that the patient may have toward the analyst or part of the transference. It allows the patient's longings to persist and serve as driving forces for analytical work and motivation to change. Freud advised that the analyst proceeds through the analytical treatment in a state of renunciation. The analyst must deny the patient who is longing for love the satisfaction he or she craves.

LIMITATIONS.   At present, the predominant treatment constraints are often economic, relating to the high cost in time and money, both for patients and in the training of future practitioners. In addition, because clinical requirements emphasize such requisites as psychological mindedness, verbal and cognitive ability, and stable life situation, psychoanalysis may be unduly restricted to a diagnostically, socioeconomically, or intellectually advantaged patient population. Other intrinsic issues pertain to the use and misuse of its stringent rules, whereby overemphasis on technique may interfere with an authentic human encounter between analyst and patient, and to the major long-term risk of interminability, in which protracted treatment may become a substitute for life. The reification of the classic analytical tradition may interfere with a more open and flexible application of its tenets to meet changing needs. It may also obstruct a comprehensive view of patient care that includes a greater appreciation of other treatment modalities in conjunction with or as an alternative to psychoanalysis.

Ms. A, a 25-year-old articulate and introspective medical student began analysis complaining of mild, chronic anxiety, dysphoria, and a sense of inadequacy, despite above-average intelligence and performance. She also expressed difficulty in long-term relationships with her male peers.

Ms. A began the initial phase of analysis with enthusiastic self-disclosure, frequent reports of dreams and fantasies, and over idealization of the analyst; she tried to please him by being a compliant, good patient, just as she had been a good daughter to her father (a professor of medicine) by going to medical school.

Over the next several months, Ms. A gradually developed a strong attachment to the analyst and settled into a phase of excessive preoccupation with him. Simultaneously, however, she began dating an older psychiatrist and proceeded to complain about the analyst's coldness and unresponsiveness, even considering dropping out of the analysis because he did not meet her demands.

In the course of analysis, through dreams and associations, Ms. A recalled early memories of her ongoing competition with her mother for her father's attention and realized that failing to obtain his exclusive love, she had tried to become like him. She was also able to see how her increasing interest in becoming a psychiatrist (rather than following her original plan to be a pediatrician), as well as her recent choice of a man to date, were recapitulations of the past vis-à-vis the analyst. As this repeated pattern was recognized, the patient began to relinquish her intense erotic and dependent tie to the analyst, viewing him more realistically and beginning to appreciate how his quiet presence reminded her of her mother. She also became less disturbed by the similarities she shared with her mother and was able to disengage from her father more comfortably. By the fifth year of analysis, she was happily married to a former classmate, was pregnant, and was a pediatric chief resident. Her anxiety had attenuated and become situation-specific (i.e., she was concerned about motherhood and the termination of analysis). (Courtesy of T. Byram Karasu, M.D.)

Psychoanalytic Psychotherapy

Psychoanalytic psychotherapy, based on fundamental dynamic formulations and techniques that derive from psychoanalysis, is designed to broaden its scope. Psychoanalytic psychotherapy, in its narrowest sense, is the use of insight-oriented methods only.

As generically applied today to an ever-larger clinical spectrum, it incorporates a blend of uncovering and suppressive measures.

The strategies of psychoanalytic psychotherapy currently range from expressive (insight-oriented, uncovering, evocative, or interpretive) techniques to supportive (relationship-oriented, suggestive, suppressive, or repressive) techniques. Although those two methods may seem antithetical, their precise definitions and the distinctions between them are by no means absolute.

The duration of psychoanalytic psychotherapy is generally shorter and more variable than in psychoanalysis. Treatment may be brief, even with an initially agreed-upon or fixed time limit, or may extend to a less definite number of months or years. Brief treatment is chiefly used for selected problems or highly focused conflict, whereas more prolonged treatment may be applied for more chronic conditions or for intermittent episodes that require ongoing attention to deal with pervasive conflict or recurrent decompensation. Unlike psychoanalysis, psychoanalytic psychotherapy rarely uses the couch; instead, the patient and therapist sit face to face. This posture helps to prevent regression because it encourages the patient to look at the therapist as a real person from whom to receive direct cues, even though transference and fantasy will continue. The couch is unnecessary because the free-association method is rarely used, except when the therapist wishes to gain access to fantasy material or dreams to enlighten a particular issue.

Expressive Psychotherapy

INDICATIONS AND CONTRAINDICATIONS.   Diagnostically, psychoanalytic psychotherapy in its expressive mode is suited to a range of psychopathology with mild to moderate ego weakening, including neurotic conflicts, symptom complexes, reactive conditions, and the whole realm of nonpsychotic character disorders, including those disorders of the self that are among the more transient and less profound on the severity-of-illness spectrum, such as narcissistic personality disorders. It is also one of the treatments recommended for patients with borderline personality disorders (BPDs), although special variations may be required to deal with the associated turbulent personality characteristics, primitive defense mechanisms, tendencies toward regressive episodes, and irrational attachments to the analyst.

Ms. B, an intelligent and verbal 34-year-old divorced woman, presented with complaints of being unappreciated at work. Always angry and irritable, she considered quitting her job and even leaving the city. Her social life was also being negatively affected; her boyfriend had threatened to leave her because of her extremely hostile, clinging behavior (the same reason her ex-husband had given when he left her 9 years earlier after only 16 months of marriage). Her past included promiscuity and experimentation with various drugs, and, currently, she indulged in heavy drinking on weekends and occasionally smoked marijuana. She had held many jobs and had lived in various cities.

The eldest of three children of a middle-class family, she came from an unhappy and unstable home: her brother had been in and out of psychiatric hospitals; her sister had left home at the age of 16 after becoming pregnant and being forced to marry; and her overly controlling parents had subjected their children to psychological (and occasionally physical) abuse, alternating between heated arguments and passionate reconciliations.

Initially, Ms. B attempted to contain her rage in treatment, but it frequently surfaced and alternated with child-like helplessness; she interrogated the psychiatrist regarding his credentials, ridiculed psychodynamic concepts, constantly challenged statements, and would demand practical advice but then denigrate or fail to follow the guidance given. The psychiatrist remained unprovoked by her aggression and explored with her the need to engage him negatively. Her response was to question and test his continued concern.

When her boyfriend left her, she attempted suicide (she cut her wrists superficially), was briefly hospitalized, and, on discharge, was placed on a selective serotonin reuptake inhibitor (SSRI) for 6 months for her minor, but protracted, depression. The psychiatrist maintained their regular frequency of sessions despite her greater demands. Although she was puzzled by the steadiness of his interest, she gradually felt safe enough to express her vulnerabilities. As they explored her lack of full commitment to work, friends, and therapy, she began to understand the meaning of her anger in terms of the early abusive relationship with her parents and her tendency to bring it into contemporary relationships. With the psychiatrist's encouragement, she also began to seek work and make small strides in relationship-oriented efforts. By the end of her second year of treatment, she decided to remain in the city, to stay at her place of employment, and to continue therapy. She needed to experience and practice her somewhat fragile new self, which included greater intimacy in relationships, additional mastery of work skills, and a more cohesive sense of self. (Courtesy of T. Byram Karasu, M.D.)

The persons best suited for the expressive psychotherapy approach have reasonably well-integrated egos and the capacity to both sustain and detach from a bond of dependency and trust. They are, to some degree, psychologically minded and self-motivated, and they are generally able, at least temporarily, to tolerate doses of frustration without decompensating. They must also have the ability to manage the rearousal of painful feelings outside the therapy hour without additional contact. Patients must have some capacity for introspection and impulse control, and they should be able to recognize the cognitive distinction between fantasy and reality.

GOALS. The overall goals of expressive psychotherapy are to increase the patient's self-awareness and to improve object relations through the exploration of current interpersonal events and perceptions. In contrast to psychoanalysis, expressive psychotherapy modifies major structural changes in ego function and defenses in light of patient limitations. The aim is to achieve a more limited and, thus, select and focused understanding of one's problems. Rather than uncovering deeply hidden and past motives and tracing them back to their origins in infancy, the major thrust is to deal with preconscious or conscious derivatives of conflicts as they became manifest in present interactions. Although the therapy seeks insight, it is less extensive; instead of delving to a genetic level, greater emphasis is on clarifying recent dynamic patterns and maladaptive behaviors in the present.

MAJOR APPROACH AND TECHNIQUES. The primary modus operandi involves the establishment of a therapeutic alliance and early recognition and interpretation of negative transference. Only limited or controlled regression is encouraged, and positive transference manifestations are generally left unexplored unless they are impeding therapeutic progress; even here, the emphasis is on shedding light on current dynamic patterns and defenses.

LIMITATIONS. A general limitation of expressive psychotherapy, as of psychoanalysis, is the problem of emotional integration of cognitive awareness. The primary danger for patients who are at the more disorganized end of the diagnostic spectrum, however, may have less to do with the over intellectualization that is sometimes seen in neurotic patients than with the threat of decompensation from or acting out of, deep or frequent interpretations that the patient is unable to integrate properly.

Some therapists fail to accept the limitations of a modified insight-oriented approach and so apply it inappropriately to modulate the techniques and goals of psychoanalysis. Overemphasis on dreams and fantasies, zealous efforts to use the couch, indiscriminate deep interpretations, and continual focus on the analysis of transference may have less to do with the patient's needs than with those of a therapist who is unwilling or unable to be flexible.

Ms. S was an attractive 30-year-old unmarried woman working as a secretary when she presented for consultation. Her chief complaints at the time were feeling "only anger and tension" and an inability to apply herself to studying voice, "which is one of the most important things to me."

In obtaining a history, the therapist noted that Ms. S had never completed anything: she had dropped out of college, never pursued a music degree, and switched from job to job, and even city to city. What initially seemed like a woman with diverse interests (e.g., jobs as a research assistant; freelance copyeditor; part-time radio announcer; manager of data entry for a software company; and, most recently, secretary) actually reflected a woman with a chaotic lifestyle and serious difficulties committing to anyone or anything. Although obviously intelligent, Ms. S presented with unrealistic expectations regarding her consultation. For example, after the first consultative session, Ms. S said she felt good afterward but felt there were "no revelations yet." Because of Ms. S's inability to commit and her somewhat disorganized life, the therapist recommended a course of psychotherapy, beginning twice a week, rather than something more intense like psychoanalysis. The therapist also realized throughout the consultation that Ms. S would have difficulty with free association without getting disorganized. The therapist also thought that Ms. S might regress unproductively on the couch without visual contact with the therapist.

Ms. S was the second oldest of four children—two brothers and a younger sister, with whom she was most competitive and who seemed the mother's favorite. She described her mother as a successful professor who was demanding and critical as if she had a "raised eyebrow" in disapproval. For example, much to her mother's chagrin, Ms. S had once wanted a sandwich "with everything on it." Ms. S was also disappointed when she received one piece of luggage rather than a complete set for a Christmas gift. She was able to accept the therapist's interpretation that she felt "part of a set" by being one of four siblings. Ms. S initially idealized her father, who was active in the family church, but eventually saw him as disappointing and rejecting.

Ms. S's ideal therapist would be "flexible," by which she meant a therapist who might do hypnosis one session, psychotherapy the next, and, maybe, analysis another session. In fact, within the first week of beginning therapy, Ms. S had simultaneously consulted a hypnotherapist, which she mentioned in passing only weeks later, for her neck pain and tension. Although she did not pursue hypnosis, she did maintain a chiropractor for most of her therapy, also something she mentioned many months after beginning therapy. She did speak of wanting to be "on best behavior" and "follow the rules." Her tremendous sense of entitlement, however, was evident: she expected "cut-rate prices" on everything from haircuts and car repairs to doctors' visits. Her initial fee was a much reduced one, which she paid late and begrudgingly.

Although she had therapy only twice a week, Ms. S developed intense feelings for her therapist. Mostly she experienced rage when she saw evidence of the therapist's other patients, such as footprints on the waiting room floor after a snowstorm or a coat hanger turned around. She expressed the wish to keep some of her things, like bobby pins and hairspray, in the therapist's bathroom. She vacillated between feelings she wanted to move in and feelings that the therapist did not exist. For example, before she took a plane flight, she wondered who would tell her therapist if something happened to her. She had never given the therapist's name to anyone, nor did she have her name in her weekly appointment book. The therapist interpreted that she had a simultaneous wish to devalue her and not to share her with anyone else.

Associations to a dream with an image of a string of baroque pearls led to thoughts that these pearls—irregular and imperfect—defective and even lopsided, represented how she viewed herself.

Over the next few years, Ms. S was able to commit to regularly coming to therapy, although the course was somewhat tumultuous, with many threats of quitting and much withholding of information. At one point, she even tried to provoke the therapist by seeking a consultation with another therapist in order to "tattle" on her, just as she had tattled on her siblings. Her therapist remained unprovoked and continued to provide a safe environment for Ms. S to explore her ambivalence to the therapist and the therapeutic situation. The therapist was also able to contain Ms. S's tendency to regress, particularly with separations, by providing her with the therapist's telephone number.

She had actually entered therapy with an unconscious wish to become a world-famous singer who would win her mother's approval and praise. Her narcissism and sense of entitlement made it difficult for her to give up on that fantasy despite repeated evidence that she did not have sufficient talent. She was finally able to settle on a compromise: she began to work diligently and closely as a research assistant to her mother, who was writing a book, and as Ms. S became more focused and organized over time, she even thought she might write a book about the church. (Courtesy of T. Byram Karasu, M.D. and S. R. Karasu, M.D.)

Supportive Psychotherapy.

Supportive psychotherapy aims at the creation of a therapeutic relationship as a temporary buttress or bridge for the deficient patient. It has roots in virtually every therapy that recognizes the ameliorative effects of emotional support and a stable, caring atmosphere in the management of patients. As a nonspecific attitude toward mental illness, it predates scientific psychiatry, with foundations in 18th-century moral treatment, whereby for the first time, patients received understanding and kindness in a humane, interpersonal treatment environment free from mechanical restraints.

Supportive psychotherapy has been the primary form used in the general practice of medicine and rehabilitation, frequently to augment other measures, such as prescriptions of medication to suppress symptoms, rest to remove the patient from excessive stimulation, or hospitalization to provide a structured therapeutic environment, protection, and control of the patient. It can serve as primary or ancillary treatment. The global perspective of supportive psychotherapy (often part of a combined treatment approach) places major etiologic emphasis on external rather than intrapsychic events, particularly on stressful environmental and interpersonal influences on a severely damaged self.

INDICATIONS AND CONTRAINDICATIONS. Supportive psychotherapy is generally indicated for those patients for whom classic psychoanalysis or insight-oriented psychoanalytic psychotherapy is typically contraindicated—those who have poor ego strength and whose potential for decompensation is high. Amenable patients fall into the following major areas: (1) individuals in acute crisis or a temporary state of disorganization and inability to cope (including those who might otherwise be well functioning) whose intolerable life circumstances have produced extreme anxiety or sudden turmoil (e.g., individuals going through grief reactions, illness, divorce, job loss, or who were victims of crime, abuse, natural disaster, or accident); (2) patients with chronic severe pathology with fragile or deficient ego functioning (e.g., those with latent psychosis, impulse disorder, or severe character disturbance); (3) patients whose cognitive deficits and physical symptoms make them particularly vulnerable and, thus, unsuitable for an insight-oriented approach (e.g., certain psychosomatic or medically ill persons); and (4) individuals

who are psychologically unmotivated, although not necessarily characterologically resistant to a depth approach (e.g., patients who come to treatment in response to family or agency pressure and are interested only in immediate relief or those who need assistance in very specific problem areas of social adjustment as a possible prelude to more exploratory work).

Mr. C, a 50-year-old married man with two sons, the owner of a small construction company, was referred by his internist after recovery from bypass surgery because of frequent, unfounded physical complaints. He was taking minor tranquilizers in increasing doses, not adhering to his daily regimen, avoiding sexual contact with his wife, and had dropped out of group therapy for postsurgical patients after one session.

He came to his first appointment 20 minutes late, after having "forgotten" two previous appointments. He was extremely anxious, often lost in his train of thought, and was semi-delusional about his wife and sons, suggesting that they might want to have him locked up. He briefly told his life history, which included his coming from a strict and hard-working but caring middle-class family and the death of his mother when he was only 11 years old. He had joined his father's business (taking over after his father's death 2 years earlier), with both of his sons as associates. Describing himself as successful in work and marriage, he claimed that "the only test I ever failed was the stress test."

Mr. C explained his lack of adherence to dietary restrictions as a lack of will and his constant contact with the internist as his having real physical problems not yet diagnosed; he rejected the idea of addiction to tranquilizers, insisting that he could quit any time. He had no fantasy life, remembered no dreams, made it clear that he had entered treatment on his internist's instruction only, and started each session by stating that he had nothing to discuss.

After suggesting that Mr. C was coming to sessions just to pass the "sanity test" and that there was no reason to have him locked up, the psychiatrist encouraged the patient to join him in figuring out the real reasons for his anxiety. Initial sessions were devoted to discussing the patient's medical condition and providing factual information about heart and bypass surgery. The therapist likened the patient's condition to that of an older house getting new plumbing, trying to allay his unrealistic fears of impending death. As Mr. C's anxiety declined, he became less defensive and more psychologically accessible. As the therapist began to explore his difficulty in accepting help, Mr. C was able to talk about his inability to admit problems (i.e., weaknesses). The therapist's explicit recognition of the patient's strength in admitting his weaknesses encouraged the patient to reveal more about himself—how he had welcomed his father's death and his belief that perhaps his illness was punishment. The psychiatrist also encouraged him to speak about his unrealistic guilt and, at the same time, helped him recognize his suspicion of his sons as the reflection of his own wishes concerning his father and his lack of commitment to his medical regimen as a wish to die to expiate guilt. After steady urging by the therapist, Mr. C returned to work. He agreed to meet monthly with the psychiatrist and to taper off his use of tranquilizers. He even agreed that he might see the psychiatrist for "deep analysis" in the future because his wife now jokingly complained of his obsessive dieting, his uncompromising exercise regimens, and his regularly scheduled sexual activities. (Courtesy of T. Byram Karasu, M.D.)

Because support forms a tacit part of every therapeutic modality, it is rarely contraindicated as such. The typical attitude regards better-functioning patients as unsuitable not because a supportive approach will harm them, but because they will not be sufficiently benefited by it. In aiming to maximize the patient's potential for further growth and change, supportive therapy is relatively restricted and superficial and, thus, is not recommended as the treatment of choice if the patient is available for, and capable of, a more in-depth approach.

GOALS. The general aim of supportive treatment is the amelioration or relief of symptoms through behavioral or environmental restructuring within the existing psychic framework. Supportive therapy helps the patient to adapt better to problems and to live more comfortably with his or her psychopathology. To restore the disorganized, fragile, or decompensated patient to a state of relative equilibrium, the therapist's primary goal is to suppress or control symptomatology and to stabilize the patient in a protective and reassuring benign atmosphere that militates against overwhelming external and internal pressures. The ultimate goal is to maximize the integrative or adaptive capacities so that the patient increases the ability to cope while decreasing vulnerability by reinforcing assets and strengthening defenses.

MAJOR APPROACH AND TECHNIQUES. Supportive therapy uses several methods, either singly or in combination, including warm, friendly, strong leadership; partial gratification of dependency needs; support in the ultimate development of legitimate independence; help in developing pleasurable activities (e.g., hobbies); adequate rest and diversion; removal of excessive strain, when possible; hospitalization, when indicated; medication to alleviate symptoms; and guidance and advice in dealing with current issues. This therapy uses techniques to help patients feel secure, accepted, protected, encouraged, safe, and not anxious.

LIMITATIONS. To the extent that much supportive therapy is spent on practical, everyday realities and on dealing with the external environment of the patient, it may be viewed as more mundane and superficial than depth approaches. Because those patients attend therapy sessions intermittently and less frequently, the interpersonal commitment may not be as compelling on the part of either the patient or the therapist. Greater severity of illness (and possible psychoses) also makes such treatment potentially more erratic, demanding, and frustrating. The need for the therapist to deal with other family members, caretakers, or agencies (auxiliary treatment, hospitalization) can become an additional complication because the therapist comes to serve as an ombudsman to negotiate with the outside world of the patient and with other professional peers. Finally, the supportive therapist must be able to accept personal limitations and the patient's limited psychological resources and to tolerate the often unrewarded efforts until the patient makes small gains.

Mr. W was a 42-year-old widowed businessman who was referred by his internist because of the sudden death of his wife, who had had an intracranial hemorrhage, about 2 months earlier. Mr. W had two children, a boy and a girl, ages 10 and 8 years, respectively.

Mr. W had never been to a psychiatrist before, and when he arrived, he admitted he was not sure what a psychiatrist could do for him. He just had to get over his wife's death. He was not sure how talking about anything could help. He had been married for 15 years. He admitted to having difficulty sleeping, particularly awakening in the middle of the night with considerable anxiety about the future. One of his relatives had given him some of her clonazepam for his anxiety, which helped tremendously, but he feared getting dependent on it. He was also drinking more than he thought he should. He was most concerned about raising his children alone and felt somewhat overwhelmed by the responsibility. He was beginning to appreciate just how wonderful a mother his wife had been and now saw how critical he had been of her for spending so much time with the children. "It really does take a lot of effort," he said.

Mr. W did admit to feelings of guilt. For one thing, he admitted to some sense that he could now start over. He had been somewhat restless in the marriage recently before his wife's death and had been unfaithful for a brief period early in the marriage. He also felt some guilt that had he been awake the night of his wife's hemorrhage, and maybe he could have saved his wife. In reality, there was nothing he could have done.

Mr. W agreed to come for a few sessions to talk about his wife. At this point, only 2 months after her death, he seemed to have an uncomplicated mourning reaction. Although he talked easily in session, he was clearly worried that he might like "being here too much." The therapist chose not to interpret his dependency conflicts. Mr. W seemed to have good coping skills and used humor as a high-functioning defense. For example, in giving a eulogy for his wife (who had been a very popular member of their congregation), he looked around at the enormous crowd of people at the church service and said he had never seen so many people attending church before, adding, "Sorry, Reverend."

After about four sessions, Mr. W said that he felt better and no longer saw the need for further sessions. He was sleeping better and had stopped drinking excessively. The therapist suggested that he might want to continue to talk more about his guilt and his life as he went forward without his wife. The therapist was also reassuring that there seemed to be nothing else Mr. W could have done to save his wife. He also encouraged the patient to begin dating when he felt ready, something that Mr. W's in-laws were not encouraging. For now, however, Mr. W was not interested in any further therapy. He was appreciative of the therapist and felt that talking about his wife's death had been helpful. The therapist accepted his wish to discontinue their sessions but encouraged Mr. W to keep in touch to let him know how he was doing. (Courtesy of T. Byram Karasu, M.D. and S. R. Karasu, M.D.)

CORRECTIVE EMOTIONAL EXPERIENCE. The relationship between therapist and patient allows a therapist to display behavior different from the destructive or unproductive behavior of a patient's parent. At times, such experiences seem to neutralize or reverse some effects of the parents' mistakes. If the patient had overly authoritarian parents, the therapist's friendly, flexible, nonjudgmental, nonauthoritarian—but at times firm and limit setting—attitude allows the patient to adjust to, be led by, and identify with a new parent figure. Franz Alexander described this process as a corrective emotional experience. It draws on elements of both psychoanalysis and psychoanalytic psychotherapy.

BRIEF PSYCHODYNAMIC PSYCHOTHERAPY

Brief psychodynamic psychotherapy has gained widespread popularity, partly because of the great pressure on health care professionals to contain treatment costs. It is also easier to evaluate treatment efficacy by comparing groups of persons who have had short-term therapy for mental illness with control groups than it is to measure the results of long-term psychotherapy. Thus, short-term therapies have been the subject of much research, especially on outcome measures, which have found them to be effective. Other short-term methods include interpersonal therapy and cognitive-behavioral therapy (CBT, discussed later in this chapter).

Brief psychodynamic psychotherapy is a time-limited treatment (10 to 12 sessions) based on psychoanalysis and psychodynamic theory. It is useful in helping persons with depression, anxiety, and posttraumatic stress disorder (PTSD), among others. There are several methods, each having its own treatment technique and specific criteria for selecting patients; however, they are more similar than different.

In 1946, Franz Alexander and Thomas French identified the basic characteristics of brief psychodynamic psychotherapy. They described a therapeutic experience designed to put patients at ease, to manipulate the transference, and to use trial interpretations flexibly. Alexander and French conceived psychotherapy as a corrective emotional experience capable of repairing traumatic events of the past and convincing patients that new ways of thinking, feeling, and behaving are possible. At about the same time, Eric Lindemann established a consultation service at Massachusetts General Hospital in Boston for persons experiencing a crisis. He developed new treatment methods to deal with these situations and eventually applied these techniques to persons who were not in crisis, but who were experiencing various kinds of emotional distress. Since then, the field has been influenced by many workers such as David Malan in England, Peter Sifneos in the United States, and Habib Davanloo in Canada.

Types

Brief Focal Psychotherapy (Tavistock–Malan).

Brief focal psychotherapy was originally developed in the 1950s by the Balint team at the Tavistock Clinic in London. Malan, a member of the team, reported the results of the therapy. Malan's selection criteria for treatment included eliminating absolute contraindications, rejecting patients for whom certain dangers seemed inevitable, clearly assessing patients' psychopathology, and determining patients' capacities to consider problems in emotional terms, face disturbing material, respond to interpretations, and endure the stress of the treatment. Malan found that high motivation invariably correlated with a successful outcome. Contraindications to treatment were serious suicide attempts, substance dependence, chronic alcohol abuse, incapacitating chronic obsessional symptoms, incapacitating chronic phobic symptoms, and gross destructive or self-destructive acting out.

REQUIREMENTS AND TECHNIQUES.   In Malan's routine, therapists should identify the transference early and interpret it and the negative transference. They should then link the transferences to patients' relationships with their parents. Both patients and therapists should be willing to become deeply involved and to bear the ensuing tension. Therapists should formulate a circumscribed focus and set a termination date in advance, and patients should work through grief and anger about termination. An experienced therapist should allow about 20 sessions as an average length for the therapy; a trainee should allow about 30 sessions. Malan himself did not exceed 40 interviews with his patients.

Time-Limited Psychotherapy (Boston University–Mann).

A psychotherapeutic model of exactly 12 interviews focusing on a specified central issue was developed at Boston University by James Mann and his colleagues in the early 1970s. In contrast with Malan's emphasis on clear-cut selection and rejection criteria, Mann was not as explicit about the appropriate candidates for time-limited psychotherapy. Mann considered the major emphases of his theory to be determining a patient's central conflict reasonably correctly and exploring young persons' maturational crises with many psychological and somatic complaints. Mann's exceptions, similar to his rejection criteria, include persons with major depressive disorder that interferes with the treatment agreement, those with acute psychotic states, and desperate patients who need, but cannot tolerate, object relations.

REQUIREMENTS AND TECHNIQUES.   Mann's technical requirements included strict limitation to 12 sessions, positive transference predominating early, specification and strict adherence to a central issue involving transference, positive identification, making separation a maturational event for patients, absolute prospect of termination to avoid development of dependence, clarification of present and past experiences and resistances, active therapists who support and encourage patients, and education of patients through direct information, reeducation, and manipulation. The conflicts likely to be encountered included independence versus dependence, activity versus passivity, unresolved or delayed grief, and adequate versus inadequate self-esteem.

Short-Term Dynamic Psychotherapy (McGill University–Davanloo).

As conducted by Davanloo at McGill University, short-term dynamic psychotherapy encompasses nearly all varieties of brief psychotherapy and crisis intervention. Davanloo's series classified patients treated as those whose psychological conflicts are predominantly oedipal, those whose conflicts are not oedipal, and those whose conflicts have more than one focus. Davanloo also devised a specific psychotherapeutic technique for patients with severe, long-standing neurotic problems, specifically those with incapacitating obsessive-compulsive disorders (OCDs) and phobias.

Davanloo's selection criteria emphasize evaluating those ego functions of primary importance to psychotherapeutic work: the establishment of a psychotherapeutic focus; the psychodynamic formulation of the patient's psychological problems; the ability to interact emotionally with evaluators; a history of give-and-take relationships with a significant person in the patient's life; the patient's ability to experience and tolerate anxiety, guilt, and depression; the patient's motivations for change, psychological mindedness, and an ability to respond to interpretation and to link evaluators with persons in the present and past. Both Malan and Davanloo emphasized a patient's responses to interpretation as an essential selection and prognostic criterion.

REQUIREMENTS AND TECHNIQUES.   The highlights of Davanloo's psychotherapeutic approach are flexibility (therapists should adapt the technique to the patient's needs), control, the patient's regressive tendencies, active intervention to avoid having the patient develop overdependence on a therapist, and the patient's intellectual insight and emotional experiences in the transference. These emotional experiences become corrective as a result of the interpretation.

Ana, a divorced 60-year-old woman, sought psychiatric help following a severe depressive episode lasting several months. This episode, which was one of many in her life, was especially severe in terms of loss of energy, interest, motivation, and the intensity of her sadness and wish to die. Only her profound religious convictions protected her from acting on these wishes. Ana had lost much weight, had trouble sleeping, experienced many nightmares, and had difficulty with concentration. Pervasive feelings of hatred for her mother plagued Ana; her mother was very old, ill, and dependent on Ana, who was unable to forgive her for abandoning her in an orphanage when she was 5 or 6 years of age.

After an extensive assessment, the dynamic formulation of Ana's problem was:

1. *Life problems:* Recurrent depressive episodes plagued by feelings of guilt and self-reproach; problems with men involving choosing partners who are commonly cold, distant, or otherwise unavailable; involuntary and painful emotional distance from her children, friends, and other close relationships; and unproductive and unrewarding work life, despite considerable intellectual gifts.

2. *Dynamics:* Ambivalent relationship with her mother, whom she blames for most of the tragedies of her life; guilt and need for punishment concerning her unrelenting hatred for her mother; and pathologic grief reaction for the loss of an idealized and more optimal relationship with her mother, the one she remembers she had before her orphanage placement. From this focus, there flows a melancholic conviction of the inevitable failure of human relationships.

3. *Pathogenic foci:* Grief and inability to mourn the loss of her mother after going to live in the orphanage, with attendant rage and guilt; pathologic grief for the loss of her father, who, because of severe alcoholism, abandoned the family first, a move that caused the mother to place her children in an orphanage in order to be able to work and ultimately recover their care. Unconsciously, she blamed her mother for the family catastrophe, thus "protecting" an idealized view of her father, to whom she was profoundly attached.

For Ana, the initial phase of treatment focused on the clarification and the experience of her destructive impulses toward her mother, which, as they were worked through, made possible the appearance of a modicum of empathy with her mother's painful life situation around the time she placed Ana and her sisters in the orphanage. Next, the therapy focused on Ana's father. She experienced deep feelings of idealization, disappointment, anger, and grief with increasing clarity and intensity, frequently via displaced feelings in the transference and after overcoming considerable resistance. The last phase of treatment permitted the development of realistic feelings of empathy and appreciation for her mother, now without anger or emotional distancing, and the reawakening within Ana of feelings of joy and hope, as well as professional ambition. (Courtesy of M. Trujillo, M.D.)

Short-Term Anxiety-Provoking Psychotherapy (Harvard University–Sifneos).

Sifneos developed short-term anxiety-provoking psychotherapy at the Massachusetts General Hospital in Boston during the 1950s. He used the following criteria for selection: a circumscribed chief complaint (implying a patient's ability to select one of a variety of problems to be given top priority and the patient's desire to resolve the problem in treatment), one meaningful or give-and-take relationship during early childhood, the ability to interact flexibly with an evaluator and to express feelings appropriately, above-average psychological sophistication (implying not only above-average intelligence but also an ability to respond to interpretations), a specific psychodynamic formulation (usually a set of psychological conflicts underlying a patient's difficulties and centering on an oedipal focus), a contract between therapist and patient to work on the specified focus and the formulation of minimal expectations of outcome, and good to excellent motivation for change, not just for symptom relief.

Chris, a 31-year-old single man, sought help for a moderate depressive episode precipitated by the loss of his relationship with his girlfriend, Joanna. She had broken off the relationship after approximately 1 year, tired of Chris's erratic work ethic and emotional instability and discouraged by his fear of commitment to the future of their relationship. This cycle of infatuation, increasing fear of commitment, and relationship loss had become a pattern in Chris's interpersonal life. His work life experienced similar problems. He frequently lost jobs because of serious conflict and threatening confrontations with his superiors. As conflicts arose at both work and home, Chris typically suffered increasing anxiety and episodic panic attacks. After the loss of each relationship, Chris usually confronted moderate depressive feelings, at times accompanied by suicidal ideation.

After an assessment, the dynamic hologram for Chris was:

1. *Life problems:* Recurrent episodes of anxiety and depression; work problems; unstable interpersonal relationships; conflict with

authority figures; antagonism toward, and emotional distance from, his father, brother, and male friends; and fears of heterosexual intimacy and commitment.

2. *Dynamic forces:* Ongoing hostility and envy toward males, authority figures, and successful people, and compulsive and possessive seeking of female love objects with a serious inability to consider, fulfill, or tolerate their independent needs.

3. *Genetic pathogenic foci:* Unconscious loss of maternal objects precipitated by birth of a brother when Chris was age 2 years; uncontrolled grief for that loss with a compulsive drive to experience child-like possession of love objects; and compulsive hostility toward others perceived as rivals.

The therapist's active inquiry yielded additional confirmation of the persistence of repressed sexual feelings toward his mother and the presence of hostile feelings toward all rivals for his mother's affection. A memory suffused with very visceral feelings emerged in this phase as a result of the therapist's active inquiry. In this memory, Chris saw himself in his mother's arms in a dark room. He remembered the intense pleasure of contact with his mother's warm skin, the texture of her clothes, and the smell of her perfume vividly. While narrating this memory to the therapist, Chris became so absorbed in the experience that he blushed intensely. He also described the painful termination of this moment of pleasure by his father's sudden and disruptive opening of the door and the flood of light that disturbed his pleasurable absorption. This sequence gave way to experiencing grief at the loss of the intense and exclusive bond with his mother after his brother's birth and a reexperiencing of anger, impotence, and loneliness. These feelings were all too familiar in his present life when his romantic attachments would be threatened or lost. The affective link between this childhood experience and his intimacy problems in the present became very obvious to Chris, and the acceptance of this link enhanced his capacity to work through this essential component of his pathology. A parallel conflict appeared in the transference as the patient resented the "intrusion" of the inquiring therapist into the zealously guarded privacy of this primal fantasy of material possession. (Courtesy of M. Trujillo, M.D.)

REQUIREMENTS AND TECHNIQUES. Treatment includes four major phases: patient–therapist encounter, early therapy, height of treatment, and evidence of change and termination. Therapists use the following techniques during the four phases.

Patient–Therapist Encounter. A therapist establishes a working alliance by using the patient's quick rapport with, and positive feelings for, the therapist that appear in this phase. The judicious use of open-ended and forced-choice questions enables the therapist to outline and concentrate on a therapeutic focus. The therapist specifies the minimal expectations of outcome to be achieved by the therapy.

Early Therapy. Transference involves clarifying feelings for the therapist as soon as they appear, a technique that establishes a true therapeutic alliance.

Height of the Treatment. Height of treatment emphasizes active concentration on the oedipal conflicts that have been chosen as the therapeutic focus; repeated use of anxiety-provoking questions and confrontations; avoidance of pregenital characterologic issues, which the patient uses defensively to avoid dealing with the therapist's anxiety-provoking techniques; avoidance at all costs of a transference neurosis; repetitive demonstration of the patient's neurotic ways or maladaptive patterns of behavior; concentration on the anxiety-laden material, even before the defense mechanisms have been clarified; repeated demonstrations of parent-transference links by the use of properly timed interpretations based on material given by the patient; establishment of a corrective emotional experience; encouragement and support of the patient, who becomes anxious while struggling to understand the conflicts; new learning and problem-solving patterns; and repeated presentations and recapitulations of the patient's psychodynamics until the defense mechanisms used in dealing with oedipal conflicts are understood.

Evidence of Change and Termination of Psychotherapy. The final phase of therapy emphasizes the tangible demonstration of change in the patient's behavior outside therapy, evidence that the patient is using adaptive patterns of behavior, and initiation of talk about terminating the treatment.

Overview and Results

The shared techniques of all the brief psychotherapies described above outdistance their differences. They share the therapeutic alliance or dynamic interaction between therapist and patient, the use of transference, the active interpretation of a therapeutic focus or central issue, the repetitive links between parental and transference issues, and the early termination of therapy.

The outcomes of these brief treatments have undergone extensive investigation. Contrary to prevailing ideas that the therapeutic factors in psychotherapy are nonspecific, controlled studies and other assessment methods (e.g., interviews with unbiased evaluators, patients' self-evaluations) point to the importance of the specific techniques used. The capacity for genuine recovery in certain patients is far greater than was thought. A certain type of patient receiving brief psychotherapy can benefit greatly from a practical working through of his or her nuclear conflict in the transference. Such patients can be recognized in advance through a process of dynamic interaction because they are responsive, motivated, and able to face disturbing feelings and because they have a circumscribed focus formulated for them. The more radical the technique in terms of transference, depth of interpretation, and the link to childhood, the more radical the therapeutic effects will be. For some disturbed patients, a carefully chosen partial focus can be therapeutically effective.

GROUP PSYCHOTHERAPY, COMBINED INDIVIDUAL AND GROUP PSYCHOTHERAPY, AND PSYCHODRAMA

Group psychotherapy is a modality that employs a professionally trained leader who selects, composes, organizes, and leads a collection of members to work together toward the maximal attainment of the goals for each individual in the group and for the group itself. Certain properties present in groups, such as mutual support, can be harnessed in the service of providing relief from psychological suffering and supply peer support to counter isolation experienced by many who seek psychiatric help. Similarly, homogeneously composed small groups are ideal settings for the dissemination of accurate information about a condition shared by group members. Medical illness, substance use disorders, and chronic and persistent severe psychiatric conditions, including schizophrenia and major affective disorders, are cases in point.

A widely accepted psychiatric treatment modality, group psychotherapy uses therapeutic forces within the group, constructive interactions among members, and interventions of a trained leader to change the maladaptive behaviors, thoughts, and feelings of emotionally distressed individuals. Group therapy applies to inpatient and outpatient settings, institutional work, partial hospitalization units, halfway houses, community settings, and private

practice. Group psychotherapy is also widely used by those who are not mental health professionals in the adjuvant treatment of physical disorders. Application of group psychotherapy principles has also found success in the business and education fields in the form of training, sensitivity, and role-playing.

Group psychotherapy is a treatment in which carefully selected persons who are emotionally ill meet in a group guided by a trained therapist and help one another effect personality change. By using a variety of technical maneuvers and theoretical constructs, the leader directs group members' interactions to bring about changes.

Classification

Group therapy, at present, has many approaches. Many individually derived forms of psychotherapy have their group counterparts. A representative sample of major theoretical orientations toward group therapy can be broadly subsumed under the psychodynamic, interpersonal, and cognitive-behavioral schools of thought. Table 23-4 illustrates some of the similarities and differences among representative group formats.

Patient Selection

To determine a patient's suitability for group psychotherapy, a therapist needs to gather a great deal of information in a screening interview. The psychiatrist should take a psychiatric history and perform a mental status examination to obtain certain dynamic, behavioral, and diagnostic information.

> Robert entered therapy seeking to understand why he was unable to maintain close or lasting relationships. A handsome and successful businessman, he had made a painful and courageous transition away from self-centered, dysfunctional parents early in his life. Although Robert made good initial impressions in his jobs, he was always puzzled and disappointed when his superiors gradually lost interest in him, and his colleagues avoided him. In one-on-one therapy, he was charming and entertaining, but perceived narcissistic slights caused him to become angry and attack. His therapist recommended group psychotherapy when the patient's transference feelings remained intense, and therapy was at a seeming impasse. Initially, Robert charmed the group and strove to be the center of attention. Visibly annoyed whenever he felt the group leader was paying more attention to other members, Robert was especially critical and hostile toward older people in the group and displayed little empathy for others. After repeated and forceful confrontations from the group about his antagonistic behavior, he gradually realized that he was repeating childhood patterns in his family of desperately seeking the attention of unloving parents and then entering violent rages when they lost interest. (Courtesy of Normund Wong, M.D.)

Diagnosis. The diagnosis of patients' disorders is essential in determining the best therapeutic approach and in evaluating patients' motivations for treatment, capacities for change, and personality structure strengths and weaknesses. Few contraindications exist for group therapy. Antisocial patients generally do poorly in a heterogeneous group setting because they cannot adhere to group standards, but if the group is composed of other antisocial patients, they may respond better to peers than to perceived authority figures. Depressed patients profit from group therapy after they have established a trusting relationship with the therapist. Patients who are actively suicidal or severely depressed should not be treated solely in a group setting. Patients who are manic are disruptive but, once under pharmacologic control, do well in the group setting.

Table 23-4
Comparison of Major Group Therapy Orientations

	Supportive	Psychodynamic	Self-Help	Cognitive/Behavioral
	Group therapy	Group therapy	Groups	Group therapy
Frequency	1–5 times/wk	1–2 times/wk	7 days/wk	1–3 times/wk
Individual screening	Usually	Always	None	Always
Group size	8–15 members	5–9 members	No size limits	5–10 members
Goals	Better adaptation for daily living	Reconstruction of personality dynamics	Social support	Relief of specific symptoms
Indications	Crisis situations; severe emotional	Neuroses; mild personality disorders	Shared life experiences	Phobias; anxiety disorders
Group composition	Homogeneous for level of psychopathology	Balance of similarities and differences	Homogeneous	Homogeneous for similar symptoms
Group focus	"Here and now"; family, vocational, environmental factors	Past and present; intragroup and extragroup dynamics	Education; emotional "sharing"	Training in methods that control symptoms
Use of confrontation	No	Yes	No	Rarely
Therapist activity	Actively structures and leads the group	Active around interpretation	No formal group leader	Very active in teaching skills to patient
Extragroup contacts	Encouraged	Prohibited or discouraged	Encouraged; formal peer sponsorship	Discouraged
Transference	Not analyzed	Utilized extensively	Not analyzed	Not relevant to the group work
Therapeutic factors	Cohesion; universality; reality testing instillation of hope imparting information	Cohesion; catharsis; family replay; interpersonal learning	Cohesion; universality; education; peer support	Cohesion; universality; education; reinforcement

Therapists should exclude patients who are delusional and who may incorporate the group into their delusional system, as well as patients who pose a physical threat to other members because of uncontrollable aggressive outbursts.

Preparation

Patients prepared by a therapist for a group experience tend to continue in treatment longer and report less initial anxiety than those who are not prepared. The preparation consists of having a therapist explain the procedure in as much detail as possible and answer the patient's questions before the first session.

Size. Group therapy has been successful with as few as 3 members and as many as 15, but most therapists consider 8 to 10 members the optimal size. Interaction may be insufficient with fewer members unless they are especially verbal, and with more than 10 members, the interaction may be too great for the members or the therapist to follow.

Frequency and Length of Sessions. Most group psychotherapists conduct group sessions once a week. Maintaining continuity in sessions is essential. When there are alternate sessions, the group meets twice a week, once with and once without the therapist. Group sessions generally last anywhere from 1 to 2 hours, but the time limit should be constant.

Marathon groups were most popular in the 1970s but are much less common today. In time-extended therapy (marathon group therapy), the group meets continuously for 12 to 72 hours.

Enforced interactional proximity and, during the most prolonged time-extended sessions, sleep deprivation break down certain ego defenses, release affective processes, and theoretically promote open communication. Time-extended sessions, however, can be dangerous for patients with weak ego structures, such as persons with schizophrenia or BPD.

Homogeneous versus Heterogeneous Groups. Most therapists believe that groups should be as heterogeneous as possible to ensure maximal interaction. Members with different diagnostic categories and varied behavioral patterns, from all races, social levels, and educational backgrounds, and of varying ages and both sexes, should be brought together. Patients between the ages of 20 and 65 years can be included effectively in the same group. Age differences help in developing parent–child and brother–sister models, and patients have the opportunity to relive and rectify interpersonal difficulties that may have appeared insurmountable.

Both children and adolescents benefit the most in groups comprising mostly persons in their age groups. Some adolescent patients are capable of assimilating the material of an adult group, regardless of content, but they may benefit significantly from a constructive peer experience that they might otherwise not have.

Open versus Closed Groups. Closed groups have a set number and composition of patients. If members leave, no new members are accepted. In open groups, membership is more fluid, and new members join whenever old members leave.

Mechanisms

Group Formation.   Each patient approaches group therapy differently, and, in this sense, groups are microcosms. Patients use typical adaptive abilities, defense mechanisms, and ways of relating, and when these tactics are ultimately reflected back to them by the group, they learn to be introspective about their personality functioning. A process inherent in group formation requires that patients suspend their previous ways of coping. In entering the group, they allow their executive ego functions—reality testing, adaptation to and mastery of the environment, and perception—to be assumed, to some degree, by the collective assessment provided by the total membership, including the leader.

Therapeutic Factors.   Table 23-5 outlines 20 significant therapeutic factors that account for change in group psychotherapy.

Table 23-5
Therapeutic Factors

Factor	Definition
Abreaction	A process by which repressed material, particularly a painful experience or conflict, is brought back to consciousness. During the process, the person not only recalls, but also relives the material, which is accompanied by the appropriate emotional response; insight usually results from the experience.
Acceptance	The feeling of being accepted by other members of the group; differences are tolerated, and there is an absence of censure.
Altruism	The act of one member's being of help to another; putting another person's need before one's own and learning that there is value in giving to others. The term was originated by Auguste Comte (1798–1857), and Freud believed it was a major factor in establishing group cohesion and community feeling.
Catharsis	The expression of ideas, thoughts, and suppressed material that is accompanied by an emotional response that produces a state of relief in the patient.
Cohesion	The sense that the group is working together toward a common goal; also referred to as a sense of we-ness; believed to be the most important factor related to positive therapeutic effects.
Consensual validation	Confirmation of reality by comparing one's own conceptualizations with those of other group members; interpersonal distortions are thereby corrected. The term was introduced by Harry Stack Sullivan. Trigant Burrow had used the phrase consensual observation to refer to the same phenomenon.
Contagion	The process in which the expression of emotion by one member stimulates the awareness of a similar emotion in another member.
Corrective familial experience	The group recreates the family of origin for some members who can work through conflicts psychologically through group interaction (e.g., sibling rivalry, anger toward parents).
Empathy	A capacity of a group member to put himself or herself into the psychological frame of reference of another group member and, thereby, understand his or her thinking, feeling, or behavior.
Identification	An unconscious defense mechanism in which the person incorporates the characteristics and qualities of another person or object into his or her ego system.
Imitation	The conscious emulation or modeling of one's behavior after that of another (also called role modeling); also known as "spectator therapy," as one patient learns from another.
Insight	Conscious awareness and understanding of one's own psychodynamics and symptoms of maladaptive behavior. Most therapists distinguish two types: (1) intellectual insight—knowledge and awareness without any changes in maladaptive behavior and (2) emotional insight—awareness and understanding leading to positive changes in personality and behavior.
Inspiration	The process of imparting a sense of optimism to group members; the ability to recognize that one has the capacity to overcome problems; also known as installation of hope.
Interaction	The free and open exchange of ideas and feelings among group members; effective interaction is emotionally charged.
Interpretation	The process during which the group leader formulates the meaning or significance of a patient's resistance, defenses, and symbols; the result is that the patient develops a cognitive framework within which to understand his or her behavior.
Learning	Patients acquire knowledge about new areas, such as social skills and sexual behavior; they receive advice, obtain guidance, and attempt to influence and are influenced by other group members.
Reality testing	Ability of the person to evaluate objectively the world outside the self; includes the capacity to perceive oneself and other group members accurately.
Transference	Projection of feelings, thoughts, and wishes onto the therapist, who has come to represent an object from the patient's past. Such reactions, although perhaps appropriate for the condition prevailing in the patient's earlier life, are inappropriate and anachronistic when applied to the therapist in the present. Patients in group therapy may also direct such feelings toward one another, a process called multiple transferences.
Universalization	The awareness of the patient that he or she is not alone in having problems; others share similar complaints or difficulties in learning; the patient is not unique.
Ventilation	The expression of suppressed feelings, ideas, or events to other group members; the sharing of personal secrets that ameliorates a sense of sin or guilt (also referred to as self-disclosure).

Role of the Therapist

Although opinions differ about how active or passive a group therapist should be, the consensus is that the therapist's role is primarily facilitative. Ideally, the group members themselves are the primary source of cure and change. The climate produced by the therapist's personality is a potent agent of change. The therapist is more than an expert applying techniques; he or she exerts a personal influence that taps such variables as empathy, warmth, and respect.

Inpatient Group Psychotherapy

Group therapy is an integral part of hospitalized patients' therapeutic experiences. Group organization can take many forms on a ward. In a community meeting, an entire inpatient unit meets with all the staff members (e.g., psychiatrists, psychologists, and nurses). In team meetings, 15 to 20 patients and staff members meet; a regular or small group comprising 8 to 10 patients may meet with 1 or 2 therapists, as in traditional group therapy. Although the goals of each group vary, they all have common purposes: to increase patients' awareness of themselves through their interactions with the other group members, who provide feedback about their behavior; to provide patients with improved interpersonal and social skills; to help the members adapt to an inpatient setting; and, to improve communication between patients and staff. In addition, one type of group meeting is attended only by inpatient hospital staff in order to improve communication among the staff members and to provide mutual support and encouragement in their day-to-day work with patients. Community meetings and team meetings are more helpful for dealing with patient treatment problems than they are for providing insight-oriented therapy, which is the province of the small-group therapy meeting.

Group Composition.   Two critical factors of inpatient groups common to all short-term therapies are the heterogeneity of the members and the rapid turnover of patients. Outside the hospital, therapists have large caseloads from which to select patients for group therapy. On the ward, therapists have a limited number of patients to choose from and have restrictions in terms of those patients who are both willing to participate and suitable for a small-group experience. In certain settings, group participation may be mandatory (e.g., in substance use disorder units), but mandatory attendance does not usually apply in a general psychiatry unit. Most group experiences are more productive when the patients themselves choose to enter them.

More sessions are preferable to fewer. During patients' hospital stays, groups may meet daily to allow interactional continuity and the carryover of themes from one session to the next. A new group member can be brought up to date quickly, either by the therapist in an orientation meeting or by another group member. A newly admitted patient has often learned many details about the small-group program from another patient before actually attending the first session. The less frequently the group sessions are held, the greater the need for a therapist to structure the group and be active in it.

Inpatient versus Outpatient Groups.   Although the therapeutic factors that account for change in small inpatient groups are similar to those in the outpatient settings, there are qualitative differences. For example, the relatively high turnover of patients in inpatient groups complicates the process of cohesion. However, the fact that all the group members are together in the hospital aids cohesion, as do the therapists' efforts to foster the process. Sharing of information, universalization, and catharsis are the main therapeutic factors at work in inpatient groups. Although insight more likely occurs in outpatient groups because of their long-term nature, some patients can obtain a new understanding of their psychological makeup within the confines of a single group session. A unique quality of inpatient groups is the patients' extra-group contacts, which are extensive because they live together on the same ward. Verbalizing their thoughts and feelings about such contacts in the therapy sessions encourages interpersonal learning. In addition, conflicts between patients or between patients and staff members can be anticipated and resolved.

Twelve former psychiatric inpatients who attended the monthly medication clinic would meet for 1 hour before their individual appointments with the psychiatrist to review their current social situation and medications. All received treatment from the same ward doctor and had known one another while on the inpatient service. The psychiatrist who performed the medication reviews also served as the group leader. Periodically, a staff member who was also familiar with the patients assisted with the group. Coffee was available, and the patients often brought pastries from home. The patients socialized with one another during the hour and frequently exchanged helpful ideas and tips about job opportunities. Those without cars shared rides with other members. The group was open-ended and well attended. Most of the patients were single and had a long history of psychotic illness. For most, this meeting was their only opportunity to socialize and be among peers. Frequently, when a member entered the hospital again, many in the group would visit their colleague on the ward. (Courtesy of Normund Wong, M.D.)

Self-Help Groups

Leaderless or self-help group experiences, usually homogeneously composed of participants with a common issue, represent an additional use of the group setting as a vehicle for change. Although these groups are not strictly considered a form of psychotherapy, they do share several parameters and can have therapeutic benefits for participants. Perhaps the best-known examples are the Twelve Step groups of Alcoholics Anonymous (AA), Al-Anon, Adult Children of Alcoholics (ACoA), and other substance use disorder centered groups. In addition, many self-help groups develop around health and illness, loss, or shared life experience. Cancer support groups, groups for widows or widowers, parents without partners, and bipolar support groups are but a few well-known self-help groups.

Combined Individual and Group Psychotherapy

In combined individual and group psychotherapy, patients see a therapist individually and also take part in group sessions. The therapist for the group and individual sessions is usually the same person. Groups can vary in size from 3 to 15 members, but the most helpful size is 8 to 10. Patients must attend all group sessions. Attendance at individual sessions is also essential, and the therapeutic process should examine failure to attend either group or individual sessions.

Combined therapy is a particular treatment modality, not a system by which to augment individual therapy by an occasional group session or a group therapy in which a participant meets alone with a therapist from time to time. Instead, it is an ongoing plan in which meaningful integration of the group experience with the individual sessions yields reciprocal feedback to help form an integrated therapeutic experience. Although the one-to-one doctor–patient relationship makes an in-depth examination of the transference reaction possible for some patients, it may not provide other patients with the corrective emotional experiences necessary for therapeutic change. The group gives patients a variety of persons with whom they can have transferential reactions. In the microcosm of the group, patients can relive and work through familial and other important influences.

Techniques. The combined therapy format may include different techniques based on varying theoretical frameworks. Some clinicians increase the frequency of individual sessions to encourage the emergence of the transference neurosis. In the behavioral model, individual sessions occur regularly, but they tend to be less frequent than in other approaches. Whether patients use a couch or a chair during individual sessions depends on a therapist's orientation. Other techniques include alternate meetings or "after-sessions" without the therapist present. A combined therapy approach called *structured interactional group psychotherapy* has a different group member as the focus of each weekly group session who is discussed in depth by the other members.

Results. Most workers in the field believe that combined therapy has the advantages of both dyadic and group settings, without sacrificing the qualities of either. Generally, the dropout rate in combined therapy is lower than that in group therapy alone. In many cases, combined therapy appears to bring problems to the surface and to resolve them more quickly than might be possible with either method alone.

Psychodrama

Psychodrama is a method of group psychotherapy originated by the Viennese-born psychiatrist Jacob Moreno that explores personality makeup, interpersonal relationships, conflicts, and emotional problems through special dramatic methods. Therapeutic dramatization of emotional problems includes the protagonist or patient, the person who acts out problems with the help of auxiliary egos, persons who enact varying aspects of the patient, and the director, psychodramatist, or therapist, the person who guides those in the drama toward the acquisition of insight.

Roles

DIRECTOR. The director is the leader or therapist and so must be an active participant. He or she has a catalytic function by encouraging the members of the group to be spontaneous. The director must also be available to meet the group's needs without superimposing his or her values. Of all the group psychotherapies, psychodrama requires the most participation from the therapist.

PROTAGONIST. The protagonist is the patient in conflict. The patient chooses the situation to portray in the dramatic scene, or the therapist chooses it if the patient so desires.

AUXILIARY EGO. An auxiliary ego is another group member who represents something or someone in the protagonist's experience. The auxiliary egos help account for the great range of therapeutic effects available in psychodrama.

GROUP. The members of the psychodrama and the audience make up the group. Some are participants, and others are observers, but all benefit from the experience to the extent that they can identify with the ongoing events. The concept of spontaneity in psychodrama refers to the ability of each group member, especially the protagonist, to experience the thoughts and feelings of the moment and to communicate emotion as authentically as possible.

Techniques. The psychodrama can focus on any particular area of functioning (a dream, a family, or a community situation), a symbolic role, an unconscious attitude, or an imagined future situation. The group can also act out such symptoms as delusions and hallucinations. Techniques to advance the therapeutic process and to increase productivity and creativity include the soliloquy (a recital of overt and hidden thoughts and feelings), role reversal (the exchange of the patient's role for the role of a significant person), the double (an auxiliary ego acting as the patient), the multiple double (several egos acting as the patient did on varying occasions), and the mirror technique (an ego imitating the patient and speaking for him or her). Other techniques include the use of hypnosis and psychoactive drugs to modify the acting behavior in various ways.

Ethical and Legal Issues

Confidentiality. Except where the law requires disclosure, the group therapist legally and ethically gives information about the group members to others only after obtaining appropriate patient consent. The therapist is obligated to take appropriate steps to be responsible to society, as well as to patients, when patients pose a danger to themselves or others. The guidelines for ethics of the American Group Psychotherapy Association state that therapists must obtain specific permission to confer with the referring therapist or with the individual therapist when the patient is in conjoint therapy.

Although the group members, as well as the therapist, should protect the identity of the members and maintain confidentiality, the group members are not legally bound to do so. During the preparation of patients for group psychotherapy, therapists should routinely instruct the prospective members to keep all material discussed in the group confidential. Theoretically, in a legal case, one member of a group can be asked to testify against another, but such a situation is likely to be rare.

A therapist must exercise clinical judgment and caution in placing a patient in a group if he or she thinks that the burdens of maintaining secrets will be too great for some potential members or if a prospective group patient harbors a secret of such magnitude or notoriety that membership in a group would not be wise.

Violence and Aggression. Although reports of violence and aggression are rare, the potential exists that a group member may physically attack another patient or a therapist. The attack may occur within the group or outside the group. Careful selection of group members can diminish the likelihood of such an event. Patients with a demonstrated history of assaultive behavior and psychotic patients who pose a potential for violence should not participate in a group. In institutional settings, in which group therapy is common, sufficient safeguards must be in place to discourage any physical danger to others—for example, guards or attendants can act as observers.

Sexual Behavior. For therapists, sexual intercourse with a patient or a former patient is unethical; in many states, such behavior is considered a criminal act. The issue is complicated in group psychotherapy, however, because members may engage in sexual activities with one another. The issues of pregnancy, rape, and sexually transmitted infections by group members are open questions. If an injury results from sexual activity by group members, the therapist could be held accountable for not preventing such behavior. The therapist should advise prospective group members that each patient is responsible for reporting any sexual contact between members. The therapist cannot anticipate every group sexual encounter or prevent sexual relationships from developing, but he or she is obligated to provide patients with guidelines of acceptable behavior. The therapist should identify sexual, vulnerable, or exploitive patients in the selection and preparation of patients for the group. Explicitly inform sociopathic patients who sexually exploit others that such behavior is not acceptable in the group and should be verbalized rather than acted out. The therapist must not encourage or tacitly allow sexual activity in the conduct of the group. Patients with AIDS are encouraged to reveal that they harbor the virus.

FAMILY THERAPY AND COUPLES THERAPY

Family Therapy

The family is the foundation of most societies. The study of families in different cultures has been a subject of fascination and scientific interest from viewpoints as diverse as sociology, group dynamics, anthropology, ethnicity, race, evolutionary biology, and, of course, the mental health field. The confluence of information gleaned from family studies has set the backdrop against which the contemporary practice of family therapy has evolved.

Family therapy is any psychotherapeutic endeavor that explicitly focuses on altering the interactions between or among family members and seeks to improve the functioning of the family as a unit. Both family therapy and couple therapy aim at some change in relational functioning. In most cases, they also aim at some other change, typically in the functioning of specific individuals in the family. Family therapy meant to heal a rift between parents and their adult children is an example of the use of family therapy centered on relationship goals. Family therapy aimed at increasing the family's coping with schizophrenia and at reducing the family's expressed emotion is an example of family therapy aimed at individual goals (in this case, the functioning of the person with schizophrenia), as well as family goals. In the early years of family therapy, experts viewed change in the family system as sufficient to produce individual change. More recent treatments aimed at change in individuals, as well as in the family system, tend to supplement the interventions that focus on interpersonal relationships with specific strategies that focus on individual behavior.

Indications.   The presence of a relational difficulty is a clear indication for family and couple therapy. Couples and family therapies are the only treatments with evidence to support their use for such problems as marital maladjustment, and other methods, such as individual therapy, often have deleterious effects in these situations. Couples and family therapy also have a clear and important role in the treatment of numerous specific psychiatric disorders, often as a component within a multimethod treatment.

Of course, as with any therapy, the indications for family and couple therapy are broad and vary from case to case. Family therapy is a therapeutic collage of ideas regarding the underpinnings of family and individual stability and change, psychopathology, and problems in living, as well as relational ethics. Family

therapy might better be called *systemically sensitive therapy*, and, in this sense, reflects a basic worldview as much as a clinical treatment methodology. For therapists thus inclined, then, all clinical problems involve salient interactional components; thus, some kind of family (or other functionally significant other's) involvement in therapy is always indicated, even in treatment that emphasizes individual problems.

An impressive array now exists of common clinical disorders and problems, including child, adolescent, and adult disorders, for which research has demonstrated family or couple treatment methods to be effective. In a few instances, couple and family interventions are probably even the treatment of choice, and for several disorders, the research argues for family intervention to be an essential part of treatment.

Techniques

INITIAL CONSULTATION.   Family therapy is familiar enough to the general public for families with a high level of conflict to request it specifically. When the initial complaint is about an individual family member, however, pretreatment work may be needed. Underlying resistance to a family approach typically includes fears by parents that the therapist will blame them for their child's difficulties, that the entire family will be pronounced sick, that a spouse will object, and that open discussion of one child's misbehavior will have a negative influence on siblings. Refusal by an adolescent or young adult patient to participate in family therapy is frequently a disguised collusion with the fears of one or both parents.

INTERVIEW TECHNIQUE.   The unique quality of a family interview springs from two important facts. A family comes to treatment with its history and dynamics firmly in place. To a family therapist, the established nature of the group, more than the symptoms, constitutes the clinical problem. Family members usually live together and, at some level, depend on one another for their physical and emotional well-being. Whatever transpires in the therapy session is known to all. Central principles of technique also derive from these facts. For example, the therapist must carefully channel the catharsis of anger by one family member toward another. The person who is the object of the anger will react to the attack, and the anger may escalate into violence and fracture relationships, with one member or more withdrawing from therapy. For another example, free association is inappropriate in family therapy because it can encourage one person to dominate a session. Thus, therapists must always control and direct the family interview.

FREQUENCY AND LENGTH OF TREATMENT.   Unless an emergency arises, sessions occur no more than once a week. Each session, however, may require as much as 2 hours. Extended sessions can include an intermission to give the therapist time to organize the material and plan a response. A flexible schedule is necessary when geography or personal circumstances make it physically difficult for the family to get together. The length of treatment depends both on the nature of the problem and on the therapeutic model. Therapists who use problem-solving models exclusively may accomplish their goals in a few sessions, whereas therapists using growth-oriented models may work with a family for years and may schedule sessions at long intervals.

Schools of Family Therapy.

Many schools of family therapy exist, none of which is superior to the others. The particular model used depends on the training received, the context in which therapy occurs, and the personality of the therapist. Table 23-6 outlines the

Table 23-6
Schools of Family and Couple Therapy

Therapeutic Approach (Examples)	Core Concepts	Typical Goals	Common Strategies and Techniques	Comments
Behavioral/cognitive-behavioral (James Alexander, Neil Jacobson, Donald Baucom, Gerald Patterson)	Functional analysis Social learning theory Communication and problem solving Attributional style	Resolution of presenting problem Enhanced communication and problem-solving skills Balance between change and acceptance	Communication and problem-solving training Acceptance training/reattribution techniques Parent management, emphasis on behavior/consequences Therapist as educator	Functional analysis, not treatment techniques, is defining characteristic Arguably the most empirically supported of all family and couple methods
Bowen family systems (Murray Bowen, Philip Guerin, Michael Kerr, Monica McGoldrick)	Differentiation of self Triangulation Emotional cutoffs Family emotional system Sibling position	Increased differentiation Detriangulation Cutoffs resolved Improved ability to manage anxiety	Use of genogram Therapist as "coach" Education about multigenerational family processes	Often conducted with only a single patient Influence continues but has waned since Bowen's death
Experiential–humanistic (Susan Johnson and Leslie Greenberg, Virginia Satir, Carl Whitaker)	Communication styles (e.g., placater–blamer) Psychotherapy of the absurd Attachment theory	Fostering creativity (comfort with "craziness") Increased family cohesion Personal growth, self-esteem Tolerance for conflict	Resolving the battle for structure and the battle for initiative Frequent use of cotherapists Family sculpture Use of self Family reconstruction	Since Whitaker's death, symbolic–experiential approach receding in visibility Emotionally focused therapy one of few nonbehavioral or psychodynamic couple methods increasing in influence
Integrative (Alan Gurman, William Pinsof, Douglas Snyder, Froma Walsh)	Importance of and relationships among multiple levels of experience Theoretical and technical eclecticism	Improved communication and problem solving Enhanced interactional insight Presenting problems	Combinations of cognitive-behavioral and psychodynamic methods, in general systems context	Along with behavioral and psychoeducational methods, the most sensitive to research findings Attempts to match interventions to problem and family
Mental Research Institute brief therapy (Don Jackson, John Weakland, Paul Watzlawick)	Distinction between "difficulties" and "problems" Communication processes Symptom as communication First- and second-order change	Resolution of presenting problem Second-order change	Reframing Therapist maneuverability	Historically overlaps strategic, but with important differences (e.g., "function" of symptoms)
Feminist (Virginia Goldner, Rachel Hare-Mustin, Betty Carter)	Raising gender consciousness Underlying effect of gender	Gender equality Recognizing gender inequities	Raising consciousness Identifying and challenging culturally constructed narratives	Not so much a way of intervening as a set of issues to address; has had a pervasive effect on family and couple therapy
Narrative (David Epston, Michael White, Harlene Anderson)	Constructivism "Languaging" "Stories" socially created Problem-saturated descriptions	Resolution of presenting problem Enhancing undiscovered parts of self	Externalization of problems Focusing on "unique outcomes" Creation of new meaning via "restorying" Therapeutic letters	Currently very popular but rarely acknowledges overlaps with cognitive and behavioral theory
Psychodynamic–psychoanalytic (Nathan Ackerman, Henry Dicks, Clifford Sager, Jill Scharff and David Scharff)	Object relations Projective identification Splitting Scapegoating	Improved insight Genetic (historical) awareness Enhanced empathy De-emphasize presenting problem Disentangle interlocking pathologies	Transference, resistance, and countertransference analysis Creation of holding environment Interpretation Emphasis on therapeutic alliance	Probably influences family therapists' clinical work more than is usually acknowledged

(continued)

Table 23-6
Schools of Family and Couple Therapy (*Continued*)

Therapeutic Approach (Examples)	Core Concepts	Typical Goals	Common Strategies and Techniques	Comments
Psychoeducational (Carol Anderson, Ian Falloon, William McFarlane, David Miklowitz)	Biopsychosocial theory Stress-diathesis Expressed emotion	Enhanced family coping skills Improved communication and problem-solving skills Relapse prevention	Survival skills workshops Family management Family information and education Concurrent use of psychopharmacology	Without doubt, the most effective family-based approach for families with a member with major psychiatric disorder
Solution focused (Steve de Shazer and Insoo Berg, William O'Hanlon, Michele Weiner-Davis)	Focus on solutions, not problems Unimportance of problem etiology Disbelief in resistance	Resolution of presenting problem Creation of solutions	Scaling questions Miracle questions Exception questions Client empowerment Coping questions Inquire about changes made since deciding to take action ("pre-session changes")	Grows out of basic Mental Research Institute philosophy, emphasizing solutions more than problems. Has made extraordinary claims of effectiveness
Strategic (Milton Erickson, Jay Haley, Cloe Madanes, James Keim)	Power and control Family life cycle Symptom-maintaining sequences Function of problems	Resolve presenting problem Disruption of problem-maintaining sequences	Persuasion Paradoxical injections Insight downplayed Pretend and ordeal techniques	Unfortunate de-emphasis on biology, psychiatric diagnosis, and personality theory
Structural (Harry Aponte, Salvador Minuchin, Jose Szapocznik)	Boundaries Hierarchies Coalitions and alliances Complementarity Engagement–enmeshment	Increased flexibility Adaptability to developmental change Balance between connectedness and differentiation Subsystem functioning	Unbalancing Enactment Joining	Arguably the most influential family therapy approach
Transgenerational (Ivan Boszormenyi-Nagy, James Framo, Laura Roberto-Forman)	Invisible loyalties Ledgers and debts Family mourning Personal authority	More universal than family-specific goals Increased trust Repair ruptured relationships	Multidirected partiality Family-of-origin sessions Use of cotherapy	Almost all multi-/transgenerational methods have significant psychodynamic underpinnings

major schools of family therapy, the influential practitioners of each method, and the focus of each technique.

Modifications of Techniques

FAMILY GROUP THERAPY.   Family group therapy combines several families into a single group. Families share mutual problems and compare their interactions with those of the other families in the group. Treatment of families impacted by schizophrenia has been effective in multiple family groups. Parents of disturbed children may also meet together to share their situations.

SOCIAL NETWORK THERAPY.   In social network therapy, the social community or network of a disturbed patient meets in group sessions with the patient. The network includes those with whom the patient comes into contact in daily life, not only the immediate family but also relatives, friends, tradespersons, teachers, and coworkers.

PARADOXICAL THERAPY.   With the paradoxical therapy approach, which evolved from the work of Gregory Bateson, a therapist suggests that the patient intentionally engage in the unwanted behavior (called the paradoxical injunction) and, for example, avoid a phobic object or perform a compulsive ritual. Although paradoxical therapy and the use of paradoxical injunctions seem to be counterintuitive, the therapy can create new insights for

some patients. It is used in individual therapy as well as in family therapy.

REFRAMING.   Reframing, also known as *positive connotation*, is a relabeling of all negatively expressed feelings or behavior as positive. When the therapist attempts to get family members to view behavior from a new frame of reference, "This child is impossible," becomes "This child is desperately trying to distract and protect you from what he or she perceives as an unhappy marriage." Reframing is an important process that allows family members to view themselves in new ways that can produce change.

Goals.   Family therapy has several goals: to resolve or reduce pathogenic conflict and anxiety within the matrix of interpersonal relationships; to enhance the perception and fulfillment by family members of one another's emotional needs; to promote appropriate role relationships between the sexes and generations; to strengthen the capacity of individual members and the family as a whole to cope with destructive forces inside and outside the surrounding environment; to influence family identity and values to orient members toward health and growth. The therapy ultimately aims to integrate families into the large systems of society, extended family, and community groups and social systems, such as schools, medical facilities, and social, recreational, and welfare agencies.

Couples (Marital) Therapy

Couples or marital therapy is a form of psychotherapy designed to psychologically modify the interaction of two persons in conflict with each other over one parameter or a variety of parameters—social, emotional, sexual, or economic. In couples therapy, a trained person establishes a therapeutic contract with a patient-couple and, through definite types of communication, attempts to alleviate the disturbance, to reverse or change maladaptive patterns of behavior, and to encourage personality growth and development.

Marriage counseling may be considered more limited in scope than marriage therapy: the focus is only surrounding a particular familial conflict, and the counseling is primarily task-oriented, geared to solving a specific problem, such as child-rearing. Marriage therapy, by contrast, emphasizes restructuring a couple's interaction and sometimes explores the psychodynamics of each partner. Both therapy and counseling emphasize helping marital partners cope effectively with their problems. Most important is the definition of appropriate and realistic goals, which may involve extensive reconstruction of the union or problem-solving approaches or a combination of both.

Types of Therapies

INDIVIDUAL THERAPY. In individual therapy, the partners may consult different therapists, who do not necessarily communicate with each other and indeed may not even know each other. The goal of treatment is to strengthen each partner's adaptive capacities. At times, only one of the partners is in treatment, and, in such cases, it is often helpful for the person who is not in treatment to visit the therapist. Not only can the visiting partner provide data about the patient that the therapist might otherwise overlook, but the therapist can identify and deal with overt or covert anxiety in the visiting partner resulting from change in the patient, correct irrational beliefs about treatment events, and examine conscious or unconscious attempts by the partner to sabotage the patient's treatment.

INDIVIDUAL COUPLES THERAPY. In individual couples therapy, each partner is in therapy, which is either concurrent, with the same therapist, or collaborative, with each partner seeing a different therapist.

CONJOINT THERAPY. In conjoint therapy, the most common treatment method in couples therapy, either one or two therapists treat the partners in joint sessions. Cotherapy with therapists of both sexes prevents a particular patient from feeling ganged up on when confronted by two members of the opposite sex.

FOUR-WAY SESSION. In a four-way session, each partner is seen by a different therapist, with regular joint sessions in which all four persons participate. A variation of the four-way session is the roundtable interview, developed by William Masters and Virginia Johnson for the rapid treatment of sexually dysfunctional couples. Two patients and two opposite-sex therapists meet regularly.

GROUP PSYCHOTHERAPY. Group therapy for couples allows a variety of group dynamics to affect the participants. Groups usually consist of three to four couples and one or two therapists. The couples identify with one another and recognize that others have similar problems; each gains support and empathy from fellow group members of the same or opposite sex. They explore sexual attitudes and have an opportunity to gain new information from their peer groups, and each receives specific feedback about his or her behavior, either negative or positive, which may have more meaning and be better assimilated coming from a neutral, nonspouse member, for example, than from the spouse or the therapist.

During the middle phase of a couples group comprising four couples, the theme of whether to have children arose. One couple had just come from a visit to the gynecologist, who informed them that they were running out of time because of the wife's age. The woman in the couple did not want to have children, but her husband did. His complaint about the marriage was that his wife never was demonstrative in showing her loving feelings for him. He felt her to be detached, distant, and sexually inhibited.

The prevailing sentiment among the other couples who had children was that children only added additional stress to an already stressed relationship. One other couple, however, voiced their different view by describing how their children had enriched their lives.

As the talk about going forward and getting pregnant progressed, the group leader noted the nonverbal communication between the ambivalent couple. Whenever the tone of the group leaned toward having children, the wife would reach out and grasp the hand of her husband tenderly. This action invariably had the effect of stopping him from pursuing the topic for fear of the withdrawal of her affection. All this occurred without words. Once identified, this repetitive nonverbal pattern was available for examination in the group, and the supportive elements provided by other members and the leader encouraged a frank, direct, and open conversation between the partners, who eventually chose to go forward and attempt to have a child. (Courtesy of H. I. Spitz, M.D. and S. Spitz, ACSW.)

COMBINED THERAPY. Combined therapy refers to all or any of the preceding techniques used concurrently or in combination. Thus, a particular patient-couple may begin treatment with one or both partners in individual psychotherapy, continue in conjoint therapy with the partner, and terminate therapy after a course of treatment in a married couples' group. The rationale for combined therapy is that there is no evidence to support that a single approach to marital problems is superior to another. Familiarity with a variety of approaches thus allows therapists flexibility that provides maximal benefit for couples in distress.

Indications. Whatever the specific therapeutic technique, initiation of couples therapy is appropriate when individual therapy has failed to resolve the relationship difficulties, when the onset of distress in one or both partners is clearly a relational problem, and when a couple in conflict requests couples therapy. Problems in communication between partners are a prime indication for couples therapy. In such instances, one spouse may be intimidated by the other, may become anxious when attempting to tell the other about thoughts or feelings, or may project unconscious expectations onto the other. The therapy works toward enabling each partner to see the other realistically.

Conflicts in one or several areas, such as the partners' sexual life, are also indications for treatment. Similarly, difficulty in establishing satisfactory social, economic, parental, or emotional roles implies that a couple needs help. Clinicians should evaluate all aspects of the marital relationship before attempting to treat only one problem, which could be a symptom of a pervasive marital disorder.

Contraindications. Contraindications for couples therapy include patients with severe forms of psychosis, particularly patients with paranoid elements and those in whom the marriage's homeostatic mechanism is a protection against psychosis, marriages in which one or both partners really want to divorce, marriages in which one spouse refuses to participate because of anxiety or fear, and when there is a threat of domestic violence.

Goals.   Nathan Ackerman defined the aims of couples therapy as follows: the goals of therapy for partner relational problems are to alleviate emotional distress and disability and to promote the levels of well-being of both partners together and of each as an individual. Ideally, therapists move toward these goals by strengthening the shared resources for problem-solving, by encouraging the substitution of adequate controls and defenses for pathogenic ones, by enhancing both the immunity against the disintegrative effects of emotional upset and the complementarity of the relationship, and by promoting the growth of the relationship and of each partner.

Part of a therapist's task is to persuade each partner in the relationship to take responsibility for understanding the psychodynamic makeup of personality. The emphasis is on each person's accountability for the effects of behavior on his or her own life, the life of the partner, and the lives of others in the environment. The result is often a deep understanding of the problems that created marital discord.

Couples therapy does not ensure the maintenance of any marriage or relationship. Indeed, in certain instances, it may show the partners that they are in a nonviable union and should consider dissolution. In these cases, couples may continue to meet with therapists to work through the difficulties of separating and obtaining a divorce, a process referred to as *divorce therapy.*

DIALECTICAL BEHAVIOR THERAPY

Dialectical behavior therapy (DBT) is the psychosocial treatment that has received the most empirical support for patients with BPD. Put simply, the overarching goal of DBT is to help create a life worth living for patients who often suffer tremendously from chronic and pervasive problems across many areas of their lives. DBT is a type of psychotherapy initially developed for chronically self-injurious patients with BPD and parasuicidal behavior. In recent years, its use has extended to other forms of mental illness. The method is eclectic, drawing on concepts derived from supportive, cognitive, and behavioral therapies. Some elements trace back to Franz Alexander's view of therapy as a corrective emotional experience and other elements from certain Eastern philosophical schools (e.g., Zen).

Weekly visits aim to improve interpersonal skills and decrease self-destructive behavior using techniques involving advice, metaphor, storytelling, and confrontation, among others. Patients with BPD especially are helped to deal with the ambivalent feelings that are characteristic of the disorder. Marsha Linehan, Ph.D., developed the treatment method based on her theory that such patients cannot identify emotional experiences and cannot tolerate frustration or rejection. As with other behavioral approaches, DBT assumes all behavior (including thoughts and feelings) is learned and that patients with BPD behave in ways that reinforce or even reward their behavior, regardless of how maladaptive it is.

Functions of DBT

As described by its originator, there are five essential "functions" in treatment: (1) to enhance and expand the patient's repertoire of skillful behavioral patterns; (2) to improve patient motivation to change by reducing reinforcement of maladaptive behavior, including dysfunctional cognition and emotion; (3) to ensure that new behavioral patterns generalize from the therapeutic to the

natural environment; (4) to structure the environment so that effective behaviors, rather than dysfunctional behaviors, are reinforced; and (5) to enhance the motivation and capabilities of the therapist so that the treatment rendered is effective. Figure 23-1 illustrates how DBT breaks the cycle of problem behavior being used to avoid emotional distress.

The four modes of treatment in DBT are as follows: (1) group skills training, (2) individual therapy, (3) phone consultations, and (4) consultation team. Descriptions of these modes of treatment are below. Other ancillary treatments used are pharmacotherapy and hospitalization when needed.

Group Skills Training.   In group format, patients learn specific behavioral, emotional, cognitive, and interpersonal skills. Unlike traditional group therapy, observations about others in the group are discouraged. Instead, DBT takes a didactic approach, using specific exercises from a skills training manual, many of which emphasize control of emotional dysregulation and impulsive behavior.

Individual Therapy.   Sessions in DBT occur weekly, generally for 50 to 60 minutes, in which review of skills learned during group training takes place, along with examination of life events from the previous week. Therapists note episodes of pathologic behavioral patterns that could have been corrected if learned skills had been put into effect. Patients are encouraged to record their thoughts, feelings, and behaviors on diary cards, which therapists analyze in the session.

Telephone Consultation.   Therapists are available for phone consultation 24 hours per day. Patients are encouraged to call when they feel themselves heading toward some crisis that might lead to injurious behavior to themselves or others. Calls are intended to be brief and usually last about 10 minutes.

Consultation Team.   Therapists meet in weekly meetings to review their work with their patients. By doing so, they provide support for one another and maintain motivation in their work. The meetings enable them to compare the techniques used and to validate those that are most effective (Table 23-7).

Results

Several studies evaluating the effect of DBT for patients with BPD found that such therapy was positive. Patients had a low dropout rate from treatment, the incidence of parasuicidal behaviors

Table 23-7
Consultation Team Agreements in Dialectical Behavior Therapy

1. Meet weekly for 1–2 hr
2. Discuss cases according to the treatment hierarchy (i.e., self-injurious/life-threatening behavior, treatment-interfering behavior, and quality-of-life–interfering behavior)
3. Accept a dialectical philosophy
4. Consult with the patient on how to interact with other therapists, and do not tell other therapists how to interact with the patient
5. Do not expect consistency of therapists with one another (even across the same patient)
6. Allow all therapists to observe their own limits without fear of judgmental reactions from other consultation group members
7. Search for nonpejorative, empathic interpretation of patient's behavior
8. Acknowledge that all therapists are fallible

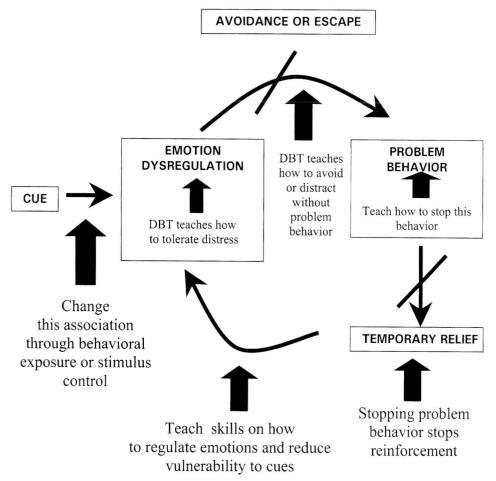

FIGURE 23-1
How dialectical behavior therapy (DBT) works.

declined, self-report of angry affect decreased, and social adjustment and work performance improved. The method is now being applied to other disorders, including substance use disorders, eating disorders, schizophrenia, and PTSD.

BIOFEEDBACK

Biofeedback involves the recording and display of small changes in the physiologic levels of the feedback parameter. The display can be visual, such as a big meter or a bar of lights, or auditory. Therapists instruct patients to change the levels of the parameter, using the feedback from the display as a guide. The basis of biofeedback is the idea that the autonomic nervous system can come under voluntary control through operant conditioning. Biofeedback can be used by itself or in combination with relaxation. For example, patients with urinary incontinence use biofeedback alone to regain control over the pelvic musculature. The rehabilitation of neurologic disorders also uses biofeedback. The relaxation that patients learn to facilitate may augment the benefits of biofeedback.

Theory

Neal Miller demonstrated the medical potential of biofeedback by showing that the normally involuntary autonomic nervous system is susceptible to operant conditioning by the use of appropriate feedback. Utilizing instruments, patients acquire information about the status of involuntary biologic functions, such as skin temperature and electrical conductivity, muscle tension, blood pressure, heart rate, and brain wave activity. Patients then learn to regulate one or more of these physiologic states that affect symptoms. For example, a person can learn to raise the temperature of his or her hands to reduce the frequency of migraines, palpitations, or angina pectoris. Presumably, patients lower the sympathetic activation and voluntarily self-regulate arterial smooth muscle vasoconstrictive tendencies.

Methods

Instrumentation.   The feedback instrument used depends on the patient and the specific problem. The most effective instruments are the electromyogram (EMG), which measures the electrical potentials of muscle fibers; the electroencephalogram (EEG), which measures alpha waves that occur in relaxed states; the galvanic skin response (GSR) gauge, which shows decreased skin conductivity during a relaxed state; and the thermistor, which measures skin temperature (which drops during tension because of peripheral vasoconstriction). Patients are attached to one of the instruments that measure a physiologic function and translate the measurement into an audible or visual signal that patients use to gauge their responses. For example, in the treatment of bruxism, an EMG is attached to the masseter muscle. The EMG emits a high tone when the muscle contracts and a low tone when at rest.

Patients can learn to alter the tone to indicate relaxation. Patients receive feedback about the masseter muscle, the tone reinforces the learning, and the condition ameliorates—all of these events interacting synergistically.

Many less-specific clinical applications (e.g., treating insomnia, dysmenorrhea, and speech problems; improving athletic performance; treating volitional disorders; achieving altered states of consciousness; managing stress; and supplementing psychotherapy for treating anxiety associated with somatic symptom and related disorders) use a model in which frontalis muscle EMG biofeedback is combined with thermal biofeedback and verbal instructions in progressive relaxation.

Relaxation Therapy.   Muscle relaxation is used as a component of treatment programs (e.g., systematic desensitization) or as a treatment in its own right (relaxation therapy). Relaxation involves (1) immobility of the body, (2) control over the focus of attention, (3) low muscle tone, and (4) cultivation of a specific frame of mind, described as contemplative, nonjudgmental, detached, or mindful.

Edmund Jacobson developed progressive relaxation in 1929. Jacobson observed that when an individual lies "relaxed," in the ordinary sense, the following clinical signs reveal the presence of residual tension: respiration is slightly irregular in time or force; the pulse rate, although often normal, is in some instances moderately increased as compared with later tests; voluntary or local reflex activities are evident in such slight marks as wrinkling of the forehead, frowning, movements of the eyeballs including frequent or rapid winking, restless shifting of the head, a limb, or even a finger; and finally, the mind continues to be active, and once started, worry or oppressive emotion will persist. It is incredible that a faint degree of tension can be responsible for all of this.

Learning relaxation, therefore, involves cultivating a muscle sense. To develop the muscle sense further, patients learn to isolate and contract specific muscles or muscle groups, one at a time. For example, patients flex the forearm while the therapist holds it back to observe tenseness in the biceps muscle. (Jacobson used the word "tenseness" rather than "tension" to emphasize the patient's role in tensing the muscles.) Once the patient reports this sensation, Jacobson would say, "This is your doing! What we wish is the reverse of this—simply not doing." The therapist repeatedly reminds the patient that relaxation involves no effort. In fact, "making an effort is being tense and therefore is not to relax." As the session progresses, the therapist instructs the patient to let go further and further, even past the point when the body part seems perfectly relaxed.

Patients would work in this fashion with different muscle groups, often over more than 50 sessions. For example, an entire session might involve relaxing the biceps muscle. Another feature of Jacobson's method was to give instructions tersely so they would not interfere with a patient's focus on muscle sensations; suggestions commonly used today (e.g., *"Your arm is becoming limp"*) were avoided. Patients were also frequently left alone, while the therapist attended to other patients.

In psychiatry, relaxation therapy is primarily a component of multifaceted broad-spectrum programs. Its use in desensitization was mentioned previously. Relaxing breathing exercises are often helpful for patients with panic disorder, especially when considered to be related to hyperventilation. In the treatment of patients with anxiety disorders, relaxation can serve as an occasion-setting stimulus (i.e., as a context of safety in which to try other specific

Table 23-8
Example Relaxation Techniques

Technique	Approach
Autogenic training	The patient is instructed to concentrate on feelings of warmth, heaviness, and relaxation throughout their body.
Biofeedback-assisted relaxation	The patient uses real-time biofeedback data to concentrate on certain physiologic functions, such as muscle tension.
Deep breathing/ breathing exercises	The patient focuses on taking slow, deep, even breaths.
Guided imagery	The patient is taught to focus on pleasant images as a replacement for negative ones.
Progressive relaxation/ progressive muscle relaxation	The patient is instructed to tighten and relax various muscle groups.
Self-hypnosis	The patient is taught to produce a relaxation response when prompted by a suggestion (usually a phrase or a nonverbal cue).

Adapted from National Center for Complementary and Integrative Health. Relaxation technique for health. https://www.nccih.nih.gov/health/relaxation-techniques-for-health

interventions confidently). Table 23-8 describes some common relaxation techniques.

Later Adaptation of Progressive Muscular Relaxation. Joseph Wolpe chose progressive relaxation as a response incompatible with anxiety when designing his systematic desensitization treatment (discussed below). For this purpose, Jacobson's original method was too lengthy to be practical. Wolpe abbreviated the program to 20 minutes during the first six sessions (devoting the remainder of these sessions to other things, such as behavioral analysis). In a later modification of progressive relaxation, patients completed work with all the principal muscle groups in one session. Once patients have mastered this procedure (typically after three sessions), they learn to combine these groups into larger groups. Finally, patients practice relaxation by recall (i.e., without tensing the muscles).

Autogenic Training.   Autogenic training is a method of self-suggestion that originated in Germany. It involves the patients directing their attention to specific bodily areas and hearing themselves think certain phrases reflecting a relaxed state. In the original German version, patients progressed through six themes over many sessions. Table 23-9 contains a list of these six areas, along with representative autogenic phrases. Autogenic relaxation is an American modification of autogenic training, in which one session covers all six areas.

Applied Tension.   Applied tension is a technique that is the opposite of relaxation; applied tension can counteract the fainting response. The treatment extends over four sessions. In the first session, patients learn to tense the muscles of the arms, legs, and torso for 10 to 15 seconds (as if they were bodybuilders). The tension is maintained long enough for a sensation of warmth to develop in the face. The patients then release the tension but do not progress to a state of relaxation. The maneuver is repeated five times

Table 23-9
Sample Autogenic Phrases

Theme	Examples of Self-Statements
Heaviness	"My left arm is heavy."
Warmth	"My left arm is warm."
Cardiac regulation	"My heartbeat is calm and regular."
Breathing adjustment	"It breathes me."
Solar plexus	"My solar plexus is warm."
Forehead	"My forehead is cool."

at half-minute intervals. Feedback of the patient's blood pressure during the muscle contraction can augment this method; increased blood pressure suggests the achievement of appropriate muscle tension. The patients continue to practice the technique five times a day. An adverse effect of treatment that sometimes develops is headache. In this case, the patient reduces the intensity of the muscle contraction and the frequency of treatment.

Patients with blood and injury phobia show a unique, biphasic response when exposed to a phobic stimulus. The first phase is associated with increased heart rate and blood pressure. In the second phase, however, blood pressure suddenly falls, and the patient faints. To treat the problem, the therapist shows the patient a series of slides that are provocative (e.g., mutilated bodies). The patient learns to identify early warning signs of fainting, such as queasiness, cold sweats, or dizziness, and to apply the learned muscle tension response quickly, contingent on these warning signs. Patients can also perform applied tension while donating blood or watching a surgical operation. The technique of isometric tension raises blood pressure, which prevents fainting.

Applied Relaxation.   Applied relaxation involves eliciting a relaxation response in the stressful situation itself. The previous discussion showed that this is not advisable right away because of the possible ironic effects of relaxation. Therefore, patients should first practice relaxation in nonstressful circumstances. The method developed by Lars-Göran Öst and coworkers in Sweden has been proven efficacious for panic disorder and generalized anxiety disorder. Establishing the relaxation response in the patient's natural environment consists of seven phases of one to two sessions each: progressive relaxation, release-only relaxation, cue-controlled relaxation, differential relaxation, rapid relaxation, application training, and maintenance. Table 23-10 provides details.

Results

Biofeedback, progressive relaxation, and applied tension are effective treatment methods for a broad range of disorders. They form one basis of behavioral medicine in which the patient changes (or learns how to change) behavior that contributes to illness. They form a basis on which many complementary and alternative medical procedures are effective (e.g., yoga and Reiki) in which relaxation is a critical component. Relaxation also informs more mainstream treatments, such as hypnosis.

COGNITIVE THERAPY

Cognitive therapy, developed by Aaron T. Beck, MD, is based on the cognitive model, which has been widely studied and has received substantial empirical support. The cognitive model posits that it is not situations that directly impact one's reaction (emotional, behavioral, and physiologic). Rather, it is one's automatic *perception* of the situation that is more closely associated with the reaction. A depressed individual, for example, who is reading this chapter

Table 23-10
Steps in Applied Relaxation

Technique	Instructions
Progressive relaxation	Session 1: hands, arms, face, neck, and shoulders. Session 2: back, chest, stomach, breathing, hips, legs, and feet.
Release-only relaxation	As with progressive relaxation, except that the tension phase is omitted; when release-only relaxation is mastered, the patient can relax within 5–7 min.
Cue-controlled relaxation	A stimulus—the word *relax*—is presented just before exhalation; patients focus on their breathing while already in a relaxed state; the therapist says the word *inhale* just before each inhalation and the word *relax* just before each exhalation; after approximately five cycles, the patient mentally says these words (optionally dropping the *inhale*).
Differential relaxation	Patients can remain relaxed and move at the same time by differentially keeping muscles unrelated to the movement in a relaxed state; after achieving a relaxed state, patients lift an arm or a leg or look around in the room, while keeping movements and tension in other body parts at a minimum; patients also perform differential relaxation in other settings, including sitting in different chairs, sitting at a desk while writing, talking on the phone, and walking.
Rapid relaxation	Patients relax by taking one to three breaths with slow exhalations, thinking the word *relax* before each exhalation and scanning their bodies for areas of tension; with this practice, relaxation is shortened to 20–30 s; patients are instructed to relax in this manner 15–20 times per day at certain predetermined events in their natural environment (e.g., when they look at a watch or make a telephone call. As a reminder, colored dots might be taped on the watch or phone. After some time, the dots are changed to a different color to keep their reminding power fresh).
Application training	Patients relax just before entering the target situation; they stay in the situation for 10–15 min, using their relaxation skills as a coping technique; patients may initially be accompanied by the therapist; alternatively, if the patient's problem is panic attacks or generalized anxiety, imagery or physical exercise is used to induce fearful sensations, which then are used for application training.

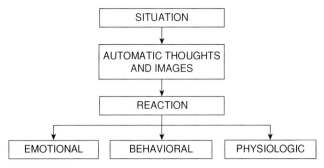

FIGURE 23-2
Cognitive model.

(situation), might think, "I can't concentrate. There is something seriously wrong with me. I'll never get better" ("automatic thoughts"). As a result, his sadness and hopelessness increase (emotional reaction); he stops reading altogether (behavioral reaction); and he feels a weight in his chest (physiologic reaction). On the other hand, another individual might think, "I don't want to read this. I don't want to know anything about this topic, but I have to." She then feels annoyed, her body becomes somewhat tense, and she skims the pages instead of reading the article carefully. One important component of cognitive therapy involves teaching patients to identify the thoughts that lead to distress or dysfunction, to evaluate their thinking, and to effectively respond to these cognitions. Figure 23-2 depicts the cognitive model.

A strong therapeutic alliance is essential for effective treatment, and the relationship is collaborative. Both patients and clinicians are active in solving problems, evaluating cognitions, and modifying behavior. Cognitive therapy is educative; clinicians teach patients how to use the techniques at home that they have employed in session. The clinician's stated goal is to help patients become their own therapists. They emphasize that the way patients get better is to apply what they have learned in session to make small changes in their thinking and behavior every day.

Originally designed as a short-term treatment for depression, cognitive therapy has evolved over the years. Patients with straightforward cases of anxiety and depression, who were relatively psychologically healthy before the onset of their disorder, often benefit from a short course of treatment, perhaps 6 to 12 sessions. At the other end of the spectrum are patients whose disorders are chronic or complex, or those for whom standard treatment needs to be varied due to personality disorders. They may need many more sessions over a significantly longer period of time. Those with recurrent episodes or with serious mental illnesses may require intermittent treatment through their lifetime.

Cognitive Theory of Depression

According to the cognitive theory of depression, cognitive dysfunctions are the core of depression, and affective and physical changes and other associated features of depression are consequences of cognitive dysfunctions. For example, apathy and low energy result from a person's expectation of failure in all areas. Similarly, paralysis of will stems from a person's pessimism and feelings of hopelessness. From a cognitive perspective, depression can be explained by the cognitive triad, which explains that negative thoughts are about the self, the world, and the future.

The goal of therapy is to alleviate depression and to prevent its recurrence by helping patients to identify and test negative cognitions, to develop alternative and more flexible schemas, and to

rehearse both new cognitive and behavioral responses. Changing the way a person thinks can alleviate the psychiatric disorder.

Strategies and Techniques

The goal of cognitive therapy is to facilitate remission and prevent or reduce relapse by teaching skills patients can use for their lifetime, within a highly supportive, collaborative relationship. Both patients and clinicians are active participants, jointly solving current problems, evaluating patients' cognitions in specific situations, and working toward needed behavior change. As a result, patients' symptoms decrease and their mood and day-to-day functioning improves.

As with other psychotherapies, therapists' attributes are important to successful therapy. Therapists must exude warmth, understand the life experience of each patient, and be genuine and honest with themselves and with their patients. They must be able to relate skillfully and interactively with their patients. Cognitive therapists set the agenda at the beginning of each session, assign homework between sessions, and teach new skills. The therapist and patient collaborate actively. There are several techniques utilized in cognitive therapy; three common components are described below.

Didactic Aspects.   The therapy's didactic aspects include explaining to patients the cognitive triad, schemas, and faulty logic. Therapists must tell patients that they will formulate hypotheses together and test them throughout the treatment. Cognitive therapy requires a full explanation of the relation between symptoms and thinking, affect, and behavior, as well as the rationale for all aspects of treatment. This explanation contrasts with psychoanalytically oriented therapies, which require little explanation.

Cognitive Techniques.   The therapy's cognitive approach includes four processes: eliciting automatic thoughts, testing automatic thoughts, identifying maladaptive underlying assumptions, and testing the validity of maladaptive assumptions.

ELICITING AUTOMATIC THOUGHTS.   Automatic thoughts, also called *cognitive distortions,* are cognitions that intervene between external events and a person's emotional reaction to the event. For example, the belief that "people will laugh at me when they see how badly I bowl" is an automatic thought that occurs to someone who receives an invitation to go bowling and responds negatively. Another example is the thought, "She doesn't like me," when someone passes in the hall without saying, "Hello." Examples of cognitive distortions are illustrated in Figure 23-3.

TESTING AUTOMATIC THOUGHTS.   Acting as a teacher, a therapist helps a patient test the validity of automatic thoughts. The goal is to encourage the patient to reject inaccurate or exaggerated automatic thoughts after careful examination. Patients often blame themselves when things that are outside their control go awry. The therapist reviews the entire situation with the patient and helps reassign the blame or cause of the unpleasant events. Generating alternative explanations for events is another way of undermining inaccurate and distorted automatic thoughts.

IDENTIFYING MALADAPTIVE ASSUMPTIONS.   As the patient and therapist continue to identify automatic thoughts, patterns usually become apparent. The patterns represent rules or maladaptive general assumptions that guide a patient's life. Samples of such rules are, "In order to be happy, I must be perfect," and, "If anyone doesn't like me, I'm not lovable." Such rules inevitably lead to

All-or-nothing thinking *(also called black-and-white, polarized, or dichotomous thinking)*: You view a situation in only two categories instead of on a continuum. Example: "If I'm not a total success, I'm a failure."

Catastrophizing *(also called fortune-telling)*: You predict the future negatively without considering other, more likely outcomes. Example: "I'll be so upset, I won't be able to function at all."

Disqualifying or discounting the positive: You unreasonably tell yourself that positive experiences, deeds, or qualities do not count. Example: "I did that project well, but that doesn't mean I'm competent; I just got lucky."

Emotional reasoning: You think something must be true because you "feel" (actually believe) it so strongly, ignoring or discounting evidence to the contrary. Example: "I know I do a lot of things okay at work, but I still feel like I'm a failure."

Labeling: You put a fixed, global label on yourself or others without considering that the evidence might more reasonably lead to a less disastrous conclusion. Example: "I'm a loser. He's no good."

Magnification/minimization: When you evaluate yourself, another person, or a situation, you unreasonably magnify the negative and/or minimize the positive. Example: "Getting a mediocre evaluation proves how inadequate I am. Getting high marks doesn't mean I'm smart."

Mental filter *(also called selective abstraction)*: You pay undue attention to one negative detail instead of seeing the whole picture. Example: "Because I got one low rating on my evaluation [which also contained several high ratings] it means I'm doing a lousy job."

Mind reading: You believe you know what others are thinking, failing to consider other, more likely possibilities. Example: "He's thinking that I don't know the first thing about this project."

Overgeneralization: You make a sweeping negative conclusion that goes far beyond the current situation. Example: "[Because I felt uncomfortable at the meeting] I don't have what it takes to make friends."

Personalization: You believe others are behaving negatively because of you, without considering more plausible explanations for their behavior. Example: "The repairman was curt to me because I did something wrong."

"Should" and "must" statements *(also called imperatives)*: You have a precise, fixed idea of how you or others should behave, and you overestimate how bad it is that these expectations are not met. Example: "It's terrible that I made a mistake. I should always do my best."

Tunnel vision: You only see the negative aspects of a situation. Example: "My son's teacher can't do anything right. He's critical and insensitive and lousy at teaching."

FIGURE 23-3
Cognitive distortions. (From Beck JS. *Cognitive Behavior Therapy: Basics and Beyond.* 2nd ed; 2011. Reprinted with permission of Guilford Press.)

disappointments and failure and, ultimately, to psychiatric symptoms such as depression. See Figure 23-4 for a sample automatic thought record.

TESTING THE VALIDITY OF MALADAPTIVE ASSUMPTIONS. Testing the accuracy of maladaptive assumptions is similar to testing the validity of automatic thoughts. In a particularly effective test, therapists ask patients to defend the validity of their assumptions. For example, patients may state that they should always work up to their potential, and a therapist may ask, "*Why is that so important to you?*" Table 23-11 gives examples of some interventions designed to elicit, identify, test, and correct the cognitive distortions that lead to depressive and other painful affects.

A woman presented for therapy with anger control problems. Before therapy, she sent a slew of hostile voicemail and e-mail messages to a colleague, alienated her neighbors with her noise complaints, and received a request to leave her bowling league after two physical altercations with members of other teams. A careful review of the patient's thoughts and beliefs surrounding these situations revealed a common denominator of a sense of *mistrust* and *entitlement*. In each situation, she believed that others had gone out of their way to mistreat her.

Furthermore, she had an exaggerated sense of self-importance represented by beliefs such as, "Nobody has the right to treat me that way," "I shouldn't have to deal with these people and their stupidity," and "I have to show them they can't ever push me around." To this patient, her anger was justified, as she was trying to defend herself from the misbehavior of others. However, to the outside observer, the patient was a "loose cannon" who took offense at the drop of a hat and whose behavior was outrageous and indefensible. In therapy, the patient at first was not open to viewing her anger problem in the manner just described. However, as she learned to recognize the activation of her schemas of *mistrust* and *entitlement*, she became more willing to consider ways in which she could modify her viewpoints and behaviors. This positive change was facilitated by the therapist's empathic responses to the patient's more credible stories of mistreatment she had received from her family, whose abusive behavior gave her the message that she should never trust anyone, and that she should never put up with being mistreated again. (Courtesy of C. F. Newman, Ph.D. and A. T. Beck, M.D.)

Behavioral Techniques. Behavioral and cognitive techniques go hand in hand; behavioral techniques test and change maladaptive and inaccurate cognitions. The overall purposes of such

AUTOMATIC THOUGHT RECORD

Directions: When you notice your mood getting worse, ask yourself, **"What's going through my mind right now?"** and as soon as possible jot down the thought or mental image in the Automatic Thoughts column.

DATE/TIME	SITUATION	AUTOMATIC THOUGHT(S)	EMOTION(S)	ALTERNATIVE RESPONSE	OUTCOME
	1. What event, daydream, or recollection led to the unpleasant emotion? 2. What (if any) distressing physical sensations did you have?	1. What thought(s) and/or image(s) went through your mind? 2. How much did you believe each one at the time?	1. What emotion(s) (sad, anxious, angry, etc.) did you feel at the time? 2. How intense (0–100%) was the emotion?	1. (optional) What cognitive distortion did you make? (e.g., all-or-nothing thinking, mind-reading, catastrophizing) 2. Use questions at bottom to compose a response to the automatic thought(s). 3. How much do you believe each response?	1. How much do you now believe each automatic thought? 2. What emotion(s) do you feel now? How intense (0–100%) is the emotion? 3. What will or did you do?
Friday 7:30 PM	I called Sally to go out, as we talked about. I got her answering machine. Felt a sinking sensation.	1) They have all gone out and forgotten about me, because I'm not important to them anymore. (90% believable) 2) I'm left out again. (90% believable) 3) I'm going to have to spend another Friday night alone. (100% believable) 4) I just don't fit in anywhere in this world. (70% believable)	1) Angry (60% intensity) 2) Lonely (95% intensity) 3) Depressed (95% intensity)	I'm engaging in arbitrary inference, overgeneralization, personalization, and catastrophization. 1) It could all be an innocent misunderstanding. (40% believable) 2) I have spent a lot of time with Sally and the others and I know they like me. (60% believable) 3) Being at home alone is not the end of the world. (50% believable)	1) 30% 2) 10% 3) 50% 4) 0% Angry (5%) Lonely (40%) Depressed (20%) Calm (70%) I will call back in an hour if I don't hear from Sally.

Questions to help compose an alternative response: (1) What is the evidence that the automatic thought is true? Not true? (2) Is there an alternative explanation? (3) What's the worst that could happen? Could I live through it? What's the best that could happen? What's the most realistic outcome? (4) What's the effect of my believing the automatic thought? What could be the effect of changing my thinking? (5) What should I do about it? (6) If _____ (friend's name) was in the situation and had this thought, what would I tell him/her?

© J.S. Beck, Ph.D., 1996

FIGURE 23-4

Sample automatic thought record.

techniques are to help patients understand the inaccuracy of their cognitive assumptions and learn new strategies and ways of dealing with issues.

Among the behavioral techniques in cognitive therapy are scheduling activities, mastery and pleasure, graded task assignments, cognitive rehearsal, self-reliance training, role-playing, and diversion techniques. One of the first tasks in therapy is to schedule activities on an hourly basis. Patients keep records of the activities and review them with the therapist. In addition to scheduling activities, patients rate the amount of mastery and pleasure their

Table 23-11
Cognitive Errors Derived from Assumptions

Cognitive Error	Assumption	Intervention
Overgeneralizing	If it's true in one case, it applies to any case that is even slightly similar.	Exposure of faulty logic. Establish criteria of which cases are similar to what degree.
Selective abstraction	The only events that matter are failures, deprivation, etc. Should measure self by errors, weaknesses, etc.	Use log to identify successes patient forgot.
Excessive responsibility (assuming personal causality)	I am responsible for all bad things, failures, etc.	Disattribution technique.
Assuming temporal causality (predicting without sufficient evidence)	If it has been true in the past, it's always going to be true.	Expose faulty logic. Specify factors that could influence outcome other than past events.
Self-references	I am the center of everyone's attention—especially my bad performances. I am the cause of misfortunes.	Establish criteria to determine when patient is the focus of attention and also the probable facts that cause bad experiences.
Catastrophizing	Always think of the worst. It's almost likely to happen to you.	Calculate real probabilities. Focus on evidence that the worst did not happen.
Dichotomous thinking	Everything is either one extreme or another (black or white, good or bad).	Demonstrate that events may be evaluated on a continuum.

From Beck AT, Rush AJ, Shaw BF, Emery G. *Cognitive Therapy of Depression*. New York: Guilford; 1979:48, with permission.

activities bring them. Patients often express surprise that they have much more mastery of activities and enjoy them more than they had thought.

To simplify the situation and allow mini-accomplishments, therapists often break tasks into subtasks, as in graded task assignments, to show patients that they can succeed. In cognitive rehearsal, patients imagine and rehearse the various steps in meeting and mastering a challenge.

Patients (especially inpatients) are encouraged to become self-reliant by doing such simple things as making their own beds, doing their own shopping, and preparing their own meals. This process is called self-reliance training. Role-playing is a particularly powerful and useful technique to elicit automatic thoughts and to learn new behaviors. Diversion techniques are effective in helping patients get through difficult times and include physical activity, social contact, work, play, and visual imagery.

Imagery or thought stoppage can treat impulsive or obsessive behavior. For instance, patients imagine a stop sign with a police officer nearby or another image that evokes inhibition at the same time that they recognize an impulse or obsession that is alien to the ego. Similarly, obesity can be treated by having patients visualize themselves as thin, athletic, trim, and well-muscled, and then training them to evoke this image whenever they have an urge to eat. Hypnosis or autogenic training can enhance such imagery. In a technique called guided imagery, therapists encourage patients to have fantasies that can be interpreted as wish fulfillments or attempts to master disturbing affects or impulses.

Indications

Cognitive therapy may be used to (1) eliminate or moderate the symptoms of a psychiatric disorder or psychological distress as an independent treatment or in combination with medication; (2) modify underlying beliefs and schemas that contribute to the development and maintenance of disorders; (3) address psychosocial problems (e.g., marital discord, job stress, caregiver burnout) that may have preceded, coincided with, or been caused by the disorder; (4) reduce the likelihood of relapse or recurrence of a disorder after symptoms have resolved; (5) increase adherence to recommended medical treatment (e.g., medication, weight loss, diabetes management); or moderate the impact of a medical condition on level of functioning (e.g., chronic pain, cancer).

BEHAVIOR THERAPY

The term *behavior* in *behavior therapy* refers to a person's observable actions and responses. Behavior therapy involves changing the behavior of patients to reduce dysfunction and to improve quality of life. Behavior therapy includes a methodology, referred to as *behavior analysis,* for the strategic selection of behaviors to change, and a technology to bring about behavior change, such as modifying antecedents or consequences or giving instructions. Behavior therapy has not only influenced mental health care but, under the rubric of behavioral medicine, it has also made inroads into other medical specialties.

Behavior therapy represents clinical applications of the principles developed in learning theory. Behavioral psychology, or behaviorism, arose in the early 20th century in reaction to the method of introspection that dominated psychology at the time. John B. Watson, the father of behaviorism, had initially studied animal psychology. This background made it a small conceptual leap to argue that psychology should concern itself only with publicly

observable phenomena (i.e., overt behavior). According to behavioristic thinking, because mental content is not publicly observable, it cannot be subjected to rigorous scientific inquiry. Consequently, behaviorists developed a focus on overt behaviors and their environmental influences.

Today, different behavioral schools continue to share a focus on verifiable behavior. Behavioral views differ from cognitive views in holding that physical, rather than mental, events control behavior. According to behaviorism, mental phenomena or speculations about them are of little or no scientific interest.

History

As early as the 1920s, scattered reports about the application of learning principles to the treatment of behavioral disorders began to appear, but they had little effect on the mainstream of psychiatry and clinical psychology. Not until the 1960s did behavior therapy emerge as a systematic and comprehensive approach to psychiatric (behavioral) disorders; at that time, it arose independently on three continents. Joseph Wolpe and his colleagues in Johannesburg, South Africa, used Pavlovian techniques to produce and eliminate experimental neuroses in cats. From this research, Wolpe developed systematic desensitization, the prototype of many current behavioral procedures for the treatment of maladaptive anxiety produced by identifiable stimuli in the environment. At about the same time, a group at the Institute of Psychiatry of the University of London, particularly Hans Jurgen Eysenck and M. B. Shapiro, stressed the importance of an empirical, experimental approach to understanding and treating individual patients, using controlled, single-case experimental paradigms and modern learning theory. The third origin of behavior therapy was work inspired by the research of Harvard psychologist B. F. Skinner. Skinner's students began to apply his operant-conditioning technology, developed in animal-conditioning laboratories, to human beings in clinical settings.

Systematic Desensitization

The foundation of systematic desensitization is the behavioral principle of counterconditioning, whereby a person overcomes maladaptive anxiety elicited by a situation or an object by approaching the feared situation gradually, in a psychophysiological state that inhibits anxiety. In systematic desensitization, patients attain a state of complete relaxation and are then exposed to the stimulus that elicits the anxiety response. The relaxed state inhibits the negative reaction of anxiety, a process called *reciprocal inhibition.* Rather than using actual situations or objects that evoke fear, patients and therapists prepare a graded list or hierarchy of anxiety-provoking scenes associated with a patient's fears. Treatment systematically pairs the learned relaxation state and the anxiety-provoking scenes. Thus, systematic desensitization consists of three steps: relaxation training, hierarchy construction, and desensitization of the stimulus.

Relaxation Training. Relaxation produces physiologic effects opposite to those of anxiety: slow heart rate, increased peripheral blood flow, and neuromuscular stability. A variety of relaxation methods exist. Some, such as yoga and Zen, have been known for centuries. Most methods use the so-called progressive relaxation, discussed above. Patients relax major muscle groups in a fixed order, beginning with the small muscle groups of the feet and working cephalad or vice versa. Some clinicians use hypnosis to facilitate relaxation or use tape-recorded exercises to allow patients to practice relaxation on their own. Mental imagery is a relaxation method in which patients imagine themselves in a place associated with pleasant, relaxed memories. Such images allow patients to enter a relaxed state or experience (as Herbert Benson termed it) the *relaxation response.*

The physiologic changes that take place during relaxation are the opposite of those induced by the adrenergic stress responses that are part of many emotions. Muscle tension, respiration rate, heart rate, blood pressure, and skin conductance decrease. Finger temperature and blood flow to the finger usually increase. Relaxation increases respiratory heart rate variability, an index of parasympathetic tone.

Hierarchy Construction.   When constructing a hierarchy, clinicians determine all the conditions that elicit anxiety, and then patients create a hierarchy list of 10 to 12 scenes in order of increasing anxiety. For example, an acrophobic hierarchy may begin with a patient imagining standing near a window on the second floor and end with being on the roof of a 20-story building, leaning on a guard rail and looking straight down.

Desensitization of the Stimulus.   In the final step, called *desensitization,* patients proceed systematically through the list from the least to the most anxiety-provoking scene while in a deeply relaxed state. Their responses to the stimuli determine the rate at which patients progress through the list. When patients can vividly imagine the most anxiety-provoking scene of the hierarchy with equanimity, they experience little anxiety in the corresponding real-life situation.

ADJUNCTIVE USE OF DRUGS.   Clinicians have used various drugs to hasten relaxation, but drugs should be used cautiously and only by clinicians trained and experienced in potential adverse effects. Either the ultra-rapidly acting barbiturate sodium methohexital or diazepam is given intravenously in subanesthetic doses. By implementing the procedural details carefully, almost all patients find the procedure pleasant, with few unpleasant side effects. The advantages of pharmacologic desensitization are a shortening of preliminary training in relaxation, the ability for nearly all patients to relax adequately, and a more rapid progression of treatment than without the drugs.

INDICATIONS.   Systematic desensitization works best in cases of a clearly identifiable anxiety-provoking stimulus. Phobias, obsessions, compulsions, and certain sexual disorders have been treated successfully with this technique.

Therapeutic-Graded Exposure

Therapeutic-graded exposure is similar to systematic desensitization, except that relaxation training is not involved, and treatment usually occurs in a real-life context. The individual must be brought in contact with (i.e., be exposed to) the warning stimulus to learn firsthand that no dangerous consequences will ensue. Exposure is graded according to a hierarchy. Patients afraid of cats, for example, might progress from looking at a picture of a cat to holding one.

Flooding

Flooding (sometimes called *implosion*) is similar to graded exposure in that it involves exposing the patient to the feared object in vivo; however, there is no hierarchy. The basis of flooding is the premise that escaping from an anxiety-provoking experience reinforces the anxiety through conditioning. Thus, clinicians can

extinguish the anxiety and prevent the conditioned avoidance behavior by not allowing patients to escape the situation. Clinicians encourage patients to confront feared situations directly, without a gradual buildup, as in systematic desensitization or graded exposure. No relaxation exercises are used, as in systematic desensitization. Patients experience fear, which gradually subsides after a time. The success of the procedure depends on having patients remain in the fear-generating situation until they are calm and feel a sense of mastery. Prematurely withdrawing from the situation or prematurely terminating the fantasized scene is equivalent to an escape, which then reinforces both the conditioned anxiety and the avoidance behavior and produces the opposite of the desired effect. In a variant, called *imaginal flooding,* the feared object or situation is confronted only in the imagination, not in real life. Many patients refuse flooding because of the psychological discomfort involved. Contraindications include situations when intense anxiety would be hazardous to a patient (e.g., those with heart disease or fragile psychological adaptation). The technique works best with specific phobias. The case study below presents an example of in vivo flooding.

> The patient was a 33-year-old woman with social fears of eating in public. In particular, she was afraid of being observed by others when chewing and swallowing, particularly at dinner parties. The therapist arranged a contrived situation in which the patient came to the session with a prepared meal and drink. She entered a conference room in which five persons in professional attire were already seated at a table. The therapist instructed the patient to eat her meal in front of these individuals. Between bites, she was instructed to look at them often, and they had been coached to avoid staring contests. She was not to distract herself from her anxiety symptoms. She was to eat her meal slowly, paying attention to the behavior of the observers and to her anxiety symptoms (e.g., dry mouth or difficulty swallowing). No conversation between the patient and the observers was permitted. The observers would look at her and observe her chewing and swallowing behaviors, at times writing comments in a notebook. Occasionally, observers would communicate by whispering to each other, exchanging written notes, or giving knowing glances and smiles.
>
> The only other communication occurred between the patient and therapist, and this was limited to the patient providing her subjective units of distress rating. The session lasted 90 minutes. Note: this situation may seem quite traumatizing. Because the exposure session is long and continues until ratings decline, the patient becomes desensitized. (Courtesy of Rolf G. Jacob, M.D. and William H. Pelham, M.D.)

In most cases, flooding (exposure) is accompanied by response prevention. Response prevention involves discontinuing all avoidance and other anxiety-reducing behaviors. In order for exposure to produce extinction, avoidance behaviors that typically reduce fear need to be prevented (e.g., looking at the floor when talking can reduce social anxiety; during exposure, therefore, to incorporate response prevention, the patient looks directly at people and not at the floor). Over time, while the patient remains in the fear-producing situation, the anxious emotional response will decrease. *Exposure and response prevention* (ERP) is actually the treatment of choice for obsessive compulsive disorder. In ERP, patients are exposed to feared stimuli and obsessions while rituals, which typically serve to reduce anxiety, are prevented.

Participant Modeling

In participant modeling, patients learn a new behavior by imitation, primarily by observation, without having to perform the behavior until they feel ready. Just as a person can acquire irrational fears by learning, a person may unlearn them by observing a fearless model confront the feared object. The technique is effective with phobic children who observe other children of their own age and sex who approach the feared object or situation. With adults, a therapist may describe the feared activity in a calm manner that a patient can identify. Or, the therapist may act out the process of mastering the feared activity with a patient. Sometimes a hierarchy of activities is established, and the patient tackles the least anxiety-provoking activity first. The participant-modeling technique is successful in treating agoraphobia by having a therapist accompany a patient into the feared situation. In a variant of the procedure, called *behavior rehearsal,* the patient acts out real-life problems under a therapist's observation or direction.

The following is a self-report by a patient with a contamination phobia, who is afraid to touch objects for fear of being infected or contaminated. She describes her reactions.

[The therapist] started touching everything very slowly. I was told to follow behind and touch everything she touched. It was like we were spreading the contamination. She touched doorknobs, light switches, walls, pictures, and woodwork. She opened drawers in each bedroom and touched the contents. She opened closets and touched clothes hanging on the rods. She touched the towels and sheets in the linen closet. She went through the children's rooms, touching dolls, stuffed animals, models, Star Wars figures, Transformers, and books.

[The therapist] kept talking to me quietly and calmly all the time we went along. I had been anxious when we started, but as we continued, my anxiety level decreased. At one point, when I had begun to think the worst was over, she pointed to the attic door and said we were going inside. I said, "No, that's where the mice were." She told me I didn't want to have a place in my home that was off-limits. I agreed but became very anxious. It was very hard for me to go inside. I began touching the boxes too, but I was very upset. Then, she put her hands down on the floor and wanted me to do the same. I said, "I can't. I just can't." [The therapist] said, "Yes, you can."

[The therapist] spent several hours with me that day. Before she left, she made a list of things for me to do by myself. Twice a day, I was to go through the house, touching everything the way she had done with me. I was to invite my friend who had a pet to come and visit, as well as friends of my children who had pets. (Courtesy of Rolf G. Jacobs, M.D. and William H. Pelham, M.D.)

Exposure to Stimuli Presented in Virtual Reality

Advances in computer technology have made it possible to present environmental cues in virtual reality for exposure treatment. Beneficial effects have been reported with virtual reality exposure of patients with height phobia, fear of flying, spider phobia, and claustrophobia. Much experimental work is ongoing. One model uses an avatar of the patient walking through a crowded supermarket filled with other avatars (including one of the therapist) as a way of conquering agoraphobia.

Assertiveness Training

Assertiveness is assertive behavior that enables a person to act in his or her own best interest, to stand up for herself or himself without undue anxiety, to express honest feelings comfortably, and to exercise personal rights without denying the rights of others.

Two types of situations frequently call for assertive behaviors: (1) setting limits on pushy friends or relatives and (2) commercial situations, such as countering a sales pitch or being persistent

when returning defective merchandise. Early assertiveness training programs tended to define specific behaviors as assertive or nonassertive. For example, individuals were encouraged to assert themselves if somebody got in front of them in a supermarket checkout line. Context has received increasing attention; that is, what would be assertive behavior in this situation depends on circumstances.

Social Skills Training

The negative symptoms in patients with schizophrenia constitute behavioral deficits that go beyond difficulties with assertiveness. These patients have inadequate expressive behaviors and inappropriate stimulus control of their social behaviors (i.e., they do not pick up social cues). Similarly, patients with depression often experience a lack of social reinforcement because of a lack of social skills, and studies have found social skills training to be efficacious for depression. Patients with social phobia similarly often have not acquired adolescents' social skills. In fact, their social defensive behaviors (e.g., avoiding eye contact, making brief statements, and minimizing self-disclosure) increase the probability of the rejection that they fear.

Social skills training programs for patients with schizophrenia cover skills in the following areas: conversation, conflict management, assertiveness, community living, friendship and dating, work and vocation, and medication management. Each of these skills has several components. For example, assertiveness skills include making requests, refusing requests, making complaints, responding to complaints, expressing unpleasant feelings, asking for information, making apologies, expressing fear, and refusing alcohol and street drugs. Each component involves specific steps. For example, conflict management includes skills in negotiating, compromising, tactful disagreeing, responding to untrue accusations, and leaving overly stressful situations. A situation in which a patient would use conflict management skills could be when the patient and a friend decide to go to a movie, and their choice of movie differs.

Negotiating and compromising, for example, involves the following steps:

1. Explain one's viewpoint briefly.
2. Listen to the other person's viewpoint.
3. Repeat the other person's viewpoint.
4. Suggest a compromise.

At his initial appointment, Phillip described severe symptoms of obsessive-compulsive disorder (OCD). He was 23 years old and living at home because he was no longer able to work or go to school. His days were consumed with behaviors related to checking, repeating, and hoarding. Phillip was unable to throw away anything—he saved junk mail, used tissues and napkins, old papers and magazines, and any kind of receipt for fear that he might lose something important. Phillip spent many hours checking his trash, his car, and his home to be sure that he had not thrown away anything important. He also checked everything he wrote (e.g., checks, school exams and papers, letters and e-mails) to be sure that he had not made a mistake, and he read and reread books, magazines, and articles to be sure he understood the written material adequately. Phillip constantly worried that he had done something wrong and would disappoint his parents. He was also depressed because he was unable to function well in life, and he had tremendous social anxiety that had plagued him for many years, making it difficult to make and keep friends.

By the end of Phillip's second session, his therapist was beginning to get a good idea of the general nature and severity of his symptoms and some of the maintaining factors. However, to plan the treatment

Table 23-12
Daily Monitoring of Rituals

Each day, record the amount of time spent doing rituals in the morning, afternoon, and evening.

	Tuesday	Wednesday	Thursday	Friday	Saturday	Sunday	Monday
Morning	2 hr	1.5 hr					
Afternoon	3 hr	2 hr					
Evening	1.5 hr	3 hr					

Once a day, record the following details about an episode of rituals:

Day	Time	Situation	Feelings	Thoughts (Obsessions)	Type of Ritual	Feelings After Rituals
Saturday	8 AM	Finished breakfast	Afraid Scared Worried	Shouldn't have thrown away my napkin Might have left something under my plate What if I lost something important?	Checking through trash Looking under plate Staring to see if I lost something	Better For now, I think I have not lost anything
Sunday	2 PM	At the store; signed a check	Worried Anxious	Did I sign my name correctly? Did I write the correct amount? What if I give them the check and it is wrong?	Staring at the check Tracing the lines I wrote Standing there	Anxious because I couldn't finish checking

Courtesy of M. A. Stanley, Ph.D. and D. C. Beidel, Ph.D.

in more detail and to get a better idea of how the symptoms occurred during his daily life, she asked Phillip to keep daily records over the next week using a form that she had prepared for him. The form had a place for recording the amount of time he spent in rituals each morning, afternoon, and evening, as well as another place to record more details about at least one episode of rituals each day (e.g., what was happening before, during, and after the rituals; see Table 23-12).

Phillip's therapist determined that his difficulties with obsessions, rituals, depression, and social fears reflected a core fear of negative evaluation. Phillip was overly concerned with making mistakes, being imperfect, and disappointing others. Even as a child, Phillip was worried about not doing well enough, and he had difficulty making friends for fear that others would not like him. His highly anxious parents provided much adulation when Phillip did things well (e.g., learned to ride a bike, got good grades in school), and they spent a great deal of time instructing him on improving his performance when an activity or grade was not perfect. As Phillip took on more responsibility at school and with part-time work, he became more concerned about doing things right. He learned that going back and checking his work relieved his anxiety. He also learned that saving his papers for future checking reassured him that he would be able to fix any unrecognized mistakes at a later time. His parents helped him to reduce his anxiety when he was uncertain about his work by reassuring him that he was doing okay. As Phillip progressed from elementary school to middle school to high school, his workload and anxiety gradually increased, but he was able to manage things with some moderate checking and saving. When he began attending college, however, the workload increased extensively, and he found himself doing even more checking and hoarding to reduce his fears about making mistakes. Phillip began to feel that these behaviors were getting out of control, but he could not stop them. He had to check and recheck to be sure that he was not making mistakes. The cycle of anxiety to ritual to reduced anxiety was so powerfully reinforcing that he could not stop. He needed help to break this cycle and to address his persistent fear of negative evaluation.

Phillip's therapist decided to begin treatment with a course of exposure and response prevention (ERP) to get his obsessions and rituals under control and begin to address his core fear of making mistakes and being evaluated negatively. Given that Phillip's depression had grown from the disability associated with his OCD, the therapist expected that a successful course of ERP might also help to reduce his depressive

symptoms. ERP for Phillip began with a home visit, where the therapist helped him to complete common daily activities with adherence to his RP plan, which included the following:

- No more checking: After eating, leave the table immediately without inspecting your plate and the surrounding areas (including under the table and chair) for lost items. Leave the restroom immediately after using it, without checking the toilet, trash, and sink for lost items. When leaving the car, do not check seats, floors, and windows. Write everything (papers, checks, etc.) only once; no checking to be sure that letters and words are correct.
- No more repeating: No more rereading books. No staring repeatedly at items to ensure that nothing is lost.
- No more saving. Throw tissues away immediately after using them. Discard trash and junk mail immediately. Do not look into the trash can for lost items.

Phillip's parents also were asked to stop reassuring him and to discontinue doing rituals for him. This session was very difficult for Phillip and his family, but they understood the logic of ERP, and they were willing to try anything.

For the next 3 weeks, Phillip and his therapist met three times a week to conduct in vivo exposure sessions that helped him to face his core fears. For many of these sessions, the therapist asked Phillip to bring hoarded items from home and to discard all unnecessary items during the therapy session. At first, this created tremendous anxiety, but over time, Phillip was able to throw things away with less fear of losing something important. He also developed the ability to conduct self-directed exposure at home. Other exposure sessions involved writing letters and mailing them without checking, reading passages from magazines and books only once, and sorting through junk mail to make quick decisions about what to save or discard. As Phillip was able to take on more responsibility for home-based exposure, session frequency decreased to two times per week, and then to once per week. After 3 months of treatment, Phillip's scores on the YBOCS (Yale-Brown Obsessive-Compulsive Scale) and BDI (Beck Depression Inventory) had decreased to 20 and 19, respectively, demonstrating significant improvement in obsessive-compulsive symptoms and depression. His SPAI (Social Phobia and Anxiety Inventory) score, however, remained relatively unchanged, suggesting that he was still experiencing significant social anxiety.

Next, while Phillip worked on maintaining the gains he had made following ERP, he and his therapist conducted some role-plays to evaluate his social skills. It was apparent that Phillip had extreme difficulty with initiating and maintaining conversations. His eye contact also was quite poor in social interactions. Thus, the therapist devised a plan for teaching and practicing new skills, which also involved additional exposure to Phillip's core fears as the therapist asked him to resume contact with old friends and identify activities where he could meet new people. He practiced new behaviors first in session with his therapist and then developed a hierarchy of feared social situations in which he could practice his new behaviors. These practice exercises also involved a form of exposure, as the therapist asked Phillip to make social contact, which produced fears of negative evaluation. After another 3 months of treatment focused on social skills training (and associated exposure), Phillip's scores on the YBOCS and BDI had decreased further (YBOCS = 15; BDI = 13), and his SPAI score had decreased to 100. Phillip had gone back to school to take one class, he was spending small amounts of time with old friends, and he was volunteering a few hours each week at his church. (Courtesy of M. A. Stanley, Ph.D. and D. C. Beidel, Ph.D.)

Aversion Therapy

When a noxious stimulus (punishment) is presented immediately after a specific behavioral response, theoretically, the response is eventually inhibited and extinguished. Aversion therapy can use many types of noxious stimuli: electric shocks, substances that induce vomiting, corporal punishment, and social disapproval. The therapist pairs the negative stimulus with the behavior, resulting in suppression of the behavior. The unwanted behavior may disappear after a series of such sequences. Aversion therapy has been used for alcohol abuse, paraphilias, and other behaviors with impulsive or compulsive qualities, but this therapy is controversial for many reasons. For example, punishment does not always lead to the expected decreased response and can sometimes be positively reinforcing.

Eye Movement Desensitization and Reprocessing

Saccadic eye movements are rapid oscillations of the eyes that occur when a person tracks an object that is moved back and forth across the line of vision. Several studies have demonstrated that inducing saccades while a person is imagining or thinking about an anxiety-producing event can yield a positive thought or image that results in decreased anxiety. Eye movement desensitization and reprocessing therapy is effective in the treatment of PTSDs and phobias.

Positive Reinforcement

When a generally rewarding event, such as food or praise, follows a behavioral response, the response tends to be strengthened and to occur more frequently than before the reward. This principle can be applied to a variety of situations. On inpatient hospital wards, patients with mental disorders receive a reward for performing a desired behavior, such as tokens that they can use to purchase luxury items or certain privileges. The process, known as *token economy,* has successfully altered behavior.

Behavioral Activation

Based on behavioral theory, depression persists because: (a) reinforcement for nondepressed (healthy) behavior is low or nonexistent, (b) depressed behavior produces positive (e.g., sympathy from others) or negative reinforcement (decrease in responsibilities or avoidance of undesirable situations), (c) exposure to aversive or unpleasant life experiences is significant, or (d) some combination of these factors. Severely depressed mood leads to behavioral withdrawal, which in turn results in loss of reinforcement from pleasurable events or activities.

Behavioral activation emphasizes structured attempts to increase overt behaviors that bring patients into contact with reinforcing environmental contingencies and corresponding improvements in thoughts, mood, and quality of life. Patients begin by engaging in a self-monitoring (or daily diary) exercise to examine already occurring daily activities to provide a baseline measurement and to provide some potential activities to target during treatment. For each behavior, they indicate their levels of reward, difficulty, and importance. Emphasis then shifts to identifying patients' values and goals within life areas that include family, social, and intimate relationships, education, employment/career, hobbies/recreation, volunteer work/charity, physical/health issues, spirituality, and anxiety-eliciting situations. An activity hierarchy is constructed, where activities are rated from "easiest" to "most difficult" to accomplish. Patients progressively move through the hierarchy, moving from easier behaviors to the more difficult.

Charles was a 70-year-old retired business executive. Throughout his life, his work consumed him. Although he married and had a family, his job was his primary focus. He went to the office early and came home late. He enjoyed what he did—it was stimulating and made him feel important and useful. But as he got older, his performance was not what it used to be, and he decided it was time to retire. However, his mood was pretty low when he no longer had a job. He did not have the energy to get more involved in his church or to develop other hobbies, so he sat around all day, without any social contacts. His wife and best friend encouraged him to talk to someone. The therapist suggested that they try behavioral activation. Charles was somewhat skeptical, as it seemed too simple, but he needed to do something. The therapist spent some time with Charles talking about the kinds of activities that used to make him feel good and some of the things he used to enjoy. They then put together a list of things he might be able to do—even if he did not feel much like it—just to see what would happen. The list included looking for volunteer work where he could use his job skills, spending more time with his wife in some of the activities they once had enjoyed (e.g., watching movies, taking walks), and rejuvenating an old hobby from his college days—fishing. Charles initially agreed to do some easy activities—go to one movie a week, take one walk a week, and contact his church activity leader about possible volunteer activities. He was surprised to find that even these "baby steps" helped him feel better. He had the chance to talk with other people and began to see that, even in retirement, he could find useful and fun things to do. (Courtesy of M. A. Stanley, Ph.D. and D. C. Beidel, Ph.D.)

Results

Behavior therapy has a wide range of applications and is useful for a wide variety of psychiatric disorders (e.g., anxiety, depression, schizophrenia, and bipolar disorder), psychological problems (e.g., marital discord, school refusal, and stress), and medical problems (e.g., adjustment to chronic illness, medication adherence, and healthy behaviors). Behavioral treatments have also been administered effectively with individual patients, couples, families, and groups, and they are useful in a range of treatment settings, including inpatient, outpatient, day treatment, and community settings.

HYPNOSIS

The concept of hypnosis conjures up myriad perceptions among clinicians and the lay public. Even the term *hypnosis* can be misleading, coming as it does from the Greek root *hypnos* (meaning "sleep"). In reality, hypnosis is not sleeping. It is more likely a complex process that requires alert focus and receptive attention. Hypnosis is a powerful means of directing innate capabilities of imagination, imagery, and attention. Many also believe the myth that the clinician projects the hypnotic trance onto the patient or has the power to influence the patient. In reality, it is the patient who has the hypnotic gift, and the clinician's role is to assess the patient's capacity to capitalize on this asset and to help the patient discover and use it effectively. Patient motivation, personality style, and biologic predisposition may contribute to the manifestation of this talent.

The hypnotic trance enhances focal attention and imagination and simultaneously decreases peripheral awareness. A hypnotist may induce this trance through formalized induction procedures, but it can also occur spontaneously. The capacity to be hypnotized and, relatedly, the occurrence of spontaneous trance states, is a trait that varies among individuals but is relatively stable throughout a person's life cycle.

History

Descriptions of trance states, ecstatic states, and spontaneous dissociative states abound in the Eastern and Western religious, literary, and philosophical traditions. Anton Franz Anton Mesmer (1734–1815) first formally described hypnosis as a therapeutic modality in the 18th century and believed it to be the result of magnetic energy or an invisible fluid that the therapist channels into the patient to correct imbalances, restoring health. James Braid (1795–1860), an English physician and surgeon, used eye fixation and closure to induce trance states. Later, Jean Martin Charcot (1825–1893) theorized the hypnotic state to be a neurophysiologic phenomenon that was a sign of mental illness. Contemporaneously, Hippolyte Bernheim (1840–1919) believed it to be a function of the normal brain.

Early in his career, Sigmund Freud (1856–1939) used hypnosis as part of his psychoanalysis and noticed that patients in a trance could relive traumatic events, a process called *abreaction*. Later, Freud switched from hypnosis to free association because he wanted to minimize the transference that sometimes accompanies the trance state. Importantly, the switch did not eliminate the occurrence of spontaneous trance during the analysis.

World War I produced many shell-shocked soldiers, and Ernst Simmel (1882–1947), a German psychoanalyst, developed a technique for accessing repressed material that he named *hypnoanalysis*. During World War II, hypnosis played a prominent role in the treatment of pain, combat fatigue, and neurosis. Formal recognition of hypnosis as a therapeutic modality did not occur, however, until the 1950s. The British Medical Society recommended its teaching in medical schools in 1955, and the American Medical Association and American Psychiatric Association officially stated its safety and efficacy in 1958.

Definition

The current understanding of hypnosis is that it is a normal activity of a normal mind through which attention is more focused, critical judgment is partially suspended, and peripheral awareness is diminished. The trance state, being a function of the subject's mind, cannot be forcibly projected by an outside person. The hypnotist, however, may aid in the achievement of the state and use its uncritical, intense focus to facilitate the acceptance of new thoughts and feelings, thereby accelerating therapeutic change. For the subject, hypnosis typically involves a sense of involuntariness, and movements seem automatic.

Trait of Hypnotizability

A person's degree of hypnotizability is a trait that is relatively stable throughout the life cycle and is measurable. The process of hypnosis takes the hypnotizability trait and transforms it into the hypnotized state. Experiencing the hypnotic concentration state requires a convergence of three essential components: absorption, dissociation, and suggestibility.

Absorption is an ability to reduce peripheral awareness that results in greater focal attention. A metaphorical description is that of a psychological zoom lens that increases attention to the given thought or emotion to the increasing exclusion of all contexts, even including orientation to time and space.

Dissociation is the separating out from consciousness elements of the patient's identity, perception, memory, or motor response as the hypnotic experience deepens. The result is that components of self-awareness, time, perception, and physical activity can occur without being known to the patient's consciousness and so may seem involuntary.

Suggestibility is the tendency of the hypnotized patient to accept signals and information with a relative suspension of normal critical judgment; it is controversial whether a person can completely suspend critical judgment. This trait will vary from an almost compulsive response to input in the highly hypnotizable to a sense of automaticity in the less hypnotizable individual.

Quantification of Hypnotizability.   Quantifying a patient's degree of hypnotizability is useful in a clinical setting because it predicts the effectiveness of hypnosis as a therapeutic modality. Quantification also provides useful information about the way patients relate to themselves and the social environment. Highly hypnotizable patients have an increased incidence of spontaneous trance-like states and so may be unduly influenced by ideas and emotions that are not being appropriately self-critiqued.

Induction

Many different induction protocols follow the same basic principles and pattern but may be better suited to patients with different levels of hypnotizability.

> *Doctor:* Take a long, deep breath—inhale and exhale; now close your eyes and relax. Pay particular attention to the muscles in and about your eyes—relax them to the point that they just won't work. Are you trying to do that? Good. If you really have them relaxed, right at this very moment, no matter how hard you try, they just won't open. Test them. The harder you try, the faster they stick together, just as if they were glued together. That's fine!
>
> Now you can open your eyes; that's good. When I tell you to and not before, open and close your eyes once more, and, when you close them this time, you will be ten times as relaxed as you are right now. Go ahead, open and close, and feel that surge of relaxation go through your whole body, from the top of your head to the tip of your toes. Very good!

Now once again, open and close your eyes, and this time, when you close them, you will double the relaxation that you currently have. Fine.

If you have followed my suggestions, right at this very moment, when I lift your hand and let it drop into your lap, it will drop like a wet cloth, heavy and limp. That's very, very good.

You now have good physical relaxation, but medical hypnosis consists of two phases: physical, which you currently have, and mental, which I will now show you how to achieve.

When I ask you to, and not before, I want you to start counting backward from 100. I know you can count; that is not what we're after. I just want you to relax mentally. As you say each number, pause momentarily until you feel a wave of relaxation cover your whole body, from the top of your head to the tip of your toes. When you feel this wave of relaxation, then say the next number, and each time you say a number, you will double the relaxation you had before you said the number. If you do this properly, an interesting thing will happen—as you say the numbers and relax, the succeeding numbers will start to disappear and vanish from your mind. Command your mind to dispel these numbers. Now, aloud and slowly, start counting backward from 100.

Patient: One hundred.

Doctor: Very good.

Patient: Ninety-nine.

Doctor: Make them start to disappear now.

Patient: Ninety-eight.

Doctor: Now they're fading away, and after the next number, they'll all be gone. Make them disappear. Let the numbers go.

Patient: Ninety-seven.

Doctor: And now they're all gone. Are they gone? Fine. If there are any numbers still lurking in your mind, when I lift your hand and drop it, they will all disappear.

(Courtesy of William Holt, M.D.)

Indications

A patient's degree of hypnotizability and the technique of hypnosis are clinically useful in diagnosis and treatment, respectively. The existence of spontaneous, trance-like states in everyday life and the potential of individuals to uncritically accept emotions and information in these states make a person's degree of hypnotizability a factor in the way the world is viewed and processed.

Therapeutically, hypnosis's effectiveness in facilitating acceptance of new thoughts and feelings makes it useful in treating habitual problems and also with symptom management. Smoking, overeating, phobias, anxiety, conversion symptoms, and chronic pain are all indications for hypnosis. They can often be treated in a single session, in which a patient learns to perform self-hypnosis. Hypnosis can also aid in psychotherapy, notably for PTSD, and may also be useful for memory retrieval.

A 32-year-old man presented to the emergency department with a severe headache. He was a chronic migraine sufferer and was unable to control the pain on this occasion with his propranolol. The emergency department recognized that he had a high hypnotic capacity. The physician suggested imagery of an icepack resting on his forehead. Initially, they placed some real ice on his forehead to help. The patient was able to control his pain completely with this imagery. He did not require narcotics, as he had on previous visits. On follow-up several weeks later, the patient reported being able to use this strategy to control, as well as prevent, migraine attacks, and he no longer had to rely on frequent emergency department visits for pain relief. (Courtesy of A. D. Axelrad, M.D., D. Brown, Ph.D., and H. J. Wain, Ph.D.)

A 22-year-old male patient presented to the emergency room with bilateral blindness. An evaluation by ophthalmology revealed that the blindness was psychogenic. The emergency physician referred the patient to psychiatry. After an initial evaluation and the development of a therapeutic alliance, the psychiatrist used hypnosis to take the patient to a safe place and then back to the time immediately before the blindness. After two sessions, the patient described seeing his wife in an adulterous relationship. At that moment, the patient vocalized a desire to harm his wife and her suitor. Immediately after this vocalization, he became amnesic for the event and blind. On describing this under hypnosis, the therapist suggested that, when he became alert, "He would only remember what he felt comfortable remembering." After the patient became alert, he had no idea what had occurred, and each day after initiation of the hypnotic intervention, the patient's anger was reframed. When the patient felt comfortable, he then confronted his wife. The patient became aware that the amnesia was being used to prevent him from acting out. The use of a psychodynamic, cognitive reframing approach with a hypnotic milieu helped this patient to gain control and understanding of his symptoms. The therapist referred the patient and his wife for marital counseling. (Courtesy of A. D. Axelrad, M.D., D. Brown, Ph.D., and H. J. Wain, Ph.D.)

A 29-year-old woman presented for evaluation and treatment of ongoing facial pain that was not responding to traditional methods of intervention. The neurologic evaluation showed no objective physical correlations. Initially, hypnotic intervention controlled the pain, but it returned 24 hours later. Her self-hypnotic technique ceased to be effective. The therapist decided to explore more completely the meaning of the pain. Using age regression under hypnosis, the patient regressed to a time before the pain. She related that her brother had been injured by a car while he was running in the street. The patient was babysitting at the time, and her father was so angry that he hit her. Recently her friend's dog ran away, and she felt responsible. As she began to recognize her need to punish herself because of her guilt over what occurred, she was able to understand her feelings and reframe her thoughts more productively. An "affect bridge" was also used, and the patient went back to a previous time when she felt guilty and received punishment. She then described her feelings of being hit by her alcoholic, abusive father. She continued to gain insight and mastery over the past and was able to ablate her pain. (Courtesy of A. D. Axelrad, M.D., D. Brown, Ph.D., and H. J. Wain, Ph.D.)

A 42-year-old married mother of three children was kidnapped and locked in a large packing trunk. After she freed herself and broke out, her abductors stabbed her multiple times, tied her up, put her back in the trunk, and threw her down a cliff. She eventually managed to break out and crawl to safety. Eventually, a passerby called 911, and paramedics transported her to a hospital. She reported that others saw her lying on the road and appeared frightened to approach her.

Following medical stabilization, she was discharged from the hospital and found herself developing nightmares, reexperiencing avoidance, and having hyperarousal symptoms. Her internist referred her for treatment. The psychiatrist initiated sertraline. She was found to be a mid- to high-range hypnotic subject. She learned to go to a safe place and to use a split-screen technique. The therapist also gave her permission to describe her nightmares, reexperiences, and overwhelming anxieties and fears that she faced while being captive, as well as her feelings of abandonment while lying on the road. The therapist reinforced her ingenuity in breaking out of the trunk. She responded to a reframing of the feeling of blame for her capture while under hypnosis. She learned to calm herself and to reframe her negative feelings about her helplessness. Hypnotic age regression helped her master her experiences and facilitate their becoming like a bad movie. Initially, her startle response was a signal for her to go to her comfort zone. Age progression helped her to rehearse the future. The treatment used the milieu of hypnosis along with exposure, cognitive reframing, psychodynamic approaches, and pharmacology. (Courtesy of A. D. Axelrad, M.D., D. Brown, Ph.D., and H. J. Wain, Ph.D.)

Contraindications

No intrinsic dangers to the hypnotic process exist. Because of the increased dependence that the hypnotized patient has toward the therapist, a strong transference may occur, however, in which the patient exhibits feelings for the therapist that are inappropriate in regard to their relationship. Strong attachments may occur, and these must be respected and properly interpreted. Negative emotions may also surface in the patient, especially in those who are emotionally fragile or who have poor reality testing. To minimize the likelihood of this negative transference, the therapist must use caution when choosing patients who have problems with basic trust, such as those who are paranoid or who require high levels of control. The hypnotized patient also has a reduced ability to evaluate hypnotic suggestions critically and, thus, the hypnotist must have a strong ethical value system. Controversy exists about whether patients can perform acts during a trance state that they would otherwise find repugnant or that run contrary to their moral system.

INTERPERSONAL THERAPY

Interpersonal psychotherapy (ITP) is a time-limited treatment for major depressive disorder developed by Gerald L. Klerman and Myrna Weissman in the 1970s. The initial formulation of ITP was an attempt to represent the current practice of psychotherapy for depression. It assumes that the development and maintenance of some psychiatric illnesses occur in a social and interpersonal context and that interpersonal relations between the patient and significant others influence the onset, response to treatment, and outcomes of these illnesses. The overall goal of ITP is to reduce or eliminate psychiatric symptoms by improving the quality of the patient's current interpersonal relations and social functioning.

The typical course of ITP lasts 12 to 20 sessions over a 4- to 5-month period. ITP moves through three defined phases: (1) the initial phase identifies the problem area that will be the target for treatment; (2) the intermediate phase works on the target problem area(s); and (3) the termination phase focuses on consolidating gains made during treatment and preparing the patients for future work on their own (Table 23-13).

Techniques

Individual Interpersonal Psychotherapy

INITIAL PHASE.   Sessions one through five typically constitute the initial phase of ITP. After assessing the patient's current psychiatric symptoms and obtaining a history of these symptoms, the therapist gives the patient a formal diagnosis. The therapist and patient then discuss the diagnosis, as well as what to expect from treatment. Assignment of the sick role during this phase serves the dual function of granting the patient both the permission to recover and the responsibility to recover. The therapist explains the rationale of ITP, underscoring that therapy will focus on identifying and altering dysfunctional interpersonal patterns related

Table 23-13
Phases of Time-Limited Interpersonal Psychotherapy

Initial Phase: Sessions 1–5
Give the syndrome a name; provide information about the prevalence and characteristics of the disorder
Describe the rationale and nature of the therapy
Conduct the interpersonal inventory to identify the current interpersonal problem area(s) associated with the onset or maintenance of the psychiatric symptoms
Review significant relationships, past and present
Identify interpersonal precipitants of episodes of psychiatric symptoms
Select and reach consensus about the interpersonal problem area(s) and treatment plan with patient

Intermediate Phase: Sessions 6–15
Implement strategies specific to the identified problem area(s)
Encourage and review work on goals specific to the problem area
Illuminate connections between symptoms and interpersonal events during the week
Work with the patient to identify and manage negative or painful affects associated with his or her interpersonal problem area

Termination Phase: Sessions 16–20
Discuss termination explicitly
Educate the patient about the end of treatment as a potential time of grieving; encourage the patient to identify associated emotions
Review progress to foster feelings of accomplishment and competence
Outline goals for remaining work; identify areas and warning signs of anticipated future difficulty
Formulate specific plans for continued work after termination of treatment

to psychiatric symptomatology. To determine the precise focus of treatment, the therapist conducts an interpersonal inventory with the patient and develops an interpersonal formulation based on this. In the interpersonal formulation, the therapist links the patient's psychiatric symptomatology to one of the four interpersonal problem areas—grief, interpersonal deficits, interpersonal role disputes, or role transitions. The patient's concurrence with the therapist's identification of the problem area and agreement to work on this area are essential before beginning the intermediate treatment phase.

INTERMEDIATE PHASE.   The intermediate phase—typically sessions 6 to 15—constitutes the "work" of the therapy. An essential task throughout the intermediate phase is to strengthen the connections the patient makes between the changes in his or her interpersonal life and the changes in psychiatric symptoms. During the intermediate phase, the therapist implements the treatment strategies specific to the identified problem area, as specified in Table 23-14.

TERMINATION PHASE.   In the termination phase (usually, sessions 16 through 20), the therapist discusses termination explicitly with the patient and assists him or her in understanding that the end of treatment is a potential time of grief. During this phase, the therapist encourages patients to describe specific changes in their psychiatric symptoms, especially as they relate to improvements in the identified problem area(s). The therapist also assists the patient in evaluating and consolidating gains, detailing plans for maintaining improvements in the identified interpersonal problem area(s), and outlining remaining work for the patient to continue on his or her own. The therapist also encourages patients to identify early warning signs of symptom recurrence and to identify plans of action.

Table 23-14
Interpersonal Problem Areas: Description, Goals, and Strategies

Problem Area	Description	Goals	Strategies
Grief	Complicated bereavement after death of a loved one	Facilitate the mourning process Help the patient to establish interest in new activities and relationships to substitute for what has been lost	Reconstruct the patient's relationship with the deceased Explore associated feelings (negative and positive) Consider ways of becoming reinvolved with others
Interpersonal deficits	A history of social impoverishment, inadequate or unsustaining interpersonal relationships	Reduce patient's social isolation Enhance quality of any existing relationships Encourage the formation of new relationships	Review past significant relationships, including negative and positive aspects Explore repetitive patterns in relationships Note problematic interpersonal patterns in the session and relate them to similar patterns in the patient's life
Interpersonal role disputes	Conflicts with a significant other—a partner, other family member, coworker, or close friend	Identify the nature of the dispute Explore options to resolve dispute Modify expectations and faulty communication to bring about a satisfactory resolution If modification is unworkable, encourage patient to reassess the expectations for the relationship and to generate options to either resolve it or dissolve it and mourn its loss	Determine the stage of the dispute: renegotiation (calm down participants to facilitate resolution); impasse (increase disharmony to reopen negotiation); dissolution (assist mourning and adaptation) Understand how nonreciprocal role expectations relate to the dispute Identify available resources to bring about change in the relationship
Role transitions	Economic or family change—the beginning or end of a relationship or career, a move, promotion, retirement, graduation, diagnosis of a medical illness	Mourn and accept the loss of the old role Recognize the positive and negative aspects of the new role and assets and liabilities of the old role Restore self-esteem by developing a sense of mastery regarding the demands of the new role	Review positive and negative aspects of old and new roles Explore feelings about what is lost Encourage development of social support system and new skills called for in new role

Reprinted with permission from Wilfley D, Stein R, Welch R. Interpersonal psychotherapy. In: Treasure J, van Furth E, Schmidt U, eds. *Handbook of Eating Disorders*. 2nd ed. Hoboken, NJ: Wiley; 2003:253.

Ms. G is a 51-year-old woman who presented for treatment of binge eating disorder. She is college-educated, has her own business, and is a divorced mother of one adult son in his early 20s. Before treatment, she had a body mass index (BMI) of 42, and her binge eating occurred approximately 10 to 15 days per month over the past 8 years. Along with her current diagnosis of binge eating disorder, Ms. G struggled with recurrent major depression.

During the initial phase, Ms. G and her therapist began to review her history and the interpersonal events that were associated with her binge eating. Ms. G shared that she began overeating and gaining weight at age 14. When she was 18 years of age, she moved to a foreign country with her parents. Soon after the move, Ms. G's father left her and her mother to return to the United States. Ms. G was enraged at her father for leaving them and still gets very tearful and angry when discussing the separation. She and her mother decided to stay abroad because she had started university, and her mother was working. Both had developed strong social ties and felt comfortable in their new home. During this time, Ms. G continued to gain weight and started dieting. Shortly after graduating from university, Ms. G met and married a foreign national and, at the age of 28, delivered their only son. Two years later, she and her husband went through a very bitter divorce. Although Ms. G described this as a terrible time in her life, she maintained close ties with her friends and her mother. During this time, she began to diet and reached her lowest adult weight. At the age of 35, when her mother died of a heart condition, Ms. G had her first episode of major depression, which was treated and resolved with antidepressants and

a brief course of psychotherapy. Although she had previous cycles of weight loss and weight regain, she did not evidence any sign of eating disturbance at this point. She continued to maintain close social ties and enjoyed her close relationship with her son. When Ms. G was in her early 40s, an economic downturn in her adopted country forced her to return to the United States. Having lost all of her savings, she struggled financially while she looked for work. During this time, she started binge eating and gaining weight. Within 1 year of this move, Ms. G's son decided to return to live with his father (who was very wealthy). Ms. G felt angry and betrayed. Yet, when her son would visit, she would assume a subservient role with him, because she was afraid of losing his affection. He, in turn, became quite demanding and critical of her. Before seeking treatment, her heightened feelings of isolation and loneliness were leading to increased binge eating, depression, and weight gain.

By session three of the initial phase, Ms. G's therapist began to consider which problem area would be the focus of the remainder of treatment. Ms. G had a history of important relationship losses and subsequent grief—the loss of her father, her husband, her mother, and, most recently, her son. However, none of these losses led to the development of binge eating problems (although her dieting clearly linked to her feelings of anger after the divorce from her husband, and her depression intimately related to her mother's death). Ms. G's anger at her son for returning to live with the enemy was clearly a role dispute, yet her binge eating had begun 2 years before his departure (although it clearly worsened after he left). Because neither of these problem areas directly linked to the onset of the eating disorder, Ms. G's therapist decided that the focus of treatment would be to assist her in managing her role transition. Her move back to the United States, with the subsequent loss of her support and friendship networks, was clearly associated with the onset and continued maintenance of her binge eating. During session four of the initial phase, Ms. G's therapist shared her formulation of the problem area with her: "From what you have described, your binge eating really began after you returned to the United States. After that transition, you felt more isolated and alone than you have ever been. It seems that binge eating was a way for you to manage that transition and the subsequent feelings of isolation and loneliness. Your transition has also negatively impacted your relationship with your son. Even though you are a very social person and enjoy the company of others, you have yet to develop the kind of support that you had before you moved. Although you have struggled with some very significant issues throughout your life—your father leaving, the pain of the divorce, and the death of your mother—your friends and support systems sustained you. If we work together to help you find and develop more intimate and supportive relationships here, I believe you will be much less likely to turn to food and binge eating as a source of support or comfort."

Ms. G agreed with the formulation and worked with her therapist to establish some treatment goals to help her resolve the problem area. First, the therapist encouraged her to become more aware of her feelings (notably isolation and loneliness) when she was binge eating and of how binge eating seemed to be the way she managed those feelings. A second goal was for her to take steps to increase her social contacts and develop more friendships. The third goal, which was a secondary problem area, centered on helping Ms. G resolve the role dispute with her son. Specifically, the therapist developed a goal with her to help her establish a clearer parental role with her son.

During the intermediate phase, the therapist helped Ms. G to grieve the loss of her previous role and the extensive support that she once had. Ms. G and her therapist worked to identify several sources of support and friendships of which she had not been aware. Soon after, Ms. G reported significant progress in initiating and establishing relationships with others. This change appeared to help give her confidence in her new roles. In fact, she began to receive a few social invitations. She became more attuned to the ways that she would rely on food, especially when she felt lonely or felt that she was not receiving enough time from others. The connection between the lack of supportive contacts and binge eating was becoming very clear to her in these intermediate sessions. During this phase, the therapist also

assisted her in setting appropriate limits in her relationship with her adult son and in recognizing his adult-like responses in return. By the termination phase, Ms. G reported that she no longer felt so lonely and isolated and that her binge eating had all but disappeared. She remarked how the quality of her relationship with her son had changed dramatically. He was more supportive and respectful, visited more frequently, and stayed with her for more extended periods. In the final sessions, she talked about her need to let go of the past and move on with her life as it is now, assuming her new roles more fully. She worked closely with her therapist to develop a plan to maintain the gains that she made in treatment and used the final session to review the important work that she accomplished. (Courtesy of D. E. Wilfley, Ph.D. and R. W. Guynn, M.D.)

Interpersonal Psychotherapy Delivered in a Group Format.   ITP delivered in a group format has many potential benefits in comparison with individual treatment. For example, a group format based on members' diagnostic similarity (e.g., depression, social phobia, eating disorders) can help alleviate patients' concerns that they are the only one with a particular psychiatric disorder, while offering a social environment for patients who are isolated, withdrawn, or disconnected from others. Given the number and different types of interpersonal interactions in a group setting, the interpersonal skills that develop may be more readily transferable to the patient's outside social life than are the relationship patterns that develop in a one-on-one setting. Moreover, a group modality has therapeutic features not present in individual psychotherapy (e.g., interpersonal learning). The group format also facilitates the identification of problems common to many patients and provides a cost-effective alternative to individual treatment. Table 23-15 links the phases of ITP to the stages of group development.

TIMELINE AND STRUCTURE OF TREATMENT.   The typical course of group ITP lasts 20 sessions over 5 months. The recommended group size ranges from six to nine members, with one or two group leaders, depending on resources and training needs. Three individual meetings (pregroup, midgroup, and postgroup), sequenced to correspond with critical time points in the three phases of ITP, in combination with other techniques, maintain the exclusive and strategic focus on individual patients' interpersonal problem areas—the hallmark of ITP.

Table 23-15
Linking the Phases of Interpersonal Psychotherapy to the Stages of Group Development

Phases/Tasks	Group Stages	Members' Work	Therapist Interventions
Initial: Sessions 1–5; identify problem areas	Engagement: Sessions 1–2	Members look for structure as they grapple with the anxiety of being in a group and sharing their problems	Establish a structure that encourages appropriate self-disclosure; facilitate norms for effective communication
	Differentiations: Sessions 3–5	Members work to manage negative feelings over interpersonal differences as they emerge in the group	Help members to understand their reactions in the context of interpersonal differences in their outside social lives
Middle: Sessions 6–15; work on goals	Work: Sessions 6–15	Members work out differences and strive toward common goals	Facilitate connections among members as they share their work with each other; encourage practice of newly acquired interpersonal skills in and outside of the group
Final: Sessions 15–20; consolidate treatment	Terminations: Sessions 16–20	Members struggle with how to manage the impending loss of connection with other group members	Help members to consolidate their work and to plan continued work; assist members in grieving the loss of the group

Reprinted with permission from Wilfley DE, MacKenzie KR, Welch RR, Ayers VE, Weissman MM. *Interpersonal Psychotherapy for Group*. New York: Basic Books; 2000:20.

PREGROUP MEETING. The pretreatment meeting is crucial for facilitating a patient's individualized work in the first phase of group ITP. The focus of the 2-hour pretreatment meeting is to identify interpersonal problem areas, establish an explicit treatment contract to work on problem areas, and prepare patients for group treatment. After identifying a patient's interpersonal problem(s) (i.e., interpersonal deficits, role disputes, role transitions, or grief), the therapist works collaboratively with the patient to formulate concrete prescriptions for change, in addition to the specific steps the patient will take to improve social relationships and patterns of relating. The therapist expresses these goals of treatment in language that is as specific and personally meaningful to the patient as possible. Before the start of the group, each group member receives a written summary of his or her goals and instructions that these goals will guide his or her work in the group.

Another important element of the pregroup meeting involves adequately preparing patients for group treatment. That is, the therapist encourages patients to think of the group as an "interpersonal laboratory" in which they can experiment with new approaches to handle challenging interpersonal situations. In this regard, patients hear about the important interpersonal skills that they will learn while participating in a group (e.g., interpersonal confrontation, honest communication, expression of feelings) and receive encouragement to learn from others as they see changes occur. The therapist stresses to patients the importance of keeping their work in the group focused on changing their current interpersonal situations or intensifying important existing relationships and not using the group as a substitute social network.

INITIAL PHASE. The first five sessions of the group treatment comprise the initial phase in group ITP. During this phase, the therapist works to cultivate positive group norms and group cohesion, while emphasizing the commonality of symptoms among members and how the group context will address these. During this phase, group members review their goals with the group and begin to make some initial changes in their respective interpersonal problem areas. As members begin to experiment with the changes outlined in their goals, the therapist works collaboratively with each group member to refine and make any alterations in the target areas before the beginning of the intermediate phase.

INTERMEDIATE PHASE. During the intermediate "work" phase of group ITP (sessions 6 through 15), the therapist works to facilitate connections among members as they share the work on their goals with one another. In contrast to other interactive group approaches, the group interpersonal psychotherapist is much less likely to focus on intragroup processes and relationships unless they are specific to the work on a member's interpersonal problem area (e.g., interpersonal deficits). The therapist, however, consistently and continuously encourages group members to practice newly acquired interpersonal skills both inside and, most importantly, outside the group. As is the case with individual ITP, an essential task throughout the intermediate phase is to strengthen the connections the group members make between difficulties in their interpersonal lives and their psychiatric problems.

MIDTREATMENT MEETING. The midtreatment meeting is held midway (usually between sessions 10 and 11) through the intermediate phase. This meeting provides an opportunity to conduct a detailed review of each group member's progress on his or her individual problems and to refine interpersonal goals. The therapist recontracts with group members during this meeting to outline and emphasize the work that remains, both inside and outside of the group, before treatment concludes.

TERMINATION PHASE. In the termination phase (sessions 16 through 20), the therapist discusses termination explicitly with the group members and begins to help them recognize that the end of treatment is a time of possible grief and loss. The therapist helps members recognize their own progress and the progress made by other group members. During this phase, group members describe the specific changes in their psychiatric symptoms, especially as they relate to improvements in the identified problem area(s) and relationships. Although it is common for group members to want to keep meeting on their own or to have frequent reunions, the therapist encourages group members to use this phase of the group to formally say goodbye to one another and the therapist. The therapist also uses this time to encourage members to detail their plans for maintaining improvements in their identified interpersonal problem area(s) and to outline their remaining work.

POSTTREATMENT MEETING. The posttreatment meeting occurs within 1 week after the final group session. The therapist uses this final individual meeting to develop an individualized plan for each group member's continued work on his or her interpersonal goals. The therapist reviews the group experience and the changes the patient has made in his or her interpersonal problem area and significant relationships.

NARRATIVE PSYCHOTHERAPY

More than anything else psychiatrists do, they listen to stories. These stories so saturate the clinical encounter that it would be impossible to imagine a clinical encounter without them. In the very first meeting between psychiatrist and patient, the psychiatrist begins with an open-ended invitation to a story: "*What brings you here?*" or "*What seems to be the problem?*" Patients respond to these questions by telling psychiatrists about their lives, their troubles, when the troubles began, what seems to have caused them, how they create difficulty, and what kinds of problem-solving they have tried. Such stories may be rudimentary, they may be only partially worked out, and they may even be baffled and confused. The patient may also be perplexed enough to answer, "I don't know why I came," or "I'm not really sure what's wrong; my family sent me." Nonetheless, the patient's response to the psychiatrist's initial questions always involves a story.

Narrative psychotherapy emerges out of this increased interest in clinical stories. The two main tributaries that lead to narrative psychotherapy come from the two different sides of psychiatry: narrative medicine and narrative psychotherapy. Narrative psychiatrists are psychiatrists who combine the wisdom of these two domains. Following the lead of narrative medicine, narrative psychiatrists recognize that psychiatric patients, like medical patients, come to clinics with intense stories to tell. Contemporary narrative medicine has developed from 30 years of work in bioethics and medical humanities devoted to humanizing the clinical encounter through a better understanding of patient stories. The term *narrative medicine* comes from Rita Charon, an internist and literary scholar, who used it to describe an approach to medicine that uses narrative approaches to augment scientific understandings of illness. Narrative medicine brings together insights from human-centered medical models, such as George Engel's biopsychosocial model and Eric Cassel's person-centered model, with research and insights from phenomenology, the humanities, and interpretive social sciences.

Narrative medicine uses these resources to understand the illness experience better, "to recognize, absorb, interpret, and be moved by the stories of illness." As Charon argued, when clinicians possess narrative competency, they can enter the clinical setting with a nuanced capacity for "attentive listening…, adopting alien perspectives, following the narrative thread of the story of another, being curious about other people's motives and experiences, and tolerating the uncertainty of stories." She further argued that doctors "*need* rigorous and disciplined training" in narrative reading and writing not just for their own sake (helping them to deal with the strains and traumas of clinical work), but also "*for the sake of their practice.*" Without such narrative competency, clinicians lack the ability to understand their client's experience of illness fully. For Charon and others in narrative medicine, narrative study is not a mere adornment to a doctor's medical training; it is a crucial and basic science that physicians should master for medical practice.

A major task of narrative medicine, and therefore narrative psychotherapy, is to be a good listener and to connect empathically with the patient's story. A narrative psychiatrist, like a narrative physician, seeks to understand the patient first and foremost. This understanding brings patient and clinician together into a shared experience of the patient's world. This narrative understanding is much more than a causal explanation of problem A or problem B that the patient might have. It does not simply abstract from the person's situation a categorical label that groups problems under a well-known abstract grid. Instead, narrative understanding tunes in to the uniqueness of the individual and the unrepeatability of their experience and difficulties. Narrative understanding, in short, is a deep appreciation of the person as a whole—what it feels like for this person, in this particular context, going through these particular problems.

In addition to following the lead of narrative medicine colleagues, narrative psychiatrists also follow the lead of contemporary colleagues in narrative psychotherapy. The history of narrative psychotherapy goes back to Sigmund Freud's early work at the inception of psychoanalysis. At that time, Freud lamented how his case histories sounded more like narrative fiction than hard science.

Contemporary narrative psychotherapy's motivation for returning to the role of narrative comes partly from the broader turn to narrative in humanities, psychology, and social science and partly from the history of psychotherapy since Freud. The past century of psychotherapy has been a century of strife, with one faction after another splitting off from psychoanalysis. Leading alternatives to psychoanalysis included behavioral, humanistic, family, cognitive, feminist, and interpersonal, just to name some. These splits are characterized by further splits within splits, fragmenting the field of psychotherapy to the point of more than 400 approaches to psychotherapy. Narrative approaches emerge at this particular moment as part of an important trend away from further fragmentation and toward psychotherapy reintegration. Narrative approaches are invaluable for psychotherapy integration because they provide a metatheoretical orientation from which to understand and practice psychotherapy.

Metaphor

Metaphor performs this function by allowing us to understand and experience one thing in terms of something else. The metaphor selects, accentuates, and backgrounds aspects of two systems of ideas so that they come to be seen as similar: "Men are seen to be more like wolves after the wolf metaphor is used, and wolves seem to be more human."

In narrative psychotherapy, understanding metaphor connects to broader work in continental linguistic philosophy, and that work, as a whole, attempts to shift standard ideas about truth and objectivity. It sidesteps the binary concepts of relativism (anything goes) and realism (there is only one correct or true way to describe the world). Rather than using the binary distinction between true and false, narrative psychotherapy instead uses a postmodern language of semiotic realism and pluridimensional consequences.

Plot

Plot works like metaphor in that it also orders experiences and provides form for narratives. Plot, or the process of emplotment, adds to metaphor two key dimensions: (1) it brings together what would otherwise be separate and heterogeneous elements, and (2) it organizes understanding and experience or time, or what could be called temporal perception.

The critical function of plot for narrative is that plot creates a narrative synthesis between multiple individual events and brings them together into a single story, making an intelligible connection between them. Remarkably, plot can create a synthesis between events and elements that are surprisingly incongruous or heterogeneous—events that do not seem to fit together.

Plot also configures these multiple elements into a temporal order. This temporal order is of two sorts. First, each plot comprises a discrete series of incidents, of theoretically infinite *nows*. Second, each plot takes these infinite nows, proceeding one after another in succession, and organizes them into a humanly manageable experience.

Character

In narrative theory, the concept of character connects directly to contemporary controversy surrounding the related and, some may argue, more basic concept of identity. The controversy around identity may be understood as a tension between essentialist and nonessentialist approaches. Essentialist notions of identity tell us that each person has a fixed personality, perhaps biologically stamped, that authentically belongs to that person and is at the core of that person's being. This "true self" or "core self" may be distorted or covered over, but it is nonetheless there for the discovery if individuals apply themselves patiently and persistently to the task. Nonessentialist critiques, however, have deconstructed this ideal of identity and its notion of an integral, originary, and unified self. One of the most productive ways to navigate the tension between essentialist and nonessentialist understandings of identity is to draw a comparison between identity (in life) and character (in fiction). Rather than adopting a linear logic that understands identity as a more fundamental concept to character, this approach uses a circular logic to argue that people understand themselves in the same way they understand characters.

Narrative approaches to identity allow people to navigate the tension between essentialist and nonessentialist identities because narrative identity allows for a kind of continuity over time, a relative stability of self, without implying a substantial or essentialist core to this stability. People's interpretations of themselves use the cultural stories surrounding them to tell a story of self that escapes the two poles of random change and absolute identity. In this way, a narrative identity is also a cultural identification. A person's identification may seem original, but he or she narrates them with the resources of history, language, and culture.

Narrative Psychiatry

With this brief introduction to narrative medicine, narrative psychotherapy, and narrative theory, it is possible further to draw out the meaning of narrative for psychiatry.

Fortunately, one of the most helpful aspects of narrative theory for psychiatry is that it provides an overarching, or metatheoretical, rationale for understanding how these many psychotherapies work. From a narrative perspective, all therapies involve a process of storytelling and story retelling. No matter which style of psychotherapy one uses, the process of therapy involves an initial presentation of problems that the client is unable to resolve. The client and therapist work together to bring additional perspectives to these problems, allowing the client to understand them in a new way. These additional perspectives vary greatly depending on the style of psychotherapy used. It matters, in other words, whether the therapy is psychodynamic, cognitive, humanistic, feminist, spiritual, or expressive. From the vantage point of narrative theory, however, what these different approaches all have in common is that they rework, or "reauthor," the patient's initial story into a new story. This new story allows new degrees of flexibility for understanding the past and provides new strategies for moving into the future.

Future Directions

Recent work in narrative medicine, narrative psychotherapy, and narrative theory has opened the door for the development of narrative psychiatry. This development provides a critical corrective to contemporary psychiatric practice that helps self-correct from an overreliance on biologic models without falling into a morass of antipsychiatry and without throwing away the bioscience baby with the bathwater. When psychiatrists take a narrative turn, they do not throw out their other skills and knowledge. The shift to narrative is, as much as anything else, an attitude shift and an opening out to additional sources of information. It starts by bringing to the foreground that the clinical encounter is a human encounter, and it follows by opening out to colleagues in the humanities, interpretive social sciences, and the arts to help to understand this human encounter better.

Most of all, narrative psychotherapy joins with other contemporary efforts in psychiatry—such as the recovery movement—to make clinical encounters much more client-focused and collaborative. Narrative psychotherapy, at its core, recognizes that there are many ways to tell the story of one's life. The choice among these different options is a key way in which people create their identity. These choices should not be reduced to expert choices or scientific choices because they are always also personal and ethical choices. In the end, they are choices about what kind of life one wants to live.

Furthermore, clinicians must come to understand the value of biography, autobiography, and literature for developing a repertoire of narrative frames and options. In the end, narrative competency in psychiatry means a tremendous familiarity with the many possible stories of psychic pain and psychic difference. The more stories clinicians know, the more likely they are to help their clients to find a narrative frame that works for them.

For patients and potential service users, a narrative understanding means that there is a range of possible therapists and healing solutions that might be helpful. An approach that is right for one person may not be right for another. There must be a fit between the person and the approach, and people should feel empowered to take their intuitions and feelings seriously. If the person getting help does not feel this fit, he or she is likely right. There may well be another approach that would work better with the person's proclivities. Like everything else, however, judgment is critical. Therapeutic experiences of all kinds can be frustrating, slow, and uncertain. How, for example, does one know when an approach misses his or her needs and when it is something that will take time, patience, and perseverance to be helpful? From a narrative perspective, there can be no gold standard or simple answers. Only judgment, wisdom, and trial and error can decide.

COMBINED PSYCHOTHERAPY AND PHARMACOTHERAPY

The use of psychotropic drugs, in combination with psychotherapy, has become widespread. It has become the standard of care for many patients seen by psychiatrists. In this therapeutic approach, the use of pharmacologic agents augments psychotherapy. It should not be a system in which the therapist meets with the patient only on an occasional or irregular basis to monitor the effects of medication, to make notations on a rating scale to assess progress, or to assess side effects. Instead, it should be a system in which both therapies are integrated and synergistic. In many cases, studies demonstrate that the results of combined therapy are superior to either type of therapy used alone. The term *pharmacotherapy-oriented psychotherapy* is used by some practitioners to refer to the combined approach. The methods of psychotherapy used can vary immensely, and all can be combined with pharmacotherapy when indicated.

Indications for Combined Therapy

A major indication for using medication when conducting psychotherapy, particularly for those patients with major mental disorders such as schizophrenia or bipolar disorder, is that psychotropics reduce anxiety and hostility. This improves the patient's capacity to communicate and to participate in the psychotherapeutic process. Another indication for combined therapy is to relieve distress when the signs and symptoms of the patient's disorder are so prominent that they require more rapid amelioration than psychotherapy alone may be able to offer. In addition, each technique may facilitate the other; psychotherapy may enable the patient to accept a much-needed pharmacologic agent, and the psychoactive drug may allow the patient to overcome resistance to entering or continuing psychotherapy (Table 23-16).

The reduction of symptoms, especially anxiety, does not decrease the patient's motivation for psychoanalysis or other insight-oriented psychotherapy. In practice, drug-induced symptom reduction improves communication and motivation. All therapies have a cognitive base, and anxiety generally interferes with the patient's ability to gain a cognitive understanding of the illness. Drugs that decrease anxiety facilitate cognitive understanding. They can improve attention, concentration, memory, and learning in patients who suffer from anxiety disorders.

Number of Treating Clinicians

Any number of clinicians can be involved in the treatment of a psychiatric disorder. In *one-person therapy,* the psychiatrist provides

Table 23-16
Benefits of Combined Therapy

Improved medication adherence
Better monitoring of clinical status
Decreased number and length of hospitalizations
Decreased risk of relapse
Improved social and occupational functioning

individual psychotherapy and medication treatment. Multiperson therapy is a form of treatment in which one clinician conducts psychotherapy while the other clinician prescribes medications. Other therapists may oversee marriage or family therapy or group therapy. The terms *cotherapy* or *triangular therapy* also describe permutations of multiperson therapy.

Communication among Therapists

Whenever more than one clinician is involved in treatment, there should be regular exchanges of information. Some patients split the transference between the two; the patient may view one therapist as giving and nurturing and may view the other as withholding and aloof. Similarly, countertransference issues, such as one therapist's identifying with the patient's idealized or devalued image of the other therapist, can interfere with therapy. Therapists must address those issues with the patient, and the cotherapists must be compatible and respectful of each other's orientation so that the therapy program can succeed.

A therapist may have some concerns about the quality of the psychopharmacology or a need to reevaluate the existing regimen. For example, a patient may not be doing well on medication, experiencing significant side effects, or showing a lack of sufficient improvement. Some patients may also be taking many different medications. When and if it is deemed in the patient's interest to question the medication regimen or the prescriber's skill, these misgivings should not be shared with the patient without first conferring with the prescribing physician.

If the therapist or pharmacologist, after a good-faith effort to understand the methods and course of treatment, still has misgivings about treatment, he or she should inform his or her counterpart that a second opinion would be useful. The therapist can then suggest to the patient that he or she consider a second opinion without raising undue alarm. Communication between treating clinicians should take place as frequently as needed. No standard exists for how frequent that should be.

Orientations of Treating Clinicians

The orientation of the treating psychiatrist or other clinician can influence the therapeutic process during combination treatment. Clinicians invariably bring a theoretical bias to the treatment setting. Some, for example, are oriented, by preference and training, to practice a specific form of psychotherapy, such as psychoanalysis, CBT, or group therapy. These clinicians view psychotherapy as the primary treatment modality, with pharmacologic agents being an adjunct to treatment. Conversely, psychopharmacologically oriented psychiatrists view psychotherapy as augmenting the use of medication. Although disagreement may arise on which approach represents the most active ingredient in clinical response, the optimal use of both modalities should complement each other.

In addition to having extensive training in one or more psychoanalytic or psychotherapeutic techniques, the psychiatrist who practices pharmacotherapy-oriented psychotherapy must have a comprehensive knowledge of psychopharmacology. That knowledge must include a thorough understanding of the indications for the use of each drug, the contraindications, the pharmacokinetics and pharmacodynamics, the drug–drug interactions (with all pharmacologic agents, not only the psychoactive agents), and the adverse effects of medications. The psychiatrist must be able both to identify adverse effects and to treat them.

Nonpsychiatric physicians often use psychoactive agents inaccurately (too small or too large a dose for too short or too long a course), because they lack the requisite psychopharmacological knowledge, training, and experience. Psychotherapists who work with primary care physicians instead of psychiatrists should understand the limitations in depth of knowledge that these practitioners have and should seek a consultation with a psychiatrist if a patient is not responding to, or tolerating, medication. In some situations, the same clinician should deliver both psychotherapy and pharmacotherapy; however, this is often not possible for a variety of reasons, including therapist availability, time limitations, and economic restraints, among others.

Therapist Attitudes.   Psychiatrists trained primarily as psychotherapists may prescribe medication more reluctantly than those more oriented toward biologic psychiatry. Conversely, those who view medication as the preferred intervention for most psychiatric disorders may be reluctant to refer patients for psychotherapy. Therapists who are pessimistic about the value of psychotherapy or who misjudge the patient's motivation may prescribe medications because of their own beliefs; others may withhold medication if they overvalue psychotherapy or undervalue pharmacologic treatments. When a patient is in psychotherapy with someone other than the clinician prescribing medication, it is essential to recognize treatment bias and to avoid contentious turf battles that put the patient in the middle of such conflict.

Linkage Phenomenon.   At some point, patients may view the improvement achieved in therapy as the result of a conscious or unconscious linkage between the psychopharmacological agent and the therapist. In fact, after being weaned from medication, patients often carry a pill with them for reassurance. In that sense, the pill acts as a transitional object between the patient and the therapist. Some patients with anxiety disorders, for example, may carry a single benzodiazepine tablet, which they take when they think they are about to have an anxiety attack. Then, the patient may report that the medication aborted the attack—before the medication could even have entered the bloodstream. In other cases, the patient never takes the pill because the patient knows that the pill is available and gains reassurance from that fact. The linkage phenomenon is usually not seen unless the patient is in a positive transference to the therapist. Indeed, the therapist may use this phenomenon to his or her advantage by suggesting that the patient carry medication to use as needed. Eventually, the behavior has to be analyzed, and patients frequently attribute magical properties to the therapist and then transfer those properties to the medication. Some clinicians believe this effect results from conditioning. After repeated trials, the sight of the medicine can decrease anxiety. The positive transference may also cause *transference cure* or *flight into health,* in which the patient feels better in an unconscious attempt to meet the presumed expectations of the prescribing physician. Therapists should consider this phenomenon if the patient reports rapid improvement well before a particular medication may reach its therapeutic level.

Rachel, a 25-year-old woman, presented with depressive symptoms and abdominal pain. After an extensive psychiatric and medical evaluation, she received a diagnosis of major depression of moderate severity and irritable bowel disorder. She began a course of CBT targeting her negative attributional style and low self-esteem, and she learned relaxation and distraction techniques for her pain. After a

12-week trial, she experienced only partial remission of her symptoms, and the psychiatrist offered her an antidepressant, citalopram at 20 mg per day. Her depressive symptoms remitted within 1 month, and she was able to function better at work but socially remained hesitant to engage with her peers. Her abdominal pain persisted, and she began to exhibit a pattern of disordered eating, severely restricting her intake to 500 calories per day due to the "pain." She experienced a 15-lb weight loss over the next several months. An intensive behavioral plan to target eating was begun, as well as continued probing of her negative cognitions relating to eating, pain, and newly emerging concerns that she would regain the weight too quickly and would become "fat." She did not meet the criteria for anorexia nervosa, although her cognitive distortions about her body image were significant. These new concerns resulted in a relapse of her depressive symptoms, including suicidal ideation, and the psychiatrist increased her citalopram to 40 mg/day. She reported severe akathisia on this dose and refused to take any more medication, including an antidepressant of another class. Rachel did agree to intensify her therapy to twice weekly, and this allowed her to explore some of the conflicts, feelings, and thoughts that fostered her treatment-refractory illness. The psychiatrist used a combination of psychotherapy and hypnosis for this work. Over the next 6 months, Rachel revealed a history of sexual abuse as a child, and this made her feel that she did not "deserve" to live or to eat and that the pain served to "punish" her for being bad. She also admitted that she resisted the medication "psychologically" because she felt that she did not deserve to get well. Her newly found insight, as well as the coping skills she developed in therapy, resulted in a reduction of her depressive symptoms, marked improvement in her eating habits with normalization of her weight, and decreased abdominal pain. She maintained these gains over the next year, including the normalization of her daily functioning, a promotion at work, and the ability to tolerate the intimacy of a boyfriend. (Courtesy of E. M. Szigethy, M.D., Ph.D. and E. S. Friedman, M.D.)

Adherence and Patient Education

Adherence.   Adherence is the degree to which a patient carries out the recommendations of the treating physician. A positive doctor–patient relationship fosters adherence, and the patient's refusal to take medication may provide insight into a negative transferential situation. In some cases, the patient acts out hostilities by nonadherence, rather than by becoming aware of, and ventilating, such negative feelings toward the doctor. Medication nonadherence may provide the psychiatrist with the first clue that a negative transference is present in an otherwise adherent patient who had appeared to be agreeable and cooperative.

Education.   Patients should know the target signs and symptoms that the drug is supposed to reduce, the length of time they will be taking the drug, the expected and unexpected adverse effects, and the treatment plan to be followed if the current drug is unsuccessful. Although some psychiatric disorders interfere with patients' abilities to comprehend that information, the psychiatrist should relay as much of the information as possible. The clear presentation of such material is often less frightening than are patients' fantasies about drug treatment. The psychiatrist should tell patients when they may expect to begin receiving benefits from the drug. That information is most critical when the patient has a mood disorder and may not observe any therapeutic effects for 3 to 4 weeks.

Some patients' ambivalent attitudes toward drugs often reflect the confusion about drug treatment that exists in the field of psychiatry. Patients often believe that taking a psychotherapeutic medication means they are not in control of their lives, or they may become addicted to the drug and have to take it forever. Psychiatrists should

explain the difference between drugs of abuse that affect the normal brain and psychiatric medications that treat emotional disorders. They should also point out to patients that antipsychotics, antidepressants, and antimanic drugs are not addictive in the way in which, for example, heroin is addictive. The psychiatrist's straightforward and honest explanation of how long the patient should take the drug helps the patient adjust to the idea of chronic maintenance medication if that is the treatment plan. In some cases, the psychiatrist may appropriately give the patient increasing responsibility for adjusting the medications as the treatment progresses. Doing so often helps the patient feel less controlled by the drug and supports a collaborative role with the therapist.

Attribution Theory

Attribution theory is concerned with how persons perceive the causes of behavior. According to attribution theory, persons are likely to attribute changes in their own behavior to external events but are likely to attribute another's behavior to internal dispositions, such as that person's personality traits. Research on drug effects by attribution theorists has shown that, when patients take medication and their behaviors change, they attribute it to the drug and not to any changes that occur within themselves. Accordingly, it may be unwise to describe a drug as extremely strong or effective, because if it does have the desired effect, the patient may believe that is the only reason he or she got better. If the drug does not work, the patient may assume his or her condition is incurable. Therapists do best by presenting the use of drugs and psychotherapy as complementary or adjunctive, as neither standing alone and both being needed for improvements or cure to occur.

Mental Disorders

Depressive Disorders.   Some patients and clinicians fear that medication covers over the depression and impedes psychotherapy. Instead, clinicians should view medication as a facilitator in overcoming the anergia that can inhibit the communication process between doctor and patient. The psychiatrist should explain to the patient that depression interferes with interpersonal activity in a variety of ways. For instance, depression produces withdrawal and irritability, which alienate significant others who may otherwise gratify the strong dependency needs that make up much of depressive psychodynamics.

When the patient is no longer taking medication, the psychiatrist should be alert for signs and symptoms of a recurrent major depressive episode. The psychiatrist may need to reinstitute medication. Before doing so, however, carefully review any stress, especially rejections, that could have precipitated recurrent major depressive disorder. A new episode of depression may occur because the patient is in a stage of negative transference, and the psychiatrist must try to elicit negative feelings. In many cases, the ventilation of angry feelings toward the therapist without an angry response can serve as a corrective emotional experience and can forestall a major depressive episode necessitating medication. Depressed patients are generally maintained on their medication for 6 months or longer after clinical improvement. The cessation of pharmacotherapy before that time is likely to result in a relapse.

Combined treatment is superior to either therapy used alone in the treatment of major depression. It is associated with improved social and occupational functioning and enhanced quality of life compared with either therapy alone.

Bipolar I Disorder.   Patients taking lithium or other treatments for bipolar I disorder are usually medicated for an indefinite period to prevent episodes of mania or depression. Most psychotherapists insist that patients with bipolar I disorder take medication before starting any insight-oriented therapy. Without such premedication, most patients with bipolar I disorder are unable to make the necessary therapeutic alliance. When those patients are depressed, their abulia seriously disrupts their flow of thoughts, and the sessions are less productive. When they are manic, their flow of associations can be rapid, and their pressured speech can flood the therapist with material and prevent him or her from making appropriate interpretations or assimilating the material into the patient's disrupted cognitive framework.

Combined therapy for bipolar disorder increases adherence, decreases relapse, and reduces the need for hospitalization.

Substance Use Disorders.   Patients with substance use disorders present the most difficult challenge in combined therapy. They are often impulsive, and, although they may promise not to use a substance, they may do so repeatedly. In addition, they frequently withhold information from the psychiatrist about episodes of substance use. For that reason, some psychiatrists do not prescribe any medication to such patients, especially not those substances with high abuse potential, such as benzodiazepines, barbiturates, and amphetamines. Drugs with no abuse potential, such as antidepressants, have an important role in treating the anxiety or depression that frequently accompanies substance-related disorders. The psychiatrist conducting psychotherapy with such patients should have no reservations about sending the patient to a laboratory for random urine toxicologic tests.

Anxiety, Obsessive-Compulsive, and Trauma-Related Disorders.   These disorders encompass OCD, PTSD, generalized anxiety disorder, phobic disorders, and panic disorder with or without agoraphobia. Many drugs are effective in managing distressing signs and symptoms. As the medication controls patients' symptoms, patients are reassured and develop confidence that the disorder will not incapacitate them. That effect is particularly strong in panic disorder, which is often associated with anticipatory anxiety about the attack. Depression can also complicate the symptom picture in patients with anxiety disorders and requires pharmacologic and psychotherapeutic intervention. Studies have shown that patients with anxiety disorders who receive ongoing psychotherapy are less likely to experience relapse compared with patients who receive medication alone.

Schizophrenia and Other Psychotic Disorders.   Included in the group of schizophrenia and other psychotic disorders are schizophrenia, delusional disorder, schizoaffective disorder, schizophreniform disorder, and brief psychotic disorder. Drug treatment for those disorders is always indicated, and hospitalization is often necessary for diagnostic purposes, to stabilize medication, to prevent danger to self or others, and to establish a psychosocial treatment program that may include individual psychotherapy. In attempting individual psychotherapy, the therapist must establish a treatment relationship and a therapeutic alliance with the patient. The patient with schizophrenia defends against closeness and trust and often becomes suspicious, anxious, hostile, or regressed in therapy. Before the advent of psychotropics, many psychiatrists were fearful for their safety when working with such patients. Indeed, many assaults occurred.

Individual psychotherapy for schizophrenia is labor-intensive, expensive, and not often attempted. The recognition that combined psychotherapy and pharmacotherapy have a greater chance of success than either type of therapy alone may reverse that situation. The psychiatrist who conducts such combined therapy must be especially empathic and must be able to tolerate the bizarre manifestations of the illness. The patient with schizophrenia is exquisitely sensitive to rejection, and the therapist should never start individual psychotherapy unless he or she is willing to make a total commitment to the process.

Other Issues

Evidence suggests that therapy can induce physical changes in the nervous system. Eric Kandel has provided elegant proof, winning the Nobel Prize for demonstrating that environmental stimuli produce lasting changes in the synaptic architecture of living organisms. Imaging studies have shown that patients who exhibit clinical improvement from psychotherapy show changes in brain metabolism that are similar to those seen in patients successfully treated with medications.

Still, some patients do well on only one form of treatment. Even with identical diagnoses, not all patients respond to the same treatment regimens. Success may be as dependent on the knowledge and quality of the clinician as on the potential benefit of a particular drug.

A real dilemma when combining treatment is the additional direct costs of two treatments. Although successful treatment results in reduced costs to society, the cost of treatment is usually narrowly defined by the patient as out-of-pocket expenses and by insurance and managed care companies as payments to the physician or hospital. Restrictions placed on the frequency and cost of visits to mental health professionals by managed care organizations, however, encourage the use of medication rather than psychotherapy.

MENTALIZATION-BASED TREATMENT

Mentalizing is the social cognitive ability to understand actions by other people and oneself in terms of mental states, including thoughts, feelings, wishes, and desires; it is a very human capability that underpins everyday interactions. In nontechnical language, it is attentiveness to thinking and feeling in oneself and others. It is beyond question that mental states influence behavior. Beliefs, wishes, feelings, and thoughts, whether within or outside people's awareness, always influence what people do. Mentalizing involves a whole spectrum of capacities: critically, this includes the ability to experience one's *own* behavior as coherently organized by mental states, and to differentiate oneself psychologically from others. Individuals with a personality disorder, who lose cognitive and emotional coherence, particularly at moments of interpersonal (relational) stress, have reduced mentalizing capacities. Mentalization-based treatment (MBT) is a psychotherapy developed for BPD that focuses specifically on the mentalizing vulnerabilities of the patient in the context of an understanding of the attachment process, which is the developmental context in which individuals initially acquire mentalizing.

Techniques

MBT is a group and individual treatment. It is anticipated that, at times, the patient will experience strong affect while focusing on identified problems in treatment sessions, and their mentalizing will be limited or failing, and/or the patient's understanding of the way mental states link to behavior is inadequate.

The clinician addresses this by a structured process (the sessional intervention trajectory) of: (1) empathy and validation about problem areas; (2) clarification, exploration, and where necessary, challenge; (3) following a structured process to gently expand mentalizing and encourage the patient to identify the mental states previously outside their awareness.

The process is primarily in the here and now of the session, but increasingly, as the patient's mentalizing improves, it comes to concern core attachment relationships, including how these are activated with the clinician and key figures in the patient's life and how they influence mentalizing itself. Gradually, improvements in mentalizing serve to enable the patient to address their distorted representations of personal and social relationships.

The assessment and introductory process in MBT facilitates the alliance between patient and clinician (see Table 23-17) and introduces the patient to the treatment frame. An MBT-Introductory group of 10 to 12 sessions assists in the development of the formulation and facilitates the alliance. This psychoeducational intervention covers all areas of mentalizing, attachment processes, personality disorder, emotion management, and the treatment itself. This preparatory work aims to ensure patients know what they are facing in trying to address their problems and are fully aware of the method and focus of treatment.

MBT is collaborative. Nothing can occur without joint discussion, taking into account the mental experiences and ideas of both patient and clinician. The process of mentalizing requires an authentic desire to understand the mental processes of oneself and others. This applies as much to the clinician as to the patient. The therapeutic process has to become a shared endeavor aimed at extending the influence of explicit, reflective, cognitive, internally focused mentalizing. Initial goals, on the road to improved mentalizing, are jointly developed and given focus. The goals cannot solely be those of the patient, although the patient's aims take priority unless they are antithetical to the whole process of treatment. The sharing of responsibility for the therapeutic process is at the core of the effectiveness of the treatment approach in the pursuit of improved mental state understanding.

Assessment involves delineation of the patient's mentalizing vulnerabilities and mentalizing profile, identification of nonmentalizing cycles, and a shared formulation, which includes specific detail of attachment patterns and areas of vulnerability to emotional dysregulation. This has to be understood by the patient and is for both patient and clinician. The formulation identifies common relational fears, for example, abandonment, which stimulate the patient's attachment system and result in the use of maladaptive attachment strategies in interpersonal interactions. In brief, the pattern of the patient's relationships informs an understanding of the relationship in treatment, and the relationship in treatment is used

to reappraise the relationships in life outside treatment. Finally, it is important that the patient and clinician consider establishing a goal of improving social function. This goal will include work, social activity, voluntary work, education, and other constructive life-affirming activity.

Indications

MBT is effective in treatment for severe BPD. Patients in the early studies of the intervention had made serious suicide attempts, been admitted to a psychiatric hospital for risk, and/or had acted on thoughts of self-harm. Trials involved both men and women, and patients showed high levels of comorbidity. Analysis of the data suggested that patients with comorbidity for a number of personality disorders, including antisocial personality disorder, did preferentially better in MBT than comparison treatment. At a clinical level, patients with marked interpersonal problems who have a personality disorder rooted in mentalizing vulnerability and attachment problems may benefit from MBT.

Contraindications

MBT is a generic treatment constructed to optimize access both by creating a low-demand treatment protocol and by facilitating access to training by a range of professionals. Individuals who have problems with mentalizing rooted in nonattachment contexts—for example, those with psychosis—may not benefit from MBT; if they do, the mechanism of change is likely to be different from that in BPD. Individuals with relatively simple problems, such as phobias or uncomplicated depression, may do better with more direct approaches, such as CBT. Even within a population of patients with BPD, patients with more complex presentations (more than one personality disorder diagnosis) are more likely to require MBT than those with a single BPD diagnosis, who may do as well in structured clinical management.

PSYCHOEDUCATIONAL INTERVENTIONS

Psychoeducation is the process of helping individuals to understand a psychiatric illness affecting them or their loved ones. Through this process, patients and/or family members learn about common signs and symptoms of the disease, treatment options, and prognosis for recovery. Psychoeducation moves beyond merely providing information and includes teaching individuals problem-solving skills, coping strategies, support resources, and tools to improve communication. Essentially, psychoeducational interventions provide strategies to support patients and families as they adjust to living with and managing a psychiatric illness.

Psychoeducation can be delivered individually or in a group setting. Interventions can be brief and incorporated into other treatment modalities (e.g., medication management, inpatient hospitalization, outpatient psychotherapy) or they can be structured and take place across several weeks or months. Common areas addressed by psychoeducation include treatment adherence, identifying signs of relapse, lifestyle factors relevant to the illness, and management of crises.

Individuals and families dealing with serious mental illnesses, such as schizophrenia and bipolar disorder, often benefit from psychoeducation. However, psychoeducation may be useful for a variety of disorders, including, for example, major depression, anxiety, autism, dementia, personality disorders, eating disorders, and substance use disorders.

Table 23-17
Alliance Building in MBT

Identification of patient's mentalizing vulnerabilities in an
    understandable form
Formulation of problems—agreed between patient and clinician
Identification of patient's risk profile and crisis management
    strategies
Agreement of short- and long-term goals

Effectiveness of Psychoeducational Interventions

Psychoeducational interventions have been shown to improve outcomes for patients and families, particularly for those dealing with serious or chronic mental illness. A Cochrane review demonstrated that individuals with schizophrenia who participated in psychoeducation had improved medication adherence and lower relapse rates as compared to those without psychoeducational intervention. Individuals with bipolar disorder who participate in psychoeducation are also reported to have improved treatment adherence and reduced relapse, particularly reduced manic/hypomanic relapse. In addition, psychoeducational interventions for depression have been associated with better illness prognosis and reduced psychosocial burden for family members.

References

Psychoanalysis and Psychoanalytic Psychotherapy

Brent BK, Holt DJ, Keshavan MS, Seidman LJ, Fonagy P. Mentalization-based treatment for psychosis: linking an attachment-based model to the psychotherapy for impaired mental state understanding in people with psychotic disorders. *Isr J Psychiatry Relat Sci*. 2014;51(1)17–24.

Buckley P. Revolution and evolution. A brief intellectual history of American psychoanalysis during the past two decades. *Am J Psychother*. 2003;57(1):1–17.

Canestri J. Some reflections on the use and meaning of conflict in contemporary psychoanalysis. *Psychoanal Q*. 2005;74(1):295–326.

Dodds J. Minding the ecological body: Neuropsychoanalysis and ecopsychoanalysis. *Front Psychol*. 2013;4:125.

Joannidis C. Psychoanalysis and psychoanalytic psychotherapy. *Psychoanal Psychother*. 2006;20(1):30–39.

Kandel ER. *Psychiatry, Psychoanalysis, and the New Biology of Mind*. Washington, DC: American Psychiatric Publishing; 2005.

Karasu SR. Psychoanalysis and psychoanalytic psychotherapy. In: Sadock BJ, Sadock VA, Ruiz P, eds. *Kaplan & Sadock's Comprehensive Textbook of Psychiatry*. 10th ed. Philadelphia, PA: Wolters Kluwer; 2017:2638–2675.

Karasu TB. *The Art of Serenity*. New York: Simon and Schuster; 2003.

McWilliams N. *Psychoanalytic Psychotherapy: A Practitioner's Guide*. New York: Guilford; 2004.

Person ES, Cooper AM, Gabbard GO, eds. *The American Psychiatric Publishing Textbook of Psychoanalysis*. Washington, DC: American Psychiatric Publishing; 2005.

Roseneil S. Beyond 'the relationship between the individual and society': broadening and deepening relational thinking in group analysis. *Group Anal*. 2013;46(2):196–210.

Shulman DG. The analyst's equilibrium, countertransferential management, and the action of psychoanalysis. *Psychoanal Rev*. 2005;92(3):469–478.

Siegel E. Psychoanalysis as a traditional form of knowledge: An inquiry into the methods of psychoanalysis. *Int J Appl Psychoanal Stud*. 2006;2(2):146–163.

Strenger C. *The Designed Self: Psychoanalysis and Contemporary Identities*. Hillsdale, NJ: Analytic Press; 2005.

Tummala-Narra P. Psychoanalytic applications in a diverse society. *Psychoanal Psychol*. 2013;30(3):471–487.

Varvin S. Which patients should avoid psychoanalysis, and which professionals should avoid psychoanalytic training?: a critical evaluation. *Scand Psychoanal Rev*. 2003;26(26):109–122.

Brief Psychodynamic Psychotherapy

Beutel ME, Höflich A, Kurth RA, Reimer CH. Who benefits from inpatient short-term psychotherapy in the long run? Patients' evaluations, outpatient after-care and determinants of outcome. *Psychol Psychother*. 2005;78(2):219–234.

Bianchi-DeMicheli F, Zutter AM. Intensive short-term dynamic sex therapy: a proposal. *J Sex Marital Ther*. 2005;31(1):57–72.

Book HE. *How to Practice Brief Psychodynamic Psychotherapy*. Washington, DC: American Psychological Association; 2003.

Davanloo H. *Basic Principles and Technique of Short Term Dynamic Psychotherapy*. New York: Spectrum; 1978.

Fonagy P, Roth A, Higgitt A. Psychodynamic psychotherapies: evidence-based practice and clinical wisdom. *Bull Menninger Clin*. 2005;69(1):1–58.

Heidari S, Lewis AJ, Allahyari A, Azadfallah P, Bertino MD. A pilot study of brief psychodynamic psychotherapy for depression and anxiety in young Iranian adults: The effect of attachment style on outcomes. *Psychoanal Psychol*. 2013;30(3):381–393.

Hersoug AG. Assessment of therapists' and patients' personality: relationship to therapeutic technique and outcome in brief dynamic psychotherapy. *J Pers Assess*. 2004; 83(3):191–200.

Keefe JR, McCarthy KS, Dinger U, Zilcha-Mano S, Barber JP. A meta-analytic review of psychodynamic therapies for anxiety disorders. *Clin Psychol Rev*. 2014; 34(4):309–323.

Leichsenring F, Rabung S, Leibing E. The efficacy of short-term psychodynamic psychotherapy in specific psychiatric disorders: a meta-analysis. *Arch Gen Psychiatry*. 2004;61(12):1208–1216.

McCullough L, Osborn KA. Short term dynamic psychotherapy goes to Hollywood: the treatment of performance anxiety in cinema. *J Clin Psychol*. 2004;60(8): 841–852.

Peretz J. Treating affect phobia: a manual for short-term dynamic psychotherapy. *Psychother Res*. 2004;14(2):261–263.

Powers TA, Alonso A. Dynamic psychotherapy and the problem of time. *J Contemp Psychother*. 2004;34(2):125–139.

Price JL, Hilsenroth MJ, Callahan KL, Petretic-Jackson PA, Bonge D. A pilot study of psychodynamic psychotherapy for adult survivors of childhood sexual abuse. *Clin Psychol Psychother*. 2004;11(6):378–391.

Scheidt CE, Waller E, Endorf K, Schmidt S, König R, Zeeck A, Joos A, Lacour M. Is brief psychodynamic psychotherapy in primary fibromyalgia syndrome with concurrent depression an effective treatment? A randomized controlled trial. *Gen Hosp Psychiatry*. 2013;35(2):160–167.

Svartberg M, Stiles TC, Seltzer MH. Randomized, controlled trial of the effectiveness of short-term dynamic psychotherapy and cognitive therapy for cluster C personality disorders. *Am J Psychiatry*. 2004;161(5):810–817.

Trujillo M. Intensive short-term dynamic psychotherapies. In: Sadock BJ, Sadock VA, Ruiz P, eds. *Kaplan & Sadock's Comprehensive Textbook of Psychiatry*. 10th ed. Philadelphia, PA: Wolters Kluwer; 2017:2796-2815.

Group Psychotherapy, Combined Individual and Group Psychotherapy, and Psychodrama

Billow RM. Bonding in group: the therapist's contribution. *Int J Group Psychother*. 2003;53(1):83–110.

Burlingame GM, Fuhriman A, Mosier J. The differential effectiveness of group psychotherapy: a meta-analytic perspective. *Group Dynamics Thor Res Prac*. 2003;7(1): 3–12.

Friedman R. Individual or group therapy? Indications for optimal therapy. *Group Anal*. 2013;46(2):164–170.

Higaki Y, Ueda S, Hatton H, Arikawa J, Kawamoto K, Kamo T, Kawasima M. The effects of group psychotherapy in the quality of life of adult patients with atopic dermatitis. *J Psychosom Res*. 2003;55(2):162.

Ogrodniczuk JS, Piper WE, Joyce AS. Treatment compliance in different types of group psychotherapy: exploring the effect of age. *J Nerv Ment Dis*. 2006;194(4): 287–293.

Paparella LR. Group psychotherapy and Parkinson's disease: when members and therapist share the diagnosis. *Int J Group Psychother*. 2004;54(3):401–409; discussion 411–418.

Scheidlinger S. Group psychotherapy and related helping groups today: an overview. *Am J Psychother*. 2004;58(3):265–280.

Segalla R. Selfish and unselfish behavior: scene stealing and scene sharing in group psychotherapy. *Int J Group Psychother*. 2006;56(1):33–46.

Spitz HI. Group psychotherapy. In: Sadock BJ, Sadock VA, Ruiz P, eds. *Kaplan & Sadock's Comprehensive Textbook of Psychiatry*. 10th ed. Philadelphia, PA: Wolters Kluwer; 2017:2735–2748.

Tyminski R. Long-term group psychotherapy for children with pervasive developmental disorders: evidence for group development. *Int J Group Psychother*. 2005; 55(2):189–210.

van der Spek N, Vos J, van Uden-Kraan CF, Breitbart W, Cuijpers P, Knipscheer-Kuipers K, Willemsen V, Tollenaar RA, van Asperen CJ, Verdonck-de Leeuw IM. Effectiveness and cost-effectiveness of meaning-centered group psychotherapy in cancer survivors: protocol of a randomized controlled trial. *BMC Psychiatry*. 2014;14(1):22.

Zoger S, Suedland J, Holgers K. Benefits from group psychotherapy in treatment of severe refractory tinnitus. *J Psychosom Res*. 2003;55:134.

Family Therapy and Couples Therapy

Dattilio FM, Piercy FP, Davis SD. The divide between "evidenced-based" approaches and practitioners of traditional theories of family therapy. *J Marital Fam Ther*. 2014;40(1):5–16.

Goldenberg I, Goldenberg H. *Family Therapy: An Overview*. 6th ed. Pacific Grove, CA: Brooks/Cole; 2004.

Gurman AS. Brief integrative marital therapy. In: Gurman AS, Jacobson NS, eds. *Clinical Handbook of Couple Therapy*. 3rd ed. New York: Guilford; 2003:180.

Gurman AS, Jacobson NS, eds. *Clinical Handbook of Couple Therapy*. 3rd ed. New York: Guilford; 2003.

Johnson SM, Greenman PS. The path to a secure bond: emotionally focused couple therapy. *J Clin Psychol*. 2006;62(5):597–609.

Johnson SM, Whiffen VE, eds. *Attachment Processes in Couple and Family Therapy*. New York: Guilford; 2003.

McGoldrick M, Giordano J, Garcia-Preto N, eds. *Ethnicity and Family Therapy*. 3rd ed. New York: Guilford; 2005.

Nichols MP, Schwartz RC. *Family Therapy: Concepts and Methods*. 6th ed. Boston, MA: Allyn & Bacon; 2004.

Nichols M, Tafuri S. Techniques of structural family assessment: a qualitative analysis of how experts promote a systemic perspective. *Fam Process*. 2013;52(2):207–215.

Snyder DK, Whisman MA, eds. *Treating Difficult Couples*. New York: Guilford; 2003.

Spitz HI, Spitz ST. Family and couples therapy. In: Sadock BJ, Sadock VA, Ruiz P, eds. *Kaplan & Sadock's Comprehensive Textbook of Psychiatry*. 10th ed. Philadelphia, PA: Wolters Kluwer; 2017:2748–2760.

Walker MD. When clients want your help to "pray away the gay": implications for couple and family therapists. *J Fem Fam Ther*. 2013;25(2):112–1134.

Dialectical Behavior Therapy

Bedics JD, Korslund KE, Sayrs JH, McFarr LM. The observation of essential clinical strategies during an individual session of dialectical behavior therapy. *Psychotherapy*. 2013;50(3):454–457.

Brown MZ, Comtois KA, Linehan MM. Reasons for suicide attempts and nonsuicidal self-injury in women with borderline personality disorder. *J Abnorm Psychol*. 2002;111(1):198–202.

Hadjiosif M. From strategy to process: validation in dialectical behaviour therapy. *Counsel Psychol Rev*. 2013;28(1):72–80.

Harned MS, Korslund KE, Linehan MM. A pilot randomized controlled trial of Dialectical Behavior Therapy with and without the Dialectical Behavior Therapy Prolonged Exposure protocol for suicidal and self-injuring women with borderline personality disorder and PTSD. *Behav Res Ther*. 2014;55:7–17.

Krause ED, Mendelson T, Lynch TR. Childhood emotion invalidation and adult psychological distress: the mediating role of inhibition. *Child Abuse Negl*. 2003; 27(2):199–213.

Lynch TL, Morse JQ, Mendelson T, Robins CJ. Dialectical behavior therapy for depressed older adults: a randomized pilot study. *Am J Geriatr Psychiatry*. 2003; 11(1):33–45.

Rizvi SL, Steffel LM, Carson-Wong A. An overview of dialectical behavior therapy for professional psychologists. *Prof Psychol*. 2013;44(2):73–80.

Rosenthal MZ, Rodriguez MA. Dialectical behavior therapy. In: Sadock BJ, Sadock VA, Ruiz P, eds. *Kaplan & Sadock's Comprehensive Textbook of Psychiatry*. 10th ed. Philadelphia, PA: Wolters Kluwer; 2017:2784–2795.

Biofeedback

Enger T, Gruzelier JH. EEG biofeedback of low beta band components: frequency-specific effects on variables of attention and event-related brain potentials. *Clin Neurophysiol*. 2004;115(1):131–139.

Enriquez-Geppert S, Huster RJ, Herrmann CS. Boosting brain functions: improving executive functions with behavioral training, neurostimulation, and neurofeedback. *Int J Psychophysiol*. 2013;88(1):1–16.

Hopko DR, Clark CG, Shorter R. Behavior therapy. In: Sadock BJ, Sadock VA, Ruiz P, eds. *Kaplan & Sadock's Comprehensive Textbook of Psychiatry*. 10th ed. Philadelphia, PA: Wolters Kluwer; 2017:2682–2705.

Manko G, Olszewski H, Krawczynski M, Tlokinski W. Evaluation of differentiated neurotherapy programs for patients recovering from severe TBI and long term coma. *Acta Neuropsychol*. 2013;11(1):9–18.

Mitani S, Fujita M, Sakamoto S, Shirakawa T. Effect of autogenic training on cardiac autonomic nervous activity in high-risk fire service workers for posttraumatic stress disorder. *J Psychosom Res*. 2006;60(5):439–444.

Nanke A, Rief W. Biofeedback in somatoform disorders and related syndromes. *Curr Opin Psychiatry*. 2004;17(2):133–138.

Othmer S, Pollock V, Miller N. The subjective response to neurofeedback. In: Earleywine M, ed. *Mind-Altering Drugs: The Science of Subjective Experience*. New York: Oxford University Press; 2005:345.

Purohit MP, Wells RE, Zafonte R, Davis RB, Yeh GY, Phillips RS. Neuropsychiatry symptoms and the use of mind-body therapies. *J Clin Psychiatry*. 2013;74(6): e520–e526.

Ritz T, Dahme B, Roth WT. Behavioral interventions in asthma: biofeedback techniques. *J Psychosom Res*. 2004;56(6):711–720.

Schoenberg PL, David AS. Biofeedback for psychiatric disorders: a systematic review. *Appl Psychophysiol Biofeedback*. 2014;39(2):109–135.

Schwartz MS, Andrasik F, eds. *Biofeedback: A Practitioner's Guide*. 3rd ed. New York: Guilford; 2003.

Scott WC, Kaiser D, Othmer S, Sideroff SI. Effects of an EEG biofeedback protocol on a mixed substance abusing population. *Am J Drug Alcohol Abuse*. 2005;31(3):455–469.

Seo JT, Choe JH, Lee WS, Kim KH. Efficacy of functional electrical stimulation-biofeedback with sexual cognitive-behavioral therapy as treatment of vaginismus. *Urology*. 2005;66(1):77–81.

Thornton KE, Carmody DP. Electroencephalogram biofeedback for reading disability and traumatic brain injury. *Child Adolesc Psychiatric Clin North Am*. 2005;14(1):137–162, vii.

Yucha C, Gilbert C. *Evidence-Based Practice in Biofeedback and Neurofeedback*. Wheat Ridge, CO: Association for Applied Psychophysiology and Biofeedback; 2004.

Cognitive Therapy

Beck AT, Freeman A, Davis DD. *Cognitive Therapy of Personality Disorders*. 2nd ed. New York: Guilford; 2003.

Beck JS, Hindman R. Cognitive therapy. In: Sadock BJ, Sadock VA, Ruiz P, eds. *Kaplan & Sadock's Comprehensive Textbook of Psychiatry*. 10th ed. Philadelphia, PA: Wolters Kluwer; 2017:2760–2775.

Coelho HF, Canter PH, Ernst E. Mindfulness-based cognitive therapy: evaluating current evidence and informing future research. *J Consult Clin Psychol*. 2007;75(6):1000–1005.

Dobson KS. The science of CBT: toward a metacognitive model of change. *Behav Ther*. 2013;44(2):224–227.

Ehde DM, Dillworth TM, Turner JA. Cognitive-behavioral therapy for individuals with chronic pain: efficacy, innovations, and directions for research. *Am Psychol*. 2014;69(2):153–166.

Hollon SD. Does cognitive therapy have an enduring effect. *Cognit Ther Res*. 2003;27:71–75.

Leahy RL, ed. *Contemporary Cognitive Therapy: Theory, Research, and Practice*. New York: Guilford; 2004.

Mulder R, Chanen AM. Effectiveness of cognitive analytic therapy for personality disorders. *Br J Psychiatry*. 2013;202(2):89–90.

Reinecke MA, Clark DA. *Cognitive Therapy Across the Lifespan: Evidence and Practice*. Cambridge, UK: Cambridge University Press; 2003.

Behavior Therapy

Fjorback LO, Arendt M, Ornbol E, Walach H, Rehfeld E, Schröder A, Fink P. Mindfulness therapy for somatization disorder and functional somatic syndromes: randomized trial with one-year follow-up. *J Psychosom Res*. 2013;74(1):31–40.

Fjorback LO, Carstensen T, Arendt M, Ornbøl E, Walach H, Rehfeld E, Fink P. Mindfulness therapy for somatization disorder and functional somatic syndromes: analysis of economic consequences alongside a randomized trial. *J Psychosom Res*. 2013;74(1):41–48.

Gilbert C. Clinical applications of breathing regulation. Beyond anxiety management. *Behav Modif*. 2003;27(5):692–709.

Hanley GP, Iwata BA, McCord BE. Functional analysis of problem behavior: a review. *J Appl Behav Anal*. 2003;36(2):147–185.

Hans E, Hiller W. Effectiveness of and dropout from outpatient cognitive behavioral therapy for adult unipolar depression: a meta-analysis of nonrandomized effectiveness studies. *J Consult Clin Psychol*. 2013;81(1):75–88.

Harmon-Jones E. Anger and the behavioral approach system. *Pers Indiv Differ*. 2003;35:995–1005.

Harvey AG, Bélanger L, Talbot L, Eidelman P, Beaulieu-Bonneau S, Fortier-Brochu E, Ivers H, Lamy M, Hein K, Soehner AM, Mérette C, Morin CM. Comparative efficacy of behavior therapy, cognitive therapy, and cognitive behavior therapy for chronic insomnia: a randomized controlled trial. *J Consult Clin Psychol*. 2014;82(4):670–683.

Harvey AG, Bryant RA, Tarrier N. Cognitive behaviour therapy for posttraumatic stress disorder. *Clin Psychol Rev*. 2003;23(3):501–522.

Haug TT, Blomhoff S, Hellstrom K, Holme I, Humble M, Madsbu HP, Wold JE. Exposure therapy and sertraline in social phobia: 1-year follow-up of a randomised controlled trial. *Br J Psychiatry*. 2003;182:312–318.

Havermans RC, Jansen ATM. Increasing the efficacy of cue exposure treatment in preventing relapse of addictive behavior. *Addict Behav*. 2003;28(5):989–994.

Hayes SC, Strosahl KD, Wilson KG. *Acceptance and Commitment Therapy: An Experiential Approach to Behavior Change*. New York: Guilford; 2003.

Hopko DR, Clark CG, Shorter R. Behavior therapy. In: Sadock BJ, Sadock VA, Ruiz P, eds. *Kaplan & Sadock's Comprehensive Textbook of Psychiatry*. 10th ed. Philadelphia, PA: Wolters Kluwer; 2017:2682–2705.

Moulds ML, Nixon RD. In vivo flooding for anxiety disorders: proposing its utility in the treatment of posttraumatic stress disorder. *J Anxiety Disord*. 2006;20(4): 498–509.

van der Valk R, van de Waerdt S, Meijer CJ, van den Hout I, de Haan L. Feasibility of mindfulness-based therapy in patients recovering from a first psychotic episode: a pilot study. *Early Intervent Psychiatry*. 2013;7(1):64–70.

Hypnosis

Altshuler KZ, Brenner AM. Other methods of psychotherapy. In: Sadock BJ, Sadock VA, Ruiz P, eds. *Kaplan & Sadock's Comprehensive Textbook of Psychiatry*. 9th ed. Vol. 2. Philadelphia, PA: Lippincott Williams & Wilkins; 2009:2911.

Axelrad AD, Brown DP, Wain HJ. Hypnosis. In: Sadock BJ, Sadock VA, Ruiz P, eds. *Kaplan & Sadock's Comprehensive Textbook of Psychiatry*. 10th ed. Philadelphia, PA: Wolters Kluwer; 2017:2705-2735.

Faymonville ME, Roediger L, Del Fiore G, Delgueldre C, Phillips C, Lamy M, Luxen A, Maquet P, Laureys S. Increased cerebral functional connectivity underlying the antinociceptive effects of hypnosis. *Brain Res Cogn Brain Res*. 2003;17(2):255–262.

Finkelstein S. Rapid hypnotic inductions and therapeutic strategies in the dental setting. *Int J Clin Exp Hypn*. 2003;51(1):77–85.

Ginandes C, Brooks P, Sando W, Jones C, Aker J. Can medical hypnosis accelerate post-surgical wound healing? Results of a clinical trial. *Am J Clin Hypn*. 2003;45(4):333–351.

Gullickson T. Hypnosis and hypnotherapy with children. *PsycCRITIQUES*. 2004.

Liossi C, Hatira P. Clinical hypnosis in the alleviation of procedure-related pain in pediatric oncology patients. *Int J Clin Exp Hypn*. 2003;51(1):4–28.

Montgomery GH, David D, Kangas M, Green S, Sucala M, Bovbjerg DH, Hallquist MN, Schnur JB. Randomized controlled trial of a cognitive-behavioral therapy plus hypnosis intervention to control fatigue in patients undergoing radiotherapy for breast cancer. *J Clin Oncol*. 2014;32(6):557–563.

Patterson DR, Jensen MP. Hypnosis and clinical pain. *Psychol Bull*. 2003;129(4): 495–521.

Ploghaus A, Becerra L, Borras C, Borsook D. Neural circuitry underlying pain modulation: expectation, hypnosis, placebo. *Trend Cogn Sci*. 2003;7(5):197–200.

Raz A, Landzberg KS, Schweizer HR, Zephrani ZR, Shapiro T, Fan J, Posner MI. Posthypnotic suggestion and the modulation of Stroop interference under cycloplegia. *Conscious Cogn*. 2003;12(3):332–346.

Santarcangelo EL, Busse K, Carli G. Frequency of occurrence of the F wave in distal flexor muscles as a function of hypnotic susceptibility and hypnosis. *Brain Res Cogn Brain Res*. 2003;16(1):99–103.

Spiegel D. Negative and positive visual hypnotic hallucinations: attending inside and out. *Int J Clin Exp Hypn*. 2003;51(2):130–146.

Spiegel H, Spiegel D. *Trance and Treatment: Clinical Uses of Hypnosis*. 2nd ed. Washington, DC: American Psychiatric Press; 2004.

Interpersonal Therapy

Binder JL, Betan EJ. Essential activities in a session of brief dynamic/interpersonal psychotherapy. *Psychotherapy*. 2013;50(3):428–432.

Bolton P, Bass J, Neugebauer R, Verdeli H, Clougherty KF, Wickramaratne P, Speelman L, Ndogoni L, Weissman M. Group interpersonal psychotherapy for depression in rural Uganda: a randomized controlled trial. *JAMA*. 2003;289(23):3117–3124.

Gilbert SE, Gordon KC. Interpersonal psychotherapy informed treatment for avoidant personality disorder with subsequent depression. *Clin Case Stud*. 2013;12(2):111–127.

Guynn RW. Interpersonal psychotherapy. In: Sadock BJ, Sadock VA, Ruiz P, eds. *Kaplan & Sadock's Comprehensive Textbook of Psychiatry*. 10th ed. Philadelphia, PA: Wolters Kluwer; 2017:2775–2784.

Huibers MJ, van Breukelen G, Roelofs J, Hollon SD, Markowitz JC, van Os J, Arntz A, Peeters F. Predicting response to cognitive therapy and interpersonal therapy, with or without antidepressant medication, for major depression: a pragmatic trial in routine practice. *J Affect Disord*. 2014:152–154:146–154.

Markowitz JC. Interpersonal psychotherapy for chronic depression. *J Clin Psychol*. 2003;59(8):847–858.

Miller MD, Frank E, Cornes C, Houck PR, Reynolds CF 3rd. The value of maintenance interpersonal psychotherapy (IPT) in older adults with different IPT foci. *Am J Geriatr Psychiatry*. 2003;11(1):97–102.

Spinelli MG, Endicott J. Controlled clinical trial of interpersonal psychotherapy versus parenting education program for depressed pregnant women. *Am J Psychiatry*. 2003;160(3):555–562.

Swartz HA, Frank E, Shear MK, Thase ME, Fleming MA, Scott J. A pilot study of brief interpersonal psychotherapy for depression among women. *Psychiatr Serv*. 2004;55(4):448–450.

Narrative Psychotherapy

Adler JM, Harmeling LH, Walder-Biesanz I. Narrative meaning making is associated with sudden gains in psychotherapy clients' mental health under routine clinical conditions. *J Consult Clin Psychol*. 2013;81(5):839–845.

Alves D, Fernández-Navarro P, Baptista J, Ribeiro E, Sousa I, Gonçalves MM. Innovative moments in grief therapy: the meaning reconstruction approach and the processes of self-narrative transformation. *Psychother Res*. 2014;24(1):25–41.

Boudreau JD, Liben S, Fuks A. A faculty development workshop in narrative-based reflective writing. *Perspect Med Educ*. 2013;1(3):143–154.

Cassel E. The nature of suffering and the goals of medicine. *N Engl J Med*. 1982;306(11):639–645.

Charon R. Narrative and medicine. *N Engl J Med*. 2004;350(9):862–864.

Charon R. Narrative medicine: attention, representation, affiliation. *Narrative*. 2005;13(3):261–270.

Charon R. *Narrative Medicine: Honoring the Stories of Illness*. Oxford, UK: Oxford University Press; 2006.

Frank AW. Narrative psychiatry: how stories can shape clinical practice (review). *Lit Med*. 2012;30(1):193–197.

Gaines A, Schillace B. Meaning and medicine in a new key: trauma, disability, and embodied discourse through cross-cultural narrative modes. *Cult Med Psychiatry*. 2013;37(4):580–586.

Hansen J. From hinge narrative to habit: self-oriented narrative psychotherapy meets feminist phenomenological theories of embodiment. *Philos Psychiatry Psychol*. 2013;20(1):69–73.

Hazelton L. Improving clinical care through the stories we tell. *CMAJ*. 2012;184(10):1178.

Launer J. Narrative diagnosis. *Postgrad Med J*. 2012;88(1036):115–116.

Lewis B. *Moving Beyond Prozac, DSM, and the New Psychiatry: The Birth of Postpsychiatry*. Ann Arbor, MI: University of Michigan Press; 2006.

Lewis B. Narrative psychiatry. In: Sadock BJ, Sadock VA, Ruiz P, eds. *Kaplan & Sadock's Comprehensive Textbook of Psychiatry*. 10th ed. Philadelphia, PA: Wolters Kluwer; 2017:2830–2841.

Teichman Y. Echoes of the trauma: relational themes and emotions in children of Holocaust survivors. *Psychother Res*. 2013;23(1):117–119.

Combined Psychotherapy and Pharmacotherapy

Anton RF, O'Malley SS, Ciraulo DA, Cisler RA, Couper D, Donovan DM, Gastfriend DR, Hosking JD, Johnson BA, LoCastro JS, Longabaugh R, Mason BJ, Mattson ME, Miller WR, Pettinati HM, Randall CL, Swift R, Weiss RD, Williams LD, Zweben A, COMBINE Study Research Group. Combined pharmacotherapies and behavioral interventions for alcohol dependence: the COMBINE study: a randomized controlled trial. *JAMA*. 2006;295(17):2003–2017.

Arean PA, Cook BL. Psychotherapy and combined psychotherapy/pharmacotherapy for late life depression. *Biol Psychiatry*. 2002;52(3):293–303.

Beitman BD, Blinder BJ, Thase ME, Riba M, Safer DL. *Integrating Psychotherapy and Pharmacotherapy: Dissolving the Mind-Brain Barrier*. New York: Norton; 2003.

Blais MA, Malone JC, Stein MB, Slavin-Mulford J, O'Keefe SM, Renna M, Sinclair SJ. Treatment as usual (TAU) for depression: a comparison of psychotherapy, pharmacotherapy, and combined treatment at a large academic medical center. *Psychotherapy (Chic)*. 2013;50(1):110–118.

Brent DA, Birmhaher B. Adolescent depression. *N Engl J Med*. 2002;347:667–671.

Burnand Y, Andreoli A, Kolatte E, Venturini A, Rosset N. Psychodynamic psychotherapy and clomipramine in the treatment of major depression. *Psychiatr Serv*. 2002;53(5):585–590.

Friedman MA, Detweiler-Bedell JB, Leventhal HE, Horne R, Keitner GI, Miller IW. Combination psychotherapy and pharmacotherapy for the treatment of major depressive disorder. *Clin Psychol*. 2004;11(1):47–68.

Karon BP. *Effective Psychoanalytic Therapy of Schizophrenia and Other Severe Disorders*. Washington, DC: American Psychological Association; 2002.

Otto MW, Smits JAJ, Reese HE. Combination psychotherapy and pharmacotherapy for mood and anxiety disorders in adults: Review and analysis. *Clin Psychol*. 2005;12(1):72–86.

Overholser JC. Where has all the psyche gone? Searching for treatments that focus on psychological issues. *J Contemp Psychother*. 2003;33(1):49–61.

Peeters F, Huibers M, Roelofs J, van Breukelen G, Hollon SD, Markowitz JC, van Os J, Arntz A. The clinical effectiveness of evidence-based interventions for depression: a pragmatic trial in routine practice. *J Affect Disord*. 2013;145(3):349–355.

Preskorn SH. Psychopharmacology and psychotherapy: what's the connection? *J Psychiatr Pract*. 2006;12(1):41–45.

Ray WA, Daugherty JR, Meador KG. Effect of a mental health "carve-out" program on the continuity of antipsychotic therapy. *N Engl J Med*. 2003;348(19):1885–1894.

Schmidt NB. Combining psychotherapy and pharmacological service provision for anxiety pathology. *J Cogn Psychother*. 2005;19(4):307.

Szigethy EM, Friedman ES. Combined psychotherapy and pharmacology. In: Sadock BJ, Sadock VA, Ruiz P, eds. *Kaplan & Sadock's Comprehensive Textbook of Psychiatry*. 9th ed. Vol. 2. Philadelphia, PA: Lippincott Williams & Wilkins; 2009:2923.

Szuhany KL, Kredlow MA, Otto MW. Combination psychological and pharmacological treatments for panic disorder. *Int J Cogn Ther*. 2014;7(2):122–135.

Ver Eecke W. In understanding and treating schizophrenia: a rejoinder to the PORT report's condemnation of psychoanalysis. *J Am Acad Psychanal*. 2003;31:11–29.

Mentalization-Based Treatment

Allen JG. *Mentalizing in the Development and Treatment of Attachment Trauma*. London, UK: Karnac Books; 2013.

Allen JG, Fonagy P, Bateman AW. *Mentalizing in Clinical Practice*. Washington, DC: American Psychiatric Publishing; 2008.

Asen E, Fonagy P. Mentalization-based therapeutic interventions for families. *J Fam Ther*. 2012;34(4):347–370.

Bateman AW. Treating borderline personality disorder in clinical practice. *Am J Psychiatry*. 2012;169(6):560–563.

Bateman A, Bolton R, Fonagy P. Antisocial personality disorder: a mentalizing framework. *FOCUS*. 2013;11(2):178–186.

Bateman A, Fonagy P. 8-year follow-up of patients treated for borderline personality disorder: mentalization-based treatment versus treatment as usual. *Am J Psychiatry*. 2008;165(5):631–638.

Bateman A, Fonagy P. Mentalization-based treatment. In: Sadock BJ, Sadock VA, Ruiz P, eds. *Kaplan & Sadock's Comprehensive Textbook of Psychiatry*. 10th ed. Philadelphia, PA: Wolters Kluwer; 2017:2894–2904.

Bateman A, Fonagy P. Randomized controlled trial of outpatient mentalization-based treatment versus structured clinical management for borderline personality disorder. *Am J Psychiatry*. 2009;166(12):1355–1364.

Bateman AW, Fonagy P, eds. *Handbook of Mentalizing in Mental Health Practice*. Washington, DC: American Psychiatric Publishing; 2012.

Bateman A, Fonagy P, eds. *Mentalization-Based Treatment for Personality Disorders: A Practical Guide*. Oxford, UK: Oxford University Press; 2016.

Bateman AW, Gunderson J, Mulder R. Treatment of personality disorder. *Lancet*. 2015;385(9969):735–743.

Bateman A, Krawitz R. *Borderline Personality Disorder: An Evidence-Based Guide for Generalist Mental Health Professionals*. Oxford, UK: Oxford University Press; 2013

Bateman A, O'Connell J, Lorenzini N, Gardner T, Fonagy P. A randomised controlled trial of mentalization-based treatment versus structured clinical management for patients with comorbid borderline personality disorder and antisocial personality disorder. *BMC Psychiatry*. 2016;16(1):304.

Bevington D, Fuggle P, Fonagy P. Applying attachment theory to effective practice with hard-to-reach youth: the AMBIT approach. *Attach Hum Dev*. 2015;17(2):157–174.

Fonagy P, Luyten P. A multilevel perspective on the development of borderline personality disorder. In: Cicchetti D, ed. *Developmental Psychopathology*. 3rd ed. New York: John Wiley & Sons; 2016.

Fonagy P, Luyten P, Allison E. Epistemic petrification and the restoration of epistemic trust: a new conceptualization of borderline personality disorder and its psychosocial treatment. *J Pers Disord*. 2015;29(5):575–609.

Gergely G. Ostensive communication and cultural learning: the natural pedagogy hypothesis. In: Metcalfe J, Terrace HS, eds. *Agency and Joint Attention*. Oxford, UK: Oxford University Press; 2013.

Ha C, Sharp C, Ensink K, Fonagy P, Cirino P. The measurement of reflective function in adolescents with and without borderline traits. *J Adolesc*. 2013;36(6):1215–1223.

National Institute for Health and Clinical Excellence. *Antisocial Personality Disorder: Treatment, Management and Prevention*. London: The British Psychological Society and the Royal College of Psychiatrists; 2010.

Robinson P, Hellier J, Barrett B, et al. The NOURISHED randomised controlled trial comparing mentalisation-based treatment for eating disorders (MBT-ED) with specialist supportive clinical management (SSCM-ED) for patients with eating disorders and symptoms of borderline personality disorder. *Trials*. 2016;17(1):549.

Rossouw TI, Fonagy P. Mentalization-based treatment for self-harm in adolescents: a randomized controlled trial. *J Am Acad Child Adolesc Psychiatry*. 2012;51(12):1304–1313.

Sharp C, Fonagy P. Practitioner review: borderline personality disorder in adolescence—recent conceptualization, intervention, and implications for clinical practice. *J Child Psychol*. 2015;56(12):1266–1288.

Sharp C, Ha C, Carbone C, Kim S, Perry K, Williams L, Fonagy P. Hypermentalizing in adolescent inpatients: treatment effects and association with borderline traits. *J Pers Disord.* 2013;27(1):3–18.

Sharp C, Venta A. Mentalizing problems in children and adolescents. In: Midgley N, Vrouva I, eds. *Minding the Child: Mentalization-Based Interventions with Children, Young People and Their Families.* London, UK: Routledge; 2012.

Psychoeducational Interventions

Bond K, Anderson IM. Psychoeducation for relapse prevention in bipolar disorder: a systematic review of efficacy in randomized controlled trials. *Bipolar Disorder.* 2015;17(4):349–362.

Colom F. Keeping therapies simple: psychoeducation in the prevention of relapse in affective disorders. *Br J Psychiatry.* 2011;198(5):338–340.

Tursi MF, Baes Cv, Camacho FR, Tofoli SM, Juruena MF. Effectiveness of psychoeducation for depression: a systematic review. *Aust N Z J Psychiatry.* 2013;47(11): 1019–1031.

Vreeland B. An evidence-based practice of psychoeducation for schizophrenia: a practical intervention for patients and their families. *Psychiatric Times.* 2012;29(2): 34–40.

Zhao S, Sampson S, Xia J, Jayaram MB. Psychoeducation (brief) for people with serious mental illness. *Cochrane Database Syst Rev.* 2015;4(9): CD010823.

24 ▲

Psychiatric Rehabilitation and Other Interventions

PSYCHIATRIC REHABILITATION

Psychiatric rehabilitation denotes a wide range of interventions designed to help people with disabilities caused by mental illness improve their functioning and quality of life by enabling them to acquire the skills and supports needed to be successful in usual adult roles and the environments of their choice. Normative adult roles include living independently, attending school, working in competitive jobs, relating to family, having friends, and having intimate relationships. Psychiatric rehabilitation emphasizes independence rather than reliance on professionals, community integration rather than isolation in segregated settings for persons with disabilities, and patient preferences rather than professional goals.

Vocational Rehabilitation

In the late 1980s, the emphasis of vocational rehabilitation began to shift to place-and-train models, termed supported employment, which were borrowed from the field of developmental disabilities. According to the federal definition, supported employment involves "competitive work in integrated settings…consistent with the strengths, resources, priorities, concerns, abilities, capabilities, interests, and informed choice of the individuals, for individuals with the most significant disabilities for whom competitive employment has not traditionally occurred; or for whom competitive employment has been interrupted or intermittent as a result of a significant disability." In contrast to other vocational approaches, supported employment programs (a) did not screen people for work readiness but helped anyone who says they wanted to work; (b) did not provide intermediate work experiences, such as prevocational work units, transitional employment, or sheltered workshops; (c) actively facilitated job acquisition, often accompanying clients on interviews; and (d) provided ongoing support once the person is employed.

Antonio is a 45-year-old man who has been a client of a mental health agency for more than 10 years. He attended the rehabilitative day treatment program until it was converted to a supported employment program. His case manager encouraged him to think about the possibility of working part-time. Antonio told his case manager that he could not work because of his schizophrenia and because he was helping to raise his two kids and needed to be home at 3 PM when they returned from school every day. The case manager explained to Antonio that getting a job does not necessarily mean working 40 hours a week and that lots of people in the agency's supported employment program were working in part-time jobs, even jobs that only require a few hours a week.

Antonio agreed to meet one of the employment specialists to discuss the possibility of work. Over the next couple of weeks, the employment specialist met with Antonio several times, read his clinical record, and talked with his case manager and psychiatrist. The employment specialist learned that Antonio loved to drive his car. He also learned that Antonio had attendance problems in past jobs because he felt unappreciated. The employment specialist found Antonio to be a sociable and likable person.

Antonio told the employment specialist that he was willing to do any job. He did not have one specific job in mind. After discussing options with Antonio and with the team, the employment specialist suggested a job at Meals on Wheels as a driver for the lunch delivery. Antonio was hired and loved it right from the start. Absenteeism was never a problem because he liked driving around and knew that people were counting on him for their meals. The hours were perfect (10 AM to 2 PM), so Antonio could be at home when his kids returned from school. He became good friends with the other workers. He told his case manager that it was wonderful to be bringing home a paycheck again. Moreover, best of all, he said, was that his kids saw him going to work just like their friends' dads. (Courtesy of Robert E. Drake, M.D., Ph.D. and Alan S. Bellack, Ph.D.)

Social Skills Rehabilitation

Social dysfunction is a defining characteristic of schizophrenia. People with the illness have difficulty fulfilling social roles, such as worker, spouse, and friend, and they have difficulty meeting their needs when social interaction is required (e.g., negotiating with merchants, requesting assistance to solve problems). Social dysfunction is semi-independent of symptomatology and plays an essential role in the course and outcome of the illness. As shown in Table 24-1, social competence involves three component skills: (1) social perception or receiving skills; (2) social cognition, or processing skills; and (3) behavioral response, or expressive skills. Social perception is the ability to read or decode social inputs accurately, including accurate detection of affect cues, such as facial expressions and nuances of voice, gesture, and body posture, as well as verbal content and contextual information. Social cognition involves an effective analysis of the social stimulus, integration of current information with historical information, and planning an adequate response. *Social problem-solving* is another term to describe this domain.

Methods. The primary modality of social skills training is the role-play of simulated conversations. The trainer first provides instructions on how to perform the skill and then models the behavior to demonstrate its performance. After identifying a relevant social situation in which the skill might be appropriate, the patient engages in role-playing with the trainer. The trainer next provides

Table 24-1
Components of Social Skill

Expressive behaviors
Speech content
Paralinguistic features
Voice volume
Speech rate
Pitch
Intonation
Nonverbal behaviors
Eye contact (gaze)
Posture
Facial expression
Proxemics
Kinesics
Receptive skills (social perception)
Attention to and interpretation of relevant cues
Emotion recognition
Processing skills
Analysis of the situation demands
Incorporation of relevant contextual information
Social problem solving
Interactive behaviors
Response timing
Use of social reinforcers
Turn taking
Situational factors
Social "intelligence" (knowledge of social mores and the demands
of the specific situation)

feedback and positive reinforcement, which are followed by suggestions for how the response can be improved. The sequence of role-playing followed by feedback and reinforcement repeats until the patient can perform the response adequately. Training typically occurs in small groups (six to eight patients), in which case patients each practice role-playing for three to four trials and provide feedback and reinforcement to one another. The therapist tailors the teaching to the individual—for example, a highly impaired group member might simply practice saying "no" to a simple request, whereas a less cognitively impaired peer might learn to negotiate and compromise.

Richard was a single white man first diagnosed with schizophrenia at age 22 when he was in college. He was hospitalized briefly but was unable to return to school and moved back home with his parents. He attended a day treatment program intermittently over the next 6 years before he received a referral for help with getting a job and dating.

Richard had missed out on a critical period of adult development and had never learned dating skills or the social skills needed to get or maintain a job. He was appropriately groomed and did not present himself as a patient, but he seemed quite uncomfortable in social interactions. He scarcely made eye contact, staring at the floor when he spoke, and did not initiate conversation, responding to questions with brief answers.

Richard joined a social skills training group for 3 months with six other patients. The focus of the group was employment skills. Patients were taught critical social skills for getting and maintaining a job, such as how to participate in job interviews; how to approach a supervisor to understand how to do a job or for help with work-related problems; how and when to make requests or explain problems, such as getting to work late because of traffic or needing to leave early to go to a doctor's appointment; and socializing with coworkers. Simultaneously,

Richard enrolled in a supported employment program and worked with a case manager to find a job as a computer support person. He found a 24-hour-per-week job at a small company and continued to attend the skills group, using the sessions to work on interpersonal issues at work, including engaging in casual conversation with coworkers and dealing with unreasonable requests from people.

When the vocational skills group ended, Richard joined a dating group with seven other male and female patients who had similar interests. This group focused on finding someone to date, dating etiquette, asking someone out (or being asked out), appropriate conversation for dates, sexual interactions, and safe sex practices. In addition to role play and discussion, the group shared ideas on how to meet people and what to do on dates.

Richard responded well to treatment. He had maintained the computer job at follow-up, 6 months after he concluded the dating skills group. His case manager also reported that he had a girlfriend, a woman whom he had met at his church group. He had also expressed an interest in enrolling in college classes at night. He was still living at home with his parents, but, for the first time, was seriously considering what he would need to do to move out. (Courtesy of Robert E. Drake, M.D., Ph.D. and Alan S. Bellack, Ph.D.)

Goals. In a treatment setting, there are four major goals of social skills training: (1) improved social skills in specific situations, (2) moderate generalization of acquired skills to similar situations, (3) acquisition or relearning of social and conversational skills, and (4) decreased social anxiety. Learning, however, is tedious or almost nonexistent when patients are floridly ill with positive symptoms and high levels of distractibility.

Some findings limit the applicability of social skills training. It is more challenging to teach complex conversational skills than to teach briefer, more discrete verbal and nonverbal responses in social situations. Because complex behaviors are more critical for generating social support in the community, therapy includes methods to improve the learning and durability of conversational skills. These training methods, focusing on training in social skills and information-processing skills, are discussed below.

Training in Social Perception Skills. There is a need for strategies for training patients in affect and social cue recognition. Patients with chronic psychotic disorders, such as schizophrenia, often have difficulty perceiving and interpreting the subtle affective and cognitive cues that are critical elements of communication. Social perception abilities are considered the first step in effective interpersonal problem solving; difficulties in this area are likely to lead to a cascade of deficits in social behavior. Training skills in social perception address these deficits and help provide a foundation for developing more specific social and coping skills.

Despite attending several social gatherings, Matt felt apart from the rest of the group. He reported that these events seemed like "a jumble of sights and sounds." His therapist, recognizing Matt's difficulty with social perception, gave him a series of questions designed to help him organize and give meaning to the social stimuli he encountered. For example, when Matt was confused about a conversation someone was having with him, he would ask himself, "What is this person's short-term goal? At what level of disclosure should I be? Should I be talking now or listening?" Identifying the rules and goals of a particular social interaction provided a template for Matt to recognize and react to a greater variety of social cues, thus enhancing his behavioral repertoire. (Courtesy of Robert Paul Liberman, M.D., Alex Kopelowicz, M.D., and Thomas E. Smith, M.D.)

INFORMATION-PROCESSING MODEL OF TRAINING. Methods of training that follow a cognitive perspective teach patients to use a set of generative rules that can be adapted for use in various situations. For example, a six-step problem-solving strategy has developed as an outline for helping patients overcome interpersonal dilemmas: (1) adopt a problem-solving attitude, (2) identify the problem, (3) brainstorm alternative solutions, (4) evaluate solutions and pick one to implement, (5) plan the implementation and carry it out, and (6) evaluate the efficacy of the effort and, if ineffective, choose another alternative. Although the step-wise, structured, linear process of problem-solving occurs intuitively, without conscious awareness in normal persons, it can be a useful interpersonal crutch to help cognitively impaired mental patients cope with the information needed to fill their social and personal needs.

Milieu Therapy

The locus of milieu is a living, learning, or working environment. The defining characteristics of treatment are the use of a team to provide treatment and the time the patient spends in the environment. Recent adaptations of milieu therapy include 24-hour-a-day programs situated in community locales frequented by patients, which provide in vivo support, case management, and training in living skills.

Most milieu therapy programs emphasize group and social interaction; peer pressure mediates rules and expectations for normalization of adaptation. When clinical staff views patients as responsible human beings, the patient role becomes blurred. Milieu therapy stresses a patient's rights to goals and to have freedom of movement and informal relationship with staff; it also emphasizes interdisciplinary participation and goal-oriented, clear communication.

Token Economy. The use of tokens, points, or credits as secondary or generalized reinforcers normalizes a mental hospital or day hospital environment with a program mimicking society's use of money to meet instrumental needs. Token economies establish the rules and culture of a hospital inpatient unit or partial hospitalization program, offering coherence and consistency to the interdisciplinary team as it struggles to promote therapeutic progress with challenging patients. These programs are challenging to establish, however, and their widespread dissemination has suffered because of the organizational prerequisites and the additional resources and rewards needed to create a truly positively reinforcing environment.

Cognitive Rehabilitation

Increased recognition of the prevalence and importance of neurocognitive deficits over the past decade has stimulated a growing interest in remediation strategies. Much of the work in this area has focused on psychopharmacological approaches, especially on the new-generation antipsychotics. New-generation medications appear to have a positive effect on neurocognitive test performance. However, the effect size for any of the medications is small to medium, and little evidence indicates that these medications have a clinically meaningful impact on neurocognitive functioning in the community. As a result, a parallel interest has arisen in the potential for *rehabilitation* or *cognitive remediation*. This body of work is distinct from cognitive-behavioral therapy and cognitive therapy, which focus on reducing psychotic symptoms.

Ethical Issues

The ethics of conducting rehabilitation strategies are generally the same as for conducting other psychotherapies. Two issues come up regularly, however: avoiding infantilization and maintaining confidentiality. The first issue concerns the risk of viewing the patient as unable to make adult choices, such as whether to participate in rehabilitation, where to live, whether or not to work, and whether or not to use drugs and alcohol. Although it may be more of a value than an ethical standard, psychiatric rehabilitation assumes that the practitioner and the patient are in a partnership to facilitate recovery and improve quality of life. The basic model involves collaboration and shared decision-making and does not portray the practitioner as an authority or parental figure. When patients make what appear to be bad choices, the practitioner must consider the patient's right to choose and whether the choice is dangerous versus merely not the choice the practitioner would make. If the choice is potentially harmful, a collaborative process of considering alternatives is more likely to produce good quality choices than an authoritative, admonitory approach.

Failure to consider the patient as a partner also leads to violations of confidentiality. Practitioners sometimes assume that they are the primary arbiters of what information to share with parents, other clinicians, and other agencies. In fact, in most circumstances that do not involve the safety of patients or others, the patient should be the arbiter of what information to share with whom. For example, in supported employment, the patients always determine whether to disclose information about their illnesses to employers.

GENETIC COUNSELING

Medical geneticists and specially trained and qualified genetic counselors have traditionally provided genetic counseling to patients in need of such help. Many psychiatrists, however, are also well placed to provide genetic education and counseling because they often have knowledge of their patient's needs and family histories and have ongoing therapeutic relationships. The ideal approach for providing psychiatric genetic counseling is through a multidisciplinary team approach, with collaboration between genetics and mental health professionals. Genetic professionals are available for consultation with psychiatry regarding advanced risk assessment, collection and construction of complicated family medical history (FMH), and the availability and limitations of genomic testing. Precision medicine is evolving to include the use of panels of genetic variants and genome sequencing to assess the origins of conditions in families where multiple individuals are affected, or psychiatric symptoms accompany signs of rare disorders.

Definitions

Genetic counseling is the process of helping people to understand and adapt to the medical, psychological, and familial implications of genetic contributions to disease. According to the National Society of Genetic Counseling, it integrates three factors: (1) interpretation of family and medical histories to assess the chance of disease occurrence or recurrence; (2) education about inheritance, testing, management, prevention, resources, and research; and (3) counseling to promote informed choices and adaptation to the risk or condition. The process aims to minimize distress and facilitate adaptation, to increase one's feeling of personal control, and to facilitate informed decision-making and life planning.

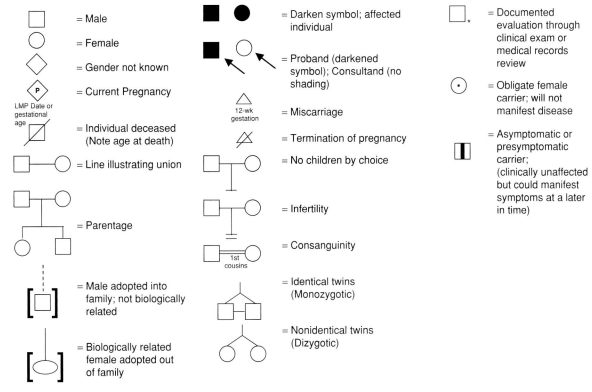

FIGURE 24-1
Standard symbols used in pedigree construction. LMP, last menstrual period.

Although the term *genetic counseling* suggests a primary focus on the genetic contributions to disease, it is not limited to that domain. Genetic counseling entails risk assessment, education, and counseling for common, complex diseases and necessarily considers both *genetic* and *environmental* components of the presenting illness. The growing awareness of the complex interplay between genes and the environment dictates a comprehensive approach to care.

To facilitate comprehension and application of the material in this section, Figure 24-1 demonstrates standard symbols used in pedigree construction, and Figure 24-2 illustrates a complex FMH presented in the form of a pedigree.

Genetics and Psychiatric Disorders

It is widely accepted that psychiatric illnesses tend to run in families (Table 24-2). Disorders can recur in families for several

Table 24-2
Examples of Psychiatric Disorders Recognized as Having a Genetic Component to Their Etiology

Psychotic disorders: Schizophrenia, schizoaffective disorder
Mood disorders: Bipolar disorder, recurrent unipolar depression
Personality disorders: Antisocial personality disorder, schizotypal disorder
Anxiety disorders: Generalized anxiety disorder, obsessive-compulsive disorder, panic disorder, phobia
Substance-related disorders: Substance dependence and abuse
Eating disorders: Anorexia nervosa, bulimia
Childhood disorders: Attention-deficit/hyperactivity disorder, autism, chronic tic disorders, including Tourette syndrome
Memory disorders: Alzheimer disease

reasons, including the functioning of the genome (rarely, due to one genomic variation with a large effect on susceptibility, or more commonly due to multiple variations that each have a small effect on susceptibility) or shared environmental exposures. Thus, genetic counseling for a complex disorder entails discussion around *both* genetic and environmental risk factors. For example, consider a case in which a father with obsessive-compulsive disorder (OCD) has concerns about symptoms developing in his children. Genetic counseling may focus on the following: (1) the family history, indicative of both genetic and shared environmental risk in the family; (2) risk factors for the children, stemming from those genetic and environmental factors; (3) early symptom identification and early intervention (aiming to modify the environment and thus affect genetically mediated disease progression); (4) a discussion of the benefits and limitations of environmental modifications aimed at reducing the risk or minimizing emerging symptoms.

The concept of complex disease (which has replaced *multifactorial* as an etiologic category for common disorders) not only takes into account the interplay of the genome and the environment but also includes the broader biologic and physiologic mechanisms of evolution and development that operate with societies and cultures. The onset of most cases of psychiatric disease, like the onset of other common disorders, is thought to arise when an individual has several risk-increasing genomic variants and has experienced one or more environmental triggers; development, growth, and maturation influence the overall risk. The modern perception that psychiatric symptomatology causes disadvantageous "disease" is related to the effects of the symptoms on the ability of the individual to interact successfully with his or her social and cultural environment.

The first evidence that genetic factors were operating in psychiatric disorders came from the analysis of families with multiple affected members, twin studies, and adoption studies.

FIGURE 24-2
Pedigree of a family with velocardiofacial (VCF) syndrome. ADHD, attention-deficit/hyperactivity disorder; Dx, diagnosed; MR, mental retardation. (From Sadock BJ, Sadock VA, Ruiz P, eds. *Kaplan & Sadock's Comprehensive Textbook of Psychiatry*. 9th ed. Philadelphia: Lippincott Williams & Wilkins; 2009, with permission.)

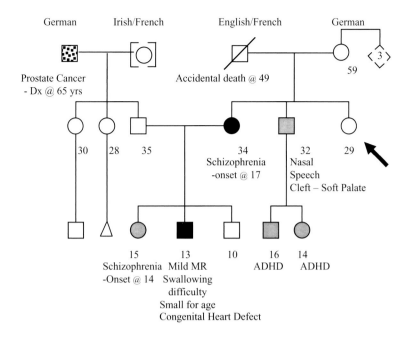

Family Medical History of Sarah Smith
Date Collected: 11/22/2002
Informant: Sarah Smith
Collected by: Jane Doe, MD

Family studies indicated familial etiology, although the relative contributions of genes and environmental factors were unclear. Twin and adoption studies provided insights into the relative contributions of etiologic risk factors, and for all major psychiatric disorders, consistently indicated the importance of genes and environment. Family, twin, and adoption studies also provided insight into the genetic heterogeneity and phenotypic variability of mental disorders.

Priorities of Psychiatric Genetic Counseling

Requests for genetic counseling often arise from the patient's or relatives' questions about the disorder that is present in the family. One can conceptualize the provision of information on the potential genomic origins of the condition and the options for genome testing or assessment of the family as shared decision-making. Patient preference dictates risk assessment and genome testing. It is important to weigh how much the patient prefers to pursue and for what purpose against the estimated likelihood that useful information will come from testing. Table 24-3 outlines the essential components of genetic counseling.

Obtaining the Data Needed for Risk Assessment. The FMH is used to assess the likely etiology of the disorder and estimate risks for recurrence in the family. Confirmation or clarification of the diagnosis or diagnoses in the family is essential to the provision of valid information.

Topics that are specific to psychiatric disorders and are essential to include in the FMH are: (1) any psychiatric diagnosis, whether

Table 24-3
Steps and Process of Genetic Counseling

Solicit and clarify the client's presenting questions and goals for genetic counseling.

Explore client's existing explanation for cause of illness.

Collect and review medical and family medical history.

Identify support systems.

Verify diagnoses in proband and other affected family members when possible.

Address issues and concerns identified through the genetic counseling process.

Assess the client's emotional and intellectual capacity before proceeding to determine the approach to the provision of education and counseling.

Provide information at cognitively appropriate levels.

Note that the processing of emotional reactions is intertwined with the provision of information.

Assess the personal meaning of the information and the client's willingness to negotiate various risks and burdens.

When applicable, assist the client in arriving at a decision by discussing available options; discuss benefits and limitations of each alternative.

Assist the client with adapting to the risk status in the family.

Assist in formulating a plan that the client is able to carry out.

Provide follow-up counseling and support. Continue to assess the client's and family's understanding of the information and the effect of the information, risks, or decisions.

childhood, adult, postpartum, or geriatric; (2) age at symptom onset and diagnosis; (3) subjective assessment of illness severity and treatment response; (4) potentially significant environmental exposures (e.g., obstetrical complications, cannabis use, head injury); (5) symptomatic, undiagnosed individuals or undiagnosed individuals treated with psychiatric medication; (6) developmental history (e.g., has the individual achieved typical milestones for age, such as independent living and employment for adults?); (7) social history; (8) substance abuse; (9) suicide and self-harm; (10) congenital disabilities, intellectual disability or learning disabilities, and unusual medical conditions; (11) the age and sex of at-risk family members.

As mental health providers will be aware, challenges to collecting the psychiatric FMH may include guilt and stigma that limit knowledge of diagnoses among family members, the frequency of undiagnosed psychiatric illness, and the dynamic nature of emerging psychiatric symptoms that may result in diagnostic change over time.

Risk Communication.   Different clients seek different types of risk counseling, and they should be queried about their preferences before risk communication begins. Some may seek broad information about the underpinnings of risk for psychiatric disorders, while others prefer a qualitative discussion of the risk magnitude. These individuals may not welcome or benefit from receiving numerical risk information. For others who prefer a detailed numerical estimation of risk for recurrence, risks based on FMH should be presented as a range to reflect the ambiguity of the estimates. In some cases, it may be possible to suggest that one end of the range is more appropriate for a specific client than midrange.

Psychosocial Counseling and Support

Genetic counseling integrates psychological and social issues that result from living with a psychiatric condition in the family with FMH and increasingly will also include genomic risk information. Historically, genetic counseling has been nondirective, which is deemed particularly appropriate within the context of reproductive decisions and presymptomatic testing for untreatable disorders, such as Huntington disease. However, nondirectiveness is challenging to practice and has been replaced with a person-centered approach, as improved treatments and risk behaviors realize health benefits. The following case exemplifies the personal experiences and meaning of psychiatric disorders.

A couple in their mid-30s with a 10-year history of infertility had been trying to adopt a child for several years. Recently, the adoption agency they were working with told them of a baby who was being placed for adoption because the biologic mother was affected with bipolar disorder and did not feel that she could provide adequate care for the baby. The FMH collected on the newborn baby did not identify others in his family with psychiatric disorders. The recurrence risk for bipolar disorder to the newborn was, therefore, estimated to be between 5 and 20 percent, with additional risks for other psychiatric disorders. The couple individually reacted quite disparately to the estimated risks. In attempting to help them clarify the factors contributing to their feelings regarding the risks, the husband shared his experience with a childhood neighbor who had "some kind of mental illness" and detailed the "torment and agony" that the child brought to the family. Retorting, the woman shared the fact that her coworker also had bipolar disorder and did "just fine" at work with the help of medication. She, therefore, did not feel that the risks for psychiatric disorders were of concern. The

psychiatrist facilitated the couple's discussion of the spectrum and meaning of mental illness, along with recurrence risks in the context of a genetic education and counseling session. Although the couple did not agree during that meeting over the potential for adopting the child, they did feel that the information and sharing of experiences and perspectives about psychiatric disorders were beneficial. They agreed to return in 1 week after further considering the issues to decide on the adoption. (Courtesy of Holly L. Peay, M.S. and Donald W. Hadley, M.S.)

Challenges Posed by Presymptomatic and Susceptibility Genetic Testing

As genomic technologies continue to improve and knowledge about variants that can increase vulnerability for psychiatric illness grows, we will more commonly identify individuals at a higher risk for psychiatric illness. Appropriate applications of such developments need careful consideration from both economic and ethical perspectives but may have critical clinical uses.

Psychiatrists will be on the front line for receiving requests for genetic counseling and testing because of their established relationship between patients and families with psychiatric disorders. The clinical identification of genomic risks will most likely occur before most individuals have access to preventative options. The option of knowing risks without preventative options raises concerns regarding the impact of such knowledge on the individual's mood, anxiety, distress, self-image, reproductive decisions, career decisions, family relationships, insurability, employment, and, potentially, other areas.

Across many disease indications, the majority of persons undergoing genomic testing and receiving their identified risk status do not experience long-term adverse effects. However, those receiving results indicating increased disease risk may experience elevated levels of disease-related anxiety and depression soon after receiving results, and a small number have prolonged difficulty in adjusting to their results. Supportive counseling should be available to facilitate adjustment.

The pursuit of genomic counseling and testing by an individual has clear and profound implications for other family members. Helping the client understand the potential reactions and effect that his or her decision to pursue genomic testing could have on close family members is an important consideration. The health professional can play a role in assisting the client in considering ways to share the information with selected significant others. Similarly, the effect of such information on the spouse or significant other requires consideration.

Ethical, Legal, and Social Considerations

Although there are many benefits of genomics knowledge, scientists and the lay public have worried, from the beginning of genetic research, about the potential for harmful consequences of knowing one's genetic makeup. How will family members, neighbors, communities, employers, health care providers, and insurance companies react to such information? Might health care providers request that those at increased genomic risk take psychiatric medications prophylactically? Might employers limit job opportunities for those with increased risk for psychiatric illness, keeping them in positions with lower levels of stress? Will persons at increased risk be pressured not to have children? Might providing such risk information induce significant enough anxiety/stress to trigger the onset of illness? Furthermore, how will families and the public be educated about the availability of susceptibility testing for psychiatric illness?

Some individuals and families may experience significant levels of stigma associated with the identification of a genetic disorder, a situation already familiar to individuals and families with psychiatric illness. The added knowledge of a hereditary component may heighten stigmatization. Conversely, having an identified, biologic basis may supplant current public perceptions that mental illness is somehow a personal or family failure in moral, spiritual, or attitudinal perspectives.

References

Aatre RD, Day SM. Psychological issues in genetic testing for inherited cardiovascular diseases. *Circ Cardiovasc Genet*. 2011;4(1):81–90.

Alcalay RN, Caccappolo E, Mejia-Santana H, Tang MX, Rosado L, Ross BM, Verbitsky M, Kisselev S, Louis ED, Comella C, Colcher A, Jennings D, Nance MA, Bressman SB, Scott WK, Tanner C, Mickel S, Andrews H, Waters C, Fahn S, Cote L, Frucht S, Ford B, Rezak M, Novak K, Friedman JH, Pfeiffer R, Marsh L, Hiner B, Siderowf A, Ottman R, Marder K, Clark LN. Frequency of known mutations in early-onset Parkinson disease: implication for genetic counseling: the consortium on risk for early onset Parkinson disease study. *Arch Neurol*. 2010;67(9): 1116–1122.

Beattie MS, Copeland K, Fehniger J, Cheung E, Joseph G, Lee R, Luce J. Genetic counseling, cancer screening, breast cancer characteristics, and general health among a diverse population of BRCA genetic testers. *J Health Care Poor Underserved*. 2013;24(3):1150–1166.

Becker DR, Drake RE. *A Working Life for People with Severe Mental Illness*. New York: Oxford University Press; 2003.

Blau G, Surges Tatum D, Goldberg CW, Viswanathan K, Karnik S, Aaronson W. Psychiatric rehabilitation practitioner perceptions of frequency and importance of performance domain scales. *Psychiatr Rehabil J*. 2014;37(1):24–30.

Costain G, Esplen MJ, Toner B, Hodgkinson KA, Bassett AS. Evaluating genetic counseling for family members of individuals with schizophrenia in the molecular age. *Schizophr Bull*. 2014;40(1):88–99.

Drake RE, Bond GR, Ben-Zeev D. Psychiatric rehabilitation. In: Sadock BJ, Sadock VA, Ruiz P, eds. *Kaplan & Sadock's Comprehensive Textbook of Psychiatry*. 10th ed. Philadelphia, PA: Wolters Kluwer; 2017:1531–1538.

Finucane B. Genetic counseling for women with intellectual disabilities. In: LeRoy BS, Veach PM, Bartels DM, eds. *Genetic Counseling Practice: Advanced Concepts and Skills*. Hoboken, NJ: Wiley; 2010;281.

Ganju V. Implementation of evidence-based practices in state mental health systems: implications for research and effectiveness studies. *Schizophr Bull*. 2003;29(1):125–131.

Goldman JS, Hahn SE, Catania JW, Larusse-Eckert S, Butson MB, Rumbaugh M, Strecker MN, Roberts JS, Burke W, Mayeux R, Bird T, American College of Medical Genetics and the National Society of Genetic Counselors. Genetic counseling and testing for Alzheimer disease: joint practice guidelines of the American College of Medical Genetics and the National Society of Genetic Counselors. *Genet Med*. 2011;13(6):597–605.

Hodgson J, Gaff C. Enhancing family communication about genetics: ethical and professional dilemmas. *J Genet Couns*. 2013;22(1):16–21.

Klitzman R, Chung W, Marder K, Shanmugham A, Chin LJ, Stark M, Leu CS, Appelbaum PS. Attitudes and practices among internists concerning genetic testing. *J Genet Couns*. 2013;22(1):90–100.

Lawrence RE, Appelbaum PS. Genetic testing in psychiatry: a review of attitudes and beliefs. *Psychiatry*. 2011;74(4):315–331.

Mitchell PB, Meiser B, Wilde A, Fullerton J, Donald J, Wilhelm K, Schofield PR. Predictive and diagnostic genetic testing in psychiatry. *Psych Clin North Am*. 2010;33(1):225–243.

Monaco LC, Conway L, Valverde K, Austin JC. Exploring genetic counselors' perceptions of and attitudes towards schizophrenia. *Public Health Genomics*. 2010;13(1):21–26.

Moran GS, Nemec PB. Walking on the sunny side: what positive psychology can contribute to psychiatric rehabilitation concepts and practice. *Psychiatric Rehab J*. 2013;36(3):202–208.

Moseley KL, Nasr SZ, Schuette JL, Campbell AD. Who counsels parents of newborns who are carriers of sickle cell anemia or cystic fibrosis? *J Genet Couns*. 2013; 22(2):218–225.

Mueser KT, Noordsy DL, Drake RE, Fox L. *Integrated Treatment for Dual Disorders: Effective Intervention for Severe Mental Illness and Substance Abuse*. New York: Guilford; 2003.

Peay HL, Biesecker BB, Austin JC. Genetic counseling for psychiatric conditions. In: Sadock BJ, Sadock VA, Ruiz P, eds. *Kaplan & Sadock's Comprehensive Textbook of Psychiatry*. 10th ed. Philadelphia, PA: Wolters Kluwer; 2017:2525–2537.

Potokar DN, Stein CH, Darrah OA, Taylor BC, Sponheim SR. Knowledge and attitudes about personalized mental health genomics: narratives from individuals coping with serious mental illness. *Comm Ment Health J*. 2012;48(5):584–591.

Rudnick A, Eastwood D. Psychiatric rehabilitation education for physicians. *Psychiatric Rehab J*. 2013;36(2):126–127.

Twamley EW, Jeste DV, Bellack AS. A review of cognitive training in schizophrenia. *Schizophr Bull*. 2003;29(2):359–382.

Zisman-Ilani Y, Roe D, Flanagan EH, Rudnick A, Davidson L. Psychiatric diagnosis: what the recovery movement can offer the DSM-5 revision process. *Psychosis*. 2013;5(2):144–153.

## 25

Consultation to Other Disciplines

Psychiatrists are often asked to consult with other doctors and health professionals to help with the psychiatric issues in their patients. Consultation-Liaison Psychiatry is devoted to this role. However, several other subspecialties have large consultative roles. These include geriatric psychiatrists, who may work in multidisciplinary settings with diseases that cross all disciplines (such as the dementias) or forensic psychiatrists who consult with other doctors, lawyers, and the courts. Much of the forensic psychiatrists' expertise concerns legal and ethical issues, and we discuss these in Chapters 27 and 28. Psychiatrists also work in the emergency department to help assess and treat psychiatric emergencies. In some larger hospitals, Emergency Psychiatry exists as a separate division with its own location. However, in most hospitals, psychiatrists consult in the general emergency setting. Some child psychiatrists may work in a consultative setting as well, particularly emergency settings. In this chapter, we cover the consultative role of consultation-liaison psychiatrists, geriatric psychiatrists, and both general and child psychiatrists working in the emergency setting.

▲ 25.1 Consultation-Liaison Psychiatry

Consultation-Liaison Psychiatry and the field of Psychosomatic Medicine have been a specific area of concern within psychiatry for more than 50 years. The term *psychosomatic* is derived from the Greek words *psyche* (soul) and *soma* (body). The term refers to how the mind affects the body. Unfortunately, it has come to be used, at least by the lay public, to describe an individual with medical complaints that have no physical cause and are "all in your head." For this and related reasons, in 2018, the Academy of Psychosomatic Medicine changed its name to the Academy of Consultation-Liaison Psychiatry. Before that, the DSM deleted the nosologic term psychophysiological (or psychosomatic) disorders and replaced it with psychological factors affecting physical conditions.

Nonetheless, the term continues to be used by researchers and is in the title of significant journals in the field (e.g., *Psychosomatic Medicine,* and the *Journal of Psychosomatic Research*). It is also used by some major national organizations in the field (the American Psychosomatic Society) as well as international organizations (e.g., the European Association for Consultation-Liaison Psychiatry and Psychosomatics). In 2003 the American Board of Medical Specialties and the American Board of Psychiatry and Neurology approved the specialty of Psychosomatic Medicine and in 2017 they changed the name to Consultation-Liaison psychiatry.

HISTORY

As Edward Shorter discusses in detail in his summary of the history of psychosomatic illness, ways of presenting illness vary over history because patients unconsciously select symptoms that are thought to represent actual somatic illnesses. Psychosomatic presentations have thus varied throughout recent history. Before 1800, physicians did not conduct clinical evaluations and could not distinguish somatic from psychogenic illness. As a result, the diagnoses of hysteria and hypochondriasis could easily be made in the presence of genuine medical illnesses and did not suggest any specific disease.

Sigmund Freud helped to bring psyche and soma together. He demonstrated the importance of emotions in producing mental disturbances and somatic disorders. His early psychoanalytic formulations detailed the role of psychic determinism in somatic conversion reactions. Using Freud's insight, several workers in the early decades of the 20th century tried to expand the understanding of the interrelationship of psyche and soma. Karl Abraham proposed the influence on adult organ tissue of various unresolved pregenital impulses in 1927. Sándor Ferenczi described the application of the idea of conversion reaction to organs under the control of the autonomic nervous systems in 1926, and Georg Groddeck suggested the attaching of symbolic meaning to fever and hemorrhage in 1929.

The field of consultation-liaison psychiatry has existed for many decades, and George W Henry described the practice in the United States in the 1920s. Divisions of consultation-liaison psychiatry began springing up in various academic departments, as did fellowship programs. The American Board of Psychiatry and Neurology offered the first examination for the subspecialty in 2005.

In Europe, particularly in Germany, pioneers such as Thure von Uexküll saw psychosomatic medicine more broadly, and not merely a subspecialty of psychiatry. The field was understood as central to the concept of all medical diseases. Diseases were conceived as being multifactorial, with both organic and psychological etiologies. It is notable that in Europe, most departments of psychosomatic medicine are independent of departments of psychiatry.

CURRENT TRENDS

The practice of Consultation-Liaison psychiatry has evolved considerably since its early clinical origins and has come to focus on psychiatric illnesses that occur in the setting of physical health care. In large part, this evolution has occurred as a result of the increased complexity of medicine, the increased understanding of the relationship of medical illness to psychiatric illness, and the greater appreciation of mind and body as one. Clinical care is now

Table 25-1
Summary of Clinical Problems in Psychosomatic Medicine

Type of Clinical Problem	Example
Psychiatric symptoms secondary to medical conditions	Delirium, dementia
Psychiatric symptoms as a reaction to medical conditions or treatments	Anxiety related to chemotherapy, depression related to limb amputation
Psychiatric complications of medical conditions and treatments	Depression secondary to interferon treatment
Psychological factors precipitating medical symptoms	Somatic Symptom and related disorders
Medical complications of psychiatric conditions or treatments	Neuroleptic malignant syndrome, acute withdrawal from alcohol or another substance
Co-occurring medical and psychiatric conditions	Recurrence of depressive disorder in the setting of cancer treatment (conditions occur independently); schizophrenia in a patient with end-stage renal disease
Psychiatric/psychosocial assessment	Capacity evaluation; evaluation prior to organ transplantation

delivered in a variety of health care settings and utilizes an ever-expanding set of diagnostic tools, as well as many effective somatic and psychotherapeutic interventions. Research in the area has progressed to include a greater understanding of the relationship between chronic medical conditions and psychiatric disorders. It has examined the pathophysiologic relationships, the epidemiology of comorbid medical and psychiatric disorders, and the role that specific interventions play in physiologic, clinical, and economic outcomes (Table 25-1).

Psychiatric morbidity is prevalent in patients with medical conditions, with a prevalence ranging from 20 to 67 percent, depending on the illness and setting. Patients in the general hospital have the highest rate of psychiatric disorders when compared with community samples or patients in ambulatory primary care. For example, compared with community samples, depressive disorders in the general hospital are more than twice as prevalent, and substance abuse is two to three times as common. Delirium occurs in 18 percent of patients. Similarly, increased rates are seen in primary and long-term care.

Psychiatric morbidity has severe effects for medically ill patients and is often a risk factor for their medical conditions. It is well established that depression is both a risk factor and a poor prognostic indicator in coronary artery disease. Psychiatric illness worsens cardiac morbidity and mortality in patients with a history of myocardial infarction, diminishes glycemic control in patients with diabetes, and decreases return to functioning in patients experiencing a stroke. Depressive and anxiety disorders compound the disability associated with stroke. In the context of neurodegenerative diseases such as Parkinson's or Alzheimer's, depression, psychosis, and behavioral disturbances are significant predictors of functional decline, institutionalization, and caregiver burden. Hospitalized patients with delirium are significantly less likely to improve in function compared with patients without delirium. Delirium is

associated with worse outcomes after surgery, even after controlling for the severity of medical illness.

Also, depression and other mental disorders significantly impact the quality of life and the ability of patients to adhere to treatment regimens (e.g., in patients with diabetes mellitus or cancer). Psychiatric disorders are linked to nonadherence with antiretroviral therapy, adversely affecting the survival of human immunodeficiency virus (HIV)-infected patients. Psychiatric disorders are also linked to nonadherence with safe sex guidelines and with the use of sterile needles in HIV-infected injection drug users, thus having significant public health implications.

EVALUATION PROCESS IN PSYCHOSOMATIC MEDICINE

Psychiatric assessment in the medical setting includes a standard psychiatric assessment as well as a particular focus on the medical history and context of physical health care. In addition to obtaining a complete psychiatric history, including history, family history, developmental history, and a review of systems, the medical history and current treatment should be reviewed and documented. A full mental status examination, including a cognitive examination, should be completed, and components of a neurologic and physical examination may be indicated depending on the nature of the presenting problem.

Another essential objective of the psychiatric evaluation is to gain an understanding of the patient's experience of his or her illness. In many cases, this becomes the central focus for both the psychiatric assessment and interventions. It is often helpful to develop an understanding of the patient's developmental and personal history as well as critical dynamic conflicts, which in turn may help to make the patient's experience with illness more comprehensible. Such an evaluation can include the use of the concepts of stress, personality traits, coping strategies, and defense mechanisms. Observations and hypotheses that are developed can help to guide a patient's psychotherapy aimed at diminishing distress and may also be helpful for the primary medical team in their interactions with the patient.

Finally, a full report synthesizing the information should be completed and include specific recommendations for additional evaluations and intervention. Ideally, the report should be accompanied by a discussion with the referring physician.

TREATMENTS USED IN PSYCHOSOMATIC MEDICINE

A host of interventions have been successfully utilized in psychosomatic medicine. Specific consideration must be given to medical illness and treatments when making recommendations for psychiatric medications. Psychotherapy also plays a vital role in psychosomatic medicine and may vary in its structure and outcomes as compared with therapy that occurs in mental health practice.

Psychopharmacologic recommendations need to consider several essential factors. In addition to targeting a patient's active symptoms, considering the history of illness and treatments, and weighing the particular side-effect profile of a particular medication, several other factors must be considered that relate to the patient's medical illness and treatment. It is critical to evaluate potential drug–drug interactions and contraindications to the use of potential psychiatric agents. Because the majority of psychiatric medications used are metabolized in the liver, awareness of liver function is essential. General appreciation of side effects, such as weight gain, risk of developing diabetes, and cardiovascular risk, must be considered in the choice of medications. Also, it is critical to incorporate knowledge of recent data that outlines the effectiveness and specific risks involved for patients with co-occurring psychiatric and physical disorders. For example, a greater understanding of the side effects of antipsychotic medications has raised concerns about the use of these medications in patients with dementia.

The use of psychosocial interventions also requires adaptation when used in this population. The methods and the goals of psychosocial interventions used in the medically ill are often determined by the consideration of disease onset, etiology, course, prognosis, treatment, and understanding of the nature of the presenting psychiatric symptoms in addition to an understanding of the patient's existing coping skills and social support networks. However, there are ample data that psychosocial interventions are effective in addressing a series of identified problems and that such interventions, in many cases, are associated with a variety of positive clinical outcomes.

Common C-L Problems

Suicide Attempt or Threat.   Suicide rates are higher in persons with medical illness than in those without medical or surgical problems. High-risk factors for suicide are men over 45 years of age, no social support, alcohol dependence, previous suicide attempt, and incapacitating or catastrophic medical illness, especially if accompanied by severe pain. If suicide risk is present, the patient should be transferred to a psychiatric unit or started on 24-hour nursing care.

Depression.   Suicidal risk must be assessed in every depressed patient. Depression without suicidal ideation is not uncommon in hospitalized patients, and treatment with antidepressant medication can be started if necessary. A careful assessment of drug–drug interactions must be made before prescribing, which should be undertaken in collaboration with the patient's primary physician.

Agitation.   Agitation is often related to the presence of a cognitive disorder or associated with withdrawal from drugs (e.g., opioids, alcohol, sedative-hypnotics). Antipsychotic medications may be beneficial for excessive agitation. Physical restraints should be used with great caution and only as a last resort as sedation is preferable and safer. The patient should be examined for command hallucinations or paranoid ideation to which they are responding in an agitated manner. Toxic reactions to medications that cause agitation should always be ruled out.

Hallucinations.   A common cause of hallucinations in the general hospital setting is delirium tremens, which usually begin 3 to 4 days after hospitalization. Patients in intensive care units (ICUs) who experience sensory isolation may respond with hallucinatory activity. Conditions such as brief psychotic disorder, schizophrenia, and neurocognitive disorders are associated with hallucinations, and they respond rapidly to antipsychotic medication. Fornication, in which the patient believes that bugs are crawling over the skin, is often associated with cocaine use.

Sleep–Wake Disorders.   A common cause of insomnia in hospitalized patients is pain, which, when treated, solves the sleep problem. Early morning awakening is associated with depression, and difficulty falling asleep is associated with anxiety. Depending on the cause, antianxiety or antidepressant agents may be prescribed. Early substance withdrawal as a cause of insomnia should be considered in the differential diagnosis.

Confusion.   Delirium is the most common cause of confusion or disorientation among hospitalized patients in general hospitals. The causes are myriad and relate to metabolic status, neurologic findings, substance abuse, and mental illness, among many others. Small doses of antipsychotics may be used when significant agitation occurs in conjunction with the confused state; however, sedatives, such as benzodiazepines, can worsen the condition and cause sundowner syndrome (ataxia, disorientation). If sensory deprivation is a contributing factor, the environment can be modified so that the patient has sensory cues (e.g., radio, clock, no curtains around the bed). Table 25-2 lists the probable causes of confusional states that require urgent attention.

Noncompliance or Refusal to Consent to Procedure.   The relationship between the patient and their doctor may be a critical underlying factor when patients are noncompliant or refuse to consent to a procedure. A negative transference toward the physician is a common cause of noncompliance. Patients who fear medication or a procedure may respond to education and reassurance. Patients whose refusal to give consent is related to impaired judgment can be declared incompetent, but only by a judge. The leading cause of impaired judgment in hospitalized patients is cognitive disorders.

No Physiologic Basis for Symptoms.   The C-L psychiatrist is often called when the physician cannot find evidence of medical or surgical disease to account for the patient's symptoms. In these instances, several psychiatric conditions must be considered, including conversion disorder, somatization disorder, factitious disorders, and malingering. Glove and stocking anesthesia with autonomic nervous system symptoms is seen in conversion disorder; multiple bodily complaints are present in somatization disorder; the wish to be in the hospital occurs in factitious disorder, and apparent secondary gain is observed in patients who are malingering (e.g., compensation cases).

C-L Psychiatry in Special Situations

Intensive Care Units.   All ICUs deal with patients who experience anxiety, depression, and delirium. ICUs also impose extraordinarily high stress on staff and patients, which is related to the intensity of the problems. Patients and staff members alike frequently observe cardiac arrests, deaths, and medical disasters, which leave them all autonomically aroused and psychologically defensive. ICU nurses and their patients experience exceptionally high levels of anxiety and depression. As a result, nurse burnout and high turnover rates are frequent.

The problem of stress among ICU staff receives much attention, especially in the nursing literature. Much less attention is given to the house staff, especially those on the surgical services. All persons in ICUs must be able to deal directly with their feelings about their extraordinary experiences and challenging emotional and physical circumstances. Regular support groups in which persons can discuss their feelings are recommended for the ICU staff and the house staff. Such support groups protect staff members from the otherwise predictable psychiatric morbidity that some may experience and also protect their patients from the loss of concentration, decreased energy, and psychomotor-retarded communications that some staff members otherwise exhibit.

Table 25-2
Some Clues to Causes of Delirium Demanding Urgent Attention

Metabolic Disorders

1. Hypoglycemia: history of diabetes or alcoholism; reduced level of consciousness, shaky, sweaty, perhaps combative
2. Hyperglycemia: history of diabetes; complaints of increased thirst, urination, or flulike symptoms
3. Hyponatremia: underlying illness like lung cancer, recent stroke, chronic pulmonary infections, heart failure, cirrhosis, diuretic use
4. Hypernatremia: dehydration from inadequate fluid intake or excessive fluid loss without replacement
5. Hypercalcemia: underlying disorder such as cancer metastatic to bone, sarcoidosis, lung and renal cell cancer, multiple myeloma, and/or prolonged immobilization
6. Hypoxia: inadequate oxygen supplied to the brain because of poor pulmonary or cardiac function or carbon monoxide poisoning
7. Hypercarbia: history of chronic lung disease characterized by carbon dioxide retention; may use oxygen at home
8. Hepatic encephalopathy: history of chronic liver disease or alcoholism; probably jaundiced; ascites
9. Uremia: history of kidney disease, enlarged prostate, recent inability to pass urine
10. Thiamine deficiency (Wernicke encephalopathy): variable degrees of ophthalmoplegia, ataxia, and mental disturbance; history of nutritional deficiency secondary to alcoholism, particularly of thiamine; since remaining thiamine in the body is rapidly used when the patient is given intravenous glucose, any patient with alcoholism should immediately receive intramuscular thiamine before glucose infusion to prevent precipitating this encephalopathy; untreated, the disorder rapidly progresses to a permanent memory disorder (Korsakoff syndrome) and, in some advanced cases, death
11. Hypothyroidism: history of progressive fatigue, constipation, sensitivity to cold, weight gain, coarsening of hair and skin, mental slowing; examination shows abnormally low temperature and enlarged heart and slow pulse; may be precipitated by the effects of lithium on thyroid function
12. Hyperthyroidism: patient may be either hyperactive or apathetic; history may reveal rapid weight loss, diarrhea, heat intolerance, and emotional instability; examination shows goiter, silky fine hair, warm moist skin, proptosis and wide-eyed stare, fine tremor, rapid or irregular pulse; in elderly patients, muscle weakness and heart failure may be most apparent

Systemic Illness

1. Decreased cardiac output from various causes, such as congestive heart failure, arrhythmia, pulmonary embolus, and myocardial infarction; acute myocardial infarction presents with confusion as the major symptom in 13% of elderly patients; aged patients do not complain of typical pain; often they complain of indigestion; vital signs may be abnormal, and patient may look ill (ashen coloring, weak, nauseated, sweaty) and be confused
2. Pneumonia: recent history of a cold, becoming bedridden and aspirating; fever may not be apparent, but tachycardia or hypotension are evident on vital signs
3. Urinary tract infection: especially in patients with indwelling urinary catheters, prostatic hypertrophy, diabetes, neurogenic bladder
4. Anemia: especially with acute blood loss (injury, intestinal bleeding), chronic illness, occult gastrointestinal malignancy
5. Acute surgical emergencies: infarction of the bowel, appendicitis, and volvulus are common and often present only with confusion and no other complaints
6. Hypertension: sustained or rapid increase in blood pressure may cause encephalopathy; often has history of elevated blood pressure; may occur in patient on MAO inhibitor antidepressants who has eaten food containing tyramine
7. Vasculitides: e.g., systemic lupus erythematosus; confusion arises from cerebral involvement or treatment with steroids
8. Any febrile illness and infection can cause confusion in the aged

Central Nervous System Disorders

1. Subdural or epidural hematoma: may or may not have history of head trauma; fluctuating mental status often present; may have no focal neurologic signs
2. Seizure: unwitnessed seizure may be suggested if patient was found on floor with evidence of incontinence or vomiting; history of seizure disorder or alcoholism
3. Stroke: history of transient ischemic attacks or strokes; may have no signs except confusion
4. Infection: meningitis (bacterial, fungal, or tuberculous), viral encephalitis
5. Tumor, primary or metastatic: with a growing mass, raised intracranial pressure may cause local compression of vital structures or herniation of the brain; in the elderly, brain atrophy allows for greater space inside the skull so that symptoms may not appear until the mass is quite large
6. Normal pressure hydrocephalus: presents with triad of gait disturbance, incontinence, dementia; surgery may be curative

Drugs and Medication

1. Almost all drugs are capable of causing confusion in the elderly; the most commonly implicated drugs include those with strong anticholinergic effects (antidepressants, antipsychotics, and antiparkinsonian drugs, and many over-the-counter preparations), sedative-hypnotics (barbiturates, benzodiazepines), cardiac medications (digoxin, propranolol, lidocaine, quinidine), antihypertensives, anticonvulsants, cimetidine, nonnarcotic and narcotic analgesics, and corticosteroids
2. Alcohol: intoxication and withdrawal syndromes occur as in young patients, but poor health in the elderly may put geriatric patients at greater risk
3. Drug abuse: far less common in elderly persons, but chronic intoxication with bromides, prescription tranquilizers occurs

From Minden SL. Elderly psychiatric emergency patients. In: Bassuk EL, Birk AW, eds. *Emergency Psychiatry*. New York: Plenum; 1984:360, with permission.

Hemodialysis Units. Hemodialysis units present a paradigm of complicated modern medical treatment settings. Patients are coping with lifelong, debilitating, and limiting disease; they are dependent on a multiplex group of caretakers for access to a machine controlling their well-being. Dialysis is scheduled three times a week and takes 4 to 6 hours; thus, it disrupts patients' previous living routines.

In this context, patients first and foremost fight the disease. Invariably, however, they also must come to terms with a level of dependence on others probably not experienced since childhood. Predictably, patients entering dialysis struggle for their independence; regress to childhood states; show denial by acting out against doctor's orders (by breaking their diet or by missing sessions); show anger directed against staff members; bargain and plead; or become infantilized and obsequious; however, most often they are accepting and courageous. The determinants of patients' responses to entering dialysis include personality styles and previous experiences with this or another chronic illness. Patients who have time to react and adapt to their disease are less challenged by the need to adapt to new circumstances. Those with recent renal failure and machine dependence may have more difficulty.

Although little has been written about social factors, the effects of culture in reaction to dialysis and the management of the dialysis unit are known to be necessary. Units are run with a firm hand, which is consistent in dealing with patients; clear contingencies are in place for behavioral failures; and adequate psychological support is available for staff members, which tend to produce the best results.

Complications of dialysis treatment can include psychiatric problems, such as depression, and suicide is not rare. Sexual problems can be neurogenic, psychogenic, or related to gonadal dysfunction and testicular atrophy. Dialysis dementia is a rare condition that includes loss of memory, disorientation, dystonias, and seizures. The disorder occurs in patients who have been receiving dialysis treatment for many years. Although not entirely understood, the leading cause is probably aluminum toxicity, and reducing dialysate aluminum levels and minimizing aluminum intake decreases the incidence of the disease. Chelating agents, such as deferoxamine, may also help if given early. However, it should be used sparingly because of its serious adverse effects.

The psychological treatment of dialysis patients falls into two areas. First, careful preparation before dialysis, including the work of adaptation to chronic illness, is essential, especially in dealing with denial and unrealistic expectations. Before dialysis, all patients should have a psychosocial evaluation. Second, once in a dialysis program, patients need periodic specific inquiries about adaptation that do not encourage dependence or the sick role. Staff members should be sensitive to the likelihood of depression and sexual problems. Group sessions function well for support, and patient self-help groups restore a useful social network, self-esteem, and self-mastery. When needed, antidepressants can be used for dialysis patients. Psychiatric care is most effective when brief and problem-oriented.

The use of home dialysis units has improved attitudes toward treatment. Patients treated at home can integrate the treatment into their daily lives more efficiently, and they feel more autonomous and less dependent on others for their care than do those who are treated in the hospital.

Surgical Units. Some surgeons believe that patients who expect to die during surgery are more likely to die. This belief now seems less superstitious than it once did. Some patients who are scheduled for surgery and show evident depression or anxiety but deny it have a higher risk for morbidity and mortality than those who can express it. Even better results occur in those with a positive attitude toward impending surgery. The factors that contribute to an improved outcome for surgery are informed consent and education so that patients know what they can expect to feel, where they will be (e.g., it is useful to show patients the recovery room), what loss of function to expect, what tubes and gadgets will be in place, and how to cope with the anticipated pain. If patients will not be able to talk or see after surgery, it is helpful to explain before surgery what they can do to compensate for these losses. If postoperative states such as confusion, delirium, and pain can be predicted, they should be discussed with patients in advance, so they do not experience them as unwarranted or as signs of danger. Constructive family support members can help both before and after surgery.

Transplantation Issues. Transplantation programs have expanded over the past decade, and C-L psychiatrists play an essential role in helping patients and families deal with the many psychosocial issues involved: (1) which and when patients on a waiting list will receive organs, (2) anxiety about the procedure, (3) fear of death, (4) organ rejection, and (5) adaptation to life after successful transplantation. After the transplant, patients require complicated aftercare, and achieving compliance with medication may be difficult without supportive psychotherapy. This challenge is particularly relevant to patients who have received liver transplants as a result of hepatitis C brought on by promiscuous sexual behavior and patients with a history of substance use disorder who used contaminated needles.

Group therapy with patients who have had similar transplantation procedures benefits members who can support one another and share information and feelings about particular stressors related to their disease. Groups may be conducted or supervised by the psychiatrist. Psychiatrists must be especially concerned about psychiatric complications. Within 1 year of transplant, almost 20 percent of patients experience major depression or an adjustment disorder with depressed mood. In such cases, evaluation for suicidal ideation and risk is essential. In addition to depression, another 10 percent of patients experience signs of posttraumatic stress disorder, with nightmares and anxiety attacks related to the procedure. Other issues concern whether or not the transplanted organ came from a cadaver or from a living donor who may or may not be related to the patient. Pretransplant consulting sessions with potential organ donors help them to deal with fears about surgery and concerns about who will receive their donated organ. Sometimes, both the recipient and donor may be counseled together, as with a family member donating a kidney. Peer support groups with both donors and recipients have also been used to facilitate coping with transplantation issues.

PSYCHO-ONCOLOGY

Psycho-oncology seeks to study both the impact of cancer on psychological functioning and the role that psychological and behavioral variables may play in cancer risk and survival. A hallmark of psycho-oncology research has been intervention studies that attempt to influence the course of illness in patients with cancer. A landmark study by David Spiegel found that women with metastatic breast cancer who received weekly group psychotherapy survived an average of 18 months longer than control patients randomly assigned to routine care. In another study, patients with malignant melanoma who received structured group intervention exhibited a statistically significant lower recurrence of cancer and a lower mortality rate than patients who did not receive such therapy. Patients with malignant melanoma who received the group intervention also exhibited significantly more large granular lymphocytes and natural killer (NK) cells as well as indications of increased NK cell activity, suggesting an increased immune response. Another study used a group behavioral intervention (relaxation, guided imagery, and biofeedback training) for patients with breast cancer, who demonstrated higher NK cell activity and lymphocyte mitogen responses than the controls.

Because new treatment protocols, in many cases, have transformed cancer from an incurable to frequently chronic and often curable disease, the psychiatric aspects of cancer—the reactions to both the diagnosis and the treatment—are increasingly important. At least half of the persons who contract cancer in the United States each year are alive 5 years later. Currently, an estimated 3 million cancer survivors have no evidence of the disease.

About half of all cancer patients have mental disorders. The largest groups are those with adjustment disorder (68 percent), and major depressive disorder (13 percent) and delirium (8 percent) are the next most common diagnoses. Most of these disorders are thought to be reactive to the knowledge of having cancer.

When persons learn that they have cancer, their psychological reactions include fear of death, disfigurement, and disability; fear of abandonment and loss of independence; fear of disruption in relationships, role functioning, and financial standings; and denial, anxiety, anger, and guilt. Although suicidal thoughts and wishes are frequent in persons with cancer, the actual incidence of suicide is only slightly higher than that in the general population.

Psychiatrists should make a careful assessment of psychiatric and medical issues in every patient. Particular attention should be given to family factors, in particular, preexisting intrafamily conflicts, family abandonment, and family exhaustion.

▲ 25.2 Geriatric Psychiatry

PSYCHIATRIC PROBLEMS OF OLDER PERSONS

Despite the ubiquity of loss in old age, the prevalence of major depressive disorder and dysthymia is less than in younger age groups. Several explanations for this phenomenon have been proposed: rarity of late-onset depression, higher mortality among persons with depression, and a general decrease in disorders caused by emotional upheavals or substance abuse in older persons. Depression may, however, be underrecognized in the elderly as it sometimes presents differently than in younger persons. Depression in old persons is often accompanied by physical symptoms or cognitive changes that may mimic dementia.

The incidence of suicide among older persons is high (40 per 100,000 population) and is highest for older white men. The suicide of older persons is perceived differently by surviving friends and family members based on gender: men are thought to have been physically ill, and women are thought to have been mentally ill.

The relation between good mental and good physical health is apparent in older persons. Adverse effects on the course of chronic medical illness are correlated with emotional problems.

MENTAL DISORDERS OF OLD AGE

The National Institute of Mental Health's Epidemiologic Catchment Area (ECA) program found that the most common mental disorders of old age are depressive disorders, cognitive disorders, phobias, and alcohol use disorders. Older adults also have a high risk of suicide and drug-induced psychiatric symptoms. Many mental disorders of old age can be prevented, ameliorated, or even reversed. Of particular importance are the reversible causes of delirium and dementia; if not diagnosed accurately and treated in a timely fashion, however, these conditions can progress to an irreversible state. Table 25-3 lists the general cognitive domains assessed in neuropsychological evaluation, with the tests used to measure that skill and a description of the specific behaviors measured by each test. The tests listed in the table constitute a comprehensive test battery generally appropriate for use with a geriatric population. The use of a comprehensive battery is preferable for confident determination of the presence and type of dementia or other cognitive disorder in elderly persons; in some

Table 25-3
Cognitive Domains

Gross Cognitive Functioning
  Mini-Mental State Examination: *orientation, repetition, following commands, naming, constructional skill, written expression, memory, mental flexibility, and calculations*

Intelligence
  Wechsler Adult Intelligence Scale-Revised (WAIS-R) or Wechsler Intelligence Scale-III (WAIS-III): *verbal and nonverbal intelligence*

Basic Attention
  WAIS-R or WAIS-III Digit Span: *repetition of digits forward and backward*

Information-Processing Speed
  WAIS-R or WAIS-III Digit Symbol: *rapid graphomotor tracking*
  Trailmaking Part A: *rapid graphomotor tracking*
  Stroop A and B: *rapid word reading and color naming*

Motor Dexterity
  Finger tapping: *right and left index finger dexterity*

Language
  Boston Naming Test: *word retrieval*
  WAIS-R or WAIS-III Vocabulary: *vocabulary range*

Visual Perceptual/Spatial
  WAIS-R or WAIS-III Picture Completion: *visual perception*
  WAIS-R or WAIS-III Block Design: *constructional ability*
  Rey–Osterrieth Complex Figure Test: *paper-and-pencil copy of complex design*
  Beery Developmental Test of Visual Motor Integration: *paper-and-pencil copy of simple-to-complex designs*

Learning and Memory
  An 8- to 10-item word list learning task: *learning and recall of rote verbal information*
  Wechsler Memory Scale-Revised (WMS-R) or Wechsler Memory Scale-III (WMS-III)
    Logical Memory subtest: *immediate and delayed recall of paragraph information*
    Visual Reproduction subtest: *immediate and delayed recall of visual designs*
  Rey–Osterrieth Complex Figure Test and Recognition Trial: *3-minute immediate recall and 30-minute delayed recall of a complex design*

Executive Functions
  Trailmaking Part B: *rapid alternation between tasks*
  Stroop C: *inhibition of an overlearned response*
  Wisconsin Card Sorting Test: *categorization and mental flexibility*
  Verbal fluency (FAS and category): *rapid word generation*
  Design fluency: *rapid generation of novel designs*

Courtesy of Kyle Brauer Boone, Ph.D.

circumstances, however, administering a several-hour battery is not possible.

Several psychosocial risk factors also predispose older persons to mental disorders. These risk factors include loss of social roles, loss of autonomy, the deaths of friends and relatives, declining health, increased isolation, financial constraints, and decreased cognitive functioning.

Many drugs can cause psychiatric symptoms in older adults. These symptoms can result from age-related alterations in drug absorption, a prescribed dosage that is too large, not following instructions and taking too large a dose, sensitivity to the medication, and conflicting regimens presented by several physicians. Drugs can cause almost the entire spectrum of mental disorders.

Dementing Disorders

Only arthritis is a more common cause of disability among adults age 65 and older than dementia, a generally progressive and irreversible impairment of the intellect, the prevalence of which increases with age. About 5 percent of persons in the United States older than age 65 have severe dementia, and 15 percent have mild dementia. Of persons older than age 80, about 20 percent have severe dementia. Known risk factors for dementia are age, family history, and female sex.

In contrast to intellectual disability, the intellectual impairment of dementia develops over time—that is, previously achieved mental functions are lost gradually. The characteristic changes of dementia involve cognition, memory, language, and visuospatial functions, but behavioral disturbances are common as well and include agitation, restlessness, wandering, rage, violence, shouting, social and sexual disinhibition, impulsiveness, sleep disturbances, and delusions. Delusions and hallucinations occur during the dementias in nearly 75 percent of patients.

Cognition is impaired by many conditions, including brain injuries, cerebral tumors, acquired immune deficiency syndrome (AIDS), alcohol, medications, infections, chronic pulmonary diseases, and inflammatory diseases. Although dementias associated with advanced age typically are caused by primary degenerative central nervous system (CNS) disease and vascular disease, many factors contribute to cognitive impairment; in older persons, mixed causes of dementia are common.

About 10 to 15 percent of all patients who exhibit symptoms of dementia have potentially treatable conditions. The treatable conditions include systemic disorders, such as heart disease, renal disease, and congestive heart failure; endocrine disorders, such as hypothyroidism; vitamin deficiency; medication misuse; and primary mental disorders, most notably depressive disorders.

Depending on the site of the cerebral lesion, dementias are classified as cortical and subcortical. Subcortical dementia occurs in Huntington disease, Parkinson disease, normal pressure hydrocephalus, vascular dementia, and Wilson disease. The subcortical dementias are associated with movement disorders, gait apraxia, psychomotor retardation, apathy, and akinetic mutism, which can be confused with catatonia. Table 25-4 lists some potentially reversible conditions that may resemble dementia. The cortical dementias occur in dementia of the Alzheimer type, Creutzfeldt–Jakob disease (CJD), and Pick disease, which frequently manifests aphasia, agnosia, and apraxia. In clinical practice, the two types of dementias overlap, and, in most cases, an accurate diagnosis can be made only by autopsy. Human prion diseases result from coding mutations in the prion protein gene (*PRNP*) and may be inherited, acquired, or sporadic. They include familial CJD, Gerstmann–Sträussler–Scheinker syndrome, and fatal familial insomnia. These are inherited as autosomal-dominant mutations. The acquired diseases include kuru and iatrogenic CJD. Kuru was an epidemic prion disease of the Fore people of Papua, New Guinea, caused by cannibalistic funeral rituals, which peaked in incidence in the 1950s. Iatrogenic disease is rare and is caused, for example, by the use of contaminated dura mater and corneal grafts and treatment with human cadaveric pituitary-derived growth hormone and gonadotropin. Sporadic CJD accounts for 85 percent of the human prion diseases and occurs worldwide, with a uniform distribution and an incidence of about 1 in 1 million per annum, with a mean age at onset of 65 years. It is exceedingly rare in individuals under 30 years of age.

Depressive Disorders

Depressive symptoms are present in about 15 percent of all older adult community residents and nursing home patients. Age itself

Table 25-4
Some Potentially Reversible Conditions that May Resemble Dementia

Substance
  Anticholinergic agents
  Antihypertensives
  Antipsychotics
  Corticosteroids
  Digitalis
  Narcotics
  Nonsteroidal anti-inflammatory agents
  Phenytoin
  Polypharmacotherapy
  Sedative hypnotics

Psychiatric Disorders
  Anxiety
  Depression
  Mania
  Delusional disorders

Metabolic and Endocrine Disorders
  Addison disease
  Cushing syndrome
  Hepatic failure
  Hypercarbia (chronic obstructive pulmonary disease)
  Hypernatremia
  Hyperparathyroidism
  Hyperthyroidism
  Hypoglycemia
  Hyponatremia
  Hypothyroidism
  Renal failure
  Volume depletion

Miscellaneous Conditions
  Fecal impaction
  Hospitalization
  Impaired hearing or vision

Courtesy of Gary W. Small, M.D.

is not a risk factor for the development of depression, but being widowed and having a chronic medical illness are associated with vulnerability to depressive disorders. High rates of recurrence characterize late-onset depression.

The common signs and symptoms of depressive disorders include reduced energy and concentration, sleep problems (especially early morning awakening and multiple awakenings), decreased appetite, weight loss, and somatic complaints. The presenting symptoms may be different in older depressed patients from those seen in younger adults because of an increased emphasis on somatic complaints in older persons. Older persons are particularly vulnerable to major depressive episodes with melancholic features, characterized by depression, hypochondriasis, low self-esteem, feelings of worthlessness, and self-accusatory trends (especially about sex and sinfulness) with paranoid and suicidal ideation. A geriatric depression scale is given in Table 25-5.

Cognitive impairment in depressed geriatric patients is referred to as depression-related cognitive dysfunction (sometimes misleadingly called pseudodementia), which can be confused easily with nonreversible dementias. In common dementias such as that caused by Alzheimer disease, intellectual performance usually is global, and impairment is consistently poor; in depression-related cognitive dysfunction, deficits in attention and concentration are variable. Compared with patients who have neurodegenerative dementias,

Table 25-5
Geriatric Depression Scale (Short Version)

Answers indicating depression are boldfaced. Each answer counts one point; scores greater than 5 indicate probable depression.

1. Are you basically satisfied with your life?	Yes/**No**
2. Have you dropped many of your activities and interests?	**Yes**/No
3. Do you feel that your life is empty?	**Yes**/No
4. Do you often get bored?	**Yes**/No
5. Are you in good spirits most of the time?	Yes/**No**
6. Are you afraid that something bad is going to happen to you?	**Yes**/No
7. Do you feel happy most of the time?	Yes/**No**
8. Do you often feel helpless?	**Yes**/No
9. Do you prefer to stay at home, rather than going out and doing new things?	**Yes**/No
10. Do you feel you have more problems with memory than most?	**Yes**/No
11. Do you think it is wonderful to be alive now?	Yes/**No**
12. Do you feel pretty worthless the way you are now?	**Yes**/No
13. Do you feel full of energy?	Yes/**No**
14. Do you feel that your situation is hopeless?	**Yes**/No
15. Do you think that most people are better off than you are?	**Yes**/No

Special Instructions. The scale can be used as a self-rating or observer-rated metric. It has also been used as an observer-rated scale in mildly demented subjects.

From Yesavage JA. Geriatric depression scale. *Psychopharmacol Bull.* 1988;24:709, with permission.

patients with depression-related cognitive dysfunction are less likely to have language impairment and to confabulate; when uncertain, they are more likely to say "I don't know"; and their memory difficulties are more limited to free recall than to recognition on cued recall tests. Depression-related cognitive dysfunction occurs in about 15 percent of depressed older patients, and 25 to 50 percent of patients with neurodegenerative dementias are depressed.

Schizophrenia

Schizophrenia usually begins in late adolescence or young adulthood and persists throughout life. Although the first episodes diagnosed after age 65 are rare, a late-onset type beginning after age 45 has been described. Women are more likely to have a late onset of schizophrenia than men. Another difference between early-onset and late-onset schizophrenia is the greater prevalence of paranoid schizophrenia in the late-onset type. About 20 percent of persons with schizophrenia show no active symptoms by age 65; 80 percent show varying degrees of impairment. Psychopathology becomes less marked as patient's age.

The residual type of schizophrenia occurs in about 30 percent of persons with schizophrenia. It primarily presents with negative symptoms, including emotional blunting, social withdrawal, eccentric behavior, and illogical thinking. Delusions and hallucinations are uncommon. Because most persons with residual schizophrenia cannot care for themselves, long-term hospitalization is required.

Older persons with schizophrenic symptoms respond reasonably well to antipsychotic drugs. Medication must be administered judiciously, and lower-than-usual dosages often are useful for older adults.

Delusional Disorder

The age of onset of delusional disorder usually is between ages 40 and 55, but it can occur at any time during the geriatric period. Delusions can take many forms; the most common are persecutory—patients believe that they are being spied on, followed, poisoned, or harassed in some way. Persons with delusional disorder may become violent toward their supposed persecutors. Some persons lock themselves in their rooms and live reclusive lives. Somatic delusions, in which persons believe they have a fatal illness, also can occur in older persons. In one study of persons older than 65 years of age, pervasive persecutory ideation was present in 4 percent of persons sampled.

Among those who are vulnerable, delusional disorder can occur under physical or psychological stress. The death of a spouse can precipitate it, loss of a job, retirement, social isolation, adverse financial circumstances, debilitating medical illness or surgery, visual impairment, and deafness. Delusions also can accompany other disorders—such as dementia of the Alzheimer type, alcohol use disorders, schizophrenia, depressive disorders, and bipolar I disorder—which need to be ruled out. Delusional syndromes also can result from prescribed medications or be early signs of a brain tumor. The prognosis is fair to good in most cases; the best results are achieved through a combination of psychotherapy and pharmacotherapy.

Persecutory delusions characterize a late-onset delusional disorder called *paraphrenia*. It develops over several years and is not associated with dementia. Some workers believe that the disorder is a variant of schizophrenia that first becomes manifest after age 60. Patients with a family history of schizophrenia show an increased rate of paraphrenia.

Anxiety Disorders

Anxiety disorders usually begin in early or middle adulthood, but some appear for the first time after age 60. The initial onset of panic disorder in older persons is rare but can occur. The ECA study determined that the 1-month prevalence of anxiety disorders in persons age 65 and older is 5.5 percent. By far, the most common disorders are phobias (4 to 8 percent). The rate for panic disorder is 1 percent.

The signs and symptoms of phobia in older adults are less severe than those that occur in younger persons, but the effects are equally, if not more, debilitating for older patients. Existential theories help explain anxiety when no specifically identifiable stimulus exists for a chronically anxious feeling. Older persons must come to grips with death. The person may deal with the thought of death with a sense of despair and anxiety, rather than with equanimity and Erikson's "sense of integrity." The fragility of the autonomic nervous system in older persons may account for the development of anxiety after a significant stressor. Because of concurrent physical disability, older persons react more severely to PTSD than younger persons.

Obsessive-Compulsive Disorders

Obsessions and compulsions may appear for the first time in older adults, although older adults with obsessive-compulsive disorder

(OCD) usually had demonstrated evidence of the disorder (e.g., being orderly, perfectionistic, punctual, parsimonious) when they were younger. When symptomatic, patients become excessive in their desire for orderliness, rituals, and sameness. They may become generally inflexible and rigid and have compulsions to check things again and again. OCD (in contrast to obsessive-compulsive personality disorder) is characterized by ego-dystonic rituals and obsessions and may begin late in life.

Somatic Symptom Disorders

Disorders characterized by physical symptoms resembling medical diseases are relevant to geriatric psychiatry because somatic complaints are common among older adults. More than 80 percent of persons over 65 years of age have at least one chronic disease—usually arthritis or cardiovascular problems. After age 75, 20 percent have diabetes, and an average of four diagnosable chronic illnesses that require medical attention.

Hypochondriasis is common in persons over 60 years of age, although the peak incidence is in those 40 to 50 years of age. The disorder usually is chronic, and the prognosis guarded. Repeated physical examinations help reassure patients that they do not have a fatal illness, but invasive and high-risk diagnostic procedures should be avoided unless medically indicated.

Telling patients that their symptoms are imaginary is counterproductive and usually engenders resentment. Clinicians should acknowledge that the complaint and pain are real to the patient, and a psychological or psychopharmacological approach to the problem is indicated.

Alcohol and Other Substance Use Disorder

Older adults with alcohol dependence usually give a history of excessive drinking that began in young or middle adulthood. They usually are medically ill, primarily with liver disease, and are either divorced, widowed, or are men who never married. Many have arrest records and are numbered among homeless persons. A large number have a chronic dementing illness, such as Wernicke encephalopathy or Korsakoff syndrome. Of nursing home patients, 20 percent have alcohol dependence.

Overall, alcohol and other substance use disorders account for 10 percent of all emotional problems in older persons, and dependence on such substances as hypnotics, anxiolytics, and narcotics is more common in old age than is generally recognized. Substance-seeking behavior characterized by crime, manipulativeness, and antisocial behavior is rarer in older than in younger adults. Older patients may abuse anxiolytics to allay chronic anxiety or to try to help sleep. The maintenance of chronically ill cancer patients with narcotics prescribed by a physician produces dependence, but the need to provide pain relief takes precedence over the possibility of narcotic dependence and is justified.

The clinical presentation of older patients with alcohol and other substance use disorders varies and includes confusion, poor personal hygiene, depression, malnutrition, and the effects of exposure and falls. The sudden onset of delirium in older persons hospitalized for medical illness is most often caused by alcohol withdrawal. Alcohol abuse also should be considered in older adults with chronic gastrointestinal (GI) problems.

Older persons may misuse over-the-counter substances, or nicotine and caffeine. Over-the-counter analgesics are used by 35 percent of older persons, and 30 percent use laxatives. Unexplained GI, psychological, and metabolic problems should alert clinicians to over-the-counter substance abuse.

Sleep Disorders

Advanced age is the single most important factor associated with the increased prevalence of sleep disorders. Sleep-related phenomena reported more frequently by older than by younger adults are sleeping problems, daytime sleepiness, daytime napping, and the use of hypnotic drugs. Clinically, older persons experience higher rates of breathing-related sleep disorder and medication-induced movement disorders than younger adults.

In addition to altered regulatory and physiologic systems, the causes of sleep disturbances in older persons include primary sleep disorders, other mental disorders, general medical disorders, and social and environmental factors. Among the primary sleep disorders, dyssomnias are the most frequent, mainly primary insomnia, nocturnal myoclonus, restless legs syndrome, and sleep apnea. Of the parasomnias, rapid eye movement (REM) sleep behavior disorder occurs almost exclusively among older men. The conditions that commonly interfere with sleep in older adults also include pain, nocturia, dyspnea, and heartburn. The lack of a daily structure and social or vocational responsibilities contributes to poor sleep.

As a result of the decreased length of their daily sleep–wake cycle, older persons without daily routines, especially patients in nursing homes, may experience an advanced sleep phase, in which they go to sleep early and awaken during the night.

Even modest amounts of alcohol can interfere with the quality of sleep and can cause sleep fragmentation and early morning awakening. Alcohol can also precipitate or aggravate obstructive sleep apnea. Many older persons use alcohol, hypnotics, and other CNS depressants to help them fall asleep, but data show that these persons experience more early morning awakening than trouble falling asleep. When prescribing sedative-hypnotic drugs for older persons, clinicians must monitor the patients for unwanted cognitive, behavioral, and psychomotor effects, including memory impairment (anterograde amnesia), residual sedation, rebound insomnia, daytime withdrawal, and unsteady gait.

Changes in sleep structure among persons over 65 years of age involve both REM sleep and nonrapid eye movement (NREM) sleep. The REM changes include the redistribution of REM sleep throughout the night, more REM episodes, shorter REM episodes, and less total REM sleep. The NREM changes include the decreased amplitude of delta waves, a lower percentage of stages 3 and 4 sleep, and a higher percentage of stages 1 and 2 sleep. Also, older persons experience increased awakening after sleep onset.

Altered timing and consolidation of the sleep account for much of the deterioration in the quality of sleep. This is due, in part, to decreasing melatonin and alternated responses to the adenosine system with age. With advanced age, persons have a lower amplitude of circadian rhythms, a 12-hour sleep-propensity rhythm, and shorter circadian cycles.

SUICIDE RISK

Elderly persons have a higher risk of suicide than any other population. The suicide rate for white men over the age of 65 is five times higher than that of the general population. One-third of elderly persons report loneliness as the principal reason for considering suicide. Approximately 10 percent of elderly individuals with suicidal ideation report financial problems, poor medical health, or depression as reasons for suicidal thoughts. Suicide victims differ demographically from individuals who attempt suicide. About 60 percent of those who commit suicide are men; 75 percent of those who attempt suicide are women. Suicide victims, as a rule, use guns or hang themselves, whereas 70 percent of suicide attempters take a drug overdose, and 20 percent cut or slash themselves. Psychological autopsy studies suggest that most elderly persons who commit suicide have had a psychiatric disorder, most commonly depression. Psychiatric disorders of suicide victims, however, often do not receive medical or psychiatric attention. More elderly suicide victims are widowed, and fewer are single, separated, or divorced than is true of younger adults. Violent methods of suicide are more common in the elderly, and alcohol use and psychiatric histories appear to be less frequent. The most common precipitants of suicide in older individuals are physical illness and loss, whereas problems with employment, finances, and family relationships are more frequent precipitants in younger adults. Many elderly persons who commit suicide communicate their suicidal thoughts to family or friends before the act of suicide.

Older patients with significant medical illnesses or a recent loss should be evaluated for depressive symptomatology and suicidal ideation or plans. Thoughts and fantasies about the meaning of suicide and life after death may reveal information that the patient cannot share directly. There should be no reluctance to question patients about suicide because no evidence indicates that such questions increase the likelihood of suicidal behavior.

OTHER CONDITIONS OF OLD AGE

Vertigo

Feelings of vertigo or dizziness, a common complaint of older adults, cause many older adults to become inactive because they fear falling. The causes of vertigo vary and include anemia, hypotension, cardiac arrhythmia, cerebrovascular disease, basilar artery insufficiency, middle ear disease, acoustic neuroma, benign postural vertigo, and Ménière disease. Most cases of vertigo have a vital psychological component, and clinicians should ascertain any secondary gain from the symptom. The overuse of anxiolytics can cause dizziness and daytime somnolence. Treatment with meclizine, 25 to 100 mg daily, has been successful in many patients with vertigo.

Syncope

The sudden loss of consciousness associated with syncope results from a reduction of cerebral blood flow and brain hypoxia. A thorough medical workup is required to rule out potential causes. Causes of syncope are listed in Table 25-6.

Hearing Loss

About 30 percent of persons over age 65 have significant hearing loss (presbycusis). After age 75, that figure rises to 50 percent. The causes vary. Clinicians should be sensitive to hearing loss in patients who complain they can hear but cannot understand what is being said or who asks that questions be repeated. Most elderly persons with hearing loss can be treated with hearing aids.

Elder Abuse

An estimated 10 percent of persons above 65 years of age are abused. The American Medical Association defines elder abuse as "an act or omission which results in harm or threatened harm to the health or welfare of an elderly person." Mistreatment includes abuse and neglect—physically, psychologically, financially, and

Table 25-6
Causes of Syncope

Cardiac Disorders
 Anatomical/valvular
  Aortic stenosis
  Mitral prolapse and regurgitation
  Hypertrophic cardiomyopathy
  Myxoma
 Electrical
  Tachyarrhythmia
  Bradyarrhythmia
  Heart block
  Sick sinus syndrome
 Functional
  Ischemia and infarct

Situational Hypotension
 Dehydration (diarrhea, fasting)
 Orthostatic hypotension
 Postprandial hypotension
 Micturition, defecation, coughing, swallowing

Abnormal Cardiovascular Reflexes
 Carotid sinus syndrome
 Vasovagal syncope

Drugs
 Vasodilators
 Calcium channel blockers
 Diuretics
 β-Blockers

Central Nervous System Abnormalities
 Cerebrovascular insufficiency
 Seizures

Metabolic Abnormalities
 Hypoxemia
 Hypoglycemia or hyperglycemia
 Anemia

Pulmonary Disorders
 Chronic obstructive pulmonary disease
 Pneumonia
 Pulmonary embolus

materially. Sexual abuse does occur. Acts of omission include withholding food, medicine, clothing, and other necessities.

Family conflicts and other problems often underlie elder abuse. The victims tend to be very old and frail. They often live with their assailants, who may be financially dependent on the victims. Both the victim and the perpetrator tend to deny or minimize the presence of abuse. Interventions include providing legal services, housing, and medical, psychiatric, and social services.

SPOUSAL BEREAVEMENT

Demographic data suggest that 51 percent of women and 14 percent of men over the age of 65 will be widowed at least once. Spousal loss is among the most stressful of all life experiences. As a group, older adults appear to have a more favorable outcome than expected following the death of a spouse. Depressive symptoms peak within the first few months after death but decline significantly within a year. A relationship exists between spousal loss and subsequent mortality. Elderly survivors of spouses who committed suicide are especially vulnerable, as are those with psychiatric illness.

PSYCHOPHARMACOLOGICAL TREATMENT OF GERIATRIC DISORDERS

Specific guidelines should be followed regarding the use of all drugs in older adults. A pretreatment medical evaluation is essential, including an electrocardiogram (ECG). It is especially useful to have the patient or a family member bring in all currently used medications because multiple drug use could be contributing to the symptoms.

Most psychotropic drugs should be given in equally divided doses three or four times over 24 hours. Older patients may not be able to tolerate a sudden rise in drug blood levels resulting from one sizeable daily dose. Any changes in blood pressure and pulse rate and other side effects should be watched. For patients with insomnia, however, giving the significant portion of an antipsychotic or antidepressant at bedtime takes advantage of its sedating and soporific effects. Liquid preparations are useful for older patients who cannot or will not swallow tablets. Clinicians should frequently reassess all patients to determine the need for maintenance medication, changes in dosage, and development of adverse effects. If a patient is taking psychotropic drugs at the time of the evaluation, the clinician should discontinue these medications, if possible, and, after a washout period, reevaluate the patient during a drug-free baseline state.

Adults over 65 years of age use the most significant number of medications of any age group; 25 percent of all prescriptions are written for them. Adverse drug reactions caused by medications result in the hospitalization of nearly 250,000 persons in the United States each year. Psychiatric drugs are among the most commonly prescribed, along with cardiovascular and diuretic medications; 40 percent of all hypnotics dispensed in the United States each year are to those older than 75 years of age, and 70 percent of older persons use over-the-counter medications, compared with only 10 percent of young adults.

Principles

The primary goals of the pharmacologic treatment of older persons are to improve the quality of life, maintain persons in the community, and delay or avoid their placement in nursing homes. The individualization of dosage is the basic tenet of geriatric psychopharmacology.

Alterations in drug dosages are required because of the physiologic changes that occur as we age. Renal disease is associated with a decreased renal clearance of drugs; liver disease results in a decreased ability to metabolize drugs; cardiovascular disease and reduced cardiac output can affect both renal and hepatic drug clearance. GI disease and decreased gastric acid secretion also influence drug absorption. As a person ages, the ratio of lean to fat body mass also changes. With normal aging, lean body mass decreases, and body fat increases. Changes in the ratio of lean to fat body mass that accompany aging affect the distribution of drugs. Many lipid-soluble psychotropic drugs are distributed more widely in fat than in lean tissue, so a drug's action can be unexpectedly prolonged in older persons. Similarly, changes in end-organ or receptor-site sensitivity must be taken into account. In older persons, the increased risk of orthostatic hypotension from psychotropic drugs is related to reduced functioning of blood pressure–regulating mechanisms.

As a general rule, the lowest possible dose should be used to achieve the desired therapeutic response. Clinicians must know the pharmacodynamics, pharmacokinetics, and biotransformation of each drug prescribed and the effects of the interaction of the drug with other drugs that a patient is taking. An adage in geriatric medicine regarding the use of drugs is: Start low, go slow.

PSYCHOTHERAPY FOR GERIATRIC PATIENTS

The standard psychotherapeutic interventions—such as insight-oriented psychotherapy, supportive psychotherapy, cognitive therapy, group therapy, and family therapy—should be available to geriatric patients. According to Sigmund Freud, persons older than 50 years are not suited for psychoanalysis because their mental processes lack elasticity. In the view of many who followed Freud, however, psychoanalysis is possible after age 50. Advanced age certainly limits the plasticity of the personality, but as Otto Fenichel stated, "It does so in varying degrees and at very different ages so that no general rule can be given." Insight-oriented psychotherapy may help remove a specific symptom, even in older persons. It is of most benefit when patients have possibilities for libidinal and narcissistic gratification, but it is contraindicated if it would bring only the insight that life has been a failure and that the patient has no opportunity to make up for it.

Common age-related issues in therapy involve the need to adapt to recurrent and diverse losses (e.g., the deaths of friends and loved ones), the need to assume new roles (e.g., the adjustment to retirement and the disengagement from previously defined roles), and the need to accept mortality. Psychotherapy helps older persons to deal with these issues and the emotional problems surrounding them and to understand their behavior and the effects of their behavior on others. In addition to improving interpersonal relationships, psychotherapy increases self-esteem and self-confidence, decreases feelings of helplessness and anger, and improves the quality of life.

Psychotherapy helps relieve tensions of biologic and cultural origins and helps older persons work and play within the limits of their functional status and as determined by their past training, activities, and self-concept in society. In patients with impaired cognition, psychotherapy can produce remarkable gains in both physical and mental symptoms. In one study conducted in a nursing home, 43 percent of the patients receiving psychotherapy showed less urinary incontinence, improved gait, greater mental alertness, improved memory, and better hearing than before psychotherapy.

Therapists must be more active, supportive, and flexible in conducting therapy with older than with younger adults, and they must be prepared to act decisively at the first sign of an incapacity that requires the active involvement of another physician, such as an internist or that requires consulting with, or enlisting the aid of, a family member.

Older persons usually seek therapy for a therapist's unqualified and unlimited support, reassurance, and approval. Patients often expect a therapist to be all-powerful, all-knowing, and able to effect a magical cure. Most patients eventually recognize that the therapist is human and that they are engaged in a collaborative effort. In some cases, however, the therapist may have to assume the idealized role, especially when the patient is unable or unwilling to test reality effectively. With the help of the therapist, the patient deals with problems that had been avoided previously. As the therapist offers direct encouragement, reassurance, and advice, the patient's self-confidence increases as conflicts are resolved.

▲ 25.3 Psychiatric Emergencies

A psychiatric emergency is any disturbance in thoughts, feelings, or actions for which immediate therapeutic intervention is necessary. For a variety of reasons—such as the growing incidence of violence, the increased appreciation of the role of medical disease in altered mental status, and the epidemic of alcoholism and other substance use disorders—the number of emergency psychiatry patients is on the rise. The widening scope of emergency psychiatry goes beyond general psychiatric practice to include such specialized problems as the abuse of substances, children, and spouses; violence in the form of suicide, homicide, and rape; and such social issues as homelessness, aging, and competence. The emergency psychiatrist must be up to date on medicolegal issues and managed care. This section provides an overview of psychiatric emergencies in general and in adults in particular. Psychiatric emergencies in children is covered later in this chapter.

TREATMENT SETTINGS

Nonpsychiatrists do most emergency psychiatric evaluations in a general medical emergency room setting, but specialized psychiatric services are increasingly favored. Regardless of the type of setting, an atmosphere of safety and security must prevail. An adequate number of staff members—including psychiatrists, nurses, aides, and social workers—must be present at all times. Additional personnel to help out in times of overcrowding should be available. Specific responsibilities, such as the use of restraints, should be clearly defined and practiced by the entire emergency team. Clear communication and lines of authority are essential. The organization of the staff into multidisciplinary teams is desirable.

Children and young adolescents are best served in a pediatric setting. Unless there is a risk of behavioral problems or of their leaving the hospital against advice, they need not be sent to the adult psychiatric emergency service.

Immediate access to the medical emergency department and appropriate diagnostic services is necessary because one-third of medical conditions present with psychiatric manifestations. The full spectrum of psychopharmacological options should be available to the psychiatrist.

Violence in the emergency service cannot be condoned or tolerated. The code of conduct expected of staff members and patients must be posted and understood from the time of the patient's arrival in the emergency room. Security is best managed as a clinical issue by the clinical staff, not by law enforcement personnel. Whenever possible, agitated and threatening patients should be sequestered from the nonagitated. Seclusion and restraint rooms should be located close to the nursing station for close observation.

The entire staff must understand that patients in physical and emotional distress are fragile and that various expectations and fantasies, often unrealistic, influence their responses to treatment. For example, a man with impaired reality testing who is brought in by the police against his will may not understand that the clinician is interested in helping him. Other patients, influenced by previous unsatisfactory treatment experiences, may be hostile. Some patients believe that psychiatrists can read minds or are only interested in admitting patients to lock them away. Such people see little point in openly discussing their problems. Many people have an inaccurate understanding of their rights as patients. All clinical interventions must take those expectations and attitudes into account to minimize the possibility of misunderstanding and consequent problems.

EPIDEMIOLOGY

Psychiatric emergency rooms are used equally by men and women and more by single than by married persons. About 20 percent of these patients are suicidal, and about 10 percent are violent. The most common diagnoses are depressive disorders, manic episodes, schizophrenia, and alcohol dependence. About 40 percent of all patients seen in psychiatric emergency rooms require hospitalization. Most visits occur during the night hours, but usage difference is not based on the day of the week or the month of the year. Contrary to popular belief, studies have not found that the use of psychiatric emergency rooms increases during the full moon or the Christmas season.

EVALUATION

The primary goal of an emergency psychiatric evaluation is the timely assessment of the patient in crisis. To that end, the physician must make an initial diagnosis, identify the precipitating factors and immediate needs, and begin treatment or refer the patient to the most appropriate treatment setting. Given the unpredictable nature of emergency medicine work, with many patients presenting both physical and emotional complaints, and because of the limited space and the competition for ancillary services, a pragmatic approach to the patient is required. Sometimes, moving the patient out of the emergency department into the most appropriate diagnostic or treatment setting is best for the patient. Medical emergencies are generally better managed elsewhere in the system. Keeping the number of emergency patients in one place to a minimum reduces the chance of agitation and violence.

The standard psychiatric interview—consisting of a history, a mental status examination, and, when appropriate and depending on the rules of the emergency department, a full physical examination and ancillary tests—is the cornerstone of the emergency psychiatry evaluation. The emergency department psychiatrist, however, must be ready to introduce modifications as needed. For example, the emergency psychiatrist may have to structure the interview with a rambling manic patient, medicate or restrain an agitated patient, or forgo the usual rules of confidentiality to assess an adolescent's risk of suicide. In general, any strategy introduced in the emergency department to accomplish the goal of assessing the patient is considered consistent with good clinical practice as long as the rationale for the strategy is documented in the medical record.

What constitutes a psychiatric emergency is highly subjective. The emergency department has increasingly come to serve as an admitting area, a holding area, a detoxification center, and a private medical office. Such medical conditions as head traumas, acute intoxications, withdrawal states, and AIDS encephalopathies may present with acute psychiatric manifestations. The emergency psychiatrists must rapidly assess and distinguish the genuine emergency psychiatric patients from those who are less acutely ill and from nonpsychiatric emergencies. A triage system using psychiatrists, nurses, and psychiatric social workers is an efficient and effective way to identify emergency, urgent, and nonurgent patients, who can then be prioritized for care (Fig. 25-1).

In one model, every patient who comes to the emergency department is assessed by a triage nurse on arrival to ascertain the patient's chief complaint, clinical condition, and vital signs. The psychiatrist then briefly meets with the patient and other significant people involved in the case—family members, emergency medical service technicians, and police—to assign the patient to one of the three categories—emergency, urgent, and nonurgent—or to refer the patient to an appropriate treatment setting, such as the medical emergency medicine service. Having a senior clinician perform that task ensures rapid identification of the most urgent and troublesome cases, an appropriate allocation of resources, and an answer to the most common question heard in the emergency department: "When am I going to see a doctor?"

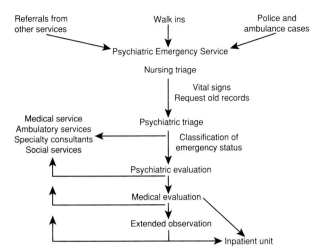

FIGURE 25-1
Evaluation and treatment of psychiatric emergencies.

The psychiatrist then assigns clinical responsibility for each patient to the appropriate personnel. As the evaluation often stretches over more than one shift, a careful procedure to transfer responsibility and to pass along information from shift to shift must be built into the system by using visual, oral, and written communications. A request for old records should be made automatically for every patient who is evaluated in the emergency department. Each emergency should be judged on its own merits. However, information from previous records and workers in the field and family members can be of crucial importance in assessing patients, especially patients who are psychotic, frightened, or otherwise unable or unwilling to cooperate in giving a good history.

The psychiatrist should have access to multilingual staff and other translation services. The use of the patient's friends or family members as translators is not desirable because of the possibility of unconscious or deliberate denial or distortion of the clinical picture stemming from their involvement with the patient.

An initial assessment of the patient's total biopsychosocial needs is optimal, but the patient's emergency status, other patients, waiting to be seen, and the constraints of the emergency setting often make such a full assessment a moot point. At a minimum, the emergency evaluation should address the following five questions before any disposition is decided on: (1) Is it safe for the patient to be in the emergency department? (2) Is the problem physiologic, functional, or a combination? (3) Is the patient psychotic? (4) Is the patient suicidal or homicidal? (5) To what degree is the patient capable of self-care? Table 25-7 provides a general strategy for evaluating patients.

Patient Safety

Physicians should consider the question of the patient's safety before evaluating every patient. The answer must address the issues of the emergency department physical layout, staffing patterns and communication, and patient population. Psychiatrists must then take stock of themselves: Are they in the proper frame of mind to conduct an evaluation? Do any issues in the case spark countertransference reactions? The self-assessment should go on throughout the evaluation. The physical and emotional safety of the patient takes priority over all other considerations. If verbal interventions fail or are contraindicated, the use of medication or restraints must be considered and, if necessary, ordered. Careful

Table 25-7
General Strategy in Evaluating the Patient

I. Self-protection
  A. Know as much as possible about the patients before meeting them.
  B. Leave physical restraint procedures to those who are trained.
  C. Be alert to risks of impending violence.
  D. Attend to the safety of the physical surroundings (e.g., door access, room objects).
  E. Have others present during the assessment if needed.
  F. Have others in the vicinity.
  G. Attend to developing an alliance with the patient (e.g., do not confront or threaten patients with persecutory psychoses).

II. Prevent harm
  A. Prevent self-injury and suicide. Use whatever methods are necessary to prevent patients from hurting themselves during the evaluation.
  B. Prevent violence toward others. During the evaluation, briefly assess the patient for the risk of violence. If the risk is deemed significant, consider the following options:
    1. Inform the patient that violence is not acceptable.
    2. Approach the patient in a nonthreatening manner.
    3. Reassure, calm, or assist the patient's reality testing.
    4. Offer medication.
    5. Inform the patient that restraint or seclusion will be used if necessary.
    6. Have teams ready to restrain the patient.
    7. When patients are restrained, always closely observe them, and frequently check their vital signs. Isolate restrained patients from surrounding agitating stimuli. Immediately plan a further approach—medication, reassurance, medical evaluation.

III. Rule out nonpsychiatric etiologies.

IV. Rule out impending psychosis.

attention to the possible outbreak of agitation or disruptive behavior beyond acceptable limits is often the best insurance against untoward occurrences.

Medical or Psychiatric?

The most important question for the emergency psychiatrist to address is whether the problem is medical, psychiatric, or both. Medical conditions—such as diabetes mellitus, thyroid disease, acute intoxications, withdrawal states, AIDS, and head traumas—can present with prominent mental status changes that mimic common psychiatric illnesses. Such conditions may be life-threatening if not treated promptly. Generally, the treatment of medical illness is more definitive, and the prognosis is better than for a functional psychiatric disorder. The psychiatrist must consider all casual possibilities.

Once patients are labeled psychiatric, their complaints may not be taken seriously by nonmental health professionals. However, such patients' conditions may deteriorate. Because of such factors as deinstitutionalization, homelessness, and chronic alcoholism, the mentally ill are at significant risk of tuberculosis, vitamin deficiencies, and other easily overlooked but easily treated conditions. Symptoms such as paranoia, internal preoccupation, and acute psychosis can make a routine medical diagnosis exceedingly tricky. Each patient must be assessed for the possibility that a nonpsychiatric medical illness is combined with an underlying psychiatric illness. A young man who comes to the emergency department intoxicated or in alcohol withdrawal two or three times a month may one day come with a subdural

Table 25-8
Features that Point to a Medical Cause of a Mental Disorder

Acute onset (within hours or minutes, with prevailing symptoms)
First episode
Older age
Current medical illness or injury
Significant substance abuse
Nonauditory disturbances of perception
Neurologic symptoms—loss of consciousness, seizures, head injury, change in headache pattern, change in vision
Classic mental status signs—diminished alertness, disorientation, memory impairment, impairment in concentration and attention, dyscalculia, concreteness
Other mental status signs—speech, movement, or gait disorders
Constructional apraxia—difficulties in drawing clock, cube, intersecting pentagons, Bender–Gestalt test

hematoma as a result of a fall. Table 25-8 lists feature that point to a medical cause of a mental disorder.

SPECIFIC INTERVIEW SITUATIONS

Psychosis

Whether the patient is psychotic refers less to diagnosis and more to the severity of symptoms and life disruption. The patient's degree of withdrawal from objective reality, level of affectivity, intellectual functioning, and degree of regression are other important parameters. Impairment in any of those areas may lead to difficulties in conducting an evaluation. Agitated, assaultive behavior or failure to comply with treatment recommendations may also result. A paranoid, hypervigilant patient may misperceive a staff member's offer of help as an attack and may lash out in self-defense. Command auditory hallucinations may cause a patient to deny symptoms and to throw prescriptions in the garbage immediately after leaving the emergency department. The psychiatrist should be alert to the complications that can arise with patients whose reality testing is impaired, and the psychiatrist should modify the approach accordingly.

All communication with patients must be straightforward. All clinical interventions should be briefly explained using language the patient can understand. Psychiatrists should not assume that the patient trusts or believes them or even wants their help. Clinicians must be prepared to structure or to terminate an interview to limit the potential for agitation and regression.

Depression and Potentially Suicidal Patients

The clinician should always ask about suicidal ideas as part of every mental status examination, especially if the patient is depressed. The patient may not realize that such symptoms as waking during the night and increased somatic complaints are related to depressive disorders. The patient should be asked directly, "*Are you or have you ever been suicidal?*" "*Do you want to die?*" "*Do you feel so bad that you might hurt yourself?*" Eight of 10 persons who eventually kill themselves give warnings of their intent. If the patient admits to a plan of action, that is a particularly dangerous sign. If a patient who has been threatening suicide becomes quiet and less agitated than before, that may be an ominous sign. The clinician should be primarily concerned with the factors listed in Table 25-9.

Table 25-9
History, Signs, and Symptoms of Suicidal Risk

1. Previous attempt or fantasized suicide
2. Anxiety, depression, exhaustion
3. Availability of means of suicide
4. Concern for effect of suicide on family members
5. Verbalized suicidal ideation
6. Preparation of a will, resignation after agitated depression
7. Proximal life crisis, such as mourning or impending surgery
8. Family history of suicide
9. Pervasive pessimism or hopelessness

A suicide note, a family history of suicide, or previous suicidal behavior on the part of the patient increases the risk of suicide. Evidence of impulsivity or pervasive pessimism about the future also places the patient at risk. If the physician decides that the patient is in imminent risk for suicidal behavior, the patient must be hospitalized or otherwise protected. A difficult situation arises when the risk does not seem to be immediate, but the potential for suicide is present as long as the patient remains depressed. If the psychiatrist decides not to hospitalize the patient immediately, the doctor should insist that the patient promise to call whenever the suicidal pressure mounts.

Violent Patients

Patients may be violent for many reasons, and the interview with a violent patient must attempt to ascertain the underlying cause of violent behavior because cause determines intervention. The differential diagnosis of violent behavior includes psychoactive substance-induced organic mental disorder, antisocial personality disorder, catatonia, medical infections, cerebral neoplasms, decompensating obsessive-compulsive personality disorder, dissociative disorders, impulse control disorders, sexual disorders, alcohol idiosyncratic intoxication, delusional disorder, paranoid personality disorder, schizophrenia, temporal lobe epilepsy, bipolar disorder, and uncontrollable violence secondary to interpersonal stress. The psychiatric interview must include questions that attempt to sort out the differential for violent behavior and questions directed toward the prediction of violence.

The best predictors of violent behavior are (1) excessive alcohol intake; (2) a history of violent acts, with arrests or criminal activity; and (3) a history of childhood abuse. Table 25-10 lists some of the most significant factors in assessing and predicting violence.

Rape and Sexual Abuse

Rape is the forceful coercion of an unwilling victim to engage in a sexual act, usually sexual intercourse, although anal intercourse and fellatio can also be acts of rape. As with other acts of violence, rape is a psychiatric emergency that requires immediate, appropriate intervention. Rape victims may suffer sequelae that persist for a lifetime. Rape is a life-threatening experience, and the victim has almost always been threatened with physical harm, often with a weapon. In addition to rape, other forms of sexual abuse include genital manipulation with foreign objects, infliction of pain, and forced sexual activity.

Most rapists are male, and most victims are female. Male rape does occur, however, often in institutions where men are detained (e.g., prisons). Women between the ages of 16 and 24 years are in the highest risk category, but female victims as young as 15 months and as old as 82 years have been raped. More than a third of all rapes are committed by rapists known to the victim, 7 percent by close

Table 25-10
Assessing and Predicting Violent Behavior

1. Signs of impending violence
   a. Very recent acts of violence, including property violence
   b. Verbal or physical threats (menacing)
   c. Carrying weapons or other objects that may be used as weapons (e.g., forks, ashtrays)
   d. Progressive psychomotor agitation
   e. Alcohol or drug intoxication
   f. Persecutory ideation in a psychotic patient
   g. Command violent auditory hallucinations—some but not all patients are at high risk
   h. Mental disorders due to a medical condition, global or with frontal lobe findings; less commonly with temporal lobe findings (controversial)
   i. Patients with catatonic excitement
   j. Certain patients with mania
   k. Certain patients with agitated depression
   l. Personality disorder patients prone to rage, violence, or impulse dyscontrol
2. Assess the risk of violence
   a. Consider violent ideation, wish, intention, plan, availability of means, implementation of plan, wish for help.
   b. Consider demographics—sex (male), age (15–24), socioeconomic status (low), social supports (few).
   c. Consider past history: violence, nonviolent antisocial acts, impulse dyscontrol (e.g., gambling, substance abuse, suicide or self-injury, psychosis).
   d. Consider overt stressors (e.g., marital conflict, real or symbolic loss).

relatives. About one-quarter of rapes involve more than one rapist (gang rape).

Typical reactions in both rape and sexual abuse victims include shame, humiliation, anxiety, confusion, and outrage. Many victims wonder whether they are partly responsible and somehow invited the assault. Victim behavior is less critical in precipitating a rape than it is in precipitating a homicide or a robbery. Rape and sexual abuse victims are often confused after the assault. Clinicians should be reassuring, supportive, and nonjudgmental. Inform the patient about the availability of medical and legal services and about rape crisis centers that provide multidisciplinary services.

If possible, a female clinician should evaluate the patient because the victim may find it easier to talk with a woman than with a man. The evaluation should take place in private. When rape or sexual abuse has not been acknowledged openly, it is usually because many victims hesitate to discuss the assault and thus avoid the topic. If the patient appears to be anxious when questioned about sexual history and avoids the discussion, it is vital to validate the patient's avoidance. Recognize that the rape victim has undergone unanticipated, life-threatening stress. It is legally and therapeutically essential to take a detailed and complete history of the attack.

With the patient's written consent, collect evidence, such as semen and pubic hair, that may be used to identify the rapist. Take photographs of the evidence, if possible. The medical record may be used as evidence in criminal proceedings; therefore, meticulous objective documentation of all aspects of the evaluation is essential.

TREATMENT OF EMERGENCIES

Psychotherapy

In an emergency psychiatric intervention, all attempts are made to help patients' self-esteem. Empathy is critical to healing in a

psychiatric emergency. The acquired knowledge of how biogenetic, situational, developmental, and existential forces converge at one point to create a psychiatric emergency is tantamount to the maturation of skill in emergency psychiatry. Adjustment disorder in all age groups may result in tantrum-like outbursts of rage. These outbursts are particularly common in marital quarrels, and police are often summoned by neighbors distressed by the sounds of a violent altercation. Such family quarrels should be approached with caution because they may be complicated by alcohol use and the presence of dangerous weapons. The warring couple frequently turns their combined fury on an unwary outsider. Wounded self-esteem is a significant issue, and clinicians must avoid patronizing or contemptuous attitudes and try to communicate an attitude of respect and an authentic peacemaking concern.

In family violence, psychiatrists should note the unique vulnerability of selected close relatives. A wife or husband may have a curious masochistic attachment to the spouse and can provoke violence by taunting and otherwise undermining a partner's self-esteem. Such relationships often end in the murder of the provoking partner and sometimes in the suicide of the other partner—the dynamics behind most so-called suicide pacts. As with many suicidal patients, many violent patients require hospitalization and usually accept the offer of inpatient care with a sense of relief.

More than one psychotherapist or type of psychotherapy is frequently used in emergency therapy. For example, a 28-year-old man, depressed and suicidal after a colostomy for intractable colitis, whose wife was threatening to leave him because of his irritability and their constant altercations, may be referred to a psychiatrist for supportive psychotherapy and antidepressant medication, to a marital therapist with his wife to improve their marital functioning, and to a colostomy support group to learn ways of coping with a colostomy. Emergency psychiatric clinicians are pragmatic; they use every necessary mode of therapeutic intervention available to resolve the crisis and facilitate value exploration and growth, with less concern than usual about diluting a therapeutic relationship. Emergency therapy emphasizes how various psychiatric modalities act synergistically to enhance recovery.

No single approach is appropriate for all persons in similar situations. What should a doctor say to a patient and family experiencing an emergency, such as a suicide attempt or a schizophrenic break? For some, a genetic rationale helps; the information that an illness has a vital biologic component relieves some persons. For others, however, this approach underlines a lack of control and increases depression and anxiety. All feel helpless because neither the family nor the patient can alter the behavior to minimize the likelihood of recurrence. Some persons may benefit from an explanation of family or individual dynamics. Others only want someone to listen to them; in time, they reach their understanding.

In an emergency, as in any other psychiatric situation, when a clinician does not know what to say, the best approach is to listen. Persons in crisis reveal how much they need support, denial, ventilation, and words to conceptualize the meaning of their crisis and to discover paths to resolution.

Pharmacotherapy

The primary indications for the use of psychotropic medication in an emergency room include violent or assaultive behavior, massive anxiety or panic, and extrapyramidal reactions, such as dystonia and akathisia as adverse effects of psychiatric drugs. Laryngospasm is a rare form of dystonia, and psychiatrists should be prepared to maintain an open airway with intubation if necessary.

Persons who are delusional or in a state of catatonic excitement require tranquilization. Episodic outbursts of violence may respond to antipsychotics (haloperidol, second-generation antipsychotics), benzodiazepines and antihistamines. If history suggests a seizure disorder, use clinical studies to confirm the diagnosis and evaluation to ascertain the cause. If the findings are positive, anticonvulsant therapy is initiated, or appropriate surgery is provided (e.g., in the case of a cerebral mass). Conservative measures may suffice for intoxication from drugs of abuse. Sometimes, drugs such as haloperidol (5 to 10 mg every half-hour to an hour) are needed until a patient is stabilized. Benzodiazepines may be used instead of, or in addition to, antipsychotics (to reduce the antipsychotic dosage). When a recreational drug has strong anticholinergic properties, benzodiazepines are more appropriate than antipsychotics.

Violent, struggling patients are subdued most effectively with an appropriate sedative or antipsychotic. Diazepam (5 to 10 mg) or lorazepam (2 to 4 mg) may be given slowly intravenously (IV) over 2 minutes. Clinicians must give IV medication with great care to avoid respiratory arrest. Patients who require IM medication can be sedated with haloperidol (5 to 10 mg IM). If the furor is caused by alcohol or is part of a postseizure psychomotor disturbance, the sleep produced by a relatively small amount of an IV medication may go on for hours. On awakening, patients are often entirely alert and rational and typically have complete amnesia about the violent episode.

If the disturbance is part of an ongoing psychotic process and returns as soon as the IV medication wears off, continuous medication may be given. It is sometimes better to use small IM or oral doses at half-hour to 1-hour intervals (e.g., haloperidol, 2 to 5 mg, or diazepam, 20 mg) until the patient is controlled than to use large dosages initially, which can result in an overmedicated patient. As the disturbing behavior is brought under control, successively smaller and less frequent doses should be used. During the preliminary treatment, a patient's blood pressure and other vital signs should be monitored.

Restraints

Restraints are used when patients are so dangerous to themselves or others that they pose a severe threat that cannot be controlled in any other way. Patients may be restrained temporarily to receive medication or for long periods if we cannot use medications. Usually, patients in restraints quiet down after a time. On a psychodynamic level, such patients may even welcome the control of their impulses provided by restraints. Table 25-11 provides a summary of the use of restraints.

Disposition

In some cases, the usual option of admitting or discharging the patient is not considered optimal. Suspected toxic psychoses, brief decompensations in a patient with a personality disorder, and adjustment reactions to traumatic events, for example, may be best managed in an extended-observation setting. Allowing the patient more time in a secure environment can result in sufficient improvement or clarification of the issues to make traditional inpatient treatment unnecessary. It can also spare the patient the trauma and stigma of psychiatric admission and can free up bed space for needier patients. Crisis intervention for victims of rape and other traumas can also be done in an extended-observation setting.

When the decision is to admit the patient to the hospital, it is preferable to do so voluntarily. Allowing patients that option gives them a sense of control over their lives and of participation in the

Table 25-11
Use of Restraints

Recommended principles for physical restraint use
- Use only after nonphysical approaches fail
- Maintain the privacy and dignity of the patient throughout the intervention
- The limitation on movement should be as nonrestrictive as safely possible
- Medical personnel should be properly trained for in how to use and monitor this intervention
- The ED should set appropriate and consistent guidelines for restraint, including
  - what treatments should be given
  - what monitoring is necessary
  - how the patient will be evaluated for ending the restraint
- The patient should be explicitly and continuously observed by the treatment team
- The use of physical restraint should be consistent with all standards and rules

Adapted from: American College of Emergency Physicians (ACEP). Use of patient restraints. Policy statement. *Ann Emerg Med*. 2014;64(5):574.

treatment decisions. Patients who meet involuntary admission criteria based on dangerousness to themselves or others cannot leave the hospital without further review and can always be converted to involuntary status if warranted.

Because the initial evaluation is often inconclusive, definitive treatment is best deferred until the patient can be further assessed in the inpatient unit or the outpatient department. When the diagnosis is clear, however, and the patient's response to previous treatment is known, nothing is gained by delay. For example, a patient with chronic schizophrenia that has decompensated after discontinuing the usual regimen of antipsychotic medication is best served by a prompt resumption of treatment.

Even if patients feel comfortable coming to the emergency department in times of need, the emergency psychiatrist should always direct or redirect them to the most appropriate treatment setting. Patients in the psychopharmacology clinic who have missed their regular appointments should be given only enough medication to sustain them until they can be seen in the clinic. Feedback to others treating them should be a matter of course.

The emergency department is often the gateway to the department of psychiatry or the general hospital. First impressions carry a great deal of weight. The kind of attention and concern showed to patients on arrival in the emergency room strongly affects how they will respond to staff members and treatment recommendations and even their treatment compliance long after they have left the emergency room.

Documentation

In the interests of good care, respect for patients' rights, cost control, and medicolegal concerns, documentation has become a central focus for the emergency physician. The medical record should convey a concise picture of the patient, highlighting all pertinent positive and negative findings. Gaps in information and their reason should be mentioned. The names and the telephone numbers of interested parties should be noted. A provisional diagnosis or differential diagnosis must be made. An initial treatment plan or recommendations should follow from the findings of the patient's history, mental status examination and other diagnostic tests, and the medical evaluation. The writing must be legible. The emergency physician has unusual latitude under the law to perform an adequate initial assessment; however, all interventions and decisions must be thought out, discussed, and documented in the patient's record.

Specific Psychiatric Emergencies

Table 25-12 outlines common psychiatric emergencies in alphabetical order. Readers are referred to the index and relevant chapters of this textbook for a thorough discussion of each disorder.

PSYCHIATRIC EMERGENCIES IN CHILDREN

Few children or adolescents seek psychiatric intervention on their own, even during a crisis; thus, most of their emergency evaluations are initiated by parents, relatives, teachers, therapists, physicians,

and child protective service workers. Some referrals are for the evaluation of life-threatening situations for the child or others, such as suicidal behavior, physical abuse, and violent or homicidal behavior. Other urgent but non–life-threatening referrals pertain to children and adolescents with exacerbations of clear-cut serious psychiatric disorders, such as mania, depression, florid psychosis, and school referral. Less diagnostically obvious situations occur when children and adolescents present with a history of a wide range of disruptive, aberrant behaviors and are accompanied by an overwhelmed, anxious, and distraught adult who perceives the child's actions as an emergency, despite the absence of life-threatening behavior of an evident psychiatric disorder. In those cases, the spectrum of contributing factors is not immediately apparent, and the emergency psychiatrist must assess the entire family or system

Table 25-12
Common Psychiatric Emergencies

Syndrome	Emergency Manifestations	Treatment Issues
Abuse of child or adult	Signs of physical trauma	Management of medical problems; psychiatric evaluation; report to authorities
Acquired immune deficiency syndrome (AIDS)	Changes in behavior secondary to medical causes; changes in behavior secondary to fear and anxiety; suicidal behavior	Management of neurologic illness; management of psychological concomitants; reinforcement of social support
Adolescent crises	Suicidal attempts and ideation; substance abuse, truancy, trouble with law, pregnancy, running away; eating disorders; psychosis	Evaluation of suicidal potential, extent of substance abuse, family dynamics; crisis-oriented family and individual therapy; hospitalization if necessary; consultation with appropriate extrafamilial authorities
Agoraphobia	Panic; depression	Alprazolam, 0.25–2 mg; antidepressant medication
Agranulocytosis (clozapine induced)	High fever, pharyngitis, oral and perianal ulcerations	Discontinue medication immediately; administer granulocyte colony-stimulating factor
Akathisia	Agitation, restlessness, muscle discomfort; dysphoria	Reduce antipsychotic dosage; propranolol (30–120 mg a day); benzodiazepines; diphenhydramine orally or IV; benztropine IM
Alcohol-Related Emergencies		
Alcohol delirium	Confusion, disorientation, fluctuating consciousness and perception, autonomic hyperactivity; may be fatal	A benzodiazepine; haloperidol for psychotic symptoms may be added if necessary
Alcohol intoxication	Disinhibited behavior, sedation at high doses	With time and protective environment, symptoms abate
Alcohol-persisting amnestic disorder	Confusion, loss of memory even for all personal identification data	Hospitalization; hypnosis; rule out organic cause
Alcohol-persisting dementia	Confusion, agitation, impulsivity	Rule out other causes for dementia; no effective treatment; hospitalization if necessary
Alcohol psychotic disorder with hallucinations	Vivid auditory (at times visual) hallucinations with affect appropriate to content (often fearful); clear sensorium	Haloperidol for psychotic symptoms
Alcohol seizures	Grand mal seizures; rarely status epilepticus	Diazepam, phenytoin; prevent by using chlordiazepoxide during detoxification
Alcohol withdrawal	Irritability, nausea, vomiting, insomnia, malaise, autonomic hyperactivity, shakiness	Fluid and electrolytes maintained; sedation with benzodiazepines; restraints; monitoring of vital signs; 100 mg thiamine IM
Idiosyncratic alcohol intoxication	Marked aggressive or assaultive behavior	Generally no treatment required other than protective environment
Korsakoff syndrome	Alcohol stigmata, amnesia, confabulation	No effective treatment; institutionalization often needed
Wernicke encephalopathy	Oculomotor disturbances, cerebellar ataxia; mental confusion	Thiamine, 100 mg IV or IM, with $MgSO_4$ given before glucose loading
Amphetamine (or related substance) intoxication	Delusions, paranoia; violence; depression (from withdrawal); anxiety, delirium	Antipsychotics; restraints; hospitalization if necessary; no need for gradual withdrawal; antidepressants may be necessary

(continued)

Table 25-12
Common Psychiatric Emergencies (*Continued*)

Syndrome	Emergency Manifestations	Treatment Issues
Anorexia nervosa	Loss of 25% of body weight of the norm for age and sex	Hospitalization; electrocardiogram (ECG), fluid and electrolytes; neuroendocrine evaluation
Anticholinergic intoxication	Psychotic symptoms, dry skin and mouth, hyperpyrexia, mydriasis, tachycardia, restlessness, visual hallucinations	Discontinue drug, IV physostigmine, 0.5–2 mg, for severe agitation or fever, benzodiazepines; antipsychotics contraindicated
Anticonvulsant intoxication	Psychosis; delirium	Dosage of anticonvulsant is reduced
Benzodiazepine intoxication	Sedation, somnolence, and ataxia	Supportive measures; flumazenil, 7.5–45 mg a day, titrated as needed, should be used only by skilled personnel with resuscitative equipment available
Bereavement	Guilt feelings, irritability; insomnia; somatic complaints	Must be differentiated from major depressive disorder; antidepressants not indicated; benzodiazepines for sleep; encouragement of ventilation
Borderline personality disorder	Suicidal ideation and gestures; homicidal ideations and gestures; substance abuse; micropsychotic episodes; burns, cut marks on body	Suicidal and homicidal evaluation (if great, hospitalization); small dosages of antipsychotics; clear follow-up plan
Brief psychotic disorder	Emotional turmoil, extreme lability; acutely impaired reality testing after obvious psychosocial stress	Hospitalization often necessary; low dosage of antipsychotics may be necessary but often resolves spontaneously
Bromide intoxication	Delirium; mania; depression; psychosis	Serum levels obtained (>50 mg a day); bromide intake discontinued; large quantities of sodium chloride IV or orally; if agitation, paraldehyde or antipsychotic is used
Caffeine intoxication	Severe anxiety, resembling panic disorder; mania; delirium; agitated depression; sleep disturbance	Cessation of caffeine-containing substances; benzodiazepines
Cannabis intoxication	Delusions; panic; dysphoria; cognitive impairment	Benzodiazepines and antipsychotics as needed; evaluation of suicidal or homicidal risk; symptoms usually abate with time and reassurance
Catatonia	Marked psychomotor disturbance (either excitement or stupor); exhaustion; can be fatal	Rapid tranquilization with benzodiazepines or antipsychotics; monitor vital signs
Cimetidine psychotic disorder	Delirium; delusions	Reduce dosage or discontinue drug
Clonidine withdrawal	Irritability; psychosis; violence; seizures	Symptoms abate with time, but antipsychotics may be necessary; gradual lowering of dosage
Cocaine intoxication and withdrawal	Paranoia and violence; severe anxiety; manic state; delirium: schizophreniform psychosis; tachycardia, hypertension, myocardial infarction, cerebrovascular disease; depression and suicidal ideation	Antipsychotics and benzodiazepines; antidepressants or electroconvulsive therapy (ECT) for withdrawal depression if persistent; hospitalization
Delirium	Fluctuating sensorium; suicidal and homicidal risk; cognitive clouding; visual, tactile, and auditory hallucinations; paranoia	Evaluate all potential contributing factors and treat each accordingly; reassurance, structure, clues to orientation; benzodiazepines and low-dosage, high-potency antipsychotics must be used with extreme care because of their potential to act paradoxically and increase agitation
Delusional disorder	Most often brought into emergency department involuntarily; threats directed toward others	Antipsychotics if patient will comply (IM if necessary); intensive family intervention; hospitalization if necessary
Dementia	Unable to care for self; violent outbursts; psychosis; depression and suicidal ideation; confusion	Small dosages of high-potency antipsychotics; clues to orientation; organic evaluation, including medication use; family intervention
Depressive disorders	Suicidal ideation and attempts; self-neglect; substance abuse	Assessment of danger to self; hospitalization if necessary, nonpsychiatric causes of depression must be evaluated

Table 25-12
Common Psychiatric Emergencies (*Continued*)

Syndrome	Emergency Manifestations	Treatment Issues
L-Dopa intoxication	Mania; depression; schizophreniform disorder, may induce rapid cycling in patients with bipolar I disorder	Lower dosage or discontinue drug
Dystonia, acute	Intense involuntary spasm of muscles of neck, tongue, face, jaw, eyes, or trunk	Decrease dosage of antipsychotic; benztropine or diphenhydramine IM
Group hysteria	Groups of people exhibit extremes of grief or other disruptive behavior	Group is dispersed with help of other health care workers; ventilation, crisis-oriented therapy; if necessary, small dosages of benzodiazepines
Hallucinogen-induced psychotic disorder with hallucinations	Symptom picture is result of interaction of type of substance, dose taken, duration of action, user's premorbid personality, setting; panic; agitation; atropine psychosis	Serum and urine screens; rule out underlying medical or mental disorder; benzodiazepines (2–20 mg) orally; reassurance and orientation; rapid tranquilization; often responds spontaneously
Homicidal and assaultive behavior	Marked agitation with verbal threats	Seclusion, restraints, medication
Hypertensive crisis	Life-threatening hypertensive reaction secondary to ingestion of tyramine-containing foods in combination with monoamine oxidase inhibitors (MAOIs); headache, stiff neck, sweating, nausea, vomiting	Antihypertensive medications as per emergency medicine team make sure symptoms are not secondary to hypotension (side effect of MAOIs alone)
Hyperthermia	Extreme excitement or catatonic stupor or both; extremely elevated temperature; violent hyperagitation	Hydrate and cool; may be drug reaction, so discontinue any drug; rule out infection
Hyperventilation	Anxiety, terror, clouded consciousness; giddiness, faintness; blurring vision	Shift alkalosis by having patient breathe into paper bag; patient education; antianxiety agents
Hypothermia	Confusion; lethargy; combativeness; low body temperature and shivering; paradoxical feeling of warmth	IV fluids and rewarming, cardiac status must be carefully monitored; avoidance of alcohol
Incest and sexual abuse of child	Suicidal behavior; adolescent crises; substance abuse	Corroboration of charge, protection of victim; contact social services; medical and psychiatric evaluation; crisis intervention
Insomnia	Depression and irritability; early morning agitation; frightening dreams; fatigue	Hypnotics only in short term; treat any underlying mental disorder; rules of sleep hygiene
Intermittent explosive disorder	Brief outbursts of violence; periodic episodes of suicide attempts	Benzodiazepines or antipsychotics for short term; long-term evaluation with computed tomography (CT) scan, sleep-deprived electroencephalogram (EEG), glucose tolerance curve
Jaundice	Uncommon complication of low-potency phenothiazine use (e.g., chlorpromazine)	Change drug to low dosage of a low-potency agent in a different class
Leukopenia and agranulocytosis	Side effects within the first 2 mo of treatment with antipsychotics	Patient should call immediately for sore throat, fever, etc., and obtain immediate blood count; discontinue drug; hospitalize if necessary
Lithium toxicity	Vomiting; abdominal pain; profuse diarrhea; severe tremor, ataxia; coma; seizures; confusion; dysarthria; focal neurologic signs	Lavage with wide-bore tube; osmotic diuresis; medical consultation; may require intensive care unit treatment
Major depressive episode with psychotic features	Major depressive episode symptoms with delusions; agitation, severe guilt; ideas of reference; suicide and homicide risk	Antipsychotics plus antidepressants; evaluation of suicide and homicide risk; hospitalization and ECT if necessary
Manic episode	Violent, impulsive behavior; indiscriminate sexual or spending behavior; psychosis; substance abuse	Hospitalization; restraints if necessary; rapid tranquilization with antipsychotics; restoration of lithium levels

(continued)

Table 25-12
Common Psychiatric Emergencies (*Continued*)

Syndrome	Emergency Manifestations	Treatment Issues
Marital crises	Precipitant may be discovery of an extramarital affair, onset of serious illness, announcement of intent to divorce, or problems with children or work; one or both members of the couple may be in therapy or may be psychiatrically ill; one spouse may be seeking hospitalization for the other	Each should be questioned alone regarding extramarital affairs, consultations with lawyers regarding divorce, and willingness to work in crisis-oriented or long-term therapy to resolve the problem; sexual, financial, and psychiatric treatment histories from both, psychiatric evaluation at the time of presentation; may be precipitated by onset of untreated mood disorder or affective symptoms caused by medical illness or insidious-onset dementia; referral for management of the illness reduces immediate stress and enhances the healthier spouse's coping capacity; children may give insights available only to someone intimately involved in the social system
Migraine	Throbbing, unilateral headache	Sumatriptan 6 mg IM
Mitral valve prolapse	Associated with panic disorder; dyspnea and palpitations; fear and anxiety	Echocardiogram; alprazolam or propranolol
Neuroleptic malignant syndrome	Hyperthermia; muscle rigidity; autonomic instability; parkinsonian symptoms; catatonic stupor; neurologic signs; 10% to 30% fatality; elevated creatine phosphokinase (CPK)	Discontinue antipsychotic; IV dantrolene; bromocriptine orally; hydration and cooling; monitor CPK levels
Nitrous oxide toxicity	Euphoria and light-headedness	Symptoms abate without treatment within hours of use
Nutmeg intoxication	Agitation; hallucinations; severe headaches; numbness in extremities	Symptoms abate within hours of use without treatment
Opioid intoxication and withdrawal	Intoxication can lead to coma and death; withdrawal is not life-threatening	IV naloxone, narcotic antagonist; urine and serum screens; psychiatric and medical illnesses (e.g., AIDS) may complicate picture
Panic disorder	Panic, terror; acute onset	Must differentiate from other anxiety-producing disorders, both medical and psychiatric; ECG to rule out mitral valve prolapse; short-acting benzodiazepines for symptomatic management; long-term management may include an antidepressant
Parkinsonism	Stiffness, tremor, bradykinesia, flattened affect, shuffling gait, salivation, secondary to antipsychotic medication	Oral antiparkinsonian drug for 4 wk to 3 mo; decrease dosage of the antipsychotic
Perioral (rabbit) tremor	Perioral tumor (rabbit-like facial grimacing) usually appearing after long-term therapy with antipsychotics	Decrease dosage or change to a medication in another class
Phencyclidine (or phencyclidine-like intoxication)	Psychosis; can lead to death; acute danger to self and others	Serum and urine assay; benzodiazepines may interfere with excretion; antipsychotics may worsen symptoms because of anticholinergic side effects; medical monitoring and hospitalization for severe intoxication
Phenelzine-induced psychotic disorder	Psychosis and mania in predisposed people	Reduce dosage or discontinue drug
Phenylpropanolamine toxicity	Psychosis; paranoia; insomnia; restlessness; nervousness; headache	Symptoms abate with dosage reduction or discontinuation (found in over-the-counter diet aids and oral and nasal decongestants)
Phobias	Panic, anxiety; fear	Treatment same as for panic disorder
Photosensitivity	Easy sunburning secondary to use of antipsychotic medication	Patient should avoid strong sunlight and use high-level sunscreens
Pigmentary retinopathy	Reported with dosages of thioridazine of 800 mg a day or above	Remain below 800 mg a day of thioridazine
Postpartum psychosis	Childbirth can precipitate schizophrenia, depression, reactive psychoses, mania, and depression; affective symptoms are most common; suicide risk is reduced during pregnancy but increased in the postpartum period	Danger to self and others (including infant) must be evaluated and proper precautions taken; medical illness presenting with behavioral aberrations is included in the differential diagnosis and must be sought and treated; care must be paid to the effects on father, infant, grandparents, and other children
Posttraumatic stress disorder	Panic, terror; suicidal ideation; flashbacks	Reassurance; encouragement of return to responsibilities; avoid hospitalization if possible to prevent chronic invalidism; monitor suicidal ideation

Table 25-12
Common Psychiatric Emergencies (*Continued*)

Syndrome	Emergency Manifestations	Treatment Issues
Priapism (trazodone induced)	Persistent penile erection accompanied by severe pain	Intracorporeal epinephrine; mechanical or surgical drainage
Propranolol toxicity	Profound depression; confusional states	Reduce dosage or discontinue drug; monitor suicidality
Rape	Not all sexual violations are reported; silent rape reaction is characterized by loss of appetite, sleep disturbance, anxiety, and, sometimes, agoraphobia; long periods of silence, mounting anxiety, stuttering, blocking, and physical symptoms during the interview when the sexual history is taken; fear of violence and death and of contracting a sexually transmitted disease or being pregnant	Rape is a major psychiatric emergency; victim may have enduring patterns of sexual dysfunction; crisis-oriented therapy, social support, ventilation, reinforcement of healthy traits, and encouragement to return to the previous level of functioning as rapidly as possible; legal counsel; thorough medical examination and tests to identify the assailant (e.g., obtaining samples of pubic hairs with a pubic hair comb, vaginal smear to identify blood antigens in semen); if a woman, methoxyprogesterone or diethylstilbestrol orally for 5 days to prevent pregnancy; if menstruation does not commence within 1 wk of cessation of the estrogen, all alternatives to pregnancy, including abortion, should be offered; if the victim has contracted a venereal disease, appropriate antibiotics; witnessed written permission is required for the physician to examine, photograph, collect specimens, and release information to the authorities; obtain consent, record the history in the patient's own words, obtain required tests, record the results of the examination, save all clothing, defer diagnosis, and provide protection against disease, psychic trauma, and pregnancy; men's and women's responses to rape affectively are reported similarly, although men are more hesitant to talk about homosexual assault for fear they will be assumed to have consented
Reserpine intoxication	Major depressive episodes; suicidal ideation; nightmares	Evaluation of suicidal ideation; lower dosage or change drug; antidepressants of ECT may be indicated
Schizoaffective disorder	Severe depression; manic symptoms; paranoia	Evaluation of dangerousness to self or others; rapid tranquilization if necessary; treatment of depression (antidepressants alone can enhance schizophrenic symptoms); use of antimanic agents
Schizophrenia	Extreme self-neglect; severe paranoia; suicidal ideation or assaultiveness; extreme psychotic symptoms	Evaluation of suicidal and homicidal potential; identification of any illness other than schizophrenia; rapid tranquilization
Schizophrenia in exacerbation	Withdrawn; agitation; suicidal and homicidal risk	Suicide and homicide evaluation; screen for medical illness; restraints and rapid tranquilization if necessary; hospitalization if necessary; reevaluation of medication regimen
Sedative, hypnotic, or anxiolytic intoxication and withdrawal	Alterations in mood, behavior, thought—delirium; derealization and depersonalization; untreated, can be fatal; seizures	Naloxone to differentiate from opioid intoxication; slow withdrawal with benzodiazepine; hospitalization
Seizure disorder	Confusion; anxiety; derealization and depersonalization; feelings of impending doom; gustatory or olfactory hallucinations; fugue-like state	Immediate EEG; admission and sleep-deprived and 24-hr EEG; rule out pseudoseizures; anticonvulsants
Substance withdrawal	Abdominal pain; insomnia, drowsiness; delirium; seizures; symptoms of tardive dyskinesia may emerge; eruption of manic or schizophrenic symptoms	Symptoms of psychotropic drug withdrawal disappear with time or disappear with reinstitution of the substance; symptoms of antidepressant withdrawal can be successfully treated with anticholinergic agents, such as atropine; gradual withdrawal of psychotropic substances over 2–4 wk generally obviates development of symptoms
Sudden death associated with antipsychotic medication	Seizures; asphyxiation; cardiovascular causes; postural hypotension; laryngeal–pharyngeal dystonia; suppression of gag reflex	Specific medical treatments
Sudden death of psychogenic origin	Myocardial infarction after sudden psychic stress; voodoo and hexes; hopelessness, especially associated with serious physical illness	Specific medical treatments; folk healers
Suicide	Suicidal ideation; hopelessness	Hospitalization, antidepressants
Sympathomimetic withdrawal	Paranoia; confusional states; depression	Most symptoms abate without treatment; antipsychotics; antidepressants if necessary

(continued)

Table 25-12
Common Psychiatric Emergencies (*Continued*)

Syndrome	Emergency Manifestations	Treatment Issues
Tardive dyskinesia	Dyskinesia of mouth, tongue, face, neck, and trunk; choreoathetoid movements of extremities; usually but not always appearing after long-term treatment with antipsychotics, especially after a reduction in dosage; incidence highest in the elderly and brain damaged; symptoms are intensified by antiparkinsonian drugs and masked but not cured by increased dosages of antipsychotic	No effective treatment reported; may be prevented by prescribing the least amount of drug possible for as little time as is clinically feasible and using drug-free holidays for patients who need to continue taking the drug; decrease or discontinue drug at first sign of dyskinetic movements
Thyrotoxicosis	Tachycardia; gastrointestinal dysfunction; hyperthermia; panic, anxiety, agitation; mania; dementia; psychosis	Thyroid function test (T_3, T_4, thyroid-stimulating hormone [TSH]); medical consultation
Toluene abuse	Anxiety; confusion; cognitive impairment	Neurologic damage is nonprogressive and reversible if toluene use in discontinued early
Vitamin B_{12} deficiency	Confusion; mood and behavior changes; ataxia	Treatment with vitamin B_{12}
Volatile nitrates	Alternations of mood and behavior; light-headedness; pulsating headache	Symptoms abate with cessation of use

involved with the child. Familial stressors and parental discord can contribute to the evolution of a crisis for a child. For example, immediate evaluations are sometimes legitimately indicated for a child caught in the crossfire of feuding parents or a seemingly irreconcilable conflict between a set of parents and a school, therapist, or protective service worker regarding the needs of the child (Table 25-13).

An emergency setting is often the site of an initial evaluation of chronic problem behavior. For example, an identified problem—such as severe tantrums, violence, and destructive behavior in a child—may have been present for months or even years. Nevertheless, the initial contact with the mental health system in the emergency room or private office may be the first opportunity for the child or adolescent to disclose underlying stressors, such as physical or sexual abuse.

Given the integral relation of severe family dysfunction to childhood behavioral disturbance, the emergency psychiatrist must assess familial discord and psychiatric disorder in family members during an urgent evaluation. One way to make the assessment is to interview the child and the individual family members, both alone and together, and to obtain a history from informants outside the family whenever possible. Noncustodial parents, therapists, and teachers may add valuable information regarding the child's daily functioning. Many families, especially those with mental illness and severe dysfunction, may have little or no inclination to seek psychiatric help on a nonurgent basis; therefore, the emergency evaluation becomes the only way to engage them in an extensive psychiatric treatment program.

Table 25-13
Familial Risk Factors

Physical and sexual abuse
Recent family crisis: loss of a parent, divorce, loss of job, family move
Severe family dysfunction, including parental mental illness

Life-Threatening Emergencies

Suicidal Behavior

ASSESSMENT. Suicidal behavior is the most common reason for an emergency evaluation in adolescents. Despite the minimal risk for a complete suicide in a child less than 12 years of age, suicidal ideation or behavior in a child of any age must be carefully evaluated, with particular attention to the psychiatric status of the child and the ability of the family or the guardians to provide the appropriate supervision. The assessment must determine the circumstances of the suicidal ideation or behavior, its lethality, and the persistence of the suicidal intention. An evaluation of the family's sensitivity, supportiveness, and competence must be done to assess their ability to monitor the child's suicidal potential. Ultimately, during an emergency evaluation, the psychiatrist must decide whether the child may return home to a safe environment and receive outpatient follow-up care or whether hospitalization is necessary. A psychiatric history, a mental status examination, and an assessment of family functioning help establish the general level of risk.

MANAGEMENT. When self-injurious behavior has occurred, the adolescent likely requires hospitalization in a pediatric unit for treatment of the injury or the observation of medical sequelae after toxic ingestion. If the adolescent is medically clear, the psychiatrist must decide whether the adolescent needs psychiatric admission. If the patient persists in suicidal ideation and shows signs of psychosis, severe depression (including hopelessness), or marked ambivalence about suicide, psychiatric admission is indicated. An adolescent who is taking drugs or alcohol should not be released until an assessment can be done when the patient is not intoxicated. Patients with high-risk profiles—such as late-adolescent males, especially those with substance abuse and aggressive behavior disorders, and those who have severe depression or who have made prior suicide attempts, particularly with lethal weapons—warrant hospitalization. Young children who made suicide attempts, even when the attempt had a low lethality, need psychiatric admission if the family is so chaotic, dysfunctional, and incompetent that follow-up treatment is unlikely.

Violent Behavior and Tantrums

ASSESSMENT. The first task in an emergency evaluation of a violent child or adolescent is to make sure that both the child and the staff members are physically protected so that nobody gets hurt. If the child appears to be calming down in the emergency area, the clinician may indicate to the child that it would be helpful if the child recounted what happened and may ask whether the child feels in sufficient control to do so. If the child agrees and the clinician judges the child to be in reasonable control, the clinician may approach the child with the appropriate backup close at hand. If not, the clinician may either give the child several minutes to calm down before reassessing the situation or, with an adolescent, suggest that medication may help the adolescent relax.

If the adolescent is combative, physical restraint may be necessary before anything else is attempted. Some rageful children and adolescents brought to an emergency setting by overwhelmed families can regain control of themselves without the use of physical or pharmacologic restraint. Children and adolescents are most likely to calm down if approached calmly in a nonthreatening manner and given a chance to tell their side of the story to a nonjudgmental adult. At this time, the psychiatrist should look for any underlying psychiatric disorder that may be mediating the aggression. The psychiatrist should speak to family members and others who have been witnessing the episode to understand the context in which it occurred and the extent to which the child has been out of control.

MANAGEMENT. Prepubertal children, in the absence of major psychiatric illness, rarely require medication to keep them safe, because they are generally small enough to be physically restrained if they begin to hurt themselves or others. It is not immediately necessary to administer medication to a child or an adolescent who was in a rage but is in a calm state when examined. Adolescents and older children who are assaultive, extremely agitated, or overtly self-injurious and who may be difficult to subdue physically may require medication before a dialogue can take place.

Children who have a history of repeated, self-limited, severe tantrums may not require admission to a hospital if they can calm down during the evaluation. However, the pattern, no doubt, will reoccur unless ongoing outpatient treatment for the child and the family is arranged. For adolescents who continue to pose a danger to themselves or others during the evaluation period, admission to a hospital is necessary.

Fire Setting

ASSESSMENT. A sense of emergency and panic often surrounds the parents of a child who has set a fire. Parents or teachers often request an emergency evaluation, even for a very young child who has accidentally lit a fire. Many children, during normal development, become interested in fire, but in most cases, a school-aged child who has set a fire has done so accidentally while playing with matches and seeks help to put it out. When a child has a strong interest in playing with matches, the level of supervision by family members must be clarified so that no further accidental fires occur. The clinician must distinguish between a child who accidentally or even impulsively sets a single fire and a child who engages in repeated fire setting with premeditation and subsequently leaves the fire without making any attempt to extinguish it. In repeated fire setting, the risk is more significant than in a single occurrence, and the psychiatrist must determine whether underlying psychopathology

exists in the child or the family members. The psychiatrist should also evaluate family interactions because any factors that interfere with adequate supervision and communication—such as high levels of marital discord and harsh, punitive parenting styles—can impede appropriate intervention.

Fire setting is one of a triad of symptoms—enuresis, cruelty to animals, and fire setting—that were believed, some years ago, to be typical of children with conduct disorders; however, no evidence indicates that the three symptoms are genuinely linked, although conduct disorder is the most frequent psychiatric disorder that occurs with pathologic fire setting.

MANAGEMENT. The critical component of management and treatment for firesetters is to prevent further incidents while treating any underlying psychopathology. In general, fire setting alone is not an indication for hospitalization, unless a continued direct threat exists that the patient will set another fire. The parents of children with a pattern of fire setting must be emphatically counseled that the child must not be left alone at home and should never be left to take care of younger siblings without direct adult supervision. Children who exhibit a pattern of concurrent aggressive behaviors and other forms of destructive behavior are likely to have a poor outcome. Outpatient treatment should be arranged for children who repeatedly set fires. Behavioral techniques that involve both the child and the family help decrease the risk for further fire setting, as is positive reinforcement for alternate behaviors.

Child Abuse: Physical and Sexual

Assessment. Physical and sexual abuse occurs in girls and boys of all ages, in all ethnic groups, and at all socioeconomic levels. The abuses vary widely for severity and duration, but any form of continued abuse constitutes an emergency for a child. No single psychiatric syndrome is a sine qua non of physical or sexual abuse, but fear, guilt, anxiety, depression, and ambivalence regarding disclosure commonly surround the child who has been abused.

Young children who are being sexually abused may exhibit precocious sexual behavior with peers and present detailed sexual knowledge that reflects exposure beyond their developmental level. Often, children who endure sexual or physical abuse display sadistic and aggressive behaviors themselves. Abused children are likely to be threatened with severe and frightening consequences by the perpetrator if they reveal the situation to anyone. Frequently, an abused child who is victimized by a family member is placed in the irreconcilable position of having to choose between enduring the abuse or risk destroying the family, not being believed or being abandoned.

In cases of suspected abuse, the child and other family members must be interviewed individually to give each member a chance to speak privately. If possible, the clinician should observe the child with each parent individually to get a sense of the spontaneity, warmth, fear, anxiety, or other prominent features of the relationships. One observation is generally not sufficient to make a final judgment about the family relationship. However, abused children almost always have mixed emotions toward abusive parents.

Physical indicators of sexual abuse in children include sexually transmitted diseases (e.g., gonorrhea); pain, irritation, and itching of the genitalia and the urinary tract; and discomfort while sitting and walking. In many instances of suspected sexual abuse, however, physical evidence is not present. Thus, a careful history is essential. The physician should speak directly about the issues without leading the child in any direction, because already frightened children may be easily influenced to endorse what they think the examiner wants to hear. Furthermore, children who have been abused often retract all or part of what has been disclosed during an interview.

The use of anatomically correct dolls in the assessment of sexual abuse can help the child identify body parts and show what has happened, but no conclusive evidence supports sexual play with dolls as a means of validating abuse.

Neglect: Failure to Thrive

Assessment. In child neglect, a child's physical, mental, or emotional condition has been impaired because of the inability of a parent or caretaker to provide adequate food, shelter, education, or supervision. Similar to abuse, any form of continued neglect is an emergency for the child. Parents who neglect their children range widely and may include parents who are very young and ignorant about the emotional and concrete needs of a child, parents with depression and significant passivity, substance-abusing parents, and parents with a variety of incapacitating mental illnesses.

In its extreme form, neglect can contribute to failure to thrive—that is, an infant, usually under 1 year of age, becomes malnourished in the absence of an organic cause. Failure to thrive typically occurs under circumstances in which adequate nourishment is available, but a disturbance within the relationship between the caretaker and the child results in a child who does not eat sufficiently to grow and develop. A negative pattern may exist between the mother and the child in which the child refuses feedings, and the mother feels rejected and eventually withdraws. She may then avoid offering food as frequently as the infant needs it. Observation of the mother and the child together may reveal a nonspontaneous, tense interaction, with withdrawal on both sides, resulting in a seeming apathy in the mother. Both the mother and the child may seem depressed.

A rare form of failure to thrive in children who are at least several years old and are not necessarily malnourished is the syndrome of psychosocial dwarfism. In that syndrome, marked growth retardation and delayed epiphyseal malnutrition accompany a disturbed relationship between the parent and the child, along with bizarre social and eating behaviors in the child. Those behaviors sometimes include eating from garbage cans, drinking toilet water, binging and vomiting, and diminished outward response to pain. Half of the children with the syndrome have decreased growth hormone. Once the children are removed from the troubled environment and placed in another setting, such as a psychiatric hospital with appropriate supervision and guidance regarding meals, the endocrine abnormalities normalize, and the children begin to grow at a more rapid rate.

Management. In cases of child neglect, as with physical and sexual abuse, the most crucial decision to be made during the initial evaluation is whether the child is safe in the home environment. Whenever neglect is suspected, it must be reported to the local child protective service agency. In mild cases, the decision to refer the family for outpatient services, as opposed to hospitalizing the child, depends on the clinician's conviction that the family is cooperative and willing to be educated and to enter into treatment and that the child is not in danger. Before a neglected child is released from an emergency setting, a follow-up appointment must be made.

Education for the family must begin during the evaluation; the family must be told, in a nonthreatening manner, that failure to thrive can become life-threatening, that the entire family needs to monitor the child's progress, and that they will receive some help in overcoming the many possible obstacles interfering with the child's emotional and physical well-being.

Anorexia Nervosa

Anorexia nervosa occurs in females about 10 times as often as in males. It is characterized by the refusal to maintain body weight, leading to weight at least 15 percent below the expected weight, by a distorted body image, by a persistent fear of becoming fat, and by the absence of at least three menstrual cycles. The disorder usually begins after puberty, but it has occurred in children of 9 to 10 years of age, in whom expected weight gain does not occur, rather than a loss of 15 percent of body weight. The disorder reaches medical emergency proportions when the weight loss approaches 30 percent of body weight or when metabolic disturbances become severe. Hospitalization then becomes necessary to control the ongoing process of starvation, potential dehydration, and the medical complications of starvation, including electrolyte imbalances, cardiac arrhythmias, and hormonal changes.

Acquired Immune Deficiency Syndrome

Assessment. AIDS, which is caused by the human immunodeficiency virus (HIV), occurs in neonate through perinatal transmission from an infected mother, in children and adolescents secondary to sexual abuse by an infected person, and adolescents through intravenous drug abuse with an infected person or intravenous drug abuse with infected needles and sexual activities with infected partners. Child and adolescent hemophiliac patients may contract AIDS through tainted blood transfusions.

Children and adolescents may present for emergency evaluations at the urging of a family member of a peer; in some cases, they take the initiative themselves when they are faced with anxiety or panic about high-risk behavior. Early screening of high-risk persons may lead to the treatment of asymptomatic infected patients with such drugs as azidothymidine (AZT) and possibly other new medications that may slow the course of the disease. During the assessment of the risks for HIV infection, the doctor can start to educate the patient and family so that an adolescent who is not infected but exhibits high-risk behavior can be counseled about that behavior and safe-sex practices.

In children, the brain is often a primary site for HIV infection; encephalitis, decreased brain development, and such neuropsychiatric symptoms as impairment in memory, concentration, and attention span may be present before the diagnosis is made. The virus can be present in the cerebrospinal fluid before it shows up in the bloodstream. Changes in cognitive function, frontal lobe disinhibition, social withdrawal, slowed information processing, and apathy constitute some common symptoms of the AIDS dementia complex. Mood disorders, personality changes, and frank psychosis can also occur in patients infected with HIV.

Munchausen Syndrome by Proxy

Assessment. Munchausen syndrome by proxy, essentially, is a form of child abuse in which a parent, usually the mother, or a caretaker repeatedly fabricates or inflicts injury or illness in a child for whom the medical intervention is then sought, often in an emergency setting. Although it is a rare scenario, mothers who inflict injury often have some prior knowledge of medicine, leading to sophisticated symptoms; the mothers sometimes engage in inappropriate camaraderie with the medical staff regarding the treatment of the child. Careful observation may reveal that the mothers often do not exhibit appropriate signs of distress on hearing the details of the child's medical symptoms. Prototypically, such mothers tend to present themselves as highly accomplished professionals in ways that seem inflated or blatantly untrue.

The illnesses appearing in the child can involve any organ system, but specific symptoms are commonly presented: bleeding from one or many sites, including the GI tract, the genitourinary system, and the respiratory system; seizures; and CNS depression. At times, the illness is simulated, rather than inflicted.

Urgent Non–Life-Threatening Situations

School Refusal

ASSESSMENT. Refusal to go to school may occur in a young child who is first entering school or in an older child or adolescent who is making a transition into a new grade or school, or it may emerge in a vulnerable child without an apparent external stressor. In any case, school refusal requires immediate intervention, because the longer the dysfunctional pattern continues, the more difficult it is to interrupt.

School refusal is generally associated with separation anxiety, in which the child's distress is related to the consequences of being separated from the parent, so the child resists going to school. School refusal can also occur in children with school phobia, in which the school is the target of fear and distress. In either case, a severe disruption of the child's life occurs. Although mild separation anxiety is universal, particularly among very young children who are first facing the school, treatment is required when a child actually cannot attend school. Severe psychopathology, including anxiety and depressive disorders, is often present when school refusal occurs for the first time in an adolescent. Children with separation anxiety disorder typically present extreme worries that catastrophic events will befall their mothers, attachment, or themselves as a result of the separation. Children with separation anxiety disorder may also exhibit many other fears and symptoms of depression, including such somatic complaints such as headaches, stomachaches, and nausea. Severe tantrums and desperate pleas may ensue when preoccupation that a parent will be harmed during the separation is frequently verbalized; in adolescents, the stated reasons for refusing to go to school are often physical complaints.

As part of an urgent assessment, the psychiatrist must ascertain the duration of the patient's absence from school and must assess the parents' ability to participate in a treatment plan that will undoubtedly involve firm parental guidelines to ensure the child's return to school. The parents of a child with separation anxiety disorder often exhibit excessive separation anxiety or other anxiety disorders themselves, thereby compounding the child's problem. When the parents are unable to participate in a treatment program from home, hospitalization should be considered.

MANAGEMENT. When school refusal caused by separation anxiety is identified during an emergency evaluation, the underlying disorder can be explained to the family, and an intervention can be started immediately. In severe cases, however, a multidimensional, long-term family-oriented treatment plan is necessary. Whenever possible, a separation-anxious child should be brought back to school the next school day, despite the distress, and a contact person within the school (counselor, guidance counselor, or teacher) should be involved to help the child stay in school while praising the child for tolerating the school situation.

When school refusal has been going on for months or years or when the family members are unable to cooperate, a treatment program to move the child back to school from the hospital should be considered. When the child's anxiety is not diminished by behavioral methods alone, antidepressants are helpful. Medication is generally prescribed not at the initial evaluation, but after a behavioral intervention has been tried.

Other Childhood Disturbances

Posttraumatic Stress Disorder. Children who have been subjected to a severe catastrophic or traumatic event may present for a prompt evaluation because they have extreme fears of the specific trauma occurring again or sudden discomfort with familiar places, people, or situations that previously did not evoke anxiety. Within weeks of a traumatic event, a child may recreate the event in play, in stories, and in dreams that directly replay the terrifying situation. A sense of reliving the experience may occur, including hallucinations and flashback (dissociative) experiences, and intrusive memories of the event come and go. Many traumatized children, over time, go on to reproduce parts of the event through their victimization behaviors toward others, without being aware that those behaviors reflect their own traumatic experiences.

Dissociative Disorders. Dissociative states—including the extreme form, multiple personality disorder—are believed most likely to occur in children who have been subjected to severe and repetitive physical, sexual, or emotional abuse. Children with dissociative symptoms may be referred for evaluation because family members or teachers observe that the children sometimes seem to be spaced out or distracted or act like different persons. Dissociative states are occasionally identified during the evaluation of violent and aggressive behavior, particularly in patients who honestly do not remember chunks of their behavior.

When a child who dissociates is violent or self-destructive or endangers others, hospitalization is necessary. A variety of psychotherapy methods have been used in the complex treatment of children with dissociative disorders, including play techniques and, in some cases, hypnosis.

References

Consultation-Liaison Psychiatry

Ader R, ed. *Psychoneuroimmunology*. 4th ed. New York: Elsevier; 2007.

Alexander F. *Psychosomatic Medicine: Its Principles and Application*. New York: Norton; 1950.

Cannon WB. *The Wisdom of the Body*. New York: Norton; 1932.

Chaturvedi SK, Desai G. Measurement and assessment of somatic symptoms. *Int Rev Psychiatry*. 2013;25(1):31–40.

Copello A, Walsh K, Graham H, Tobin D, Griffith E, Day E, Birchwood M. A consultation-liaison service on integrated treatment: A program description. *J Dual Diagn*. 2013;9(2):149–157.

Dew MA, DiMartini AD, De Vito Dabbs A, Myaskovsky L, Steel J. Rates and risk factors for nonadherence to the medical regimen after adult solid organ transplantation. *Transplantation*. 2007;83(7):858–873.

DiMartini A, Crone C, Fireman M, Dew MA. Psychiatric aspects of organ transplantation in critical care. *Crit Care Clin*. 2008;24:949–981.

Dobbels F, Verleden G, Dupont L, Vanhaecke J, De Geest S. To transplant or not? The importance of psychosocial and behavioural factors before lung transplantation. *Chronic Respir Dis*. 2006;3(1):39–47.

Escobar J. Somatoform disorders. In: Sadock BJ, Sadock VA, eds. *Kaplan & Sadock's Comprehensive Textbook of Psychiatry*. 9th ed. Vol. 1. Philadelphia, PA: Lippincott Williams & Wilkins; 2009:1927.

Fava GA, Sonino N. The clinical domains of psychosomatic medicine. *J Clin Psychiatry*. 2005;66:849–858.

Goodwin RD, Olfson M, Shea S, Lantigua RA, Carrasquilo O, Gameroff MJ, Weissman MM. Asthma and mental disorders in primary care. *Gen Hosp Psychiatry*. 2004;25:479–483.

Hamilton JC, Eger M, Razzak S, Feldman MD, Hallmark N, Cheek S. Somatoform, factitious, and related diagnoses in the National Hospital Discharge Survey: Addressing the proposed DSM-5 revision. *Psychosomatics*. 2013;54(2): 142–148.

Kaplan HI. History of psychosomatic medicine. In: Sadock BJ, Sadock VA, eds: *Kaplan and Sadock's Comprehensive Textbook of Psychiatry*. 8th ed. Philadelphia, PA: Lippincott Williams & Wilkins; 2005:2105.

Lesperance F, Frasure-Smith N, Theroux P, Irwin M. The association between major depression and levels of soluble intercellular adhesion molecule 1, interleukin-6, and C-reactive protein in patients with recent acute coronary syndromes. *Am J Psychiatry*. 2004;161:271–277.

Lipsitt DR. Consultation-liaison psychiatry and psychosomatic medicine: The company they keep. *Psychosom Med*. 2001;63(6):896–909.

Matthews KA, Gump BB, Harris KF, Haney TL, Barefoot JC. Hostile behaviors predict cardiovascular mortality among men enrolled in the multiple risk factor intervention trial. *Circulation*. 2004;109:66–70.

Palta P, Samuel LJ, Miller ER, Szanton SL. Depression and oxidative stress: Results from a meta-analysis of observational studies. *Psychosom Med*. 2014;76(1): 12–19.

Schrag AE, Mehta AR, Bhatia KP, Brown RJ, Frackowiak RS, Trimble MR, Ward NS, Rowe JB. The functional neuroimaging correlates of psychogenic versus organic dystonia. *Brain*. 2013;136(3):770–781.

Shorter E. *From Paralysis to Fatigue: A History of Psychosomatic Illness in the Modern Era*. New York: Free Press; 1992.

Geriatric Psychiatry

Balzer DG, Steffens DC. *Essentials of Geriatric Psychiatry*. 2nd ed. Arlington: American Psychiatric Association; 2012.

Bartels SJ, Naslund JA. The underside of the silver tsunami—older adults and mental health care. *N Engl J Med*. 2013;368(6):493–496.

Cohen CI, Ibrahim F. Serving elders in the public sector. In: McQuistion HL, Sowers WE, Ranz JM, Feldman JM, eds. *Handbook of Community Psychiatry*. New York: Springer Science+Business Media; 2012:485.

Colarusso CA. Adulthood. In: Sadock BJ, Sadock VA, Ruiz P, eds. *Kaplan & Sadock's Comprehensive Textbook of Psychiatry*. 9th ed. Philadelphia, PA: Lippincott Williams & Wilkins; 2009:3909.

de Waal MWM, van der Weele GM, van der Mast RC, Assendelft WJJ, Gussekloo J. The influence of the administration method on scores of the 15-item geriatric depression scale in old age. *Psychiatry Res*. 2012;197(3):280–284.

Høiseth G, Kristiansen KM, Kvande K, Tanum L, Lorentzen B, Refsum H. Benzodiazepines in geriatric psychiatry. *Drugs Aging*. 2013;30(2):113–118.

Jeste D. Geriatric psychiatry: Introduction. In: Sadock BJ, Sadock VA, Ruiz P, eds. *Kaplan & Sadock's Comprehensive Textbook of Psychiatry*. 9th ed. Philadelphia, PA: Lippincott Williams & Wilkins; 2009:3932.

McDonald WM, Kellner CH, Petrides G, Greenberg RM. Applying research to the clinical use of ECT in geriatric mood disorders. *Am J Geriatr Psychiatry*. 2013; 21:S7.

McDonald WM, Reynolds CF, Ancoli-Israel S, McCall V. Understanding sleep disorders in geriatric psychiatry. *Am J Geriatr Psychiatry*. 2013;21:S38.

Miller MD, Solai LK, eds. *Geriatric Psychiatry*. New York: Oxford University Press; 2013.

Ng B, Atkins M. Home assessment in old age psychiatry: A practical guide. *Adv Psychiatry Treat*. 2012;18:400.

Reifler BV, Colenda CC, Juul D. Geriatric psychiatry. In: Aminoff MJ, Faulkner LR, eds. *The American Board of Psychiatry and Neurology: Looking Back and Moving Ahead*. Arlington: American Psychiatric Publishing; 2012:135.

Steinberg M, Hess K, Corcoran C, Mielke MM, Norton M, Breitner J, Green R, Leoutsakos J, Welsh-Bohmer K, Lyketsos C, Tschanz J. Vascular risk factors and neuropsychiatric symptoms in Alzheimer's disease: The Cache County Study. *Int J Geriatr Psychiatry*. 2014;29(2):153–159.

Thakur ME, Blazer DG, Steffens DC, eds. *Clinical Manual of Geriatric Psychiatry*. Arlington: American Psychiatric Publishing; 2014.

Thorp S, Stein MB, Jeste DV, Patterson TL, Wetherell JL. Prolonged exposure therapy for older veterans with posttraumatic stress disorder: A pilot study. *Am J Geriatr Psychiatry*. 2012;20(3):276–280.

Emergency Psychiatry

Agar L. Recognizing neuroleptic malignant syndrome in the emergency department: A case study. *Perspect Psychiatr Care*. 2010;46(2):143–151.

Ballard ED, Stanley IH, Horowitz LM, Cannon EA, Pao M, Bridge JA. Asking youth questions about suicide risk in the pediatric emergency department: Results from a qualitative analysis of patient opinions. *Clin Pediatr Emerg Med*. 2013; 14(1):20–27.

Baron DA, Dubin WR, Ning A. Other psychiatric emergencies. In: Sadock BJ, Sadock VA, eds. *Kaplan & Sadock's Comprehensive Textbook of Psychiatry*. 9th ed. Vol. 2. Philadelphia, PA: Lippincott Williams & Wilkins; 2009:2732.

Bienvenu OJ, Neufeld KJ, Needham DM. Treatment of four psychiatric emergencies in the intensive care unit. *Crit Care Med*. 2012;40(9):2662–2670.

Bruckner TA, Yonsu K, Chakravarthy B, Brown TT. Voluntary psychiatric emergencies in Los Angeles County after funding of California's Mental Health Services Act. *Psychiatr Serv*. 2012;63(8):808–814.

Cashman M, Pasic J. Pediatric psychiatric disorders in the emergency department. In: Zun LS, ed. *Behavioral Emergencies for the Emergency Physician*. New York: Cambridge University Press; 2013:211.

Ceballos-Osorio J, Hong-McAtee I. Failure to thrive in a neonate: A life-threatening diagnosis to consider. *J Pediatr Heath Care*. 2013;27(1):56–61.

Dolan MA, Fein JA. Pediatric and adolescent mental health emergencies in the emergency medical services system. *Pediatrics*. 2011;127(5):e1356–e1366.

D'Onofrio G, Jauch E, Jagoda A, Allen MH, Anglin D, Barsan WG, Berger RP, Bobrow BJ, Boudreaux ED, Bushnell C, Chan YF, Currier G, Eggly S, Ichord R, Larkin GL, Laskowitz D, Neumar RW, Newman-Toker DE, Quinn J, Shear K, Todd KH, Zatzick D. NIH roundtable on opportunities to advance research on neurologic and psychiatric emergencies. *Ann Emerg Med*. 2010;56(5):551–564.

Douglass AM, Luo J, Baraff LJ. Emergency medicine and psychiatry agreement on diagnosis and disposition of emergency department patients with behavioral emergencies. *Acad Emerg Med*. 2011;18(4):368–373.

Flaherty LT. Models of psychiatric consultation to schools. In: Weist MD, Lever NA, Bradshaw CP, Owens JS, eds. *Handbook of School Mental Health: Issues in Clinical Child Psychology*. 2nd ed. New York: Springer Science+Business Media; 2014:283.

Frosch E, Kelly P. Issues in pediatric psychiatric emergency care. *Emerg Psychiatry*. 2013:193.

Georgieva I, Mulder CL, Wierdsma A. Patients' preference and experiences of forced medication and seclusion. *Psychiatr Q*. 2012;83(1):1–13.

Gilbert SB. Beyond acting out: Managing pediatric psychiatric emergencies in the emergency department. *Adv Emerg Nurs J*. 2012;34(2):147–163.

Ginnis KB, White EM, Ross AM, et al. Family-based crisis intervention in the emergency department: A new model of care. *J Child Fam Stud*. 2015;24:172–179.

Grupp-Phelan J, Delgado SV. Management of the suicidal pediatric patient: An emergency medicine problem. *Clin Pediatr Emerg Med*. 2013;14(1):12–19.

Hamm MP, Osmond M, Curran J, Scott S, Ali S, Hartling L, Gokiert R, Cappelli M, Hnatko G, Newton AS. A systematic review of crisis interventions used in the emergency department: Recommendations for pediatric care and research. *Pediatr Emerg Care*. 2010;26(12):952–962.

Jaffee SR. Family violence and parent psychopathology: Implications for children's socioemotional development and resilience. In: Goldstein S, Brooks RB, eds. *Handbook of Resilience in Children*. 2nd ed. New York: Springer Science+Business Media; 2013:127.

Kalb LG, Stuart EA, Freedman B, Zablotsky B, Vasa R. Psychiatric-related emergency department visits among children with an autism spectrum disorder. *Pediatr Emerg Care*. 2012;28(12):1269–1276.

Lin M-T, Burgess JF Jr, Carey K. The association between serious psychological distress and emergency department utilization among young adults in the USA. *Soc Psychiatry Psychiatr Epidemiol*. 2012;47(6):939–947.

Magallón-Neri EM, Canalda G, De la Fuente JE, Forns M, García R, González E, Castro-Fornieles J. The influence of personality disorders on the use of mental health services in adolescents with psychiatric disorders. *Compr Psychiatry*. 2012; 53(5):509–515.

Maunder RG, Halpern J, Schwartz B, Gurevich M. Symptoms and responses to critical incidents in paramedics who have experienced childhood abuse and neglect. *Emerg Med J*. 2012;29(3):222–227.

Miller AB, Esposito-Smythers C, Weismoore JT, Renshaw KD. The relation between child maltreatment and adolescent suicidal behavior: A systematic review and critical examination of the literature. *Clin Child Fam Psychol Rev*. 2013;16(2):146–172.

Ougrin D, Tranah T, Leigh E, Taylor L, Asarnow JR. Practitioner review: Self-harm in adolescents. *J Child Psychol Psychiatry*. 2012;53(4):337–350.

Polevoi SK, Shim JJ, McCulloch CE, Grimes B, Govindarajan P. Marked reduction in length of stay for patients with psychiatric emergencies after implementation of a comanagement model. *Acad Emerg Med*. 2013;20(4):338–343.

Reading R. Weight faltering and failure to thrive in infancy and early childhood. *Child Care Health Devel*. 2013;39:151.

Rodnitzky RL. Movement disorder emergencies. In: Roos KL, ed. *Neurology Emergencies*. New York: Springer Science+Business Media; 2012:259.

Simpson SA, Joesch JM, West II, Pasic J. Risk for physical restraint or seclusion in the psychiatric emergency service (PES). *Gen Hosp Psychiatry*. 2014;36(1): 113–118.

Tenenbein M. Urine drug screens in pediatric psychiatric patients. *Pediatr Emerg Care*. 2014;30(2):136–137.

Weiss AP, Chang G, Rauch SL, Smallwood JA, Schechter M, Kosowsky J, Hazen E, Haimovici F, Gitlin DF, Finn CT, Orav EJ. Patient- and practice-related determinants of emergency department length of stay for patients with psychiatric illness. *Ann Emerg Med*. 2012;60(2):162–171.e5.

Ziaei M, Massoudifar A, Rajabpour-Sanati A, Pourbagher-Shahri AM, Abdolrazaghnejad A. Management of Violence and Aggression in Emergency Environment; a Narrative Review of 200 Related Articles. *Adv J Emerg Med*. 2018;3(1):e7.

Zun LS, ed. *Behavioral Emergencies for the Emergency Physician*. New York: Cambridge University Press; 2013.

## 26

Level of Care

Before the 1960s in the United States, most psychiatric care for serious mental illnesses took place in hospitals. The rest was individual therapy with a psychiatrist or psychologist or other highly trained professionals; this treatment was reserved mainly for patients considered "neurotic" and having the means to pay for hourly sessions that would often occur several days a week.

Several forces changed this. The community mental health movement was motivated by social justice, occurring at a time defined by the civil rights movement. Experts argued that the housing of seriously mentally ill patients in a public hospital was unjust. The treatment there emphasized long-term custodial care rather than rehabilitation, and few patients improved. Visionaries such as Walter Barton, then medical director for the American Psychiatric Association, argued that the federal government must lead the way to develop alternatives to the current system of institutionalization. The result was The Mental Retardation Facilities and Community Mental Health Centers Construction Act of 1963, championed by President Kennedy, who proposed a "wholly new emphasis and approach to care for the mentally ill."

The act and the amendments that followed it under President Johnson initiated the federal government's role in mental health care, something previously left to the states. It established a grant program for states to establish local mental health centers, under the overview of the National Institutes of Health. The purpose was to build a robust network of mental health centers for community-based care as an alternative to long-term institutionalization.

Only about half of the proposed centers were built, and funding for these sites has been chronically inadequate. Thus, the movement was more successful at deinstitutionalizing mental health care than it has been at offering quality alternatives. Part of the reason for this is another crucial force in the US health care system, the rise of managed care. Managed care emphasizes seeking the lowest level of care possible and the use of lower-cost professionals as a way of saving money.

The result is that we now have a myriad of treatment settings, services, and options. Most rely on grants and third-party payers, although some require considerable patient expenditures. The details and terminology differ by institution and region. However, they roughly fall into several categories. In this chapter, we briefly describe these options as well as the requirements and goals for each treatment. Our purpose is to help the reader navigate these options with an emphasis on choosing the treatment that is best for the patient. Although analogous services exist for children and adolescents, this chapter focuses on adult levels of care.

Table 26-1 summarizes the main levels of care that we should consider for most psychiatric patients.

INPATIENT ADMISSION

Inpatient admission units are usually specializing in intensive psychiatric care. The patients may voluntarily agree to hospitalization, or clinicians may hospitalize them against their will in a manner consistent with state law. The units are usually locked and equipped to restrain or seclude patients when required. Nurses and other staff are present around the clock. Physicians are present on the unit at least 5 days a week, and a covering physician is always available.

The hospitalization allows an intense treatment, with regular observation throughout a day and robust treatments, including medical adjustments, group, and individual psychotherapies, case management, and milieu treatments. Previously the most common form of psychiatric care, inpatient hospitalization is now reserved for patients who are unsafe in or unlikely to benefit from other treatments.

The patient's risk of illness or severity is usually high. Many patients are hospitalized because they are at high risk of imminently harming themselves or others. Alternatively, their disorder may be so impairing that they cannot function adequately outside the hospital or attend to even basic activities of daily living (ADLs).

Usually, the treatments required are ones that clinicians cannot safely or practically give in other settings. These include treatments that require daily observation for serious side effects. They may be given with such frequency, such as some intense psychotherapies, that other settings are not practical. In the latter case, the clinicians have often already tried other settings and have decided that the patient is likely to deteriorate should they continue the attempts to treat the patient in another setting.

In some cases, the practicality of alternative treatments arises from a patient's poor insight or inability to cooperate with treatment. Such patients may require involuntary hospitalization, and an inpatient unit is the only setting that would be appropriate to hold them against their will until the treatment allows them an ability to make their ordinary appropriate judgments. In the most severe cases, staff may have to restrain a violent or self-harming patient physically.

Except for some specialized care facilities, the goals of treatment are short term. Treatments aim to manage the crisis and stabilize the patient to the point that treatment can continue in a less restrictive setting for the patient. Crisis interventions, intense and frequent therapy, and medications are usual treatments. Longer-term treatments may begin in this setting, but usually to continue the treatments following the hospitalization.

The length of stay varies widely. A 2010 Centers for Disease Control and Prevention (CDC) survey reported the average length of stay for patients with schizophrenia as about 7.2 days, and for major depressive disorder, about 10.6 days. This number varies significantly by regional practice. Internationally, it varies by health care system, economic resources, and many other factors. Figure 26-1 gives some example comparisons of the average lengths of stay in 2010 for various countries.

The goal of treatment is to return the patient to a safe and functional state so that the team can then transition the patient to a lower level of care. This goal includes reducing the patient's threat

Table 26-1
Main Levels of Care

	Inpatient Hospitalization	Partial Hospital	Intensive Outpatient Treatment	Outpatient	Residential Care
Risk	High: risk of imminent danger to self/others	Moderate but not imminent risk	No imminent risk	Low risk of harm	Moderate risk
Disease severity	Severe symptoms	Moderate	Moderate	Mild to moderate	Moderately severe
Functioning, activities of daily living (ADLs)	Poor, cannot attend to basic ADLs without assistance	Moderate dysfunction	Mild to moderate dysfunction	Adequate to attend to ADLs independently or with some assistance	Severe
Treatments	Require around-the-clock administration, regular observation for side effects or adjustment, or are given at a frequency making other settings impractical	Fully staffed unit offering a range of services similar to inpatient, however, limited to the working day and given daily, usually 5 days a week	May vary from several times a week to weekly or monthly, depending on the level of severity and treatment. Includes both psychotherapies and medications	May vary from several times a week to weekly or monthly, depending on the level of severity and treatment. Includes both psychotherapies and medications	Psychosocial treatments and medication management, although not necessarily at the level of an inpatient unit
Patient cooperation	Voluntary or involuntary	Voluntary	Voluntary	Voluntary	Voluntary or court-ordered
Need for restraints	May need restraining for safety purposes to prevent violence or injury	None	None	None	None
Goals of treatment	Reduce safety concern, reduce symptoms, restore functioning	Improvements in symptoms and functioning to transition the patient to a less restrictive treatment	Achieve and maintain the usual premorbid level of functioning	Achieve and maintain the usual premorbid level of functioning	Improvement in symptoms and functioning to a level where the patient can live in a less restrictive setting

to themselves or others, decreasing the symptoms of the disorder, and improving the patient's functional level.

Discharge planning usually begins on day one of the hospitalization. It helps to identify early on the likely next step in treatment, should it be back home, to a transitional setting or, less often, to long-term custodial care.

PARTIAL HOSPITAL TREATMENT

Partial hospitals are facilities that provide a near hospital level of care, the exception being that the care takes place for about 6 to 8 hours a day, after which the patients can go home. The service is fully staffed in a manner typical to a psychiatric hospital unit,

FIGURE 26-1
Average lengths of stay (LOS) for mental health disorders for selected countries in 2010. (Source: Organisation for Economic Co-Operation and Development [OECD.Stat].)

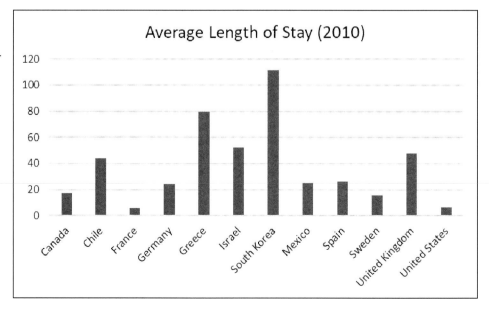

however only during the day. The units usually offer a full range of treatment from various psychotherapies and psychosocial options to medication management. The patient usually attends daily, for 5 days a week.

Appropriate patients for a partial hospital program include patients who may be at significant risk for harm to themselves or others. However, the treatment team assesses that the patient is sufficiently stable such that the reinforcement of the intensive treatment is sufficient to prevent such harm. Thus, the patient is not an imminent risk or is not too impulsive to be trusted to be independent during the evening.

The patients are usually of moderate severity in symptoms. Similarly, they often have moderate dysfunction such that their self-care may be substandard. They often have ongoing trouble maintaining normal relationships.

The program usually offers a variety of psychotherapy treatments, often in a group setting. They have the benefit of milieu therapy in the unit environment. Case management is also available. Psychiatrists are present and help manage the patient's medication and overall treatment plan.

The average length of treatment is from 1 to a few weeks, although in some cases it may be longer. The treatment should continue until the patient is sufficiently stable for a less intensive mode of treatment.

INTENSIVE OUTPATIENT TREATMENT

Intensive outpatient treatment (IOP) is a treatment in the outpatient setting that involves 3 to 4 hours of psychosocial treatment for between 1 and 4 days of treatment, with an average of 6 to 12 hours of treatment per week.

This care is usually appropriate when the level of danger is sufficiently stable so as not to be at imminent risk of harming themselves or others. Patients usually have moderate symptoms and mild to moderate functioning. For example, their self-care may be mildly below what we would expect for them. However, they should be sufficiently functional to be able to live independently or with assistance from a caregiver.

Although sufficiently stable to live independently, the psychiatrist should be sure that the patient's home environment is sufficiently safe and without illness triggers to allow for improvement with treatment.

The treatments emphasize a group format but often include some individual psychotherapy treatments or medication management. Psychotherapies may include cognitive behavioral therapy, interpersonal therapy, or other therapies in a group format.

The length of treatment varies widely and depends on the illness, but usually lasts 1 to several weeks. The goal is to address the patient's symptoms sufficiently that a less intensive model of care is feasible.

OUTPATIENT CARE

Outpatient care is pharmacologic or psychosocial management, provided by a health care professional, usually in an office setting.

This care is usually appropriate when the danger to the patient is considered reasonably low risk. Patients need not be free of all thoughts of harm to themselves or others; however, this risk should be low, and the clinician should have a reasonable belief that the patient can warn them should their situation worsen.

Also, the patient's disorder should be likely to improve with outpatient care. This situation, fortunately, includes most psychiatric disorders. The modes of treatment may include psychotherapy or medication or a combination of both.

Patients are voluntary and require some level of motivation for their treatment, sufficient so that they can show up regularly for their appointments. At times of symptomatic worsening, family members or other caretakers may assist with providing some external motivation until the patient can resume on their own.

The length of treatment varies widely depending on the disorder. The frequency of treatment also varies. In the case of an acute illness, such as an episode of major depressive disorder, a manic episode, or a worsening of anxiety, the treatment may occur weekly or more frequently. Generally, the frequency of treatment will decrease as the patient improves, but as many disorders are chronic, patients often require ongoing medication or therapy to maintain remission. For patients who have been stable for an extended time, twice a year follow-ups may be reasonable. However, the clinician should work out with the patient a plan for increasing the follow-ups when necessary, as it less likely the clinician will catch a pending recurrence of the illness early.

RESIDENTIAL CARE

Residential care is a 24-hour facility that offers a level of treatment less intensive than traditional inpatient treatment. It generally does not have the level of security typical of an inpatient unit. Although medical and nursing staff are available, the units do not have the same level of staffing, and the treatments are not as frequent as an inpatient unit.

Patients may be at some risk of harming themselves or others, but not at imminent risk and thus not requiring the level of observation or restraint available in an inpatient unit. Their symptoms are moderately severe, as they can have severe functional limitations such that they cannot safely live independently. The patients are usually voluntary, although they may be court-ordered for treatment; however, in those cases, they are willfully participating. The units are usually not locked.

The facilities offer a variety of treatments, often in a group setting. The units differ from long-term rehabilitation units, such as nursing homes, in that the goals are improvement in symptoms and functioning and return to a lower level of care.

References

American Association of Community Psychiatrists. Level of care utilization system for psychiatric and addiction services (LOCUS). Accessed August 31, 2020. Available at https://sites.google.com/view/aacp123/resources/locus

Barton WE. Trends in community mental health programs. *Psychiatr Serv.* 2000; 51(5):611–615.

Breland JY, Asch SM, Slightam C, Wong A, Zulman DM. Key ingredients for implementing intensive outpatient programs within patient-centered medical homes: a literature review and qualitative analysis. *Healthc (Amst).* 2016;4(1):22–29.

Centers for Disease Control and Prevention. FastStats. Accessed August 4, 2020. Available at https://www.cdc.gov/nchs/fastats/mental-health.htm

Centers for Disease Control and Prevention. National Hospital Discharge Survey—Publications and Reports. Accessed January 22, 2020. Available at https://www.cdc.gov/nchs/nhds/nhds_publications.htm

Centers for Disease Control and Prevention. Number, rate, and average length of stay for discharges from short-stay hospitals, by age, region, and sex: United States, 2010. Accessed August 31, 2020. Available at https://www.cdc.gov/nchs/data/nhds/1general/2010gen1_agesexalos.pdf

Marshall M, Crowther R, Sledge WH, Rathbone J, Soares-Weiser K. Day hospital versus admission for acute psychiatric disorders. *Cochrane Database Syst Rev.* 2011;2011(12):CD004026.

Nurjannah I, Mills J, Usher K, Park T. Discharge planning in mental health care: An integrative review of the literature. *J Clin Nurs.* 2014;23(9–10):1175–1185.

Organisation for Economic Co-Operation and Development (OECD). OECD statistics. Accessed August 31,2020. Available at https://stats.oecd.org/Index.aspx?ThemeTreeId=9

Sharfstein SS. Whatever happened to community mental health? *Psychiatr Serv.* 2000;51(5):616–20.

U.S. Department of Health and Human Services, Substance Abuse and Mental Health Services Administration. Behavioral health, United States, 2012. Accessed August 31, 2020. Available at https://www.samhsa.gov/data/sites/default/files/2012-BHUS.pdf

27

Ethics and Professionalism

Ethical guidelines and knowledge of ethical principles help psychiatrists avoid *ethical conflicts* (which are tensions between what one wants to do and what is ethically right to do) and think through *ethical dilemmas* (conflicts between ethical perspectives or values).

Ethics deal with the relations between people in different groups and often entail balancing rights. *Professional ethics* refers to the appropriate way to act when in a professional role. Professional ethics derive from a combination of morality, social norms, and the parameters of the relationship people have agreed to have.

PROFESSIONAL CODES

Most professional organizations and many business groups have codes of ethics that reflect a consensus about the general standards of appropriate professional conduct. The American Medical Association's (AMA's) *Principles of Medical Ethics* and the American Psychiatric Association's (APA's) *Principles of Medical Ethics with Annotations Especially Applicable to Psychiatry* articulate ideal standards of practice and professional virtues of practitioners. These codes include exhortations to use skillful and scientific techniques; to self-regulate misconduct within the profession; and to respect the rights and needs of patients, families, colleagues, and society.

BASIC ETHICAL PRINCIPLES

Four ethical principles that psychiatrists ought to weigh in their work are respect for autonomy, beneficence, nonmaleficence, and justice. At times, the principles conflict, and we must make decisions concerning how to balance them.

Respect for Autonomy

Autonomy requires that a person act intentionally after being given sufficient information and time to understand the benefits, risks, and costs of all reasonable options. It may mean honoring an individual's right not to hear every detail and even choosing someone else (e.g., family or doctor) to decide the best course of treatment.

Psychiatrists need to provide patients with a rational understanding of their disorder and options for treatment. Patients need conceptual understanding; the psychiatrist should not merely state isolated facts. Patients also need time to think and to talk with friends and family about their decision. Finally, if a patient is not in a state of mind to make decisions for himself or herself, the psychiatrist should consider mechanisms for alternative decision-making, such as guardianship, conservators, and health care proxy.

A young adult experienced a schizophrenic episode in which his religious fervor turned into psychotic delusions. After being involuntarily hospitalized because he became suicidal, he insistently refused medication, claiming that his physicians were trying to poison him. His psychiatrist decided to respect his refusal of medication as long as he could control his suicidal tendencies. As his mental suffering became more intense, in 1 week, the patient changed his mind about medication and agreed to try it. The therapeutic relationship with his psychiatrist deepened, and the patient left the hospital willing to continue with both antipsychotic medication and psychotherapy. Although not all cases work out so well, this one illustrates the benefits of negotiation about treatment even when hospitalization is involuntary.

Beneficence

The requirement for psychiatrists to act with beneficence derives from their fiduciary relationship with patients and the profession's belief that they also have an obligation to the society. As a result of the role obligation of trust, psychiatrists must heed their patients' interests, even to the neglect of their own.

The expression of the principle is called *paternalism*, the use of the psychiatrist's judgment about the best course of action for the patient or research subject. *Weak paternalism* is acting beneficently when the patient's impaired faculties prevent an autonomous choice. *Strong paternalism* is acting beneficently despite the patient's intact autonomy.

There are times when it is appropriate to permit beneficence to overrule patient autonomy. For example, when the patient faces substantial harm or risk of harm, we would choose the paternalistic act to ensure the optimal combination of maximal harm reduction, low added risk, and minimal necessary infringement on patient autonomy.

Nonmaleficence

To adhere to the principle of nonmaleficence (*primum non nocere* or *first, do no harm*), psychiatrists must be careful in their decisions and actions and must ensure that they have had adequate training for what they do. They also need to be open to seeking second opinions and consultations. They need to avoid creating risks for patients by an action or inaction.

Justice

The concept of justice concerns the issues of reward and punishment and the equitable distribution of social benefits. Relevant issues include whether resources should be distributed equally to those in greatest need, whether they should go to where they can have the most significant impact on the well-being of each individual served, or to where they will ultimately have the highest impact on society.

SPECIFIC ISSUES

From a practical point of view, several specific issues most frequently involve psychiatrists. These include (1) sexual boundary violations, (2) nonsexual boundary violations, (3) violations of confidentiality, (4) mistreatment of the patient (incompetence, double agentry), and (5) illegal activities (insurance, billing, insider stock trading).

Sexual Boundary Violations

For a psychiatrist to engage a patient in a sexual relationship is unethical. Furthermore, legal sanctions against such behavior make the ethical question moot. Psychiatrists who violate this ethical principle are subject to various criminal law statutes. Rape charges have been used against such psychiatrists; sexual assault and battery charges also have been used to convict psychiatrists.

Also, patients who have been victimized sexually by psychiatrists and other physicians have won damages in malpractice suits. Insurance carriers for the APA and the AMA no longer insure against patient–therapist sexual relations, and the carriers exclude liability for any such sexual activity.

The issue of whether sexual relations between an ex-patient and a therapist violate an ethical principle, however, remains controversial. Proponents of the view that "Once a patient, always a patient," insist that any involvement with an ex-patient—even if it leads to marriage—is unethical. They maintain that a transferential reaction that always exists between the patient and the therapist prevents a rational decision about their emotional or sexual union. Others insist that, if a transferential reaction still exists, the therapy is incomplete and that as autonomous human beings, ex-patients should not be subjected to paternalistic moralizing by physicians. Accordingly, they believe that no sanctions should prohibit emotional or sexual involvement by ex-patients and their psychiatrists. Some psychiatrists maintain that a reasonable time should elapse before such a liaison. The length of the "reasonable" period remains controversial: some have suggested 2 years. Other psychiatrists maintain that any period of prohibited involvement with an ex-patient is an unnecessary restriction. The majority of psychiatrists, as well as the APA, believe that it is always unethical, and their code of ethics states: "Sexual activity with a current or *former* patient is unethical."

Although not spelled out in *The Principles,* sexual activity with a patient's family member is also unethical. This principle is most important when the psychiatrist is treating a child or adolescent. Most training programs in child and adolescent psychiatry emphasize that the parents are patients too and that the ethical and legal proscriptions apply to parents (or parent surrogates) as well as to the child. Nevertheless, some psychiatrists misunderstand this concept. Sexual activity between a doctor and a patient's family member is also unethical.

As an example of an egregious violation, the *Medical Board of California Action Report* (July 2006) reported on a psychiatrist who had a 7-year affair with a patient who had schizophrenia. The doctor not only had sex with the patient but also had her procure prostitutes with whom he and the patient had group sex. He paid for their services by providing them with prescriptions for controlled substances and went so far as to bill Medi-Cal for these encounters as group therapy. The state revoked the physician's license, and he was also criminally convicted of fraud.

Nonsexual Boundary Violations

The *doctor–patient relationship* is the relationship between a doctor and a patient to provide and obtain treatment. That relationship has boundaries both around it and within it. Either person may cross the boundary.

Not all boundary-crossings are boundary violations. For example, a patient may say to a doctor, "I left my money at home, can you lend me cash for the parking garage?" The patient has invited the doctor to cross the doctor–patient boundary and set up a lender–borrower relationship as well. Depending on the doctor's theoretical orientation, the clinical situation with the patient, and other factors, the doctor may elect to cross the boundary. Whether the boundary-crossing is also a boundary violation is debatable. A *boundary violation* is a boundary-crossing that is exploitative. It gratifies the doctor's needs at the expense of the patient. The doctor is responsible for preserving the boundary and for ensuring that they hold boundary-crossings to a minimum and that exploitation does not occur.

> A supervisor told a psychiatry resident never to accept gifts from patients. In the course of treating a young girl with schizophrenia, the patient offered her a modest Christmas gift (a cotton scarf), which she refused to accept. The resident explained, gently, that this was against the "rules of the hospital." The next day the patient attempted suicide. She experienced the resident's refusal to accept the gift as a profound rejection, which she could not tolerate. The case illustrates the need to understand the dynamics of gift-giving and the transferential meaning to the patients of rejecting (or accepting) the gift.
>
> There is a story (possibly apocryphal) of how Freud, who was an inveterate cigar smoker, was offered a box of difficult-to-find Havana cigars by a patient during his analysis. Freud accepted the cigars and then proceeded to ask his patient to explore his motivations in offering the gift. Freud's reasons for accepting the cigars are more evident than the patient's unconscious motivation for giving them, about which no information is available.

Harm to the patient is not a component of a boundary violation. For example, using information supplied by the patient (e.g., a stock tip) is an unethical boundary violation, although no apparent harm may come to the patient. For purposes of discussion, nonsexual boundary violations come in several arbitrary (overlapping and not mutually exclusive) categories.

Business. Almost any business relationship with a former patient is problematic, and almost any business relationship with a current patient is unethical. Naturally, the circumstance and location may play a significant role in this admonition. In a rural area or a small community, a doctor might be treating the only pharmacist (or plumber or couch upholsterer) in town; then, when doing business with the pharmacist-patient, the doctor tries to keep boundaries in check. Ethical psychiatrists try to avoid doing business with a patient or a patient's family member or asking a patient to hire one of their family members. Ethical psychiatrists avoid investing in a patient's business and collaborating with a patient in a business deal.

Ideologic Issues. Ideologic issues can cloud judgment and may lead to ethical lapses. Any clinical decision should reflect what is best for the patient; the psychiatrist's ideology should not be a factor in the decision. A psychiatrist who is consulted by a patient with an illness should tell the patient what forms of treatment are available to treat the illness and allow the patient to decide on a course of treatment. Naturally, psychiatrists should recommend the treatment that they feel is in the best interest of the patient, but ultimately, the patient should be free to choose.

Social.   We should consider the particular locale and circumstances in any discussion of the behavior of an ethical psychiatrist in social situations. The overarching principle is that the boundaries of the psychiatrist–patient relationship should be respected. Furthermore, if options exist, they should be exercised in favor of the patient. Problems often arise in treatment situations when friendships develop between the psychiatrist and the patient. Objectivity is compromised, therapeutic neutrality is impaired, and factors outside the consciousness of either party may play a destructive role. During treatment, the psychiatrist should avoid such a friendship. Similarly, psychiatrists should not treat their social friends for the same set of reasons. Obviously, in an emergency, a person does what a person must.

Financial.   For psychiatrists who practice in the private sector, dealing with the patient about money is a part of treatment. Issues surrounding setting the fee, collecting the fee, and other financial matters are grist for the mill. Even so, they must observe ethical concerns. *The Principles* advises the doctor on such matters as charging for missed appointments and other contractual problems. Financial issues are a frequent source of ethics complaints against doctors. The doctor must recognize the power that these issues have in the therapeutic relationship. Because the psychotherapeutic relationship is so much like a social relationship—the office looks like a living room; the doctor wears regular clothes; some patients might, without recognizing it, assume that a friendship exists that forgives payment of a fee. When they receive the bill, their feelings, even though they are unconscious, are ruffled. We cannot sufficiently emphasize the point that psychiatrists dispense their services in a contractual context. Early in their careers, psychiatrists are often reluctant to discuss fees openly out of a sense of embarrassment over discussing money or a sense of protecting the patient.

How an ethical psychiatrist handles the situation when a patient temporarily or permanently runs out of money is essential. Many options are available—some more problematic than others. The psychiatrist can undoubtedly lower the fee, but caution is needed because a fee lowered to the point of inadequate compensation for the treatment may evoke countertransference resentment. The number of patients receiving a reduced fee is a similar consideration. Running up a bill can also be a problem. Is there an expectation of eventually being paid? Ultimately, the psychiatrist may have to alter the frequency of sessions. Any psychiatrist who sees private patients will eventually face these problems.

Confidentiality

Confidentiality refers to the therapist's responsibility not to release information learned in the course of treatment to third parties. *Privilege* refers to the patient's right to prevent disclosure of information from treatment in judicial hearings. Psychiatrists must maintain confidentiality because it is an essential ingredient of psychiatric care; it is a prerequisite for patients to be willing to speak freely to therapists. Violating confidentiality by gossiping embarrasses people and violates nonmaleficence. Violation of confidentiality also breaks the promise that a psychiatrist has explicitly or implicitly made to keep material confidential.

Confidentiality must also give way to the responsibility to protect others when a patient makes a credible threat to harm someone. The situation becomes complicated when the risk is not to a particular individual, such as when a doctor is impaired, or someone's mental state adversely affects his or her performance of a dangerous job, such as police work, firefighting, or use of dangerous machinery. Erosion has also arisen from the demands of an insurance company for detailed information. Psychiatrists should tell patients if they are going to release their information, under what circumstances, and when they do. They are not required to warn a patient when they report the abuse of a child or a threat to others.

There are various settings in which we may use patient data ethically. The general rule for doing so is to disclose only that information that is truly necessary. In teaching, research, and supervision, we should avoid using personal information that might allow others to identify a patient unless it is necessary. In ward rounds and case conferences, in which one presents patient material, we should remind those present that what they hear should not be repeated.

Confidentiality endures after death, with the ethical obligation to withhold information unless the next of kin provides consent. A subpoena is not an automatic license to release the entire record. A psychiatrist can petition the judge for an in-camera (private) review to define what precise information they must disclose.

Ethics in Managed Care

Psychiatrists have specific responsibilities toward patients treated in managed care settings, including the responsibilities to disclose all treatment options, exercise appeal rights, continue emergency treatment, and cooperate reasonably with utilization reviewers.

Responsibility to Disclose.   Psychiatrists have a continuing responsibility to the patient to obtain informed consent for treatments or procedures. The psychiatrist should disclose all the treatment options, even those not covered under the terms of a managed care plan. Most states have enacted legislation making gag rules illegal that limit information about treatment provided to patients under managed care.

Responsibility to Appeal.   The AMA Council on Ethical and Judicial Affairs states that physicians have an ethical obligation to advocate for any care that they believe will materially benefit their patients, regardless of any allocation guidelines or gatekeeper directives.

Responsibility to Treat.   Physicians are liable for failure to treat their patients within the defined standard of care. The treating physician has the sole responsibility to determine what is medically necessary. Psychiatrists must be careful not to discharge suicidal or violent patients prematurely merely because a managed care company does not approve continued coverage of benefits.

Responsibility to Cooperate with Utilization Review.   The psychiatrist should cooperate with utilization reviewers' requests for information on proper authorization from the patient. When the company denies benefits, it is crucial to understand and follow grievance procedures carefully, return telephone calls from review agencies, and provide documented justification for continued treatment.

With the advent of managed care and the need to send periodic progress reports and documentation of signs and symptoms to third-party reviewers to pay for treatment, some psychiatrists may diminish or exaggerate symptomatology. The following case report and discussion illustrate the ethical difficulties psychiatrists face in dealing with managed care.

Mrs. P admitted herself to the hospital because she was afraid she might kill herself. She was experiencing a major depressive episode, but she improved markedly during the first weeks in Dr. A's ward. Although Dr. A believed that Mrs. P was no longer suicidal, he thought she would benefit significantly from continued hospitalization. Because he knew that Mrs. P could not afford to pay for hospitalization and that the insurance company would only pay if the patient were suicidally depressed, he decided not to document Mrs. P's improvement. He noted in the chart that "the patient continues to have a risk of suicide."

Does Dr. A engage in deception? Yes, he intentionally misleads by what he writes and what he omits writing in the chart. Although what he writes is true in some literal sense, his statement is misleading in the context of treatment. Mrs. P is not suicidally depressed in the way that she was.

What Dr. A omits from the chart is also deceptive. Whether a particular omission is deceptive depends, in part, on the roles and expectations of the people involved. Not telling a colleague that one dislikes his tie is not a deception. It is merely polite unless the role or relationship involves the expectation that one offers a candid opinion. Dr. A's case is different. His professional role is to document the patient's course, and the expectation is that he will note any significant improvement. Thus, his failure to document Mrs. P's progress accurately is a kind of deception.

The second and more difficult question is whether deception is justified in this instance. The answer depends on the reasons for and against the deception and the alternatives available. The reasons for this deception are apparent. Dr. A's aim and primary obligation are to help the patient. He believes that Mrs. P would benefit significantly from continued hospitalization that she cannot afford. He may also believe that it is unfair for the insurance company to refuse to pay for the inpatient treatment of nonsuicidal depression and that his deception rectifies that unfair practice.

Important reasons also exist against this deception. The first concerns honesty and social trust. It is a good thing if people can rely on what others say and write. Without some honesty and trust, many social exchanges and practices would be impossible. Deception, even for beneficent purposes, has real potential to damage social trust. A risk exists that deception may damage people's trust in the profession of psychiatry and even patients' trust in their psychiatrists. Damage to trust may, in turn, compromise treatment.

The second reason concerns future medical treatment. If Mrs. P seeks medical treatment in the future, the physicians who attend her will read the misleading notes. If they believe that the notes are an accurate account of the previous treatment, they may suggest an inappropriate treatment for the present problem. Even if they doubt the record's accuracy, the psychiatrist has deprived their colleagues of an accurate history and report. In either case, the prior deception can hinder treatment.

The third reason concerns obligations and coverage policies. Dr. A seems to ignore the obligation that he has to the population that is covered by the insurance policy. He shifts a burden onto this population by forcing the insurance company to pay for treatment that it did not agree to cover. Perhaps the insurance company should pay for inpatient treatment in cases such as Mrs. P's; perhaps its policies are unreasonable and unfair. However, Dr. A's deception does not challenge the insurance company and pressure it to change its policy, nor does his deception encourage patients and their families to contest the company's policies. The use of deception simply circumvents, in an ad hoc way, a policy that should be challenged and discussed.

Dr. A also seems to ignore his obligation to future patients. By introducing an inaccuracy into the chart, he compromises the value of medical records research. His deception works, in a small way, to deprive future patients of the benefit of the research that relies on medical records.

One should also consider alternatives to deception. One alternative is to tailor the chart. Another alternative is to describe Mrs. P's response accurately and to discharge her to outpatient care. However, a third alternative exists. Dr. A can accurately document the patient's course and can recommend continued hospitalization. He can petition the insurance company for coverage. If the insurance company decides not to approve further inpatient care for the patient, Dr. A can appeal that decision. This alternative is more time consuming, and nothing guarantees that it will succeed, but it avoids all the problems associated with the use of deception.

Impaired Physicians

A physician may become impaired as the result of psychiatric or medical disorders or the use of mind-altering and habit-forming substances (e.g., alcohol and drugs). Many illnesses can interfere with the cognitive and motor skills required to provide competent medical care. Although the legal responsibility to report an impaired physician varies, depending on the state, the ethical responsibility remains universal. We should report an incapacitated physician to an appropriate authority, and the reporting physician is required to follow the specific hospital, state, and legal procedures. A physician who treats an impaired physician should not be required to monitor the impaired physician's progress or fitness to return to work. An independent physician or group of physicians who have no conflicts of interest should perform the monitoring.

Most states have a division that investigates professional misconduct, usually overseen by their board of health. The definitions of professional misconduct differ by state but invariably include practicing while impaired. Professional misconduct complaints derive mainly from the public in addition to insurance companies, law enforcement agencies, and doctors, among others. Many states also have a physician health committee, often independent of the disciplinary board, which helps to ensure that impaired physicians receive appropriate treatment and monitoring.

Physicians in Training

It is unethical to delegate authority for patient care to anyone who is not appropriately qualified and experienced, such as a medical student or a resident, without adequate supervision from an attending physician. Residents are physicians in training and, as such, must provide a good deal of patient care. Within a healthy, ethical teaching environment, residents and medical students may care for many ill patients. However, this care should be supervised and supported by highly trained and experienced physicians. Patients have the right to know the level of training of their care providers and should be informed about the resident's or medical student's level of training. Residents and medical students should know and acknowledge their limitations and should ask for supervision from experienced colleagues as necessary.

Physician Charter on Professionalism

In 2001, a movement to clarify the concept of "professionalism" was begun by the American Board of Internal Medicine. A set of principles called the *Physician Charter on Professionalism* was developed, which describes what it means for physicians to perform at their highest and most ethical level. Table 27-1 lists the principles and commitments of professional behaviors in the *Physician Charter on Professionalism* to which all physicians (including psychiatrists) should adhere.

Table 27-2 considers some common ethical questions that psychiatrists may face.

Table 27-1
Physician Charter on Professionalism

Fundamental Principles
- **Primacy of patient welfare.** Altruism contributes to the trust central to doctor–patient relationships. Market forces, societal pressures, and administrative exigencies must not compromise this principle.
- **Patient autonomy.** Physicians must be honest with patients and empower them to make informed decisions about treatment.
- **Social justice.** Physicians should work actively to eliminate discrimination in health care, whether based on race, gender, socioeconomic status, ethnicity, religion, or any other social category.

A Set of Commitments
- **Professional competence.** Physicians must be committed to lifelong learning. The profession as a whole must strive to see that all of its members are competent.
- **Honesty with patients.** Physicians must ensure that patients are completely and honestly informed before consenting to a treatment; they must be empowered to decide about the course of therapy. Physicians should also acknowledge that medical errors that injure patients sometimes occur. If a patient is injured through error, he or she should be informed promptly because failure to do so seriously compromises patient and societal trust.
- **Patient confidentiality.** Fulfilling the commitment to confidentiality is more pressing now than ever before given the widespread use of electronic information systems for compiling patient data.
- **Maintaining appropriate relations with patients.** Physicians should never exploit patients for any sexual advantage, personal financial gain, or other private purpose.
- **Improving quality of care.** This commitment entails both maintaining clinical competence and working collaboratively with other professionals to reduce medical error, increase patient safety, minimize overuse of health care resources, and optimize the outcomes of care.
- **Improving access to care.** Physicians must individually and collectively strive to reduce barriers to equitable health care.
- **Just distribution of finite resources.** Physicians should be committed to working with other physicians, hospitals, and payers to develop guidelines for cost-effective care. The physician's professional responsibility for appropriate allocation of resources requires scrupulous avoidance of superfluous tests and procedures.
- **Scientific knowledge.** Physicians have a duty to uphold scientific standards, to promote research, and to create new knowledge and ensure its appropriate use.
- **Maintaining trust by managing conflicts of interest.** Physicians have an obligation to recognize, disclose to the general public, and address conflicts of interest. Relationships between industry and opinion leaders should be disclosed.
- **Professional responsibilities.** Physicians are expected to participate in the process of self-regulation, including remediation and discipline of members who have failed to meet professional standards.

Table 27-2
Ethical Questions and Answers

Topic	Question	Answer
Abandonment	How can psychiatrists avoid being charged with patient abandonment on retirement?	Retiring psychiatrists are not abandoning patients if they provide their patients with sufficient notice and make every reasonable effort to find follow-up care for the patients.
	Is it ethical to provide only outpatient care to a seriously ill patient who may require hospitalization?	This could constitute abandonment unless the outpatient practitioner or agency arranges for their patients to receive inpatient care from another provider.
Bequests	A dying patient bequeaths his or her estate to his or her treating psychiatrist. Is this ethical?	No. Accepting the bequest seems improper and exploitational of the therapeutic relationship. However, it may be ethical to accept a token bequest from a deceased patient who named his or her psychiatrist in the will without that psychiatrist's knowledge.
Competency	Is it ethical for psychiatrists to perform vaginal examinations? Hospital physical examinations?	Psychiatrists may provide nonpsychiatric medical procedures if they are competent to do so and if the procedures do not preclude effective psychiatric treatment by distorting the transference. Pelvic examinations carry a high risk of distorting the transference and would be better performed by another clinician.
	Can ethics committees review issues of physician competency?	Yes. Incompetency is an ethical issue.
Confidentiality	Must confidentiality be maintained after the death of a patient?	Yes. Ethically, confidences survive a patient's death. Exceptions include protecting others from imminent harm or proper legal compulsions.
	Is it ethical to release information about a patient to an insurance company?	Yes, if the information provided is limited to that which is needed to process the insurance claim.
	Can a videotaped segment of a therapy session be used at a workshop for professionals?	Yes, if informed, uncoerced consent has been obtained, anonymity is maintained, the audience is advised that editing makes this an incomplete session, and the patient knows the purpose of the videotape.
	Should a physician report mere suspicion of child abuse in a state requiring reporting of child abuse?	No. A physician must make several assessments before deciding whether to report suspected abuse. One must consider whether abuse is ongoing, whether abuse is responsive to treatment, and whether reporting will cause potential harm. Check specific statutes. Make safety for potential victims the top priority.

(continued)

Table 27-2
Ethical Questions and Answers (*Continued*)

Topic	Question	Answer
Conflict of interest	Is there a potential ethical conflict if a psychiatrist has both psychotherapeutic and administrative duties in dealing with students or trainees?	Yes. You must define your role in advance to the trainees or students. Administrative opinions should be obtained from a psychiatrist who is not involved in a treatment relationship with the trainee or student.
Diagnosis without examination	Is it ethical to offer a diagnosis based only on review of records to determine, for insurance purposes, if suicide was the result of illness?	Yes.
	Is it ethical for a supervising psychiatrist to sign a diagnosis on an insurance form for services provided by a supervisee when the psychiatrist has not examined the patient?	Yes, if the psychiatrist ensures that proper care is given and the insurance form clearly indicates the role of supervisor and supervisee.
Exploitation (also see Bequests)	What constitutes exploitation of the therapeutic relationship?	Exploitation occurs when the psychiatrist uses the therapeutic relationship for personal gain. This includes adopting or hiring a patient as well as sexual or financial relationships.
Fee splitting	What is fee splitting?	Fee splitting occurs when one physician pays another for a patient referral. This would also apply to lawyers giving a forensic psychiatrist referrals in exchange for a percentage of the fee. Fee splitting may occur in an office setting if the psychiatrist takes a percentage of his or her office mates' fees for supervision or expenses. Costs for such items or services must be arranged separately. Otherwise, it would appear that the office owner could benefit from referring patients to a colleague in the office. Fee splitting is illegal.
Informed consent	Is it ethical to refuse to divulge information about a patient who has agreed to give this information to those requesting it?	No. It is the patient's decision, not the therapist's.
	Is informed consent needed when presenting or writing about case material?	Not if the patient is aware of the supervisory or teaching process and confidentiality is preserved.
Moonlighting	Can psychiatric residents ethically "moonlight"?	They can if their duties are not beyond their ability, if they are properly supervised, and if the moonlighting does not interfere with their residency training.
Reporting	Should psychiatrists expose or report unethical behavior of a colleague or colleagues? Can a spouse bring an ethical complaint?	Psychiatrists are obligated to report colleagues' unethical behavior. A spouse with knowledge of unethical behavior can bring an ethical complaint as well.
Research	How can ethical research be performed with subjects who cannot give informed consent?	Consent can be given by a legal guardian or via a living will. Incompetent persons have the right to withdraw from the research project at any time.
Retirement	See Abandonment.	
Supervision	What are the ethical requirements when a psychiatrist supervises other mental health professionals?	The psychiatrist must spend sufficient time to ensure that proper care is given and that the supervisee is not providing services that are outside the scope of his or her training. It is ethical to charge a fee for supervision.
Taping and recording	Can videotapes of patient interviews be used for training purposes on a national level (e.g., workshops, board examination preparation)?	Appropriate and explicit informed consent must be obtained. The purpose and scope of exposure of the tape must be emphasized in addition to the resulting loss of confidentiality.

Table by Eugene Rubin, M.D. Data derived from the American Medical Association's Principles of Medical Ethics.

Military Psychiatry

Psychiatrists in the military face unique ethical problems because confidentiality does not exist under the military code of conduct. Psychiatrists, when treating military patients, are obligated to warn them regarding these limits. The reasoning is related to concepts of military necessity; however, many experts have pointed out the problems with this rule, as many soldiers may avoid needed care rather than risk exposure. Given the concerns about the rates of suicide in the military, there is growing pressure to revise this standard. Anecdotally many military psychiatrists choose to use their judgment as to what they are required to reveal to a patient's superiors.

References

Blass DM, Rye RM, Robbins BM, Miner MM, Handel S, Carroll JL Jr, Rabins PV. Ethical issues in mobile psychiatric treatment with homebound elderly patients: The psychogeriatric assessment and treatment in city housing experience. *J Am Geriatr Soc.* 2006;54(5):843–848.

Cervantes AN, Hanson A. Dual agency and ethics conflicts in correctional practice: Sources and solutions. *J Am Acad Psychiatry Law.* 2013;41(1):72–78.

DuVal G. Ethics in psychiatric research: Study design issues. *Can J Psychiatry.* 2004;49(1):55–59.

Fleischman AR, Wood EB. Ethical issues in research involving victims of terror. *J Urban Health.* 2002;79:315–321.

Green SA. The ethical commitments of academic faculty in psychiatric education. *Acad Psychiatry.* 2006;30(1):48–54.

Kaldjian LC, Weir RF, Duffy TP. A clinician's approach to clinical ethical reasoning. *J Gen Intern Med.* 2005;20:306–311.

Kipnis K. Gender, sex, and professional ethics in child and adolescent psychiatry. *Child Adolesc Psychiatr Clin N Am*. 2004;13(3):695–708.

Kontos N, Freudenreich O, Querques J. Beyond capacity: Identifying ethical dilemmas underlying capacity evaluation requests. *Psychosomatics*. 2013;54(2):103–110.

Marrero I, Bell M, Dunn LB, Roberts LW. Assessing professionalism and ethics knowledge and skills: Preferences of psychiatry residents. *Acad Psychiatry*. 2013; 37(6):392–397.

Merlino JP. Psychoanalysis and ethics–relevant then, essential now. *J Am Acad Psychoanal Dyn Psychiatry*. 2006;34(2):231–247.

Parker M. Judging capacity: Paternalism and the risk-related standard. *J Law Med*. 2004;11(4):482–491.

Roberts LW. Ethical philanthropy in academic psychiatry. *Am J Psychiatry*. 2006; 163(5):772–778.

Schneider PL, Bramstedt KA. When psychiatry and bioethics disagree about patient decision making capacity (DMC). *J Med Ethics*. 2006;32:90–93.

Simon L. Psychotherapy as civics: The patient and therapists as citizens. *Ethical Hum Psychol Psychiatry*. 2005;7(1):57–64.

Strebler A, Valentin C. Considering ethics, aesthetics and the dignity of the individual. *Cult Med Psychiatry*. 2014;38(1):35–59.

Wada K, Doering M, Rudnick A. Ethics education for psychiatry residents. A mixed-design retrospective evaluation of an introductory course and a quarterly seminar. *Camb Q Healthc Ethics*. 2013;22(04):425–435.

Weiss LW. Ethics in psychiatry. In: Sadock BJ, Sadock VA, Ruiz P, eds. *Kaplan & Sadock's Comprehensive Textbook of Psychiatry*. 10th ed. Vol. 2. Philadelphia, PA: Lippincott Williams & Wilkins; 2017.

28 ▲

Forensic and Legal Issues

"Forensic" is from Latin and means "of the forum." In Rome, criminal cases were presented in a public forum, hence the modern connotation of the term is relating to courts of law. At various times, psychiatry and the law intersect. Forensic psychiatry is the branch of psychiatry that examines this intersection. This chapter considers some of the legal aspects of psychiatry.

MEDICAL MALPRACTICE

Medical malpractice is a tort or civil wrong. It is a wrong resulting from a physician's negligence. Simply put, negligence means doing something that a physician with a duty to care for the patient should not do, or not doing something they should, as defined by current medical practice. Usually, expert witnesses help to establish the standard of care. Also, journal articles; professional textbooks, such as the *Kaplan and Sadock's Comprehensive Textbook of Psychiatry;* professional practice guidelines; and ethical practices promulgated by professional organizations all help to establish the standard of care.

To prove malpractice, the plaintiff (e.g., patient, or family) must establish by a preponderance of evidence that (1) a doctor–patient relationship existed that created a *duty* of care, (2) a *deviation* from the standard of care occurred, (3) the patient was *damaged,* and (4) the deviation *directly* caused the damage.

These elements of a malpractice claim are sometimes called the *4 Ds* (duty, deviation, damage, and direct causation).

Each of the four elements of a malpractice claim must be present, or there can be no finding of liability. For example, a psychiatrist whose negligence is the direct cause of harm to an individual (physical, psychological, or both) is not liable for malpractice if no doctor–patient relationship existed to create a duty of care. Psychiatrists are not likely to be successfully sued if they advise on a radio program, particularly if they begin with the caveat that there is no doctor–patient relationship intended from the general advice-giving. No malpractice claim will be sustained against a psychiatrist if a patient's worsening condition is unrelated to negligent care. Not every adverse outcome is the result of negligence. Psychiatrists cannot guarantee correct diagnoses and treatments. When the psychiatrist provides due care, they may make mistakes without necessarily incurring liability. Most psychiatric cases are complicated. Psychiatrists make judgment calls when selecting a particular treatment course among the many options that may exist. In hindsight, the decision may prove wrong but not be a deviation in the standard of care.

In addition to negligence suits, patients can sue psychiatrists for the intentional torts of assault, battery, false imprisonment, defamation, fraud or misrepresentation, invasion of privacy, and intentional infliction of emotional distress. In an intentional tort, wrongdoers intend harm to another person or realize, or should have realized, that such harm is likely to result from their actions. For example, telling a patient

that sex with the therapist is therapeutic perpetrates a fraud. Most malpractice policies do not provide coverage for intentional torts.

Negligent Prescription Practices

Negligent prescription practices usually include exceeding recommended dosages and then failing to adjust the medication level to therapeutic levels, unreasonable mixing of drugs, prescribing medications that are not indicated, prescribing too many drugs at one time, and failing to disclose medication effects. Elderly patients frequently take a variety of drugs prescribed by different physicians. We should only prescribe multiple psychotropic medications with special care because of possible harmful interactions and adverse effects. We should also carefully document our reasons for prescribing multiple medications.

Psychiatrists who prescribe medications must explain the diagnosis, risks, and benefits of the drug within reason and as circumstances permit (Table 28-1). Obtaining informed consent can be problematic if a psychiatric patient has diminished cognitive capacity because of mental illness or chronic brain impairment. In these cases, a substitute health care decision maker may need to provide consent.

We should obtain informed consent each time we change a medication and introduce a new drug. If a medication injures a patient and the doctor did not inform them of this risk, there may be sufficient grounds for a malpractice action.

The question is often asked: How frequently should patients be seen for medication follow-up? The answer is that we should see patients according to their clinical needs. There is no stock answer about the frequency of visits. The longer the time interval between visits, however, the higher the likelihood of adverse drug reactions and clinical developments. Patients taking medications should probably not go beyond 6 months for follow-up visits. Managed care policies that do not reimburse for frequent follow-up appointments can result in a psychiatrist prescribing large amounts of medications. The psychiatrist is duty-bound to provide appropriate treatment to the patient, quite apart from managed care or other payment policies.

There are several other areas of negligence involving medication that may result in malpractice actions. A psychiatrist may fail to treat adverse effects that they have, or should have, recognized. They may also fail to monitor a patient's compliance with prescription limits or fail to prescribe the appropriate amount of medication. Prescribing addictive drugs to a vulnerable patient creates a risk, as can failing to seek appropriate consultation when indicated. Finally, stopping a medication inappropriately can be a cause of a malpractice action.

Split Treatment

In split treatment, the psychiatrist provides medication, and a nonmedical therapist conducts the psychotherapy. The following vignette illustrates a possible complication.

Table 28-1
Informed Consent: Reasonable Information to Be Disclosed

Although there exists no consistently accepted standard for information disclosure for any given medical or psychiatric situation, as a rule of thumb, five areas of information are generally provided:
1. Diagnosis—description of the condition or problem
2. Treatment—nature and purpose of proposed treatment
3. Consequences—risks and benefits of the proposed treatment
4. Alternatives—viable alternatives to the proposed treatment, including risks and benefits
5. Prognosis—projected outcome with and without treatment

Table by RI Simon, M.D.

A psychiatrist provided medications for a depressed 43-year-old woman. A master's level counselor saw the patient for outpatient psychotherapy. The psychiatrist saw the patient for 20 minutes during the initial evaluation and prescribed a tricyclic drug, and the patient was prescribed sufficient drugs for follow-up in 3 months. The psychiatrist initially diagnosed recurrent major depression. The patient denied suicidal ideation but had markedly diminished appetite and sleep. The patient had a long history of recurrent depression with suicide attempts. There were no further discussions between the psychiatrist and the counselor, who saw the patient once a week for 30 minutes in psychotherapy. Within 3 weeks, after a failed romantic relationship, the patient stopped taking her antidepressant medication, started to drink heavily, and committed suicide with an overdose of alcohol and antidepressant drugs. The patient's family sued the counselor and psychiatrist for negligent diagnosis and treatment.

Psychiatrists must do an adequate evaluation, obtain prior medical records, and understand that no such thing as a partial patient exists. Split treatments are potential malpractice traps because patients can "fall between the cracks" of fragmented care. The psychiatrist retains full responsibility for the patient's care in a split-treatment situation. This responsibility does not preempt the responsibility of the other mental health professionals involved in the patient's treatment. Section V, annotation 3 of the *Principles of Medical Ethics with Annotations Especially Applicable to Psychiatry,* states: "When the psychiatrist assumes a collaborative or supervisory role with another mental health worker, he/she must expend sufficient time to assure that proper care is given."

In managed care or other settings, a marginalized role of merely prescribing medication apart from a working doctor–patient relationship does not meet generally accepted standards of good clinical care. The psychiatrist must be more than just a medication technician. Fragmented care in which the psychiatrist only dispenses medication while remaining uninformed about the patient's overall clinical status constitutes substandard treatment that may lead to a malpractice action. At a minimum, such a practice diminishes the efficacy of the drug treatment itself or may even lead to the patient's failure to take the prescribed medication.

Split-treatment situations require that the psychiatrist remain fully informed of the patient's clinical status as well as the nature and quality of treatment the patient is receiving from the nonmedical therapist. In a collaborative relationship, the psychiatrist and therapist share the responsibility for the patient's care according to their qualifications and limitations. The responsibilities of each discipline do not diminish those of the other disciplines. The treatment team should explain the separate responsibilities of each discipline to the patient. The psychiatrist and the nonmedical therapist must

periodically evaluate the patient's clinical condition and requirements to determine whether the collaboration should continue. On termination of the collaborative relationship, both parties treating the patient should inform the patient either separately or jointly. In split treatments, if the patient sues the nonmedical therapist, the collaborating psychiatrist will likely be sued also and vice versa.

Psychiatrists who prescribe medications in a split-treatment arrangement should be able to hospitalize a patient if it becomes necessary. If the psychiatrist does not have admitting privileges, they should make prearrangements with other psychiatrists who can hospitalize patients if emergencies arise. Many community mental health organizations, group psychiatry practices, and managed care companies rely on split treatment, and this is a potential malpractice minefield.

PRIVILEGE AND CONFIDENTIALITY

Privilege

Privilege is the right to maintain secrecy or confidentiality in the face of a subpoena. Privileged communications are statements made by certain persons within a relationship—such as husband–wife, priest–penitent, or doctor–patient—that the law protects from forced disclosure on the witness stand. In the case of the doctor–patient relationship, the right of privilege belongs to the patient, not to the physician so that the patient can waive the right.

Psychiatrists, who are licensed to practice medicine, may claim medical privilege, but privilege has some qualifications. For example, this privilege does not exist in military courts, regardless of whether the physician is in the military. Also, the state where the trial takes place is irrelevant even if the state recognizes such privilege as military courts are not under the jurisdiction of the states.

In 1996, the United States Supreme Court recognized a psychotherapist–patient privilege in *Jaffee v. Redmon.* Emphasizing the critical public and private interests served by the psychotherapist–patient privilege, the court wrote:

Because we agree with the judgment of the state legislatures and the Advisory Committee that a psychotherapist-patient privilege will serve a "public good transcending the normal predominant principle utilizing all rational means for ascertaining truth"… we hold that confidential communications between a licensed psychotherapist and her patients in the course of diagnosis or treatment are protected from compelled disclosure under Rule 501 of the Federal Rules of Evidence.

Confidentiality

A long-held premise of medical ethics binds physicians to hold secret all information given by patients. This professional obligation is called *confidentiality.* Confidentiality applies to certain populations and not to others; a group that is within the circle of confidentiality shares information without receiving specific permission from a patient. Such groups include, in addition to the physician, other staff members treating the patient, clinical supervisors, and consultants.

A subpoena can force a psychiatrist to breach confidentiality, and courts must be able to compel witnesses to testify for the law to function adequately. A subpoena ("under penalty") is an order to appear as a witness in court or at a deposition. Physicians usually are served with a *subpoena duces tecum,* which requires that they also produce their relevant records and documents. Although the power to issue subpoenas belongs to a judge, they are routinely issued at the request of an attorney representing a party to an action.

In bona fide emergencies, we can release information in as limited a way as feasible to carry out necessary interventions. We should try, time allowing, to obtain the patient's permission, and we should always debrief the patient after an emergency as to what information we released.

As a rule, clinical information may be shared with the patient's permission—preferably written permission, although oral permission suffices with proper documentation. Each release is good for only one piece of information, and the psychiatrist should obtain permission for each subsequent release, even to the same party. Permission overcomes only the legal barrier, not the clinical one; the release is permission, not an obligation. If a clinician believes that the information may be destructive, they should discuss this with the patient, and they can refuse the release, with some exceptions.

Third-Party Payers and Supervision.   Increased insurance coverage for health care is precipitating a concern about confidentiality and the conceptual model of psychiatric practice. Today, insurance covers about 70 percent of all health care bills. An insurance carrier must be able to obtain information with which it can assess the administration and costs of various programs to provide coverage.

Quality control of care necessitates that confidentiality is not absolute; it also requires a review of individual patients and therapists. The therapist in training must breach a patient's confidence by discussing the case with a supervisor. Institutionalized patients who have been ordered by a court to get treatment must have their individualized treatment programs submitted to a mental health board.

Discussions about Patients.   In general, psychiatrists have multiple loyalties: to patients, to society, and the profession. Through their writings, teaching, and seminars, they can share their acquired knowledge and experience and provide information that may be valuable to other professionals and the public. It is not easy to write or talk about a psychiatric patient without breaching the confidentiality of the relationship. Unlike physical ailments, which we can usually discuss without anyone recognizing the patient, a psychiatric history usually entails a discussion of distinguishing characteristics. Psychiatrists have an obligation not to disclose identifiable patient information (and, perhaps, any descriptive patient information) without appropriate informed consent. Failure to obtain informed consent could result in a claim based on breach of privacy, defamation, or both.

The Internet and Social Media.   Psychiatrists and other mental health professionals must be aware of the legal implications of discussing patients over the Internet. Internet communications about patients are not confidential, are subject to hacking, and are open to legal subpoenas. Some psychiatrists have blogged about patients thinking they were sufficiently disguised only to find that others do recognize them, including the involved patient. Some professional organizations have electronic mailing lists in which they ask advice about patients from their colleagues or make referrals and, in so doing, provide detailed information about the patient, which others can trace. Similarly, using social media to communicate about patients is equally risky.

Child Abuse.   In many states, all physicians must take a course on child abuse for medical licensure. All states now legally require that psychiatrists (along with others), when suspecting child abuse, must immediately report this to an appropriate agency. In this situation, confidentiality is decisively limited by legal statute because potential or actual harm to vulnerable children outweighs the value of confidentiality in a psychiatric setting. Although many complex psychodynamic nuances accompany the required reporting of suspected child abuse, such reports generally are considered ethically justified.

HIGH-RISK CLINICAL SITUATIONS

Tardive Dyskinesia

It is estimated that at least 10 to 20 percent of patients and perhaps as high as 50 percent of patients treated with first-generation antipsychotics for more than 1 year exhibit some tardive dyskinesia. These figures are even higher for elderly patients. Despite the possibility for many tardive dyskinesia–related suits, relatively few psychiatrists have been sued. Also, patients who develop tardive dyskinesia may not have the physical energy and psychological motivation to pursue litigation. Allegations of negligence involving tardive dyskinesia occur when there is a failure to evaluate a patient properly, a failure to obtain informed consent, a negligent diagnosis of a patient's condition, and a failure to monitor.

Suicidal Patients

Psychiatrists may face legal action when their patients commit suicide. This is particularly true when psychiatric inpatients kill themselves. Psychiatrists are assumed to have more control over inpatients, making the suicide preventable.

The evaluation of suicide risk is one of the most complex, dauntingly difficult clinical tasks in psychiatry. Suicide is a rare event. In our current state of knowledge, clinicians cannot accurately predict when or if a patient will commit suicide. No professional standards exist for predicting who will or will not commit suicide. Professional standards do exist for assessing suicide risk, but at best, only the degree of suicide risk can be judged clinically after a comprehensive psychiatric assessment.

A review of the case law on suicide reveals that certain affirmative precautions should be taken with a suspected or confirmed suicidal patient. For example, failing to perform a reasonable assessment of a suicidal patient's risk for suicide or implement an appropriate precautionary plan will likely render a practitioner liable. The law tends to assume that suicide is preventable if it is foreseeable. Courts carefully scrutinize suicide cases to determine if a patient's suicide was foreseeable. *Foreseeability* is a deliberately vague legal term that has no comparable clinical counterpart, a common sense rather than a scientific construct. It does not (and should not) imply that clinicians can predict suicide. Foreseeability should not be confused with preventability, however. In hindsight, many suicides seem preventable that were not foreseeable.

Violent Patients

Psychiatrists who treat violent or potentially violent patients may be sued for failure to control aggressive outpatients and for the discharge of violent inpatients. Psychiatrists could be sued for failing to protect society from the violent acts of their patients if it was reasonable for the psychiatrist to have known about the patient's violent tendencies and if the psychiatrist could have done something that could have safeguarded the public. In the landmark case *Tarasoff v. Regents of the University of California,* the California Supreme Court ruled that mental health professionals have a duty to protect identifiable, endangered third parties from imminent threats of serious harm made by their outpatients. Since then, courts and state legislatures have increasingly held psychiatrists to a fictional standard of having to predict future behavior (dangerousness) of their potentially violent patients. Research has consistently demonstrated that psychiatrists cannot predict future violence with any dependable accuracy.

The duty to protect patients and endangered third parties is primarily a professional and moral obligation and, only secondarily, a legal duty. Most psychiatrists acted to protect both their patients and others threatened by violence long before *Tarasoff*.

If a patient threatens harm to another person, most states require that the psychiatrist perform some intervention that might prevent the harm from occurring. In states with duty-to-warn statutes, the states define the options available to psychiatrists and psychotherapists. In states offering no such guidance, health care providers should use their clinical judgment and act to protect endangered third persons. Typically, a variety of options to warn and protect are clinically and legally available, including voluntary hospitalization, involuntary hospitalization (when meeting civil commitment requirements), warning the intended victim of the threat, notifying the police, adjusting medication, and seeing the patient more frequently. Warning others of danger, by itself, is usually insufficient. Psychiatrists should consider the *Tarasoff* duty to be a national standard of care, even if they practice in states that do not have a duty to warn and protect.

Tarasoff I.   The 1976 case *Tarasoff v. Regents of the University of California* (now known as *Tarasoff I*) raised the issue of the legal duty to warn. In this case, Prosenjit Poddar, a student and a voluntary outpatient at the mental health clinic of the University of California, told his therapist that he intended to kill a student readily identified as Tatiana Tarasoff. Realizing the seriousness of the intention, the therapist, with the concurrence of a colleague, decided to commit Poddar for observation under a 72-hour emergency psychiatric detention provision of the California commitment law. The therapist notified the campus police, both orally and in writing that Poddar was dangerous and should be committed.

Concerned about the breach of confidentiality, the therapist's supervisor vetoed the recommendation and ordered all records relating to Poddar's treatment destroyed. At the same time, the campus police temporarily detained Poddar but released him on his assurance that he would "stay away from that girl." Poddar stopped going to the clinic when he learned from the police about his therapist's recommendation to commit him. Two months later, he carried out his previously announced threat to kill Tatiana. The young woman's parents thereupon sued the university for negligence.

As a consequence, the California Supreme Court, which deliberated the case for an unprecedented time of about 14 months, ruled that a physician or a psychotherapist who has reason to believe that a patient may injure or kill someone should warn the potential victim.

The discharge of the duty imposed on the therapist to warn intended victims against danger may take one or more forms, depending on the case. Therefore, stated the court, it may call for the therapist to notify the intended victim or others likely to notify the victim of the danger, to notify the police, or to take whatever other steps are reasonably necessary under the circumstances.

The *Tarasoff I* ruling does not require therapists to report a patient's fantasies; instead, it requires them to report an intended homicide. The therapist must exercise sound judgment to decide when this is the case.

Tarasoff II.   In 1982, the California Supreme Court issued a second ruling in the case of *Tarasoff v. Regents of the University of California* (now known as *Tarasoff II*), which broadened its earlier ruling, extending the duty to warn, to include the duty to protect.

The *Tarasoff II* ruling has stimulated intense debates in the medicolegal field. Lawyers, judges, and expert witnesses argue the definition of protection, the nature of the relationship between the therapist and the patient, and the balance between public safety and individual privacy.

Clinicians argue that the duty to protect hinders treatment because a patient may not trust a doctor if confidentiality is not maintained. Furthermore, because it is not easy to determine whether a patient is sufficiently dangerous to justify long-term incarceration, unnecessary involuntary hospitalization may occur because of a therapist's defensive practices.

As a result of such debates in the medicolegal field, since 1976, the state courts have not made a uniform interpretation of the *Tarasoff II* ruling (the duty to protect). In general, clinicians should note whether a specific identifiable victim seems to be in imminent and probable danger from the threat of an action contemplated by a mentally ill patient. The imminent harm should also be potentially serious or severe. Usually, the patient must be a danger to another person and not to property; the therapist should take clinically reasonable action.

HOSPITALIZATION

All states provide for some form of involuntary hospitalization. Such action usually is taken when psychiatric patients present a danger to themselves or others in their environment to the extent that their urgent need for treatment in a closed institution is evident. Individual states allow involuntary hospitalization when patients are unable to care for themselves adequately.

The doctrine of *parens patriae* allows the state to intervene and to act as a surrogate parent for those who are unable to care for themselves or who may harm themselves. In English common law, *parens patriae* ("father of his country") dates to the time of King Edward I and originally referred to a monarch's duty to protect the people. The U.S. common law transformed the doctrine into a paternalism in which the state acts for persons who are mentally ill and for minors.

The statutes governing hospitalization of persons who are mentally ill generally have been designated commitment laws, but psychiatrists have long considered the term to be undesirable. *Commitment* legally means a warrant for imprisonment. The American Bar Association and the American Psychiatric Association have recommended that state governments replace the term *commitment* with the less offensive and more accurate term *hospitalization,* which most states have adopted. Although this change does not correct past mistakes, the emphasis on hospitalization is in keeping with psychiatrists' interest in treatment rather than punishment.

Procedures of Admission

Four procedures of admission to psychiatric facilities have been endorsed by the American Bar Association to safeguard civil liberties and to make sure that no one can capriciously force a person into a mental hospital. Although each of the 50 states has the power to enact its laws on psychiatric hospitalization, the procedures outlined here are gaining much acceptance.

Informal Admission. Informal admission operates on the general hospital model, in which the procedure for a psychiatric admission is the same as that for other patients. Under such circumstances, the ordinary doctor–patient relationship applies, with the patient free to enter and to leave, even against medical advice.

Voluntary Admission. In cases of voluntary admission, patients apply in writing for admission to a psychiatric hospital. They may come to the hospital on the advice of a personal physician, or they may seek help on their own. In either case, we would admit patients if an examination reveals the need for hospital treatment. The patient is free to leave, even against medical advice.

Temporary Admission. We may use a temporary admission for patients who are so senile or so confused that they require hospitalization and are not able to make decisions on their own and for patients who are so acutely disturbed that they must be admitted immediately to a psychiatric hospital on an emergency basis. Under the procedure, a hospital would admit a person on the written recommendation of one physician. After admitting the patient, a psychiatrist or the hospital staff must confirm the need for hospitalization. The procedure is temporary because we cannot hold these patients against their will for more than a set time, usually 15 days.

Involuntary Admission. Involuntary admission involves the question of whether patients are suicidal and, thus, a danger to themselves or homicidal and thus a danger to others. Because these persons lack insight into their illness, a relative or friend may make the application for admission to a hospital. After making the application, at least two physicians must examine the patient, and if both physicians confirm the need for hospitalization, the hospital can admit the patient.

Involuntary hospitalization involves an established procedure for written notification of the next of kin. Furthermore, the patients have access at any time to legal counsel, who can bring the case before a judge. If the judge does not think that there is an indication for hospitalization, that judge can order the patient's release.

Involuntary admission allows us to hospitalize a patient for a set time, usually defined by the state and often in the range of 60 days. After this time, if the patient is to remain hospitalized, the case must be reviewed periodically by a board consisting of psychiatrists, nonpsychiatric physicians, lawyers, and other citizens not connected with the institution.

Involuntarily hospitalized persons who believe that they should be released have the right to file a petition for a writ of habeas corpus. Under the law, those who believe that they have been illegally deprived of liberty can proclaim a writ of habeas corpus. The legal procedure asks a court to decide whether a patient was hospitalized without due process of law. The courts must hear this case immediately, regardless of how the motion is filed. Hospitals are obligated to submit the petitions to the court immediately.

RIGHT TO TREATMENT

Among the rights of patients, the right to the standard quality of care is fundamental. This right has been litigated in highly publicized cases under the slogan of "right to treatment."

In 1966, Judge David Bazelon, speaking for the District of Columbia Court of Appeals in *Rouse v. Cameron,* noted that the purpose of involuntary hospitalization is treatment and concluded that the absence of treatment draws into question the constitutionality of the confinement. Treatment in exchange for liberty is the

logic of the ruling. In this case, the patient was discharged on a writ of habeas corpus, the basic legal remedy to ensure liberty. Judge Bazelon further held that if alternative treatments that infringe less on personal liberty are available, involuntary hospitalization cannot take place.

Alabama Federal Court judge Frank Johnson was more venturesome in the decree he rendered in 1971 in *Wyatt v. Stickney.* The *Wyatt* case was a class-action proceeding brought under newly developed rules that sought not release but treatment. Judge Johnson ruled that persons civilly committed to a mental institution have a constitutional right to receive such individual treatment as will give them a reasonable opportunity to be cured or to have their mental condition improved. Judge Johnson set out minimum requirements for staffing, specified physical facilities, and nutritional standards and required individualized treatment plans.

The new codes, more detailed than the old ones, include the right to be free from excessive or unnecessary medication; the right to privacy and dignity; the right to the least restrictive environment; the unrestricted right to be visited by attorneys, clergy, and private physicians; and the right to refuse lobotomies, electroconvulsive treatments, and other procedures without fully informed consent. Patients can be required to perform therapeutic tasks but not hospital chores unless they volunteer for them and receive the federal minimum wage as payment. This requirement is an attempt to eliminate the practice of peonage, in which state hospitals forced psychiatric patients to work at menial tasks, without payment, for the benefit of the state.

In several states today, medication or electroconvulsive therapy cannot be forcibly administered to a patient without first obtaining court approval, which may take as long as 10 days.

RIGHT TO REFUSE TREATMENT

The right to refuse treatment is a legal doctrine that holds that, except in emergencies, we cannot force patients to accept treatment against their will. An "emergency" is a condition in clinical practice that requires immediate intervention to prevent death or severe harm to the patient or another person or to prevent deterioration of the patient's clinical state.

In the 1976 case of *O'Connor v. Donaldson,* the Supreme Court of the United States ruled that harmless mentally ill patients cannot be confined against their will without treatment if they can survive outside. According to the Court, a finding of mental illness alone cannot justify a state's confining persons in a hospital against their will. Instead, involuntarily confined patients must be considered dangerous to themselves or others or possibly so unable to care for themselves that they cannot survive outside. As a result of the 1979 case of *Rennie v. Klein,* patients have the right to refuse treatment and to use an appeal process. As a result of the 1981 case of *Roger v. Oken,* patients have an absolute right to refuse treatment, but a guardian may authorize treatment.

Many rightly question psychiatrists' ability to predict dangerousness. Also, many psychiatrists worry about the risk entailed by involuntarily hospitalizing a patient if the patient can then sue them for monetary damages for infringing on the patient's civil rights.

CIVIL RIGHTS OF PATIENTS

Because of several clinical, public, and legal movements, criteria for the civil rights of persons who are mentally ill, apart from their rights as patients, have been both established and affirmed.

Least Restrictive Alternative

The principle of *least restrictive alternative* holds that patients have the right to receive the least restrictive means of treatment for the requisite clinical effect. Therefore, if it is possible to treat a patient as an outpatient, we should not pursue commitment. Similarly, if it is safe to treat a patient in an open ward, we should not seclude them.

Although reasonably straightforward on first reading, the difficulty arises when clinicians attempt to apply the concept to choose among involuntary medication, seclusion, and restraint as the intervention of choice. Distinguishing among these interventions based on restrictiveness proves to be a purely subjective exercise fraught with personal bias. Moreover, each of these three interventions is both more and less restrictive than each of the other two. Nevertheless, we should make an effort to think in terms of restrictiveness when deciding how to treat patients.

Visitation Rights

Patients have the right to receive visitors and to do so at reasonable hours (customary hospital visiting hours). Hospitals have to allow for the fact that at certain times, a patient's clinical condition may not permit visits. We should document when this is the case, as we should not suspend such rights without good reason.

Specific categories of visitors are not limited to the regular visiting hours; these include a patient's attorney, private physician, and members of the clergy—all of whom, broadly speaking, have unrestricted access to the patient, including the right to privacy in their discussions. Even here, a bona fide emergency may delay such visits. Again, the patient's needs come first. Under similar reasoning, we should curtail specific noxious visits (e.g., a patient's relative bringing drugs into the ward).

Communication Rights

Patients should generally have free and open communication with the outside world by telephone or mail, but this right varies regionally to some degree. Some jurisdictions charge the hospital administration with responsibility for monitoring the communications of patients. In some areas, hospitals must make available reasonable supplies of paper, envelopes, and stamps for patient's use.

Specific circumstances affect communication rights. A patient hospitalized with an associated criminal charge of making harassing or threatening phone calls should not have unrestricted access to the telephone, and similar considerations apply to mail. As a rule, however, patients should be allowed private telephone calls, and we should not invade their privacy by listening in or opening their mail.

Private Rights

Patients have several rights to privacy. In addition to confidentiality, they are allowed private bathroom and shower space, secure storage space for clothing and other belongings, and adequate floor space per person. They also have the right to wear their clothes and to carry their own money.

Economic Rights

Apart from special considerations related to incompetence, psychiatric patients generally are permitted to manage their financial

Table 28-2
Indications and Contraindications for Seclusion and Restraint

Indications
Prevent clear, imminent harm to the patient or others
Prevent significant disruption to treatment program or physical surroundings
Assist in treatment as part of ongoing behavior therapy
Decrease sensory overstimulation[a]
Patient's voluntary reasonable request

Contraindications
Extremely unstable medical and psychiatric conditions[b]
Delirious or demented patients who are unable to tolerate decreased stimulation[b]
Overtly suicidal patients[b]
Patients with severe drug reactions or overdoses or who require close monitoring of drug dosages[b]
For punishment or convenience of staff

[a]Seclusion only.
[b]Unless close supervision and direct observation are provided.
Data from *The Psychiatric Uses of Seclusion and Restraint (Task Force Report No. 22)*. Washington, DC: American Psychiatric Association.

affairs. One feature of this fiscal right is the requirement that we pay patients if they work in the institution (e.g., gardening or preparing food). This right often creates tension between the valid therapeutic need for activity, including jobs, and exploitive labor. A consequence of this tension is that some hospitals have had to eliminate valuable occupational, vocational, and rehabilitative programs because of the failure of legislatures to supply the funding to pay wages to patients who participate in these programs.

SECLUSION AND RESTRAINT

Seclusion and restraint raise complex legal issues. Seclusion and restraint have both indications and contraindications (Table 28-2). Seclusion and restraint have become increasingly regulated over the past decade.

Legal challenges to the use of restraints and seclusion have been brought on behalf of institutionalized persons with psychiatric illnesses or cognitive disabilities. Typically, these lawsuits do not stand alone but are part of a challenge to a wide range of alleged abuses.

In general, courts hold, or consent decrees provide that hospitals can only implement restraints and seclusion when a patient creates a risk of harm to self or others, and no less restrictive alternative is available. Table 28-3 lists additional restrictions.

Table 28-3
Restrictions for Seclusion and Restraint

Restraints and seclusion can be implemented only when a patient creates a risk of harm to self or others and no less restrictive alternative is available.
Restraint and seclusion can only be implemented by a written order from an appropriate medical official.
Orders are to be confined to specific, time-limited periods.
A patient's condition must be regularly reviewed and documented.
Any extension of an original order must be reviewed and reauthorized.

INFORMED CONSENT

Lawyers representing an injured claimant now invariably add to a claim of negligent performance of procedures (malpractice) an informed consent claim as another possible area of liability. Ironically, this is one claim under which there is no requirement for expert testimony. The usual claim of medical malpractice requires the litigant to produce an expert to establish that the defendant physician departed from accepted medical practice. However, in a case in which the physician did not obtain informed consent, the fact that the treatment was technically well performed, was in accord with the generally accepted standard of care, and effected a complete cure is immaterial. As a practical matter, however, unless the treatment had adverse consequences, a complainant will not get far with a jury for actions based solely on an allegation that the doctor performed treatment without consent.

In the case of minors, the parent or guardian must give consent to medical treatment. By statute, most states, however, list specific diseases and conditions that a minor can consent to have treated—including venereal disease, pregnancy, substance dependence, alcohol abuse, and contagious diseases. In an emergency, a physician can treat a minor without parental consent. The trend is to adopt the so-called mature minor rule, which allows minors to consent to treatment under ordinary circumstances. As a result of the Supreme Court's 1967 *Gault* decision, all juveniles must now be represented by counsel, must be able to confront witnesses, and must be given proper notice of any charges. Emancipated minors have the rights of an adult when they can show that they are living as adults with control over their own lives.

Consent Form

The essential elements of a consent form should include a fair explanation of the procedures and their purposes. The form should identify those procedures that are experimental. Also, the form should describe any attendant discomforts and risks than can be expected, as well as the benefits that are reasonable to expect. The form should also disclose appropriate alternative procedures that may be advantageous to the patient with an offer to answer any inquiries concerning the procedures. Finally, the form should explain that the patient is free to withdraw patient consent and to discontinue participation in the project or activity at any time without prejudice.

Some theorists suggest that a standardized discussion that covers the issues noted above can substitute for a form. In such a case, it would be essential to document the discussion.

CHILD CUSTODY

The action of a court in a child custody dispute centers on the child's best interests. The maxim reflects the idea that a natural parent does not have an inherent right to be named a custodial parent, but the presumption, although a bit eroded, remains in favor of the mother in the case of young children. As a rule, the courts presume that the welfare of a child of tender years generally is best served by maternal custody when the mother is a good and fit parent. Giving the mother custody may also serve her best interest, as many parents may not otherwise ever resolve the pain of losing a child, but her best interest is not to be equated ipso facto with the best interest of the child. Care and protection proceedings are the court's interventions in the welfare of a child when the parents are unable to care for the child.

More fathers are asserting custodial claims. In about 5 percent of all cases, fathers are named custodians. With more women going to work outside the home, and more men assuming the primary role in child care, the traditional rationale for maternal custody has less force today than it did in the past.

Currently, every state has a statute allowing a court, usually a juvenile court, to assume jurisdiction over a neglected or abused child and to remove the child from parental custody. It usually orders that a welfare or probation department supervise the care and custody of the child.

TESTAMENTARY AND CONTRACTUAL CAPACITY AND COMPETENCE

Courts may ask psychiatrists to evaluate patients' testamentary capacities or their competence to make a will. Three psychological abilities are necessary to prove this competence. Patients must know the nature and the extent of their bounty (property), the fact that they are making a bequest, and the identities of their natural beneficiaries (spouse, children, and other relatives).

When probating a will, one of the heirs or another person may challenge its validity. Judgment in such cases must rely on reconstruction, using data from documents and from expert psychiatric testimony, of the testator's mental state at the time they wrote the will. When someone cannot, or chooses not, to write a will, all states provide for the distribution of property to the heirs. If there are no heirs, the estate goes to the public treasury.

Witnesses at the signing of a will, which might include a psychiatrist, may attest that the testator was rational at the time of executing the will. In unusual cases, a lawyer may videotape the signing to safeguard the will from attack. Ideally, persons who are thinking of making a will and believe that there may be questions about their testamentary competence should hire a forensic psychiatrist to perform a dispassionate examination antemortem to validate and record their capacity.

An incompetence proceeding and the appointment of a guardian may be necessary when a family member is spending the family's assets, and the property is in danger of dissipation, as in the case of patients who are elderly, have cognitive disabilities, are dependent on alcohol, or have psychosis. An issue is whether such persons are capable of managing their affairs. A guardian appointed to take control of the property of one deemed incompetent, however, cannot make a will for the ward (the incompetent person).

We determine competence based on a person's ability to make a sound judgment—to weigh, to reason, and to make reasonable decisions. Competence is task-specific, not general; the capacity to weigh decision-making factors (competence) often is best demonstrated by a person's ability to ask pertinent and knowledgeable questions after explaining the risks and benefits. Although physicians (especially psychiatrists) often give opinions on competence, only a judge's ruling converts the opinion into a finding; a patient is not competent or incompetent until the court so rules. The diagnosis of a mental disorder is not, in itself, sufficient to warrant a finding of incompetence. Instead, the mental disorder must cause impairment in judgment for the specific issues involved. After they have been declared incompetent, persons lose specific rights: they cannot make contracts, marry, start a divorce action, drive a vehicle, handle their property, or practice their professions. A formal courtroom proceeding decides incompetence, and the court usually appoints a guardian who will best serve a patient's interests. Another hearing is necessary to declare a patient competent. Admission to a mental hospital, even involuntarily, does not automatically mean that a person is incompetent.

Competence also is essential in contracts because a contract is an agreement between parties to do a specific act. A contract is invalid if, when it was signed, one of the parties was unable to comprehend the nature and effect of his or her act. The marriage contract is subject to the same standard and thus can be voided if either party did not understand the nature, duties, obligations, and other characteristics entailed at the time of the marriage. In general, however, the courts are unwilling to declare a marriage void based on incompetence.

Whether competence is related to wills, contracts, or the making or breaking of marriages, the fundamental concern is a person's state of awareness and capacity to comprehend the significance of the particular commitment made.

Durable Power of Attorney

A modern development that permits persons to make provisions for their anticipated loss of decision-making capacity is called a *durable power of attorney*. The document permits the advance selection of a substitute decision maker who can act without the necessity of court proceedings when the signatory becomes incompetent through illness or progressive dementia.

CRIMINAL LAW

Competence to Stand Trial

The Supreme Court of the United States stated that the prohibition against trying someone who is mentally incompetent is fundamental to the US system of justice. Accordingly, the court, in *Dusky v. the United States,* approved a test of competence that seeks to ascertain whether a criminal defendant "has sufficient present ability to consult with his lawyer with a reasonable degree of rational understanding—and whether he has a rational as well as factual understanding of the proceedings against him."

Competence to Be Executed

One of the new areas of competence to emerge in the interface between psychiatry and the law is the question of a person's competence to be executed. The requirement for competence in this area is believed to rest on three general principles. First, a person's awareness of what is happening is supposed to heighten the retributive element of the punishment. Punishment is meaningless unless the person is aware of it and knows the punishment's purpose. Second, a competent person who is about to be executed is believed to be in the best position to make whatever peace is appropriate with his or her religious beliefs, including confession and absolution. Third, a competent person who is about to be executed preserves, until the end, the possibility (admittedly slight) of recalling a forgotten detail of the events or the crime that exonerate the person.

The need to preserve competence was supported recently in the Supreme Court case of *Ford v. Wainwright.* However, no matter the outcome of legal struggles with this question, most medical bodies have gravitated toward the position that it is unethical for any clinician to participate, no matter how remotely, in state-mandated executions; a physician's duty to preserve life transcends all other competing requirements. Major medical societies, such as the American Medical Association (AMA), believe that doctors should not participate in the death penalty. A psychiatrist who agrees to examine a patient slated for execution may find the person incompetent based on a mental disorder and may recommend a treatment plan, which, if implemented, would ensure the person's fitness to be executed. Although room exists for a difference of opinion regarding whether or not a psychiatrist should become involved, the authors of this text agree with the AMA.

Criminal Responsibility

According to criminal law, committing a socially harmful act is not the sole criterion of whether a crime has been committed. Instead, the objectionable act must have two components: voluntary conduct (*actus reus*) and evil intent (*mens rea*). An evil intent cannot exist when an offender's mental status is so deficient, so abnormal, or so diseased to have deprived the offender of the capacity for rational intent. The law can be invoked only when an illegal intent is implemented. Neither behavior, however harmful, nor the intent to harm is, in itself, a ground for criminal action.

M'Naghten Rule. The precedent for determining legal responsibility was established in 1843 in the British courts. The so-called M'Naghten rule, which, until recently, has determined criminal responsibility in most of the United States, holds that persons are not guilty by reason of insanity if they labored under a mental disease such that they were unaware of the nature, the quality, and the consequences of their acts or if they were incapable of realizing that their acts were wrong. Moreover, to absolve persons from punishment, a delusion used as evidence must be one that, if true, would be an adequate defense. If the delusional idea does not justify the crime, such persons are presumably held responsible, guilty, and punishable. The M'Naghten rule is known commonly as the right–wrong test.

The M'Naghten rule derives from the famous M'Naghten case of 1843. When Daniel M'Naghten murdered Edward Drummond, the private secretary of Robert Peel, M'Naghten had been suffering from delusions of persecution for several years, had complained to many persons about his "persecutors," and finally had decided to correct the situation by murdering Robert Peel. When Drummond came out of Peel's home, M'Naghten shot Drummond, mistaking him for Peel. The jury, as instructed under the prevailing law, found M'Naghten not guilty by reason of insanity. In response to questions about what guidelines could be used to determine whether a person could plead insanity as a defense against criminal responsibility, the English chief judge wrote:

1. To establish a defense on the ground of insanity, it must be clearly proved that, at the time of committing the act, the party accused was laboring under such a defect of reason, from disease of the mind, as not to know the nature and quality of the act he was doing, or if he did know it, he did not know he was doing what was wrong.
2. Where a person labors under partial delusions only and is not in other respects insane and as a result commits an offense, he must be considered in the same situation regarding responsibility as if the facts with respect to which the delusion exists were real.

According to the M'Naghten rule, the question is not whether the accused knows the difference between right and wrong in general, instead, it is whether the defendant understood the nature and the quality of their act and whether they knew the difference between right and wrong—specifically whether the defendant knew the act was wrong or perhaps thought the act was correct, a delusion causing the defendant to act in legitimate self-defense.

Jeffery Dahmer killed 17 young men and boys between June 1978 and July 1991. Most of his victims were either gay or bisexual. He would meet and select his prey at gay bars or bathhouses and then lure them by offering them money for posing for photographs or simply to enjoy some beer and videos. Then he would drug them, strangle them, masturbate on the body or have sex with the corpse, dismember the body, and dispose of it. Sometimes he would keep the skull or other body parts as souvenirs.

On July 13, 1992, Dahmer changed his plea to guilty by means of insanity. The jury, however, decided that Dahmer's meticulous murder plans and the systematic way that he disposed of his victims' bodies was evidence that Dahmer could control his behavior. All of the testimony bolstered the notion that, as with most serial killers, Dahmer knew what he was doing and knew right from wrong. Finally, the jury did not accept the defense that Dahmer experienced a mental illness to the degree that it had disabled his thinking or behavioral controls. Dahmer was sentenced to 15 consecutive life terms or a total of 957 years in prison. An inmate killed him on November 28, 1994.

Irresistible Impulse. In 1922, a committee of jurists in England reexamined the M'Naghten rule. The committee suggested broadening the concept of insanity in criminal cases to include the irresistible impulse test, which rules that a person charged with a criminal offense is not responsible for an act if the act was committed under an impulse that the person was unable to resist because of mental disease. The courts interpret this concept such that it has been called the *policeman-at-the-elbow law.* In other words, the court grants an impulse to be irresistible only when it can be determined that the accused would have committed the act even if a policeman had been at the accused person's elbow. To most psychiatrists, this interpretation is unsatisfactory because it covers only a small, select group of those who are mentally ill.

Durham Rule. In the case of *Durham v. the United States,* Judge Bazelon handed down a decision in 1954 in the District of Columbia Court of Appeals. The decision resulted in the product rule of criminal responsibility, namely that an accused person is not criminally responsible if his or her unlawful act was the product of mental disease or mental defect. In the Durham case, Judge Bazelon expressly stated that the purpose of the rule was to get good and complete psychiatric testimony. He sought to release the criminal law from the theoretical straitjacket of the M'Naghten rule, but judges and juries in cases using the *Durham* rule became mired in confusion over the terms *product, disease,* and *defect.* In 1972, some 18 years after the rule's adoption, the Court of Appeals for the District of Columbia, in *United States v. Brawner* discarded the rule. The court—all nine members, including Judge Bazelon—decided in a 143-page opinion to throw out its *Durham* rule and to adopt in its place the test recommended in 1962 by the American Law Institute in its model penal code, which is the law in the federal courts today.

Model Penal Code. In its model penal code, the American Law Institute recommended the following test of criminal responsibility: Persons are not responsible for criminal conduct if, at the time of such conduct, as a result of mental disease or defect, they lacked substantial capacity either to appreciate the criminality (wrongfulness) of their conduct or to conform their conduct to the requirement of the law. The term *mental disease or defect* does not include an abnormality manifested only by repeated criminal or otherwise antisocial conduct.

Subsection 1 of the American Law Institute rule contains five operative concepts: mental disease or defect, lack of substantial capacity, appreciation, wrongfulness, and conformity of conduct to the requirements of law. The rule's second subsection, stating that repeated criminal or antisocial conduct is not, of itself, to be taken as mental disease or defect, aims to keep the sociopath or psychopath within the scope of criminal responsibility.

Guilty but Mentally Ill. Some states have established an alternative verdict of guilty but mentally ill. Under guilty but mentally ill statutes, this alternative verdict is available to the jury if the defendant pleads not guilty by reason of insanity. Under an insanity plea, four outcomes are possible: not guilty, not guilty by reason of insanity, guilty but mentally ill, and guilty.

The problem with finding someone guilty but mentally ill is that it is an alternative verdict without a difference. It is the same as finding the defendant just plain guilty. The court must still impose a sentence on the convicted person. Although the convicted person supposedly receives psychiatric treatment, if necessary, this treatment provision is available to all prisoners.

OTHER AREAS OF FORENSIC PSYCHIATRY

Emotional Damage and Distress

A rapidly rising trend in recent years is to sue for psychological and emotional damage, both secondary to physical injury or as a consequence of witnessing a stressful act and from the suffering endured under the stress of such circumstances as concentration camp experiences. The German government heard many of these claims from persons detained in Nazi camps during World War II. In the United States, the courts have moved from a conservative to a liberal position in awarding damages for such claims. Psychiatric examinations and testimony are sought in these cases, often by both the plaintiffs and the defendants.

Recovered Memories

Patients alleging recovered memories of abuse have sued parents and other alleged perpetrators. In several instances, the alleged victimizers have sued therapists who, they claim, negligently induced false memories of sexual abuse. In an about-face, some patients have recanted and joined forces with others (usually their parents) to sue therapists.

Courts have handed down multimillion-dollar judgments against mental health practitioners. A fundamental allegation in these cases is that the therapist abandoned a position of neutrality to suggest, persuade, coerce, and implant false memories of childhood sexual

Table 28-4
Risk Management Principles for Cases of Recovered Memories of Abuse in Psychotherapy

1. Maintain therapist neutrality: Do not suggest abuse.
2. Stay clinically focused: Provide adequate evaluation and treatment for patients presenting problems and symptoms.
3. Carefully document the memory-recovery process.
4. Manage personal bias and countertransference.
5. Avoid mixing treater and expert witness roles.
6. Closely monitor supervisory and collaborative therapy relationships.
7. Clarify nontreatment roles with family members.
8. Avoid special techniques (e.g., hypnosis or sodium amobarbital [Amytal]) unless clearly indicated; obtain consultation first.
9. Stay within professional competence: Do not take cases that you cannot handle.
10. Distinguish between narrative truth and historical truth.
11. Obtain consultation in problematic cases.
12. Foster patient autonomy and self-determination: Do not suggest lawsuits.
13. In managed care settings, inform patients with recovered memories that more than brief therapy may be required.
14. When making public statements, distinguish personal opinions from scientifically established facts.
15. Stop and refer, if uncomfortable with a patient who is recovering memories of childhood abuse.
16. Do not be afraid to ask about abuse as part of a competent psychiatric evaluation.

abuse. The guiding principle of clinical risk management in recovered memory cases is the maintenance of therapist neutrality and the establishment of sound treatment boundaries. Table 28-4 lists the risk management principles that should be considered when evaluating or treating a patient who recovers memories of abuse in psychotherapy.

Worker's Compensation

The stresses of employment can cause or accentuate mental illness. Patients are entitled to be compensated for their job-related disabilities or to receive disability retirement benefits. A psychiatrist is often called on to evaluate such situations.

Civil Liability

Psychiatrists who sexually exploit their patients are subject to civil and criminal actions in addition to ethical and professional licensure revocation proceedings. Malpractice is the most common legal action (Table 28-5).

Table 28-5
Sexual Exploitation: Legal and Ethical Consequences

Civil lawsuit
  Negligence
  Loss of consortium
Breach-of-contract action
Criminal sanctions (e.g., statutory, adultery, sexual assault, rape)
Civil action for intentional tort (e.g., battery, fraud)
License revocation
Ethical sanctions
Dismissal from professional organizations

Table by RI Simon, M.D.

Table 28-6
Patients' Rights under the Privacy Rule

Physicians must give the patient a written notice of his or her privacy rights; the privacy policies of the practice; and how patient information is used, kept, and disclosed. A written acknowledgment should be taken from the patient verifying that he or she has seen such notice.

Patients should be able to obtain copies of their medical records and to request revisions to those records within a stated amount of time (usually 30 days). Patients do not have the right to see psychotherapy notes.

Physicians must provide the patient with a history of most disclosures of their medical history on request. Some exceptions exist. The APA Committee on Confidentiality has developed a model document for this requirement.

Physicians must obtain authorization from the patient for disclosure of information other than for treatment, payment, and health care operations (these three are considered to be routine uses, for which consent is not required). The APA Committee on Confidentiality has developed a model document for this requirement.

Patients may request another means of communication of their protected information (e.g., request that the physician contact them at a specific phone number or address).

Physicians cannot generally limit treatment to obtaining patient authorization for disclosure of their information for nonroutine uses.

Patients have the right to complain about Privacy Rule violations to the physician, their health plan, or to the Secretary of HHS.

APA, American Psychiatric Association; HHS, Department of Health and Human Services.

Health Insurance Portability and Accountability Act

The Health Insurance Portability and Accountability Act (HIPAA) was passed in 1996 to address the medical delivery system's mounting complexity and its rising dependence on electronic communication. The act orders that the federal Department of Health and Human Services (HHS) develop rules protecting the transmission and confidentiality of patient information, and all units under HIPAA must comply with such rules.

The Privacy Rule, administered by the Office for Civil Rights (OCR) at HHS, protects the confidentiality of patient information (Table 28.6).

References

Adshead G. Evidence-based medicine and medicine-based evidence: The expert witness in cases of factitious disorder by proxy. *J Am Acad Psychiatry Law.* 2005;33:99–105.

Andreasson H, Nyman M, Krona H, Meyer L, Anckarsäter H, Nilsson T, Hofvander B. Predictors of length of stay in forensic psychiatry: The influence of perceived risk of violence. *Int J Law Psychiatry.* 2014;37(6):635–642.

Arboleda-Flórez JE. The ethics of forensic psychiatry. *Curr Opin Psychol.* 2006;19(5):544–546.

Baker T. *The Medical Malpractice Myth.* Chicago, IL: University of Chicago Press; 2005.

Billick SB, Ciric SJ. Role of the psychiatric evaluator in child custody disputes. In: Rosner R, ed. *Principles and Practice of Forensic Psychiatry.* 2nd ed. New York: Chapman & Hall; 2003.

Bourget D. Forensic considerations of substance-induced psychosis. *J Am Acad Psychiatry Law.* 2013;41(2):168–173.

Chow WS, Priebe S. Understanding psychiatric institutionalization: A conceptual review. *BMC Psychiatry.* 2013;13:169.

Koh S, Cattell GM, Cochran DM, Krasner A, Langheim FJ, Sasso DA. Psychiatrists' use of electronic communication and social media and a proposed framework for future guidelines. *J Psychiatr Pract.* 2013;19(3):254–263.

Meyer DJ, Price M. Forensic psychiatric assessments of behaviorally disruptive physicians. *J Am Acad Psychiatry Law.* 2006;34(1):72–81.

Reid WH. Forensic practice: A day in the life. *J Psychiatr Pract.* 2006;12(1):50–54.

Rogers R, Shuman DW. *Fundamentals of Forensic Practice: Mental Health and Criminal Law*. New York: Springer; 2005.

Rosner R, ed. *Principles and Practice of Forensic Psychiatry*. 2nd ed. New York: Chapman & Hall; 2003.

Simon RI, ed. *Posttraumatic Stress Disorder in Litigation*. 2nd ed. Washington, DC: American Psychiatric Publishing; 2003.

Simon RI, Gold LH. *The American Psychiatric Publishing Textbook of Forensic Psychiatry*. Washington, DC: American Psychiatric Publishing; 2004.

Simon RI, Shuman DW. Clinical-legal issues in psychiatry. In: Sadock BJ, Sadock VA, Ruiz P, eds. *Kaplan & Sadock's Comprehensive Textbook of Psychiatry*. 9th ed. Vol. 2. Philadelphia, PA: Lippincott Williams & Wilkins; 2009:4427.

Studdert DM, Mello MM, Gawande AA, Gandhi TK, Kachalia A, Yoon C, Puopolo AL, Brennan TA. Claims, errors, and compensation payments in medical malpractice litigation. *N Engl J Med*. 2006;354(19):2024–2033.

Wecht CH. The history of legal medicine. *J Am Acad Psychiatry Law*. 2005;33(2):245–251.

29 ▲

End-of-Life Issues and Palliative Care

▲ 29.1 Death, Dying, and Bereavement

DEATH AND DYING

Definitions

The terms *death* and *dying* require definition: Whereas *death* may be considered the absolute cessation of vital functions, *dying* is the process of losing these functions. Dying may also be seen as a developmental concomitant of living, a part of the birth-to-death continuum. Living may entail numerous mini-deaths—the end of growth and its potential, health-compromising illnesses, multiple losses, decreasing vitality and growing dependency with aging, and dying. Dying, and the individual's awareness of it, imbues humans with values, passions, wishes, and the impetus to make the most of the time.

Two terms that have been used with increased frequency in recent years refer to the quality of living as death comes near. A *good death* is one that is free from avoidable distress and suffering for patients, families, and caregivers and is reasonably consistent with clinical, cultural, and ethical standards. A *bad death,* in contrast, is characterized by needless suffering, a dishonoring of the patient or family's wishes or values, and a sense among participants or observers that norms of decency have been offended.

Uniform Determination of Death Act. The President's Commission for the Study of Ethical Problems in Medicine and Biomedical and Behavioral Research published its definition of death in 1981. Working with the American Bar Association, the American Medical Association (AMA), and the National Conference of Commissioners on Uniform State Laws, the commission established that one who has sustained either (1) irretrievable cessation of circulatory and respiratory functions or (2) irretrievable cessation of all functions of the entire brain, including the brainstem, is dead. The determination of death must be per accepted medical standards.

Generally accepted criteria for determining brain death require a series of neurologic and other assessments. For children, particular guidelines apply. They generally specify two assessments separated by an interval of at least 48 hours for those between the ages of 1 week and 2 months, 24 hours for those between the ages of 2 months and 1 year, and 12 hours for older children; additional confirmatory tests may also be advisable under some circumstances. Brain death criteria usually are not applied to infants younger than 7 days. Table 29-1 lists the clinical criteria for brain death in adults and children.

Legal Aspects of Death

According to law, physicians must sign the death certificate, which attests to the cause of death (e.g., congestive heart failure or pneumonia). They must also attribute the death to natural, accidental, suicidal, homicidal, or unknown causes. A medical examiner, coroner, or pathologist must examine anyone who dies unattended by a physician and perform an autopsy to determine the cause of death. In some cases, a psychological autopsy is performed: A person's sociocultural and psychological background is examined retrospectively by interviewing friends, relatives, and doctors to determine whether mental illness, such as a depressive disorder, was present. For example, a determination can be made that a person died because he or she was pushed (murder) or because he or she jumped (suicide) from a high building. Each situation has clear medical and legal implications.

Stages of Death and Dying

Elisabeth Kübler-Ross, a psychiatrist and thanatologist, made a comprehensive and useful organization of reactions to impending death. A dying patient seldom follows a regular series of responses that can be identified; no established sequence applies to all patients. Nevertheless, the following five stages proposed by Kübler-Ross are widely encountered.

Stage 1: Shock and Denial. On being told that they are dying, persons initially react with shock. They may appear dazed at first and then may refuse to believe the diagnosis; they may deny that anything is wrong. Some persons never pass beyond this stage and may go from doctor to doctor until they find one who supports their position. The degree to which denial is adaptive or maladaptive appears to depend on whether a patient continues to obtain treatment even while denying the prognosis. In such cases, physicians must communicate to patients and their families, respectfully and directly, necessary information about the illness, its prognosis, and the options for treatment. For effective communication, physicians must allow for patients' emotional responses and reassure them that they will not be abandoned.

Stage 2: Anger. Persons become frustrated, irritable, and angry at being ill. They commonly ask, "Why me?" They may become angry at God, their fate, a friend, or a family member; they may even blame themselves. They may displace their anger onto the hospital staff members and the doctor, whom they blame for the illness. Patients in the stage of anger are challenging to treat. Doctors who have difficulty understanding that anger is a predictable reaction and is a displacement may withdraw from patients or transfer them to other doctors' care.

Table 29-1
Clinical Criteria for Brain Death in Adults and Children

Coma
Absence of motor responses
Absence of pupillary responses to light and pupils at midposition
  with respect to dilatation (4–6 mm)
Absence of corneal reflexes
Absence of caloric responses
Absence of gag reflex
Absence of coughing in response to tracheal suctioning
Absence of sucking and rooting reflexes
Absence of respiratory drive at a $Paco_2$ that is 60 or 20 mm Hg
  above normal baseline values
Interval between two evaluations, according to patient's age
  Term to 2 mo old, 48 hr
  >2 mo to 1 yr old, 24 hr
  >1 yr to <18 yr old, 12 hr
  ≥18 yr old, interval optional
Confirmatory tests
  Term to 2 mo old, two confirmatory tests
  >2 mo to 1 yr old, one confirmatory test
  >1 yr to <18 yr old, optional
  ≥18 yr old, optional

$Paco_2$, partial pressure of arterial carbon dioxide.
Reprinted from Wijdicks EF. The diagnosis of brain death. *N Engl J Med.* 2001;344: 1215–1221, with permission.

Physicians treating angry patients must realize that the anger being expressed cannot be taken personally. An empathic, nondefensive response can help defuse patients' anger and can help them refocus on their deep feelings (e.g., grief, fear, loneliness) that underlie the anger. Physicians should also recognize that anger may represent patients' desire for control in a situation in which they feel completely out of control.

Stage 3: Bargaining.   Patients may attempt to negotiate with physicians, friends, or even God; in return for a cure, they promise to fulfill one or many pledges, such as giving to charity and attending church regularly. Some patients believe that if they are good (compliant, nonquestioning, cheerful), the doctor will make them better. The treatment of such patients involves making it clear that they will be taken care of to the best of the doctor's abilities and that everything that can be done will be done, regardless of any action or behavior on the patients' part. Patients must also be encouraged to participate as partners in their treatment and to understand that being a good patient means being as honest and straightforward as possible.

Stage 4: Depression.   In the fourth stage, patients show clinical signs of depression—withdrawal, psychomotor retardation, sleep disturbances, hopelessness, and, possibly, suicidal ideation. The depression may be a reaction to the effects of the illness on their lives (e.g., loss of a job, economic hardship, helplessness, hopelessness, and isolation from friends and family) or it may be in anticipation of the loss of life that will eventually occur. A major depressive disorder with vegetative signs and suicidal ideation may require treatment with antidepressant medication or electroconvulsive therapy (ECT). All persons feel some sadness at the prospect of their death, and normal sadness does not require biologic intervention. However, major depressive disorder and active suicidal ideation can be alleviated and should not be accepted as normal reactions to impending death. A person who suffers from major depressive disorder may be unable to sustain hope, which can enhance the dignity and quality of life and even prolong longevity.

Studies have shown that some terminally ill patients can delay their death until after a loved one's significant event, such as the graduation of a grandson from college.

Stage 5: Acceptance.   In the stage of acceptance, patients realize that death is inevitable, and they accept the universality of the experience. Their feelings can range from a neutral to a euphoric mood. Under ideal circumstances, patients resolve their feelings about the inevitability of death and can talk about facing the unknown. Those with strong religious beliefs and a conviction of life after death sometimes find comfort in the ecclesiastical maxim, "Fear not death; remember those who have gone before you and those who will come after."

Near-Death Experiences

Near-death descriptions are often strikingly similar. They often involve an out-of-body experience of viewing one's body and overhearing conversations, feelings of peace, hearing a distant noise, entering a dark tunnel, leaving the body behind, meeting dead loved ones, witnessing beings of light, returning to life to complete unfinished business, and deep sadness on leaving this new dimension. This pattern of sensations and perceptions is usually described as peaceful and loving; it feels real to participants, who distinguish it from dreams or hallucinations. These experiences provoke sweeping lifestyle changes, such as fewer material concerns, a heightened sense of purpose, a belief in God, joy of life, compassion, less fear of death, an enhanced approach to life, and intense feelings of love. In a similar vein, hospice nurses have described experiences among terminally ill patients of visions that may include a sense of the presence of departed loved ones, of spiritual beings, of bright light, or of being in a particular place, often described with a sense of warmth and love. Although such "visions" do not readily lend themselves to scientific investigation and thus are not legitimized, patients may benefit from discussing them with clinicians. A term to describe this experience is *unio mystica,* which refers to an oceanic feeling of mystic unity with infinite power.

Life Cycle Considerations about Death and Dying

The clinical diversity of death-related attitudes and behaviors between children and adults has its roots in developmental factors and age-dependent differences in causes of death. As opposed to adults, who usually die from chronic illness, children are apt to die from sudden, unexpected causes. Almost half of the children who die between the ages of 1 and 14 years and nearly 75 percent of those who died in late adolescence and early adulthood die from accidents, homicides, and suicides. With their characteristics of violence, suddenness, and mutilation, such unnatural causes of death are extraordinary stressors for grieving survivors. Bereaved parents and siblings of dead young children and teenagers often feel victimized and traumatized by their losses; their grief reactions resemble posttraumatic stress disorder (PTSD). Devastating family disruptions can occur, and surviving siblings risk having their emotional needs put on the back burner, ignored, or completely unnoticed.

Children.   Children's attitudes toward death mirror their attitudes toward life. Although they share with adolescents, adults, and elderly adults similar fears, anxieties, beliefs, and attitudes about dying, some of their interpretations and reactions are age specific. None welcome it without ambivalence, and all temper their acceptance with healthy doses of denial and avoidance. Dying children are often aware of their condition and want to discuss it. They often have more sophisticated views about dying than their medically well counterparts, engendered by their failing health, separation from parents, subjection to painful procedures, and the deaths of hospital chums.

At the preschool, preoperational stage of cognitive development, death is seen as a temporary absence, incomplete and reversible, like departure or sleep. Separation from the primary caretaker(s) is the main fear of preschool-age children. This fear surfaces as an increase in nightmares, more aggressive play, or concern about the deaths of others rather than direct discourse. Terminally ill children may assume responsibility for their death, feeling guilty for dying. Preschool children may be unable to relate the treatment to the illness, instead of viewing treatment as punishment and family separation as rejection. They need reassurance that they are loved, have done nothing wrong, are not responsible for their illness, and will not be abandoned.

School-age children manifest concrete-operational thinking and recognize death as a final reality. They, however, view death as something that happens to older people, not to them. Between the ages of 6 and 12 years, children have active fantasies of violence and aggression, often dominated by themes of death and killing. School-age children ask questions about serious illness and death if encouraged to do so; however, if they receive cues that the subject is taboo, they may withdraw and participate less fully in their care. Facilitating open discussion and updating children with relevant information, including prognostic changes, can be very helpful. Also, children may need help coping with peers and school demands. Teachers should be informed and updated. Classmates may need education and assistance to help them understand the situation and respond appropriately.

Adolescents. Capable of formal cognitive operations, adolescents understand that death is inevitable and final but may not accept that their death is possible. The significant fears of dying teenagers parallel those of all teenagers. These include losing control, being imperfect, and being different. Concerns about body image, hair loss, or loss of bodily control can generate resistance to continuing treatment. Alternating emotions of despair, rage, grief, bitterness, numbness, terror, and joy are typical. The potential for withdrawal and isolation is high because teenagers may equate parental support with loss of independence or may deny their fears of abandonment by actually repulsing friendly gestures. Teenagers must be included in all decision-making processes surrounding their deaths. Many are capable of great courage, grace, and dignity in facing death.

Adults. Some of the most often expressed fears of adult patients entering hospice care, listed in the approximate order of frequency, include fears of (1) separation from loved ones, homes, and jobs; (2) becoming a burden to others; (3) losing control; (4) what will happen to dependents; (5) pain or other worsening symptoms; (6) being unable to complete life tasks or responsibilities; (7) dying; (8) being dead; (9) the fears of others (reflected fears); (10) the fate of the body; and (11) the afterlife. Problems in communication arise out of trepidation, making it essential for those involved in health care to provide environments of trust and safety in which people can begin to talk about uncertainties, anxieties, and concerns.

Late-age adults often accept that their time has come. Their main fears include long, painful, and disfiguring deaths; prolonged vegetative states; isolation; and loss of control or dignity. Elderly

patients may talk or joke openly about dying and sometimes welcome it. In their 70s and beyond, they rarely harbor illusions of indestructibility—most have already had several close calls: Their parents have died, and they have gone to funerals of friends and relatives. Although they may not be happy to die, they can be reconciled to it.

According to Erik Erikson, the eighth and final stage in the life cycle brings a sense of either integrity or despair. As elderly adults enter the last phase of their lives, they reflect on their pasts. When they have taken care of their affairs, have been relatively successful, and have adapted to the triumphs and disappointments of life, they can look back with satisfaction and only a few regrets. The integrity of the self allows people to accept inevitable disease and death without fear of succumbing helplessly. If elderly individuals look back on life as a series of missed opportunities or personal misfortunes, however, they feel a sense of bitter despair, a preoccupation with what might have been if only this or that had happened. Then death is fearsome because it symbolizes emptiness and failure.

Management

Caring for a dying patient is highly individual. Caretakers need to deal with death honestly, tolerate wide ranges of affects, connect with suffering patients and bereaved loved ones, and resolve routine issues as they arise. Although each therapeutic relationship between a patient and health provider has a uniqueness derived from the patient's and health provider's gender, constitution, life experience, age, stage of life, resources, faith, culture, and other considerations, major themes confront all health providers caring for dying patients.

BEREAVEMENT, GRIEF, AND MOURNING

Bereavement, grief, and *mourning* are terms that apply to the psychological reactions of those who survive a significant loss. Grief is the subjective feeling precipitated by the death of a loved one. The term is used synonymously with mourning, although, in the strictest sense, mourning is the process by which grief is resolved; it is the societal expression of post bereavement behavior and practices. Bereavement means the state of being deprived of someone by death and refers to being in the state of mourning. Regardless of the fine points that differentiate these terms, the experiences of grief and bereavement have sufficient similarities to warrant a syndrome that has signs, symptoms, a demonstrable course, and an expected resolution.

Normal Bereavement Reactions

The first response to loss, *protest,* is followed by a more extended period of *searching* behavior. As hope to reestablish the attachment bond diminishes, searching behaviors give way to *despair* and *detachment* before bereaved individuals eventually *reorganize* themselves around the recognition that the lost person will not return. Although the bereaved ultimately learn to accept the reality of death, they also find psychological and symbolic ways of keeping the memory of the deceased person very much alive. Grief work allows the survivor to redefine his or her relationship to the deceased person and to form new but enduring ties.

Duration of Grief. Most societies mandate modes of bereavement and time for grieving. In contemporary America, bereaved individuals are expected to return to work or school in a few weeks, to establish equilibrium within a few months, and to be capable of pursuing new relationships within 6 months to 1 year. Ample evidence suggests that the bereavement process does not end within a prescribed interval; certain aspects persist indefinitely for many otherwise high-functioning, typical individuals.

The most lasting manifestation of grief, especially after spousal bereavement, is loneliness. Often present for years after the death of a spouse, loneliness may, for some, be a daily reminder of the loss. Other common manifestations of protracted grief occur intermittently. For example, a man who has lost his wife may experience elements of acute grief every time he hears her name or sees her picture on the nightstand. Usually, these reactions become increasingly short-lived over time, dissipating within minutes and become tinged with positive and pleasant affects. Such bittersweet memories may last a lifetime. Thus, most grief does not fully resolve or permanently disappear; instead, grief becomes circumscribed and submerged only to reemerge in response to specific triggers.

Anticipatory Grief

In *anticipatory grief*, grief reactions are brought on by the slow dying process of a loved one through injury, illness, or high-risk activity. Although anticipatory grief may soften the blow of the eventual death, it can also lead to premature separation and withdrawal while not necessarily mitigating later bereavement. At times, the intensification of intimacy during this period may heighten the actual sense of loss even though it prepares the survivor in other ways.

Anniversary Reactions.   When the trigger for an acute grief reaction is a special occasion, such as a holiday or birthday, the rekindled grief is called an *anniversary reaction*. It is not unusual for anniversary reactions to occur each year on the same day the person died or, in some cases, when the bereaved individual becomes the same age the deceased person was at the time of death. Although these anniversary reactions tend to become relatively mild and brief over time, they can be experienced as the reliving of one's original grief and prevail for hours or days.

Mourning

From earliest history, every culture records its own beliefs, customs, and behaviors related to bereavement. Specific patterns include rituals for mourning (e.g., wakes or Shiva), for disposing of the body, for invocation of religious ceremonies, and periodic official remembrances. The funeral is the prevailing public display of bereavement in contemporary North America. The funeral and burial service acknowledge the real and final nature of the death, countering denial; they also garner support for the bereaved, encouraging tribute to the dead, uniting families, and facilitating community expressions of sorrow. If cremation replaces burial, ceremonies associated with the dissemination of the ashes perform similar functions. Visits, prayers, and other ceremonies allow for continuing support, coming to terms with reality, remembering, emotional expression, and concluding unfinished business with the deceased. Several cultural and religious rituals provide purpose and meaning, protect the survivors from isolation and vulnerability, and set limits on grieving. Subsequent holidays, birthdays, and anniversaries serve to remind the living of the dead and may elicit grief as real and fresh as the original experience; over time, these anniversary grievings become attenuated but often remain in some form.

Bereavement

Because bereavement often evokes depressive symptoms, it may be necessary to demarcate normal grief reactions from major depressive disorder (Table 29-2). DSM-5 took a significant step from DSM-IV in that it removed the bereavement exclusion from a major depressive disorder so that we can diagnose individuals experiencing a recent loss as having major depression if we believe that is the case. To acknowledge that some persons may have a syndrome of disabling grief that is not depression, DSM-5 proposed criteria for persistent complex bereavement, which they included as a condition for further study. ICD-10 considers this an adjustment disorder and includes the grief reaction as a category of that disorder. Table 29-3 summarizes the criteria for each approach.

Complicated Bereavement

Complicated bereavement has a confusing array of terms to describe it—*abnormal, atypical, distorted, morbid, traumatic,* and *unresolved,* to name a few types. Three patterns of complicated, dysfunctional grief syndromes have been identified—chronic, hypertrophic, and delayed grief. These are not diagnostic categories within DSM-5 but are descriptive syndromes that, if present, may be prodromal of a major depressive disorder.

Table 29-2
Differentiating the Depressive Symptoms Associated with Bereavement from Major Depression

Bereavement	Major Depressive Disorder
Symptoms may meet syndromal criteria for major depressive episode, but the survivor rarely has morbid feelings of guilt and worthlessness, suicidal ideation, or psychomotor retardation	Any symptoms as defined by DSM-5
Considers self-bereaved	May consider self-weak, defective, or bad
Dysphoria often triggered by thoughts or reminders of the deceased	Dysphoria is often autonomous and independent of thoughts or reminders of the deceased
Onset is within the first 2 mo of bereavement	Onset at any time
Duration of depressive symptoms is less than 2 mo	Depression often becomes chronic, intermittent, or episodic
Functional impairment is transient and mild	Clinically significant distress or impairment
No family or personal history of major depression	Family or personal history of major depression

Table 29-3
Approaches to Diagnosing Bereavement

	DSM-5	ICD-10
Diagnostic name	Persistent Complex Bereavement Disorder (list under "conditions for further study")	Adjustment Disorder, Grief Reaction
Duration	Experiences symptoms from each group of symptoms below, more days than not, for 12 mo (adults) or 6 mo (children)	Occurs while adapting to a period of life change
Symptoms	Since the death of someone close to them, experiencing following symptoms, out of proportion or inconsistent with sociocultural norms (Symptom group B) • Longing for the deceased • Sorry/pain about the death • Preoccupied with the lost person • Preoccupied with the circumstances surrounding the death (Symptom group C) • Difficulty accepting the death • Cannot believe or is numb to the loss • Difficulty thinking about positive memories • Bitter or angry about the loss • Self-blame • Avoids things that remind them of the lost person • Wants to die to be with the person • Cannot trust others • Feels alone/detached • Feels empty or unable to function without the lost person • Trouble seeing their purpose independent of the lost person • Trouble/reluctance pursuing other interests	Distress/Emotional disturbance • Depression • Anxiety • Worry • Difficulty coping • Difficulty planning • Difficulty carrying out daily routines • Disturbance of conduct (adolescents)
Required number of symptoms	Symptom group B: 1 symptom Symptom group C: 6 symptoms	Any combination of the above
Psychosocial consequences of symptoms	Distress of functional impairment	Usually interferes with functioning
Symptoms specifiers	With traumatic bereavement: the death was violent (homicide, suicide), and the bereaved is preoccupied with the suffering that preceded death	

Chronic Grief. The most common type of complicated grief is chronic grief, often highlighted by bitterness and idealization of the dead person. Chronic grief is most likely to occur when the relationship between the bereaved and the deceased had been extremely close, ambivalent, or dependent; or when social supports are lacking, and friends and relatives are not available to share the sorrow over the extended time needed for most mourners.

Hypertrophic Grief. Most often seen after a sudden and unexpected death, bereavement reactions are extraordinarily intense in hypertrophic grief. Customary coping strategies are ineffectual to mitigate anxiety, and withdrawal is frequent. When one family member is experiencing a hypertrophic grief reaction, disruption of family stability can occur. Hypertrophic grief frequently takes on a long-term course, albeit one attenuated over time.

Delayed Grief. Absent or inhibited grief when one usually expects to find overt signs and symptoms of acute mourning is referred to as delayed grief. This pattern is marked by prolonged denial; anger and guilt may complicate its course.

Traumatic Bereavement. Traumatic bereavement refers to grief, which is both chronic and hypertrophic. This syndrome is characterized by recurrent, intense pangs of grief with persistent yearning, pining, and longing for the deceased; recurrent intrusive images of the death; and a distressing admixture of avoidance and preoccupation with reminders of the loss. Positive memories are often blocked or excessively sad, or they are experienced in prolonged states of reverie that interfere with daily activities. A history of psychiatric illness appears to be frequent in this condition, as is a very close, identity-defining relationship with the deceased person.

Medical or Psychiatric Illnesses Associated with Bereavement. Medical complications include exacerbations of existing diseases and vulnerability to new ones; fear for one's health and more trips to the doctor; and an increased mortality rate, especially in men. The highest relative mortality risk is found immediately after bereavement, particularly from ischemic heart disease. The greatest effect of bereavement on mortality is for men younger than 65 years. Higher mortality rates in bereaved men than in bereaved women are due to increase in the relative risk of death by suicide, accident, cardiovascular disease, and some infectious diseases. In widows, the relative risk of death from cirrhosis and suicide may increase. In both sexes, bereavement appears to exacerbate health-compromising behaviors, such as increased alcohol consumption, smoking, and the use of over-the-counter medications.

Psychiatric complications of bereavement include an increased risk for major depressive disorder, prolonged anxiety, panic, and posttraumatic stress–like syndrome; increased alcohol, drug, and cigarette consumption; and an increased risk of suicide. Because of their psychosocial, emotional, and cognitive immaturity, bereaved children may be especially vulnerable to psychopathology.

Bereavement and Depression. Although symptoms overlap, grief can be distinguished from a full depressive episode. Most bereaved individuals experience intense sadness, but only a few meet DSM-5 criteria for a major depressive episode. Grief is a complex experience in which positive emotions take their place beside the negative ones. Grief is fluid and changing, an evolving state in which emotional intensity gradually lessens, and positive, comforting aspects of the lost relationship come to the fore. Pangs of grief are stimulus bound, related to internal and external reminders of the deceased person. This condition differs from depression, which is more pervasive and characterized by significant difficulties experiencing self-validating, positive feelings. Grief is a fluctuating state with individual variability, in which cognitive and behavioral adjustments are progressively made until the bereaved individual can hold the deceased person in a comfortable place in memory, and a satisfying life can be resumed. By contrast, a major depressive episode consists of a recognizable and stable cluster of debilitating symptoms accompanied by a protracted, enduring low mood. Major depressive episode tends to be persistent and associated with poor work and social functioning, pathologic psychoneuroimmunological function, and other neurobiologic changes unless treated.

Bereavement and Posttraumatic Stress Disorder. Unnatural and violent deaths, such as homicide, suicide, or death in the context of terrorism, are much more likely to precipitate PTSD in surviving loved ones than are natural deaths. In such circumstances, themes of violence, victimization, and volition (i.e., the choice of death over life, as in the case of suicide) are intermixed with other aspects of grief, and traumatic distress marked by fear, horror, vulnerability, and disintegration of cognitive assumptions ensues. Disbelief, despair, anxiety symptoms, preoccupation with the deceased person, and the circumstances of the death, withdrawal, hyperarousal, and dysphoria are more intense and more prolonged than they are under nontraumatic circumstances, and an increased risk may exist for other complications. Although treatment studies in survivors of sudden death are few and far between, most experts agree that initial attention should be focused on traumatic distress, that a role is seen for both pharmacotherapy and psychotherapy, and that self-help support groups can be enormously beneficial.

Biologic Perspectives

Grief is both a physiologic and emotional response. During acute grief (as with other stressful events), persons may experience disruption of biologic rhythms. Grief is also accompanied by impaired immune functioning, including decreased lymphocyte proliferation and impaired functioning of natural killer cells. Whether the immune changes are clinically significant has not been established, but the mortality rate for widows and widowers following the death of a spouse is higher than that in the general population. Widowers appear to be at risk longer than widows.

Phenomenology of Grief. Bereavement reactions include intense feeling states; invoke a variety of coping strategies; and lead to alterations in interpersonal relationships, biopsychosocial

Table 29-4
Phases of Grief

Shock and denial (min, days, wk)
  Disbelief and numbness
  Searching behaviors: pining, yearning, and protest
Acute anguish (wk, mo)
  Waves of somatic distress
  Withdrawal
  Preoccupation
  Anger
  Guilt
Lost patterns of conduct
  Restless and agitated
  Aimless and amotivational
  Identification with the bereaved
Resolution (mo, yr)
  Have grieved
  Return to work
  Resume old roles
  Acquire new roles
  Reexperience pleasure
  Seek companionship and love of others

functioning, self-esteem, and world view that can last indefinitely. Manifestations of grief reflect the individual's personality, previous life experiences, and past psychological history; the significance of the loss; the nature of the bereaved person's relationship with the deceased person; the existing social network; intercurrent life events; health; and other resources. Despite individual variations in the bereavement process, investigators have proposed grieving process models, which include at least three partially overlapping phases or states: (1) initial shock, disbelief, and denial; (2) an intermediate period of acute discomfort and social withdrawal; and (3) a culminating period of restitution and reorganization. As with Kübler-Ross' stages of dying, the grieving stages do not prescribe a correct course of grief; instead, they are general guidelines describing an overlapping and fluid process that varies with the survivors (Table 29-4).

LIFE CYCLE PERSPECTIVES ABOUT BEREAVEMENT

Bereavement during Childhood and Adolescence

Approximately 4 percent of North American children lose one or both parents by the age of 15 years; sibling death is the second most commonly experienced bereavement. Grief reactions are colored by developmental levels and concepts of death and may not resemble adult reactions. Children may display minimal grief at the time of death and experience the full effect of the loss later. Grieving children may not withdraw and dwell on the person who died, but instead, may throw themselves into activities. Indifference, anger, or misbehavior may be displayed rather than the sadness; behaviors can be erratic and labile. Strong feelings of anger and fears of abandonment or death may show up in the behavior of grieving children. Children often play death games as a way of working out their feelings and anxieties. These games are familiar to the children and provide safe opportunities to express their feelings. Although they may seem to show grief only occasionally and briefly, in reality, a child's grief often lasts longer than that of an adult.

Mourning in children may need to be addressed again and again as the child ages. Children will think about the loss repeatedly, especially during critical times in their lives, such as going to camp, graduating from school, getting married, or giving birth to their children. A child's grief can be influenced by his or her age, personality, developmental stage, earlier experiences with death, and relationship with the deceased person. The surroundings, cause of death, and family members' ability to communicate with one another and to continue as a family after death can also affect grief. The child's ongoing need for care, his or her opportunity to share feelings and memories, the parent's ability to cope with stress, and the child's steady relationships with other adults are other factors that may influence grief. Even older children frequently feel abandoned or rejected when a parent dies and may show hostility toward the deceased or the surviving parent, now perceived as one who might also "abandon" them. They may feel responsible because of earlier misbehavior or because they said or wished that that person would die at some time.

Children younger than 2 years may show loss of speech or diffuse distress. Children younger than 5 years are apt to respond with eating, sleeping, and bowel and bladder dysfunctions. Intense feelings of sadness, fear, and anxiety can occur, but these feelings are not persistent and tend to alternate between longer lasting normal states. School-age children may become phobic or hypochondriacal, withdrawn, or pseudomature, and school performance and peer relations often suffer. Adolescents, as with adults, run the gamut in expressing bereavement, ranging from behavioral problems, somatic symptoms, and erratic moods to stoicism. Whereas adolescent boys losing a parent may become delinquent, girls may turn to a sexual pattern for comfort and reassurance. Behavioral disturbances and depression are familiar at all ages. Rates of depressive episodes in bereaved children and adolescents are as high as in bereaved adults.

Bereaved children must be treated in a manner that considers their levels of emotional and cognitive maturity. They need to be told that death is real and irreversible and that they are blameless. Feelings and concerns should be expressed, and questions should be invited and answered with simplicity, candor, and clarity. Children, as with adults, need rituals to commemorate their loved ones; attendance at the funeral and participation in mourning may be beneficial first steps.

Bereavement during Adulthood

No consensus exists on which type of loss is associated with the most severe reactions. Although the death of a spouse is often ranked as the most stressful life event, some have argued that losing a child is even more profound. The death of a child is a particular sorrow, a lifelong loss for surviving mothers, fathers, brothers, sisters, grandparents, and other family members. A child's death is a life-altering experience. The deaths of parents and siblings in adult life have not achieved much systematic study, but they are generally considered relatively mild compared with the loss of a spouse or child.

Grief appears most intense for the mother in late perinatal losses (stillbirths or neonatal deaths rather than miscarriages) and often is reexperienced during subsequent pregnancies. Sudden infant death syndrome is particularly problematic in that death is sudden and unexpected. Parents may experience extra guilt or blame each other, often resulting in subsequent marital difficulties.

The surviving family members, friends, or lovers of individuals who have died from acquired immunodeficiency syndrome (AIDS) are uniquely challenged. The illness carries with it the stigmata of the illness itself and the gay community in general; it carries with it caretakers' fear of contracting the illness, and it is most prevalent in people who are in the prime of life. Asymptomatic infection

may permit the infected person and those close to him or her time to adapt to the diagnosis. When a person who is human immunodeficiency virus (HIV) positive begins to manifest symptoms of opportunistic infection or associated cancer; however, the illness again becomes a threat. Coping with emotional reality is arduous and complicated. Often caretakers, as well as HIV-positive patients, wish for death, which can evoke feelings of guilt. For bereaved lovers, their own HIV status, multiple losses, and other concurrent stressors can complicate recovery. Gay men who have lost lovers to AIDS may be more depressed, consider suicide more often, and be more vulnerable to illicit drug use than are other bereaved individuals.

Elderly adults face more losses than individuals at other phases of the life cycle, and intense loneliness may be a lasting memorial to those who have died. For highly impaired elders who lose a spouse they depended on for daily functions or who was their sole source of companionship, bereavement reactions are profound.

Grief Therapy

Persons in normal grief seldom seek psychiatric help because they accept their reactions and behaviors as appropriate. Accordingly, a bereaved person should not routinely see a psychiatrist or psychologist unless a markedly divergent reaction to the loss is noted. For example, under usual circumstances, a bereaved person does not make a suicide attempt; if someone seriously contemplates suicide, psychiatric intervention is indicated.

When professional assistance is sought, it usually involves a request for sleeping medication from a family physician. A mild sedative to induce sleep may be useful in some situations, but antidepressant medication or antianxiety agents are rarely indicated in normal grief. Bereaved persons may have to go through the mourning process, however painful it is, for a successful resolution to occur. Narcotizing patients with drugs interferes with the normal process that ultimately can lead to a desired outcome.

Because grief reactions can develop into a depressive disorder or pathologic mourning, specific counseling sessions for bereaved individuals are often valuable. Grief therapy is an increasingly important skill. In regularly scheduled sessions, grieving persons are encouraged to talk about feelings of loss and about the person who has died. Many bereaved persons have difficulty recognizing and expressing angry or ambivalent feelings toward a deceased person, and they must be reassured that these feelings are normal.

Grief therapy need not be conducted only on a one-to-one basis; group counseling is also useful. Self-help groups also have great value in some instances. About 30 percent of widows and widowers report that they become isolated from friends, withdraw from social life, and thus experience feelings of isolation and loneliness. Self-help groups offer companionship, social contacts, and emotional support; they eventually enable their members to reenter society in a meaningful way. Bereavement care and grief therapy have been most effective with widows and widowers. The necessity for this therapy stems, in part, from the contraction of the family unit; extended family members are no longer available to provide the needed emotional support and guidance during the mourning period.

▲ 29.2 Palliative Care

Psychological symptoms are nearly universal at the end of life. Psychiatric syndromes occur with an increased but definable frequency and have different age and gender distribution. For example, anxiety and depression are as common in men as in women. Psychiatric classification remains an essential framework on which to base clinical observations, but it was not designed with dying patients in mind. Hence, for such patients, it is pragmatically useful to think of a few syndromes for which this exists. The most common ones are anxiety states, depressive states, and confusional states. These frequently coexist and overlap. Rarely, specific phobias of needles, enclosures, and the like may interfere with comfort and should be addressed, adapting the usual treatments to the patient's medical status. Occasionally, an emotional crisis or exacerbation of symptoms can be identified as an adjustment disorder, but it is occurring against the backdrop of other severe symptoms, so technically, it does not meet diagnostic criteria. However, this should not prevent the consultant from identifying the precipitating factor and defusing the response in the usual ways. Major psychotic disorders become submerged by the increasing symptomatology of the active dying process and only require specific attention when the patient is not actively dying and when the psychotic symptoms are separated from and superimposed on the symptoms of the illness.

PREVALENCE

Much of the research on prevalence has been done in cancer and AIDS and shows a marked increase in psychiatric conditions near the end of life. Severe depressive symptoms were found in from 25 to 77 percent in a sample of hospitalized cancer patients, although stricter criteria find 15 percent with major depression and another 15 percent having severe depressive symptoms. The prevalence of delirium rises from a range from 25 to 40 percent to as high as 85 percent with increasingly advanced disease. The association of psychiatric symptoms with pain was demonstrated in one of several consistent studies in which 39 percent of patients with a psychiatric diagnosis reported significant pain compared with 19 percent for those without a psychiatric diagnosis. In a sample of inpatients with AIDS, 65 percent had an organic mental disorder, and 27 percent had major depression. The financial cost of psychiatric disorders can be inferred from a study in which patients with a psychiatric diagnosis remained in the hospital 60 days longer than those without a psychiatric diagnosis.

Most commonly, terminally ill patients demonstrate an intertwining of anxiety and depression. These are difficult to tease apart, and the term *negative affect* has been suggested to define them as a symptom complex. It is hard not to feel grief at what is being lost and fear about the ultimate unknown. Individuals whose deep faith in an afterlife animates their spirit are an exception, and, even among them, many describe coexisting regret at the loss of their temporal life and its furnishings.

GENERAL TREATMENT PRINCIPLES

Because the improved quality of life is the primary goal, pharmacologic treatment and any other measures that bring symptom relief should be instituted rapidly while an integrated plan for psychological and family interventions is being designed and set into motion. Psychiatric syndromes in this group are often secondary to medical conditions; hence, an etiologic diagnosis often yields useful clues to prevention and improved management. It should be sought simultaneously as long as the search is in line with treatment goals.

ANXIETY IN PATIENTS WITH ADVANCED DISEASE

Anxiety can be the presenting symptom for almost all medical disorders and can occur as a side effect from many medications. However, in patients with advanced disease, it usually presents with somatic symptoms, such as restlessness, hyperactivity, tachycardia, gastrointestinal (GI) distress, nausea, insomnia, shortness of breath, numbness, or tremor. It lowers the threshold for pain, worsens functional impairment, and increases the distress experienced in all comorbid conditions. It often interferes with the patient's ability to cooperate with other treatments or to relate optimally with loved ones. Patients refer to fear, worry, apprehension, or ruminations more often than to anxiety per se.

> Mr. S, a 50-year-old physical therapist with newly diagnosed advanced lung cancer, was noted by his family to be anxious to the point of having panic symptoms when his wife would leave his bedside to attend to chores. He would start hyperventilating, would feel short of breath, would become restless and unable to concentrate on anything, and would be overwhelmed with morbid ruminations about his future. He was upset and felt guilty at having become overly dependent on his wife. He was taught relaxation and breathing exercises and was treated with clonazepam, which brought about a marked resolution of his anxiety. Mr. S felt more relaxed, less anxious, and more resilient and became able to withstand periods of solitude without difficulty. (Courtesy of Marguerite Lederberg, M.D.)

DEPRESSION IN PATIENTS WITH ADVANCED DISEASE

Depressive symptoms are also common in advanced disease and are associated with the same existential factors found with anxiety. Studies have found a prevalence ranging from 9 percent, using the strictest criteria, to 58 percent, with less demanding ones. Risk factors include a previous history or family history. Having a way of differentiating somatic effects of disease from the neurovegetative criteria of major depression is especially daunting in terminally ill patients.

Table 29-5 describes the Endicott Substitution Criteria, which have been found to perform as well as the DSM criteria for depression and go further in that they also reflect the clinical observation which classically described that depressive thoughts and feelings are not universal in terminally ill patients and, when present, reflect depression just as they do in physically healthy patients.

Table 29-5
Endicott Substitution Criteria for Depression

Physical-Somatic Symptoms	Psychological Symptom Substitute
Changes in appetite or weight, or both	Tearfulness, depressed appearance
Sleep disturbance	Social withdrawal, decreased talkativeness
Fatigue, loss of energy	Brooding, self-pity, pessimism
Memory and concentration deficits, indecisiveness	Lack of reactivity

Although there are not many studies on the treatment of depression in terminally ill individuals, the available studies and a large body of clinical experience with medically ill patients show that the pharmacologic treatment of depression can be useful even when definable medical causes exist and even in the last days of life.

A patient with diabetes and end-stage renal disease who had been on dialysis for 2 years was diagnosed with depression with marked insomnia and was started on 15 mg by mouth every day of mirtazapine, which helped her sleep immediately and showed an antidepressant effect within 3 weeks. Four weeks later, she was admitted to the hospital in congestive heart failure for what was to be her terminal admission. She did not wish to give up the antidepressant but now felt oversedated and wished that she could be more alert during the day to interact with her loved ones. She was started on methylphenidate 5 mg by mouth twice daily, after which she was more alert, engaged, and communicative with her family. On her death, her family was grateful to have been able to connect with her until the end.

CONFUSIONAL STATES IN PATIENTS WITH ADVANCED DISEASE

The prevalence of delirium rises to 85 percent in patients with advanced disease. If one includes the last hours of life, it nears 100 percent unless the patient lapses rapidly into a coma or dies of an acute event, such as pulmonary embolus. Acute events are always unexpected and traumatize the survivors even though they knew full well that the patient was near the end of life. Some patients slip into an irreversible coma, leaving families in a bedside vigil, which may give them a period of adaptation before the final instant of death. However, for some 75 to 85 percent of patients, death is associated with a period of delirium.

Patients frequently experience some disorientation, impaired memory, concentration, and altered arousal as they become increasingly ill. These symptoms may remain mild or may be the harbingers of full delirium. Clinicians should be aware that mild and early signs of delirium are often mistaken for depression, anxiety, and poor coping.

A psychiatric consultation was sought to evaluate depression in a 56-year-old practicing attorney with pancreatic cancer. His moderately severe back pain was being treated with morphine. The patient was noted by the inpatient staff to be more withdrawn, disengaged, and quiet, making poor eye contact and sleeping most of the day.

On examination, the psychiatric consultant found Mr. K to have disturbed arousal and to be mildly confused and disoriented. His speech was slow and his thought process disorganized. Mr. K admitted to intermittently experiencing visual hallucinations that he had been too embarrassed to report earlier to the nursing staff.

Mr. K was diagnosed with a hypoactive delirium secondary to opioid medications. He was treated with a low dose of olanzapine, 2.5 mg at bedtime. Mr. K's sensorium improved dramatically. He became alert, fully oriented, and better related, without any perceptual disturbances or thought disorder. This treatment was accomplished without needing to decrease his much-needed pain medications.

DISEASE-SPECIFIC CONSIDERATIONS

Different illnesses bring special issues. For example, a patient on dialysis can opt for death three times a week and is more vulnerable to acting on feelings of depression, anger, hopelessness, and

reactions to family neglect or conflict. Patients with cancer must acknowledge possible death while hoping for a cure or remission. Treatment decisions in the face of a disease that is less and less treatable become increasingly difficult and can cause acute anxiety. Stem cell transplant patients experience high levels of anxiety and depression because they are getting a last chance with high stakes and high risks. The availability of organ transplants has created a large population of patients who wait, knowing that they may die while waiting for a cure that could be just around the corner. Neurodegenerative disorders are associated with increased physical disability and dependence. When there is associated loss of cognitive faculties, the problems may be behavioral. Otherwise, depression is frequent, although not an inevitable problem. Many patients state that they will not tolerate complete immobility and dependence, yet when the time comes, they go on life supports and stay on them. It has been shown in several settings that as patients become increasingly ill, they accept an increasingly limited quality of life as worth living and opt for more onerous, less promising treatments if they offer even a small chance of help.

PATIENT–FAMILY UNIT

The intensity of family relationships becomes even more significant during the terminal period. The response of family members can be a conspiracy of silence. Nothing is sadder than a bedside where family members are tense and silent because they want to protect the patient by not talking about dying, and the patient is tense and silent because he or she is protecting the family by not talking about things that will upset them. Instead of closeness, expressions of gratitude, apologies, reminiscences, and farewells, there is a distance, and the patient is dying alone even though others physically surround the patient.

The psychiatrist can use family sessions to open patient–family dialogues. He or she can identify discrepant views of the illness, can deal with conflicts regarding treatment, and can explore concerns regarding an absent member, all of which undermine patient support and medical management. A major crisis, such as the imminent loss of a member, destabilizes the family structure, creating an opportunity for the psychiatrist to promote adaptive change and reconstitution. *Family-centered grief therapy,* which initially includes the patient and continues after the patient's death, provides a natural setting for such interventions.

When an older adolescent dropped out of college to take over her dying mother's duties, the family subtly discouraged her return to school after her mother's death. Psychiatric intervention allowed the patient to play a part in reorganizing family roles in a way that made it more possible for her daughter to continue her studies.

DECISION POINTS, ADVANCE DIRECTIVES, PROXIES, AND SURROGATES

This section reviews the transitions and decisions that characterize the end of life.

Transition to Palliative Care

The transition to palliative care is not always clear. As soon as a diagnosis of an incurable disease is made, a cure is no longer the goal of care. However, if death is distant or even if some life extension can still be obtained, the patient and family focus on this positive goal. The physician is under no illusion about the future but has the delicate task of promoting short-term gains without obliterating the awareness of what lies ahead. Only when the nearness of death is acknowledged can thoughtful decisions be made about palliative care.

Where to Die?

Unattended Deaths.   Many traumatic or unexpected deaths become known from a catastrophic phone call. The traumatized family then needs help to absorb the loss, to cope with the circumstances, and to come to some kind of closure. It is not realized how much the experience of living through the illness, death, and the funeral rites is crucial to the normal resolution of the mourning process.

An unexpected death, even an understandable one, such as a heart attack, leaves an aching sense of unfinished business over and above the expected grief. If the person was the victim of a crime, obsessive thoughts might be difficult to repress, and grief may turn to unquenchable anger with profound psychological disruption. It is also difficult, if not impossible, for survivors to make peace with suicide.

Emergency departments, police departments, and religious and community institutions should be equipped with a list of referral resources to help survivors of traumatic deaths. Psychiatric input can include program development and consultation to a wide range of professionals and individuals. Families must be helped to construct their ritual whereby they acknowledge to themselves and others the finality of their loss and perhaps create a place, if not a grave, around which to center their memorializing.

Attended Deaths.   Patients can die in an acute hospital, in nursing homes, in hospices, and at home, with or without hospice support.

Most patients still die in acute care hospitals, having received active care until shortly before they die. This may occur because death is sudden or because the family or patient needed to be in a place where "everything is being done." Fortunately, a growing number of hospitals have palliative care teams that provide appropriate care in the acute hospital setting.

Many patients die in nursing homes without the benefit of special care. This unfortunate situation could be remedied by bringing formal hospice care into nursing homes, but funding sources and turf issues need to be settled before it can become routine practice.

Inpatient hospice care was the first model of care to be developed and is warmly remembered by grateful families whose multiple human needs and those of their loved ones had been met in ways that they had not been trained to expect. As hospice gained acceptance, the insufficiency of inpatient beds encouraged the development of home hospice. Its existence has, in turn, encouraged more families to elect to keep dying patients at home.

In a home hospice program, the patient is evaluated and accepted in the usual manner but stays at home. The patient and family receive extensive instruction about what to expect. They are helped to obtain necessary materials, taught how to use them, and helped to obtain as much home help as they need. All the while, they receive medical supervision, nursing care, and emotional support with 24-hour phone availability and routine daily contacts.

Without this kind of help, a good death at home can be challenging to achieve. With it, patients feel safe from the abandonment that is so commonly feared, and families feel safe from the terror of

an unmanageable event. The families of these patients work hard, but they are more likely to feel competent and in control. They experience more of a sense of achievement and less of the gnawing sense of inadequacy that is otherwise common.

CARING FOR THE DYING PATIENT

Marguerite S. Lederberg, M.D., at Memorial Sloan Kettering Cancer Center in New York makes the following observation:

A dying human being whose physical, social, emotional, and spiritual needs are being effectively attended to seldom demands to be helped to commit suicide, and the family members—given proper help and support—derive a deep sense of peace from having helped their loved one to die feeling loved and secure.

One of the most critical tasks for a physician caring for a dying patient is to determine when the time for curative care has ceased. It is only then that palliative care can begin. Some physicians are so upset by death that they are reluctant to use palliative methods; instead, they continue to treat the patient knowing that efforts are futile. Alternatively, they resort to using so-called heroic methods that do not prevent death, and that may produce needless suffering. Ideally, physicians should strive to extend the patient's life and decrease suffering; at the same time, they must accept death as a defining characteristic of life. Some physicians, however, develop dysfunctional attitudes about death, which they reinforce throughout their lives in their experiences and training. It has been postulated that doctors are more frightened of death than members of other professional groups and that many enter the study of medicine so they may gain control of their mortality using the defense mechanism of intellectualization. Risk factors that can interfere with a physician's ability to care optimally for dying patients are listed in Table 29-6. These factors range from overidentifying with the patient to being fearful of death, as mentioned.

Physicians able to deal with death and dying can communicate effectively in several areas: diagnosis and prognosis, the nature of the terminal illness, advance directives about life-sustaining treatment, hospice care, legal and ethical issues, grief and bereavement, and psychiatric care. Also, palliative care physicians must be skilled in pain management, especially in the use of potent opioids—the gold standard of drugs used for pain relief. In 1991, the American

Table 29-6
Risk Factors for the Development of Aversive Reactions in Physicians

The physician:
  Identifies with the patient: looks, profession, age, character, and so on.
  Identifies the patient with someone in his or her own life.
  Is currently dealing with a sick family member.
  Is recently bereaved or dealing with unresolved loss or grief issues.
  Feels professionally insecure.
  Is fearful of death and disability.
  Is unconsciously reflecting feelings felt or expressed by the patient or family.
  Cannot tolerate high and protracted levels of ambiguity or uncertainty.
  Carries a psychiatric diagnosis, such as depression or substance abuse.

Adapted from Meier DE, Back AL, Morrison RS The inner life of physicians and care of the seriously ill. *JAMA.* 2001;286:3007–3014, with permission.

Board of Pain Medicine was established to ensure that physicians treating patients in pain were both qualified to do so and were kept up to date on the latest advances in the field.

COMMUNICATION

After a diagnosis and prognosis have been made, physicians need to talk to the patient and the patient's family. Formerly, doctors subscribed to a conspiracy of silence, believing that their patient's chances for recovery would improve if they knew less, because news of impending death might bring despair. The standard of care is to be honest and open toward a patient. The question is no longer whether to tell a patient, but when and how. In 1972, the American Hospital Association drafted the Patient's Bill of Rights, declaring that patients have the "right to obtain complete, current information regarding diagnosis, treatment, and prognosis in terms the patient can be reasonably expected to understand."

Breaking Bad News

When breaking news of impending death to the patient, as when relating any bad news, diplomacy and compassion should be the guiding principles. Often, the bad news is not entirely related during one meeting but instead is absorbed gradually over a series of separate conversations. Preparations, including scheduling sufficient time for the visit, researching pertinent information such as test results and facts about the case, and even arranging furniture can help make the patient feel comfortable.

If possible, these conversations should take place in a private, suitable space with the patient on equal terms with the physician (i.e., the patient dressed and the physician seated). If it is possible and desired by the patient, the patient's spouse or partner should be present. The treating physician should explain the current situation to the patient in clear, simple language even when speaking to highly educated patients. Information need to be repeated, or additional meetings may be necessary to communicate all of the information. A gentle, sensible approach will help modulate the patient's denial and acceptance. At no time should physicians take their patient's angry comments personally, and they should never criticize the patient's response to the bad news.

Physicians can signal their availability for honest communication by encouraging and answering questions from patients. Estimates on how long a patient has to live are usually inaccurate and thus should not be given, or given with that caveat. Also, physicians should make it clear to their patients that they are willing to see them through until death occurs. Ultimately, physicians must choose how much information to give and when based on each patient's needs and capacities.

The same general approaches apply as physicians seek to comfort members of the patient's family. Helping family members deal with feelings about the patient's illness can be just as important as comforting the patient because family members are often the primary source of emotional support for patients.

Telling the Truth

Tactful honesty is the doctor's most valuable aid. Honesty, however, need not preclude hope or guarded optimism. It is essential to be aware that if 85 percent of patients with a particular disease die in 5 years, 15 percent are still alive after that time. When deciding when and what to tell a patient about their prognosis, we should consider our commitment to the principle of "do no harm." In general, most patients want to know the truth about their condition. Various studies of patients with malignancies show that 80 to 90 percent want to know their diagnosis.

Doctors, however, should ask patients how much they want to know because some persons do not want to know all the facts about their illness. Such patients, if told the truth, deny that they ever were told, and they cannot participate in end-of-life decisions, such as the use of life-sustaining equipment. The patients who openly request that they not be given "bad news" are often those who most fear death. Physicians should deal with these fears directly, but if the patient still cannot bear to hear the truth, someone closely related to the patient must be informed.

Informed Consent

In the United States, informed consent is legally required for both conventional and experimental treatment. Patients must be given sufficient information about their diagnosis, prognosis, and treatment options to make knowledgeable decisions. This information includes a discussion of potential risks and benefits, available alternative treatments, and the results of not receiving treatment. This approach may come at some psychological cost; severe anxiety and occasional psychiatric decompensation can occur when patients feel overburdened by demands to make decisions. Nevertheless, patients respond best to doctors who explain the various options in detail. Physicians must be prepared to deal with difficult questions posed by patients. Some of them are listed in Table 29-7.

End-of-life discussions are challenging, mainly because they can influence how patients make informed choices.

TERMINAL CARE DECISIONS

Modern society is poorly equipped to cope with the life-and-death decisions spawned by technology. When it first emerged, cardiopulmonary resuscitation was enthusiastically supported by the medical profession. It was endowed with magical power and eventually became a ritualized rite rather than an optional medical treatment. That practice played into the therapeutic activism characteristic of many physicians. By the end of the 20th century, however, a countermovement began. First, the right to refuse treatment was established, mostly because of synergy between the consumer movement and the bioethics movement, with its emphasis on patient autonomy. Next, the legality of DNR orders and the moral equivalence of stopping and not starting treatment were established. The medical profession was less enthusiastic than the public about these changes, perhaps because practitioners know too well the emotional ambiguities that surround death and must repeatedly experience them.

Table 29-7
Some Difficult Questions from Patients

"Why me?"
"Why didn't you catch this earlier? Did you make a mistake?"
"How long do I have?"
"What would you do in my shoes?"
"Should I try experimental therapy?"
"Should I go to a 'medical mecca' for treatment or a second opinion?"
"If my suffering gets really bad, will you help me die?"
"Will you work with me all the way through to my death, no matter what?"

From Quill TF. Perspectives on care at the close of life. Initiating end-of-life discussions with seriously ill patients: Addressing the "elephant in the room". *JAMA.* 2000;284:2502–2507, with permission.

Table 29-8
Persistent Vegetative State

No evidence of awareness of self or environment; no interaction with others
No meaningful response to stimuli
No receptive or expressive language
Return of sleep–wake cycles, arousal, even smiling, frowning, yawning
Preserved brainstem or hypothalamic autonomic functions to permit survival
Bowel and bladder incontinence
Variably preserved cranial nerve and spinal reflexes

Brain Death and Persistent Vegetative State

In an attempt to deal with these ambiguities, the concept of brain death emerged. Brain death is associated with the loss of higher brain functions (e.g., cognition) and all brain stem functions (e.g., pupillary and reflex eye movement), respiration, and gag and corneal reflexes. Determination of brain death is a generally accepted criterion for death. Some clinicians advocate an absence of brain waves on electroencephalography (EEG) to confirm the diagnosis.

The American Academy of Neurology defined the persistent vegetative state as a condition in which no awareness exists of self or environment associated with severe neurologic damage (Table 29-8). The medical treatment provides no benefits to patients in a persistent vegetative state, and after the diagnosis is established, DNR and do-not-intubate (DNI) orders can be followed and life-sustaining methods (e.g., feeding tubes, ventilators) can be removed.

In 1976, the case of Karen Ann Quinlan made international headlines when her parents sought the assistance of a judge to discontinue the use of a ventilator in their daughter, who was in a persistent vegetative state. Ms. Quinlan's physician had refused her parents' request to remove the ventilator because they said they feared that they might be held civilly or even criminally liable for her death. The New Jersey Supreme Court ruled that competent persons have a right to refuse life-sustaining treatment and that this right should not be lost when a person becomes incompetent. Because the court believed that the physicians were unwilling to withdraw the ventilator because of the fear of legal liability, not precepts of medical ethics, it devised a mechanism to grant the physicians prospective legal immunity for taking this action. The New Jersey Supreme Court ruled that after a prognosis, confirmed by a hospital ethics committee, that "no reasonable possibility of a patient returning to a cognitive, sapient state," exists, life-sustaining treatment can be removed, and no one involved, including the physicians, can be held civilly or criminally responsible for the death.

The publicity surrounding the Quinlan case motivated two independent developments: It encouraged states to enact "living will" legislation that provided legal immunity to physicians who honored patients' written "advance directives," specifying how they would want to be treated if they ever became incompetent. It also encouraged hospitals to establish ethics committees that could attempt to resolve similar treatment disputes without going to court. (Courtesy of Annas GJ. "Culture of Life" politics at the bedside—the case of Terri Schiavo. *N Eng J Med.* 2005;352:1710–1715.)

Advance Directives

Advance directives are wishes and choices about medical intervention when the patient's condition is considered terminal. Advance directives, which are legally binding in all 50 states, include three types: living will, health care proxy, and DNR and DNI orders.

Living Will.   In a living will, a mentally competent patient gives specific instructions that doctors must follow when the patient cannot communicate with them because of illness. These instructions may include rejection of feeding tubes, artificial airways, and any other measures to prolong life.

Health Care Proxy.   Also known as a *durable power of attorney,* the health care proxy gives another person the power to make medical decisions if the patient cannot do so. That person, also known as the surrogate, is empowered to make all decisions about terminal care based on what he or she thinks the patient would want.

Do-Not-Resuscitate and Do-Not-Intubate Orders.   These orders prohibit doctors from attempting to resuscitate (DNR) or intubate (DNI) the patient who is in extremis. DNR and DNI orders are made by the patient who is competent to do so. They can be made part of the living will or expressed by the health care proxy. Figure 29-1 is an infographic that includes a checklist of important items to consider when making an advanced directive.

The Uniform Rights of the Terminally Ill Act, drafted by the National Conference of Commissioners on Uniform State Laws was approved and recommended for enactment in all states. This act authorizes an adult to control the decisions regarding the administration of life-sustaining treatment by executing a declaration instructing a physician to withhold or to withdraw life-sustaining treatment if the person is in a terminal condition and cannot participate in medical treatment decisions. In 1991, the Federal Patient Self-Determination Act became law in the United States. It required that all health care facilities (1) provide each patient admitted to a hospital with written information about the right to refuse treatment, (2) ask about advance directives, and (3) keep written records of whether the patient has an advance directive or has designated a health care proxy.

Today, patients who have left no advance directives or who are legally incompetent to do so have access to hospital ethics committees that hold active legal and ethical debates about these issues. These ethics committees are also of help to doctors, who can gain both legal and moral support when recommending that no further treatment occur. It is much easier for all parties, however, if the patient has advance directives or a proxy. Ideally, physicians should initiate discussions with patients about advance directives and proxies early even while the patient is healthy. The patient should be reminded that these early formulations can be modified but that even having preliminary advance directives will ensure that treating physicians observe the patient's wishes in the event of an emergency.

CARING FOR THE FAMILY

Family members play an essential role as caregivers to terminally ill patients and have needs of their own that often go unrecognized. Their responsibilities can be overwhelming, especially if only one family member is available or if family members themselves are infirm or elderly. Table 29-9 lists some family caregiving tasks. Many of these tasks require long hours of work or supervision that can lead to physical and emotional fatigue. One study of caregivers reports that 25 to 30 percent lost their jobs, and more than half moved to lower-paying jobs to accommodate the need for flexibility. The highest stress level was found in families who cared for a terminally ill patient at home, mainly when the death occurred in the home and realized in retrospect that they would have preferred an environment in which death occurs in the presence of skilled caretakers.

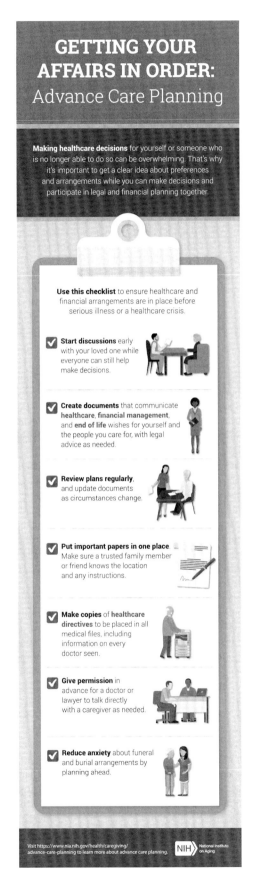

FIGURE 29-1

Advance Care planning checklist. (Source: National Institute on Aging, https://www.nia.nih.gov/health/infographics/getting-your-affairs-order-advance-care-planning.)

Table 29-9
Tasks of Family Members of Dying Individuals

1. Administering medications
2. Dealing with adverse effects of medications
3. Providing help with, or actually performing, activities of daily living
4. Changing wound dressing
5. Managing ambulatory infusion pumps or other equipment
6. Providing symptom management (e.g., for pain, nausea and vomiting, shortness of breath, seizures, and terminal agitation)
7. Notifying the nurse or doctor when they are needed
8. Shopping for needed items and picking up prescriptions
9. Providing a presence and companionship
10. Attending to spiritual and religious needs
11. Carrying out advance directives
12. Managing financial matters

Dying at Home

Depending on the patient's wishes and the specific disease, the choice to die at home is one that should be explored. Although it is more burdensome on a family than dying in a hospital or hospice, death at home can be a welcome alternative for the patient and family seeking to spend quality time together. A home care team can assess a home for its suitability and suggest ways to facilitate activities of daily living, including modifications to furniture; hospital bed leasing; and installation of assistive devices, such as handrails and commodes. The family's care can be supplemented with house calls by physicians, nurses, therapists, and chaplains. In any case, the family must know what their responsibilities are and must be well prepared to care for the patient. Recently, hospice home care was approved by Medicare and is being more widely used.

Family therapy sessions allow family members to explore feelings about death and dying. They serve as a forum in which anticipatory grief and mourning can take place. The ability to share feelings can be cathartic, especially if guilt is involved. Family members often have to deal with feelings of guilt about past interactions with the dying patient. Family sessions also help to achieve consensus about the patient's advance directives. If family members disagree about the patient's wishes, the medical staff may be unable to act. In such cases, legal action may be needed to resolve family disputes about what course of action to pursue.

PALLIATIVE CARE

Palliative care is the most critical part of end-of-life care. It refers to providing relief from the suffering caused by pain or other symptoms of a terminal disease. Although this is most commonly associated with analgesic drug administration, many other medical interventions and surgical procedures fall under the umbrella of palliative care because they can make the patient more comfortable. Monitors and their alarms, peripheral and central lines, phlebotomy, measurement of signs, and even supplemental oxygen are usually discontinued to allow the patient to die peacefully. Relocating the patient to a quiet, private room (as opposed to an intensive care unit) and allowing family members to be present is another critical palliative care modality.

The shift from active, curative treatment to palliative care is sometimes the first tangible sign that the patient will die, a transition that is emotionally difficult for everyone concerned about the patient to accept. The discontinuation of machines and measurements, which, up until this point, have been an integral part of the hospital experience, can be extremely disconcerting to the patient, family members, and even other physicians. Indeed, if these parties are not active in planning this transition, it can easily seem that persons have given up on the patient.

Because of this difficulty, palliative care is sometimes avoided altogether (i.e., curative treatment is continued until the patient dies). This approach is likely to cause problems if it is adopted merely to avoid the reality of impending death. A well-negotiated transition to palliative care often decreases anxiety after the patient and family go through an appropriate anticipatory grief reaction. Furthermore, a positive emotional outcome is much more likely if the physician and staff project a conviction that palliative care will be an active, involved process, without a hint of withdrawal or abandonment. When this does not occur or when the family cannot tolerate the transition, the ensuing stress frequently results in a need for psychiatric consultation.

> A 36-year-old physician with end-stage leukemia was seen in psychiatric consultation because he reported seeing the "angel of death" at the foot of his hospital bed. He described the experience as frightening and inexplicable. The consultant asked the patient, "Are you afraid that you are going to die?" That was the first time anyone had mentioned death or dying in any context to the patient. He welcomed the opportunity to talk openly about his fears to the medical staff and his family and eventually died a peaceful death.

Psychiatric consultation is indicated for patients who become severely anxious, suicidal, depressed, or overtly psychotic. In each instance, appropriate psychiatric medication can be prescribed to provide relief. Patients who are suicidal do not always have to be transferred to a psychiatric service. An attendant or nurse can be assigned to the patient on a 24-hour basis (one-on-one coverage). In such instances, the relationship that develops between the observer and the patient may have therapeutic overtones, especially with patients whose depression is related to a sense of abandonment. Patients who are terminal and who are at high risk for suicide are usually in pain. When pain is relieved, suicidal ideation is likely to diminish. A careful evaluation of suicide potential is required for all patients. A premorbid history of past suicide attempts is a high-risk factor for suicide in terminally ill patients. In patients who become psychotic, impaired cognitive function secondary to metastatic lesions to the brain must always be considered. Such patients respond to antipsychotic medications, and psychotherapy may also be of use.

PAIN MANAGEMENT

Types of Pain

Dying patients are subject to several different kinds of pain, as summarized in Table 29-10. The distinctions are important because they call for different treatment strategies; whereas somatic and visceral pain is responsive to opiates, neuropathic and sympathetically maintained pain may require adjuvant medications in addition to opiates. Most patients with advanced cancer, for example, have more than one kind of pain and require complex treatment regimens.

Treatment of Pain

It cannot be overemphasized that pain management should be aggressive, and treatment should be multimodal. A good pain regimen may require several drugs or the same drug used in different ways and administered via different routes. For example, intravenous morphine can be supplemented by self-administered

Table 29-10
Types of Pain

Nociceptive Pain	
Somatic pain	Usually, but not always constant, aching, gnawing, and well localized (e.g., bone metastases)
Visceral pain	Usually, but not always constant, deep, squeezing, poorly localized, with possible cutaneous referral (e.g., pleural effusion leading to deep chest pain, diaphragmatic irritation referred to the shoulder)
Neuropathic pain	Burning dysesthetic pain with shock-like paroxysms associated with direct damage to peripheral receptors, afferent fibers, or the central nervous system, leading to loss of central inhibitory modulation and spontaneous firing (e.g., phantom limb pain; can involve sympathetic somatic afferents)
Psychogenic pain	Variable characteristics secondary to psychological factors in the absence of medical factors; rare as a pure phenomenon in patients with cancer but often an additional factor in the presence of organic pain

Courtesy of Marguerite S. Lederberg, M.D. and Jimmie C. Holland, M.D.

oral "rescue" doses, or intravenous bolus doses can supplement a continuous epidural drip. Transdermal patches may provide baseline concentrations in patients for whom intravenous or oral intake is difficult. Patient-controlled analgesia systems for intravenous opiate administration result in better pain relief with lower amounts dispensed than in staff-administered dosing.

Opioids commonly cause delirium and hallucinations. A frequent mechanism of psychotoxicity is the accumulation of drugs or metabolites whose durations of analgesia are shorter than their plasma half-lives (morphine, levorphanol, and methadone). The use of drugs such as hydromorphone, which have half-lives closer to their analgesic duration, can relieve the problem without loss of pain control. Cross-tolerance is incomplete between opiates; hence, several should be tried in any patient with the dosage lowered when switching drugs. Table 29-11 lists opioid analgesics.

The benefits of maintenance analgesia administration in terminally ill patients compared with as-needed administration cannot be overemphasized. Maintenance dosing improves pain control, increases drug efficiency, and relieves patient anxiety, but as-needed orders allow pain to increase while waiting for the drug to be given. Moreover, as-needed analgesia administration perversely sets up the patient for staff complaints about drug-seeking behavior. Even when maintenance treatment is used, extra doses of medication should be available for breakthrough pain, and repeated use of these medications should signal the need to raise the maintenance dose. Depending on their previous experiences with opioid analgesics and their weight, it is not unusual for some patients to require 2 g or more of morphine per day for relief of symptoms.

Knowing doses of different drugs and different routes of administration is essential to avoid accidental undermedication. For example, when changing a patient from intramuscular to oral morphine use, the intramuscular dose must be multiplied by 6 to avoid causing the patient pain and provoking drug-seeking behavior. Many adjuvant drugs used for pain are psychotropic with which psychiatrists are familiar, but in some cases, their analgesic effect is separate from their primary psychotropic effect. Commonly used adjuvants include antidepressants, mood stabilizers (e.g., gabapentin) phenothiazines, butyrophenones, antihistamines,

Table 29-11
Opioid Analgesics for Management of Pain

Drug and Equianalgesic Dose Relative Potency	Dose (mg IM or Oral)	Plasma Half-Life (hr)[a]	Starting Oral Dose[b] (mg)	Available Commercial Preparations
Morphine	10 IM 60 oral	3–4	30–60	Oral: tablet, liquid, slow-release tablet Rectal: 5–30 mg Injectable: SC, IM, IV, epidural, intrathecal
Hydromorphone	1.5 IM 7.5 oral	2–3	2–18	Oral: tablets: 1, 2, 4 mg Injectable: SC, IM, IV 2 mg/mL, 3 mg/mL, and 10 mg/mL
Methadone	10 IM 20 oral	12–24	5–10	Oral: tablets, liquid Injectable: SC, IM, IV
Levorphanol	2 IM 4 oral	12–16	2–4	Oral: tablets Injectable: SC, IM, IV
Oxymorphone	1	2–3	NA	Rectal: 10 mg Injectable: SC, IM, IV
Heroin	5 IM 60 oral	3–4	NA	NA
Meperidine	75 IM 300 oral	3–4 (normeperidine 12–16)	75	Oral: tablets Injectable: SC, IM, IV
Codeine	130 oral 200 oral	3–4	60	Oral: tablets in combination with acetylsalicylic acid, acetaminophen, liquid
Oxycodone[c]	15 oral 30 oral	—	5	Oral: tablets, liquid, oral formulation in combination with acetaminophen (tablet and liquid) and aspirin (tablet)

IM, intramuscular; IV, intravenous; NA, not applicable; SC, subcutaneous.
[a]The time of peak analgesia in nontolerant patients ranges from ½ to 1 hour and the duration from 4 to 6 hours. The peak analgesic effect is delayed, and the duration is prolonged after oral administration.
[b]Recommended starting IM doses; the optimal dose for each patient is determined by titration, and the maximal dose is limited by adverse effects.
[c]A long-acting sustained-release form of oxycodone (Oxycontin) has been abused by drug addicts, and its use has been criticized because of this; however, it is a very useful preparation available in 10-, 20-, 40-, and 160-mg doses that need to be taken once every 12 hours. It is used as a maintenance therapy for severe persistent pain.
Adapted from Foley K. Management of cancer pain. In: DeVita VT, Hellman S, Rosenberg SA, eds. *Cancer: Principles and Practice of Oncology.* 4th ed. Philadelphia, PA: JB Lippincott; 1993:936, with permission.

amphetamines, and steroids. They are particularly crucial in neuropathic and sympathetically maintained pain, for which they can be the mainstay of treatment.

Other developments in pain management include more intrusive procedures, such as nerve blocks or the use of continuous epidural infusions. Additionally, radiation therapy, chemotherapy, and even surgical resection can be considered as pain management modalities in palliative care. Short courses of radiotherapy or chemotherapy can be used to shrink tumors or manage metastatic lesions that cause pain or impairment. In patients with end-stage Hodgkin disease, for example, systemic chemotherapy can improve the patient's quality of life by decreasing tumor burden. Surgical resection of invasive tumors, most notably breast carcinomas, can be useful for the same reason.

PALLIATION OF OTHER SYMPTOMS

Symptom management is a high priority in palliative care. Patients are often more concerned about the day-to-day distress of their symptoms than they are about their impending death, which may not be as real to them. Table 29-12 lists common end-of-life symptoms. A comprehensive approach to palliation involves attending to these end-of-life symptoms as well as pain. Sources of distress include psychiatric symptoms, such as anxiety and physical symptoms. Foremost among physical symptoms are those involving the GI system, including diarrhea, constipation, anorexia, nausea, vomiting, and

bowel obstruction. Other significant symptoms include insomnia, confusion, mouth sores, dyspnea, cough, pruritus, decubitus ulcers, and urinary frequency or incontinence. Caretakers should follow these symptoms carefully and establish appropriate early and aggressive care for these symptoms before they become burdensome.

An effective treatment for nausea and vomiting associated with chemotherapy is the use of Δ-tetrahydrocannabinol (THC), the active ingredient of marijuana. The oral synthetic cannabinoid, dronabinol (Marinol), is used in 1- to 2-mg doses every 8 hours. The use of marijuana cigarettes to deliver THC is believed to be more effective than pills. Proponents say that its absorption is faster and antiemetic properties are more potent via the pulmonary system. Repeated attempts to legalize marijuana cigarettes for medical use have met with only limited success in this country.

A 47-year-old man with incurable lung cancer who had been treated unsuccessfully with chemotherapy and radiotherapy had been suffering from intractable dyspnea for 1 week. His family, nursing, and other staff were increasingly upset by his difficulty breathing and his pleas for relief. The attending physician refused to prescribe anything more substantial than codeine. The palliative care team at the hospital intervened at the family's request. Relief was obtained with the use of 5 to 10 mg of an intravenous bolus of morphine every 15 minutes. When the patient became comfortable, a continuous drip of intravenous morphine was instituted, complemented by subcutaneous morphine as needed.

Table 29-12
Common End-of-Life Symptoms/Signs

Symptom/Sign	Comments	Management/Care
Cachexia	All terminal disease states are associated with cachexia secondary to anorexia and dehydration	Feeding tubes useful in some cases; small sips of water of help
Delusions	Common in terminal state	Antipsychotic medication useful
Delirium/Confusion	Occurs in nearly 90% of all terminal patients but is reversible in over 50%	Can be reversed if cause is found and treatable; may respond to antipsychotic and/or pain medication
Depression or anxiety	Psychological factors, e.g., fear of death, abandonment and/or physiologic factors, e.g., pain, hypoxia	Antianxiety and antidepressant medication of use; opioids have strong antianxiety effects
Dysphagia	Seen in neurologic disease, e.g., multiple sclerosis, amyotrophic lateral sclerosis	Attention to oral care, e.g., ice chips, lip balm; adjust to upright position when feeding
Dyspnea or cough	Associated with severe anxiety; fear of suffocation in extreme case; common in lung cancer patients	Opioids, supplemental oxygen, bronchodilators of use
Fatigue	Most common occurrence in terminal illness	Psychostimulants can be used for relief
Incontinence	Associated with radiation induced fistulas	Keep patient clean and dry; use indwelling or condom catheter if necessary
Nausea or vomiting	Side effect of radiation and chemotherapy	Antiemetics, e.g., metoclopramide, prochlorperazine; marijuana of use
Loss of skin integrity	Decubiti most common on weight-bearing areas	Turn body frequently; elbow and hip pads; inflating mattresses
Pain	Pain medications can be administered orally, sublingually, by injection or infusion, or via skin patch	Opioids are the gold standard

Data from National Coalition on Health Care (NCHC) and the Institute for Healthcare Improvement (IHI). Promises to Keep: Changing the Way We Provide Care at the End of Life, release, October 12, 2000.

The AMA supports the position that patients with a terminal condition require substantial doses of opioids regularly and should not be denied drugs for fear of producing physical dependence.

HOSPICE CARE

In 1967, the founding of St. Christopher's Hospice in England by Cicely Saunders launched the modern hospice movement. Several factors in the 1960s propelled the development of hospices, including concerns about inadequately trained physicians, inept terminal care, gross inequities in health care, and neglect of elderly adults. Life expectancy had increased, and heart disease and cancer were becoming more common. Saunders emphasized an interdisciplinary approach to symptom control, care of the patient and family as a unit, the use of volunteers, continuity of care (including home care), and follow-up with family members after a patient's death. The first hospice in the United States, Connecticut Hospice, opened in 1974. By 2000, more than 3,000 hospices were open in the United States. Round-the-clock pain control with opioids is an essential component of hospice management.

In 1983, Medicare began reimbursing hospice care. Medicare hospice guidelines emphasize home care, with benefits provided for a broad spectrum of physician, nursing, psychosocial, and spiritual services at home or, if necessary, in a hospital or nursing home. The patient is eligible for these services if the physician certifies them as having 6 months or less to live. By electing hospice care, patients agree to receive palliative rather than curative treatment. Many hospice programs are hospital-based, sometimes in separate units and sometimes in the form of hospice beds interspersed throughout the facility. Other program models include free-standing hospices and programs, hospital-affiliated hospices, nursing home hospice care, and home care programs.

Nursing homes are the site of death for many elderly patients with incurable chronic illness, yet dying nursing home residents have limited access to palliative and hospice care. Families generally express satisfaction with their involvement in hospice care. Savings with hospice care vary, but home care programs generally cost less than conventional institutional care, particularly in the final months of life. Hospice patients are less likely to receive diagnostic studies or such intensive therapy as surgery or chemotherapy; however, a new trend is to allow treatment programs to continue while the patient remains in the hospice. Hospice care is a proven, viable alternative for patients who elect a palliative approach to terminal care. Also, hospice goals of dignified, comfortable death for terminally ill patients and care for patients and families together have been increasingly adopted in mainstream medicine.

NEONATAL AND INFANT END-OF-LIFE CARE

Advances in reproductive medicine have increased the number of infants born prematurely as well as the number of multiple births. These advances have increased the need for life-sustaining methods of care and have made decisions about when to use palliative care more complicated. Some bioethicists believe that withholding life-sustaining interventions is appropriate under certain circumstances; others maintain that life-sustaining methods should not be used at all. An extensive study of attitudes among neonatologists about end-of-life decisions found no consensus about if and when to terminate life.

For newborns, the decision to forego life-sustaining procedures is usually limited to those children whose death is imminent. Even if their future quality of life is determined to be bleak, most physicians believe that some life is better than no life at all. Physicians who support withholding intensive care consider the following quality-of-life issues: (1) extent of bodily damage (e.g., severe neurologic impairment), (2) the burden that a disabled child will place on the family, and (3) the ability of the child to derive some pleasure from existence (e.g., having an awareness of being alive and being able to form relationships).

The American Academy of Pediatrics permits nontreatment decisions for newborns when the infant is irreversibly comatose or when treatment would be futile and only prolong the process of dying. These standards do not permit the parents to have any input in the decision-making process. In a well-publicized case in England in 2000, doctors decided to surgically separate conjoined twins, even though one would die from the procedure. This procedure occurred despite the objections of the parents, who believed that nature should take its course. Neonatal end-of-life decisions remain in a state of limbo. No clear-cut criteria exist about which patients should receive intensive care and which should receive palliative care.

CHILD END-OF-LIFE CARE

After accidents, cancer is the second most common cause of death in children. Although many childhood cancers are treatable, palliative care is necessary for children with cancers that are not. Children require more support than adults in coping with death. On average, a child does not view death as permanent until the age of about 10 years. Before then, death is viewed as sleep or separation. Therefore, children should be told what they can understand. If they are capable, they should be involved in the decision-making process about treatment plans. Assurances that patients are pain-free and physically comfortable are just as crucial for children as they are for adults.

A unique aspect of end-of-life care in children involves addressing their fear of being separated from their parents. It is helpful to have parents participate in end-of-life care tasks within their capacities. Family sessions with the child in attendance allow feelings to emerge and questions to be answered.

SPIRITUAL ISSUES

There is increasing awareness of the importance of this area to patients, families, and many staff members as well. Several studies have shown that religious beliefs are often associated with mature and active coping methods, and the field of psychological and spiritual interfaces in terminally ill patients is spawning a whole new area of psychological research within the traditional medical establishment. The psychiatric consultant should inquire about faith, its meaning, associated religious practices, and impact on the coping response. It can be a source of strength or guilt at all stages of the disease, ranging from the earliest "What did I do to cause this?" through "Will God give me only what I can carry?" to the poignant life review of the late stage. It is often a primary factor in the reactions to suicidality and attitudes toward terminal care decisions. Mental health professionals should deal with these areas in an unselfconscious and noncondescending manner and work to help patients fully integrate this aspect of their personality into their current crisis. The professional should also work in harmony with the patient's spiritual guide if one is available. Sometimes an experienced chaplain working with the appropriate patient can achieve positive results more directly than any psychotherapy. The following case exemplifies how creative pastoral care can relieve suffering.

A young woman was admitted to Calvary Hospital in a terminal state. She was experiencing a severe depression, which she attributed to not being able to see her oldest daughter receive her first communion. Arrangements were made for a ceremonial communion for her daughter to take place at Calvary Hospital. After the ceremony, the patient's mood improved markedly as one of her fears was alleviated, and a religious need was satisfied. As her mood improved, she was able to address other unresolved issues and had quality visits with her children in her remaining days. (From O'Neil MT. Pastoral care. In: Cimino JE, Brescia MJ, eds. *Calvary Hospital Model for Palliative Care in Advanced Cancer*. Bronx, NY: Palliative Care Institute; 1998, with permission.)

ALTERNATIVE AND COMPLEMENTARY MEDICINE

Many patients, when they are told they are terminally ill, seek alternative treatments, ranging from innocuous programs aimed at enhancing general health to more aggressive, harmful, or fraudulent regimens. Although most patients combine the alternative and the traditional, a substantial number favor complementary medicine as the only treatment for their disease.

Complementary methods to cure terminal illness, especially cancer, emphasize a holistic approach, involving purification of the body, detoxification through internal cleansing, and attention to nutritional and emotional well-being. Despite their widespread appeal, not one of these methods has been demonstrated to cure cancer or prolong life, yet all have strong followings bolstered by anecdotal accounts of their efficacy. The popular metabolic therapy attributes cancer and other potentially fatal illnesses to toxins and waste materials accumulating in the body; treatment is based on reversing this process by diet, vitamins, minerals, enzymes, and colonic irrigations. Another approach includes macrobiotic diets or megavitamins to enhance the body's capacity to destroy malignancy. In 1987, the National Research Council recommended minimizing carcinogenic substances and fat in the diet and increasing whole-grain, fruit, and vegetable consumption as preventive guidelines. Psychological approaches cite maladaptive personality and coping styles as contributors to fatal diseases; treatment consists of shaping a positive attitude. Spiritual approaches aim at achieving harmony between the patient and nature. Some groups use spirituality as a way to ward off illness, which is sometimes seen as an external evil to be exorcised. Immunotherapies have gained popularity in recent years; cancer is attributed to a defective immune system, and restoration of immunocompetency is seen as the cure. Many patients find increased strength to endure the suffering of terminal illness with the help of alternative medicine even though the course of the disease may not be affected. (For a further discussion of alternative medicine, see Chapter 21.)

▲ 29.3 Euthanasia and Physician-Assisted Suicide

EUTHANASIA

From the Greek term for a good death, *euthanasia* means compassionately allowing, hastening, or causing the death of another. Generally, someone resorts to euthanasia to relieve suffering, maintain dignity, and shorten the course of dying when death is inevitable.

Euthanasia can be *voluntary* if the patient has requested it or *involuntary* if the decision is made against the patient's wishes or without the patient's consent. Euthanasia can be *passive*—simply withholding heroic lifesaving measures—or *active*—deliberately taking a person's life. Euthanasia assumes that the physician intends to aid and abet the patient's wish to die.

Arguments for euthanasia revolve around patient autonomy and dignified death. One of the most dramatic ways patients can exercise their right to self-determination is by asking that life-sustaining treatment to be withdrawn. If the patient is mentally competent, physicians must respect such wishes. Proponents of active, voluntary euthanasia argue that the same rights should be extended to patients who are not on life-sustaining treatment but also choose to have their physicians help them die.

Opponents of euthanasia also provide strong ethical and medical justification for their position. First, active euthanasia, even if the patient voluntarily requests it, is a form of killing and should never be sanctioned. Second, many patients who request aid in dying may be suffering from depression, which, when treated, will change the patient's mind about wanting to die.

Most medical, religious, and legal groups in the United States are against euthanasia. Both the American Psychiatric Association (APA) and the AMA condemn active euthanasia as illegal and contrary to medical ethics; however, few individuals have been convicted of euthanasia. Most physicians and medical groups in other parts of the world also oppose legalizing euthanasia. In the United Kingdom, for example, the British Medical Association believes that euthanasia is "alien to the traditional ethos and moral focus of medicine" and, if legalized, "would irrevocably change the context of health care for everyone, but especially for the most vulnerable."

The World Medical Association issued the following declaration on euthanasia in October 2019:

The WMA is firmly opposed to euthanasia and physician-assisted suicide... no physician should be forced to participate in euthanasia or assisted suicide, nor should any physician be obliged to make referral decisions to this end.

Separately, the physician who respects the basic right of the patient to decline medical treatment does not act unethically in forgoing or withholding unwanted care, even if respecting such a wish results in the death of the patient. (*Adopted by the 70th WMA General Assembly, Tbilisi, Georgia, October 2019,* https://www.wma.net/policies-post/declaration-on-euthanasia-and-physician-assisted-suicide/)

Similarly, the New York State Committee on Bioethical Issues issued a statement declaring its opposition to euthanasia. The committee stated that physicians are obligated to relieve pain and suffering for the dying patient, even at the risk of hastening a patient's death. Physicians, however, should not perform active euthanasia or participate in assisted suicide. The Committee believed that support, comfort, respect for patient autonomy, good communication, and adequate pain control would dramatically decrease the demand for euthanasia and assisted suicide. They argued that the societal risks of involving physicians in medical interventions to cause a patient's death were too significant to condone active euthanasia or physician-assisted suicide. In response to shifting public opinion and lobbying groups with different views, state laws that banned physician-assisted death in Washington State and New York were sent to the United States Supreme Court, challenging the constitutionality of these prohibitions. In June 1997, the Court unanimously held that terminally ill patients do not have the right to physician aid in dying. The ruling, however, left room for continuing debate and future policy initiatives at the state level.

PHYSICIAN-ASSISTED SUICIDE

In the United States, most of the debate centers on physician-assisted suicide rather than on euthanasia. Some have argued that physician-assisted suicide is a humane alternative to active euthanasia in that the patient maintains more autonomy, remains the actual agent of death, and may be less likely to be coerced. Others believe that the distinctions are capricious in that the intent in both cases is to bring about a patient's death. Indeed, it may be difficult to justify providing a lethal dose of medication to a terminally ill patient (physician-assisted suicide) while ignoring the desperate pleas of another patient who may be even more ill and distressed but who cannot complete the action because of problems with swallowing, dexterity, or strength.

Several degrees are seen to which a physician may assist the suicidal patient to end his or her life. Physician-assisted suicide can involve providing information on ways of committing suicide, supplying a prescription for a lethal dose of medication or a means of inhaling a lethal amount of carbon monoxide, or perhaps even providing a suicide device that the patient can operate.

The controversy over physician-suicide came to national attention surrounding the activities of retired pathologist Jack Kevorkian, who, in 1989, provided his suicide machine to a 54-year-old woman with probable Alzheimer disease. After the woman killed herself with his device, Kevorkian was charged with first-degree murder. The charges were later dismissed because Michigan had no law against physician-assisted suicide. Since that first case, Kevorkian assisted in several more suicides, often for persons he met on only a few occasions and frequently for persons who did not have a terminal illness. Claiming to have helped more than 130 people take their lives, Kevorkian was sent to prison in 1999, was released in 2006, and died in 2011. His attorneys and followers applauded his courage in easing pain and suffering; his detractors countered that he was a serial mercy killer. Opponents of Kevorkian's methods charged that, without safeguards, consultations, and thorough psychiatric evaluations, patients might search out suicide not because of terminal illness or intractable pain but because of untreated depressive disorders. They argued that suicide rarely occurs in the absence of psychiatric illness. Finding more effective treatments for pain and depression, rather than inventing more sophisticated devices to help desperate patients kill themselves, defines compassionate and effective physician care.

In 1994, Oregon passed a ballot initiative legalizing physician-assisted suicide (Death with Dignity Act), making Oregon the first state in the United States to permit assisted suicides (Table 29-13). An assessment of the first 4 years revealed the following: Patients dying from physician-assisted suicide represent approximately eight of 10,000 deaths. The most common underlying illnesses were cancer, amyotrophic lateral sclerosis, and chronic lower respiratory disease. The three most common end-of-life concerns were loss of autonomy (85 percent), a decreasing ability to participate in activities that made life enjoyable (77 percent), and losing control of bodily functions (63 percent). Eighty percent of the patients were enrolled in hospice programs, and 91 percent died at home. The prescribing physician was present in 52 percent of the cases.

In 2001, Attorney General John Ashcroft attempted to prosecute Oregon doctors who helped terminally ill patients die, claiming that doctor-assisted suicide is not a legitimate medical purpose. The case was brought to the Supreme Court, which in 2006 supported the Oregon law and said the "authority claimed by the attorney general is both beyond his expertise and incongruous with the statutory purposes and design." Since 2001, three other states—Washington

Table 29-13
Oregon's Assisted Suicide Law

The patient must be terminally ill and expected to die within 6 mo; mentally competent; fully informed about his or her diagnosis, prognosis, risks, and alternatives, such as comfort care; and be making a voluntary choice.

A second doctor must agree that the patient is terminally ill, acting on his or her own free will, fully informed, and capable of making health care decisions.

If either doctor thinks that the patient is suffering from any form of mental illness that could affect his or her judgment, they must refer the patient for counseling.

The patient must make one written request and two spoken requests.

The doctor must ask the patient to tell the next of kin, but the patient may decide not to do so.

The patient is free to change his or her mind at any time.

There is a 15-day waiting period between the patient making the request and the doctor writing the prescription.

All information must be written down in the medical records.

Only people who normally live in Oregon may use the Act.

Mercy killing, lethal injection, and active euthanasia are not permitted.

Pharmacists must be told of the prescribed medication's ultimate use.

Physicians, pharmacists, and health care systems are under no obligation to participate in the Death with Dignity Act.

Table 29-14
The AMA's Recommended Approach to Requests of Physician-Assisted Suicide

1. Evaluation of the patient for depression or other psychiatric conditions that could cause disordered thought
2. Evaluation of the patient's "decision-making competence"
3. Discussion with the patient about his or her goals for care
4. Evaluation and response to the patient's "physical, mental, social, and spiritual suffering"
5. Discussion with the patient about the full range of treatment and care options
6. Consultation by the attending physician with other professional colleagues
7. Assurance that care plans chosen by the patient are being followed, including removal of unwanted treatment and the provision of adequate pain and symptom relief
8. Discussion with the patient explaining why physician-assisted suicide is to be avoided and why it is not compatible with the principled nature of the care protocol

(2008), Montana (2009), and Vermont (2011)—have passed laws similar to the one in Oregon.

Despite the abhorrence that many physicians and medical ethicists express regarding physician-assisted suicide, poll after poll shows that as many as two-thirds of Americans favor the legalization of physician-assisted suicide in certain circumstances, and evidence even indicates that the formerly uniform opposition to physician-assisted suicide within the medical community has eroded. Consistent with their positions on active euthanasia, the AMA, APA, and American Bar Association, however, continue to oppose physician-assisted suicide. Recently, the American College of Physicians-American Society of Internal Medicine (ACP-ASIM) expressed its commitment to improving care for patients at the end of life while recommending against the legalization of physician-assisted suicide. The ACP-ASIM believes physician-assisted suicide raises grave ethical concerns, undermines the physician–patient relationship, and the trust necessary to sustain it alters the medical profession's role in society, and endangers the values American society places on life, especially on the lives of disabled, incompetent, and vulnerable individuals.

The American Association of Suicidology in its 1996 *Report of the Committee on Physician-Assisted Suicide and Euthanasia* concluded that involuntary euthanasia could never be condoned; the report also stated, however, that "intolerable, prolonged suffering of persons in extremis should never be insisted upon, against their wishes, in single-minded efforts to preserve life at all cost." This position acknowledges that patients can die as a result of treatment given to them for the explicit purpose of relieving suffering. However, death associated with palliative care differs significantly from physician-assisted suicide in that death is not the goal of treatment and is not intentional.

How to Deal with Requests for Suicide

To help guide clinicians facing requests for physician-assisted suicide, the AMA's Institute for Ethics proposed an eight-step clinical protocol. Table 29-14 lists these steps.

Psychiatrists view suicide as an irrational act that is the product of mental illness, usually depression. In almost every case in which a patient asks to be put to death, a triad exists of depression associated with an incurable medical condition that causes intolerable pain. In these instances, every effort should be made to provide antidepressants or psychostimulants for depression and opioids for pain. Psychotherapy, spiritual counseling, or both may also be needed. Also, family therapy to help with the stress of dealing with a dying patient may be necessary. Family therapy is also useful because some patients may ask to be put to death because they do not wish to be a burden to their families; others may feel coerced by their families into believing that they are, or will be, a burden and may choose death as a result. Currently, no professional codes countenance euthanasia or assisted suicide in the United States. Therefore, psychiatrists must stand on the side of responsible rescue and treatment.

A distinction also is needed between major depression and suffering. Psychiatrists have not sufficiently studied the nature of suffering. It remains the province of theologians and philosophers. Suffering is a complex mix of spiritual, emotional, and physical factors that transcends pain and other symptoms of a terminal illness. Physicians are more skilled at dealing with depression than with suffering. Anatole Broyard, who chronicled his death in his book *Intoxicated by My Illness,* wrote the following:

> I see no reason or need for my doctor to love me nor would I expect him to suffer with me. I wouldn't demand a lot of my doctor's time; I just wish he would brood on my situation for perhaps 5 minutes, that he would give me his whole mind just once, be bonded with me for a brief space, survey my soul as well as my flesh, to get at my illness, for each man is ill in his own way.

FUTURE DIRECTIONS

Advances in technology bring more complex medical, legal, moral, and ethical controversies regarding life, death, euthanasia, and physician-assisted suicide. Some forms of euthanasia have found a place in modern medicine, and expansion of the boundaries of patients' rights and their ability to choose the way they live and die is inevitable. Both patients and physicians need to be better educated about depression, pain management, palliative care, and quality of life. Medical schools and residency training programs need to give the topics of death, dying, and palliative care the attention they deserve. Society must ensure that economics, ageism, and racism do not get in the way of adequate and humane management of patients with chronic terminal illnesses. Finally, a national health care policy must provide adequate insurance coverage, home care, and hospice services to all appropriate patients. If these mandates are followed, the argument for physician assistance in dying will lose much of its impact.

References

Bachman B. The development of a sustainable, community-supported children's bereavement camp. *Omega (Westport)*. 2013;67:21–35.

Bolton JM, Au W, Walld R, Chateau D, Martens PJ, Leslie WD, Enns MW, Sareen J. Parental bereavement after the death of an offspring in a motor vehicle collision: A population-based study. *Am J Epidemiol*. 2014;179(2):177–185.

Broeckaert B. Palliative sedation, physician-assisted suicide, and euthanasia: "Same, same but different"? *Am J Bioethics*. 2011;11:62–64.

Canetto SS. Physician-assisted suicide in the United States: Issues, challenges, roles and implications for clinicians. In: Qualls SH, Kasl-Godley JE, eds. *End-of-Life Issues, Grief, and Bereavement: What Clinicians Need to Know*. Hoboken, NJ: John Wiley & Sons; 2011:263.

Carvalho TB, Rady MY, Verheijde JL, Robert JS. Continuous deep sedation in end-of-life care: Disentangling palliation from physician-assisted death. *Am J Bioethics*. 2011;11:60–62.

Corr CA, Corr DM. *Death & Dying, Life & Living*. 7th ed. Belmont, CA: Wadsworth; 2013.

Deschepper R, Distelmans W, Bilsen J. Requests for euthanasia/physician-assisted suicide on the basis of mental suffering: Vulnerable patients or vulnerable physicians? *JAMA Psychiatry*. 2014;71(6):617–618.

Fahy BN. Palliative care in the acute care surgery setting. In: Moore LJ, Turner KL, Todd SR, eds. *Common Problems in Acute Care Surgery*. New York: Springer; 2013:477.

Gamliel E. To end life or not to prolong life: The effect of message framing on attitudes towards euthanasia. *J Health Psychol*. 2013;18:693.

Hui D, Elsayem A, De la Cruz M, Berger A, Zhukovsky DS, Palla S, Evans A, Fadul N, Palmer JL, Bruera E. Availability and integration of palliative care at US cancer centers. *JAMA*. 2010;303(11):1054–1061.

Jaiswal R, Alici Y, Breitbart W. A comprehensive review of palliative care in patients with cancer. *Int Rev Psychiatry*. 2014;26(1):87–101.

Kaplow JB, Saunders J, Angold A, Costello EJ. Psychiatric symptoms in bereaved versus nonbereaved youth and young adults: A longitudinal epidemiological study. *J Am Acad Child Adol Psych*. 2010;49:1145–1154.

Kaspers PJ, Pasman H, Onwuteaka-Philipsen BD, Deeg DJ. Changes over a decade in end-of-life care and transfers during the last 3 months of life: A repeated survey among proxies of deceased older people. *Palliat Med*. 2013;27:544–552.

Kelley AS, Meier DE. Palliative care–a shifting paradigm. *N Eng J Med*. 2010;363:781–782.

Kimsma GK. *Physician-Assisted Death in Perspective*. New York: Cambridge University Press; 2012.

King M, Vasanthan M, Petersen I, Jones L, Marston L, Nazareth I. Mortality and medical care after bereavement: A general practice cohort study. *PLoS One*. 2013;8:e52561.

Kraemer F. Ontology or phenomenology? How the LVAD challenges the euthanasia debate. *Bioethics*. 2013;27:140–150.

Lederberg MS. End-of-life and palliative care. In: Sadock BJ, Sadock VA, Ruiz P, eds. *Kaplan & Sadock's Comprehensive Textbook of Psychiatry*. 9th ed. Philadelphia, PA: Lippincott, Williams & Wilkins; 2009:2353.

Lerning MR, Dickinson GE. *Understanding Death, Dying and Bereavement*. 7th ed. Stamford, CT: Cengage Learning; 2010.

Lichtenthal WG, Neimeyer RA, Currier JM, Roberts K, Jordan N. Cause of death and the quest for meaning after the loss of a child. *Death Stud*. 2013;37:311–342.

Maple M, Edwards HE, Minichiello V, Plummer D. Still part of the family: The importance of physical, emotional, and spiritual memorial places and spaces for parents bereaved through the suicide death of their son or daughter. *Mortality*. 2013;18:54.

Matzo M, Sherman MW, eds. *Palliative Care Nursing: Quality Care to End of Life*. 3rd ed. New York: Springer Publishing Company; 2013.

Meier DE, Issacs SL, Hughes RG, eds. *Palliative Care: Transforming the Care of Serious Illness*. San Francisco, CA: Jossey-Bass; 2010.

Moore RJ, ed. *Handbook of Pain and Palliative Care*. New York: Springer; 2013

Neimeyer RA, ed. *Techniques of Grief Therapy: Creative Practices for Counseling the Bereaved*. New York: Routledge; 2012.

Nuckols TK, Anderson L, Popescu I, Diamant AL, Doyle B, Capua PD, Chou R. Opioid prescribing: A systematic review and critical appraisal of guidelines for chronic pain. *Ann Intern Med*. 2014;160(1):38–47.

Penman J, Oliver M, Harrington A. The relational model of spiritual engagement depicted by palliative care clients and caregivers. *Int J Nursing Pract*. 2013;19:39–46.

Perper JA, Cina SJ. *When Doctors Kill: Who, Why and How*. New York: Springer; 2010:159.

Qualls SH, Kasl-Godley JE, eds. *End-of-Life Issues, Grief, and Bereavement: What Clinicians Need to Know*. Hoboken, NJ: John Wiley & Sons; 2011.

Rady MY, Verheijde JL. Continuous deep sedation until death: Palliation or physician-assisted death? *Am J Hosp Palliat Med*. 2010;27:205–214.

Raus K, Sterckx S, Mortier F. Is continuous sedation at the end of life an ethically preferable alternative to physician-assisted suicide? *Am J Bioeth*. 2011;11:32–40.

Risse GB, Balboni MJ. Shifting hospital-hospice boundaries: Historical perspectives on the institutional care of the dying. *Am J Hosp Palliat Med*. 2013;19:325–330.

Rys S, Deschepper R, Mortier F, Deliens L, Atkinson D, Bilsen J. The moral difference or equivalence between continuous sedation until death and physician-assisted death: Word games or war games? *J Bioeth Inq*. 2012;9:171–183.

Saaty TL, Vargas LG. *Models, Methods, Concepts & Applications of the Analytic Hierarchy Process*. New York: Springer; 2012:249.

Schachter SR, Holland JC. Loss, grief, and bereavement: Implications for family caregivers and health care professionals of the mentally ill. In: Talley RC, Fricchione GL, Druss BG, eds. *The Challenges of Mental Health Caregiving*. New York: Springer; 2014:145.

Servaty-Seib HL, Taub DJ. Bereavement and college students: The role of counseling psychology. *Counseling Psychol*. 2010;38:947.

Smith TJ, Temin S, Alesi ER, Abernethy AP, Balboni TA, Basch EM, Ferrell BR, Loscalzo M, Meier DE, Paice JA, Peppercorn JM, Somerfield M, Stovall E, Von Roenn JH. American Society of Clinical Oncology provisional clinical opinion: The integration of palliative care into standard oncology care. *J Clin Oncol*. 2012;30:880–887.

Stroebe M, Schut H, van den Bout J, eds. *Complicated Grief: Scientific Foundations for Health Care Professionals*. New York: Routledge; 2013.

Temel JS, Greer JA, Muzikansky A, Gallagher ER, Admane S, Jackson VA, Dahlin CM, Blinderman CD, Jacobsen J, Pirl WF, Billings JA, Lynch TJ. Early palliative care for patients with metastatic non-small-cell lung cancer. *N Eng J Med*. 2010;363:733–742.

Vadivelu N, Kaye AD, Berger JM, eds. *Essentials of Palliative Care*. New York: Springer; 2013.

Westefeld JS, Casper D, Lewis AM. Physician-assisted death and its relationship to the human service professions. *J Loss Trauma*. 2013;18:539–555.

Zisook S, Shear MK, Irwin SA. Death, dying, and bereavement. In: Sadock BJ, Sadock VA, Ruiz P, eds. *Kaplan & Sadock's Comprehensive Textbook of Psychiatry*. 9th ed. Philadelphia, PA: Lippincott Williams & Wilkins; 2009:2378.

INTRODUCTION

The subject area of public psychiatry embodies a fundamental core of experience and tradition. In the context of the reexamination of American health care initiated by the effect of managed care and the health care reform, the experience of public psychiatry is poised to serve as the foundation for a transformation of behavioral health care.

The term *public* can refer to psychiatric programs, treatments, or institutions paid for by public funds or as objects of public policy, whether paid for or not. The traditional concept of public psychiatry has been expanded to include medical and psychosocial initiatives directed for the public good, whether funded by public or private funds and directed in particular to those who are economically disadvantaged.

The care and treatment offered under public psychiatry are delivered in a variegated mosaic of inpatient and community-based services that are more or less integrated into a coherent network sponsored by public agencies. Funding for public psychiatric services tends to be provided by federally legislated appropriations that are passed through the state, county, and municipal government agencies (such as departments of mental health; substance use treatment services; children, youth, and family services; and public health, social services, education, adult corrections, and juvenile justice agencies). Ultimately, most public psychiatry and community services are provided by not-for-profit community mental health, substance use treatment, child guidance, or health care organizations that are either funded by or subcontracted to government agencies. Thus, the very existence of public and community psychiatric services and the policies and resources determining how they are delivered are dependent on legislative mandates and fiscal appropriations from all levels of public government.

CONTEMPORARY PUBLIC AND COMMUNITY PSYCHIATRY

There are five themes around which the discussion of contemporary public and community psychiatry is structured: public health, public agencies, evidence-based psychiatry, roles for psychiatrists, and delivery systems.

Public Health

Public health is not merely publicly funded health care but is instead a specific discipline and tradition. It is a complicated field that historically has been defined negatively by the dominance of *personal health,* that is, the health care delivery systems that take care of individual patients. Until the advent of managed care in the 1990s, U.S. health care was an industry mainly organized in terms of individual doctor-entrepreneurs. Each jurisdiction uniquely defined and organized its public health programs, and the particular pattern of personal health practices had a substantial influence—hence

the wide variation in public health programs. Nonetheless, as a discipline and tradition, public health's mission is to assure the conditions in which people can be healthy. Public health consists of organized community efforts aimed at the prevention of disease and the promotion of health. It involves many disciplines but rests on the scientific core of epidemiology. It provides an essential template for contemporary public and community psychiatry.

The Surgeon General's report on mental health underscored the necessity of a public health approach to care and rehabilitation for people experiencing mental illness that is "broader in focus than medical models that concentrate on diagnosis and treatment." Although diagnosis and treatment are core areas of expertise for all psychiatrists, the Surgeon General recommended that even when psychiatric diagnosis or treatment is the primary focus for practitioners, researchers, or educators, they should ground their professional activities in a vision and knowledge base that is "*population-based...* encompass[ing] a focus on epidemiologic surveillance, health promotion, disease prevention, and access to services." These fundamental public health functions define the public health perspective in public and community psychiatry. In the discussion that follows, these four public health components are framed in current terms of health care reform to define a coherent "public health" strategy for public and community psychiatry.

Health Promotion

Psychiatric professionals can contribute substantially to the promotion of public health by working with primary health care professionals and educators to identify and provide front-line treatment and referrals to adults and children who have undetected psychiatric symptoms, subthreshold syndromes, and psychiatric disorders. Collaborative care models bring psychiatric professionals into primary care and school settings as consultants for medical, nursing, and education professionals. These professionals work in those settings, as well as for educators and direct treatment providers to at-risk or psychiatrically impaired individuals.

Furthermore, people with identified mental illness or addictive disorders can benefit from enhanced physical and mental health care, as well as from the alleviation or management of psychiatric symptoms. Achieving or regaining physical or mental health (i.e., recovery) depends not only on genetic and biologic factors but also on a person's or family's access to social and psychological resources and integration into supportive social networks. Illness management (also known as *disease management* or *chronic illness care management*) is a framework that has been adapted from medicine to guide mental health professionals in delivering services that go beyond traditional diagnostic treatment to promote the health and recovery of people with mental illness or addiction. *Illness management* has been defined as "professional-based interventions designed to help people collaborate with professionals in the treatment of their mental illness, reduce their susceptibility to relapses, and cope more effectively with their symptoms... [to] improve self-efficacy and self-esteem and to foster skills that help people pursue their personal goals." Several approaches to illness management have been scientifically and clinically evaluated and have been found to enhance standard psychiatric treatment.

Prevention.   Psychiatric disorders most often follow a course over time that begins with an often lengthy period in which prodromal or subthreshold symptoms or functional problems precede the full onset of a disorder with marked impairment. Intervention with adults, adolescents, or children who are not clinically impaired but who are at high risk or who are manifesting preclinical symptoms or functional problems is an approach to prevention that is cost-effective because it targets a relatively small group of individuals promptly. Examples of high-risk patients include those with a family history of psychiatric or addictive disorders or exposure to extreme stressors, such as violence, neglect, or antisocial behavior. Also, prodromal symptoms and behaviors that would argue for early intervention include periodic or pervasive dysphoria, problems with separation from caregivers, or involvement with deviant peers.

Application of the traditional public health concepts of *primary, secondary,* and *tertiary psychiatry* has been confusing in psychiatry. *Primary prevention* involves addressing the root causes of illness with healthy individuals, to prevent illness before it occurs. *Secondary prevention* involves the early identification and early treatment of individuals with acute or subclinical disorders or *high-risk* persons to reduce morbidity. *Tertiary prevention* attempts to reduce the effects of a disorder on an individual through rehabilitation and chronic illness care management. The Institute of Medicine, to help clarify different aspects of prevention, developed a classification system with three different categories. *Universal* interventions are those intended for the general public, such as immunizations or media campaigns, providing information about illnesses, early warning signs, and resources for health promotion and timely treatment. *Selective* interventions focus on individuals at higher-than-average risk (e.g., persons with prodromal symptoms or a family history of psychiatric disorders) to reduce morbidity by enhancing resilience and preventing the onset of illness. *Indicated interventions* target individuals who are experiencing impairment as a result of illness as early as possible in the course of the illness, to reduce the burden of the illness on the individual, family, community, and treatment system. Psychiatric services most often take the form of indicated interventions, but the smaller number of psychiatric practitioners and researchers who conduct and evaluate selective or universal interventions in public and community settings is making a substantial contribution to the broader health of society.

Prevention interventions are effective with adults with a variety of risk factors or preclinical problems. For example, women who have been raped are less likely to develop posttraumatic stress disorder (PTSD) if they receive a five-session cognitive-behavioral treatment than if their recovery is left to chance. People with subthreshold symptoms of depression who are identified early by their primary care providers are less likely to develop the full syndrome if their medical treatment includes education about depression and learning skills for coping actively with depressive symptoms or stressors. Prevention with adults must be judiciously designed to address the specific factors that place a person at risk for illness or that enhance the person's ability to cope effectively. For example, brief supportive meetings with people who have experienced a traumatic stressor

(e.g., a mass disaster or life-threatening accident) tend to have little benefit and may inadvertently intensify posttraumatic stress. In contrast, a focused cognitive-behavioral approach to teaching skills for coping with traumatic memories and stress symptoms is effective in preventing posttraumatic stress and depressive disorders with adult and child disaster or accident survivors.

Several prevention programs have been developed and evaluated to address physical and mental health risks in childhood and adolescence, incorporating several elements that influence intervention effectiveness. Their broad and systematic implementation, however, has been halting. Some states have made an effort to implement *school-based* interventions involving teachers and the peer group. These tend to be more effective than programs exclusively relying on intervening with parents or children alone. Such interventions in middle childhood have been successful in influencing peer group norms regarding alcohol and substance use, violence and bullying, and depression, thus achieving the dual outcome of reducing immediate initiation of alcohol and substance use and increasing the long-term support within the peer group for sustained abstinence into adolescence. Thus, systems-based *multimodal* interventions simultaneously targeting and developing enhanced relationships among the child, peer group, school personnel, parents, and the wider community tend to be most effective as universal or selected approaches to early prevention of what otherwise may become lifelong behavioral, legal, academic, and addictive problems.

Access to Effective Mental Health Care.   Access is a significant problem for most people with severe mental illness or addictions. In the United States, the National Comorbidity Survey (NCS) and the National Comorbidity Survey-Replication (NCS-R) found that fewer than 40 percent of people with severe psychiatric disorders had received any mental health treatment in the previous year, and fewer than one in six (15 percent) had received minimally adequate mental health services. Young adults, African Americans, people residing in specific geographical areas, people with psychotic disorders, and patients treated by medical but not mental health providers were at the highest risk for inadequate psychiatric treatment. Although income was not a predictor of inadequate treatment, many of the people who did not receive adequate mental health services were likely to be uninsured or underinsured. Such people often cannot access mental health care other than through a primary care provider or clinic or in the public mental health system.

Even when mental illness is identified, people with socioeconomic adversities often do not, or cannot, get adequate mental health services in their communities. For example, although it is estimated that more than 200,000 incarcerated adults in the United States have psychiatric disorders, few were detected or received treatment until they reached jail or prison. Federal and state correctional systems have instituted mental health screening and treatment programs to address psychiatric disorders as a health problem for incarcerated adults and to manage the problematic behavior that can occur in controlled settings as a result of mental illness. On returning to the community, the vast majority of prisoners with psychiatric disorders cease to receive more than minimal mental health services: A recent study found that fewer than one in six (16 percent—strikingly similar to the NCS finding) received steady mental health services, and only one in 20 with addictions received steady substance abuse recovery services. Thus, access to mental health and addiction treatment services is far better *in prison* than in the community! This disparity has caused great concern because of the possibility that correctional facilities may be a de facto system of care for low-income people (often of minority backgrounds) with serious mental illness.

Evidence of severe and pervasive barriers to accessing mental health care can be found in several social crises. Impoverished children and adults increasingly are deferring physical and mental health care until illnesses become chronic and severe and then often do not know or cannot gain entry into any setting for services except public hospital emergency departments. Children with severe psychiatric or behavioral disorders are being held in emergency department facilities for days and even weeks because the staff cannot locate any available treatment facilities with an appropriate level of care, especially if they are underinsured. People who cannot afford private services thus face daunting obstacles when seeking appropriate mental health care as a result of a severe underfunding of practitioners and programs. The public policy dilemmas that are driven by the ever-increasing cost of health care bear directly on the field of public psychiatry. It also tragically affects the lives of tens or hundreds of thousands of people who do not receive adequate care.

Psychiatry and Public Agencies

Psychiatry's relationship to public sector agencies has, with some specific exceptions, been one of detachment because of the dominance of the private practice models before the advent of managed care and also mainly because of the nature and structure of U.S. social welfare programs. This separation is a divide that often begins during academic preparation, in that many psychiatry training programs eschew meaningful rotations in public sector settings. In contrast to most industrial nations in which comprehensive social welfare reforms have been initiated, U.S. social welfare programs grew incrementally and categorically, that is, one category of service at a time. Large-scale initiatives, such as President Johnson's War on Poverty, have been implemented in piecemeal fashion by fragmented federal, state, and local government bureaucracies and have been vastly reduced through subsequent initiatives, such as the recent changes in federal regulations to "end welfare as we know it." Various social service agencies have been created through a process, and set of alliances called the *iron triangle*. Advocates form an organization to champion a particular cause. Example causes may include blindness, developmental disabilities, primary care, or mental health, among others. The advocates then find key legislative sponsors to advance the cause through legislation and appropriation. This creates a bureaucracy and bureaucrats that join the alliance. Through successive legislative sessions, the alliance of advocates, lawmakers, and bureaucrats builds a more durable and more reliable categorical agency, for example, adults and families with dependent children or people with biologically based severe mental illness. From the 1930s through the end of the twentieth century, U.S. social welfare agencies were created on this pattern; the system has resulted in generous funding but a hopeless fragmentation of services at local service delivery levels in which each agency depends on separate funding silos that also deliver conflicting rules and regulations.

It has been said that "mental health is not a place." Psychiatrists have a role at the receiving end of every categorical silo, as the clients in each agency experience mental illness. Services for children with severe emotional, mental, or behavioral disturbances are a dramatic case. Five categorical agencies—child welfare, education, primary health, substance abuse, and juvenile justice—all have a responsibility to care for these children (and, indirectly, for their caregivers, including parents and families). Especially for the children with the most severe disabilities, the protective service worker taking a child into court, the special education teacher working day to day with the child, the juvenile probation officer, the substance abuse counselor, and the child's pediatrician all need the consultation and support of a skilled psychiatrist. The situation is similar for adults with severe mental illness, for whom case managers, vocational rehabilitation counselors, basic needs benefits specialists, social workers, psychotherapists, substance abuse counselors, parole or probation officers, legal conservators, visiting nurses, peer specialists, and physicians all may be mandated to deliver services.

Workforce Influences on Contemporary Practice

Shortages in the ranks of psychiatry have been well documented historically, and some project this to continue. However, as the field of psychiatry connects with its science and evidence base (e.g., neuroscience, genetics, pharmacology, outcomes science) while retaining its strength in the meaningful connection with patients and their families, some would argue that the reversal of the shortage trend has begun. The National Institutes of Health (NIH) sponsored Decade of the Brain (the 1990s), and Decade of the Mind (the 2000s) contributed to this change. Medical students are increasingly stimulated to enter the field by recognizing the importance of psychiatry to health care in general, realizing that this is still a field in which the practitioner (and by extension, the interdisciplinary team) is an instrument of change through integration of contemporary knowledge, skillful learned interactions with patients, and a willingness to commit to providing value. The national aggregate numbers, however, cannot adequately capture the extreme variations that exist geographically; rural and frontier sites are dramatically more likely to experience shortages than more urban environments.

Because subsets of the public sector populations have special needs, responses to their needs have to be correspondingly tailored:

▶ Children and family needs are expressed differently than those for adults and require different responses.
▶ Mental illnesses have culturally driven ways of presenting, and interventions must be culturally competent.
▶ Issues of language (including American Sign Language with deaf and hard of hearing individuals) can complicate diagnosis and treatment.
▶ The rapidly expanding elderly population will pose significant new challenges for effective treatment.

Just these few examples suggest the sophistication with which education and training must be engineered to meet the existing and changing demands of people in need of services.

Contemporary Evidence Base for Effective Public and Community Psychiatry

Since the 1980s, several structured interventions have been developed to address the gap between what historically has been taught in most psychiatry training programs—typically, an office-, clinic-, or hospital-based approach focusing on diagnoses and pharmacotherapy supplemented by psychotherapy—and the competencies required to deliver or to support the delivery of the full array of psychiatric rehabilitation services. Public and community approaches to psychiatric rehabilitation involve not only pharmacotherapy but also an array of complementary services. These services must be coordinated to assist people with severe mental illness or behavioral disorders. The services much also help patient's families and support systems. Patient's and their loved ones need help with managing symptoms, accessing resources, and using these resources effectively. The goal of this support is to help patients gain the highest degree of autonomy in the least restrictive setting possible. The competencies required to effect these interventions go beyond the scope of psychiatry, thus requiring that psychiatrists effectively collaborate with other rehabilitation and mental health specialists. Although psychiatrists rarely implement the educational psychotherapy and other interventions involved, psychiatrists should be aware of them and understand how to reinforce them. Hence, familiarity with the manuals that describe how to implement these interventions with fidelity is strongly advised—and increasingly incorporated into psychiatry training.

Evidence-Based Manualized Interventions for Child Psychiatric Rehabilitation. Children with severe emotional disturbances and adolescents with severe behavioral disorders traditionally have been removed from their families and placed in restrictive psychiatric or juvenile justice settings (e.g., psychiatric inpatient wards, residential group homes, and juvenile detention centers). These placements separate the child from the natural family, school, peer group, and community environments, which may provide some benefit by reducing the child's exposure to addiction, conflict, violence, or deviant behavior. However, the placements also deprive the child and family of the opportunity to build better relationships with one another and with other children, families, teachers, and community groups. The second key ingredient to effective public and community child psychiatry comprises interventions that complement pharmacotherapy. Since the 1970s, several rehabilitative approaches for children with severe disorders (and their families) have been developed, tested, and disseminated in replicable manuals and training programs.

Implementation of evidence-based practices is not always easy. It rarely occurs even in clinics and practice groups that are well trained and motivated to use evidence-based treatment models, given that most current systems of payment and service delivery were not designed to accommodate or support the use of science-based interventions such as those highlighted here. Also, evidence-based dissemination and implementation strategies must be deliberately designed to support the initial adoption and sustained use of evidence-based mental health treatment models. For example, a recent study of the implementation of one of the most widely disseminated evidence-based mental health interventions for children and families, multisystemic therapy (MST), demonstrated that initial training yielded a very positive early rate of adoption of the program with reasonable fidelity to the model. However, only teams that were provided with regular ongoing supervision and support (for supervisors as well as therapists) from expert consultants were able to sustain the initial successes.

Roles of Psychiatrists in Public and Community Psychiatry Multidisciplinary Teams

Psychiatrists in the public sector rarely work in isolation. Most often, psychiatrists work within a team of professionals. The team includes many disciplines, including psychology, social work, nursing, occupational therapy, rehabilitation or addiction counseling, social services, housing, and employment specialists. It also includes nondegreed direct care workers, such as bachelor's degree-level counselors or case managers, high school graduate indigenous outreach workers, peer-support specialists, and family advocates. Each of these members brings unique skills and experience to address the needs of people with severe and persistent mental illnesses. The team, rather than any single provider, assumes responsibility for the ongoing care of each patient across the many levels of services and often for many years. Its success is based on effective communication. Every communication should be explicitly focused on the *client's* (i.e., patient and family) *stated goals,* as

well as on the team's technical and logistical issues, to maximize the client's motivation to participate actively and productively in all services by ensuring that the services indeed are patient-centered and collaborative.

Psychiatrists play three primary roles in multidisciplinary psychiatric rehabilitation teams: Conducting psychiatric evaluations, providing pharmacotherapy, and serving as the team's medical director (and, at times, as the administrative supervisor or team leader).

Psychiatric Evaluation and Diagnosis. As with any practice setting, the sine qua non in the public and community setting is a thorough evaluation. This involves a complete history and examination leading to an accurate diagnosis. The goal of evaluation and diagnosis is to develop the most clinically useful individualized approach to treatment and rehabilitation for each patient. Psychiatric evaluations in public and community settings must include a careful review of the individual's psychosocial strengths and resources. The focus on strengths and resources often is lost or obscured when systemic factors (e.g., eligibility regulations for government funded services or benefits) emphasize disability. It can also limit the individual's or family's access to services or benefits (e.g., welfare-to-work regulations that place a time or other eligibility restrictions on types of temporary aid, such as food stamps or vouchers for household supplies or housing).

Pharmacotherapy. The psychiatrist's most visible role usually is providing pharmacotherapy. The most difficult challenge in public sector mental health settings often is not the technical formulation of an effective medication regimen but instead the arranging of a plan of care so that the patient reliably follows the prescribed regimen (i.e., *adherence* or *compliance*). A recent review of interventions designed to enhance adherence to psychotropic medication regimens by patients with schizophrenia found that education alone often was the only strategy used. This is true despite evidence showing that the optimal strategy includes such approaches as concrete problem solving, motivational techniques, and practical assistant (reminders or cues for example). Although the psychiatrist must address technical, medical issues around diagnosis and treatment, effective pharmacotherapy largely depends on providing practical assistance. This approach includes helping patients manage the stresses and problems that might affect adherence. Such practical assistance might be direct, as in encounters with patients, or indirect, by working closely with nonpsychiatric mental health professionals and nondegreed care workers.

Team Leadership. The psychiatrist also often plays a leadership role as the project or program medical director—with the attendant responsibilities of monitoring the medical safety and well-being of all patients and establishing or supporting management and clinical procedures that support the quality of care and a cohesive treatment team. As the team leader or only as a team member, the psychiatrist serves as a role model for compassionate and professional behavior in relation not only to patients but also to all other team members. Formal or informal leadership is especially important when psychiatry residents and medical students work on a team as a training experience. The team psychiatrist serves not only as a mentor and a role model for the core aspects of psychiatric practice but also to demonstrate the values and skills necessary to integrate psychiatry within the framework of multimodal community-based longitudinal psychosocial interventions.

Psychiatrists who work in these settings and desire a leadership role must go beyond their prescription pads to acquire more expertise. This expertise requires gaining the knowledge, attitudes, and skills relevant to the contemporary practice guidelines for psychiatric rehabilitation. It also includes respecting and supporting other team members and earning their respect and support in return. Also, the psychiatrist must cope with large caseloads, and collaborate with agencies and programs to ensure continuity, consistency, and coordination of care. If psychiatrists can incorporate these attitudes and skills, they can expect reciprocity and cohesion from other team members, and clients will benefit. Surveys of psychiatrists in the public sector indicate that those who embrace the rehabilitation perspective by expanding their roles to be consultants and teachers for patients, families, trainees, and colleagues from other mental health disciplines are more satisfied professionally than those who focus on diagnosis and treatment alone.

New Paradigms.   Virtually all health care should be integrated and coordinated to deliver practical, rational, and cost-efficient care. The broader, contemporary definition of care must include public health. Linking public health models with acute care management, which, in turn, is coupled with chronic illness care management, rehabilitation, or recovery models, represents the continuum for an integrated system.

However, this continuum is insufficient without four other components: (1) the application of new research to improve care and the application of bench-to-bedside models to translational research, (2) meaningful involvement of patients and families in a shared decision-making paradigm, (3) integration with primary and specialty care systems, and (4) the development of the clinical system as a system of advocacy. Training preprofessionals in such a model is one approach to introduce meaningful and sustained change to health care and its delivery and is already operational in some systems.

New Models for Service Delivery and Treatment

Organized Systems of Care.   The focus of reform has moved increasingly to coherent, efficient, and accountable delivery systems. The basic idea of the *system of care* for children with severe emotional disturbances can be described in two ways—in terms of interagency structures and clinical processes. Five categorical agencies in a given community form a *strong consortium* that targets a specific population of children (and their families) to whose needs none of the agencies can adequately respond on their own. The consortium agencies commit themselves to treat the child and family with a *common plan of care* and to find ways to pool their resources to do so appropriately. This care often requires that in the central bureaucracies at the state level, a parallel interagency commitment be in place that supports the local system of care initiative, resolves any regulatory conflicts that may arise, and gives permission to innovative aspects of the delivery system. The collaborative interagency structure provides the resources and flexibility for effective clinical work.

From the viewpoint of *clinical processes,* the system of care provides a full enactment of the traditional clinical practice that meets the requirements of medical quality assurance. What is different is that it is carried out in-home and community settings, and it involves participants from different disciplines—child welfare, special education, and juvenile justice—in one standardized treatment methodology. The center of the system of care is the *child and family team* that is made up of the child and family, clinicians and agency representatives involved in the case, and significant supportive individuals identified by the child and family. Current

issues are reviewed—strengths, problems, and needs—diagnostic issues are considered, clinical goals are articulated, and appropriate treatment strategies are identified. The expected outcome of each intervention is specified, and progress toward it is systematically charted. The system of care requires a full array of flexible services. The essential *starters* include clinical diagnostic services, care coordination or case management, crisis intervention services, and a flexible essential supportive service—child care specialists who can be assigned to support the child and family in any situation. Particularly effective systems of care have relied on substantial community organization and collaboration or innovative funding models, or both, that blend or braid funding streams to focus on clear assignment of responsibility for a particular child and family, as well as adequate resources.

The basic model for community support for adults was called *assertive community treatment* (ACT). ACT was implemented with multidisciplinary teams with psychiatrists, nurses, psychologists, social workers, psychiatric aides, and paraprofessionals. The ACT team would assume the care of a designated number of adult patients with severe and persistent mental illness and would be available around the clock, 7 days a week. The team would help find housing, manage money, organize household routines, find social contacts, find work, and support the individual's adjustment to workplace settings. Concurrently, medications would be managed and help provided to facilitate an individual adjusting to community living. At the heart of the program was the necessary clinical process that developed and maintained an individualized treatment plan, which was adjusted continuously to the changing needs of each client. The ACT model has been modified in various ways as it has been implemented in different states. Innovative funding models have been developed in several states by using bundled rates and case rates, which make it easier to implement and to sustain than traditional fee-for-service payment systems.

In contemporary managed care terms, ACT teams are *disease and disability management models* that assign accountability to provide systems that may not assume risk in managing community support of persons with disabling conditions. The National Alliance on Mental Illness (NAMI) has developed program models and protocols for the Program for Assertive Community Treatment (PACT) to encourage public agencies to contract for ACT services.

Effective Treatment Models.   The previous discussions have outlined the various treatment models that have been introduced since the 1980s to establish an evidence base for the effectiveness of specific interventions and approaches to care. The attention to *evidence-based* treatment models has been a response to the call for quality and accountability for service outcomes demanded from health care services in general by purchasers and policymakers and part of an effort to cope with the difficulties of evaluating service delivery models or systems of care.

The movement to evidence-based services is necessary to break down components of the service delivery system to determine the relative effectiveness of specific service interventions using the evaluative tools and methods that are available. Eventually, the case will be made to address the broader policy questions concerning the value of coherent and rationally organized service delivery in mitigating the effects of mental disability on the development of the child and enabling the recovery process for adults with severe and persistent mental illness.

Table 30-1 summarizes some of the evidence-based treatments used in adult psychiatric rehabilitation, and Table 30-2 summarizes treatment for children.

Table 30-1
Evidence-Based Manualized Interventions for Adult Psychiatric Rehabilitation

Modality	Goals and Targeted Areas	Results of Evaluation Research
Social and independent living skills	Teaches skills for managing symptoms and preventing relapse (mental illness and addictions), improving social communication with providers, peers, and family, and choosing and engaging in activities that match the person's abilities, limitations, and interests	Social and independent living skills evaluated in randomized, clinical trials show positive outcome, with increased successful community living and reduced rehospitalization
Assertive community treatment (ACT)	Provides ongoing care coordination and case management to increase ability to live independently in the community and prevent/manage psychiatric crises	Randomized effectiveness trials with adults and adolescents with serious and persistent mental illness and co-occurring addictive disorders demonstrate increased psychiatric, residential, and vocational stability
Cognitive-behavior therapy (CBT)	Teaches skills for recognizing and modifying thoughts and beliefs that increase or prolong distress, and strengthening thoughts and beliefs that are self-affirming and interpersonally assertive	Meta-analyses support CBT's efficacy in reducing the severity of anxiety disorders, somatoform disorders, bulimia, anger control problems, and generalized stress reactions, and offer modest support for CBT as an adjunctive treatment with addictive disorders and serious mental illness
Dialectical behavior therapy	Teaches skills for regulating intense emotions, tolerating extreme emotional distress, achieving interpersonal effectiveness, and developing mindfulness Originally developed for adults with borderline personality disorder, but has been adapted for use with a wide range of Axis I disorders in which extreme dysregulation and poor impulse control are problematic	Evaluated in randomized clinical trials with parasuicidal adult patients with borderline personality disorder, resulting in reduced behavioral and psychiatric crises greater than that achieved by expert psychiatrists' treatment Randomized clinical trials and observational studies show positive psychosocial outcomes with adults with severe and persistent mental illness and chronic addictions and with adolescents who are suicidal or self-harming, including those who have substance abuse or posttraumatic stress disorders (PTSDs)
Acceptance and commitment therapy	Teaches skills for identifying and managing (rather than avoiding and feeling controlled by) the symptoms of psychosis, affective, anxiety, eating, traumatic stress, and addictive disorders. Acceptance of symptoms facilitated by explanation that psychotic symptoms are extreme versions of normal perception and cognitive phenomena (private experiences)	Randomized clinical trials show evidence of increased awareness but reduced distress and impairment due to psychiatric symptoms across a variety of psychiatric disorders in outpatient and inpatient treatment settings
Relapse prevention therapy	Teaches skills for identifying the warning signs of potential or actual resumption of substance use or psychiatric symptoms Uses cognitive-behavioral skills for proactively modifying patterns of thought and behavior that are likely to escalate into a full relapse	Randomized clinical trials show efficacy in delaying, reducing the severity of, and preventing substance use relapse with adults with chronic addictions and co-occurring or comorbid psychiatric disorders
Interpersonal psychotherapy	Teaches skills for interacting and communicating effectively in close relationships, with a particular focus on overcoming four core interpersonal problems: unresolved grief, role conflict (e.g., dissatisfaction with parenting), role transition (e.g., marital separation), and interpersonal deficits (e.g., isolation and anger management)	Randomized clinical trials show evidence of reduced severity and risk of relapse of moderate to severe depression, PTSD, anxiety disorders, and eating disorders
Behavioral therapy	Provides systematic reinforcement contingencies to increase adaptive behavior and to extinguish maladaptive behavior	Randomized effectiveness trials show evidence of reduced alcohol, drug, and other addictive behaviors
Motivational enhancement therapy	Teaches skills for recognizing and aligning choices and behavior with personal motivations	Randomized effectiveness trials show evidence of reduced alcohol, drug, and other addictive behaviors
Trauma-focused CBT for PTSD	Teaches skills for safely recalling rather than avoiding troubling memories of traumatic events and for recognizing and managing PTSD symptoms, such as intrusive memories or flashbacks, emotional numbing, dissociation, and distress (e.g., guilt, grief), and problems with sleep or anger, or concentration problems due to hyperarousal or hypervigilance	Randomized clinical trials of seven approaches with adults (prolonged exposure therapy, cognitive processing therapy, eye movement desensitization and reprocessing, narrative exposure therapy, seeking safety, skills training for affect/interpersonal regulation with modified prolonged exposure, and emotion-focused trauma therapy) show evidence of safety and efficacy for adults with severe PTSD, co-occurring addictive disorders, problems with anger, dissociation, grief, and guilt, including one study with adults with chronic mental illness
Self-regulation focused CBT for PTSD	Teaches emotion regulation skills for recognizing and modulating traumatic stress symptoms without requiring reworking of traumatic memories	Randomized effectiveness trials of three approaches with adults (trauma affect regulation: guide for education and therapy, patient-centered therapy, and skills training in affect/interpersonal regulation) show evidence of safety and efficacy for adults with severe PTSD, co-occurring addictive disorders, problems with anger, dissociation, grief, and guilt, including in individuals with comorbid serious mental illness, and incarcerated women

Table 30-2
Evidence-Based Manualized Intervention for Child Psychiatric Rehabilitation

Modality	Goals and Targeted Areas	Results of Evaluation
Problem-solving skills training (PSST)	Teaches children skills and supports parents in helping children with self-monitoring, prosocial goal setting, developing peer positive environments, setting limits with friends, and developing problem-solving and communication skills	Randomized, clinical trials show evidence of improved problem-solving and interpersonal skills and modest reductions in oppositional and inattentive behavior
Cognitive-behavior therapy	Teaches skills for recognizing and modifying thoughts and beliefs that increase or prolong distress, and strengthening thoughts and beliefs that are self-affirming and interpersonally prosocial and assertive	Meta-analyses demonstrate efficacy in reducing children's anxiety and depressive symptoms
Parent behavior/Teacher classroom management training	Parent management training focuses on classroom strategies to help teachers and parents manage problematic child behavior and promote social, emotional, and academic competence	Randomized effectiveness studies with two approaches (Incredible Years; Oregon PMT) demonstrate reduced antisocial, oppositional, impulsive behavior, extending to adolescence for children with severe early antisocial problems
Brief strategic family therapy (BSFT)	A short-term, problem-focused intervention with an emphasis on modifying maladaptive patterns of interactions. It focuses on ways to help families interact more effectively	In a randomized, clinical trial with inner-city families whose children had a variety of behavior problems and varying degrees of juvenile justice involvement, BSFT was superior to usual community care services
Functional family therapy (FFT)	FFT teaches skills for problem solving and behavior management and delivers to parents and children together	Randomized and quasi-experimental studies show reduced juvenile recidivism for youths receiving FFT
Multidimensional family therapy (MDFT)	MDFT identifies family interaction patterns and restructures them to increase trust, cooperation, and emotional support among all members of the family; MDFT has evolved from a primarily clinic-based intervention to delivering services in the home and community settings to enhance youth engagement and the immediacy of services; MDFT is developing a variant for traumatized youth incorporating trauma affect regulation: guide for education and therapy (TARGET)	Randomized clinical trials of MDFT across a variety of ethnocultural and socioeconomic subpopulations have shown that it is associated with reduced youth substance abuse and legal problems and enhanced family functioning and school involvement
Multisystemic therapy (MST)	MST involves up to 6 mo of individualized, community-based contact by an M.A. or Ph.D. level therapist, supported by a 24-hr backup team; MST addresses all relevant environments by empowering parents with the skills and resources needed to independently prevent and manage crises and maintain family rules; variants of MST are under development for sexual offending youth, youth in psychiatric crisis, and youth who have experienced childhood maltreatment	In randomized clinical trials, MST has been shown to reduce juvenile delinquent recidivism and crime severity, psychiatric symptoms, out-of-home placements, and drug use while improving family functioning and school attendance; large-scale dissemination studies in the United States, Canada, and Scandinavia show that MST is superior to usual services on some, but not all, psychosocial outcomes
Intensive in-home child and adolescent psychiatric services (IICAPS)	IICAPS provides assistance in the home for families who have children with serious emotional disorders using a clinical team consisting of clinicians and counselors who are supervised by a child and adolescent psychiatrist	One randomized effectiveness trial and observational studies with a system of community agencies treating psychiatrically impaired, socioeconomically disadvantaged children demonstrate reduced psychiatric morbidity
Trauma-informed affect regulation therapies for posttraumatic stress disorder (PTSD)	Dyadic therapies for young children and their primary caregivers, and group and individual therapies for adolescents, teach children and caregivers skills for affect regulation to reduce PTSD-related emotional and behavioral problems	Randomized controlled trials with young traumatized children (child–parent psychotherapy, parent–child interaction therapy) and youth (trauma affect regulation: guide for education and therapy; trauma and grief components therapy for adolescents) demonstrate improvements in parent–child relationships and child/youth emotional, behavioral, and interpersonal functioning
Multidimensional treatment foster care (MTFC)	MTFC provides training and ongoing support, parent education, family therapy, and youth mentoring to enable foster parents to maintain a structured therapeutic environment for teaching children skills, setting limits, and modeling communication and problem-solving strategies	Three randomized controlled trials showed that MTFC reduced adolescents' psychiatric rehospitalization, arrests and incarceration, running away, and drug use while improving vocational and educational outcome
Cognitive-behavioral intervention for trauma in the schools (CBITS)	CBITS provides 10-session groups in school mental health or counseling settings for preadolescents or adolescents with PTSD due to family or community violence; CBITS includes education about traumatic stress, skills for anxiety management, and desensitization of trauma memories	Two randomized, controlled trials with inner-city children (one with Spanish-speaking youth) showed CBITS to be associated with reductions in PTSD and depression but not in teacher-reported behavioral or emotional problems
Trauma-focused cognitive–behavioral therapy (TF-CBT)	TF-CBT guides traumatized children and their parents in recognizing and managing PTSD symptoms and in desensitizing trauma memories	Randomized, controlled trials with sexually and physically abused children and children who experienced traumatic losses, disasters, or violence showed reductions in PTSD and depression and improvements in social functioning, but no improvement in disruptive or oppositional behavior

Chronic Illness Care Model: Psychiatry in the Context of Primary Care. Finally, the care of persons with long-term mental health problems is included in innovative developments in the provision of primary health care for persons with chronic illnesses (http://www.improvingchroniccare.org). The Health Resources Services Administration (HRSA), the federal agency responsible for the community health centers or Federally Qualified Health Centers (FQHCs), has adopted the chronic illness care model in its training and technical assistance efforts for community health centers. The model grows out of the current concern for the quality of care and accountability for health care delivery systems for effective outcomes. Depression management is one of the four chronic health conditions that the HRSA has selected for its training collaboratives.

The model begins with the assumption that the health care delivery system is part of a community context and must be responsive in its interactions with the community. Four areas of focus are essential in implementing the model in the health care delivery system: self-management support, delivery system design, decision support, and clinical tracking system. *Self-management support* gives patients a central role in determining their care, fostering a sense of responsibility for their health. Patients collaborate with the primary care team to establish goals, create treatment plans, and solve problems along the way. *Delivery system design* requires a reorganization of how the health system operates so that up-to-date information about a given patient is centralized, and follow-up responsibility is assigned as a standard procedure, and so on. *Decision support* requires that treatment decisions are based on explicit, proven practice guidelines supported by at least one defining study. Guidelines are discussed with patients and providers, and treatment team members are trained continuously in the latest proven methods. Finally, *clinical tracking systems* track individual patients and populations of patients with similar problems. These systems must be practical and operational—able to check an individual's treatment at any point to confirm that the treatment conforms to recommended guidelines. The real integration of psychiatric care into primary care is an important innovation to consider that would improve physical health care for individuals with psychiatric disorders and eliminate the separation imposed by placing individuals with psychiatric problems into community mental health centers.

THE ROLE OF PUBLIC AND COMMUNITY PSYCHIATRY IN TWENTY-FIRST CENTURY HEALTH CARE

Public psychiatry emerged historically as an attempt to provide humane care for people with severe mental disabilities who did not have the resources to be protected from the stigma and approbation that shielded so-called "eccentrics" and "black sheep" fortunate enough to have been born into the wealthier social strata. Community psychiatry evolved as an answer to concerns that public psychiatric treatment was a de facto form of marginalization and oppression, if not inhumane exile and imprisonment, of economically disadvantaged persons with mental illness. The best ideas from community and public psychiatry are sometimes lost amidst the competition for scarce resources. The spirit and skills of advocacy that sparked the development and continue to characterize the best practices of public and community psychiatry, as well as the dedication to bring demonstrably effective services to the people who are most in need but are least served, have never been more needed by the entire mental health field.

References

Abualenain J, Frohna WJ, Shesser R, Ding R, Smith M, Pines JM. Emergency department physician-level and hospital-level variation in admission rates. *Ann Emerg Med.* 2013;61(6):638–643.

Agrawal S, Edwards M. Personal Accounts: Upside down: The consumer as advisor to a psychiatrist. *Psychiatr Serv.* 2013;64(4):301–302.

Andrade LH, Alonso J, Mneimneh Z, Wells JE, Al-Hamzawi A, Borges G, Bromet E, Bruffaerts R, de Girolamo G, de Graaf R, Florescu S, Gureje O, Hinkov HR, Hu C, Huang Y, Hwang I, Jin R, Karam EG, Kovess-Masfety V, Levinson D, Matschinger H, O'Neill S, Posada-Villa J, Sagar R, Sampson NA, Sasu C, Stein DJ, Takeshima T, Viana MC, Xavier M, Kessler RC. Barriers to mental health treatment: Results from the WHO World Mental Health surveys. *Psychol Med.* 2014;44(6): 1303–1317.

Appelbaum PS. Public safety, mental disorders, and guns. *JAMA Psychiatry.* 2013; 70(6):565–566.

Conrad EJ, Lavigne KM. Psychiatry consultation during disaster preparedness: Hurricane Gustav. *South Med J.* 2013;106(1):99–101.

Coors ME. Genetic research on addiction: Ethics, the law, and public health. *Am J Psychiatry.* 2013;170(10):1215–1216.

Elbogen EB, Wagner HR, Johnson SC, Kinneer P, Kang H, Vasterling JJ, Timko C, Beckham JC. Are Iraq and Afghanistan veterans using mental health services? New data from a national random-sample survey. *Psychiatr Serv.* 2013;64(2): 134–141.

Evans-Lacko S, Henderson C, Thornicroft G. Public knowledge, attitudes and behaviour regarding people with mental illness in England 2009–2012. *Br J Psychiatry Suppl.* 2013;55:s51–s57.

Holzinger A, Matschinger H, Angermeyer MC. What to do about depression? Help-seeking and treatment recommendations of the public. *Epidemiol Psychiatr Sci.* 2011;20(2):163–169.

Huey LY, Ford JD, Cole RF, Morris JA. Public and community psychiatry. In: Sadock BJ, Sadock VA, Ruiz P, eds. *Kaplan & Sadock's Comprehensive Textbook of Psychiatry.* 9th ed. Vol. 2. Philadelphia, PA: Lippincott Williams & Wilkins; 2009:4259.

Kornblith LZ, Kutcher ME, Evans AE, Redick BJ, Privette A, Schecter WP, Cohen MJ. The "found down" patient: A diagnostic dilemma. *J Trauma Acute Care Surg.* 2013;74(6):1548–1552.

LeMelle S, Arbuckle MR, Ranz JM. Integrating systems-based practice, community psychiatry, and recovery into residency training. *Acad Psychiatry.* 2013;37(1): 35–37.

Malmin M. Warrior culture, spirituality, and prayer. *J Relig Health.* 2013;52(3): 740–758.

Pandya A. A review and retrospective analysis of mental health services provided after the September 11 attacks. *Can J Psychiatry.* 2013;58(3):128–134.

31 ▲

Global and Cultural Issues in Psychiatry

Mental disorders are highly prevalent in all regions of the world and represent a significant source of disability and social burden worldwide. Treatments for all these disorders are available and are efficacious in both developed and developing countries. However, mental disorders are remarkably undertreated worldwide, especially in low-income countries. National mental health policies are lacking in several countries, especially low-income ones. Resources for mental health care are scarce and unequally distributed. World psychiatry focuses on these and other issues, such as the stigma attached to mental disorders, the relationships between mental and physical diseases, and the ethics of mental health care.

PREVALENCE AND BURDEN OF MENTAL DISORDERS WORLDWIDE

The World Health Organization (WHO) estimates that more than 25 percent of individuals worldwide develop one or more mental disorders during their lifetime. Among people seen by primary health care professionals, more than 20 percent have one or more current mental disorders. In a study carried out by the WHO at 14 sites in Africa, Asia, the Americas, and Europe, the average current prevalence of any mental disorder was 24 percent, without consistent differences between low- and high-income countries. The most common diagnoses were those of depression (average, 10.4 percent) and generalized anxiety disorder (average, 7.9 percent). Female rates were 1.89 times higher than male rates for depression, but male rates were higher for alcohol-related disorders so that there was no sex difference in the proportion of people having at least one mental disorder. Physical ill-health and educational disadvantage were both significantly associated with a diagnosis of mental disorder.

To quantify the burden of the various diseases and injuries, the WHO, in collaboration with the Harvard School of Public Health and the World Bank, introduced the disability-adjusted life year (DALY). DALY for a given disease or injury is the sum of the years of life lost due to premature mortality plus the years lost due to disability for incident cases of that disease or injury in the general population. In the original estimates for the year 1990, mental and neurologic disorders accounted for 10.5 percent of the total DALYs lost due to all diseases and injuries. The estimate for the year 2000 was 12.3 percent, with two mental disorders (depression and alcohol use disorders) and suicide ranking in the top 20 causes of DALYs for all ages.

In the estimates for the year 2005, mental and neurologic disorders accounted for 13.5 percent of all DALYs in the world, and is the main contributor to burden among noncommunicable diseases (Table 31-1).

Table 31-2 summarizes the global burden of disease for mental and substance use disorders at various times in the last few decades.

By 2030, mental and neurologic disorders will likely account for 14.4 percent of all global DALYs and 25.4 percent of those due to noncommunicable diseases. Depression will rank number 2 in the percentage of total DALYs in that year (5.7 percent), following HIV/AIDS and preceding ischemic heart disease (Table 31-3). It will be number 1 in high-income countries (9.8 percent), number 2 in middle-income countries (6.7 percent), and number 3 in low-income countries (4.7 percent).

The WHO estimates that one of four families worldwide has at least one member with a mental disorder. The objective and subjective burden related to caring for people with severe mental disorders (in terms of disruption of family relationships; constraints in social, leisure, and work activities; financial difficulties; detrimental effects on physical health; feelings of loss, depression, and embarrassment in social situations; and the stress of coping with disturbing behaviors) is substantial and significantly higher than that related to caring for people with long-term physical diseases such as diabetes and heart, kidney, or lung diseases. Cross-cultural differences exist in some dimensions of family burden.

Suicide is among the 10 leading causes of death for all ages in most of the countries for which information is available. In some countries (e.g., China), it is the leading cause of death for people between 15 and 34 years of age.

According to WHO estimates, about 849,000 people died from suicide worldwide in the year 2001. In that year, the number of suicide deaths overtook the number of deaths by violence (500,000) and war (230,000). In 2020, approximately 1.53 million people will die from suicide worldwide, based on current trends, and 10 to 20 times more people will attempt suicide. Reported suicide rates vary considerably across countries; for instance, in many Eastern and Central European countries, the annual suicide rates are between 48.0 and 79.3 per 100,000. In contrast, many Islamic and Latin American countries report rates of less than 4.0 per 100,000. More than 85 percent of suicides occur in low- or middle-income countries. However, this figure may represent an underestimate due to the low reliability of official statistics in those countries: for example, when epidemiologists used a verbal autopsy in South India, the observed rates for suicide exceeded official national estimates 10-fold. In the Asia-Pacific region, perhaps 300,000 cases of suicide per year occur by self-poisoning with pesticides.

Suicide rates are higher in men than in women (3.2:1 in 1950, 3.6:1 in 1995, and an estimated 3.9:1 in 2020). China is the only country where suicide rates in women are consistently higher than those in men, especially in rural areas. Over the past few decades, suicide rates are generally stable worldwide, but there is a rising trend among young men ages 15 to 19 years. A systematic review covering 15,629 cases in the general population worldwide estimated that 98 percent of those who committed suicide had a diagnosable mental disorder, with mood disorders accounting for

Table 31-1
Disorder-Specific Global Sheehan Disability Scale Ratings for Commonly Occurring Mental and Chronic Physical Disorders in Developed and Developing WMH Countries

| | Proportion Rated Severely Disabling | | | |
| | Developed | | Developing | |
	%	(SE)	%	(SE)
I. Physical Disorders				
Arthritis	23.3	(1.5)	22.8	(3.0)
Asthma	8.2	(1.4)	26.9	(5.4)
Back/Neck	34.6	(1.5)	22.7	(1.8)
Cancer	16.6	(3.2)	23.9	(10.3)
Chronic pain	40.9	(3.6)	24.8	(3.8)
Diabetes	13.6	(3.4)	23.7	(6.1)
Headaches	42.1	(1.9)	28.1	(2.1)
Heart disease	26.5	(3.9)	27.8	(5.2)
High blood pressure	5.3	(0.9)	23.8	(2.6)
Ulcer	15.3	(3.9)	18.3	(3.6)
II. Mental Disorders				
ADHD	37.6	(3.6)	24.3	(7.4)
Bipolar	68.3	(2.6)	52.1	(4.9)
Depression	65.8	(1.6)	52.0	(1.8)
GAD	56.3	(1.9)	42.0	(4.2)
IED	36.3	(2.8)	27.8	(3.6)
ODD	34.2	(6.0)	41.3	(10.3)
Panic disorder	48.4	(2.6)	38.8	(4.7)
PTSD	54.8	(2.8)	41.2	(7.3)
Social phobia	35.1	(1.4)	41.4	(3.6)
Specific phobia	18.6	(1.1)	16.2	(1.6)

35.8 percent, substance-related disorders for 22.4 percent, personality disorders for 11.6 percent, and schizophrenia for 10.6 percent of cases.

TREATMENT GAP AND PROJECTED POPULATION-LEVEL TREATMENT EFFECTIVENESS WORLDWIDE

Clinical trials have convincingly proved the efficacy of pharmacologic and psychosocial treatments for mood, anxiety, psychotic, and substance-related disorders carried out in low- and middle-income, as well as in high-income countries. However, the treatment gap is substantial for all mental disorders worldwide, particularly in low-income countries.

In the World Mental Health Surveys, failure and delays in treatment seeking were generally higher in low-income countries, older cohorts, men, and cases with earlier ages of onset. People with mood disorders had earlier treatment contact than other mental disorders, this is likely because many countries have targeted this disorder, with screening campaigns and public informational campaigns.

RESOURCES FOR MENTAL HEALTH CARE WORLDWIDE

According to the *Mental Health Atlas 2005,* only 62.1 percent of countries worldwide, accounting for 68.3 percent of the world population, have a mental health policy (i.e., a document of the government or ministry of health specifying the goals for improving the mental health situation of the country, the priorities among those goals, and the main directions for attaining them). Mental health policies are present in 58.8 percent of low-income and 70.5 percent of high-income countries. In Africa, only 50 percent of countries have a mental health policy. In Southeast Asia, only about half of countries have a mental health policy, and only about a quarter of the population are affected by these policies (Table 31-4).

Community care facilities exist in only 68.1 percent of the countries (51.7 percent of low-income and 93 percent of high-income countries). Only 60.9 percent of the countries report providing treatment facilities for severe mental disorders at the primary care level (55.2 percent of low-income and 79.5 percent of high-income countries). About one-fourth of low-income countries do not provide even rudimentary antidepressant medications in primary care settings. In many others, the supply does not cover all regions of the country or is very irregular. Because medicines are often not available in health care facilities, patients and families must pay for them out of pocket.

Whereas 61.5 percent of European countries spend more than 5 percent of their health budget on mental health care, 70 percent of countries in Africa and 50 percent of countries in Southeast Asia spend less than 1 percent. Out-of-pocket payment is the most important method of financing mental health care in 38.6 percent of countries in Africa and 30 percent of countries in Southeast Asia, but it is not the primary method of financing mental health care in any European country (Table 31-5). All countries with out-of-pocket payment as the dominant method of financing mental health care belong to low-income or lower-middle-income categories, but almost all countries with social insurance as the dominant method of financing belong to high-income or upper-middle-income categories.

The median number of psychiatrists per 100,000 population ranges from 0.04 in Africa and 0.2 in Southeast Asia to 9.8 in Europe (Table 31-6). It is 0.1 in low-income countries compared with 9.2 in high-income countries. Two-thirds of low-income countries have less than one psychiatrist per 100,000 population. Chad, Eritrea, and Liberia (with populations of 9, 4.2, and 3.5 million, respectively) each have just one psychiatrist per 100,000 population. Afghanistan, Rwanda, and Togo (with populations of 25, 8.5, and 5 million respectively) each have just two psychiatrists per 100,000 population. Large-scale migration of psychiatrists from low- and middle-income to high-income countries, as part of the larger picture of migration of health professionals in general, has been consistently documented. India and some sub-Saharan African countries are the most important contributors to the mental health workforce in the United Kingdom, although the United Kingdom has 110 psychiatrists per million population. However, India has 2 per million and sub-Saharan Africa less than 1 per million. The median number of psychologists working in mental health care per 100,000 population ranges from 0.03 in Southeast Asia and 0.05 in Africa to 3.1 in Europe. Approximately 69 percent of low-income countries have less than one psychologist per 100,000 population. The median number of psychiatric nurses per 100,000 population ranges from 0.1 in Southeast Asia and 0.2 in Africa to 24.8 in Europe.

**Table 31-2
Global Burden of Disease: Mental and Substance Use Disorders**

Mental Disorders	Substance Use Disorders	Before 1998	1998–2005	2006–2013	Total
All causes		100.0%	100.0%	100.0%	100.0%
Mental and substance use disorders		37.8%	58.5%	35.6%	67.6%
Schizophrenia		17.0%	9.0%	3.7%	19.1%
Alcohol use disorders		19.7%	28.7%	14.9%	31.4%
Drug use disorders		20.7%	47.3%	26.1%	51.6%
	Opioid use disorders	12.8%	17.6%	2.7%	19.7%
	Cocaine use disorders	6.9%	31.9%	5.9%	34.6%
	Amphetamine use disorders	6.4%	23.9%	8.0%	27.7%
	Cannabis use disorders	16.0%	42.0%	20.7%	46.8%
	Other drug use disorders	—	—	—	—
Depressive disorders		19.7%	23.9%	11.2%	33.0%
	Major depressive disorder	19.7%	23.9%	11.2%	33.0%
	Dysthymia	9.0%	13.8%	5.3%	18.6%
Bipolar disorder		8.5%	16.0%	3.7%	18.6%
Anxiety disorders		12.8%	21.8%	5.3%	26.1%
Eating disorders		10.6%	12.2%	4.3%	14.9%
	Anorexia nervosa	10.1%	12.2%	4.3%	14.4%
	Bulimia nervosa	8.5%	11.7%	3.2%	14.9%
Autistic spectrum disorders		5.3%	5.9%	3.7%	9.6%
	Autism	5.3%	5.3%	3.7%	9.6%
	Asperger syndrome	1.6%	4.8%	1.6%	5.3%
Attention-deficit or hyperactivity disorder		10.6%	10.1%	4.8%	19.1%
Conduct disorder		5.9%	6.4%	1.6%	11.2%
Idiopathic intellectual disability		6.4%	3.2%	1.1%	7.4%
Other mental and substance use disorders		0.5%	0.5%	0.0%	1.1%

**Table 31-3
Leading Causes of Disability-Adjusted Life Year (DALY) Worldwide as Estimated for the Year 2030**

Disease or Injury	Percent of Total
1. HIV/AIDS	12.1
2. Unipolar depressive disorders	5.7
3. Ischemic heart disease	4.7
4. Road traffic accidents	4.2
5. Perinatal conditions	4.0
6. Cerebrovascular disease	3.9
7. Chronic obstructive pulmonary disease	3.1
8. Lower respiratory infections	3.0
9. Hearing loss, adult onset	2.5
10. Cataracts	2.5

From Mathers CD, Loncar D. Projections of global mortality and burden of disease from 2002 to 2030. *PLoS Med.* 2006;3(11):e442.

**Table 31-4
Presence of a Mental Health Policy in Countries of Each Region of the World Health Organization (WHO)**

WHO Region	Percent of Countries	Percent of Population Coverage
Africa	50.0	69.4
Americas	72.7	64.2
Eastern Mediterranean	72.7	93.8
Europe	70.6	89.1
Southeast Asia	54.5	23.6
Western Pacific	48.1	93.8

From *World Health Organization: Mental Health Atlas 2005.* Geneva: World Health Organization; 2005.

Table 31-5
Countries in Which Out-of-Pocket Payment Is the Most Common Method of Financing Mental Health Care in Each Region of the World Health Organization (WHO)

WHO Region	Percent of Countries
Africa	38.6
Americas	12.9
Eastern Mediterranean	15.8
Europe	0
Southeast Asia	30.0
Western Pacific	18.5

From *World Health Organization: Mental Health Atlas 2005*. Geneva: World Health Organization; 2005.

From these figures, it is clear that resources for mental health care are grossly inadequate compared with the needs, and that inequalities across countries are substantial, especially between low- and high-income countries. Moreover, resources tend to be concentrated in urban areas, especially in low-income countries, leaving vast regions without any form of mental health care.

Even worse is the situation concerning child and adolescent mental health care. According to the WHO, only 7 percent of countries worldwide have a specific child and adolescent mental health policy. In less than one-third of all countries, is it possible to identify an institution or a governmental entity with overall responsibility for child mental health. School-based services are almost exclusively present in high-income countries; and even in Europe, only 17 percent of countries have a sufficient number of these services. There are no pediatric beds for mental health identified in low-income countries, but such beds exist in 50 percent of high-income countries. In all African countries outside South Africa, there are as little as 10 psychiatrists trained to work with children. In European countries, the number of child psychiatrists ranges from one per 5,300 to one per 51,800. In more than 70 percent of countries worldwide, there is no list of essential psychotropic medications for children. In 45 percent of countries worldwide, psychostimulants are either prohibited or unavailable for use in children with attention-deficit/hyperactivity disorder.

Table 31-6
Median Number of Mental Health Professionals per 100,000 Population in Each Region of the World Health Organization (WHO)

WHO Region	Psychiatrists	Psychiatric Nurses	Psychologists Working in Mental Health
Africa	0.04	0.20	0.05
Americas	2.00	2.60	2.80
Eastern Mediterranean	0.95	1.25	0.60
Europe	9.80	24.80	3.10
Southeast Asia	0.20	0.10	0.03
Western Pacific	0.32	0.50	0.03

From *World Health Organization: Mental Health Atlas 2005*. Geneva: World Health Organization; 2005.

PRINCIPLES FOR MENTAL HEALTH PROGRAM DEVELOPMENT AND BARRIERS TO CHANGE WORLDWIDE

According to the WHO, the development of mental health programs worldwide should adhere to the following principles: (1) providing treatment in primary care; (2) making psychotropic medications available; (3) giving care in the community; (4) educating the public; (5) involving communities, families, and consumers; (6) establishing national policies and legislation; (7) developing human resources; (8) linking with other relevant sectors; (9) monitoring community mental health; and (10) supporting more research.

The guiding principles proposed for the prevention of suicide worldwide include (1) reducing access to means of suicide (e.g., pesticides, firearms), (2) treating people with mental disorders, (3) improving media portrayal of suicide, (4) training primary health care personnel, (5) implementing school-based programs, and (6) developing hotlines and crisis centers.

The most significant barriers to the implementation of the preceding principles worldwide, according to the WHO, include the following: (1) some stakeholders may be resistant to the changes; (2) health authorities may not believe in the effectiveness of mental health interventions; (3) there may be no consensus among the country's stakeholders about how to formulate or implement the new policy; (4) financial and human resources may be scarce; (5) other essential health priorities may compete with mental health care for funding; (6) primary care teams may feel overburdened by their workload and refuse to accept the introduction of the new policy; and (7) many mental health specialists may not want to work in community facilities or with primary care teams, preferring to remain in hospitals. The suggested solutions include (1) adopting an "all-winners approach" that ensures countries take into account the needs of all stakeholders, (2) developing pilot projects and evaluating their effect on health and consumer satisfaction, (3) asking for technical reports from international experts, (4) focusing the implementation of the mental health policy on a demonstration area and performing cost-effectiveness studies, (5) linking mental health programs to other health priorities, and (6) showing primary care practitioners that people with mental disorders are already a hidden part of their burden and that the burden will decrease if they identify and treat these disorders.

STIGMATIZING ATTITUDES TOWARD PEOPLE WITH MENTAL DISORDERS

Stigmatizing attitudes toward people with mental disorders are widespread in the general public and even among mental health professionals. Although stigma may be less severe in some Asian and African countries, a study carried out in India within the Stigma Programme of the World Psychiatric Association (WPA), in which the investigators interviewed 463 persons with schizophrenia and 651 family members in four cities, reported that two-thirds of the respondents had experienced discrimination. Women and people living in urban areas were the most stigmatized. Whereas men experienced more significant discrimination in the job area, women experienced more problems in the family and social areas.

Unlike people with physical disabilities, those with mental disorders are often perceived by the public to be in control of their disabilities and responsible for causing them. The view that "weakness," "laziness," or "lack of willpower" contributes to the development of mental disorders still exists in many countries. The stigmatization of people with mental disorders may result in public avoidance, systematic discrimination, and reduced help-seeking behavior. In a survey carried out in 1996 in a probability sample of 1,444 adults in the United States, more than half of the respondents were unwilling to spend an evening socializing with, work next to, or have a family member marry a person with mental illness. Although most countries have some provision for disability benefits, people with mental illness are often explicitly excluded from such entitlements. Moreover, mental disorders are frequently not considered in social and private insurance schemes for health care. Shame is one of the main barriers to seeking help for mental disorders in both developed and developing countries.

We can subdivide the strategies for addressing the stigmatization of people with mental disorders into three groups: protest, education, and contact. There is some evidence that protest campaigns may be useful in reducing stigmatizing behaviors against people with mental disorders. Education may promote a better understanding of mental illness, and educated people may be less likely to endorse stigma and discrimination. There is an inverse relationship between having contact with a person with mental illness and endorsing stigmatizing behavior.

RELATIONSHIPS BETWEEN MENTAL AND PHYSICAL DISEASES

People with severe mental disorders have higher mortality from physical illnesses compared with the general population. In a follow-up study carried out in the United Kingdom, the standardized mortality ratio (SMR) for natural causes in people with schizophrenia was 2.32 (i.e., death was more than twice higher than in the general population). The SMR for causes "avoidable by appropriate treatment" was 4.68. The highest SMRs were those for endocrine, nervous, respiratory, circulatory, and gastrointestinal diseases. There is also an increased nonsuicide all-cause mortality for bipolar disorder (SMR 1.9 for men and 2.1 for women) and dementia (relative risk [RR] 2.63; 95 percent confidence interval [CI] 2.17 to 3.21). A meta-analysis of 15 population-based studies of the effect of a diagnosis of depression on subsequent all-cause mortality yielded a pooled odds ratio of 1.7 (CI 1.5 to 2.0). Evidence from low-income countries is limited, but a large population study conducted in Ethiopia found high mortality rates for major depression (SMR 3.55, 95 percent CI 1.97 to 6.39) and schizophrenia (almost 5 percent per year).

People with mental disorders also have a higher prevalence of several physical diseases compared with the general population. In a study carried out in the United States, people with psychotic disorders were more likely than other people to develop diabetes, hypertension, heart disease, asthma, gastrointestinal disorders, skin infections, malignant neoplasms, and acute respiratory disorders. This high rate remained true even when only considering patients without a concomitant substance use disorder. In a study conducted in Nigeria, 55.2 percent of persons with schizophrenia-spectrum disorders referred for the first time to a psychiatric clinic had at least one physical disease, but in persons with neurotic disorders, the rate was 11.8 percent. A strong prospective association exists between depression and coronary heart disease outcomes, including fatal myocardial infarction; on the other hand, the incidence of depression is increased after myocardial infarction, especially in the first month after the event. Depression also increases the risk of type II diabetes. In South Asia, there are reports of an association between maternal perinatal depression and infant malnutrition and stunting at 6 months.

People with severe mental disorders are at increased risk of contracting HIV infection, although prevalence rates vary substantially worldwide. A large multicenter study conducted in sub-Saharan Africa, Asia, Latin America, Europe, and the United States reported a higher prevalence of the depressive disorder among symptomatic HIV-seropositive people than in asymptomatic HIV-seropositive cases and seronegative control participants. Evidence from both developed and developing countries shows that adherence to highly active antiretroviral therapy (HAART) is negatively affected by depression, cognitive impairment, and substance abuse.

In a study carried out in the United Kingdom, people with severe mental illness were significantly more likely to be obese (body mass index higher than 30) and morbidly obese (body mass index higher than 40) than the general population; the respective figures were 35.0 versus 19.4 percent and 3.7 versus 1.3 percent. When these figures were broken down by age and sex, 28.7 percent of men with severe mental illness between 18 and 44 years of age were obese compared with 13.6 percent in the general population, and 3.7 versus 0.4 percent were morbidly obese. Even more striking were the figures concerning women of the same age; 50.6 versus 16.6 percent and 7.4 versus 2.0 percent, respectively.

A meta-analysis of worldwide studies confirmed that there is a highly significant association between schizophrenia and current smoking. The weighted average odds ratio was 5.9; it was 7.2 in men and 3.3 in women. The association remained significant when controls with severe mental illness were used (odds ratio, 1.9). Heavy smoking and high nicotine dependence were also more frequent in people with schizophrenia than in the general population.

The quality of physical health care received by patients with severe mental illness is often worse than the general population. A study conducted in the United States found that adverse events during medical and surgical hospitalizations were significantly more frequent in patients with schizophrenia than in the other people, including infections due to medical care, postoperative respiratory failure, postoperative deep venous thrombosis or pulmonary embolism, and postoperative sepsis. All of these adverse events were associated with a significantly increased odds of admission to an intensive care unit and of death.

The decreased access of people with mental disorders to medical services relates to several factors concerning the health care system. There is a well-documented effect of lack of insurance and the cost of care. In a study carried out in the United States, people with mental disorders were twice as likely as those without mental disorders to have been denied insurance because of a preexisting condition (odds ratio, 2.18). Having a mental disorder conferred a higher risk of having delayed seeking care because of cost (odds ratio, 1.76) and of having been unable to obtain needed medical care (odds ratio, 2.30).

Even when a doctor sees people with mental illness, their physical diseases often remain undiagnosed. Primary care providers may misperceive the medical complaints of people with mental disorders as "psychosomatic" or be unskilled or feel uncomfortable in dealing with this population. Underlying stigmatization may be involved. Moreover, during hospitalizations in medical and surgical wards, health care professionals may not be experienced in dealing with the unique needs of patients with schizophrenia, may minimize or misinterpret their somatic symptoms, and may make inappropriate use of restraints or sedative drugs or fail to consider possible interactions of psychotropic drugs with other medications. On the other hand, many psychiatrists are unable or unwilling to perform physical and even neurologic examinations or are not up to date on the management of even common physical diseases.

The first step is raising awareness of the problem among mental health care professionals, primary care providers, and patients with schizophrenia and their families. Education and training of mental health professionals and primary care providers is a further essential step. We should train mental health professionals to perform at least basic medical tasks. They should understand the importance of recognizing physical illness in people with severe mental disorders and become familiar with the most common reasons for underdiagnosis or misdiagnosis of physical illness in these patients. On the other hand, primary care providers should overcome their reluctance to treat people with severe mental illness and learn practical ways to interact and communicate with them; it is not only an issue of knowledge and skills but also most of all one of attitudes.

A well-identified professional should be responsible for physical health care in each person with a severe mental disorder. Mental health services should be able to provide at least a standard routine assessment of their patients to identify or at least suspect the presence of physical health problems. Guidelines about the management of patients receiving antipsychotic drugs should be known and applied by all mental health services. Patients should be involved as much as possible; for instance, mental health professionals should encourage patients to monitor and chart their weight. Mental health services should routinely provide dietary and exercise programs. Flexible smoking cessation programs, which have shown some degree of success, could be considered in some settings.

ETHICAL ISSUES IN MENTAL HEALTH CARE

The protection and promotion of the human rights of people with mental disorders are emerging as a priority worldwide. In 1991, the United Nations (UN) issued Resolution 46/119 for the Protection of Persons with Mental Illness and the Improvement of Mental Health Care. In that resolution, the UN codified the human rights of people with mental disorders, and their right to treatment. The 25 principles covered the following areas: definition of mental illness; protection of confidentiality; standards of care and treatment, including involuntary admission and consent to treatment; rights of persons with mental disorders in mental health facilities; protection of minors; provision of resources for mental health facilities; the role of community and culture; review mechanisms providing for the protection of the rights of offenders with mental disorders; and procedural safeguards protecting rights of persons with mental disorders. The UN encouraged national governments to promote the principles of the resolution by appropriate legislative, juridical, administrative, educational, and other provisions. However, violations of the human rights of people with mental disorders still exist in many countries, and in a substantial number of low- and middle-income countries, patients in mental hospitals are physically restrained or secluded for long periods.

In Latin America, an influential document has been the Declaration of Caracas, adopted in 1990 by the Regional Conference on Restructuring Psychiatric Care in Latin America, which states that resources, care, and treatment for people with mental disorders should safeguard their dignity and human and civil rights and strive to maintain them in their communities. The Declaration also states that mental health legislation should safeguard the human rights of people with mental disorders and that countries should organize services so that they can enforce these rights.

In Africa, the Banjul Charter on Human and Peoples' Rights, a legally binding document supervised by the African Commission on Human and Peoples' Rights, in Article 5 addresses the right to respect for the dignity inherent in human beings and the prohibition of all forms of degradation, including cruel, inhuman, or degrading treatment.

According to the WHO, mental health legislation should cover the following issues: access to fundamental mental health care, least restrictive care, informed consent to treatment, voluntary and involuntary admission to treatment, competence issues, periodical review mechanism, confidentiality, rehabilitation, accreditation of professionals and facilities, and rights of families and caregivers. Specific legislation in the field of mental health is present in 74 percent of low-income countries versus 92.7 percent of high-income countries.

In 1996, the WPA released the Madrid Declaration, which contains the ethical principles by which all national psychiatric societies should abide. The declaration includes seven general guidelines focusing on the aims of psychiatry: (1) psychiatrists must serve patients by providing the best therapy available, consistent with accepted scientific knowledge and ethical principles, and should devise therapeutic interventions that are the least restrictive to the freedom of the patient; (2) it is the duty of psychiatrists to keep abreast of scientific developments of their specialty and to convey updated knowledge to others; (3) the patient should be accepted as a partner by right in the therapeutic process, and the therapist–patient relationship must be based on mutual trust and respect, to allow the patient to make free and informed decisions; (4) treatment must always be in the best interest of the patient, and no treatment should be provided against the patient's will, unless withholding treatment would endanger life of the patient or those who surround him or her; (5) when psychiatrists are requested to assess a person, it is their duty to inform the person being assessed about the purpose of the intervention; (6) information contained in the therapeutic relationship should be kept in confidence and used exclusively for the purpose of improving the mental health of the patient; and (7) because psychiatric patients are particularly vulnerable research subjects, extra caution should be taken to safeguard their autonomy, as well as their mental and physical integrity.

INTERNATIONAL ORGANIZATIONS ACTIVE IN THE MENTAL HEALTH FIELD

Many international organizations are active in the mental health field. They include the WHO, which is the world's leading public health agency; some professional associations, among which the largest is the WPA, representing the psychiatric profession worldwide; and several organizations with a membership of users and families (such as the World Fellowship for Schizophrenia and Allied Disorders and the Global Alliance of Mental Illness Advocacy Networks [GAMIAN]) or both mental health professionals and users and families (such as the World Federation for Mental Health [WFMH]).

The WHO is a UN agency that is funded by 192 member states. It has six regional groupings: Africa, the Americas, Eastern Mediterranean, Europe, Southeast Asia, and Western Pacific. The Department of Mental Health and Substance Abuse is in Geneva, and it has advisors for mental health in each of its regional offices. Its main functions are direction and coordination of international health work and technical cooperation with countries. Among the numerous recent WHO activities in the mental health field, of particular interest, are the release of the *World Health Report 2001* and the development of the report *Mental Health: New Understanding, New Hope,* which was devoted entirely to mental health. It provided a summary of the current and projected impact of mental disorders and the principles of mental health policy and service provision, as well as a set of recommendations for future action that countries can adapt to their various needs and resources. Project Atlas aims to collect information on mental health resources across the world. Global and regional analyses of those resources were first published in 2001 and updated in 2005. Reports from the project focus, for example, on resources for child and adolescent mental health and psychiatric education and training worldwide (the latter in collaboration with the WPA).

The WPA is an association of national psychiatric societies aimed at increasing the knowledge and skills necessary for work in the field of mental health and the care for the mentally ill. Its member societies number 134, and it spans 122 countries and represents more than 200,000 psychiatrists. The WPA organizes the World Congress of Psychiatry every 3 years. It also organizes international and regional congresses and meetings and thematic conferences. It has 65 scientific sections, which disseminate information and promoting collaborative work in specific domains of psychiatry. It has produced several educational programs, books, and consensus statements (including the Declaration of Madrid on ethical principles for psychiatric practice). It has an official journal, *World Psychiatry,* which is in English, Spanish, and Chinese and is indexed in PubMed and Current Contents and reaches more than 33,000 psychiatrists worldwide.

The WFMH is a multidisciplinary advocacy and education organization aimed at promoting the advancement of mental health awareness, prevention, advocacy, and best-practice recovery-focused interventions worldwide. Among its activities is the organization of the World Mental Health Day, observed every year on October 10, each time with a different theme.

FUTURE PERSPECTIVES

There are several statements from various groups and organizations about the priorities for future action in the mental health field at the international level. Of particular interest is a document produced by 39 leaders comprising the Lancet Commission on global mental health and sustainable development, or the Global Mental Health Commission. This document identifies five main goals: (1) placing mental health on the public health priority agenda, (2) improving the organization of mental health services, (3) integrating the availability of mental health into general health care, (4) developing human resources for mental health, and (5) strengthening public mental health leadership.

Among the strategies proposed to place mental health on the public health priority agenda are the development and use of uniform and understandable messages for mental health advocacy and the education of decision-makers within governments and donor agencies on the evidence concerning the public health significance of mental disorders and the cost-effectiveness of mental health care. Strategies suggested to improve the organization of mental health services include, among others, the provision of incentive arrangements to overcome vested interests blocking change and the organization of international technical support to learn from countries that have experienced successful mental health reforms. The authors proposed that mental health professionals be appointed and trained specially to support and supervise primary health care staff, to help integrate mental and general health care. It is also crucial that we increase and diversify the professional and specialist workforce is increased and diversified and improve the quality of mental health training to ensure that it is practical and widely practiced in community or primary care settings.

References

Belsky J, Hartman S. Gene-environment interaction in evolutionary perspective: Differential susceptibility to environmental influences. *World Psychiatry*. 2014;13(1): 87–89.

Biglu MH. 2565–Global attitudes towards forensic psychiatry (2006–2012). *Eur Psychiatry*. 2013;28:1.

Golhar TS, Srinath S. Global child and adolescent mental health needs: Perspectives from a national tertiary referral center in India. *Adolesc Psychiatry*. 2013;3(1): 82–86.

Kirmayer LJ, Raikhel E, Rahimi S. Cultures of the Internet: Identity, community and mental health. *Transcult Psychiatry*. 2013;50(2):165–191.

Leckman JF. What's next for developmental psychiatry? *World Psychiatry*. 2013; 12(2):125–126.

Maj M. World aspects of psychiatry. In: Sadock BJ, Sadock VA, Ruiz P, eds. *Kaplan & Sadock's Comprehensive Textbook of Psychiatry*. 9th ed. Vol. 2. Philadelphia, PA: Lippincott Williams & Wilkins; 2009:4510.

Malhi GS, Coulston CM, Parker GB, Cashman E, Walter G, Lampe LA, Vollmer-Conna U. Who picks psychiatry? Perceptions, preferences and personality of medical students. *Aust N Z J Psychiatry*. 2011;45(10):861–870.

Marienfeld C, Rohrbaugh RM. Impact of a global mental health program on a residency training program. *Acad Psychiatry*. 2013;37(4):276–280.

Pargament KI, Lomax JW. Understanding and addressing religion among people with mental illness. *World Psychiatry*. 2013;12(1):26–32.

Pitel L, Geckova AM, Kolarcik P, Halama P, Reijneveld SA, van Dijk JP. Gender differences in the relationship between religiosity and health-related behaviour among adolescents. *J Epidemiol Community Health*. 2012;66(12):1122–1128.

Robinson JA, Bolton JM, Rasic D, Sareen J. Exploring the relationship between religious service attendance, mental disorders, and suicidality among different ethnic groups: Results from a nationally representative survey. *Depress Anxiety*. 2012; 29(11):983–990.

White R. The globalisation of mental illness. *The Psychologist*. 2013;26(3):182–185.

Contributions from the Sciences and Social Sciences to Psychiatry

32

Normal Development and Aging

▲ 32.1 Infant, Child, and Adolescent Development

The transactional nature of development in infancy, childhood, and adolescence, consisting of a continuous interplay between biologic predisposition and environmental experiences, forms the basis of current conceptualizations of development. There is much evidence that observed developmental outcomes evolve from interactions between particular biologic substrates and specific environmental events. For example, the serotonin transporter gene sensitizes a child with early adverse experiences of abuse or neglect to increased risk for later development of a depressive disorder. Also, the degree of resilience and adaptation, that is, the ability to withstand adversity without damaging effects, is likely to be mediated by endogenous glucocorticoids, cytokines, and neurotrophins. Thus, allostasis, the process of achieving stability in the face of adverse environmental events, results from interactions between specific environmental challenges and particular genetic backgrounds that combine to result in a response. Adverse childhood experiences (ACEs) are likely to alter the trajectory of development in a given individual and that during early development, the brain is especially vulnerable to injury. Future studies may uncover windows of plasticity in older children and adolescents that affect vulnerability as well. Acquiring subtle social skills, for example, relates to changes in the adolescent brain. Adolescents' keen abilities, competencies, and interests in a host of technologic advances—including the Internet, social media sites, and smartphones, to name a few—shed some light on their potential to adapt to new and challenging demands.

PRENATAL, INFANT, AND CHILD

The phases of development described in this section are defined as follows: prenatal is the time frame from conception to 8 weeks; the fetus, from 8 weeks to birth; infancy, from birth to 15 months; the toddler period, from 15 months to 2½ years; the preschool period, from 2½ years to 6 years; and the middle years, from 6 to 12 years.

PRENATAL

Historically, the analysis of human development began with birth. The influence of endogenous and exogenous in utero factors, however, now requires that developmental schemes consider intrauterine events. The infant is not a tabula rasa, a smooth slate upon which outside influences etch patterns. On the contrary, myriad factors within the womb have already influenced the newborn. For example, the studies of

Stella Chess and Alexander Thomas (described later) have demonstrated a wide range of temperamental differences among newborns. Maternal stress, through the production of adrenal hormones, also influences the behavioral characteristics of newborns.

The time frame in which the development of the embryo and fetus occurs is known as the prenatal period. After implantation, the egg begins to divide and is known as an embryo. Growth and development occur at a rapid pace; by the end of 8 weeks, the shape is recognizably human, and the embryo has become a fetus. Figure 32-1 illustrates a sonogram of a 9-week and 15-week fetus in utero.

The fetus maintains an internal equilibrium that, with variable effects, interacts continuously with the intrauterine environment. In general, most disorders that occur are multifactorial—the result of a combination of effects, some of which can be cumulative. Damage at the fetal stage usually has a more global impact than damage after birth, because rapidly growing organs are the most vulnerable. Boys are more vulnerable to developmental damage than girls are; geneticists recognize that in humans and animals, female fetuses show a propensity for greater biologic vigor than male fetuses, possibly because of the second X chromosome in the female.

Prenatal Life

Much biologic activity occurs in utero. A fetus is involved in a variety of behaviors that are necessary for adaptation outside the womb. For example, a fetus sucks on thumb and fingers; folds and unfolds its body, and eventually assumes a position in which its occiput is in an anterior vertex position, which is the position in which fetuses usually exit the uterus.

Behavior. Pregnant women are extraordinarily sensitive to fetal movements. They describe their unborn babies as active or passive, as kicking vigorously or rolling around, as quiet when the mothers are active, but as kicking as soon as the mothers try to rest.

Women usually detect fetal movements 16 to 20 weeks into the pregnancy; the fetus can be artificially set into total body motion by in utero stimulation of its ventral skin surfaces by the 14th week. The fetus may be able to hear by the 18th week, and it responds to loud noises with muscle contractions, movements, and an increased heart rate. A bright light flashed on the abdominal wall of the 20-week pregnant woman causes changes in fetal heart rate and position. The retinal structures begin to function at that time. Eyelids open at 7 months. Smell and taste develop then, and the fetus can respond to substances injected into the amniotic sac, such as contrast medium. Some reflexes present at birth exist in utero: the grasp reflex, which appears at 17 weeks; the Moro

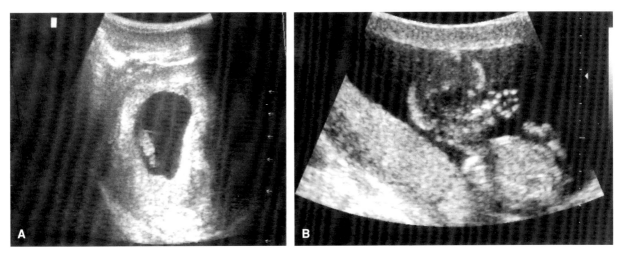

FIGURE 32-1
A: Sonogram of fetus at 9 weeks. **B:** Same fetus at 15 weeks. (Courtesy K.C. Attwell, M.D.)

(startle) reflex, which appears at 25 weeks; and the sucking reflex, which appears at about 28 weeks.

Nervous System.   The nervous system arises from the neural plate, which is a dorsal ectodermal thickening that appears on

about day 16 of gestation. By the sixth week, part of the neural tube becomes the cerebral vesicle, which later becomes the cerebral hemispheres (Fig. 32-2).

The cerebral cortex begins to develop by the 10th week, but layers do not appear until the sixth month of pregnancy; the sensory

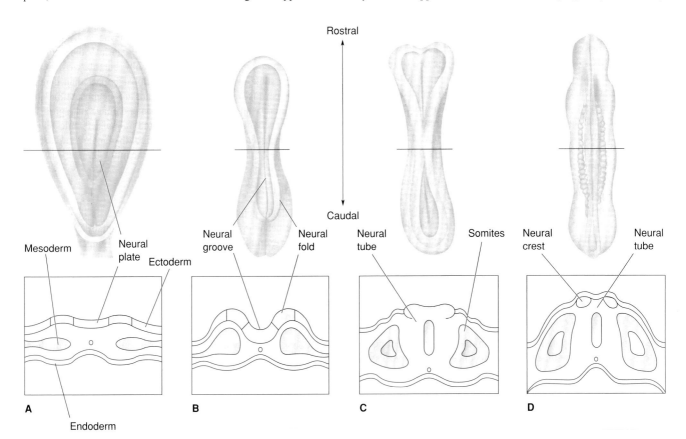

FIGURE 32-2
Formation of the neural tube and neural crest. These schematic illustrations follow the early development of the nervous system in the embryo. The drawings above are dorsal views of the embryo; those below are cross sections. **A:** The primitive embryonic central nervous system (CNS) begins as a thin sheet of ectoderm. **B:** The first important step in the development of the nervous system is the formation of the neural groove. **C:** The walls of the groove, called neural folds, come together and fuse, forming the neural tube. **D:** The bits of neural ectoderm that are pinched off when the tube rolls up are called the neural crest, from which the peripheral nervous system (PNS) will develop. The somites are mesoderm that will give rise to much of the skeletal system and the muscles. (Reprinted from Bear MF, Conners BW, Paradiso MA, eds. *Neuroscience: Exploring the Brain*. 2nd ed. Philadelphia, PA: Lippincott Williams & Wilkins; 2001:179, with permission.)

cortex and the motor cortex form before the association cortex. Some brain function has been detected in utero by fetal encephalographic responses to sound. The human brain weighs about 350 g at birth and 1,450 g at full adult development, a fourfold increase, mainly in the neocortex. This increase is almost entirely because of the growth in the number and branching of dendrites establishing new connections. After birth, the number of new neurons is negligible. Uterine contractions can contribute to fetal neural development by causing the developing neural network to receive and transmit sensory impulses.

Pruning.   Pruning refers to the programmed elimination during the development of neurons, synapses, axons, and other brain structures from the original number, present at birth, to a lesser number. Thus, the developing brain contains structures and cellular elements that are absent in the older brain. The fetal brain generates more neurons than it will need for adult life. For example, in the visual cortex, neurons increase in number from birth to 3 years of age, at which point they diminish in number. The adult brain contains fewer neural connections than were present during the early and middle years of childhood. About twice as many synapses are present in certain parts of the cerebral cortex during early postnatal life than during adulthood.

Pruning occurs to rid the nervous system of cells that have served their function in the development of the brain. Some neurons, for example, exist to produce neurotrophic or growth factors and are programmed to die once they complete their task, a process called *apoptosis.*

These observations imply that the immature brain can be vulnerable in locations that lack sensitivity to injury later on. The developing white matter of the human brain before 32 weeks of gestation is especially sensitive to damage from hypoxic and ischemic injury and metabolic insults. Neurotransmitter receptors located on synaptic terminals are subject to injury from excessive stimulation by excitatory amino acids, (e.g., glutamate, aspartate), a process referred to as excitotoxicity. This process may be relevant to the etiology of disorders such as schizophrenia.

Maternal Stress

Maternal stress correlates with high levels of stress hormones (epinephrine, norepinephrine, and adrenocorticotropic hormone) in the fetal bloodstream, which act directly on the fetal neuronal network to increase blood pressure, heart rate, and activity level. Mothers with high levels of anxiety are more likely to have babies who are hyperactive, irritable, and of low birth weight, and who have problems feeding and sleeping than are mothers with low anxiety levels. Fever in the mother causes the fetus's temperature to rise.

Genetic Disorders

In many cases, genetic counseling depends on prenatal diagnosis. The diagnostic techniques used include amniocentesis (transabdominal aspiration of fluid from the amniotic sac), ultrasound examinations, x-ray studies, fetoscopy (direct visualization of the fetus), fetal blood and skin sampling, chorionic villus sampling, and α-fetoprotein screening. In about 2 percent of women tested, the results are positive for some abnormality, including X-linked disorders, neural tube defects (detected by high levels of α-fetoprotein), chromosomal disorders (e.g., trisomy 21), and various inborn errors of metabolism (e.g., Tay–Sachs disease and the lipoidoses). Figure 32-3 illustrates hypertelorism of the eyes.

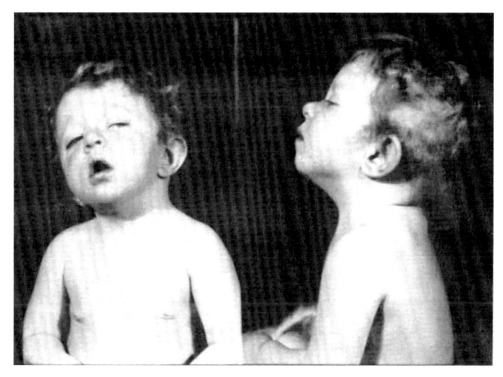

FIGURE 32-3
Hypertelorism. Note the wide distance between the eyes, flat nasal bridge, and external strabismus. (Courtesy of Michael Malone, M.D. Children's Hospital, Washington, DC.)

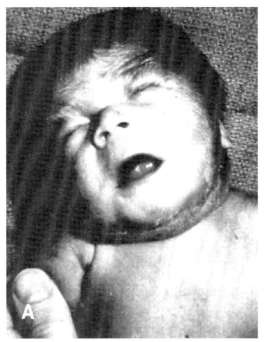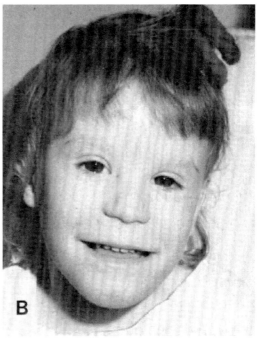

FIGURE 32-4
Photographs of children with "fetal-alcohol syndrome." **A:** Severe case. **B:** Slightly affected child. Note in both children the short palpebral fissures and hypoplasia of the maxilla. Usually, the defect includes other craniofacial abnormalities. Cardiovascular defects and limb deformities are also common symptoms of the fetal alcohol syndrome. (From Langman J. *Medical Embryology.* 7th ed. Philadelphia, PA: Williams & Wilkins; 1995:108, with permission.)

Some diagnostic tests carry a risk; for instance, about 5 percent of women who undergo fetoscopy miscarry. Amniocentesis, usually performed between the 14th and 16th weeks of pregnancy, causes fetal damage or miscarriage in less than 1 percent of women tested. Fully 98 percent of all prenatal tests in pregnant women reveal no abnormality in the fetus. Women older than 35 years of age and those with a family history of a congenital disability should have prenatal testing.

Parental reactions to congenital disabilities can include feelings of guilt, anxiety, or anger. The loss of the fantasized perfect child may cause depression. Some women may choose to terminate a pregnancy because of a known or suspected congenital malformation.

Maternal Drug Use

Alcohol.   Alcohol use in pregnancy is a significant cause of severe physical and mental congenital disabilities in children. Each year, up to 40,000 babies are born with some degree of alcohol-related damage. The National Institute on Drug Abuse (NIDA) reports that 19 percent of pregnant women used alcohol during their pregnancy, the highest rate being among white women.

Fetal alcohol syndrome (Fig. 32-4) affects about one-third of all infants born to alcoholic women. Table 32-1 lists the characteristics of the disorder. The incidence of infants born with fetal alcohol syndrome is about 0.5 per 1,000 live births.

Some studies suggest that alcohol use during pregnancy may also contribute to attention-deficit/hyperactivity disorder (ADHD).

Smoking.   Smoking during pregnancy may cause both premature births and below-average infant birth weight. Some reports have associated sudden infant death syndrome (SIDS) with mothers who smoke.

Other Substances.   Chronic marijuana use is associated with low infant birth weight, prematurity, and withdrawal-like symptoms, including excessive crying, tremors, and hyperemesis (severe and chronic vomiting). Crack cocaine use by women during pregnancy may cause behavioral abnormalities such as increased

 Table 32-1
Characteristics of Fetal Alcohol Syndrome

Growth retardation of prenatal origin (height, weight)
Facial Dysmorphism
   Microcephaly (head circumference below the third percentile)
   Hypertelorism (large distance between eyes)
   Microphthalmia (small eyeballs)
   Short palpebral fissures
   Inner epicanthal folds
   Midface hypoplasia (underdevelopment)
   Smooth or short philtrum
   Thin upper lip
   Short, turned up nose
Cardiac Defects
Central nervous system (CNS) manifestations
   Delayed development
   Hyperactivity
   Attention deficits
   Learning disabilities
   Intellectual deficits
   Seizures

Table 32-2
Causes of Human Malformations Observed During the First Year of Life

Suspected Cause	% of Total
Genetic	
Autosomal genetic disease	15–20
Cytogenic (chromosomal abnormalities)	5
Unknown	
Polygenic	
Multifactorial (genetic–environmental interactions)	
Spontaneous error of development	
Synergistic interactions of teratogens	
Environmental	
Maternal conditions: diabetes; endocrinopathies; nutritional deficiencies, starvation; drug and substance addictions	4
Maternal infections: rubella, toxoplasmosis, syphilis, herpes, cytomegalic inclusion disease, varicella, Venezuelan equine encephalitis, parvovirus B19	3
Mechanical problems (deformations): abnormal cord constrictions, disparity in uterine size and uterine contents	1–2
Chemicals, drugs, radiation, hyperthermia	<1
Preconception exposures (excluding mutagens and infectious agents)	<1

Reprinted from Brent RL, Beckman DA. Environmental teratogens. *Bull NY Acad Med.* 1990;66(2):123–163, with permission.

irritability and crying and decreased desire for human contact. Infants born to mothers dependent on narcotics go through a withdrawal syndrome at birth.

Prenatal exposure to various prescribed medications can also result in abnormalities. Common drugs with teratogenic effects include antibiotics (tetracyclines), anticonvulsants (valproate, carbamazepine, phenytoin), progesterone-estrogens, lithium, and warfarin. Table 32-2 outlines the etiologies of malformations that may emerge during the first year of life.

INFANCY

The average newborn weighs about 3,400 g (7.5 lb). Small fetuses (birth weight below the 10th percentile for their gestational age) occur in about 7 percent of all pregnancies. From the 26th to the 28th week of gestation, the prematurely born fetus has a good chance of survival. Arnold Gesell described developmental landmarks that are widely used in both pediatrics and child psychiatry. These landmarks outline the sequence of children's motor, adaptive, and personal–social behavior from birth to 6 years (Table 32-3).

Premature infants are born before 34 weeks or weigh less than 2,500 g (5.5 lb). Such infants are at increased risk for learning disabilities, such as dyslexia, emotional and behavioral problems, mental retardation, and child abuse. With each 100 g increment of weight, beginning at about 1,000 g (2.2 lb), infants have a progressively better chance of survival. A 36-week-old fetus has less chance of survival than a 3,000 g (6.6 lb) fetus born close to term. Figure 32-5 gives examples of some differences between full-term and premature infants.

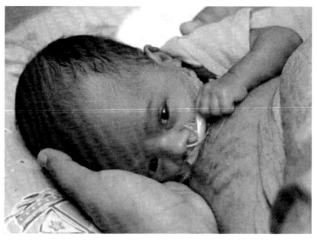

FIGURE 32-5
Premature baby at breast during a gavage feed. (Photo courtesy of Mike McCarter, Connecticut Children's Medical Center.)

Postmature infants are born 2 weeks or more beyond the expected date of birth. The incidence of postmaturity is high if based on menstrual history alone. The postmature baby typically has long nails, scanty lanugo, more scalp hair than usual, and increased alertness.

Developmental Milestones in Infants

Reflexes and Survival Systems at Birth. Primitive reflexes are present at birth. They include the rooting reflex (puckering of the lips in response to perioral stimulation), the grasp reflex, the plantar (Babinski) reflex, the knee reflex, the abdominal reflexes, the startle (Moro) reflex (Fig. 32-6), and the tonic neck reflex. In healthy children, the grasp reflex, the startle reflex, and the tonic neck reflex disappear by the fourth month. The Babinski reflex usually disappears by the 12th month.

Survival systems—breathing, sucking, swallowing, and circulatory and temperature homeostasis—are relatively functional

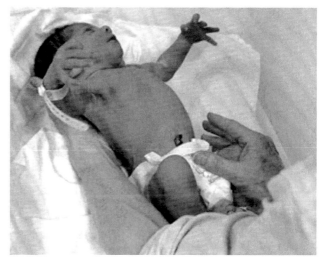

FIGURE 32-6
The Moro reflex. The head is allowed to fall backward. The arms abduct and extend.

Table 32-3
Landmarks of Normal Behavioral Development

Age	Motor and Sensory Behavior	Adaptive Behavior	Personal and Social Behavior
Birth to 4 wk	Hand-to-mouth reflex, grasping reflex Rooting reflex (puckering lips in response to perioral stimulation), Moro reflex (digital extension when startled), sucking reflex, Babinski reflex (toes spread when sole of foot is touched) Differentiates sounds (orients to human voice) and sweet and sour tastes Visual tracking Fixed focal distance of 8 in Makes alternating crawling movements Moves head laterally when placed in prone position	Anticipatory feeding-approach behavior at 4 days Responds to sound of rattle and bell Regards moving objects momentarily	Responsiveness to mother's face, eyes, and voice within first few hours of life Endogenous smile Independent play (until 2 yr) Quiets when picked up Impassive face
4 wk	Tonic neck reflex positions predominate Hands fisted Head sags but can hold head erect for a few seconds Visual fixation, stereoscopic vision (12 wk)	Follows moving objects to the midline Shows no interest and drops object immediately	Regards face and diminishes activity Responds to speech Smiles preferentially to mother
16 wk	Symmetrical postures predominate Holds head balanced Head lifted 90 degrees when prone on forearm Visual accommodation	Follows a slowly moving object well Arms activate on sight of dangling object	Spontaneous social smile (exogenous) Aware of strange situations
28 wk	Sits steadily, leaning forward on hands Bounces actively when placed in standing position	One-hand approach and grasp of toy Bangs and shakes rattle Transfers toys	Takes feet to mouth Pats mirror image Starts to imitate mother's sounds and actions
40 wk	Sits alone with good coordination Creeps Pulls self to standing position Points with index finger	Matches two objects at midline Attempts to imitate scribble	Separation anxiety manifest when taken away from mother Responds to social play, such as pat-a-cake and peek-a-boo Feeds self cracker and holds own bottle
52 wk	Walks with one hand held Stands alone briefly	Seeks novelty	Cooperates in dressing
15 mo	Toddles Creeps up stairs		Points or vocalizes wants Throws objects in play or refusal
18 mo	Coordinated walking, seldom falls Hurls ball Walks up stairs with one hand held	Builds a tower of three or four cubes Scribbles spontaneously and imitates a writing stroke	Feeds self in part, spills Pulls toy on string Carries or hugs a special toy, such as a doll Imitates some behavioral patterns with slight delay
2 yr	Runs well, no falling Kicks large ball Goes up and down stairs alone Fine motor skills increase	Builds a tower of six or seven cubes Aligns cubes, imitating train Imitates vertical and circular strokes Develops original behaviors	Pulls on simple garment Domestic mimicry Refers to self by name Says "no" to mother Separation anxiety begins to diminish Organized demonstrations of love and protest Parallel play (plays side by side but does not interact with other children)
3 yr	Rides tricycle Jumps from bottom steps Alternates feet going up stairs	Builds tower of 9 or 10 cubes Imitates a three-cube bridge Copies a circle and a cross	Puts on shoes Unbuttons buttons Feeds self well Understands taking turns
4 yr	Walks down stairs one step to a tread Stands on one foot for 5–8 s	Copies a cross Repeats four digits Counts three objects with correct pointing	Washes and dries own face Brushes teeth Associative or joint play (plays cooperatively with other children)
5 yr	Skips, using feet alternately Usually has complete sphincter control Fine coordination improves	Copies a square Draws a recognizable person with a head, a body, and limbs Counts 10 objects accurately	Dresses and undresses self Prints a few letters Plays competitive exercise games
6 yr	Rides two-wheel bicycle	Prints name Copies triangle	Ties shoelaces

Adapted from Arnold Gessell, M.D., Ph.D. and Stella Chess, M.D.

Table 32-4
Language Development

Age and Stage of Development	Mastery of Comprehension	Mastery of Expression
0–6 mo	Shows startle response to loud or sudden sounds; Attempts to localize sounds, turning eyes or head; Appears to listen to speakers, may respond with smile; Recognizes warning, angry, and friendly voices; Responds to hearing own name	Has vocalizations other than crying; Has differential cries for hunger, pain; Makes vocalizations to show pleasure; Plays at making sounds Babbles (a repeated series of sounds)
7–11 mo Attending-to-Language	Shows listening selectivity (voluntary control over responses to sounds); Listens to music or singing with interest; Recognizes "no," "hot," own name; Looks at pictures being named for up to 1 min; Listens to speech without being distracted by other sounds	Responds to own name with vocalizations; Imitates the melody of utterances; Uses jargon (own language); Has gestures (shakes head for no); Has exclamation ("oh-oh"); Plays language games (pat-a-cake, peekaboo)
12–18 mo Single-Word	Shows gross discriminations between dissimilar sounds (bells vs. dog vs. horn vs. mother's or father's voice); Understands basic body parts, names of common objects; Acquires understanding of some new words each week; Can identify simple objects (baby, ball, etc.) from a group of objects or pictures; Understands up to 150 words by age 18 mo	Uses single words (mean age of first word is 11 mo; by age 18 mo, child is using up to 20 words); "Talks" to toys, self, or others using long patterns of jargon and occasional words; Approximately 25% of utterances are intelligible; All vowels articulated correctly; Initial and final consonants often omitted
12–24 mo Two-Word Messages	Responds to simple directions ("Give me the ball") Responds to action commands ("Come here," "Sit down") Understands pronouns (me, him, her, you) Begins to understand complex sentences ("When we go to the store, I'll buy you some candy")	Uses two-word utterances ("Mommy sock," "all gone," "ball here"); Imitates environmental sounds in play ("moo," "mmm, mmm," etc.); Refers to self by name, begins to use pronouns; Echoes two or more last words of sentences; Begins to use three-word telegraphic utterances ("all gone ball," "me go now"); Utterances 26–50% intelligible; Uses language to ask for needs
24–36 mo Grammar Formation	Understands small body parts (elbow, chin, eyebrow); Understands family name categories (grandma, baby) Understands size (little one, big one) Understands most adjectives Understands functions (why do we eat, why do we sleep)	Uses real sentences with grammatical function words (can, will, the, a); Usually announces intentions before acting "Conversations" with other children, usually just monologues Jargon and echolalia gradually drop from speech Increased vocabulary (up to 270 words at 2 yr, 895 words at 3 yr); Speech 50–80% intelligible P, b, m articulated correctly; Speech may show rhythmic disturbances
36–54 mo Grammar Development	Understands prepositions (under, behind, between) Understands many words (up to 3,500 at 3 yr, 5,500 at 4 yr) Understands cause and effect (What do you do when you're hungry? cold?) Understands analogies (Food is to eat, milk is to ____)	Correct articulation of n, w, ng, h, t, d, k, g; Uses language to relate incidents from the past; Uses wide range of grammatical forms: plurals, past tense, negatives, questions; Plays with language: rhymes, exaggerates; Speech 90% intelligible, occasional errors in the ordering of sounds within words; Able to define words; Egocentric use of language rare; Can repeat a 12-syllable sentence correctly; Some grammatical errors still occur
55 mo on True Communication	Understands concepts of number, speed, time, space; Understands left and right; Understands abstract terms; Is able to categorize items into semantic classes	Uses language to tell stories, share ideas, and discuss alternatives; Increasing use of varied grammar; spontaneous self-correction of grammatical errors; Stabilizing of articulation f, v, s, z, l, r, th, and consonant clusters; Speech 100% intelligible

Reprinted from Rutter M, Hersov L, eds. *Child and Adolescent Psychiatry*. London: Blackwell; 1985, with permission.

at birth, but the sensory organs are still developing. Further differentiation of neurophysiologic functions depends on an active process of stimulatory reinforcement from the external environment, such as persons touching and stroking the infant. The newborn infant is awake for only a short period each day; rapid eye movement (REM) and non-REM sleep are present at birth. Other spontaneous behaviors include crying, smiling, and penile erection in males. Infants 1 day old can detect the smell of their mother's milk, and those 3 days old distinguish their mother's voice.

Language and Cognitive Development. At birth, infants can make noises, such as crying, but they do not vocalize until about 8 weeks. At that time, guttural or babbling sounds occur spontaneously, especially in response to the mother. The persistence and further evolution of children's vocalizations depend on parental reinforcement. Language development occurs in well-delineated stages, as outlined in Table 32-4.

By the end of infancy (about 2 years), infants have transformed reflexes into voluntary actions that are the building blocks of cognition. They begin to interact with the environment, to experience

Table 32-5
Piaget's Stages of Cognitive Development

Period of Development	Cognitive Spatial Stages and Associated Concepts	Cognitive Achievements
Gestational		Fetus can "learn" sounds and respond differentially to them after birth
Infancy: Birth–2 yr	**Sensorimotor**	Infants "think" with their eyes, ears, and senses
Birth–1 mo	Reflective; egocentric (newer research refutes this)	Newborns can learn to associate stroking with sucking
4–8 mo	Secondary circular: looks for objects partially hidden	Newborns can learn to suck to produce certain visual displays or music
8–12 mo	Secondary circulation coordinated: peek-a-boo, finds hidden objects	Can remember for 1-mo periods Can play with parent by looking for partially hidden objects
12–18 mo	Tertiary circular: explores properties and drops objects	Memory improves
18 mo–2 yr	Mental representation, make-believe play; memory of objects	Body parts used as objects Can stack one object within another Remembers hidden objects Drops objects over crib Knows animal sounds; names objects Knows body parts and familiar pictures Can understand causes not visible
Early Childhood: 2–7 yr 2–7 yr	**Preoperational** Egocentrism: "I want you to eat this too." Animistic: "I'm afraid of the moon." Lack of hierarchy: "Where do these blocks go?" Centration: "I want it now, not after dinner." Irreversibility: "I don't know how to go back to that room."	Preschoolers use symbols Development of language and make-believe No sign of logic 3-yr-olds can count 2–3 objects; know colors and age 4-yr-olds can fantasize without concrete props
2–5 yr	Transductive reasoning: "We have to go this way because that's the way Daddy goes."	5–6-yr-olds get humor; understand good and bad; can do some chores 7–11-yr-olds have good memory; recall; can solve problems
Middle Childhood: **7–11 yr**	**Concrete operational** Hierarchical classification—arranges cars by types Reversibility—can play games backward and forward (e.g., checkers, triple kings) Conservation—lose two dimes and look for same Decentration—worry about small details, obsessive Spatial operations—likes models for directions Horizontal decalage—conservation of weight, logic Transitive inference—syllogisms; compare everything, brand names important	Children begin to think logically Understand conservation of matter Frozen milk same amount as melted Can organize objects into hierarchies Children seem rational and organized
Adolescence: 11–19 yr 11 yr onward	**Formal operational** Hypothetical-deductive reasoning; adolescent quick thinking or excuses Imaginary audience—everyone is looking at them Personal fable—inflated opinion of themselves Propositional thinking—logic	Abstraction and reason Can think of all possibilities

feedback from their bodies, and to become intentional in their actions. By the end of the second year of life, children begin to use symbolic play and language.

Jean Piaget (1896–1980), a Swiss psychologist, observed the growing capacity of young children (including his own) to think and to reason. Table 32-5 outlines Piaget's stages of cognitive development.

Emotional and Social Development.   By the age of 3 weeks, infants imitate the facial movements of adult caregivers. They open their mouths and thrust out their tongues in response to adults who

do the same. By the third and fourth months of life, we can easily elicit these behaviors. These imitative behaviors are likely the precursors of the infant's emotional life. The smiling response occurs in two phases: the first phase is endogenous smiling, which occurs spontaneously within the first 2 months and is unrelated to external stimulation; the second phase is exogenous smiling, usually stimulated by the mother, and occurs by the 16th week.

The stages of emotional development parallel those of cognitive development. The caregiving person provides the primary stimulus for both aspects of mental growth. Human infants depend totally on adults for survival. Through warm and predictable interactions, an

Table 32-6
Emotional Development

Stages First Seen	Emotional Skills	Emotional Behavior
Gestational–Infancy: 0–2 yr		
0–2 mo onward	Love, evoked by touching	Social smile and joy shown
	Fear, evoked by loud noise	Responds to emotions of others
	Rage, evoked by body restrictions	All emotions there
	Brain pathways for emotion forming	
3–4 mo onward	Self-regulation of emotions starts; brain pathways of emotion growing	Laughter possible and more control over smiles; anger shown
7–12 mo	Self-regulation of emotion grows	Able to elicit more responsiveness
	Increased intensity of basic three	Denies to cope with stress
1–2 yr	Shame and pride appear; envy, embarrassment appear	Some indications of empathy starting; expressions of feeling: "I like you, Daddy" "I'm sorry"
	Displaces onto other children	Likes attention and approval; enjoys play alone or next to peers
Early Childhood: 2–5 yr		
3–6 yr	Can understand causes of many emotions	Empathy increases with understanding
	Can begin to find ways for regulating emotions and for expressing them Identifies with adult to cope	More response and less reaction; self-regulation: "Use your words to say that you are angry with him"
		Aggression becomes competition
		By age 5, shows sensitivity to criticism and cares about feelings of others
Middle Childhood: 5–11 yr		Ego rules until age 6
7–11 yr	Can react to the feelings of others	Empathy becomes altruism: "I feel so bad about their fire, I'm going to give them some of my things"
	More aware of other's feelings	Superego dominates

infant's social and emotional repertoire expands with the interplay of caregivers' social responses (Table 32-6).

In the first year, infants' moods are highly variable and intimately related to internal states such as hunger. Toward the second two-thirds of the first year, infants' moods grow increasingly related to external social cues; a parent can get even a hungry infant to smile. When the infant is internally comfortable, a sense of interest and pleasure in the world and its primary caregivers should prevail. Prolonged separation from the mother (or other primary caregivers) during the second 6 months of life can lead to depression that may persist into adulthood as part of an individual's character.

Temperamental Differences

Infants vary in their autonomic reactivity and temperament. Chess and Thomas identified nine behavioral dimensions in which reliable differences among infants can be observed (Table 32-7).

In studies of temperament, most temperamental dimensions of individual children remain stable through adulthood, but some do not persist. This is likely due to genetic and environmental effects on personality. A complex interplay exists among the initial characteristics of infants, the mode of parental interactions, and children's subsequent behavior. Observations of the stability and plasticity of certain temperamental traits support the importance of interactions between genetic endowment (nature) and environmental experience (nurture) in behavior.

Attachment

Bonding is the term used to describe the intense emotional and psychological relationship a mother develops for her baby. Attachment is the relationship the baby develops with its caregivers. Infants in

the first months after birth become attuned to social and interpersonal interaction. They show a rapidly increasing responsivity to the external environment and an ability to form a special relationship with significant primary caregivers—that is, to form an attachment. Table 32-8 lists the commonly observed attachment styles.

Harry Harlow. Harry Harlow studied social learning and the effects of social isolation on monkeys. Harlow placed newborn rhesus monkeys with two types of surrogate mothers—one a wire-mesh surrogate with a feeding bottle and the other a wire-mesh surrogate covered with terry cloth. The monkeys preferred

Table 32-7
Temperament—Newborn to 6 Years

Dimension	Description
Activity level	Percent of time spent in activities
Distractibility	Degree to which stimuli are allowed to alter behavior
Adaptability	Ease moving into change
Attention span	Amount of time spent on attending
Intensity	Energy level
Threshold of responsiveness	Intensity required for response
Quality of mood	Amount positive compared to amount negative behavior
Rhythmicity	Regulation of functions
Approach/withdrawal	Response to new situations

Table 32-8 Types of Attachment	
Secure Attachment	Children show fewer adjustment problems; however, these children have typically received more consistent and developmentally appropriate parenting for most of their life. The parents of securely attached children are likely better able to maintain these aspects of parenting through a divorce. Given that the family factors that lead to divorce also impact the children, there could be fewer securely attached children in divorcing families
Insecure/Avoidant Attachment	Children become anxious, clinging, and angry with the parent. These children typically come from families with adults who were also insecurely attached to their families and, thus, were unable to provide the kind of consistency, emotional responsiveness, and care that securely attached parents could offer. Such parents have a more difficult time with divorce, and are more likely to become rejecting.
Insecure/ Ambivalent Attachment	Children generally are raised with disorganized, neglecting, and inattentive parenting. The parents are even less able to provide stability and psychological strength for them after a divorce and, as a result, the children are even more likely to become clinging but inconsolable in their distress, as well as to act out, suffer mood swings, and become oversensitive to stress.

the terry-cloth surrogates, which provided contact and comfort, to the feeding surrogate. (When hungry, the infant monkeys would go to the feeding bottle but then would quickly return to the terry-cloth surrogate.) When frightened, monkeys raised with terry-cloth surrogates showed intense clinging behavior and appeared to be comforted, whereas those raised with wire-mesh surrogates gained no comfort and appeared to be disorganized. The results of Harlow's experiments suggest that infant attachment is not merely the result of feeding.

Both types of surrogate-reared monkeys were subsequently unable to adjust to life in a monkey colony and had extraordinary difficulty learning to mate. When impregnated, the female monkeys failed to mother their young.

John Bowlby.   John Bowlby studied the attachment of infants to mothers and concluded that early separation of infants from their mothers had severe adverse effects on children's emotional and intellectual development. He described attachment behavior, which develops during the first year of life, as the maintenance of physical contact between the mother and child when the child is hungry, frightened, or in distress.

Mary Ainsworth.   Mary Ainsworth expanded on Bowlby's observations and found that the interaction between mother and baby during the attachment period influences the baby's current and future behavior significantly. Many observers believe that patterns of infant attachment affect future adult emotional relationships. Patterns of attachment vary among babies; for example, some babies signal or cry less than others. Sensitive responsiveness to infant signals, such as cuddling the baby when it cries, causes

infants to cry less in later months. Close bodily contact with the mother when the baby signals for her fosters self-reliance, rather than clinging dependence. Unresponsive mothers produce anxious babies.

Ainsworth also confirmed that attachment serves to reduce anxiety. What she called the secured base effect enables a child to move away from the attachment figure and explore the environment. Inanimate objects, such as a teddy bear or a blanket (called the transitional object by Donald Winnicott), also serve as a secure base, one that often accompanies children as they investigate the world. A growing body of literature derived from direct observation of mother–infant interactions and longitudinal studies has expanded on and refined Ainsworth's original descriptions. Maternal sensitivity and responsiveness are the main determinants of secure attachment. However, when the attachment is insecure, the type of insecurity (avoidant, anxious, or ambivalent) is determined by infant temperament. Overall, male infants are less likely to have secure attachments and are more vulnerable to changes in maternal sensitivity than are female infants.

The birth of a second child decreases the attachment of the firstborn child. This decrease is most notable when the firstborn is 2 to 5 years of age as opposed to younger. Not surprisingly, the extent of the decrease also depends on the mother's sense of security, confidence, and mental health.

Social Deprivation Syndromes and Maternal Neglect. Investigators, especially René Spitz, have long documented the severe developmental retardation that accompanies maternal rejection and neglect. Infants in institutions characterized by low staff-to-infant ratios and frequent turnover of personnel tend to display marked developmental retardation, even with adequate physical care and freedom from infection. The same infants, placed in adequate foster or adoptive care, exhibit marked acceleration in development.

Fathers and Attachment.   Babies become attached to fathers as well as to mothers, but the attachment is different. Generally, mothers hold babies for caregiving, and fathers hold babies for purposes of play. Given a choice of either parent after separation, infants usually go to the mother, but if the mother is unavailable, they turn to the father for comfort. Babies raised in extended families or with multiple caregivers can establish many attachments.

Stranger Anxiety.   A developmentally expected fear of strangers first appears in infants at about 26 weeks of age and is more fully developed by 32 weeks. At the approach of a stranger, infants cry and cling to their mothers. Babies exposed to only one caregiver are more likely to have stranger anxiety than babies exposed to a variety of caregivers. Stranger anxiety likely results from a baby's growing ability to distinguish caregivers from all other persons.

Separation anxiety, which occurs between 10 and 18 months of age, is related to stranger anxiety but is not identical to it. Separation from the person to whom the infant is attached precipitates separation anxiety. Stranger anxiety, however, occurs even when the infant is in the mother's arms. The infant learns to separate as it starts to crawl and move away from the mother, but the infant continually looks back and frequently returns to the mother for reassurance.

Margaret Mahler (1897–1985) proposed a theory to describe how young children acquire a sense of identity separate from that of their mothers'. Her observations of children and their mothers lead to her theory of separation-individuation. Table 32-9 lists Mahler's stages of separation-individuation.

Table 32-9
Stages of Separation-Individuation Proposed by Mahler

1. Normal autism (birth–2 mo)
   Periods of sleep outweigh periods of arousal in a state reminiscent of intrauterine life.
2. Symbiosis (2–5 mo)
   Developing perceptual abilities gradually enable infants to distinguish the inner from the outer world; mother–infant is perceived as a single fused entity.
3. Differentiation (5–10 mo)
   Progressive neurologic development and increased alertness draw infants' attention away from self to the outer world. Physical and psychological distinctiveness from the mother is gradually appreciated.
4. Practicing (10–18 mo)
   The ability to move autonomously increases children's exploration of the outer world.
5. Rapprochement (18–24 mo)
   As children slowly realize their helplessness and dependence, the need for independence alternates with the need for closeness. Children move away from their mothers and come back for reassurance.
6. Object constancy (2–5 yr)
   Children gradually comprehend and are reassured by the permanence of mother and other important people, even when not in their presence.

Infant Care

Clinicians are now beginning to view infants as important actors in the family drama, ones who partly determine its course. Infants' behavior controls mothers' behavior, just as mothers' behavior modulates infants' behavior. A calm, smiling, predictable infant is a powerful reward for tender maternal care. A jittery, irregular, irritable infant tries a mother's patience. When a mother's capacity for giving is marginal, such infant traits may cause her to turn away from her child and thus complicate the child's already-troubled beginnings.

Parental Fit

Parental fit describes how well the mother or father relates to the newborn or developing infant; the idea takes into account the temperamental characteristics of both parent and child. Each newborn has innate psychophysiological characteristics, which are known collectively as temperament. Chess and Thomas identified a range of standard temperamental patterns, from the difficult child at one end of the spectrum to the easy child at the other end.

Difficult children, who make up 10 percent of all children, have a hyperalert physiologic makeup. They overreact to stimuli (cry easily at loud noises), sleep poorly, eat at unpredictable times, and are difficult to comfort. Easy children, who make up 40 percent of all children, are regular in eating, eliminating, and sleeping; they are flexible, can adapt to change and new stimuli with a minimum of distress, and are easily comforted when they cry. The other 50 percent of children are mixtures of these two types. The difficult child is harder to raise and places higher demands on the parent than the easy child. Chess and Thomas used the term *goodness of fit* to characterize the harmonious and consonant interaction between a mother and a child in their motivations, capacities, and styles of behavior. Poor fit is likely to lead to distorted development and maladaptive functioning. A difficult child must be recognized because parents of such infants often have feelings of inadequacy and believe that they are doing something wrong to account for the child's difficulty in sleeping and eating and their problems

comforting the child. Also, most difficult children have emotional disturbances later in life.

Good-Enough Mothering. Winnicott believed that infants begin life in a state of nonintegration, with unconnected and diffuse experiences, and that mothers provide the relationship that enables infants' incipient selves to emerge. Mothers supply a holding environment in which infants are contained and experienced. During the last trimester of pregnancy and for the first few months of a baby's life, the mother is in a state of primary maternal preoccupation, absorbed in fantasies about, and experiences with, her baby. The mother need not be perfect, but she must provide good-enough mothering. She plays a vital role in bringing the world to the child and offering empathic anticipation of the infant's needs. If the mother can resonate with the infant's needs, the baby can become attuned to its bodily functions and drives that are the basis for the gradually evolving sense of self.

TODDLER PERIOD

Accelerated motor and intellectual development occur in the second year. The ability to walk gives toddlers some control over their actions; this mobility enables children to determine when to approach and when to withdraw. The acquisition of speech profoundly extends their horizons. Typically, children learn to say "no" before they learn to say "yes." Toddlers' negativism is vital to the development of independence, but if it persists, oppositional behavior connotes a problem.

Learning language is a crucial task in the toddler period. Vocalizations become distinct, and toddlers can name a few objects and make needs known in one or two words. Near the end of the second year and into the third year, toddlers sometimes use short sentences. The pace of language development varies considerably from child to child, and although a small number of children are genuinely late developers, most child experts recommend a hearing test if the child is not making two-word sentences by age 2.

Developmental Milestones in Toddlers

Language and Cognitive Development. Toddlers begin to listen to explanations that can help them tolerate delay. They create new behaviors from old ones (originality) and engage in symbolic activities, for instance, using words and playing with dolls when the dolls represent something, such as a feeding sequence. Toddlers have varied capacities for concentration and self-regulation.

Emotional and Social Development. In the second year, pleasure and displeasure become further differentiated. Social referencing is often apparent at this age; the child looks to parents and others for emotional cues about how to respond to novel events. Toddlers show exploratory excitement, assertive pleasure, and pleasure in discovery and in developing new behavior (e.g., new games), including teasing and surprising or fooling the parent (e.g., hiding). The toddler has capacities for an organized demonstration of love, as when the toddler runs up and hugs, smiles, and kisses the parent at the same time, and of protest when the toddler turns away, cries, bangs, bites, hits, yells, and kicks. Comfort with family and apprehension with strangers may increase. Anxiety appears to be related to disapproval and the loss of a loved caregiver and can be disorganizing.

Sexual Development. Sexual differentiation is evident from birth when parents start dressing and treating infants differently because of the expectations evoked by sex typing. Through imitation, reward, and coercion, children assume the behaviors that their cultures define as appropriate for their sexual roles. Children exhibit curiosity about anatomical sex. When their curiosity is recognized as healthy and elicits age-appropriate replies, children acquire a sense of the wonder of life and are comfortable with their roles. If the subject of sex is taboo and parents rebuff children's questions, shame and discomfort may result.

Gender identity, the conviction of being male or female, begins to manifest at 18 months of age and is often fixed by 24 to 30 months. It was once widely believed that gender identity was primarily a function of social learning. John Money reported on children with ambiguous or damaged external genitalia who were raised as the sex opposite to their chromosomal sex. Long-term follow-up of those individuals suggests that the major part of gender identity is innate and that rearing may not affect the genetic diathesis.

Gender role describes the behavior that society deems appropriate for one sex or another, and it is not surprising that significant cultural differences exist. There may be different expectations for boys and girls in what and with whom they play, their tone of voice, the expression of emotions, and how they dress. Nevertheless, some generalizations are possible. Boys are more likely than girls to engage in rough and tumble play. Mothers talk more to girls than to boys, and by the time the child is 2 years of age, fathers generally pay more attention to boys. Many educated, middle-class parents determined to raise nonsexist children are startled to see their children's determined preference for sex-stereotyped toys: girls want to play with dolls and boys with guns.

Toilet Training.   The second year of life is a period of increasing social demands on children. Toilet training serves as a paradigm of the family's general training practices; that is, the parent who is overly severe in the area of toilet training is likely to be punitive and restrictive in other areas also. Control of daytime urination is usually complete by the age of 2½, and control of nighttime urination is usually complete by the age of 4 years. Since 1900, the pendulum has swung between extremes of permissiveness and control in toilet training. The trend in the United States has been toward delayed training, but in the last few years, this trend appears to be shifting back to early training.

Toddlers may have sleep difficulties related to fear of the dark, which may be helped with a nightlight. Most toddlers generally sleep about 12 hours a day, including a 2-hour nap. Parents must be aware that children of this age may need reassurance before going to bed and that the average 2-year-old takes about 30 minutes to fall asleep.

Parenting Challenges.   In infancy, the primary responsibility for parents is to meet the infant's needs sensitively and consistently. The parental task in the toddler stage requires firmness about the boundaries of acceptable behavior and encouragement of the child's progressive emancipation. Parents must be careful not to be too authoritarian at this stage; children must be allowed to operate for themselves and to learn from their mistakes and must be protected and assisted when challenges are beyond their abilities.

During the toddler period, children are likely to struggle for the exclusive affection and attention of their parents. They may compete with siblings or one or another parent for the starring role in the family. Although children are beginning to be able to share, they do so reluctantly. When the demands for exclusive possession are not resolved effectively, the result is likely to be jealous competitiveness in relationships with peers and lovers. The fantasies aroused by the struggle lead to fear of retaliation and displacement of fear onto external objects. In an equitable, loving family, a child elaborates on a moral system of ethical rights. Parents need to balance between punishment and permissiveness and set realistic limits on a toddler's behavior.

PRESCHOOL PERIOD

Marked physical and emotional growth occurs during the preschool period. Generally, between 2 and 3 years of age, children reach half their adult height. The 20 baby teeth are in place at the beginning of the stage, and by the end, they begin to fall out. Children are ready to enter school by the time the stage ends at age 5 or 6. They have mastered the tasks of primary socialization—to control their bowels and urine, to dress and feed themselves, and to control their tears and temper outbursts, at least most of the time.

The term preschool for the age group of 2½ to 6 years may be a misnomer; many children are already in school-like settings, such as preschool nurseries and daycare centers, where working mothers must often place their children. Preschool education can be valuable, but stressing academic advancement too far beyond a child's capabilities can be counterproductive.

Developmental Milestones in Preschoolers

Language and Cognitive Development.   In the preschool period, children's use of language expands, and they use sentences. Individual words have regular and consistent meanings at the beginning of the period, and children begin to think symbolically. In general, however, their thinking is egocentric; they cannot place themselves in the position of another child and are incapable of empathy. Children think intuitively and prelogically and do not understand causal relations.

Emotional and Social Behavior.   At the start of the preschool period, children can express such complex emotions as love, unhappiness, jealousy, and envy, both preverbally and verbally. Their emotions are still easily influenced by somatic events, such as tiredness and hunger. Although they still think mostly egocentrically, children's capacity for cooperation and sharing is emerging. Various losses, such as of a loved person or approval, may cause anxiety. Although still potentially disorganizing, preschool children can tolerate anxiety better than when they were younger. Four-year-olds are learning to share and to have concern for others and may express feelings of tenderness.

By the end of the preschool period, children have many relatively stable emotions. The child balances expansiveness, curiosity, pride, and gleeful excitement related to the self and the family with coyness, shyness, fearfulness, jealousy, and envy. Shame and humiliation are evident. Capacities for empathy and love are developed but are fragile and quickly lost if competitive or jealous strivings intervene. Anxiety and fears are related to bodily injury and loss of respect, love, and emerging self-esteem. Guilt feelings are possible.

Children between the ages of 3 and 6 years are aware of their bodies and differences between the sexes. Their physical awareness extends beyond genitalia. Children may be preoccupied with illness or injury, and some call this the "the Band-Aid phase." Every injury must be examined and taken care of by a parent.

Children develop a division between what they want and what others tell them to do. The division increases until a gap grows between their set of expanded desires, their exuberance at unlimited growth, and their parents' restrictions; they gradually turn parental values into self-obedience, self-guidance, and self-punishment.

At the end of the preschool stage, the child's conscience is evolving. The development of a conscience sets the tone for the moral sense of "right and wrong." Until about 7 years of age, children typically experience rules as "absolute" and as existing for their own sake. They do not understand that more than one point of view on a moral issue may exist; a violation of the rules calls for absolute retribution—that is, children have the notion of immanent justice.

SIBLING RIVALRY. In the preschool period, children relate to others in new ways. The birth of a sibling (a common occurrence during this time) tests a preschool child's capacity for further cooperation and sharing but may also evoke sibling rivalry, which is most likely to occur at this time. Sibling rivalry depends on child-rearing practice. Favoritism, for any reason, commonly aggravates such rivalry. Children who get special treatment because they are gifted, are defective in some way, or have a preferred gender are likely to receive angry feelings from their siblings. Experiences with siblings can influence growing children's relationships with peers and authority; for example, a problem may result if the needs of a new baby prevent the mother from attending to a firstborn child's needs. If not handled properly, the displacement of the firstborn can be a traumatic event.

PLAY. In the preschool years, children begin to distinguish reality from fantasy, and play reflects this growing awareness. Pretend games are popular and playfully help test real-life situations. Dramatic play in which children act out a role is typical. One-to-one play relationships advance to complicated patterns with rivalries, secrets, and two-against-one intrigues. Children's play behavior reflects their level of social development.

Between 2½ and 3 years, children commonly engage in parallel play, solitary play alongside another child with no interaction between them. By age 3, play is often associative, that is, playing with the same toys in pairs or small groups, but still with no real interaction among them. By age 4, children are usually able to share and engage in cooperative play. Real interactions and taking turns become possible.

Between 3 and 6 years of age, drawings may trace growth. A child's first drawing of a human being is a circular line with marks for the mouth, nose, and eyes; they add ears and hair later; arms and stick-like fingers appear next, and then legs appear. Last to appear is a torso in proportion to the rest of the body. Intelligent children can deal with details in their art. Drawings express creativity throughout a child's development: They are representational and formal in early childhood, make use of perspective in middle childhood, and become abstract and affect-laden in adolescence. Drawings also reflect children's body image concepts and sexual and aggressive impulses.

IMAGINARY COMPANIONS. Imaginary companions most often appear during preschool years, usually in children with above-average intelligence and usually in the form of persons. Imaginary companions may also be things, such as anthropomorphized toys. Some studies suggest that up to 50 percent of children between the ages of 3 and 10 years have imaginary companions at one time or another. Their significance is not clear, but these figures are usually friendly, relieve loneliness, and reduce anxiety. In most instances, imaginary companions disappear by age 12, but they can occasionally persist into adulthood.

MIDDLE YEARS

The period between age 6 and puberty is the middle years. During this time, children enter elementary school. The formal demands for academic learning and accomplishment become significant determinants of further personality development.

Developmental Milestones in School-Age Children

Language and Cognitive Development. In the middle years, language expresses complex ideas with relations among several elements. Logical exploration tends to dominate fantasy, and children show an increased interest in rules and orderliness and an increased capacity for self-regulation. During this period, children's conceptual skills develop, and thinking becomes organized and logical. The ability to concentrate is well established by age 9 or 10, and by the end of the period, children begin to think in abstract terms. Improved gross motor coordination and muscle strength enable children to write fluently and draw artistically. They are also capable of complex motor tasks and activities, such as tennis, gymnastics, golf, baseball, and skateboarding.

Recent evidence has shown that changes in thinking and reasoning during the middle years result from maturational changes in the brain. Children are now capable of increased independence, learning, and socialization. Theorists consider moral development a gradual, stepwise process spanning childhood, adolescence, and young adulthood.

In the middle years, both girls and boys make new identifications with other adults, such as teachers and counselors. These identifications may so influence girls that their goals of wanting to marry and have babies, as their mothers did, may be combined with a desire for a career or may be postponed or abandoned entirely.

Girls who cannot identify with their mothers or whose fathers are overly attached may become fixated at about a 6-year-old level; as a result, they may fear men or women or both or become seductively close to them. A similar situation can occur in boys who have been unable to identify successfully with fathers who were aloof, brutal, or absent. As a result, boys may enter this period with a variety of problems. They may be fearful of men, unsure of their sense of masculinity, or unwilling to leave their mothers (sometimes manifested by a school phobia); they may lack initiative and be unable to master school tasks, thus incurring academic problems.

The school-age period is a time when peer interaction assumes significant importance. Interest in relationships outside the family takes precedence over those within the family. Nevertheless, a special relationship exists with the same-sex parent, with whom children identify and who is now an ideal and a role model.

Empathy and concern for others begin to emerge early in the middle years; by the time children are 9 or 10, they have well-developed capacities for love, compassion, and sharing. They have a capacity for long-term, stable relationships with family, peers, and friends, including best friends. Emotions about sexual differences begin to emerge as either excitement or shyness with the opposite sex. School-age children prefer to interact with children of the same sex. Although the middle years have sometimes been referred to as a latency period—a moratorium on psychosexual exploration and play until the eruption of sexual impulses with puberty—it is now recognized that a considerable amount of sexual interest continues through these years. Sex play and curiosity are typical, especially among boys, but also among girls. Boys compare genitals and sometimes engage in group or mutual masturbation. Interest in anal humor and toilet jokes is also typical. Children this age often start using sexual and excretory words as expletives.

BEST FRIEND. Harry Stack Sullivan postulated that a buddy, or best friend, is an influential phenomenon during the school years. By about 10 years of age, children develop a close same-sex relationship, which Sullivan believed is necessary for further healthy psychological growth. Moreover, Sullivan believed that the absence of a close friend during the middle years of childhood is an early harbinger of schizophrenia.

SCHOOL REFUSAL. Some children refuse to go to school at this time, generally because of separation anxiety. A fearful mother may transmit her fear of separation to a child, or a child who has not resolved dependence needs panics at the idea of separation. School refusal is usually not an isolated problem; children with the problem typically avoid many other social situations.

Sex Role Development

Persons' sex roles are similar to their gender identity; persons see themselves as male or female. The sex-role also involves identification with culturally acceptable masculine or feminine ways of behaving, but changing expectations in society (particularly in the United States) of what constitutes masculine and feminine behavior can create ambiguity.

Parents react differently to their male and female children. Independence, physical play, and aggressiveness are encouraged in boys; dependence, verbalization, and physical intimacy are encouraged in girls. Nowadays, however, boys are encouraged to verbalize their feelings and to pursue interests traditionally associated with girls, whereas girls are encouraged to pursue careers traditionally dominated by men and to participate in competitive sports. As society grows more tolerant in its expectations of the sexes, roles become less rigid, and opportunities for boys and girls enlarge and broaden.

Biologically, boys are more physically aggressive than girls; and parental expectations, particularly the expectations of fathers, reinforce this trait. Differences also exist between boys and girls in the influence of persons outside the family. Girls tend to respond to the expectations and opinions of girls and teachers of either sex but to ignore boys. Boys, on the other hand, tend to respond to other boys but to ignore girls and teachers.

Dreams and Sleep

Children's dreams can have a profound effect on behavior. During the first year of life, when reality and fantasy are not yet fully differentiated, dreams may be experienced as if they were, or could be, real. At age 3, many children believe dreams are shared directly by more than one person, but most 4-year-olds understand that dreams are unique to each person. Children view dreams either with pleasure or, as is most often reported, with fear. The dream content depends on the children's life experience, developmental stage, mechanisms used during dreaming, and sex.

Disturbing dreams are most common when children are 3, 6, and 10 years of age. Two-year-old children may dream about being bitten or chased; at the age of 4, they may have many animal dreams and also dream of persons who either protect or destroy. At age 5 or 6, dreams of being killed or injured, of flying and being in cars, and of ghosts become prominent; the role of conscience, moral values, and increasing conflicts are concerned with these themes. In early childhood, aggressive dreams rarely seem to occur; instead, dreamers are

in danger, a state that perhaps reflects children's dependent position. By about the age of 5, children realize that their dreams are not real; before then, they believed them to be real events. By age 7, children know that they create their dreams themselves.

Between the ages of 3 and 6 years, children usually want to keep their bedroom door open or to have a nightlight, so that they can either maintain contact with their parents or view the room in a realistic, nonfearful way. At times, children resist going to sleep to avoid dreaming. Disorders associated with falling asleep, therefore, are often connected with dreaming. Children often create rituals to protect themselves in the withdrawal from the world of reality into the world of sleep. Parasomnias, such as sleepwalking, sleep talking, enuresis (bed-wetting), and night terrors, are common at this age. They usually occur during stage 4 sleep when dreaming is minimal, and they do not indicate emotional trouble or underlying psychopathology. Most children grow out of parasomnias by adolescence.

Periods of REM occur about 60 percent of the time during the first few weeks of life, a period when infants sleep two-thirds of the time. Premature babies sleep even longer than full-term babies, and a higher proportion of their sleep is REM sleep. The sleep-wake cycle of newborns is about 3 hours long. Adults spend about 20 percent of sleep dreaming. Even newborns have brain activity similar to that of the dreaming state.

Birth Spacing

For women in the United States, 10 percent of conceptions that lead to live births are considered unwanted, and 20 percent are wanted but considered ill-timed.

Children born close together have higher rates of premature or underweight births and malnutrition; they develop more slowly and are at increased risk of contracting and dying from childhood infectious diseases. Studies have shown that a mother and child's health risks are reduced when the child is born 3 to 5 years after a previous birth. Compared with 24- to 29-month intervals, children born in 36- to 41-month intervals have a 28 percent reduction in stunting and a 29 percent reduction of low birth weight. Women who have children at 27- to 32-month intervals are 1.3 times more likely to avoid anemia, 1.7 times more likely to avoid third-trimester bleeding, and 2.5 times more likely to survive childbirth.

Birth Order

The effects of birth order vary. Firstborn children may be more highly valued or given more attention than subsequent children. Firstborn children appear to be more achievement-oriented and motivated to please their parents than subsequent children born to the same parents. Some studies show that people in certain competitive occupational areas, such as architecture, accounting, and engineering, tend to be firstborn children.

Second and third children have the advantage of their parents' previous experience. Younger children also learn from their older siblings. For example, they may show a more sophisticated use of pronouns at an earlier age than firstborns did. When spacing children too tightly, however, there may not be enough time for each child. The arrival of new children in the family affects not only the parents but also the siblings. Firstborn children may resent the birth of a new sibling, who threatens their sole claim on parental attention. In some cases, regressive behavior, such as enuresis or thumb-sucking, occurs.

Some researchers have suggested that there is a relationship between birth order and personality. However, extensive multicohort analyses have not supported this.

Children and Divorce

Many children live in homes in which divorce has occurred. Approximately 30 to 50 percent of all children in the United States live in homes in which one parent (usually the mother) is the sole head of the household, and 61 percent of all children born in any given year can expect to live with only one parent before they reach the age of 18 years. A child's age at the time of the parents' divorce affects the child's reaction to the divorce. Immediately after a divorce, an increase in behavioral and emotional disorders appears in all age groups. Infants do not understand anything about separation or divorce; however, they do notice changes in their parents' responses to them and may experience changes in their eating or sleeping patterns; have bowel problems; and seem more fretful, fearful, or anxious. Children 3 to 6 years of age may not understand what is happening, and those who do understand often assume that they are somehow responsible for the divorce. Older children, especially adolescents, comprehend the situation and may believe that they could have prevented the divorce had they intervened in some way, but they are still hurt, angry, and critical of their parents' behavior.

Some children harbor the fantasy that their parents will reunite. Such children may show animosity toward a parent's real or potential new mate. Adaptation to the effects of divorce in children typically takes several years; however, up to about one-third of children from divorced homes may have lasting psychological trauma. Among boys, physical aggression is a common sign of distress. Adolescents tend to spend more time away from the parental home after the divorce. Children who adapt best to divorce are typically in a situation in which both parents make genuine efforts to spend time and relate to the child despite the child's potential anger about the divorce. The pre-divorce stability of the household is another influence, as are economic factors. To facilitate adaptation in children, a divorced couple who are amicable and avoid arguing with one another is most likely to succeed. Table 32-10 lists the potential psychological effects of divorce on children.

Table 32-10
Effects of Divorce on Children

- Children in homes with absent fathers are more likely to suffer from antisocial personality disorder, child conduct disorder, and attention-deficit hyperactivity disorder.
- The divorce rate of children of divorced parents doubles that of children from stable families.
- Children of divorce are far more likely to be delinquent, engage in premarital sex, and bear children out of wedlock during adolescence and young adulthood.
- Children from divorced homes function more poorly than children from continuously married parents across a variety of domains, including academic achievement, social relations, and conduct problems.
- Children from divorced homes have more psychological problems than those from homes disrupted by the death of a parent.
- Children from disrupted marriages experience greater risk of injury, asthma, headaches, and speech defects than children from intact families.
- Children of divorce tend to be impulsive, irritable, socially withdrawn, lonely, unhappy, anxious, and insecure.
- Children of divorce, especially boys, are more aggressive than children whose parents stayed married.
- Suicide rates for children of divorce are much higher than for children from intact families.
- Twenty to 25% have significant adjustment problems as teenagers

Data adapted from Americans for Divorce Reform, Arlington, Virginia. Table by Nitza Jones.

Table 32-11
Types of Step-Families

Neo-Traditional Families	• Resembles "traditional" families • Absent biologic parent is included at times. • Discipline, boundaries and limits, and expectations are discussed openly. • Family coalitions and "side-taking" are better avoided.
Romantic Families	• Expect to be a "traditional family" immediately • The absent biologic parent is expected to disappear and is often criticized. • Stepparent/stepchild difficulties are common. • Stress is unbearable. • Few open and frank discussions about problems
Matriarchal Families	• Run by a highly competent mom and her companion follows • Companion is a "buddy" to the children, not to the parent. • Birth of a step-sibling causes problems.

Stepparents.   Although many possible scenarios that may occur after a divorce and remarriage, several potential scenarios have been outlined in Table 32-11. These include (1) Neo-traditional, (2) Romantic, and (3) Matriarchal. When remarriage occurs, children must learn to adapt to the stepparent and the "blended" family. Adaptation is often challenging, especially when a child feels that a stepparent is nonsupportive, resents the stepchild, or favors his or her natural children. Of step-families, 25 percent tend to dissolve within the first 2 years, whereas 75 percent grow to find a new balance in their blended family. A biologic child born to a new couple with a stepchild already in the home may receive more attention than the stepchild, leading to sibling rivalry. After 5 years, about 20 percent of adolescents in step-families suggest that they move out and try living with their other biologic parent.

Family Factors in Child Development

Family Stability.   Parents and children living under the same roof in harmonious interaction is the expected cultural norm in Western society. Within this framework, childhood development presumably proceeds most expeditiously. Deviations from the norm, such as divorced- and single-parent families, are associated with a broad range of problems in children, including low self-esteem, increased risk of child abuse, and increased incidence of divorce when they eventually marry, and increased incidence of mental disorders, particularly depressive disorders and antisocial personality disorder as adults. Why some children from unstable homes are less affected than others (or even immune to these deleterious effects) is of great interest. Michael Rutter postulates that sex (boys are more affected than girls), age (older children are less vulnerable than younger ones), and inborn personality characteristics influence vulnerability. For example, children who have a placid temperament are less likely to be victims of abuse within a family than are hyperactive children; they may be less affected by the emotional turmoil surrounding them.

Adverse Events.   It is now well known that significant adverse events, especially in early childhood, such as sexual and physical abuse, neglect, or loss of a parent, interact with genetic background in a given child and influences the trajectory of development. For example, as mentioned earlier, early severe maltreatment such as sexual abuse increases the risk of multiple psychosocial difficulties and the emergence of many psychiatric disorders. Among young maltreated children, those with particular genetics, that is, who have the "short" variant of the serotonin transporter gene (short 5-HTTLPR polymorphism), may be more vulnerable to chronic depression in adulthood. This example of specific gene–environment interaction plays a vital role in a child's development as well as in the risk for future psychopathology. Current investigations are also seeking insight into what factors lead to resilience in youth exposed to adverse events, yet maintain allostasis, that is, stability in the face of stressful events. Hormones of the adrenal glands, thyroid, gonads, as well as metabolic hormones, play a role in the brain's ability to maintain stability upon exposure to stress, and the prefrontal cortex, hippocampus, and amygdala play critical roles in regulating emotionality, aggression, and resilience.

Daycare Centers. The role of daycare centers for children is under continuous investigation, and various studies have produced different results. One study found that children placed in daycare centers before the age of 5 are less assertive and less adequately toilet trained than home-reared children. Another study found that children in daycare to be more advanced in social and cognitive development than children who were not in daycare. The National Institute of Child Health and Human Development reported that 4½-year-olds who had spent more than 30 hours a week in child care were more demanding, more aggressive, and more noncompliant than those raised at home and showed higher cognitive skills, particularly in math and reading. These same children continued to score higher in math and reading skills but had more poor work habits and social skills in third grade. The researchers were careful to note that this behavior was within the normal range, however.

All studies of daycare must take into account the quality of both the daycare center and the homes from which children come. For example, a child from a disadvantaged home may be better off at a daycare center than a child from an advantaged home. Similarly, a woman who wishes to leave home to work for financial or other reasons and cannot do so may resent remaining in the home in a child-rearing role, which may adversely affect the child.

Parenting Styles. How children are raised, vary considerably between and within cultures. Rutter has clustered this diversity into four general styles. Subsequent research has confirmed that certain styles tend to correlate with particular behavior in the children, although the outcomes are by no means absolute. The authoritarian style, characterized by strict, inflexible rules, can lead to low self-esteem, unhappiness, and social withdrawal. The indulgent-permissive style, which includes little or no limit setting coupled with unpredictable parental harshness, can lead to low self-reliance, poor impulse control, and aggression. The indulgent-neglectful style, one of noninvolvement in the child's life and rearing, puts the child at risk for low self-esteem, impaired self-control, and increased aggression. The authoritative-reciprocal style, marked by firm rules and shared decision-making in a warm, loving environment, is believed to be the style most likely to result in self-reliance, self-esteem, and a sense of social responsibility.

Development and Expression of Psychopathology

The expression of psychopathology in children can be related to both age and developmental level. Specific developmental

disorders, particularly developmental language disorders, often are diagnosed in the preschool years. Delayed development of language is a common parental concern. Children who do not use words by 18 months or phrases by 2½ to 3 years may need assessment, particularly if they do not appear to understand typical verbal cues or much language at all. Mild mental retardation or specific learning problems often are not diagnosed until after the child begins elementary school. Disruptive behavior disorder will become apparent at that time as the child begins to interact with peers. Similarly, attention-deficit disorders may only be apparent in school with its need for sustained attention. Other conditions, particularly schizophrenia and bipolar disorder, are rare in preschool and school-aged children.

ADOLESCENCE

Adolescence, marked by the physiologic signs and surging sexual hormones of puberty, is the period of maturation between childhood and adulthood. Adolescence is a transitional period in which peer relationships deepen, autonomy in decision-making grows, and they seek intellectual pursuits and social belonging. Adolescence is mostly a time of exploration and making choices, a gradual process of working toward an integrated concept of self. Adolescents are "works in progress," characterized by increasing ability for mastery over complex challenges of academic, interpersonal, and emotional tasks while searching for new interests, talents, and social identities. A body of growing literature of the specific mechanisms of brain development in adolescence has increased our understanding of broadening social skills in adolescents, in addition to the three expected developmental changes in adolescence: increased risk-taking, increased sexual behavior, and a move toward peer affiliation rather than a primary family attachment. The total cortical gray matter is at its peak at about age 11 years in girls and 13 years in boys, which enhances the ability to understand subtle social situations, control impulses, make long-range plans, and think ahead. White matter volume increases throughout childhood and adolescence, which may allow for increased "connectivity," thereby enhancing the abilities of adolescents to acquire new competencies, such as those needed to master today's technology.

What Is Normal Adolescence?

The concept of normality in adolescent development refers to the degree of psychological adaptation an adolescent achieves while navigating the hurdles and meeting the milestones characteristic of this period of growth. For up to approximately 75 percent of youth, adolescence is a period of successful adaptation to physical, cognitive, and emotional changes, mostly continuous with their previous functioning. Psychological maladjustment, self-loathing, disturbance of conduct, substance abuse, affective disorders, and other impairing psychiatric disorders emerge in approximately 20 percent of the adolescent population.

Adolescent adjustment is continuous with previous psychological function; thus, psychologically disturbed children are at higher risk for psychiatric disorders during adolescence. Adolescents with psychiatric disorders are at increased risk for more significant conflicts with families and for feeling alienated from their families. Although up to 60 percent of adolescents endorse occasional distress or a psychiatric symptom, this group of adolescents functions well academically and with peers and describes themselves as generally satisfied with their lives.

The developmentalist Erik Erikson characterizes the normative task of adolescence as identity versus role confusion. The integration of past experiences with current changes takes place in what Erikson calls *ego identity*. Adolescents explore various aspects of their psychological selves by becoming fans of heroes or other well-known musical or political idols. Some adolescents appear consumed by their identification with a particular idol, whereas others are more moderate in their expression. Adolescents who feel accepted by a peer group and are involved in a variety of activities are less likely to become consumed by adoration of an idol. Socially isolated adolescents, feel socially rejected and become overly identified with an idol to the exclusion of all other activities, are at higher risk for serious emotional problems, and require psychiatric intervention.

Erickson uses the term moratorium to describe the interim period between the concrete thinking of childhood and a more evolved complex ethical development. Erikson defines identity crisis as a normative part of adolescence in which adolescents pursue alternative behaviors and styles and, then, successfully mold these different experiences into a stable identity. A failure to do so would result in identity diffusion, or role confusion, in which the adolescent lacks a cohesive or confident sense of identity. Adolescence is the time to bond with peers, experiment with new beliefs and styles, fall in love for the first time, and explore creative ideas for future endeavors.

Most adolescents go through this developmental process with optimism, develop good self-esteem, maintain good peer relationships, and sustain harmonious relationships with their families.

Stages of Adolescence

Early Adolescence.   Early adolescence, from 12 to 14 years of age, is the period in which the most striking initial changes occur—physically, attitudinally, and behaviorally. Growth spurts often begin in these years for boys, whereas girls may have already had rapid growth for 1 to 2 years. At this stage, boys and girls begin to criticize usual family habits, insist on spending time with peers with less supervision, have a greater awareness of style and appearance, and may question previously accepted family values. A new awareness of sexuality may be displayed by increased modesty and embarrassment with their current physical development or may exhibit itself in an increased interest in the opposite sex.

Early adolescents engage in subtle or overt displays of their growing desire for autonomy, sometimes with challenging behaviors toward authority figures, including teachers and school administrators, and exhibit disdain for rules themselves. At this age, some adolescents begin to experiment with cigarettes, alcohol, and marijuana.

During early adolescence, there is a normal variation in when new defining behaviors are acquired. Overall, although many early adolescents make new friends and modify their public image, most maintain positive connections to family members, old friends, and their family's values. However, for some, early adolescence can a time of overwhelming turmoil, during which there is a dramatic rejection of family, friends, and lifestyle, resulting in a powerful alienation of the adolescent.

Jake, a 13-year-old adolescent, had just started the 8th grade. In the past, he has been a jovial, fun-loving, and cooperative student, but this year he found the school rules increasingly irritating and felt that his teachers were too strict. He had always been a good student while putting in a minimum of work. His older brother Sean, now in 11th grade, had established himself as a compliant, well-liked, and well-behaved student who always put maximal effort into school projects in the same school, so Jake was compared with his brother regularly by many teachers. Jake resented these comparisons because, unlike his brother, whom Jake felt was a "nerd," Jake was more rebellious, took more risks, and made friends with more popular peers. To distinguish himself from his older brother in school and at home, Jake began to challenge the rules at school, stating that they were "stupid" and "meaningless." Jake began to cut classes, to stay out late, and to experiment with alcohol and marijuana. He rejected his best friends from sixth and seventh grade and began to hang out with more daring peers. When Jake was at home, he was able to relate to his older brother Sean only when they played basketball and video games.

Jake's grades began to deteriorate only slightly, but his parents noticed that on his report cards, his teachers rated his effort and behavior as unsatisfactory. During the second month of school, Jake's parents received a phone call that Jake was going to be suspended due to possession of a small amount of marijuana on the school grounds during recess. During a subsequent meeting with the assistant principal and school counselor, Jake argued that the suspension was unfair because his grades were still good, and did not understand why his marijuana possession had triggered a suspension. When confronted with the fact that he had broken not only the school rules, but also violated the law, and that he was fortunate because the school did not involve the police, Jake became angry and continued to insist that they were mistreating him. He also blurted out that all of his teachers and his parents favored his older brother Sean and treated him like a second-class citizen. The school suspended Jake for 5 days but indicated that they would report the incident to the police unless Jake and his family initiated immediate counseling.

Jake begrudgingly began psychotherapy and entered into a weekly therapy group specializing in substance use for teens. Jake's parents also sought therapy to work on becoming more unified in their parenting. Jake remained in psychotherapy for the next 1½ years, during which time his attitude and reasoning style changed and evolved considerably. At age 15, Jake was able to understand why his school had suspended him for possession of marijuana and came to appreciate their willingness to give him the chance to seek counseling, rather than be turned over to the police. Over time, Jake was able to admit the dangers of using drugs and took responsibility for his ill-advised behaviors. Alcohol and drug use continued to be a focus of his therapy and, by 15, Jake had virtually lost interest in alcohol, and admitted to smoking marijuana rarely at parties. Jake became more open to making friends with a variety of peers, and he disclosed that he liked himself better now than when he was 13. He now treated his brother respectfully when alone or with friends, and he felt that his parents appreciated him for "who he was." (Courtesy of Caroly S. Pataki, M.D.)

Middle Adolescence.   During the middle phase of adolescence (roughly between the ages of 14 and 16), adolescents' lifestyles may reflect their efforts to pursue their own stated goals of being independent. Their abilities to combine abstract reasoning with realistic decision-making and judgment are put to the test. In this phase, sexual behavior intensifies, making romantic relationships more complicated, and self-esteem becomes a pivotal influence on positive and negative risk-taking behaviors.

In this phase of development, adolescents tend to identify with a group of peers who become highly influential in their choices of activities, styles, music, idols, and role models. Adolescents' underestimation of the risks associated with a variety of recreational behaviors and their sense of "omnipotence," mixed with their drive to be autonomous, frequently cause some conflict with parental requests and expectations. Most teens can achieve the challenge of defining themselves as unique and different from their families while still connected with family members.

Jenna, a 16-year-old junior in high school, had just gotten her driver's license. She realized that she was lucky to have been given a brand new car at 16 because many of her friends did not yet have cars. Jenna was upset that her parents disapproved of her agreement to drive all of her friends to places that she did not even want to go. Jenna was an attractive and well-liked adolescent who had always been an "A" and "B" student, and never had school conflicts. She played the flute in the school's orchestra and was not involved in any team sports. Jenna started "going out" with a boy in her grade at school, Brett, who was also 16 years old, shortly after getting her license, and even though they did not know each other that well, Jenna felt that they had a close relationship. Since he did not yet have a car, she was the "identified driver" whenever they went out or to parties. Jenna was glad about this because she did not like alcohol and was relieved that Brett would not be driving, given that he drank quite a bit at parties. Jenna got along reasonably well with her parents, who were considered very "easygoing" by her friends, and she felt that she and her parents had similar values and ideas.

Things were going well until Brett began to pressure her to go further in their sexual relationship. When Jenna told him that she was not ready, Brett hounded her more. When the subject of sex had come up with her parents "hypothetically" in the past, they had dismissed the subject, indicating that when it was the right time for her, Jenna would know. Jenna knew that she was not ready to have sex, although many of her classmates were sexually active. Jenna was not an impulsive person and liked to plan things carefully so that they would feel right to her. Jenna realized that she could not agree with Brett's request, but she was confident that she could make him understand. One of Jenna's friends suggested that Brett might break up with her as a result, but Jenna was willing to take that risk. Jenna carefully told Brett that she loved him, but she was not yet ready for sex. Jenna was slightly surprised that instead of pressuring her more or breaking up with her, Brett accepted her decision. He seemed a little relieved.

Jenna and Brett continued their relationship into their senior year of high school, and, toward the end of her senior year, Jenna desired to be sexually active with him. They decided to go to a community clinic known for its positive attitude toward adolescents, to learn about birth control methods, and pick one without including their parents. Jenna and Brett took the time to learn about a variety of birth control methods and chose to use condoms. When they left the clinic, Jenna and Brett felt closer than they had before and realized how they had both grown in their relationship. Jenna and Brett both felt that they were doing the right thing. (Courtesy of Caroly S. Pataki, M.D.)

Late Adolescence. Late adolescence (between the ages of 17 and 19) is a time when continued exploration of academic pursuits, musical and artistic tastes, athletic participation, and social bonds lead a teen toward a greater definition of self and a sense of belonging to specific groups or subcultures within mainstream society. Well-adjusted adolescents can be comfortable with current choices of activities, tastes, hobbies, and friendships, yet remain aware that they will continue to refine their "identities" during young adulthood.

Joey was a second-semester freshman in college, living away from home, and had just turned 18 years of age. He reflected on the fact that he was no longer a "minor" and could make almost any decision for himself without involving his parents.

Joey felt liberated, but at the same time, he was confused and a little lost. Since 10th grade, Joey had planned to pursue a career in medicine like his father, so he had taken a heavy load of science courses in the first semester, all of which he had despised. This semester, however, Joey signed up for liberal arts classes. He did not mention this to his father. He then added classes that ranged from art history to architectural drafting to sociology, philosophy, and music. He had

been influenced, he believed, by his roommate Tony, who was in the architecture program, and by his girlfriend, Lisa, who was majoring in studio art.

As the semester progressed, Joey found that his favorite course was the drafting class. Joey could not help but wonder whether he liked the drafting class so much because of how much he idolized Tony, or because he enjoyed the class. Joey talked this over with Lisa, who suggested that he chill out and not figure out the rest of his life right now. She recommended that he take at least two more semesters of varied classes, including those in the architecture curriculum, before making a final decision about a career. Joey realized that Lisa's approach to college and life was so relaxed, the opposite of his approach, following his parents' pressure to plan, make commitments early, and see them through, regardless of how it felt. Lisa's approach left more room for reflecting on experiences and then making a choice, rather than jumping into what he was "supposed" to do. Joey took her advice and allowed himself another year to try out majors and then decide on a career. After experiencing courses in many varied subjects, Joey decided that he did truly enjoy architecture and was able to switch his focus from premed to architecture. (Courtesy of Caroly S. Pataki M.D.)

Components of Adolescence

Physical Development. Puberty is the process by which adolescents develop physical and sexual maturity, along with reproductive ability. The first signs of the pubertal process are an increased rate of growth in both height and weight. This process begins in girls by approximately 10 years of age. By the age of 11 or 12, many girls noticeably tower over their male classmates, who do not experience a growth spurt, on average, until they reach 13 years of age. By age 13, many girls have experienced menarche, and most have developed breasts and pubic hair.

Wide variation exists in the normal range of onset and timing of pubertal development and its components. A set sequence occurs, however, in the order in which pubertal development proceeds. Thus, secondary sexual characteristics in boys, such as increased length and width of the penis, for example, will occur after the release of androgens from developed enlarged testes.

Sexual maturity ratings (SMRs), also referred to as Tanner Stages, range from SMR 1 (prepuberty) to SMR 5 (adult). The SMR ratings include stages of genital maturity in boys and breast development in girls, as well as pubic hair development. Table 32-12 outlines SMRs for boys and girls.

The primary female sex characteristic is ovulation, the release of eggs from ovarian follicles, approximately once every 28 days. When adolescent girls reach SMR 3 to 4, ovarian follicles are producing enough estrogen to result in menarche, the onset of menstruation. When adolescent girls reach SMR 4 to 5, an ovarian follicle matures monthly, and ovulation occurs. Estrogen and progesterone promote sexual maturation, including further development of fallopian tubes and breasts.

For adolescent boys, the primary sex characteristic is the development of sperm by the testes. In boys, sperm development occurs in response to follicle-stimulating hormone acting on the seminiferous tubules within the testes. The pubertal process in boys consists of the growth of the testes stimulated by luteinizing hormone. An adolescent boy's ability to ejaculate generally emerges within 1 year of reaching SMR 2. Secondary sexual characteristics in boys include thickening of the skin, broadening of the shoulders, and the development of facial hair.

Cognitive Maturation. Cognitive maturation in adolescence encompasses a wide range of expanded abilities that fall within the

Table 32-12
Sexual Maturity Ratings for Male and Female Adolescents

Sexual Maturity Rating	Girls	Boys
Stage 1	Preadolescent, papilla elevated No pubic hair	Penis, testes, scrotum preadolescent No pubic hair
Stage 2	Breast bud, small mound; areola diameter increased Sparse long pubic hair, mainly along labia	Penis size same, testes and scrotum enlarged, with scrotal skin reddened Sparse long pubic hair, mainly at the base of penis
Stage 3	Breast and areola larger; no separation of contours Pubic hair darker and coarser; spread over pubic area	Penis elongated, with increased size of testes and scrotum Pubic hair darker and coarser; spread over pubic area
Stage 4	Breast size increased Areola and papilla raised Pubic hair coarse and thickened; covers less area than in adults, does not extend to thighs	Penis increased in length and width Testes and scrotum larger Pubic hair coarse and thickened; covers less area than in adults, does not extend to thighs
Stage 5	Breasts resemble adult female breast; areola has recessed to breast contour Pubic hair increased in density; area extends to thighs	Penis, testes, scrotum appear mature Pubic hair increased in density; area extends to thighs

global category of executive functions of the brain. These include the transition from concrete thinking to more abstract thinking, an increased ability to draw logical conclusions in scientific pursuits, with peer interactions, and in social situations; and new abilities for self-observation and self-regulation. Adolescents acquire increased awareness of their intellectual, artistic, and athletic gifts and talents, yet it often takes many more years into young adulthood to establish a practical application for these abilities.

The central cognitive change that occurs gradually during adolescence is the shift from concrete thinking (concrete operational thinking, according to Jean Piaget) to the ability to think abstractly (formal operational thinking, in Piaget's terminology). This evolution occurs as an adaptation to stimuli that demand an adolescent to produce hypothetical responses, as well as in response to the adolescent's expanded abilities to provide generalizations from specific situations. The development of abstract thinking is not a sudden epiphany but, rather, a gradual process of expanding logical deductions beyond concrete experiences and achieving the capacity for idealistic and hypothetical thinking based on everyday life.

Adolescents often use an omnipotent belief system that reinforces their sense of immunity from danger, even when confronted with logical risks. Some degree of child-like magical thinking continues to coexist with more mature abstract thinking in many adolescents. Despite the persistence of magical thinking into adolescence, adolescent cognition departs from that of younger children insofar as the increased ability for self-observation and development of strategies to promote strengths and compensate for weaknesses.

One of the essential cognitive tasks in adolescence is to identify and gravitate toward those pursuits that seem to match the adolescent's cognitive strengths, in academic courses, and in thinking about future aspirations. Piaget believed that cognitive adaptation in adolescence is profoundly influenced by social relationships and the dialogue between adolescents and peers, making social cognition an integral part of cognitive development in adolescence.

Socialization.   Socialization in adolescence encompasses the ability to find acceptance in peer relationships, as well as the development of more mature social cognition. The skills to develop a sense of belonging to a peer group are of central importance to a sense of well-being. Being viewed as socially competent by peers is a critical component in building good self-esteem for most early adolescents. Peer influences are powerful and can foster positive social interactions, as well as apply pressure in less socially accepted behaviors or even high-risk behavior. Belonging to a peer group is, in general, a sign of adaptation and a developmentally appropriate step in separating from parents and turning the focus of loyalty toward friends. Children between the ages of 6 and 12 can engage in exchanges of ideas and opinions and acknowledge feelings of peers, but the relationships often wax and wane in a discontinuous way based on altercations and good times. Friendships deepen with repeated good times, but, for some school-aged children, a variety of peers are often interchangeable—that is, a child may seek a companion when that child has free time, rather than out of a desire to spend time with a specific friend. As adolescence ensues, friendships become more individualized, and adolescents may share personal secrets with a friend rather than a family member. The adolescent may achieve a comfort level with one or several early adolescent peers, and the group may "stick together," spending most of their free time together. In early adolescence, a blend of the above two social modes may emerge, small "cliques" arise, and, even within the cliques, competition and jealousies regarding which dyads are "preferred" or higher ranked within the clique may result in some discontinuities in the relationships. In later adolescence, the peer group solidifies, leading to increased stability in the friendships and a greater mutuality in the quality of the interactions.

Moral Development.   Morality is a set of values and beliefs about codes of behavior that conform to those shared by others in society. Adolescents, as do younger children, tend to develop patterns of behaviors characteristic of their family and educational environments and by imitation of specific peers and adults whom they admire. Moral development does not strictly follow chronologic age but, instead, is an outgrowth from cognitive development.

Piaget described moral development as a gradual process parallel to cognitive development, with expanded abilities in differentiating the best interests for society from those of individuals occurring during late adolescence. Preschool children simply follow the rules set forth by the parents; in the middle years, children accept rules but show an inability to allow for exceptions; and during adolescence, young persons recognize rules in terms of what is good for the society at large.

Lawrence Kohlberg integrated Piaget's concepts and described multiple stages of moral development within three significant levels of morality. The first level is preconventional morality, in which punishment and obedience to the parent are the determining factors. The second level is the morality of conventional role-conformity, in which children try to conform to gain approval and to maintain good relationships with others. The third and highest level is the morality of self-accepted moral principles, in which children voluntarily comply with rules based on a concept of ethical principles and make exceptions to rules in certain circumstances.

Although Kohlberg's and Piaget's notions of moral development focus on a unified theory of cognitive maturation for both sexes, Carol Gilligan emphasizes the social context of moral development leading to divergent patterns in moral development. Gilligan points out that, in women, compassion and the ethics of caring are dominant features of moral decision-making, whereas, for men, predominant features of moral judgments are related more to a perception of justice, rationality, and a sense of fairness. Although influential, many psychologists and scholars criticize Gilligan's work as primarily observational and lacking scientific rigor. Feminist scholars note that Gilligan rarely considers the role of societal expectations in influencing gender-based behavior.

Modern psychologists have incorporated insights from cognitive psychology and suggest that moral development goes beyond the rationality of Piaget and Kolberg. Psychologists such as Jonathan Haidt emphasize the role of intuition and preconceived beliefs based on the fundamental moral foundations found in a society. He suggests that the logical explanations one gives to justify one's actions are post hoc rationalizations meant to justify one's emotional (i.e., irrational) reactions to the moral dilemmas we face in society.

Self-Esteem.   Self-esteem is a measure of one's sense of self-worth based on perceived success and achievements, as well as a perception of how much one is valued by peers, family members, teachers, and society in general. The most important correlates of good self-esteem are one's perception of attractive physical appearance and high value to peers and family. Secondary features of self-esteem relate to academic achievement, athletic abilities, and unique talents. Adolescent self-esteem is mediated, to a significant degree, by the positive feedback received from a peer group and family members, and adolescents often seek out a peer group that offers acceptance, regardless of negative behaviors associated with that group. Adolescent girls have more of a problem maintaining self-esteem than do boys. Girls continued to rate themselves with generally lower self-esteem into adulthood.

Current Environmental Influences and Adolescence

Adolescent Sexual Behavior.   Sexual experimentation in adolescents often begins with fantasy and masturbation in early adolescence, followed by noncoital genital touching with the opposite sex or, in some cases, same-sex partners, oral sex with partners, and initiation of sexual intercourse at a later point in development. By high school, most male adolescents report experience with masturbation, and more than half of adolescent girls report masturbation. The balance between healthy adolescent sexual experimentation and emotionally and physically safe sexual practices is one of the significant challenges for society.

Estimates vary, but about 50 percent of 9th- to 12th-grade students reported having had sexual intercourse. The median age at first intercourse is about 16 years for boys and 17 years for girls. Boys generally have more sexual partners than do girls, and boys are less likely than girls to seek emotional attachments with their sexual partners.

FACTORS INFLUENCING ADOLESCENT SEXUAL BEHAVIOR.   Factors that affect sexual behavior in adolescents include personality traits, gender, cultural and religious background, racial factors, family attitudes, and sexual education and prevention programs.

Personality factors are associated with sexual behavior, as well as sexual risk-taking. Higher levels of impulsivity are associated with a younger age at the first experience of sexual intercourse; a higher number of sexual partners; sexual intercourse without the use of contraception, including condoms; and a history of a sexually transmitted disease (STD, chlamydia).

Historically, male adolescents have initiated sexual intercourse at a younger age than female adolescents. The younger a teenage girl is when she has sex for the first time, the more likely she is to have had unwanted sexual activity. Close to four of ten girls who had first intercourse at 13 or 14 years of age report it was either not voluntary or unwanted. Three of four girls and over half of boys report that girls who have sex do so because their boyfriends want them to. In general, adolescents who initiate sexual intercourse at younger ages are also more likely to have a higher number of sexual partners.

The additive effects of more highly educated families, social and religious youth groups, and school-based educational programs can decrease high-risk sexual behavior among adolescents. Female empowerment strategies can play an essential role in decreasing unwanted sexual behavior and teenage pregnancies. The primary reason that teenage girls who have never had intercourse give for abstaining from sex is that having sex would be against their religious or moral values. Other reasons include the desire to avoid pregnancy, fear of contracting a STD, and not having met the appropriate partner.

CONTRACEPTIVES.   Currently, 98 percent of teenagers 15 to 19 years are using at least one method of birth control. The two most common methods are condoms and birth control pills. STDs, despite the use of condoms, are still at high levels in teens—approximately one in four sexually active teens contracts an STD every year. Approximately half of all new human immunodeficiency virus (HIV) infections occur in people younger than age 25.

PREGNANCY.   Each year 750,000 to 850,000 teenage girls younger than age 19 become pregnant. Of this number, 432,000 give birth, a 19 percent decline from 532,000 in 1991; the rest (418,000) obtain abortions. The largest decline in teen pregnancy by race is for black women. Hispanic teen births have declined 20 percent, but continue to have the highest teen birth rates compared with other races.

Teenage pregnancy creates a plethora of health risks for both mother and child. Children born to teenage mothers have a higher chance of dying before the age of 5 years. Those who survive are more likely to perform poorly in school and are at higher risk of abuse and neglect. Teenage mothers are less likely to gain adequate weight during pregnancy, increasing the risk of premature births and low–birth-weight infants. Low–birth-weight babies are more likely to have organs that are not fully developed, resulting in bleeding in the brain, respiratory distress syndrome, and intestinal problems. Teenage mothers are also less likely to seek regular prenatal care and to take recommended daily multivitamins, and they are more likely to smoke, drink, or use drugs during pregnancy. Only one-third of teenage mothers obtain high school diplomas, and only 1.5 percent have a college degree by the age of 30.

The average adolescent mother who cannot care for her child has the child either placed in foster care or raised by the teenager's already overburdened parents or other relatives. Few teenage mothers marry the fathers of their children; the fathers, usually teenagers, cannot care for themselves, much less the mothers of their children. If the two do marry, they usually divorce. Many are more likely to end up on welfare.

ABORTION. Nearly four of ten teen pregnancies end in abortion. Almost all the girls are unwed mothers from low socioeconomic groups; their pregnancies result from sex with boys to whom they felt emotionally attached. Most (61 percent) teenagers elect to have abortions with their parents' consent, but laws of mandatory parental consent put two rights into a competition: a girl's claim to privacy and a parent's need to know. Most adults believe that teenagers should have parental permission for an abortion, but when parents refuse to give their consent, most states prohibit parents from vetoing the teenager's decision.

The abortion rate in many European countries tends to be far lower than that in the United States. The Control and Prevention (CDC) reports that the abortion rate in the United States for girls between the ages of 15 and 19 is about 30 per 1,000. In France, about 10.5 of every 1,000 girls under the age of 20 had an abortion, according to World Health Organization statistics. The rate of abortion in Germany was 6.8; in Italy, 6.3; and in Spain, 4.5. Britain has a higher rate, 18.5. Family planning experts believe that more sex education and the availability of contraceptive devices help keep the number of abortions down. In Holland, where contraceptives are freely available in schools, the teenage pregnancy rate is among the lowest in the world.

Risk-Taking Behavior. Reasonable risk-taking is a necessary endeavor in adolescence, leading to confidence both in forming new relationships and in sports and social situations. High-risk behaviors among adolescents are associated with severe negative consequences, however, and can take many forms, including drug and alcohol use, unsafe sexual practices, self-injurious behaviors, and reckless driving.

Drug Use

ALCOHOL. About 30 percent of 12th graders report having five or more drinks in a row within 2 weeks. The average age when youths first try alcohol is 11 years for boys and 13 years for girls. The national average age at which Americans begin regular drinking is 15.9 years of age. People ages 18 to 25 show the highest prevalence of binge and heavy drinking. Drunk driving has declined since 2002. Alcohol dependence, along with other drugs, is associated with depression, anxiety, oppositional defiant disorder, antisocial personality disorder, and an increased rate of suicide.

NICOTINE. The number of young American smokers has declined since 1990. However, the rate of smoking among teenagers is still as high as or higher than that of adults. According to the American Cancer Society, on average more than one of five students have smoked cigarettes. Each day, more than 4,000 teenagers try their first cigarette, and another 2,000 become regular, daily smokers. Cigarette smokers are more likely to get into fights, carry weapons, attempt suicide, suffer from mental health problems such as depression, and engage in high-risk sexual behaviors. One of three will eventually die from smoking-related diseases. Cigarettes are the

most common type of tobacco used among middle-school students, followed by cigars, smokeless tobacco, and pipes.

CANNABIS. Marijuana is the most popular illicit drug, with 14.6 million people using it (6.2 percent of the population), two-thirds being under the age of 18. Its use, however, is slowly declining. About 6 percent of 12th graders report daily use of marijuana.

One of the primary reasons for such prevalence of marijuana use among teenagers is because many find that marijuana is easier to get than alcohol or cigarettes. This belief has declined in recent years. Once teenagers are dependent on marijuana, they often tumble into truancy, crime, and depression.

COCAINE. About 13 percent of high school seniors use cocaine, exceeding the national average of 3.6 percent. Also, about 1 percent of 12th graders admit to using phencyclidine (PCP). Crystal methamphetamine (ice) has an annual prevalence in 12th graders of about 2 percent.

OPIOIDS. In recent years, the number of teens using prescription pain relievers for nonmedical reasons has increased. Prescription drug abuse by people ages 18 to 25 has increased by 15 percent. Drugs of specific concern are the pain relievers oxycodone and hydrocodone. Oxycodone has gained ground among high school students since its emergence in 2001, with 5 percent of 12th graders, 3.5 percent of 10th graders, and 1.7 percent of 8th graders reporting use. About 9 percent of 12th graders use hydrocodone, 6 percent of 10th graders, and 2.5 percent of 8th graders.

HEROIN. Heroin use is prevalent among adolescents, although less so than cocaine. The average age of use is 19, but almost 2 percent of 12th graders use it. The nasal route (snorting) is the most common method of use.

Violence. Although rates of violent crime have decreased throughout the United States in recent years, violent crimes by young offenders are on the increase. Homicides are the second leading cause of death among people aged 15 to 25. (Accidents are first; suicides are third.) Black male teenagers are far more likely to be murder victims than are boys from any other racial or ethnic group or girls of any race. The factor most strongly associated with violence among adolescent boys is growing up in a household without a father or father surrogate; this factor aside, race, socioeconomic status, and education show no effect on the propensity toward violence.

BULLYING. *Bullying* is the use of one's strength or status to intimidate, injure, or humiliate another person of lesser strength or status. It can be physical, verbal, or social. Physical bullying involves physical injury or threat of injury to someone. Verbal bullying refers to teasing or insulting someone. Social bullying refers to the use of peer rejection or exclusion to humiliate or isolate a victim.

About 30 percent of 6th- through 10th-grade students experience moderate-to-frequent bullying, as a bully, a target, or both. Approximately 1.7 million children within this age group bully other children. Boys are more likely to be involved in bullying and violent behavior than girls. Girls tend to use verbal bullying rather than physical.

An estimated 160,000 students miss school each day because of fear of attack or intimidation from peers; some may drop out. Stresses of "victimization" can interfere with student's engagement and learning in school. Children who bully other children are at risk for engaging in more violent severe behaviors, such as frequent fighting and carrying a weapon.

Cyberbullying. During the last decade, electronic or internet bullying has become of great concern to adolescents. Cyberbullying is defined broadly to convey the use of electronic means to intimidate or harm someone intentionally. The reported prevalence of cyberbullying is variable, reports ranging from 1 to 62 percent of youth reporting that they were victims of cyber victimization. A study of about 700 Australian students, recruited at age 10 years, and followed until ages 14 to 15 years, found that 15 percent had engaged in cyberbullying, 21 percent had engaged in traditional bullying, and 7 percent had engaged in both. Another study of self-reported information collected from 399 teens in the 8th to 10th grades found that involvement in cyberbullying, either as a victim or a bully, specifically contributed to the prediction of depressive symptoms and suicidal ideation. This correlation between cyberbullying and depressive symptomatology is more reliable than the association of traditional bullying and affective disorder.

Gangs.   Gang violence is a problem throughout the United States. There are 2,000 different youth gangs around the country, with more than 200,000 teens and young adults as members. Most members are between the ages of 12 and 24 years, with an average of 17 to 18 years. Gang membership is a brief phase for many teenagers; one-half to two-thirds leave the gang by the 1-year mark. Boys are more likely to join gangs than girls; however, female gang membership may be underrepresented. Female gang members are more likely to be found in small cities and rural areas and tend to be younger than male gang members. Female gang members are also involved in less delinquent or criminal activity than males and commit fewer violent crimes.

WEAPONS.   Each day, on average, nearly 10 American children younger than the age of 18 years are killed in handgun suicides, homicides, and accidents. Many more are wounded. One in five youths in grades 9 to 12 carries a weapon: knife, gun, or club.

By law, anyone younger than 18 years cannot purchase a firearm. Two-thirds of students in grades 6 to 12 say that they can get a firearm within 24 hours, however. More than 22 million children live in a home with a firearm. In 40 percent of these homes, at least one gun is not locked, and 13 percent are unlocked and loaded. Two of three students involved in school shootings acquired their guns from their own home or that of a relative. At least 60 percent of suicide deaths in teens involve the use of a handgun.

SCHOOL VIOLENCE.   According to the CDC, of all youth homicides in 2010, about 2 percent occurred in schools. Approximately 7 percent of teachers report they have been threatened with injury or physically attacked by a student from their school. Also, among students in grades 9 through 12, about 6 percent reported carrying a weapon on school property on one or more days in the 30 days before the survey.

Many factors can lead to violent acts in teenagers. Some inherited traits include impulsivity, learning difficulties, low IQ, or fearlessness. A correlation also exists between witnessing violent acts and involvement in violence. Children who witness violent acts are more aggressive and grow up more likely to become involved in violence—either as a victimizer or as a victim. Table 32-13 lists some of the early and imminent warning signs of school violence.

On April 20, 1999, two teenage boys, ages 17 and 18 years, went on a shooting rampage through Columbine High School of Littleton, Colorado. Armed with shotguns, a semiautomatic rifle, and a pistol, they laughed and shouted as they shot classmates and teachers at

Table 32-13
Warning Signs of School Violence

Early Warning Signs
  Social withdrawal
  Excessive feelings of isolation and being alone
  Excessive feelings of rejection
  Being a victim of violence
  Feelings of being picked on and persecuted
  Expression of violence in writings and drawings
  Uncontrolled anger
  Patterns of impulsive and chronic hitting, intimidating, and
    bullying behaviors
  History of discipline problems
  History of violent and aggressive behavior
  Intolerance for differences and prejudicial attitudes
  Drug and alcohol use
  Affiliation with gangs
  Inappropriate access to, possession of, and use of firearms
  Serious threats of violence

Imminent Warning Signs
  Serious physical fighting with peers or family members
  Severe destruction of property
  Severe rage for seemingly minor reasons
  Detailed threats of lethal violence
  Possession and/or use of firearms and other weapons
  Other self-injurious behaviors or threats of suicide

point-blank range while hurling homemade explosives. Fifteen were killed, including the 2 gunmen, who also injured 25 people.

The gunmen were members of the "trench coat mafia" at the high school, a clique of social misfits who stood out at the school for their gothic style of dress and nihilistic attitude. The two gunmen were obsessed with violent video games and intrigued with Nazi culture, even though one was part Jewish. They chose the date of the attack to coincide with Adolf Hitler's birthday.

On March 21, 2005, a 16-year-old boy went on a shooting rampage at Red Lake High School on the Red Lake Indian Reservation in far northern Minnesota. He began his shooting spree by killing his grandfather and the grandfather's companion. He then donned his grandfather's police-issue gun belt and bulletproof vest before heading to the school, where he killed a security guard, a teacher, five students, and then himself. About 15 others were injured.

The gunman had a troubled childhood; his father committed suicide in 1997, and his mother suffered head injuries in an auto accident. He expressed admiration for Adolf Hitler on a neo-Nazi website, using the handle "Todesengel," which is German for "Angel of Death." He had bouts of depression, suicide ideation and was taking fluoxetine. He was a member of a clique of about five students known as "The Darkers," who wore black clothes and chains, spiked or dyed their hair, and loved heavy-metal music. The gunman usually wore a long black trench coat, eyeliner, and combat boots. Peers described him as a quiet teenager.

SEXUAL OFFENSE.   Adolescents younger than age 18 years account for 20 percent of arrests for all sexual offenses (excluding prostitution), 20 to 30 percent of rape cases, 14 percent of aggravated sexual assault offenses, and 27 percent of child sexual homicides. These adolescent offenders account for the victimization of approximately one-half of boys and one-fourth of girls who are molested or sexually abused. Most instances have involved adolescent male perpetrators.

There appear to be two types of juvenile sex offenders: those who target children and those who offend against peers or adults.

Table 32-14
Juvenile Sex Offender Subtypes

Juvenile Offenders Who Sexually Offend against Peers or Adults
    Predominantly assault females and strangers or casual
        acquaintances
    Sexual assaults occur in association with other types of criminal
        activity (e.g., burglary)
    Have histories of nonsexual criminal offenses, and appear more
        generally delinquent and conduct   disordered
    Commit their offenses in public areas
    Display higher levels of aggression and violence in the
        commission of their sexual crimes
    More likely to use weapons and to cause injuries to their victims

Juvenile Offenders Who Sexually Offend against Children
    Most victims are male and are related to them, either siblings or
        other relatives
    Almost half of the offenders have had at least one male victim
    The sexual crimes tend to reflect a greater reliance on
        opportunity and guile than injurious force. This appears to
        be particularly true when their victim is related to them.
        These youths may "trick" the child into complying with the
        molestation, use bribes, or threaten the child with loss of the
        relationship
    Within the overall population of juveniles who sexually
        assault children are certain youths who display high levels
        of aggression and violence. Generally, these are youths who
        display more severe levels of personality and/or psychosexual
        disturbances, such as psychopathy, sexual sadism, and so on
    Suffer from deficits in self-esteem and social competency
    Many show evidence of depression

Characteristics Common to Both Groups
    High rates of learning disabilities and academic dysfunction
        (30–60%)
    The presence of other behavioral health problems, including
        substance abuse, and disorders of conduct (up to 80% have
        some diagnosable psychiatric disorder)
    Observed difficulties with impulse control and judgment

The age difference between the victim and the offender is the main difference between the two groups. Table 32-14 lists the differences and similarities between these two groups.

Etiologic factors of juvenile sex offending include maltreatment experiences, exposure to pornography, substance abuse, and exposure to aggressive role models. A significant number of offending adolescents have a childhood history of physical abuse (25 to 50 percent) or sexual abuse (10 to 80 percent). Half of the adolescent offenders lived with both parents and one other juvenile at the time of their offending. Evidence also suggests that most juvenile sex offenders are likely to become adult sex offenders. The most common psychosocial deficits of adolescent sexual offenders include low self-esteem, few social skills, minimal assertive skills, and poor academic performance. The most common psychiatric diagnoses are conduct disorder, substance abuse disorder, adjustment disorder, ADHD, specific phobia, and mood disorders. Male offenders are more often diagnosed with paraphilias and antisocial behavior, whereas female offenders are more likely to be diagnosed with mood disorders and engage in self-mutilation.

Prostitution.   Teenagers constitute a large portion of all prostitutes, with estimates ranging up to 1 million teenagers involved in prostitution. The average age of a recruit is 13 years; however, some are young as 9 years of age. Most adolescent prostitutes are girls, but boys may become same-sex prostitutes. Most teenagers who enter a life of prostitution come from broken homes; however, a growing number of teenage prostitutes come from middle- to upper-middle-class homes. Many have been victims of rape or abuse as children. Most teenagers ran away from home and were taken in by pimps and substance abusers; the adolescents themselves then became substance abusers. Twenty-seven percent of teenage prostitution occurs in large cities, and incidents usually take place at an outside location, such as highways, roads, alleys, fields, woods, or parking lots. Teenage prostitutes are at high risk for acquired immunodeficiency syndrome (AIDS), and many (up to 70 percent in some studies) have HIV.

As many as 17,500 individuals are smuggled into the United States each year as "sex slaves." They arrive under the pretenses of a better life and job opportunities, but once they are in the United States, they are forced into prostitution, making little money while traffickers make thousands of dollars from their services. Many times they are raped and abused.

Tattoos and Body Piercing.   Body piercing and tattoos have become more prevalent among adolescents since the 1980s. In the general population, approximately 10 to 13 percent of adolescents have tattoos. Of the more than 500 adolescents surveyed in a study, 13.2 percent report at least one tattoo, and 26.9 percent report at least one body piercing, other than in their ear lobe, at some point in their lives. Both tattoos and body piercing are more common in girls than in boys. Adolescents who endorsed possession of at least one tattoo or body piercing are more likely to endorse the use of gateway drugs (cigarettes, alcohol, marijuana), as well as experience with hard drugs (cocaine, crystal methamphetamine, and ecstasy).

▲ 32.2 Adulthood

INTRODUCTION

For most of the history of developmental psychology, the predominant theory held that development ended with childhood and adolescence. Adults were considered to be finished products in whom the ultimate developmental states had been reached. Beyond adolescence, the developmental point of view was relevant only insofar as success or failure to reach adult levels or to maintain them determined the maturity or immaturity of the adult personality.

In contradistinction were the long-recognized ideas that adult experiences, such as pregnancy, marriage, parenthood, and aging, had an obvious and significant impact on mental processes and experience in the adult years. This view of adulthood suggests that the patient, of any age, is still in the process of ongoing development, as opposed to merely having a past that influences mental processes and is the primary determinant of current behavior. Although the debate continues, the idea that development continues throughout life is increasingly accepted.

Development in adulthood, as in childhood, is always the result of the interaction among body, mind, and environment, never exclusively the result of any one of the three variables. Most adults are forced to confront and adapt to similar circumstances: establishing an independent identity, forming a marriage or other partnership, raising children, building and maintaining careers, and accepting the disability and death of one's parents.

In modern Western societies, adulthood is the most prolonged phase of human life. Although the exact age of consent varies from person to person, adulthood can be divided into three main parts: young or early adulthood (ages 20 to 40), middle adulthood (ages 40 to 65), and late adulthood or old age.

YOUNG ADULTHOOD (20 TO 40 YEARS OF AGE)

Usually considered to begin at the end of adolescence (about age 20) and to end at age 40, early adulthood is characterized by peaking biologic development, the assumption of major social roles, and the evolution of an adult self and life structure. The successful passage into adulthood depends on the satisfactory resolution of childhood and adolescent crises.

During late adolescence, young persons generally leave home and begin to function independently. Sexual relationships become serious, and the quest for intimacy begins. The 20s are spent, for the most part, exploring options for occupation and marriage or alternative relationships and making commitments in various areas.

Early adulthood requires choosing new roles (e.g., husband, father) and establishing an identity congruent with those new roles. It involves asking and answering the questions "Who am I?" and "Where am I going?" The choices made during this time may be tentative; young adults may make several false starts.

Transition from Adolescence to Young Adulthood

The transition from adolescence to young adulthood is characterized by real and intrapsychic separation from the family of origin and the engagement of new, phase-specific tasks (Table 32-15). It involves many important events, such as graduating from high school, starting a job or entering college, and living independently. During these years, the individual resolves the issue of childhood dependency sufficiently to establish self-reliance and begins to formulate new, young-adult goals that eventually result in the creation of new life structures that promote stability and continuity.

Developmental Tasks

Establishing a self that is separate from parents is a significant task of young adulthood. For most individuals, the emotional detachment from parents that takes place in adolescence and young adulthood is followed by a new inner definition of themselves as comfortably alone and competent, able to care for themselves in the real world. This shift away from the parents continues long after marriage, and parenthood results in the formation of new relationships that replace the progenitors as the most influential individuals in the young adult's life.

Psychological separation from the parents is followed by the synthesis of mental representations from the childhood past and the young-adult present. The psychological separation from parents in adolescence has been called the *second individuation,* and the continued elaboration of these themes in young adulthood has been called the *third individuation.* The continuous process of

Table 32-15
Development Tasks of Young Adulthood

To develop a young-adult sense of self and other: the third individuation
To develop adult friendships
To develop the capacity for intimacy; to become a spouse
To become a biologic and psychological parent
To develop a relationship of mutuality and equality with parents while facilitating their midlife development
To establish an adult work identity
To develop adult forms of play
To integrate new attitudes toward time

Table 32-16
Psychological Development Concepts

Concept	Definition	Example
Transition	The bridge between two successive stages	Late adolescence
Normative crisis	A period of rapid change or turmoil that strains a person's adaptive capacities	Midlife crisis
Stage	Period of consolidation of skills and capacities	Mature adulthood
Plateau	Period of developmental stability	Adulthood up to midlife
Rite of passage	Social ritual that facilitates a transition	Graduation; marriage

Adapted from Wolman T, Thompson T. Adult and later-life development. In: Stoudemire A, ed. *Human Behavior.* Philadelphia, PA: Lippincott-Raven; 1998, with permission.

elaboration of self and differentiation from others that occurs in the developmental phases of young and middle age continues to influence our meaningful adult relationships.

Several different models have been proposed for understanding adult development. They are all theoretical and somewhat idealized. They all use metaphors to describe complex social, psychological, and interpersonal interactions. The models are heuristic: They provide a conceptual framework for thinking about important common experiences. They are descriptive rather than prescriptive; that is, they offer a useful way of looking at what many persons do, not a formula for what all persons should do. Some of the terms and concepts commonly used are explained in Table 32-16. These periods involve individuation, that is, leaving the family of origin and becoming one's own man or woman, passing through midlife, and preparing in middle adulthood for the transition into late adulthood.

Work Identity.   The transition from learning and play to work may be gradual or abrupt. Socioeconomic group, gender, and race affect the pursuit and development of particular occupational choices. Blue-collar workers generally enter the workforce directly after high school; white-collar workers and professionals usually enter the workforce after college or professional school. Depending on the choice of career and opportunity, work may become a source of ongoing frustration or activity that enhances self-esteem. Symptoms of job dissatisfaction are a high rate of job changes, absenteeism, mistakes at work, accident proneness, and even sabotage.

UNEMPLOYMENT.   The effects of unemployment transcend those of loss of income; the psychological and physical tolls are enormous. The incidence of alcohol dependence, homicide, violence, suicide, and mental illness rises with unemployment. One's core identity, which is often tied to occupation and work, is seriously damaged when a job is lost, whether through firing, attrition, or early or sometimes even regular retirement.

A young adult female patient had much enjoyed her 5 years in college, and only reluctantly accepted a job with a large real estate firm. During college, she had limited interest in her appearance, and she began work in clothing borrowed from family and friends. She scoffed when her boss began to criticize her dress and gave her an advance to buy an upscale wardrobe, but she then began to enjoy the fine clothing and the respect engendered by her appearance and position. As her income began to rise, work became a source of pleasure and self-esteem and the way to acquire some of the trappings of adulthood. (Courtesy of Calvin Colarusso, M.D.)

Developing Adult Friendships.

In late adolescence and young adulthood, before marriage and parenthood, friendships are often the primary source of emotional sustenance. Roommates, apartment-mates, sorority sisters, and fraternity brothers, as indicated by the names used to describe them, are substitutes for parents and siblings, temporary stand-ins until more permanent replacements are found.

Friendships mostly meet the emotional needs of closeness and confidentiality. All major developmental issues are discussed with friends, particularly those in similar circumstances. As marriages occur and children are born, the central emotional importance of friendships diminishes. Some friendships are abandoned at this point because the spouse objects to the friend, recognizing at some level that they are competitors. Gradually, there is a movement toward a new form of friendship, couples friendships. They reflect the newly committed status but are more difficult to form and to maintain because four individuals must be compatible, not just two.

As children begin to move out of the family into the community, parents follow. Dance classes and Little League games provide the progenitors with a new focus and the opportunity to make friends with others who are at the same point developmentally and who are receptive to the formation of relationships that help explain and cushion the pressures of young adult life.

Sexuality and Marriage.

The developmental shift from sexual experimentation to the desire for intimacy is experienced in young adulthood as intense loneliness, resulting from the awareness of an absence of committed love similar to that experienced in childhood with their parents. Brief sexual encounters in short-lived relationships no longer significantly boost self-esteem. Increasingly, the desire is for emotional involvement in a sexual context. The young adult who fails to develop the capacity for intimate relationships runs the risk of living in isolation and self-absorption in midlife.

For most individuals in Western culture, the experience of intimacy increases the desire for marriage. Most persons in the United States marry for the first time in their mid-to-late 20s. The median age of first marriage has been rising steadily since 1950 for both men and women, and the number of persons who never marry has been increasing. Today, approximately 50 percent of all adults ages 18 and older are not married, compared with only 28 percent in 1960. The proportion of 30- to 34-year-olds who never married has almost tripled, and the ratio of never-married 35- to 39-year-olds doubled.

INTERRACIAL MARRIAGE. Mixed-race marriages were banned in 19 states until a U.S. Supreme Court decision in 1967. In 1970, such marriages accounted for only 2 percent of all marriages. The trend has been steadily upward. Currently, interracial marriages account for about 1.5 million marriages in the United States.

Despite the trend toward more interracial marriages, they remain a small proportion of all marriages. Most persons are more likely to marry someone from the same racial and ethnic background. Marriages between Hispanic whites and non-Hispanic whites and between Asians and whites are more common than those between blacks and whites.

SAME-SEX MARRIAGE. Same-sex marriage is recognized as legal by many states in the United States and by the U.S. Supreme Court, as well as in several countries around the world (e.g., France and Denmark). It differs from same-sex civil unions granted by states, which do not provide the same federal protections or benefits as marriage. No reliable estimates are available for the number of same-sex marriages in the United States; however, in 2013, it was estimated to be about 80,000. There is growing consensus in the United States and around the world that gay and lesbian persons should be allowed the same marital rights and privileges as straight adults. Same-sex marriage can be subject to more stress than heterosexual marriage because of continued prejudice toward such unions among certain conservative political or religious groups who oppose such unions.

MARITAL PROBLEMS. Although marriage tends to be regarded as a permanent tie, unsuccessful unions can be terminated, as indeed they are in most societies. Nevertheless, many marriages that do not end in separation or divorce are disturbed. In considering marital problems, clinicians are concerned with both the persons involved and with the marital unit itself. How any marriage works relates to the partner selected, the personality organization or disorganization of each, the interaction between them, and the original reasons for the union. Persons marry for a variety of reasons—emotional, social, economic, and political, among others. One person may look to the spouse to meet unfulfilled childhood needs for good parenting. Another may see the spouse as someone to be saved from an otherwise unhappy life. Irrational expectations between spouses increase the risk of marital problems.

MARRIAGE AND COUPLES THERAPY. When families consist of grandparents, parents, children, and other relatives living under the same roof, assistance for marital problems can sometimes be obtained from a member of the extended family with whom one or both partners have rapport. With the contraction of the extended family in recent times, however, this source of informal help is no longer as accessible as it once was. Similarly, religion once played a more important role than it does now in the maintenance of family stability. Wise religious leaders are available to provide counseling. Still, they are not sought out to the extent they once were, which reflects the decline in religious influence among large segments of the population. Traditionally, a couple's extended family and their religion guided them during distressing times. In addition to these supports, social pressure helped to prevent the dissolution of marriages. As family, religious, and societal pressures have been relaxed, legal procedures for relatively easy separation and divorce have expanded. Concurrently, the need for formalized marriage counseling services has developed.

Marital therapy is a form of psychotherapy for married persons in conflict with each other. A trained person establishes a professional contract with the patient-couple and, through definite types of communication, attempts to alleviate the disturbance, to reverse or change maladaptive patterns of behavior, and to encourage personality growth and development.

In *marriage counseling,* only a particular conflict related to the immediate concerns of the family is discussed; marriage counseling is conducted much more superficially by persons with less psychotherapeutic training than is marital therapy. *Marital therapy* places greater emphasis on restructuring the interaction between the couple, including, at times, exploration of the psychodynamics of each partner. Both therapy and counseling emphasize helping marital partners cope effectively with their problems.

Parenthood.   Parenthood intensifies the relationship between new parents. Through their physical and emotional union, the couple has produced a fragile, dependent being that needs them in the interlocking roles of father and mother. This recognition expands their internal images of each other to include thoughts and feelings emanating from the role of parent. As they live together as a family, the lovers' relationship with each other changes. They become parents relating to one another and their children.

Parent–child problems do arise, however. In addition to the economic burden of raising a child (estimated to be $250,000 for a middle-class family whose child goes to college), there are emotional costs. Children may reawaken conflicts that parents themselves had as children, or children may have chronic illnesses that challenge families' resources. In general, men have been more concerned with their work and occupational advancement than with child-rearing, and women have been more concerned about their role as mothers than with advancement in their occupation. However, this emphasis is changing dramatically for both sexes. A small but growing number of couples are choosing to split a job (or work at two part-time jobs) and share child-rearing duties.

Parenting has been described as a continuing process of letting go. Children must be allowed to separate from parents and, in some cases, must be encouraged to do so. Letting go involves separation from children who are starting school. School phobias and school refusal syndromes that are accompanied by extreme separation anxiety may have to be handled. Often, a parent who cannot let go of a child accounts for this situation; some parents want their children to remain tightly bound to them emotionally. Family therapy that explores these dynamics may be needed to resolve such problems.

As children get older and enter adolescence, the process of establishing identity assumes great importance. Peer relationships become crucial to a child's development, and overprotective parents who keep a child from developing friendships or having the freedom to experiment with friends that the parents disapprove of can interfere with the child's passage through adolescence. Parents need not refrain from exerting influence over their children; guidance and involvement are crucial. But they must recognize that adolescents especially require parental approval. However, rebellious on the surface, adolescents are much more tractable than they appear, provided parents are not overbearing or generally punitive.

SINGLE-PARENT FAMILIES.   More than 10 million single-parent families exist with one or more children under the age of 18; of these families, 20 percent are single-parent homes in which a woman is the sole head of the household. The increase in the number of single-parent families has risen by almost 200 percent since 1980.

ALTERNATIVE LIFESTYLE PARENTING.   Single, partnered, and married gay men and women are choosing to raise children. In most cases, such children are obtained through adoption. Some, however, may be born to a lesbian through artificial insemination or obtained from a willing mother surrogate. The number of such family units is increasing. The data about the development of children in these homes indicate that they are at no greater risk for emotional problems (or for a gay orientation) than children raised in conventional households.

ADOPTION.   Since the turn of the century, adoption or foster placement has replaced institutional care as the preferred way to raise children who are neglected, unwanted, or abandoned. Many couples who are unable to conceive (and some couples who already have children) turn to adoption.

In addition to the full range of typical parent–child developmental issues, adoptive parents face particular problems. They must decide how and when to tell the child about the adoption. They must deal with the child's possible desire for information about his or her biologic parents. Adopted children are more likely to develop conduct disorders, problems with drug abuse, and antisocial personality traits. It is unclear whether these problems result from the process of adoption or whether parents who give up children for adoption are more likely to pass along a genetic predisposition for these behaviors.

With the widespread use of birth control and access to safe abortions, the number of infants available for adoption has declined steeply. Wealthy parents may prefer to arrange for private adoption rather than wait many uncertain years for institutional adoption. (In private adoptions, a biologic mother is paid for her legal and medical expenses but not for the baby. Baby selling is a felony in all states.) International adoptions (especially from Bosnia, Latin America, Eastern Europe, and China) have also become more common. Questionable regulation in these countries has raised concerns that some infants put up for adoption in developing countries may not be orphans but are being sold by impoverished mothers.

MIDDLE ADULTHOOD (40 TO 65 YEARS OF AGE)

Middle adulthood is the golden age of adulthood, similar to the latency years in childhood, but much longer. Physical health, emotional maturity, competence, and power in the work situation, and gratifying relationships with spouse, children, parents, friends, and colleagues all contribute to a normative sense of satisfaction and well-being. Concerning occupation, many persons begin to experience the gap between early aspirations and current achievements. They may wonder whether the lifestyle and the commitments they chose in early adulthood are worth continuing; they may feel that they would like to live their remaining years in a different, more satisfying way, without knowing exactly how. As children grow up and leave home, parental roles change, and persons redefine their roles as husbands and wives.

Significant gender-specific changes occur in middle adulthood. Many women who no longer need to nurture young children can release their energy into independent pursuits that require assertiveness and a competitive spirit, traits that were traditionally considered masculine. Alternatively, men in middle adulthood may develop qualities that enable them to express their emotions and recognize their dependency needs, traits that were usually considered feminine. With the new balance of the masculine and the feminine, a person may now be able to relate more effectively to someone of the other sex than in the past.

Transition from Young to Middle Adulthood

The transition from young adulthood to middle adulthood is slow and gradual, with no sharp physical or psychological demarcation. The aging process picks up speed and becomes a powerful organizing influence on intrapsychic life, but the change is gradual, unlike during adolescence. Mental change is experienced similarly, slow and imperceptible, without a sense of disruption.

Development in young adulthood is embedded in close relationships. Intimacy, love, and commitment are related to the mastery of the relationships most immediate to personal experience. The transition from young adulthood to middle age includes widening

Table 32-17
Features Salient to Middle Adulthood

Issues	Positive Features	Negative Features
Prime of life	Responsible use of power; maturity; productivity	Winner–loser view; competitiveness
Stock taking: what to do with the rest of one's life	Possibility; alternatives; organization of commitments; redirection	Closure; fatalism
Fidelity and commitments	Commitment to self, others, career, society; filial maturity	Hypocrisy; self-deception
Growth-death (to grow is to die); juvenescence and rejuvenation fantasies	Naturality regarding body, time	Obscene or frenetic efforts (e.g., to be youthful); hostility and envy of youth and progeny; longing
Communication and socialization	Matters understood; continuity; picking up where left off; large social network; rootedness of relationships, places, and ideas	Repetitiveness; boredom; impatience; isolation; conservatism; confusion; rigidity

Adapted from Robert N. Butler, M.D.

concern for the more extensive social system and differentiation of one's own social, political, and historical system from others. Authors have described middle adulthood in terms of generativity, self-actualization, and wisdom.

Developmental Theorists

Robert Butler described several underlying themes in middle adulthood that appear to be present regardless of marital and family status, gender, or economic level (Table 32-17). These themes include aging (as changes in bodily functions are noticed in middle adulthood); taking stock of accomplishments and setting goals for the future; reassessing commitments to family, work, and marriage; dealing with parental illness and death, and attending to all the developmental tasks without losing the capacity to experience pleasure or to engage in playful activities.

Erik Erikson. Erikson described middle adulthood as characterized either by generativity or by stagnation. Erikson defined *generativity* as the process by which persons guide the oncoming generation or improve society. This stage includes having and raising children, but wanting or having children does not ensure generativity. A childless person can be generative by (1) helping others, (2) being creative, and (3) contributing to society. Parents must be secure in their own identities to raise children successfully: They cannot be preoccupied with themselves and act as if they were, or wished to be, the child in the family.

To be *stagnant* means that a person stops developing. For Erikson, stagnation was anathema, and he referred to adults without any impulses to guide the new generation or to those who produce children but don't care for them as being "within a cocoon of self-concern and isolation." Such persons are in great danger. Because they are unable to negotiate the developmental tasks of middle adulthood, they are unprepared for the next stage of the life cycle, old age, which places more demands on the psychological and physical capacities than all the preceding stages.

George Vaillant. In his longitudinal study of 173 men who were interviewed at 5-year intervals after they graduated from Harvard, Vaillant found a strong correlation between physical and emotional health in middle age. Also, those with the most deficient psychological adjustment during college years had a high incidence

of physical illness in middle age. No single factor in childhood accounted for adult mental health, but an overall sense of stability in the parental home predicted well-adjusted adulthood. A close sibling relationship during college years was correlated with emotional and physical well-being in middle age. In another study, Vaillant found that childhood and adult work habits were related and that adult mental health and good interpersonal relationships were associated with the capacity to work in childhood. Vaillant's studies are ongoing and represent the most extended continuous study of adulthood ever performed.

Calvin Colarusso and Robert Nemiroff. Based on their experience as clinicians and psychoanalysts, Calvin Colarusso and Robert Nemiroff propose a broad theoretical foundation for adult development by suggesting that the developmental process is the same in the adult as in the child because, like the child, the adult is always in the midst of an ongoing dynamic process, continually influenced by a constantly changing environment, body, and mind. Whereas child development focuses primarily on the formation of psychic structure, adult development is concerned with the continuing evolution of existing psychic structure and with its use. Although the fundamental issues of childhood continue in altered form as central aspects of adult life, attempts to explain all adult behavior and pathology in terms of the experiences of childhood are considered reductionistic. The adult past must be taken into account in understanding adult behavior in the same way that the childhood past is considered. The aging body is understood to have a profound influence on psychological development in adulthood, as is the growing midlife recognition and acceptance of the finiteness of time and the inevitability of personal death.

Developing Midlife Friendships

Unlike friendships in latency and adolescence and, to some extent, in young adulthood, midlife friendships do not usually have a sense of urgency or the need for the frequent or nearly constant physical presence of the friend. Midlife individuals have neither the need to build a new psychic structure (as do latency-age children and adolescents) nor the pressing need to find new relationships (as do young adults). They may have many sources of gratification available through relationships with spouses, children, and colleagues.

As their firstborn sons progressed through high school, two women in their mid-40s became fast friends. In addition to raising money for the school activities in which their sons were involved, thus maintaining a close involvement with the boys, they spent many hours talking about the boys' activities, girlfriends, and college plans. Their husbands, who liked each other, became acquaintances, not friends. They directed their feelings about their sons into other relationships. After the boys left for college, the intensity of the friendship diminished, tending to peak again during vacation periods. (Courtesy of Calvin Colarusso, M.D.)

Because of their unique position in the life cycle, midlife adults are easily able to initiate and sustain friendships with individuals of different ages, as well as chronologic peers. In the face of a disrupted marriage or intimacy or the pressure of other midlife developmental themes, friendships may quickly become vehicles for the direct expression of impulses.

Reappraising Relationships. Midlife is a time of serious reappraisal of marriage and committed relationships. In the process, individuals struggle with the question of whether to settle for what they have or to search for greater perfection with a new partner. For some, the conflict rages internally and is kept from others; others express it through actions that take the form of affairs, trial separations, and divorce.

Recent research on happy marriage indicates that these couples, despite internal and real conflict, have found or achieved a special *goodness-of-fit* between their individual needs, wishes, and expectations. In the eyes of these couples, marital success is based on the ongoing, successful engagement of several psychological tasks. Among the most important are providing a safe place for conflict and difference, holding a double vision of the other, and maintaining a satisfying sexual life.

The decision to leave a long-standing, committed relationship has great consequences, not only for the two individuals involved but also for their friends and loved ones. The effect on children, in particular, is especially profound, extending far beyond childhood. The impact on the abandoned spouse, parents, and close relatives may be nearly as severe.

Various forms of therapeutic intervention, such as marital counseling, individual psychotherapy, and psychoanalysis, can be extremely effective in helping uncertain individuals decide what to do or in helping those who leave deal with the consequences of their decision on the abandoned partner, children, and other loved ones. Problems relating to intimacy, love, and sex can occupy a prominent position in an outpatient practice.

The four case studies presented here by Calvin Colarusso, M.D., illustrate some of the issues described above.

A couple in their late 50s sought treatment to decide their marriage. Both had been unhappy for years and wanted to divorce, feeling that they had to act now while there was still time to begin new relationships that would fulfill them. Their concerns were for their children and grandchildren. How would they react? Would they respect their decision to end a relationship of more than 30 years or attempt to stop the separation? As the work progressed, they decided that seeking happiness in the hopefully 20 or 30 years that they had left to live had to come ahead of the feelings of their loved ones. The fact that their decision was a mutual one facilitated their family's gradual acceptance of the divorce.

A 43-year-old patient, Mr. S, was continually preoccupied with his marriage during this 4-year psychoanalysis. Sexually inhibited during adolescence, he "married the only girl in the world who knew less about sex than I did." Both were virgins on their wedding night. As the marriage progressed, the couple gradually developed a "satisfactory" sex life, but the patient always wondered what he had missed. As his sexual inhibitions were explored, Mr. S's sense of having "missed out on a lot of opportunities" lead to visits to massage parlors and prostitutes. Eventually, such behavior ceased because of the recognition that his wife was a wonderful mother and loving wife and not the cause of the lack of sexual experience that he brought into the marriage. "I'll always feel that I missed out when I was young, but I've got so much going for me now, I'm not going to mess it up over something that I can't change."

A 38-year-old woman entered therapy after her husband discovered that she was having sexual relations with men in their early and middle 20s. She explained that she loved her husband, but he seemed to take her for granted. He no longer made her feel attractive and wanted. As the therapy progressed, it became clear that she felt that as long as she could attract younger men, she was still young and sexually desirable. Struggling with the early signs of physical aging, the realization that the young men were only using her to satisfy their own sexual needs was sobering and distressing. As she began to see that such behavior was self-destructive, she approached her husband about starting marital therapy.

Fifty-year-old Mrs. T left her "wonderful" husband because "I've missed something. I just have to get out on my own." Married at 18 years of age, "after going from my parents' home to his home," she recognized that her rage at her husband for "not being all the other men I could have married, for closing off all the living I could have done" was irrational but uncontrollable. "I have to live on my own for a while to see if I can do it before it's too late." Fully intending to return to her husband, she continued exploring the infantile and adult issues that precipitated the separation, leaving the future of the marriage in doubt.

Sexuality

Whereas the young adult is preoccupied with developing the capacity for intimacy, the midlife individual is focused on maintaining intimacy in the face of deterring physical, psychological, and environmental pressures. In a long-standing relationship, these pressures include real and imaginary concerns about diminished sexual capability, emotional withdrawal because of preoccupation with developmental tasks, and the realistic pressures related to work and providing for dependent children and, sometimes, elderly parents as well. In relationships that begin in midlife, the maintenance of intimacy can be compromised by the absence of a common past, age and generational differences in interests and activities, and the difficulties involved in forming a stepfamily.

For sexual intimacy to continue, the participants must (1) accept the appearance of the partner's middle-aged body, (2) continue to find it sexually stimulating, and (3) accept the normative changes that occur in sexual functioning. For those who master these developmental issues, the partner's body remains sexually stimulating. Diminished sexual ability is compensated for by feelings of love and tenderness generated over the years by a satisfying relationship.

Those who cannot accept the changes in the partner's body or their stop having sex, begin affairs or leave the relationship, usually in search of a younger partner.

Normative changes in midlife sexual functioning include diminished sexual drive and an increase in mechanical problems. Men have greater difficulty getting and sustaining erections and experience a longer refractory period after ejaculation. Because of diminished estrogen production, women experience a thinning of the vaginal mucosa, a decrease in secretions, and fewer contractions at the time of orgasm. Women do not reach their sexual prime until their mid-30s; consequently, they have a greater capacity for orgasm in middle adulthood than in young adulthood. Women, however, are more vulnerable than men to narcissistic blows to their self-esteem as they lose their youthful appearance, which is overvalued in today's society. During middle adulthood, they may feel less sexually desirable than in early adulthood and, thus, feel less entitled to adequate sex life. An inability to deal with changes in body image prompts many women and men to undergo cosmetic surgery to maintain their youthful appearance.

The demands of raising children interfere with the privacy and emotional equilibrium required for intimacy, as do the pressures and responsibilities of work. Fatigue and diminished interest are common denominators in these circumstances. Patients with deeply rooted problems with sexuality or relationships may use aging, work, and relationships with children or elderly parents as a means of rationalizing their conflicts and refusing to analyze them.

Climacterium

Middle adulthood is the time of the male and female climacterium, the period in a life characterized by decreased biologic and physiologic functioning. For women, the menopausal period is considered the climacterium, and it may start anywhere from the 40s to the early 50s. Bernice Neugarten studied this period and found that more than 50 percent of women described menopause as an unpleasant experience. Still, a significant portion believed that their lives had not changed in any meaningful way, and many women experienced no adverse effects. Because they no longer had to worry about becoming pregnant, some women report feeling sexually freer after menopause than before its onset. Generally, the female climacterium has been stereotyped as a sudden or radical psychophysiological experience. Still, it is more often a gradual experience as estrogen secretion decreases with changes in the flow, timing, and eventual cessation of the menses. Vasomotor instability (hot flashes) can occur, and menopause can extend over several years. Some women experience anxiety and depression, but women who have a history of poor adaptation to stress are more predisposed to the menopausal syndrome.

For men, the climacterium has no clear demarcation; male hormones stay reasonably constant through the 40s and 50s and then begin to decline. Nevertheless, men must adapt to a decline in biologic functioning and overall physical vigor. About age 50, a slight decrease in healthy sperm and seminal fluid occurs, not sufficient, however, to preclude insemination. Coincident with a decreased testosterone level may be fewer and less firm erections and decreased sexual activity generally. Some men experience a so-called midlife crisis during this period. The crisis can be mild or severe, characterized by a sudden drastic change in work or marital relationships, severe depression, increased use of alcohol or drugs, or a shift to an alternate lifestyle.

Midlife Transition and Crisis

The *midlife transition* has been defined as an intensive reappraisal of all aspects of life precipitated by the growing recognition that life is finite and approaching an end. It is characterized by mental turmoil, not action. For most people, the reappraisal results in decisions to keep most life structures, such as marriages and careers, which have been painstakingly built over time. When significant changes are made, they are thoughtful and considered, even when they include major shifts, such as divorce or a job change. The developmentally aware clinician recognizes that every patient in this age group is engaged in a midlife transition (whether the patient is talking about it or not) and facilitates the process by making it conscious and verbal.

A true *midlife crisis* is a major, revolutionary turning point in life, involving changes in commitments to career or spouse, or both, and accompanied by significant, ongoing emotional turmoil for the individual and others. It is an upheaval of substantial proportions. A flurry of impulsive actions follows a period of internal agitation, for example, leaving spouse and children, becoming involved with a new sexual partner, and quitting a job, all within days or weeks of each other. Although unrecognized warning signs may have existed, those who are left behind are often shocked by the suddenness and abruptness of the change.

Efforts by family members or therapists to get the individual to stop and to reconsider usually fall on deaf ears. The overwhelming need is to avoid anyone who counsels restraint and to ignore therapists who recommend examining motivations and feelings before making such major decisions. Usually, during the crisis, the therapist is left with the painful job of helping those who have been left to deal with their shock and grief.

Empty-Nest Syndrome.   Another phenomenon described in middle adulthood has been called the *empty-nest syndrome,* a depression that occurs in some men and women when their youngest child is about to leave home. Most parents, however, perceive the departure of the youngest child as a relief rather than stress. If no compensating activities have been developed, particularly by the mother, some parents become depressed. This is especially true of women whose predominant role in life has been mothering or of couples who decided to stay in an otherwise unhappy marriage "for the sake of the children."

Other Tasks of Middle Adulthood

As persons approach the age of 50, they clearly define what they want from work, family, and leisure. Men who have reached their highest level of advancement in work may experience disillusionment or frustration when they realize they can no longer anticipate new work challenges. For women who have invested themselves entirely in mothering, this period leaves them with no suitable identity after the children leave home. Sometimes, social rules become rigidly established; lack of freedom in lifestyle and a sense of entrapment can lead to depression and a loss of confidence. Also, unique financial burdens can occur in middle age, produced by pressures to care for aged parents at one end of the spectrum and children at the other end.

Daniel Levinson described a transitional period between the ages of 50 and 55, during which a developmental crisis may occur when persons feel incapable of changing an intolerable life structure. Although no single event characterizes the transition, the physiologic changes that begin to appear may have a dramatic effect on a person's sense of self. For example, a person may experience a decrease in cardiovascular efficiency that accompanies aging. Chronologic age and physical infirmity are not linear; however, those who exercise regularly, who do not smoke, and who eat and drink in moderation can maintain their physical health and emotional well-being.

Middle adulthood is when persons frequently feel overwhelmed by too many obligations and duties, but it is also a time of great satisfaction for most persons. They have developed a wide array of acquaintances, friendships, and relationships, and the satisfaction they express about their network of friends predicts positive mental health. Some social ties, however, may be a source of stress when demands either cannot be met or assault a person's self-esteem. Middle-aged persons most generally possess power, leadership, wisdom, and understanding, and if their health and vitality remain intact, it is indeed the prime of life.

DIVORCE

Divorce is a significant crisis in life. Spouses often grow, develop, and change at different rates; one spouse may discover that the other is not the same as when they first married. In truth, both partners have changed and evolved, not necessarily in complementary directions. Frequently, one spouse blames a third person for alienation of affections and refuses to examine his or her role in the marital problems. Certain aspects of marital deterioration and divorce seem to be related to specific qualities of middle life—the need for change, weariness with acting responsibly, fear of facing up to oneself.

Types of Separation

Paul Bohannan, an anthropologist with expertise in marriage and divorce, described the types of separations that take place at the time of divorce.

Psychic Divorce. In psychic divorce, the love object is given up, and a grief reaction about the death of the relationship occurs. Sometimes a period of anticipatory mourning sets in before the divorce. Separating from a spouse forces a person to become autonomous, to change from a position of dependence. The separation may be difficult to achieve, mainly if both are used to being dependent on each other (as happens typically in marriage) or if one was so dependent as to be afraid or incapable of becoming independent. Most persons report such feelings as depression, ambivalence, and mood swings at the time of divorce. Studies indicate that recovery from divorce takes about 2 years; by then, the ex-spouse may be viewed neutrally, and each spouse accepts his or her new identity as a single person.

Legal Divorce. Legal divorce involves going through the courts so that each of the parties is remarriageable. Of divorced women and divorced men, 75 percent and 80 percent, respectively, remarry within 3 years of divorce. No-fault divorce, in which neither person is judged to be the guilty party, has become the most widely used legal mechanism for divorce.

Economic Divorce. Economic divorce involves significant concerns about the division of the couple's property between them and economic support for the wife. Many men who are ordered by the courts to pay alimony or child support flout the law and create a major social problem.

Community Divorce. The social network of the divorced couple changes markedly. A few relatives and friends are retained from the community, and new ones are added. The task of meeting new friends is often tricky for divorced persons, who may realize how dependent they were on their spouses for social exchanges.

Coparental Divorce. Coparental divorce is the separation of a parent from the child's other parent. Being a single parent differs from being a married parent.

Custody

The parental right doctrine is a legal concept that awards custody to the more fit natural parent and attempts to ensure that the best interests of the child are served. In the past, mothers were almost always awarded custody, but custody is now given to fathers in about 15 percent of cases. Custodial fathers are likely to be white, married, older, and better educated than custodial mothers. Women who are granted custody have a better chance of being awarded child support and of actually receiving payment than do men who are given custody. Nevertheless, women who accept payments still have lower incomes than men who receive compensation.

The types of custody include *joint custody,* in which a child spends equal time with each parent, an increasingly common practice; *split custody,* in which siblings are separated and each parent has custody of one or more of the children; and *single custody,* in which the children live solely with one parent and the other parent has rights of visitation that may be limited in some way by the court. Child support payments are more likely to be made when parents have joint custody or when the noncustodial parent is given visitation rights.

Problems can surface in the parent–child relationship with the custodial or the noncustodial parent. The absence of the noncustodial parent in the home represents the reality of the divorce, and the custodial parent may become the target of the child's anger about the divorce. The parent under such stress may not be able to deal with the child's increased needs and emotional demands.

The noncustodial parent must cope with limits placed on time spent with the child. This parent loses the day-to-day gratification and the responsibilities involved with parenting. Emotional distress is common in parent and child. Joint custody offers a solution with some advantages, but it requires substantial maturity on the part of the parents and can present some problems. Parents must separate their child-rearing practices from their postdivorce resentments, and they must develop a spirit of cooperation about rearing the child. They must also be able to tolerate frequent communication with the ex-spouse.

Reasons for Divorce

Divorce tends to run in families, and rates are highest in couples who marry as teenagers or come from different socioeconomic backgrounds. Every marriage is psychologically unique, and so is each divorce. If a person's parents were divorced, he or she might choose to resolve a marital problem in the same way, through a divorce. Expectations of the spouse may be unrealistic: One partner may expect the other to act as an all-giving mother or a magically protective father. The parenting experience places the most significant strain on a marriage. In surveys of couples with and without children, those without children reported getting more pleasure from their spouse than those with children. Illness in the child creates the greatest strain of all and more than 50 percent of marriages in which a child has died through illness or accident end in divorce.

Other causes of marital distress are problems with sex and money. Both areas may be used as a means of control, and withholding sex or money is a means of expressing aggression. Also, less social pressure to remain married currently exists. As discussed above, the easing of divorce laws and the declining influence of religion and the extended family make divorce an acceptable course of action today.

Intercourse Outside of Marriage. Adultery is defined as voluntary sexual intercourse between a married person and someone other than his or her spouse. For men, the first extramarital affair is often associated with the wife's pregnancy, when coitus may be interdicted. Most of these incidents are kept secret from the spouse and, if known, rarely account for divorce. Nevertheless, the infidelity can serve as the catalyst for basic dissatisfactions in the marriage to the surface, and these problems may then lead to its dissolution. Adultery may decline, as potentially fatal STDs such as acquired immune deficiency syndrome (AIDS) serve as sobering deterrents.

ADULT MATURITY

Success and happiness in adulthood are made possible by achieving a modicum of maturity—a mental state, not an age. The capacity for maturity, however, is a direct outgrowth of the engagement and mastery of the developmental tasks of young and middle adulthood. From a developmental perspective, maturity can be defined as a mental state found in healthy adults that is characterized by detailed knowledge of the parameters of human existence, a sophisticated level of self-awareness based on an honest appraisal of one's own experience within those basic parameters, and the ability to use this intellectual and emotional knowledge and insight caringly concerning one's self and others.

The achievement of maturity in midlife leads to the emergence of the capacity for wisdom. Those who possess wisdom have learned from the past and are fully engaged in life in the present. Just as important, they anticipate the future and make the necessary decisions to enhance prospects for health and happiness. In other words, a philosophy of life has been developed that includes understanding and acceptance of the person's place in the order of human existence. Unfortunately, the joys of midlife do not last forever. Old age lies ahead. Although the hope and statistical expectation is for many years of mental competence and independence, physical and mental decline, increased dependence, and, eventually, death must be anticipated. Late adulthood has its great pleasure, when there is a focus on continued mental and physical activity, a dominant preoccupation with the present and the future, and involvement with and facilitation of the young. Then, death can be met with feelings of satisfaction and acceptance, the natural endpoint of human existence that follows a life lived and well loved.

▲ 32.3 Old Age

When we progress from youth to old age, the focus may change from pursuing wealth to maintaining health. In late adulthood, the aging body increasingly becomes a central concern, replacing the midlife preoccupations with career and relationships. This change is so because of diminution in function, altered physical appearance, and the increased incidence of physical illness. Despite these occurrences, the body in late adulthood can still be a source of considerable pleasure and can convey a sense of competence, particularly when giving attention to regular exercise, a healthy diet, adequate

Table 32-18
Developmental Tasks of Late Adulthood

To maintain the body image and physical integrity
To conduct the life review
To maintain sexual interests and activities
To deal with the death of significant loved ones
To accept the implications of retirement
To accept the genetically programmed failure of organ systems
To divest oneself of the attachment to possessions
To accept changes in the relationship with grandchildren

rest, and preventive maintenance medical care. The normal state in the aged is physical and mental health, not illness and debilitation. The developmental tasks of late adulthood that lead to mental health are listed in Table 32-18.

Old age, or late adulthood, usually refers to the stage of the life cycle that begins at age 65. Gerontologists—those who study the aging process—divide older adults into two groups: young-old, ages 65 to 74, and old-old, ages 75 and beyond. Some use the term oldest-old to refer to those over 85. Older adults can also be described as well-old (healthy persons) and sick-old (persons who have an infirmity that interferes with functioning and requires medical or psychiatric attention). The health needs of older adults have grown enormously as the population ages, and geriatric physicians and psychiatrists play significant roles in treating this population.

DEMOGRAPHICS

The number of individuals over age 65 is rapidly expanding. In 1900, for example, 4 percent of the US population was older than 65 years. By 2012 it was 13.7 percent, and by 2050, it is projected to be about 20 percent. That increase far exceeds the general population growth—tenfold compared with just over threefold between 1900 and 2000—and is projected to continue (e.g., 2.5 times vs. just over 1.5 times between 1990 and 2050) (Table 32-19).

Table 32-19
Aging Population of the United States: 1900–2050

Year	Median Age	Mean Age	All Ages (N)	65 and Over (N)	65 and Over (%)	85 and Over (N)	85 and Over (%)
				Population, in Millions and as a Percentage of Total Population			
1900			76.0	3.1	4.1	0.1	0.1
1950			150.1	12.3	8.2	0.6	0.4
1990			248.7	31.1	12.5	3.0	1.2
2000	35.7	36.5	276.2	35.3	12.8	4.3	1.6
2010	37.2	37.8	300.4	40.1	13.3	6.0	2.0
2030	38.5	39.9	350.0	70.2	20.1	8.8	2.5
2050	38.1	40.3	392.0	80.1	20.4	18.9	4.8

Population: U.S. Bureau of the Census. Current Population Reports, Special Studies, P23-190, 65+ in the United States. Washington, DC: U.S. Government Printing Office; 1996.
Mean/Median Age, 2000–2050: Day JC. Population projections of the United States by age, sex, race, and Hispanic origin: 1995 to 2050. In: U.S. Bureau of the Census, Current Population Reports, P25–1130. Washington, DC: U.S. Government Printing Office; 1996.

The life expectancy for women at birth is projected to continue to exceed that for men by 7 years until 2050. By 2050, the composition of the US population by age and sex is estimated to differ markedly from that today. Such changes are bound to influence income and marital statistics, the percentage of elderly persons living alone or in long-term care facilities, and other aspects of the social network. A summary of demographic highlights of the aged is given in Table 32-20.

The accuracy of these projections, however, depends on the accuracy of other predications such as birth rates, immigration, and emigration—all of which are more difficult to gauge for the future than the remaining variables, death rates, or life expectancies. Projections concerning life expectancy, for example, can change substantially within a single decade.

BIOLOGY OF AGING

The aging process, or senescence (from the Latin *senescere,* "to grow old"), is characterized by a gradual decline in the functioning of all of the body's systems—cardiovascular, respiratory, genitourinary, endocrine, and immune, among others. However, the belief that old age is invariably associated with profound intellectual and physical infirmity is a myth. Many older persons retain their cognitive abilities and physical capacities to a remarkable degree.

An overview of the biologic changes that accompany old age is given in Table 32-21. The various decrements listed do not occur linearly in all systems. Not all organ systems deteriorate at the same rate, nor do they follow a similar pattern of decline for all persons. Each person is genetically endowed with one or more vulnerable systems, or a system may become vulnerable because of environmental stressors or intentional misuse, such as excessive ultraviolet exposure, smoking, or alcohol use. Moreover, not all organ systems deteriorate at the same time. Any one of several organ systems begins to deteriorate, and this deterioration then leads to illness or death.

Aging generally means the aging of cells. In the most commonly held theory, each cell has a genetically determined life span, during which it can replicate itself a limited number of times before it dies. Structural changes occur in cells with age. In the central nervous system, for example, age-related cell changes occur in neurons, which show signs of degeneration. In senility (characterized by severe memory loss and a loss of intellectual functioning), signs of degeneration are much more severe. An example is the neurofibrillary degeneration seen most commonly in dementia of the Alzheimer's type.

Structural changes and mutations in deoxyribonucleic acid (DNA) and ribonucleic acid (RNA) are also found in aging cells; these have been attributed to genotypic programming, x-rays, chemicals, and food products, among others. Probably no single cause of aging exists, and all areas of the body are affected to some degree. Genetic factors have been implicated in disorders that commonly occur in older persons, such as hypertension, coronary artery disease, arteriosclerosis, and neoplastic disease. Family studies indicate inheritance factors for breast and stomach cancer, colon polyps, and certain mental disorders of old age. Huntington disease shows an autosomal dominant mode of inheritance with complete penetrance. The average age of onset is between 35 and 40 years, but cases have occurred as late as 70 years.

Longevity

Longevity has been studied since the beginning of recorded history and has always been a topic of great interest. The research about longevity reveals that a family history of longevity is the best indicator of a long life; of persons who live past 80, half of their

**Table 32-20
Demographic Highlights of the Aged**

- The older population (65+) numbered 4.04 million in 2010, an increase of 5.4 million for 15.3 since 2000.
- The number of Americans aged 45–64—who will reach 65 over the next two decades—increased by 31% during this decade.
- Over one in every eight, or 13.1%, of the population is an older American.
- Persons reaching age 65 have an average life expectancy of an additional 18.8 yr (20 yr for females and 17.3 for males).
- Older women outnumber older men at 23 million older women to 17.5 million older men.
- In 2010, 20% of persons 65+ were minorities—8.4% were African American.[a] Persons of Hispanic origin (who may be of any race) represented 6.9% of the older population. About 3.5% were Asian or Pacific Islanders,[a] and less than 1% were American Indian or Native Alaskan.[a]
- In addition, 0.8% of persons 65+ identified themselves as being of two or more races.
- Older men were much more likely to be married than older women—72% of men vs. 42% of women. In 2010, 40% older women were widows.
- About 29% (11.3 million) of noninstitutionalized older persons live alone (8.1 million women, 3.2 million men).
- Almost half of older women (47%) age 75+ live alone.
- About 485,000 grandparents aged 65 or more had the primary responsibility for their grandchildren who lived with them.
- The population 65 and over has increased from 35 million in 2000 to 40 million in 2010 (a 15% increase) and is projected to increase up to 55 million in 2020 (a 36% increase for that decade).
- The 85+ population is projected to increase from 5.5 million in 2010 and then 6.6 million in 2020 (19%) for that decade.
- Minority populations have increased from 5.7 million in 2000 (16.3% of the elderly population) to 8.1 million in 2010 (20% of the elderly) and are projected to increase to 13.1 million in 2020 (24% of the elderly).
- The median income of older persons in 2010 was $25,704 for males and $15,072 for females. Median money income (after adjusting for inflation) of all households headed by older people fell 1.5% (not statistically significant) from 2009 to 2010. Households containing families headed by person 65+ reported a median income in 2010 of $45,763.
- The major sources of income as reported by older persons in 2009 were Social Security (reported by 87% of older persons), income from assets (reported by 53%), private pensions (reported by 28%), government employee pensions (reported by 14%), and earnings (reported by 26%).
- Social Security constituted 90% or more of the income received by 35% of beneficiaries in 2009 (22% married couples and 43% of nonmarried beneficiaries).
- Almost 3.5 million elderly persons (9.0%) were below the poverty level in 2010. This poverty rate is not statistically different from the poverty rate in 2009 (8.9%). During 2011, the U.S. Census Bureau also released a new Supplemental Poverty Measure (SPM) that takes into account regional variations in the living costs, noncash benefits received, and nondiscretionary expenditures but does not replace the official poverty measure. The SPM shows a poverty level for older persons of 15.9%, an increase of over 75% over the official rate of 9% mainly due to medical out-of-pocket expenses.
- About 11% (3.7 million) of older Medicare enrollees received personal care from a paid or unpaid source in 1999.

---

[a]Principle source data for the profile are from the U.S. Census Bureau, the National Center for Health Statistics, and the Bureau of Labor Statistics. The profile incorporates the latest data (2010) available but not all items are updated on an annual basis.

fathers also lived past 80. Nevertheless, many conditions leading to a shortened life can be prevented, ameliorated, or delayed with effective intervention. Heredity is but one factor—one beyond a person's control. Predictors of longevity that are within a person's

Table 32-21
Biologic Changes Associated with Aging

Cellular Level
Change in cellular DNA (deoxyribonucleic acid) and RNA (ribonucleic acid) structures: intracellular organelle degeneration
Neuronal degeneration in central nervous system, primarily in superior temporal precentral and inferior temporal gyri; no loss in brainstem nuclei
Receptor sites and sensitivity altered
Decreased anabolism and catabolism of cellular transmitter substances
Intercellular collagen and elastin increase

Immune System
Impaired T-cell response to antigen
Increase in function of autoimmune bodies
Increased susceptibility to infection and neoplasia
Leukocytes unchanged, T lymphocytes reduced
Increased erythrocyte sedimentation (nonspecific)

Musculoskeletal
Decrease in height because of shortening of spinal column (2-in loss in both men and women from the second to the seventh decades)
Reduction in lean muscle mass and muscle strength; deepening of thoracic cage
Increase in body fat
Elongation of nose and ears
Loss of bone matrix, leading to osteoporosis
Degeneration of joint surfaces may produce osteoarthritis
Risk of hip fracture is 10–25% by age 90
Continual closing of cranial sutures (parietomastoid suture does not attain complete closure until age 80)
Men gain weight until about age 60, then lose; women gain weight until age 70, then lose

Integument
Graying of hair results from decreased melanin production in hair follicles (by age 50, 50% of all persons male and female are at least 50% gray; pubic hair is last to turn gray)
General wrinkling of skin
Less active sweat glands
Decrease in melanin
Loss of subcutaneous fat
Nail growth slowed

Genitourinary and Reproductive
Decreased glomerular filtration rate and renal blood flow
Decreased hardness of erection, diminished ejaculatory spurt
Decreased vaginal lubrication
Enlargement of prostate
Incontinence

Special Senses
Thickening of optic lens, reduced peripheral vision
Inability to accommodate (presbyopia)
High-frequency sound hearing loss (presbyacusis)—25% show loss by age 60, 65% by age 80
Yellowing of optic lens
Reduced acuity of taste, smell, and touch
Decreased light-dark adaption

Neuropsychiatric
Takes longer to learn new material, but complete learning still occurs
Intelligence quotient (IQ) remains stable until age 80
Verbal ability maintained with age
Psychomotor speed declines

Memory
Tasks requiring shifting attentions performed with difficulty
Encoding ability diminishes (transfer of short- to long-term memory and vice versa)
Recognition of right answer on multiple-choice tests remains intact
Simple recall declines

Neurotransmitters
Norepinephrine decreases in central nervous system
Increased monoamine oxidase and serotonin in brain

Brain
Decrease in gross brain weight, about 17% by age 80 in both sexes
Widened sulci, smaller convolutions, gyral atrophy
Ventricles enlarge
Increased transport across blood–brain barrier
Decreased cerebral blood flow and oxygenation

Cardiovascular
Increase in size and weight of heart (contains lipofuscin pigment derived from lipids)
Decreased elasticity of heart valves
Increased collagen in blood vessels
Increased susceptibility to arrhythmias
Altered homeostasis of blood pressure
Cardiac output maintained in absence of coronary heart disease

Gastrointestinal (GI) System
At risk for atrophic gastritis, hiatal hernia, diverticulosis
Decreased blood flow to gut, liver
Diminished saliva flow
Altered absorption from GI tract (at risk for malabsorption syndrome and avitaminosis)
Constipation

Endocrine
Estrogen levels decrease in women
Adrenal androgen decreases
Testosterone production declines in men
Increase in follicle-stimulating hormone (FSH) and luteinizing hormone (LH) in postmenopausal women
Serum thyroxine (T_4) and thyroid-stimulating hormone (TSH) normal, triiodothyronine (T_3) reduced
Glucose tolerance test result decreases

Respiratory
Decreased vital capacity
Diminished cough reflex
Decreased bronchial epithelium ciliary action

control include regular medical checkups, minimal or no caffeine or alcohol consumption, work gratification, and a perceived sense of the self as being socially useful in an altruistic role, such as a spouse, teacher, mentor, parent, or grandparent. Healthy eating and adequate exercise are also associated with health and longevity.

Life Expectancy

In the United States, the average life expectancy has increased throughout the last century—from 48 years in 1900 to 77.4 years for men and 82.2 years for women in 2013. The projected life expectancy at birth, and age 65 is indicated in Table 32-22. Changes in morbidity and mortality have also occurred. Over the past 30 years, for example, a 60 percent decline has occurred in mortality from cerebrovascular disease and a 30 percent decline in mortality from coronary artery disease. In contrast, mortality from cancer, which rises steeply with age, has increased, especially cancer of the lung, colon, stomach, skin, and prostate.

The oldest-old, persons over 85 years of age, is the most rapidly growing segment of the older population. Over the past

Table 32-22
Projected Life Expectancy at Birth and Age 65, by Sex: 1990–2050 (in Years)

	At Birth			At Age 65		
Year	Men	Women	Difference	Men	Women	Difference
1990	72.1	79.0	6.9	15.0	19.4	4.4
2000	73.5	80.4	6.9	15.7	20.3	4.6
2010	74.4	81.3	6.9	16.2	21.0	4.8
2020	74.9	81.8	6.9	16.6	21.4	4.8
2030	75.4	82.3	6.9	17.0	21.8	4.8
2040	75.9	82.8	6.9	17.3	22.3	5.0
2050	76.4	83.3	6.9	17.7	22.7	5.0

Data from U.S. Bureau of the Census, Washington, DC.

25 years, the population of all older persons increased by 100 percent, compared with 45 percent for the entire US population, but the increase for the 85 and older group exceeded 275 percent. It is expected that by 2050, the oldest-old will make up about 25 percent of the elderly population and 5 percent of the total population in the United States. Figure 32-7 gives projected percentages for the average annual growth rate of the elderly population to 2050.

The leading causes of death among older persons are heart disease, cancer, and stroke. Accidents are among the leading causes of death of persons over 65. Most fatal accidents are caused by falls, pedestrian incidents, and burns. Falls are most commonly the result of cardiac arrhythmias and hypotensive episodes.

Some gerontologists consider death in very old persons (over 85) to result from an aging syndrome characterized by diminished elastic-mechanical properties of the heart, arteries, lungs, and other organs. Death results from trivial tissue injuries that would not be fatal to a younger person; accordingly, senescence is viewed as the cause of death.

Ethnicity and Race

The proportion of older persons in the black, Hispanic, and Asian populations is smaller than that in the white population, but it is increasing rapidly. By 2050, 20 percent of older persons will be nonwhite. The proportion of older persons who are Hispanic will increase from 4 percent to approximately 14 percent over the same period. According to the U.S. Census Bureau, Hispanic refers to persons "whose origins are Mexican, Puerto Rican, Cuban, Central or South American, and other Hispanic or Latino, regardless of race" (Fig. 32-8).

Sex Ratios

On average, women live longer than men and are more likely than men to live alone. The number of men per 100 women decreases sharply from ages 65 to 85 (Fig. 32-9).

Geographic Distribution

The most populous states have the largest number of older persons. California has the most (3.3 million), followed by New York, Pennsylvania, Texas, Michigan, Illinois, Florida, and Ohio, each with more than 1 million. States with high proportions of older persons include Pennsylvania, Florida, Nebraska, and North Dakota. Florida's high percentage of older adults related its popularity as a retirement locale. In other states, the reason is usually more young persons leaving.

Exercise, Diet, and Health

Diet and exercise play a role in preventing or ameliorating chronic diseases of older persons, such as arteriosclerosis and hypertension. Hyperlipidemia, which correlates with coronary artery disease, can be controlled by reducing body weight, decreasing the intake of saturated fat, and limiting the intake of cholesterol. Increasing the daily intake of dietary fiber can also help decrease serum lipoprotein levels. A daily intake of 1 oz (about 30 mL) of alcohol has been correlated with longevity and elevated high-density lipoproteins (HDLs). Studies have also clearly demonstrated that statin drugs that reduce cholesterol have a dramatic effect on reducing cardiovascular disease in persons with diet-resistant or exercise-resistant hyperlipidemia.

Low salt intake (less than 3 g a day) is associated with a lowered risk of hypertension. Hypertensive geriatric patients can often correct their condition by moderate exercise and decreased salt intake without the addition of drugs.

A regimen of moderate daily exercise (walking for 30 minutes a day) has been associated with a reduction in cardiovascular

FIGURE 32-7
Average annual growth rate of the elderly population. (Data from U.S. Bureau of the Census.)

(In percent)

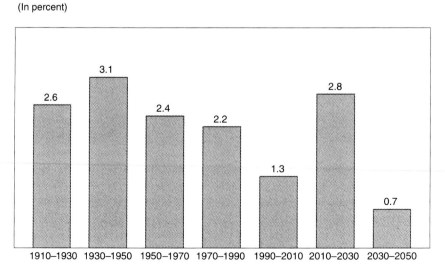

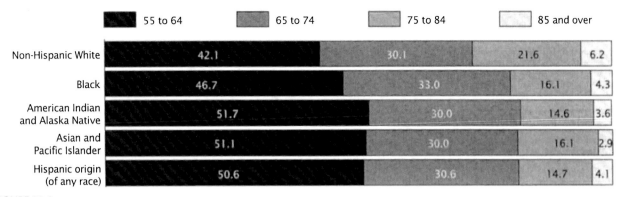

FIGURE 32-8

Percent distribution of people 55 years and over by race, Hispanic origin, and age: 2002. (Data from U.S. Bureau of the Census.)

disease, decreased incidence of osteoporosis, improved respiratory function, the maintenance of ideal weight, and a general sense of well-being. Exercise has been shown to improve strength and function even among the very old. In many cases, a disease process has been reversed and even cured by diet and exercise, without additional medical or surgical intervention.

Table 32-23 lists the biologic changes associated with diet and exercise. A comparison with Table 32-19 reveals that almost every biologic change associated with aging is positively affected by diet and exercise.

STAGE THEORIES OF PERSONALITY DEVELOPMENT

Early personality theorists proposed that development was completed by the end of childhood or adolescence. One of the first development theorists to propose that personality continues to develop and grow over the life span was Erik Erikson. Erikson believed that development proceeded through a series of psychosocial stages, each with its conflict that is resolved by the individual with greater or lesser success. Erikson termed the crisis of the last epoch of life integrity versus despair and believed that successful resolution of this crisis involved a process of life review and achieving a sense of peace and wisdom through coming to terms with how one's life was lived. For example, Erikson proposed that successful resolution of this crisis would be characterized by a sense of having lived one's life well, whereas a less successful resolution would be characterized by feeling that life was too short, that one did not choose wisely, and bitterness that one will not have a chance to live life over.

Table 32-23
Positive and Healthy Physiologic Effects of Exercise and Nutrition

Increases
Strength of bones, ligaments, and muscles
Muscle mass and body density
Articular cartilage thickness
Skeletal muscle ATP (adenosine triphosphatase), CRP (C-reactive protein), K^+ (potassium), and myoglobin
Skeletal muscle oxidative enzyme content and mitochondria
Skeletal muscle arterial collaterals and capillary density
Heart volume and weight
Blood volume and total circulating hemoglobin
Cardiac stroke volume
Myocardial contractility
Maximal CO_2 (A-V)
Maximal blood lactate concentration
Maximal pulmonary ventilation
Maximal respiratory work
Maximal oxygen diffusing capacity
Maximal exercise capacity as measured by the maximal oxygen intake, exercise time, and distance
Serum high-density lipoprotein concentration
Anaerobic threshold
Plasma insulin concentration with submaximal exercise

Decreases
Heart rate at rest and during submaximal exercise
Blood lactate concentration during submaximal exercise
Pulmonary ventilation during submaximal work
Respiratory quotient during submaximal work
Serum triglyceride concentration
Body fatness
Serum low-density lipoprotein concentration
Systolic blood pressure
Core temperature threshold for initiation of sweating
Sweat sodium and chloride content
Plasma epinephrine and norepinephrine with submaximal exercise
Plasma glucagon and growth hormone concentrations with submaximal exercise
Relative hemoconcentration with submaximal exercise in the heat

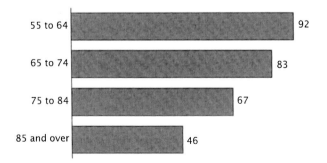

(Men per 100 women)

FIGURE 32-9

Sex ratio of people 55 years and over by age: 2002. (Data from U.S. Bureau of the Census.)

Reprinted from Buskirk ER. In: White PL, Monderka T, eds. *Diet and Exercise: Synergism in Health Maintenance.* Chicago: American Medical Association; 1982:133, with permission.

Normal Development and Aging **917**

Table 32-24
Old Age Developmental Theorists

Sigmund Freud	Increasing control of the ego and id with aging results in increased autonomy. Regression may permit primitive modes of functioning to reappear.
Erik Erikson	The central conflict in old age is between integrity, the sense of satisfaction people feel reflecting on a life lived productively, and despair, the sense that life has little purpose or meaning. Contentment in old age comes only with getting beyond narcissism and into intimacy and generativity.
Heinz Kohut	Old people must continually cope with narcissistic injury as they attempt to adapt to the biologic, psychological, and social losses associated with the aging process. The maintenance of self-esteem is a major task of old age.
Bernice Neugarten	The major conflict of old age relates to giving up the position of authority and evaluating achievements and former competence. It is a time of reconciliation with others and resolution of grief over the death of others and the approaching death of self.
Daniel Levinson	Ages 60–65 is a transition period ("the late adult transition"). People who are narcissistic and too heavily invested in body appearance are liable to become preoccupied with death. Creative mental activity is a normal and healthy substitute for reduced physical activity.

Several studies have attempted to validate aspects of Erikson's theory. In one study, a sample of more than 400 men was studied prospectively, and the highest Eriksonian life stage each achieved was rated according to data gathered on the circumstances of his life. For example, if a man had achieved independence from his family of origin and was self-sufficient but was unable to develop an intimate relationship, the highest life stage achieved would be the identity stage, not the intimacy stage. This study found that Eriksonian stages are passed through in sequential order, although often not at the same age for every individual, and that the stages are surprisingly universal in populations that are ethnically and socioeconomically diverse.

A longitudinal study of approximately 500 subjects from two age cohorts found that the earlier age cohort scored significantly higher on integrity than the latter age cohort, and scores for both age cohorts on integrity had declined significantly by the final time of testing. These data suggest that the conflict of integrity versus despair may have a more favorable outcome in earlier age cohorts than in later ones, raising the possibility that changing societal values have hurt the struggle for integrity. Another study found that wisdom, a construct related to integrity, bore a more substantial relation to life satisfaction in elderly adults than other variables, including finances, health, and living situation.

A survey of theories of development in old age is given in Table 32-24.

Personality Over the Life Span: Stability or Change?

Although Erikson and other stage theorists focused on unique developmental tasks and stages central to each phase of life, other theorists focused on defining core personality traits within the individual and determining their course over the life span. For example, do those who are gregarious or extroverted during early childhood and adolescence remain extroverted through midlife and old age? Several well-designed longitudinal studies that have followed individuals over periods ranging from 10 to 50 years have found strong evidence for stability in five essential personality traits: extroversion, neuroticism, agreeableness, openness to experience, and conscientiousness. Some studies found slight decreases in extroversion and slight increases in agreeableness as individuals move into the oldest-old category, which contrasts with early theories that proposed that personality rigidifies as individuals age.

Is the fact that personality appears to have considerable stability over time inconsistent with the basic tenets of stage theories? Perhaps not. It may be that although individuals are consistent over time in their basic personality structure, the themes and conflicts with which they struggle change considerably over the life span, from concerns about developing identity and a stable sense of self to finding a life partner, to issues related to life review, as hypothesized by the stage theories. Also, in developing theories about personality change, few studies have examined the impact of significant historical events on personality; thus, how these events may result in personality change have not been studied systematically.

PSYCHOSOCIAL ASPECTS OF AGING

Social Activity

Healthy older persons usually maintain a level of social activity that is only slightly changed from that of earlier years. For many, old age is a period of continued intellectual, emotional, and psychological growth. In some cases, however, physical illness or the death of friends and relatives may preclude continued social interaction. Moreover, as persons experience an increased sense of isolation, they may become vulnerable to depression. Growing evidence indicates that maintaining social activities is valuable for physical and emotional well-being. Contact with younger persons is also essential. Old persons can pass on cultural values and provide care services to the younger generation and thereby maintain a sense of usefulness that contributes to self-esteem.

Ageism

Ageism, a term coined by Robert Butler, refers to discrimination toward old persons and to the negative stereotypes about old age that are held by younger adults. Old persons may themselves resent and fear other old persons and discriminate against them. In Butler's scheme, persons often associate old age with loneliness, poor health, senility, and general weakness or infirmity. The experience of older persons, however, does not consistently support this attitude. For example, although 50 percent of young adults expect poor health to be a problem for those over 65 years old, 75 percent of persons 65 to 74 years of age describe their health as good. Two-thirds of persons 75 and older feel the same way. Health problems, when they do exist, more often involve chronic than acute conditions. More than four of five persons over the age of 65 have at least one chronic condition (Table 32-25).

Good health, however, is not the sole determinant of a good quality of life in old age. Surveys of old persons show that social contacts are at least as highly valued. The factors affecting good aging appear to be multidimensional. Aging "robustly" means considering aging in terms of productive involvement, affective status, functional status, and cognitive status. These four indicators are only minimally correlated. The most robustly aging individuals

Table 32-25
Top Ten Chronic Conditions for People 65+, by Age and Race (Number Per 1,000 People)

Condition	Age				Race (65+)		
	65+	45–64	65–74	75+	White	Black	Black as of White
Arthritis	483.0	253.8	437.3	554.5	483.2	522.6	108
Hypertension	380.6	229.1	383.8	375.6	367.4	517.7	141
Hearing impairment	286.5	127.7	239.4	360.3	297.4	174.5	59
Heart disease	278.9	118.9	231.6	353.0	286.5	220.5	77
Cataracts	156.8	16.1	107.4	234.3	160.7	139.8	87
Deformity or orthopedic impairment	155.2	155.5	141.4	177.0	156.2	150.8	97
Chronic sinusitis	153.4	173.5	151.8	155.8	157.1	125.2	80
Diabetes	88.2	58.2	89.7	85.7	80.2	165.9	207
Visual impairment	81.9	45.1	69.3	101.7	81.1	77.0	95
Varicose veins	78.1	57.8	72.6	86.6	80.3	64.0	80

Data from National Center for Health Statistics, Washington, DC.

report more significant social contact, better health and vision, and fewer significant life events in the past 3 years than their less robustly aging counterparts. A linear, age-related decrease occurs in robustness, but it can still be found among the oldest-old.

George Vaillant followed up a group of Harvard freshmen into old age and found the following about emotional health at age 65: Having been close to brothers and sisters during college correlated with emotional well-being; undergoing early traumatic life experiences, such as the death of a parent or parental divorce, did not correlate with poor adaptation in old age; being depressed at some point between ages 21 and 50 predicted emotional problems at age 65, and possessing the personality traits of pragmatism and dependability as a young adult was associated with a sense of well-being at age 65.

Transference

Several forms of transference, some of them unique to adulthood, are present in older adults. First is the well-recognized parental transference, in which the patient reacts to the therapist as a child to a parent. Peer or sibling transference, expressions of experiences from a variety of nonparental relationships, is also common. In this form of transference, the patient looks to the therapist to share experiences with siblings, spouses, friends, and associates. At first, therapists may be surprised by older patients' ability to ignore their age in creating such transferences.

In son or daughter transference, quite common in middle-aged individuals and the elderly, the therapist is cast in the role of the patient's child, grandchild, or son-in-law or daughter-in-law. The themes expressed in this form of transference are multiple and often center on defenses against dependency feelings, activity and dominance versus passivity and submission, and attempts to rework unsatisfying aspects of relationships with children before time runs out. Finally, sexual transferences in older individuals are frequent and intense, and the therapist needs to be able to accept them and manage his or her countertransference responses.

Countertransference

Older individuals are dealing with illness and signs of aging, the loss of spouses and friends, and the constant awareness of time limitation and the nearness of death. These are painful issues that are just beginning to come into focus for younger therapists who would prefer not to confront them with great intensity daily.

The second source of countertransference responses centers on the older patient's sexuality. The presence of a vivid fantasy life, masturbation, and intercourse is disconcerting in and of themselves if the therapist has not had much experience in working with individuals who are the same age as their parents and grandparents. Consider the experience presented in the case study of a 31-year-old female therapist who was treating a 62-year-old man.

Early in the treatment process, Mr. E's sexual feelings emerged. His well-groomed appearance and adolescent-like nervousness caused the therapist discomfort. Her concern was how to engender respect and develop a therapeutic alliance with a patient who approached each session as a date, mainly because he was old enough to be her grandfather. At first shocked by his open expression of sexual interest in her, with the help of supervision and her therapy, she was able to recognize that she and the patient had similar conflicts to resolve, despite the 30-year age difference between them. She had hoped that Mr. E would be "all grown up," devoid of issues that she was grappling with also. She came to recognize that failure to help him understand the relation between his past and still vibrant sexuality would do the patient a great disservice. It would spring from her a lack of understanding of late-life sexual development and her countertransference reaction to him based on her conflicted attitudes toward the sexuality of her parents and grandparents. (Courtesy of Calvin A. Colarusso, M.D.)

Socioeconomics

The economics of old age is of paramount importance to older persons themselves and society at large. The past 30 years have seen a dramatic decline in the proportion of the US elderly population who are poor, primarily as a result of the availability of Medicare, Social Security, and private pensions. In 1959, 35.2 percent of persons over 65 lived below the poverty line, but by 2012 this figure had declined to 9.1 percent. Persons over age 65 make up 12 percent of the population, but they include only 9 percent of those living at low socioeconomic levels. Women are more likely than men to be impoverished. Income sources vary for persons age 65 and older. Despite overall economic gains, many older persons are so preoccupied with money worries that their enjoyment of life is lessened. Obtaining proper medical care may be incredibly difficult when personal funds are not available or are insufficient.

Medicare (Title 18) provides both hospital and medical insurance for those over age 65. About 150 million medical bills are reimbursed under the Medicare program each year, but only about 40 percent of all medical expenses incurred by older persons are covered under Medicare. The rest is paid by private insurance, state insurance, or personal funds. Some services—such as outpatient psychiatric treatment, skilled nursing care, physical rehabilitation, and preventive physical examinations—are covered minimally or not at all.

In addition to Medicare, the Social Security program pays benefits to persons over age 65 (over age 67 in 2027) and pays benefits at reduced rates starting at age 62. To qualify for benefits, a person must have worked long enough to become insured: A worker must have worked for 10 years to be eligible for benefits. Benefits are also paid to widows, widowers, and dependent children if those receiving benefits or contributing to Social Security die (survivor benefits). Social Security is not a pension scheme but a pay-as-you-go income supplement to prevent mass destitution among older persons. Benefits are paid by those currently working to those who are retired. Serious difficulties for Social Security are forecast for the next three decades when the number of baby boomers reaching old age will significantly exceed the number of younger workers paying into the plan.

Retirement

For many older persons, retirement is a time for the pursuit of leisure and freedom from the responsibility of previous working commitments. For others, it is a time of stress, mainly when retirement results in economic problems or a loss of self-esteem. Ideally, employment after age 65 should be a matter of choice. With the passage of the Age Discrimination in Employment Act of 1967 and its amendments, forced retirement at age 70 has been virtually eliminated in the private sector, and it is not legal in federal employment.

Most of those who retire voluntarily reenter the workforce within 2 years, for a variety of reasons, including adverse reactions to being retired, feelings of being unproductive, economic

hardship, and loneliness. The amount of time spent in retirement has increased as the life span has nearly doubled since 1900. Currently, the number of years spent in retirement is almost equal to the number of years spent working.

Sexual Activity

The frequency of orgasm, from coitus or masturbation, decreases with age in men and women. The most critical factors in determining the level of sexual activity with age are the health and survival of the spouse, one's health, and the level of past sexual activity. Although some degree of declining sexual interest and function is inevitable with age, social and cultural factors appear to be more responsible for the sexual changes observed than for the psychological changes of aging per se. Although satisfying sexual activity is possible for reasonably healthy elderly, many do not actualize this potential. The widely held notion that the elderly are essentially asexual is often a self-fulfilling prophecy.

Long-Term Care

Many older persons who are infirm require institutional care. Although only 5 percent are institutionalized in nursing homes at any one time, about 35 percent of older persons require care in a long-term facility at some time during their lives (Fig. 32-10). Older nursing home residents are mainly widowed women, and about 50 percent are over age 85.

Medicare does not cover nursing home care costs; they range from $20,000 to $1 million a year. About 20,000 long-term nursing care institutions are available in the United States. This number is not enough to meet the need. Those older persons who do not require skilled nursing care can be managed in other types of health-related facilities, such as centers they attend during the daytime hours, but the need for care far exceeds the availability of such centers.

Besides institutions, the older person's children tend to care for them. The most common caregivers are daughters and daughters-in-law, wives, and other women (Fig. 32-11). More than 50 percent of these women caregivers also work, and about 40 percent also care for their children. In general, women end up as caregivers more often than men because of cultural and societal expectations. According to the American Association of Retired Persons,

FIGURE 32-10

People age 65 or older in need of long-term care: 1980–2040. (Reprinted from Manton B, Saldo J. *Dynamics of Health Changes in the Oldest Old: New Perspectives and Evidence.* Milbank Q; 1985;63:12, with permission.)

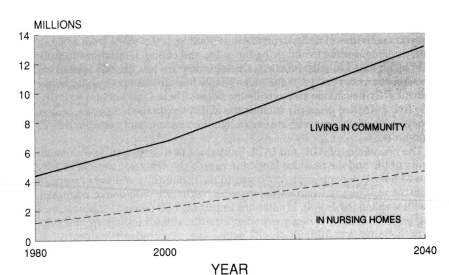

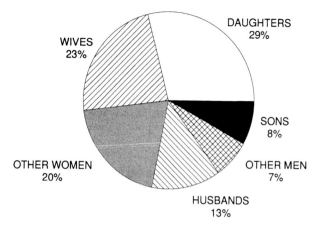

FIGURE 32-11
Caretakers and their relationship to the elderly care recipient. (Data from Select Committee on Aging, U.S. House of Representatives.)

daughters with jobs spend an average of 12 hours a week providing care and currently spend about $150 a month for travel, telephone calls, special foods, and medication for older persons.

References

Infant, Child, and Adolescent Development

Blackmore SJ. Development of the social brain in adolescence. *J R Soc Med.* 2012; 105(3):111–116.

Blair C, Raver CC. Child development in the context of adversity: experiential canalization of brain and behavior. *Am Psychol.* 2012;67(4):309–318.

Bonanno RA, Hymel S. Cyber bullying and internalizing difficulties: above and beyond the impact of traditional forms of bullying. *J Youth Adolesc.* 2013;42(5):685–697.

Briggs GG. *Drugs in Pregnancy and Lactation: A Reference Guide to Fetal and Neonatal Risk.* Philadelphia, PA: Lippincott Williams & Wilkins; 2005.

Brown GW, Ban M, Craig TKJ, Harris TO, Herbert J, Uher R. Serotonin transporter length polymorphism, childhood maltreatment and chronic depression: a specific gene-environment interaction. *Depress Anxiety.* 2013;30(1):5–13.

Burgess AW, Garbarino C, Carlson MI. Pathological teasing and bullying turned deadly: shooters and suicide. *Victims & Offenders.* 2006;1(1):1–14.

Burnett S, Sebastian C, Kadosh KC, Blakemore SJ. The social brain in adolescence: evidence from functional magnetic resonance imaging and behavioural studies. *Neurosci Biobehav Rev.* 2011;35(8):1654–1664.

Doyle AB, Markiewicz D. Parenting, marital conflict and adjustment from early- to mid-adolescence: mediated by adolescent attachment style. *J Youth Adolesc.* 2005; 34(2):97–110.

Giedd JN. The digital revolution and adolescent brain evolution. *J Adolesc Health.* 2012;51(2):101–105.

Gordon MF. Normal child development. In: Sadock BJ, Sadock VA, Ruiz P, eds. *Kaplan & Sadock's Comprehensive Textbook of Psychiatry.* 9th ed. Vol. 2. Philadelphia, PA: Lippincott Williams & Wilkins; 2009:3338.

Hemphill SA, Kotevski A, Tollit M, Smith R, Herrenkohl TI, Toumbourou JW, Catalano RF. Longitudinal predictors of cyber and traditional bullying perpetration in Australian secondary school students. *J Adolesc Health.* 2012;51(1):59–65.

Karatoreos IN, McEwen BS. Annual research review: the neurobiology and physiology of resilience and adaptation across the life course. *J Child Psychol Psychiatry.* 2013;54(4):337–347.

Ladouceur CD, Peper JS, Crone EA, Dahl RE. White matter development in adolescence: the influence of puberty and implications for affective disorders. *Dev Cogn Neurosci.* 2012;2(1):36–54.

Obradovic J. How can the study of physiological reactivity contribute to our understanding of adversity and resilience processes in development? *Dev Psychopathol.* 2013;24(2):371–387.

Pataki CS. Adolescent development In: Sadock BJ, Sadock VA, Ruiz P, eds. *Kaplan & Sadock's Comprehensive Textbook of Psychiatry.* 9th ed. Vol. 2. Philadelphia, PA: Lippincott Williams & Wilkins; 2009:3356.

Van den Bergh BR, Mulder EJ, Mennes M, Glover V. Antenatal maternal anxiety and stress and the neurobehavioural development of the fetus and child: Links and possible mechanisms. A review. *Neurosci Biobehav Rev.* 2005;29(2):237–258.

Willoughby T, Good M, Adachi PJC, Hamza C, Tavernier R. Examining the link between adolescent brain development and risk taking form a social-developmental perspective. *Brain and Cogn.* 2013;83(3):315–323.

Wright MF, Li Y. Kicking the digital dog: a longitudinal investigation of young adults' victimization and cyber-displaced aggression. *Cyberpsychol Behav Soc Netw.* 2012; 15(9):448–454.

Adulthood

Baxter J, Haynes M, Hewitt B. Pathways into marriage: cohabitation and the domestic division of labor. *J Fam Issues.* 2010;31(11):1507–1529.

Bottiroli S, Cavallini E, Fastame MC, Hertzog C. Cultural differences in rated typicality and perceived causes of memory changes in adulthood. *Arch Gerontol Geriatr.* 2013;57(3):271–281.

Colarusso CA. Adulthood. In: Sadock BJ, Sadock VA, Ruiz P, eds. *Kaplan & Sadock's Comprehensive Textbook of Psychiatry.* 9th ed. Vol. 2. Philadelphia, PA: Lippincott Williams & Wilkins; 2009:3909.

Diehl M, Chui H, Hay EL, Lumley MA, Grühn D, Labouvie-Vief G. Change in coping and defense mechanisms across adulthood: longitudinal findings in a European American sample. *Dev Psychol.* 2014;50(2):634–648.

Gager CT, Yabiku ST. Who has the time? The relationship between household labor time and sexual frequency. *J Fam Issues.* 2010;31(2):135–163.

Goldberg AE, Sayer A. Lesbian couples' relationship quality across the transition to parenthood. *J Marriage Fam.* 2006;68(1):87–100.

Goldberg AE, Smith JZ. Predictors of psychological adjustment in early placed adopted children with lesbian, gay, and heterosexual parents. *J Fam Psychol.* 2013; 27(3):431–432.

Howlin P, Moss P, Savage S, Rutter M. Social outcomes in mid- to later adulthood among individuals diagnosed with autism and average nonverbal IQ as children. *J Am Acad Child Adolesc Psychiatry.* 2013;52(6):572–581.e1.

Jones PB. Adult mental health disorders and their age at onset. *Br J Psychiatry Suppl.* 2013;202(s54:s5–s10.

Joyner K, Kao G. Interracial relationships and the transition to adulthood. *Am Sociol Rev.* 2005;70(4):563–581.

Kornrich S, Brines J, Leupp K. Egalitarianism, housework, and sexual frequency in marriage. *Am Sociol Rev.* 2013;78(1):26–50.

Kwon P. Resilience in lesbian, gay, and bisexual individuals. *Person Soc Psychol Rev.* 2013;17(4):371–383.

Masarik AS, Conger RD, Martin MJ, Donnellan M, Masyn KE, Lorenz FO. Romantic relationships in early adulthood: influences of family, personality, and relationship cognitions. *Person Relation.* 2013;20(2):356–373.

Nelson LJ, Barry CM. Distinguishing features of emerging adulthood: the role of self-classification as an adult. *J Adolesc Res.* 2005;20(2):242–262.

Perrig-Chiello P, Perren S. Biographical transitions from a midlife perspective. *J Adult Dev.* 2005;12(4):169–181.

Schwartz SJ, Côté JE, Arnett J. Identity and agency in emerging adulthood: two developmental routes in the individualization process. *Youth Soc.* 2005;37(2):201–229.

Tasker F. Lesbian mothers, gay fathers, and their children: a review. *J Dev Behav Pediatr.* 2005;26(3):224–240.

Turk JK. The division of housework among working couples: distinguishing characteristics of egalitarian couples. *Contemp Perspect Fam Res.* 2012;6:235–258.

Old Age

Colarusso CA. Adulthood. In: Sadock BJ, Sadock VA, Ruiz P, eds. *Kaplan & Sadock's Comprehensive Textbook of Psychiatry.* 9th ed. Vol. 2. Philadelphia, PA: Lippincott Williams & Wilkins; 2009:3909.

Reifler BV, Colenda CC, Juul D. Geriatric psychiatry. In: Aminoff MJ, Faulkner LR, eds. *The American Board of Psychiatry and Neurology: Looking Back and Moving Ahead.* Arlington, TX: American Psychiatric Publishing; 2012:135.

33 ◭

Contributions from the Neurosciences

The human brain is responsible for our cognitive processes, emotions, and behaviors—that is, everything we think, feel, and do. Although the early development and adult function of the brain are shaped by multiple factors (e.g., epigenetic, environmental, and psychosocial experiences), the brain is the final integrator of these influences. Despite the many advances in neural sciences, there has not been a genuine transformational advance in the treatment of mental disorders for more than half a century. The most apparent reason for the absence of more progress is the profound complexity of the human brain. A perhaps less apparent reason is the current practice of psychiatric diagnosis, which, for most clinicians, is based on syndrome-based classification systems.

The purpose of this chapter is to introduce the neural sciences sections, which describe the anatomy and function of the human brain, and then to discuss how an evolution of thinking toward a brain-based or biologically based diagnostic system for mental illness might facilitate our efforts to advance brain research, to develop better treatments, and to improve patient care.

In other fields of medicine, diagnosis is based on physical signs and symptoms, a medical history, and results of laboratory and radiologic tests. In psychiatry, a diagnosis is based primarily on the clinician's impression of the patient's interpretation of his or her thoughts and feelings. The patient's symptoms are then cross-referenced to a diagnostic or classification manual (e.g., *Diagnostic and Statistical Manual of Mental Disorders* [DSM-5], *International Statistical Classification of Diseases and Related Health Problems* [ICD]) containing hundreds of potential syndromes, and one or more diagnoses are applied to the particular patient. These standard classification systems represent significant improvements in reliability over previous diagnostic systems, but there is little reason to believe that these diagnostic categories are valid, in the sense that they represent discrete, biologically distinct entities. Although a patient with no symptoms or complaints can be diagnosed as having diabetes, cancer, or hypertension based on blood tests, x-rays, or vital signs, a patient with no symptoms cannot be diagnosed with schizophrenia, for example, because there are no currently recognized objective, independent assessments.

The goals of clinicians and researchers are to reduce human suffering by increasing our understanding of diseases, developing new treatments to prevent or cure diseases, and caring for patients optimally. If the brain is the organ of focus for mental illnesses, then it may be time to be more ambitious in building the classification of patients with mental illnesses directly from our understanding of biology, rather than only from the assessment of a patient's symptoms.

THE HUMAN BRAIN

The following neural sciences sections each address a field of brain biology. Each of these fields could be relevant to the pathophysiology and treatment of mental illnesses. Although the complexity of the human brain is daunting compared with other organs of the body, progress can only be made if one approaches this complexity consistently, methodically, and bravely.

The neuronal and glial cells of the human brain are organized in a characteristic manner, which has been increasingly clarified through modern neuroanatomical techniques. Also, our knowledge of normal human brain development has become more robust in the last decade. The human brain evolved from the brains of lower animal species, allowing inferences to be made about the human brain from animal studies. Neurons communicate with one another through chemical and electrical neurotransmission. The major neurotransmitters are the monoamines, amino acids, and neuropeptides. Other chemical messengers include neurotrophic factors and an array of other molecules, such as nitric oxide. Electrical neurotransmission occurs through a wide range of ion channels. Chemical and electrical signals received by a neuron subsequently initiate various molecular pathways within other neurons that regulate the biology and function of individual neurons, including the expression of individual genes and the production of proteins.

Also, to the central nervous system (CNS), the human body contains two other systems that have complex internal communicative networks: the endocrine system and the immune system. The recognition that these three systems communicate with each other has given birth to the fields of psychoneuroendocrinology and psychoneuroimmunology. Another property shared by the CNS, the endocrine system, and the immune system is the regular changes they undergo with time (e.g., daily, monthly), which is the basis of the field of chronobiology.

Psychiatry and the Human Brain

In the first half of the 20th century, our emphasis on psychodynamic and social psychiatry divorced psychiatric research from the study of the human brain. Since the 1950s, the appreciation of the effectiveness of medications in treating mental disorders and the mental effects of illicit drugs have reestablished a biologic view of mental illness, which had already been seeded by the introduction of electroconvulsive therapy (ECT) and James Papez's description of the limbic circuit in the 1930s. This biologic view has been reinforced further by the development of brain imaging techniques that have helped reveal how the brain performs in normal and abnormal conditions. During this period, countless discoveries have been made in basic neural science research using experimental techniques to assess the development, structure, biology, and function of the CNS of humans and animals.

Psychopharmacology. The effectiveness of drugs in the treatment of mental illness has been a significant feature of the last half-century of psychiatric practice. The first five editions of this textbook divided psychopharmacological treatment into four chapters on antipsychotic, antidepressant, antianxiety, and mood-stabilizing drugs. The prior division of psychiatric drugs into four classes is less valid now than it was in the past for the following reasons: (1) Many drugs of one class are used to treat disorders previously assigned to another class; (2) drugs from all four categories are used to treat disorders not previously treatable by drugs (e.g., eating disorders, panic disorders, and impulse control disorders); and (3) drugs such as clonidine, propranolol, and verapamil can effectively treat a variety of psychiatric disorders and do not fit easily into the other categories of psychiatric drugs.

The primary motivation for this change was that the variety and application of the drug treatments no longer fit a division of disorders into psychosis, depression, anxiety, and mania. In other words, the clinical applications of biologically based treatments did not neatly align with our syndrome-based diagnostic system. An implication of this observation could be that drug response might be a better indicator of underlying biologic brain dysfunction than any particular group of symptoms. For example, although the DSM-5 distinguishes major depressive disorder from generalized anxiety disorder, most clinicians are aware that these are often overlapping symptoms and conditions in clinical practice. Moreover, the same drugs are used to treat both conditions.

The animal models that are used to identify new drug treatments may also have affected our ability to advance research and treatment. Many major classes of psychiatric drugs were discovered serendipitously. Specifically, the drugs were developed originally for nonpsychiatric indications, but observant clinicians and researchers noted that psychiatric symptoms improved in some patients, which led to a focused study of these drugs in psychiatric patients. The availability of these effective drugs, including monoaminergic antidepressants and antipsychotics, led to the development of animal models that could detect the effects of these drugs (e.g., tricyclic antidepressants [TCAs] increase the time mice spend trying to find a submerged platform in a "forced swim" test). These animal models were then used to screen new compounds in an attempt to identify drugs that were active in the same animal models. The potential risk of this overall strategy is that these animal models are merely a method for detecting a particular molecular mechanism of action (e.g., increasing serotonin concentrations), rather than a model for a true behavioral analog of human mental illness (e.g., behavioral despair in a depressed patient).

Endophenotypes.   A possible diagnosis-related parallel to how this textbook separated the four classes of psychotropic drugs into approximately 30 different categories is the topic of *endophenotypes* in psychiatric patients. An endophenotype is an internal phenotype, which is a set of objective characteristics of an individual that are not visible to the unaided eye. Because there are so many steps and variables that separate a particular set of genes from the final functioning of a whole human brain, it may be more tractable to consider intermediate assessments such as endophenotypes. This hypothesis is based on the assumption that the number of genes that are involved in an endophenotype might be fewer than the number of genes involved in causing what we would conceptualize as a disease. For psychiatry, an endophenotype is based on neuropsychological, cognitive, neurophysiologic, neuroanatomical, biochemical, and brain imaging data. Such an endophenotype, for example, might include specific cognitive impairments as just one of its objectively measured features. This endophenotype would not be limited to patients with a diagnosis of schizophrenia because it

might also be found in some patients with depression or bipolar disorder.

The potential role of an endophenotype can be further clarified by stating what it is not. An endophenotype is not a symptom, and it is not a diagnostic marker. A classification based on the presence or absence of one or more endophenotypes would be based on objective biologic and neuropsychological measures with specific relationships to genes and brain function. A classification based on endophenotypes might also be a productive approach toward the development of more relevant animal models of mental illnesses, and thus the development of novel treatments.

Psychiatry and the Human Genome

Perhaps 70 to 80 percent of the 25,000 human genes are expressed in the brain, and because most genes code for more than one protein, there may be 100,000 different proteins in the brain. Perhaps 10,000 of these are known proteins with somewhat identified functions, and no more than 100 of these are the targets for existing psychotherapeutic drugs.

The study of families with the use of population genetic methods over the last 50 years has consistently supported a genetic, heritable component to mental disorders. More recent techniques in molecular biology have revealed that specific chromosomal regions and genes are associated with particular diagnoses. A potentially compelling application of these techniques has been to study transgenic models of behavior in animals. These transgenic models can help us understand the effects of individual genes as well as discover completely novel molecular targets for drug development.

It may be a natural response to resist "simple" genetic explanations for human features. Nonetheless, research on humans generally has found that approximately 40 to 70 percent of aspects of cognition, temperament, and personality are attributable to genetic factors. Because these are the very domains that are affected in mentally ill patients, it would not be surprising to discover a similar level of genetic influence on mental illness, mostly if we were able to assess this impact at a more discrete level, such as with endophenotypes.

Individual Genes and Mental Disorders.   Several types of data and observations suggest that any single gene is likely to have only a modest effect on the development of a mental disorder and that when a mental disorder is present in an individual, it represents the effects of multiple genes, speculatively on the order of five to ten genes. This hypothesis is also supported by our failure to find single genes with significant effects on mental illnesses. Some researchers, however, still consider it a possibility that genes with significant effects will be identified.

"Nature" and "Nurture" within the CNS.   In 1977, George Engel, at the University of Rochester, published a paper that articulated the biopsychosocial model of disease, which stressed an integrated approach to human behavior and disease. The biologic system refers to the anatomical, structural, and molecular substrates of disease; the psychological system refers to the effects of psychodynamic factors; and the social system examines cultural, environmental, and familial influences. Engel postulated that each system affects and is affected by the others.

The observation that a significant percentage of identical twins are discordant for schizophrenia is one example of the type of data that supports the understanding that there are many significant interactions between the genome and the environment (i.e., the biologic basis of the biopsychosocial concept). Studies in animals have also demonstrated that many factors—including activity, stress, drug exposure, and environmental toxins—can regulate the expression of genes and the development and functioning of the brain.

Mental Disorders Reflect Abnormalities in Neuroanatomical Circuits and Synaptic Regulation. Although genes lead to the production of proteins, the actual functioning of the brain needs to be understood at the level of regulation of complex pathways of neurotransmission and intraneuronal signaling, and networks of neurons within and between brain regions. In other words, the downstream effects of abnormal genes are modifications in discrete attributes such as axonal projections, synaptic integrity, and specific steps in intraneuronal molecular signaling.

Why Not a Genetic-Based Diagnostic System? Some researchers have proposed moving psychiatry toward a completely genetic-based diagnostic system. This proposal, however, seems premature based on the complexity of the genetic factors presumably involved in psychiatric disorders, the current absence of sufficient data to make these genetic connections, and the importance of epigenetic and environmental influences on the final behavioral outcomes resulting from an individual's genetic information.

Lessons from Neurology

Clinical and research neurologists seem to have been able to think more than psychiatrists about their diseases of interest and their causes, perhaps because the symptoms are generally nonbehavioral. Neurologists have biologically grounded differential diagnoses and treatment choices. This clarity of approach has helped lead to significant advances in neurology in the last two decades, for example, clarification of the amyloid precursor protein abnormalities in some patients with Alzheimer disease, the presence of trinucleotide repeat mutations in Huntington disease and spinocerebellar ataxia, and the appreciation of alpha-synucleinopathies, such as Parkinson disease and Lewy body dementia.

The continued separation of psychiatry from neurology is, in itself, a potential impediment to good patient care and research. Many neurologic disorders have psychiatric symptoms (e.g., depression in patients following a stroke or with multiple sclerosis or Parkinson disease), and several of the most severe psychiatric disorders have been associated with neurologic symptoms (e.g., movement disorders in schizophrenia). This overlap is not surprising given that the brain is the organ shared by psychiatric and neurologic diseases, and the division between these two disease areas is arbitrary. For example, patients with Huntington disease are at much greater risk for a wide range of psychiatric symptoms and syndromes, and thus many different DSM-5 diagnoses. Because we know that Huntington disease is an autosomal dominant genetic disorder, the observation that it can manifest with so many different DSM-5 diagnoses does not speak to a reliable biologic distinction among the existing DSM-5 categories.

Examples of Complex Human Behaviors

The goal to understand the human brain and its normal and abnormal functioning is genuinely one of the last frontiers for humans to explore. Trying to explain why a particular individual is the way he or she is, or what causes schizophrenia, for example, will remain too large a challenge for some decades. It is more approachable to consider more discrete aspects of human behavior.

It is not the role of textbooks to set policies or to write diagnostic manuals, but rather to share knowledge, generate ideas, and encourage innovation. The authors believe, however, that it is time to reap the insights of decades of neural science and clinical brain research and to build the classification of mental illnesses on fundamental principles of biology and medicine. Regardless of official diagnostic systems, however, clinicians and researchers should fully understand the biologic component of the biopsychosocial model, and not let research or patient care suffer because of a diagnostic system that is not founded on biologic principles.

FUNCTIONAL NEUROANATOMY

The sensory, behavioral, affective, and cognitive phenomena and attributes experienced by humans are mediated through the brain. It is the organ that perceives and affects the environment and integrates past and present. The brain is the organ of the mind that enables persons to sense, do, feel, and think.

Sensory systems create an internal representation of the external world by processing external stimuli into neuronal impulses. A separate map is formed for each sensory modality. *Motor systems* enable persons to manipulate their environment and to influence the behavior of others through communication. In the brain, sensory input, representing the external world, is integrated with internal drivers, memories, and emotional stimuli in *association units,* which in turn drive the actions of motor units. Although psychiatry is concerned primarily with the brain's association function, an appreciation of information processing of the sensory and motor systems is essential for sorting logical thought from the distortions introduced by psychopathology.

Brain Organization

The human brain contains approximately 86 billion *neurons* (nerve cells) and approximately 85 billion *glial cells.* Neurons most classically consist of a *soma,* or cell body, which contains the nucleus; usually multiple *dendrites,* which are processes that extend from the cell body and receive signals from other neurons; and a single *axon,* which extends from the cell body and transmits signals to other neurons. Connections between neurons are made at *axon terminals;* there, the axons of one neuron generally contact the dendrite or cell body of another neuron. Neurotransmitter release occurs within axon terminals and is one of the central mechanisms for intraneuronal communications, and also for the effects of psychotropic drugs.

There are three types of glial cells, and although they have often been thought of as having only a supportive role for neuronal functioning, glia has been increasingly appreciated as potentially involved in brain functions that may contribute more directly to both normal and disease mental conditions. The most common type of glial cells are *astrocytes,* which have several functions, including the nutrition of neurons, deactivation of some neurotransmitters, and integration with the blood–brain barrier (BBB). The *oligodendrocytes* in the CNS and the *Schwann cells* in the peripheral nervous system wrap their processes around neuronal axons, resulting in *myelin sheaths* that facilitate the conduction of electrical signals. The third type of glial cells, the *microglia,* which are derived from macrophages, are involved in removing cellular debris following neuronal death.

The neurons and glial cells are arranged in regionally distinct patterns within the brain. Neurons and their processes form groupings in many different ways, and these patterns of organization, or architecture, can be evaluated by several approaches. The pattern of distribution of nerve cell bodies, called *cytoarchitecture,* is revealed by aniline dyes called Nissl stains that stain ribonucleotides in the nuclei and the cytoplasm of neuronal cell bodies. The Nissl stains show the relative size and packing density of the neurons and, consequently, reveal the organization of the neurons into the different layers of the cerebral cortex.

Sensory Systems

The external world offers an infinite amount of potentially relevant information. In this overwhelming volume of sensory information in the environment, the sensory systems must both detect and discriminate stimuli; they winnow relevant information from the mass of confounding input by applying filtration at all levels. Sensory systems first transform external stimuli into neural impulses and then filter out irrelevant information to create an internal image of the environment, which serves as a basis for reasoned thought. Feature extraction is the quintessential role of sensory systems, which achieve this goal with their hierarchical organizations, first by transforming physical stimuli into neural activity in the primary sense organs and then by refining and narrowing the neural activity in a series of higher cortical processing areas. This neural processing eliminates irrelevant data from higher representations and reinforces crucial features. At the highest levels of sensory processing, neural images are transmitted to the association areas to be acted on in the light of emotions, memories, and drives.

Somatosensory System. The *somatosensory system,* an intricate array of parallel point-to-point connections from the body surface to the brain, was the first sensory system to be understood in anatomical detail. The six somatosensory modalities are light touch, pressure, pain, temperature, vibration, and proprioception (position sense). The organization of nerve bundles and synaptic connections in the somatosensory system encodes spatial relationships at all levels so that the organization is strictly *somatotopic* (Fig. 33-1).

Within a given patch of skin, various receptor nerve terminals act in concert to mediate distinct modalities. The mechanical properties of the skin's mechanoreceptors and thermoreceptors generate neural impulses in response to dynamic variations in the environment while they suppress static input. Nerve endings are either fast or slow responders; their depth in the skin also determines their sensitivity to sharp or blunt stimuli. Thus the representation of the external world is significantly refined at the level of the primary sensory organs.

The receptor organs generate coded neural impulses that travel proximally along the sensory nerve axons to the spinal cord. These far-flung routes are susceptible to varying systemic medical conditions and pressure palsies. Pain, tingling, and numbness are the typical presenting symptoms of peripheral neuropathies.

All somatosensory fibers project to and synapse in the thalamus. The thalamic neurons preserve the somatotopic representation by projecting fibers to the somatosensory cortex, located immediately posterior to the Sylvian fissure in the parietal lobe. Despite the considerable overlap, several bands of cortex roughly parallel to the Sylvian fissure are segregated by a somatosensory modality. Within each band is the sensory "homunculus," the culmination of the careful somatotopic segregation of the sensory fibers at the lower levels. The clinical syndrome of *tactile agnosia (astereognosis)* is defined by the inability to recognize objects based on touch, although the primary somatosensory modalities—light touch, pressure, pain, temperature, vibration, and proprioception—are intact.

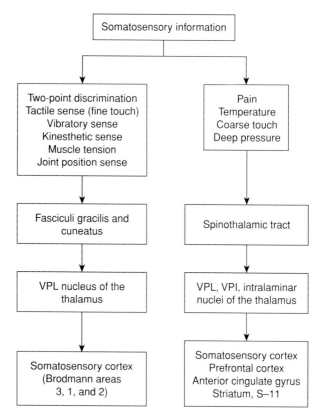

FIGURE 33-1

Pathway of somatosensory information processing. (Adapted from Patestas MA, Gartner LP. *A Textbook of Neuroanatomy.* Malden, MA: Blackwell; 2006:149.)

This syndrome, localized at the border of the somatosensory and association areas in the posterior parietal lobe, appears to represent an isolated failure of only the highest order of feature extraction, with preservation of the more basic levels of the somatosensory pathway.

Reciprocal connections are a critical anatomical feature of crucial importance to conscious perception—as many fibers project down from the cortex to the thalamus as project up from the thalamus to the cortex. These reciprocal fibers play a critical role in filtering sensory input. In normal states, they facilitate the sharpening of internal representations, but in pathologic states, they can generate false signals or inappropriately suppress sensation. Such cortical interference with sensory perception is thought to underlie many psychosomatic syndromes, such as the hemisensory loss that characterizes conversion disorder.

The prenatal development of the strict point-to-point pattern that characterizes the somatosensory system remains an area of active study. Patterns of sensory innervation result from a combination of axonal guidance by particular molecular cues and pruning of exuberant synaptogenesis based on an organism's experience. Leading hypotheses weigh contributions from a genetically determined molecular map—in which the arrangement of fiber projections is organized by fixed and diffusible chemical cues—against contributions from the modeling and remodeling of projections based on coordinated neural activity. Thumbnail calculations suggest that the 30,000 to 40,000 genes in human deoxyribonucleic acid (DNA) are far too few to completely encode the position of all the trillions of synapses in the brain. Genetically determined positional cues probably steer growing fibers toward the general target, and activity-dependent mechanisms fine-tune the pattern of projections. Recent data suggest that well-established adult thalamocortical sensory projections can be gradually remodeled as a result of a reorientation of coordinated sensory input or in response to the loss of part of the somatosensory cortex, for instance, in stroke.

DEVELOPMENT OF THE SOMATOSENSORY SYSTEM.

A strict somatotopic representation exists at each level of the somatosensory system. During development, neurons extend axons to connect to distant brain regions; after arriving at the destination, a set of axons must therefore sort itself to preserve the somatotopic organization. A classic experimental paradigm for this developmental process is the representation of a mouse's whiskers in the somatosensory cortex. The murine somatosensory cortex contains a barrel field of cortical columns, each of which corresponds to one whisker. When mice are inbred to produce fewer whiskers, fewer somatosensory cortex barrels appear. Each barrel is expanded in area, and the entire barrel field covers the same area of the somatosensory cortex as it does in normal animals. This experiment demonstrates that specific higher cortical structures can form in response to peripheral input and that different input complexities determine different patterns of synaptic connectivity. Although the mechanisms by which peripheral input molds cortical architecture are mostly unknown, animal model paradigms are beginning to yield clues. For example, in a mutant mouse that lacks monoamine oxidase A and, thus, has exceptionally high cortical levels of serotonin, barrels fail to form in the somatosensory cortex. This result indirectly implicates serotonin in the mechanism of barrel field development.

In adults, the classic mapping studies of Wilder Penfield suggested the existence of a homunculus, an immutable cortical representation of the body surface. More recent experimental evidence from primate studies and stroke patients, however, has promoted a more plastic conception than that of Penfield. Minor variations exist in the cortical pattern of ordinary individuals, yet dramatic shifts in the map can occur in response to the loss of cortex from stroke or injury. When a stroke ablates a significant fraction of the somatosensory homunculus, the homuncular representation begins to contract and shift proportionally to fill the remaining intact cortex.

Moreover, the cortical map can be rearranged solely in response to a change in the pattern of tactile stimulation of the fingers. The somatotopic representation of the proximal and distal segments of each finger typically forms a contiguous map, presumably because both segments contact surfaces simultaneously. However, under experimental conditions in which the distal segments of all fingers are simultaneously stimulated while contact of the distal and proximal parts of each finger is separated, the cortical map gradually shifts 90 degrees to reflect the new sensory experience. In the revised map, the cortical representation of the proximal segment of each finger is no longer contiguous with that of the distal segment.

These data support the notion that the internal representation of the external world, although static in gross structure, can be continuously modified at the level of synaptic connectivity to reflect relevant sensory experiences. The cortical representation also tends to shift to fit entirely into the available amount of cortex.

These results also support the notion that cortical representations of sensory input, or memories, may be holographic rather than spatially fixed: The pattern of activity, rather than the physical structure, may encode information. In sensory systems, this plasticity of cortical representation allows recovery from brain lesions; the phenomenon may also underlie learning.

Visual System. Visual images are transduced into neural activity within the retina and are processed through a series of brain cells, which respond to increasingly complex features, from the eye to the higher visual cortex. The neurobiologic basis of feature extraction is best understood in the finest detail in the visual system. Beginning with classic work in the 1960s, research in the visual pathway has produced two main paradigms for all sensory systems. The first paradigm, mentioned earlier for the somatosensory system, evaluates the contributions of genetics and experience—or nature and nurture—in the formation of the final synaptic arrangement. Transplantation experiments, resulting in an accurate point-to-point pattern of connectivity, even when the eye was surgically inverted, have suggested an innate, genetically determined mechanism of synaptic pattern formation. The crucial role of early visual experience in establishing the adult pattern of visual connections, on the other hand, crystallized the hypothesis of the activity-dependent formation of synaptic connectivity. The final adult pattern is the result of both factors.

The second central paradigm, most revealed in the visual system, is that of highly specialized brain cells that respond exclusively to particular stimuli. Recent work, for example, has identified cells in the inferior temporal cortex that respond only to faces viewed at a specific angle. An individual's response to a particular face requires the activity of large neural networks and may not be limited to a single neuron. Nevertheless, the cellular localization of specific feature extraction is of critical importance in defining the boundary between sensory and association systems, but only in the visual system has this significant question been posed experimentally.

In the primary visual cortex, columns of cells respond specifically to lines of a specific orientation. The cells of the primary visual cortex project to the secondary visual cortex. There the cells respond specifically to particular movements of lines and angles. In turn, these cells project to two association areas, where additional features are extracted and conscious awareness of images forms.

The inferior temporal lobe detects the shape, form, and color of the object—the *what* questions; the posterior parietal lobe tracks the location, motion, and distance—the *where* questions. The posterior parietal lobe contains distinct sets of neurons that signal the intention either to look into a specific part of visual space or to reach for a particular object. In the inferior temporal cortices (ITCs), adjacent cortical columns respond to complex forms. Responses to facial features tend to occur in the left ITC, and responses to complex shapes tend to occur in the right ITC. The brain devotes specific cells to the recognition of facial expressions and the aspect and position of faces of others for the individual.

The crucial connections between the feature-specific cells and the association areas involved in memory and conscious thought remain to be delineated. Much elucidation of feature recognition is based on invasive animal studies. In humans, the clinical syndrome of *prosopagnosia* describes the inability to recognize faces in the presence of preserved recognition of other environmental objects. Based on the pathologic and radiologic examination of individual patients, prosopagnosia is thought to result from the disconnection of the left ITC from the visual association area in the left parietal lobe. Such lesional studies are useful in identifying necessary components of a mental pathway, but they may be inadequate to define the entire pathway. One noninvasive technique that is still being perfected and is beginning to reveal the full anatomical relation of the human visual system to conscious thought and memory is functional neuroimaging.

As is valid for language, there appears to be a hemispheric asymmetry for individual components of visuospatial orientation. Although both hemispheres cooperate in perceiving and drawing complex images, the right hemisphere, especially the parietal lobe, contributes the overall contour, perspective, and right-left orientation, and the left hemisphere adds internal detail, embellishment, and complexity. The brain can be fooled in optical illusions.

Neurologic conditions such as strokes and other focal lesions have permitted the definition of several disorders of visual perception. *Apperceptive visual agnosia* is the inability to identify and draw items using visual cues, with preservation of other sensory modalities. It represents a failure of transmission of information from the higher visual sensory pathway to the association areas and is caused by bilateral lesions in the visual association areas. *Associative visual agnosia* is the inability to name or use objects despite the ability to draw them. It is caused by bilateral medial occipitotemporal lesions and can occur along with other visual impairments. Color perception may be ablated in lesions of the dominant occipital lobe that include the splenium of the corpus callosum. *Color agnosia* is the inability to recognize a color despite being able to match it. *Color anomia* is the inability to name a color despite being able to point to it. *Central achromatopsia* is a complete inability to perceive color.

Anton syndrome is a failure to acknowledge blindness, possibly owing to the interruption of fibers involved in self-assessment. It is seen with bilateral occipital lobe lesions. The most common causes are hypoxic injury, stroke, metabolic encephalopathy, migraine, herniation resulting from mass lesions, trauma, and leukodystrophy. *Balint syndrome* consists of a triad of optic ataxia (the inability to direct optically guided movements), *oculomotor apraxia* (inability to direct gaze rapidly), and *simultanagnosia* (inability to integrate a visual scene to perceive it as a whole). Balint syndrome is seen in bilateral parietooccipital lesions. *Gerstmann syndrome* includes agraphia, calculation difficulties (acalculia), right-left disorientation, and finger agnosia. It has been attributed to lesions of the dominant parietal lobe.

DEVELOPMENT OF THE VISUAL SYSTEM. In humans, the initial projections from both eyes intermingle in the cortex. During the development of visual connections in the early postnatal period, there is a window of time during which binocular visual input is required for the development of ocular dominance columns in the primary visual cortex. Ocular dominance columns are stripes of cortex that receive input from only one eye, separated by stripes innervated only by fibers from the other eye. Occlusion of one eye during this critical period eliminates the persistence of its fibers in the cortex and allows the fibers of the active eye to innervate the entire visual cortex. In contrast, when normal binocular vision is allowed during the critical development window, the usual dominance columns form, occluding one eye after the completion of innervation of the cortex, produces no subsequent alteration of the ocular dominance columns. This paradigm crystallizes the importance of early childhood experience on the formation of adult brain circuitry.

Auditory System. Sounds are instantaneous, incremental changes in ambient air pressure. The pressure changes cause the ear's tympanic membrane to vibrate; the vibration is then transmitted to the ossicles (malleus, incus, and stapes) and thereby to the endolymph or fluid of the cochlear spiral. Vibrations of the endolymph move cilia on hair cells, which generate neural impulses. The hair cells respond to sounds of different frequencies in a tonotopic manner

within the cochlea, like an extended, spiral piano keyboard. Neural impulses from the hair cells travel in a tonotopic arrangement to the brain in the fibers of the cochlear nerve. They enter the brainstem cochlear nuclei, are relayed through the lateral lemniscus to the inferior colliculi, and then to the medial geniculate nucleus (MGN) of the thalamus. MGN neurons project to the primary auditory cortex in the posterior temporal lobe. Dichotic listening tests, in which different stimuli are presented to each ear simultaneously, demonstrate that most of the input from one ear activates the contralateral auditory cortex and that the left hemisphere tends to be dominant for auditory processing.

Sonic features are extracted through a combination of mechanical and neural filters. The representation of sound is roughly tonotopic in the primary auditory cortex, whereas *lexical processing* (i.e., the extraction of vowels, consonants, and words from the auditory input) occurs in higher language association areas, especially in the left temporal lobe. The syndrome of *word deafness,* characterized by intact hearing for voices but an inability to recognize speech, may reflect damage to the left parietal cortex. This syndrome is thought to result from the disconnection of the auditory cortex from Wernicke area. A rare, complementary syndrome, *auditory sound agnosia,* is defined as the inability to recognize nonverbal sounds, such as a horn or a cat's meow, in the presence of intact hearing and speech recognition. Researchers consider this syndrome to be the right hemisphere correlate of pure word deafness.

DEVELOPMENT OF THE AUDITORY SYSTEM. Some children are unable to process auditory input and therefore have impaired speech and comprehension of spoken language. Studies on some of these children have determined that they can discriminate speech if the consonants and vowels—the phonemes—are slowed two- to fivefold by a computer. Based on this observation, a tutorial computer program was designed that initially asked questions in a slowed voice and, as subjects answered questions correctly, gradually increased the rate of phoneme presentation to approximate typical rates of speech. Subjects gained some ability to discriminate routine speech over 2 to 6 weeks and appeared to retain these skills after the tutoring period was completed. This finding probably has therapeutic applicability to 5 to 8 percent of children with speech delay, but ongoing studies may expand the eligible group of students. This finding, moreover, suggests that neuronal circuits required for auditory processing can be recruited and be made more efficient long after language is usually learned, provided that the circuits are allowed to finish their task correctly, even if this requires slowing the rate of input. Circuits thus functioning with high fidelity can then be trained to speed their processing.

A recent report has extended the age at which language acquisition may be acquired for the first time.

A boy who had intractable epilepsy of one hemisphere was mute because the uncontrolled seizure activity precluded the development of organized language functions. At the age of 9 years, he had the abnormal hemisphere removed to cure epilepsy. Although up to that point in his life he had not spoken, he initiated an accelerated acquisition of language milestones beginning at that age and ultimately gained language abilities only a few years delayed relative to his chronologic age.

Researchers cannot place an absolute upper limit on the age at which language abilities can be learned, although acquisition at ages beyond the usual childhood period is usually incomplete.

Anecdotal reports document the acquisition of reading skills after the age of 80 years.

Olfaction.   Odorants, or volatile chemical cues, enter the nose, are solubilized in the nasal mucus, and bind to odorant receptors displayed on the surface of the sensory neurons of the olfactory epithelium. Each neuron in the epithelium displays a unique odorant receptor, and cells displaying a given receptor are arranged randomly within the olfactory epithelium. Humans possess several hundred distinct receptor molecules that bind the massive variety of environmental odorants; researchers estimate that humans can discriminate 10,000 different odors. Odorant binding generates neural impulses, which travel along the axons of the sensory nerves through the cribriform plate to the olfactory bulb. Within the bulb, all axons corresponding to a given receptor converge onto only 1 or 2 of 3,000 processing units called *glomeruli.* Because each odorant activates several receptors that activate a characteristic pattern of glomeruli, the identity of external chemical molecules is represented internally by a spatial pattern of neural activity in the olfactory bulb.

Each glomerulus projects to a unique set of 20 to 50 separate columns in the olfactory cortex. In turn, each olfactory cortical column receives projections from a unique combination of glomeruli. The connectivity of the olfactory system is genetically determined. Because each odorant activates a unique set of several receptors and thus a unique set of olfactory bulb glomeruli, each olfactory cortical column is tuned to detect a different odorant of some evolutionary significance to the species. Unlike the signals of the somatosensory, visual, and auditory systems, olfactory signals do not pass through the thalamus but project directly to the frontal lobe and the limbic system, especially the pyriform cortex. The connections to the limbic system (amygdala, hippocampus, and pyriform cortex) are significant. Olfactory cues stimulate strong emotional responses and can evoke powerful memories.

Olfaction, the most ancient sense in evolutionary terms, is tightly associated with sexual and reproductive responses. A related chemosensory structure, the vomeronasal organ, is thought to detect *pheromones,* chemical cues that trigger unconscious, stereotyped responses. In some animals, ablation of the vomeronasal organ in early life may prevent the onset of puberty. Recent studies have suggested that humans also respond to pheromones in a manner that varies according to the menstrual cycle. The structures of higher olfactory processing in phylogenetically more primitive animals have evolved in humans into the limbic system, the center of the emotional brain, and the gate through which experience is admitted into memory according to emotional significance. The elusive basic animal drives with which clinical psychiatry constantly grapples may, therefore, originate from the ancient centers of higher olfactory processing.

DEVELOPMENT OF THE OLFACTORY SYSTEM.   During normal development, axons from the nasal olfactory epithelium project to the olfactory bulb and segregate into about 3,000 equivalent glomeruli. If an animal is exposed to a single dominant scent in the early postnatal period, then one glomerulus expands massively within the bulb at the expense of the surrounding glomeruli. Thus, as discussed earlier concerning the barrel fields of the somatosensory cortex, the size of brain structures may reflect the environmental input.

Taste.   Soluble chemical cues in the mouth bind to receptors in the tongue and stimulate the gustatory nerves, which project to the nucleus solitarius in the brainstem. The sense of taste is believed to discriminate only in broad classes of stimuli: sweet, sour, bitter, salty and umami. Each modality is mediated through a unique set of cellular receptors and channels, of which several may be expressed in each taste neuron. The detection and the discrimination of foods, for example, involve a combination of the senses of taste, olfaction, touch, vision, and hearing. Taste fibers activate the medial temporal lobe, but the higher cortical localization of taste is only poorly understood.

Autonomic Sensory System.   The autonomic nervous system (ANS) monitors the essential functions necessary for life. The activity of visceral organs, blood pressure, cardiac output, blood glucose levels, and body temperature are all transmitted to the brain by autonomic fibers. Most autonomic sensory information remains unconscious; if such information rises to conscious levels, it is only as a vague sensation, in contrast to the capacity of the primary senses to transmit sensations rapidly and precisely.

Alteration of Conscious Sensory Perception through Hypnosis.   *Hypnosis* is a state of heightened suggestibility attainable by a certain proportion of the population. Under a state of hypnosis, gross distortions of perception in any sensory modality and changes in the ANS can be achieved instantaneously. The anatomy of the sensory system does not change, yet the same specific stimuli may be perceived with opposed emotional value before and after induction of the hypnotic state. For example, under hypnosis, a person may savor an onion as if it were a luscious chocolate truffle, only to reject the onion as abhorrently pungent seconds later when the hypnotic suggestion is reversed. The localization of the hypnotic switch has not been determined, but it presumably involves both sensory and association areas of the brain. Experiments tracing neural pathways in human volunteers via functional neuroimaging have demonstrated that shifts in attention in an environmental setting determine changes in the regions of the brain that are activated on an instantaneous time scale. Thus the organizing centers of the brain may route conscious and unconscious thoughts through different sequences of neural processing centers, depending on a person's ultimate goals and emotional state. These attention-mediated variations in synaptic utilization can occur instantaneously, much like the alteration in the routing of associational processing that may occur in hypnotic states.

Motor Systems

Body muscle movements are controlled by the lower motor neurons, which extend axons—some as long as 1 m—to the muscle fibers. Lower motor neuron firing is regulated by the summation of upper motor neuron activity. In the brainstem, primitive systems produce gross coordinated movements of the entire body. Activation of the rubrospinal tract stimulates flexion of all limbs, whereas activation of the vestibulospinal tract causes all limbs to extend. Newborn infants, for example, have all limbs tightly flexed, presumably through the dominance of the rubrospinal system. The movements of an anencephalic infant, who completely lacks a cerebral cortex, may be indistinguishable from the movements of an average newborn. In the first few months of life, the flexor spasticity is gradually mitigated by the opposite actions of the vestibulospinal fibers, and more limb mobility occurs.

At the top of the motor hierarchy is the corticospinal tract, which controls fine movements and which eventually dominates the brainstem system during the first years of life. The upper motor neurons of the corticospinal tract reside in the posterior frontal lobe, in a section of the cortex known as the *motor strip.* Planned movements are conceived in the association areas of the brain, and in consultation with the basal ganglia and cerebellum, the motor cortex directs their smooth execution. The importance of the corticospinal system becomes immediately evident in strokes, in which spasticity returns as the cortical influence is ablated, and the actions of the brainstem motor systems are released from cortical modulation.

Basal Ganglia.   The *basal ganglia,* a subcortical group of gray matter nuclei, appear to mediate postural tone. The four functionally distinct ganglia are the striatum, the pallidum, the substantia nigra, and the subthalamic nucleus. Collectively known as the corpus striatum, the caudate and putamen harbor components of both motor and association systems. The caudate nucleus plays a vital role in the modulation of motor acts. Anatomical and functional neuroimaging studies have correlated decreased activation of the caudate with obsessive-compulsive behavior. When functioning correctly, the caudate nucleus acts as a gatekeeper to allow the motor system to perform only those acts that are goal-directed. When it fails to perform its gatekeeper function, extraneous acts are performed, as in obsessive-compulsive disorder (OCD) or the tic disorders, such as Tourette disorder. Overactivity of the striatum owing to lack of dopaminergic inhibition (e.g., in parkinsonian conditions) results in *bradykinesia,* an inability to initiate movements. The caudate, in particular, shrinks dramatically in Huntington disease. This disorder is characterized by rigidity, on which is gradually superimposed choreiform, or "dancing," movements. Psychosis may be a prominent feature of Huntington disease, and suicide is not uncommon. The caudate is also thought to influence associative or cognitive processes.

The globus pallidus contains two parts linked in series. In a cross-section of the brain, the internal and external parts of the globus pallidus are nested within the concavity of the putamen. The globus pallidus receives input from the corpus striatum and projects fibers to the thalamus. This structure may be severely damaged in Wilson disease and in carbon monoxide poisoning, which are characterized by dystonic posturing and flapping movements of the arms and legs.

The substantia nigra is named the black substance because the presence of melanin pigment causes it to appear black to the naked

eye. It has two parts, one of which is functionally equivalent to the globus pallidus interna. The other part degenerates in Parkinson disease. Parkinsonism is characterized by rigidity and tremor and is associated with depression in more than 30 percent of cases.

Finally, lesions in the subthalamic nucleus yield ballistic movements, sudden limb jerks of such velocity that they are compared to projectile movement.

Together, the nuclei of the basal ganglia appear capable of initiating and maintaining the full range of useful movements. Investigators have speculated that the nuclei serve to configure the activity of the overlying motor cortex to fit the purpose of the association areas. Also, they appear to integrate proprioceptive feedback to maintain an intended movement.

Cerebellum.   The cerebellum consists of a simple six-cell pattern of circuitry that is replicated roughly 10 million times. Simultaneous recordings of the cerebral cortex and the cerebellum have shown that the cerebellum is activated several milliseconds before a planned movement. Moreover, the ablation of the cerebellum renders intentional movements coarse and tremulous. These data suggest that the cerebellum carefully modulates the tone of agonistic and antagonistic muscles by predicting the relative contraction needed for smooth motion. This prepared motor plan is used to ensure that precisely the right amount of flexor and extensor stimuli is sent to the muscles. Recent functional imaging data have shown that the cerebellum is active, even during the mere imagination of motor acts when no movements ultimately result from its calculations. The cerebellum harbors two, and possibly more, distinct "homunculi" or cortical representations of the body plan.

Motor Cortex.   Penfield's groundbreaking work defined a motor homunculus in the precentral gyrus, Brodmann area 4 (Fig. 33-2), where a somatotopic map of the motor neurons is found. Individual cells within the motor strip cause contraction of single muscles. The brain region immediately anterior to the motor strip is called the *supplementary motor area,* Brodmann area 6. This region contains cells that, when individually stimulated, can trigger more complex movements by influencing a firing sequence of motor strip cells. Recent studies have demonstrated a broad representation of motor movements in the brain.

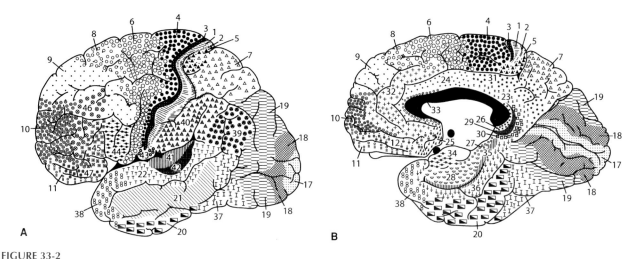

FIGURE 33-2

Drawing of the lateral view (**A**) and medial view (**B**) of the cytoarchitectonic subdivisions of the human brain as determined by Brodmann. (From Sadock BJ, Sadock VA, Ruiz P. *Kaplan & Sadock's Comprehensive Textbook of Psychiatry.* 9th ed. Philadelphia, PA: Lippincott Williams & Wilkins; 2009.)

The skillful use of the hands is called *praxis,* and deficits in skilled movements are termed *apraxias.* The three levels of apraxia are limb-kinetic, ideomotor, and ideational. *Limb-kinetic apraxia* is the inability to use the contralateral hand in the presence of preserved strength; it results from isolated lesions in the supplementary motor area, which contains neurons that stimulate functional sequences of neurons in the motor strip.

Ideomotor apraxia is the inability to perform an isolated motor act on command, despite preserved comprehension, strength, and spontaneous performance of the same act. Ideomotor apraxia simultaneously affects both limbs and involves functions so specialized that they are localized to only one hemisphere. Conditions in two separate areas can produce this apraxia. Disconnection of the language comprehension area, Wernicke area, from the motor regions causes an inability to follow spoken commands, and lesions to the left premotor area may impair the actual motor program as the higher-order motor neurons generate it. This program is transmitted across the corpus callosum to the right premotor area, which directs the movements of the left hand. A lesion in this callosal projection can also cause isolated ideomotor apraxia in the left hand. This syndrome implies the representation of specific motor acts within discrete sections of the left premotor cortex. Thus just as some cells respond selectively to specific environmental features in the higher sensory cortices, some cells in the premotor cortex direct specific complex motor tasks.

Ideational apraxia occurs when the individual components of a sequence of skilled acts can be performed in isolation, but the entire series cannot be organized and executed as a whole. For example, the sequence of opening an envelope, removing the letter, unfolding it, and placing it on the table cannot be performed in order, even though the individual acts can be performed in isolation. The representation of the concept of a motor sequence may involve several areas, specifically the left parietal cortex, but it likely also relies on the sequencing and executive functions of the prefrontal cortex. This apraxia is a typical finding of diffuse cortical degeneration, such as Alzheimer disease.

Autonomic Motor System.   The *autonomic system* is divided into a sensory component (described earlier) and a motor component. The *autonomic motor system* is divided into two branches: the sympathetic and the parasympathetic. As a rule, organs are innervated by both types of fibers, which often serve antagonistic roles. The *parasympathetic system* slows the heart rate and begins the process of digestion. In contrast, the *sympathetic system* mediates the fight or flight response, with increased heart rate, shunting of blood away from the viscera, and increased respiration. The sympathetic system is highly activated by sympathomimetic drugs, such as amphetamine and cocaine, and may also be activated by withdrawal from sedating drugs such as alcohol, benzodiazepines, and opioids. Investigators who have found an increased risk of heart attacks in persons with high levels of hostility have suggested that chronic activation of the sympathetic fight or flight response, with the elevated secretion of adrenaline, may underlie this association.

The brain center that drives the autonomic motor system is the *hypothalamus,* which houses a set of paired nuclei that appear to control appetite, rage, temperature, blood pressure, perspiration, and sexual drive. For example, lesions to the ventromedial nucleus, the satiety center, produce a voracious appetite and rage. In contrast, lesions to the upper region of the lateral nucleus, the hunger center, produce a profound loss of appetite. Numerous research groups are making intense efforts to define the biochemical

regulation of appetite and obesity and frequently target the role of the hypothalamus.

In the regulation of sexual attraction, the role of the hypothalamus has also become an area of active research. In the 1990s, three groups independently reported neuroanatomical differences between some of the hypothalamic nuclei of straight and gay men. Researchers interpreted this finding to suggest that human sexual orientation has a neuroanatomical basis, and this result has stimulated several follow-up studies of the biologic basis of sexual orientation. At present, however, these controversial findings are not accepted without question (including by some of the original authors), and no clear consensus has emerged about whether the structure of the hypothalamus consistently correlates with sexual orientation. In animal studies, early nurturing and sexual experiences consistently alter the size of specific hypothalamic nuclei.

Primitive Reflex Circuit.   Sensory pathways function as extractors of specific features from the overwhelming multitude of environmental stimuli, whereas motor pathways carry out the wishes of the organism. These pathways may be linked directly, for example, in the spinal cord, where a primitive reflex arc may mediate the brisk withdrawal of a limb from a painful stimulus, without immediate conscious awareness. In this loop, the peripheral stimulus activates the sensory nerve, the sensory neuron synapses on and directly activates the motor neuron, and the motor neuron drives the muscle to contract. This response is strictly local and all-or-none. Such primitive reflex arcs, however, rarely generate an organism's behaviors. In most behaviors, sensory systems project to association areas, where sensory information is interpreted in terms of internally determined memories, motivations, and drives. The exhibited behavior results from a plan of action determined by the associated components and carried out by the motor systems.

Localization of Brain Functions.   Many theorists have subdivided the brain into functional systems. Brodmann defined 47 areas based on cytoarchitectonic distinctions, a cataloging that has been remarkably durable as the functional anatomy of the brain has been elucidated. Various distinct functions, based on data from lesion studies and functional neuroimaging, have been assigned to nearly all Brodmann areas. At the other extreme, individual experts have distinguished only three processing blocks: The brainstem and the thalamic reticular activating system provide arousal and set up attention; the posterior cortex integrates perceptions and generates language; and, at the highest level, the frontal cortex generates programs and executes plans like an orchestra conductor.

Hemispheric lateralization of function is a crucial feature of higher cortical processing. The primary sensory cortices for touch, vision, hearing, smell, and taste are represented bilaterally, and the first level of abstraction for these modalities is also usually represented bilaterally. The highest levels of feature extraction, however, are generally unified in one brain hemisphere only. For example, recognition of familiar and unfamiliar faces seems localized to the left inferior temporal cortex, and cortical processing of olfaction occurs in the right frontal lobe.

Hypotheses about the flow of thought in the brain are based on few experimental data, although this scarcity of findings has not impeded numerous theoreticians from speculating about functional neuroanatomy. Several roles have been tentatively assigned to specific lobes of the brain, based on the functional deficits resulting from the localized injury. These data indicate that some areas of the cortex may be necessary for a specific function, but they do not define the complete set of structures that suffices for a complicated task. Anecdotal evidence from surface electrocorticography for the study of epilepsy, for example, suggests that a right parietal seizure impulse may shoot immediately to the left frontal lobe and then to the right temporal lobe before spreading locally to the remainder of the parietal lobe. This evidence illustrates the limitations of naively assigning a mental function to a single brain region. Functional neuroimaging studies frequently reveal the simultaneous activation of disparate brain regions during the performance of even a simple cognitive task. Nevertheless, particularly in the processing of vision and language, fairly well-defined lobar syndromes have been confirmed.

Language. The clearest known example of hemispheric lateralization is the localization of language functions to the left hemisphere. Starting with the work of Pierre Broca and Karl Wernicke in the 19th century, researchers have drawn a detailed map of language comprehension and expression.

At least eight types of aphasias in which one or more components of the language pathway are inured have been defined. *Prosody,* the emotional and affective components of language, or "body language," appears to be localized in a mirror set of brain units in the right hemisphere.

Because of the significant role of verbal and written language in human communication, the neuroanatomical basis of language is the most wholly understood association function. Language disorders, also called *aphasias,* are readily diagnosed in routine conversation, whereas perceptual disorders may escape notice, except during detailed neuropsychological testing, although these disorders may be caused by injury of an equal volume of the cortex. Among the earliest models of cortical localization of function were Broca's 1865 description of a loss of fluent speech caused by a lesion in the left inferior frontal lobe and Wernicke's 1874 localization of language comprehension to the left superior temporal lobe. Subsequent analyses of patients rendered aphasic by strokes, trauma, or tumors have led to the definition of the entire language association pathway from sensory input through the motor output.

Language most demonstrates hemispheric localization of function. In most persons, the hemisphere dominant for language also directs the dominant hand. Ninety percent of the population is right-handed, and 99 percent of right-handers have left hemispheric dominance for language. Of the 10 percent who are left-handers, 67 percent also have left-hemispheric language dominance; the other 33 percent have either mixed or right-hemispheric language dominance. This innate tendency to lateralization of language in the left hemisphere is positively associated with an asymmetry of the planum temporale, a triangular cortical patch on the superior surface of the temporal lobe that appears to harbor Wernicke area. Patients with mixed hemispheric dominance for language lack the expected asymmetry of the planum temporale. That asymmetry has been observed in prenatal brains suggests a genetic determinant. Indeed, the absence of asymmetry runs in families, although both genetic and intrauterine influences probably contribute to the final pattern.

Language comprehension is processed at three levels. First, in *phonologic processing,* individual sounds, such as vowels or consonants, are recognized in the inferior gyrus of the frontal lobes. Phonologic processing improves if lip reading is allowed, if speech is slowed, or if contextual clues are provided. Second, *lexical processing* matches the phonologic input with recognized words or sounds in the individual's memory. Lexical processing determines whether a sound is a word. Recent evidence has localized lexical

processing to the left temporal lobe, where the representations of lexical data are organized according to the semantic category. Third, *semantic processing* connects the words to their meaning. Persons with an isolated defect in semantic processing may retain the ability to repeat words in the absence of an ability to understand or spontaneously generate speech. Semantic processing activates the middle and superior gyri of the left temporal lobe, whereas the representation of the conceptual content of words is widely distributed in the cortex. Language production proceeds in the opposite direction, from the cortical semantic representations through the left temporal lexical nodes to either the oromotor phonologic processing area (for speech) or the graphomotor system (for writing). Each of these areas can be independently or simultaneously damaged by stroke, trauma, infection, or tumor, resulting in a specific type of aphasia.

The garbled word salad or illogic utterances of an aphasic patient leave little uncertainty about the diagnosis of left-sided cortical injury, but the right hemisphere contributes a somewhat more subtle, but equally important, affective quality to language. For example, the phrase "I feel good" may be spoken with an infinite variety of shadings, each of which is understood differently. The perception of prosody and the appreciation of the associated gestures, or "body language," appear to require an intact right hemisphere. Behavioral neurologists have mapped an entire pathway for prosody association in the right hemisphere that mirrors the language pathway of the left hemisphere. Patients with right hemisphere lesions, who have impaired comprehension or expression of prosody, may find it difficult to function in society despite their intact language skills.

Developmental dyslexia is defined as an unexpected difficulty with learning in the context of adequate intelligence, motivation, and education. Whereas speech consists of the logical combination of 44 basic phonemes of sounds, reading requires a broader set of brain functions and, thus, is more susceptible to disruption. The awareness of specific phonemes develops at about the ages of 4 to 6 years. It appears to be a prerequisite to the acquisition of reading skills. The inability to recognize distinct phonemes is the best predictor of a reading disability. Functional neuroimaging studies have localized the identification of letters to the occipital lobe adjacent to the primary visual cortex. Phonologic processing occurs in the inferior frontal lobe, and semantic processing requires the superior and middle gyri of the left temporal lobe. A recent finding of uncertain significance is that phonologic processing in men activates only the left inferior frontal gyrus, whereas phonologic processing in women activates the inferior frontal gyrus bilaterally. Careful analysis of an individual's particular reading deficits can guide remedial tutoring efforts that can focus on weaknesses and thus attempt to bring the reading skills up to the general level of intelligence and verbal skills.

In children, developmental nonverbal learning disorder is postulated to result from right hemisphere dysfunction. A nonverbal learning disorder is characterized by poor fine-motor control in the left hand, deficits in the visuoperceptual organization, problems with mathematics, and incomplete or disturbed socialization.

Patients with nonfluent aphasia, who cannot complete a simple sentence, may be able to sing an entire song, apparently because many aspects of music production are localized to the right hemisphere. Music is represented predominantly in the right hemisphere, but the full complexity of musical ability seems to involve both hemispheres. Trained musicians appear to transfer many musical skills from the right hemisphere to the left as they gain proficiency in musical analysis and performance.

Arousal and Attention. Arousal, or the establishment and maintenance of an awake state, appears to require at least three brain regions. Within the brainstem, the ascending reticular activating system (ARAS), a diffuse set of neurons, appears to set the level of consciousness. The ARAS projects to the intralaminar nuclei of the thalamus, and these nuclei, in turn, project widely throughout the cortex. Electrophysiologic studies show that both the thalamus and the cortex fire rhythmical bursts of neuronal activity at rates of 20 to 40 cycles per second. During sleep, these bursts are not synchronized. During wakefulness, the ARAS stimulates the thalamic intralaminar nuclei, which in turn coordinate the oscillations of different cortical regions. The greater the synchronization, the higher the level of wakefulness. The absence of arousal produces stupor and coma. In general, small discrete lesions of the ARAS can produce a stuporous state, whereas, at the hemispheric level, large bilateral lesions are required to cause the same depression in alertness. One particularly unfortunate but instructive condition involving extensive, permanent, bilateral cortical dysfunction is the persistent vegetative state. Sleep–wake cycles may be preserved, and the eyes may appear to gaze, but the external world does not register, and no evidence of conscious thought exists. This condition represents the expression of the isolated actions of the ARAS and the thalamus.

The maintenance of attention appears to require an intact right frontal lobe. For example, a widely used test of persistence requires scanning and identifying only the letter A from a long list of random letters. Healthy persons can usually maintain the performance of such a task for several minutes, but in patients with right frontal lobe dysfunction, this capacity is severely curtailed. Lesions of similar size in other regions of the cortex usually do not affect persistence tasks. In contrast, the more generally adaptive skill of maintaining a coherent line of thought is diffusely distributed throughout the cortex. Many medical conditions can affect this skill and may produce acute confusion or delirium.

One widely diagnosed disorder of attention is attention-deficit/hyperactivity disorder (ADHD). No pathologic findings have been consistently associated with this disorder. Functional neuroimaging studies, however, have variously documented either frontal lobe or right hemisphere hypometabolism in patients with ADHD, compared with normal controls. These findings strengthen the notion that the frontal lobes—especially the right frontal lobe—are essential to the maintenance of attention.

Memory. The clinical assessment of memory should test three periods, which have distinct anatomical correlates. *Immediate memory* functions over seconds; *recent memory* applies on a scale of minutes to days, and *remote memory* encompasses months to years. Immediate memory is implicit in the concept of attention and the ability to follow a train of thought. This ability has been divided into phonologic and visuospatial components, and functional imaging has localized them to the left and right hemispheres, respectively. A related concept, incorporating immediate and recent memory, is *working memory,* which is the ability to store information for several seconds, whereas other, related cognitive operations take place on this information. Recent studies have shown that single neurons in the dorsolateral prefrontal cortex not only record features necessary for working memory but also record the certainty with which the information is known and the degree of expectation assigned to the permanence of a particular environmental feature. Some neurons fire rapidly for an item that is eagerly awaited but may cease firing if hopes are dashed unexpectedly. The encoding of the emotional value of an item contained in the working memory may be of great usefulness in determining goal-directed behavior. Some researchers localize working memory predominantly to the left frontal cortex. Clinically, however, bilateral prefrontal cortex lesions are required for severe impairment of working memory. Other types of memory have been described: episodic, semantic, and procedural.

Three brain structures are critical to the formation of memories: the medial temporal lobe, specific diencephalic nuclei, and the basal forebrain. The *medial temporal lobe* houses the *hippocampus,* an elongated, highly repetitive network. The *amygdala* is adjacent to the anterior end of the hippocampus. The amygdala has been suggested to rate the emotional importance of experience and to activate the level of hippocampal activity accordingly. Thus an emotionally intense experience is indelibly etched in memory, but neutral stimuli are quickly disregarded.

Animal studies have defined a hippocampal place code, a pattern of cellular activation in the hippocampus that corresponds to the animal's location in space. When the animal is introduced to a novel environment, the hippocampus is broadly activated. As the animal explores and roams, the firing of certain hippocampal regions begins to correspond to specific locations in the environment. In about 1 hour, a highly detailed internal representation of the external space (a "cognitive map") appears in the form of specific firing patterns of the hippocampal cells. These patterns of neuronal firing may bear little spatial resemblance to the environment they represent; instead, they may seem randomly arranged in the hippocampus. If the animal is manually placed in a particular part of a familiar space, only the corresponding hippocampal regions show intense neural activity. When recording continues into sleep periods, firing sequences of hippocampal cells outlining a coherent path of navigation through the environment are registered, even though the animal is motionless. If the animal is removed from the environment for several days and then returned, the previously registered hippocampal place code is immediately reactivated. A series of animal experiments have dissociated the formation of the hippocampal place code from either visual, auditory, or olfactory cues, although each of these modalities may contribute to place code generation. Other factors may include internal calculations of distances based on counting footsteps or other proprioceptive information. Data from targeted genetic mutations in mice have implicated both the N-methyl-D-aspartate (NMDA) glutamate receptors and the calcium-calmodulin kinase II (CaMKII) in the proper formation of hippocampal place fields. These data suggest that the hippocampus is a significant site for the formation and storage of immediate and recent memories. Although no data yet support the notion, it is conceivable that the hippocampal cognitive map is inappropriately reactivated during a *déjà vu* experience.

The most famous human subject in the study of memory is H. M., a man with intractable epilepsy, who had both his hippocampi and amygdalae surgically removed to alleviate his condition. The epilepsy was controlled, but he was left with a complete inability to form and recall memories of facts. H. M.'s learning and memory skills were relatively preserved, which led to the suggestion that declarative or factual memory may be separate within the brain from procedural or skill-related memory. A complementary deficit in procedural memory with preservation of declarative memory may be seen in persons with Parkinson disease, in whom dopaminergic neurons of the nigrostriatal tract degenerate. Because this deficit in procedural memory can be ameliorated with treatment with levodopa, which is thought to potentiate dopaminergic neurotransmission in the nigrostriatal pathway, a role has been postulated for dopamine in procedural memory.

Additional case reports have further implicated the amygdala and the afferent and efferent fiber tracts of the hippocampus as essential to the formation of memories. Also, lesional studies have suggested mild lateralization of hippocampal function in which the left hippocampus is more efficient at forming verbal memories, and the right hippocampus tends to form nonverbal memories. After unilateral lesions in humans, however, the remaining hippocampus may compensate to a large extent. Medical causes of amnesia include alcoholism, seizures, migraine, drugs, vitamin deficiencies, trauma, strokes, tumors, infections, and degenerative diseases.

The motor system within the cortex receives directives from the association areas. The performance of a novel act requires constant feedback from the sensory and association areas for completion, and functional neuroimaging studies have demonstrated widespread activation of the cortex during unskilled acts. Memorized motor acts initially require activation of the medial temporal lobe. With practice, however, the performance of ever-larger segments of an act necessary to achieve a goal become encoded within discrete areas of the premotor and parietal cortices, particularly the left parietal cortex, with the result that a much more limited activation of the cortex is seen during highly skilled acts, and the medial temporal lobe is bypassed. This process is called the *corticalization of motor commands.* In lay terms, the process suggests a neuroanatomical basis for the adage "practice makes perfect."

Within the diencephalon, the dorsal medial nucleus of the thalamus and the mammillary bodies appear necessary for memory formation. These two structures are damaged in thiamine deficiency states usually seen in chronic alcoholics, and their inactivation is associated with Korsakoff syndrome. This syndrome is characterized by severe inability to form new memories and a variable inability to recall remote memories.

Alzheimer disease is the most common clinical memory disorder. Alzheimer disease is characterized pathologically by the degeneration of neurons and their replacement by senile plaques and neurofibrillary tangles. Clinicopathologic studies have suggested that cognitive decline is best correlated with the loss of synapses. Initially, the parietal and temporal lobes are affected, with relative sparing of the frontal lobes. This pattern of degeneration correlates with the early loss of memory, which is mostly a temporal lobe function. Also, syntactical language comprehension and visuospatial organization, functions that rely heavily on the parietal lobe, are impaired early in the course of Alzheimer disease.

In contrast, personality changes, which reflect frontal lobe function, are relatively late consequences of Alzheimer disease. A rarer, complementary cortical degeneration syndrome, Pick disease, first affects the frontal lobes while sparing the temporal and parietal lobes. In Pick disease, disinhibition and impaired language expression, which are signs of frontal dysfunction, appear early, with relatively preserved language comprehension and memory.

Memory loss can also result from disorders of the subcortical gray matter structures, specifically the basal ganglia and the brainstem nuclei, from the disease of the white matter, or from disorders that affect both gray and white matter.

Emotion. Individual emotional experiences occupy the attention of all mental health professionals. Emotion derives from basic drives, such as feeding, sex, reproduction, pleasure, pain, fear, and aggression, which all animals share. The neuroanatomical basis for these drives appears to be centered in the limbic system. Distinctly human emotions, such as affection, pride, guilt, pity, envy, and resentment, are primarily learned and most likely are represented in the cortex. The regulation of drives appears to require an intact frontal cortex. The complex interplay of the emotions, however, is far beyond the understanding of functional neuroanatomists. Where, for example, are the representations of the id, the ego, and the superego? Through what pathway are ethical and moral judgments shepherded? What processes allow beauty to be in the eye of the beholder? These philosophical questions represent a real frontier of human discovery.

Several studies have suggested that within the cortex exists a hemispheric dichotomy of emotional representation. The left hemisphere houses the analytical mind but may have a limited emotional repertoire. For example, lesions to the right hemisphere, which cause profound functional deficits, may be noted with indifference by the intact left hemisphere. The denial of illness and of the inability to move the left hand in cases of right hemisphere injury is called *anosognosia.* In contrast, left hemisphere lesions, which cause profound aphasia, can trigger a catastrophic depression, as the intact right hemisphere struggles with the realization of the loss. The right hemisphere also appears dominant for affect, socialization, and body image.

Damage to the left hemisphere produces intellectual disorder and loss of the narrative aspect of dreams. Damage to the right hemisphere produces affective disorders, loss of the visual aspects of dreams, and a failure to respond to humor, shadings of metaphor, and connotations. In dichotic vision experiments, two scenes of varied emotional content were displayed simultaneously to each half of the visual field and were perceived separately by each hemisphere. A more intense emotional response attended the scenes displayed to the left visual field that was processed by the right hemisphere. Moreover, hemisensory changes representing conversion disorders have been repeatedly noted to involve the left half of the body more often than the right, an observation that suggests an origin in the right hemisphere.

Within the hemispheres, the temporal and frontal lobes play a prominent role in emotion. The temporal lobe exhibits a high frequency of epileptic foci, and temporal lobe epilepsy (TLE) presents an exciting model for the role of the temporal lobe in behavior. In studies of epilepsy, abnormal brain activation is analyzed, rather than the deficits in activity analyzed in classic lesional studies. TLE is of particular interest in psychiatry because patients with temporal lobe seizures often manifest bizarre behavior without the classic grand mal shaking movements caused by seizures in the motor cortex. A proposed TLE personality is characterized by hyposexuality, emotional intensity, and a perseverative approach to interactions termed *viscosity.* Patients with left TLE may generate references to personal destiny and philosophical themes and display a humorless approach to life. In contrast, patients with right TLE may display excessive emotionality, ranging from elation to sadness. Although patients with TLE may display excessive aggression between seizures, the seizure itself may evoke fear.

The inverse of a TLE personality appears in persons with bilateral injury to the temporal lobes after head trauma, cardiac arrest, herpes simplex encephalitis, or Pick disease. This lesion resembles the one described in the Klüver–Bucy syndrome, an experimental model of temporal lobe ablation in monkeys. Behavior in this syndrome is characterized by hypersexuality, placidity, a tendency to explore the environment with the mouth, inability to recognize the emotional significance of visual stimuli, and continually shifting attention, called *hypermetamorphosis.* In contrast to the aggression-fear spectrum sometimes seen in patients with TLE, complete experimental ablation of the temporal lobes appears to produce a uniform, bland reaction to the environment, possibly because of an inability to access memories.

The prefrontal cortices influence mood in a complementary way. Whereas activation of the left prefrontal cortex appears to lift the mood, activation of the right prefrontal cortex causes depression. A lesion to the left prefrontal area, at either the cortical or the subcortical level, abolishes the typical mood-elevating influences and produces depression and uncontrollable crying. In contrast, a comparable lesion to the right prefrontal area may produce laughter, euphoria, and *witzelsucht,* a tendency to joke and make puns. Effects opposite to those caused by lesions appear during seizures, in which occurs abnormal, excessive activation of either prefrontal cortex. A seizure focus within the left prefrontal cortex can cause gelastic seizures, for example, in which the ictal event is laughter. Functional neuroimaging has documented left prefrontal hypoperfusion during depressive states, which normalized after the depression was treated successfully.

Limbic System Function.
James Papez delineated the limbic system in 1937. The Papez circuit consists of the hippocampus, the fornix, the mammillary bodies, the anterior nucleus of the thalamus, and the cingulate gyrus (Fig. 33-3). The boundaries of the limbic system were subsequently expanded to include the amygdala, septum, basal forebrain, nucleus accumbens, and orbitofrontal cortex.

Although this schema creates an anatomical loop for emotional processing, the specific contributions of the individual components other than the hippocampus or even whether a given train of neural impulses travels along the entire pathway is unknown.

The amygdala appears to be a critically important gate through which internal and external stimuli are integrated. Information from the primary senses is interwoven with internal drives, such as hunger and thirst, to assign emotional significance to sensory experiences. The amygdala may mediate learned fear responses, such as anxiety and panic, and may direct the expression of certain emotions by producing a particular affect. Neuroanatomical data suggest that the amygdala exerts a more powerful influence on the cortex, to stimulate or suppress cortical activity than the cortex exerts on the amygdala. Pathways from the sensory thalamic

relay stations separately send sensory data to the amygdala and the cortex, but the subsequent effect of the amygdala on the cortex is the more potent of the two reciprocal connections.

In contrast, damage to the amygdala has been reported to ablate the ability to distinguish fear and anger in other persons' voices and facial expressions. Persons with such injuries may have a preserved ability to recognize happiness, sadness, or disgust. The limbic system appears to house the emotional association areas, which direct the hypothalamus to express the motor and endocrine components of the emotional state.

Fear and Aggression.
The electrical stimulation of animals throughout the subcortical area involving the limbic system produces rage reactions (e.g., growling, spitting, and arching of the back). Whether the animal flees or attacks depends on the intensity of the stimulation.

Limbic System and Schizophrenia.
The limbic system has been particularly implicated in neuropathologic studies of schizophrenia. Eugen Bleuler's well-known four A's of schizophrenia—affect, associations, ambivalence, and autism—refer to brain functions served in part by limbic structures. Several clinicopathologic studies have found a reduction in the brain weight of the gray matter but not of the white matter in persons with schizophrenia. In pathologic as well as in magnetic resonance imaging (MRI) reports, persons with schizophrenia may have reduced the volume of the hippocampus, amygdala, and parahippocampal gyrus. Schizophrenia may be a late sequela of a temporal epileptic focus, with some studies reporting an association in 7 percent of patients with TLE.

Functional neuroimaging studies have demonstrated decreased activation of the frontal lobes in many patients with schizophrenia, particularly during tasks requiring willed action. A reciprocal increase in activation of the temporal lobe can occur during willed actions, such as finger movements or speaking, in persons with schizophrenia. Neuropathologic studies have shown a decreased density of neuropil, the intertwined axons, and dendrites of the neurons in the frontal lobes of these patients. During development, the density of neuropil is highest around age 1 year and then is

FIGURE 33-3

Schematic drawing of the major anatomic structures of the limbic system. The cingulate and parahippocampal gyri form the "limbic lobe," a rim of tissue located along the junction of the diencephalon and the cerebral hemispheres. (Adapted from Hendelman WJ. *Student's Atlas of Neuroanatomy*. Philadelphia, PA: WB Saunders; 1994:179.)

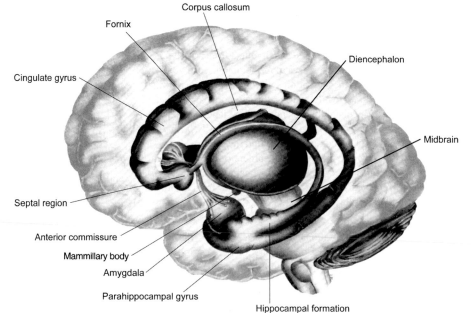

reduced somewhat through synaptic pruning; the density plateaus throughout childhood and is further reduced to adult levels in adolescence. One hypothesis of the appearance of schizophrenia in the late teenage years is that excessive adolescent synaptic pruning occurs and results in too little frontolimbic activity. Some experts have suggested that hypometabolism and paucity of interneuronal connections in the prefrontal cortex may reflect inefficiencies in working memory, which permits the disjointed discourse and loosening of associations that characterize schizophrenia. At present, the molecular basis for the regulation of the density of synapses within the neuropil is unknown. Other lines of investigation aimed at understanding the biologic basis of schizophrenia have documented inefficiencies in the formation of cortical synaptic connections in the middle of the second trimester of gestation, which may result from a viral infection or malnutrition. Neurodevelopmental surveys administered during childhood found an increased incidence of subtle neurologic abnormalities before the appearance of the thought disorder in persons who subsequently exhibited signs of schizophrenia.

In one intriguing study, positron emission tomography (PET) scanning was used to identify the brain regions that are activated when a person hears spoken language. A consistent set of cortical and subcortical structures demonstrated increased metabolism when speech was processed. The researchers then studied a group of patients with schizophrenia who were experiencing active auditory hallucinations. They found that the same brain areas that were activated when actual sounds were playing were activated while the patients were hallucinating. This included the primary auditory cortex. At the same time, decreased activation was seen of areas thought to monitor speech, including the left middle temporal gyrus and the supplementary motor area. This study raises the questions of what brain structure is activating the hallucinations, and by what mechanism do neuroleptic drugs suppress the hallucinations. Functional imaging has much to tell about the neuroanatomical basis of schizophrenia.

Frontal Lobe Function. The *frontal lobes,* the region that determines how the brain acts on its knowledge, constitute a category unto themselves. In comparative neuroanatomical studies, the massive size of the frontal lobes is the main feature that distinguishes the human brain from that of other primates, and that lends it uniquely human qualities. There are four subdivisions of the frontal lobes. The first three—the motor strip, the supplemental motor area, and Broca area—are mentioned in the preceding discussion of the motor system and language. The fourth, most anterior, division is the prefrontal cortex. The prefrontal cortex contains three regions in which lesions produce distinct syndromes: the *orbitofrontal,* the *dorsolateral,* and the *medial.* Dye-tracing studies have defined dense reciprocal connections between the prefrontal cortex and all other brain regions. Therefore, to the extent that anatomy can predict function, the prefrontal cortex is ideally connected to allow sequential use of the entire palette of brain functions in executing the goal-directed activity. Indeed, frontal lobe injury usually impairs the executive functions: motivation, attention, and sequencing of actions.

Bilateral lesions of the frontal lobes are characterized by changes in personality—how persons interact with the world. The *frontal lobe syndrome,* which is most commonly produced by trauma, infarcts, tumors, lobotomy, multiple sclerosis, or Pick disease, consists of slow thinking, poor judgment, decreased curiosity, social withdrawal, and irritability. Patients typically display apathetic indifference to experience that can explode into impulsive

disinhibition. Unilateral frontal lobe lesions may be mostly unnoticed because the intact lobe can compensate with high efficiency.

Frontal lobe dysfunction may be challenging to detect using highly structured, formal neuropsychological tests. Intelligence, as reflected in the intelligence quotient (IQ), may be average, and functional neuroimaging studies have shown that the IQ seems to require mostly parietal lobe activation. For example, during the administration of the Wechsler Adult Intelligence Scale-Revised (WAIS-R), the highest levels of increased metabolic activity during verbal tasks occurred in the left parietal lobe, whereas the highest levels of increased metabolic activity during performance skills occurred in the right parietal lobe. In contrast, frontal lobe pathology may become apparent only under unstructured, stressful, real-life situations.

> A famous case illustrating the result of frontal lobe damage involves Phineas Gage, a 25-year-old railroad worker. While he was working with explosives, an accident drove an iron rod through Gage's head. He survived, but both frontal lobes were severely damaged. After the accident, his behavior changed dramatically. The case was written up by J. M. Harlow, M.D., in 1868, as follows: [George] is fitful, irreverent, indulging at times in the grossest profanity (which was not previously his custom), manifesting but little deference for his fellows, impatient of restraint or advice when it conflicts with his desires…His mind was radically changed, so decidedly that his friends and acquaintances said he was "no longer Gage" (see Fig. 33-4).

In one study of right-handed males, lesions of the right prefrontal cortex eliminated the tendency to use internal, associative memory cues and led to an extreme tendency to interpret the task at hand in terms of its immediate context. In contrast, right-handed males who had lesions of the left prefrontal cortex produced no context-dependent interpretations and interpreted the tasks entirely

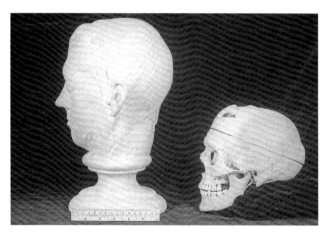

FIGURE 33-4
The life mask and skull of Phineas Gage. Note damage to the frontal region. "A famous case illustrating the result of frontal lobe damage involves Phineas Gage, a 25-year-old railroad worker. While he was working with explosives, an accident drove an iron rod through Gage's head. He survived, but both frontal lobes were severely damaged. After the accident, his behavior changed dramatically. The case was written up by J.M. Harlow, M.D., in 1868, as follows: [Gage] is fitful, irreverent, indulging at times in the grossest profanity (which was not previously his custom), manifesting but little deference for his fellows, impatient of restraint or advice when it conflicts his desires… His mind was radically changed, so decidedly that his friends and acquaintances said he was 'no longer Gage'." (Courtesy of Anthony A. Walsh, Ph.D.)

in terms of their internal drives. A mirror image of the functional lateralization appeared in left-handed subjects. This test thus revealed the most precise known association of higher cortical functional lateralization with the subjects' dominant hand. Future experiments in this vein will attempt to reproduce these findings with functional neuroimaging. If corroborated, these studies suggest a remarkable complexity of functional localization within the prefrontal cortex and may also have implications for the understanding of psychiatric diseases in which prefrontal pathology has been postulated, such as schizophrenia and mood disorders.

The massive innervation of the frontal lobes by dopamine-containing nerve fibers is of interest because of the action of antipsychotic medications. At the clinical level, antipsychotic medications may help to organize the rambling associations of a patient with schizophrenia. At the neurochemical level, most typical antipsychotic medications block the actions of dopamine at the D_2 receptors. The frontal lobes, therefore, may be a significant therapeutic site of action for antipsychotic medications.

Development

The nervous system is divided into central and peripheral nervous systems (CNS and PNS). The CNS consists of the brain and spinal cord; the PNS refers to all the sensory, motor, and autonomic fibers and ganglia outside the CNS. During development, both divisions arise from the neural tube. The neural tube forms through the folding of the neural plate, a specialization of the ectoderm (the outermost of the three embryonic layers). During embryonic development, the neural tube itself becomes the CNS; the ectoderm immediately superficial to the neural tube becomes the neural crest, which gives rise to the PNS. The formation of these structures requires chemical communication between the neighboring tissues in the form of cell surface molecules and diffusible chemical signals.

In many cases, an earlier-formed structure, such as the notochord, is said to *induce* the surrounding ectoderm to form a later structure, in this case, the neural plate. The identification of the chemical mediators of tissue induction is an active area of research. Investigators have begun to examine whether failures of the interactions of these mediators and their receptors could underlie errors in brain development that cause psychopathology.

Neuronal Migration and Connections.   The life cycle of a neuron consists of a cell birth, migration to the adult position, extension of an axon, elaboration of dendrites, synaptogenesis, and, finally, the onset of chemical neurotransmission. Individual neurons are born in proliferative zones, generally located along the inner surface of the neural tube. At the peak of neuronal proliferation in the middle of the second trimester, 250,000 neurons are born each minute. Postmitotic neurons migrate outward to their adult locations in the cortex, guided by radially oriented astrocytic glial fibers. Glia-guided neuronal migration in the cerebral cortex occupies much of the first 6 months of gestation. For some neurons in the prefrontal cortex, migration occurs over a distance 5,000 times the diameter of the neuronal cell body. Neuronal migration requires a complex set of cell-cell interactions and is susceptible to errors in which neurons fail to reach the cortex and instead reside in ectopic positions. A group of such incorrectly placed neurons is called a *heterotopia*. Neuronal heterotopias have been shown to cause epilepsy and are positively associated with mental retardation. In a neuropathologic study of the planum temporale of four consecutive patients with dyslexia, heterotopias were a common finding.

Recently, heterotopic neurons within the frontal lobe have been postulated to play a causal role in some cases of schizophrenia.

Many neurons lay down an axon as they migrate, whereas others do not initiate axon outgrowth until they have reached their cortical targets. Thalamic axons that project to the cortex initially synapse on a transient layer of neurons called the *subplate neurons.* In normal development, the axons subsequently detach from the subplate neurons and proceed superficially to synapse on the actual cortical cells. The subplate neurons then degenerate. Some brains from persons with schizophrenia reveal an abnormal persistence of subplate neurons, suggesting a failure to complete axonal pathfinding in the brains of these persons. This finding does not correlate with the presence of schizophrenia in every case, however. A characteristic branched dendritic tree elaborates once the neuron has completed migration. Synaptogenesis occurs at a furious rate from the second trimester through the first 10 years or so of life. The peak of synaptogenesis occurs within the first 2 postnatal years when as many as 30 million synapses form each second. Ensheathment of axons by myelin begins prenatally; it is mostly complete in early childhood but does not reach its full extent until late in the third decade of life. Myelination of the brain is also sequential.

Neuroscientists are tremendously interested in the effect of experience on the formation of brain circuitry in the first years of life. As noted earlier, many examples are seen of the impact of early sensory experience on the wiring of cortical sensory processing areas. Similarly, early movement patterns are known to reinforce neural connections in the supplemental motor area that drive specific motor acts. Neurons rapidly form a fivefold excess of synaptic connections; then, through a Darwinian process of elimination, only those synapses that serve a relevant function persist. This synaptic pruning appears to preserve input in which the presynaptic cell fires in synchrony with the postsynaptic cell, a process that reinforces repeatedly activated neural circuits. One molecular component that is thought to mediate synaptic reinforcement is the postsynaptic NMDA glutamate receptor. This receptor allows the influx of calcium ions only when activated by glutamate at the same time as the membrane in which it sits is depolarized. Thus, glutamate binding without membrane depolarization or membrane depolarization without glutamate binding fails to trigger calcium influx. NMDA receptors open in dendrites that are exposed to repeated activation, and their activation stimulates the stabilization of the synapse. Calcium is a crucial intracellular messenger that initiates a cascade of events, including gene regulation and the release of trophic factors that strengthen particular synaptic connections. Although less experimental evidence exists for the role of experience in modulating synaptic connectivity of association areas than has been demonstrated in sensory and motor areas, neuroscientists assume that similar activity-dependent mechanisms may apply in all areas of the brain.

Adult Neurogenesis.   A remarkable recent discovery has been that new neurons can be generated in specific brain regions (notably the dentate gyrus of the hippocampus) in adult animals, including humans. This discovery is in marked contrast to the previous belief that no neurons were produced after birth in most species. This discovery has a potentially profound impact on our understanding of normal development, incorporation of experiences, as well as the ability of the brain to repair itself after various types of injuries.

Neurologic Basis of Development Theories.   In the realm of emotion, early childhood experiences have been suspected to be at the root of psychopathology since the earliest theories of Sigmund Freud. Freud's psychoanalytic method aimed at tracing the threads of a patient's earliest childhood memories. Franz Alexander added the goal of allowing the patient to relive these memories in a less pathologic environment, a process known as a *corrective emotional experience.* Although neuroscientists have no data demonstrating that this method operates at the level of neurons and circuits, emerging results reveal a profound effect of early caregivers on an adult individual's emotional repertoire. For example, the concept of attunement is defined as the process by which caregivers "playback a child's inner feelings." If a baby's emotional expressions are reciprocated consistently and sensitively, specific emotional circuits are reinforced. These circuits likely include the limbic system, in particular, the amygdala, which serves as a gate to the hippocampal memory circuits for emotional stimuli. In one anecdote, for example, a baby whose mother repeatedly failed to mirror her level of excitement emerged from childhood a too passive girl, who was unable to experience a thrill or a feeling of joy.

The relative contributions of nature and nurture are perhaps nowhere more indistinct than in the maturation of emotional responses, partly because the localization of emotion within the adult brain is only poorly understood. It is reasonable to assume, however, that the reactions of caregivers during a child's first 2 years of life are eventually internalized as distinct neural circuits, which may be only incompletely subject to modification through subsequent experience. For example, axonal connections between the prefrontal cortex and the limbic system, which probably play a role in modulating basic drives, are established between the ages of 10 and 18 months. Recent work suggests that a pattern of terrifying experiences in infancy may flood the amygdala and drive memory circuits to be specifically alert to threatening stimuli, at the expense of circuits for language and other academic skills. Thus infants raised in a chaotic and frightening home may be neurologically disadvantaged for the acquisition of complex cognitive skills in school.

An adult correlate to this cascade of detrimental overactivity of the fear response is found in posttraumatic stress disorder (PTSD), in which persons exposed to an intense trauma involving death or injury may have feelings of fear and helplessness for years after the event. A PET scanning study of patients with PTSD revealed abnormally high activity in the right amygdala while the patients were reliving their traumatic memories. The researchers hypothesized that the stressful hormonal milieu present during the registration of the memories might have served to burn the memories into the brain and to prevent their erasure by the usual memory modulation circuits. As a result, the traumatic memories exerted a pervasive influence and led to a state of constant vigilance, even in safe, familiar settings.

Workers in the related realms of mathematics have produced results documenting the organizing effects of early experiences on internal representations of the external world. Since the time of Pythagoras, music has been considered a branch of mathematics. A series of studies have shown that groups of children who were given 8 months of intensive classical music lessons during preschool years later had significantly better spatial and mathematical reasoning in school than a control group. Nonmusical tasks, such as navigating mazes, drawing geometric figures, and copying patterns of two-color blocks, were performed significantly more skillfully by the musical children. Early exposure to music, thus, may be ideal preparation for later acquisition of complex mathematical and engineering skills.

These tantalizing observations suggest a neurologic basis for the developmental theories of Jean Piaget, Erik Erikson, Margaret Mahler, John Bowlby, Sigmund Freud, and others. Erikson's epigenetic theory states that normal adult behavior results from the successful, sequential completion of each of several infantile and childhood stages. According to the epigenetic model, failure to complete an early stage is reflected in subsequent physical, cognitive, social, or emotional maladjustment. By analogy, the experimental data just discussed suggest that early experience, particularly during the critical window of opportunity for establishing neural connections, primes the necessary circuitry for language, emotions, and other advanced behaviors. Miswiring of an infant's brain may lead to severe handicaps later when the person attempts to relate to the world as an adult. These findings support the vital need for adequate public financing of Early Intervention and Head Start programs, programs that may be the most cost-effective means of improving persons' mental health.

NEURAL DEVELOPMENT AND NEUROGENESIS

The human brain is a structurally and functionally complex system that exhibits ongoing modification in response to both experience and disease. The anatomical and neurochemical systems that underlie the cognitive, social, emotional and sensorimotor functions of the mature nervous system emerge from neuronal and glial cell populations that arise during the earliest periods of development.

An understanding of molecular and cellular mechanisms mediating nervous system development is critical in psychiatry because abnormalities of developmental processes contribute to many brain disorders. Although a developmental basis may not be surprising in early childhood disorders, such as autism, fragile X mental retardation, and Rett syndrome, even mature diseases, including schizophrenia and depression, reflect ontogenetic factors. For example, evidence from brain pathology and neuroimaging indicates that there are reductions in forebrain region volumes, neuron and glial cell numbers, and some classes of interneurons in schizophrenia that are apparent at the time of diagnosis. Similarly, in autism, early brain growth is abnormally increased, and abnormalities of the cellular organization are observed that reflect disturbances in the fundamental processes of cell proliferation and migration. When there is abnormal regulation of early brain development, a foundation of altered neuron populations that may differ in cell types, numbers, and positions is laid down. They may also develop abnormal connections, which also have consequences for interacting glial populations. With progressive postnatal development, the maturing brain systems call upon component neurons to achieve increasing levels of complex information processing, which may be deficient should initial conditions be disturbed. New neural properties emerge during maturation as neuron populations elaborate additional functional networks based on and modified by ongoing experience. Given the brain's dynamic character, we may expect that developmental abnormalities in neural populations and systems, caused by genetic as well as environmental factors, will manifest at diverse times in a person's life.

Overview of Nervous System Morphologic Development

In considering brain development, several overarching principles need to be considered. First, different brain regions and neuron populations are generated at distinct times of development and exhibit specific temporal schedules. This pattern has implications for the consequences of specific developmental insults, such as the production of autism following fetal exposure to the drug thalidomide only during days 20 to 24 of gestation. Second, the sequence of cellular processes comprising ontogeny predicts that abnormalities in early events necessarily lead to differences in subsequent stages, although not all abnormalities may be accessible to our clinical tools. For example, a deficit in the number of neurons will likely lead to reductions in axonal processes and ensheathing white matter in the mature brain. However, at the clinical level, since glial cells outnumber neurons 8 to 1, the glial cell population, the oligodendrocytes, and their myelin appear as an altered white matter on neuroimaging with little evidence of a neuronal disturbance. Third, it is clear that specific molecular signals, such as extracellular growth factors and cognate receptors or transcription factors, play roles at multiple developmental stages of the cell. For example, both insulin-like growth factor I (IGF-I) and brain-derived neurotrophic factor (BDNF) regulate multiple cellular processes during the developmental generation and mature function of neurons, including cell proliferation, survival promotion, neuron migration, process outgrowth, and the momentary synaptic modifications (plasticity) underlying learning and memory. Thus changes in expression or regulation of a ligand or its receptor, by experience, environmental insults, or genetic mechanisms, will have effects on multiple developmental and mature processes.

The Neural Plate and Neurulation. The nervous system of the human embryo first appears between 2½ and 4 weeks of gestation. During development, the emergence of new cell types, including neurons, results from interactions between neighboring layers of cells. On gestational day 13, the embryo consists of a sheet of cells. Following gastrulation (days 14 to 15), which forms a two-cell–layered embryo consisting of ectoderm and endoderm, the neural plate region of the ectoderm is delineated by the underlying mesoderm, which appears on day 16. The mesoderm forms by cells entering a midline cleft in the ectoderm called the primitive streak. After migration, the mesodermal layer lies between

the ectoderm and endoderm and induces the overlying ectoderm to become a neural plate. Induction usually involves the release of soluble growth factors from one group of cells, which in turn bind receptors on neighboring cells, eliciting changes in nuclear transcription factors that control downstream gene expression. In some cases, cell–cell contact-mediated mechanisms are involved. In the gene-patterning section below, the critical roles of soluble growth factors and transcription factor expression are described.

The neural plate, the induction of which is complete by 18 days, is a sheet of columnar epithelium and is surrounded by ectodermal epithelium. After formation, the edges of the neural plate elevate, forming the neural ridges. Subsequently, changes in intracellular cytoskeleton and cell-extracellular matrix attachment cause the ridges to merge in the midline and fuse, a process termed neurulation, forming the neural tube, with a central cavity presaging the ventricular system (Fig. 33-5). Fusion begins in the cervical region at the hindbrain level (medulla and pons) and continues rostrally and caudally. Neurulation occurs at 3 to 4 weeks of gestation in humans, and its failure results in anencephaly rostrally and spina bifida caudally. Neurulation defects are well known following exposure to retinoic acid in dermatologic preparations and anticonvulsants, especially valproic acid, as well as diets deficient in folic acid.

Another product of neurulation is the neural crest, the cells of which derive from the edges of the neural plate and dorsal neural tube. From this position, neural crest cells migrate dorsolaterally under the skin to form melanocytes and ventromedially to form dorsal root sensory ganglia and sympathetic chains of the peripheral nervous system and ganglia of the enteric nervous system. However, neural crest gives rise to diverse tissues, including cells of neuroendocrine, cardiac, mesenchymal, and skeletal systems, forming the basis of many congenital syndromes involving the brain and other organs. The neural crest origin at the border of neural and epidermal ectoderm and its generation of melanocytes forms the basis of the neurocutaneous disorders, including tuberous sclerosis and neurofibromatosis. Finally, another nonneuronal structure

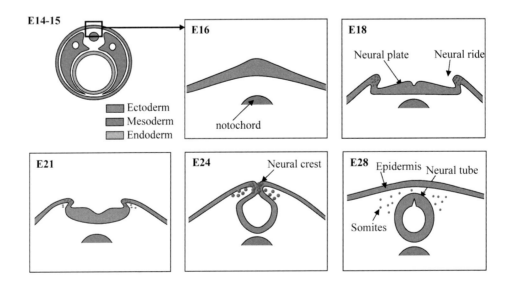

FIGURE 33-5

Mechanisms of neurulation. Neurulation begins with the formation of a neural plate in response to soluble growth factors released by the underlying notochord. The neural plate originates as a thickening of the ectoderm that results from cuboidal epithelial cells becoming columnar in shape. With further changes in cell shape and adhesion, the edges of the plate fold and rise, meeting in the midline to form a tube. Cells at the tips of the neural folds come to lie between the neural tube and overlying epidermis, forming the neural crest that gives rise to the peripheral nervous system and other structures. (From Sadock BJ, Sadock VA, Ruiz P. *Kaplan & Sadock's Comprehensive Textbook of Psychiatry.* 9th ed. Philadelphia, PA: Lippincott Williams & Wilkins; 2009:44.)

of mesodermal origin formed during neurulation is the notochord found on the ventral side of the neural tube. As we will describe later in this chapter, the notochord plays a critical role during neural tube differentiation, since it is a signaling source of soluble growth factors, such as sonic hedgehog (Shh), which affect gene patterning and cell determination.

Regional Differentiation of the Embryonic Nervous System.

After closure, the neural tube expands differentially to form major morphologic subdivisions that precede the major functional divisions of the brain. These subdivisions are important developmentally because different regions are generated according to specific schedules of proliferation and subsequent migration and differentiation. The neural tube can be described in three dimensions, including longitudinal, circumferential, and radial. The longitudinal dimension reflects the rostrocaudal (anterior–posterior) organization, which mostly consists of the brain and spinal cord. Organization in the circumferential dimension, tangential to the surface, represents two significant axes: In the dorsoventral axis, cell groups are uniquely positioned from top to bottom.

On the other hand, in the medial to the lateral axis, there is mirror-image symmetry, consistent with the right-left symmetry of the body. Finally, the radial dimension represents the organization from the innermost cell layer adjacent to the ventricles to the outermost surface and exhibits region-specific cell layering. At 4 weeks, the human brain is divided longitudinally into the prosencephalon (forebrain), mesencephalon (midbrain), and rhombencephalon (hindbrain). These three subdivisions or "vesicles" divide further into five divisions by 5 weeks, consisting of the prosencephalon, which forms the telencephalon (including cortex, hippocampus, and basal ganglia) and diencephalon (thalamus and hypothalamus), the mesencephalon, (midbrain), and the rhombencephalon, yielding

metencephalon (pons and cerebellum) and myelencephalon (medulla). Morphologic transformation into five vesicles depends on the region-specific proliferation of precursor cells adjacent to the ventricles, the so-called ventricular zones (VZs). As discussed later, proliferation intimately depends on soluble growth factors made by proliferating cells themselves or released from regional signaling centers. In turn, growth factor production and cognate receptor expression also depend on region-specific patterning genes. We now know that VZ precursors, which appear morphologically homogeneous, express a checkerboard array of molecular genetic determinants that control the generation of specific types of neurons in each domain (Fig. 33-6).

In the circumferential dimension, the organization begins very early and extends over many rostrocaudal subdivisions. In the spinal cord, the majority of tissue comprises the lateral plates, which later divide into dorsal or alar plates, composed of sensory interneurons, and motor or basal plates, consisting of ventral motor neurons. Two other diminutive plates, termed the roof plate and floor plate, are virtually absent in maturity; however, they play critical regulatory roles as growth factor signaling centers in the embryo. Indeed, the floor plate, in response to Shh from the ventrally located notochord, produces its own Shh, which in turn induces neighboring cells in the ventral spinal cord and brainstem to express region-specific transcription factors that specify cell phenotype and function. For example, in combination with other factors, floor plate Shh induces midbrain precursors to differentiate into dopamine-secreting neurons of the substantia nigra.

Similarly, the roof plate secretes growth factors, such as bone morphogenetic proteins (BMPs), which induce dorsal neuron cell fate in the spinal cord. In the absence of a roof plate, dorsal structures fail to form, such as the cerebellum, and midline hippocampal structures are missing. Finally, in the radial dimension, the

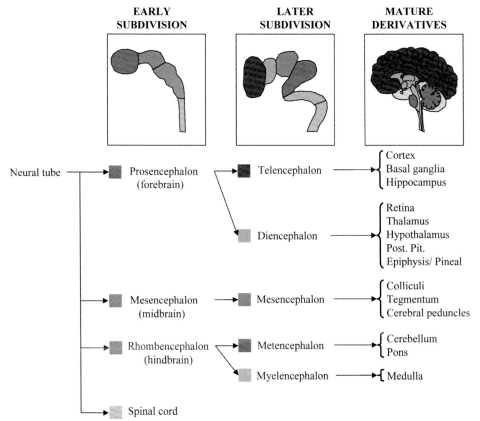

FIGURE 33-6

Progression of brain regional differentiation. Early after neurulation, the neural tube differentiates into four regions (forebrain, midbrain, hindbrain, and spinal cord) that give rise following later divisions and maturation to the different brain structures. (From Sadock BJ, Sadock VA, Ruiz P. *Kaplan & Sadock's Comprehensive Textbook of Psychiatry*. 9th ed. Philadelphia, PA: Lippincott Williams & Wilkins; 2009:45.)

organization of layers is subdivision specific, produced by differential proliferation of VZ precursors and cell migration, as described later.

The Ventricular and Subventricular Proliferative Zones.

The distinct patterns of precursor proliferation and migration in different regions generate the radial organization of the nervous system. In each longitudinal subdivision, the final population size of a brain region depends on the interplay of regulated neurogenesis with programmed cell death. Traditional concepts had suggested that there was excess cell production everywhere and that final cell number regulation was achieved primarily after neurogenesis through selective cell death mediated by target-derived survival (trophic) factors. We now know that the patterning genes discussed later play significant roles in directing regional precursor proliferation that is coordinated with final structural requirements, and that programmed cell death occurs at multiple stages. Consequently, in diseases characterized by brain regions smaller than usual, such as schizophrenia, there may be a failure to generate neurons initially, as opposed to normal generation with subsequent cell loss.

Radial and Tangential Patterns of Neurogenesis and Migration.

Of interest to psychiatry, the cerebral cortex is the paradigmatic model of inside-to-outside neurogenesis. A large number of studies now relate specific genetic mutations to distinct cortical malformations that alter neurogenesis, migration, and cellular organization, thereby increasing our knowledge of both normal and pathophysiologic cortical development. The characteristic six-cell layers represent a common cytoarchitectural and physiologic basis for the neocortical function and are derived from the embryonic forebrain telencephalic vesicles. Within each layer, neurons exhibit related axodendritic morphologies, use common neurotransmitters, and establish similar afferent and efferent connections. In general, pyramidal neurons in layer 3 establish synapses within and between cortical hemispheres, whereas deeper layer 5/6 neurons project primarily to subcortical nuclei, including the thalamus, brainstem, and spinal cord. The majority of cortical neurons originate from the forebrain VZ. At the earliest stages, the first postmitotic cells migrate outward from the VZ to establish a superficial layer termed the preplate. Two consequential cell types comprise the preplate— Cajal–Retzius cells, which form outermost layer one or marginal zone, and subplate neurons, which lay beneath future layer 6. These distinct regions form when later-born cortical plate neurons migrate within and divide the preplate in two (Fig. 33-7).

A recent discovery, postulated for years, has changed the view of the origins of cortical neuron populations involved in human brain disease. Neuron tracing experiments in culture and in vivo demonstrate that the neocortex, a dorsal forebrain derivative, is also populated by neurons generated in the ventral forebrain (see Fig. 33-7). Molecular studies of patterning genes, especially *Dlx*, strongly support this model (see below). In contrast to excitatory pyramidal neurons, the overwhelming majority of inhibitory

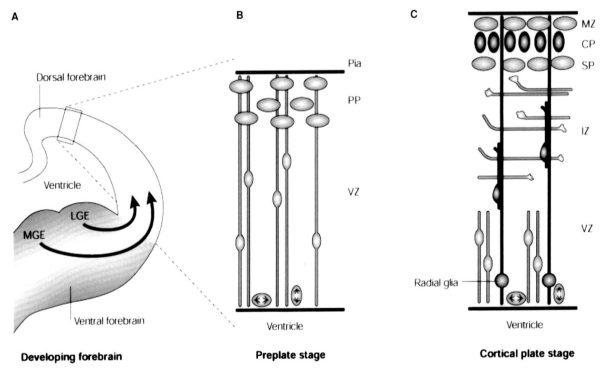

FIGURE 33-7

Schematic drawing of radial and tangential migration during cerebral cortex development. **A:** A coronal section of one-half of the developing rat forebrain. The dorsal forebrain gives rise to the cerebral cortex. Medial ganglionic eminences (MGEs) and lateral ganglionic eminences (LGEs) of the ventral forebrain generate neurons of the basal ganglia and the cortical interneurons. The arrows indicate the tangential migration route for γ-aminobutyric acid (GABA) interneurons to the cortex. The boxed area (enlarged in B and C) shows the developing cortex at early and late stages. **B:** In the dorsal forebrain, the first cohort of postmitotic neurons migrate out from the ventricular zone (VZ) and create a preplate (PP) below the pial surface. **C:** Subsequent postmitotic neurons will migrate along radial glia through the intermediate zone (IZ) and take position in the middle of the preplate, creating a cortical plate (CP) between the outer marginal zone (MZ) and inner subplate (SP). Ultimately, the CP will be composed of six layers that are born sequentially, migrating in an inside-to-outside pattern. Horizontal processes in the IZ represent axon terminals of thalamic afferents. (From Nadarajah B, Parnavelas JG. Modes of neuronal migration in the developing cerebral cortex. *Nat Neurosci.* 2002;3:423, with permission.)

γ-aminobutyric acid (GABA)-secreting interneurons originate from mitotic precursors of the ganglionic eminences that generate the neurons of the basal ganglia. Subsets of interneurons also secrete neuropeptides, such as neuropeptide Y (NPY) and somatostatin, and express nitrous oxide (NOS)-generating enzyme. Not associated with cortical VZ radial glia, these GABA interneurons reach the cortical plate by migrating tangentially, in either the superficial marginal zone or a deep position above the VZ, the subplate region where thalamic afferents are also growing. Significantly, in brains from patients with schizophrenia, the prefrontal cortex exhibits a reduced density of interneurons in layer 2. Also, there is upregulation of GABA$_A$-receptor binding, a potential functional compensation, as well as a relative deficiency of NOS-expressing neurons. These observations have led to the hypothesis that schizophrenia is due to reduced GABAergic activity. The origin of GABA interneurons from the ganglionic eminences and their association with specific patterning genes raises new genetic models of disease causation and possible strategies for disease intervention. Thus, more broadly, normal cortical development depends on a balance of two principal patterns of neurogenesis and migration, consisting of radial migration of excitatory neurons from the dorsal forebrain VZ and tangential migration of inhibitory neurons from the ventral forebrain.

In contrast to inside-to-outside neurogenesis observed in the cortex, phylogenetically older regions, such as the hypothalamus, spinal cord, and hippocampal dentate gyrus, exhibit the reverse order of cell generation. First-formed postmitotic neurons lie superficially, and last-generated cells localize toward the center. Although this outside-to-inside pattern might reflect passive cell displacement, radial glia, and specific migration signaling molecules are involved. Furthermore, cells do not always lie in direct extension from their locus of VZ generation. Instead, some groups of cells migrate to specific locations, as observed for neurons of the inferior olivary nuclei.

Of prime importance in psychiatry, the hippocampus demonstrates both radial and nonradial patterns of neurogenesis and migration. The pyramidal cell layer, Ammon's horn Cornu Ammonis (CA) 1 to 3 neurons, is generated in a typical outside-to-inside fashion in the dorsomedial forebrain for a discrete period, from 7 to 15 weeks of gestation, and exhibits intricate migration patterns. In contrast, the other significant population, dentate gyrus granule neurons, start appearing at 18 weeks and exhibits prolonged postnatal neurogenesis, originating from several migrating secondary proliferative zones. In rats, for instance, granule neurogenesis starts at embryonic day 16 (E16) with proliferation in the forebrain VZ. At E18, an aggregate of precursors migrates along a subpial route into the dentate gyrus. There, they generate granule neurons in situ. After birth, there is another migration, localizing proliferative precursors to the dentate hilus, which persists until 1 month of life. After that, granule precursors move to a layer just under the dentate gyrus, termed the subgranular zone (SGZ), which produces neurons throughout life in adult rats, primates, and humans. In rodents, SGZ precursors proliferate in response to cerebral ischemia, tissue injury, and seizures, as well as growth factors. Finally, the diminished hippocampal volume reported in schizophrenia raises the possibility that disordered neurogenesis plays a role in pathogenesis, as either a basis for dysfunction or a consequence of brain injuries, consistent with associations of gestational infections with disease manifestation.

Finally, a different combination of radial and nonradial migration is observed in the cerebellum, which is a brain region that plays an essential function in nonmotor tasks, with particular significance

for autism spectrum disorders (ASDs). Except for granule cells, the other significant neurons, including Purkinje and deep nuclei, originate from the primary VZ of the fourth ventricle, coincident with other brainstem neurons. In rats, this occurs at E13 to E15, and in humans, at 5 to 7 weeks of gestation. The granule neurons, as well as the basket and stellate interneurons, originate in the secondary proliferative zone, the external germinal cell layer (EGL), which covers the newborn cerebellum at birth. EGL precursors originate in the fourth ventricle VZ and migrate dorsally through the brainstem to reach this superficial position. The rat EGL proliferates for 3 weeks, generating more neurons than in any other structure, whereas, in humans, EGL precursors exist for at least 7 weeks and up to 2 years. When an EGL precursor stops proliferating, the cell body sinks below the surface and grows bilateral processes that extend transversely in the molecular layer, and then the soma migrates further down into the internal granule layer (IGL). Cells reach the IGL along specialized Bergmann glia, which serve guidance functions similar to those of the radial glia. However, in this case, cells originate from a secondary proliferative zone that generates neurons exclusively of the granule cell lineage, indicating a restricted neural fate. Clinically, this postnatal population in infants makes cerebellar granule neurogenesis vulnerable to infectious insults of early childhood and an undesirable target of several therapeutic drugs, such as steroids, well known to inhibit cell proliferation. Also, proliferative control of this stem cell population is lost in the common childhood brain tumor, medulloblastoma (see Fig. 33-8).

Developmental Cell Death. During nervous system development, cell elimination is required to coordinate the proportions of interacting neural cells. Developmental cell death is a reproducible,

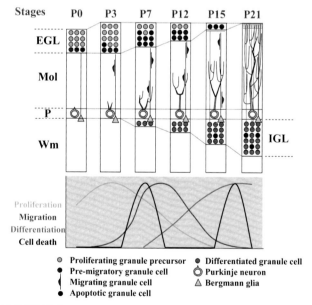

FIGURE 33-8

Neurogenesis, migration, and differentiation of granule cells during cerebellar development. Granule cell precursors proliferate in the external germinal layer. After exiting the cell cycle, they migrate through the molecular layer and past the Purkinje neurons to reach the internal granule layer where they differentiate and make synapses. Neurons that do not migrate properly or that do not establish proper synaptic connections undergo apoptosis. EGL, external germinal cell layer; Mol, molecular layer; P, Purkinje cell layer; IGL, internal granule cell layer; Wm, white matter. (From Sadock BJ, Sadock VA, Ruiz P. *Kaplan & Sadock's Comprehensive Textbook of Psychiatry.* 9th ed. Philadelphia, PA: Lippincott Williams & Wilkins; 2009:48.)

spatially, and temporally restricted death of cells that occurs during the organism's development. Three types of developmental cell death have been described: (1) phylogenetic cell death that removes structures in one species that served evolutionarily earlier ones, such as the tail or the vomeronasal nerves; (2) morphogenetic cell death, which sculpts the fingers from the embryonic paddle and is required to form the optic vesicles, as well as the caudal neural tube; and (3) histogenetic cell death, a widespread process that allows the removal of select cells during development of specific brain regions. Numerous studies have focused on histogenetic cell death, the impact of which varies among brain regions but can affect 20 to 80 percent of neurons in some populations. A significant role for developmental cell death was proposed in the 1980s based on the paradigm of nerve growth factor, suggesting that following neurogenesis, neurons compete for trophic factors. In this model, the survival of differentiating neurons depended absolutely on establishing axonal connections to the correct targets in order to obtain survival-promoting (trophic) growth factors, such as the neurotrophins. Otherwise, they would be eliminated by programmed cell death. This competitive process was thought to ensure the proper matching of new neuronal populations with the size of its target field. Although such interactions are involved in controlling cell degeneration, this model is overly simplistic: Developmental cell death also occurs in neural precursors and immature neurons, before any synaptic contacts are established.

APOPTOSIS.   Apoptotic cell death, or apoptosis, is the primary type of developmental cell degeneration. Apoptosis or "programmed cell death" involves specific molecules that possess enzymatic activities such as cysteine-containing aspartate-specific proteases, also called "caspases," which participate in complex intracellular mechanisms. A large number of signals (both proapoptotic and antiapoptotic) converge to regulate common signaling pathways. Of importance for psychiatry, both developmental as well as pathologic cell death, involves many of the same signaling cascades. A failure to inhibit apoptosis is involved in cancers and autoimmune diseases (multiple sclerosis), whereas excess stimulation of apoptosis is observed in neurodegenerative diseases during both development (Huntington disease, lysosomal diseases, and leukodystrophy) and aging (Alzheimer and Parkinson diseases). Massive apoptotic cell death is also observed during acquired developmental brain injuries such as hypoxia-ischemia, fetal alcohol syndrome, and exposure to ionizing radiations and neurotoxicants. Thus dysregulation of apoptotic cell death during development can lead to severe brain abnormalities, which may only manifest later as mature functional impairments.

Programmed cell death is a necessary process during neurodevelopment, as genetic deletion of caspases in embryonic mice produces enlarged and disorganized brains with marked regional specificity. Programmed cell death occurs at multiple stages of nervous system development, interacting with neurogenesis and differentiation with precise and complex mechanisms. As many neuropathologies also involve dysregulation of apoptosis, future studies hold promise for elucidation and treatment of neurologic diseases.

The Concept of Neural Patterning

Principles of Function.   The morphologic conversion of the nervous system through the embryonic stages, from the neural plate through the neural tube to brain vesicles, is controlled by interactions between extracellular factors and intrinsic genetic programs. In many cases, extracellular signals are soluble growth factors secreted from regional signaling centers, such as the notochord, floor, or roof plates, or surrounding mesenchymal tissues. The precursor's ability to respond (competence) depends on cognate receptor expression, which is determined by patterning genes whose proteins regulate gene transcription. The remarkable new observation is that the subdivisions of the embryonic telencephalon that were initially based on mature differences in morphology, connectivity, and neurochemical profiles are also distinguished embryonically by distinct patterns of gene expression. Classical models had suggested that the cerebral cortex was generated as a reasonably homogeneous structure, unlike most epithelia, with individual functional areas specified relatively late, after cortical layer formation, by the ingrowth of afferent axons from the thalamus. In marked contrast, recent studies indicate that proliferative VZ precursors themselves display regional molecular determinants, a "protomap," which the postmitotic neurons carry with them as they migrate along radial glia to the cortical plate.

Consequently, innervating thalamic afferents may serve to modulate only intrinsic molecular determinants of the protomap. Indeed, in two different genetic mutants, *Gbx2* and *Mash1*, in which thalamocortical innervation is disrupted, expression of cortical patterning genes proceeds unaltered. On the other hand, thalamic afferent growth may be directed by patterning genes and subsequently play roles in modulating regional expression patterns. Thus experience-dependent processes may contribute less to cortical specialization than initially postulated.

The term patterning genes connotes families of proteins that serve primarily to control transcription of other genes, the products of which include other transcription factors or proteins involved in cellular processes, such as proliferation, migration, or differentiation. Characteristically, transcription factor proteins contain two principal domains, one that binds DNA promoter regions of genes and the other that interacts with other proteins, either transcription factors or components of intracellular second messengers. Notably, transcription factors form multimeric protein complexes to control gene activation. Therefore, a single transcription factor will play diverse roles in multiple cell types and processes, according to what other factors are present, the so-called cellular environment. The combinatorial nature of gene promoter regulation leads to a diversity of functional outcomes when a single patterning gene is altered.

Furthermore, because protein interactions depend on protein–protein affinities, there may be complex changes as a single factor's expression level is altered. This process may be a critical mechanism of human variation and disease susceptibility, since polymorphisms in gene promoters, known to be associated with human disease, can alter levels of gene protein products. A transcription factor may associate primarily with one partner at a low concentration but with another at a higher titer. The multimeric nature of regulatory complexes allows a single factor to stimulate one process while simultaneously inhibiting another. During development, a patterning gene may thus promote one event, say the generation of neurons, by stimulating one gene promoter, while simultaneously sequestering another factor from a different promoter whose activity is required for an alternative phenotype, such as glial cell fate. Finally, the factors frequently exhibit cross-regulatory functions, where one factor negatively regulates the expression of another. This activity leads to the establishment of tissue boundaries, allowing the formation of regional subdivisions, such as basal ganglia and cerebral cortex in the forebrain.

Also, to combinatorial interactions, patterning genes exhibit distinct temporal sequences of expression and function, acting hierarchically. Functional hierarchies were established experimentally by using genetic approaches, either deleting a gene (loss of function) or over-/ectopically expressing it (gain of function), and defining developmental consequences. At the most general level, genetic analyses indicate that regionally restricted patterning genes participate in specifying the identity, and therefore function, of cells in which they are expressed. Subdivisions of the brain and cerebral cortex specifically, are identified by regionalized gene expression in the proliferative VZ of the neural tube, leading to subsequent differentiation of distinct types of neurons in each mature (postmitotic) region. Thus the protomap of the embryonic VZ predicts the cortical regions it will generate and may instruct the hierarchical temporal sequence of patterning gene expression. It appears that the different genes underlie multiple stages of brain development, including the following: (1) determining that ectoderm will give rise to the nervous system (as opposed to the skin); (2) defining the dimensional character of a region, such as positional identity in dorsoventral or rostrocaudal axes; (3) specifying cell class, such as neuron or glia; (4) defining when proliferation ceases, and differentiation begins, (5) determining specific cell subtype, such as GABA interneuron, as well as projection pattern; and (6) defining laminar position in the region, such as cerebral cortex. Although investigations are ongoing, studies indicate that these many steps depend on interactions of transcription factors from multiple families. Furthermore, a single transcription factor plays regulatory roles at multiple stages in the developmental life of a cell, yielding complex outcomes, for instance, in genetic loss of function studies and human disease.

Recent advances in molecular biology have led to the identification of another principle of nervous system organization, which, if sustained by further studies, may provide a molecular basis for brain system diseases, such as Parkinson disease and autism. Using molecular techniques to permanently identify cells that had expressed during the development of a specific gene, in this case, the soluble growth factor, Wnt3a, investigators were able to determine where cells originated embryonically and could trace their path of migration along the neuraxis during development. These genetic-fate mapping studies indicate that cells that expressed Wnt3a migrated widely from the dorsal midline into the dorsal regions of the brain and spinal cord, thereby contributing to diverse adult structures in the diencephalon, midbrain, and brainstem, and rostral spinal cord. Of interest, most of these structures were linked into a functional neural network, specifically the auditory system. The observation that a single functional system emerges from a specific group of fated cells would allow for restricted neurologic system–based disorders, such as deficits in dopamine or catecholamine neurons, or for the dysfunction of inter-related brain regions that subserve social cognition and interaction, a core symptom of the ASDs. Other adult system degenerations may also be considered. This new observation may change the way that we consider temporal changes in patterning gene expression of specific brain regions during development.

Finally, patterning gene expression in nervous system subdivisions is not insensitive to environmental factors. On the contrary, the expression is intimately regulated by growth factors released from regional signaling centers. Indeed, although a century of classical experimental embryology described the induction of new tissues between neighboring cell layers morphologically, we have only recently defined molecular identities of soluble protein morphogens and cell response genes underlying development. Signaling molecules from discrete centers establish tissue gradients that provide positional information (dorsal or ventral), impart

cell specification, or control regional growth. Signals include the BMPs, the Wingless-Int proteins (Wnts), Shh, fibroblast growth factors (FGFs), and epidermal growth factors (EGFs), to name a few. These signals set up developmental domains characterized by expression of specific transcription factors, which in turn control further regional gene transcription and developmental processes. The importance of these mechanisms for cerebral cortical development is only now emerging, altering our concepts of the roles of subsequent thalamic innervation and experience-dependent processes. In light of the temporal and combinatorial principles discussed earlier, brain development can be viewed as a complex and evolving interaction of extrinsic and intrinsic information.

Specific Inductive Signals and Patterning Genes in Development

Induction of the CNS begins at the neural plate stage when the notochord, underlying mesenchyme, and surrounding epidermal ectoderm produce signaling molecules that affect the identity of neighboring cells. Specifically, the ectoderm produces BMPs that prevent neural fate determination by promoting and maintaining epidermal differentiation. In other words, neural differentiation is a default state that manifests unless it is inhibited. In turn, neural induction proceeds when inhibitory proteins block BMP's epidermis-inducing activity, such as noggin, follistatin, and chordin, which are secreted by Hensen's node (homologous to the amphibian Spemann organizer), a signaling center at the rostral end of the primitive streak. Once the neural tube closes, the roof plate and floor plate become new signaling centers, organizing dorsal and ventral neural tube, respectively. The same ligand/receptor system is used sequentially for multiple functions during development. BMPs are a case in point since they prevent neural development at the neural plate stage, whereas after neurulation, the factors are produced by the dorsal neural tube itself to induce sensory neuron fates.

The Spinal Cord. The spinal cord is a prime example of the interaction of soluble signaling factors with intrinsic patterning gene expression and function. The synthesis, release, and diffusion of inductive signals from signaling sources produce concentration gradients that impose distinct neural fates in the spinal cord (Fig. 33-9). The notochord and floor plate secrete Shh, which induces motoneurons and interneurons ventrally, whereas the epidermal ectoderm and roof plate release several BMPs that impart neural crest and sensory relay interneuron fates dorsally. Growth factor inductive signals act to initiate discrete regions of transcription factor gene expression. For instance, high concentrations of Shh induce winged-helix transcription factor *Hnf3β* gene in floor plate cells and *Nkx6.1* and *Nkx2.2* in the ventral neural tube, whereas the expression of more dorsal genes, *Pax6, Dbx1/2, Irx3,* and *Pax7,* is repressed. In response to Shh, ventral motoneurons express transcription factor gene *Isl1,* whose protein product is essential for neuron differentiation. Subsequently, ventral interneurons differentiate, expressing *En1* or *Lim1/2* independent of Shh signaling.

In contrast, the release of BMPs by dorsal cord and roof plate induces a distinct cascade of patterning genes to elicit sensory interneuron differentiation. In aggregate, the coordinated actions of Shh and BMPs induce the dorsoventral dimension of the spinal cord. Similarly, other inductive signals determine the rostrocaudal organization of the CNS, such as retinoic acid, an upstream regulator of *hox* patterning genes, anteriorly, and the FGFs posteriorly. The overlapping and unique expression of the many *hox* gene

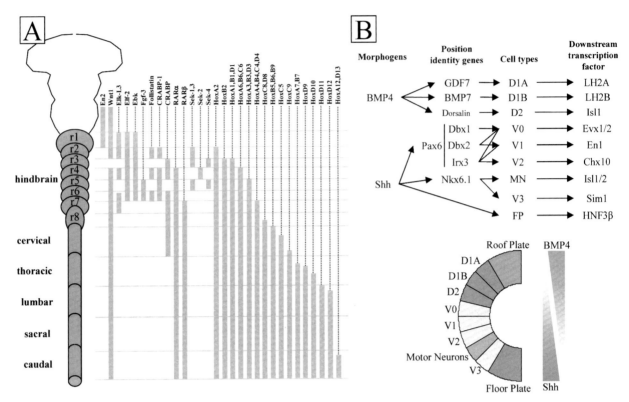

FIGURE 33-9

Patterning genes in the spinal cord. **A:** Diagram illustrating the localization of gene expression in the developing "trunk." Rhombomere boundaries are specified by specific combinations of transcription factors. (Modified from Darnell, 2005.) **B:** Morphogen induction of spinal cord cell fate. Dorsoventral gradients of sonic hedgehog (Shh) and bone morphogenetic protein (BMP) induce expression of several position identity genes. Combinatorial effects of these factors establish progenitor domains and result in the expression of specific downstream molecular markers. D, dorsal neurons; V, ventral neurons. (From Sadock BJ, Sadock VA, Ruiz P. *Kaplan & Sadock's Comprehensive Textbook of Psychiatry*. 9th ed. Philadelphia, PA: Lippincott Williams & Wilkins; 2009:51.)

family members are essential for establishing the segmental pattern in the anterior–posterior axis of the hindbrain and spinal cord, now-classic models well described in previous reviews.

Recent advances in spinal cord transcription factor expression and function reinforce that these factors play roles at multiple developmental cell stages. This is likely due to their participation in diverse protein regulatory complexes: The transcription factors Pax6, Olig2, and Nkx2.2, which define the positional identity of multipotent progenitors early in development, also play crucial roles in controlling the timing of neurogenesis and gliogenesis in the developing ventral spinal cord.

The Cerebral Cortex.   Recent evidence suggests that forebrain development also depends on inductive signals and patterning genes, as observed in more caudal neural structures. In the embryo, the dorsal forebrain structures include the hippocampus medially, the cerebral cortex dorsolaterally, and the entorhinal cortex ventrolaterally, whereas in the basal forebrain, the globus pallidus lies medially and the striatum laterally. Based on gene expression and morphologic criteria, it has been hypothesized that the forebrain is divided into a checkerboard-like grid pattern of domains generated by the intersection of longitudinal columns and transverse segments, perpendicular to the longitudinal axis. The columns and segments (prosomeres) exhibit restricted expression of patterning genes, allowing for unique combinations of factors within each embryonic subdivision. Many of these genes, including *Hnf3β, Emx2, Pax6,* and *Dlx2,* are first expressed even before neurulation in the neural plate. They are then maintained, providing the

"protomap" determinants of the VZ described earlier. As in the spinal cord, initial forebrain gene expression is influenced by a similar array of signaling center soluble factors—Shh, BMP, and retinoic acid. As the telencephalic vesicles form, signaling centers localize to the edges of the cortex. In the dorsal midline, there is the anterior neural ridge, anterior cranial mesenchyme secreting FGF8, the roof plate, and, at the junction of the roof plate with the telencephalic vesicle, the cortical hem (Fig. 33-10). Other factors originate laterally from the dorsal–ventral forebrain junction, as well as from basal forebrain structures themselves.

Do molecular studies identify how different cortical regions interact with thalamic neurons to establish specific functional modalities, such as vision and sensation? Moreover, once regional identity is established, can later developmental events modify it? It has been proposed that initially, there are no functional distinctions in the cortex but that they are induced by the ingrowth of extrinsic thalamic axons, which convey positional and functional specifications, the so-called "protocortex model." However, in contrast, the abundant molecular evidence provided earlier suggests that intrinsic differences are established early in the neuroepithelium by molecular determinants that regulate areal specification, including the targeting of thalamic axons, termed the "protomap" model. Experimental tests indicate that neither model is entirely correct. Although there is early molecular regionalization of the cortex, the initial targeting of thalamic axons to the cortex is independent of these molecular differences. In the rodent, thalamic afferents first target to their usual cortical regions prenatally in the late embryo. However, once thalamic afferents reach the cortex, which occurs

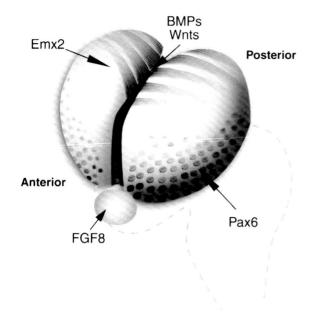

BMPs
Wnts
Emx2
Posterior
Anterior
Pax6
FGF8

FIGURE 33-10

Patterning genes and signaling centers in the developing cerebral cortex. This schematic diagram shows a lateral–superior view of the two cerebral hemispheres of the embryonic mouse, sitting above the midbrain and hindbrain (*broken lines*). The anterior–lateral extent of *Pax6* gene expression is indicated by circles. The posterior–medial domain of *Emx2* expression is indicated by stripes. The genes exhibit continuous gradients of expression that decrease as they extend to opposite poles. The signaling factor fibroblast growth factor 8 (FGF8) is produced by and released from mesenchymal tissue in the anterior neural ridge, which regulates *Pax6* and *Emx2* expression. In the midline, bone morphogenetic proteins (BMPs) and Wingless-Int proteins (Wnts) are secreted from other signaling centers, including the roof plate and the cortical hems. (Courtesy of E. DiCicco-Bloom and K. Forgash.)

several days after birth, interactions of thalamic axon branches with local, regional cues lead to modifications of initial outgrowth and the establishment of connections that conform to areal molecular identities. Furthermore, the developing cortex exhibits a remarkable and unexpected level of flexibility in mediating modality-specific functions: In the ferret, surgical elimination of visual pathway (lateral geniculate nucleus) in postnatal pups results in the transfer of visual signaling to the auditory cortex, which successfully mediates vision! Thus the animal's visual information is effectively processed by their auditory cortex.

The Hippocampus. The hippocampus is a region of significant importance in schizophrenia, depression, autism, and other disorders, and defining mechanisms regulating hippocampal formation may provide clues to the developmental bases of these disorders. In mice, the hippocampus is located in the medial wall of the telencephalic vesicle. Where it joins the roof plate, the future roof of the third ventricle, there is a newly defined signaling center, the cortical hem, which secretes BMPs, Wnts, and FGFs (see Fig. 33-10). Genetic experiments have defined patterning genes localized to the cortical hem and hippocampal primordia, whose deletions result in a variety of morphogenetic defects. In mice lacking Wnt3a, which is expressed in the cortical hem, the hippocampus is either completely missing or significantly reduced, whereas the neighboring cerebral cortex is mainly preserved. A similar phenotype is produced by deleting an intracellular factor downstream to Wnt receptor activation, the *Lef1* gene, suggesting that the Wnt3a-*Lef1* pathway is

required for hippocampal cell specification or proliferation, issues remaining to be defined. When another cortical hem gene, *Lhx5*, is deleted, mice lack both the hem and neighboring choroid plexus, both sources of growth factors. However, in this case, the cortical hem cells may proliferate in excess, and the hippocampal primordia may be present but disorganized, exhibiting abnormalities in cell proliferation, migration, and differentiation. A related abnormality is observed with *Lhx2* mutation. Finally, a sequence of bHLH transcription factors plays roles in hippocampal neurogenesis: Dentate gyrus differentiation is defective in *NeuroD* and *Mash1* mutants. Significantly, expression of all these hippocampal patterning genes is regulated by factors secreted by anterior neural ridge, roof plate, and the cortical hem, including FGF8, Shh, BMPs, and Wnts. Moreover, the basal forebrain region secretes an EGF-related protein, transforming growth factor α (TGF-α), which can stimulate expression of the classical limbic marker protein, lysosomal-associated membrane protein (LAMP). These various signals and genes now serve as candidates for disruption in human diseases of the hippocampus.

The Basal Ganglia. Also, to the motor and cognitive functions, the basal ganglia take on new importance in neocortical function, since they appear to be the embryonic origin of virtually all adult GABA interneurons, reaching the neocortex through tangential migration. Gene expression studies have identified several transcription factors that appear in precursors originating in the ventral forebrain ganglionic eminences, allowing interneurons to be followed as they migrate dorsally into the cortical layers. Conversely, genetic deletion mutants exhibit diminished or absent interneurons, yielding results consistent with other tracing techniques. These transcription factors, including *Pax6, Gsh2,* and *Nkx2.1,* establish boundaries between different precursor zones in the ventral forebrain VZ, through mechanisms involving mutual repression. As a simplified model, the medial ganglionic eminence (MGE) expresses Nkx2.1 primarily and gives rise to most GABA interneurons of the cortex and hippocampus, whereas the lateral ganglionic eminence (LGE) expresses *Gsh2* and generates GABA interneurons of the SVZ and olfactory bulb. The boundary between the ventral and dorsal forebrain then depends on LGE interaction with the dorsal neocortex, which expresses *Pax6*. When *Nkx2.1* is deleted, LGE transcription factor expression spreads ventrally into the MGE territory, and there is a 50 percent reduction in neocortical and striatal GABA interneurons.

In contrast, the deletion of *Gsh2* leads to ventral expansion of the dorsal cortical molecular markers and concomitant decreases in olfactory interneurons. Finally, *Pax6* mutation causes both MGE and LGE to spread laterally and into dorsal cortical areas, yielding increased interneuron migration. The final phenotypic changes are involved, as these factors exhibit unique and overlapping expression and interact to control cell fate.

Neuronal Specification. As indicated for basal ganglia, throughout the nervous system, transcription factors participate in decisions at multiple levels, including determining the generic neural cell, such as a neuron or glial cell, as well as neuron subtypes. *Mash1* can promote a neuronal fate over a glial fate as well as induce the GABA interneuron phenotype. However, another bHLH factor, *Olig1/2,* can promote oligodendrocyte development, whereas it promotes motor neuron differentiation elsewhere, indicating that the variety of factors expressed in a specific cell leads to combinatorial effects and thus diverse outcomes for cell differentiation. The bHLH inhibitory factor, *Id,* is expressed at

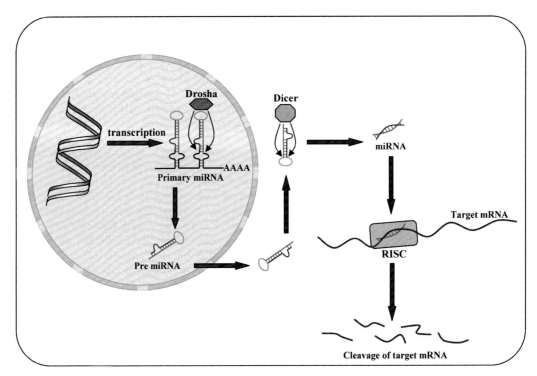

FIGURE 33-11
Processing and function of micro RNA (miRNA). After transcription, the primary miRNA forms a hairpin conformation. This structure allows the enzyme Drosha to cleave the transcript, producing a pre-miRNA that then exits the nucleus through nuclear pores. In the cytoplasm, Dicer cleaves the pre-miRNA stem loop, resulting in the formation of two complementary short RNA molecules. Only one of these molecules is integrated in the RNA-induced silencing complex (RISC) and serves as a guide strand that allows recognition and specificity for target RNA due to its sequence complementarity. After integration into the RISC complex, the miRNA matches with the complementary mRNA strand and induces mRNA duplex degradation by the argonaute protein, the catalytic enzyme of the RISC complex. (From Sadock BJ, Sadock VA, Ruiz P. *Kaplan & Sadock's Comprehensive Textbook of Psychiatry*. 9th ed. Philadelphia, PA: Lippincott Williams & Wilkins; 2009:55.)

the transition from somatosensory to the motor cortex, implying the roles of family members in areal characteristics. In the hippocampus, granule neuron fate is dependent on *NeuroD* and *Math1*, with deficient cell numbers when either one is deleted. The role of specific factors in cortical cell layer determination remains an area of active investigation but likely includes *Tbr1*, *Otx1*, and *Pax6*.

A New Mechanism for Regulating Gene Expression: miRNAs

Over the last decade, a new mechanism for regulating messenger ribonucleic acid (mRNA) has been explored in a simple to complex organisms that involve microRNAs (miRNAs). We now know that miRNAs contribute not only to normal development and brain function but also to brain disorders, such as Parkinson and Alzheimer diseases, tauopathies, and brain cancer. miRNAs can affect the regulation of RNA transcription, alternative splicing, molecular modifications, or RNA translation. miRNAs are 21- to 23-nucleotide-long single-strand RNA molecules. Unlike mRNAs that encode the instructions for ribosome complex translation into proteins, miRNAs are noncoding RNAs that are not translated but are instead processed to form loop structures. miRNAs exhibit a sequence that is partially complementary to one or several other cellular mRNAs. By binding to target mRNA transcripts, the miRNAs serve to interfere with their function, thereby downregulating the expression of these gene products. This gene silencing involves a complex mechanism: The larger miRNA primary transcript is first processed by the Microprocessor, an enzymatic complex consisting of the nuclease Drosha and the double-stranded RNA binding protein

Pasha. The mature miRNA binds to its complementary RNA and then interacts with the endonuclease Dicer that is part of the RNA-induced silencing complex (RISC), resulting in the cleavage of the target mRNA and gene silencing (Fig. 33-11).

Currently, 475 miRNAs have been identified in humans, and their total number is estimated to be between 600 and 3,441. Potentially, up to 30 percent of all genes might be regulated by miRNAs, a whole new layer of molecular complexity. A connection between miRNAs and several brain diseases has already been made. For example, miR-133b, which is expressed explicitly in midbrain dopaminergic neurons, is deficient in midbrain tissue from patients with Parkinson disease. Furthermore, the miRNAs encoding miR-9, miR-124a, miR-125b, miR-128, miR-132, and miR-219 are abundantly represented in the fetal hippocampus, are differentially regulated in the aged brain, and are altered in Alzheimer disease hippocampus. Similar RNA species termed short-interfering RNAs (siRNAs) have been discovered in plants where they prevent the transcription of viral RNA. The mechanisms involved in these effects are closely related to those of miRNA. Thus siRNAs are now being used in both basic and clinical research to downregulate specific cellular gene products, thereby advancing the study of pathways involved in neurodevelopment and providing new selective tools to regulate disease-causing genes or therapeutic molecular targets.

Regulation of Neurodevelopment by Extracellular Factors

The interaction of extracellular factors with intrinsic genetic determinants controlling region-specific neurogenesis includes signals

Table 33-1
Regulation of Neurodevelopment by Extracellular Factors

Extracellular Factors	Proliferation		Migration		Differentiation		Survival	
bFGF	↑	Cortex Cerebellum Hippocampus	—	—	↑	Nigrostriatum Cortex	↑	Nigrostriatum Cerebellum Cortex
IGF-1	↑	Cortex Cerebellum	—	—	↑	Spinal neurons Cerebellum	↑	Cortex Cerebellum
EGF	↑	Cortex Adult SVZ	—	—	↑	Cortex	—	—
TGF-β	↓	Cortex Cerebellum	—	—		—	↓	Cortex Cerebellum
Shh	↑	Cortex Cerebellum	↑	Cerebellum	—	—	—	—
PACAP	↓	Cortex Cerebellum	↓	Cerebellum	↑	Cerebellum	↑	Cerebellum
GABA	↓	Cortex	↑	Cortex	—	—	—	—
Glutamate	↓	Cortex	↑	Cortex Cerebellum	↓ ↑	Pyramidal neurons Granule neurons	↑ ↓	Immature neurons Mature neurons
TNF-α	↓	Neurons	—	—	—	—	↓	Neurons
BDNF	—	—	↑	Cerebellum	↑	Cortex Adult SVZ	↑	Cortex Cerebellum
Wnt	↑	Embryonic stem cells Hippocampus	—	—	↑	Axon guidance Spinal cord	—	—
NT3	↓	Cortical stem cells	↑	Cortex	↑	Cortex	↑	Cortex
LIF/CNTF/gp130	↑	Cortex Embryonic Stem cells	—	—	↑	Astrocytes	—	—

From Sadock BJ, Sadock VA, Ruiz P. *Kaplan & Sadock's Comprehensive Textbook of Psychiatry*. 9th ed. Philadelphia, PA: Lippincott Williams & Wilkins;2009:55.

that regulate cell proliferation, migration, differentiation, and survival (Table 33-1). Patterning genes control the expression of growth factor receptors and the molecular machinery of the cell division cycle. Extracellular factors are known to stimulate or inhibit the proliferation of VZ precursors and originate from the cells themselves, termed autocrine, neighboring cells/tissues, or paracrine, or from the general circulation, as in endocrine, all sources known to affect proliferation in the prenatal and postnatal developing brain. Although defined initially in cell culture, several mitogenic growth factors are now well-characterized in vivo, including those stimulating proliferation, such as basic FGF (bFGF), EGF, IGF-I, Shh, and signals inhibiting cell division, such as pituitary adenylate-cyclase–activating polypeptide (PACAP), GABA and glutamate, and members of the TGF-β superfamily. However, in addition to stimulating reentry of cells into the cell cycle, termed a mitogenic effect, extracellular signals also enhance proliferation by promoting survival of the mitotic population, a trophic action. Stimulation of both pathways is necessary to produce maximal cell numbers. These mitogenic and trophic mechanisms during development parallel those identified in carcinogenesis, reflecting roles of c-myc and bcl-2, respectively. Several of the neurotrophins, especially BDNF and neurotrophin-3 (NT3), promote the survival of mitotic precursors as well as the newly generated progeny.

The developmental significance of extracellular mitogens is demonstrated by the expression of the factors and their receptors in regions of neurogenesis. It is also demonstrated by the profound and permanent consequences of altering their activities during development. For example, by administering growth factors to developing embryos or pups, one can induce changes in proliferation in prenatal cortical VZ, postnatal cerebellar EGL, and hippocampal dentate gyrus that produce lifelong modifications in brain region population size and cell composition. Such changes may be relevant to structural differences observed in neuropsychiatric disorders, such as depression, schizophrenia, and autism. Precisely, in the cerebral cortex VZ of the embryonic rat, proliferation is controlled by promitogenic bFGF and antimitogenic PACAP, which are expressed as autocrine/paracrine signals. Positive and negative effects were shown in living embryos in utero by performing intracerebroventricular (ICV) injections of the factors or antagonists. ICV injection of bFGF produced a larger adult cortex composed of 87 percent more neurons, which employed glutamate, thus increasing the ratio of excitatory pyramidal neurons to GABA inhibitory neurons, which were unchanged.

Conversely, embryonic PACAP injection inhibited the proliferation of cortical precursors by 26 percent, reducing the number of labeled layer 5/6 neurons in the cortical plate 5 days later. A similar reduction was accomplished by genetically deleting promitogenic bFGF or leukocyte inhibitory factor (LIF)/ciliary neurotrophic factor (CNTF)/gp130 signaling, diminishing cortical size. Furthermore, the effects of mitogenic signals depended critically on the stage-specific program of regional development, since bFGF injection at later ages when gliogenesis predominates affected glial numbers selectively. Thus developmental dysregulation of mitogenic pathways due to genetic or environmental factors (hypoxia, maternal/fetal infection, or drug or toxicant exposure) will likely produce subtle changes in the size and composition of the developing cortex. Other signals likely to play proliferative roles include Wnt's, TGF-α, IGF-I, and BMPs. Although interactions between intrinsic cortical programs and extrinsic factors remain to be defined, a remarkable new study of mouse embryonic stem cells suggests that embryonic mammalian forebrain specification may be a developmentally ancestral intrinsic program that emerges in the absence of extrinsic signals. In specific culture conditions that block endogenous Shh signaling, mouse embryonic stem cells can sequentially generate the various types of neurons that display the most salient features of genuine cortical pyramidal neurons. When grafted into the cerebral cortex, these cells differentiate into neurons that project to select cortical (visual and limbic regions) and subcortical targets, corresponding to a wide range of pyramidal layer neurons. Insight into precision control of neuronal differentiation will open new avenues to perform neuronal grafts in humans for cellular replacement in various acquired and neurodegenerative diseases.

Similar to the cerebral cortex, later generated populations of granule neurons, such as in the cerebellum and hippocampal dentate gyrus, are also sensitive to growth factor manipulation, which is especially relevant to therapies administered intravenously to premature and newborn infants in the neonatal nursery. Like in humans, cerebellar granule neurons are produced postnatally in rats, but for only 3 weeks, whereas in both species, dentate gyrus neurons are produced throughout life. Remarkably, a single peripheral injection of bFGF into newborn rat pups rapidly crossed into the cerebrospinal fluid (CSF) and stimulated proliferation in the cerebellar EGL by 30 percent as well as hippocampal dentate gyrus by twofold by 8 hours, consistent with an endocrine mechanism of action. The consequence of mitogenic stimulation in the cerebellum was a 33 percent increase in the number of internal granule layer neurons and a 22 percent larger cerebellum. In the hippocampus, mitotic stimulation elicited by a single bFGF injection increased the absolute number of dentate gyrus granule neurons by 33 percent at 3 weeks, defined stereologically, producing a 25 percent larger hippocampus containing more neurons and astrocytes, a change that persisted lifelong. Conversely, genetic deletion of bFGF resulted in smaller cerebellum and hippocampus at birth and throughout life, indicating that levels of the growth factor were critical for normal brain region formation. Other proliferative signals regulating cerebellar granule neurogenesis include Shh and PACAP, the disruption of which contributes to human medulloblastoma, whereas in the hippocampus, the Wnt family may be involved.

Clinical Implications.   There are several clinical implications of these surprising growth factor effects observed in newborns. First, we may need to investigate possible neurogenetic effects of therapeutic agents we administer in the newborn nursery for long-term consequences. Second, because bFGF is as effective in stimulating adult neurogenesis (see subsequent text) as in newborns because of specific transport across the mature BBB, there is the possibility that other protein growth factors are also preferentially transported into the brain and alter ongoing neurogenesis. Indeed, in rats, IGF-I also stimulates mature hippocampal dentate gyrus neurogenesis. Third, other therapeutics cross the BBB efficiently due to their lipid solubility, such as steroids, which inhibit neurogenesis across the age spectrum. Steroids are frequently used perinatally to promote lung maturation and treat infections and trauma, but effects on human brain formation have not been examined. Fourth, it is well known that neurologic development may be delayed in children who experience a severe systemic illness that is associated with numerous inflammatory cytokines. One may wonder to what degree this reflects an interference with neurogenesis and concomitant processes, potentially producing long-term differences in cognitive and motor functional development. Finally, maternal infection during pregnancy is a known risk factor for schizophrenia, and cytokines that cross the placental barrier may directly affect fetal brain cell proliferation and differentiation as well as cell migration, target selection, and synapse maturation, as shown in animal models, eventually leading to multiple brain and behavioral abnormalities in the adult offspring.

Cell Migration

Throughout the nervous system, newly generated neurons naturally migrate away from proliferative zones to achieve final destinations. If this process is disrupted, abnormal cell localization and function result. In humans, more than 25 syndromes with disturbed neuronal migration have been described. As noted earlier, neurons migrate in both radial and tangential fashions during development and may establish cell layers that are inside-to-outside, or the reverse, according to region. In the developing cerebral cortex, the most well-characterized mechanism is radial migration from underlying VZ to appropriate cortical layers in an inside-to-outside fashion. Also, however, the inhibitory GABA interneurons that are generated in ventrally located medial ganglionic eminences reach the cortex through tangential migration in the intermediate zone along with axonal processes or other neurons. The neurons in the developing cerebellum also exhibit both radial and tangential migration. Purkinje cells leave the fourth ventricle VZ and exhibit radial migration, whereas other precursors from the rhombic lip migrate tangentially to cover the cerebellar surface, establishing the EGL, a secondary proliferative zone. From EGL, newly generated granule cells migrate radially inward to create the internal granule cell layer. Finally, granule interneurons of the olfactory bulb exhibit a different kind of migration, originating in the SVZ of the lateral ventricles overlying the striatum. These neuroblasts divide and migrate simultaneously in the rostral migratory stream in transit to the bulb, on a path comprising chains of cells that support forward movements. The most commonly recognized disorders of human neuronal migration are the extensive lissencephalies (see subsequent text), although incomplete migration of more restricted neuron aggregates (heterotopias) frequently underlies focal seizure disorders.

Animal models have defined molecular pathways involved in neuronal migration. Cell movement requires signals to start and stop migration, adhesion molecules to guide migration, and functional cytoskeleton to mediate cell translocation. The best-characterized mouse model of aberrant neuronal migration is reeler, a spontaneous mutant in which cortical neuron laminar position is inverted, being generated in outside-to-inside fashion. Reelin is a large, secreted extracellular glycoprotein produced embryonically by the earliest neurons in the cortical preplate, Cajal–Retzius cells, and hippocampus and cerebellum. Molecular and genetic analysis has established a signaling sequence in reelin activity that includes at least two receptors, the very low-density lipoprotein receptor (VLDLR) and the apoprotein E receptor 2 (ApoER2), and the intracellular adapter protein, disabled 1 (Dab1), initially identified in the scrambler mutant mouse, a reelin phenocopy. Current thoughts consider the reelin system as one mediator of radial glia-guided neuron migration, although its specific functions in starting or stopping migration remain controversial. The roles of the VLDL and

ApoE2 receptors are intriguing for their possible contributions to Alzheimer disease risk. Recent studies have found human reelin gene (*RELN*) mutations associated with autosomal recessive lissencephaly with cerebellar hypoplasia, exhibiting a markedly thickened cortex with pachygyria, abnormal hippocampal formations, and severe cerebellar hypoplasia with absent folia. Additional studies suggest that reelin polymorphisms may contribute to ASD risk as well.

Concerning cytoskeletal proteins, studies of the filamentous fungus *Aspergillus nidulans* surprisingly provided insight into the molecular machinery underlying the human migration disorder, Miller–Dieker syndrome, lissencephaly associated with abnormal chromosome 17q13.3. Lissencephaly is a diverse disorder characterized by a smooth cortical surface lacking in gyri and sulci, with markedly reduced brain surface area. The absence of convolutions results from a migration defect: the majority of neurons fail to reach their final destinations. In classical lissencephaly (type I), the cerebral cortex is thick and usually four-layered, whereas, in cobblestone lissencephaly (type II), the cortex is chaotically organized with a partly smooth and partly pebbled surface and deficient lamination. The most severely affected parts of the brain are the cerebral cortex and hippocampus, with the cerebellum less affected. In fungus, the gene *NudF* was found to be essential for intracellular nuclear distribution, a translocation process also involved in mammalian cell migration. The human homolog of *NudF* is LIS-1 or PAFAH1B1, a mutation of which accounts for up to 60 percent of lissencephaly cases of type I pathology. The LIS-1 gene product interacts with microtubules and related motor components dynein and dynactin as well as doublecortin (DCX), which may regulate microtubule stability. Mutations in the DCX gene result in X-linked lissencephaly in males and bands of heterotopic neurons in white matter in females, appearing as a "double cortex" on imaging studies, producing severe mental retardation and epilepsy. Other migratory defects occur when proteins associated with the actin cytoskeleton are affected, such as a mutation in the filamin 1 gene responsible for periventricular nodular heterotopias in humans and mutations of a regulatory phosphokinase enzyme, the CDK5/p35 complex.

Cell migration also depends on molecules mediating cellular interactions, which provide cell adhesion to establish neuron–neuron and neuron–glia relationships or induce attraction or repulsion. Astrotactin is a major glial protein involved in neuronal migration on radial glial processes, whereas neuregulins and their receptors, ErbB2-4, play roles in neuronal–glial migratory interactions. Recent genetic studies associate neuregulin polymorphisms with schizophrenia, suggesting that this developmental disease may depend on altered oligodendrocyte numbers and activities and synaptic functions. Furthermore, some work suggests that early appearing neurotransmitters themselves, GABA and glutamate, and platelet-derived growth factor (PDGF) regulate migration speed. In contrast to radial migration from cortical VZ, GABA interneurons generated in ganglionic eminences employ different mechanisms to leave the ventral forebrain and migrate dorsally into the cerebral cortex. Several signaling systems have been identified, including the Slit protein and Robo receptor, the semaphorins and their neuropilin receptors, and hepatocyte growth factor and its c-Met receptor, all of which appear to repel GABA interneurons from the basal forebrain, promoting tangential migration into the cortex. Significantly, the c-Met receptor has recently been associated with ASDs, suggesting that altered GABA interneuron migration into the cortex and deficits in inhibitory signaling may contribute to the phenotype, including seizures and abnormal cognitive

processing. Finally, several human forms of congenital muscular dystrophy with severe brain and eye migration defects result from gene mutations in enzymes that transfer mannose sugars to serine/threonine -OH groups in glycoproteins, thereby interrupting interactions with several extracellular matrix molecules and producing type II cobblestone lissencephalies.

Differentiation and Neuronal Process Outgrowth

After newly produced neurons and glial cells reach their final destinations, they differentiate into mature cells. For neurons, this involves outgrowth of dendrites and extension of axonal processes, the formation of synapses, and the production of neurotransmitter systems, including receptors and selective reuptake sites. Most axons will become insulated by myelin sheaths produced by oligodendroglial cells. Many of these events occur with a peak period from 5 months of gestation onward. During the first several years of life, many neuronal systems exhibit exuberant process growth and branching, which is later decreased by selective "pruning" of axons and synapses, dependent on experience. In contrast, myelination continues for several years after birth and into adulthood.

Although there is tremendous synapse plasticity in the adult brain, a fundamental feature of the nervous system is the point-to-point or topographic mapping of one neuron population to another. During development, neurons extend axons to innervate diverse distant targets, such as the cortex and spinal cord. The structure that recognizes and responds to cues in the environment is the growth cone, located at the axon tip. The axonal process is structurally supported by microtubules that are regulated by numerous microtubule-associated proteins (MAPs), whereas the terminal growth cone exhibits a transition to actin-containing microfilaments. The growth cone has rod-like extensions called filopodia that bear receptors for specific guidance cues present on cell surfaces and in the extracellular matrix. Interactions between filopodial receptors and environmental cues cause growth cones to move forward, turn, or retract. Recent studies have identified the actin-modulating proteins and kinases involved in rapid growth cone movements, such as LIMK kinase that causes the language phenotype associated with Williams syndrome. Perhaps surprising is that activation of growth cone receptors leads to local mRNA translation to produce synaptic proteins, whereas traditional concepts assumed that all proteins were transported to axon terminals from distant neuronal cell somas. The region-specific expression of extracellular guidance molecules, such as cadherins, regulated by patterning genes *Pax6* and *Emx2*, results in the highly directed outgrowth of axons, termed axonal pathfinding. These molecules affect the direction, speed, and fasciculation of axons, acting through either positive or negative regulation. Guidance molecules may be soluble extracellular factors or may be bound to extracellular matrix or cell membranes. In the latter class of signal is the newly discovered family of transmembrane proteins, the ephrins. Ephrins act via the largest known family of tyrosine kinase receptors in the brain, Eph receptors, and play a significant role in topographic mapping between neuron populations and their targets. Ephrins frequently serve as chemorepellent cues, negatively regulating growth by preventing developing axons from entering incorrect target fields. For example, the optic tectum expresses ephrins A2 and A5 in a gradient that decreases along the posterior to the anterior axis, whereas innervating retinal ganglion cells express a gradient of Eph receptors. Ganglion cell axons from the posterior retina, which possess high Eph A3 receptor levels, will preferentially innervate the anterior tectum because the low-level ephrin expression does not activate the Eph kinase that causes growth cone retraction. In the category of soluble molecules, netrins serve primarily as chemoattractant proteins secreted, for instance, by the spinal cord floor plate to stimulate spinothalamic sensory interneurons to grow into the anterior commissure. In contrast, Slit is a secreted chemorepulsive factor that, through its roundabout (Robo) receptor, regulates midline crossing and axonal fasciculation and pathfinding.

The Neurodevelopmental Basis of Psychiatric Disease

An increasing number of neuropsychiatric conditions are considered to originate during brain development, including schizophrenia, depression, autism, and ADHD. Defining when a condition begins helps direct attention to underlying pathogenic mechanisms. The term neurodevelopmental suggests that the brain is abnormally formed from the very beginning due to disruption of fundamental processes, in contrast to a normally formed brain that is injured secondarily or that undergoes degenerative changes. However, the value of the term neurodevelopmental needs to be reconsidered because of different use by clinicians and pathologists. Also, given that the same molecular signals function in both development and maturity, altering an early ontogenetic process by changes in growth factor signaling, for instance, probably means that other adult functions exhibit ongoing dysregulation as well. For example, clinical researchers of schizophrenia consider the disorder neurodevelopmental because at the time of onset and diagnosis, the prefrontal cortex and hippocampus are smaller and ventricles enlarged already at adolescent presentation.

In contrast, the neuropathologist uses the term neurodevelopmental for specific morphologic changes in neurons. If a brain region exhibits a normal cytoarchitecture, but with neurons of smaller than the normal diameter, reminiscent of "immature" stages, then this may be considered an arrest of development. However, if the same cellular changes are accompanied by inflammatory signs, such as gliosis and white blood cell infiltrate, then this is termed neurodegeneration. These morphologic and cellular changes may no longer be adequate to distinguish disorders that originate from development versus adulthood, especially given the roles of glial cells, including astrocytes, oligodendrocytes, and microglia, as sources of neurotrophic support during both periods of life. Thus abnormalities in glial cells may occur in both epochs to promote disease or act as mechanisms of repair. Many neurodegenerative processes, such as in Alzheimer and Parkinson diseases, are associated with microglial cells.

On the other hand, neuronal dysfunction in adulthood, such as cell shrinkage, may occur without inflammatory changes. In animal models, interruption of BDNF neurotrophic signaling in the adult brain results in neuron and dendrite atrophy in the cerebral cortex without eliciting glial cell proliferation. Thus finding small neurons without gliosis in the brains of patients with schizophrenia or autism does not necessarily mean that the condition is only or primarily developmental in origin. In turn, several etiologic assumptions about clinical brain conditions may require reexamination.

Because the same processes that mediate development, including neurogenesis, gliogenesis, axonal growth and retraction, synaptogenesis, and cell death, also function during adulthood, a new synthesis has been proposed. All of these processes, although perhaps in more subtle forms, contribute to adaptive and pathologic processes. Successful aging of the nervous system may require precise regulation of these processes, allowing the brain to adapt appropriately and counteract the numerous intrinsic and extrinsic events that could potentially lead to neuropathology. For example, adult neurogenesis and synaptic plasticity are necessary to maintain neuronal circuitry and ensure proper cognitive functions. Programmed cell death is crucial to prevent tumorigenesis that can occur as cells accumulate mutations throughout life. Thus dysregulation of these ontogenetic processes in adulthood will lead to disruption of brain homeostasis, expressing itself as various neuropsychiatric diseases.

Schizophrenia.   The neurodevelopmental hypothesis of schizophrenia postulates that etiologic and pathogenetic factors occurring before the formal onset of the illness, that is, during gestation, disrupt the course of normal development. These subtle early alterations in specific neurons, glia, and circuits confer vulnerability to other later developmental factors, ultimately leading to malfunctions. Schizophrenia is a multifactorial disorder, including both genetic and environmental factors. Clinical studies using risk assessment have identified some relevant factors, including prenatal and birth complications (hypoxia, infection, or substance and toxicant exposure), family history, body dysmorphia, especially structures of neural crest origin, and presence of mild premorbid deficits in social, motor, and cognitive functions. These risk factors may affect ongoing developmental processes such as experience-dependent axonal and dendritic production, programmed cell death, myelination, and synaptic pruning. An intriguing animal model using human influenza-induced pneumonia of pregnant mice shows that the inflammatory cytokine response produced by the mother may directly affect the offspring's brain development, with no evidence of the virus in the fetus or placenta.

Neuroimaging and pathology studies identify structural abnormalities at disease presentation, including smaller prefrontal cortex and hippocampus and enlarged ventricles, suggesting abnormal development. More severely affected patients exhibit a more significant number of affected regions with more considerable changes. In some cases, ventricular enlargement and cortical gray matter atrophy increase with time. These ongoing progressive changes should lead us to reconsider the potential role of active degeneration in schizophrenia, whether due to the disease or its consequences, such as stress or drug treatment. However, classic signs of neurodegeneration with inflammatory cells are not present.

Structural neuroimaging strongly supports the conclusion that the hippocampus in schizophrenia is significantly smaller, perhaps by 5 percent. In turn, brain morphology has been used to assess the etiologic contributions of genetic and environmental factors. Comparisons of concordance for schizophrenia in monozygotic and dizygotic twins support roles for both factors. Among monozygotic twins, only 40 to 50 percent of both twins have the illness, indicating that the genetic constitution alone does not ensure disease and suggesting that the embryonic environment also contributes. Neuroimaging, pharmacologic, and pathologic studies suggest that some genetic factors allow for susceptibility and that secondary insults, such as birth trauma or perinatal viral infection, provide the other. This model is consistent with imaging studies showing small hippocampus in both affected and unaffected monozygotic twins.

Moreover, healthy, genetically at-risk individuals show hippocampal volumes (smaller) more similar to affected probands than normal controls. Thus hippocampal volume reduction is not pathognomonic of schizophrenia but instead may represent a biologic marker of genetic susceptibility. It is not difficult to envision roles for altered developmental regulators in producing a smaller hippocampus, which in turn limits functional capacity. A smaller hippocampus may result from subtle differences in the levels of transcription factors, such as *NeuroD, Math1,* or *Lhx,* signaling by Wnt3a and downstream mediator *Lef1,* or proliferative control mediated by bFGF, the family members of which exhibit altered expression levels in schizophrenia brain samples. Such genetic limitations may only become manifest following another developmental challenge, such as gestational infection, stressors, or toxicant exposure.

A regional locus of schizophrenia pathology remains uncertain but may include the hippocampus, entorhinal cortex, multimodal association cortex, limbic system, amygdala, cingulate cortex, thalamus, and medial temporal lobe. Despite size reductions in specific regions, attempts to define changes in cell numbers have been unrewarding since most studies do not quantify the entire cell population but assess only regional cell density. Without assessing a region's total volume, cell density measures alone are limited in revealing population size. Most studies have found no changes in cell density in diverse regions. A single study successfully examining total cell number in the hippocampus found normal neuron density and a 5 percent volume reduction on the left and 2 percent on the right, yielding no significant change in total cell number.

In contrast to total neuron numbers, using neuronal cell-type–specific markers, many studies have found a decreased density of nonpyramidal GABA interneurons in the cortex and hippocampus. In particular, parvalbumin-expressing interneurons are reduced, whereas calretinin-containing cells are normal, suggesting a deficiency of an interneuron subtype. These morphometric data are supported by molecular evidence for decreased GABA neurons, including reduced mRNA and protein levels of the GABA-synthesizing enzyme, GAD67, in the cortex and hippocampus. Another product of the adult GABA-secreting neurons, reelin, which initially appears in Cajal–Retzius cells in the embryonic brain, is reduced 30 to 50 percent in schizophrenia and bipolar disorder with psychotic symptoms. Such a deficiency, leading to diminished GABA signaling, may underlie a potential compensatory increase in $GABA_A$ receptor binding detected in hippocampal CA 2 to 4 fields by both pyramidal and nonpyramidal neurons, apparently selective since benzodiazepine binding is unchanged. More generally, deficiency in a subpopulation of GABA interneurons raises intriguing new possibilities for schizophrenia etiology. As indicated in the preceding gene patterning section, different subpopulations of forebrain GABA interneurons originate from distinct precursors located in the embryonic basal forebrain. Thus cortical and hippocampal GABA interneurons may derive primarily from the MGE under control of the patterning gene *Nkx2.1,* whereas SVZ and olfactory neurons derive from *Gsh2*-expressing LGE precursors.

Furthermore, the timing and sequence of GABA interneuron generation may depend on a regulatory network, including *Mash1, Dlx1/2,* and *Dlx5/6,* all gene candidates for schizophrenia risk. Indeed, *DLX1* gene expression is reduced in the thalamus of patients with psychosis. Thus abnormal regulation of these factors may diminish selectively GABA interneuron formation, which in turn may represent a genetically determined vulnerability and may contribute to diminished regional brain size or function.

The most compelling neuropathologic evidence for a developmental basis is the finding of aberrantly localized or clustered neurons, especially in lamina II of the entorhinal cortex and in the white matter underlying prefrontal cortex and temporal and parahippocampal regions. These abnormalities represent alterations of developmental neuronal migration, survival, and connectivity. Also, in the hippocampus and neocortex, pyramidal neurons appear smaller in many studies, exhibiting fewer dendritic arborizations and spines with reduced neuropil, findings that are associated with reductions in neuronal molecules, including MAP2, spinophilin, synaptophysin, and SNAP25. Although the genes associated with

schizophrenia are reviewed extensively in other chapters, worth mentioning here is a particularly intriguing candidate gene, *DISC1,* whose protein has roles during development, including regulating cell migration, neurite outgrowth, and neuronal maturation as well as in the adult brain, where it modulates cytoskeletal function, neurotransmission, and synaptic plasticity. DISC1 protein interacts with many other proteins intimately involved in neuronal cell migration and forms a protein complex with Lis1 and NudEL that is downstream of reelin signaling.

Autism Spectrum Disorders. Another condition that is neurodevelopmental in origin is ASDs, a complex and heterogeneous group of disorders characterized by abnormalities in social interaction and communication and the presence of restricted or repetitive interests and activities. In the last edition of DSM (DSM-IV), the ASDs included classic autistic disorder, Asperger syndrome, and pervasive developmental disorder not otherwise specified. These three disorders were grouped due to their common occurrence in families, indicating related genetic factors and shared signs and symptoms. Recent conceptualizations of ASDs propose that there are multiple "autisms" differing in underlying pathogenetic mechanisms and manifestations. The different core symptom domains (or other endophenotypes) will likely be more heritable than the syndromic diagnosis, which was constructed to be inclusive. The broad diversity of ASD signs and symptoms reflects the multiplicity of abnormalities observed in pathologic and functional studies and includes both forebrain and hindbrain regions. Forebrain neurons in the cerebral cortex and limbic system play critical roles in social interaction, communication, and learning and memory. For example, the amygdala, which connects to prefrontal and temporal cortices and fusiform gyrus, plays a prominent role in social and emotional cognition. In ASDs, the amygdala and fusiform gyrus demonstrate abnormal activation during facial recognition and emotional attribution tasks. Some investigators hypothesize that ASDs reflect dysfunctions in specific neural networks, such as the social network.

On the other hand, neurophysiologic tests of evoked cortical potentials and oculomotor responses indicate a standard perception of primary sensory information but disturbed higher cognitive processing. The functional impairments in higher-order cognitive processing and neocortical circuitry suggest a developmental disorder involving synaptic organization, a mechanism that may be uniformly present throughout the brain, a model in distinct contrast to abnormalities of specific neural networks. The earlier reference to the expression of Wnt3a in cells that migrated widely during development and appear in auditory systems is one example of how developmental changes may affect single functional networks. In contrast, changes in common and widely expressed synaptic molecules, such as the neuroligins, would represent the other mechanism.

The most important recent discovery in ASD pathogenesis has been the widely reported and replicated brain growth phenotype: The brain starts with, most likely, average size at birth increases in volume at an accelerated rate by the end of the first year compared to the typically developing child, and this process continues from ages 2 to 4 years. These data derive from both neuroimaging studies as well as measures of head circumference performed by multiple labs. It is not known whether this reflects an acceleration of normal developmental processes or a disease-specific aberration in postnatal development, including changes in cell numbers, neuronal processes, synapse formation, and modifications, or glial cell dysfunction, to name a few. The most prominent differences are observed in the frontal and parietal cortex, cerebellar hemispheres, as well as the amygdala. These findings are also consistent with recent reports of macrocephaly in up to ~20 percent of ASD cases in brain and DNA banks. These findings raise many questions to be addressed by developmental neuroscientists.

Functional neuroimaging studies indicate broad forebrain but also cerebellar dysfunctions in ASD, and classical pathologic studies have suggested abnormalities restricted to limbic and cerebellar structures. However, classical studies were hampered by small sample sizes, poor control for comorbidities such as epilepsy and mental retardation that affect neuroanatomy, and the use of tissue cell density measures as opposed to unbiased stereologic methods to estimate regional neuron numbers. Although previous studies described increased densities of small neurons in interconnecting limbic nuclei, including CA fields, septum, mammillary bodies, and amygdala, these results have not been replicated by other laboratories. In contrast, the most consistent neuropathology has been observed in the cerebellum (21 of 29 brains), showing reductions in the number of Purkinje neurons without signs of acquired postnatal lesions, such as gliosis, empty baskets, and retrograde loss of afferent inferior olive neurons, suggesting prenatal origins.

A more recent study identifies widespread and nonuniform abnormalities, suggesting dysregulation of many processes, including neuron proliferation, migration, survival, organization, and programmed cell death. Four of six brains were macrocephalic, consistent with an increased size defined by numerous pathology and neuroimaging studies. In the cerebral cortex, there was thickened or diminished gray matter, disorganized laminar patterns, misoriented pyramidal neurons, ectopic neurons in both superficial and deep white matter, and increased or decreased neuron densities. This evidence of abnormal cortical neurogenesis and migration accords well with the deficits in cognitive functions. In the brainstem, neuronal disorganization appeared as discontinuous and malpositioned neurons in olivary and dentate nuclei, ectopic neurons in medulla and cerebellar peduncles, and aberrant fiber tracts. There were widespread patchy or diffuse decreases of Purkinje neurons, sometimes associated with increased Bergmann glia, or ectopic Purkinje neurons in the molecular layer. Hippocampal neuronal atrophy was not observed, and quantitative stereology found no consistent change in neuron density or number. Moreover, a single recent neuropathologic study using multiple immunologic indices has reported increased levels of immune cytokines in the CSF of patients and brain tissues as well as astrocytes expressing high levels of glial fibrillary acidic protein in the frontal and cingulated cortex, white matter, and cerebellum, all suggesting potential immune activation without evidence of an inflammatory process. We await confirmation of these critical findings.

Although seemingly incompatible, these various data support a model of developmental abnormalities occurring at different times, altering regions according to specific schedules of neurogenesis and differentiation. It is notable that a similar range of abnormalities was found in classical studies but was excluded since these abnormalities did not occur in every brain examined. Moreover, in 15 children exposed to the teratogen thalidomide during days 20 to 24 of gestation, when cranial and Purkinje neurogenesis occurs in the brainstem, four cases exhibited autism. Based on these data, autism is associated with insults at 3 weeks for thalidomide, 12 weeks when inferior olivary neurons are migrating, and ~30 weeks when olivary axons make synapses with Purkinje cells. These diverse abnormalities in cell production, survival, migration, organization, and differentiation in both the hindbrain and forebrain indicate disturbed brain development over a range of stages. Recent genetic studies have defined two genetic polymorphisms associated reproducibly with ASD in several datasets, both of which influence brain developmental processes. The first is *ENGRAILED-2*, the cerebellar patterning gene whose dysregulation causes deficits in Purkinje and granule neurons in animal models and acts to control proliferation and differentiation. The second is the hepatocyte growth factor receptor *cMET*, whose function affects tangential migration of GABA interneurons from the ventral forebrain ganglionic eminences, potentially leading to imbalances of excitatory and inhibitory neurotransmission.

Furthermore, although the cellular derangements may be directly responsible for the core symptoms of autism, there is an alternative hypothesis: Disturbed regulation of developmental processes produces an as-yet-unidentified biochemical, cellular lesion that may be associated with autism. This proposal is supported by the currently known genetic causes of autism that account for 10 percent of cases, including tuberous sclerosis, neurofibromatosis, Smith–Lemli–Opitz syndrome, Rett syndrome, and fragile X mental retardation. These genetic etiologies interfere with cell proliferation control, cholesterol biosynthesis and Shh function, and synaptic and dendrite protein translation and function, fundamental processes in the sequence of development. An intriguing potential link in these monogenetic causes of autism symptoms is their participation in protein synthesis in the synapse, mainly as regulated via the PI3K/Akt signaling pathway and the mammalian target of rapamycin (mTOR) complex, an area of active research.

The Remarkable Discovery of Adult Neurogenesis

In the last decade, there has been a fundamental shift in paradigm regarding the limits of neurogenesis in the brain, with important implications for neural plasticity, mechanisms of disease etiology and therapy, and possibilities of repair. Until recently, it has generally been maintained that we do not produce new neurons in the brain after birth (or soon after that, considering cerebellar EGL); thus, brain plasticity and repair depend on modifications of a numerically static neural network. We now have strong evidence to the contrary: new neurons are generated throughout life in certain regions, well documented across the phylogenetic tree, including birds, rodents, primates, and humans. As an area of intense interest and investigation, we may expect rapid progress over the next two decades, likely altering models described herein.

The term neurogenesis has been used inconsistently in different contexts, indicating sequential production of neural elements during development, first neurons then glial cells, but frequently connoting only neuron generation in the adult brain, in contrast to gliogenesis. For this discussion, we use the first, more general meaning, and distinguish cell types as needed. The first evidence of mammalian neurogenesis in the adult hippocampus was reported in the 1960s in which ^{3}H-thymidine-labeled neurons were documented. As a standard marker for cell production, these studies used nuclear incorporation of ^{3}H-thymidine into newly synthesized DNA during chromosome replication, which occurs before cells undergo division. After a delay, cells divide, producing two ^{3}H-thymidine-labeled progeny. Cell proliferation is defined as an absolute increase in cell number, which occurs only if cell production is not balanced by cell death. Because there is currently little evidence for a progressive increase in brain size with age, except perhaps for rodent hippocampus, most neurogenesis in the adult brain is compensated for by cell loss. More recent studies of neurogenesis employ the more convenient thymidine analog BrdU, which can be injected into living animals and then detected by immuno-histochemistry.

During embryonic development, neurons are produced from almost all regions of the ventricular neuroepithelium. Neurogenesis in the adult, however, is mostly restricted to two regions: the SVZ lining the lateral ventricles and a narrow proliferative zone underlying the dentate gyrus granule layer (subgranular zone) in the hippocampus. In mice, rodents, and monkeys, newly produced neurons migrate from the SVZ in an anterior direction into the olfactory bulb to become GABA interneurons. The process has been elegantly characterized at both ultrastructural and molecular levels. In the SVZ, the neuroblasts (A cells) on their way to the olfactory bulb create chains of cells and migrate through a scaffold of glial cells supplied by slowly dividing astrocytes (B cells). Within this network of cell chains, there are groups of rapidly dividing neural precursors (C cells). Evidence suggests that the B cells give rise to the C cells, which in turn develop into the A cells, the future olfactory bulb interneurons. The existence of a sequence of precursors with progressively restricted abilities to generate diverse neural cell types makes defining mechanisms that regulate adult neurogenesis in vivo a significant challenge.

As in the developing brain, adult neurogenesis is also subject to regulation by extracellular signals that control precursor proliferation and survival and, in many cases, the very same factors. After the initial discovery of adult neural stem cells generated under EGF stimulation, other regulatory factors were defined, including bFGF, IGF-I, BDNF, and LIF/CNTF. Although the hallmark of neural stem cells includes the capacity to generate neurons, astrocytes, and oligodendroglia, termed multipotentiality, specific signals appear to produce relatively different profiles of cells that may migrate to distinct sites. Intraventricular infusion of EGF promotes primarily gliogenesis in the SVZ, with cells migrating to the olfactory bulb, striatum, and corpus callosum, whereas bFGF favors the generation of neurons destined for the olfactory bulb. Both factors appear to stimulate mitosis directly, with differential effects on the cell lineage produced. In contrast, BDNF may increase neuron formation in SVZ as well as striatum and hypothalamus, though effects may be primarily through promoting survival of newly generated neurons that otherwise undergo cell death. Finally, CNTF and related LIF may promote gliogenesis or support the self-renewal of adult stem cells rather than enhancing a specific cell category.

Remarkably, in addition to direct intraventricular infusions, adult neurogenesis is also affected by peripheral levels of growth factors, hormones, and neuropeptides. Peripheral administration of both bFGF and IGF-I stimulate neurogenesis, increasing selectively mitotic labeling in the SVZ and hippocampal subgranular zone, respectively, suggesting that there are specific mechanisms for factor transport across the BBB. Of interest, elevated prolactin levels, induced by peripheral injection or natural pregnancy, stimulate proliferation of progenitors in the mouse SVZ, leading to increased olfactory bulb interneurons, potentially playing roles in learning new infant scents. This process may be relevant to changes in prolactin seen in psychiatric disease. Conversely, in behavioral paradigms of social stress, such as territorial challenge by male intruders, activation of the hypothalamic–pituitary–adrenal (HPA) axis with increased glucocorticoids leads to reduced neurogenesis in the hippocampus, apparently through local glutamate signaling. Inhibition is also observed after peripheral opiate administration, a model for substance abuse. Thus neurogenesis may be one target process affected by changes of hormones and neuropeptides associated with several psychiatric conditions.

The discovery of adult neurogenesis naturally leads to questions about whether new neurons can integrate into the complex cytoarchitecture of the mature brain and speculation about its functional significance, if any. In rodents, primates, and humans, new neurons are generated in the dentate gyrus of the hippocampus, an area important for learning and memory. Some adult-generated neurons in humans have been shown to survive for at least 2 years. Furthermore, newly generated cells in the adult mouse hippocampus indeed elaborate extensive dendritic and axonal arborizations appropriate to the neural circuit and display functional synaptic inputs and action potentials. From a functional perspective, the generation or survival of new neurons correlates strongly with multiple instances of behavioral learning and experience. For example, the survival of newly generated neurons is markedly enhanced by hippocampal-dependent learning tasks and by an enriched, behaviorally complex environment. Of perhaps greater importance, a reduction in dentate gyrus neurogenesis impairs the formation of trace memories, that is when an animal must associate stimuli that are separated in time, a hippocampal-dependent task. Finally, in songbirds, neurogenesis is activity-dependent and is increased by foraging for food and learning a new song, whether it occurs seasonally or is induced by steroid hormone administration.

From clinical and therapeutic perspectives, fundamental questions are whether changes in neurogenesis contribute to disease and whether newly formed neurons undergo migration to and integration into regions of injury, replacing dead cells and leading to functional recovery. A neurogenetic response has now been shown for multiple conditions in the adult, including brain trauma, stroke, and epilepsy. For instance, ischemic stroke in the striatum stimulates adjacent SVZ neurogenesis, with neurons migrating to the injury site. Furthermore, in a highly selective paradigm not involving local tissue damage, degeneration of layer three cortical neurons elicited SVZ neurogenesis and cell replacement. These studies raise the possibility that newly produced neurons typically participate in recovery and may be stimulated as a novel therapeutic strategy. However, in contrast to potential reconstructive functions, neurogenesis may also play roles in pathogenesis: In a kindling model of epilepsy, newly generated neurons were found to migrate to incorrect positions and participate in aberrant neuronal circuits, thereby reinforcing the epileptic state.

Conversely, reductions in neurogenesis may contribute to several conditions that implicate dysfunction or degeneration of the hippocampal formation. Dentate gyrus neurogenesis is inhibited by increased glucocorticoid levels observed in aged rats. It can be reversed by steroid antagonists and adrenalectomy, observations potentially relevant to the correlation of elevated human cortisol levels with reduced hippocampal volumes, and the presence of memory deficits. Similarly, stress-induced increases in human glucocorticoids may contribute to decreased hippocampal volumes seen in schizophrenia, depression, and PTSD.

A potential role for altered neurogenesis in disease has gained the most support in recent studies of depression. Several studies in animals and humans suggest a correlation of decreased hippocampal size with depressive symptoms, whereas clinically significant antidepressant therapy elicits increased hippocampal volume and enhanced neurogenesis, with causal relationships still being defined. For example, postmortem and brain imaging studies indicate cell loss in corticolimbic regions in bipolar disorder and major depression. Significantly, mood stabilizers, such as lithium and valproic acid, as well as antidepressants and ECT, activate intracellular pathways that promote neurogenesis and synaptic plasticity. Furthermore, in a useful primate model, the adult tree shrew, the chronic psychosocial stress model of depression elicited ~15 percent reductions in brain metabolites and a 33 percent decrease in neurogenesis (BrdU mitotic labeling), effects that were prevented by coadministration of antidepressant, tianeptine. More importantly, although stress exposure elicited small reductions in hippocampal volumes, stressed animals treated with antidepressants exhibited increased hippocampal volumes. Similar effects have been found in rodent models of depression.

Also, to the previous structural relationships, recent evidence has begun defining the roles of relevant neurotransmitter systems to antidepressant effects on behavior and neurogenesis. In a most exciting finding, a causal link between antidepressant-induced neurogenesis and a positive behavioral response has been demonstrated. In the serotonin 1A receptor null mouse, fluoxetine, a selective serotonin reuptake inhibitor [SSRI], produced neither enhanced neurogenesis nor behavioral improvement. Furthermore, when hippocampal neuronal precursors were selectively reduced (85 percent) by X-irradiation, neither fluoxetine nor imipramine induced neurogenesis or behavioral recovery. Finally, one study using hippocampal cultures from normal and mutant rodents strongly supports a neurogenetic role for endogenous NPY, which is contained in dentate gyrus hilar interneurons. NPY stimulates precursor proliferation selectively via the Y1 (not Y2 or Y5) receptor, a finding consistent with the receptor-mediating antidepressive effects of NPY in animal models and the impact of NPY levels on both hippocampal-dependent learning and responses to stress. In aggregate, these observations suggest that volume changes observed with human depression and therapy may directly relate to alterations in ongoing neurogenesis. More generally, the discovery of adult neurogenesis has led to significant changes in our perspectives on the regenerative capacities of the human brain.

NEUROPHYSIOLOGY AND NEUROCHEMISTRY

The study of chemical interneuronal communication is called neurochemistry, and in recent years there has been an explosion of knowledge in understanding chemical transmission between neurons and the receptors affected by those chemicals. It also influences our understanding of brain physiology. This section chapter focuses on the complex heterogeneity of both these areas to help explain the complexity of thoughts, feelings, and behaviors that make up the human experience.

Monoamine Neurotransmitters

The monoamine neurotransmitters and acetylcholine have been historically implicated in the pathophysiology and treatment of a wide variety of neuropsychiatric disorders. Each monoamine neurotransmitter system modulates many different neural pathways, which themselves subserve multiple behavioral and physiologic processes. Conversely, each CNS neurobehavioral process is likely modulated by multiple interacting neurotransmitter systems, including monoamines.

This complexity poses a significant challenge to understanding the precise molecular, cellular, and systems-level pathways through which various monoamine neurotransmitters affect neuropsychiatric disorders. However, recent advances in human genetics and genomics, as well as in experimental neuroscience, have shed light on this question. Molecular cloning has identified a large number of genes that regulate monoaminergic neurotransmissions, such as the enzymes, receptors, and transporters that mediate the synthesis, cellular actions, and cellular reuptake of these neurotransmitters,

respectively. Human genetics studies have provided evidence of tantalizing links between allelic variants in specific monoamine-related genes and psychiatric disorders and trait abnormalities. In contrast, the ability to modify gene function and cellular activity in experimental animals has clarified the roles of specific genes and neural pathways in mediating behavioral processes.

Monoamines act on target cells by binding to specific cell-surface receptors. There are multiple receptor subtypes for each monoamine, which are expressed in diverse regions and subcellular locales and which engage a variety of intracellular signaling pathways. This panoply of receptors thus allows each monoamine neurotransmitter to modulate target cells in many ways; the same molecule may activate some cells while inhibiting others, depending on which receptor subtype is expressed by each cell. The various monoamines are discussed below.

Serotonin.   Although only one in a million CNS neurons produces serotonin, these cells influence virtually all aspects of CNS function. The cell bodies of these serotonergic neurons are clustered in the midline raphe nuclei of the brainstem; the rostral raphe nuclei send ascending axonal projections throughout the brain, whereas the descending caudal raphe nuclei send projections into the medulla, cerebellum, and spinal cord (Fig. 33-12). The descending serotonergic fibers that innervate the dorsal horn of the spinal cord have been implicated in the suppression of nociceptive pathways, a finding that may relate to the pain-relieving effects of some antidepressants. The tonic firing of CNS serotonin neurons varies across the sleep–wake cycle, with an absence of activity during rapid eye movement (REM) sleep. Increased serotonergic firing is observed during rhythmic motor behaviors and suggests that serotonin modulates some forms of motor output.

Most serotonergic innervation of the cortex and limbic system arises from the dorsal and median raphe nuclei in the midbrain; the serotonergic neurons in these areas send projections through the medial forebrain bundle into target forebrain regions. The median raphe provides most of the serotonergic fibers that innervate the limbic system, whereas the dorsal raphe nucleus provides most of the serotonergic fibers that innervate the striatum and thalamus.

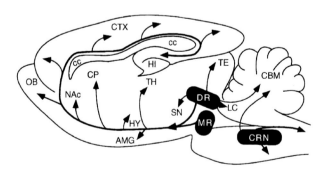

FIGURE 33-12

Brain serotonergic pathways (in rats). Serotonergic neurons are located in brainstem midline raphe nuclei and project throughout the neuraxis. (There is an approximate similarity between monoamine pathways in rats and in humans.) AMG, amygdala; CBM, cerebellum; cc, corpus callosum; CP, caudate putamen; CRN, caudal raphe nuclei; CTX, neocortex; DR, dorsal raphe nucleus; HI, hippocampus; HY, hypothalamus; LC, locus ceruleus; MR, median raphe nucleus; NAc, nucleus accumbens; OB, olfactory bulb; SN, substantia nigra; TE, tectum; TH, thalamus; TM, tuberomammillary nucleus of hypothalamus. (From Sadock BJ, Sadock VA, Ruiz P. *Kaplan & Sadock's Comprehensive Textbook of Psychiatry*. 9th ed. Philadelphia, PA: Lippincott Williams & Wilkins; 2009:65.)

Also, to the different target fields of these serotonergic nuclei, there are cellular differences between their constituent neurons. Dorsal raphe serotonergic fibers are fine, with small vesicle-coated swellings called varicosities, whereas median raphe fibers have large spherical or beaded varicosities. It is unclear to what extent serotonin acts as a true synaptic or "private" neurotransmitter versus action as a local endocrine hormone or "social transmitter," or whether its roles differ depending on the fiber type from which it is released. These fibers show differential sensitivity to the neurotoxic effects of the amphetamine analog 3,4-methylenedioxymethamphetamine (MDMA, "ecstasy"), which lesions the fine axons of the dorsal raphe while sparing the thick beaded axons of the median raphe. The significance of these morphologic differences is unclear, although recent work has identified functional differences between the serotonergic neurons of the dorsal and median raphe nuclei.

Dopamine.   Dopamine neurons are more widely distributed than those of other monoamines, residing in the midbrain substantia nigra and ventral tegmental area (VTA) and the periaqueductal gray, hypothalamus, olfactory bulb, and retina. In the periphery, dopamine is found in the kidney, where it functions to produce renal vasodilation, diuresis, and natriuresis. Three dopamine systems are highly relevant to psychiatry: The nigrostriatal, mesocorticolimbic, and tuberohypophyseal system (Fig. 33-13). Degeneration of the nigrostriatal system causes Parkinson disease and has led to an intense research focus on the development and function of dopamine neurons in the midbrain substantia nigra nuclei. Dopamine cell bodies in the pars compacta division of this region send ascending projections to the dorsal striatum (especially to the caudate and putamen) and thereby modulate motor control. The extrapyramidal effects of antipsychotic drugs are thought to result from the blockade of these striatal dopamine receptors.

The midbrain VTA lies medial to the substantia nigra and contains dopaminergic neurons that give rise to the mesocorticolimbic dopamine system. These neurons send ascending projections that innervate limbic structures, such as the nucleus accumbens and amygdala; the mesoaccumbens pathway is a central element in the neural representation of reward, and intense research has been devoted to this area in recent years. All known drugs of abuse activate the mesoaccumbens dopamine pathway, and plastic changes in this pathway are thought to underlie drug addiction. The mesolimbic projection is believed to be a significant target for the antipsychotic properties of dopamine receptor antagonist drugs in controlling the positive symptoms of schizophrenia, such as hallucinations and delusions.

VTA dopamine neurons also project to cortical structures, such as the prefrontal cortex, and modulate working memory and attention; decreased activity in this pathway is proposed to underlie negative symptoms of schizophrenia. Thus antipsychotic drugs that decrease positive symptoms by blocking dopamine receptors in the mesolimbic pathway may simultaneously worsen these negative symptoms by blocking similar dopamine receptors in the mesocortical pathway. The decreased risk of extrapyramidal side effects seen with clozapine (Clozaril; vs. other typical antipsychotic medications) is thought to be due to its relatively selective effects on this mesocortical projection. The tuberohypophyseal system consists of dopamine neurons in the hypothalamic arcuate and paraventricular nuclei that project to the pituitary gland and thereby inhibit prolactin release. Antipsychotic drugs that block dopamine receptors in the pituitary may thus disinhibit prolactin release and cause galactorrhea.

Norepinephrine and Epinephrine.   The postganglionic sympathetic neurons of the ANS release norepinephrine, resulting in widespread peripheral effects, including tachycardia and elevated blood pressure. The adrenal medulla releases epinephrine, which produces similar effects; epinephrine-secreting pheochromocytoma tumors produce bursts of sympathetic activation, central arousal, and anxiety.

Norepinephrine-producing neurons are found within the brain in the pons and medulla in two major clusterings: The locus ceruleus (LC) and the lateral tegmental noradrenergic nuclei (Fig. 33-14). Noradrenergic projections from both of these regions extensively ramify as they project throughout the neuraxis. In humans, the LC is found in the dorsal portion of the caudal pons and contains approximately 12,000 tightly packed neurons on each side of the brain. These cells provide the central noradrenergic projections to the neocortex, hippocampus, thalamus, and midbrain tectum. The activity of LC neurons varies with the animal's level of wakefulness. Firing rates are responsive to novel or stressful stimuli, with the largest responses to stimuli that disrupt ongoing behavior and reorient attention. Altogether, physiologic studies indicate a role for this structure in the regulation of arousal state, vigilance, and

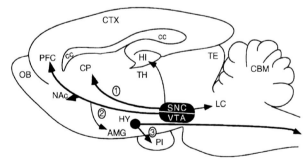

FIGURE 33-13

Brain dopaminergic pathways (in rats). The three principal dopaminergic pathways: (*1*) nigrostriatal pathway, (*2*) mesocorticolimbic pathway, and (*3*) tuberohypophyseal pathway. AMG, amygdala; CBM, cerebellum; cc, corpus callosum; CP, caudate putamen; CTX, neocortex; HI, hippocampus; HY, hypothalamus; LC, locus ceruleus; NAc, nucleus accumbens; OB, olfactory bulb; PFC, prefrontal cortex; PI, pituitary; SNC, substantia nigra pars compacta; TE, tectum; TH, thalamus; VTA, ventral tegmental area. (From Sadock BJ, Sadock VA, Ruiz P. *Kaplan & Sadock's Comprehensive Textbook of Psychiatry*. 9th ed. Philadelphia, PA: Lippincott Williams & Wilkins; 2009:66.)

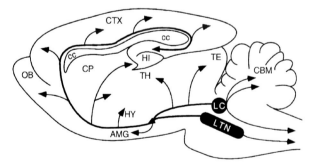

FIGURE 33-14

Brain noradrenergic pathways (in rats). Projections of noradrenergic neurons located in the locus ceruleus (LC) and lateral tegmental noradrenergic nuclei (LTN). AMG, amygdala; CBM, cerebellum; cc, corpus callosum; CP, caudate putamen; CTX, neocortex; HI, hippocampus; HY, hypothalamus; OB, olfactory bulb; TE, tectum; TH, thalamus. (From Sadock BJ, Sadock VA, Ruiz P. *Kaplan & Sadock's Comprehensive Textbook of Psychiatry*. 9th ed. Philadelphia, PA: Lippincott Williams & Wilkins; 2009:66.)

stress response. The projections from lateral tegmental nucleus neurons, which are loosely scattered throughout the ventral pons and medulla, partially overlap those of the LC. Fibers from both cell groups innervate the amygdala, septum, and spinal cord. Other regions, such as the hypothalamus and lower brainstem, receive adrenergic inputs predominantly from the lateral tegmental nucleus. The relatively few neurons that utilize epinephrine as a neurotransmitter are located in the caudal pons and medulla, intermingled with noradrenergic neurons. Projections from these groups ascend to innervate the hypothalamus, LC, and visceral efferent and afferent nuclei of the midbrain.

Histamine.   Histamine is perhaps best known for its role in allergies. It is an inflammatory mediator stored in mast cells and released upon cellular interaction with allergens. Once released, histamine causes vascular leakage and edema and other facial and topical allergy symptoms. In contrast, central histaminergic neural pathways have only more recently been characterized by immunocytochemistry using antibodies to the synthetic enzyme histidine decarboxylase and histamine. Histaminergic cell bodies are located within a region of the posterior hypothalamus termed the tuberomammillary nucleus. The activity of tuberomammillary neurons is characterized by firing that varies across the sleep–wake cycle, with the highest activity during the waking state, slowed firing during slow-wave sleep, and absence of firing during REM sleep. Histaminergic fibers project diffusely throughout the brain and spinal cord (Fig. 33-15). Ventral ascending projections course through the medial forebrain bundle and then innervate the hypothalamus, diagonal band, septum, and olfactory bulb. Dorsal ascending projections innervate the thalamus, hippocampus, amygdala, and rostral forebrain. Descending projections travel through the central midbrain gray to the dorsal hindbrain and spinal cord. The fibers have varicosities that are seldom associated with classical synapses, and histamine has been proposed to act at a distance from its sites of release, like a local hormone. The hypothalamus receives the densest histaminergic innervation, consistent with a role for this transmitter in the regulation of autonomic and neuroendocrine processes. Also, muscular histaminergic innervation is seen in monoaminergic and cholinergic nuclei.

Acetylcholine.   Within the brain, the axonal processes of cholinergic neurons may either project to distant brain regions

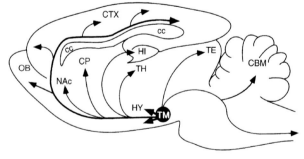

FIGURE 33-15

Brain histaminergic pathways (in rats). Histaminergic neurons are located in the tuberomammillary nucleus of the caudal hypothalamus (TM) and project to the hypothalamus (HY) and more distant brain regions. CBM, cerebellum; cc, corpus callosum; CP, caudate putamen; CTX, neocortex; HI, hippocampus; NAc, nucleus accumbens; OB, olfactory bulb; TE, tectum; TH, thalamus. (From Sadock BJ, Sadock VA, Ruiz P. *Kaplan & Sadock's Comprehensive Textbook of Psychiatry.* 9th ed. Philadelphia, PA: Lippincott Williams & Wilkins; 2009:67.)

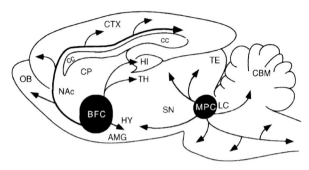

FIGURE 33-16

Brain cholinergic projection pathways (in rats). The majority of cholinergic projection neurons are located in the basal forebrain complex (BFC) and the mesopontine complex (MPC). AMG, amygdala; CBM, cerebellum; cc, corpus callosum; CP, caudate putamen; CTX, neocortex; HI, hippocampus; HY, hypothalamus; LC, locus ceruleus; NAc, nucleus accumbens; OB, olfactory bulb; SN, substantia nigra; TE, tectum; TH, thalamus. (From Sadock BJ, Sadock VA, Ruiz P. *Kaplan & Sadock's Comprehensive Textbook of Psychiatry.* 9th ed. Philadelphia, PA: Lippincott Williams & Wilkins; 2009:67.)

(projection neurons) or contact local cells within the same structure (interneurons). Two large clusters of cholinergic projection neurons are found within the brain: The basal forebrain complex and the mesopontine complex (Fig. 33-16). The basal forebrain complex provides most of the cholinergic innervation to the nonstriatal telencephalon. It consists of cholinergic neurons within the nucleus basalis of Meynert, the horizontal and vertical diagonal bands of Broca, and the medial septal nucleus. These neurons project to widespread areas of the cortex and amygdala, to the anterior cingulate gyrus and olfactory bulb, and the hippocampus, respectively. In Alzheimer disease, there is significant degeneration of neurons in the nucleus basalis, leading to a substantial reduction in cortical cholinergic innervation. The extent of neuronal loss correlates with the degree of dementia, and the cholinergic deficit may contribute to the cognitive decline in this disease, consistent with the beneficial effects of drugs that promote acetylcholine signaling in this disorder.

The mesopontine complex consists of cholinergic neurons within the pedunculopontine and laterodorsal tegmental nuclei of the midbrain and pons and provides cholinergic innervation to the thalamus and midbrain areas (including the dopaminergic neurons of the VTA and substantia nigra) and descending innervation to other brainstem regions such as the LC, dorsal raphe, and cranial nerve nuclei. In contrast to central serotonergic, noradrenergic, and histaminergic neurons, cholinergic neurons may continue to fire during REM sleep and have been proposed to play a role in REM sleep induction. Acetylcholine is also found within interneurons of several brain regions, including the striatum. The modulation of striatal cholinergic transmission has been implicated in the antiparkinsonian actions of anticholinergic agents. Within the periphery, acetylcholine is a prominent neurotransmitter, located in motoneurons innervating skeletal muscle, preganglionic autonomic neurons, and postganglionic parasympathetic neurons. Peripheral acetylcholine mediates the characteristic postsynaptic effects of the parasympathetic system, including bradycardia and reduced blood pressure, and enhanced digestive function.

Monoamine Synthesis, Storage, and Degradation

Also, to neuroanatomic similarities, monoamines are synthesized, stored, and degraded in similar ways (Fig. 33-17). Monoamines are synthesized within neurons from common amino acid precursors

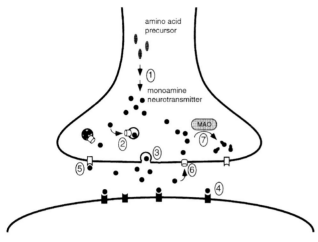

FIGURE 33-17

Schematic diagram of a monoaminergic synapse. Steps involved in synaptic transmission are described in the text. MAO, monoamine oxidase. (From Sadock BJ, Sadock VA, Ruiz P. *Kaplan & Sadock's Comprehensive Textbook of Psychiatry*. 9th ed. Philadelphia, PA: Lippincott Williams & Wilkins; 2009:68.)

(Fig. 33-17, step 1) and taken up into synaptic vesicles by way of a vesicular monoamine transporter (Fig. 33-17, step 2). On stimulation, vesicles within nerve terminals fuse with the presynaptic terminal and release the neurotransmitter into the synaptic cleft (Fig. 33-17, step 3). Once released, the monoamines interact with postsynaptic receptors to alter the function of postsynaptic cells (Fig. 33-17, step 4), and they may also act on presynaptic autoreceptors on the nerve terminal to suppress further release (Fig. 33-17, step 5). Also, released monoamines may be taken back up from the synaptic cleft into the nerve terminal by plasma membrane transporter proteins (Fig. 33-17, step 6), a process known as reuptake. Reuptake plays an essential role in limiting the total magnitude and temporal duration of monoamine signaling. Once monoamines are taken up, they may be subject to enzymatic degradation (Fig. 33-17, step 7), or they may be protected from degradation by uptake into vesicles. The processing of acetylcholine differs from this scheme and is described later in this section.

Serotonin

The CNS contains less than 2 percent of the serotonin in the body; peripheral serotonin is located in platelets, mast cells, and enterochromaffin cells. More than 80 percent of all the serotonin in the body is found in the gastrointestinal system, where it modulates motility and digestive functions. Platelet serotonin promotes aggregation and clotting through a most unusual mechanism: The covalent linkage of serotonin molecules to small GTP-binding proteins, which can then activate these proteins, is a process termed "serotonylation." Peripheral serotonin cannot cross the BBB, so serotonin is synthesized within the brain as well. Serotonin is synthesized from the amino acid tryptophan, which is derived from the diet. The rate-limiting step in serotonin synthesis is the hydroxylation of tryptophan by the enzyme tryptophan hydroxylase to form 5-hydroxytryptophan (4-HT) (Fig. 33-18). Two isoforms of tryptophan hydroxylase exist—one isoform is found mainly in the periphery, whereas the second isoform is restricted to the CNS.

Under normal circumstances, tryptophan concentration is rate-limiting in serotonin synthesis. Therefore, much attention has focused on the factors that determine tryptophan availability.

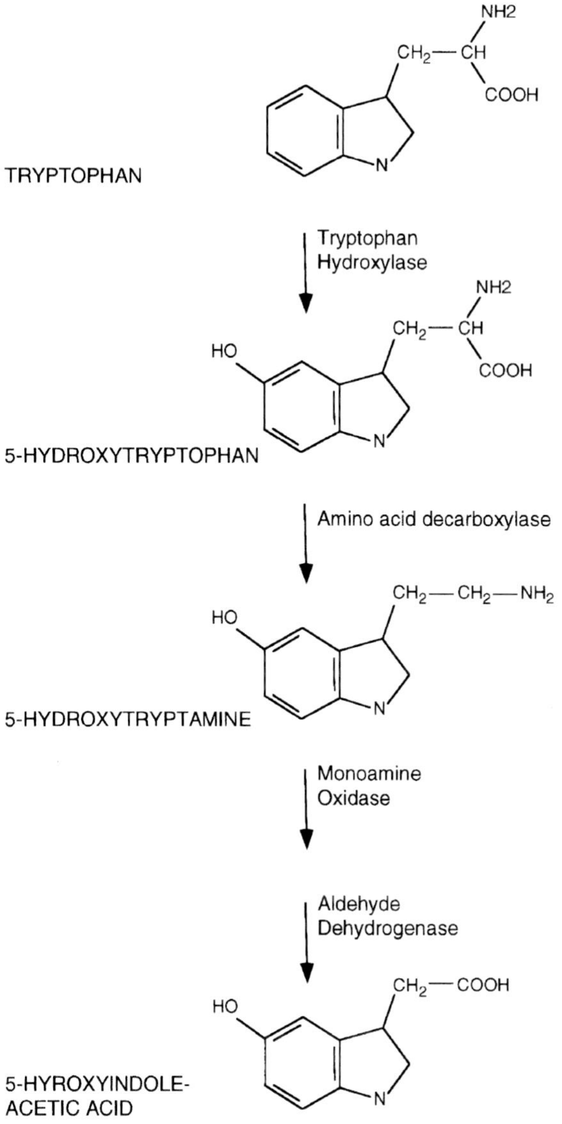

FIGURE 33-18

Synthesis and catabolism of serotonin. (From Sadock BJ, Sadock VA, Ruiz P. *Kaplan & Sadock's Comprehensive Textbook of Psychiatry*. 9th ed. Philadelphia, PA: Lippincott Williams & Wilkins; 2009:68.)

Unlike serotonin, tryptophan is taken up into the brain by way of a saturable active carrier mechanism. Because tryptophan competes with other large neutral amino acids for transport, brain uptake of this amino acid is determined both by the amount of circulating tryptophan and by the ratio of tryptophan to other large neutral amino acids. This ratio may be elevated by carbohydrate intake, which induces insulin release and the uptake of many sizeable neutral amino acids into peripheral tissues.

Conversely, high-protein foods tend to be relatively low in tryptophan, thus lowering this ratio. Moreover, the administration of specialized low tryptophan diets produces significant declines in brain serotonin levels. After tryptophan hydroxylation, 5-hydroxytryptophan is rapidly decarboxylated by aromatic amino acid decarboxylase (an enzyme also involved in dopamine synthesis) to form serotonin.

The first step in the degradation of serotonin is mediated by monoamine oxidase type A (MAO_A), which oxidizes the amino group to form an aldehyde. MAO_A is located in mitochondrial membranes and is nonspecific in its substrate specificity; in addition to serotonin, it oxidizes norepinephrine. The elevation of serotonin levels by MAO inhibitors (MAOIs) is believed to underlie the antidepressant efficacy of these drugs. After oxidation by MAO_A, the resulting aldehyde is further oxidized to 5-hydroxyindoleacetic acid (5-HIAA). Levels of 5-HIAA are often measured as a correlate of serotonergic system activity, although the relationship of these levels to serotonergic neuronal activity remains unclear.

Catecholamines. The catecholamines are synthesized from the amino acid tyrosine, which is taken up into the brain via an active transport mechanism (Fig. 33-19). Within catecholaminergic neurons, tyrosine hydroxylase catalyzes the addition of a hydroxyl group to the meta position of tyrosine, yielding L-dopa. This rate-limiting step in catecholamine synthesis is subject to inhibition by high levels of catecholamines (end-product inhibition). Because tyrosine hydroxylase usually is saturated with substrate, manipulation of tyrosine levels does not readily affect the rate of catecholamine synthesis. Once formed, L-dopa is rapidly converted to dopamine by dopa decarboxylase, which is located in the cytoplasm. It is now recognized that this enzyme acts not only on L-dopa but also on all naturally occurring aromatic L-amino acids, including tryptophan, and thus it is more appropriately termed aromatic amino acid decarboxylase. In noradrenergic and adrenergic neurons, dopamine is actively transported into storage vesicles, where it is oxidized by dopamine β-hydroxylase to form norepinephrine. In adrenergic neurons and the adrenal medulla, norepinephrine is converted to epinephrine by phenylethanolamine N-methyltransferase (PNMT), which is located within the cytoplasmic compartment.

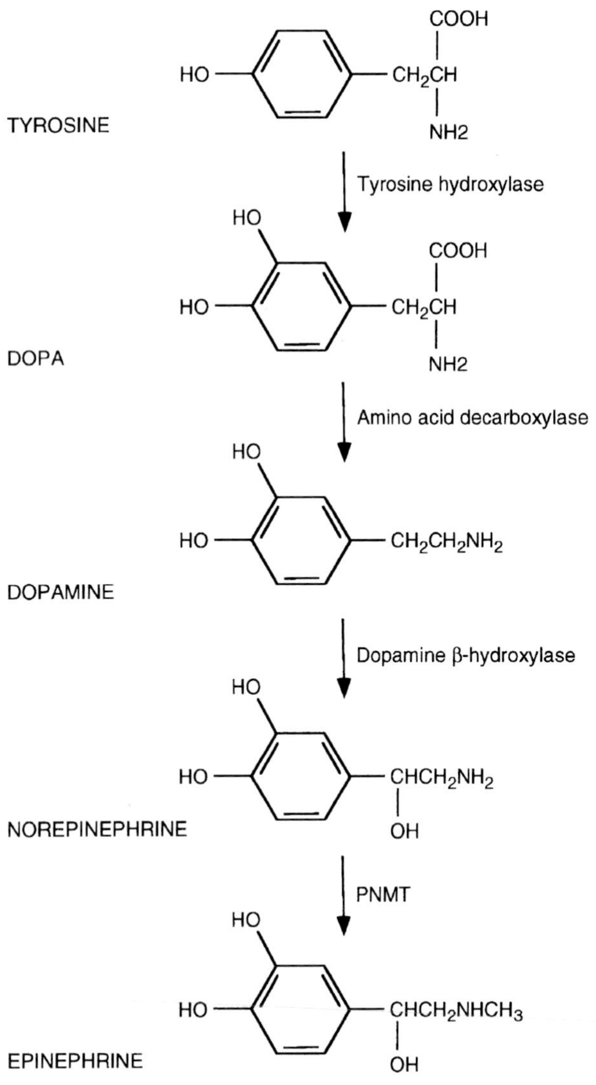

Two enzymes that play significant roles in the degradation of catecholamines are monoamine oxidase and catechol-O-methyltransferase (COMT). MAO is located on the outer membrane of mitochondria, including those within the terminals of adrenergic fibers, and oxidatively deaminates catecholamines to their corresponding aldehydes. Two MAO isozymes with differing substrate specificities have been identified: MAO_A, which preferentially deaminates serotonin and norepinephrine, and MAO type B (MAO_B), which deaminates dopamine, histamine, and a broad spectrum of phenylethylamines. Neurons contain both MAO isoforms. The blockade of monoamine catabolism by MAO inhibitors produces elevations in brain monoamine levels. MAO is also found in peripheral tissues such as the gastrointestinal tract and liver, where it prevents the accumulation of toxic amines. For example, peripheral MAO degrades dietary tyramine, an amine that can displace norepinephrine from sympathetic postganglionic nerve endings, producing hypertension if tyramine is present in sufficient quantities. Thus patients treated with MAO inhibitors are cautioned to avoid pickled and fermented foods that typically have high levels of tyramine. Catechol-O-methyltransferase (COMT) is located in the cytoplasm and is widely distributed throughout the brain and peripheral tissues, although little to none is found in adrenergic neurons. It has a broad substrate specificity, catalyzing the transfer of methyl groups from S-adenosyl methionine to the m-hydroxyl group of most catechol compounds. The catecholamine metabolites produced by these and other enzymes are frequently measured as indicators of the activity of catecholaminergic systems. In humans, the predominant metabolites of dopamine and norepinephrine are homovanillic acid (HVA) and 3-methoxy-4-hydroxyphenylglycol (MHPG), respectively.

Histamine. As is the case for serotonin, the brain contains only a small portion of the histamine found in the body. Histamine is distributed throughout most tissues of the body, predominantly in mast cells. Because it does not readily cross the BBB, it is believed that histamine is synthesized within the brain. In the brain, histamine is formed by the decarboxylation of the amino acid histidine by a specific L-histidine decarboxylase. This enzyme is not typically saturated with substrate, so synthesis is sensitive to histidine levels. This is consistent with the observation that the peripheral administration of histidine elevates brain histamine levels. Histamine is metabolized in the brain by histamine N-methyltransferase, producing methylhistamine. In turn, methylhistamine undergoes oxidative deamination by MAO_B.

Acetylcholine. Acetylcholine is synthesized by the transfer of an acetyl group from acetyl coenzyme A (ACoA) to choline in a reaction mediated by the enzyme choline acetyltransferase (ChAT). The majority of choline within the brain is transported from the blood rather than being synthesized de novo. Choline is taken up into cholinergic neurons by a high-affinity active transport mechanism, and this uptake is the rate-limiting step in acetylcholine synthesis.

FIGURE 33-19

Synthesis of catecholamines. (From Sadock BJ, Sadock VA, Ruiz P. *Kaplan & Sadock's Comprehensive Textbook of Psychiatry.* 9th ed. Philadelphia, PA: Lippincott Williams & Wilkins; 2009:69.)

The rate of choline transport is regulated, such that increased cholinergic neural activity is associated with enhanced choline uptake. After synthesis, acetylcholine is stored in synaptic vesicles through the action of a vesicular acetylcholine transporter. After vesicular release, acetylcholine is rapidly broken down by hydrolysis by acetylcholinesterase, located in the synaptic cleft. Much of the choline produced by this hydrolysis is then taken back into the presynaptic terminal via the choline transporter. Although acetylcholinesterase is primarily in cholinergic neurons and synapses, a second class of cholinesterase, butyrylcholinesterase, is primarily in the liver and plasma as well as in glia. In the treatment of Alzheimer disease, strategies aimed at enhancing cholinergic function, primarily through the use of cholinesterase inhibitors to prevent usual degradation of acetylcholine, have shown moderate efficacy in ameliorating cognitive dysfunction as well as behavioral disturbances. Cholinesterase inhibitors are also used in the treatment of myasthenia gravis, a disease characterized by weakness due to blockade of neuromuscular transmission by autoantibodies to acetylcholine receptors.

Transporters. A great deal of progress has been made in the molecular characterization of the monoamine plasma membrane transporter proteins. These membrane proteins mediate the reuptake of synaptically released monoamines into the presynaptic terminal. This process also involves cotransport of Na^+ and Cl^- ions and is driven by the ion concentration gradient generated by the plasma membrane Na^+/K^+ ATPase. Monoamine reuptake is an essential mechanism for limiting the extent and duration of activation of monoaminergic receptors. Reuptake is also a primary mechanism for replenishing terminal monoamine neurotransmitter stores. Moreover, transporters serve as molecular targets for several antidepressant drugs, psychostimulants, and monoaminergic neurotoxins. Whereas transporter molecules for serotonin (SERT), dopamine (DAT), and norepinephrine (NET) have been well characterized, transporters selective for histamine and epinephrine have not been demonstrated.

Among drugs of abuse, cocaine binds with high affinity to all three known monoamine transporters, although the stimulant properties of the drug have been attributed primarily to its blockade of DAT. This view has been recently supported by the absence of cocaine-induced locomotor stimulation in a strain of mutant mice engineered to lack this molecule. Psychostimulants produce a paradoxical locomotor suppression in these animals that has been attributed to their blockade of the serotonin transporter. The rewarding properties of cocaine have also been attributed primarily to dopamine transporter inhibition, although other targets mediate these effects as well since cocaine still has rewarding effects in mice lacking the dopamine transporter. It appears that serotonergic as well as dopaminergic mechanisms, may be involved. Transporters may also provide routes that allow neurotoxins to enter and damage monoaminergic neurons; examples include the dopaminergic neurotoxin 1-methyl-4-phenyl-1,2,3,6-tetrahydropyridine (MPTP) and the serotonergic neurotoxin MDMA.

Vesicular Monoamine Transporter. Also, to the reuptake of monoamines into the presynaptic nerve terminal, a second transport process serves to concentrate and store monoamines within synaptic vesicles. The transport and storage of monoamines in vesicles may serve several purposes: (1) to enable the regulated release of the transmitter under appropriate physiologic stimulation, (2) to protect monoamines from degradation by MAO, and (3) to protect neurons from the toxic effects of free radicals produced by the oxidation of cytoplasmic monoamines. In contrast with the plasma membrane transporters, a single type of vesicular monoamine transporter is believed to mediate the uptake of monoamines into synaptic vesicles within the brain. Consistent with this, blockade of this vesicular monoamine transporter by the antihypertensive drug reserpine (Serpasil) has been found to deplete brain levels of serotonin, norepinephrine, and dopamine and to increase the risk of suicide and affective dysfunction.

Receptors

Ultimately, the effects of monoamines on CNS function and behavior depend on their interactions with receptor molecules. The binding of monoamines to these plasma membrane proteins initiates a series of intracellular events that modulate neuronal excitability. Unlike the transporters, multiple receptor subtypes exist for each monoamine neurotransmitter (Table 33-2).

Serotonin Receptors. The 5-hydroxytryptophan type 1 (5-HT$_1$) receptors comprise the largest serotonin receptor subfamily, with human subtypes designated 5-HT$_{1A}$, 5-HT$_{1B}$, 5-HT$_{1D}$, 5-HT$_{1E}$, and 5-HT$_{1F}$. All five 5-HT$_1$ receptor subtypes display intronless gene structures, high affinities for serotonin, and adenylate cyclase inhibition. The most intensively studied of these has been the 5-HT$_{1A}$ receptor. This subtype is found on postsynaptic membranes of forebrain neurons, primarily in the hippocampus, cortex, and septum, and on serotonergic neurons, where it functions as an inhibitory somatodendritic autoreceptor. There is a significant interest in the 5-HT$_{1A}$ receptor as a modulator of both anxiety and depression. The downregulation of 5-HT$_{1A}$ autoreceptors by the chronic administration of serotonin reuptake inhibitors has been implicated in their antidepressant effects, and SSRIs may produce some behavioral effects via increases in hippocampal neurogenesis mediated by postsynaptic 5-HT$_{1A}$ receptor activation. Also, partial 5-HT$_{1A}$ receptor agonists such as buspirone display both anxiolytic and antidepressant properties.

Much recent attention has focused on the contributions of 5-HT$_{2A/C}$ receptors to the actions of atypical antipsychotic drugs such as clozapine, risperidone, and olanzapine. Analysis of the receptor-binding properties of these drugs has led to the hypothesis that 5-HT$_{2A}$ receptor blockade correlates with the therapeutic effects of atypical antipsychotics. The 5-HT$_{2A}$ receptor also influences working memory, which is likely impaired in schizophrenia.

The 5-HT$_{2C}$ receptor is expressed at high levels in many CNS regions, including the hippocampal formation, prefrontal cortex, amygdala, striatum, hypothalamus, and choroid plexus. Stimulation of 5-HT$_{2C}$ receptors has been proposed to produce anxiogenic effects as well as anorectic effects, which may result from interactions with the hypothalamic melanocortin and leptin pathways. 5-HT$_{2C}$ receptors may also play a role in the weight gain and development of type 2 diabetes mellitus associated with atypical antipsychotic treatment. Indeed, a line of mice lacking this receptor subtype exhibits an obesity syndrome associated with overeating and enhanced seizure susceptibility, suggesting that this receptor regulates neuronal network excitability. A variety of antidepressant and antipsychotic drugs antagonize 5-HT$_{2C}$ receptors with high affinity.

Conversely, hallucinogens such as lysergic acid diethylamide (LSD) display agonist activity at 5-HT$_2$ (and other) serotonin receptor subtypes. 5-HT$_{2C}$ receptor transcripts also undergo RNA editing, producing isoforms of the receptor with significantly altered basal versus serotonin-induced activity. Alterations in 5-HT$_{2C}$ receptor mRNA editing have been found in the brains of suicide victims with a history of major depression, and SSRIs have been shown to alter these editing patterns.

Table 33-2
Monoamine Receptors: Overview

Transmitter	Subtype	Primary Effector	Proposed Clinical Relevance
Histamine	H_1	↑ PI Turnover	Antagonists used as antiallergenic and anti-inflammatory agents, also promote sedation, weight gain
	H_2	↑ AC	Antagonists used to treat peptic ulcers, GI reflux, and GI bleeding
	H_3	↓ AC	Antagonists proposed to treat sleep disorders, obesity, dementia
	H_4	↓ AC	Possible role for antagonists as anti-inflammatory agents
Epinephrine/ Norepinephrine	$\alpha_{1A,B,D}$	↑ PI Turnover	Antagonists used in management of prostate disease
	$\alpha_{2A,B,C}$	↓ AC	Agonists sedative and hypertensive
	β_1	↑ AC	Regulation of cardiac function, antagonists may be anxiolytic
	β_2	↑ AC	Agonists used as bronchodilators
	β_3	↑ AC	Possible role for agonists to treat obesity
Serotonergic	$5HT_{1A,1B,1D,1E,1F}$	↓ AC, ↑ GIRK currents	Partial agonists (buspirone) anxiolytic, role in hippocampal neurogenesis; 5-HT1B/D antagonists used as antimigraine agents (triptans)
	$5\text{-}HT_{2A}$, $5\text{-}HT_{2B}$, $5\text{-}HT_{2C}$	↑ PI Turnover	2A antagonists → antipsychotic effects, 2A agonists → hallucinogens; 2B agonism → cardiac valvulopathy 2C agonists → under development as anorexigens, antiepileptics?
	$5\text{-}HT_3$	Na⁺ channel, cell membrane depolarization	Agonists (ondansetron) are antiemetics.
	$5\text{-}HT_4$	↑ AC	Partial agonists used in IBS (tegaserod)
	$5\text{-}HT_5$, $5\text{-}HT_6$, $5\text{-}HT_7$	↑ AC	Unclear Unclear Antagonists may have antidepressant potential
Dopaminergic	D_1-like family (D_1, D_5)	↑ AC	D_1 agonists used in Parkinson disease
	D_2-like family (D_2, D_3, D_4)	↓ AC	D_2 antagonists are antipsychotics (e.g., haloperidol) D_3 agonists used in Parkinson disease, restless legs syndrome (e.g., pramipexole)

From Sadock BJ, Sadock VA, Ruiz P. *Kaplan & Sadock's Comprehensive Textbook of Psychiatry.* 9th ed. Philadelphia, PA: Lippincott Williams & Wilkins; 2009:71.

Dopamine Receptors. In 1979, it was recognized that the actions of dopamine are mediated by more than one receptor subtype. Two dopamine receptors, termed D_1 and D_2, were distinguished based on differential binding affinities of a series of agonists and antagonists, distinct effector mechanisms, and distinct distribution patterns within the CNS. It was subsequently found that the therapeutic efficacy of antipsychotic drugs correlated strongly with their affinities for the D_2 receptor, implicating this subtype as an essential site of antipsychotic drug action. Recent molecular cloning studies have identified three additional dopamine receptor genes encoding the D_3, D_4, and D_5 dopamine receptors. Based on their structure, pharmacology, and primary effector mechanisms, the D_3 and D_4 receptors are considered to be "D_2-like," and the D_5 receptor "D_1-like." The functional roles of the recently discovered subtypes remain to be definitively elucidated.

The D_1 receptor was initially distinguished from the D_2 subtype by its high affinity for the antagonist SCH 23390 and relatively low affinity for butyrophenones such as haloperidol (Haldol). Whereas D_1 receptor activation stimulates cyclic adenosine monophosphate (cAMP) formation, D_2 receptor stimulation produces the opposite effect.

Adrenergic Receptors. As for the α_1 receptors, the functions of α_2 receptor subtypes (designated α_{2A}, α_{2B}, and α_{2C}) have been challenging to determine due to a lack of selective agonists and antagonists; α_2 receptors display both presynaptic autoreceptor and postsynaptic actions, and all appear to inhibit the cAMP formation and to activate potassium channels with resultant membrane hyperpolarization. These receptors regulate neurotransmitter release from peripheral sympathetic nerve endings. The stimulation of central α_2 autoreceptors (likely the α_{2A} subtype) inhibits firing of the noradrenergic neurons of the LC, which are implicated in arousal states.

This mechanism has been proposed to underlie the sedative effects of the α_2 receptor agonist clonidine (Catapres). Also, the stimulation of brainstem α_2 receptors has been proposed to reduce sympathetic and to augment parasympathetic nervous system activity. This action may relate to the utility of clonidine in lowering blood pressure and in suppressing the sympathetic hyperactivity associated with opiate withdrawal. Activation of α_2 receptors inhibits the activity of serotonin neurons of the dorsal raphe nucleus, whereas activation of local α_1 receptors stimulates the activity of these neurons, and this is thought to be a significant activating input to the serotonergic system.

Histamine Receptors. Histaminergic systems have been proposed to modulate arousal, wakefulness, feeding behavior, and neuroendocrine responsiveness. Four histaminergic receptor subtypes have been identified and termed H_1, H_2, H_3, and H_4. The H_4 receptor was identified recently and is detected predominantly in the periphery, in regions such as the spleen, bone marrow, and leukocytes. The other three histamine receptors have a prominent expression in the CNS. H_1 receptors are expressed throughout the body, particularly in the smooth muscle of the gastrointestinal tract and bronchial walls, as well as on vascular endothelial cells. H_1 receptors are widely distributed within the CNS, with exceptionally high levels in the thalamus, cortex, and cerebellum. H_1 receptor activation is associated with G_q activation and stimulation of phosphoinositide turnover and tends to increase excitatory neuronal responses. These receptors are the targets of classical antihistaminergic agents used in the treatment of allergic rhinitis and conjunctivitis. The sedative effects of these compounds derive from their actions in the CNS and implicate histamine in the regulation of arousal and the sleep–wake cycle. Accordingly, a line of mutant mice lacking histamine displays deficits in waking and attention. Also, the sedation and weight gain produced by several antipsychotic and antidepressant drugs have been attributed to H_1 receptor antagonism. Conversely, H_1 receptor agonists stimulate arousal and suppress food intake in animal models.

Cholinergic Receptors.   M1 receptors are the most abundantly expressed muscarinic receptors in the forebrain, including the cortex, hippocampus, and striatum. Pharmacologic evidence has suggested their involvement in memory and synaptic plasticity, and recent evaluation of mice lacking the M1 receptor gene revealed deficits in memory tasks believed to require interactions between the cortex and the hippocampus.

Nicotinic receptors have been implicated in cognitive function, especially working memory, attention, and processing speed. Cortical and hippocampal nicotinic acetylcholine receptors appear to be significantly decreased in Alzheimer disease, and nicotine administration improves attention deficits in some patients. The acetylcholinesterase inhibitor galantamine used in the treatment of Alzheimer disease also acts to modulate nicotinic receptor function positively. The α_7 nicotinic acetylcholine receptor subtype has been implicated as one of many possible susceptibility genes for schizophrenia, with lower levels of this receptor being associated with impaired sensory gating. Some rare forms of the familial epilepsy syndrome autosomal dominant nocturnal frontal lobe epilepsy (ADNFLE) are associated with mutations in the α_4 or β_2 subunits of the nicotinic acetylcholine receptor. Finally, the reinforcing properties of tobacco use are proposed to involve the stimulation of nicotinic acetylcholine receptors located in mesolimbic dopaminergic reward pathways.

Amino Acid Neurotransmitters

For more than 50 years, biogenic amines have dominated thinking about the role of neurotransmitters in the pathophysiology of psychiatric disorders. However, over the last decade, evidence has accumulated from postmortem, brain imaging, and genetic studies that the amino acid neurotransmitters, in particular glutamic acid and GABA, play an important, if not central, role in the pathophysiology of a broad range of psychiatric disorders including schizophrenia, bipolar disorder, major depression, Alzheimer disease, and anxiety disorders.

Glutamic Acid.   Glutamate mediates fast excitatory neurotransmission in the brain and is the transmitter for approximately 80 percent of brain synapses, particularly those associated with dendritic spines. The repolarization of neuronal membranes that are depolarized by glutamatergic neurotransmission may explain perhaps 80 percent of the brain's energy expenditure. The concentration of glutamate in the brain is 10 mM, the highest of all amino acids, of which approximately 20 percent represents the neurotransmitter pool of glutamate.

Two families of receptors mediate the postsynaptic effects of glutamate. The first are the glutamate-gated cation channels that are responsible for fast neurotransmission. The second type of glutamate receptor are the metabotropic glutamate receptors (mGluR), which are G-protein–coupled receptors like α-adrenergic receptors and dopamine receptors. The mGluRs primarily modulate glutamatergic neurotransmission.

MAJOR GLUTAMATERGIC PATHWAYS IN THE BRAIN.   All primary sensory afferent systems appear to use glutamate as their neurotransmitter, including retinal ganglion cells, cochlear cells,

trigeminal nerve, and spinal afferents. The thalamocortical projections that distribute afferent information broadly to the cortex are glutamatergic. The pyramidal neurons of the corticolimbic regions, the primary source of intrinsic, associational, and efferent excitatory projections from the cortex, are glutamatergic. A temporal lobe circuit that figures significantly in the development of new memories is a series of four glutamatergic synapses: The perforant path innervates the hippocampal granule cells that innervate CA3 pyramidal cells that innervate CA1 pyramidal cells. The climbing fibers innervating the cerebellar cortex are glutamatergic, as well as the corticospinal tracks.

IONOTROPIC GLUTAMATE RECEPTORS.   Three families of ionotropic glutamate receptors have been identified based on selective activation by conformationally restricted or synthetic analogs of glutamate. These include α-amino-3-hydroxy-5-methyl-4-isoxazole propionic acid (AMPA), kainic acid (KA), and N-methyl-D-aspartic acid (NMDA) receptors. Subsequent cloning revealed 16 mammalian genes that encode structurally related proteins, which represent subunits that assemble into functional receptors. Glutamate-gated ion channel receptors appear to be tetramers, and subunit composition affects both the pharmacologic and the biophysical features of the receptor.

METABOTROPIC GLUTAMATE RECEPTORS.   These receptors are so designated because G proteins mediate their effects. All mGluRs are activated by glutamate, although their sensitivities vary remarkably. To date, eight mGluRs have been cloned. These genes encode for seven membrane-spanning proteins that are members of the superfamily of G-protein–coupled receptors.

THE ROLE OF ASTROCYTES.   Specialized end-feet of the astrocyte surround glutamatergic synapses. The astrocyte expresses the two Na^+-dependent glutamate transporters that play the primary role in removing glutamate from the synapse, thereby terminating its action: EAAT1 and EAAT2 (*excitatory amino acid transporter*). The neuronal glutamate transporter, EAAT3, is expressed in upper motor neurons, whereas EAAT4 is expressed primarily in cerebellar Purkinje cells and EAAT5 in the retina. Mice homozygous for null mutations of either EAAT1 or EAAT2 exhibit elevated extracellular glutamate and excitotoxic neurodegeneration. Notably, several studies have described the loss of EAAT2 protein and transport activity in the ventral horn in amyotrophic lateral sclerosis.

The astrocytes express AMPA receptors so that they can monitor synaptic glutamate release. GlyT1, which maintains subsaturating concentrations of glycine in the synapse, is expressed on the astrocyte plasma membrane. GlyT1 transports three Na^+ out for each molecule of glycine transported into the astrocyte. This stoichiometry results in a robust reversal of the direction of transport when glutamate released in the synapse activates the AMPA receptors on the astrocyte, thus depolarizing the astrocyte. Thus glycine release in the synapse by GlyT1 is coordinated with glutamatergic neurotransmission.

Similarly, activation of the astrocyte AMPA receptors causes GRIP to dissociate from the AMPA receptor and bind to serine racemase, activating it to synthesize D-serine. D-Serine levels are also determined by D-amino acid oxidase (DAAO) with low D-serine levels in the cerebellum and brainstem where DAAO expression is high, and high D-serine levels are found in corticolimbic brain regions where DAAO expression is relatively low. In contrast, the expression of GlyT1 is highest in the cerebellum and brainstem. This distribution suggests that D-serine is the primary modulator of the NMDA receptor in the forebrain, whereas glycine is more prominent in the brainstem and cerebellum.

PLASTICITY IN GLUTAMATERGIC NEUROTRANSMISSION. The extinction of conditioned fear is an active process mediated by the activation of NMDA receptors in the amygdala. Treatment of rats with NMDA receptor antagonists prevents the extinction of conditioned fear, whereas treatment with the glycine modulatory site partial agonist D-cycloserine facilitates the extinction of conditioned fear. (D-Cycloserine is an antibiotic used to treat tuberculosis that has 50 percent of the efficacy of glycine at the NMDA receptor.) Patients with acrophobia were administered either placebo or a single dose of D-cycloserine along with cognitive-behavioral therapy (CBT) to determine whether the phenomenon generalizes to humans. D-Cycloserine plus CBT resulted in a highly significant reduction in acrophobic symptoms that persisted for at least 3 months as compared to placebo plus CBT. Other placebo-controlled clinical trials support the notion that D-cycloserine is a robust enhancer of CBT, suggesting that pharmacologically augmenting neural plasticity may be used to bolster psychological interventions.

Fragile X mental retardation protein (FMRP), which is deficient in individuals with fragile X syndrome, appears to be synthesized locally within the spine during times of NMDA receptor activation and also plays a role in transporting specific mRNAs to the spine for translation. Notably, mice in which the FMRP gene has been inactivated through a null mutation, as well as patients with fragile X syndrome have fewer dendritic spines, the preponderance of which have an immature morphology. Loss of FMRP exaggerates responses of mGluR5, which stimulates dendritic protein synthesis, and treatment with an mGluR5 antagonist reverses the fragile-X–like phenotype in mice with the FMRP gene inactivated.

EXCITOTOXICITY. In the early 1970s, it was shown that the systemic administration of large amounts of monosodium glutamate to immature animals resulted in the degeneration of neurons in brain regions where the BBB was deficient.

Excitotoxicity is also implicated as a proximate cause of neuronal degeneration in Alzheimer disease. Most evidence points to the toxic consequences of aggregates of β-amyloid, especially β-amyloid$_{1-42}$. The β-amyloid fibrils depolarize neurons, resulting in loss of the Mg^{2+} block and enhanced NMDA receptor sensitivity to glutamate. The fibrils also impair glutamate transport into astrocytes, thereby increasing the extracellular concentration of glutamate. β-Amyloid directly promotes oxidative stress through inflammation that further contributes to neuronal vulnerability to glutamate. Thus, several mechanisms contribute to neuronal vulnerability to NMDA-receptor–mediated excitotoxicity in Alzheimer disease. Memantine, a recently approved treatment for mild to moderate Alzheimer disease, is a weak noncompetitive inhibitor of NMDA receptors. It reduces the tonic sensitivity of NMDA receptors to excitotoxicity but does not interfere with "phasic" neurotransmission, thereby attenuating neuronal degeneration in Alzheimer disease.

Inhibitory Amino Acids: GABA.

GABA is the major inhibitory neurotransmitter in the brain, where it is broadly distributed and occurs in millimolar concentrations. Given its physiologic effects and distributions, it is not surprising that the dysfunction of GABAergic neurotransmission has been implicated in a broad range of neuropsychiatric disorders, including anxiety disorders, schizophrenia, alcohol dependence, and seizure disorders. Chemically, GABA differs from glutamic acid, the major excitatory neurotransmitter, only by the removal of a single carboxyl group from the latter.

GABA is synthesized from glutamic acid by glutamic acid decarboxylase (GAD), which catalyzes the removal of the α-carboxyl group. In the CNS, the expression of GAD appears to be restricted to GABAergic neurons, although in the periphery, it is expressed in pancreatic islet cells. Two distinct but related genes encode GAD. GAD65 is localized to nerve terminals, where it is responsible for synthesizing GABA that is concentrated in the synaptic vesicles. Consistent with its role in fast inhibitory neurotransmission, mice homozygous for a null mutation of GAD65 have an elevated risk for seizures. GAD67 appears to be the primary source for neuronal GABA because mice homozygous for a null mutation of GAD67 die at birth, have a cleft pallet, and exhibit significant reductions in brain GABA.

GABA is catabolized by GABA transaminase (GABA-T) to yield succinic semialdehyde. Transamination generally occurs when the parent compound, α-ketoglutarate, is present to receive the amino group, thereby regenerating glutamic acid. Succinic semialdehyde is oxidized by succinic semialdehyde dehydrogenase (SSADH) into succinic acid, which reenters the Krebs cycle. GABA-T is a cell surface, a membrane-bound enzyme expressed by neurons and glia, which is oriented toward the extracellular compartment. As would be anticipated, drugs that inhibit the catabolism of GABA have anticonvulsant properties. One of the mechanisms of action of valproic acid is the competitive inhibition of GABA-T. γ-Vinyl-GABA is a suicide substrate inhibitor of GABA-T that is used as an anticonvulsant in Europe (vigabatrin [Sabril]).

The synaptic action of GABA is also terminated by high-affinity transport back into the presynaptic terminal as well as into astrocytes. Four genetically distinct GABA high-affinity transporters have been identified with differing kinetic and pharmacologic characteristics. They all share homology with other neurotransmitter transporters with the characteristic of 12 membrane-spanning domains. The active transport is driven by the sodium gradient so that upon depolarization, transportation of GABA out of the neuron is favored. GABA transported into astrocytes is catabolized by GABA-T and ultimately converted to glutamic acid and then to glutamine, which is transported back into the presynaptic terminal for GABA synthesis. Tiagabine (Gabitril) is a potent GABA transport inhibitor that is used to treat epilepsy. Preliminary results suggest that it also may be useful in panic disorder.

GABA$_A$ RECEPTORS. GABA$_A$ receptors are distributed throughout the brain. The GABA$_A$ complex, when activated, mediates an increase in membrane conductance with an equilibrium potential near the resting membrane potential of −70 mV (Fig. 33-20). In the mature neuron, this typically results with an influx of Cl^-, causing membrane hyperpolarization. Hyperpolarization is inhibitory because it increases the threshold for generating an action potential. In immature neurons, which have unusually high levels of intracellular Cl^-, activating the GABA$_A$ receptor can counterintuitively cause depolarization. For this reason, anticonvulsants that act by enhancing GABA$_A$ receptor activity may exacerbate seizures in the neonatal period.

Barbiturates such as phenobarbital and pentobarbital are noted for their sedative and anticonvulsant activities. Barbiturates allosterically increase the affinities of the binding sites for GABA and benzodiazepines at pharmacologically relevant concentrations. Barbiturates also affect channel dynamics by markedly increasing the extended open state and reducing the short open state, thereby increasing Cl^- inhibition. Chemically modified analogs of progesterone and corticosterone have been shown in behavioral studies to have sedative and anxiolytic effects through their interaction with the GABA$_A$ receptor complex. They share features with barbiturates, although they act at a distinctly different site. Thus, they

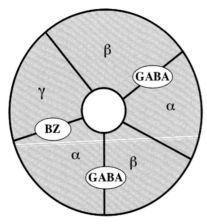

FIGURE 33-20

Schematic representation of the GABA$_A$ receptor. The receptor-channel complex is a heteropentamer. The GABA binding site is at the interface of the α and β subunits. The benzodiazepine binding site is at the interface between the γ and α subunits. (From Sadock BJ, Sadock VA, Ruiz P. *Kaplan & Sadock's Comprehensive Textbook of Psychiatry*. 9th ed. Philadelphia, PA: Lippincott Williams & Wilkins; 2009:81.)

allosterically enhance agonist ligand binding to the receptor and increase the duration of chloride channel opening. A variety of behavioral effects associated with steroid administration or fluctuation of endogenous steroids and sex-specific effects of GABAergic drugs have been linked to the action of endogenous neurosteroids.

Concerning GABA$_A$ receptor antagonists, picrotoxin, like the barbiturates, alters channel dynamics but in the opposite direction by reducing long open states and favoring the briefest open state. The proconvulsant pentylenetetrazol also acts by reducing chloride channel permeability. Penicillin, which at high concentrations is proconvulsant, binds to the positively charged residues in the channel, thereby occluding it. As a general class, anesthetics, including barbiturates, steroids, and volatile anesthetics, increase chloride conductance, thereby inhibiting neurotransmissions. Amino acids in the membrane-spanning domain of the GABA receptor subunits confer sensitivity to anesthetics. The precise mechanism whereby ethanol enhances GABA$_A$ receptor function remains unclear due to inconsistent results, suggesting that subunit composition may be necessary. However, recent studies suggest that ethanol increases the response of the tonic GABA-activated currents, which contain the δ subunit and exhibit remarkably high affinity to GABA.

Recently, recombinant DNA strategies exploiting site-directed mutagenesis have permitted the identification of sites on the specific subunits that mediate the pharmacologic action of drugs such as the benzodiazepines. Removal of the binding ability for benzodiazepines has established that the α_1 subunit plays a significant role in the sedative and amnestic effects of benzodiazepines, whereas inactivating the benzodiazepine site on the α_2 subunit eliminates the anxiolytic effect of benzodiazepines

GABA$_B$ RECEPTORS. The GABA$_B$ receptors are distinguished pharmacologically from GABA$_A$ receptors by the fact that they are insensitive to the canonical GABA$_A$ receptor antagonist bicuculline and that they are potently activated by baclofen [β-(4-chlorophenyl)-GABA], which is inactive at GABA$_A$ receptors. They are members of the G-protein–coupled superfamily of receptors but are highly unusual, as they are made of a dimer of two seven-transmembrane–spanning subunits. GABA$_B$ receptors are widely distributed throughout the nervous system and are localized both

presynaptically and postsynaptically. The postsynaptic GABA$_B$ receptors cause a long-lasting hyperpolarization by activating potassium channels. Presynaptically, they act as autoreceptors and heteroreceptors to inhibit neurotransmitter release.

GLYCINE AS A NEUROTRANSMITTER. Glycine is an inhibitory neurotransmitter primarily in the brainstem and spinal cord, although the expression of glycine receptor subunits in the thalamus, cortex, and hippocampus suggests a broader role. Glycine is a nonessential amino acid that is synthesized in the brain from L-serine by serine hydroxymethyltransferase. Glycine is concentrated within synaptic vesicles by H$^+$-dependent vesicular inhibitory amino acid transporter (VIAAT or VGAT), which also transports GABA. Termination of the synaptic action of glycine is through reuptake into the presynaptic terminal by the glycine transporter II (GlyT2), which is quite distinct from GlyT1 that is expressed in astrocytes and modulates NMDA receptor function.

The inhibitory effects of glycine are mediated by a ligand-gated chloride channel, which can also respond to β-alanine, taurine, L-alanine, L-serine, and proline, but not to GABA. The canonical antagonist for the glycine receptor is the plant alkaloid strychnine. The receptor was first identified through the specific binding of [^{3}H] strychnine. [^{3}H]Glycine binds to two sites: One that is displaceable by strychnine and represents the glycine A receptor and a second that is insensitive to strychnine and is designated the glycine B receptor, representing the glycine modulatory site on the NMDA receptor.

Neuropsychiatric Implications of Amino Acid Transmitters

SCHIZOPHRENIA. Evidence accumulating from postmortem, pharmacologic, and genetic studies is shifting the focus of the pathophysiology of schizophrenia from dopamine to glutamate and GABA. Indeed, after the use of D$_2$ receptor antagonists as the sole treatment of schizophrenia for the last 50 years, more than two-thirds of the treated patients remain substantially disabled. Early postmortem studies indicated a reduction in the activity of GAD in the cortex in patients with schizophrenia as compared to suitable controls. With the advent of immunocytochemistry and gene expression techniques, it has been possible to define the GABAergic deficit in schizophrenia more precisely. It appears that the parvalbumin-positive GABAergic interneurons in the intermediate layers of the cortex bear the brunt of the pathology, which includes reduced expression of GAD67, parvalbumin, and the GABA transporter (GAT). The finding that GABA$_A$ receptors are upregulated, as measured by autoradiography or with antibodies, supports the theory that these changes reflect the hypofunction of the presynaptic GABAergic neurons. These particular GABAergic interneurons, which include the chandelier cells, play an essential role in negative feedback inhibition to the pyramidal cells in the cortex. Despite this highly reproducible neuropathology, genes related to GABAergic function have not figured prominently in genome-wide searches, suggesting that GABAergic deficits may be a downstream consequence of some more proximal genetic defects.

The theory that hypofunction of NMDA receptors is an etiologic factor in schizophrenia initially arose from the observation that phencyclidine (PCP) and related dissociative anesthetics that block NMDA receptors produce a syndrome that can be indistinguishable from schizophrenia (Fig. 33-21). Dissociative anesthetics are so named because they prevent the acquisition of new memories while the patient is conscious. In fact, under laboratory conditions, low-dose infusion of ketamine can produce positive symptoms, negative symptoms, and specific cognitive deficits associated with schizophrenia in clear consciousness. Subsequent

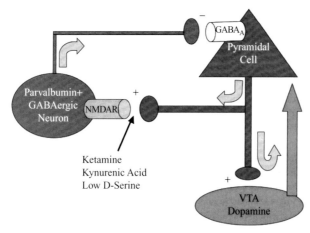

FIGURE 33-21

Pathologic circuit in schizophrenia. The NMDA receptors on the rapidly firing parvalbumin (PV) expressing GABAergic interneurons in the intermediate levels of the cortex are disproportionately sensitive to antagonists or loss of the coagonist, d-serine. NMDA receptor hypofunction causes reduced expression of PV, GAD67, and the GABA transporter and upregulation of GABA$_A$ receptors on pyramidal neurons. Disinhibition of the pyramidal neurons causes cognitive dysfunction and negative symptoms and drives excessive subcortical dopamine release resulting in psychosis. (From Sadock BJ, Sadock VA, Ruiz P. *Kaplan & Sadock's Comprehensive Textbook of Psychiatry*. 9th ed. Philadelphia, PA: Lippincott Williams & Wilkins; 2009:83.)

studies indicated that low-dose ketamine could also cause enhanced amphetamine-induced subcortical dopamine release as is observed in schizophrenia, as well as abnormal cortical event-related potentials (ERPs) and disruption of prepulse inhibition in experimental animals.

Several putative risk genes for schizophrenia are closely associated with the NMDA receptor function. DAAO, which encodes a protein that activates D-amino acid oxidase, has been repeatedly linked to the risk of schizophrenia. D-Amino acid oxidase itself has been associated with increased risk. Recently an allelic variant of serine racemase in the promoter region has also been associated with the risk for schizophrenia. Each of these gene variants could reduce the availability of D-serine in the cortex, thereby impairing the NMDA receptor function. Notably, CSF and blood levels of D-serine are significantly reduced in patients with schizophrenia. Neuregulin 1 appears to be a convincing risk gene and interacts directly with NMDA receptors. Dysbindin, another risk gene, is expressed in glutamatergic terminals. mGluR3, which downregulates glutamate release, has also been associated with schizophrenia.

Recent findings have provided a link between the GABAergic neuropathology and NMDA receptor hypofunction. Chronic treatment of rats with NMDA receptor antagonists causes downregulation of GAD67, parvalbumin, and GAT. The sensitive subpopulation of GABAergic neurons are interneurons that fire rapidly and provide the perisomatic innervation of the pyramidal cells. Their NMDA receptors appear to be much more sensitive to antagonists than those less active GABAergic neurons and pyramidal cells. The subtly reduced GABAergic inhibition results in a disinhibition of the glutamatergic pyramidal output. This degradation of the inhibitory feedback could account for the cognitive deficits and negative symptoms in schizophrenia, and the disinhibited output also results in elevated subcortical dopamine release and psychosis. Thus psychosis would be considered a downstream event resulting from a disruption in critical glutamatergic-GABAergic synaptic function in the cerebral cortex.

ANXIETY AND DEPRESSION. GABAergic dysfunction has been associated with anxiety disorders, especially panic disorder, as well as with major depressive disorder. Clinically, there is considerable comorbidity between anxiety and affective disorders. Decreased levels of the GABA$_A$ receptor modulators, the three α-reduced neuroactive steroids, have been found both in plasma and in CSF in major depressive disorder. Effective treatment with SSRIs increases the neurosteroid levels. In contrast, in patients with panic disorder, the plasma neurosteroid levels were significantly elevated, perhaps as a compensatory mechanism. Magnetic resonance spectroscopy (MRS) has disclosed significant reductions in GABA levels in the anterior cingulate and the basal ganglia of medicated patients with panic disorder. PET scanning reveals a highly selective reduction in benzodiazepine receptor sites bilaterally in the insular cortex in panic disorder. A genome-wide screen has shown significant linkage at 15q in a region containing GABA$_A$ receptor subunit genes and panic disorder. MRS reveals significant reductions in both GABA and glutamate/glutamine (Glx) in the prefrontal cortex in major depressive disorder. Postmortem studies indicate upregulation of the GABA$_A$ receptor α_1 and β_3 subunits in the cerebral cortices of depressed patients who committed suicide, consistent with a reduction in GABAergic neurotransmission. The reduced levels of GABA in the occipital cortex in episodes of major depressive disorder normalized with effective treatment with SSRI or with ECT.

Glutamatergic dysfunction has also been implicated in depression. NMDA receptor antagonists have antidepressant effects in several animal models of depression, including forced swim, tail suspension, and learned helplessness. A single injection of ketamine protects the induction of behavioral despair in rats for up to 10 days. Chronic treatment with antidepressants alters the expression of NMDA receptor subunits and decreases glycine receptor B binding. Two placebo-controlled clinical trials have shown that a single dose of ketamine can produce a rapid, substantial, and persistent reduction in symptoms in patients with major depressive disorder.

ALCOHOLISM. Ethanol at concentrations associated with intoxication has a dual action of enhancing GABAergic receptor function and attenuating the NMDA receptor function. The GABA receptor effects may be associated with the anxiolytic effects of ethanol. Persistent abuse and dependency on ethanol result in a downregulation of GABA$_A$ receptors and an upregulation of NMDA receptors such that acute discontinuation of ethanol results in a hyperexcitable state characterized by delirium tremens. Furthermore, supersensitive NMDA receptors in the context of thiamine deficiency may contribute to the excitotoxic neuron degeneration of Wernicke–Korsakoff syndrome.

Acamprosate is a derivative of homotaurine that was developed as an agent to reduce alcohol consumption, craving, and relapse in alcoholic patients, for which it exhibits moderate efficacy in clinical trials. Because taurine resembles GABA, it was thought that acamprosate acted via GABA$_A$ receptors, but electrophysiologic studies found little evidence to support this hypothesis. Subsequent studies demonstrated that it inhibited NMDA receptor responses in cortical slices and recombinant NMDA receptors. The precise mechanism whereby acamprosate alters NMDA receptor function, however, remains unclear.

Fetal alcohol syndrome is the most common preventable cause of mental retardation. Convincing evidence has been developed that the microencephaly associated with fetal alcohol exposure results from inhibition of NMDA receptor function, resulting in widespread neuronal apoptosis in the immature cortex. NMDA receptor activation is essential for immature neuronal survival and differentiation.

Neuropeptides

Neuropeptides represent the most diverse class of signaling molecules in the CNS. Initially discovered for their role in the hypothalamic regulation of pituitary hormone secretion, the complex role of peptides in brain function has emerged over the last 30 years. Many neuropeptides and their receptors are widely distributed within the CNS, where they have an extraordinary array of direct or neuromodulatory effects, ranging from modulating neurotransmitter release and neuronal firing patterns to the regulation of emotionality and complex behaviors. More than 100 unique biologically active neuropeptides have been identified in the brain, a subset of which is presented in Table 33-3. Adding to the complexity of neuropeptide systems in the CNS, the actions of many peptides are mediated via multiple receptor subtypes localized in different brain regions. The discovery of new peptides and receptor subtypes has outpaced our understanding of the roles of these peptides in normal or aberrant CNS function. Pharmacologic, molecular, and genetic approaches are now leading the way in our understanding of the contribution of neuropeptide systems in psychiatric disorders.

Neuropeptides have been implicated in the regulation of a variety of behavioral and physiologic processes, including thermoregulation, food and water consumption, sex, sleep, locomotion, learning and memory, responses to stress and pain, emotion, and social cognition. Involvement in such behavioral processes suggests that neuropeptidergic systems may contribute to the symptoms and behaviors exhibited in major psychiatric illnesses such as psychoses, mood disorders, dementia, and ASDs.

Investigating Neuropeptide Function. The roles of neuropeptides in CNS function and behavior have been examined using a multitude of experimental techniques. The levels of analysis include the following: Molecular structure and biosynthesis of the peptide and its receptor(s), the neuroanatomical localization of the peptide and its receptor(s), the regulation of the expression and release of the peptide, and the behavioral effects of the peptide. Most information on neuropeptide biology is derived from laboratory animal studies; however, there is a growing database on the localization, activity, and potential psychiatric relevance of several neuropeptide systems in humans.

Most neuropeptide structures have been identified based on the chemical analysis of purified biologically active peptides, leading ultimately to the cloning and characterization of the genes encoding them. Characterization of the gene structure of peptides and their receptors has provided insight into the molecular regulation of these systems, and their chromosomal localization is useful in genetic studies examining the potential roles of these genes in psychiatric disorders. Structural characterization permits the production of immunologic and molecular probes that are useful in determining peptide distribution and regulation in the brain. Quantitative radioimmunoassays on microdissected brain regions or immunocytochemistry on brain sections are typically used to localize the distribution of peptide within the brain. Both techniques use specific antibodies generated against the neuropeptide to detect the presence of the peptide. Immunocytochemistry allows researchers to visualize the precise cellular localization of peptide-synthesizing cells as well as their projections throughout the brain, although the technique is generally not quantitative. With molecular probes homologous to the mRNA encoding the peptides or receptor, in situ hybridization can be used to localize and quantify gene expression in brain sections. This technique is a powerful way to examine the molecular regulation of neuropeptide synthesis with a precise neuroanatomical resolution, which is impossible for other classes of nonpeptide neurotransmitters that are not derived directly from the translation of mRNAs, such as dopamine, serotonin, and norepinephrine.

Generally, the behavioral effects of neuropeptides are initially investigated by infusions of the peptide directly into the brain. Unlike many nonpeptide neurotransmitters, most neuropeptides do not penetrate the BBB in amounts sufficient enough to produce CNS effects. Furthermore, serum and tissue enzymes tend to degrade the peptides before they reach their target sites. The degradation is usually the result of the cleavage of specific amino acid sequences targeted by a specific peptidase designed for that purpose. Thus, intracerebroventricular (ICV) or site-specific infusions of the peptide in animal models are generally required to probe for the behavioral effects of peptides. However, there are examples of the delivery of neuropeptides via intranasal infusions in human subjects, which may help the peptide access the brain.

One of the most significant impediments for exploring the roles and potential therapeutic values of neuropeptides is the inability of the peptides or their agonists/antagonists to penetrate the BBB. Thus the behavioral effects of most peptides in humans are mostly uninvestigated, except for a few studies utilizing intranasal delivery. However, in some instances, small-molecule, nonpeptide agonists/antagonists have been developed that can be administered peripherally and permeate the BBB in sufficient quantities to affect receptor activation.

Table 33-3
Selected Neuropeptide Transmitters

Adrenocorticotropic hormone (ACTH)
Angiotensin
Atrial natriuretic peptide
Bombesin
Calcitonin
Calcitonin gene-related peptide (CGRP)
Cocaine and amphetamine regulated transcript (CART)
Cholecystokinin (CCK)
Corticotropin-releasing factor (CRF)
Dynorphin
β-Endorphin
Leu-enkephalin
Met-enkephalin
Galanin
Gastrin
Gonadotropin-releasing hormone (GnRH)
Growth hormone
Growth hormone-releasing hormone (GHRH; GRF)
Insulin
Motilin
Neuropeptide S
Neuropeptide Y (NPY)
Neurotensin
Neuromedin N
Orphanin FQ/Nociceptin
Orexin
Oxytocin
Pancreatic polypeptide
Prolactin
Secretin
Somatostatin (SS; SRIF)
Substance K
Substance P
Thyrotropin-releasing hormone (TRH)
Urocortin (1, 2, and 3)
Vasoactive intestinal polypeptide (VIP)
Vasopressin (AVP; ADH)

From Sadock BJ, Sadock VA, Ruiz P. *Kaplan & Sadock's Comprehensive Textbook of Psychiatry.* 9th ed. Philadelphia, PA: Lippincott Williams & Wilkins; 2009:84.

The use of pretreatment and posttreatment CSF samples or of samples obtained during the active disease state versus when the patient is in remission addresses some of the limitations in study design. For such progressive diseases as schizophrenia or Alzheimer disease, serial CSF samples may be a valuable indicator of disease progression or response to treatment. Even with these constraints, significant progress has been made in describing the effects of various psychiatric disease states on neuropeptide systems in the CNS.

Biosynthesis.   Unlike other neurotransmitters, neuropeptide biosynthesis involves mRNA transcription from a specific gene, translation of an mRNA-encoded polypeptide preprohormone, and posttranslational processing involving proteolytic cleavage of the preprohormone. Over the last 25 years, the gene structures and biosynthetic pathways of many neuropeptides have been elucidated. The gene structure of selected neuropeptides is illustrated in Figure 33-22. Neuropeptide genes are generally composed of multiple exons that encode a protein preprohormone. The N-terminus of the preprohormone contains a signal peptide sequence, which guides the growing polypeptide to the rough endoplasmic reticulum (RER) membrane. The single preprohormone molecule often contains the sequences

of multiple peptides that are subsequently separated by proteolytic cleavage by specific enzymes. For example, translation of the gene encoding NT yields a preprohormone, which upon enzymatic cleavage produces both NT and neuromedin N.

Distribution and Regulation.   Although many neuropeptides were initially isolated from the pituitary and peripheral tissues, the majority of neuropeptides were subsequently found to be widely distributed throughout the brain. Those peptides involved in regulating pituitary secretion are concentrated in the hypothalamus. Hypothalamic releasing and inhibiting factors are produced in neurosecretory neurons adjacent to the third ventricle that send projections to the median eminence where they contact and release peptide into the hypothalamohypophysial portal circulatory system. Peptides produced in these neurons are often subject to regulation by the peripheral hormones that they regulate. For example, thyrotropin-releasing hormone (TRH) regulates the secretion of thyroid hormones, and thyroid hormones negatively feedback on TRH gene expression. However, neuropeptide-expressing neurons and their projections are found in many other brain regions, including limbic structures, midbrain, hindbrain, and spinal cord.

FIGURE 33-22

Schematics illustrating the gene structure, preprohormone messenger RNA (mRNA), and processed neuropeptides of thyrotropin-releasing hormone (TRH), corticotropin-releasing factor (CRF), oxytocin (OT), arginine vasopressin (AVP), and neurotensin (NT). *Boxed regions* indicate the locations of the exons in the respective genes. *Shaded or hatched regions* indicate coding regions. Each preprohormone begins with a signal peptide (SP) sequence. *Black boxes* indicate the locations of the sequences encoding the neuropeptide. (From Sadock BJ, Sadock VA, Ruiz P. *Kaplan & Sadock's Comprehensive Textbook of Psychiatry.* 9th ed. Philadelphia, PA: Lippincott Williams & Wilkins; 2009:87.)

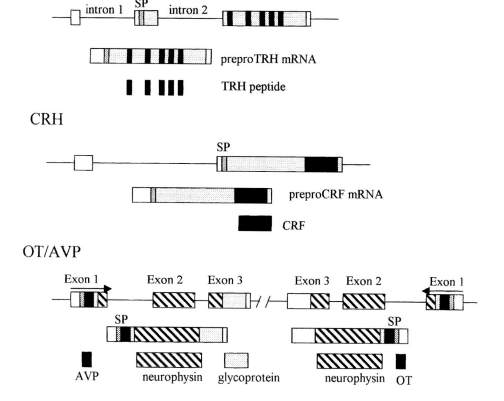

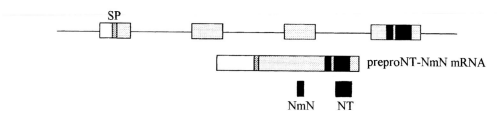

Neuropeptide Signaling.   Neuropeptides may act as neurotransmitters, neuromodulators, or neurohormones. Neurotransmitters are typically released from axonal terminals into a synapse where they change the postsynaptic membrane potential, either depolarizing or hyperpolarizing the cell. For classical neurotransmitters, this often involves direct modulation of voltage-gated ion channels. In contrast, neuromodulators and neurohormones do not directly affect the firing of the target cell itself but may alter the response of the cell to other neurotransmitters through the modulation of second messenger pathways. Neuropeptide release is not restricted to synapses or axon terminals but may occur throughout the axon or even from dendrites.

Specific neuropeptide receptors mediate the cellular signaling of neuropeptides. Thus understanding neuropeptide receptor function is essential for understanding neuropeptide biology. Neuropeptide receptors have undergone the same process of discovery and characterization that receptors for other neurotransmitters have enjoyed. Most neuropeptide receptors are G-protein–coupled, seven-transmembrane domain receptors belonging to the same family of proteins as the monoamine receptors.

Molecular technology has made it possible to clone and characterize neuropeptide receptor genes and complementary DNAs (cDNAs). This process is most often accomplished in one of three ways. First, the neuropeptide receptor protein is biochemically purified and partially sequenced, which allows the development of oligonucleotide probes that can be used to isolate the cDNA encoding the protein from a cDNA library. A second approach involves producing expression libraries in which cells containing the receptor cDNA can be isolated based on their ability to bind to a radiolabeled peptide ligand. Finally, many neuropeptide receptors are now isolated based on their sequence homology with other known peptide receptors. Once the cDNA of the receptor has been isolated, it can be used to produce purified receptor protein for structural and functional studies. By mutation of specific amino acids in the receptor structure and determination of relative binding affinities of peptides with various amino acid substitutions, it is possible to elucidate the nature of the ligand–receptor interaction. This information facilitates the development of drugs that specifically modulate receptor function, including nonpeptide drugs, leading to the ability to manipulate peptide systems in ways that are currently enjoyed by the more classic neurotransmitters. The availability of cDNAs encoding the receptor also permits the neuroanatomical mapping of the receptor-producing cells in the brain, which is critical for understanding the neural circuits modulated by the peptide. Finally, with the cloned receptor in hand, it is possible to use transgenic techniques, such as targeted gene overexpression or gene knockouts, to elucidate the functions of these receptors further. siRNA techniques now allow the targeted synthesis disruption of specific receptor populations, allowing researchers to examine the roles of these receptor populations on physiology and behavior.

The following three factors determine the biologic roles of a neuropeptide hormone: (1) the temporal-anatomical release of the peptide, (2) functional coupling of the neuropeptide receptor to intracellular signaling pathways, and (3) the cell type and circuits in which the receptor is expressed. Genetic studies have demonstrated that regulatory sequences flanking the receptor coding region determine the expression pattern of the receptor and thus the physiologic and behavioral response to the neuropeptide.

Peptidases.   Unlike monoamine neurotransmitters, peptides are not actively taken up by presynaptic nerve terminals. Instead, released peptides are degraded into smaller fragments, and eventually into single amino acids by specific enzymes termed peptidases.

The enzymes may be found bound to presynaptic or postsynaptic neural membranes or in solution in the cytoplasm and extracellular fluid, and they are distributed widely in peripheral organs and serum as well as in the CNS. As a result, neuropeptides generally have half-lives on the order of minutes once released.

Specific Neuropeptides as Prototypes of Neuropeptide Biology

THYROTROPIN-RELEASING HORMONE.   In 1969, TRH, a pyroglutamylhistidylprolinamide tripeptide (Table 33-4), became the first of the hypothalamic releasing hormones to be isolated and characterized. The discovery of the structure of this hormone led to the conclusive demonstration that peptide hormones secreted from the hypothalamus regulate the secretion of hormones from the anterior pituitary. The gene for TRH in humans resides on chromosome 3q13.3–q21. In the rat, it consists of three exons (coding regions) separated by two introns (noncoding sequences) (see Fig. 33-22). The first exon contains the 5′ untranslated region of the mRNA encoding the TRH preprohormone, the second exon contains the signal peptide (SP) sequence and much of the remaining N-terminal end of the precursor peptide, and the third contains the remainder of the sequence, including five copies of the TRH precursor sequence, the C-terminal region, and the 3′ untranslated region. The 5′ flanking of the gene, or promoter, contains sequences homologous to the glucocorticoid receptor and the DNA-binding sites for thyroid hormone, providing a mechanism for the regulation of this gene by cortisol and negative feedback by thyroid hormone. Enzymatic processing of TRH begins with excision of the progenitor peptides by carboxypeptidases, amidation of the C-terminal proline, and cyclization of the N-terminal glutamine to yield five TRH molecules per prohormone molecule. TRH is widely distributed in the CNS with TRH immunoreactive neurons being located in the olfactory bulbs, entorhinal cortices, hippocampus, extended amygdala, hypothalamus, and midbrain structures. As is the case for most neuropeptides, the TRH receptor is also a member of the seven-transmembrane domain, G-protein–coupled receptor family.

Hypothalamic TRH neurons project nerve terminals to the median eminence; there, they release TRH into the hypothalamohypophyseal portal system where it is transported to the adenohypophysis, causing the release of thyroid-stimulating hormone (TSH) into the systemic circulation. TSH subsequently stimulates the release of the thyroid hormones triiodothyronine (T_3) and thyroxine (T_4)

Table 33-4
Selected Neuropeptide Structures

Name	Amino Acid Sequence
Thyrotropin-releasing hormone (TRH)	pE-H-P-NH$_2$
Corticotropin-releasing factor (CRF)	S-E-E-P-P-I-S-L-D-L-T-F-H-L-L-R-E-V-L-E-M-A-R-A-E-Q-L-A-Q-Q-A-H-S-N-R-K-L-M-E-I-I-NH$_2$
Arginine vasopressin (AVP)	C-Y-I-Q-N-C-P-L-G-NH$_2$
Oxytocin (OT)	C-Y-F-Q-N-C-P-R-G-NH$_2$
Neurotensin (NT)	pE-L-Y-E-N-K-P-R-R-P-Y-I-L-OH

Note the cyclized glutamines at the N-termini of TRH and NT indicated by pE-, the cysteine–cysteine disulfide bonds of AVP and OT, and the amidated C-termini of TRH, CRF, AVP, and OT.

From Sadock BJ, Sadock VA, Ruiz P. *Kaplan & Sadock's Comprehensive Textbook of Psychiatry.* 9th ed. Philadelphia, PA: Lippincott Williams & Wilkins; 2009:85.

from the thyroid gland. TRH neurons in the paraventricular nucleus (PVN) contain thyroid hormone receptors and respond to increases in thyroid hormone secretion with a decrease in TRH gene expression and synthesis. This negative feedback of thyroid hormones on the TRH-synthesizing neurons was first demonstrated by a decrease in TRH content in the median eminence, but not in the PVN of the hypothalamus after thyroidectomy. This effect can be reversed with exogenous thyroid hormone treatment. The treatment of normal rats with exogenous thyroid hormone decreases TRH concentration in the PVN and the posterior nucleus of the hypothalamus. With a probe against the TRH preprohormone mRNA, in situ hybridization studies have demonstrated that TRH mRNA is increased in the PVN 14 days after thyroidectomy. The ability of thyroid hormones to regulate TRH mRNA can be superseded by other stimuli that activate the hypothalamic–pituitary–thyroid (HPT) axis. In that regard, repeated exposure to cold (which releases TRH from the median eminence) induces increases in the levels of TRH mRNA in the PVN despite concomitantly elevated concentrations of thyroid hormones.

Further evidence of the different levels of communication of the HPT axis is seen in the ability of TRH to regulate the production of mRNA for the pituitary TRH receptor. It is also seen for TRH concentrations to regulate the mRNA coding for both the α and β subunits of the thyrotropin (TSH) molecule. Also, TRH-containing synaptic boutons have been observed in contact with TRH-containing cell bodies in the medial and periventricular subdivisions of the paraventricular nucleus, thus providing anatomical evidence for ultrashort feedback regulation of TRH release. Negative feedback by thyroid hormones may be limited to the hypothalamic TRH neurons because negative feedback on TRH synthesis by thyroid hormones has not been found in extrahypothalamic TRH neurons.

The early availability of adequate tools to assess HPT axis function (i.e., radioimmunoassays and synthetic peptides), coupled with observations that primary hypothyroidism is associated with depressive symptomatology, ensured extensive investigation of the involvement of this axis in affective disorders. Early studies established the hypothalamic and extrahypothalamic distribution of TRH. This extrahypothalamic presence of TRH quickly led to speculation that TRH might function as a neurotransmitter or neuromodulator. Indeed, a large body of evidence supports such a role for TRH. Within the CNS, TRH is known to modulate several different neurotransmitters, including dopamine, serotonin, acetylcholine, and opioids. TRH has been shown to arouse hibernating animals and counteracts the behavioral response and hypothermia produced by a variety of CNS depressants, including barbiturates and ethanol.

The use of TRH as a provocative agent for the assessment of the HPT axis function evolved rapidly after its isolation and synthesis. Clinical use of a standardized TRH stimulation test, which measures negative feedback responses, revealed blunting of the TSH response in approximately 25 percent of euthyroid patients with major depression. These data have been widely confirmed. The observed TSH blunting in depressed patients does not appear to be the result of excessive negative feedback due to hyperthyroidism because thyroid measures such as basal plasma concentrations of TSH and thyroid hormones are generally in the normal range in these patients. TSH blunting may be a reflection of pituitary TRH receptor downregulation due to median eminence hypersecretion of endogenous TRH. Indeed, the observation that CSF TRH concentrations are elevated in depressed patients as compared to those of controls supports the hypothesis of TRH hypersecretion but does not elucidate the regional CNS origin of this tripeptide. TRH mRNA expression in the PVN of the hypothalamus is decreased in patients with major depression. However, it is not clear whether

the altered HPT axis represents a causal mechanism underlying the symptoms of depression or only a secondary effect of depression-associated alterations in other neural systems.

CORTICOTROPIN-RELEASING FACTOR (CRF) AND UROCORTINS. There is convincing evidence to support the hypothesis that CRF and the urocortins play an intricate role in integrating the endocrine, autonomic, immunologic, and behavioral responses of an organism to stress.

Although it was initially isolated because of its functions in regulating the HPA axis, CRF is widely distributed throughout the brain. The PVN of the hypothalamus is the primary site of CRF-containing cell bodies that influence anterior pituitary hormone secretion. These neurons originate in the parvocellular region of the PVN and send axon terminals to the median eminence, where CRF is released into the portal system in response to stressful stimuli. A small group of PVN neurons also projects to the brainstem and spinal cord, where they regulate autonomic aspects of the stress response. CRF-containing neurons are also found in other hypothalamic nuclei, the neocortex, the extended amygdala, brainstem, and spinal cord. Central CRF infusion into laboratory animals produces physiologic changes and behavioral effects similar to those observed following stress, including increased locomotor activity, increased responsiveness to an acoustic startle, and decreased exploratory behavior in an open field.

The physiologic and behavioral roles of the urocortins are less understood, but several studies suggest that urocortins 2 and 3 are anxiolytic and may dampen the stress response. This research has led to the hypothesis that CRF and the urocortins act in opposition, but this is likely an oversimplification. Urocortin 1 is primarily synthesized in the Edinger–Westphal nucleus, lateral olivary nucleus, and supraoptic hypothalamic nucleus. Urocortin 2 is synthesized primarily in the hypothalamus, while urocortin three-cell bodies are found more broadly in the extended amygdala, perifornical area, and preoptic area.

Hyperactivity of the HPA axis in major depression remains one of the most consistent findings in biologic psychiatry. The reported HPA axis alterations in major depression include hypercortisolemia, resistance to dexamethasone suppression of cortisol secretion (a measure of negative feedback), blunted adrenocorticotropic hormone (ACTH) responses to intravenous CRF challenge, increased cortisol responses in the combined dexamethasone/CRF test, and elevated CSF CRF concentrations. The exact pathologic mechanism(s) underlying HPA axis dysregulation in major depression and other affective disorders remains to be elucidated.

Mechanistically, two hypotheses have been advanced to account for the ACTH blunting following exogenous CRF administration. The first hypothesis suggests that pituitary CRF receptor downregulation occurs as a result of hypothalamic CRF hypersecretion. The second hypothesis postulates the altered sensitivity of the pituitary to glucocorticoid negative feedback. Substantial support has accumulated favoring the first hypothesis. However, neuroendocrine studies represent a secondary measure of CNS activity; the pituitary ACTH responses principally reflect the activity of hypothalamic CRF rather than that of the corticolimbic CRF circuits. The latter of the two is more likely to be involved in the pathophysiology of depression.

Of particular interest is the demonstration that the elevated CSF CRF concentrations in drug-free depressed patients are significantly decreased after successful treatment with ECT, indicating that CSF CRF concentrations, like hypercortisolemia, represent a state rather than a trait marker. Other recent studies have confirmed this normalization of CSF CRF concentrations following successful treatment with fluoxetine. One group demonstrated a significant reduction of elevated CSF CRF concentrations in 15 female patients with major depression who remained depression-free for at least 6 months following antidepressant treatment, as compared to little significant treatment effect on CSF CRF concentrations in 9 patients who relapsed in these 6 months. This finding suggests that elevated or increasing CSF CRF concentrations during antidepressant treatment may be the harbinger of an inadequate response in major depression despite early symptomatic improvement. Of interest, treatment of normal subjects with desipramine or, as noted above, of individuals with depression with fluoxetine is associated with a reduction in CSF CRF concentrations.

If CRF hypersecretion is a factor in the pathophysiology of depression, then reducing or interfering with CRF neurotransmission might be an effective strategy to alleviate depressive symptoms. Over the last several years, several pharmaceutical companies have committed considerable effort to the development of small-molecule CRF_1 receptor antagonists that can effectively penetrate the BBB. Several compounds have been produced with reportedly promising characteristics.

OXYTOCIN (OT) AND VASOPRESSIN (AVP).   The vasopressor effects of posterior pituitary extracts were first described in 1895, and the potent extracts were named AVP. OT and AVP mRNAs are among the most abundant messages in the hypothalamus, being heavily concentrated in the magnocellular neurons of the PVN and the supraoptic nucleus of the hypothalamus, which send axonal projections to the neurohypophysis. These neurons produce OT and AVP, which is released into the bloodstream, where these peptides act like hormones on peripheral targets. OT and AVP are generally synthesized in separate neurons within the hypothalamus. OT released from the pituitary is most often associated with functions associated with female reproduction, such as regulating uterine contractions during parturition and the milk ejection reflex during lactation. AVP, also known as antidiuretic hormone, regulates water retention in the kidney and vasoconstriction through interactions with vasopressin V2 and V1a receptor subtypes, respectively. AVP is released into the bloodstream from the neurohypophysis following a variety of stimuli, including plasma osmolality, hypovolemia, hypertension, and hypoglycemia. The actions of OT are mediated via a single receptor subtype (oxytocin receptor, OTR), which is distributed in the periphery and within the limbic CNS.

In contrast to the OTR, there are three vasopressin receptor subtypes, V1a, V1b, and V2 receptors, each of which is a G-protein–coupled seven-transmembrane domain receptor. The V2 receptor is localized in the kidney and is not found in the brain. The V1a receptor is distributed widely in the CNS and is thought to mediate most of the behavioral effects of AVP. The V1b receptor is concentrated in the anterior pituitary, and some reports describe V1b receptor mRNA in the brain, although its function is unknown.

Neurotensin (NT).   Although NT is found in several brain regions, it has been most thoroughly investigated in terms of its association with other neurotransmitter systems, particularly the mesolimbic dopamine system, and has gained interest in research on the pathophysiology of schizophrenia. There are several lines of evidence suggesting that NT and its receptors should be considered as potential targets for pharmacologic intervention in this disorder. First, the NT system is positioned anatomically to modulate the neural circuits implicated in schizophrenia. Second, peripheral administration of antipsychotic drugs has been shown to modulate NT systems consistently. Third, there is evidence that central NT systems are altered in patients with schizophrenia.

NT was first shown to interact with dopamine systems while undergoing characterization of its potent hypothermic-potentiating and sedative-potentiating activities. Subsequent work indicated that NT possessed many properties that were also shared by antipsychotic drugs, including the ability to inhibit avoidance, but not escape responding in a conditioned active avoidance task; the ability to block the effects of indirect dopamine agonists or endogenous dopamine in the production of locomotor behavior; and the ability to elicit increases in dopamine release and turnover. Perhaps most importantly, both antipsychotic drugs and NT neurotransmission enhance sensorimotor gating. Sensorimotor gating is the ability to screen or filter relevant sensory input, deficits in which may lead to involuntary flooding of indifferent sensory data. Increasing evidence suggests that deficits in sensorimotor gating are a cardinal feature of schizophrenia. Both dopamine agonists and NT antagonists disrupt performance on tasks designed to gauge sensorimotor gating. Unlike antipsychotic drugs, NT is not able to displace dopamine from its receptor. As noted earlier, NT is colocalized in specific subsets of dopamine neurons and is coreleased with dopamine in the mesolimbic and medial prefrontal cortex dopamine terminal regions that are implicated as the sites of dopamine dysregulation in schizophrenia. Antipsychotic drugs that act at D_2 and D_4 receptors increase the synthesis, concentration, and release of NT in those dopamine terminal regions but not in others. That effect of antipsychotic drugs in increasing NT concentrations persists after months of treatment and is accompanied by the expected increase in NT mRNA concentrations as well as expression of the "immediate early gene" c-fos within hours of initial drug treatment. The altered regulation of NT expression by antipsychotic drugs extends to the peptidases that degrade the peptide because recent reports have revealed decreased NT metabolism in rat brain slices 24 hours after the acute administration of haloperidol. When administered directly into the brain, NT preferentially opposes dopamine transmission in the nucleus accumbens but not the caudate-putamen. In the nucleus accumbens, NT receptors are located predominantly on GABAergic neurons, which release GABA on dopamine terminals, thereby inhibiting release.

Decreased CSF NT concentrations have been reported in several populations of patients with schizophrenia when compared to those of controls or other psychiatric disorders. Although treatment with antipsychotic drugs has been observed to increase NT concentrations in the CSF, it is not known whether this increase is causal or merely accompanies the decrease in psychotic symptoms seen with successful treatment. Postmortem studies have shown an increase in NT concentrations in the dopamine-rich Brodmann area 32 of the frontal cortex, but that result may have been confounded by premortem antipsychotic treatment. Other researchers have found no postmortem alterations in NT concentrations of a broad sampling of subcortical regions. Decreases in NT receptor densities in the entorhinal cortex have been reported in entorhinal cortices of schizophrenic postmortem samples. A critical test of the hypothesis that NT may act as an endogenous antipsychotic-like substance awaits the development of an NT receptor agonist that can penetrate the BBB.

Other Neuropeptides.   Several other neuropeptides have been implicated in the pathophysiology of psychiatric disorders. These include, but are not limited to, cholecystokinin (CCK), substance P, and neuropeptide Y.

CCK initially discovered in the gastrointestinal tract, and its receptors are found in areas of the brain associated with emotion, motivation, and sensory processing (e.g., cortex, striatum, hypothalamus, hippocampus, and amygdala). CCK is often colocalized with dopamine in the VTA neurons that comprise the mesolimbic and mesocortical dopamine circuits. Like NT, CCK decreases dopamine release. Infusions of a CCK fragment have been reported to induce panic in healthy individuals, and patients with panic disorder exhibit increased sensitivity to the CCK fragment compared to that of normal controls. Pentagastrin, a synthetic CCK agonist, dose-dependently produced increased blood pressure, pulse, HPA activation, and physical symptoms of panic. Recently, a CCK receptor gene polymorphism has been associated with panic disorder.

The undecapeptide substance P is localized in the amygdala, hypothalamus, periaqueductal gray, LC, and parabrachial nucleus and is colocalized with norepinephrine and serotonin. Substance P serves as a pain neurotransmitter, and administration to animals elicits behavioral and cardiovascular effects resembling the stress response. More recent data suggest a role for substance P in major depression and PTSD. Both depressed and PTSD patients had elevated CSF substance P concentrations. Furthermore, in PTSD patients, marked increases in CSF substance P concentrations were detected following precipitation of PTSD symptoms. One study has indicated that a substance P receptor (termed the neurokinin 1 [NK1] receptor) antagonist capable of passing the BBB is more effective than a placebo and as useful as paroxetine in patients with major depression with moderate to severe symptom severity. However, subsequent studies have been unable to confirm these findings.

Neuropeptide Y (NPY) is a 36 amino acid peptide found in the hypothalamus, brainstem, spinal cord, and several limbic structures and is involved in the regulation of appetite, reward, anxiety, and energy balance. NPY is colocalized with serotonergic and noradrenergic neurons and is thought to facilitate the containment of adverse effects following exposure to stress. Suicide victims with a diagnosis of major depression are reported to have a pronounced reduction in NPY levels in the frontal cortex and caudate nucleus. Furthermore, CSF NPY levels are decreased in depressed patients. Chronic administration of antidepressant drugs increases neuropeptide Y concentrations in the neocortex and hippocampus in rats. Plasma NPY levels were found to be elevated in soldiers subjected to the "uncontrollable stress" of interrogation, and NPY levels were correlated with the feelings of dominance and confidence during the stress. Also, low NPY response to stress has been associated with increased vulnerability to depression and PTSD.

Novel Neurotransmitters

Nitric Oxide. The discovery that gases could function as neurotransmitters revealed that highly atypical modes of signaling existed between neurons. In the early 1990s, nitric oxide was the first gas to be ascribed a neurotransmitter function and proved to be an atypical neurotransmitter for several reasons. First, it was not stored in or released from synaptic vesicles, as it was a small gas it could freely diffuse into the target neuron. Second, its target was not a specific receptor on the surface of a target neuron, but intracellular proteins whose activity could directly be modulated by nitric oxide, leading to neurotransmission. Nitric oxide also lacks a reuptake mechanism to remove it from the synapse. Although enzymatic inactivation of it is postulated to exist, nitric oxide appears to have a very short half-life of a few seconds.

Nitric oxide was initially discovered as a bactericidal compound released from macrophages, and as an endothelial cell, it derived relaxation factor allowing for the dilation of blood vessels. A role for nitric oxide in the brain followed, revealing a role for the gas in neurotransmission, learning and memory processes, neurogenesis, and neurodegenerative disease.

NITRIC OXIDE AND BEHAVIOR.   Nitric oxide neurotransmission can play a role in behavior, as neuronal nitric oxide synthase (nNOS)-deficient male mice display exaggerated aggressive tendencies and increased sexual activity. In female mice, the contrary is true, as they have reduced aggression. As manic bipolar patients may show both hypersexuality and aggression, the nitric oxide pathway may participate in the psychopathology of affective states.

In the periphery, nNOS localizes to neurons that innervate blood vessels of the penis, including the corpus cavernosa. Stimulation of these nerves releases nitric oxide, leading to cyclic guanosine monophosphate (cGMP) formation, blood vessel wall relaxation and vasodilation, penile engorgement, and initial erection. The sustained phase of erection also depends on nitric oxide; turbulent blood flow leads to phosphorylation of eNOS and sustained nitric oxide production. Drugs used in the treatment of erectile dysfunction—sildenafil (Viagra), tadalafil (Cialis), and vardenafil (Levitra)—act to inhibit phosphodiesterase type 5 (PDE5), an enzyme that degrades cGMP in the penis (Fig. 33-23), thereby potentiating nitric oxide neurotransmission and penile erection.

Numerous lines of evidence have suggested a role for nitric oxide in the regulation of sleep–wake cycles. nNOS expressing neurons occur in several areas that initiate REM sleep, including the pons, dorsal raphe nucleus, laterodorsal tegmentum, and pedunculopontine tegmentum. In animal models, microinjection of compounds that release nitric oxide decreases wakefulness and increases slow-wave sleep compared with controls. Consistent with this, NOS inhibitors show a trend toward decreasing slow-wave and REM sleep. Studies of NOS-deficient mice suggest that nitric oxide may serve a more involved role than merely promoting sleep. nNOS-deficient animals also show reduced REM sleep; however, inducible nitric oxide synthase (iNOS)-deficient mice demonstrate the reverse, suggesting a complex interplay between NOS enzymatic isoforms.

NITRIC OXIDE AND MOOD DISORDERS.   NOS-expressing neurons are well represented in areas implicated in depression, including the dorsal raphe nucleus and prefrontal cortex. A role for nitric oxide has been suggested in antidepressant response, as SSRI antidepressants can directly inhibit NOS activity. Moreover, in animal studies such as the forced swim test, NOS and soluble guanylyl cyclase inhibitors can achieve antidepressant-like effects. Plasma nitric oxide levels were elevated in patients with bipolar disorder compared to healthy controls. However, in depressed subjects, studies have found decreased nitric oxide levels and increased plasma nitrite, a byproduct of nitric oxide. Reduced NOS has also been described in the paraventricular nucleus of patients with schizophrenia and depression compared to controls.

Nitric oxide has been questioned as to its ability to regulate neurotransmission at serotonin, norepinephrine, and dopamine nerve termini. However, there has been no clear consensus, and nitric oxide appears to be able to increase or decrease activity at these neurons depending on the timing of its activation and the region of the brain studied.

NITRIC OXIDE AND SCHIZOPHRENIA.   Nitric oxide has been investigated as a candidate molecule contributing to symptoms of schizophrenia. Two genetic studies have identified schizophrenia-associated single nucleotide polymorphisms (SNPs) in CAPON, a protein that associates with nNOS. SNPs in nNOS itself have been associated with schizophrenia, although others have not been able to reproduce such findings. Changes in NOS levels have been reported in postmortem brain samples of individuals with schizophrenia. Abnormalities have been noted in the cortex, cerebellum, hypothalamus, and brainstem, although no specific trend can be

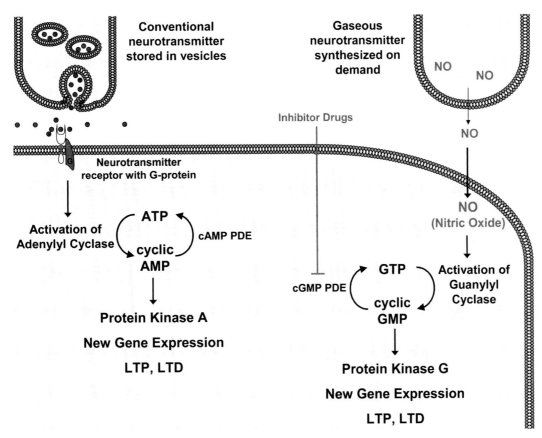

FIGURE 33-23

Neurotransmitter and signaling functions of nitric oxide (NO) via production of cyclic guanosine monophosphate (cGMP). Gaseous nitric oxide is enzymatically generated and freely diffuses into an adjacent neuron (*upper right*). In comparison to traditional neurotransmitters (*upper left*), nitric oxide (NO) does not act via a specific neurotransmitter receptor on the surface membrane of a neuron. In contrast, NO freely diffuses across the neuronal membrane and activates the enzyme, guanylyl cyclase, which converts guanosine 5'-triphosphate (GTP) into the second messenger, cGMP. Nitric oxide effects are mediated, in part, by cGMP activation of neuronal protein kinases, new gene expression, and effects on neuronal long-term potentiation (LTP) and long-term depression (LTD). ATP, adenosine triphosphate. (From Sadock BJ, Sadock VA, Ruiz P. *Kaplan & Sadock's Comprehensive Textbook of Psychiatry*. 9th ed. Philadelphia, PA: Lippincott Williams & Wilkins; 2009:104.)

discerned. Elevated NOS activity has been noted in platelets from drug-naive and drug-treated individuals with schizophrenia. Some investigators find increased nitric oxide activity and others the reverse. In autopsy samples, schizophrenic patients were found to have abnormally localized NOS expressing neurons in the prefrontal cortex, hippocampus, and lateral temporal lobe, consistent with abnormal migration of these neuronal types during development. In a rat model, prenatal stress led to reduced NOS expressing neurons in the fascia dentate and hippocampus.

NEUROPATHOLOGIC ROLES OF NITRIC OXIDE. Abundant evidence exists that nitric oxide is a direct participant in a variety of neuropathic events. Superoxide, a byproduct of cellular metabolism, can react with nitric oxide to form peroxynitrite (chemical formula $ONOO^-$). This labile and toxic compound forms chemical adducts with protein tyrosine residues, a process termed *protein nitration,* and DNA, leading to cellular dysfunction.

Cell loss resulting from ischemic stroke is mediated in part by overstimulation of the glutamate NMDA receptor, a process termed *excitotoxicity.* Nitric oxide produced by NMDA activation appears to mediate a significant portion of this excitotoxic neuronal death, and stroke damage is reduced in mice with a genetic deletion of nNOS.

S-Nitrosylation has also been implicated in pathologic processes in the brain. Mutations in the Parkin protein are associated with early-onset Parkinson disease. Parkin is an E3 ubiquitin ligase, adding ubiquitin molecules to proteins and targeting them for destruction in the cell proteasome. In sporadic Parkinson disease (i.e., without the early-onset mutation), nitric oxide can nitrosylate the Parkin protein and inhibit its protective E3 ubiquitin ligase function. An overabundance of nitric oxide signaling may thus predispose to the dysfunction and cell death of dopaminergic neurons in Parkinson disease by interfering with proteins essential for cell functioning. In Alzheimer disease, excess oxidation of brain protein, lipids, and carbohydrates has long been appreciated, but nitrosative stress from excess nitric oxide also appears to participate in the disease. Protein disulfide isomerase (PDI) is a cellular protective protein that may help combat the accumulation of misfolded proteins, such as the amyloid fibrils occurring in the disease. In both Alzheimer and Parkinson disease brains, PDI appears to be S-nitrosylated in a harmful way that impedes its cellular protective function.

The discovery that nitric oxide participates in neurodegenerative processes raises the possibility for improved diagnostic processes, such as detecting damage to cellular components produced by nitric oxide before the onset of full-blown symptoms. Also, drugs may be designed to attenuate the damage to crucial neuronal proteins that protect against disease onset. However, entirely and nonspecifically inhibiting or stimulating

NOS is likely to produce significant side effects because of its wide-ranging activities throughout the body.

Carbon Monoxide.

Although carbon monoxide (CO) is most well known as an air pollutant derived from combustion reactions, it is produced physiologically in a great variety of organisms ranging from human to bacterium. Once thought to be a toxic byproduct of metabolic reactions, carbon monoxide is increasingly recognized to play an essential role in regulating a variety of physiologic processes in the brain and other organs. These varied effects include regulation of olfactory neurotransmission, blood vessel relaxation, smooth muscle cell proliferation, and platelet aggregation.

Carbon monoxide is far better known for its toxic effects than its activities at physiologic concentrations. It binds tightly to heme molecules within hemoglobin, forming carboxyhemoglobin, which can no longer transport oxygen to tissues. One- to two-pack per day smokers typically have 3 to 8 percent of their hemoglobin as carboxyhemoglobin, with nonsmokers having less than 2 percent. Following acute carbon monoxide poisoning, 5 to 10 percent of carboxyhemoglobin is associated with impaired alertness and cognition, and 30 to 50 percent of carboxyhemoglobin leads to significant drops in oxygen transport to tissues.

CARBON MONOXIDE AND NEUROTRANSMISSION. Carbon monoxide appears to participate in the neurotransmission of odorant perception. Odorants lead to carbon monoxide production and subsequent cGMP synthesis that promotes long-term adaptation to odor stimuli. Carbon monoxide has the potential to regulate a variety of perceptual and cognitive processes that are yet untested. Similarly, in the rat retina, long periods of light exposure led to increased HO1 expression, carbon monoxide production, and cGMP signaling. Carbon monoxide may also participate in adaptation to chronic pain. HO2-deficient animals manifest reduced hyperalgesia and allodynia after exposure to chronic pain stimuli. Carbon monoxide may thus set the threshold for pain perception, although it is unclear whether the effect occurs in the central or peripheral nervous system. Aside from its role in promoting cGMP production, carbon monoxide may also directly bind to and open the calcium-activated big potassium (BK_{Ca}) channel, leading to as yet uncharacterized effects on neurotransmission.

In the gastrointestinal (GI) nervous system, carbon monoxide serves as a neurotransmitter to relax the internal anal sphincter in response to nonadrenergic noncholinergic (NANC) nerve stimulation and vasoactive intestinal peptide (VIP).

Carbon monoxide has been implicated in the development of hippocampal LTP, although lines of evidence are contradictory. Carbon monoxide and tetanic stimulation of nerves lead to increased excitatory postsynaptic potentials (EPSPs). HO inhibitors that block carbon monoxide production lead to impaired induction of LTP and reduced calcium-dependent release of glutamate neurotransmitter. However, HO_2-deficient animals fail to manifest any differences in LTP. These disparate findings may be explained by a role for HO_1 in LTP, or an ability of HO inhibitors to block some other processes necessary to LTP induction nonspecifically.

At toxic levels, carbon monoxide is well known to impair oxygen transport by binding to hemoglobin with a higher affinity than oxygen. Amazingly, carbon monoxide itself plays a physiologic role in the mechanism by which the carotid body senses oxygen. HO, expressed in glomus cells of the carotid body, uses oxygen as a substrate in the production of carbon monoxide (Fig. 33-24). When oxygen levels

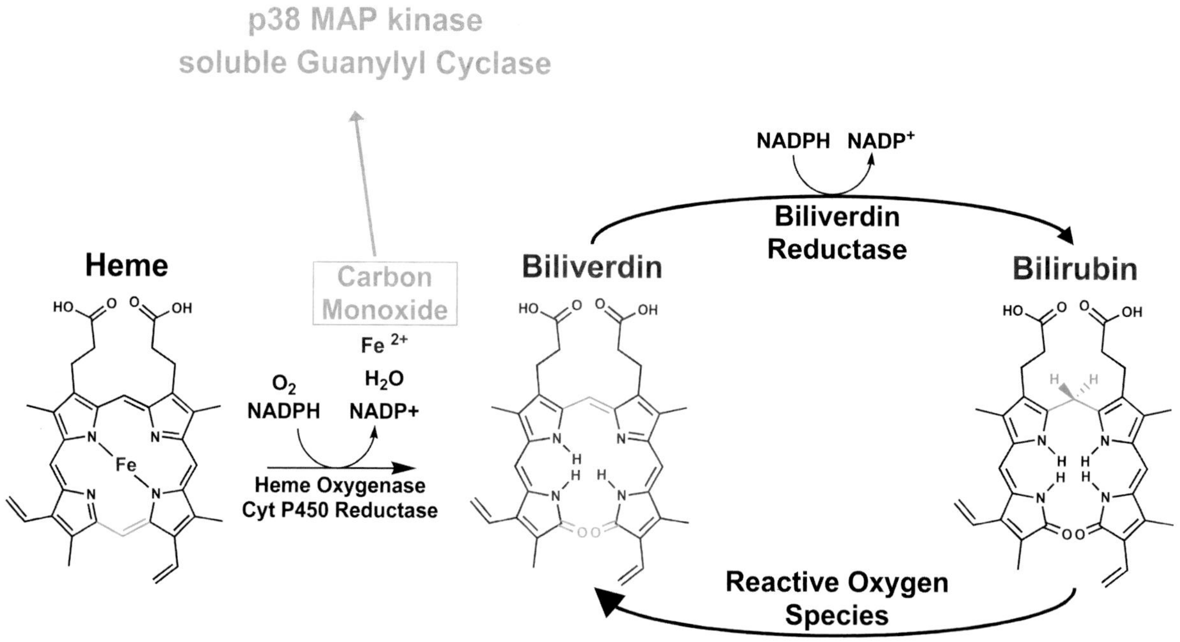

FIGURE 33-24

Synthesis of carbon monoxide (CO), an unexpected neurotransmitter. Gaseous carbon monoxide is enzymatically synthesized in neurons by way of the enzyme heme oxygenase, also converting heme into the molecule biliverdin and liberating free iron (Fe). Similar to nitric oxide, CO is not stored in neuronal vesicles and can freely diffuse across neuronal membranes. CO also similarly activates soluble guanylyl cyclase, and leads to activation of multiple intracellular signaling molecules such as p38 MAP kinase. CO exerts its neurotransmitter and signaling functions at concentrations far below that at which classical CO toxicity occurs. The significance of this pathway in neurons is underlined by the existence of two distinct heme oxygenase enzymes, one of which is predominantly expressed in the brain. Biliverdin is converted to bilirubin via the enzyme biliverdin reductase. Similar to CO, bilirubin is no longer relegated to the status of toxic byproduct and may be an important antioxidant. (From Sadock BJ, Sadock VA, Ruiz P. *Kaplan & Sadock's Comprehensive Textbook of Psychiatry.* 9th ed. Philadelphia, PA: Lippincott Williams & Wilkins; 2009:107.)

drop, so does carbon monoxide production, leading to a resetting of the threshold in which the carotid body senses oxygen. The molecular mechanism may occur via carbon monoxide regulation of the carotid body BK ion channel.

Endocannabinoids: From Marijuana to Neurotransmission.

Whether known as cannabis, hemp, hashish, ma-fen, or a variety of slang terms, marijuana has been cultivated and utilized by human populations for thousands of years. Despite a long debate about risks and benefits, it has only been in recent decades that we have started to learn how marijuana exerts its effects on the brain. The "high" users experience, euphoria and tranquility, relates to cannabis acting on a neural pathway involving cannabinoids endogenous to the human brain, or endocannabinoids.

The first described medicinal use of cannabis dates to approximately 2700 BC in the pharmacopeia of Chinese Emperor Shen Nung, who recommended its use for a variety of ailments. At this time, adverse properties were also apparent, and large amounts of the fruits of hemp could lead to "seeing devils," or a user might "communicate with spirits and lightens one's body." For centuries, cannabis was employed in India as an appetite stimulant; habitual marijuana users remain well acquainted with "the munchies."

For many years the mechanisms by which the active components of marijuana, *cannabinoids,* exerted their psychoactive effects remained a mystery. Chemists sought to isolate the psychoactive components of cannabis from the many components of the plant oil (Table 33-5).

Table 33-5
Selected Discoveries in Cannabinoid Research

1899	Cannabinol isolated from cannabis resin
1940	Identification of cannabinol structure
1964	Discovery of the structure of δ-9-tetrahydrocannabinol (THC), the most psychoactive component of cannabis
1988	Specific THC-binding sites identified in brain
1990	Identification of a brain cannabinoid receptor, CB1
1992	Discovery of the first endogenous brain endocannabinoid, anandamide
1993	Identification of a second cannabinoid receptor, CB2
1994	Rimonabant (Acomplia), a CB1 receptor blocker is developed
1995	Report of a second endocannabinoid, 2-AG
1996	Fatty acid amide hydrolase (FAAH), an endocannabinoid degrading enzyme, is discovered
2003	FAAH inhibitors reduce anxiety-like behaviors in animal studies
2003	Identification of enzymes that synthesize endocannabinoids
2006	Monoacylglycerol lipase (MAGL), a second endocannabinoid-degrading enzyme, is found
2006	Rimonabant approved for use in Europe for weight loss
2007	Rimonabant meta-analysis finds increased anxiety and depressive symptoms in humans without a history of psychiatric illness

From Sadock BJ, Sadock VA, Ruiz P. *Kaplan & Sadock's Comprehensive Textbook of Psychiatry.* 9th ed. Philadelphia, PA: Lippincott Williams & Wilkins; 2009:109.

DISCOVERY OF THE BRAIN ENDOCANNABINOID SYSTEM. Estimates suggest that 20 to 80 μg of tetrahydrocannabinol (THC) reaches the brain after one smokes a marijuana cigarette (i.e., "joint"). This quantity is comparable to the 100 to 200 μg of norepinephrine neurotransmitter present in the entire human brain. Thus the effects of THC might be explained by the effects on neurotransmitter systems. In the 1960s, there were at least two schools of thought on how THC exerted its psychoactive effects. One held that THC worked like that of the inhaled volatile anesthetics (i.e., no specific receptor existed), and it might have a generalized effect on neuronal membranes or widespread actions on neurotransmitter receptors. A competing school of thought speculated that specific receptors for cannabinoids existed in the brain, but they were difficult to identify due to the lipophilic nature of these chemicals. Novel cannabinoids were synthesized that were more water-soluble, and in the late 1980s, this allowed for the discovery of a specific cannabinoid receptor, CB1.

Several additional endocannabinoids were soon discovered, 2-arachidonylglycerol (2-AG), *N*-arachidonyldopamine (NADA), 2-arachidonoylglycerol ether (noladin ether), and virodhamine (Fig. 33-25). The different endocannabinoids have differing affinities for the cannabinoid receptors, CB1 and CB2. Anandamide appears to have the highest selectivity for the CB1 receptor, followed by NADA and noladin ether. In contrast, virodhamine prefers CB2 receptors and has only partial agonist activity at CB1. 2-AG appears not to discriminate between CB1 and CB2.

BIOSYNTHESIS OF ENDOCANNABINOIDS. Arachidonic acid is utilized as a building block for the biosynthesis of endocannabinoids, prostaglandins, and leukotrienes and is found within cellular phospholipids of the plasma membrane and other intracellular membranes. The synthesis of anandamide requires the sequential action of two enzymes (Fig. 33-26). In the first reaction, the enzyme *N*-acetyltransferase (NAT) transfers an arachidonic acid side chain from a phospholipid to phosphatidylethanolamine (PE), generating NAPE (*N*-arachidonyl-phosphatidylethanolamine). In the second reaction, the enzyme *N*-arachidonyl-phosphatidylethanolamine phospholipase (NAPD-PLD) converts NAPE to anandamide. Because NAPE is already a natural component of mammalian membranes, it is the second step that generates anandamide, which is most crucial to neurotransmission.

Endocannabinoids are not stored in synaptic vesicles for later use but are synthesized on-demand, as is done for the gaseous neurotransmitters. An essential criterion for a signaling molecule to be considered a neurotransmitter is that neuronal depolarization should lead to its release. Depolarization leads to increases in cellular calcium, which in turn promotes the synthesis of the endocannabinoids and their release. The mechanism is explained in part by calcium activation of NAPE-PLD and DAGL, leading to augmented biosynthesis of anandamide and 2-AG, respectively.

Endocannabinoids generated in a neuron must cross the synaptic cleft to act on cannabinoid receptors. Similar to THC, endocannabinoids are highly lipophilic and thus poorly soluble in CSF. It is hypothesized that a specific endocannabinoid transporter exists to allow endocannabinoids to cross the synaptic cleft and allow entry into the target neuron.

INACTIVATION OF ENDOCANNABINOIDS. Neurotransmitters are typically inactivated either by reuptake from the neurons that release them or by degradation by highly specific enzymes, such as the example of acetylcholine being hydrolyzed by acetylcholinesterase. At least two enzymes exist to target the destruction of endocannabinoids and attenuate their neurotransmission. Fatty acid

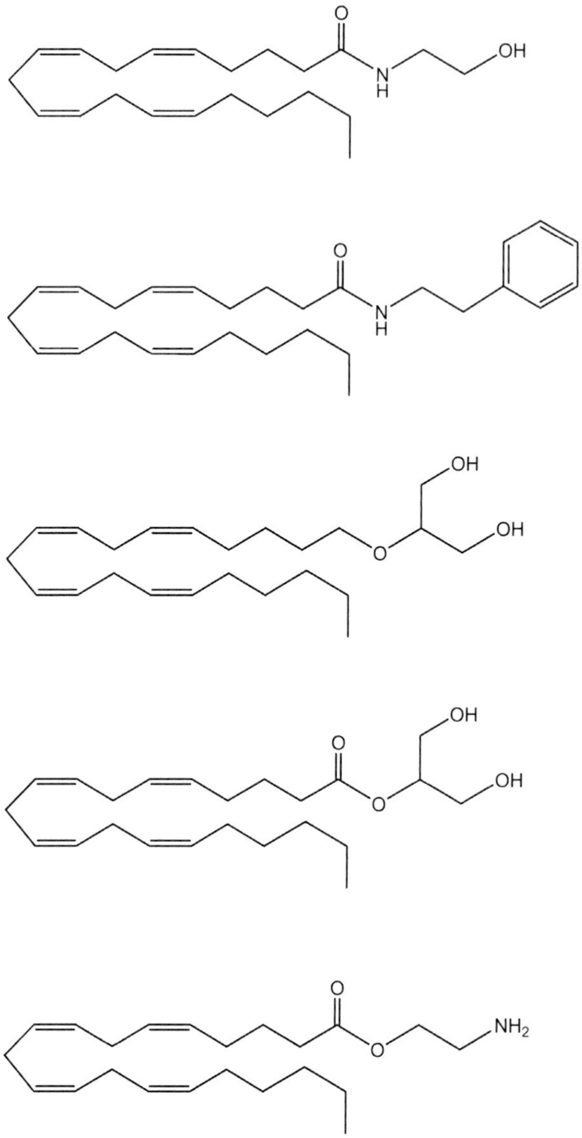

FIGURE 33-25
Endogenous cannabinoids. At least
five endocannabinoids exist in the
mammalian brain, each differing in
affinity for CB1 and CB2 cannabinoid receptors. All are derived
from the essential omega-6 fatty
acid, arachidonic acid, which is
also a substrate in the formation of
prostaglandins and leukotrienes.
(From Sadock BJ, Sadock VA, Ruiz P.
*Kaplan & Sadock's Comprehensive
Textbook of Psychiatry*. 9th ed. Philadelphia, PA: Lippincott Williams &
Wilkins; 2009:111.)

Endogenous Cannabinoids

Anandamide

CB1>>CB2

N-Arachidonoyl dopamine
(NADA)

CB1>CB2

2-Arachidonoylglycerol ether
(Noladin)

CB1>CB2

2-Arachidonoylglycerol
(2-AG)

CB1=CB2

Virodhamine

CB2>CB1

amide hydrolase (FAAH) converts anandamide to arachidonic acid
and ethanolamine (Fig. 33-26). FAAH is found in regions of the
brain where CB1 receptors are predominant and localize to postsynaptic neurons where anandamide is made. Rapid degradation
of anandamide in part explains its relatively low potency compared
to THC. Confirming the role of FAAH in anandamide inactivation,
knockout mice without FAAH exhibit a 15-fold increase of anandamide, but not 2-AG. These mice have more significant behavioral
responses to exogenous anandamide, owing to its decreased degradation. The endocannabinoid 2-AG is inactivated by FAAH, but
also by a monoacylglycerol lipase (MAGL) located in presynaptic
neurons.

Pharmacologic inhibitors of FAAH have analgesic effects and
reduce anxiety in animal models, but do not have the undesirable
effects of THC such as immobility, lowered body temperature, or
greater appetite. Such a pharmacologic strategy would be analogous to MAOIs and COMT inhibitors (COMTIs). MAOIs used to
treat depression, slow the breakdown of serotonin and other monoamines, thereby increasing serotonin, whereas COMTIs serves an

analogous role in blocking the destruction of dopamine and other
catecholamines.

CANNABINOID RECEPTORS.   CB1 receptors are possibly the most
abundant G-protein–coupled receptors in the brain. They occur at
the highest density in the basal ganglia, cerebellum, hippocampus,
hypothalamus, anterior cingulate cortex, and cerebral cortex, particularly the frontal cortex. Humans or animals that receive large
doses of THC develop catalepsy, a reduction of spontaneous movement, and freeze in bizarre and unnatural postures. The action of
cannabinoids in the basal ganglia and cerebellum may be associated with these behaviors, which may prove relevant in understanding catatonic symptoms in schizophrenia.

CB1 receptors are predominantly found on axons and nerve termini, with little presence on neuronal dendrites and the cell body.
CB1 receptors localize to the presynaptic rather than the postsynaptic side of the neuronal cleft, suggesting a role in the regulation
of neurotransmission. A second cannabinoid receptor, CB2, is predominantly expressed on the surface of white blood cells of the

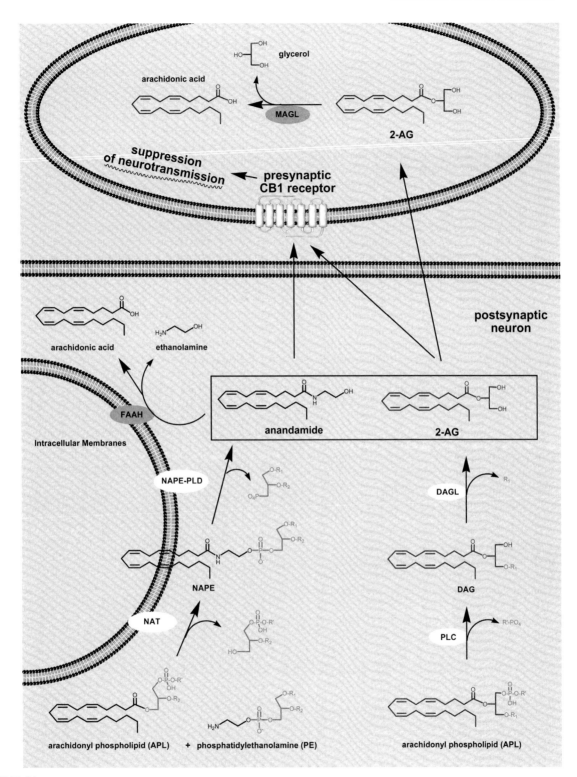

FIGURE 33-26

Retrograde neurotransmission of the endocannabinoids, anandamide, and 2-arachidonylglycerol (2-AG). Anandamide is synthesized on demand for neurotransmission via a two-step process. The enzyme NAT transfers the arachidonic acid chain from a phospholipid (APL) to phosphati-dylethanolamine (PE), thereby producing NAPE. A second enzyme, NAPE-PLD, generates anandamide. 2-AG is similarly synthesized in two steps by the enzymes PLC and DAGL. The endocannabinoids made in a postsynaptic neuron cross the synapse and activate presynaptic CB1 receptors, and suppress neurotransmission of the presynaptic neuron (although activation of the presynaptic neuron occurs in some cases). 2-AG is predominantly inactivated in the presynaptic neuron by MAGL, whereas anandamide is destroyed in the postsynaptic neuron by FAAH. PE, phosphatidylethanolamine; APL, arachidonyl phospholipids; NAT, N-acyltransferase; NAPE, N-arachidonyl-phosphatidylethanolamine; NAPE-PLD, N-arachidonyl-phosphatidylethanolamine phospholipase D; FAAH, fatty acid amide hydrolase; MAGL, monoacylglycerol lipase; PLC, phospholipase C; DAG, diacylglycerol; DAGL, diacylglycerol lipase; R_1-R_3, various acyl or akyl side chains of phospholipids; R′, side chain of phospholipid head group. (From Sadock BJ, Sadock VA, Ruiz P. *Kaplan & Sadock's Comprehensive Textbook of Psychiatry*. 9th ed. Philadelphia, PA: Lippincott Williams & Wilkins; 2009:112.)

immune system, but small amounts appear to be present in the brainstem.

Effects on Neurotransmission. The cannabinoid CB1 receptor is associated with G proteins that mediate its intracellular signaling, in part, through inhibition of adenylyl cyclase. This action leads to a decrease in levels of the essential second messenger, cyclic adenosine monophosphate. Activation of the CB1 receptor also leads to the activation of potassium channels and inhibition of N-type calcium channels. Because calcium is integral to neurotransmitter release, cannabinoids can block neurotransmission through this mechanism. Cannabinoid receptors also activate mitogen-activated protein kinases.

With the use of cell culture models and slices of the brain, cannabinoids have been shown to block the release of a variety of neurotransmitters, including GABA, norepinephrine, and acetylcholine. Norepinephrine and acetylcholine tend to be excitatory neurotransmitters, and cannabinoid inhibition of their release would be expected to have an overall inhibitory effect. However, GABA is an inhibitory neurotransmitter, and cannabinoid inhibition of it would lead to overall excitatory effects, demonstrating that cannabinoids can have complex effects on neurotransmission depending on the specific context. Cannabinoids also appear to increase the release of brain endorphin neurotransmitters and increase dopamine release in the nucleus accumbens, a "reward center" relevant to addiction and learning. The endocannabinoids have been implicated in a variety of forms of synaptic plasticity, including LTP and long-term depression (LTD).

ENDOCANNABINOIDS IN ANXIETY AND MOOD. Endocannabinoid neurotransmission may be an essential regulator of anxiety, and cannabis users regularly describe a tranquilizing effect of THC. The loss of signaling by the endocannabinoid system appears to promote anxiety-like states in animal studies. CB1 receptor-deficient animals exhibit more pronounced anxiety behavior when exposed to stress or new environs.

The endocannabinoid pathway may represent an attractive target in understanding posttraumatic stress responses and phobias. Although one cannot yet safely measure endocannabinoid levels in human subjects, this model is supported by clinical trials of the cannabinoid receptor blocker, rimonabant (Acomplia), which may offer promise as a strategy for weight loss (see below). A frequent adverse reaction to the drug is increased anxiety and depression.

Addiction. The endocannabinoid system may be an attractive target for understanding addiction. Mice deficient in CB1 receptors are unsurprisingly resistant to the behavioral effects of cannabinoids; they also appear to have reduced addiction to and withdrawal from opiates. Further interaction has also been found between the opioid and cannabinoid systems, as cannabinoids appear to increase the release of dopamine in the nucleus accumbens, a key reward area of the brain implicated in addiction. This dopamine release appears to require μ-opioid receptors, as pharmacologic inhibition of these receptors blocks the ability of cannabinoids to increase dopamine release. Rats with a preference for alcohol have decreased FAAH activity, suggestive of higher cannabinoid signaling. CB1 receptor antagonists dampen their alcohol consumption, whereas inhibiting FAAH increases their alcohol consumption. Furthermore, CB1-deficient animals also appear to have reduced alcohol intake. A single amino acid mutation in human FAAH is associated with drug abuse, and this abnormal enzyme appears to be less stable than its wild-type counterpart.

ENDOCANNABINOIDS IN PSYCHOSIS. Heavy use of cannabis can produce psychotic symptoms in individuals with no prior history of psychiatric disorder, although it is unclear whether this is solely due to the drug or an underlying vulnerability to psychosis in such persons. Cannabis use often worsens psychosis in schizophrenia, and heavy use has been associated with developing schizophrenia, although some suggest that this association is an accelerated development of symptoms in those who would eventually manifest schizophrenia. Nonetheless, the endocannabinoid system has implications for the pathophysiology of schizophrenia, as cannabinoid signaling appears to increase the release of dopamine. Medications that act as antagonists of D_2 receptors will likely remain a component of schizophrenia treatment for some time.

Feeding. Following drug ingestion, THC users develop an increased appetite ("the munchies"), and cannabis has been utilized as an appetite stimulant for centuries. This effect may depend on CB1 receptors present in the hypothalamus. Endocannabinoid levels increase in the hypothalamus and limbic system when animals are deprived of food. Mice genetically deficient in CB1 receptors become resistant to developing obesity after being given a high-fat diet. Similarly, the CB1 receptor antagonist, rimonabant, appears to facilitate weight loss by blocking cannabinoid signaling. In a clinical trial of more than 3,000 obese patients, those treated with 20 mg/day of rimonabant lost 6.3 kg at 1 year, compared to 1.6 kg in the placebo group. Nausea was the most common side effect reported. A 2007 meta-analysis of clinical trials reported an overall 4.7 kg weight loss with rimonabant treatment, besting the weight-loss drugs orlistat (2.9 kg) and sibutramine (4.2 kg).

EFFECTS ON BRAIN INJURY AND PAIN. In mouse models of traumatic brain injury, 2-AG appears neuroprotective, reducing brain edema, infarct size, and cell death, while improving functional outcomes. Anandamide is also protected against brain injury in a model of multiple sclerosis (MS), and human patients with the disease have increased production of anandamide. A study of cannabinoid agonist, HU-211, led to more rapid clinical improvement following head trauma. FAAH inhibitors improved motor symptoms in a mouse model of Parkinson disease, likely via cannabinoids increasing dopamine neurotransmission.

There is increasing evidence that neurotransmission via the endocannabinoid pathway regulates pain perception. THC and cannabinoid agonists have proven effective in animal models of acute and chronic pain, ranging from burn injury to nerve damage and inflammation. The CB1 receptor plays an essential role in these effects, as the analgesic effects of cannabinoid drugs are lost when CB1 antagonist rimonabant is given. Similarly, the analgesic effect of THC is lost in mice that are genetically deficient in the CB1 receptor.

Stress has long been associated with diminished pain perception, such as in cases of injured military personnel who demonstrate remarkable pain tolerance, a phenomenon known as *stress-induced analgesia.* The endocannabinoid system may mediate these effects. Animal models reveal anandamide and 2-AG production after stress, and stress-induced analgesia is blocked by the CB1 blocker, rimonabant, in these animals.

Endocannabinoid regulation of pain perception appears to be distinct from that of the endogenous opiate system, but the two pathways may share overlapping neural pathways. Evidence for this has been provided using CB1 blocker, rimonabant, and naloxone (Narcan), which blocks opiate receptors. Rimonabant attenuates analgesia provided by THC and cannabinoids, but only partially blocks the response to morphine. However, the opposite is true for opiates: Naloxone blocks morphine-induced analgesia but also partially blocks the analgesia of THC and cannabinoid drugs. Combinations of cannabinoid and opiate drugs evince synergistic analgesic effects in animal models.

Although it was initially assumed that cannabinoids exert their analgesic effects via the CNS, in animal models, it has been shown that localized administration of cannabinoids may also be useful, including drugs selective for the CB2 receptor, whose expression is minimal in the CNS.

Endocannabinoids may also influence pain sensitivity by mechanisms that do not involve the CB1 and CB2 receptors. Both anandamide and NADA can also activate a calcium channel known as the vanilloid receptor (also known as transient receptor potential vanilloid type 1 [TRPV-1]) that is found on sensory nerves. This same receptor is also famous for being activated by capsaicin, which causes the hot sensation after eating chili peppers. Thus endocannabinoids can exert opposing functions: Promoting analgesia through the CB1 and CB2 receptors but potentially increasing pain via TRP channels. Although CB2 receptors are primarily expressed in the periphery, postmortem analyses reveal an upregulation in the brain from those with Alzheimer disease.

The rapid development of novel cannabinoid drugs may allow for targeting of specific symptoms, rather than elicit all of the typical effects of THC. For instance, ajulemic acid demonstrates analgesic and anti-inflammatory properties but may offer a benefit of limited psychoactive side effects. In a randomized clinical trial of this compound, Mathias Karst and colleagues found efficacy in reducing chronic neuropathic pain.

EFFECTS IN THE PERIPHERY.   Cannabinoids lead to direct relaxation of vascular smooth muscle by local CB1 receptors. This vasodilation extends to the conjunctiva, leading to a "bloodshot" appearance in some cannabis users. Relaxation of ocular arteries by cannabinoids may offer utility as a treatment for glaucoma, a condition of high intraocular pressure, and activation of CB1 receptors in the kidney can improve renal blood flow. A role in generalized blood pressure regulation is unproven, and blood pressure is unaltered in persons treated with rimonabant or animals deficient in CB1 receptors. Cannabinoid signaling may also be relevant to ectopic pregnancy, as CB1-deficient mice retain many embryos in the oviduct.

Nonpsychoactive Cannabinoids.   Although THC is the principal psychoactive component of cannabis, the many nonpsychoactive cannabinoids also have intriguing properties and may regulate neurotransmission.

Cannabidiol may offer potential therapeutic effects and appears to stimulate TRPV-1 receptors and influence endocannabinoid degradation. Also, cannabidiol demonstrated a protective effect in a mouse model of inflammatory arthritis. Although results have been mixed, purified cannabidiol may also exert antipsychotic activity, although the net effect of plant cannabis use typically exacerbates schizophrenia symptoms owing to THC. Tetrahydrocannabivarin is a plant cannabinoid that antagonizes CB1 receptors. It is a candidate marker to distinguish whether a patient has been using plant-derived cannabis or prescription THC, which contains no tetrahydrocannabivarin.

Eicosanoids

OVERVIEW.   Clinical findings suggest that the dietary supplements omega-3 fatty acids, eicosapentaenoic acid (EPA), its ester ethyl-eicosapentaenoic (E-EPA), and docosahexaenoic acid (DHA) help relieve symptoms of depression, bipolar illness, schizophrenia, and cognitive impairment. DHA and EPA may help reduce behavioral outbursts and improve attention in children.

CHEMISTRY.   Essential fatty acids are a group of polyunsaturated fats that contain a carbon–carbon double bond in the third position from the methyl end group in the fatty acid chain. They are essential because unlike monosaturated and saturated fatty acids, polyunsaturated fatty acids cannot be synthesized de novo and can be acquired only through diet from natural fats and oils. Linoleic acid (LA) is the parent compound of omega-6 fatty acids, and α-linolenic acid (ALA) is the parent compound of omega-3 fatty acids. Both omega-3 and omega-6 groups use the same enzymes for desaturation and chain elongation. Algae and plankton synthesize Omega-3 fatty acids. Fish such as herring, salmon, mackerel, and anchovy feed on these aquatic species and become a rich dietary source of omega-3. EPA and DHA are highly unsaturated omega-3 fatty acids that contain 6 and 5 double bonds on their long structural chain, respectively. They are positioned in the cell membrane by phospholipids and play a crucial role in cell membrane signaling.

EFFECTS ON SPECIFIC ORGANS AND SYSTEMS.   The most substantial scientific evidence for treatment with fatty acid supplements comes from the cardiovascular literature. Several human trials have demonstrated that omega-3 fatty acids lower blood pressure, reduce the rate of recurrent myocardial infarction, and lower triglyceride levels. In the nervous system, fatty acids are essential components of neurons, immune cells, and glial phospholipid membrane structures. They increase cerebral blood flow, decrease platelet aggregation, and delay the progression of atherosclerosis in the cardiovascular system. Omega-6 fatty acids appear to reduce inflammation and neuronal apoptosis and decrease phosphatidylinositol second messenger activity. Omega-3 fatty acids have been suggested to alter gene expression.

In the CNS, fatty acids are selectively concentrated in neuronal membranes and involved in cell membrane structure. Omega-6 arachidonic acid has been shown to enhance glutamate neurotransmission, stimulate stress hormone secretion, and trigger glial cell activation in the setting of oxidative toxicity and neurodegeneration. The omega-3 fatty acids DHA and EPA appear to protect neurons from inflammatory and oxidative toxicities. Increases in serotonin, enhancement of dopamine, and regulation of CRF have been demonstrated in cell culture models.

In rodent models of depression, chronic EPA treatment normalized behavior in open field tests. Serotonin and norepinephrine were also increased in the limbic regions. Mice fed omega-3 poor diets had reduced memory, altered learning patterns, and more behavioral problems.

THERAPEUTIC INDICATIONS.   Clinical research with the use of fish oil for mood disorders was based on epidemiology studies where there appears to be a negative correlation between fish consumption and depressive symptoms. Countries with lower per capita fish consumption had up to 60 times increased rates of major depression, bipolar disorder, and postpartum depression. Observational studies concluded that the lower incidence of seasonal affective disorder in Iceland and Japan, rather than latitude predicted, is related to the amount of fatty acid these populations consume in their diet. A study in Norway showed that the use of cod liver oil decreased depressive symptoms. Depression after a myocardial infarction shows higher arachidonic acid to EPA ratio. Postmortem studies in the brains of patients diagnosed with major depressive disorder show reduced DHA in the orbitofrontal cortex.

The first randomized, controlled pilot study of omega-3 fatty acids focused on adjunctive treatment in both bipolar and unipolar patients with depression in addition to their standard lithium (Eskalith) or valproic acid (Depakene) treatment. The omega-3 fatty acid group had significant improvement on the Hamilton Depression Scale and a more extended period of remission than the placebo group. A subsequent more extensive study supported a benefit from treatment with E-EPA for bipolar illness. However, a study of a group of patients with either bipolar disorder or rapid cycling treated with E-EPA showed no significant difference in any outcome measure between the EPA and placebo groups. Bleeding time was also increased in the treatment group. There are no current data on monotherapy in bipolar illness or depression.

The most convincing evidence comes from early brain development and learning studies. Pregnant mothers who consumed foods rich in DHA gave birth to infants who had improved problem-solving skills but not necessarily improved memory. Visual acuity and eye development are also associated with DHA supplementation during pregnancy.

Reports of behavioral studies of prisoners in England who consumed higher amounts of seafood containing omega-3 fatty acids showed a decrease in assault rates. A Finnish study of violent criminals identified lower levels of omega-3 fatty acids in their system compared to the nonviolent offenders.

The negative and psychotic symptoms of schizophrenia may be improved with supplementation with omega-3 fatty acids. Antipsychotic medications like haloperidol (Haldol) appear to have fewer extrapyramidal side effects when combined with antioxidants and omega-3 fatty acids.

EPA and DHA have been associated with decreased dementia incidence. After reviewing the Rotterdam study of a longitudinal cohort of more than 5,300 patients, fish consumption appeared to be inversely related to the development of new cases of dementia. Later analysis of the study after 6 years demonstrated that low intake of omega-3 fatty acids was not associated with an increased risk of dementia. In contrast, the Zutphen study, also in the Netherlands, concluded that high fish consumption was inversely related to cognitive decline at a 3-year follow-up and after 5 years. Well-designed clinical trials are needed before omega-3 fatty acids can be recommended for the prevention of cognitive impairment.

PRECAUTIONS AND ADVERSE REACTIONS.   The most adverse complication of eicosanoid use is an increased risk of bleeding. Dietary sources can contain heavy metals, and there is no standard preparation for capsule formulations. Treatment studies have yielded a variety of different doses, but evidence for the therapeutic dose and clinical guidelines are almost nonexistent. The length of treatment still needs to be determined.

Neurosteroids

BACKGROUND.   Although steroids are critical for the maintenance of body homeostasis, neurosteroids are synthesized from cholesterol in the brain and independent of peripheral formation in the adrenals and gonads. Neurosteroids are produced by a sequence of enzymatic processes governed by cytochrome P450 (CYP) and non-CYP enzymes, either within or outside the mitochondria of several types of CNS and peripheral nervous system (PNS) cells.

Recent work has shown that neurosteroids can operate through a nongenomic pathway to regulate neuronal excitability through their effects on neurotransmitter-gated ion channels. Receptors are generally located in the nucleus, membrane, or microtubules of the CNS and PNS. Although steroids and neurosteroids can act on the same nuclear receptors, neurosteroids differ from steroids in their topologic distribution and regional synthesis. The most well-known effect of neurosteroids is on the GABA receptor, particularly the $GABA_A$ receptor. Neurosteroids acting primarily at this site include allopregnanolone ($3\alpha,5\alpha$-tetrahydroprogesterone), pregnanolone (PREG), and tetrahydrodeoxycorticosterone (THDOC). Dehydroepiandrosterone sulfate (DHEA-S), the most prevalent neurosteroid, acts as a noncompetitive modulator of GABA. Its precursor dehydroepiandrosterone (DHEA) has also been shown to exert inhibitory effects at the GABA receptor. Some neurosteroids may also act at the NMDA, α-amino-3-hydroxy-5-methyl-4-isoxazole-propanoic acid (AMPA), kainate, glycine, serotonin, sigma type-1, and nicotinic acetylcholine receptors. Progesterone is also considered a neurosteroid and can regulate gene expression at progesterone receptors.

NEUROSTEROIDS IN NEURODEVELOPMENT AND NEUROPROTECTION.
In general, neurosteroids stimulate axonal growth and promote synaptic transmission. Specific neuroprotective effects are unique to each neurosteroid. DHEA acts to regulate brain serotonin and dopamine levels, suppress cortisol, increase hippocampal primed burst potentiation and cholinergic function, decrease amyloid-β protein, inhibit the production of proinflammatory cytokines, and prevent free radical scavenging. DHEA and DHEA-S have both been shown to have a role in glial development and neuronal growth and to promote their survival in animals; the injection of these substances into the brains of mice promoted long-term memory while reversing amnesia. Progesterone is linked to myelinating processes like aiding in the repair of damaged neural myelination. Allopregnanolone contributes to the reduction of contacts during axonal regression.

ROLE OF NEUROSTEROIDS IN MENTAL ILLNESS.   Neurosteroids have distinct implications for the maintenance of normal neurologic function and also may contribute to neuropathology. Neurosteroids are differentially regulated in males and females and may affect the manifestation of psychological disorders in these two populations. Specifically, they play a distinct role in depression and anxiety disorders and may be targeted by psychiatric medications someday soon.

Depression.   When compared with nondepressed controls, studies show that depressed patients have lower plasma and CSF concentrations of allopregnanolone. Also, this research has elucidated an inverse relationship between allopregnanolone concentrations and the severity of depressive illness. However, there are no allopregnanolone-based therapies available for humans, so its direct efficacy is unsubstantiated. Antidepressant drugs, specifically fluoxetine (Prozac), have been shown in multiple studies to increase the levels of certain neurosteroids. Nonetheless, there is debate over the therapeutic properties of neurosteroids, prompting the investigation of neurosteroid concentrations in patients undergoing nonpharmacologic therapies. Preliminary results indicate that the lack of modifications in neurosteroid levels during nonpharmacologic treatments supports the validity of the pharmacologic properties of antidepressants, not their therapeutic action, in the elevation of neurosteroid levels in medicated populations.

Anxiety Disorders.   In patients with anxiety disorders, the primary mechanism of action is on the GABA receptor. Homeostasis characterized by regular GABAergic activity is restored after panic attacks as neurosteroids are released in response to stress. Allopregnanolone stimulates GABAergic activity with 20 times the strength of benzodiazepines and 200 times the potency of barbiturates. Both positive and negative regulation of the GABA$_A$ receptor are correlated with anxiolytic and anxiogenic action, respectively.

Psychotic Disorders.   Also, to their primary relevance to the pharmacologic treatment of mood and anxiety disorders, neurosteroids contribute to psychotic, childhood, substance abuse, eating, and postpartum disorders. DHEA and DHEA-S mediate the effect of neurosteroids on psychotic disorders such as schizophrenia. DHEA has been dispensed to decrease anxiety in patients with schizophrenia, as DHEA and DHEA-S suppress GABA inhibition and heighten the neuronal response at the NMDA and sigma receptors. DHEA and DHEA-S levels are typically elevated in the initial episode of a patient with schizophrenia, indicating the onset of psychosis upregulates neurosteroids. Because neurosteroid levels are studied across various illness stages, some questions still exist regarding the role of neurosteroids in psychosis.

Childhood Mental Illness.   In children, the clinical symptomology of ADHD is inversely correlated with DHEA and pregnenolone levels.

Substance Abuse.   Alcohol is theorized to regulate the GABA receptor and induce de novo steroid synthesis in the brain, specifically, pregnenolone, allopregnanolone, and allotetrahydrodeoxycorticosterone levels are increased in the brain and periphery in response to increases in peripheral alcohol levels. It is hypothesized that sharp increases in ethanol concentration may mimic the acute stress response and elevate neurosteroid concentrations by the HPA axis. To prevent ethanol dependence, researchers are investigating fluctuations in neurosteroid levels and in vivo neurosteroid responsiveness. Neurosteroids (increased allopregnanolone levels in particular) are associated with drug abuse. However, DHEA-S may check the acquisition of morphine tolerance. Past research has shown that DHEA-S levels were also increased in patients who abstained from cocaine use in a treatment program, and as patients relapsed, DHEA-S concentrations decreased accordingly.

Eating Disorders.   Concerning eating disorders, DHEA has been shown to diminish food intake, temper obesity, moderate insulin resistance, and lower lipids in rats with a model of youth-onset, hyperphagic, and genetic obesity. By regulating the serotonergic system, DHEA is hypothesized to promote a reduced caloric load. Although hypothetical, low levels of DHEA and DHEA-S are recorded in young women with anorexia nervosa, and 3 months of oral DHEA supplementation increased bone density and tempered the emotional problems associated with the disorder.

Postpartum and Gynecologic Disorders.   Because estrogen and progesterone levels fluctuate during pregnancy and drop markedly after delivery, neurosteroids are thought to contribute to postpartum disorders. Low postpartum DHEA concentrations have been linked to mood instability. Also, allopregnanolone levels correlated with mood disorders during pregnancy and in premenstrual syndrome (PMS). It has been noted that women with the premenstrual dysphoric disorder have higher allopregnanolone/progesterone ratios than normal controls; women treated for this disorder reported improvement as allopregnanolone levels decreased.

Neurosteroids, Memory Disorders, and Aging.   Neurosteroid levels may be irregular in neurodegenerative disorders and aging conditions such as Alzheimer disease and Parkinson disease. DHEA levels at age 70 are only about 20 percent of their maximum value recorded in the late 20s, and some researchers believe DHEA supplementation can prevent or slow the cognitive declines associated with the aging process. However, conflicting studies have indicated that DHEA administration does not improve cognitive measures in patients. Also, in patients with Alzheimer disease, DHEA concentrations are markedly decreased.

PSYCHONEUROENDOCRINOLOGY

The term *psychoneuroendocrinology* encompasses the structural and functional relationships between hormonal systems and the CNS and behaviors that modulate and are derived from both. Classically, *hormones* have been defined as the products of endocrine glands transported by the blood to exert their action at sites distant from their release. Advances in neuroscience have shown, however, that in the CNS, the brain not only serves as a target site for regulatory control of hormonal release but also has secretory functions of its own and serves as an end-organ for some hormonal actions. These complex interrelationships make classic distinctions between the origin, structure, and function of neurons and those of endocrine cells dependent on physiologic context.

Hormone Secretion

Hormone secretion is stimulated by the action of a neuronal secretory product of neuroendocrine transducer cells of the hypothalamus. Examples of hormone regulators (Table 33-6) include corticotropin-releasing hormone (CRH), which stimulates adrenocorticotropin (adrenocorticotropic hormone [ACTH]); TRH, which stimulates the release of TSH; gonadotropin-releasing hormone (GnRH), which stimulates the release of luteinizing hormone (LH) and follicle-stimulating hormone (FSH); and somatostatin (somatotropin release-inhibiting factor [SRIF]) and growth-hormone-releasing hormone (GHRH), which influence growth hormone (GH) release. Chemical signals cause the release of these neurohormones from the median eminence of the hypothalamus into the portal hypophyseal bloodstream and subsequent transport to the pituitary to regulate the release of target hormones. Pituitary hormones, in turn, act directly on target cells (e.g., ACTH on the adrenal gland) or stimulate the release of other hormones from peripheral endocrine organs. Also, these hormones have feedback actions that regulate secretion and exert neuromodulatory effects in the CNS.

Table 33-6
Examples of Regulating Hormones

Regulating Hormone	Hormone Stimulated (or Inhibited)
Corticotropin-releasing hormone	Adrenocorticotropic hormone
Thyrotropin-releasing hormone	Thyroid-stimulated hormone
Luteinizing hormone-releasing hormone	Luteinizing hormone
Gonadotropin-releasing hormone	Follicle-stimulating hormone
Somatostatin	Growth hormone (inhibited)
Growth hormone-releasing hormone	Growth hormone
Progesterone, oxytocin	Prolactin
Arginine vasopressin	Adrenocorticotropic hormone

From Sadock BJ, Sadock VA, Ruiz P. *Kaplan & Sadock's Comprehensive Textbook of Psychiatry.* 9th ed. Philadelphia, PA: Lippincott Williams & Wilkins; 2009:162.

Table 33-7
Classifications of Hormones

Structure	Examples	Storage	Lipid Soluble
Proteins, polypeptides, glycoproteins	ACTH, β-endorphin, TRH, LH, FSH	Vesicles	No
Steroids, steroid-like compounds	Cortisol, estrogen, thyroxine	Diffusion after synthesis	Yes
Functions			
Autocrine	Self-regulatory effects		
Paracrine	Local or adjacent cellular action		
Endocrine	Distant target site		

ACTH, adrenocorticotropic hormone; TRH, thyrotropin-releasing hormone; LH, luteinizing hormone; FSH, follicle-stimulating hormone.
Courtesy of Victor I Reus, M.D. and Sydney Frederick-Osborne, Ph.D.

Hormones are divided into two general classes: (1) proteins, polypeptides, and glycoproteins, and (2) steroids and steroid-like compounds (Table 33-7); these are secreted by an endocrine gland into the bloodstream and are transported to their sites of action.

Developmental Psychoneuroendocrinology

Hormones can have both organizational and activational effects. Exposure to gonadal hormones during critical stages of neural development directs changes in brain morphology and function (e.g., sex-specific behavior in adulthood). Similarly, thyroid hormones are essential for the normal development of the CNS, and thyroid deficiency during critical stages of postnatal life will severely impair growth and development of the brain, resulting in behavioral disturbances that may be permanent if replacement therapy is not instituted.

Endocrine Assessment

Neuroendocrine function can be studied by assessing baseline measures and by measuring the response of the axis to some neurochemical or hormonal challenge. The first method has two approaches. One approach is to measure a single time point—for example, morning levels of growth hormone; this approach is subject to significant error because of the pulsatile nature of the release of most hormones. The second approach is to collect blood samples at multiple points or to collect 24-hour urine samples; these measurements are less susceptible to significant errors. The best approach, however, is to perform a neuroendocrine challenge test, in which the person is given a drug or a hormone that perturbs the endocrine axis in some standard way. Persons with no disease show much less variation in their responses to such challenge studies than in their baseline measurements.

Hypothalamic–Pituitary–Adrenal Axis

Since the earliest conceptions of the stress response by Hans Selye and others, investigation of HPA function has occupied a central position in psychoendocrine research. CRH, ACTH, and cortisol levels all rise in response to a variety of physical and psychic stresses and serve as prime factors in maintaining homeostasis and developing adaptive responses to novel or challenging stimuli. The hormonal response depends on the characteristics of the stressor and how one assesses and copes with it. Aside from generalized effects on arousal, distinct effects on sensory processing, stimulus habituation and sensitization, pain, sleep, and memory storage and retrieval have been documented. In primates, social status can influence adrenocortical profiles and, in turn, be affected by exogenously induced changes in hormone concentration.

Pathologic alterations in HPA function have been associated primarily with mood disorders, PTSD, and dementia of the Alzheimer type, although recent animal evidence points toward the role of this system in substance use disorders as well. Disturbances of mood are found in more than 50 percent of patients with Cushing syndrome (characterized by elevated cortisol concentrations), with psychosis or suicidal thought apparent in more than 10 percent of patients studied. Cognitive impairments similar to those seen in major depressive disorder (principally in visual memory and higher cortical functions) are common and relate to the severity of the hypercortisolemia and possible reduction in hippocampal size. In general, reduced cortisol levels normalize mood, and mental status. Conversely, in Addison disease (characterized by adrenal insufficiency), apathy, social withdrawal, impaired sleep, and decreased concentration frequently accompany prominent fatigue. Replacement of glucocorticoid (but not of electrolyte) resolves behavioral symptomatology.

Similarly, HPA abnormalities are reversed in persons who are treated successfully with antidepressant medications. Failure to normalize HPA abnormalities is a poor prognostic sign. Alterations in HPA function associated with depression include elevated cortisol concentrations, failure to suppress cortisol in response to dexamethasone, increased adrenal size and sensitivity to ACTH, a blunted ACTH response to CRH, and, possibly, elevated CRH concentrations in the brain.

Hypothalamic–Pituitary–Gonadal Axis

The gonadal hormones (progesterone, androstenedione, testosterone, estradiol, and others) are steroids that are secreted principally by the ovary and testes, but significant amounts of androgens arise from the adrenal cortex as well. The prostate gland and adipose tissue, also involved in the synthesis and storage of dihydrotestosterone, contribute to individual variance in sexual function and behavior.

The timing and presence of gonadal hormones play a critical role in the development of sexual dimorphisms in the brain. Developmentally, these hormones direct the organization of many sexually dimorphic CNS structures and functions, such as the size of the hypothalamic nuclei and corpus callosum, neuronal density in the temporal cortex, the organization of language ability, and responsivity in Broca motor speech area. Women with congenital adrenal hyperplasia—a deficiency of the enzyme 21-hydroxylase, which leads to high exposure to adrenal androgens in prenatal and postnatal life, in some studies—are more aggressive and assertive and less interested in traditional female roles than female control subjects. Sexual dimorphisms may also reflect acute and reversible actions of relative steroid concentrations (e.g., higher estrogen levels transiently increase CNS sensitivity to serotonin).

Testosterone.   Testosterone is the primary androgenic steroid, with both androgenic (i.e., facilitating linear body growth) and somatic growth functions. Testosterone is associated with increased violence and aggression in animals and correlation studies in humans, but anecdotal reports of increased aggression with testosterone treatment have not been substantiated in investigations in humans. In hypogonadal men, testosterone improves mood and decreases irritability. Varying effects of anabolic–androgenic steroids on mood have been noted anecdotally. A prospective, placebo-controlled study of anabolic–androgenic steroid administration in normal subjects reported positive mood symptoms, including euphoria, increased energy, and sexual arousal, in addition to increases in the negative mood symptoms of irritability, mood swings, violent feelings, anger, and hostility.

Testosterone is essential for sexual desire in both men and women. In males, muscle mass and strength, sexual activity, desire, thoughts, and intensity of sexual feelings depend on normal testosterone levels, but these functions are not augmented by supplemental testosterone in those with normal androgen levels. Adding small amounts of testosterone to routine hormonal replacement in postmenopausal women has proved, however, to be as beneficial as its use in hypogonadal men.

Dehydroepiandrosterone. DHEA and DHEA sulfate (DHEA-S) are adrenal androgens secreted in response to ACTH and represent the most abundant circulating steroids. DHEA is also a neurosteroid that is synthesized in situ in the brain. DHEA has many physiologic effects, including a reduction in neuronal damage from glucocorticoid excess and oxidative stress. Behavioral interest has centered on its possible involvement in memory, mood, and several psychiatric disorders. *Adrenarche* is the prepubertal onset of adrenal production of DHEA-S and may play a role in human maturation through increasing the activity of the amygdala and hippocampus and promoting synaptogenesis in the cerebral cortex. DHEA has been shown to act as an excitatory neurosteroid and to enhance memory retention in mice, but studies of DHEA administration to humans have not consistently shown any improvement in cognition. Several trials of DHEA administration point to an improvement in well-being, mood, energy, libido, and functional status in depressed individuals. Administration of DHEA to women with adrenal insufficiency (e.g., Addison disease) has repeatedly been demonstrated to enhance mood, energy, and sexual function; effects in men remain to be assessed. Mood, fatigue, and libido improved in human immunodeficiency virus (HIV)-positive patients treated with DHEA in one study, and DHEA and DHEA-S are inversely correlated with severity in ADHD. Women diagnosed with fibromyalgia have significantly decreased DHEA-S levels, but supplementation does not improve outcomes. Several cases of possible DHEA-induced mania have been reported, and DHEA has been reported to be inversely related to extrapyramidal symptoms (EPS) in patients with schizophrenia who are treated with antipsychotics. DHEA administration, in these cases, improves EPS.

Double-blind treatment studies have shown antidepressant effects of DHEA in patients with major depression, midlife-onset dysthymia, and schizophrenia, although beneficial effects on memory have not been reliably demonstrated. A small, double-blind trial of DHEA treatment of Alzheimer disease failed to reveal significant benefit, although a near-significant improvement in cognitive function was seen after 3 months of treatment.

Animal studies suggest that DHEA may be involved in eating behavior, aggressiveness, and anxiety as well, with its effects resulting from its transformation into estrogen, testosterone, or androsterone from its antiglucocorticoid activity, or direct effects on $GABA_A$, NMDA, and σ receptors. Because of the putative antiglucocorticoid effects, the ratio of cortisol to DHEA levels may be particularly crucial in understanding adaptive responses to stress. Both cortisol and DHEA appear to be involved in fear conditioning, with the cortisol/DHEA ratio hypothesized to be an index of the degree to which an individual is buffered against the adverse effects of stress. This ratio is related to some measures of psychopathology and response to treatment, predicting the persistence of the first episode major depression and being related to the degree of depression, anxiety, and hostility in patients with schizophrenia and response to antipsychotic treatment. Patients with PTSD have higher DHEA levels and lower cortisol/DHEA ratios related to symptom severity, suggesting a role in PTSD recovery. Fear-potentiated startle is more extensive in individuals with high as compared to low cortisol/DHEA-S ratios and is positively associated with cortisol and negatively with DHEA-S. More significant DHEA response to ACTH is related to lower PTSD ratings, and the cortisol/DHEA ratio to negative mood symptoms. A genetic variation in an ACTH receptor promoter has been found to influence DHEA secretion in response to dexamethasone and may underlie some individual differences in stress response.

Estrogen and Progesterone. Estrogens can influence neural activity in the hypothalamus and limbic system directly through the modulation of neuronal excitability, and they have complex multiphasic effects on nigrostriatal dopamine receptor sensitivity. Accordingly, evidence indicates that the antipsychotic effect of psychiatric drugs can change over the menstrual cycle and that the risk of tardive dyskinesia depends partly on estrogen concentrations. Several studies have suggested that gonadal steroids modulate spatial cognition and verbal memory and are involved in impeding age-related neuronal degeneration. Increasing evidence also suggests that estrogen administration decreases the risk and severity of dementia of the Alzheimer type in postmenopausal women. Estrogen has mood-enhancing properties and can also increase sensitivity to serotonin, possibly by inhibiting monoamine oxidase. In animal studies, long-term estrogen treatment results in a decrease in serotonin 5-HT_1 receptors and an increase in 5-HT_2 receptors. In oophorectomized women, significant reductions in tritiated imipramine binding sites (which indirectly measure presynaptic serotonin uptake) were restored with estrogen treatment.

The association of these hormones with serotonin is hypothetically relevant to mood change in premenstrual and postpartum mood disturbances. In premenstrual dysphoric disorder, a constellation of symptoms resembling major depressive disorder occurs in most menstrual cycles, appearing in the luteal phase and disappearing within a few days of the onset of menses. No definitive abnormalities in estrogen or progesterone levels have been demonstrated in women with the premenstrual dysphoric disorder, but decreased serotonin uptake with premenstrual reductions in steroid levels has been correlated with the severity of some symptoms.

Most psychological symptoms associated with the menopause are reported during perimenopause rather than after complete cessation of menses. Although studies suggest no increased incidence of major depressive disorder, reported symptoms to include worry, fatigue, crying spells, mood swings, diminished ability to cope, and diminished libido or intensity of orgasm. Hormone replacement therapy (HRT) is effective in preventing osteoporosis and reinstating energy, a sense of well-being, and libido; however, its use is very controversial. Studies have shown that combined estrogen–progestin drugs (e.g., Premarin) cause small increases in breast cancer, heart attack, stroke, and blood clots among menopausal women. Studies of the effects of estrogen alone in women who have had hysterectomies (because estrogen alone increases the risk for uterine cancer) are ongoing.

Hypothalamic–Pituitary–Thyroid Axis

Thyroid hormones are involved in the regulation of nearly every organ system, mainly those integral to the metabolism of food and the regulation of temperature, and are responsible for the optimal development and function of all body tissues. Also, to its prime endocrine function, TRH has direct effects on neuronal excitability, behavior, and neurotransmitter regulation.

Thyroid disorders can induce virtually any psychiatric symptom or syndrome, although no consistent associations of specific syndromes and thyroid conditions are found. Hyperthyroidism is commonly associated with fatigue, irritability, insomnia, anxiety, restlessness, weight loss, and emotional lability; marked impairment in concentration and memory may also be evident. Such states can progress into delirium or mania, or they can be episodic. On occasion, a real psychosis develops, with paranoia as a frequent presenting feature. In some cases, psychomotor retardation, apathy, and withdrawal are the presenting features rather than agitation and anxiety. Symptoms of mania have also been reported following the rapid normalization of thyroid status in hypothyroid individuals and may covary with thyroid level in individuals with episodic endocrine dysfunction. In general, behavioral abnormalities resolve with normalization of thyroid function and respond symptomatically to traditional psychopharmacological regimens.

The psychiatric symptoms of chronic hypothyroidism are generally well recognized (Fig. 33-27). Classically, fatigue, decreased libido, memory impairment, and irritability are noted, but an actual secondary psychotic disorder or dementia-like state can also develop. Suicidal ideation is common, and the lethality of actual attempts is profound. In milder, subclinical states of hypothyroidism, the absence of gross signs accompanying endocrine dysfunction can result in its being overlooked as a possible cause of a mental disorder.

Growth Hormone

Growth hormone deficiencies interfere with growth and delay the onset of puberty. Low GH levels can result from a stressful

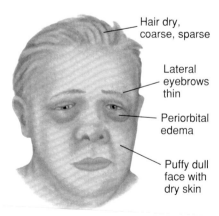

FIGURE 33-27
Myxedema: The patient with severe hypothyroidism (myxedema) has a dull, puffy facies. The edema, often particularly pronounced around the eyes, does not pit with pressure. The hair and eyebrows are dry, coarse, and thinned. The skin is dry. (From Bickley LS, Szilagyi P. *Bates' Guide to Physical Examination and History Taking*, 8th ed. Philadelphia, PA: Lippincott Williams & Wilkins; 2003.)

experience. Administration of GH to individuals with GH deficiency benefits cognitive function in addition to its more obvious somatic effects, but evidence indicates poor psychosocial adaptation in adulthood for children who were treated for GH deficiency. A significant percentage of patients with major depressive disorder and dysthymic disorder may have a GH deficiency. Some prepubertal and adult patients with diagnoses of major depressive disorder exhibit hyposecretion of GHRH during an insulin tolerance test, a deficit that has been interpreted as reflecting alterations in both cholinergic and serotonergic mechanisms. Several GH abnormalities have been noted in patients with anorexia nervosa. Secondary factors, such as weight loss, however, in both major depressive disorder and eating disorders, may be responsible for alterations in the endocrine release.

Nonetheless, at least one study has reported that GHRH stimulates food consumption in patients with anorexia nervosa and lowers food consumption in patients with bulimia. Administration of GH to older men increases lean body mass and improves vigor. GH is released in pulses throughout the day, but the pulses are closer together during the first hours of sleep than at other times.

Prolactin

Since its identification in 1970, the anterior pituitary hormone prolactin has been examined as a potential index of dopamine activity, dopamine receptor sensitivity, and antipsychotic drug concentration in studies of CNS function in psychiatric patients and as a correlate of stress responsivity. The secretion of prolactin is under direct inhibitory regulation by dopamine neurons located in the tuberoinfundibular section of the hypothalamus and is, therefore, increased by classical antipsychotic medications. Prolactin also inhibits its secretion using a short-loop feedback circuit to the hypothalamus. Also, a significant number of prolactin-releasing or prolactin-modifying factors have been identified, including estrogen, serotonin (mainly through the 5-HT$_2$ and 5-HT$_3$ receptors), norepinephrine, opioids, TRH, T$_4$, histamine, glutamate, cortisol, CRH, and oxytocin, with interaction effects possible. For example, estrogen may promote the serotonin-stimulated release of prolactin.

Prolactin is primarily involved in reproductive functions. During maturation, prolactin secretion participates in gonadal development, whereas, in adults, prolactin contributes to the regulation of the behavioral aspects of reproduction and infant care, including estrogen-dependent sexual receptivity and breast-feeding. In female rats, prolactin secretion is strongly stimulated with exposure to pups. In women, basal prolactin levels are elevated in the postpartum period before weaning, and prolactin release is stimulated by suckling. Hyperprolactinemia is associated with low testosterone in men and reduced libido in men and women. In rodents, prolactin level is increased along with corticosterone in response to such stressful stimuli as immobilization, hypoglycemia, surgery, and cold exposure and may be specifically associated with the use of passive coping in the face of a stressor. Prolactin promotes various stress-related behaviors in rats, depending on the condition, such as increasing object-directed exploration while decreasing other exploration.

Patients with hyperprolactinemia often complain of depression, decreased libido, stress intolerance, anxiety, and increased irritability. These behavioral symptoms usually resolve in parallel with decrements in serum prolactin when surgical or pharmacologic treatments are used. In psychotic patients, prolactin concentrations and prolactin-related sexual disturbances have been positively correlated with the severity of tardive dyskinesia.

Prolactin levels are also positively correlated with adverse symptoms in schizophrenia.

Melatonin

Melatonin, a pineal hormone, is derived from the serotonin molecule and it controls photoperiodically mediated endocrine events (particularly those of the hypothalamic–pituitary–gonadal axis). It also modulates immune function, mood, and reproductive performance and is a potent antioxidant and free-radical scavenger. Melatonin has a depressive effect on CNS excitability, is an analgesic, and has seizure-inhibiting effects in animal studies. Melatonin can be a useful therapeutic agent in the treatment of circadian phase disorders such as jet lag. Intake of melatonin increases the speed of falling asleep, as well as its duration and quality.

Oxytocin

Oxytocin, also a posterior pituitary hormone, is involved in osmoregulation, the milk ejection reflex, food intake, and female maternal and sexual behaviors. Oxytocin may be released during orgasm, more so in women than in men, and promote bonding between the sexes. It has been used in autistic children experimentally in an attempt to increase socialization.

Insulin

Increasing evidence indicates that insulin may be integrally involved in learning and memory. Insulin receptors occur in high density in the hippocampus and are thought to help neurons metabolize glucose. Patients with Alzheimer disease have lower insulin concentrations in the CSF than controls, and both insulin and glucose dramatically improve verbal memory. Depression is frequent in patients with diabetes, as are indexes of impaired hormonal response to stress. It is not known whether these findings represent the direct effects of the disease or are secondary, nonspecific effects. Some antipsychotics are known to dysregulate insulin metabolism.

Endocrine Variables in Psychiatric Disorders

Although it is clear that alterations in endocrine regulation are involved in the pathophysiology and treatment responses of many psychiatric disorders, incorporating these findings into clinical diagnostic assessment, and decision-making remains problematic. Large-scale longitudinal or cost-effectiveness studies are rare, despite indications that baseline alterations in glucocorticoid regulation and thyroid status (two of the best-studied abnormalities) may be useful in subtyping psychiatric disorders and prediction of outcome. Alterations in HPA/stress regulation underlie several psychiatric diagnoses and may serve as complementary independent variables in assigning treatment response and course of illness to the classical behavioral categories that have thus far defined psychiatric practice. Studying genetic polymorphisms in factors regulating hormonal response may help us better understand the influence of hormonal variability on the illness and also possible underlying differences in the illness as reflected in these genetic subtypes.

IMMUNE SYSTEM AND CENTRAL NERVOUS SYSTEM INTERACTIONS

Interactions between the immune system and the CNS play a critical role in the maintenance of bodily homeostasis and the development of diseases, including psychiatric disease. Alterations in CNS function brought about by a variety of stressors have been shown to influence both the immune system as well as diseases that involve the immune system. Moreover, many of the relevant hormonal and neurotransmitter pathways that mediate these effects have been elucidated. Of considerable interest is accumulating data that cytokines, which derive from immune cells and microglia, have profound effects on the CNS. The relative role of cytokines and their signaling pathways in the various psychiatric diseases is an area of active investigation, as is the role of infectious and autoimmune diseases in the pathophysiology of psychiatric disorders. These findings highlight the importance of interdisciplinary efforts involving the neurosciences and immunology for gaining new insights into the etiology of psychiatric disorders.

Overview of the Immune System

The immune system can protect the body from the invasion of foreign pathogens, such as viruses, bacteria, fungi, and parasites. Also, the immune system can detect and eliminate cells that have become neoplastically transformed. These functions are accomplished through highly specific receptors on immune cells for molecules derived from invading organisms and a rich intercellular communication network that involves direct cell-to-cell interactions and signaling between cells of the immune system by soluble factors called *cytokines*. The body's absolute dependence on the efficient functioning of the immune system is illustrated by the less than 1-year survival rate of untreated infants born with severe combined immunodeficiency disease and the devastating opportunistic infections and cancers that arise during untreated acquired immunodeficiency syndrome (AIDS).

Behavioral Conditioning

The fact that learning processes are capable of influencing immunologic function is an example of interactions between the immune system and the nervous system. Several classical conditioning paradigms have been associated with suppression or enhancement of the immune response in various experimental designs. The conditioning of immunologic reactivity provides further evidence that the CNS can have significant immunomodulatory effects.

Some of the first evidence for immunologic conditioning was derived from the serendipitous observation that animals undergoing extinction in a taste-aversion paradigm with cyclophosphamide, an immunosuppressive agent, had unexpected mortality. In that taste-aversion paradigm, animals were simultaneously exposed to an oral saccharin solution (the conditioned stimulus) and an intraperitoneal injection of cyclophosphamide (unconditioned stimulus). Because the animals experienced considerable physical discomfort from the cyclophosphamide injection, through the process of conditioning, they began to associate the ill effects of cyclophosphamide with the taste of the oral saccharin solution. If given a choice, the animals avoided the saccharin solution (taste aversion). Conditioned avoidance can be eliminated or extinguished if the saccharin is repeatedly presented in the absence of cyclophosphamide. However, it was observed that animals undergoing extinction of cyclophosphamide-induced taste aversion died unexpectedly, leading to the speculation that the oral saccharin solution had a specific conditioned association with the immunosuppressive effects of cyclophosphamide. Repeated exposure to the saccharin-associated conditioned immunosuppression during extinction might explain the unexpected death of animals. To test that hypothesis, researchers conditioned the animals with saccharin (conditioned stimulus) and intraperitoneal cyclophosphamide (unconditioned conditioned stimulus) and then immunized them with sheep red blood cells. At different times after immunization, the conditioned animals were re-exposed to saccharin (conditioned stimulus) and examined. The conditioned animals exhibited a significant decrease in mean antibody titers to sheep red blood cells when compared to the control animals. Thus, the evidence demonstrated that immunosuppression of humoral immunity was occurring in response to the conditioned stimulus of saccharin alone.

Stress and the Immune Response

Interest in the effects of stress on the immune system grew out of a series of animal and human studies suggesting that stressful stimuli can influence the development of immune-related disorders, including infectious diseases, cancer, and autoimmune disorders. Although stress has been historically associated with suppression of immune function, recent data indicate that such a conclusion oversimplifies the complexities of the mammalian immune response to environmental perturbation and that stress may also activate certain aspects of the immune system, particularly the innate immune response.

Stress and Illness.   Experiments conducted on laboratory animals in the late 1950s and the early 1960s indicated that a wide variety of stressors—including isolation, rotation, crowding, exposure to a predator, and electric shock—increased morbidity and mortality in response to several types of tumors and infectious diseases caused by viruses and parasites. However, as research progressed, it became increasingly clear that "stress" is too variegated a concept to have singular effects on immunity and that the effects of stress on immunity depend on several factors. Chief among these factors is whether a stressor is acute or chronic. Other critical variables include stressor severity and type, as well as the timing of stressor application and the type of tumor or infectious agent investigated. For example, mice subjected to electric grid shock 1 to 3 days before the infection of Maloney murine sarcoma virus-induced tumor cells exhibited decreased tumor size and incidence. In contrast, mice exposed to grid shock 2 days after tumor cell injection exhibited an increase in tumor size and number.

The relevance of the effects of stress on immune-related health outcomes in humans has been demonstrated in studies that have shown an association between chronic stress and increased susceptibility to the common cold, reduced antibody responses to vaccination, and delayed wound healing. Also, stress, as well as depression, through their effects on inflammation, has been linked to increased morbidity and mortality in infectious diseases, such as HIV infection, autoimmune disorders, neoplastic diseases, as well as diabetes and cardiovascular disorders, which are increasingly being recognized as diseases in which the immune system, inflammation, in particular, plays a pivotal role (Fig. 33-28).

Effects of Chronic Stress.   When challenged with a medical illness or chronic psychological stressor, complex interactions between the immune and nervous systems promote a constellation

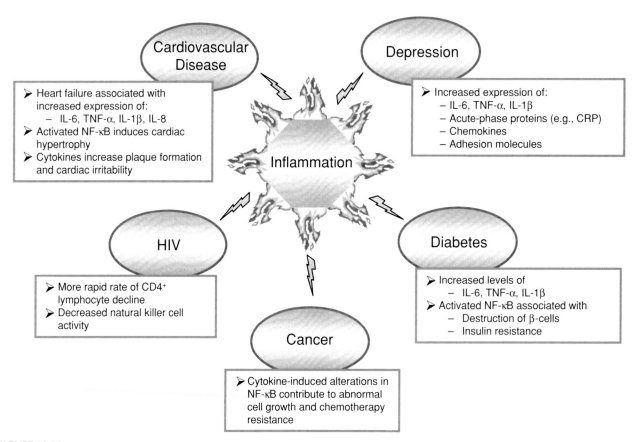

FIGURE 33-28

Inflammation and disease. IL, interleukin; TNF, tumor necrosis factor; NF-kB, nuclear factor κB; C RP, C-reactive protein. (From Cowles MK, Miller AH. Stress cytokines and depressive illness. In: Squire LR, ed. *The New Encyclopedia of Neuroscience.* Academic Press; 2009:521, with permission.)

of immune-induced behavioral changes, alternatively referred to as "sickness syndrome" or "sickness behavior." These behavioral changes include dysphoria, anhedonia, fatigue, social withdrawal, hyperalgesia, anorexia, altered sleep–wake patterns, and cognitive dysfunction. Although seen in response to infection, the full syndrome can be reproduced in humans and laboratory animals by the administration of innate immune cytokines. Blocking cytokine activity diminishes or prevents the development of sickness behavior in laboratory animals, even when such behavior develops as a result of psychological stress. Evidence that cytokine-induced behavioral toxicity is related to significant depression comes in part from studies showing that in humans and laboratory animals, antidepressants can abolish or attenuate the development of sickness behavior in response to cytokine administration.

Relevance of Immune System–CNS Interactions to Psychiatric Disorders

Major Depression. The neuropsychiatric disorder that has been best characterized in terms of the influence of the brain on the immune system and vice versa is major depression. For many years major depression was seen as the quintessential example of how stress-related disorders may decrease immunocompetence. More recently, however, it has become evident that stress also activates inflammatory pathways, even while suppressing measures of acquired immunity. Not surprisingly, studies now indicate that, in addition to immunosuppression, major depression is also frequently associated with inflammatory activation. Recent research showing that proinflammatory cytokines are capable of suppressing many of the immune measures examined in major depression may provide a mechanism to account for how chronic stress-induced inflammatory activity may give rise to depression-related suppression of in vitro functional assays, such as lymphocyte proliferation.

Bipolar Disorder. Patients with bipolar disorder evince many of the immune alterations frequently observed in the context of unipolar depression. Several studies have observed that bipolar patients, particularly when manic, demonstrate increased plasma concentrations of inflammatory cytokines. Other studies indicate that treatments for mania, such as lithium, lower plasma concentrations of several cytokines. Of interest, the available literature seems to suggest that patients in the manic phase of the disorder may be more likely than depressed patients to demonstrate increased inflammatory markers. It should not be surprising that mania—which seems the phenomenologic opposite of depression—should be associated with increased inflammation, given that mania and depression have also been reported to show identical neuroendocrine and autonomic abnormalities, such as dexamethasone non suppression and increased sympathetic activity, both of which would be expected to promote inflammatory activity.

Schizophrenia. There has been growing interest in the idea that infectious agents, particularly viruses, may underlie at least some cases of schizophrenia. Although it is well established that viral encephalitis can present clinically as psychosis, the primary focus of the "viral hypothesis" for schizophrenia has been on infections during neurodevelopment, given its congruence with the emerging consensus that prenatal or early postnatal insult is implicated in the causality of schizophrenia. Several lines of indirect evidence suggest that viral infection during CNS development may be involved in the pathogenesis of schizophrenia. The data include: (1) an excess number of patient births in the late winter and early spring, suggesting possible exposure to viral infection in utero during the fall and winter peak of viral illnesses, (2) an association between exposure to viral epidemics in utero and the later development of schizophrenia, (3) higher prevalence of schizophrenia in crowded urban areas, which have conditions that are particularly conducive to the transmission of viral pathogens, and (4) seroepidemiologic studies indicating a higher infection rate for certain viruses in schizophrenia patients or their mothers.

Also, schizophrenia has been associated with indices of immune activation, including elevations in cytokines. Although these immune findings in patients with schizophrenia may indicate evidence of immune system activation secondary to an infection, it should be noted that they might also indicate that an autoimmune process is involved in the disorder. Despite the plethora of studies pointing to abnormalities in cellular and humoral immunity in schizophrenia, the data have not been uniform or conclusive, and there is a need for more studies that account for confounding variables such as medication status and tobacco use. Moreover, attempts to isolate infectious agents from schizophrenic brain tissue or to detect viral nucleic acids in the CNS or peripheral blood of patients with schizophrenia have generally yielded negative results.

Because the initial neuronal abnormalities in schizophrenia have been proposed to arise during neurodevelopment, a perinatal viral infection could insidiously disrupt development and then be cleared by the immune system before clinical diagnosis. In such a scenario, host factors such as cytokines could be responsible for causing the developmental abnormality by interacting with growth factors or adhesion molecules. Recent animal models have identified that maternal immune activation with resultant production of interleukin 6 (IL-6) critically affects behavioral and transcriptional changes in offspring. Behavioral changes, including deficits in prepulse inhibition and latent inhibition, are consistent with behavioral abnormalities in animal models of both schizophrenia and autism. Various animal models using influenza virus, Borna disease virus, or lymphocytic choriomeningitis virus in rodents have demonstrated that prenatal or postnatal viral infections can lead to neuroanatomical or behavioral alterations that are somewhat reminiscent of schizophrenia in humans. As mentioned earlier, epidemiologic studies also support the link between infection with a teratogenic virus and the development of psychotic disorders later in life. Associations have been observed between maternal infection with rubella or influenza during gestation and the development of a schizophrenia spectrum disorder in the offspring. Similarly, maternal antibodies to the herpes simplex virus that develops during pregnancy are correlated with increased rates of psychosis during adulthood in the offspring.

Non-HIV retroviruses might also play a role in the pathogenesis of schizophrenia. Retroviruses integrate into host DNA and can disrupt the function of adjacent genes. Moreover, the genomes of all humans contain sequences of "endogenous retroviruses" that hold the capacity to alter the transcriptional regulation of host genes. If genes controlling the development or function of the brain undergo transcriptional disruption by retroviral effects, then this might lead to a cascade of biochemical abnormalities, eventually giving rise to schizophrenia.

Autism. Although a convincing case can be made for a significant immune component in autism, the relationship of immune abnormalities to the neurobehavioral symptoms of the disease remains controversial. Recent epidemiologic studies have not substantiated the claim that childhood vaccines trigger autism, and immune-based therapies for autism have not been reliably effective.

Thus, although it is tempting to speculate that the immune system holds a clue to a cure for autism, there is currently not enough data to determine whether immune anomalies cause autism, are *caused by* autism or are just adventitiously associated with the disease.

Alzheimer Disease. Although Alzheimer disease is not considered an inflammatory disease primarily, emerging evidence indicates that the immune system may contribute to its pathogenesis. The discovery that amyloid plaques are associated with acute-phase proteins, such as complement proteins and C-reactive protein, suggests the possibility of an ongoing immune response. The idea that inflammatory processes are involved in Alzheimer disease has been bolstered by recent studies showing that long-term use of nonsteroidal anti-inflammatory drugs (NSAIDs) is negatively correlated with the development of Alzheimer disease.

HIV AIDS. AIDS is an immunologic disease associated with a variety of neurologic manifestations, including dementia. HIV encephalitis results in synaptic abnormalities and loss of neurons in the limbic system, basal ganglia, and neocortex.

Multiple Sclerosis. Multiple sclerosis (MS) is a demyelinating disease characterized by disseminated inflammatory lesions of white matter. Considerable progress has been made in elucidating the immunopathology of myelin destruction that occurs in MS and the animal model for the disease, experimental allergic encephalomyelitis. Although the initial step in lesion formation has not been determined, disruption of the BBB and infiltration of T cells, B cells, plasma cells, and macrophages appear to be associated with lesion formation.

Other Disorders. Finally, several disorders are seen in which neural-immune interactions are suspected but not well documented. *Chronic fatigue syndrome* is an illness with a controversial etiology and pathogenesis. Also, to persistent fatigue, symptoms frequently include depression and sleep disturbances. Tests of immune function have found indications of both immune activation and immunosuppression. Neuroendocrine assessments indicate that patients with chronic fatigue syndrome may be hypocortisolemic because of impaired activation of the HPA axis. Although an acute viral infection frequently precedes the onset of chronic fatigue syndrome, no infectious agent has been causally associated with it.

In contrast, *Lyme disease,* in which sleep disturbances and depression are also common, is caused by infection with the tick-borne spirochete *Borrelia burgdorferi,* which can invade the CNS and cause encephalitis and neurologic symptoms. Lyme disease is remarkable because it appears to produce a spectrum of neuropsychiatric disorders, including anxiety, irritability, obsessions, compulsions, hallucinations, and cognitive deficits. Immunopathology of the CNS may be involved because symptoms can persist or reappear even after a lengthy course of antibiotic treatment, and the spirochete is frequently difficult to isolate from the brain. *Gulf War syndrome* is a controversial condition with inflammatory and neuropsychiatric features. The condition has been attributed variously to combat stress, chemical weapons (e.g., cholinesterase inhibitors), infections, and vaccines. Given the impact of stress on neurochemistry and immune responses, these pathogenic mechanisms are not mutually exclusive.

Therapeutic Implications

The bidirectional nature of CNS–immune system interactions implies the therapeutic possibility that agents known to alter stress system activity positively might benefit immune functioning and, conversely, that agents that modulate immune functioning may be of potential benefit in the treatment of neuropsychiatric disturbance, especially in the context of medical illness. Increasing evidence supports both hypotheses.

Antidepressants and the Immune System. Emerging data indicate that in animals and humans, antidepressants attenuate or abolish behavioral symptoms induced by inflammatory cytokine exposure. For example, pretreatment of rats with either imipramine or fluoxetine (a TCA and SSRI, respectively) for 5 weeks before endotoxin administration significantly attenuated endotoxin-induced decrements in saccharine preference (commonly accepted as a measure for anhedonia), as well as weight loss, anorexia, and reduced exploratory, locomotor, and social behavior. Similarly, several studies in humans suggest that antidepressants can ameliorate mood disturbances in the context of chronic cytokine therapies, especially if given prophylactically before cytokine exposure. For example, the SSRI paroxetine significantly decreased the development of major depression in patients receiving high doses of interferon-α (IFN-α) for malignant melanoma.

Behavioral Interventions and Immunity. It has been known for years that psychosocial factors can mitigate or worsen the effects of stress, not only on immune functioning but also on the long-term outcomes of medical conditions in which the immune system is known to play a role. Therefore, behavioral interventions aimed at maximizing protective psychosocial factors might be predicted to have a beneficial effect, not only in terms of mitigating the effect of stress on immune functioning but perhaps also on diminishing emotional disturbances that arise in the context of immune system dysregulation.

Two factors that have been repeatedly identified as protective against stress-induced immune alterations are social support and the ability to see stressors as being to some degree under the individual's control. One study used a genome-wide scan to assess gene expression activity in socially isolated versus nonisolated individuals. It found that social isolation was associated with increased activation of several proinflammatory cytokine-related pathways and reduced activity in anti-inflammatory cytokine pathways, as well as in the glucocorticoid receptor, which plays an essential role in the neuroendocrine control of inflammatory processes. Of interest, the two types of psychotherapy most often examined in illnesses associated with immune dysregulation are group therapy, which provides social support, and cognitive behavioral therapy, which provides cognitive reframing techniques aimed at enhancing one's sense of agency (and hence control).

NEUROGENETICS

Starting from the rediscovery of Gregor Mendel's basic concepts at the turn of the 20th century, the field of genetics has matured into an essential cornerstone not only of the biologic sciences but of all of medicine. The discovery of the basic structure and properties of DNA in the middle of the century led to an exponential acceleration in our understanding of all aspects of the life sciences, including deciphering the complete sequence of the human genome and those of myriad other species. Massive databases of such sequences now provide 21st-century biologists with the task of decoding the functional significance of all this information. In particular, researchers are trying to determine how to sequence variations contributing to the phenotypic variation between species and individuals within a species. In humans, we hope that discoveries about the relationship between genotypes and phenotypes will revolutionize our understanding of why and how some individuals but not others develop common diseases. This hope is particularly vital for psychiatry, as our knowledge of the pathogenic mechanisms of the psychiatric disease remains sparse.

Genetic mapping studies aim to identify the genes implicated in heritable diseases, based on their chromosomal location. These studies are carried out by investigating affected individuals and their families through two approaches, linkage, and association (Fig. 33-29). It is now straightforward to genetically map Mendelian traits (traits for which a specific genotype at one particular locus is both necessary and sufficient to cause the trait). Psychiatric diseases, however, do not follow simple Mendelian inheritance patterns but rather are examples of etiologically complex traits. Etiologic complexity may be due to many factors, including incomplete penetrance (expression of the phenotype in only some of the individuals carrying the disease-related genotype), the presence of phenocopies (forms of the disease that are not caused by genetic factors), locus heterogeneity (different genes associated with the same disease in different families or populations), or polygenic inheritance (risk for the disease only increases if susceptibility variants at multiple genes act in concert). Mapping a complex disorder involves several component steps, including the definition of

the phenotype to be studied, epidemiologic studies to determine the evidence for genetic transmission of that phenotype, choice of an informative study population, and determination of the appropriate experimental and statistical approaches.

Genetic Epidemiologic Approaches

Genetic epidemiologic investigations provide quantitative evidence regarding the degree to which given trait aggregates in families and can suggest to what degree such aggregation reflects a genetic contribution to the etiology of the trait. Family studies compare the aggregation of disease among the relatives of affected individuals compared to control samples. Because these studies do not differentiate between genetic and environmental contributions to such familial aggregation, they provide only indirect evidence regarding the heritability of a trait. Often these studies measure the relative risk (λ), defined as the rate of occurrence of disease among specified categories of relatives of an affected individual divided by the rate of occurrence of the disease for the general population. A relative risk of >1 suggests a genetic etiology, and the magnitude of the measure gives an estimate of the genetic contribution to the disease. Relative risks can be calculated for sibling pairs, parent–offspring pairs, and various other types of family relationships. Likely modes of transmission can be assessed by comparing the degree of relative

Gene Mapping Strategies

	Linkage Analysis		Genome Wide Association	
	Pedigree Analysis	Affected Sib Pair Analysis	Case-Control	Family-Trios
Study Subjects	Multigenerational families with multiple affected individuals	Two or more affected siblings	Affected individuals and matched unaffected controls sampled from population	Affected individual and parents
Basic Idea	Identify genetic markers that cosegregate with disease phenotype	Identify chromosomal regions shared by siblings concordant for disease.	Tests for statistical association of alleles and disease in cases versus controls.	Tests for association using nontransmitted parental chromosome as control.
Strengths	1) Can detect rare variants of large effect. 2) Gains power by incorporating information about familial relationships into the model.	1) Robust to differences in genetic composition of study population. 2) Easier to collect clinical samples compared to special pedigrees. 3) Allows incorporation of enviromental data.	1) Can detect common variants of small effect. 2) Does not require collection of family data.	1) Can detect common variants of small effect. 2) Robust to problems of population stratification.
Limitations	1) Limited power to identify common variants of small effect. 2) Cost intensive.	1) Limited power to identify common variants of small effect.	1) Increased false-positive rate in the presence of population stratification. 2) Requires large sample sizes.	1) About two-thirds as powerful as case-control designs. 2) Difficult to collect samples for late-onset diseases.

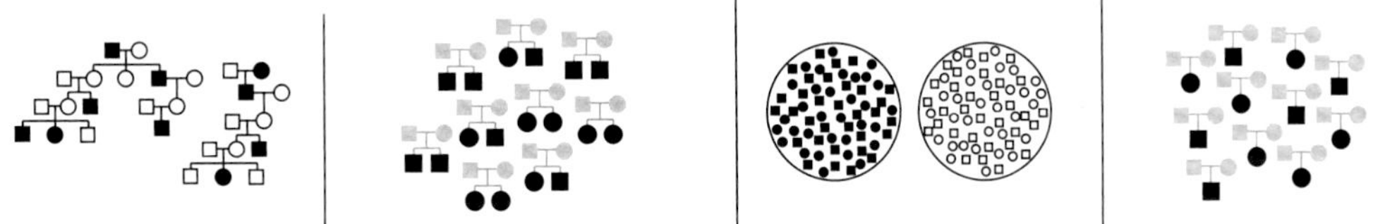

FIGURE 33-29

Comparison of gene-mapping strategies. Genetic mapping approaches can be divided into those that rely on linkage analysis and those that rely on association analysis. Linkage studies can be further categorized as either focused on investigation of pedigrees or focused on investigation of sib pairs. Association studies can be categorized as either case–control or family-based. Some of the key features as well as advantages and disadvantages of these different approaches are shown. (From Sadock BJ, Sadock VA, Ruiz P. *Kaplan & Sadock's Comprehensive Textbook of Psychiatry*. 9th ed. Philadelphia, PA: Lippincott Williams & Wilkins; 2009:321.)

risk for each type of relationship. Multiple family studies have been carried out for many of the major psychiatric disorders, including major depression, bipolar disorder, schizophrenia, and OCD. Although these studies have consistently reported familial aggregation for all of these disorders, the degree of such aggregation has varied substantially across studies, mainly reflecting differences in phenotype definition and how study samples were ascertained and assessed.

Twin studies examine the concordance rates of a particular disorder (the percentage of twin pairs where both twins have the disorder) in monozygotic (MZ) and dizygotic (DZ) twins. For a disorder that is strictly determined by genetic factors, the concordance rate should be 100 percent in MZ twin pairs (who share 100 percent of their genetic material) and 25 or 50 percent in DZ twin pairs (who are no more closely related than any siblings), depending on whether the disease is recessive or dominant, respectively. For a disorder where genetic factors play a role in disease causation but are not the exclusive cause of disease, the concordance rates should be more significant for MZ twins than those for DZ twins. The higher the degree of concordance of MZ twins, the higher the trait heritability or the evidence for a genetic contribution to disease risk. When genetic factors do not play a role, the concordance rates should not differ between the twin pairs, under the simplifying assumption that the environment for MZ twin pairs is no more similar than that for DZ twin pairs. Several twin studies that have been conducted for traits such as autism, bipolar disorder, and schizophrenia have consistently suggested high heritability and have therefore spurred efforts to map loci for each of these conditions genetically. Different twin studies may, however, generate varying point estimates for the heritability of any given disorder. When evaluating the results of twin studies, it is, therefore, essential to scrutinize how the phenotype was ascertained because, as with family studies, the different heritability estimates are likely due to differences in the mode of assessing and defining phenotypes. For example, early twin studies of psychiatric disorders often relied on their phenotypes on unstructured interviews by a single clinician.

In contrast, modern studies generally utilize standardized assessments and a review of diagnostic material by a panel of expert clinicians. Similarly, part of the apparent variation in heritability between different twin studies can be attributed to the fact that some studies employ narrow definitions of affectedness for a given phenotype. Other studies employ broader phenotype definitions (e.g., considering a twin with major depressive disorder to be phenotypically concordant with a co-twin diagnosed with bipolar disorder). Because of such differences in approach across studies, it is usually prudent to view such investigations as providing a rough estimate of the genetic contribution to trait variability. Nevertheless, even such estimates are useful in deciding which traits are likely to be mappable.

Basic Concepts of Gene Mapping

Recombination and Linkage.   Once genetic epidemiologic studies of particular phenotypes have suggested that these phenotypes are heritable, genetic mapping studies are conducted to identify the specific genetic variants that contribute to the risk of the disorder. All genetic mapping methods aim to identify disease-associated variants based on their chromosomal position and the principle of genetic linkage. All cells contain two copies of each chromosome (called homologs), one inherited from the mother and one inherited from the father. During meiosis, the parental homologs cross over, or recombine, creating unique new chromosomes

that are then passed on to the progeny. Genes that are physically close to one another on a chromosome are genetically linked, and those that are farther apart or are on different chromosomes are genetically unlinked. Unlinked genes will recombine at random (i.e., there is a 50 percent chance of recombination with each meiosis). Genetic loci that are linked will recombine less frequently than expected by random segregation, with the degree of recombination proportional to the physical distance between them. The principle of linkage underlies the use of genetic markers, segments of DNA of known chromosomal locations that contain variations or polymorphisms (described in more detail later). Strategies to map disease genes are based on identifying genetic marker alleles that are shared—to a greater extent than expected by chance—by affected individuals. It is presumed that such sharing reflects linkage between a disease locus and a marker locus, that is, the alleles at both loci are inherited "identical by descent" (IBD), from a common ancestor, and that this linkage pinpoints the chromosomal site of the disease locus.

The evidence for linkage between two loci depends on the recombination frequency between them. Recombination frequency is measured by the recombination fraction (Θ). It is equal to the genetic distance between the two loci (1 percent recombination equals 1 centimorgan [cM] in the genetic distance and, on average, covers a physical distance of about 1 megabase [mB] of DNA). A recombination fraction of 0.5 or 50 percent indicates that two loci are not linked but rather that they are segregating independently. A LOD (logarithm of the odds) score is calculated to determine the likelihood that two loci are linked at any particular genetic distance. The LOD score is calculated by dividing the likelihood of acquiring the data if the loci are linked at a given recombination fraction by the likelihood of acquiring the data if the loci are unlinked ($\Theta = 0.5$). This step gives an odds ratio, and the log (base 10) of this odds ratio is the LOD score. A LOD score can be obtained for various values of the recombination fraction, from $\Theta = 0$ (completely linked) to $\Theta = 0.5$ (unlinked). The value of Θ that gives the largest LOD score is considered to be the best estimate of the recombination fraction between the disease locus and the marker locus. This recombination fraction can then be converted into a genetic map distance between the two loci.

Linkage Disequilibrium.   Linkage disequilibrium (LD) is a phenomenon that is used to evaluate the genetic distance between loci in populations rather than in families. When alleles at two loci occur together in the population more often than would be expected given the allele frequencies at the two loci, those alleles are said to be in LD. When strong LD is observed between two loci, it usually indicates that the two loci are sited in very close physical proximity to one another on a given chromosome and is useful in mapping disease susceptibility loci because one locus can be used to predict the presence of another locus. This predictability is vital because current gene-mapping strategies can sample only a subset of the estimated 10 million common human polymorphisms. Because of the existence of LD, one can use data from a subset of genotyped polymorphisms to infer genotypes at nearby loci. Clusters of alleles that are in LD and inherited as a single unit are termed haplotypes. Thus LD mapping "consolidates" genomic information by identifying haplotypes in populations that can then be used to infer IBD sharing among unrelated individuals.

There are several methods to measure the extent of LD. One of the most commonly used measures of LD is r^2, a measure of the difference between observed and expected haplotype probabilities. Unlike D', another widely used measure of LD, r^2 values do not depend on the allele frequencies of the loci being assessed. A considerable r^2 value indicates that the observed frequency of association between two alleles is more significant than that expected by chance; that is, the alleles are in LD. LD studies have traditionally been used to complement traditional pedigree analyses, for example, to hone in on a locus that has been mapped by linkage analysis. However, LD-based association analysis has become the method of choice for whole-genome screens, particularly for diseases where traditional linkage studies have been unsuccessful. These studies have one great advantage over a traditional family analysis. Because affected individuals are chosen from an entire population, the only limit to the number of potential subjects is the population size and disease frequency. Maximizing the potential number of affected individuals that can be included in the analysis is extremely important for disorders where genetic heterogeneity or incomplete penetrance is likely to be a factor.

Genetic Markers. Mapping studies, regardless of their type, depend on the availability of genetic markers. The most widely used markers are microsatellite markers (also called simple tandem repeats [STRs], or simple sequence length polymorphisms [SSLPs]) and SNPs. SSLPs are stretches of variable numbers of repeated nucleotides two to four base pairs in length. These markers are highly polymorphic, as the number of repeat units at any given STR locus varies substantially between individuals. SNPs, as the name implies, are single base pair changes at a specific nucleotide; they are the most common form of sequence variation in the genome. SNPs are widely used for genetic mapping studies because they are distributed so widely across the genome and because they can be assessed in a high-throughput, automated fashion. Other forms of genetic variation that have been investigated for use as genetic markers include small insertion or deletion polymorphisms, termed indels, that generally range between 1 and 30 base pairs and copy number variations (CNVs), which can refer to either deletions or duplications. Recent genome-wide surveys have revealed that CNVs are common and can range in length from several base pairs to several million base pairs. CNVs may contribute to chromosomal recombination and rearrangements, thereby playing an essential role in generating genetic diversity. Also, as many of these variants are sizable, it is hypothesized that they may significantly influence the expression of genes that encompass or are adjacent to the variant.

Mapping Strategies

The genetic variants that contribute to disease susceptibility can be roughly categorized into those that are highly penetrant and those that are of low penetrance. High-penetrance variants, by definition, have a large effect on phenotype, and therefore identifying these variants usually provides fundamental insights into pathobiology. Because individuals carrying high-penetrance variants have a high probability of expressing a disease phenotype, such variants tend to be rare and to segregate in families and are generally most powerfully mapped using pedigree-based approaches (see Fig. 33-29). In contrast, low-penetrance variants have a relatively weak effect on phenotype, and therefore identification of individual low-penetrance variants may, at least initially, provide relatively little new biologic knowledge. However, because of their small effects, such variants are typically frequent, and identifying them may add to our understanding of disease risk. Because we do not expect these variants to segregate strongly with the disease phenotype in pedigrees, efforts to identify them focus on population samples.

Pedigree Analysis. A pedigree analysis, which is conducted in multigenerational families, consists of scanning the genome or a portion of the genome with a series of markers in one or more affected pedigrees, calculating a LOD score at each marker position, and identifying the chromosomal regions that show a significant deviation from what would be expected under independent assortment. The primary goal of the pedigree analysis is to determine if two or more genetic loci (i.e., a genetic marker of known location and the unknown disease loci) are cosegregating within a pedigree.

Following the successful application of pedigree analysis to map Mendelian disorders such as Huntington disease, many investigators adopted this strategy for mapping psychiatric disease genes with, at best, mixed success. In the late 1980s and mid-1990s, several pedigree-based studies reported the mapping of susceptibility loci for Alzheimer disease, bipolar disorder, and schizophrenia. Although the linkage findings for three Alzheimer disease loci were relatively quickly replicated, the findings reported for bipolar disorder and schizophrenia were ultimately determined to have been false positives. Several different explanations have been proposed for the failure of pedigree-based approaches to map psychiatric loci; however, most investigators now recognize that these studies were generally drastically underpowered, considering the apparent etiologic complexity of psychiatric disorders.

Pedigree analysis in psychiatry has increasingly turned toward an application that is more appropriately powered, namely, the mapping of quantitative trait loci (QTLs). QTLs are defined as genetic loci that contribute to the variation in continuously varying traits (as opposed to categorical traits such as disease diagnoses). QTLs are typically loci of small effect that only contribute to a portion of the observed variance of a trait in the population. It is now generally accepted that using analytical methods developed in the late 1990s, it may be possible to use pedigree studies to map a wide range of quantitative traits that are relevant for understanding psychiatric disorders. Several such studies are now being undertaken, typically with multiple phenotypes being assessed in each individual in the pedigree.

Sib-Pair Analysis. Affected sib-pair (ASP) analysis became widely used during the 1990s for the genetic mapping of complex traits, including many psychiatric disorders. Sib-pair analysis examines the frequency with which sibling pairs concordant for a trait share a particular region of the genome compared with the frequency that is expected under random segregation.

Sib-pair analysis is based on the fact that siblings share approximately 50 percent of their genomes IBD. Therefore, if a set of unrelated sib pairs affected with a given trait shares a particular area of the genome at a frequency significantly more significant than 50 percent (the proportion of sharing expected under conditions of random segregation), then that area of the genome is likely to be linked to the trait in question. In this method, siblings are genotyped, and population frequencies and parental genotypes are used to estimate the proportion of genes shared IBD at each site for each sib-pair. The linkage analysis then compares those pairs concordant and discordant for each locus.

Like pedigree studies, ASP studies have more power to locate genes of a large effect than genes of small effect. This limitation can be partially addressed by a two-tiered design that incorporates additional markers or family members after an initial linkage study in affected siblings or by an increased sample size. It generally requires less effort to identify and assess even large sets of affected sibs than to identify and assess all members of extended pedigrees, mainly when investigators can take advantage of data repositories that include samples and phenotype data from sib pairs ascertained from multiple sites. For example, the U.S. National Institute of Mental Health (NIMH) maintains such repositories for sizable collections of sib pairs affected with schizophrenia, bipolar disorder, autism, and Alzheimer disease. An additional benefit of the ASP design is that it allows for the incorporation of epidemiologic information, permitting the simultaneous examination of environmental and gene–environment interactions.

Association Studies.   In the last few years, there has been increasing acceptance of the notion that association studies are more powerful than linkage approaches for mapping the loci of relatively small effects that are thought to underlie much of the risk for complex disorders. Whereas linkage studies attempt to find cosegregation of a genetic marker and a disease locus within a family or families, association studies examine whether a particular allele occurs more frequently than expected in affected individuals within a population. As noted previously in this chapter, mapping of genes using association studies is based on the idea that specific alleles at markers closely surrounding a disease gene will be in LD with the gene; that is, these alleles will be carried in affected individuals more often than expected by random segregation, because they are inherited IBD.

There are two common approaches to association studies (see Fig. 33-29), case-control designs, and family-based designs, which typically investigate trios (mother, father, and an affected offspring). In a case-control study, allele frequencies are compared between a group of unrelated affected individuals and a matched control sample. This design is generally more powerful than a family-based design because large samples of cases and controls are more straightforward to collect than trios and are less expensive since they require the genotyping of fewer individuals. Case-control samples may be the only practical design for traits with a late age of onset (such as Alzheimer disease) for which parents of affected individuals are typically unavailable. The main drawback of the case-control approach is the potential problem of population stratification; if the cases and controls are not carefully matched demographically, then they may display substantial differences in allele frequency that reflect population differences rather than associations with the disease.

Family-based association studies are designed to ameliorate the problem of population stratification. In this design, the nontransmitted chromosomes (the copy of each chromosome that is not passed from parent to child) are used as control chromosomes, and differences between allele frequencies in the transmitted and nontransmitted chromosomes are examined, eliminating the problem of stratification, as the comparison group is by definition genetically similar to the case group. Although more robust to population stratification than a case-control study, family-based studies are only about two-thirds as powerful using the same number of affected individuals, as noted previously.

Until recently, it was not practical to conduct association studies on a genome-wide basis, as relatively few SNPs were available. Therefore, association studies focused on testing one or a few markers in candidate genes chosen based on their hypothesized function with a given disease. Recently, however, as a result of international efforts that have identified millions of SNPs distributed relatively evenly across the genome and that have developed technology for genotyping them relatively inexpensively, genome-wide association (GWA) studies are now a reality. Such studies hold much promise for the identification of common variants contributing to

common diseases. While few GWA studies of psychiatric disorders have been completed, such studies have already reported remarkable findings for complex traits such as rheumatoid arthritis, inflammatory bowel disease, and type 2 diabetes. The successful studies of these diseases have made use of extensive samples (in some cases up to several thousand cases and controls), providing further support for the hypothesis that underpowered study designs bear much of the responsibility for the disappointing results to date of psychiatric genetic investigations.

Statistical Considerations.   Scientists in other biomedical research fields are often surprised by the high level of statistical evidence that geneticists require to consider a linkage or association result to be significant. This requirement can be imagined in terms of the very low expectation that any two loci are either linked or associated with one another. The likelihood that any two given loci are linked (i.e., the prior probability of linkage) is expected to be approximately 1:50, based on the genetic length of the genome. To compensate for this low prior probability of linkage and bring the posterior (or overall) probability of linkage to about 1:20, which corresponds to the commonly accepted significance level of $p = 0.05$, a conditional probability of 1,000:1 odds in favor of linkage is required, corresponding to the traditionally accepted LOD score threshold of 3. This generally provides an acceptable false-positive rate (Fig. 33-30), but some false-positive findings have exceeded even this threshold.

Geneticists generally expect that the chance that any two loci in the genome are associated with one another is even lower than that of their being in linkage. Typically a p-value of less than about 10^{-7} is considered to indicate "genome-wide significance." This standard essentially discounts the prior probability that some investigators assign to variants in candidate genes chosen based on their hypothesized functional relevance to a given disorder or trait. GWA studies are now replicating associations with very low p-values for a wide range of complex traits, whereas most candidate gene associations

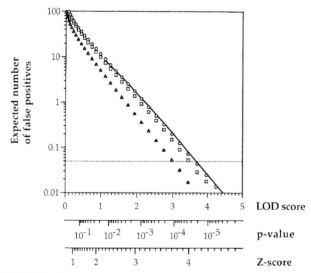

FIGURE 33-30

Number of false positives expected in a whole genome scan for a given threshold of logarithm of odds (LOD) score. *Solid line* represents the expectation for a perfect genetic map. *Symbols* represent the results for 100 sib pairs using genetic maps with markers spaced every .1 cM (*circles*), every 1 cM (*squares*), and every 10 cM (*triangles*). The *dotted line* indicates the 5 percent genome-wide significance level. (Courtesy of Dr. Eric Lander.)

(which usually report as significant much higher *p*-values) remain unreplicated. It is, therefore, increasingly apparent that genome-wide levels of significance are appropriately applied to all initial association studies for a given trait.

Defining Phenotypes for Mapping Studies

The generally disappointing results of psychiatric genetic mapping studies have focused increasing attention on the problem of defining and assessing phenotypes for such studies. Most psychiatric mapping studies to date have relied on categorical disease diagnoses, as exemplified by the *Diagnostic and Statistical Manual* (DSM-5) classification scheme. Criticisms of this approach rest on two arguments. First, diagnosis of the psychiatric disease depends on subjective clinical evaluation, a fact that underscores the difficulty in ascertaining individuals who can be considered affected with a given disease. Second, even when a psychiatric diagnosis can be established unambiguously, the menu-based system used for psychiatric classification provides the possibility that any two individuals affected with a given disorder may display mostly nonoverlapping sets of symptoms, likely reflecting distinct etiologies. Concern that the diagnosis-based approach to phenotyping may represent one of the chief obstacles to the genetic mapping of

psychiatric phenotypes has generated considerable interest in mapping heritable traits known to demonstrate continuous variation in the population. Continuous measures that are hypothesized to be related to psychiatric disorders include biochemical measures (e.g., serum or CSF levels of neurotransmitter metabolites or hormones), cognitive measures, personality assessments, structural or functional brain images, biophysical markers such as responses to evoked potentials, or molecular assays such as gene expression profiles. Critical features of categorical and continuous phenotyping strategies are shown in Figure 33-31, and each is discussed in more detail below.

Categorical Phenotypes.   The most commonly used categorical phenotypes in psychiatry are DSM diagnoses. Some studies focus on a single DSM diagnosis, whereas other studies include individuals with a range of different diagnoses. The latter approach is typically used for disorders that are hypothesized to represent a single disease spectrum, such as mood disorders. The categorical approach is designed to help us classify subjects as unambiguously as possible. Several strategies are used to accomplish this goal. The first strategy involves deciding on the appropriate diagnostic criteria for the study in question and deciding how these criteria will be applied to individuals in the study. One way of standardizing the procedures used to identify and assess potential study subjects

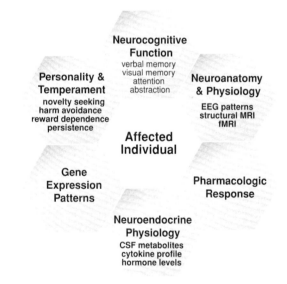

Phenotyping Strategies

A. Categorical Traits

Bipolar Disorder   **Schizophrenia**

Elevated Mood
Flight of Ideas
Pressured Speech

Disorganized Speech
Disorganized Behavior

Hallucinations
Suicidality
Delusions

Insomnia   Flat Affect
Irritability   Avolition
Impaired Concentration

Major Depression
Depressed Mood
Appetite Disturbance
Anergy
Guilt/Worthlessness

B. Continuous Traits

Neurocognitive Function
verbal memory
visual memory
attention
abstraction

Personality & Temperament
novelty seeking
harm avoidance
reward dependence
persistence

Neuroanatomy & Physiology
EEG patterns
structural MRI
fMRI

Affected Individual

Gene Expression Patterns

Pharmacologic Response

Neuroendocrine Physiology
CSF metabolites
cytokine profile
hormone levels

FIGURE 33-31

Two alternate schemes for conceptualizing psychiatric phenotypes. **A:** Categorical Traits as conceptualized by the Diagnostic and Statistical Manual (DSM-5) represent a "menu-based" approach to psychiatric disorders. Individuals are assessed for a checklist of signs and symptoms that are then used to categorize the individual as "affected" according to a specific diagnosis. Not all symptoms are present in samples of individuals who carry a particular DSM diagnosis, and many of these symptoms occur across diagnostic boundaries, as illustrated in this Venn diagram. DSM phenotypes therefore probably represent etiologically heterogeneous categories, and this fact may help to explain the limited progress thus far of genetic mapping investigations focused on these phenotypes. **B:** Alternatively, in the Continuous Traits model, "affectedness" can be conceptualized in terms of an expectation that an individual will demonstrate extreme values on a set of continuous measures that correlate with psychopathology and thus are hypothesized to underlie the disorder (as illustrated by examples of six different types of measures shown in the hexagon). Such measures may also be associated with particular components of categorical phenotypes, such as those depicted in the Venn diagram in Figure 33-31A. The justification for using continuous measures as the phenotypes for genetic mapping studies is that they are considered etiologically simpler and more reliably assessed compared to categorical phenotypes. In addition, mapping such traits combines information from all members of the study population (affected and unaffected individuals alike), which adds considerably to power. (From Sadock BJ, Sadock VA, Ruiz P. *Kaplan & Sadock's Comprehensive Textbook of Psychiatry*. 9th ed. Philadelphia, PA: Lippincott Williams & Wilkins; 2009:325.)

is to use only experienced clinicians in the diagnostic process and to train them in the administration of the instruments and the diagnostic criteria to be employed. Also, a "best estimate" procedure or a consensus diagnosis is frequently used. The best estimate process involves making use of every piece of available information, including medical records, interviews, and videotapes, to arrive at a diagnosis. For a consensus diagnosis, two or more diagnosticians independently review the material and make a diagnosis for each individual. The diagnoses are then compared, and individuals for whom an agreement in diagnosis cannot be reached are not entered as "affected" into the study.

A well-designed study makes use of all available information about the genetic epidemiology of the disorder to choose a sample of affected individuals to study. It is often the case that a subset of families carries the disorder in what appears to be a simple Mendelian pattern, whereas the inheritance pattern is less clear for other families or groups. In a disorder where there are likely to be multiple genes contributing to the phenotype, it makes sense, to begin with, a study sample where there may be significant loci. Redefining the disease phenotype can often simplify the mapping process by identifying such groups or families. For example, in the search for a genetic defect for Alzheimer disease, the process was advanced enormously by limiting the study population to those individuals who had an early age of onset (before age 65); the early-onset trait segregated in an autosomal dominant fashion. Other ways of redefining the phenotype include focusing on factors such as ethnic background, age of onset, treatment response, symptom severity, or the presence of comorbid disorders.

Narrowing the phenotype using the approaches discussed earlier may increase the chances of finding a genetic defect in complex diseases, but it can also significantly reduce the power of the study by limiting the number of available affected individuals. For this reason, it has been argued that for some disorders broadening the phenotype is an appropriate strategy. The suggestion is that for some complex diseases, the phenotype of interest may represent the end of a spectrum and that other phenotypes within the spectrum must also be included to have enough power to map genes. For example, mapping studies of bipolar disorder might include affected individuals with major depressive disorder as well as those individuals diagnosed with bipolar disorder.

Although the two approaches of narrowing the disease phenotype and broadening the disease phenotype may seem to be mutually exclusive, many groups studying complex disorders have incorporated both approaches into their study designs. One way to do this is to create stratified diagnostic categories, ranging from a narrow diagnostic category to a broad diagnostic category, and test for genetic linkage under each of these schemas. Some investigators argue that for complex diseases that are part of a spectrum, this strategy decreases the rate of false negatives, that is, of missing an existing linkage because of misspecification. Others argue that using several models and picking the one that gives the highest scores dramatically increases the rates of false positives, that is, of identifying an area of linkage where none exists. One problem that exists with the use of multiple diagnostic categories is that as more models are used (and therefore more statistical tests are performed), increasingly stringent levels of evidence are required to consider a result significant.

While categorical phenotypes remain the mainstay of psychiatric genetic studies, the limitations of DSM nosology as the basis of phenotyping for genetic studies are becoming apparent. Genetic investigations are focusing increasingly on traits that may be components of one or more DSM diagnostic categories. For example, there is growing evidence that genetic susceptibility to psychosis, broadly defined, contributes to both severe bipolar disorder and schizophrenia, and several investigative approaches are being employed to attempt to identify genes that underlie such susceptibility and even to explore possible etiologic relationships between psychiatric and nonpsychiatric disorders. For example, bioinformatics models have been employed to investigate medical records databases and have uncovered extensive pairwise correlations among a diverse list of psychiatric disorders, neurologic disorders, autoimmune disorders, and infectious diseases. Eventually, the results of such model-fitting experiments may provide a framework to design more powerful linkage and association studies that can search for alleles that contribute to susceptibility to multiple disorders.

Continuous Phenotypes. Because of the difficulties experienced in genetic mapping of categorical diagnoses, neurobehavioral geneticists are increasingly focused on investigating quantitative traits that are hypothesized to underlie a particular psychiatric diagnosis, and that may be simpler to map genetically. The rationale for efforts to map such alternative phenotypes or endophenotypes is that the genes identified through such efforts may provide clues regarding the biologic pathways that are relevant to understanding a particular disorder. Several features characterize useful endophenotypes. First, they should be state-independent; that is, they should not fluctuate as a function of the disease course or medication treatment and should show adequate test–retest stability. Second, they should be heritable; that is, there should be evidence that genetic factors are responsible for a substantial proportion of the variability of the trait within the population. Third, the endophenotype should be correlated with the disease under investigation; that is, different values of the trait measure are observed in patients compared to unrelated control subjects.

Measures of brain structure and function provide most of the traits now under investigation as endophenotypes for psychiatric disorders. For example, several features of brain morphometry (as assessed by MRI) are highly heritable (in the range of 60 to 95 percent), including total brain volume, cerebellar volume, gray and white matter density, amygdala and hippocampal volume, and regional cortical volume. Several studies show that brain structural features that are correlated in clinical samples with disorders such as schizophrenia or bipolar disorder are also abnormal in relatives of affected individuals. Physiologic measures of brain activity that have been employed as candidate endophenotypes for psychiatric disorders include electroencephalography (EEG) patterns. Several "pencil and paper" assessments have been employed to measure endophenotypes relating to neurocognitive function and temperament.

Animal Models. In contrast to categorical phenotypes, endophenotypes can be more straightforwardly related to phenotypes that can be assessed in animal models. Studies of genetic variations that affect circadian rhythms provide a good example. Variations in circadian rhythms have long been recognized as prominent features of mood disorders, and quantitative assessments of activity patterns have been proposed as endophenotypes for such disorders. Numerous studies in animal models have demonstrated that genetically controlled biologic clocks determine circadian activity and that variations in clock genes are associated with variations in such activity from bacteria to humans. Genetic mapping efforts in fruit flies starting in the early 1970s resulted in the identification of at least seven "clock genes," beginning with a *period*. Subsequent studies showed that the homologs of several of these genes play essential roles in regulating mammalian circadian rhythms. Genetic mapping studies in mice also have identified previously unknown circadian rhythm genes, beginning with the discovery and characterization in the early 1990s of a *clock*. These genetic discoveries have not only explicated the cellular networks and neurophysiologic circuits responsible for the control of mammalian circadian rhythms. However, they have also generated animal models that may shed light on the pathobiology of psychiatric syndromes such as bipolar disorder. For example, mice carrying a targeted mutation in the *clock* demonstrate abnormal activity patterns, such as hyperactivity and decreased sleep, which is modified by the administration of lithium.

Progress in the Genetics of Specific Disorders

The progress in identifying susceptibility genes for psychiatric disorders has been disappointing compared to that observed for nonpsychiatric disorders. Alzheimer disease represents the most successful application of gene-mapping strategies to complex neurobehavioral disorders, and the section on this disease provides an example of how genetic linkage studies add to the understanding of the pathogenesis of a complex trait. An overview section on autism describes genetic investigations of syndromes that have features of autism but have relatively simple inheritance patterns and discusses how these studies have provided starting points for investigations of more complex ASDs. Finally, the frustrating search for unequivocal gene findings for bipolar disorder and schizophrenia is used to illustrate the challenges that are motivating new approaches in the field of neurobehavioral genetics.

Alzheimer Disease. Alzheimer disease provides an excellent example of the power of genetics to elucidate the complex biology of a neuropsychiatric disorder. Alzheimer disease is a well-defined form of dementia characterized by progressive impairment of memory and intellectual functioning. The clinical signs and symptoms, although characteristic, are not limited to Alzheimer disease; they are also found in several other types of dementia. For this reason, the diagnosis of Alzheimer disease can only be confirmed histopathologically at autopsy. The presence of senile plaques (made up of a core of β-amyloid fibrils surrounded by dystrophic neurites), tau-rich neurofibrillary tangles, and congophilic angiopathy in the brain parenchyma and associated blood vessels are pathognomonic for Alzheimer disease.

A variable age of onset has been noted for Alzheimer disease, ranging from as early as age 35 to as late as age 95. The concordance rate for Alzheimer disease in MZ twin pairs is about 50 percent, indicating a moderately substantial genetic contribution to disease risk. It is now evident from a wide range of genetic studies that Alzheimer disease can be divided into two broad categories. These are the familial forms, which account for a tiny minority of Alzheimer disease cases and are characterized by early onset and autosomal dominant inheritance with high penetrance; and sporadic forms, in which the genetic contribution is hypothesized to be similar to that characterizing other common neuropsychiatric diseases.

The search for the genetic basis of familial Alzheimer disease began with traditional linkage studies. First, an investigation of a candidate locus on chromosome 21 in humans identified mutations in the *amyloid precursor protein* (*APP*) gene in a small number of families in which significant linkage had previously been observed to markers from this region. Transgenic mice with different *APP*

mutations were created and have been shown to produce β-amyloid deposits and senile plaques as well as to show synapse loss, astrocytosis, and microgliosis, all part of the pathology of Alzheimer disease. Mutations in the genes that encode β-APP all lead to an increase in the extracellular concentration of longer fragments of β-amyloid (Aβ42). Most of the strains of transgenic mice with mutations in APP exhibit increased rates of behavioral changes and impairment in several memory tasks, indicating dysfunction in object-recognition memory and working memory, among others. These findings represent striking evidence that mutations in the β-amyloid gene are indeed responsible for at least some of the histopathologic elements of Alzheimer disease.

Even as the preceding findings were being reported, it was clear that mutations in the β-amyloid gene could not wholly explain the etiology and pathology of Alzheimer disease, not least because it was shown that linkage to chromosome 21 was excluded in most early-onset Alzheimer disease families. Also, no neurofibrillary tangles are observed in most of the different β-amyloid transgenic mice. The subsequent search for the genetic underpinnings of Alzheimer disease using genome-wide linkage analysis of early-onset Alzheimer disease families resulted in the identification of two additional Alzheimer disease susceptibility genes: *presenilin-1* (*PS-1*) on chromosome 14q24.3 and *presenilin-2* (*PS-2*) on chromosome 1q. PS-1 and PS-2 are integral transmembrane proteins with at least seven transmembrane domains. Although their function has not yet been completely elucidated, they are involved in the pathogenesis of Alzheimer disease. Inactivation of *presenilins* in mice leads to neurodegeneration and behavioral manifestations of memory loss. Biochemical and cellular studies have implicated presenilins in several critical pathways, including apoptosis (programmed cell death) and protein processing in the endoplasmic reticulum.

These findings emphasize one of the strengths of using family-based linkage analysis. Pedigree-based studies are especially suited to identify highly penetrant disease genes that serve essential roles in critical biologic processes. Although mutations in *APP* and *presenilin* are rare, research into the biology of the expressed proteins has provided vital insights into the pathophysiology of dementia. Because these highly penetrant mutations elucidate essential biologic functions, they also provide a firm ground to design therapeutic interventions. For example, amyloid-β "vaccines" designed to induce an immunogenic response to pathogenic amyloid are now in advanced clinical trials. Unlike the current psychopharmacological treatments for Alzheimer disease that nonspecifically target cholinergic and glutaminergic neuronal systems, the amyloid-β vaccines may specifically treat the causes of Alzheimer disease by generating an immune response that may reverse the deposition of senile plaques.

SPORADIC AND LATE-ONSET ALZHEIMER DISEASE. Mutations in *APP, PS-1,* or *PS-2* are present in a majority of familial cases of early-onset Alzheimer disease but do not account for sporadic or familial late-onset Alzheimer disease. For this reason, investigators turned to other approaches to search for evidence of linkage in a large number of small families with late-onset Alzheimer disease. In 1991, the results of a nonparametric linkage study using 36 markers in late-onset Alzheimer disease families provided evidence for a susceptibility gene on the long arm of chromosome 19. In 1993, association studies revealed that the e4 allele of the *apolipoprotein E* gene was strongly associated with late-onset Alzheimer disease and that this association almost certainly was responsible for the previously observed linkage signal on chromosome 19.

There are three known alleles of this gene—e2, e3, and e4. In most populations, the e3 allele is the most common. However, in familial late-onset Alzheimer disease, the incidence of e4 is approximately 50 percent, and in sporadic late-onset Alzheimer disease, it is 40 percent, compared with about 16 percent in normal controls. Epidemiologic studies suggest that between 30 and 60 percent of late-onset Alzheimer disease cases have at least one *apoE-e4* allele. The e4 genotype appears to be a more important risk factor for Alzheimer disease in populations of European and Asian origin when compared with populations of African origin. Overall, the association of *apoE-e4* with Alzheimer disease remains probably the most robust association yet identified for a common human disease.

The establishment of *apoE-e4* as a susceptibility allele for late-onset Alzheimer disease has led to the search for additional alleles that might interact with *apoE-e4* to modify disease risk. In 2007, investigators used GWA strategies (in histologically confirmed cases and controls) to identify *GAB2* (GRB-associated binding protein 2) as an additional risk allele in *apoE-e4* carriers (but not in Alzheimer disease patients who were not e4 carriers). Initial studies suggest that carriers of both *apoE-e4* and *GAB2* risk alleles have an almost 25-fold more significant risk for Alzheimer disease than individuals who do not carry either risk allele. Larger-scale GWA studies of Alzheimer disease are in progress and will likely yield further associations; however, it is unlikely that any will have as strong an effect as *apoE*.

Autism.   Autism is a severe neurodevelopmental disorder that is characterized by three primary features: impaired language and communication; abnormal or impaired social interaction; and restricted, repetitive, and stereotyped patterns of behavior. Understanding the etiology of autism has proceeded slowly, but there is convincing evidence that alterations in specific cellular and molecular neurodevelopmental pathways are essential in its etiology. In comparison with other neuropsychiatric disorders, there is particularly strong evidence for a genetic contribution to the risk of autism and ASDs. The sibling recurrence risk for autism or ASD is between 2 and 6 percent. Given a population prevalence of about 1 in 2,000 (0.04 percent), this means that the siblings of autistic individuals are approximately 50 to 100 times more likely to develop autism than a person in the general population. Twin studies of autism show extraordinarily high heritability (as demonstrated by MZ twin concordance of 80 to 92 percent) but also demonstrate the genetic complexity of these disorders, with the DZ twin concordance rate of 1 to 10 percent suggesting a highly multigenic mode of inheritance.

Increasing interest is now focused on the possibility that individuals affected with autism may display more considerable numbers of large-scale chromosomal aberrations (5 to 10 percent in some studies) than unaffected individuals. Also, to such gross abnormalities, several recent studies have suggested that autism is associated with an unusually high prevalence of submicroscopic CNVs. For example, in 2007, the Autism Genome Project Consortium applied microarray strategies to almost 8,000 individuals from about 1,500 families, each with at least two affected family members, and found that about 10 percent of the ASD families carried CNVs, with an average size of more than 3 million base pairs, mostly consisting of duplications rather than deletions. Although the design of this study did not permit assessment of whether the frequency of CNVs is higher in patients with autism than that in controls, another study found a de novo CNV incidence of 10 percent in sporadic (no family history) cases of autism compared to an incidence of

1 percent in controls. These results, while exciting, are still considered preliminary. Even before the demonstration of high rates of de novo mutations in autism, epidemiologic studies had strongly suggested that the genetic basis of this disorder is likely complex. For example, although the risk of autism in first-degree relatives of autistic probands is high, there is a substantial falloff for second- and third-degree relatives of such probands, suggesting that multiple genetic variants must interact to increase susceptibility to this syndrome. Segregation analyses of autism also support the hypothesis that it is a heterogeneous disorder that reflects the actions of multiple genetic variants of small effect. A latent class analysis performed to study possible modes of transmission suggested an epistatic model with up to about 10 interacting loci, whereas other studies have estimated that as many as 15 such loci may be involved. Genetic studies of autism have included whole-genome screens, candidate gene studies, chromosome rearrangement studies, mutation analyses, and, most recently, comparative genomic hybridization studies. Taken together and recognizing that most findings still await adequate replication, these studies have contributed to an emerging picture of autism susceptibility that includes genes involved in three major systems: those involving synapse formation and maintenance, those involving cell migration, and those involving the excitatory/inhibitory neurotransmitter networks. Figure 33-32 shows a schematic of the currently known potential candidate genes for autism and their molecular relationships with one another.

SYNAPSE FORMATION AND MAINTENANCE.   Perhaps the most significant breakthroughs in identifying susceptibility genes for autism have come from studies of disorders that display clinical features associated with autism or ASDs but with simpler inheritance patterns, including fragile X syndrome, tuberous sclerosis, and Rett syndrome. In general, the genetic defects associated with these disorders affect synapse formation and maintenance. Fragile X, which accounts for 3 to 4 percent of autism cases, is caused by an unstable trinucleotide repeat in the 5′ region of the fragile X mental retardation 1 (*FMR1*) gene at Xq27.3. This repeat expands as it is transmitted to succeeding generations, resulting in abnormal methylation and inhibition of expression of *FMR1*. *FMR1* produces an RNA-binding protein that acts as a chaperone for the transport of RNA from the nucleus to the cytoplasm and is involved in messenger RNA (mRNA) translation at the synapse. Abnormalities in dendritic spine density (increased over normal) and anatomy (longer and thinner than normal) have been reported in individuals with fragile X as well as in mouse models of this disorder. Tuberous sclerosis, which accounts for perhaps 2 to 10 percent of autism cases (the rate of tuberous sclerosis is higher among autistic individuals with seizure disorders), results from mutations in one of two tumor suppressor genes, *TSC1* on 9q34, and *TSC2* on 16p13, both of which are involved in guanosine triphosphatase (GTPase) inactivation. Loss of a single copy of *TSC1* in mice has been shown to disrupt cytoskeletal dynamics and dendritic spine structure.

Although somewhat less well understood, the genetics of Rett syndrome, an X-linked pervasive developmental disorder (the first with a known genetic etiology), also point to abnormalities in synapse formation and maintenance in ASD and ASD-like disorders. Mutations in *MeCP2* cause Rett syndrome. The gene makes a methylated-DNA-binding protein that regulates gene expression and chromatin structure. Although little is known about the exact role of *MeCP2* in the development of Rett syndrome, the pattern of normal early development and later regression suggests that

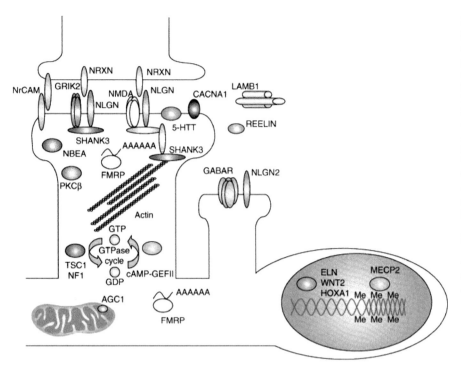

FIGURE 33-32

Schematic of the cell biology of proteins expressed from genes identified through mapping studies of autism spectrum disorders. The function of each gene product falls into three broad functional categories. Proteins involved in synapse formation and maintenance include FMR1, TSC1, TSC2, MeCP2, NLGN 3 and 4, and SHANK3. Another set of proteins is involved in neuronal migration and cell fate including REELIN, WNT2, LAMB1, and NrCAM. Proteins involved in neurotransmitter systems are also altered in some individuals with autism and include 5-HTT (serotonin transporter encoded by SLC6A4), GABAR, and the NMDA subunit encoded by GRIN2A. See text for details. (From Persico AM, Bourgeron T. Searching for ways out of the autism maze: genetic, epigenetic and environmental clues. *Trends Neurosci.* 2006;29:349, with permission.)

this gene is more likely to be involved in synapse maintenance and remodeling than in synapse development.

Neuroligin (*NLGN*) 3 and 4 and *SHANK3*, additional genes that appear to play a role in synapse formation, may be affected by chromosomal rearrangements observed in some individuals affected with autism. The neuroligin genes, sited on the X chromosome, produce cell adhesion molecules that are located on postsynaptic glutamatergic neurons. When mutated in rodents, these genes show defective trafficking and synapse induction. In nonmutated form, their expression induces the formation of normal, presynaptic terminals in axons. *SHANK3* is a binding partner of the neuroligins and regulates the structural organization of dendritic spines. Mutations in *SHANK3* have been identified in ASD-affected members of at least three families to date, and a comparative genomic hybridization study of autistic individuals, their family members, and controls recently identified a large deletion in chromosome 22q13, the region containing *SHANK3*, in at least one individual with autism.

CELL MIGRATION. Of the regions highlighted by a genome screen in autism families, chromosome 7q has provided the most consistent evidence for linkage, albeit over an extensive region. Known chromosomal rearrangements in this region in individuals affected with autism add to its interest. The linkage region on chromosome 7q contains several genes that are strong candidates for autism, most notably *RELN*, which maps to chromosome 7q22. *RELN* codes for reelin, a signaling protein secreted by Cajal–Retzius cells located in the marginal zone of the developing brain. It plays a vital role in neuronal migration as well as in the development of neural connections. Reeler mice, which have spontaneous deletions of *RELN*, have cytoarchitectonic alterations in their brains during development that are similar to those that have been described in autistic brains. The complete absence of *RELN* in humans leads to a more severe phenotype with lissencephaly and severe mental retardation but not autism. Individuals with autism show reduced levels of reelin mRNA and protein in brain and blood serum, suggesting that mutations leading to reduced

expression of *RELN* rather than its absence may be significant in ASD. Genetic association studies with *RELN* have been equivocal, suggesting that if *RELN* does contribute to the development of autism, then it may play such a role in a small subset of affected individuals. *WNT2* (wingless-type MMTV integration site family member 2) is another gene identified as a potential candidate for autism based on linkage studies. *WNT2* is located on 7q31 and is part of a family of genes that encode secreted signaling proteins implicated in several developmental processes, including the regulation of cell fate and patterning during embryogenesis. At least two families have been identified in which nonconservative coding sequence variants in *WNT2* segregate with autism. LD between an SNP in the 3′ untranslated region of *WNT2* and autism is also present in families with severe language abnormalities that accounted for most of the evidence for linkage on chromosome 7q in one of the original genome screens.

EXCITATORY/INHIBITORY NEUROTRANSMITTER SYSTEMS. Although there is little current evidence that mutations in genes encoding neurotransmitter transporters or receptors are directly responsible for the development of autism, there is some evidence that such genes might act as modifiers or susceptibility factors for autism spectrum phenotype. The evidence is perhaps most robust for the role of the GABA receptors in the development and expression of autistic disorders. These receptors occur in a cluster on chromosome 15q11–13, and duplications of this region are the most common cytogenetic abnormalities seen in autism cases (up to 6 percent of cases). GABA is an important inhibitory neurotransmitter in the CNS and is responsible for controlling excitability in mature brains. Chromosome 15q11–13 is one of the most complex regions of the genome. It has a high rate of genomic instability, including frequent duplication and deletion events, and imprinting plays a vital role in the expression of genes in this region. The 15q11–13 region is the critical region for Angelman and Prader–Willi syndromes, neurologic disorders due to deletions or mutations in this region that occur on maternally and paternally inherited chromosomes, respectively.

Despite the high rate of duplications of 15q11–13 among autistic individuals, genome screens have not shown strong support for linkage or association to this region. Candidate gene studies continue, however, in part because a rate of 6 percent of autistic individuals with duplications in this region is hard to ignore.

Bipolar Disorder.   The search for the genetic basis of bipolar disorder has been fraught with missteps and partial answers. The history of genetic mapping attempts for bipolar disorder illustrates not only the extreme complexity of psychiatric disorders but also the evolution of genetic approaches to such diseases. Bipolar disorder is an episodic illness characterized by recurrent periods of both mania and depression. Psychotic symptoms are often a part of the clinical picture, particularly in more severely affected individuals.

Numerous genetic epidemiologic investigations conducted over several decades have strongly supported a genetic contribution to risk for bipolar disorder. The definition of the bipolar disorder phenotype in these studies has varied substantially, resulting in a wide range of heritability estimates. This problem is typical of many psychogenetic studies. For example, many early studies into the genetic basis of mood disorders did not distinguish between unipolar and bipolar mood disorders. Furthermore, the diagnostic methodology used in such early studies differs substantially from that employed in current-day genetic studies. For example, a Danish twin study that suggested a very high heritability for bipolar disorder and thereby had a substantial influence on the design of initial genetic mapping studies of mood disorders employed only unstructured diagnostic interviews by a single clinician rather than the structured assessments used in current studies, which have suggested somewhat lower heritabilities.

Current estimates of the concordance for bipolar disorder range between 65 and 100 percent in MZ twins and 10 and 30 percent in DZ twins. This ratio indicates that the disorder is highly heritable (between about 60 and 80 percent). Several studies have shown that bipolar disorder is substantially more heritable than unipolar major depression, which has an estimated heritability between 30 and 40 percent.

Early family studies suggested that bipolar disorder segregation patterns were compatible with single-gene inheritance of a locus of significant effect. However, although some bipolar disorder pedigrees may segregate such a locus, mounting evidence indicates that if such pedigrees exist, they must be quite rare. Furthermore, the fact that genetic linkage studies have failed to uncover such a locus with unequivocal evidence in any pedigrees argues against this possibility. The observed rapid decrease in recurrence risk for bipolar disorder from monozygotic co-twins to first-degree relatives is also not consistent with single-gene inheritance models but instead suggests models of multiple interacting genes.

EARLY LINKAGE STUDIES.   Tremendous excitement followed the first reports of linkage to bipolar disorder on chromosomes X and 11 in 1987. Investigators noted that in several families, bipolar disorder and other affective disorders appeared to be inherited in an X-linked fashion. Likewise, these disorders appeared to cosegregate in several Israeli families with color blindness and G6PD deficiency, which map to the X chromosome. Linkage studies in these pedigrees, using color blindness or G6PD deficiency as marker loci, gave LOD scores between 4 and 9. Early studies of chromosome 11 were similar to those for chromosome X in that they reported significant linkage after testing only a few markers in a single region, in this case, in an extended Old Order Amish pedigree heavily loaded for bipolar disorder.

Not surprisingly, these findings generated a great deal of interest. Both studies showed high LOD scores and seemed to provide clear evidence for linkage. However, replication studies in other populations failed to produce positive results for either the X chromosome or chromosome 11, and evidence for linkage virtually disappeared in both chromosomal regions in the samples in which linkage was initially reported when the pedigrees were extended to include additional affected individuals and when additional markers were typed in the putative linkage regions. The most likely explanation in each case is that the original linkage results were false-positive findings and may have reflected over-optimistic interpretation of evidence that, in retrospect, was relatively scanty.

GENOME-WIDE SCREENS.   The early linkage studies of bipolar disorder evaluated only a few markers because they were all that were available. With the construction of genetic linkage maps of the genome in the 1990s, linkage studies of most complex traits, including bipolar disorder, began to search genome-wide. The advantage of genome-wide mapping studies is that they do not require *a priori* knowledge of the biologic underpinnings of a particular phenotype. Complete genome screens provide an opportunity to evaluate the evidence of linkage at all points in the genome without bias. Although genome-wide studies had greater power to detect accurate linkage than studies focused on only a few markers in arbitrary locations or around a few candidate genes, these investigations have also generally had disappointing results. The challenge of achieving replicated significant linkage results for bipolar disorder and other complex traits is apparent when one reviews the many gene-mapping studies that have suggested—but not demonstrated unequivocally—bipolar disorder susceptibility loci on chromosome 18.

CHROMOSOME 18.   The first report of linkage came from a partial genome screen that examined 11 markers on chromosome 18 and identified suggestive linkage near the centromere. Because the inheritance patterns for bipolar disorder are unknown, the results were analyzed using both recessive and dominant models. Some of the markers were positive under a recessive model in some families, some were positive under a dominant model in other families, and some markers gave positive LOD scores in a subset of families under both models. Attempts to replicate this finding in other populations have been mixed. So far, at least two groups have found no evidence for linkage to the pericentromeric region of chromosome 18 in their samples, although one other group has found evidence to support linkage to this region. Other studies have found suggestive evidence for linkage on chromosome 18, including a complete genome screen in two large Costa Rican pedigrees that gave evidence for linkage on chromosome 18q22–23 as well as in an area on 18p. The combined evidence of these several studies, although somewhat contradictory and confusing, points to at least two different susceptibility loci on chromosome 18: one on 18p and one on 18q.

IMPROVING STUDY POWER.   The equivocal findings represented by the attempts to pinpoint susceptibility loci on chromosome 18 have led investigators to implement several new strategies to map bipolar disorder genes. One such strategy is a meta-analysis, which involves combining data across multiple individual investigations to increase statistical power, and in some cases, the combined analysis points to loci not initially found in the individual studies. Several meta-analytical techniques have been used to explore gene-mapping studies for bipolar disorder. The multiple scan probability (MSP) and genome scan meta-analysis (GSMA) methods require only linkage statistics and *p*-values from each study to examine combined data. MSP was used to combine chromosomal regions with *p*-values less than 0.01 from 11 independent bipolar disorder studies and provided evidence for susceptibility loci on chromosomes 13q and 22q. Although the MSP and GSMA methods have the advantage of requiring only linkage significance data, they are not able to account for study-specific issues that will limit the extent to which multiple studies can be compared. Combining original genotype data from multiple studies can circumvent this problem. With this method, the largest meta-analysis to date combined 11 bipolar disorder genome-wide linkage scans consisting of 5,179 individuals from 1,067 families. Access to the original genotype data allowed the construction of a standardized genetic map in which the markers of each respective study were mapped onto one standard gender-averaged map. The results of this meta-analysis identified two susceptibility loci with genome-wide significance on 6q and 8q.

Another strategy that has been used to increase the power of gene-mapping studies in the formation of consortia that combine data across multiple clinical sites. A consortium combining data from the UK and Ireland led to support for linkage at 9p21 and 10p14–21. Likewise, combining data from Spanish, Romanian, and Bulgarian families provided additional support for findings on chromosomes 4q31 and 6q24. Investigators can also increase power by standardizing marker sets and clinical evaluation protocols between independent studies to permit direct comparisons between such studies. This approach was used to identify a bipolar disorder susceptibility locus on chromosome 5q31–33. The region showed suggestive nonparametric linkage results in pedigrees from the Central Valley of Costa Rica. With identical genetic markers and diagnostic criteria, the same region was highlighted in an independent analysis of a set of Colombian families who have a genetic background similar to that of the Costa Rican families. A follow-up study using additional markers in an expanded set of Colombian and Costa Rican families confirmed genome-wide significant evidence to a candidate region of 10 cM in 5q31–33. This finding is especially impressive given that the linkage peak in the bipolar studies overlaps with linkage regions for schizophrenia and psychosis, identified in a previous study of 40 families from the Portuguese Islands. These results contribute to a growing opinion that there may be substantial genetic overlap between different DSM disorders.

Schizophrenia. In the past decade we have seen exciting advances in the genetic studies of schizophrenia. Much of these are due to the several large consortia formed to investigate the disorder. These collaborative efforts allow for large samples with sufficient power to investigate the disorder.

Before these studies, family studies established a heritability of between 60 and 80 percent, however we lacked any meaningful genome-wide studies. In 2009 several of the consortia combined samples and identified an SNP in the MHC on chromosome 6p22 as a risk locus. What followed were several elegant studies, including a landmark 2016 paper from the Schizophrenia Working Group of the Psychiatric Genomics Consortium, which focused on the C4 alleles and demonstrated their role in synaptic pruning during critical developmental period. This supports the hypothesis that schizophrenia is the result of abnormalities of neurodevelopment.

Before this work, various candidate genes emerged. They spawned a diverse range of basic and clinical investigations aiming to elucidate their functional significance, for example, using mouse gene targeting and functional MRI.

The early identification of chromosome 6p24–22 as implicated in schizophrenia led to the proposal of *Dysbindin* (*DTNB1*) as a candidate gene for schizophrenia. Additional association studies of *Dysbindin* have been equivocal.

Linkage studies subsequently pointed to a region on chromosome 1 containing the candidate genes *DISC 1* and *DISC 2* (*disrupted in schizophrenia 1* and *2*) located on chromosome 1q21–22 and 1q32–42. These genes were initially identified in a large Scottish pedigree in the early 1990s. A balanced translocation between chromosomes 1 and 11 segregated in this pedigree and was possibly associated with severe mental illness. *DISC 1* and *2* were identified in the original Scottish family because of their location near the chromosomal translocation breakpoint. As with *Dysbindin,* follow-up studies of *DISC 1* and *2* have been equivocal.

Genome screens, including a screen focused on extended Icelandic kindreds, have identified a schizophrenia candidate region on chromosome 8p21–22. Fine mapping of the region narrowed the search and eventually led to the proposal of *neuregulin 1* (*NRG1*) as a schizophrenia candidate gene. Association studies again provided equivocal and difficult-to-interpret results.

Despite the equivocal genetic studies, significant resources have been channeled into molecular and neurophysiologic investigations of the functional products of *dysbindin, DISC 1* and *2,* and *neuregulin.* Mutant mice for each of the three genes are now available and have been used to demonstrate interesting biologic findings. For example, *dysbindin* is expressed in the hippocampus and dorsolateral prefrontal cortex. The dysbindin protein binds to B-dystrobrevin and has been implicated in synaptic structure and signaling. *DISC 1* has been shown to influence neurite formation in cellular studies, and mutant mice for *DISC 1* show impairments in a wide variety of tests, including learning, memory, and sociability. Neuregulin belongs to a family of growth factors that mediate numerous functions, including synapse formation, neuronal migration, and neurotransmission. Targeted disruption of *erbB4,* the postsynaptic target of neuregulin, leads to synaptic glutamatergic hypofunction. Despite the exciting biology uncovered, it remains unclear whether and to what extent any of these genes contribute to the etiology of schizophrenia in humans, and many geneticists have been cautious in their endorsement of the legitimacy of the mutant mice generated from the current list of candidate genes as models of psychiatric disorders.

APPLIED ELECTROPHYSIOLOGY

EEG is the recording of the electrical activity of the brain. It is used in clinical psychiatry principally to evaluate the presence of seizures, particularly temporal lobe, frontal lobe, and petit mal seizures (absence seizures), which can produce complex behaviors. EEG is also used during ECT to monitor the success of the stimulus in producing seizure activity and as a critical component of polysomnography used in the evaluation of sleep disorders. Quantitative electroencephalography (QEEG) and cerebral evoked potentials (EPs) represent newer EEG-based methods that provide improved research and clinical insights into brain functioning.

Electroencephalography

A brain wave is a transient difference in electrical potential (greatly amplified) between any two points on the scalp or between some electrode placed on the scalp and a reference electrode located elsewhere on the head (i.e., ear lobe or nose). The difference in electrical potential measured between any two EEG electrodes fluctuates or oscillates rapidly, usually many times per second. It is this oscillation that produces the characteristic "squiggly line" that is recognized as the appearance of "brain waves."

Brain waves reflect a change by becoming faster or slower in frequency or lower or higher in voltage, or perhaps some combination of these two responses. A routine EEG can never constitute positive proof of the absence of brain dysfunction. Even in diseases with established brain pathophysiology, such as multiple sclerosis, deep subcortical neoplasm, some seizure disorders, and Parkinson disease and other movement disorders, a substantial incidence of patients with normal EEG studies may be encountered. Nonetheless, a normal EEG can often provide convincing evidence for excluding certain types of brain pathology that may present with behavioral or psychiatric symptoms. More often, information from the patient's symptoms, clinical course and history, and other laboratory results identifies a probable cause for the EEG findings. EEG studies are often ordered when a pathophysiologic process is already suspected, or a patient experiences a sudden, unexplained change in mental status.

Electrode Placement.   The electrodes usually used to record the EEG are attached to the scalp with a conductive paste. A standard array consists of 21 electrodes. The placement of the electrodes is based on the 10/20 International System of Electrode Placement (Fig. 33-33). This system measures the distance between readily identifiable landmarks on the head and then locates electrode positions at 10 percent or 20 percent of that distance in an anterior–posterior or transverse direction. Electrodes are then designated by an uppercase letter denoting the brain region beneath that electrode and a number, with odd numbers used for the left hemisphere and with even numbers signifying the right hemisphere (the subscript Z denotes midline electrodes). Thus, the O_2 electrode is placed over the right occipital region, and the P_3 lead is found over the left parietal area.

In particular circumstances, other electrodes may be used. Nasopharyngeal (NP) electrodes can be inserted into the NP space through the nostrils and can be closer to the temporal lobe than scalp electrodes. No actual penetration of tissue occurs. These

electrodes may be contraindicated with many psychiatric patients displaying behaviors, such as confusion, agitation, or belligerence, which could pull the leads out, possibly lacerating the nasal passage. Sphenoidal electrodes use a hollow needle through which a fine electrode that is insulated, except at the tip, is inserted between the zygoma and the sigmoid notch in the mandible until it is in contact with the base of the skull lateral to the foramen ovale.

Activated EEG.   Specific activating procedures are used to increase the probability that abnormal discharges, particularly spike or spike-wave seizure discharges, will occur. Strenuous hyperventilation is one of the most frequently used activation procedures. While remaining reclined with the eyes closed, the patient is asked to over breathe through the open mouth with deep breaths for 1 to 4 minutes, depending on the laboratory (3 minutes is standard). In general, hyperventilation is one of the safest EEG-activating procedures, and, for most of the population, it presents no physical risk. It can pose a risk for patients with cardiopulmonary disease or risk factors for cerebral vascular pathophysiology, however. Photic stimulation (PS) generally involves placing an intense strobe light approximately 12 inches in front of the subject's closed eyes and flashing at frequencies that can range from 1 to 50 Hz, depending on how the procedure is carried out. Retinal damage does not occur because each strobe flash, although intense, is too brief in duration to harm the patient. When the resting EEG is normal, and a seizure disorder or behavior that is suspected to be a manifestation of a paroxysmal EEG dysrhythmia is suspected, PS can be a valuable activation method to use. EEG recording during sleep, natural or sedated, is now widely accepted as an essential technique for eliciting a variety of paroxysmal discharges, when the wake tracing is normal, or for increasing the number of abnormal discharges to permit a more definitive interpretation. It has been shown that the CNS stress produced by 24 hours of sleep deprivation alone can lead to the activation of paroxysmal EEG discharges in some cases.

Normal EEG Tracing

The normal EEG tracing (Fig. 33-34) is composed of a complex mixture of many different frequencies. Discrete frequency bands within the broad EEG frequency spectrum are designated with Greek letters.

Awake EEG.   The four basic waveforms are alpha, beta, delta, and theta. Highly rhythmic *alpha waves* with a frequency range of 8 to 13 Hz constitute the dominant brain wave frequency of the normal eyes-closed awake EEG. Alpha frequency can be increased or decreased by a wide variety of pharmacologic, metabolic, or endocrine variables. Frequencies that are faster than the upper 13 Hz limit of the alpha rhythm are termed *beta waves,* and they are not uncommon in average adult waking EEG studies, particularly over the frontal-central regions. *Delta waves* (≤3.5 Hz) are not present in the normal waking EEG but are a prominent feature of deeper stages of sleep. The presence of significant generalized or focal delta waves in the awake EEG is strongly indicative of a pathophysiologic process. Waves with a frequency of 4.0 to 7.5 Hz are collectively referred to as *theta waves.* A small amount of sporadic, arrhythmic, and isolated theta activity can be seen in many normal waking EEG studies, particularly in frontal-temporal regions. Although theta activity is limited in the waking EEG, it is a prominent feature of the drowsy and sleep tracing. Excessive theta

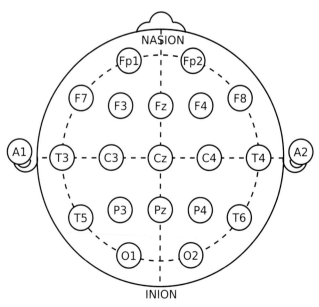

FIGURE 33-33
International 10–20 Electrode Placement System.

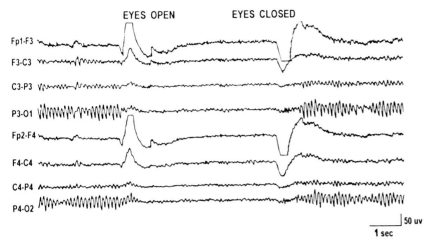

EYES OPEN   EYES CLOSED

Fp1-F3

F3-C3

C3-P3

P3-O1

Fp2-F4

F4-C4

C4-P4

P4-O2

50 uv

1 sec

FIGURE 33-34

Normal electroencephalogram (EEG) tracings in an awake 28-year-old man. (Reprinted from Emerson RG, Walesak TS, Turner CA. EEG and evoked potentials. In: Rowland LP, ed. *Merritt's Textbook of Neurology*. 9th ed. Baltimore, MD: Lippincott Williams & Wilkins; 1995:68, with permission.)

in awake EEG, generalized, or focal, suggests the operation of a pathologic process.

With maturation, EEG activity gradually goes from a preponderance of irregular medium- to high-voltage delta activity in the tracing of the infant, to greater frequency and more rhythmic pattern. Rhythmic activity in the upper theta-lower alpha range (7 to 8 Hz) can be seen in posterior areas by early childhood, and, by mid-adolescence, the EEG essentially has the appearance of an adult tracing.

Sleep EEG. The EEG patterns that characterize drowsy and sleep states are different from the patterns seen during the awake state. The rhythmic posterior alpha activity of the waking state subsides during drowsiness and is replaced by irregular low-voltage theta activity. As drowsiness deepens, slower frequencies emerge, and sporadic vertex sharp waves may appear at central electrode sites, particularly among younger persons. Finally, the progression into sleep is marked by the appearance of 14-Hz sleep spindles (also called *sigma waves*), which, in turn, gradually become replaced by high-voltage delta waves as deep sleep stages are reached.

EEG Abnormalities

Apart from some of the apparent indications for an EEG study (i.e., suspected seizures), EEG studies are not routinely performed as part of a diagnostic work-up in psychiatry. EEG, however, is a valuable assessment tool in clinical situations in which the initial presentation or the clinical course appears to be unusual or atypical (Table 33-8). Table 33-9 summarizes some common types of EEG abnormalities.

Some psychotropic medications and recreational or abused drugs produce EEG changes, yet, except for the benzodiazepines and some compounds with a propensity to induce paroxysmal EEG discharges, little, if any, the clinically relevant effect is noted when the medication is not causing toxicity. Benzodiazepines, which always generate a significant amount of diffuse beta activity, have EEG-protective effects so that they can mask alterations caused by concomitant medications (Table 33-10).

Medical and neurologic conditions produce a wide range of abnormal EEG findings. EEG studies, thus, can contribute to the detection of unsuspected organic pathophysiology influencing a psychiatric presentation (Fig. 33-35). Table 33-11 lists EEG alterations in medical disorders, and Table 33-12 lists EEG alterations associated with psychiatric disorders.

Table 33-8
Warning Signs of the Presence of Covert Medical or Organic Factors Causing or Contributing to Psychiatric Presentation

Atypical age of onset (i.e., anorexia nervosa beginning at mid-adulthood)

Complete lack of positive family history of the disorder when a positive family history is expected

Any focal or localized symptoms (i.e., unilateral hallucinations)

Focal neurologic abnormalities

Catatonia

Presence of any difficulty with orientation or memory (in general, Mini Mental State Examination should be normal)

Atypical response to treatment

Atypical clinical course

Note: Clinicians should have a high index of suspicion for underlying medical conditions and a low threshold for initiating appropriate workups.

Table 33-9
Common Electroencephalography (EEG) Abnormalities

Diffuse slowing of background rhythms	Most common EEG abnormality; nonspecific and is present in patients with diffuse encephalopathies of diverse causes
Focal slowing	Suggests localized parenchymal dysfunction and focal seizure disorder; seen with focal fluid collection, such as hematomas
Triphasic waves	Typically consist of generalized synchronous waves occurring in brief runs; approximately one-half of patients with triphasic waves have hepatic encephalopathy, and the remainder have other toxic–metabolic encephalopathies
Epileptiform discharges	Interictal hallmark of epilepsy; strongly associated with seizure disorders
Periodic lateralizing epileptiform discharges	Suggest the presence of an acute destructive cerebral lesion; associated with seizures, obtundation, and focal neurologic signs
Generalized periodic sharp waves	Most commonly seen following cerebral anoxia; recorded in about 90% of patients with Creutzfeldt–Jakob disease

Table 33-10
Electroencephalography (EEG) Alterations Associated with Medication and Drugs

Drug	Alterations
Benzodiazepines	Increased beta activity
Clozapine (Clozaril)	Nonspecific change
Olanzapine (Zyprexa)	Nonspecific change
Risperidone (Risperdal)	Nonspecific change
Quetiapine (Seroquel)	No significant changes
Aripiprazole (Abilify)	No significant changes
Lithium	Slowing or paroxysmal activity
Alcohol	Decreased alpha activity; increased theta activity
Opioids	Decreased alpha activity; increased voltage of theta and delta waves; in overdose, slow waves
Barbiturates	Increased beta activity; in withdrawal states, generalized paroxysmal activity and spike discharges
Marijuana	Increased alpha activity in frontal area of brain; overall slow alpha activity
Cocaine	Similar to marijuana
Inhalants	Diffuse slowing of delta and theta waves
Nicotine	Increased alpha activity; in withdrawal, marked decrease in alpha activity
Caffeine	In withdrawal, increase in amplitude or voltage of theta activity

Topographic Quantitative Electroencephalography (QEEG)

Unlike standard EEG interpretation, which relies on waveform recognition, QEEG involves computer analysis of data extracted from the EEG. Findings are compared with an extensive population database of subjects without any known neurologic or psychiatric disorder as well as QEEG profiles that may be characteristic

Table 33-11
Electroencephalography (EEG) Alterations Associated with Medical Disorders

Seizures	Generalized, Hemispheric, or Focal Spike, Spike-Wave Discharge, or Both
Structural lesions	Focal slowing, with possible focal spike activity
Closed head injuries	Focal slowing (sharply focal head trauma) Focal delta slowing or more widespread slowing (subdural hematomas)
Infectious disorders	Diffuse, often synchronous, high voltage slowing (acute phase of encephalitis)
Metabolic and endocrine disorders	Diffuse generalized slowing of wake frequencies Triphasic waves: 1.5–3.0 per second high-voltage slow waves, with each slow wave initiated by a blunt or rounded spike-like transient (hepatic encephalopathy)
Vascular pathophysiology	Slowed alpha frequency and increased generalized theta slowing (diffuse atherosclerosis) Focal or regional delta activity (cerebrovascular accidents)

of some defined diagnostic group. In QEEG, the analog-based electrical signals are processed digitally and converted to graphic, colored topographical displays. These images are sometimes called "brain maps."

QEEG remains primarily a research method, but it holds considerable clinical potential for psychiatry, mainly in establishing neurophysiologic subtypes of specific disorders and for identifying electrophysiologic predictors of response. Examples of some of the more promising results of QEEG research include the identification of subtypes of cocaine dependence and the subtype most likely to be associated with sustained abstinence; identification of subtypes of OCD that predict clinical responsiveness or lack of responsiveness to SSRIs; and the differentiation between normals, attention-deficit disorder and ADHD, and learning disability subpopulations. QEEG findings in ADHD show that increased theta abnormality frontally may be a strong predictor of response

FIGURE 33-35

Diffuse slowing in a 67-year-old patient with dementia. Six- to seven cycles per second (cps) activity predominates over the parieto-occipital regions. Although reactive to eye closure, the frequency of this rhythm is abnormally slow. (Reprinted from Emerson RG, Walesak TS, Turner CA. EEG and evoked potentials. In: Rowland LP, ed. *Merritt's Textbook of Neurology*. 9th ed. Baltimore, MD: Lippincott Williams & Wilkins; 1995:68, with permission.)

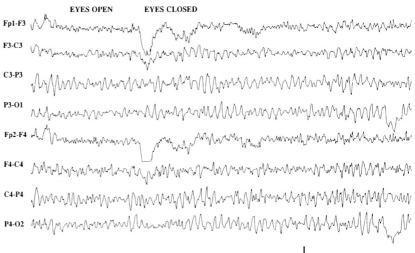

Table 33-12
Electroencephalography (EEG) Alterations
Associated with Psychiatric Disorders

Panic disorder	Paroxysmal EEG changes consistent with partial seizure activity during attack in one-third of patients; focal slowing in about 25% of patients
Catatonia	Usually normal, but EEG indicated in new patient presenting with catatonia to rule out other causes
Attention-deficit/ hyperactivity disorder (ADHD)	High prevalence (up to 60%) of EEG abnormalities versus normal controls; spike or spike-wave discharges
Antisocial personality disorder	Increased incidence of EEG abnormalities in those with aggressive behavior
Borderline personality disorder	Positive spikes: 14 and 6 per second seen in 25% of patients
Chronic alcoholism	Prominent slowing and periodic lateralized paroxysmal discharges
Alcohol withdrawal	May be normal in patients who are not delirious; excessive fast activity in patients with delirium
Dementia	Rarely normal in advanced dementia; may be helpful in differentiating pseudodementia from dementia

to methylphenidate and other psychostimulants and that favorable clinical responses may be associated with a normalization of the EEG abnormality.

Cerebral Evoked Potentials

Cerebral EPs are a series of surface (scalp) recordable waves that result from brain visual, auditory, somatosensory, and cognitive stimulation. They are abnormal in many psychiatric conditions, including schizophrenia and Alzheimer disease, thus creating difficulty in using cerebral EPs for differential diagnosis purposes.

CHRONOBIOLOGY

Chronobiology is the study of biologic time. The rotation of the Earth about its axis imposes a 24-hour cyclicity on the biosphere. Although it is widely accepted that organisms have evolved to occupy geographical niches that can be defined by the three spatial dimensions, it is less appreciated that organisms have also evolved to occupy temporal niches that are defined by the fourth dimension—time. Much like light represents a small portion of the electromagnetic spectrum, the 24-hour periodicity represents a small time domain within the spectrum of temporal biology. A broad range of frequencies exist throughout biology, ranging from millisecond oscillations in ocular field potentials to the 17-year cycle of emergence seen in the periodic cicada (*Magicicada* spp.). Although these different periodicities all fall within the realm of chronobiology, *circadian* (Latin: *circa,* about; *dies,* day) rhythms that have a period of about one day are among the most extensively studied, and best understood biologic rhythms.

A defining feature of circadian rhythms is that they persist in the absence of time cues and are not driven merely by the 24-hour environmental cycle. Experimental animals housed for several months under constant darkness, temperature, and humidity continue to

exhibit robust circadian rhythms. Maintenance of rhythmicity in a "timeless" environment points to the existence of an internal biologic timing system that is responsible for generating these endogenous rhythms.

The site of the primary circadian oscillator in mammals, including humans, is the suprachiasmatic nucleus (SCN), located in the anterior hypothalamus. The mean circadian period generated by the human SCN is approximately 24.18 hours. Like a slightly slow watch, an individual with such a period gradually comes out of synchrony with the astronomical day. In slightly more than 3 months, an ordinarily diurnal human would be in antiphase to the day–night cycle and thus would become transiently nocturnal. Therefore, a circadian clock must be reset regularly to be effective at maintaining the proper phase relationships of behavioral and physiologic processes within the context of the 24-hour day.

Although factors such as temperature and humidity exhibit daily fluctuations, the environmental parameter that most reliably corresponds to the period of Earth's rotation around its axis is the change in illuminance associated with the day–night cycle. Organisms have evolved to use this daily change in light levels as a time cue or *zeitgeber* (German: *zeit,* time; *geber,* giver) to reset the endogenous circadian clock. Regulation of the circadian pacemaker through the detection of changes in illuminance requires a photoreceptive apparatus that communicates with the central oscillator. This apparatus is known to reside in the eyes because surgical removal of the eyes renders an animal incapable of resetting its clock in response to light.

The circadian clock drives many rhythms. These include rhythms in behavior, core body temperature, sleep, feeding, drinking, and hormonal levels. One such circadian-regulated hormone is the indoleamine, melatonin. Melatonin synthesis is controlled through a multisynaptic pathway from the SCN to the pineal gland. Serum levels of melatonin become elevated at night and return to baseline during the day. The nocturnal rise in melatonin is a convenient marker of circadian phase. Exposure to light elicits two distinct effects on the daily melatonin profile. First, light acutely suppresses elevated melatonin levels, immediately decreasing them to baseline levels. Second, light shifts the phase of the circadian rhythm of melatonin synthesis. Because melatonin can be assayed easily, it provides a convenient window into the state of the circadian pacemaker. Any perturbation of the clock is reflected in the melatonin profile; thus, melatonin offers an output that can be used to study the regulation of the central circadian pacemaker.

Sleep and Circadian Rhythms

Sleep Regulation.   Restful consolidated sleep is most appreciated when sleep disturbances are experienced. Sleep is the integrated product of two oscillatory processes. The first process frequently referred to as the *sleep homeostat,* is an oscillation that stems from the accumulation and dissipation of sleep debt. The biologic substrates encoding sleep debt are not known, although adenosine is emerging as a primary candidate neuromodulator of the sleep homeostat. The second oscillatory process is governed by the circadian clock and controls a daily rhythm in sleep propensity or, conversely, arousal. These interacting oscillations can be dissociated by housing subjects in a timeless environment for several weeks.

The circadian cycle in arousal (wakefulness) steadily increases throughout the day, reaching a maximum immediately before the circadian increase in plasma melatonin (Fig. 33-36). Arousal subsequently decreases to coincide with the circadian trough in core

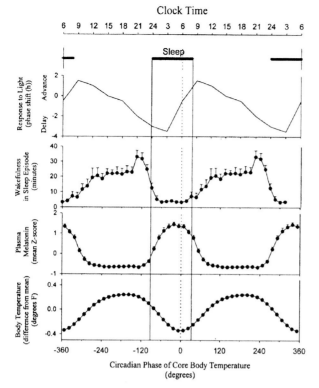

FIGURE 33-36

Relative phase relationship of sleep in young adults to other circadian phase markers. (From Dijk D-J, Lockley SW. Invited review: integration of human sleep-wake regulation and circadian rhythmicity. *J Appl Physiol*. 2002;92:852, with permission.)

body temperature. Experiments imposing forced sleep schedules throughout the circadian day have shown that an uninterrupted 8-hour bout of sleep can only be obtained if sleep is initiated approximately 6 hours before the temperature nadir. This nadir typically occurs at approximately 5:00 AM to 6:00 AM. In healthy individuals, initiating sleep between 11:00 PM and 12:00 AM affords the highest probability of getting eight solid hours of sleep.

It should be stressed that diurnal preference varies among individuals as a function of age, endogenous circadian periods, and other factors. This variability is paralleled by physiology. Clinically, diurnal preference can be quantified using the Horne-Östberg (HO) Morningness-Eveningness Questionnaire (MEQ). In qualitative terms, *morning people* or *morning larks* tend to awaken earlier and experience the core body temperature minimum at an earlier clock time relative to *night people* or *night owls*. Sleep deprivation studies have shown that the homeostatic component of sleep is remarkably similar among individuals of similar age. (It should be noted that there is a well-established age-dependent decline in sleep need.) Therefore, diurnal preference is dictated almost exclusively by the circadian component of sleep regulation.

Circadian Sleep Disorders.

Advanced sleep phase syndrome (ASPS) is a pathologic extreme of the morning lark phenotype. An autosomal-dominant familial form of ASPS (FASPS) has been genetically characterized. Afflicted family members exhibit a striking 4-hour advance of the daily sleep–wake rhythm. They typically fall asleep at approximately 7:30 PM and spontaneously awaken at approximately 4:30 AM. Affected individuals have an SNP in the gene encoding hPER2, the human homolog of the mouse *Per2* clock gene. This adenine-to-guanine nucleotide

polymorphism results in serine-to-glycine amino acid substitution that causes the mutant protein to be inefficiently phosphorylated by casein kinase Iε, an established component of the circadian molecular clockwork. Similarly, delayed sleep phase syndrome (DSPS) is influenced by genetics. A length polymorphism in a repeat region of the *hPER3* gene appears to be associated with diurnal preference in patients with DSPS, the shorter allele being associated with evening preference.

The advent of the light bulb extended the human day into night. This encroachment on the night, although increasing productivity, affects our sleep patterns (Fig. 33-37). The typical use of artificial lights results in a single, consolidated bout of sleep lasting approximately 8 hours. This pattern of sleep is uncommon among most other mammals, which typically experience more fractured sleep. Human sleep under more natural photoperiods, where the duration of the night is longer than in artificial settings, becomes decompressed. Specifically, a bimodal distribution of sleep is observed; bouts of sleep occur early and late at night. Periods of *quiet wakefulness* are interspersed between the two primary bouts of sleep. This natural sleep pattern is more similar to the sleep patterns of other mammals.

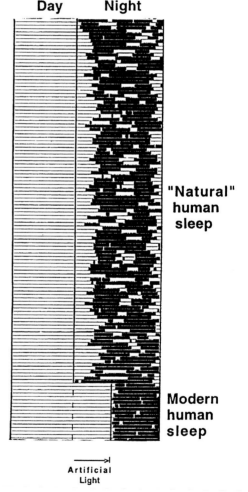

FIGURE 33-37

Change in sleep structure in response to artificial lighting. Total sleep time is reduced, and periods of quiet wakefulness are abolished by extending daytime into nighttime through artificial lighting. (From Wehr TA, Moul DE, Barbato G, Giesen HA, Seidel JA, Barker C, Bender C. Conservation of photoperiod-responsive mechanisms in humans. *Am J Physiol*. 1993;265:R846, with permission.)

Seasonality

The 24-hour period of the Earth's rotation around its axis is unchanging. However, the Earth's axis is tilted 23.45 degrees from the plane of its orbit around the sun (the ecliptic). The relative day to night proportion within day varies as the Earth proceeds through its orbit of the sun. Many organisms are capable of synchronizing physiology to the seasonal cycle to maximize survival. For example, precise seasonal cycles in reproduction are seen throughout the plant and animal kingdoms. Large mammals that typically have long gestation periods, such as sheep, conceive in the fall when the nights are long and the days are short, so birth occurs during the relatively mild season of spring. These animals are referred to as *short-day breeders.*

Conversely, mammals with gestation periods of only a few weeks, such as hamsters, conceive and give birth during spring and summer, when the days are long and the nights are short. Hence, these animals are referred to as *long-day breeders.* Like circadian rhythms, many of these yearly (circannual) rhythms tend to persist in the absence of seasonal cues with endogenous periods of approximately 1 year.

Melatonin and Seasonality. The most reliable environmental parameter providing a faithful representation of the solar day is the day–night cycle. Similarly, the most reliable environmental parameter reflecting the progression through the seasons is the change in day length, the fraction of the 24-hour day between sunrise and sunset. In seasonally breeding animals, day length is physiologically encoded through the melatonin profile. As described previously, melatonin levels are elevated during the night. A long night, such as that experienced during the short day lengths of winter, results in an elevated melatonin profile of a relatively long duration. A short summer night, by contrast, results in a short duration of elevated melatonin. This seasonal signal is interpreted by the reproductive axis, resulting in an appropriate reproductive response. Melatonin's role in transducing day length was elucidated by pinealectomizing seasonally breeding animals, thereby removing the primary endogenous source of melatonin. Melatonin was then infused in profiles mimicking long days or short days. The duration of elevated melatonin was the primary determinant of seasonal reproductive status, even when the infused profile was administered under a conflicting day length. Variations in other parameters, such as the amplitude of the melatonin profile, the amount of total melatonin synthesized, or the phase relationship of the profile to the light-dark cycle, are of limited importance in producing a humoral signal that transduces day length.

Reproductive responses to changing day length can be dramatic. A male Siberian hamster (*Phodopus sungorus*) maintained in long days is reproductively competent and typically has a testicular weight of approximately 250 mg per testis. Under short days, however, the testes regress to approximately 15 mg per testis, representing a 94 percent decrease in testicular mass. The same degree of regression is observed in response to melatonin infusions that mimic short days. Communication of the hormonally transduced day length to the reproductive axis is likely to be mediated, at least partially, through melatonin receptors in the *pars tuberalis* of the pituitary gland. The exact mechanism remains unknown, but activation of these receptors is hypothesized to regulate an unidentified factor putatively named tuberalin indirectly. Tuberalin, in turn, controls gene expression and prolactin release from lactotrophs in the adenohypophysis of the pituitary.

Seasonality in Humans. Whether humans are truly seasonal is still a point of considerable debate. Several lines of evidence exist that suggest the presence of a residual tendency toward seasonality. A peak in the rate of suicide occurs in the summer; this peak is cross-cultural. Birth rates also tend to show a seasonal variation; a small but distinguishable peak in the rate of births occurs in spring and summer. This pattern, however, is itself variable and is heavily influenced by unknown cultural and geographic factors. Of interest, the amplitude of the spring–summer birth rate peak has diminished as societies have become industrialized.

The decompressed bimodal structure of human sleep during long nights indicates that the length of natural sleep is related to the length of the night. Potentially, a two-oscillator system could function to maintain proper sleep patterns during changing photoperiods. Such a proposed system would consist of an evening oscillator that tracks the transition from day to night (dusk) and a morning oscillator that tracks the transition from night to day (dawn). The relative phase differences between these oscillators may encode the changing day lengths associated with the passing of the seasons. Biologic evidence for a two-oscillator system exists in rodents and humans.

The melatonin profile of many vertebrates, including some humans, is bimodal, with evening and morning peaks. In rodents, metabolic and electrophysiologic studies of the SCN typically have been done in brain slices cut in the coronal plane. Results of electrophysiologic studies conducted in brain slices cut in the horizontal plane have provided new insights. The action potential frequency in SCN neurons from horizontally cut preparations is bimodal, with peaks in the early and late subjective day. Furthermore, the inter-peak interval varies as a function of the photoperiod in which the animal was housed. These studies lend credence to long-standing suspicions that the SCN of seasonally breeding mammals and, perhaps, nonseasonal mammals harbor a morning and evening oscillator that interact to convey day-length information.

Effect of Aging. In general, as humans age, the circadian period shortens, the circadian phase advances resulting in earlier waking times and bedtimes, the amplitudes of most circadian rhythms decrease, and dramatic phase shifts such as those caused by jet-lag are less tolerated. Again, a mouse model has provided an interesting insight into the interaction of the aging process and the circadian clock. The effect of chronic jet-lag on aged mice has dramatic consequences on mortality. About half of aged mice forced to phase advance 6 hours once per week survive this treatment compared with an 83 percent survival rate in unshifted age-matched mice. Aged mice subjected to weekly 6-hour phase delays show an intermediate survival of 68 percent. These profound effects of phase-shifting are not observed in younger mice. The pathogenesis of chronic jet-lag remains to be determined. Of interest, these mice did not have an increased rate of tumorigenesis. It is likely that in humans, as in mice, the internal desynchrony of oscillators that result from a rotating light schedule may have dire consequences that may be exacerbated by aging.

Circadian Rhythms and Pharmacotherapy

Circadian rhythmicity can be affected by drugs, and conversely, the circadian clock can modulate the efficacy of drugs throughout the day. A better understanding of these interactions will lead to more effective pharmacotherapies. Some of the best-studied interactions between medications and the circadian clock have included the circadian effects of antidepressants. Elevated nocturnal body temperature is a common feature among depressed patients. This effect may be due to reduced amplitude of the master circadian oscillator in the hypothalamus that drives body temperature. TCAs and SSRIs reduce elevated nocturnal body temperature while simultaneously enhancing circadian amplitude. Similarly, many depressed patients exhibit a dampened amplitude in daily activity rhythms. Like body temperature, the amplitude in daily activity cycles of depressed individuals may be augmented by TCA or SSRI therapy.

The use of lithium to treat bipolar disorder has been long established. However, lithium also affects the circadian system, resulting in a lengthening of the circadian period. The molecular mechanism by which this occurs remains unknown. Glycogen synthase kinase 3β (GSK3β) has been implicated in participating within the molecular clock mechanism. Of interest, GSK3β is inhibited by lithium. In cell culture, GSK3β has been shown to stabilize the negative clockwork regulator REV-ERBα via phosphorylation. REV-ERBα typically represses the transcription of the *BMAL1* gene. With lithium, however, GSK3β is inhibited, thereby preventing the phosphorylation and stabilization of REV-ERBα, which is then targeted for proteasomal degradation. The degradation of REV-ERBα results in the de-repression of *BMAL1* transcription. Whether lithium's influence on circadian behavior is attributable to its inhibitory effect on *GSK3*β-mediated stabilization of REV-ERBα remains to be determined.

Short-acting benzodiazepines (e.g., triazolam [Halcion] and brotizolam [Lendormin]) also exert chronobiologic effects. In hamsters, triazolam or brotizolam administered during the middle of the subjective day induces circadian phase advances in activity. Brotizolam has been shown to reduce the light-induced expression of clock genes *Per1* and *Per2* in the SCN. Although benzodiazepines are allosteric modulators of γ-aminobutyric acid A receptors (GABA$_A$), several lines of evidence indicate that the circadian effects of short-acting benzodiazepines require an intact serotonergic system. When the 5-HT$_{1A/7}$ receptor agonist 8-hydroxy-2-(di-*n*-propylamino)-tetralin (8-OH-DPAT) is injected into hamsters at subjective midday, phase advances in locomotor behavior and SCN neuronal activity are observed in addition to a reduction in *Per1* and *Per2* gene expression in the SCN. Recreational drugs of abuse also affect the circadian system. 3,4-Methylenedioxymethamphetamine (MDMA), or "ecstasy," can act as a serotonin neurotoxin. Hamsters treated with MDMA showed reduced triazolam-induced phase shifts in circadian locomotor activity and a diminished ability to re-entrain rhythms posttreatment. MDMA-treated animals exhibited a reduction of serotonergic axonal terminals in the SCN, again emphasizing the importance of an intact serotonergic system in the regulation of the circadian axis. Recreational use of methamphetamine has increased dramatically. Chronic administration of methamphetamine disorganizes rodent activity rhythms. However, the administration of methamphetamine to rodents rendered arrhythmic through ablation of the SCN results in a reemergence of rhythmicity. The mechanism involved in the rescue of rhythmicity or site of action remains unknown.

The efficacy and toxicity of many pharmacotherapeutics vary as a function of the circadian phase. Daily variations in fixed-dose lethal toxicity have been appreciated in rodents for years. Many anticancer drugs, ranging in mechanism from antimetabolites to DNA intercalators to mitotic inhibitors, have 2- to 10-fold changes in tolerability in rodents over the day. Much of this difference is attributed to circadian variations in the body's ability to absorb, distribute, metabolize, and eliminate toxic compounds. These four processes are affected by underlying circadian rhythms in physiologic processes such as daily variations in gastric pH,

gastrointestinal mobility, glomerular filtration rate, and membrane viscosity. The rhythmic intake of food during traditionally timed meals also influences how the body handles therapeutic drugs. It is becoming clear that to maximize efficacy and minimize the toxicity of drugs, the circadian phase of administration must be considered. Appropriate circadian timing of the administration of multiple drugs can be a daunting challenge to infirmed individuals or their caretakers. The development of small implanted programmable pumps that can be directed to administer anticancer drugs or other therapeutics at particular times of day may provide a limited solution to this challenge. The emergence of the field of chronotherapy reflects our increased understanding of the circadian system's impact on pharmacologic treatment efficacy.

References

Introduction

Agit Y, Buzsaki G, Diamond DM, Frackowiak R, Giedd J. How can drug discovery for psychiatric disorders be improved? *Nat Rev Drug Discov.* 2007;6(3):189–201.

Cacioppo JT, Decety J. Social neuroscience: challenges and opportunities in the study of complex behavior. *Ann N Y Acad Sci.* 2011;1224(1):162–173.

Gould TD, Gottesman II. Commentary: psychiatric endophenotypes and the development of valid animal models. *Genes Brain Behav.* 2006;5(2):113–119.

Grebb JA, Carlsson A. Introduction and considerations for a brain-based diagnostic system in psychiatry. In: Sadock BJ, Sadock VA, Ruiz P, eds. *Kaplan & Sadock's Comprehensive Textbook of Psychiatry.* 9th ed. Philadelphia, PA: Lippincott Williams & Wilkins; 2009.

Hoef F, McCandliss BD, Black JM, Gantman A, Zakerani N, Hulme C, Lyytinen H, Whitfield-Gabrieli S, Glover GH, Reiss AL, Gabrieli JDE. Neural systems predicting long-term outcome in dyslexia. *Proc Natl Acad Sci U S A.* 2011;108(1):361–366.

Krummenacher P, Mohr C, Haker H, Brugger P. Dopamine, paranormal belief, and the detection of meaningful stimuli. *J Cogn Neurosci.* 2010;22(8):1670–1681.

Müller-Vahl KR, Grosskreutz J, Prell T, Kaufmann J, Bodammer N, Peschel T. Tics are caused by alterations in prefrontal areas, thalamus and putamen, while changes in the cingulate gyrus reflect secondary compensatory mechanisms. *BMC Neurosci.* 2014;15:6.

Niv Y, Edlund JA, Dayan P, O'Doherty JP. Neural prediction errors reveal a risk-sensitive reinforcement-learning process in the human brain. *J Neurosci.* 2012;32(2):551–562.

Peltzer-Karpf A. The dynamic matching of neural and cognitive growth cycles. *Nonlinear Dynamics Psychol Life Sci.* 2012;16(1):61–78.

Functional Neuroanatomy

Björklund A, Dunnett SB. Dopamine neuron systems in the brain: an update. *Trends Neurosci.* 2007;30(5):194–202.

Blond BN, Fredericks CA, Blumberg HP. Functional neuroanatomy of bipolar disorder: structure, function, and connectivity in an amygdala-anterior paralimbic neural system. *Bipolar Disord.* 2012;14(4):340–355.

Green S, Lambon Ralph MA, Moll J, Deakin JF, Zahn R. Guilt-selective functional disconnection of anterior temporal and subgenual cortices in major depressive disorder. *Arch Gen Psychiatry.* 2012;69(10):1014–1021.

Katschnig P, Schwingenschuh P, Jehna M, Svehlík M, Petrovic K, Ropele S, Zwick EB, Ott E, Fazekas F, Schmidt R, Enzinger C. Altered functional organization of the motor system related to ankle movements in Parkinson's disease: insights from functional MRI. *J Neural Transm.* 2011;118(5):783–793.

Kringelbach ML, Berridge KC. The functional neuroanatomy of pleasure and happiness. *Discov Med.* 2010;9(49):579–587.

Melchitzky DS, Lewis DA. Functional neuroanatomy. In: Sadock BJ, Sadock VA, Ruiz P, eds. *Kaplan & Sadock's Comprehensive Textbook of Psychiatry.* 9th ed. Philadelphia, PA: Lippincott Williams & Wilkins; 2009.

Morris CA. The behavioral phenotype of Williams syndrome: a recognizable pattern of neurodevelopment. *Am J Med Genet C Semin Med Genet.* 2010;154C(4):427–431.

Nguyen AD, Shenton ME, Levitt JJ. Olfactory dysfunction in schizophrenia: a review of neuroanatomy and psychophysiological measurements. *Harv Rev Psychiatry.* 2010;18(5):279–292.

Prats-Galino A, Soria G, de Notaris M, Puig J, Pedraza S. Functional anatomy of subcortical circuits issuing from or integrating at the human brainstem. *Clin Neurophysiol.* 2012;123(1):4–12.

Sapara A, Birchwood M, Cooke MA, Fannon D, Williams SC, Kuipers E, Kumari V. Preservation and compensation: the functional neuroanatomy of insight and working memory in schizophrenia. *Schizophr Res.* 2014;152:201–209.

Vago DR, Epstein J, Catenaccio E, Stern E. Identification of neural targets for the treatment of psychiatric disorders: the role of functional neuroimaging. *Neurosurg Clin N Am.* 2011;22(2):279–305.

Watson CE, Chatterjee A. The functional neuroanatomy of actions. *Neurology.* 2011; 76(16):1428–1434.

Weis S, Leube D, Erb M, Heun R, Grodd W, Kircher T. Functional neuroanatomy of sustained memory encoding performance in healthy aging and in Alzheimer's disease. *Int J Neurosci.* 2011;121(7):384–392.

Zilles K, Amunts K, Smaers JB. Three brain collections for comparative neuroanatomy and neuroimaging. *Ann N Y Acad Sci.* 2011;1225:E94–E104.

Neural Development and Neurogenesis

DiCicco-Bloom E, Falluel-Morel A. Neural development and neurogenesis. In: Sadock BJ, Sadock VA, Ruiz P, eds. *Kaplan & Sadock's Comprehensive Textbook of Psychiatry.* 9th ed. Philadelphia, PA: Lippincott Williams & Wilkins; 2009.

Eisch AJ, Petrik D. Depression and hippocampal neurogenesis: a road to remission? *Science.* 2012;338(6103):72–75.

Hsieh J, Eisch AJ. Epigenetics, hippocampal neurogenesis, and neuropsychiatric disorder: unraveling the genome to understand the mind. *Neurobiol Dis.* 2010; 39(1):73–84.

Kobayashi M, Nakatani T, Koda T, Matsumoto KI, Ozaki R, Mochida N, Keizo T, Miyakawa T, Matsuoka I. Absence of BRINP1 in mice causes increase of hippocampal neurogenesis and behavioral alterations relevant to human psychiatric disorders. *Mol Brain.* 2014;7:12.

Levenson CW, Morris D. Zinc and neurogenesis: making new neurons from development to adulthood. *Adv Nutr.* 2011;2(2):96–100.

Molina-Holgado E, Molina-Holgado F. Mending the broken brain: neuroimmune interactions in neurogenesis. *J Neurochem.* 2010;114(5):1277–1290.

Sanes DH, Reh TA, Harris WA. *Development of the Nervous System.* 3rd ed. Burlington, MA: Academic Press; 2011.

Sek T, Sawamoto K, Parent JM, Alvarez-Buylla A, eds. *Neurogenesis in the Adult Brain I: Neurobiology.* New York: Springer; 2011.

Sek T, Sawamoto K, Parent JM, Alvarez-Buylla A, eds. *Neurogenesis in the Adult Brain II: Clinical Implications.* New York: Springer; 2011.

Shi Y, Zhao X, Hsieh J, Wichterle H, Impey S, Banerjee S, Neveu P, Kosik KS. MicroRNA regulation of neural stem cells and neurogenesis. *J Neurosci.* 2010; 30(45):14931–14936.

Neurophysiology and Neurochemistry

Abi-Dargham A. The neurochemistry of schizophrenia: a focus on dopamine and glutamate. In: Charney DS, Nestler E, eds. *Neurobiology of Mental Illness.* 3rd ed. New York: Oxford University Press; 2009:321.

Berger M, Honig G, Wade JM, Tecott LH. Monoamine neurotransmitters. In: Sadock BJ, Sadock VA, Ruiz P, eds. *Kaplan & Sadock's Comprehensive Textbook of Psychiatry.* 9th ed. Philadelphia, PA: Lippincott Williams & Wilkins; 2009.

Butler JS, Foxe JJ, Fiebelkorn IC, Mercier MR, Molholm S. Multisensory representation of frequency across audition and touch: high density electrical mapping reveals early sensory-perceptual coupling. *J Neurosci.* 2012;32(44):15338–15344.

Coyle JT. Amino acid neurotransmitters. In: Sadock BJ, Sadock VA, Ruiz P, eds. *Kaplan & Sadock's Comprehensive Textbook of Psychiatry.* 9th ed. Philadelphia, PA: Lippincott Williams & Wilkins; 2009.

Ferrer I, López-Gonzalez I, Carmona M, Dalfó E, Pujol A, Martínez A. Neurochemistry and the non-motor aspects of Parkinson's disease. *Neurobiol Dis.* 2012;46:508.

Francis PT. Neurochemistry of Alzheimer's disease. In: Abou-Saleh MT, Katona CLE, Kumar A, eds. *Principles and Practice of Geriatric Psychiatry.* 3rd ed. Hoboken, NJ: Wiley-Blackwell; 2011:295.

Hallett M, Rothwell J. Milestones in clinical neurophysiology. *Mov Disord.* 2011; 26(6):958–967.

Kasala ER, Bodduluru LN, Maneti Y, Thipparaboina R. Effect of meditation on neurophysiological changes in stress mediated depression. *Complement Ther Clin Pract.* 2014;20(1):74–80.

Martinez D, Carpenter KM, Liu F, Slifstein M, Broft A, Friedman AC, Kumar D, Van Heertum R, Kleber HD, Nunes E. Imaging dopamine transmission in cocaine dependence: link between neurochemistry and response to treatment. *Am J Psychiatry.* 2011;168(6):634–641.

Posey DJ, Lodin Z, Erickson CA, Stigler KA, McDougle CJ. The neurochemistry of ASD. In: Fein D, ed. *Neuropsychology of Autism.* New York: Oxford University Press; 2011:77.

Recasens M, Guiramand J, Aimar R, Abdulkarim A, Barbanel G. Metabotropic glutamate receptors as drug targets. *Curr Drug Targets.* 2007;8(5):651–681.

Reidler JS, Zaghi S, Fregni F. Neurophysiological effects of transcranial direct current stimulation. In: Coben R, Evan JR, eds. *Neurofeedback and Neuromodulation Techniques and Applications.* New York: Academic Press; 2011:319.

Sedlack TW, Kaplin AI. Novel neurotransmitters. In: Sadock BJ, Sadock VA, Ruiz P, eds. *Kaplan & Sadock's Comprehensive Textbook of Psychiatry.* 9th ed. Philadelphia, PA: Lippincott Williams & Wilkins; 2009.

Smith SM. Resting state fMRI in the human connectome project. *Neuroimage* 2013; 80:144–158.

Young LJ, Owens MJ, Nemeroff CB. Neuropeptides: biology, regulation, and role in neuropsychiatric disorders. In: Sadock BJ, Sadock VA, Ruiz P, eds. *Kaplan & Sadock's Comprehensive Textbook of Psychiatry.* 9th ed. Philadelphia, PA: Lippincott Williams & Wilkins; 2009.

Psychoneuroendocrinology

Bartz JA, Hollander E. The neuroscience of affiliation: forging links between basic and clinical research on neuropeptides and social behavior. *Horm Behav.* 2006; 50(4):518–528.

Dubrovsky B. Neurosteroids, neuroactive steroids, and symptoms of affective disorders. *Pharmacol Biochem Behav.* 2006;84(4):644–655.

Duval F, Mokrani MC, Ortiz JA, Schulz P, Champeval C. Neuroendocrine predictors of the evolution of depression. *Dialogues Clin Neurosci.* 2005;7(3):273–282.

Goldberg-Stern H, Ganor Y, Cohen R, Pollak L, Teichberg V, Levite M. Glutamate receptor antibodies directed against AMPA receptors subunit 3 peptide B (GluR3B) associate with some cognitive/psychiatric/behavioral abnormalities in epilepsy patients. *Psychoneuroendocrinology.* 2014;40:221–231.

Martin EI, Ressler KJ, Binder E, Nemeroff CB. The neurobiology of anxiety disorders: brain imaging, genetics, and psychoneuroendocrinology. *Clin Lab Med.* 2010;30(4):865–891.

McEwen BS. Physiology and neurobiology of stress and adaptation: central role of the brain. *Physiol Rev.* 2007;87(3):873–904.

Phillips DI. Programming of the stress response: a fundamental mechanism underlying the long-term effects of the fetal environment? *J Intern Med.* 2007;261(5): 453–460.

Strous RD, Maayan R, Weizman A. The relevance of neurosteroids to clinical psychiatry: from the laboratory to the bedside. *Eur Neuropsychopharmacol.* 2006; 16(3):155–169.

Zitzmann M. Testosterone and the brain. *Aging Male.* 2006;9(4):195–199.

Immune System and Central Nervous System Interactions

Bajramovic JJ. Regulation of innate immune responses in the central nervous system. *CNS Neurol Disord Drug Targets.* 2011;10(1):4–24.

Capuron L, Miller AH. Immune system to brain signaling: neuropsychopharmacological implications. *Pharmacol Ther.* 2011;130(2):226–238.

Danese A, Moffitt TE, Pariante CM, Ambler A, Poulton R. Elevated inflammation levels in depressed adults with a history of childhood maltreatment. *Arch Gen Psychiatry.* 2008;65(4):409–415.

Dantzer R, O'Connor JC, Freund GG, Johnson RW, Kelley KW. From inflammation to sickness and depression: when the immune system subjugates the brain. *Nat Rev Neurosci.* 2008;9(1):46–56.

Raison CL, Borisov AS, Woolwine BJ, Massung B, Vogt G, Miller AH. Interferon-α effects on diurnal hypothalamic-pituitary-adrenal axis activity: relationship with proinflammatory cytokines and behavior. *Mol Psychiatry.* 2010;15(5):535–547.

Raison CL, Cowles MK, Miller AH. Immune system and central nervous system interactions. In: Sadock BJ, Sadock VA, Ruiz P, eds. *Kaplan & Sadock's Comprehensive Textbook of Psychiatry.* 9th ed. Philadelphia, PA: Lippincott Williams & Wilkins; 2009:175.

Ransohoff RM, Brown MA. Innate immunity in the central nervous system. *J Clin Invest.* 2012;122(4):1164–1171.

Steiner J, Bernstein HG, Schiltz K, Müller UJ, Westphal S, Drexhage HA, Bogerts B. Immune system and glucose metabolism interaction in schizophrenia: a chicken–egg dilemma. *Prog Neuropsychopharmacol Biol Psychiatry.* 2014;48:287–294.

Wilson EH, Weninger W, Hunter CA. Trafficking of immune cells in the central nervous system. *J Clin Invest.* 2010;120(5):1368–1379.

Yousef S, Planas R, Chakroun K, Hoffmeister-Ullerich S, Binder TM, Eiermann TH, Martin R, Sospedra M. TCR bias and HLA cross-restriction are strategies of human brain-infiltrating JC virus-specific CD4+ T cells during viral infection. *J Immunol.* 2012;189(7):3618–3630.

Neurogenetics

Craddock N, O'Donovan MC, Owen MJ. Phenotypic and genetic complexity of psychosis. Invited commentary on Schizophrenia: a common disease caused by multiple rare alleles. *Br J Psychiatry.* 2007;190:200–203.

De Luca V, Tharmalingam S, Zai C, Potapova N, Strauss J, Vincent J, Kennedy JL. Association of HPA axis genes with suicidal behaviour in schizophrenia. *J Psychopharmacol.* 2010;24(5):677–682.

Demers CH, Bogdan R, Agrawal A. The genetics, neurogenetics and pharmacogenetics of addiction. *Curr Behav Neurosci Rep.* 2014;1(1):33–44.

Farmer A, Elkin A, McGuffin P. The genetics of bipolar affective disorder. *Curr Opin Psychiatry.* 2007;20:8.

Fears SC, Mathews CA, Freimer NB. Genetic linkage analysis of psychiatric disorders. In: Sadock BJ, Sadock VA, Ruiz P, eds. *Kaplan & Sadock's Comprehensive Textbook of Psychiatry.* 9th ed. Philadelphia, PA: Lippincott Williams & Wilkins; 320.

Gianakopoulos PJ, Zhang Y, Pencea N, Orlic-Milacic M, Mittal K, Windpassinger C, White SJ, Kroisel PM, Chow EW, Saunders CJ, Minassian BA, Vincent JB. Mutations in MECP2 exon 1 in classical Rett patients disrupt MECP2_e1 transcription, but not transcription of MECP2_e2. *Am J Med Genet B Neuropsychiatr Genet.* 2012; 159B(2):210–216.

Guerrini R, Parrini E. Neuronal migration disorders. *Neurobiol Dis.* 2010;38(2): 154–166.

Kumar KR, Djarmati-Westenberger A, Grünewald A. Genetics of Parkinson's disease. *Semin Neurol.* 2011;31(5):433–440.

Novarino G, El-Fishawy P, Kayserili H, Meguid NA, Scott EM, Schroth J, Silhavy JL, Kara M, Khalil RO, Ben-Omran T, Ercan-Sencicek AG, Hashish AF, Sanders SJ, Gupta AR, Hashem HS, Matern D, Gabriel S, Sweetman L, Rahimi Y, Harris RA, State MW, Gleeson JG. Mutations in BCKD-kinase lead to a potentially treatable form of autism with epilepsy. *Science.* 2012;338(6105):394–397.

Perisco AM, Bourgeron T. Searching for ways out of the autism maze: genetic, epigenetic and environmental clues. *Trends Neurosci.* 2006;29(7):349–358.

Schizophrenia Working Group of the Psychiatric Genomics Consortium. Biological insights from 108 schizophrenia-associated genetic loci. *Nature.* 2014; 511(7510):421–427. https://doi.org/10.1038/nature13595

Sekar A, Bialas AR, de Rivera H, Davis A, Hammond TR, Kamitaki N, Tooley K, Presumey J, Baum M, Van Doren V, Genovese G, Rose SA, Handsaker RE, Daly MJ, Carroll MC, Stevens B, McCarroll SA; Schizophrenia Working Group of the Psychiatric Genomics Consortium. Schizophrenia risk from complex variation of complement component 4. *Nature.* 2016;530(7589):177–183. https://doi.org/10.1038/nature16549

Spors H, Albeanu DF, Murthy VN, Rinberg D, Uchida N, Wachowiak M, Friedrich RW. Illuminating vertebrate olfactory processing. *J Neurosci.* 2012;32(41):14102–14108.

Applied Electrophysiology

Alhaj H, Wisniewski G, McAllister-Williams RH. The use of the EEG in measuring therapeutic drug action: focus on depression and antidepressants. *J Psychopharmacol.* 2011;25(9):1175–1191.

André VM, Cepeda C, Fisher YE, Huynh MY, Bardakjian N, Singh S, Yang XW, Levine MS. Differential electrophysiological changes in striatal output neurons in Huntington's disease. *J Neurosci.* 2011;31(4):1170–1182.

Boutros NN, Arfken CL. A four-step approach to developing diagnostic testing in psychiatry. *Clin EEG Neurosci.* 2007;38:62.

Boutros NN, Galderisi S, Pogarell O, Riggio S, eds. *Standard Electroencephalography in Clinical Psychiatry: A Practical Handbook.* Hoboken, NJ: Wiley-Blackwell; 2011.

Boutros NN, Iacono WG, Galderisi S. Applied electrophysiology. In: Sadock BJ, Sadock VA, Ruiz P, eds. *Kaplan & Sadock's Comprehensive Textbook of Psychiatry.* 9th ed. Philadelphia, PA: Lippincott Williams & Wilkins; 2009:211.

Gosselin N, Bottari C, Chen JK, Petrides M, Tinawi S, de Guise E, Ptito A. Electrophysiology and functional MRI in post-acute mild traumatic brain injury. *J Neurotrauma.* 2011;28(3):329–341.

Horan WP, Wynn JK, Kring AM, Simons RF, Green MF. Electrophysiological correlates of emotional responding in schizophrenia. *J Abnorm Psychol.* 2010;119(1):18–30.

Hunter AM, Cook IA, Leuchter AF. The promise of the quantitative electroencephalogram as a predictor of antidepressant treatment outcomes in major depressive disorder. *Psychiatr Clin North Am.* 2007;30(1):105–124.

Jarahi M, Sheibani V, Safakhah HA, Torkmandi H, Rashidy-Pour A. Effects of progesterone on neuropathic pain responses in an experimental animal model for peripheral neuropathy in the rat: a behavioral and electrophysiological study. *Neuroscience.* 2014;256:403–411.

Winterer G, McCarley RW. Electrophysiology of schizophrenia. In: Weinberger DR, Harrison PJ. *Schizophrenia.* 3rd ed. Hoboken, NJ: Blackwell Publishing Ltd; 2011:311.

Chronobiology

Delezie J, Challet E. Interactions between metabolism and circadian clocks: reciprocal disturbances. *Ann N Y Acad Sci.* 2011;1243:30–46.

Dridi D, Zouiten A, Mansour HB. Depression: chronophysiology and chronotherapy. *Biol Rhyth Res.* 2014;45:77–91.

Eckel-Mahan K, Sassone-Corsi P. Metabolism and the circadian clock converge. *Physiol Rev.* 2013;93(1):107–135.

Glickman G, Webb IC, Elliott JA, Baltazar RM, Reale ME, Lehman MN, Gorman MR. Photic sensitivity for circadian response to light varies with photoperiod. *J Biol Rhythms.* 2012;27(4):308–318.

Gonnissen HK, Rutters F, Mazuy C, Martens EA, Adam TC, Westerterp-Plantenga MS. Effect of a phase advance and phase delay of the 24-h cycle on energy metabolism, appetite, and related hormones. *Am J Clin Nutr.* 2012;96(4):689–697.

Lanzani MF, de Zavalía N, Fontana H, Sarmiento MI, Golombek D, Rosenstein RE. Alterations of locomotor activity rhythm and sleep parameters in patients with advanced glaucoma. *Chronobiol Int.* 2012;29(7):911–919.

Loddenkemper T, Lockley SW, Kaleyias J, Kothare SV. Chronobiology of epilepsy: diagnostic and therapeutic implications of chrono-epileptology. *J Clin Neurophysiol.* 2011;28(2):146–153.

Provencio I. Chronobiology. In: Sadock BJ, Sadock VA, Ruiz P, eds. *Kaplan & Sadock's Comprehensive Textbook of Psychiatry.* 9th ed. Philadelphia, PA: Lippincott Williams & Wilkins; 2009:198.

Shafer SL, Lemmer B, Boselli E, Boiste F, Bouvet L, Allaouchiche B, Chassard D. Pitfalls in chronobiology: a suggested analysis using intrathecal bupivacaine analgesia as an example. *Anesth Analg.* 2010;111(4):980–985.

Wehrens SM, Hampton SM, Kerkhofs M, Skene DJ. Mood, alertness, and performance in response to sleep deprivation and recovery sleep in experienced shiftworkers versus non-shiftworkers. *Chronobiol Int.* 2012;29(5):537–548.

34

Contributions from the Behavioral and Social Sciences

The underpinnings of psychiatry span many disciplines. The previous chapter covered the neuroscience foundations of psychiatry. However, there are also contributions from the psychosocial sciences, the sociocultural sciences, and many more areas of scientific pursuit. Also, many theories and models of the mind have grown from the psychoanalytic and other theoretical schools that have had a vital influence on the practice of psychiatry, both historically and currently.

This chapter provides a brief tour through some of the significant fields that, along with the neurosciences, have helped psychiatry to grow from a purely empirical practice into a robust and evidence-based branch of medicine. Along the way, it also provides some brief biographies of some of the greatest thinkers and researchers in these fields.

▲ 34.1 Contributions from the Psychosocial Sciences

JEAN PIAGET AND COGNITIVE DEVELOPMENT

Jean Piaget (1896–1980) is considered one of the greatest thinkers of the 20th century. His contributions to the understanding of cognitive development had a paradigmatic influence in developmental psychology and had significant implications for interventions with children, both educational and clinical.

Piaget was born in Neuchatel, Switzerland, where he studied at the university and received a doctorate in biology at 22. Interested in psychology, he studied and researched several centers, including the Sorbonne in Paris, and he worked with Eugen Bleuler at the Burghöltzli Psychiatric Hospital.

Piaget created a broad theoretical system for the development of cognitive abilities; in this sense, his work was similar to that of Sigmund Freud, but Piaget emphasized how children think and acquire knowledge.

Widely renowned as a child (or developmental) psychologist, Piaget referred to himself primarily as a *genetic epistemologist;* he defined genetic epistemology as the study of the development of abstract thought based on a biologic or innate substrate. That self-designation reveals that Piaget's central project was more than articulating *developmental child psychology,* as this term is generally understood; it was an account of the progressive development of human knowledge.

Cognitive Development Stages

According to Piaget, the following four major stages lead to the capacity for adult thought (Table 34-1): (1) sensorimotor,
(2) preoperational thought, (3) concrete operations, and (4) formal operations. Each stage is a prerequisite for the following one, but the rate at which different children move through different stages varies with their native endowment and environmental circumstances.

Sensorimotor Stage (Birth to 2 Years). Piaget used the term *sensorimotor* to describe the first stage: infants begin to learn through sensory observation, and they gain control of their motor functions through activity, exploration, and manipulation of the environment. Piaget divided this stage into six substages, listed in Table 34-2.

From the outset, biology and experience blend to produce learned behavior. For example, infants are born with a sucking reflex, but a type of learning occurs when infants discover the location of the nipple and alter the shape of their mouths. A stimulus is received, and a response results, accompanied by a sense of awareness that is the first schema, or elementary concept. As infants become increasingly mobile, one schema is built on another, and new and more complex schemata are developed. Infants' spatial, visual, and tactile worlds expand during this period; children interact actively with the environment and use previously learned behavior patterns. For example, having learned to use a rattle, infants shake a new toy as they did the rattle they had already learned to use. Infants also use a rattle in new ways.

The critical achievement of this period is the development of *object permanence* or the *schema of the permanent object.* This phrase relates to a child's ability to understand that objects have an existence independent of their involvement. Infants learn to differentiate themselves from the world and maintain a mental image of an object, even when it is not visible. When an object is dropped in front of infants, they look down to the ground to search for the object; that is, they behave for the first time as though they have a reality outside themselves.

At about 18 months, infants begin to develop mental symbols and to use words, a process known as *symbolization.* Infants can create a visual image of a ball or a mental symbol of the word *ball* to stand for, or signify, the real object. Such mental representations allow children to operate on new conceptual levels. The attainment of object permanence marks the transition from the sensorimotor stage to the preoperational stage of development.

Stage of Preoperational Thought (2 to 7 Years). During the stage of preoperational thought, children use symbols and language more extensively than in the sensorimotor stage. Thinking and reasoning are intuitive; children learn without the use of reasoning. They cannot think logically or deductively, and their concepts are

Table 34-1
Stages of Intellectual Development Postulated by Piaget

Age (yr)	Period	Cognitive Developmental Characteristics
0–1.5 (to 2)	Sensorimotor	Divided into six stages, characterized by: 1. Inborn motor and sensory reflexes 2. Primary circular reaction 3. Secondary circular reaction 4. Use of familiar means to obtain ends 5. Tertiary circular reaction and discovery through active experimentation 6. Insight and object permanence
2–7	Preoperations subperiod[a]	Deferred imitation, symbolic play, graphic imagery (drawing), mental imagery, and language
7–11	Concrete operations	Conservation of quantity, weight, volume, length, and time based on reversibility by inversion or reciprocity; operations; class inclusion and seriation
11–end of adolescence	Formal operations	Combinatorial system, whereby variables are isolated and all possible combinations are examined; hypotheticodeductive thinking

[a]This subperiod is considered by some authors to be a separate developmental period.

primitive; they can name objects but not classes of objects. Preoperational thought is midway between socialized adult thought and the completely autistic Freudian unconscious. Events are not linked by logic. Early in this stage, if children drop a glass that breaks, they have no sense of cause and effect. They believe that the glass was ready to break, not that they broke the glass. Children in this stage cannot grasp the sameness of an object in different circumstances: the same doll in a carriage, a crib, or a chair is perceived to be three different objects. During this time, things are represented in terms of their function. For example, a child defines a bike as "to ride" and a hole as "to dig."

In this stage, children begin to use language and drawings in more elaborate ways. From one-word utterances, two-word phrases develop, made up of either a noun and a verb or a noun and an objective. A child may say, "Bobby eat," or "Bobby up."

Table 34-2
Piaget's Sensorimotor Period of Cognitive Development

Age	Characteristics
Birth–2 mo	Uses inborn motor and sensory reflexes (sucking, grasping, looking) to interact and accommodate to the external world
2–5 mo	Primary circular reaction: Coordinates activities of own body and five senses (e.g., sucking thumb); reality remains subjective—does not seek stimuli outside of its visual field; displays curiosity
5–9 mo	Secondary circular reaction: Seeks out new stimuli in the environment; starts both to anticipate consequences of own behavior and to act purposefully to change the environment; beginning of intentional behavior
9 mo–1 yr	Shows preliminary signs of object permanence; has a vague concept that objects exist apart from itself; plays peek-a-boo; imitates novel behaviors
1 yr–18 mo	Tertiary circular reaction: Seeks out new experiences; produces novel behaviors
18 mo–2 yr	Symbolic thought: Uses symbolic representations of events and objects; shows signs of reasoning (e.g., uses one toy to reach for and get another); attains object permanence

Children in the preoperational stage cannot deal with moral dilemmas, although they feel good and bad. For example, when asked, "Who is more guilty, the person who breaks one dish on purpose or the person who breaks ten dishes by accident?" a young child usually answers that the person who breaks ten dishes by accident is more guilty because more dishes are broken. Children in this stage have a sense of *immanent justice;* the belief that punishment for bad deeds is inevitable.

Children in this developmental stage are *egocentric:* they see themselves as the center of the universe; they have a limited point of view, and they cannot take the role of another person. Children cannot modify their behavior for someone else; for example, children are not negativistic when they do not listen to a command to be quiet because their brother has to study. Instead, egocentric thinking prevents an understanding of their brother's point of view.

During this stage, children also use magical thinking, called *phenomenalistic causality,* in which events that occur together are thought to cause one another (e.g., thunder causes lightning, and bad thoughts cause accidents). Also, children use *animistic thinking,* which is the tendency to endow physical events and objects with life-like psychological attributes, such as feelings and intentions.

SEMIOTIC FUNCTION. The semiotic function emerges during the preoperational period. With this new ability, children can represent something—such as an object, an event, or a conceptual scheme—with a signifier, representing a representative function (e.g., language, mental image, symbolic gesture). That is, children use a symbol or sign to stand for something else. Drawing is a semiotic function initially done as a playful exercise but eventually signifying something else in the real world.

Stage of Concrete Operations (7 to 11 Years). The stage of concrete operations is so named because, in this period, children operate and act on the concrete, real, and perceivable world of objects and events. Egocentric thought is replaced by *operational thought,* which involves dealing with a wide array of information outside the child. Therefore, children can now see things from someone else's perspective.

Children in this stage begin to use limited logical thought processes and can serialize, order, and group things into classes based on common characteristics. *Syllogistic reasoning,* in which a logical conclusion is formed from two premises, appears during this stage; for example, all horses are mammals (premise); all mammals are warm-blooded (premise); therefore, all horses are warm-blooded (conclusion). Children can reason and follow the rules and regulations. They can regulate themselves, and they begin to develop a moral sense and a code of values.

Children who become overly invested in rules may show obsessive-compulsive behavior; children who resist a code of values often seem willful and reactive. The most desirable developmental outcome in this stage is that a child attains healthy respect for rules and understands that there are legitimate exceptions to rules.

Conservation is the ability to recognize that, although the shape of objects may change, the objects still maintain or conserve other characteristics that enable them to be recognized as the same. For example, if a ball of clay is rolled into a long, thin sausage shape, children recognize that each form contains the same amount of clay. An inability to conserve (which is characteristic of the preoperational stage) is observed when a child believes there is more clay in the sausage-shaped piece because it is longer. *Reversibility* is the capacity to understand the relation between things and realize that one thing can turn into another and back again—for example, ice and water.

The most critical sign that children are still in the preoperational stage is that they have not achieved conservation or reversibility. The ability of children to understand concepts of quantity is one of Piaget's most influential cognitive developmental theories. Measures of quantity include measures of substance, length, number, liquids, and area (Fig. 34-1).

The 7- to 11-year-old child must organize and order occurrences in the real world. Dealing with the future and its possibilities occur in the formal operational stage.

Stage of Formal Operations (11 through the End of Adolescence).

The stage of formal operations is so named because young persons' thinking operates in a formal, highly logical, systematic, and symbolic manner. This stage is characterized by the ability to think abstractly, to reason deductively, and to define concepts, and also by the emergence of skills for dealing with permutations and combinations; young persons can grasp the concept of probabilities. Adolescents attempt to deal with all possible relations and hypotheses to explain data and events during this stage. Language use is complex; it follows formal rules of logic and is grammatically correct. Abstract thinking is shown by adolescents' interest in various issues—philosophy, religion, ethics, and politics.

HYPOTHETICODEDUCTIVE THINKING.   Hypotheticodeductive thinking, the highest organization of cognition, enables persons to make a hypothesis or proposition and to test it against reality. *Deductive reasoning* moves from the general to the particular and is a more complicated process than *inductive reasoning,* which moves from the particular to the general.

Because young persons can reflect on their own and other persons' thinking, they are susceptible to self-conscious behavior. As adolescents attempt to master new cognitive tasks, they may return to egocentric thought, but on a higher level than in the past. For example, adolescents may think that they can accomplish everything or can change events by thought alone. Not all adolescents enter the stage of formal operations at the same time or to the same degree. Depending on individual capacity and intervening experience, some may not reach the stage of formal operational thought at all and may remain in the concrete operational mode throughout life.

Psychiatric Applications

Piaget's theories have many psychiatric implications. Hospitalized children in the sensorimotor stage have not achieved object

Conservation of substance (6–7 years)

A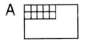

The experimenter presents two identical plasticene balls. The subject admits that the balls have equal amounts of plasticene.

B

One of the balls is deformed. The subject is asked whether the balls still contain equal amounts.

Conservation of length (6–7 years)

A

Two sticks are aligned in front of the subject. The subject admits their equality.

B

One of the sticks is moved to the right. The subject is asked whether they are still the same length.

Conservation of area (9–10 years)

A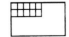

The subject and the experimenter each have identical sheets of cardboard. Wooden blocks are placed on the sheets in identical positions. The subject is asked whether each sheet has the same amount of space remaining.

B

The experimenter scatters the blocks on one of the sheets. The subject is asked the same question.

FIGURE 34-1
Some simple tests for conservation, with approximate ages of attainment. When the sense of conservation is achieved, the child answers that **B** contains the same quantity as **A**. (Modified from Lefrancois GR. *Of Children: An Introduction to Child Development.* Belmont, CA: Wadsworth; 1973:305, with permission.)

permanence and, therefore, have separation anxiety. They do best if their mothers are allowed to stay with them overnight. Children at the preoperational stage, who cannot deal with concepts and abstractions, benefit more from role-playing proposed medical procedures and situations than by having them described in detail. For example, a child who receives intravenous therapy is helped by acting out the procedure with a toy intravenous set and dolls.

Because children at the preoperational stage do not understand cause and effect, they may interpret physical illness as punishment for bad thoughts or deeds. Because they have not yet mastered the capacity to conserve and do not understand the concept of reversibility (which usually occurs during the concrete operational stage), they cannot understand that a broken bone mends or that blood loss in an accident can be replaced.

Adolescents' thinking, during the stage of formal operations, may appear overly abstract when it is, in fact, a normal developmental stage. Adolescent turmoil may not herald a psychotic process but may well result from a typical adolescent's coming to grips with newly acquired abilities to deal with the unlimited possibilities of the surrounding world.

Adults under stress may regress cognitively as well as emotionally. Their thinking can become preoperational, egocentric, and sometimes animistic.

Implications for Psychotherapy.

Piaget was not an applied psychologist and did not develop the implications of his cognitive model for psychotherapeutic intervention. Nevertheless, his work formed one of the foundations of the *cognitive revolution* in psychology. One aspect of this revolution was an increasing emphasis on the cognitive components of the therapeutic endeavor. In contrast to classical psychodynamic therapy, which focused primarily on drives and affects, and in contrast to behavior therapy, which focused on overt actions, cognitive approaches to therapy focused on thoughts, including automatic assumptions, beliefs, plans, and intentions. By including "theory theory" and "script theory," we can see additional applications to psychotherapy.

Cognitive development theory has influenced psychotherapeutic approaches in multiple ways. Some therapists have taken developmental notions from Piaget's work and developed intervention techniques. Others have developed cognitive models of treatment independent of Piaget but with heavy reliance on cognition. Others have included Piaget's concepts in a broader set of constructs to undergird new developmental approaches to psychotherapy.

First, some psychotherapists applied Piagetian notions directly to child interventions. Susan Harter, for example, discussed techniques for helping young children become aware of divergent or contradictory emotions and to integrate these complex emotions within a more abstract or higher class of emotions. One of Harter's techniques is to ask the young child to make a drawing that shows different and conflicting feelings in one person. This technique represents an application of the concrete operation of class inclusion to the realm of the emotions. Harter's work applied Piagetian findings to the common therapeutic problem of helping children to recognize, tolerate, and integrate mixed or ambivalent affects within stable object relations.

As such, it drew on cognitive theory and psychodynamic theory. Similar techniques are important in work with children who have been exposed to trauma or sexual abuse. It is an essential component of such work to assist them in labeling, differentiating, and accepting the full range of emotions stemming from these experiences.

Second, other psychotherapists developed treatment models that, although not directly dependent on Piagetian psychology,

emphasized core ideas quite similar to those Piaget discovered in his naturalistic observations of cognitive development. These models are even more closely aligned with recent developments in "theory theory." Aaron Beck, for example, developed an entire school of cognitive therapy that focuses on the role of cognitions in causing or maintaining psychopathology. Cognitive therapy is an effective treatment for problems as diverse as depression, anxiety disorders, and substance use disorders.

A core idea in cognitive therapy is that the patient has developed certain core beliefs, aspects of the self-schema, and conditional probability beliefs as a result of developmental experiences, and these contribute to emotional or behavioral problems. For example, depressed persons may have the core belief, "I am unlovable." Addicted persons may have the belief, "Unless I drink, I cannot feel happy." In cognitive therapy, the person can be assisted in identifying the negative automatic thoughts and underlying dysfunctional attitudes or beliefs that contribute to emotional distress or addictive behavior. The critical therapeutic process after identification of the maladaptive thoughts is to help the patient view these thoughts more objectively, not unquestioningly take them as veridical. Here, cognitive therapy emphasizes evidence, consistent both with Piagetian theory and "theory theory." The patient is assisted in seeking out evidence to test negative thinking; active involvement, rather than passive listening, is required.

What the cognitive therapist accomplishes through such techniques as Socratic questioning and asking if there are other ways to look at the same event is similar to what the talented teacher does in guiding children to a more adequate, more intelligent understanding of operational tasks. The notion of equilibration is relevant in both instances. By helping the individual see that previous cognitive structures are inadequate, the therapist or teacher disturbs the old cognitive structure, and the patient or student experiences a disruption that leads to the search for more-adequate structures. The compensation for external disturbance is what Piaget termed *equilibration*. New structures can be constructed only through a process of accommodation, enabling the subject to assimilate a more comprehensive array of data, a new perspective, or more complex information.

Because it requires *thinking about thinking*, cognitive therapy seems to require formal operational thinking, although this has not been empirically tested. At the least, it requires the ability to recognize and articulate affects, to recognize and label events that give rise to affects, and to translate into thought the mediating process that occurs rapidly between the event and the affect. Cognitive-behavioral models of psychotherapy include cognitive techniques and more behavioral, interactive techniques, such as increasing pleasant activities and improving communication and problem-solving skills. It is possible that the less-cognitive, more-behavioral techniques, although requiring a lower level of cognitive development, can also lead to the garnering of evidence and modification of specific expectancies, attributions, and self-schemata.

Because "script theory" or narrative approaches to cognition in psychotherapy are empirically based, generated by repetitive experiences rather than by reflective abstraction, and domain-specific, they may have even more general application to psychotherapy than classic Piagetian theories or "theory theory." For example, in dialectical behavior therapy, patients provide a "chain analysis" of events, feelings, thoughts, situational stimuli, and interpersonal factors that led to negative or self-damaging behavior. This narrative provides guidance to the patient and the therapist about where and how to intervene to prevent similar behavior.

Developmentally Based Psychotherapy. Developmentally based psychotherapy, developed by Stanley Greenspan, M.D., integrates cognitive, affective, drive, and relationship-based approaches with a new understanding of the stages of human development. The clinician first determines the level of the patient's ego or personality development and the presence or absence of deficits or constrictions. For example, can the person regulate activity and sensations, relate to others, read nonverbal affective symbols, represent experience, build bridges between representations, integrate emotional polarities, abstract feelings, and reflect on internal wishes and feelings?

From a developmental point of view, the integral parts of the therapeutic process include learning how to regulate experience; to engage more fully and deeply in relationships; to perceive, comprehend, and respond to complex behaviors and interactive patterns; and to be able to engage in the ever-changing opportunities, tasks, and challenges during life (e.g., adulthood and aging) and, throughout, to observe and reflect on one's own and others' experiences. These processes are the foundation of the ego, and more broadly, the personality. Their presence constitutes emotional health and their absence, emotional disorder. The developmental approach describes how to harness these core processes and assist the patients in mobilizing their growth.

ATTACHMENT THEORY

Attachment and Development

Attachment can be defined as the emotional tone between children and their caregivers and is evidenced by an infant's seeking and clinging to the caregiving person, usually the mother. By their first month, infants usually have begun to show such behavior, designed to promote proximity to the desired person.

Attachment theory originated in the work of John Bowlby, a British psychoanalyst (1907–1990). In his studies of infant attachment and separation, Bowlby pointed out that attachment constituted a central motivational force and that mother–child attachment was an essential medium of human interaction that had significant consequences for later development and personality functioning. Being monotropic, infants tend to attach to one person; but they can form attachments to several persons, such as the father or a surrogate. Attachment develops gradually; it results in an infant's wanting to be with a preferred person, who is perceived as stronger, wiser, and able to reduce anxiety or distress. Attachment thus gives infants feelings of security. The interaction between mother and infant facilitates the process; the amount of time together is less critical than the activity between the two.

The term *bonding* is sometimes used synonymously with attachment, but the two are different phenomena. Bonding concerns the mother's feelings for her infant and differs from attachment. Mothers generally do not rely on their infants as a source of security, as is the case in attachment behavior. Much research reveals that the bonding of mother to infant occurs when there is skin-to-skin contact between the two or when other types of contact, such as voice and eye contact, are made. Some workers have concluded that a mother who has skin-to-skin contact with her baby immediately after birth shows a stronger bonding pattern and may provide more attentive care than a mother who does not have this experience. Some researchers have even proposed a critical period immediately after birth, during which such skin-to-skin contact must occur if bonding is to occur. This concept is much disputed: many mothers are bonded to their infants and display excellent maternal care even though they did not have skin-to-skin contact immediately postpartum. Because human beings can develop representational models of their babies in utero and even before conception, this representational thinking may be as crucial to the bonding process as skin, voice, or eye contact.

Ethologic Studies. Bowlby suggested a Darwinian evolutionary basis for attachment behavior; namely, such behavior ensures that adults protect their young. Ethologic studies show that nonhuman primates and other animals exhibit attachment behavior patterns that are presumably instinctual and are governed by inborn tendencies. An example of an instinctual attachment system is *imprinting*. Certain stimuli can elicit innate behavior patterns during the first few hours of an animal's behavioral development; thus, the animal offspring becomes attached to its mother at a critical period early in its development. A similar sensitive or critical period during which attachment occurs has been postulated for human infants. The presence of imprinting behavior in humans is highly controversial, but bonding and attachment behavior during the first year of life closely approximate the critical period; in humans, however, this period occurs over years rather than hours.

HARRY HARLOW. Harry Harlow's work with monkeys is relevant to attachment theory. Harlow demonstrated the emotional and behavioral effects of isolating monkeys from birth and keeping them from forming attachments. The isolates were withdrawn, unable to relate to peers, unable to mate, and incapable of caring for their offspring.

Phases of Attachment

In the first attachment phase, sometimes called the *preattachment stage* (birth to 8 or 12 weeks), babies orient to their mothers, follow them with their eyes over a 180-degree range, and turn toward and move rhythmically with their mother's voice. In the second phase, sometimes called *attachment in the making* (8 to 12 weeks to 6 months), infants become attached to one or more persons in the environment. In the third phase, sometimes called *clear-cut attachment* (6 through 24 months), infants cry and show other signs of distress when separated from the caretaker or mother; this phase can occur as early as 3 months in some infants. On being returned to the mother, the infant stops crying and clings to gain further assurance of the mother's return. Sometimes, seeing the mother after a separation is sufficient for crying to stop. In the fourth phase (25 months and beyond), the mother figure is seen as independent, and a more complex relationship between the mother and the child develops. Table 34-3 summarizes the development of standard attachment from birth through 3 years.

Mary Ainsworth. Mary Ainsworth (1913–1999) was a Canadian developmental psychologist from the University of Toronto. She described three main types of insecure attachment: insecure-avoidant, insecure-ambivalent, and insecure-disorganized. The insecure-avoidant child, having experienced brusque or aggressive parenting, tends to avoid close contact with people and lingers near caregivers rather than approaching them directly when faced with a threat. The insecure-ambivalent child finds exploratory play difficult, even in the absence of danger, and clings to his or her inconsistent parents. Insecure-disorganized children have parents who are emotionally absent with a parental history of abuse in their childhood. These children tend to behave in bizarre ways when threatened. According to Ainsworth, disorganization is a severe form of insecure attachment and a possible precursor of severe

Table 34-3
Normal Attachment

Birth to 30 days
  Reflexes at birth
  Rooting
  Head turning
  Sucking
  Swallowing
  Hand-mouth
  Grasp
  Digital extension
  Crying—signal for particular kind of distress
  Responsiveness and orientation to mother's face, eyes, and voice
  4 days—anticipatory approach behavior at feeding
  3–4 wk—infant smiles preferentially to mother's voice
Age 30 days through 3 mo
  Vocalization and gaze reciprocity further elaborated from 1 to 3 mo; babbling at 2 mo, more with the mother than with a stranger
  Social smile
  In strange situation, increased clinging response to mother
Age 4 through 6 mo
  Briefly soothed and comforted by sound of mother's voice
  Spontaneous, voluntary reaching for mother
  Anticipatory posturing to be picked up
  Differential preference for mother intensifies
  Subtle integration of responses to mother
Age 7 through 9 mo
  Attachment behaviors further differentiated and focused specifically on mother
  Separation distress, stranger distress, strange-place distress
Age 10 through 15 mo
  Crawls or walks toward mother
  Subtle facial expressions (coyness, attentiveness)
  Responsive dialogue with mother clearly established
  Early imitation of mother (vocal inflections, facial expression)
  More fully developed separation distress and mother preference
  Pointing gesture
  Walking to and from mother
  Affectively positive reunion responses to mother after separation or, paradoxically, short-lived, active avoidance or delayed protest
Age 16 mo through 2 yr
  Involvement in imitative jargon with mother (12–14 mo)
  Head-shaking "no" (15–16 mo)
  Transitional object used during the absence of mother
  Separation anxiety diminishes
  Mastery of strange situations and persons when mother is near
  Evidence of delayed imitation
  Object permanence
  Microcosmic symbolic play
Age 25 mo through 3 yr
  Able to tolerate separations from mother without distress when familiar with surroundings and given reassurances about mother's return
  Two- and three-word speech
  Stranger anxiety much reduced
  Object consistency achieved—maintains composure and psychosocial functioning without regression in absence of mother
  Microcosmic play and social play; cooperation with others begins

Based on material by Justin Call, M.D.

Table 34-4
The Strange Situation

Episode[a]	Persons Present	Change
1	Parent, infant	Enter room
2	Parent, infant, stranger	Unfamiliar adult joins the dyad
3	Infant, stranger	Parent leaves
4	Parent, infant	Parent returns, stranger leaves
5	Infant	Parent leaves
6	Infant, stranger	Stranger returns
7	Parent, infant	Parent returns, stranger leaves

[a]All episodes are usually 3 minutes long, but episodes 3, 5, and 6 can be curtailed if the infant becomes too distressed, and episodes 4 and 7 are sometimes extended.
Reprinted from Lamb ME, Nash A, Teti DM, Bornstein MH. Infancy. In: Lewis M, ed. *Child and Adolescent Psychiatry: A Comprehensive Textbook*. 2nd ed. Philadelphia, PA: Williams & Wilkins; 1996:256, with permission.

example, some babies signal or cry less than others. Sensitive responsiveness to infant signals, such as cuddling a crying baby, causes infants to cry less in later months, rather than reinforcing crying behavior. Close bodily contact with the mother when the baby signals for her is also associated with the growth of self-reliance, rather than a clinging dependence, as the baby grows older. Unresponsive mothers produce anxious babies; these mothers often have lower intelligence quotients (IQs) and are emotionally more immature and younger than responsive mothers.

Ainsworth also confirmed that attachment serves to reduce anxiety. What she called the *secure base effect* enables children to move away from attachment figures and to explore the environment. Inanimate objects, such as a teddy bear and a blanket (called the transitional object by Donald Winnicott), also serve as a secure base, one that often accompanies them as they investigate the world.

STRANGE SITUATION. Ainsworth developed the strange situation, the research protocol for assessing the quality and security of an infant's attachment. In this procedure, the infant is exposed to escalating amounts of stress; for example, the infant and the parent enter an unfamiliar room, an unfamiliar adult then enters the room, and the parent leaves the room. The protocol has seven steps (Table 34-4). According to Ainsworth's studies, about 65 percent of infants are securely attached by 24 months.

Anxiety

Bowlby's theory of anxiety holds that a child's sense of distress during separation is perceived and experienced as anxiety and is the prototype of anxiety. Any stimuli that alarm children and cause fear (e.g., loud noises, falling, and cold blasts of air) mobilize signal indicators (e.g., crying) that cause the mother to respond in a caring way by cuddling and reassuring the child. The mother's ability to relieve the infant's anxiety or fear is fundamental to the growth of attachment in the infant. When the mother is close to the child, and the child experiences no fear, the child gains a sense of security, the opposite of anxiety. When the mother is unavailable to the infant because of physical absence (e.g., if the mother is in prison) or because of psychological impairment (e.g., severe depression), anxiety develops in the infant.

Separation anxiety is the response of a child who is isolated or separated from its mother or caretaker. It is most common at 10 to

personality disorder and dissociative phenomena in adolescence and early adulthood.

Mary Ainsworth expanded on Bowlby's observations and found that the interaction between the mother and her baby during the attachment period significantly influences the baby's current and future behavior. Patterns of attachments vary among babies; for

18 months of age and generally disappears by the end of the third year. It is usually expressed with tearfulness or irritability. Somewhat earlier (at about 8 months), stranger anxiety is an anxiety response to someone other than the caregiver appears.

Signal Indicators. Signal indicators are infants' signs of distress that prompt or elicit a behavioral response in the mother. The primary signal is crying. The three types of signal indicators are hunger (the most common), anger, and pain. Some mothers can distinguish between them, but most mothers generalize the hunger cry to represent distress from pain, frustration, or anger. Other signal indicators that reinforce attachment are smiling, cooing, and looking. The sound of an adult human voice can prompt these indicators.

Losing Attachments. Persons' reactions to the death of a parent or a spouse can be traced to the nature of their past and present attachment to the lost figure. An absence of demonstrable grief may be owing to real experiences of rejection and the lack of closeness in the relationship. The person may even consciously offer an idealized picture of the deceased. Persons who show no grief usually try to present themselves as independent and disinterested in closeness and attachment.

Sometimes, however, the severing of attachments is traumatic. The death of a parent or a spouse can precipitate a depressive disorder, and even suicide, in some persons. The death of a spouse increases the chance that the surviving spouse will experience a physical or mental disorder during the next year. The onset of depression and other dysphoric states often involves rejection by a significant figure in a person's life.

Disorders of Attachment

Attachment disorders are characterized by biopsychosocial pathology that results from maternal deprivation, a lack of care by, and interaction with, the mother or caregiver. Failure-to-thrive syndromes, psychosocial dwarfism, separation anxiety disorder, avoidant personality disorder, depressive disorders, delinquency, academic problems, and borderline intelligence have been traced to negative attachment experiences. When maternal care is deficient because (1) a mother is mentally ill, (2) a child is institutionalized for a long time, or (3) the primary object of attachment dies, children sustain emotional damage. Bowlby initially thought that the damage was permanent and invariable. However, he revised his theories to consider the time at which the separation occurred, the type and degree of separation, and the level of security that the child experienced before the separation.

Bowlby described a predictable set and sequence of behavior patterns in children who are separated from their mothers for extended periods (more than 3 months): protest, in which the child protests the separation by crying, calling out, and searching for the lost person; despair, in which the child appears to lose hope that the mother will return; and detachment, in which the child emotionally separates him- or herself from the mother. Bowlby believed that this sequence involves ambivalent feelings toward the mother; the child both wants her and is angry with her for her desertion.

Children in the detachment stage respond indifferently when the mother returns; the mother has not been forgotten, but the child is angry at her for having gone away in the first place and fears that she will go away again. Some children have affectionless personalities characterized by emotional withdrawal, little or no feeling, and a limited ability to form affectionate relationships.

Anaclitic Depression. Anaclitic depression, also known as hospitalism, was first described by René Spitz in infants who had made normal attachments but were suddenly separated from their mothers for varying times and placed in institutions or hospitals. The children became depressed, withdrawn, nonresponsive, and vulnerable to physical illness, but they recovered when their mothers returned, or surrogate mothering was available.

Child Maltreatment

Abused children often maintain their attachments to abusive parents. Studies of dogs have shown that severe punishment and maltreatment increase attachment behavior. When children are hungry, sick, or in pain, they too show clinging attachment behavior. Similarly, when children are rejected by their parents or are afraid of them, their attachment may increase; some children want to remain with an abusive parent. Nevertheless, when a choice must be made between a punishing and a nonpunishing figure, the nonpunishing person is the preferable choice, especially if they are sensitive to the child's needs.

Psychiatric Applications

The applications of attachment theory in psychotherapy are numerous. When a patient can attach to a therapist, a secure base effect is seen. The patient may then be able to take risks, mask anxiety, and practice new patterns of behavior that otherwise might not have been attempted. Patients whose impairments can be traced to never having made an attachment in early life may do so for the first time in therapy, with salutary effects.

Patients whose pathology stems from exaggerated early attachments may attempt to replicate them in therapy. Therapists must enable such patients to recognize the ways their early experiences have interfered with their ability to achieve independence.

For patients who are children and whose attachment difficulties may be more apparent than those of adults, therapists represent consistent and trusted figures who can engender a sense of warmth and self-esteem in children, often for the first time.

Relationship Disorders. A person's psychological health and sense of well-being depend significantly on the quality of his or her relationships and attachment to others, and a core issue in all close personal relationships is establishing and regulating that connection. In a typical attachment interaction, one person seeks more proximity and affection, and the other either reciprocates, rejects, or disqualifies the request. A pattern is shaped through repeated exchanges. Distinct attachment styles have been observed. Adults with an anxious-ambivalent attachment style tend to be obsessed with romantic partners, suffer from extreme jealousy, and have a high divorce rate. Persons with an avoidant attachment style are relatively uninvested in close relationships, although they often feel lonely. They seem afraid of intimacy and tend to withdraw when there is stress or conflict in the relationship. Break-up rates are high. Persons with a secure attachment style are highly invested in relationships and tend to behave without much possessiveness or fear of rejection.

LEARNING THEORY

Learning is defined as a change in behavior resulting from repeated practice. The principles of learning are always operating and always influencing human activity. Learning principles are often deeply involved in the etiology and maintenance of psychiatric disorders because so much of human behavior (including overt behavior, thought patterns, and emotion) is acquired through learning. Learning processes also strongly influence psychotherapy because human behavior changes. Thus, learning principles can influence the effectiveness of therapy. No method of therapy can be said to be immune to the effects of learning. Even the simple prescription of medication can bring learning processes into play because the patient will have opportunities to learn about the drug's effects and side effects, will need to learn to adhere to the instructions and directions for taking it, and will need to learn to overcome any resistance to adherence.

Basic Concepts and Considerations

A great deal of modern research on learning still focuses on Pavlovian (classical) and operant learning. Pavlovian conditioning, developed by Ivan Petrovich Pavlov (1849–1936), occurs when neutral stimuli are associated with a psychologically significant event. The main result is that the stimuli come to evoke a set of responses or emotions that may contribute to many clinical disorders, including (but not limited to) anxiety disorders and drug dependence. The events in Pavlov's experiment are often described using terms designed to make the experiment applicable to any situation. The food is the unconditional stimulus (*US*) because it unconditionally elicits salivation before the experiment begins. The bell is the conditional stimulus (*CS*) because it only elicits the salivary response conditional on the bell–food pairings. The new response to the bell is correspondingly called the conditional response (*CR*), and the natural response to the food itself is the unconditional response (*UR*). Modern laboratory studies of conditioning use an extensive range of CSs and USs and measure a wide range of conditioned responses.

Operant conditioning, developed by B.F. Skinner (1904–1990), occurs when a behavior (instead of a stimulus) is associated with a psychologically significant event. In the laboratory, the most famous experimental arrangement is when a rat presses a lever to earn food pellets. In this case, as opposed to Pavlov's, the behavior is an operant because it operates on the environment. The food pellet is a reinforcer—an event that increases the strength of the behavior of which it is made a consequence. A central idea behind this method is that the rat's behavior is "voluntary" in the sense that the animal is not compelled to make the response (it can perform it whenever it "wants" to). In this sense, it is similar to the thousands of operant behaviors that humans choose to commit—freely—in any day. Of course, the even larger idea is that even though the rat's behavior appears as though it is voluntary, it is lawfully controlled by its consequences: if the experimenter were to stop delivering the food pellet, the rat would stop pressing the lever, and if the experimenter were to allow the lever press to produce larger pellets, or perhaps pellets at a higher probability or rate, then the rate of the behavior might increase. The point of operant conditioning experiments, then, is mostly to understand the relation of behavior to its payoff.

Pavlovian and operant conditioning differ in several ways. One of the most fundamental differences is that the responses observed in Pavlov's experiment are *elicited* and thus controlled by presenting an antecedent stimulus. In contrast, the "response" observed in Skinner's experiment is not elicited or compelled by an antecedent stimulus in any obvious way—its consequences instead control it. This distinction between *operants* and *respondents* is essential in clinical settings. If a young patient is referred to the clinic for acting out in the classroom, an initial goal of the clinician will be to determine whether the behavior is a respondent or an operant. Then the clinician will go about changing either its antecedents or its consequences, respectively, to reduce its probability of occurrence.

Despite the academic separation of operant and respondent conditioning, they have an important common function: both learning processes allow organisms to adapt to the environment. The idea is illustrated by considering the *law of effect* (Fig. 34-2), which says that whether an operant behavior increases or decreases in strength depends on the effect it has on the environment. When the action leads to a positive outcome, the action is strengthened; conversely, when the action leads to a negative outcome, we have *punishment,* and the action is weakened. Similarly, when an action decreases the probability of a positive event, behavior also declines. (Such a procedure is now widely known as a *time-out* from reinforcement.) When an action terminates or prevents the occurrence of a negative event, the behavior will strengthen. By enabling the organism to maximize its interaction with positive events and minimize its interaction with negative ones, operant conditioning allows the organism to optimize its interaction with the environment. Reward learning also provides a framework for understanding the development of somewhat maladaptive behaviors like overeating (in which behavior is reinforced by food) and drug-taking (in which the pharmacologic effects of drugs reinforce behaviors)—cases in which reward principles lead to psychopathology.

A parallel to Figure 34-2 exists in Pavlovian conditioning, in which one can likewise think of whether the CS is associated with positive or negative events (Fig. 34-3). Although such learning can lead to a vast constellation or system of behaviors, in a very general way, it also leads to behavioral tendencies of approach or withdrawal. Thus, when a CS signals a positive US, the CS will evoke approach behaviors—called *sign tracking*. For example, an

FIGURE 34-2
The law of effect in instrumental/operant learning. Actions either produce or prevent good or bad events, and the strength of the action changes accordingly (*arrow*). "Reinforcement" refers to a strengthening of behavior. *Positive reinforcement* occurs when an action produces a positive event, whereas *negative reinforcement* occurs when an action prevents or eliminates a negative event. (Courtesy of Mark E. Bouton, PhD.)

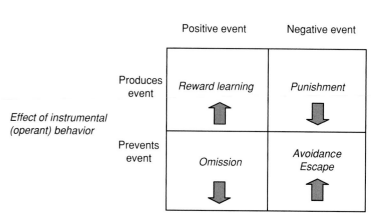

CS signals	Positive event	Negative event
Increase in Probability of event	Approach CS	Withdraw from CS
Decrease in Probability of event	Withdraw from CS	Approach CS

FIGURE 34-3

Sign tracking in Pavlovian learning. Conditional stimuli (CSs) signal either an increase or a decrease in the probability of good or bad events, and the CS generally engages approach or withdrawal behaviors accordingly. (Courtesy of Mark E. Bouton, PhD.)

organism will approach a signal for food. Analogously, when a CS signals a negative US, it will evoke behaviors that tend to move the organism away from the CS.

Conversely, CSs associated with a decrease in the probability of a good thing will elicit withdrawal behaviors, whereas CSs associated with the decrease in the probability of a bad thing can elicit an approach. An example of the latter case might be a stimulus that signals safety or decreases the probability of an aversive event, which evokes an approach in a frightened organism. In the end, these fundamental behavioral effects of both operant (see Fig. 34-2) and Pavlovian (see Fig. 34-3) learning serve to maximize the organism's contact with good things and minimize contact with bad things.

Perhaps because they have such similar functions, Pavlovian learning and operant learning are influenced by similar variables. For example, in either case, the behavior is especially strong if the magnitude of the US or reinforcer is large, or if the US or reinforcer occurs relatively close to the CS or operant response in time. In either case, the learned behavior decreases if the US or reinforcer that was once paired with the CS or the response is eliminated from the situation. This phenomenon, called *extinction,* provides a means of eliminating unwanted behaviors learned through either form of conditioning and has led to several very effective cognitive-behavioral therapies.

Pavlovian Conditioning

Effects of Conditioning on Behavior. Many laypeople have the mistaken impression that Pavlovian learning is a rigid affair in which a fixed stimulus comes to elicit a fixed response. Conditioning is considerably more complex and dynamic than that. For example, signals for food may evoke a broad set of responses that function to prepare the organism to digest food: they can elicit the secretion of gastric acid, pancreatic enzymes, and insulin along with Pavlov's famous salivary response. The CS can also elicit approach behavior (as described earlier), an increase in body temperature, and a state of arousal and excitement. When a signal for food is presented to a satiated animal or human, they may eat more food. Some of these effects may be motivational; for example, an additional effect of presenting a CS for food is that it can invigorate ongoing operant behaviors that have been reinforced with food. CSs thus have powerful behavioral potential. Signals for food evoke a whole *behavior system* that is functionally organized to find, procure, and consume food.

Pavlovian conditioning is also involved in other aspects of eating. Through conditioning, humans and other animals may learn to like or dislike certain foods. In animals like rats, flavors associated with nutrients (sugars, starches, calories, proteins, or fats) come to be preferred. Flavors associated with sweet tastes are also preferred, whereas flavors associated with bitter tastes are avoided. At least as necessary, flavors associated with illness become disliked, as illustrated by the person who gets sick drinking an alcoholic beverage and consequently learns to hate the flavor. The fact that flavor CSs can be associated with such a range of biologic consequences (USs) is essential for omnivorous animals to learn about new foods. It also has some clinical implications. For example, chemotherapy can make cancer patients sick, causing the conditioning of an aversion to a recently eaten food (or to the clinic itself). Other evidence suggests that animals may learn to dislike food that is associated with becoming sick with cancer. On the flip side, conditioning can enable external cues to trigger food consumption and craving, potentially influencing overeating and obesity.

Pavlovian conditioning also occurs when organisms ingest drugs. Whenever a drug is taken, in addition to reinforcing the behaviors that lead to its ingestion, the drug constitutes a US and may be associated with potential CSs that are present at the time (e.g., rooms, odors, injection paraphernalia). CSs that are associated with drug USs can sometimes have an interesting property: they often elicit a conditioned response that seems opposite to the unconditional effect of the drug. For example, although morphine causes a rat to feel less pain, a CS associated with morphine elicits an opposite increase, not a decrease in pain sensitivity. Similarly, although alcohol can cause a drop in body temperature, a conditioned response to a CS associated with alcohol is typically increased in body temperature. In these cases, the conditioned response is said to be *compensatory* because it counteracts the drug effect. Compensatory responses are another example of how classical (Pavlovian) conditioning helps organisms prepare for a significant US.

Compensatory conditioned responses have implications for drug abuse. First, they can cause drug tolerance, in which repeated administration of a drug reduces its effectiveness. As a drug and a CS are repeatedly paired, the compensatory response to the CS becomes stronger and more effective at counteracting the effect of the drug. The drug, therefore, has less impact. One implication is that tolerance will be lost if the drug is taken without being signaled by the usual CS. Consistent with this idea, administering a drug in a new environment can cause a loss of drug tolerance and make drug overdose more likely. A second implication stems from the fact that compensatory responses may be unpleasant or aversive. A CS associated with an opiate may elicit several compensatory responses—it may cause the drug user to be more sensitive to pain, change body temperature, and perhaps become hyperactive (the opposite of another unconditional opiate effect). The unpleasantness of these responses may motivate the user to retake the drug to get rid of them, an example of escape learning, or negative reinforcement, and a classic example of how Pavlovian and operant learning processes might readily interact. The idea is that the urge to take drugs may be strongest in the presence of CSs that have been associated with the drug. The hypothesis is consistent with self-reports of abusers, who, after a period of abstinence, are tempted to retake the drug when they are reexposed to drug-associated cues.

Pavlovian learning may potentially be involved in anxiety disorders. CSs associated with frightening USs can elicit a whole system of conditioned fear responses, broadly designed to help the organism cope. In animals, cues associated with frightening events (such as a brief foot shock) elicit changes in respiration, heart rate, and blood pressure, and even a (compensatory) decrease in sensitivity to pain. Brief CSs that occur close to the US in time can also elicit adaptively timed protective reflexes. For example, the rabbit blinks in response to a brief signal that predicts a mild electric shock near the eye. The same CS, when lengthened in duration and paired with the same US, elicits mainly fear responses, and fear elicited by a CS may potentiate the conditioned eyeblink response elicited by another CS or a startle response to a sudden noise. Once again, CSs do not merely elicit a simple reflex, but also evoke a complex and interactive set of responses.

Classical fear conditioning can contribute to phobias (in which specific objects may be associated with a traumatic US), as well as other anxiety disorders, such as panic disorder and posttraumatic stress disorder (PTSD). In panic disorder, people who have unexpected panic attacks can become anxious about having another one. In this case, the panic attack (the US or UR) may condition anxiety to the external situation in which it occurs (e.g., a crowded bus) and also internal ("interoceptive") CSs created by early symptoms of the attack (e.g., dizziness or a sudden pounding of the heart). These CSs may then evoke anxiety or panic responses. Panic disorder may begin because external cues associated with panic can arouse anxiety, which may exacerbate the next unconditional panic attack or panic response elicited by an interoceptive CS. Emotional reactions elicited by CSs may not require conscious awareness for their occurrence or development. Indeed, fear conditioning may be independent of conscious awareness.

In addition to eliciting conditioned responses, CSs also motivate ongoing operant behavior. For example, presenting a CS that elicits anxiety can increase the vigor of operant behaviors learned to avoid or escape the frightening US. Thus, an individual with an anxiety disorder will be more likely to express avoidance in the presence of anxiety or fear cues. Similar effects may occur with CSs that predict other USs (such as drugs or food)—as already mentioned. A drug-associated CS may motivate the drug abuser to take more drugs. The motivating effects of CSs may stem from the fact that CSs may be associated with both the sensory and emotional properties of USs. For example, the survivor of a traumatic train derailment might associate stimuli that occur immediately before derailment (such as the blue flash that occurs when the train separates from its overhead power supply) with both the emotional and the sensory aspects of the crash. Consequently, when the survivor later encounters another flashing blue light (e.g., the lights on a police car), the CS might evoke both emotional responses (mediated by association with the trauma's emotional qualities) and sensory associations (mediated by association with the trauma's sensory qualities). Both might play a role in the nightmares and "reexperiencing" phenomena that are characteristic of PTSD.

The Nature of the Learning Process.

Research beginning in the late 1960s began to uncover some critical details about the learning process behind Pavlovian conditioning. Several findings proved especially influential. For example, it was shown that conditioning is not an inevitable consequence of pairing a CS with a US. Such pairings will not cause conditioning if there is a second CS present that already predicts the US. This finding (known as *blocking*) suggests that a CS must provide new information about the US if learning occurs. The importance of the CS's information value is also suggested by the fact that a CS will not be treated as a signal for the US if the US occurs equally often (or is equally probable) in the presence and the absence of the CS. Instead, the organism treats the CS as a signal for the US if the probability of the US is more significant in the presence of the CS than in its absence. Also, the organism will treat the CS as a signal for "no US" if the probability of the US is less in the presence of the CS than in its absence. In the latter case, the signal is called a *conditioned inhibitor* because it will inhibit other CSs. The conditioned inhibition phenomenon is clinically relevant because inhibitory CSs may hold pathologic CRs like fear or anxiety at bay. A loss of the inhibition would allow the anxiety response to emerge.

There are also essential variants of classical conditioning. In *sensory preconditioning,* two stimuli (A and B) are first paired, and then one of them (A) is later paired with the US. Stimulus A evokes conditioned responding, of course, but so does stimulus B—indirectly, through its association with A. One implication is that exposure to a potent US like a panic attack may influence reactions to stimuli that have never been paired with the US directly; the sudden anxiety to stimulus B might seem spontaneous and mysterious. A related finding is *second-order conditioning.* Here, A is paired with a US first and then subsequently paired with stimulus B. Once again, both A and B will evoke responding. Sensory preconditioning and second-order conditioning increase the range of stimuli that can control the conditioned response. A third variant worth mentioning occurs, as indicated previously, when the onset of a stimulus becomes associated with the rest of that stimulus, as when a sudden increase in heart rate caused by the onset of a panic attack comes to predict the rest of the panic or feeling, or when the onset of a drug may predict the rest of the drug effect. Such intraevent associations may play a role in many of the body's regulatory functions, such that an initial change in some variable (e.g., blood pressure or blood glucose level) may come to signal a further increase in that variable and therefore initiate a conditioned compensatory response.

Emotional responses can also be conditioned through observation. For example, a monkey that merely observes another monkey being frightened by a snake can learn to be afraid of the snake. The observer learns to associate the snake (CS) with its emotional reaction (US/UR) to the other monkey being afraid. Although monkeys readily learn to fear snakes, they are less likely to associate other salient cues (such as colorful flowers) with fear in the same way. This is an example of *preparedness* in classical conditioning—some stimuli are especially useful signals for some USs. Another example is that tastes are easily associated with illness but not a shock, whereas auditory and visual cues are easily associated with shock but not an illness. Preparedness may explain why human phobias tend to be for particular objects (snakes or spiders) and not others (knives or electric sockets) that may as often be paired with pain or trauma.

Erasing Pavlovian Learning.

If Pavlovian learning plays a role in the etiology of behavioral and emotional disorders, a natural question concerns how to eliminate it or undo it. Pavlov studied *extinction:* conditioned responding decreases if the CS is presented repeatedly without the US after conditioning. Extinction is based on behavioral or cognitive-behavioral therapies designed to reduce pathologic conditioned responding through repeated exposure to the CS (exposure therapy). It is presumably a consequence of any form of therapy in the course of which the patient learns that previous harmful cues are no longer harmful. Another elimination procedure is *counterconditioning,* in which the CS is paired with a very different US/UR.

Counterconditioning was the inspiration for *systematic desensitization,* a behavior therapy technique in which frightening CSs are deliberately associated with relaxation during therapy.

Although extinction and counterconditioning reduce unwanted conditioned responses, they do not destroy the original learning, which remains in the brain, ready to return to behavior under the right circumstances. For example, conditioned responses that have been eliminated by extinction or counterconditioning can recover if time passes before the CS presents again (spontaneous recovery). Conditioned responses can also return if the patient returns to the context of conditioning after extinction in another context, or if the CS is encountered in a context that differs from the one in which extinction has occurred (all are examples of the renewal effect). The renewal effect is significant because it illustrates the principle that extinction performance depends on the organism being in the context in which extinction was learned. If the CS is encountered in a different context, the extinguished behavior may relapse or return. Recovery and relapse can also occur if the current context is associated again with the US ("reinstatement") or if the CS is paired with the US again ("rapid reacquisition"). One theoretical approach assumes that extinction and counterconditioning do not destroy the original learning but instead entail new learning that gives the CS a second meaning (e.g., "the CS is safe" in addition to "the CS is dangerous"). As with an ambiguous word, which has more than one meaning, responding evoked by an extinguished or counterconditioned CS depends fundamentally on the current context.

Research on context effects in animal and human learning and memory suggests that a wide variety of stimuli can play context (Table 34-5). Drugs, for example, can be very salient in this regard. When rats are given fear extinction while under the influence of a benzodiazepine tranquilizer or alcohol, fear is renewed when the CS is tested in the absence of the context provided by the drug. This is an example of *state-dependent learning,* in which the retention of information is best when tested in the same state in which it was initially learned. State-dependent fear extinction has apparent implications for combining therapy with drugs. It also has implications for the administration of drugs more generally. For example, if a person were to take a drug to reduce anxiety, the anxiety reduction would reinforce drug-taking. State-dependent extinction might

Table 34-5
Effective Contextual Stimuli Studied in Animal and Human Research Laboratories

Exteroceptive context:
   Room, place, environment, other external background stimuli

Interoceptive context:
   Drug state
   Hormonal state
   Mood state
   Deprivation state
   Recent events
   Expectation of events
   Passage of time

From Sadock BJ, Sadock VA, Ruiz P. *Kaplan & Sadock's Comprehensive Textbook of Psychiatry*. 9th ed. Philadelphia, PA: Lippincott Williams & Wilkins; 2009:652.

further preserve any anxiety that might otherwise be extinguished during natural exposure to the anxiety-eliciting cues. Thus, drug use could paradoxically preserve the original anxiety, creating a self-perpetuating cycle that could provide a possible explanation for the link between anxiety disorders and substance abuse. One point of this discussion is that drugs can play multiple roles in learning: they can be USs or reinforcers on the one hand, and CSs or contexts on the other. The possible complex behavioral effects of drugs are worth bearing in mind.

Another general message is that contemporary theory emphasizes that extinction (and other processes, such as counterconditioning) entails new learning rather than a destruction of the old. Recent psychopharmacological research has built on this idea: if extinction and therapy constitute new learning, drugs that might facilitate new learning might also facilitate the therapy process. For example, there has been considerable recent interest in D-cycloserine, a partial agonist of the *N*-methyl-D-aspartate (NMDA) glutamate receptor. The NMDA receptor is involved in long-term potentiation, a synaptic facilitation phenomenon that has been implicated in several examples of learning. Of interest, there is evidence that the administration of D-cycloserine can facilitate extinction learning in rats and possibly in humans undergoing exposure therapy for anxiety disorders. In the studies supporting this conclusion, the administration of the drug increased the amount of extinction that was apparent after a small (and incomplete) number of extinction trials. Although such findings are promising, it is essential to remember that the context-dependence of extinction, and thus the possibility of relapse with a change of context, may easily remain. Consistent with this possibility, although D-cycloserine allows fear extinction to be learned in fewer trials, it does not appear to prevent or reduce the strength of the renewal effect. Such results further underscore the importance of behavioral research—and behavioral theory—in understanding the effects of drugs on therapy. Nonetheless, the search for drugs that might enhance the *learning* that occurs in therapy situations will continue to be an essential area of research.

Another process that might theoretically modify or erase memory is illustrated by a phenomenon called *reconsolidation.* Newly learned memories are temporarily labile and easy to disrupt before they are consolidated into a more stable form in the brain. The consolidation of memory requires the synthesis of new proteins and can be blocked by administering protein synthesis inhibitors (e.g., anisomycin). Animal research suggests that consolidated memories that have recently been reactivated might also return briefly to a similarly vulnerable state; protein synthesis inhibitors can likewise block their "reconsolidation." For example, several studies have shown that the reactivation of conditioned fear by one or two presentations of the CS after a brief fear conditioning experience can allow it to be disrupted by anisomycin. When the CS is tested later, there is little evidence of fear—as if reactivation and then drug administration diminished the strength of the original memory. However, like the effects of extinction, these fear-diminishing effects do not necessarily mean that the original learning has been destroyed or erased. There is some evidence that fear of the CS that has been diminished in this way can still return over time (i.e., spontaneously recover) or with reminder treatments. This sort of result suggests that the effect of the drug is somehow able to interfere with retrieval or access to the memory rather than to be an actual "reconsolidation."

Generally speaking, eliminating a behavior after therapy should not be interpreted as the erasure of the underlying knowledge. For the time being, it may be safest to assume that, after any treatment, a part of the original learning may remain in the brain, ready to produce relapse if retrieved. Instead of trying to find treatments that destroy the original memory, another therapeutic strategy might be to accept the possible retention of the original learning and build therapies that allow the organism to prevent or cope with its retrieval. One possibility is to conduct extinction exposure in the contexts in which relapse might be most problematic to the patient and to encourage retrieval strategies (such as the use of retrieval cues like reminder cards) that might help to remind the patient of the therapy experience.

Operant/Instrumental Learning

The Relation Between Behavior and Payoff. Operant learning has many parallels with Pavlovian learning. As one example, extinction also occurs in operant learning if the reinforcer is omitted following training. Although extinction is once again a useful technique for eliminating unwanted behaviors, just as we saw with Pavlovian learning, it does not destroy the original learning—spontaneous recovery, renewal, reinstatement, and rapid reacquisition effects still obtain. Although early accounts of instrumental learning, beginning with Edward Thorndike, emphasized the role of the reinforcer as "stamping in" the instrumental action, more-modern approaches tend to view the reinforcer as a sort of guide or motivator of behavior. A modern, "synthetic" view of operant conditioning (see later discussion) holds that the organism associates the action with the outcome in much the way that stimulus–outcome learning is believed to be involved in Pavlovian learning.

Human behavior is influenced by a wide variety of reinforcers, including social ones. For example, simple attention from teachers or hospital staff members has been shown to reinforce disruptive or problematic behavior in students or patients. In either case, when the attention is withdrawn and redirected toward other activities, the problematic behaviors can decrease (i.e., undergo extinction). Human behavior is also influenced by verbal reinforcers, like praise, and, more generally, by *conditioned reinforcers,* such as money, that have no intrinsic value except for the value derived through association with more basic, "primary" rewards. Conditioned reinforcers have been used in schools and institutional settings in the so-called *token economies* in which positive behaviors are reinforced with tokens that can be used to purchase valued items. In more natural settings, reinforcers are always delivered in social relationships, in which their effects are dynamic and reciprocal. For example, the relationship between a parent and a child is full of interacting and reciprocating operant contingencies in which the delivery (and withholding) of reinforcers and punishers shapes the behavior of each. Like Pavlovian learning, operant learning is always operating and always influencing behavior.

Research on operant conditioning in the laboratory has offered many insights into how action relates to its payoff. In the natural world, few actions are reinforced every time they are performed; instead, most actions are reinforced only intermittently. In a *ratio reinforcement schedule,* the reinforcer is directly related to the amount of work or responding that the organism emits. That is, there is some work requirement that determines when the next reinforcer will be presented. In a "fixed ratio schedule," every xth action is reinforced; in a "variable ratio schedule," there is an average ratio requirement, but the number of responses required for each successive reinforcer varies. Ratio schedules, especially variable ratio schedules, can generate high rates of behavior, as seen in the behavior directed at a casino slot machine. In an *interval reinforcement schedule,* the presentation of each reinforcer depends on the organism emitting the response after some time has also elapsed.

In a "fixed interval schedule," the first response after x seconds have elapsed is reinforced. In a "variable interval schedule," there is an interval requirement for each reinforcer, but the length of that interval varies. A person checking e-mail throughout the day is being reinforced on a variable interval schedule—a new message is not present to reinforce each checking response, but the presence of a new message becomes available after variable time points throughout the day. Of interest, on interval schedules, the response rate can vary substantially without influencing the overall rate of reinforcement. (On ratio schedules, there is a more direct relationship between behavior rate and reinforcement rate.) In part because of this, interval schedules tend to generate slower response rates than ratio schedules.

Classic research on operant behavior underscores the fact that the performance of any action always involves *choice.* That is, whenever the individual performs a particular behavior, he or she chooses to engage in that action over many other possible alternatives. When a choice has been studied by allowing the organism to perform either of two different operant behaviors (paying off with their separate schedules of reinforcement), the rate of operant behavior depends not only on the behavior's rate of reinforcement but also on the rate of reinforcement of all other behaviors in the situation. Put most generally, the strength of Behavior 1 (e.g., the rate at which Behavior 1 is performed) is given by

$$B_1 = K^*R_1/(R_1 + R_O)$$

where B_1 can be seen as the strength of Behavior 1, R_1 is the rate at which B_1 has been reinforced, and R_O is the rate at which all alternative (or "other") behaviors in the environment have been reinforced; K is a constant that corresponds to all behavior in the situation and may have a different value for different individuals. This principle, known as the *quantitative law of effect,* captures several ideas that are relevant to psychiatrists and clinical psychologists. It indicates that an action can be strengthened either by increasing its rate of reinforcement (R_1) or decreasing the rate of reinforcement for alternative behaviors (R_O). Conversely, an action can be weakened either by reducing its rate of reinforcement (R_1) or increasing reinforcement for alternative behaviors (R_O). The latter point has an especially important implication: in principle, one can slow the strengthening of new, undesirable behavior by providing an environment that is otherwise rich in reinforcement (high R_O). Thus, an adolescent who experiments with drugs or alcohol would be less likely to engage in this behavior at a high rate (high B_1) if their environment were otherwise rich with reinforcers (e.g., provided by extracurricular activities or outside interests).

The choice among actions is also influenced by the size of their corresponding reinforcers and how soon the reinforcers will occur. For example, individuals sometimes have to choose between an action that yields a small but immediate reward (e.g., taking a hit of a drug) versus another that yields a larger but delayed reward (e.g., going to a class and earning credit toward a general educational development certificate). Individuals who choose the more immediate reward are often said to be "impulsive," whereas those who choose the delayed reward are said to exercise "self-control." Of interest, organisms often choose immediate small rewards over delayed larger ones, even though it may be maladaptive to do so in the long run. Such "impulsive" choices are especially difficult to resist when the reward is imminent. Choice is believed to be determined by the relative value of the two rewards, with that value being influenced by both the reinforcer's size and its delay. The bigger the reinforcer, the better is the value, and the more immediate the reinforcer, the better, too: when a reward is delayed, its value decreases or is "discounted" over time. When offered a choice, the organism will always choose the action that leads to the reward whose value is currently higher.

Theories of Reinforcement.

It is possible to use the preceding principles of operant conditioning without knowing in advance what kind of event or stimulus will be reinforcing for the individual patient. None of the reinforcement rules say much about what sorts of events in an organism's world will play a reinforcer. Skinner defined a reinforcer empirically, by considering the effect it had on operant behavior. A reinforcer was defined as any event that could be shown to increase the strength of an operant if it was made a consequence of the operant. This empirical (some would say "atheoretical") view can be valuable because it allows idiosyncratic reinforcers for idiosyncratic individuals. For instance, if a therapist works with a child who is injuring himself, the approach advises the therapist merely to search for the consequences of the behavior and then manipulate them to bring the behavior under control. So, if, for example, the child's self-injurious behavior decreases when the parent stops scolding the child for doing it, then the scold is the reinforcer, which might seem counterintuitive to everyone (including the parent who thinks that the scold should function as a punisher). On the other hand, it would also be useful to know what kind of event will reinforce an individual before the therapist has to try everything.

Several approaches allow for predictions ahead of time. Perhaps the most useful is the *Premack principle* (named for researcher David Premack), which claims that, for any individual, reinforcers can be identified by giving the individual a preference test in which he or she is free to engage in any number of activities. The individual might spend the most time engaging in activity A, the second-most time engaged in activity B, and the third-most time engaged in activity C. Behavior A can thus be said to be preferred to B and C, and B is preferred to C. The Premack principle asserts that access to a preferred action will reinforce any action that is less preferred. In the present example, if doing activity C allowed access to doing A or B, activity C will be reinforced—it will increase in strength or probability.

Similarly, activity B will be reinforced by activity A (but not C). The principle accepts large individual differences. For example, in an early study, some children given a choice spent more time eating candy than playing pinball, whereas others spent more time playing pinball then eating candy. Candy eating reinforced pinball playing in the former group. In contrast, pinball playing reinforced candy eating in the latter group. There is nothing particularly special about food (eating) or any particular kind of activity as a possible reinforcer. Any behavior that is preferred to a second behavior will theoretically reinforce the second behavior.

The principle has been refined over the years. It is now recognized that even a less-preferred behavior can reinforce a more-preferred behavior if the organism has been deprived of doing the low-preferred behavior below its ordinary level. In the preceding example, even the low-preference activity C could reinforce A or B if it were suppressed for a while below its baseline level of preference. However, the main implication is that in the long run, a person's reinforcers can be discovered by looking at how they allocate their activities when access to them is free and unconstrained.

Motivational Factors.

Instrumental action is often said to be goal-oriented. As Edward Tolman illustrated in many experiments conducted in the 1930s and 1940s, organisms may flexibly perform several actions to achieve a goal; instrumental learning thus provides a variable means to a fixed end. Tolman's perspective on

the effects of reinforcers has returned to favor. He argued that reinforcers are not necessary for learning, but instead are essential for motivating instrumental behavior. The classic illustration of this point is the *latent learning* experiment. Rats received several trials in a complex maze in which they were removed from the maze without reward once they got to a particular goal location. When arriving at the goal was suddenly rewarded, the rats suddenly began working through the maze with very few errors. Thus, they had learned about the maze without the benefit of the food reinforcer, but the reinforcer was nonetheless crucial for motivating them to get through the maze efficiently. The reinforcer was unnecessary for learning, but it gave the organism a reason to translate its knowledge into action.

Subsequent research has identified many motivating effects of reward. For example, organisms with experience receiving a small reward may show *positive contrast* when they are suddenly reinforced with a larger reward. That is, their instrumental behavior may become more vigorous than that in control subjects who have received the larger reward all along. Conversely, organisms show *negative contrast* when they are switched from a high reward to a lower reward—their behavior becomes weaker than control subjects who have received the same smaller reward all along. Negative contrast involves frustration and emotionality. Both types of contrast are consistent with the idea that the current effectiveness depends on what the organism has learned to expect; an increase from expectation causes elation, whereas a decrease from expectation causes frustration. There is a sense in which receiving a reward that is smaller than expected might seem punishing.

Negative contrast is an example of a *paradoxical reward effect*—a set of behavioral phenomena given the name because they show that reward can sometimes weaken behavior and that nonreward can sometimes strengthen it. The best known is the *partial reinforcement extinction effect,* in which actions that have been intermittently (or "partially") reinforced persist longer when reinforcers are completely withdrawn than actions that have been continuously reinforced. The finding is considered paradoxical because an action that has been reinforced (say) half as often as another action may be more persistent. One explanation is that the action that has been partially reinforced has been reinforced in the presence of some frustration—and is thus persistent in new adversity or sources of frustration. Other evidence suggests that effortfulness is a dimension of behavior that can be reinforced. That is, human and animal participants that have been reinforced for performing effortful responses learn a sort of "industriousness" that transfers to new behaviors. One implication is that new behaviors learned in therapy will be more persistent over time if a high effort has been deliberately reinforced.

The organism's current motivational state also influences the effectiveness of a reinforcer. For example, food is more reinforcing for a hungry organism, and water is more reinforcing for a thirsty one. Such results are consistent with many theories of reinforcement (e.g., the Premack principle) because the presence of hunger or thirst would undoubtedly increase the organism's preference ranking for food or water. However, recent research indicates that the effects of motivational states on instrumental actions are not this automatic. Specifically, if a motivational state is going to influence an instrumental action, the individual needs first to learn how the action's reinforcer will influence the motivational state. The process of learning about the effects the reinforcer has on the motivational state is called *incentive learning.*

An experimental example best illustrates incentive learning. In 1992, Bernard Balleine reported a study that taught trained rats that were not hungry to lever press to earn a novel food pellet. The animals were then food-deprived and tested for their lever pressing under conditions in which the lever press no longer produced the pellet. The hunger state did not affect the lever-press rate; that is, hungry rats did not lever press any more than rats that were not food-deprived. On the other hand, if the rat had been given separate experience eating the pellets while it was food-deprived, during the test, it lever pressed at a high rate. Thus, hunger invigorated the instrumental action only if the animal had previously experienced the reinforcer in that state, allowing it to learn that the specific substance influenced the state (incentive learning). The interpretation of this result, and others like it, will be developed further later in this section. The main idea is that individuals will perform an instrumental action when they know that it produces an outcome that is desirable in the current motivational state. The clinical implications are underexplored but could be significant. For example, persons who abuse drugs will need to learn that the drug makes them feel better in the withdrawal state before the withdrawal will motivate drug-seeking. Persons with anxiety might not be motivated to take a beneficial medication while anxious until they have had the opportunity to learn how the medication makes them feel when they are in the anxious state, and a person with depression may need to learn what natural reinforcers make them feel better while they are depressed. According to theory, direct experience with a reinforcer's effect on depressed mood might be necessary before the person will be interested in performing actions that help to ameliorate the depressed state.

Pavlovian and Operant Learning Together

Avoidance Learning.   Theories of the motivating effects of reinforcers have usually emphasized that Pavlovian CSs in the background are also associated with the reinforcer. The expectancy of the reinforcer (or conditioned motivational state) the CSs arouse increases the vigor of the operant response. This is *two-factor* or *two-process theory:* Pavlovian learning co-occurs and motivates behavior during operant learning.

The interaction of Pavlovian and instrumental factors is especially important in understanding avoidance learning (see Fig. 34-2). In avoidance situations, organisms learn to perform actions that prevent the delivery or presentation of an aversive event. The explanation of avoidance learning is subtle because it is difficult to identify an obvious reinforcer. Although preventing the occurrence of the aversive event is essential, how can the nonoccurrence of that event reinforce? The answer is that cues in the environment (Pavlovian CSs) come to predict the occurrence of the aversive event, and consequently, they arouse anxiety or fear. The avoidance response can, therefore, be reinforced if it escapes from or reduces that fear. Pavlovian and operant factors are thus both important: Pavlovian fear conditioning motivates and allows reinforcement of an instrumental action through its reduction. Escape from fear or anxiety is believed to play a significant role in many human behavior disorders, including anxiety disorders. Thus, the obsessive-compulsive patient checks or washes his or her hands repeatedly to reduce anxiety, the agoraphobic stays home to escape the fear of places associated with panic attacks, and the bulimic learn to vomit after a meal to reduce the learned anxiety evoked by eating the meal.

Although the two-factor theory remains an essential view of avoidance learning, excellent avoidance can be obtained in the laboratory without reinforcement: for example, if an animal is required to perform an action that resembles one of its natural and prepared fear responses—so-called *species-specific defensive reactions* (*SSDRs*). Rats will readily learn to freeze (remain motionless) or flee (run to another environment) to avoid shock, two behaviors that have evolved to escape or avoid predation. Freezing and fleeing are also respondents rather than operants; they are controlled by their antecedents (Pavlovian CSs that predict shock) rather than reinforced by their consequences (escape from fear). Thus, when the rat can use an SSDR for avoidance, the only necessary learning is Pavlovian—the rat learns about environmental cues associated with danger, and these arouse fear and evoke natural defensive behaviors including withdrawal (negative sign tracking; Fig. 34-3). To learn to perform an action that is not similar to a natural SSDR requires more feedback or reinforcement through fear reduction.

A good example is lever pressing, which is easy for the rat to learn when the reinforcer is a food pellet but challenging to learn when the same action avoids shock. More recent work with avoidance in humans suggests an essential role for CS-aversive event and response–no aversive event expectancies. The larger point is that Pavlovian learning is vital in avoidance learning; when the animal can avoid with an SSDR, it is the only learning necessary; when the required action is not an SSDR, Pavlovian learning permits the expectation of something bad.

A cognitive perspective on aversive learning is also encouraged by studies of *learned helplessness.* In this phenomenon, organisms exposed to either controllable or uncontrollable aversive events differ in their reactivity to later aversive events. For example, the typical finding is that a subject exposed to inescapable shock in one phase of an experiment is less successful at learning to escape shock with altogether new behavior in a second phase, whereas subjects exposed to escapable shock are normal. Both types of a subject are exposed to the same shock, but its psychological dimension (its controllability) creates a difference, perhaps because subjects exposed to inescapable shock learn the independence of their actions and the outcome. Although this finding (and interpretation) was once seen as a model of depression, the current view is that the controllability of stressors mainly modulates their stressfulness and negative impact. At a theoretical level, the result also implies that organisms receiving instrumental contingencies in which their actions lead to outcomes might learn something about the controllability of those outcomes.

One of the main conclusions of aversive learning is that there are biologic and cognitive dimensions to instrumental learning. The possibility that Pavlovian contingencies can control much instrumental learning is also consistent with research in which animals have learned to respond to positive reinforcers. For example, pigeons have been widely used in operant learning experiments since the 1940s. In the typical experiment, the bird learns to peck at a plastic disk on a wall of the chamber (a response "key") to earn food. Although pecking seems to be an operant response, it turns out that the pigeon's peck can be entrained by merely illuminating the key for a few seconds before presenting the reinforcer on several trials. Although there is no requirement for the bird to peck the key, the bird will begin to peck at the illuminated key—a Pavlovian predictor of food—anyway. Its consequences only weakly control the pecking response; if the experimenter arranges things so that pecks prevent the delivery of food (which is otherwise delivered on trials without pecks), the birds will continue to peck almost indefinitely on many trials. (Although the peck has a negative correlation with food, key illumination remains a weakly positive predictor of food.) Thus, this classic "operant" behavior is at least partly a Pavlovian one. Pavlovian contingencies cannot be ignored. When

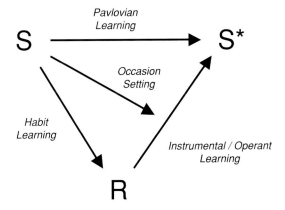

FIGURE 34-4

Any instrumental/operant learning situation permits a number of types of learning, which are always occurring all the time. R, operant behavior or instrumental action; S, stimulus in the background; S*, biologically significant event (e.g., reinforcer, US). (Courtesy of Mark E. Bouton, PhD.)

rats are punished with mild foot shock for pressing a lever that otherwise produces food, they stop lever pressing at least partly (and perhaps predominantly) because they learn that the lever now predicts shock, and they withdraw from it. A child might likewise learn to stay away from the parent who delivers punishment rather than refrain from performing the punished behavior. A great deal of behavior in operant learning settings may be controlled by Pavlovian learning and sign tracking rather than authentic operant learning.

A Synthetic View of Instrumental Action.   Then, the idea is that several hypothetical associations control behavior in any instrumental learning situation, as illustrated in Figure 34-4. Much behavior in an instrumental learning arrangement can be controlled by a Pavlovian factor in which the organism associates background cues (CSs) with the reinforcer (S*, denoting a biologically significant event). As discussed earlier, this type of learning can allow the CS to evoke a variety of behaviors and emotional reactions (and motivational states) that can additionally motivate instrumental action.

In modern terms, the instrumental factor is represented by the organism learning a direct, and similar, association between the instrumental action (R) and the reinforcer (S*). Evidence for this sort of learning comes from experiments on *reinforcer devaluation* (Fig. 34-5). In such experiments, the organism can first be trained to perform two instrumental actions (e.g., pressing a lever and pulling a chain), each paired with a different reinforcer (e.g., food pellet versus a liquid sucrose solution). In a separate second phase, one of the reinforcers (e.g., pellet) is paired with illness, which creates the conditioning of a powerful taste aversion to the reinforcer. In a final test, the organism is returned to the instrumental situation and can perform either instrumental action. No reinforcers are presented during the test. The result is that the organism no longer performs the action that produced the reinforcer that is now aversive. The organism must have (1) learned which action produced which reinforcer and (2) combined it with the knowledge that it no longer likes or values that reinforcer. The result cannot be explained by the simpler, more traditional view that reinforcers merely stamp in or strengthen instrumental actions.

Organisms also need to learn how reinforcers influence a particular motivational state called "incentive learning." Incentive

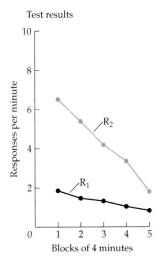

FIGURE 34-5

The reinforcer devaluation effect. Results of the test session. The result indicates the importance of the response–reinforcer association in operant learning. For the organism to perform in the way that it does during testing, it must learn which action leads to which reinforcer and then choose to perform the action that leads to the outcome it currently liked or valued. R1, R2, operant behaviors or instrumental actions. (Data from Colwill and Rescorla [1986]. From Bouton ME. *Learning and Behavior: A Contemporary Synthesis*. Sunderland, MA: Sinauer; 2007.)

learning is crucially involved in instrumental learning as a process through which the animal learns the value of the reinforcer. Thus, in the reinforcer devaluation experiment shown in Figure 34-5, an important thing that occurs in the second phase is that the organism must contact the reinforcer and learn that it does not like it. As described earlier, incentive learning is probably always involved in making outcomes (and the associated actions that produce them) more or less desirable.

Other experiments have illustrated the other associations to the stimulus that are represented in Figure 34-4. In addition to being directly associated with the reinforcer, a stimulus can signal a relation between an action and an outcome. This is called *occasion setting:* instead of eliciting a response directly, stimuli in operant situations can set the occasion for the operant response. There is good evidence that they do so by signaling a specific response–reinforcer relationship. For example, in one experiment, rats learned to lever press and chain pull in background noise and background light. When the noise was present, lever pressing yielded a pellet reinforcer, and chain pulling yielded sucrose.

In contrast, when the light was present, the relations were reversed: Lever pressing yielded sucrose, and chain pulling yielded pellet. There was evidence that the rats learned corresponding relationships. In a second phase, pellets were associated with illness, so the rat no longer valued the pellet. In a final test, rats were allowed to lever press or chain pull in extinction in noise or light present during separate tests. In the presence of the noise, the animal's chain pulled rather than lever pressed. When the light was present, the animal's lever pressed rather than chain pulled. Thus, the noise informed the rat that the lever press yielded a pellet, and the light informed the rat that the chain pull did. This is the occasion-setting function illustrated in Figure 34-4.

It is worth noting that other stimuli besides lights and noises set the occasion for operant behavior. Modern research on learning in animals has underscored the importance of other stimuli, such as temporal and spatial cues, and particular perception and memory processes. A particularly interesting example of research on the *stimulus control* of operant behavior is categorization. Pigeons can be shown images of cars, chairs, flowers, and cats on a computer screen positioned on the wall of a Skinner box. Pecking one of four keys in the presence of these images is reinforced in any picture containing a car, a chair, a flower, or a cat. Of interest, as the number of exemplars in each category increases, the pigeon makes more errors as it learns the discrimination. However, more exemplars create better learning in the sense that it is more ready to transfer to new test images—after many examples of each category, the pigeon is more accurate at categorizing (and responding accurately to) new stimuli. One implication is that training new behaviors in various settings or ways will enhance generalization to new situations.

The final association in Figure 34-4 is simple *habit learning* or a direct association between the stimulus and the response. Through this association, the background may elicit the instrumental action directly, without the intervening cognition of R–S* and the valuation of S*. Although S–R learning was once believed to dominate learning, the current view sees it as developing only after extensive and consistent instrumental training. In effect, actions that have been performed repeatedly (and repeatedly associated with the reinforcer) become automatic and routine. One source of evidence is the fact that the reinforcer devaluation effect—which implies a kind of cognitive mediation of operant behavior—no longer occurs after extensive instrumental training as if the animal reflexively engages in the response without remembering the actual outcome it produces. It seems reasonable to expect that many pathologic behaviors that come into the clinic might also be automatic and blind through repetition. Of interest, the evidence suggests that the eventual dominance of the S-R habit in behavior does not replace or destroy more cognitive mediation by learned S–S*, R–S*, or S–(R–S*) relations. Under some conditions, even a habitual response might be brought back under the control of the action–reinforcer association. The conversion of actions to habits and the relation of habit to cognition are active areas of research.

BIOLOGY OF MEMORY

The topic of memory is fundamental to the discipline of psychiatry. Memory is the glue that binds our mental life, the scaffolding for our personal history. In part, personality is an accumulation of habits that have been acquired, many very early in life, which creates dispositions and influences how we behave. In the same sense, the neuroses are often products of learning—anxieties, phobias, and maladaptive behaviors that result from particular experiences. Psychotherapy itself is a process by which new habits and skills are acquired by accumulating new experiences. In this sense, memory is at the theoretical heart of psychiatry's concern with personality, the consequences of early experience, and the possibility of growth and change.

Memory is also of clinical interest because disorders of memory and complaints about memory are common in neurologic and psychiatric illness. Memory impairment is also a side effect of specific treatments, such as electroconvulsive therapy (ECT). Accordingly, the effective clinician needs to understand something of the biology of memory, the varieties of memory dysfunction, and how memory can be evaluated.

From Synapses to Memory

Memory is a particular case of the general biologic phenomenon of *neural plasticity*. Neurons can show history-dependent activity

by responding differently as a function of prior input, and this plasticity of nerve cells and synapses is the basis of memory. In the last decade of the 19th century, researchers proposed that the persistence of memory could be accounted for by nerve cell growth. This idea has been restated many times, and current understanding of the synapse as the critical site of change is founded on extensive experimental studies in animals with simple nervous systems. Experience can lead to structural change at the synapse, including alterations in the strength of existing synapses and alterations in the number of synaptic contacts along specific pathways.

Plasticity.   Neurobiologic evidence supports two necessary conclusions: first, short-lasting plasticity, which may last for seconds or minutes depending on specific synaptic events, including an increase in neurotransmitter release; and second, long-lasting memory, which depends on new protein synthesis, the physical growth of neural processes, and an increase in the number of synaptic connections.

A significant source of information about memory has come from the extended study of the marine mollusk *Aplysia californica*. Individual neurons and connections between neurons have been identified, and the wiring diagram of some simple behaviors has been described. *Aplysia* is capable of associative learning (including classic conditioning and operant conditioning) and nonassociative learning (habituation and sensitization). *Sensitization* had been studied using the gill-withdrawal reflex, a defensive reaction in which tactile stimulation causes the gill and siphon to retract. When tactile stimulation is preceded by sensory stimulation to the head or tail, gill withdrawal is facilitated. The cellular changes underlying this sensitization begin when a sensory neuron activates a modulatory interneuron, enhancing the strength of synapses within the circuitry responsible for the reflex. This modulation depends on a second-messenger system in which intracellular molecules (including cyclic adenosine monophosphate [cAMP] and cAMP-dependent protein kinase) lead to enhanced transmitter release that lasts for minutes in the reflex pathway. Both short- and long-lasting plasticity within this circuitry are based on enhanced transmitter release. The long-lasting change uniquely requires the expression of genes and the synthesis of new proteins. Synaptic tagging mechanisms allow gene products delivered throughout a neuron to increase synaptic strength selectively at recently active synapses. Also, the long-term change, but not the short-term change, is accompanied by the growth of neural processes of neurons within the reflex circuit.

In vertebrates, memory cannot be studied as directly as in the simple nervous system of *Aplysia*. Nevertheless, it is known that behavioral manipulations can also result in measurable changes in the brain's architecture. For example, rats reared in enriched as opposed to ordinary environments show an increase in the number of synapses ending on individual neurons in the neocortex. These changes are accompanied by small increases in cortical thickness, the diameter of neuronal cell bodies, and the number and length of dendritic branches. The behavioral experience thus exerts powerful effects on the wiring of the brain.

Many of these same structural changes have been found in adult rats exposed to an enriched environment and adult rats given extensive maze training. In maze training, vision was restricted to one eye, and the corpus callosum was transected to prevent information received by one hemisphere from reaching the other hemisphere. The result was that structural changes in neuronal shape and connectivity were observed only in the trained hemisphere. This finding rules out several nonspecific influences, including motor activity, indirect effects of hormones, and overall level of arousal. Long-term memory in vertebrates is believed to be based on morphologic growth and change, including increases in synaptic strength along particular pathways.

Long-Term Potentiation. The phenomenon of *long-term potentiation* (LTP) is a candidate mechanism for mammalian long-term memory. LTP is observed when a postsynaptic neuron is persistently depolarized after a high-frequency burst of presynaptic neural firing. LTP has several properties that make it suitable as a physiologic substrate of memory. It is established quickly and then lasts for a long time. It is associative, in that it depends on the co-occurrence of presynaptic activity and postsynaptic depolarization. It occurs only at potentiated synapses, not all synapses terminating on the postsynaptic cell. Finally, LTP occurs prominently in the hippocampus, a structure that is important for memory.

The induction of LTP is known to be mediated postsynaptically and to involve activation of the NMDA receptor, which permits the influx of calcium into the postsynaptic cell. LTP is maintained by an increase in the number of α-amino-3-hydroxy-5-methyl-4-isoxazolepropionate (AMPA; non-NMDA) receptors postsynaptic cell and also possibly by increased transmitter release.

A promising method for elucidating molecular mechanisms of memory relies on introducing specific mutations into the genome. By deleting a single gene, one can produce mice with specific receptors or cell signaling molecules inactivated or altered. For example, in mice with a selective deletion of NMDA receptors in the CA1 field of the hippocampus, many aspects of CA1 physiology remain intact, but the CA1 neurons do not exhibit LTP, and memory impairment is observed in behavioral tasks. Genetic manipulations introduced reversibly in the adult are particularly advantageous, in that specific molecular changes can be induced in developmentally normal animals.

Associative Learning. The study of *classical conditioning* has provided many insights into the biology of memory. Classical conditioning has been especially well studied in rabbits, using a tone as the conditioned stimulus and an air puff to the eye (which automatically elicits a blink response) as the unconditioned stimulus. Repeated pairings of the tone and the air puff lead to a conditioned response, in that the tone alone elicits an eye blink. Reversible lesions of the deep nuclei of the cerebellum eliminate the conditioned response without affecting the unconditioned response. These lesions also prevent initial learning from occurring, and, when the lesion is reversed, rabbits usually learn. Thus, the cerebellum contains essential circuitry for the learned association. The relevant plasticity appears to be distributed between the cerebellar cortex and the deep nuclei.

An analogous pattern of cerebellar plasticity is believed to underlie motor learning in the vestibuloocular reflex and, perhaps, associative learning of motor responses in general. Based on the idea that learned motor responses depend on the coordinated control of changes in timing and strength of the response, it has been suggested that synaptic changes in the cerebellar cortex are critical for learned timing. In contrast, synaptic changes in the deep nuclei are critical for forming an association between a conditioned stimulus and an unconditioned stimulus.

Fear conditioning and fear-potentiated startle are types of learning that serve as useful models for anxiety disorders and related psychiatric conditions. For example, mice exhibit freezing behavior when returned to the same context in which aversive shock was delivered on an earlier occasion. This type of learning

depends on the encoding of contextual features of the learning environment. Acquiring and expressing this type of learning requires neural circuits that include both the amygdala and the hippocampus. The amygdala may be important for associating negative affect with new stimuli. The hippocampus may be important for representing the context. With extinction training, when the context is no longer associated with an aversive stimulus, the conditioned fear response fades. The frontal cortex is believed to play a critical role in extinction.

Cortical Organization of Memory

One fundamental question concerns the locus of memory storage in the brain. In the 1920s, Karl Lashley searched for the site of memory storage by studying the behavior of rats after removing different amounts of their cerebral cortex. He recorded the number of trials needed to relearn a maze problem that rats learned before surgery, and he found that the deficit was proportional to the amount of cortex removed. The deficit did not seem to depend on the particular location of cortical damage. Lashley concluded that the memory resulting from maze learning was not localized in any one part of the brain but instead was distributed equivalently over the entire cortex.

Subsequent research has led to reinterpretations of these results. Maze learning in rats depends on different types of information, including visual, tactile, spatial, and olfactory information. Neurons that process these various types of information are segregated into different areas of the rat cerebral cortex, and memory storage is segregated in a parallel manner. Thus, the correlation between maze-learning abilities and lesion size that Lashley observed results from progressive encroachment of larger lesions on specialized cortical areas serving the many components of information processing relevant for maze learning.

The functional organization of the mammalian cerebral cortex has been revealed through neuropsychological analyses of deficits following brain damage and physiologic studies of intact brains. The cortical areas responsible for processing and storing visual information have been studied most extensively in nonhuman primates. Nearly one-half of the primate neocortex is specialized for visual functions.

The cortical pathways for visual information processing begin in the primary visual cortex (V1) and proceed from parallel pathways or streams. One stream projects ventrally to the inferotemporal cortex and is specialized for processing information concerning the identification of visual objects. Another stream projects dorsally to the parietal cortex and is specialized for processing information about spatial location.

Specific visual processing areas in the dorsal and ventral streams, together with areas in the prefrontal cortex, register the immediate experience of perceptual processing. The results of perceptual processing are first available as *immediate memory.* Immediate memory refers to the amount of information that can be held in mind (like a telephone number) to be available for immediate use. Immediate memory can be extended in time by rehearsing or otherwise manipulating the information, in which case what is stored is said to be in *working memory.*

Regions of the visual cortex in forward portions of the dorsal and ventral streams serve as the ultimate repositories of visual memories. The inferotemporal cortex, for example, lies at the end of the ventral stream, and inferotemporal lesions lead to selective impairments in both visual object perception and visual memory. Nonetheless, such lesions do not disrupt elementary visual functions, such as acuity. Electrophysiologic studies in the monkey show that neurons in area TE, which is one part of the inferotemporal cortex, register specific and complex features of visual stimuli, such as shape, and respond selectively to patterns and objects. The inferotemporal cortex can thus be thought of as both a higher-order visual processing system and a storehouse of the visual memories that result from that processing.

In sum, memory is distributed and localized in the cerebral cortex. Memory is distributed in the sense that, as Lashley concluded, there is no cortical center dedicated solely to the storage of memories. Nonetheless, memory is localized in the sense that different aspects or dimensions of events are stored at specific cortical sites—namely, in the same regions that are specialized to analyze and process what is to be stored.

Memory and Amnesia

The principle that the functional specialization of cortical regions determines both the locus of information processing and the locus of information storage does not provide a complete account of memory in the brain. If it did, then brain injury would always include difficulty in memory for a restricted type of information and a loss of ability to process information of that same type. This kind of impairment occurs, for example, in the aphasias and the agnosias. However, there is another kind of impairment that can occur as well, called amnesia.

The hallmark of amnesia is a loss of new learning ability that extends across all sensory modalities and stimulus domains. This *anterograde amnesia* can be explained by understanding the role of brain structures critical for acquiring information about facts and events. Typically, anterograde amnesia occurs together with *retrograde amnesia,* a loss of knowledge acquired before the onset of amnesia. Retrograde deficits often have a temporal gradient, following a principle known as Ribot's law; deficits are most severe for information that was most recently learned.

A patient with a presentation of amnesia exhibits severe memory deficits in the context of the preservation of other cognitive functions, including language comprehension and production, reasoning, attention, immediate memory, personality, and social skills. The selectivity of the memory deficit in these cases implies that intellectual and perceptual functions of the brain are separated from the capacity to lay down in memory the records that ordinarily result from engaging in intellectual and perceptual work.

Specialized Memory Function. Amnesia can result from damage to the medial portion of the temporal lobe or damage to regions of the midline diencephalon. Studies of a severely amnesic patient known as HM stimulated intensive investigation of the role of the medial temporal lobe in memory.

HM became amnesic in 1953, at 27 years of age, when he sustained a bilateral resection of the medial temporal lobe to relieve severe epilepsy. The removal included approximately one-half of the hippocampus, the amygdala, and most neighboring entorhinal and perirhinal cortices (Fig. 34-6). After the surgery, HM's seizure condition was much improved, but he experienced profound forgetfulness. His intellectual functions were generally preserved. For example, HM exhibited normal immediate memory, and he could maintain his attention during conversations. After an interruption, however, HM could not remember what had recently occurred. HM's dense amnesia was permanent and debilitating. In HM's words, he felt as if he were waking from a dream because he had no recollection of what had just happened.

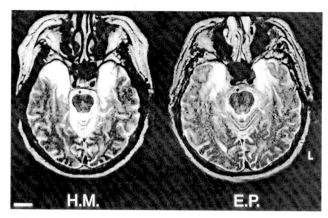

FIGURE 34-6
Structural magnetic resonance images of the brains of patients HM and EP through the level of the temporal lobe. Damaged tissue is indicated by bright signal in these T2-weighted axial images. Both patients sustained extensive damage to medial temporal structures, as the result of surgery for epilepsy in HM, and as the result of viral encephalitis in EP. Scale bar: 2 cm. L, left side of the brain. (Reprinted from Corkin S, Amaral EG, González RG, Johnson KA, Hyman BT. H. M.'s medial temporal lobe lesion: Findings from magnetic resonance imaging. *J Neurosci.* 1997;17(10):3964–3979 and Stefanacci L, Buffalo EA, Schmolck H, Squire LR. Profound amnesia after damage to the medial temporal lobe: A neuroanatomical and neuropsychological profile of patient E.P. *J Neurosci.* 2000;20(18):7024–7036, with permission.)

In monkeys, many parallels to human amnesia have been demonstrated after surgical damage to anatomical components of the medial temporal lobe. Cumulative study of the resulting memory impairment eventually identified the medial temporal structures and connections crucial for memory. These include the hippocampus, including the dentate gyrus, hippocampal fields CA1, CA2, CA3, and the subiculum—and the adjacent cortical regions, including the entorhinal, perirhinal, and parahippocampal cortices.

Another important medial temporal lobe structure is the amygdala. The amygdala is involved in the regulation of much of emotional behavior. In particular, the storage of emotional events engages the amygdala. Modulatory effects of projections from the amygdala to the neocortex are responsible for producing enhanced memory for emotional or arousing events compared to neutral events.

A detailed study of amnesic patients offers unique insights into the nature of memory and its organization in the brain. An extensive series of informative studies, for example, described the memory impairment of patient EP.

EP was diagnosed with herpes simplex encephalitis at 72 years of age. Damage to the medial temporal lobe region (see Fig. 34-6) produced persistent and profound amnesia. During testing sessions, EP was cordial and talked freely about his life experiences, but he relied exclusively on stories from his childhood and early adulthood. He would repeat the same story many times. Strikingly, his performance on tests of recognition memory was no better than would result from guessing (Fig. 34-7A). Tests involving facts about his life and autobiographical experiences revealed poor memory for the time leading up to his illness but normal memory for his childhood (Fig. 34-7B). EP also has good spatial knowledge about the town in which he lived as a child, but he was unable to learn the layout of the neighborhood where he moved to after he became amnesic (Fig. 34-7C).

Given the severity of the memory problems experienced by EP and other amnesic patients, it is noteworthy that these patients

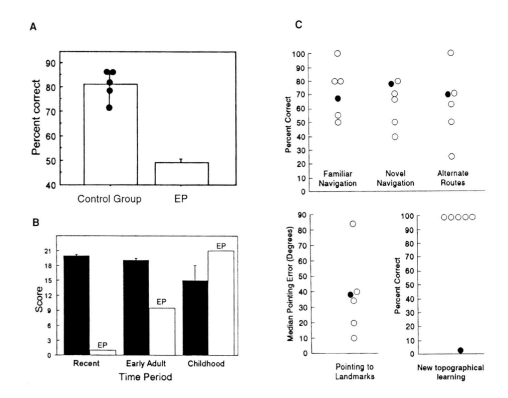

FIGURE 34-7

Formal test results for patient EP, showing severe anterograde and retrograde deficits, with intact remote memory. **A:** Scores were combined from 42 different tests of recognition memory for words given to patient EP and a group of five healthy control subjects. The testing format was either two-alternative forced choice or yes–no recognition. Brackets for EP indicate the standard error of the mean. Data points for the control group indicate each participant's mean score across all 42 recognition memory tests. EP's average performance (49.3 percent correct) was not different from chance and was approximately five standard deviations (SDs) below the average performance of control subjects (81.1 percent correct; SD, 6.3). **B:** Autobiographical remembering was quantified by using a structured interview known as the Autobiographical Memory Interview. Items assessed personal semantic knowledge (maximum score 21 for each time period). Performance for the recent time period reflects poor memory for information that could have been acquired only subsequent to the onset of his amnesia. For EP, performance for the early adult period reflects retrograde memory deficits. Performance for the childhood period reflects good remote memory. Similar results for semantic and episodic remembering were obtained from these time periods. (Data from Kopelman MD, Wilson BA, Baddeley AD. The autobiographical memory interview: A new assessment of autobiographical and personal semantic memory in amnesic patients. *J Clin Exp Neuropsychol.* 1989;5:724; and Reed JM, Squire LR. Retrograde amnesia for facts and events: Findings from four new cases. *J Neurosci.* 1998;18:3943). **C:** Assessments of spatial memory demonstrated EP's good memory for spatial knowledge from his childhood, along with extremely poor new learning of spatial information. Performance was compared to that of five individuals (*open circles*) who attended EP's high school at the same time as he did, lived in the region over approximately the same time period, and, like EP (*filled circles*), moved away as young adults. Normal performance was found for navigating from home to different locations in the area (familiar navigation), between different locations in the area (novel navigation), and between these same locations when a main street was blocked (alternative routes). Subjects were also asked to point to particular locations while imagining themselves in a particular location (pointing to landmarks), or they were asked about locations in the neighborhoods in which they currently lived (new topographical learning). EP showed difficulty only in this last test, because he moved to his current residence after he became amnesic. (Data from Teng E, Squire LR. Memory for places learned long ago is intact after hippocampal damage. *Nature.* 1999;400:675.) (Adapted from Stefanacci L, Buffalo EA, Schmolck H, Squire LR. Profound amnesia after damage to the medial temporal lobe: A neuroanatomical and neuropsychological profile of patient E. P. *J Neurosci.* 2000;20(18):7024–7036. Printed with permission.)

nonetheless perform typically on certain kinds of memory tests. The impairment selectively concerns memory for factual knowledge and autobiographical events, collectively termed *declarative memory.* Amnesia presents as a global deficit, in that it involves memory for information presented in any sensory modality, but the deficit is limited, in that it covers only memory for facts and events.

Hippocampal pathology in patients with amnesia can also be revealed using high-resolution magnetic resonance imaging (MRI). Such studies indicate that damage limited to the hippocampus results in clinically significant memory impairment. In addition to the hippocampus, other medial temporal lobe regions also make critical contributions to memory. Thus, a moderately severe memory impairment results from CA1 damage, whereas a more profound and disabling amnesia results from medial temporal lobe damage that includes the hippocampus and adjacent

cortex. Memory impairment due to medial temporal lobe damage is also typical in patients with early Alzheimer disease or amnestic mild cognitive impairment. As Alzheimer disease progresses, the pathology affects many cortical regions and produces substantial cognitive deficits and memory dysfunction.

Amnesia can also result from damage to structures of the medial diencephalon. The critical regions damaged in diencephalic amnesia include the mammillary nuclei in the hypothalamus, the dorsomedial nucleus of the thalamus, the anterior nucleus, the internal medullary lamina, and the mammillothalamic tract. However, uncertainty remains regarding which specific lesions are required to produce diencephalic amnesia. *Alcoholic Korsakoff syndrome* is the most prevalent and best-studied example of diencephalic amnesia, and in these cases, the damage is found in brain regions that may be especially sensitive to prolonged bouts of thiamine deficiency and

Table 34-6
Memory and Cognitive Deficits Associated with Frontal Damage

Test	Amnesia	Korsakoff Syndrome	Frontal Lobe Damage
Delayed recall	+	+	−
Dementia Rating Scale: Memory index	+	+	−
Dementia Rating Scale: Initiation and perseveration index	−	+	+
Wisconsin Card Sorting Test	−	+	+
Temporal order memory	+	++	++
Metamemory	−	+	+
Release from proactive interference	−	+	−

+, deficit; −, no deficit; ++, disproportionate impairment relative to item memory.
From Squire LR, Zola-Morgan S, Cave CB, Haist F, Musen G, Suzuki WA. *Memory, organization of brain systems and cognition Cold Spring Harb Symp Quant Biol.* 1990;55:1007.

alcohol abuse. Patients with alcoholic Korsakoff syndrome typically exhibit memory impairment due to a combination of diencephalic damage and frontal lobe pathology. Frontal damage alone produces characteristic cognitive deficits and specific memory problems (e.g., in effortful retrieval and evaluation); in Korsakoff syndrome, the pattern of deficits thus extends beyond what is commonly found in other amnesia cases (see Table 34-6).

The ability to remember factual and autobiographical events depends on the integrity of both the cortical regions responsible for representing the information in question and several brain regions responsible for memory formation. Thus, medial temporal and diencephalic brain areas work in concert with widespread areas of neocortex to form and to store declarative memories (Fig. 34-8).

Retrograde Amnesia

Memory loss in amnesia typically affects recent memories more than remote memories (Fig. 34-9). Temporally graded amnesia has been demonstrated retrospectively in studies of amnesic patients and prospectively in studies of monkeys, rats, mice, and rabbits. These findings have important implications for understanding the nature of the memory storage process. Memories are dynamic, not static. As time passes after learning, some memories are forgotten, whereas others become stronger due to a process of *consolidation* that depends on cortical, medial temporal, and diencephalic structures.

The study of retrograde amnesia has been important for understanding how memory changes over time. The dynamic nature of memory storage can be conceptualized as follows. An event is experienced and encoded by a collection of cortical regions involved in representing a combination of different event features. At the same time, the hippocampus and adjacent cortex receive pertinent high-level information from all sensory modalities. Later, when the original event is recalled, the same set of cortical regions is activated. If a subset of the cortical regions is activated, the hippocampus and related structures can facilitate recall by facilitating the remaining cortical regions (i.e., pattern completion). When the original event is retrieved and newly associated with other information, hippocampal–cortical networks can be modified. In this way, a gradual consolidation process occurs that changes memory storage (see Fig. 34-8). The neocortical components representing some events can become so effectively linked together that ultimately a memory can be retrieved without any contribution from the medial temporal lobe. As a result, amnesic patients can exhibit normal retrieval of remote facts and events and autobiographical memories. Distributed neocortical regions are the permanent repositories of these enduring memories.

In contrast to what is observed after damage restricted to the hippocampus, extensive retrograde impairments for facts and events from the distant past can also occur. Damage to the frontal lobes, for example, can lead to difficulty in organizing memory retrieval. Accurate retrieval often begins with activation of lifetime

FIGURE 34-8
Brain regions believed to be critical for the formation and storage of declarative memory. Medial diencephalon and medial temporal regions are critical for declarative memory storage. The entorhinal cortex is the major source of projections for the neocortex to the hippocampus, and nearly two-thirds of the cortical input to the entorhinal cortex originates in the perirhinal and parahippocampal cortex. The entorhinal cortex also receives direct connections from the cingulate, insula, orbitofrontal, and superior temporal cortices. (Adapted from Paller KA. Neurocognitive foundations of human memory. In: Medin DL, ed.: *The Psychology of Learning and Motivation.* Vol. 40. San Diego, CA: Academic Press; 2008:121 and Gluck MA, Mercado E, Myers CE. *Learning and Memory: From Brain to Behavior.* New York: Worth; 2008:109, Fig. 3-16.)

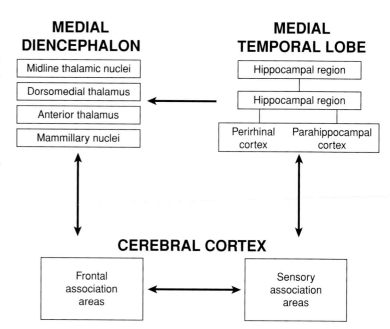

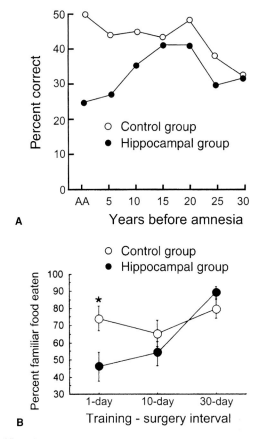

A

B

FIGURE 34-9

A: Temporally limited retrograde amnesia for free recall of 251 news events. Scores were aligned relative to the onset of amnesia in patients ($N = 6$) and to a corresponding time point in age-matched and education-matched healthy individuals ($N = 12$). The time period after the onset of amnesia is labeled AA (anterograde amnesia) to designate that this time point assessed memory for events that occurred after the onset of amnesia. Standard errors ranged from 2 to 10 percent. Brain damage in the patient group was limited primarily to the hippocampal region. **B:** Temporally limited retrograde amnesia in rats with lesions of the hippocampus and subiculum. Rats learned to prefer an odorous food as the result of an encounter with another rat with that odor on its breath. Percent preference for the familiar food was observed for three training-surgery intervals. At 1 day after learning, the control group performed significantly better than the rats with lesions ($p < 0.05$). At 30 days, the two groups performed similarly, and both groups performed well above chance. *Error bars* show standard errors of the mean. (Adapted from Manns JR, Hopkins RO, Squire LR. Semantic memory and the human hippocampus. *Neuron.* 2003;38(1):127–133 and Clark RE, Broadbent NJ, Zola SM, Squire LR. Anterograde amnesia and temporally graded retrograde amnesia for a nonspatial memory task after lesions of hippocampus and subiculum. *J Neurosci.* 2002;22(11):4663–4669, with permission.)

periods and proceeds to identify general classes of events and then more specific events, but this process becomes difficult following frontal damage. Damage to other cortical regions can also impair memory storage. Networks in the anterolateral temporal cortex, for example, are critical for retrieving stored information because these areas are essential for long-term storage itself. Patients with *focal retrograde amnesia* exhibit substantial retrograde memory impairments together with only moderately impaired new learning ability. Some capacity for new learning remains, presumably, because medial temporal lobe structures can communicate with other areas of the cortex that remain undamaged.

MULTIPLE TYPES OF MEMORY

Memory is not a single faculty of the mind but consists of various subtypes. Amnesia affects only one kind of memory, *declarative memory.* Declarative memory is what is ordinarily meant by the term *memory* in everyday language. Declarative memory supports the conscious recollection of facts and events. The classic impairment in amnesia thus concerns memory for routes, lists, faces, melodies, objects, and other verbal and nonverbal material, regardless of the sensory modality in which the material is presented.

Amnesic patients can display a broad impairment in these components of declarative memory, while several other memory abilities are preserved. The heterogeneous set of preserved abilities is collectively termed *nondeclarative memory.* Nondeclarative memory includes skill learning, habit learning, simple forms of conditioning, and priming (see next section). For these kinds of learning and memory, amnesic patients can perform normally.

In controlled laboratory settings, the acquisition of a variety of perceptual, perceptual-motor, and cognitive skills can be tested in isolation, and amnesic patients are found to acquire these skills at rates equivalent to the rates at which healthy individuals acquire the skills. For example, amnesic patients can learn to read mirror-reversed text normally, they exhibit the typical facilitation in reading speed with successive readings of ordinary prose, and they improve as rapidly as healthy individuals at a speeded reading of repeating nonwords. Also, amnesic patients can, after seeing strings of letters generated by a finite-state rule system, classify novel strings of letters as rule-based or not rule-based. Classification performance is normal even though amnesic patients are impaired at remembering the events of training or the specific items they have studied.

Priming

Priming refers to the facilitation of the ability to detect or to identify a particular stimulus based on a specific recent experience. Many tests have been used to measure priming in amnesia and show that it is intact. For example, words might be presented in a study phase and then again, after a delay, in a test phase, when a priming measure such as reading speed is obtained. Patients are instructed to read words as quickly as possible in such a test, and they are not informed that memory is being assessed.

In one priming test, patients named pictures of previously presented objects reliably faster than they named pictures of new objects, even after a delay of 1 week. This facilitation occurred at normal levels, even though the patients were markedly impaired at recognizing which pictures had been presented previously. Particularly striking examples of preserved priming come from studies of patient EP (Fig. 34-10), who exhibited intact priming for words but performed at chance levels when asked to recognize which words had been presented. This form of memory, termed *perceptual priming,* is thus a distinct class of memory independent of the medial temporal lobe regions typically damaged in amnesia.

Another form of priming reflects improved access to meaning rather than percepts. For example, subjects study a list of words, including *tent* and *belt,* and then are asked to free-associate them. Thus, they are given words such as *canvas* and *strap* and asked to produce the first word that comes to mind. The result is that subjects are more likely to produce *tent* in response to *canvas* and to produce *belt* in response to *strap* than if the words *tent* and *belt* had not been presented recently. This effect, called *conceptual priming,* is also preserved in amnesic patients, even though they fail to recognize the same words on a conventional memory test (Fig. 34-11).

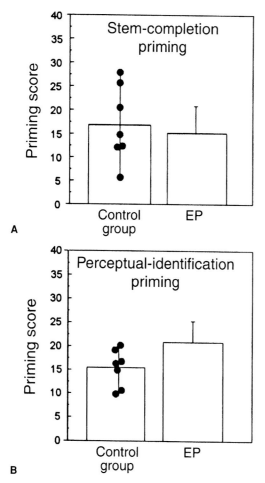

FIGURE 34-10
Preserved priming in patient EP relative to seven control subjects.
A: Stem-completion priming on six separate tests. Priming reflected
a tendency for subjects to complete three-letter stems with previously encountered words when they were instructed to produce
the first word to come to mind (e.g., MOT___ completed to form
MOTEL). Priming scores were calculated as percentage correct
for studied words minus percentage correct for baseline words
(guessing). **B:** Perceptual-identification priming on 12 separate tests.
Subjects attempted to read 48 words that were visually degraded.
Priming scores were calculated as percentage correct identification
of previously studied words minus percentage correct identification
of nonstudied words. Brackets indicate standard error of the mean.
(Data from Hamann SB, Squire LR. Intact perceptual memory in the
absence of conscious memory. *Behav Neurosci.* 1997;111:850.)
(Reprinted from Stefanacci L, Buffalo EA, Schmolck H, Squire LR.
Profound amnesia after damage to the medial temporal lobe: A
neuroanatomical and neuropsychological profile of patient E. P.
J Neurosci. 2000;20(18):7024–7036, with permission.)

Not all types of priming are preserved in amnesia. Some priming
tests have been designed to examine the formation of new associations. When priming tests are based not on preexisting knowledge
but the acquisition of new associative knowledge, priming tends
to be impaired. In other words, priming in certain complex situations can require the same type of linkage among multiple cortical
regions critical for declarative memory.

Memory Systems

Table 34-7 depicts one scheme for conceptualizing multiple types
of memory. Declarative memory depends on medial temporal

and midline diencephalic structures along with large portions of
the neocortex. This system provides for the rapid learning of facts
(*semantic memory*) and events (*episodic memory*). Nondeclarative
memory depends on several different brain systems. Habits depend
on the neocortex and the neostriatum, and the cerebellum is essential for the conditioning of skeletal musculature, the amygdala for
emotional learning, and the neocortex for priming.

Declarative memory and nondeclarative memory differ in significant ways. Declarative memory is phylogenetically more recent
than nondeclarative memory. Also, declarative memories are
available to conscious recollection. The flexibility of declarative
memory permits the retrieved information to be available to multiple response systems. Nondeclarative memory is inaccessible to
awareness and is expressed only by engaging specific processing
systems. Nondeclarative memories are stored as changes within
these processing systems—changes encapsulated such that the
stored information has limited access to other processing systems.

Semantic memory, which concerns general knowledge of the
world, has often been categorized as a separate form of memory.
Facts committed to memory typically become independent of
the original episodes in which the facts were learned. Amnesic
patients can sometimes acquire information that would ordinarily
be learned as facts, but the patients learn it by relying on a different
brain system than the system that supports declarative memory.

Consider a test requiring the concurrent learning of eight object
pairs. Healthy individuals can rapidly learn which the correct object in
each pair is, whereas severely amnesic patients like EP learn only gradually over many weeks, and at the start of each session, they cannot
describe the task, the instructions, or the objects. In patients who do
not have severe amnesia, factual information is typically acquired as
conscious declarative knowledge. In these cases, the brain structures
that remain intact within the medial temporal lobe presumably support learning. In contrast, when factual information is acquired as
nondeclarative knowledge, as in the case of EP's learning of pairs of
objects, learning likely occurs directly as a habit, perhaps supported
by the neostriatum. Humans thus appear to have a robust capacity for
habit learning that operates outside of awareness and independent of
the medial temporal lobe structures that are damaged in amnesia.

Frontal Contributions to Memory

Although amnesia does not occur after limited frontal damage, the
frontal lobes are fundamentally crucial for declarative memory.
Patients with frontal lesions have a poor memory for the context
in which information was acquired, they have difficulty in unaided
recall, and they may even have some mild difficulty on tests of item
recognition. More generally, patients with frontal lesions have difficulty implementing memory retrieval strategies and evaluating and
monitoring their memory performance.

NEUROIMAGING AND MEMORY

The understanding of memory derived from studies of amnesia has
been extended through studies using various methods for monitoring
brain activity in healthy individuals. For example, activation of posterior prefrontal regions with positron emission tomography (PET) and
functional magnetic resonance imaging (fMRI) have shown that these
regions are involved in strategic processing during retrieval and working
memory. Anterior frontal regions near the frontal poles have been linked
with functions such as evaluating the products of retrieval. Frontal
connections with posterior neocortical regions support the organization
of retrieval and the manipulation of information in working memory.

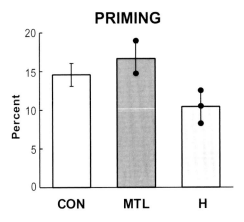
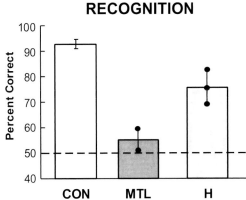

FIGURE 34-11

Preserved conceptual priming in amnesia. In the free association test, subjects studied a set of words (e.g., *lemon*) and 5 minutes later viewed cue words that included associates of the studied words (e.g., *orange*). Subjects were asked to produce the first word that came to mind in response to each cue word. Results are shown separately for the control group (CON; $n = 12$), amnesic patients with large medial temporal lobe lesions (MTL; $n = 2$), and amnesic patients with lesions believed to be limited to the hippocampal region (H; $n = 3$). The **left panel** shows conceptual priming scores computed as the percentage of studied words produced in the free association test minus a baseline measure of the likelihood of producing those words by chance. All of the groups performed similarly in the conceptual priming test. The **right panel** shows results from a yes–no recognition memory test using comparable words. Both patient groups were impaired relative to the control group. The *dashed line* indicates chance performance. The data points for the MTL and H groups show the scores of individual patients averaged across four separate tests. *Brackets* show standard errors of the mean for the control group. (Reprinted from Levy DA, Stark CEL, Squire LR. Intact conceptual priming in the absence of declarative memory. *Psychol Sci.* 2004;15(10):680–686, with permission.)

Consistent with the evidence from patients with frontal lesions, frontal–posterior networks can be viewed as instrumental in the retrieval of declarative memories and the online processing of new information.

Neuroimaging has also identified contributions to memory made by the parietal cortex. Multiple parietal regions (including inferior and superior parietal lobules, precuneus, posterior cingulate, and retrosplenial cortex) are activated in conjunction with remembering recent experiences. Although many functions have been hypothesized to explain this parietal activity, a single consensus position has not yet been reached, and it may be the case that several different functions are relevant.

Neuroimaging studies have also illuminated priming phenomena and how they differ from declarative memory. Perceptual priming appears to reflect changes in the early stages of the cortical pathways engaged during perceptual processing. For example, in the case of stem-completion priming, in which subjects study a list of words (e.g., MOTEL) and then are tested with a list of stems (e.g., MOT___) and with instructions to complete each stem with the first word to come to mind, neuroimaging and divided visual-field studies have implicated visual processing systems in extrastriate cortex, especially in the right hemisphere. In contrast, the conscious recollection of remembered words engages brain areas at later stages of processing. Neural mechanisms supporting priming and declarative memory retrieval have also been distinguished in brain electrical activity recorded from the scalp (Fig. 34-12). In

Table 34-7
Types of Memory

A. Declarative memory
  1. Facts
  2. Events

B. Nondeclarative memory
  1. Skills and habits
  2. Priming
  3. Simple classical conditioning
  4. Nonassociative learning

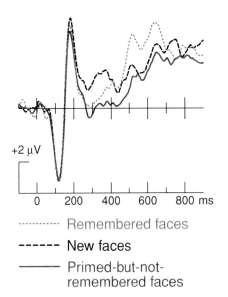

$+2\ \mu V$

0   200   400   600   800 ms

·············· Remembered faces

------ New faces

——— Primed-but-not-remembered faces

FIGURE 34-12

Brain potentials associated with perceptual priming versus declarative memory retrieval. Paller et al. (2003) studied 16 volunteers, who took a memory test involving three sorts of faces: new faces, faces they had seen recently and remembered well, and faces they had seen but did not remember because the faces had been presented too briefly to process effectively. In a companion experiment with a priming test, speeded responses were found, indicative of priming. Frontal recordings of brain waves elicited by the primed faces included negative potentials from 200 to 400 ms after face presentation that differed from the brain waves elicited by new faces. These differences were particularly robust for trials with the fastest responses (data shown were from trials with responses faster than the median reaction time). Remembered faces uniquely elicited positive brain waves that began about 400 ms after face presentation. Brain potential correlates of face recollection occurred later than those for perceptual priming and were larger over posterior brain regions. (Adapted from Paller KA, Hutson CA, Miller BB, Boehm SG. Neural manifestations of memory with and without awareness. *Neuron.* 2003;38(3):507–516, with permission.)

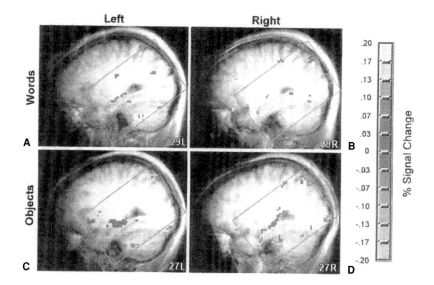

FIGURE 34-13

Activity in the left and right hippocampal regions measured with functional magnetic resonance imaging (fMRI) during declarative memory retrieval. Data were collected from 11 participants who saw words at study and test and from 11 different participants who saw pictures of namable objects at study and test. Recognition memory accuracy was 80.2 percent correct for words and 89.9 percent correct for objects. Areas of significant fMRI signal change (targets vs. foils) are typically shown in sagittal sections as color overlays on averaged structural images. The *box* indicates the area in which reliable data were available for all subjects. With words, retrieval-related activity was observed in the hippocampus on the left side (**A**) but not on the right side (**B**). With namable objects, retrieval-related activity was observed in the hippocampus on both the left side (**C**) and the right side (**D**). (Reprinted from Stark CE, Squire LR. Functional magnetic resonance imaging (fMRI) activity in the hippocampal region during recognition memory. *J Neurosci.* 2000;20(20):7776–7781, with permission.)

sum, priming differs from declarative memory in that it is signaled by brain activity that occurs earlier, and that originates in different brain regions.

Hippocampal activity associated with the formation and retrieval of declarative memories has also been investigated with neuroimaging. In keeping with the neuropsychological evidence, the hippocampus appears to be involved in the recollection of recent events (Fig. 34-13). The retrieval-related hippocampal activity has been observed in memory tests with many different types of stimuli. The hippocampus is also active during the initial storage of information. Whereas the left inferior prefrontal cortex is engaged as a result of attempts to encode a word, hippocampal activity at encoding is more closely associated with whether encoding leads to a stable memory that can later be retrieved (Fig. 34-14). These findings confirm and extend the idea that medial temporal and frontal regions are essential for memory storage and make different contributions.

SLEEP AND MEMORY

The speculation that memories are processed during sleep has a long history. Freud noted that dreams could reveal fragments of recent experiences in the form of day residues. Although many questions about how and why memories may be processed during sleep remain unresolved, recent experiments have provided new empirical support to bolster the idea that memory processing during sleep serves an adaptive function. It is now clear that memory performance can be facilitated when sleep occurs after initial learning, and that sleep-related facilitation can be observed for many different types of memory.

Memory storage appears to be aided explicitly by processing during deep sleep within a few hours after learning, especially in stages 3 and 4 (slow-wave sleep). Some results indicate that slow-wave sleep facilitates the storage of declarative memories but not nondeclarative memories. Direct evidence for this proposal has

been obtained using stimulation with olfactory stimuli (Fig. 34-15), stimulation with direct current electrical input at the approximate frequency of electroencephalographic slow waves, and other methods. Furthermore, neuronal recordings in animals have revealed a phenomenon of hippocampal replay, in which activity patterns expressed during the day are later observed during sleep. In summary, declarative memories acquired during waking can be processed again during sleep, and this processing can influence the likelihood of subsequent memory retrieval when the individual is awake. The facilitation of declarative memory is typically manifest as a reduction in the amount of forgetting that occurs, not as an improvement in memory.

ASSESSMENT OF MEMORY FUNCTIONS

A variety of quantitative methods are available to assess memory functions in neurologic and psychiatric patients. Quantitative methods are useful for evaluating and following patients longitudinally and carrying out a one-time examination to determine the status of memory function. It is desirable to obtain information about the severity of memory dysfunction, as well as to determine whether a memory is selectively affected or whether memory problems are occurring, as they often do, against a background of additional intellectual deficits. Although some widely available tests, such as the Wechsler Memory Scale, provide useful measures of memory, most single tests assess memory rather narrowly. Even general-purpose neuropsychological batteries provide for only limited testing of memory functions. A complete assessment of memory usually involves several specialized tests that sample intellectual functions, new learning capacity, remote memory, and memory self-report.

The assessment of general intellectual functions is central to any neuropsychological examination. In the case of memory testing, information about intellectual functions provides information about a patient's general test-taking ability and a way to

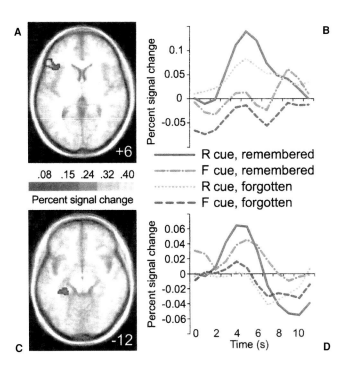

R cue, remembered

F cue, remembered

R cue, forgotten

F cue, forgotten

FIGURE 34-14

Functional activations of prefrontal and medial temporal regions that were predictive of later memory performance. Single words were presented visually, each followed by an instruction to remember (R cue) or to forget (F cue). Trials were sorted based on the remember or forget instruction and on subsequent recognition performance. Activity in the left inferior prefrontal cortex and left hippocampus was predictive of subsequent recognition but for different reasons. Left inferior prefrontal activation (**A**) was associated with the encoding attempt, in that responses were largest for trials with a cue to remember, whether or not the word was actually recognized later. The time course of activity in this region (**B**) was computed based on responses that were time locked to word onset (time 0). Left inferior prefrontal activity increased for words that were later remembered, but there was a stronger association with encoding attempt, because responses were larger for words followed by an R cue that were later forgotten than for words followed by an F cue that were later remembered. In contrast, left parahippocampal and posterior hippocampal activation (**C**) was associated with encoding success. As shown by the time course of activity in this region (**D**), responses were largest for words that were subsequently remembered, whether the cue was to remember or to forget. (Reprinted from Reber PJ, Siwiec RM, Gitelman DR, Parrish TB, Mesulam MM, Paller KA. Neural correlates of successful encoding identified using functional magnetic resonance imaging. *J Neurosci.* 2002;22(21):9541–9548, with permission.)

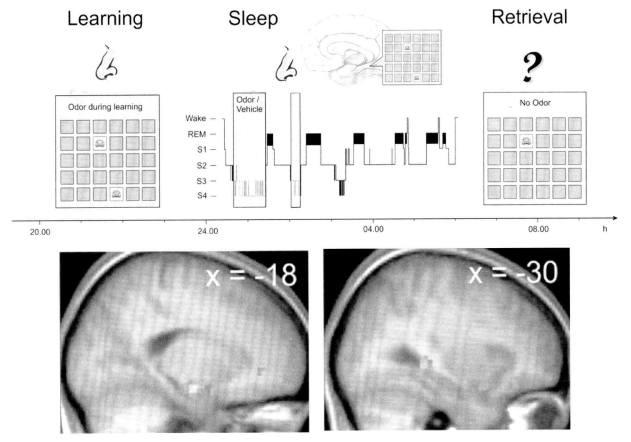

FIGURE 34-15

Evidence for memory processing during sleep. Subjects first learned object–location associations when a rose odor was present. Following learning, subjects slept wearing a device for delivering odors to the nose, and the rose odor was administered during the first two slow-wave sleep periods of the night (in 30-second periods to prevent habituation). Memory facilitation was observed when object–location associations were tested the following morning in the absence of odor stimulation. Facilitated memory was not found when stimulation occurred during slow-wave sleep but not during learning, when stimulation occurred during learning and then during rapid-eye-movement (REM) sleep, or when subjects were kept awake. Moreover, odor stimulation during slow-wave sleep was found to produce anterior and posterior hippocampal activation (**lower panels**). (Reprinted from Rasch B, Büchel C, Gais S, Born J. Odor cues during slow-wave sleep prompt declarative memory consolidation. *Science.* 2007;315(5817):1426–1429, with permission.)

assess the selectivity of memory impairment. Useful tests include the Wechsler Adult Intelligence Scale; a test of object naming, such as the Boston Naming Test; a rating scale to assess the possibility of global dementia; a test of word fluency; and specialized tests of frontal lobe function.

New Learning Capacity

Memory tests are sensitive to impaired new learning ability when they adhere to either of two critical principles. First, tests are sensitive to memory impairment when more information is presented than can be held in immediate memory. For example, one might ask patients to memorize a list of 10 faces, words, sentences, or digits, given that 10 items are more than can be held in mind. The paired-associate learning task is an especially sensitive test of this kind. In the paired-associate task, the examiner asks the patient to learn a list of unrelated pairs of words (e.g., queen–garden, office–river) and then to respond to the first word in each pair by recalling the second word.

Second, tests are sensitive to memory impairment when a delay, filled with distraction, is interposed between the learning phase and the test phase. In that case, examiners typically ask patients to learn a small amount of information and then distract them for several minutes by conversation to prevent rehearsal. Recollection is then assessed for the previously presented material. Memory can be tested by the unaided recall of previously studied material (free recall), presenting a cue for the material to be remembered (cued recall), or by testing recognition memory. In multiple-choice tests of recognition memory, the patient tries to select previously studied items from a group of studied and unstudied items. In yes–no recognition tests, patients see studied and unstudied items one at a time and are asked to say "yes" if the item was presented previously and "no" if it was not. These methods for assessing recently learned material vary in their sensitivity for detecting memory impairment, with free recall being most sensitive, cued recall intermediate, and recognition least sensitive.

The specialization of function of the two cerebral hemispheres in humans means that left and right unilateral damage is associated with different kinds of memory problems. Accordingly, different kinds of memory tests must be used when unilateral damage is a possibility. In general, damage to medial temporal or diencephalic structures in the left cerebral hemisphere causes difficulty remembering verbal material, such as word lists and stories. Damage to medial temporal or diencephalic structures in the right cerebral hemisphere impairs memory for faces, spatial layouts, and other nonverbal material that is typically encoded without verbal labels. Left medial temporal damage can lead to impaired memory for spoken and written text. Right medial temporal damage can lead to impaired learning of spatial arrays, whether the layouts are examined by vision or touch. A useful way to test for nonverbal memory is to ask a patient to copy a complex geometric figure, and then, after a delay of several minutes, without forewarning, ask the patient to reproduce it.

Remote Memory

Evaluations of retrograde memory loss should attempt to determine the severity of any memory loss and the period that it covers. Most quantitative tests of remote memory are composed of material in the public domain that can be corroborated. For example, tests have been used that concern news event, photographs of famous persons, or former one-season television programs. An advantage of these

methods is that one can sample large numbers of events and often target particular periods. A disadvantage is that these tests are not so useful for detecting memory loss for information learned during the weeks or months immediately before the onset of amnesia. Most remote memory tests sample periods rather coarsely and cannot detect a retrograde memory impairment covering only a few months.

In contrast, autobiographical memory tests can potentially provide fine-grained information about a patient's retrograde memory. In the word-probe task, first used by Francis Galton in 1879, patients are asked to recollect specific episodes from their past in response to single word cues (e.g., bird and ticket) and date the episodes. The number of episodes recalled tends to be systematically related to the time the episode is taken. Most memories naturally come from recent periods (the last 1 to 2 months). In contrast, patients with amnesia often exhibit temporally graded retrograde amnesia, drawing relatively few episodic memories from the recent past but producing as many remote autobiographical memories as normal subjects (see Fig. 34-9).

Memory Self-Reports

Patients can often supply descriptions of their memory problems that are extremely useful for understanding the nature of their impairment. Tests of the ability to judge one's memory abilities are called tests of *metamemory.* Self-rating scales are available that yield quantitative and qualitative information about memory impairment. As a result, it is possible to distinguish memory complaints associated with depression from memory complaints associated with amnesia. Depressed patients tend to rate their memory as poor in a relatively undifferentiated way, endorsing equally all of the items on a self-rating form. By contrast, amnesic patients tend to endorse some items more than others; that is, there is a pattern to their memory complaints. Amnesic patients do not report difficulty in remembering very remote events or in following what is being said to them, but they do report having difficulty remembering an event a few minutes after it happens. Indeed, self-reports can match rather closely the description of memory dysfunction that emerges from objective tests. Specifically, new-learning capacity is affected, immediate memory is intact, and very remote memory is intact. Some amnesic patients, however, tend to underestimate their memory impairment markedly. In patients with Korsakoff syndrome, for example, their poor metamemory stems from frontal lobe dysfunction. In any case, querying patients in some detail about their sense of impairment and administering self-rating scales are valuable and informative adjuncts to more formal memory testing.

Psychogenic Amnesia

Patients sometimes exhibit memory impairment that differs markedly from the typical patterns of memory loss that follow brain damage. For example, some cases of amnesia present with a sudden onset of retrograde amnesia, a loss of personal identity, and minimal anterograde amnesia. These patients may even be unable to recall their name. Given the psychological forces that prompt the onset of amnesia in these cases, they are commonly termed *psychogenic amnesia,* or sometimes *hysterical amnesia, functional amnesia,* or *dissociative amnesia.*

Differentiating psychogenic amnesia from a memory disorder that results from frank neurologic injury or disease is often straightforward. Psychogenic amnesias typically do not affect new-learning capacity. Patients enter the hospital able to record a continuing procession of daily events. By contrast, new-learning problems tend to be at the core of neurologic amnesia. The main positive symptom in psychogenic amnesia is extensive and severe retrograde amnesia. Patients may be unable to recollect pertinent information from childhood or some part of their past. Formal neuropsychological testing has shown that the pattern of memory deficits varies widely from patient to patient. This variability may reflect a patient's commonsense concepts of memory, even when symptoms are not the result of conscious attempts to simulate amnesia. Some patients may perform poorly only when asked to remember past autobiographical events. Other patients also may fail at remembering past news events. Some patients perform well when memory tests appear to assess general knowledge, such as remembering the names of celebrities or cities. Learning new material is usually intact, perhaps because such tests appear to concern the present moment, not traveling into the past. Occasionally, patients with psychogenic amnesia exhibit broad memory deficits such that they cannot perform previously familiar skills or identify everyday objects or common vocabulary words.

By contrast, patients with neurologic amnesia never forget their name, and remote memory for the events of childhood and adolescence is typically normal unless there is damage to the lateral temporal or frontal lobes. Patients with psychogenic amnesia sometimes have evidence of head trauma or brain injury, but the pattern of deficits cannot be taken as a straightforward result of neurologic insult. The clinician's challenge is not to distinguish psychogenic amnesia from neurologic amnesia, but to distinguish psychogenic amnesia from malingering. Indeed, the diagnosis of psychogenic amnesia can be difficult to substantiate and may be met with skepticism by hospital staff. Some features that argue in favor of a genuine psychogenic disorder include (1) memory test scores that are not as low

as possible, and never worse than chance levels; (2) memory access that is improved by hypnosis or amobarbital (Amytal) interview; and (3) a significant premorbid psychiatric history. In some cases, psychogenic amnesia has been observed to clear after days, but in many cases, it has persisted as a potentially permanent feature of the personality.

IMPLICATIONS

Memory Distortion

Current understanding of the biology of memory has significant implications for several fundamental issues in psychiatry. Given the selective and constructive nature of autobiographical remembering and the imperfect nature of memory retrieval more generally, it is surprising that memory is so often accurate. How much can we trust our memories? Subjective feelings of confidence are not perfect indicators of retrieval accuracy. Moreover, memory distortion can lead to unfortunate consequences, such as when mistaken eyewitness testimony harms an innocent individual.

It is possible to remember with confidence events that never happened. For example, it is possible to confuse an event that was only imagined or dreamed about with a real-life event. One factor contributing to memory distortion is that similar brain regions are essential both for visual imagery and for the long-term storage of visual memories (Fig. 34-16). Another factor contributing to memory distortion is that memory functions best in remembering the gist of an event, not the particulars from which the gist is derived. In a noted demonstration, people listen to a list of words: *Candy, sour, sugar, tooth, heart, taste, dessert, salt, snack, syrup, eat,* and *flavor.* Subsequently, when asked to write down the words they heard, 40 percent wrote down the word *sweet,* even though

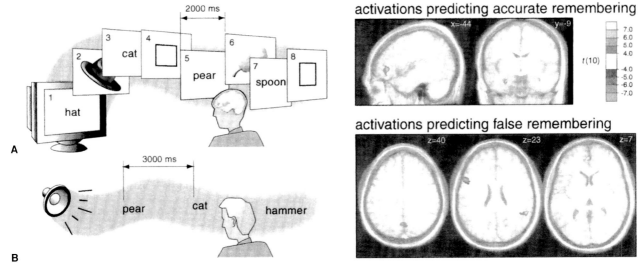

FIGURE 34-16

Neural substrates of false memories. **A:** Functional magnetic resonance imaging data were acquired in a learning phase, when subjects read names of objects and visualized the referents. One-half of the names were followed 2 seconds later by a picture of the object. **B:** In a surprise memory test given outside of the scanner, subjects listened to object names and decided whether they had seen a picture of the corresponding object. On some trials, subjects claimed to have seen a picture of an object that they had only imagined. **C:** Results showed that the left inferior prefrontal cortex and the left anterior hippocampus were more active during learning in response to pictures later remembered compared to pictures later forgotten. **D:** Several different brain areas showed a greater response to words in the learning phase that were later falsely remembered as pictures compared to words not misremembered. Activations that predicted false remembering were found in a brain network important for the generation of visual imagery in response to object names (precuneus, inferior parietal cortex, and anterior cingulate, shown in the left, middle, and right images, respectively). (Reprinted from Gonsalves B, Reber PJ, Gitelman DR, Parrish TB, Mesulam MM, Paller KA. Neural evidence that vivid imagining can lead to false remembering. *Psychol Sci.* 2004;15(10):655–660, with permission.)

it did not appear on the list. Thus, many people in this demonstration failed to discriminate between the words presented and a word strongly associated with all the words but had not itself been presented. The word *sweet* can be thought of as a gist word, a word that represents the other words, which captures the meaning of the whole list. Presumably, the words in the study list evoked a thought of the word *sweet,* either at the time of learning or during the memory test, and people then tended to confuse merely thinking of the word with actually hearing it.

The reconstructive nature of recollection means that the interpretation of eyewitness testimony is not straightforward. Whole episodes are not available in the neocortex, but rather must be pieced together based on fragmentary components and in the context of potentially misleading influences present at the time of retrieval. Studies in adults and children have documented that illusory memories can be created. Children are particularly susceptible to these effects, especially when subjected to leading questions and false suggestions.

Given these features of memory, when memory for childhood abuse is remembered after many years, it is prudent to ask whether the memory is accurate. Genuine examples of memory recovery have been documented, whereby an individual produces a veridical memory for a past traumatic event after not recalling the event for extended periods. Numerous examples of apparent memory recovery have also been subsequently discovered to be instances of false memory. Unfortunately, there is no perfect method, in the absence of independent corroboration, for determining whether a recollective experience is based on a real event.

Infantile Amnesia

The biology of memory has also provided insights relevant to the phenomenon of infantile amnesia—the apparent absence of conscious memory for experiences from approximately the first 3 years of life. Traditional views of infantile amnesia have emphasized repression (psychoanalytic theory) and retrieval failure (developmental psychology). A common assumption has been that adults retain memories of early events but cannot bring them into consciousness. However, it now appears that the capacity for declarative memory does not become fully available until approximately the third year of life, whereas nondeclarative memory emerges early in infancy (e.g., classical conditioning and skill learning). Thus, infantile amnesia results not from the adult's failure to retrieve early memories, but from the child's failure to store them adequately in the first place.

Nevertheless, studies in young infants show that a rudimentary capacity for declarative memory is present even at a few months of age. As a child develops, memories can be retained across increasingly long intervals, and what is represented becomes correspondingly richer and more full of detail. Medial temporal and diencephalic regions seem to be sufficiently developed during these early months and years. What limits the capacity for declarative memory appears to be the gradual development and differentiation of the neocortex.

As the neocortex develops, the memories represented there become more complex, language abilities allow for more elaborate verbal descriptions of events, and a developing sense of self supports autobiographical knowledge. As new strategies emerge for organizing incoming information, declarative memories become more persistent, more richly encoded, and better interconnected with other information. It is not the case that fully formed childhood memories are stored but cannot be retrieved. The perspective

consistent with the current understanding of the biology of memory is that declarative memories formed very early in life are fragmentary, simple, and tied to the specific context of an infant's understanding of the world. They are unlike typical declarative memories in adults, which are imbued with meaning and a complex understanding of events.

Memories and the Unconscious

The existence of multiple memory systems also has implications for issues central to psychoanalytic theory, including the construct of the *unconscious.* How one believes that experience influences current behavior depends on what view one takes of the nature of memory. By the traditional view, memory is a unitary faculty, and representations in memory vary mainly in strength and accessibility. Unconscious material is below some threshold of accessibility but could potentially be made available to consciousness.

The modern, biologic view begins with the distinction between a kind of memory that can be brought to mind—declarative memory—and other kinds of memory that are, by their nature, unconscious. Stored nondeclarative memories are expressed through performance without affording any conscious memory content. Nondeclarative memories shape our personalities in the form of numerous habits and conditioned responses. In this view, one's behavior is indeed affected by events from early life, but the effects of early experience persist in a nondeclarative form without necessarily including an explicit, conscious record of the events. Learned behavior can be expressed through altered dispositions, preferences, conditioned responses, habits, and skills, but exhibiting such behavior need not be accompanied by an awareness that behavior is being influenced by experience, nor is there a necessity that any particular experience has been recorded as a complete episode. That is, an influence from early experience does not require memory of any specific episode. One can be afraid of dogs without remembering being knocked down by a dog as a child. In this case, the fear of dogs is not experienced as a memory. It is experienced as a part of the personality. Furthermore, an intense fear of dogs carries with it no implication that the brain retains a specific record of any early experience that subsequently resulted in fear of dogs.

Behavioral change can occur by acquiring new habits that supersede old ones or by becoming sufficiently aware of a habit that one can to some extent isolate it, countermand it, or limit the stimuli that elicit it. However, one need not become aware of any early formative event in the same sense that one knows the content of declarative memory. The unconscious does not become conscious. Various forms of nondeclarative memory simply influence behavior without having the additional capacity for these influences to become accessible to conscious awareness.

▲ 34.2 Normality and Mental Health

There has been an implicit assumption that mental health could be defined as the antonym of mental illness. In other words, mental health was the absence of psychopathology and synonymous with *normal.* Achieving mental health by alleviating gross pathologic signs and symptoms of illness is also the definition of the mental health model strongly advocated by third-party payers. Indeed, viewing mental health as simply the absence of mental illness is at the heart of much of the debate concerning mental health policies. The great epidemiologic studies of the last half-century also focused on who was mentally ill, and not well.

DEFINING MENTAL HEALTH

Several steps are necessary for defining positive mental health. The first step is to note that "average" is not healthy; it always includes mixing in with the healthy the prevalent amount of psychopathology in the population. For example, in the general population, being of "average" weight or eyesight is unhealthy, and if all sources of biopsychosocial pathology were excluded from the population, the average IQ would be significantly greater than 100.

The second step in discussing mental health is to appreciate the caveat that what is healthy sometimes depends on geography, culture, and the historical moment. Sickle cell trait is unhealthy in New York City, but in the tropics, where malaria is endemic, the sickling of red blood cells may be lifesaving.

The third step is to make clear whether one is discussing *trait* or *state*. Who is physically healthier—an Olympic miler disabled by a temporary but straightforward (state) sprained ankle or a person with type 1 diabetes (trait) with temporarily normal blood sugar? In cross-cultural studies, such differences become especially important. Superficially, an Indian mystic in a state of trance may resemble a person with catatonic schizophrenia, but the mystic does not resemble someone in the schizophrenic condition over time.

The fourth and most crucial step is to appreciate the twofold danger of "contamination by values." On the one hand, cultural anthropology teaches us how fallacious any definition of mental health can be. Competitiveness and scrupulous neatness may be healthy in one culture and regarded as personality disorders in another. Furthermore, if mental health is "good," what is it good for? The self or society? For "fitting in" or for creativity? For happiness or survival? Furthermore, who should be the judge?

MODELS OF MENTAL HEALTH

This chapter contrasts six different empirical approaches to mental health. First, mental health can be conceptualized as *above normal* and a mental state that is objectively desirable, as in Sigmund Freud's definition of mental health, which is the capacity to work and love. Second, from the viewpoint of healthy adult development, mental health can be conceptualized as *maturity*. Third, mental health can be conceptualized in terms of *positive psychology*—as epitomized by the presence of multiple human strengths. Fourth, mental health can be conceptualized as *emotional intelligence* and successful object relations. Fifth, mental health can be conceptualized as *subjective well-being*—a mental state that is subjectively experienced as happy, contented, and desired. Sixth, mental health can be conceptualized as *resilience,* as the capacity for successful adaptation and homeostasis.

Model A: Mental Health as Above Normal

This first perspective differs from the traditional medical approach to health and illness. No manifest psychopathology equals mental health. In this medical model, if one were to put all individuals on a continuum, normality would encompass a significant portion of adults, and abnormality would be the small remainder. This definition of health correlates with the traditional role model of the doctor who attempts to free his patient from grossly observable signs of illness. In other words, in this context, health refers to a

reasonable, rather than an optimal state of functioning. However, as already pointed out, mental health is not normal; it is above average. Some believe that true mental health is the exception, not the rule. Moreover, until recently, some believed that mental health was imaginary.

Model B: Mental Health as Maturity

Unlike other organs of the body that are designed to stay the same, the brain is designed to be plastic. Therefore, just as optimal brain development requires almost a lifetime, so does assessing positive mental health. A 10-year-old's lungs and kidneys are more likely to reflect optimal function than are those of a 60-year-old, but that is not true of a 10-year-old's central nervous system. To some extent, then, adult mental health reflects a continuing process of maturational unfolding. Statistically, physically healthy 70-year-olds are mentally healthier than they were at age 30 years; for example, Laura Carstensen found through prospective studies that individuals are less depressed and show greater emotional modulation at age 70 years than they did at age 30 years.

However, if prospective studies of adult development reveal that the immature brain functions less well than the mature brain, does that mean that adolescents are mentally healthier than toddlers? Are the middle-aged mentally healthier than adolescents? The answer is both yes and no, but the question illustrates that in order to understand mental health, we must first understand what we mean by maturity.

To confirm the hypothesis that maturity and positive mental health are almost synonymous, it is necessary to study the behavior and emotional states of persons over a lifetime. Although such longitudinal studies have come to fruition only recently, all of them illustrate the association of maturity with increasing mental health. After age 50 years, of course, the association between mental health and maturity is contingent on a healthy central nervous system. The ravages of illnesses like brain trauma, major depression, arteriosclerosis, Alzheimer's, and alcoholism must all be avoided.

The association of mental health to maturity is probably mediated not only by progressive brain myelination into the sixth decade but also by the evolution of emotional and social intelligence through experience. Erik Erikson conceptualized that such development produced a "widening social radius." In such a view, life after age 50 years was no longer a staircase leading downward, as in the Pennsylvania Dutch cartoons of life-span development, but a path leading outward. In Erikson's model, the adult social radius expanded over time through the mastery of specific tasks such as "Identity versus Identity Diffusion," "Intimacy versus Isolation," "Generativity versus Stagnation," and "Integrity versus Despair."

Identity.   In such a model, the social radius of each adult developmental task fits inside the next. First, adolescents must achieve an *Identity* that allows them to become separate from their parents, for mental health and adult development cannot evolve through a false self. The task of *Identity* requires mastering the last task of childhood: sustained separation from social, residential, economic, and ideologic dependence on the family of origin. Identity is not just a product of egocentricity, of running away from home, or of marrying to get out of a dysfunctional family. There is a world of difference between the instrumental act of running away from home and the developmental task of knowing where one's family values end and one's values begin. Such separation derives as much from the identification and internalization of important adolescent friends and nonfamily mentors as it does from simple biologic maturation. For example, our accents become relatively fixed by age 16 years and reflect those of our adolescent peer group rather than the accents of our parents.

Intimacy.   Then, young adults should develop *Intimacy,* which permits them to become reciprocally, and not selfishly, involved with a partner. However, living with just one other person in an interdependent, reciprocal, committed, and contented fashion for years and years may seem neither desirable nor possible to a young adult. Once achieved, however, the capacity for intimacy may seem as effortless and desirable as riding a bicycle. Sometimes the relationship is with a person of the same gender; sometimes, it is entirely asexual; and sometimes, as in religious orders, the interdependence is with a community. Superficially, mastery of intimacy may take very different guises in different cultures and epochs, but "mating-for-life" and "marriage-type love" are developmental tasks built into the developmental repertoires of many warm-blooded species, including ours.

Career Consolidation.   *Career Consolidation* is a task that is usually mastered together with or that follows the mastery of intimacy. Mastery of this task permits adults to find a career as valuable as they once found play. On a desert island, one can have a hobby but not a career, for careers involve being of value to other people. Four crucial developmental criteria transform a "job" or hobby into a "career:" Contentment, compensation, competence, and commitment. Such a career can be "wife and mother"—or, in more recent times, "husband and father." To the outsider, the process of Career Consolidation often appears "selfish," but without such "selfishness," one becomes "selfless" and has no "self" to give away in the next stage of generativity. Persons with schizophrenia and individuals with a severe personality disorder often manifest a lifelong inability to achieve either intimacy or sustained, gratifying employment.

Generativity.   *Generativity* involves the demonstration of a clear capacity to care for and guide the next generation. Research reveals that sometime between ages 35 and 55 years, our need for achievement declines, and our need for community and affiliation increases. Depending on the opportunities that the society makes available, generativity can mean serving as a consultant, guide, mentor, or coach to young adults in the larger society. Like leadership, generativity means to be in a caring relationship in which one gives up much of the control that parents retain over young children. Good mentors learn "to hold loosely" and to share responsibility. Generativity reflects the capacity to give the self—finally completed through mastery of the first three tasks of adult development—away. Its mastery is strongly correlated with successful adaptation to old age. This is because, in old age, there are inevitable losses, and these may overwhelm us if we have not continued to grow beyond our immediate family.

Integrity.   Finally, in old age, it is common to feel that some life exists after death and that one is part of something greater than oneself. Thus, the last life task in Erikson's words is *Integrity,* achieving some sense of peace and unity with respect both to one's life and to the whole world. Erikson described integrity as "an experience which conveys some world order and spiritual sense. No matter how dearly paid for, accepting one's life cycle as something that had to be and that, by necessity, permitted no substitutions."

It must be kept in mind that mastery of one life task is not necessarily healthier than mastery of another, for adult development is neither a foot race nor a moral imperative. Instead, these sequential tasks are offered as a road map to help clinicians make sense of where they are and where their patients might be located. One can be a mature 20-year-old, that is, healthy. One can be an immature 50-year-old, which may be unhealthy. Nevertheless, acquiring a social radius that extends beyond the person by definition allows more flexibility and is usually healthier than self-preoccupation. Generativity by ages 40 to 50 years offers a powerful predictor of a contented old age.

Model C: Mental Health as Positive or "Spiritual" Emotions

This model defines mental and spiritual health as the amalgam of the positive emotions that bind us to other human beings. Love, hope, joy, forgiveness, compassion, faith, awe, and gratitude comprise the essential positive and "moral" emotions included in this model. Of great importance, these selected positive emotions all involve human connection. None of the emotions listed is just about the self. These positive emotions appear to be a common denominator of all major faiths. Omitted from the list are five other positive emotions—excitement, interest, contentment (happiness), humor, and a sense of mastery, for a person can feel these latter five emotions alone on a desert island.

Negative emotions originating in the hypothalamus, such as fear and anger, are elaborated in the human amygdala (larger in humans than in other mammals). Of tremendous importance to individual survival, the negative emotions are all about "me." In contrast, positive emotions, apparently generated in the limbic system and unique to mammals, can free the self from the self. People feel the emotions of vengeance and forgiveness deeply, but the long-term results of these two emotions are very different. Negative emotions are crucial for survival in the present time. The positive emotions are more expansive and help us to broaden and build. In the future, they widen one's tolerance for strangers, expand one's moral compass, and enhance one's creativity. Whereas negative emotions narrow attention and miss the forest for the trees, positive emotions, especially joy, make thought patterns more flexible, creative, integrative, and efficient.

The effect of positive emotion on the autonomic (visceral) nervous system has much in common with the relaxation response to meditation. In contrast to the metabolic and cardiac arousal that the fight-or-flight response of negative emotion induces in our *sympathetic* autonomic nervous system, positive emotion via our *parasympathetic* nervous system reduces basal metabolism, blood pressure, heart rate, respiratory rate, and muscle tension. fMRI studies of Kundalini yoga practitioners demonstrate that meditation increases the activity of the hippocampus and the right lateral amygdala, which in turn leads to parasympathetic stimulation and the sensation of deep peacefulness.

Positive emotions have a biologic basis, which means that they have evolved through natural selection. The prosocial emotions probably reflect adaptations that permitted the survival of relatively defenseless *Homo sapiens* and their defenseless children in the African savannah 1 to 2 million years ago.

Evidence for Positive Emotions.   It has taken recent developments in neuroscience and ethology to make positive emotions a subject fit for scientific study. For example, infantile autism, a not uncommon genetic disorder of emotional attachment, was not discovered until 1943 by a Johns Hopkins child psychiatrist, Leo Kanner—in his son. Until then, medicine could not articulate a positive emotion as basic, but as cognitively subtle, as attachment. Today, the congenital lack of empathy and difficulties of attachment in childhood autism can be recognized by any competent pediatrician.

To locate positive emotion in the mammalian limbic system has been a slow, arduous process. In 1955, James Olds, an innovative neuropsychologist, observed that 35 of 41 electrode placements within the limbic system of rats, but only 2 of 35 placements outside of the limbic system, proved sufficiently rewarding to lead to self-stimulation. Also in the 1950s, neurobiologist Paul MacLean pointed out that the limbic structures govern our mammalian capacity not only to remember (cognition), but also to play (joy), to cry out at separation (faith/trust), and to take care of our own (love). Except for rudimentary memory, reptiles express none of these qualities.

Studies using fMRI demonstrated that when individuals subjectively experience existential states of fear, sadness, or pleasure, blood flow increases in limbic areas and decreases in many higher brain areas. Various studies have located pleasurable human experiences (tasting chocolate, winning money, admiring pretty faces, enjoying music, and experiencing orgasmic ecstasy) in limbic areas—especially in the orbitofrontal region, anterior cingulate, and insula. These diverse structures are closely integrated and organized to help us to seek and to recognize all that falls under the rubric of mammalian love and human spirituality.

The *anterior cingulate gyrus* links valence and memory to create attachment. Along with the hippocampus, the anterior cingulate is the brain region most responsible for making the past meaningful. In terms of mediating attachment, the anterior cingulate receives one of the richest dopaminergic innervations of any cortical area. Thus, the cingulate gyrus provides motivational salience not only for lovers but also for drug addicts. The anterior cingulate is crucial in directing whom we should approach and whom we should avoid. Maternal touch, body warmth, and odor via the limbic system and primarily via the anterior cingulate regulate a rat pup's behavior, neurochemistry, endocrine release, and circadian rhythm. Brain imaging studies reveal that the anterior cingulate gyrus is aroused neither by facial recognition of friends per se nor by sexual arousal per se. Instead, anterior cingulate fMRI images light up when a lover gazes at a picture of a partner's face or when a new mother hears her infant's cry.

Perhaps no area of the brain is more ambiguous in its evolutionary heritage or more crucial to mental health than our *prefrontal cortex*. The prefrontal cortex is in charge of estimating rewards and punishments and plays a critical role in adapting and regulating our emotional response to new situations. Thus, the prefrontal lobes are deeply involved in emotional, "moral," and "spiritual" lives.

From an evolutionary standpoint, the human frontal lobes are not different from chimpanzees in terms of the number of neurons. Instead, it is the frontal lobe white matter (the connectivity between neurons through myelinated fibers) that accounts for larger frontal lobes of humans. This connectivity to the limbic system underscores its "executive" function, which includes the ability to delay gratification, comprehend symbolic language, and, most importantly, to establish temporal sequencing. By being able to connect memory of the past to "memory of the future," the frontal lobes establish for *Homo sapiens* predictable cause and effect.

Surgical or traumatic ablation of the ventromedial prefrontal cortex can turn a conscientious, responsible adult into a moral imbecile without any other evidence of intellectual impairment.

The *insula* is another part of the limbic system that is only beginning to be understood. The insula is a medial cortical gyrus located between the amygdala and the frontal lobe. The brain has no sensation; humans feel emotion only in their bodies. The insula helps to bring these visceral feelings into consciousness: The pain in one's heart of grief, the warmth in one's heart of love, and the tightness in one's gut from fear all make their way into consciousness through the insula.

Both the limbic anterior cingulate and insula appear to be active in the positive emotions of humor, trust, and empathy. The higher apes are set apart from other mammals by a unique neural component called the spindle cell. Humans have 20 times more spindle cells than chimps or gorillas (adult chimpanzees average about 7,000 spindle cells; human newborns have four times more, and human adults have almost 200,000 spindle cells). Monkeys and other mammals, with the possible exception of whales and elephants, are lacking in these unique cells. These large, cigar-shaped spindle or "von Economo" neurons appear to be central to the governance of social emotions and moral judgment. Spindle cells may have helped the Great Apes and humans integrate their mammalian limbic systems with their expanding neocortices. Spindle cells are concentrated in the anterior cingulate cortex, the prefrontal cortex, and the insula. More recently, scientists have discovered a particular group of "mirror neurons" in the insula and anterior cingulate. These neurons are more highly developed in humans than in primates and appear to mediate empathy—the experience of "feeling" the emotions of another.

Although the practical applications of this newest model of mental health are still many years away, these findings provide further evidence that the brain and mind are one. In several studies, the prosocial biologic activity of the anterior cingulate cortex and insula was highest in individuals with the highest social awareness (based on objectively scored tests). In other words, there are not only individual biologic differences for negative mental health, but also positive mental health.

Model D: Mental Health as Socioemotional Intelligence

High socioemotional intelligence reflects above-average mental health in the same way that a high IQ reflects above-average intellectual aptitude. Such emotional intelligence lies at the heart of positive mental health. In the *Nicomachean Ethics*, Aristotle defined socioemotional intelligence as follows: "Anyone can become angry—that is easy. However, to be angry with the right person, to the right degree, at the right time, for the right purpose, and in the right way—that is not easy."

All emotions exist to assist in basic survival. Although the exact number of primary emotions is arguable, seven emotions are currently distinguished according to characteristic facial expressions connoting anger, fear, excitement, interest, surprise, disgust, and sadness. The capacity to identify these different emotions in ourselves and others plays a vital role in mental health. The benefits of reading feelings from nonverbal cues have been demonstrated in almost a score of countries. These benefits included being better emotionally adjusted, more popular, and more responsive to others. Empathic children do better in school and are more popular than their peers without being more intelligent. The Head Start Program, a program of the United States Department of Health and Human Services that provides education and other services for low-income children and their families, found that early school success was achieved not by intelligence but by knowing what kind of behavior is expected, knowing how to rein in the impulse to misbehave, being able to wait, and knowing how to get along with other children. At the same time, the child must communicate his or her needs and turn to teachers for help.

Ethologically, emotions are critical to mammalian communication. Because such communications are not always consciously recognized, the more skillful individuals are in identifying their emotions, the more skilled the individual will be in communicating with others, and in empathically recognizing their emotions. Put differently, the more you are skilled in empathy, the more others will value you, and the greater will be your social supports, self-esteem, and intimate relationships.

The following criteria can define social and emotional intelligence:

▶ Accurate conscious perception and monitoring of one's emotions.
▶ Modification of emotions so that their expression is appropriate. This involves the capacity to self-soothe personal anxiety and to shake off hopelessness and gloom.
▶ Accurate recognition of and response to emotions in others.
▶ Skill in negotiating close relationships with others.
▶ Capacity for focusing emotions (motivation) toward the desired goal. This involves delayed gratification and adaptively displacing and channeling impulse.

Some behavioral scientists divide emotions into positive and negative as if negative emotions were unhealthy (this point of view was emphasized in Model C). This tendency is an oversimplification. As with pus, fever, and cough, the negative emotions of sadness, fear, and anger are also crucial to healthy self-preservation. On the one hand, positive emotions like joy, love, interest, and excitement are associated with subjective contentment; on the other hand, although negative emotions interfere with contentment, their expression can be equally healthy.

Advances in Studying Emotional Intelligence. Over the last 15 years, three critical empirical steps have been taken in our understanding of the relationship of socioemotional intelligence to positive mental health.

The first step is that both fMRI studies and neurophysiologic experimentation have led to advances in our understanding of integrating the prefrontal cortex with the limbic system, especially with the amygdala and its connections. As noted in the previous model, these research advances have brought us closer to understanding emotions as neurophysiologic phenomena rather than as Platonic abstractions. The prefrontal cortex is the region of the brain responsible for working memory, and the frontal lobes, through their connections to the amygdala, hippocampus, and other limbic structures, encode emotional learning in a manner quite distinct from both conventional conditioning and declarative memory.

The second step has been the slow but steady progress in conceptualizing and measuring "emotional intelligence." Over the last decade, measures of emotional intelligence have evolved rapidly.

The third advance is the use of videotape to chart emotional interaction. Videos of sustained family interactions reveal that an essential aspect of healthy infant development, of adolescent development, and marital harmony is how partners or parents respond to emotion in others. To ignore, to punish, and to be intimidated or contemptuous of how another feels spells disaster. Children of emotionally attuned parents are better at handling their own emotions and are more effective at soothing themselves when upset. Such children even manifest lower levels of stress hormones and other physiologic indicators of emotional arousal.

There are now many exercises in handling relationships that help couples, business executives, and diplomats to become more skilled at conflict resolution and negotiation. In the last decade, there has also been an increasing effort to teach schoolchildren core emotional and social competencies, sometimes called "emotional literacy." The relevance of these advances in psychology to psychiatry includes teaching emotion recognition and differentiation in eating disorders and teaching anger modulation and finding creative solutions to social predicaments for behavior disorders.

Model E: Mental Health as Subjective Well-Being

Positive mental health does not just involve being a joy to others; one must also experience subjective well-being. Long before humankind considered definitions of mental health, they pondered criteria for subjective happiness. For example, objective social support accomplishes little if, subjectively, the individual cannot feel loved. Thus, the capacity for subjective well-being becomes a vital model of mental health.

Subjective well-being is never categorical. Healthy blood pressure is the objective absence of hypotension and hypertension, but happiness is less neutral. Subjective well-being is not just the absence of misery, but the presence of positive contentment. Nevertheless, if happiness is an inescapable dimension of mental health, happiness is often regarded with ambivalence. If through the centuries, philosophers have sometimes regarded happiness as the highest good, psychologists and psychiatrists have tended to ignore it.

Subjective happiness can have maladaptive as well as adaptive facets. The search for happiness can appear selfish, narcissistic, superficial, and banal. Pleasures can come quickly and soon be gone. Happiness is often based on illusion or dissociative states. Illusory happiness is seen in the character structure associated with bipolar and dissociative disorders. Maladaptive happiness can bring temporary bliss but has no sticking power. In the Study of Adult Development, scaled measures of "happiness" had little predictive power and, often, insignificant association with other subjective and objective measures of contentment. It is because of such ambiguity of meaning that, throughout this section, the term *subjective well-being* will be substituted for happiness.

Empirical Evidence. The mental health issues involved in subjective well-being are complicated and clouded by historical relativism, value judgment, and illusion. Europeans have always been skeptical of the American concern with happiness. Only in the last decade have investigators pointed out that a primary function of positive emotional states and optimism is that they facilitate self-care. Subjective well-being makes available personal resources that can be directed toward innovation and creativity in thought and action. Thus, subjective well-being, like optimism, becomes an antidote to learned helplessness. Again, controlling for income, education, weight, smoking, drinking, and disease, happy people are only half as likely to die at an early age or become disabled as unhappy people.

A distinction can be made between *pleasure* and *gratification*. Pleasure is in the moment, is closely allied with happiness, and involves the satisfaction of impulse and biologic needs. Pleasure is highly susceptible to habituation and satiety. If pleasure involves satisfaction of the senses and emotions, gratification involves joy, purpose, and the satisfaction of "being the best you can be" and meeting aesthetic and spiritual needs.

Subjective (unhappy) distress can be healthy. As ethologically minded investigators have long pointed out, subjective negative affects (e.g., fear, anger, and sadness) can be healthy reminders to seek environmental safety and not to wallow in subjective well-being. If positive emotions facilitate optimism and contentment, fear is the first protection against the external threat; sadness protests against loss and summons help and anger signals trespass.

Clarifying Subjective Well-Being.

Since the 1970s, investigators have made a serious effort to attend to definitional and causal parameters of subjective well-being and address critical questions. One such question is: Is subjective well-being more a function of environmental good fortune or a function of an inborn, genetically based temperament? Put differently, does subjective well-being reflect trait or state? If subjective well-being reflects a safe environment and the absence of stress, it should fluctuate over time, and those individuals who are happy in one domain or time in their lives might not be happy in another.

A second question, but one related to the first, is what is a cause and what is an effect. Are happy people more likely to achieve enjoyable jobs and good marriages, or do conjugal stability and career contentment lead to subjective well-being? Or are such positive associations the result of still a third factor? For example, the absence of a genetic tendency for alcoholism, for major depression, for trait neuroticism, and even for the presence of a chronic wish to give socially desirable answers (impression management) might facilitate both subjective well-being and reports of a good marriage and career contentment.

As with physiologic homeostasis, evolution has prepared humans to make subjective adjustments to environmental conditions. Thus, one can adapt to good and bad events to not remain in a state of either elation or despair. However, humans have a more challenging time adjusting to their genes. Studies of adopted-away twins have demonstrated that half of the variance in subjective well-being is due to heritability. The subjective well-being of monozygotic twins raised apart is more similar than the subjective well-being of heterozygous twins raised together. Among the heritable factors making a significant contribution to high subjective well-being are low trait neuroticism, high trait extraversion, absence of alcoholism, and absence of major depression. In contrast to tested intelligence, when heritable variables are controlled, subjective well-being is not affected by environmental factors like income, parental social class, age, and education.

If subjective well-being were mainly due to the meeting of basic needs, then there should be a relatively low correlation between subjective well-being in work and subjective well-being in recreational settings or subjective well-being in social versus subjective well-being in solitary settings. Because women experience more objective clinical depression than men, the fact that gender is not a determining factor in subjective well-being is interesting. One explanation is that women appear to report both positive and negative affects more vividly than men. In one study, gender accounted for only 1 percent of the variance in happiness, but 13 percent of the variance in the intensity of reported emotional experiences.

Other Sources of Well-Being.

In some instances, the environment *can* be critical to subjective well-being. Young widows remain subjectively depressed for years. Even though their poverty has been endured for centuries, respondents in impoverished nations, like India and Nigeria, report lower subjective well-being than other, more prosperous nations. The loss of a child never stops aching. Although achieving concrete goals like money and fame does not lead to a sustained increase in subjective

well-being, social comparison, such as seeing a neighbor become more prosperous than you, can exert a negative effect on subjective well-being.

The maintenance of self-efficacy, agency, and autonomy make additional environmental contributions to subjective well-being. For example, elders will use their discretionary income to live independently, even though this means living alone rather than with relatives. Subjective well-being is usually higher in democracies than in dictatorships. Assuming responsibility for favorable or unfavorable outcomes (internalization) is another major factor leading to subjective well-being. Placing the blame elsewhere (externalization) significantly reduces subjective well-being. In other words, the mental mechanisms of paranoia and projection make people feel worse rather than better.

Refined methods of measurement of subjective states of mind have included the Positive and Negative Affect Scale (PANAS), which assesses both positive and negative affect, each with 10 affect items. The *Satisfaction with Life Scale* represents the most recent evolution of a general life satisfaction scale. Most recently, the widely validated Short Form 36 (SF-36) has allowed clinicians to assess the subjective cost/benefits of clinical interventions. Because short-lived environmental variables can distort subjective well-being, a consensus is emerging that naturalistic experience-sampling methods are the most valid way to assess subjective well-being. With such sampling methods, research subjects are contacted at random times during the day for several days or weeks and asked to assess their subjective well-being. Finally, to tease verbal self-report from actual subjective experience, physiologic measures of stress (e.g., measuring galvanic skin response and salivary cortisol and filming facial expression by concealed cameras) have also proven useful.

Model F: Mental Health as Resilience

There are three broad classes of coping mechanisms that humans use to overcome stressful situations. First, there is how an individual elicits help from appropriate others: Namely *consciously seeking social support*. Second, there are *conscious cognitive strategies* that individuals intentionally use to master stress. Third, there are *adaptive involuntary coping mechanisms* (often called "defense mechanisms") that distort our perception of internal and external reality to reduce subjective distress, anxiety, and depression.

Involuntary Coping Mechanisms.

Involuntary coping mechanisms reduce conflict and cognitive dissonance during sudden *changes* in internal and external reality. If such changes, in reality, are not "distorted" and "denied," they can result in disabling anxiety or depression, or both. Such homeostatic mental "defenses" shield us from sudden changes in the four lodestars of conflict: impulse (affect and emotion), reality, people (relationships), and social learning (conscience). First, such involuntary mental mechanisms can restore psychological homeostasis by ignoring or deflecting sudden increases in the lodestar of impulse—affect and emotion. Psychoanalysts call this lodestar "id," religious fundamentalists call it "sin," cognitive psychologists call it "hot cognition," and neuroanatomists point to the hypothalamic and limbic regions of the brain.

Second, such involuntary mental mechanisms can provide a mental time-out to adjust to sudden changes in *reality* and self-image, which cannot be immediately integrated. Individuals who initially responded to the television images of the sudden destruction of New York City's World Trade Center as if it were a movie provide a vivid example of the denial of an external reality that was changing too fast for voluntary adaptation. Sudden good news—the instant transition from student to a physician or winning the lottery—can evoke involuntary mental mechanisms as often as can an unexpected accident or a diagnosis of leukemia.

Third, involuntary mental mechanisms can mitigate sudden unresolvable conflict with important *people,* living or dead. People become a lodestar of conflict when one cannot live with them and cannot live without them. Death is such an example; another is an unexpected proposal of marriage. Internal representations of essential people may continue to cause conflict for decades after they are dead yet continue to evoke an involuntary mental response.

Finally, the fourth source of conflict or anxious depression is social learning or conscience. Psychoanalysts call it "superego," anthropologists call it "taboos," behaviorists call it "conditioning," and neuroanatomists point to the associative cortex and the amygdala. This lodestar is not just the result of admonitions from our parents that we absorb before age 5 years, but it is formed by our whole identification, with culture, and sometimes by irreversible learning resulting from overwhelming trauma.

Healthy Involuntary Mental Mechanisms. Longitudinal studies from both Berkeley's Institute of Human Development and Harvard's Study of Adult Development have illustrated the importance of the mature defenses to mental health.

HUMOR. Humor makes life easier. With humor, one sees all, feels much, but does not act. Humor permits the discharge of emotion without individual discomfort and unpleasant effects upon others. Mature humor allows individuals to look directly at what is painful, whereas dissociation and slapstick distract them. However, like the other mature defenses, humor requires the same delicacy as building a house of cards—timing is everything.

ALTRUISM. When used to master conflict, altruism involves an individual getting pleasure from giving to others what the individual would have liked to receive. For example, using reaction formation, a former alcohol abuser works to ban alcohol in his town and annoys his social drinking friends. Using altruism, the same former alcoholic serves as an Alcoholics Anonymous sponsor to a new member—achieving a transformative process that may be life-saving to both the giver and receiver. Many acts of altruism involve a free will, but others involuntarily soothe unmet needs.

SUBLIMATION. The sign of a successful sublimation is neither careful cost accounting nor shrewd compromise, but rather psychic alchemy. By analogy, sublimation permits the oyster to transform an irritating grain of sand into a pearl. In writing his Ninth Symphony, the deaf, angry, and lonely Beethoven transformed his pain into triumph by putting Schiller's "Ode to Joy" to music.

SUPPRESSION. Suppression is a defense that modulates emotional conflict or internal/external stressors through stoicism. Suppression minimizes and postpones but does not ignore gratification. Empirically, this is the defense most highly associated with other facets of mental health. Effective suppression is analogous to a well-trimmed sail; every restriction is precisely calculated to exploit, not hide, the winds of passion. Evidence that suppression is not merely a conscious "cognitive strategy" is provided by the fact that jails would empty if delinquents could learn just to say "No."

ANTICIPATION. If suppression reflects the capacity to keep current impulse in mind and control it, anticipation is the capacity to keep the affective response to an unbearable future event in mind in

manageable doses. The defense of anticipation reflects the capacity to perceive future danger affectively and cognitively and by this means to master conflict in small steps. Examples are that moderate amounts of anxiety before surgery promote postsurgical adaptation and that anticipatory mourning facilitates the adaptation of parents of children with leukemia.

Psychiatry needs to understand how best to facilitate the transmutation of less-adaptive defenses into more-adaptive defenses. One suggestion has been first to increase social supports and interpersonal safety and second, to facilitate the intactness of the central nervous system (e.g., rest, nutrition, and sobriety). The newer forms of integrative psychotherapies using videotape can also catalyze such change by allowing patients actually to see their involuntary coping style.

▲ 34.3 Contributions from the Sociocultural Sciences

SOCIOBIOLOGY AND ETHOLOGY

Sociobiology

The term *sociobiology* was coined in 1975 by Edward Osborne Wilson, an American biologist whose book, called *Sociobiology,* emphasized the role of evolution in shaping behavior. Sociobiology is the study of human behavior based on the transmission and modification of genetically influenced behavioral traits. It explores the ultimate question of *why* specific behaviors or other phenotypes came to be.

Evolution. Evolution is described as any change in the genetic makeup of a population. It is the foundational paradigm from which all of biology arises. It unites ethology, population biology, ecology, anthropology, game theory, and genetics. Charles Darwin (1809–1882) posited that natural selection operates via differential reproduction, in a competitive environment, whereby specific individuals are more successful than others. Given that differences among individuals are at least somewhat heritable, any comparative advantage will result in a gradual redistribution of traits in succeeding generations, such that favored characteristics will be represented in a more significant proportion over time. In Darwin's terminology, *fitness* meant reproductive success.

COMPETITION. Animals vie with one another for resources and territory, the area that is defended for the exclusive use of the animal, and that ensures access to food and reproduction. The ability of one animal to defend a disputed territory or resource is called *resource holding potential,* and the more significant this potential, the more successful the animal.

AGGRESSION. Aggression serves both to increase territory and to eliminate competitors. Defeated animals can emigrate, disperse, or remain in the social group as subordinate animals. A dominance hierarchy in which animals are associated with subtle but well-defined ways is part of every social pattern.

REPRODUCTION. Because behavior is influenced by heredity, those behaviors that promote reproduction and survival are among the most important. Men tend to have a higher variance in reproductive success than do women, thus inclining men to be competitive with other men. Male–male competition can take various forms;

for example, sperm can be thought of as competing for access to the ovum. Competition among women, although genuine, typically involves social undermining rather than overt violence. Sexual dimorphism, or different behavioral patterns for males and females, evolves to ensure the maintenance of resources and reproduction.

ALTRUISM. *Sociobiologists define altruism* as behavior that reduces the personal reproductive success of the initiator while increasing that of the recipient. According to the traditional Darwinian theory, altruism should not occur in nature because, by definition, selection acts against any trait whose effect is to decrease its representation in future generations. However, an array of altruistic behaviors occurs among free-living mammals as well as humans. In a sense, altruism is selfishness at the level of the gene rather than at the level of the individual animal. A classic case of altruism is the female worker classes of individual wasps, bees, and ants. These workers are sterile and do not reproduce, but labor altruistically for the reproductive success of the queen.

Another possible mechanism for the evolution of altruism is group selection. If groups containing altruists are more successful than those composed entirely of selfish members, the altruistic groups succeed at the expense of the selfish ones, and altruism evolves. However, within each group, altruists are at a severe disadvantage relative to selfish members; however well the group as a whole does.

IMPLICATIONS FOR PSYCHIATRY. Evolutionary theory provides possible explanations for some disorders. Some may be manifestations of adaptive strategies. For example, cases of anorexia nervosa may be partially understood as a strategy ultimately caused to delay mate selection, reproduction, and maturation in situations where males are perceived as scarce. Persons who take risks may do so to obtain resources and gain social influence. An erotomanic delusion in a single postmenopausal woman may represent an attempt to compensate for the painful recognition of reproductive failure.

Studies of Identical Twins Reared Apart: Nature versus Nurture.

Studies in sociobiology have stimulated one of the oldest debates in psychology. Does human behavior owe more to nature or to nurture? Curiously, humans readily accept that genes determine most of the behaviors of nonhumans, but tend to attribute their behavior almost exclusively to nurture. However, recent data unequivocally identify our genetic endowment as equally important, if not more important, factors.

The best "experiments of nature" permitting an assessment of the relative influences of nature and nurture are cases of genetically identical twins separated in infancy and raised in different social environments. If nurture is the most important determinant of behavior, they should behave differently. On the other hand, if nature dominates, each will closely resemble the other, despite their having never met. Several hundred pairs of twins separated in infancy, raised in separate environments, and then reunited in adulthood have been rigorously analyzed. Nature has emerged as a critical determinant of human behavior.

Laura R and Catherine S were reunited at the age of 35. They were identical twins that had been adopted by two different families in Chicago. Growing up, neither twin was aware of the other's existence. As children, each twin had a cat named Lucy, and both habitually cracked their knuckles. Laura and Catherine each began to have migraine headaches beginning at the age of 14. Both were elected valedictorian of their high school classes and majored in journalism in

college. Each sister had married a man named John and had given birth to a daughter in wedlock. Both of their marriages fell apart within 2 years. Each twin maintained a successful rose garden and took morning spin classes at their local fitness center. Upon meeting, each twin discovered that the other had also named her daughter Erin and owned a German Sheppard named Rufus. They had similar voices, hand gestures, and mannerisms.

Jack Y and Oskar S, identical twins born in Trinidad in 1933 and separated in infancy by their parents' divorce, were first reunited at age 46. His Catholic mother and grandmother raised Oskar in Nazi-occupied Sudetenland, Czechoslovakia. Jack was raised by his Orthodox Jewish father in Trinidad and spent time on an Israeli kibbutz. Each wore aviator glasses and a blue sport shirt with shoulder plackets, had a trim mustache, liked sweet liqueurs, stored rubber bands on his wrists, read books and magazines from back to front, dipped buttered toast in his coffee, flushed the toilet before and after using it, enjoyed sneezing loudly in crowded elevators to frighten other passengers, and routinely fell asleep at night while watching television. Each was impatient, squeamish about germs, and gregarious.

Bessie and Jessie, identical twins, separated at 8 months of age after their mother's death, were first reunited at age 18. Each had had a bout of tuberculosis, and they had similar voices, energy levels, administrative talents, and decision-making styles. Each had had her hair cut short in early adolescence. Jessie had a college-level education, whereas Bessie had had only 4 years of formal education, yet Bessie scored 156 on intelligence quotient testing, and Jessie scored 153. Each read avidly, which may have compensated for Bessie's sparse education; she created an environment compatible with her inherited potential.

Neuropsychological Testing Results.

The dominant influence of genetics on behavior has been documented in several sets of identical twins on the Minnesota Multiphasic Personality Inventory (MMPI). Twins reared apart generally showed the same degree of genetic influence across the different scales as twins reared together. For example, despite being reared on different continents, in countries with different political systems and different languages, two particularly fascinating identical twin pairs generated scores more closely correlated across 13 MMPI scales than the already tight correlation noted among all tested identical twin pairs, most of whom had shared similar rearing.

Reared-apart twin studies report a high correlation ($r = 0.75$) for IQ similarity. In contrast, the IQ correlation for reared-apart nonidentical twin siblings is 0.38, and for sibling pairs in general, it is in the 0.45 to 0.50 range. Strikingly, IQ similarities are not influenced by similarities in access to dictionaries, telescopes, and original artwork, in parental education and socioeconomic status, or characteristic parenting practices. These data overall suggest that tested intelligence is determined roughly two-thirds by genes and one-third by the environment.

Studies of reared-apart identical twins reveal a genetic influence on alcohol use, substance abuse, childhood antisocial behavior, adult antisocial behavior, risk aversion, and visuomotor skills, as well as on psychophysiological reactions to music, voices, sudden noises, and other stimulation, as revealed by brain wave patterns and skin conductance tests. Moreover, reared-apart identical twins show that genetic influence is pervasive, affecting virtually every measured behavioral trait. For example, many individual preferences previously assumed to be due to nurture (e.g., religious interests, social attitudes, vocational interests, job satisfaction, and work values) are strongly determined by nature.

A selected glossary of some terms used in this section and other ethologic terms is given in Table 34-8.

Table 34-8
Selected Glossary of Ethologic Terms

Action-specific energy	Energy associated with the innate releasing mechanism and specific to a particular behavior pattern, which builds up if the releasing stimulus is not present to activate the behavior pattern; conversely, it is depleted by repetition.
Aggression	Intraspecific conflict manifested by physical attack or social signaling.
Appetitive behavior	Phase of behavior involving the active seeking of sign stimuli and thought to be driven by action-specific energy accumulating through inactivity of the specific behavior pattern.
Consummatory response	Phase of behavior whereby the energy driving the appetitive phase is released. Involves the perception of sign stimuli, the activation of the innate releasing mechanism (IRM), and the performance of the fixed action pattern (FAP).
Critical period	The time during which imprinting must occur, usually shortly after birth or early in life. Also known as "sensitive period."
Displacement activity	A set of behavior patterns occurring alongside an unrelated set of behavior patterns. Originally, irrelevant movements from one behavioral system occurring in the presence of powerful but thwarted drive from another behavior system.
Ethology	The biologic study of behavior. From the Greek ethos, meaning custom, usage, manner, habit. The modern usage is attributed to Oskar Heinroth, Konrad Lorenz's teacher.
Fixed action pattern (FAP)	A genetically determined behavior pattern that is initiated by stimuli particular to the pattern and that consists of species-specific, stereotyped movements.
Imprinting	A specialized form of learning occurring early in life and often influencing behavior later in life. The exposure to the stimulus situation must occur during a particular period, the critical period, and the exposure can be of short duration and without obvious reward. The learning is particularly resistant to change.
Innate	Genetically determined behavior patterns; in theory not influenced by experience.
Innate releasing mechanism (IRM)	Sensory mechanism selectively responsive to specific external stimuli and responsible for triggering the stereotyped motor response.
Instinct	A developmental process resulting in species-typical behavior.
Redirection activity	The venting of one drive from two or more incompatible, but simultaneously activated, drives on some third animal or object.
Ritualization	Process of a behavior pattern being incorporated through evolution into a primary signaling function, frequently with exaggeration and embellishment of some of the movements.

Courtesy of William T. McKinney, Jr., M.D.

Ethology

The systematic study of animal behavior is known as ethology. In 1973, the Nobel Prize in psychiatry and medicine was awarded to three ethologists, Karl von Frisch, Konrad Lorenz, and Nikolaas Tinbergen. Those awards highlighted the particular relevance of ethology, not only for medicine but also for psychiatry.

Konrad Lorenz.   Born in Austria, Konrad Lorenz (1903–1989) is best known for his studies of imprinting. Imprinting implies that, during a specific short period of development, a young animal is highly sensitive to a specific stimulus that then, but not at other times, provokes a specific behavior pattern. Lorenz described newly hatched goslings programmed to follow a moving object and thereby become imprinted rapidly to follow it and, possibly, similar objects. Typically, the mother is the first moving object the gosling sees, but should it see something else first, the gosling follows it. For instance, a gosling imprinted by Lorenz followed him and refused to follow a goose (Fig. 34-17). Imprinting is an essential concept for psychiatrists to understand to link early developmental experiences with later behaviors.

Lorenz also studied the behaviors that function as sign stimuli—that is, social releasers—in communications between individual animals of the same species. Many signals have the character of fixed motor patterns that appear automatically; the reaction of other members of the species to the signals is equally automatic.

Lorenz is also well known for his study of aggression. He wrote about the practical function of aggression, such as territorial defense

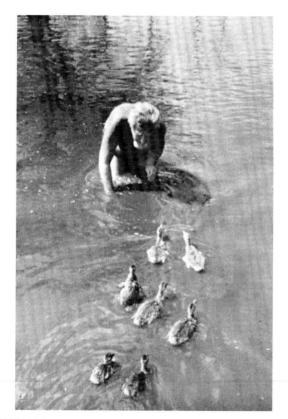

FIGURE 34-17
In a famous experiment, Konrad Lorenz demonstrated that goslings responded to him as if he were the natural mother. (Reprinted from Hess EH. Imprinting, an effect of early experience, imprinting determines later social behavior in animals. *Science.* 1959;130(3368): 133–141, with permission.)

by fish and birds. Aggression among members of the same species is common, but Lorenz pointed out that in normal conditions, it seldom leads to killing or even to serious injury. Although animals attack one another, a certain balance appears between tendencies to fight and flight, with the tendency to fight to be strongest in the center of the territory and the tendency to flight strongest at a distance from the center.

In many works, Lorenz tried to draw conclusions from his ethologic studies of animals that could also be applied to human problems. The postulation of a primary need for aggression in humans, cultivated by the pressure for selecting the best territory, is a primary example. Such a need may have served a practical purpose historically, when humans lived in small groups that had to defend themselves from other groups. Competition with neighboring groups could become an important factor in selection. Lorenz pointed out, however, that this once useful trait may be outliving its survival value, now that we live in an era with weapons that can kill not just individuals but entire populations.

Nikolaas Tinbergen. Born in the Netherlands, Nikolaas Tinbergen (1907–1988), a British zoologist, conducted a series of experiments to analyze various aspects of animal behavior. He was also successful in quantifying behavior and measuring the power or strength of various stimuli in eliciting specific behavior. Tinbergen described displacement activities, which have been studied mainly in birds. For example, in a conflict situation, when the needs for fight and flight are of roughly equal strength, birds sometimes do neither. Instead, they display behavior that appears to be irrelevant to the situation (e.g., a herring gull defending its territory can start to pick grass). Displacement activities of this kind vary according to the situation and the species concerned. Humans can engage in displacement activities when under stress.

Lorenz and Tinbergen described innate releasing mechanisms, animals' responses triggered by releasers, which are specific environmental stimuli. Releasers (including shapes, colors, and sounds) evoke sexual, aggressive, or other responses. For example, big eyes in human infants evoke more caretaking behavior than do small eyes.

In his later work, Tinbergen, along with his wife, studied early childhood autistic disorder. They began by observing the behavior of autistic and typical children when they meet strangers, analogous to the techniques used in observing animal behavior. In particular, they observed in animals the conflict between fear and the need for contact and noted that the conflict could lead to behavior similar to that of autistic children. They hypothesized that, in certain predisposed children, fear can greatly predominate and can also be provoked by stimuli that generally have a positive social value for most children. This innovative approach to studying infantile autistic disorder opened up new avenues of inquiry. Although their conclusions about preventive measures and treatment must be considered tentative, their method shows how ethology and clinical psychiatry can relate to each other.

Karl von Frisch. Born in Austria, Karl von Frisch (1886–1982) conducted studies on changes of color in fish and demonstrated that fish could learn to distinguish among several colors and that their sense of color was somewhat congruent with that of humans. He later went on to study the color vision and behavior of bees and is most widely known for his analysis of how bees communicate with one another—that is, their language, or what is known as their dances. His description of the exceedingly complex behavior of bees prompted an investigation of communication systems in other animal species, including humans.

Characteristics of Human Communication.   Communication is traditionally seen as an interaction in which a minimum of two participants—a sender and a receiver—share the same goal: exchanging accurate information. Although shared interest in accurate communication remains valid in some domains of animal signaling—notably such well-documented cases as the "dance of the bees," whereby foragers inform other workers about the location of food sources—a more selfish and, in the case of social interaction, more accurate model of animal communication has mostly replaced this concept.

Sociobiologic analyses of communication emphasize that because individuals are genetically distinct, their evolutionary interests are similarly distinct, although admittedly with significant fitness overlap, especially among kin, reciprocators, parents and offspring, and mated pairs. Senders are motivated to convey information that induces the receivers to behave in a manner that enhances the senders' fitness. Receivers, similarly, are interested in responding to communication only insofar as such a response enhances their fitness. One crucial way to enhance reliability is to make the signal costly; for example, an animal could honestly indicate its physical fitness, freedom from parasites and other pathogens, and possibly its genetic quality as well by growing elaborate and metabolically expensive secondary sexual characteristics such as the oversized tail of a peacock. Human beings, similarly, can signal their wealth by conspicuous consumption. This approach, known as the *handicap principle,* suggests that effective communication may require that the signaler engages in exceptionally costly behavior to ensure success.

Subhuman Primate Development

An area of animal research that has relevance to human behavior and psychopathology is the longitudinal study of nonhuman primates. Monkeys have been observed from birth to maturity, not only in their natural habitats and laboratory facsimiles but also in laboratory settings that involve various degrees of social deprivation early in life. Social deprivation has been produced through two predominant conditions: social isolation and separation. Socially isolated monkeys are raised in varying degrees of isolation and are not permitted to develop normal attachment bonds. Monkeys separated from their primary caretakers, thereby experience disruption of an already developed bond. Social isolation techniques illustrate the effects of an infant's early social environment on subsequent development (Figs. 34-18 and 34-19), and separation techniques illustrate the effects of loss of a significant attachment figure. The name most associated with isolation and separation studies is Harry Harlow. A summary of Harlow's work is presented in Table 34-9.

In a series of experiments, Harlow separated rhesus monkeys from their mothers during their first weeks. During this time, the monkey infant depends on its mother for nourishment and protection, and physical warmth and emotional security—*contact comfort,* as Harlow first termed it in 1958. Harlow substituted a surrogate mother made from wire or cloth for the real mother. The infants preferred the cloth-covered surrogate mother, which provided contact comfort, to the wire-covered surrogate, which provided food but no contact comfort (Fig. 34-20).

Treatment of Abnormal Behavior.   Stephen Suomi demonstrated that monkey isolates could be rehabilitated if exposed to monkeys that promote physical contact without threatening the isolates with aggression or overly complex play interactions. These

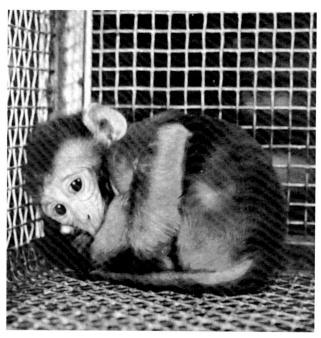

FIGURE 34-18
Social isolate after removal of isolation screen.

Table 34-9
Social Deprivation in Nonhuman Primates

Type of Social Deprivation	Effects
Total isolation (not allowed to develop caretaker or peer bond)	Self-orality, self-clasping, very fearful when placed with peers, unable to copulate. If impregnated, female is unable to nurture young (motherless mothers). If isolation goes beyond 6 mo, no recovery is possible.
Mother-only reared	Fails to leave mother and explore. Terrified when finally exposed to peers. Unable to play or to copulate.
Peer-only reared	Engages in self-orality, grasps others in clinging manner, easily frightened, reluctant to explore, timid as adult, play is minimal.
Partial isolation (can see, hear, and smell other monkeys)	Stares vacantly into space, engages in self-mutilation, stereotyped behavior patterns.
Separation (taken from caretaker after bond has developed)	Initial protest stage changing to despair 48 hours after separation; refuses to play. Rapid reattachment when returned to mother.

Adapted from work of Harry Harlow, M.D.

monkeys were called therapist monkeys. To fill such a therapeutic role, Suomi chose normal young monkeys that would play gently with the isolates and approach and cling to them. Within 2 weeks, the isolates were reciprocating the social contact, and their incidence of abnormal self-directed behaviors began to decline significantly. By the end of the 6-month therapy period, the isolates were actively initiating play bouts with both the therapists and each other, and most of their self-directed behaviors had disappeared. The isolates were observed closely for the next 2 years, and their improved behavioral repertoires did not regress over time. The results of this and subsequent monkey-therapist studies underscored the potential reversibility of early cognitive and social deficits at the human level. The studies also served as a model for developing treatments for socially retarded and withdrawn children.

Several investigators have argued that social separation manipulations with nonhuman primates provide a compelling basis for animal models of depression and anxiety. Some monkeys react to

separations with behavioral and physiologic symptoms similar to those seen in depressed human patients; both ECT and tricyclic drugs effectively reverse the symptoms in monkeys. Not all separations produce depressive reactions in monkeys, just as separation does not always precipitate depression in humans, young and old.

Individual Differences. Recent research has revealed that some rhesus monkey infants consistently display fearfulness and anxiety in situations where similarly reared peers to show normal exploratory behavior and play. These situations generally involve exposure to a novel object or situation. Once the object or situation has become familiar, any behavioral differences between the anxiety-prone, timid infants and their outgoing peers disappear, but the individual differences appear to be stable during development. Infant monkeys at 3 to 6 months of age that are at high risk for fearful or anxious reactions tend to remain at high risk for such reactions, at least until adolescence.

A long-term follow-up study of these monkeys has revealed some behavioral differences between fearful and nonfearful female monkeys when they become adults and have their first infants. Usually, fearful female monkeys who grow up in socially benign and stable environments become fine mothers, but fearful female monkeys who have reacted with depression to frequent social separations during childhood are at high risk for maternal dysfunction; more than 80 percent of these mothers either neglect or abuse their first offspring. However, nonfearful female monkeys that encounter the same number of social separations but do not react to any of these separations with depression turn out to be good mothers.

Experimental Disorders

Stress Syndromes. Several researchers, including Ivan Petrovich Pavlov in Russia and W. Horsley Gantt and Howard Scott Liddell in the United States, studied the effects of stressful environments on animals, such as dogs and sheep. Pavlov produced a phenomenon

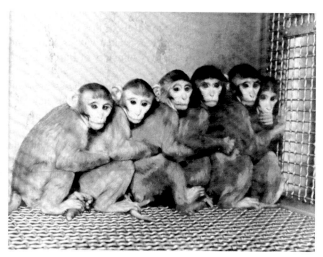

FIGURE 34-19
Choo-choo phenomenon in peer-only-reared infant rhesus monkeys.

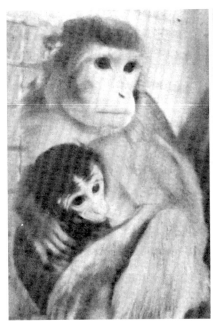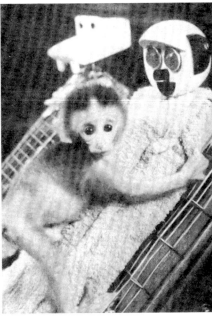

FIGURE 34-20
Monkey infant with mother (**left**) and with cloth-covered surrogate (**right**).

in dogs, which he labeled *experimental neurosis,* by using a conditioning technique that led to symptoms of extreme and persistent agitation. The technique involved teaching dogs to discriminate between a circle and an ellipse and then progressively diminishing the difference between them. Gantt used the term *behavior disorders* to describe the reactions he elicited from dogs forced into similar conflictual learning situations. Liddell described the stress response he obtained in sheep, goats, and dogs as *experimental neurasthenia,* which was produced in some cases by merely doubling the number of daily test trials in an unscheduled manner.

Learned Helplessness. The learned helplessness model of depression, developed by Martin Seligman, is an excellent example of an experimental disorder. Dogs were exposed to electric shocks from which they could not escape. The dogs eventually gave up and did not attempt to escape new shocks. The apparent giving up generalized to other situations, and eventually, the dogs always appeared to be helpless and apathetic. Because the cognitive, motivational, and affective deficits displayed by the dogs resembled symptoms common to human depressive disorders, learned helplessness, although controversial, was proposed as an animal model of human depression. In connection with learned helplessness and the expectation of inescapable punishment, research on subjects has revealed brain release of endogenous opiates, destructive effects on the immune system, and elevation of the pain threshold.

A social application of this concept involves schoolchildren who have learned that they fail in school no matter what they do; they view themselves as helpless losers, and this self-concept causes them to stop trying. Teaching them to persist may reverse the process, with excellent results in self-respect and school performance.

Unpredictable Stress. Rats subjected to chronic unpredictable stress (crowding, shocks, irregular feeding, and interrupted sleep time) show decreases in movement and exploratory behavior; this finding illustrates the roles of unpredictability and lack of environmental control in producing stress. These behavioral changes can be reversed by antidepressant medication. Animals under experimental stress (Fig. 34-21) become tense, restless, hyperirritable, or inhibited in specific conflict situations.

Dominance. Animals in a dominant position in a hierarchy have certain advantages (e.g., mating and feeding). Being more dominant than peers is associated with elation, and a fall in position in the hierarchy is associated with depression. When persons lose jobs, are replaced in organizations, or otherwise have their dominance or hierarchical status changed, they can experience depression.

Temperament. Temperament mediated by genetics plays a role in behavior. For example, one group of pointer dogs was bred for fearfulness and a lack of friendliness toward persons, and another group was bred for the opposite characteristics. The phobic dogs were extremely timid and fearful and showed decreased exploratory capacity, increased startle response, and cardiac arrhythmias. Benzodiazepines diminished these fearful, anxious responses. Amphetamines and cocaine aggravated the responses of genetically nervous dogs to a greater extent than they did the responses of stable dogs.

Brain Stimulation. Pleasurable sensations have been produced in humans and animals through self-stimulation of specific brain areas, such as the medial forebrain bundle, the septal area, and the lateral hypothalamus. Rats have engaged in repeated self-stimulation (2,000 stimulations per hour) to gain rewards. Catecholamine production increases with self-stimulation of the brain area, and drugs that decrease catecholamines decrease the process. The centers for sexual pleasure and opioid reception are closely related anatomically. Heroin addicts report that the so-called rush after intravenous injection of heroin is akin to an intense sexual orgasm.

Pharmacologic Syndromes. With the emergence of biologic psychiatry, many researchers have used pharmacologic means to produce syndrome analogs in animal subjects. Two classic examples are the reserpine (Serpasil) model of depression and the amphetamine psychosis model of paranoid schizophrenia. In the depression studies, animals given the norepinephrine-depleting drug reserpine exhibited behavioral abnormalities analogous to major depressive disorder in humans. The behavioral abnormalities produced

FIGURE 34-21
The monkey on the left, known as the executive monkey, controls whether both will receive an electric shock. The decision-making task produces a state of chronic tension. Note the more relaxed attitude of the monkey on the **right**. (From U.S. Army photographs, with permission.)

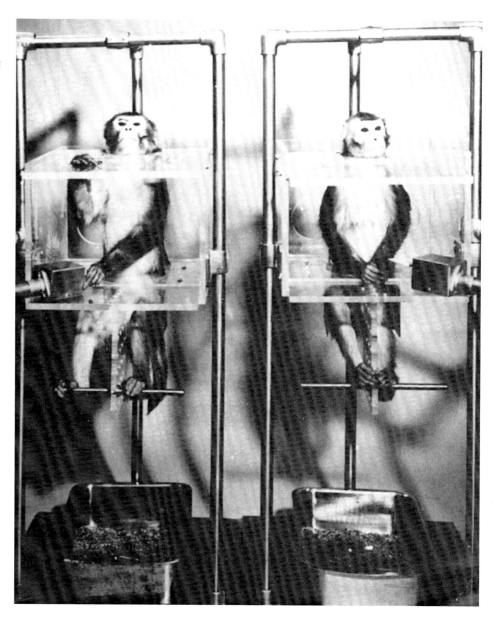

were generally reversed by antidepressant drugs. These studies tended to corroborate the theory that depression in humans is, in part, the result of diminished levels of norepinephrine. Similarly, animals given amphetamines acted in a stereotypical, inappropriately aggressive, and frightened manner that resembled paranoid psychotic symptoms in humans. These models are considered too simplistic in their concepts of cause, but they remain as early paradigms for this type of research.

Studies have also been done on the effects of catecholamine-depleting drugs on monkeys during separation and reunion periods. These studies showed that catecholamine depletion and social separation could interact in a highly synergistic fashion and yield depressive symptoms in subjects for whom mere separation or low-dose treatment alone does not suffice to produce depression.

Reserpine has produced a severe depression in humans and, as a result, is rarely used as either an antihypertensive (its original indication) or an antipsychotic. Similarly, amphetamine and its congeners (including cocaine) can induce psychotic behavior in persons who use it in overdose or over long periods.

Sensory Deprivation

The history of sensory deprivation and its potentially deleterious effects evolved from instances of aberrant mental behavior in explorers, shipwrecked sailors, and prisoners in solitary confinement. Toward the end of World War II, startling confessions, induced by the brainwashing prisoners of war, caused a rise of interest in this psychological phenomenon brought about by the deliberate diminution of sensory input.

To test the hypothesis that an essential element in brainwashing is prolonged exposure to sensory isolation, D. O. Hebb and his coworkers brought solitary confinement into the laboratory. They demonstrated that volunteer subjects—under conditions of visual, auditory, and tactile deprivation for periods of up to 7 days—reacted with increased suggestibility. Some subjects also showed characteristic symptoms of the sensory deprivation state: anxiety, tension, inability to concentrate or organize thoughts, increased suggestibility, body illusions, somatic complaints, intense subjective emotional distress, and vivid sensory imagery—usually visual and sometimes reaching the proportions of hallucinations with a delusionary quality.

Psychological Theories.

Anticipating psychological explanation, Sigmund Freud wrote: "It is interesting to speculate what could happen to ego function if the excitations or stimuli from the external world were either drastically diminished or repetitive. Would there be an alteration in the unconscious mental processes and an effect upon the conceptualization of time?"

Indeed, under conditions of sensory deprivation, the abrogation of such ego functions as perceptual contact with reality and logical thinking brings about confusion, irrationality, fantasy formation, hallucinatory activity, and wish-dominated mental reactions. In the sensory-deprivation situation, the subject becomes dependent on the experimenter and must trust the experimenter to satisfy such basic needs as feeding, toileting, and physical safety. A patient undergoing psychoanalysis may be in a kind of sensory deprivation room (e.g., a soundproof room with dim lights and a couch) in which primary-process mental activity is encouraged through free association.

COGNITIVE.

Cognitive theories stress that the organism is an information-processing machine, whose purpose is an optimal adaptation to the perceived environment. Without sufficient information, the machine cannot form a cognitive map against which the current experience is matched. Disorganization and maladaptation then result. To monitor their behavior and to attain optimal responsiveness, persons must receive continuous feedback; otherwise, they are forced to project outward idiosyncratic themes that have little relation to reality. This situation is similar to that of many psychotic patients.

Physiologic Theories.

The maintenance of optimal conscious awareness and accurate reality testing depends on a necessary state of alertness. This alert state, in turn, depends on a constant stream of changing stimuli from the external world, mediated through the ascending reticular activating system in the brainstem. In the absence or impairment of such a stream, as occurs in sensory deprivation, alertness drops away, direct contact with the outside world diminishes, and impulses from the inner body and the central nervous system may gain prominence. For example, idioretinal phenomena, inner ear noise, and somatic illusions may take on a hallucinatory character.

TRANSCULTURAL PSYCHIATRY

Culture is defined as a set of meanings, norms, beliefs, values, and behavior patterns shared by people. These values include social relationships, language, nonverbal expression of thoughts and emotions, moral and religious beliefs, rituals, technology, and economic beliefs and practices, among other items. Culture has six essential components: (1) Culture is learned; (2) culture can be passed on from one generation to the next; (3) culture involves a set of meanings in which words, behaviors, events, and symbols have meanings agreed upon by the cultural group; (4) culture acts as a template to shape and orient future behaviors and perspectives within and between generations, and to take account of novel situations encountered by the group; (5) culture exists in a constant state of change; and (6) culture includes patterns of both subjective and objective components of human behavior. Also, culture shapes which and how psychiatric symptoms are expressed; culture influences the meanings that are given to symptoms; and culture affects

the interaction between the patient and the health care system, as well as between the patient and the physician and other clinicians with whom the patient and family interact.

Race is a concept, the scientific validity of which is now considered highly questionable, by which human beings are grouped primarily by physiognomy. Its effect on individuals and groups, however, is considerable, due to its reference to physical, biologic, and genetic underpinnings, and because of the intensely emotional meanings and responses, it generates. *Ethnicity* refers to the subjective sense of belonging to a group of people with a common national or regional origin and shared beliefs, values, and practices, including religion. It is part of every person's identity and self-image.

Cultural Formulation

Culture plays a role in mental health and mental illness; therefore, a cultural assessment should be a component of every complete psychiatric assessment. The outline for cultural formulation found in the *Diagnostic and Statistical Manual of Mental Disorders* (DSM-5) is intended to give clinicians a framework for assessing the role of culture in psychiatric illness. Its purposes are (1) to enhance the application of diagnostic criteria in multicultural environments; (2) cultural conceptualizations of distress; (3) psychosocial stressors and cultural features of vulnerability and resilience; (4) to enable the clinician to systematically describe the patient's cultural and social reference groups and their relevance to clinical care; and (5) to identify the effect that cultural differences may have on the relationship between the patient and family and the treating clinician, as well as how such cultural differences affect the course and the outcome of treatment provided.

The outline for cultural formulation consists of five areas of assessment: (1) cultural identity of the individual; (2) cultural explanations of the individual's illness; (3) cultural factors related to psychosocial environment and levels of functioning; (4) cultural elements of the relationship between the individual and the clinician; and (5) overall cultural assessment for diagnosis and care.

Cultural Identity of the Individual.

Cultural identity refers to the characteristics shared by a person's cultural group. Identity allows for a self-definition. Factors that comprise an individual's cultural identity include race, ethnicity, country of origin, language use, religious beliefs, socioeconomic status, migration history, the experience of acculturation, and the degree of affiliation with the individual's group of origin. Cultural identity emerges throughout the individual's life and in a social context. It is not a fixed trait of an individual or of the group of which the individual is part. An individual may have several cultural reference groups.

The clinician should encourage the patient to describe the component aspects of their cultural identity. Evaluating the cultural identity of the patient allows identification of potential areas of strength and support that may enhance treatment effectiveness, as well as vulnerabilities that may interfere with the progress of treatment. Eliciting this data permits the identification of unresolved cultural conflicts that may be addressed during treatment. These conflicts can be between the various aspects of the patient's identity and between traditional and mainstream cultural values and behavioral expectations affecting the individual. Knowledge of the patient's cultural identity allows the clinician to avoid misconceptions based on inadequate background information or stereotypes related to race, ethnicity and other aspects of cultural identity. Also, it helps build rapport because the clinician is attempting to understand the individual as a person and not just a representative of the cultural groups that have shaped the patient's identity.

Cultural Explanations of the Individual's Illness.

The explanatory model of illness is the patient's understanding of and attempts to explain why they became ill. The explanatory model defines the culturally acceptable means of expression of the symptoms of the illness or *idioms of distress,* the particular way individuals within a specific cultural group report symptoms, and their behavioral response to them heavily influenced by cultural values. The cultural explanations of illness may also help define the sick role or behavior the patient assumes. The explanatory model of illness includes the patient's beliefs about their prognosis and the treatment options they would consider. The patient's explanatory model may be only vaguely conceptualized or may be quite clearly defined, and it may include several conceptual perspectives that could conflict with one another. Formulation of a collaborative model that is acceptable to both the clinician and the patient is the sought-for endpoint, which would include an agreed-upon set of symptoms to be treated and an outline of treatment procedures to be used.

Difficulties may arise when there are conceptual differences in the explanatory model of illness between clinician, patient, family, and community. Conflicts between the patient's and the clinician's explanatory models may lead to diminished rapport or treatment noncompliance. Conflicts between the patient's and the family's explanatory models of illness may result in a lack of support from the family and family discord. Conflicts between the patient's and the community's explanatory models could lead to social isolation and stigmatization of the patient.

Examples of the more common explanatory models of illness include the *moral model, the religious model,* the *magical* or *supernatural explanatory model,* the *medical model,* and the *psychosocial stress model.* The *moral model* implies that the patient's illness is caused by a moral defect such as selfishness or moral weakness. The *religious model* suggests that the patient is being punished for a religious failing or transgression. The *magical* or *supernatural explanatory model* may involve attributions of sorcery or witchcraft as being the cause of the symptoms. The *medical model* attributes the patient's illness primarily to a biologic etiology. The *psychosocial model* infers that overwhelming psychosocial stressors cause or are primary contributors to the illness.

Culture has both direct and indirect effects on help-seeking behavior. In many cultural groups, an individual and their family may minimize symptoms due to stigma associated with seeking assistance for psychiatric disorders. Culture affects the patient's expectations of treatment, such as whether the clinician should assume an authoritarian, paternalistic, egalitarian, or nondirective demeanor in the treatment process.

Cultural Factors Related to Psychosocial Environment and Level of Functioning.

Understanding the patient's family dynamics and cultural values are integral to assessing the patient's psychosocial environment. The definition of what constitutes a family and the roles of individuals in the family differ across cultures. This includes an understanding of the patient's cultural group and its relationship to the mainstream culture or cultures. It includes the patient's life experience of racial and ethnic discrimination. For immigrants and refugees, it includes the individual's and family's perceptions of the openness of the host society toward people of their country and region of origin, their racial, ethnic, religious, and other attributes. The patient and family may identify strongly or weakly with communal sources of support familiar from their country or region of origin, or they may identify along the same gradient with communal sources of support in the host culture.

Cultural Elements of the Relationship between the Individual and the Clinician.

The cultural identity of the clinician and the mental health team has an impact on patient care. The culture of mental health care professionals influences diagnosis and treatment. Clinicians who have an understanding of their own cultural identity may be better prepared to anticipate the cultural dynamics that may arise in interactions with people of diverse cultural backgrounds. Unacknowledged differences between the clinician's and patient's cultural identity can result in assessment and treatment that is unintentionally biased and stressful for all. Clinicians need to examine their assumptions about other cultures to be optimally effective in serving the culturally diverse patient populations that are the norm in most contemporary medical facilities.

Culture influences transference and counter-transference in the clinical relationship between people seeking psychiatric care and their treating clinicians. Transference relationships and dynamics are affected when the patient and clinician have different cultural background characteristics. A perceived social power differential between the patient and clinician could lead to overcompliance, resistance in the exploration of family and social conflict situations, or to the clinician being conceptualized as a cultural role model or stereotype.

Overall Cultural Assessment for Diagnosis and Care.

The treatment plan should include the use of culturally appropriate health care and social services. Interventions also may be focused on the family and social levels. In making a psychiatric diagnosis, the clinician should consider principles of cultural relativism and not fall prone to category fallacy. Many psychiatric disorders show cross-cultural variation. Objective evaluation of the multiple possible effects of culture on psychopathology can be a challenging task for the clinician. Diagnostic dilemmas may arise in dealing with patients of diverse cultural backgrounds. Some of these dilemmas may include problems in judging distortion from reality, problems in assessing unfamiliar behaviors and distinguishing pathologic from normal cultural behavior.

Migration, Acculturation, and Acculturative Stress

From the time of the first significant surge of immigration to the United States in the 1870s, and for the next 100 years, the predominant national sentiment toward immigrants, as in most other host countries, was that they should acculturate to the normative behaviors and values of the majority or mainstream culture of the host population. Most immigrants had the same wish to assimilate, to become part of the *melting pot.* This process of acculturative change can be seen as unidirectional, as individuals who identified themselves as part of immigrant, indigenous, and other minority groups both rejected and progressively lost distinctive aspects of their cultural heritage in favor of becoming part of the mainstream majority culture of the host country. In countries that encouraged this outcome of acculturation, people were expected to progress from unacculturated, through the gradient of minimally, moderately, and fully acculturated.

The intensity of acculturative stress experienced by immigrant and other minority groups, and the individuals comprising those groups, has been directly proportional to the openness of the host government and population. The central issue is to what extent are immigrants' and other minority groups' customs, values, and differences from the majority population of the host country accepted, encouraged, and welcomed as an enrichment of the host country instead of being seen as alien and unwelcome. The *acceptance position* encourages the cultural integration of immigrants, whereas the *rejection position* encourages either cultural exclusion or cultural assimilation.

To assess the outcome of acculturative stress, for groups and their component individuals, two determining factors need to be considered. The first is the extent to which the group and its members value and wish to preserve their cultural uniqueness, including the language, beliefs, values, and social behaviors that define the group. The second factor is the mirror-image issue of the extent to which the group and its members value and wish to increase their contact and involvement with other groups, particularly the majority culture. This conceptual framework leads to four possible outcomes of acculturative stress that are not conceptualized along the unidirectional gradient from unacculturated to wholly acculturated.

The four possible outcomes are *rejection, integration, assimilation,* and *marginalization. Rejection* is characterized by individuals' wishes, both conscious and intuitive, to maintain their cultural integrity, whether by actively resisting the incorporation of the values and social behavior patterns of another cultural group or groups with whom they have regular contact or by disengaging themselves from contact with and the influence of those other cultural groups. Some religious cults are examples of rejection.

Integration, as an outcome of acculturative stress, derives from the wish to both maintain a firm sense of one's cultural heritage and not abandon those values and behavioral characteristics that define the uniqueness of one's culture of origin. At the same time, such individuals can incorporate enough of the value system and norms of behavior of the other cultural group with which they interact closely, to feel and behave like members of that cultural group, principally the majority host culture. Accordingly, the defining feature of integration is psychological: It is the gradual process of formulation of a bicultural identity, a sense of self that intertwines the unique characteristics of two cultures.

Assimilation is the psychological process of the conscious and unconscious giving up of the unique characteristics of one's culture of origin in favor of the more or less complete incorporation of the values and behavioral characteristics of another cultural group, usually, but not always, the majority culture. Examples include involuntary migration when war and social upheaval necessitate such changes for purposes of survival. However, there are many other life circumstances, including racial, ethnic, and religious discrimination, that motivate people to overlook, suppress, or deny aspects of their cultural heritage to have a seamless fit within another group. The price of such an effort, in terms of intrapsychic conflict, can be high.

Marginalization is defined by the psychological characteristics of rejection or the progressive loss of valuation of one's cultural heritage, while at the same time rejecting, or being alienated from, the defining values and behavioral norms of another cultural group, usually that of the majority population. This is the psychological outcome of acculturative stress that is closest to the concept of identity diffusion.

Psychiatric Assessment of Immigrants and Refugees

Migration History. Mental illness among immigrants and refugees may have been present before migration, may have developed during the immigration process, such as during months or years living in refugee camps, or presented for the first time in immigration. The immigration process and premigration trauma may precipitate the manifestation of underlying symptoms or result in exacerbation of a preexisting disorder. Obtaining a thorough migration history will help understand the background and precipitating stressors and help guide the development of an appropriate treatment plan.

The premigration history includes inquiry about the patient's social support network, social and psychological functioning, and significant premigration life events. Information about the country and region of origin, the family history in the country of origin—including an understanding of family members who may have decided not to immigrate—educational and work experiences in the country of origin, and prior socioeconomic status should be obtained. Also, premigration political issues, trauma, war, and natural disaster faced by the patient and family in the country or region of origin should be explored. For those who had to escape persecution, warfare, or natural disaster, what were the means of escape, and what type of trauma was suffered before and during migration? Traumatic life events are not limited just to refugees. Immigration may result in losses of social networks, including family and friends, material losses, business, career, property, and loss of the cultural milieu, including their familiar community and religious life. Premigration planning includes reasons for immigrating, duration, and extent of planning, premigration aspirations, and beliefs about the host country. The type of migration experience, whether as voluntary immigrants or as unprepared refugees, can have profoundly different effects on migrants' mental health.

The Mental Status Examination. As with any patient, conducting a mental status examination is a central component of the psychiatric examination. However, its interpretation in culturally distinct groups and immigrant populations requires caution, as it may be culturally biased. The patient's response is molded by their culture of origin, educational level, and type of acculturative adaptation. The components of the standardized mental status examination are the following: cooperation, appearance, and behavior, speech, affect, thought process, thought content, cognition, insight, and judgment. Cultural differences are wide and varied in dress and grooming. Facial expressions and body movements used in the expression of affect may be more reflective of normal cultural manifestations than pathology. If the clinician is unfamiliar with the individual's culture and the patient's fluency in the language of the host country is limited, the clinician must use caution in interpreting disturbances of speech and thought process, perception, and affect. The presence of hallucinations, for example, can be easily misinterpreted, such as hearing encouraging or clarifying comments from deceased family members, normative experiences in many cultures. The clinician should not assume that the patient understands what the clinician is trying to communicate, and miscommunication involving interpreters is a common problem. The cognitive examination may be particularly tricky. Education and literacy have an important and biasing role. The patient may need adequate time to fully express him- or herself through repeating questions and restating questions to reduce miscommunication. Asking about the meaning of proverbs unfamiliar to the patient may be an inappropriate means of determining abstract thinking. An accurate mental status examination can be accomplished when one allows additional time for clarification of concepts.

Immigration Acculturation and Mental Health

Many countries have had difficulty coping with the surging numbers of migrants. This has led to more significant restrictions on migrant numbers, partly in response to public sentiment that the social and cultural integrity of the nation has become threatened, even undermined, by waves of migrants from other countries and cultures. During the last 10 years, fears of terrorist violence and civil disruption have led many countries to adopt increasingly restrictive and sometimes punitive policies toward legal and illegal migrants, refugees, and asylum seekers. This trend has been observed in the United States, in some countries of the European Union, and Australia.

Racial and Ethnic Differences in Psychiatric Disorders in the United States

Several community-based epidemiologic studies in the United States have examined the rates of disorders across specific ethnic groups. These studies have found a lower than expected prevalence of psychiatric disorders among disadvantaged racial and ethnic minority groups. African Americans were found to have lower rates of major depression in the Epidemiological Catchment Area study. The lifetime prevalence rates for major depression for whites was 5.1 percent; for Hispanics, 4.4 percent; and for African Americans, 3.1 percent. African Americans, however, had higher rates for all lifetime disorders combined. This finding of differential rates could be explained by adjusting for socioeconomic status.

The National Comorbidity Study (NCS) found lower lifetime prevalence rates of mental illness among African Americans than whites, and in a particular mood, anxiety, and substance use disorders. The lifetime rates for mood disorders were 19.8 percent for whites, 17.9 percent for Hispanic Americans, and 13.7 percent for African Americans. The National Health and Nutrition Examination Survey-III also found lifetime rates of major depression significantly higher among whites, 9.6 percent, than African Americans, 6.8 percent, or Mexican Americans, 6.7 percent. Although African Americans had a lower lifetime risk of mood disorders than whites, once diagnosed, they were more likely to remain persistently ill.

NCS rates for anxiety disorders were 29.1 percent among whites, 28.4 percent for Hispanic Americans, and 24.7 percent for African Americans. The rates for lifetime substance use disorders for the three groups, whites, Hispanic Americans, and African Americans, were 29.5, 22.9, and 13.1 percent. Hispanic Americans, and in particular Mexican Americans, were found to be at lower risk for substance use and anxiety disorders than whites. In an epidemiologic study conducted in Florida, substantially lower rates were observed among African Americans for depressive disorders and substance use disorders. The lower rate for substance use disorders was also found in the National Epidemiological Survey on Alcohol and Related Conditions, with whites having a prevalence rate of 1-year alcohol use disorders of 8.9 percent; Hispanic Americans, 8.9 percent; African Americans, 6.9 percent; Asian Americans, 4.5 percent; and Native Americans, 12.2 percent. This study also found lower lifetime rates for major depression among Hispanic Americans, 10.9 percent, compared to whites, 17.8 percent. In 2007, the National Survey of American Life compared rates of major depression between Caribbean blacks, African Americans, and whites. Although there were no significant differences in 1-year prevalence between the three groups, lifetime rates were highest among whites, 17.9 percent, followed by Caribbean blacks, 12.9 percent, and African Americans, 10.4 percent. The chronicity of

major depressive disorder was higher for African Americans and Caribbean blacks, approximately 56 percent, while much lower for whites, 38.6 percent. This study was consistent with findings from the NCS that concluded that members of disadvantaged racial and ethnic groups in the United States do not have an increased risk for psychiatric disorders; however, once diagnosed, they do tend to have more persistent disorders.

Although African Americans have a lower prevalence rate for mood, anxiety, and substance use disorders, this may not be the case for schizophrenia. The Child Health and Development Study found that African Americans were about threefold more likely than whites to be diagnosed with schizophrenia. The association may be partly explained by African American families having lower socioeconomic status, a significant risk factor for schizophrenia.

A more detailed examination of differences across racial groups was included in the National Comorbidity Study Replication (NCS-R). Non-Hispanic African Americans and Hispanic Americans were at significantly lower risk than non-Hispanic whites for anxiety disorders and mood disorders. Non-Hispanic African Americans had lower rates of substance use disorders than non-Hispanic whites. More specifically, both minority groups were at lower risk for depression, generalized anxiety disorder, and social phobia. Also, Hispanic Americans had a lower risk for dysthymia, oppositional-defiant disorder, and attention-deficit/hyperactivity disorder. Non-Hispanic African Americans had a lower risk for panic disorder, substance use disorders, and early-onset impulse-control disorders. The lower rates among Hispanic Americans and African Americans compared to non-Hispanic whites appear to be due to reduced lifetime risk of disorders instead of the persistence of chronic disorders. The researchers concluded that the pattern of racial–ethnic differences in risk for psychiatric disorders suggests the presence of protective factors that originate in childhood and have generalized effects, as the lower lifetime risk for both Hispanic Americans and African Americans begins before age 10 years for depression and anxiety disorders. The retention of ethnic identification and participation in communal, religious, and other activities have been suggested as protective factors that may decrease the lifetime risk for psychiatric disorders in close-knit ethnic minority communities. Cultural differences in response to psychiatric diagnostic survey items may be another possible explanation for these findings. However, disadvantaged ethnic groups usually overreport in studies measuring psychological distress, whereas these studies find lower rates.

Discrimination, Mental Health, and Service Utilization

Disparities in Mental Health Services. Studies, including recent ones, have shown that racial and ethnic minorities in the United States receive more limited mental health services than whites. Analysis of medical expenditures in the United States has shown that the mental health care system provides comparatively less care to African Americans and Hispanic Americans than to whites, even after controlling for income, education, and availability of health insurance. African Americans have about a 10 percent probability of receiving any mental health expenditure, compared to 20 percent for whites. Hispanic Americans are about 40 percent less likely than whites to receive any mental health expenditure. Total mental health expenditure for Hispanic Americans is about 60 percent less than for whites.

Also, studies conducted over the last 25 years have shown that regardless of disorder diagnosed, African American psychiatric patients are more likely than white patients to be treated as in-patients, hospitalized involuntarily, placed in seclusion or restraints without evidence of a greater degree of violence, and treated with higher doses of antipsychotic medications. These differences are not due to the greater severity of the disorders between white and African American patients. One hypothesis for this discrepancy of treatment between African American and white patients is that whites are more likely to seek mental health care voluntarily than African Americans, and African Americans are more likely to enter the mental health care system through more coercive and less voluntary referral systems. African Americans are also more likely than whites to use emergency room services, resulting in more crisis-oriented help-seeking and service utilization. Once hospitalized in an institution with predominantly white staff, African American patients may receive differential care due to discrimination. That is, service personnel who are not familiar with the illness concepts and behavioral norms of nonwhite groups tend to assess minorities as more severely ill and more dangerous than patients of their own racial or ethnic group; consequently, such patients tend more often than white patients to be hospitalized involuntarily, placed in seclusion or restrains, and treated with higher doses of antipsychotic medications.

African American patients assessed in psychiatric emergency services are more likely to be diagnosed with schizophrenia and substance abuse than matched white patients. White patients are more often diagnosed with a mood disorder. The cultural distance between the clinician and the patient can affect the degree of psychopathology inferred and the diagnosis given. These differences in diagnosis by race have also been found when comparable research diagnostic instruments have been used for patient assessment. Semistructured diagnostic instruments based on explicit diagnostic criteria do not necessarily eliminate racial disparities in diagnostic outcomes. It appears that the process that clinicians use to link symptom observations to diagnostic constructs may differ, in particular for schizophrenia, between African American and white patients. The pattern of psychotic symptoms that predicts a clinician making a diagnosis of schizophrenia in African American and white patients is different. Among African American patients, loose associations, inappropriate affect, auditory hallucinations, and vague speech increased the likelihood of a diagnosis of schizophrenia. In white patients the main predictors were vague speech and loose associations. Also, auditory hallucinations are more frequently attributed to African American patients.

African Americans are less likely to have had outpatient treatment and longer delays in seeking care, and they present more severely ill. The reason for hospitalization was also different between African Americans and whites. African American patients were more likely to be admitted for behavioral disturbance, whereas white patients were more likely to be admitted for cognitive or affective disturbances. Also, African Americans were more likely to have police or emergency service involvement, despite no racial differences in violence, suicidality, or substance use when assessed. Furthermore, African American patients are more likely, even after controlling for health insurance status, to be referred to the public rather than private in-patient psychiatric facilities, suggesting racial bias in psychiatric emergency room assessment and recommended treatment.

African American patients diagnosed with major depression are less likely to receive antidepressant medications than whites and less likely to be treated with ECT. Demographic or socioeconomic differences cannot explain these findings. One explanation may be that there are conscious or unconscious biases in psychiatrists' treatment decisions. Although both African Americans and Hispanic Americans were less likely to fill an antidepressant prescription when diagnosed with depression, once a prescription was filled, they were just as likely as whites to receive an adequate course of treatment. These findings indicate that initiating care for depression is the biggest hurdle in overcoming these disparities. African American patients are more likely to be treated with depot neuroleptics than whites after controlling for the type and severity of illness. When treated with antipsychotic drugs, African Americans are less likely to receive second-generation antipsychotics than whites, placing them at increased risk for tardive dyskinesia and dystonia. These differences in antipsychotic prescribing patterns may be due to physicians' concern over an increased risk of diabetes among African Americans compared with whites or may be due to physicians perceiving their symptoms differently. Disparities in mental health care for African Americans and Hispanic Americans have also been noted in studies conducted with adolescents.

A disparity in prescription drug use for mental illness also has been found among Hispanic Americans and Asian Indian Americans. From 1996 to 2000, Asian Indian Americans were found to use prescription drugs 23.6 percent less than whites, whereas the differences between whites and African Americans and between whites and Hispanic Americans were 8.3 and 6.1 percent, respectively. Disparities in mental health service use among Asian American immigrants may be linked to language-based discrimination, although racial bias cannot be excluded. A study of Chinese Americans found a higher level of informal services and help-seeking from friends and relatives for emotional problems. Those Chinese Americans who reported experiencing language-based discrimination had a more negative attitude toward formal mental health services.

Data on racial and ethnic differences in mental health counseling and psychotherapy are similar to the psychopharmacological studies showing disparities for minorities. A study examining visits to primary care physicians based on the National Ambulatory Medical Care Survey from 1997 to 2000 found that primary care physicians provided similar or higher rates of general health counseling to African Americans than white patients. However, the rates of mental health counseling were significantly lower for African American patients. The lower rate of mental health counseling among African Americans may be due to decreased reporting of depressive symptoms, inadequate communication between African American patients and their primary care physicians, and decreased willingness to discuss mental health issues. On the other hand, another study utilizing the Medical Expenditure Panel Survey from 2000 found that African Americans were more likely than Hispanic Americans or whites to receive an adequate course of psychotherapy for depression. These findings suggest that initiating treatment is the biggest hurdle and that once they are engaged in treatment, African Americans have high compliance with psychotherapy.

Research in Transcultural Psychiatry

There are three perspectives, among other possible approaches, that offer great promise for future research in cultural psychiatry. The first would be based on identifying specific fields in general psychiatry that could be the subject of focused research from a cultural perspective. Topics of epidemiology and neurobiology could be assessed in this way. The former would address issues primarily in the public health arena, including stigmatization, racism, and acculturation. Several cultural variables should be considered in conducting cultural psychiatry research, including language, religion, traditions, beliefs, ethics, and gender orientation.

The second would aim to explore critical concepts or instruments in culturally relevant clinical research. There are four key concepts: *idioms of distress, social desirability, ethnographic data,* and *explanatory models. Idioms of distress* are the specific ways in which different cultures or societies report ailments; behavioral responses to threatening or pathogenic factors; and the uniqueness in the style of description, nomenclature, and assessment of stress. *Social desirability* stems from the similarities or differences among cultures, vis-à-vis the actual experiencing stressful events. Members of some cultures may be more or less willing to suffer physical or emotional problems, thus showing different levels of vulnerability or resignation, resilience, or acceptance. Issues of stigma in different cultural contexts contribute to this level of desirability or rejection. Third, *ethnographic data* should be included, together with strictly clinical data and laboratory analyses or tests, and narratives of life that enrich the descriptive aspects of the condition and expand on the surrounding sociocultural and interpersonal, and environmental aspects of the experience. The fourth concept is *explanatory models.* Each culture explains the pathology of any kind in its distinctive way. The explanation includes not only the presumptive original cause but also the impact of the adduced factors and the interpersonal exchanges and interactions that lead to the culturally accepted clinical diagnosis.

A third approach attempts to combine the first two by examining different areas of research based on the clinical dimensions of cultural psychiatry. This deals with conceptual, operational, and topical issues in the field now and in the future, including their biocultural connections.

Conceptual Issues in Cultural Psychiatry.   One of the primary issues in research in cultural psychiatry is the conceptual differentiation between culture and environment. Although generally accepted as the conceptual opposite of genetic, the environment represents a very broad, polymorphic concept. It is, therefore, essential to establish that, while perhaps part of that environmental set, culture and cultural factors in health and disease are terms of a different, even unique, nature.

To what extent does culture apply to the clinical realities of psychiatry? Culture plays a role in both normality and psychopathology. The role of culture in psychiatric diagnosis is an excellent example of this conceptual issue. Furthermore, culture impacts treatment approaches based on conventional medical and psychiatric knowledge and explanatory models. Finally, cultural variables have a role in prognosis and outcome.

A conceptual debate exists between those who advocate an *evidence-based* approach to research and practice versus those who assign a *value-based* view to everything clinical, more so if influenced by cultural factors. The value-based approach invokes poverty, unemployment, internal and external migration, and natural and human-made disasters. Evidence may be found to support both positions in scientific research.

Operational Issues in Cultural Psychiatry.   The dichotomy of normality and abnormality in human behavior is a crucial operational issue. Culture plays a definitive role in shaping these approaches. This raises the notion of relativism, a strong conceptual pillar in cultural psychiatry. Normality is a relative idea; that is, it varies in different cultural contexts.

Another operational issue is that of the choice of cultural variables. Each one has a specific weight and impact on symptoms,

syndromes, or clinical entities in psychiatry. Some of them may be essential in assessing a clinical topic, namely, language, education, religion, and gender orientation. An additional operational factor is a description, assessment, and testing of the strengths and weaknesses of an individual patient. Aspects of an individual's behavior, attitudes, disposition, sociability, occupational skills, and other factors are culturally determined.

Culture plays a significant role in perceiving the severity of symptoms, the disruption of the individual's functionality, and the quality of life. The assessment of severity is also the result of the meaning attributed to causal or pathogenic factors of psychopathology. Judgments about the level of dysfunction and the quality of a patient's life involve elusive concepts such as happiness, well-being, and peace of mind.

Research on cultural psychiatry issues needs to consider the representativeness of the study populations and the generalizability of the findings. Methodologic rigor needs to be applied to collecting demographic data, delineation of and differentiation between ethnic groups or subgroups, and measurement of demographic variables, symptoms, diagnosis, and culturally specific constructs.

Many tests and questionnaires used in clinical settings and research have been developed on English-speaking Western subjects and may not be appropriate for ethnic minority patients or non–English-speaking individuals due to lack of cultural equivalence. Translating items is insufficient to achieve linguistic equivalence, as the meaning and connotation changes and idioms of expression differ between languages. Also, norms may differ between ethnic groups, and tests need to be standardized with representative patients.

The complexity of translating an instrument varies depending on how much the construct being measured differs between the two cultures. There are four different approaches to translation. An ethnocentric approach is one in which the researcher assumes that the concepts overlap entirely in the two cultures. The instrument is used with individuals who differ from the population in which the instrument was initially developed and normed. The pragmatic approach assumes that some overlap between the two cultures and attempts are made to measure the overlapping aspects of the construct, *emic* aspects. An emic plus *etic* approach goes one step further and also attempts to measure culture-specific aspects of the construct. Lastly, sometimes the translation is not possible when the concepts do not overlap at all within the two cultures.

CULTURE-BOUND SYNDROMES

Cross-cultural mental health professionals have introduced several terms to refer to and describe culture-specific forms of expressing and diagnosing emotional distress. The term *culture-bound* was used to describe patterned behaviors of distress or illness whose phenomenology appeared distinct from psychiatric categories and were considered unique to particular cultural settings. The clear implication was that Western psychiatric categories were not culture-bound, but rather universal and that proper characterization would disclose a simple translation key for non-Western syndromes. The dichotomy between syndromes that are "culture-free," emerging from Euro-American and European societies, and those that are "culture-bound," emerging from everywhere else, is, of course, patently false. Culture suffuses all forms of psychological distress, the familiar as well as the unfamiliar.

Culture-Bound Syndromes and Their Relationship to Psychiatric Diagnoses

Only a few of the many cultural forms of expressing distress have received sustained research attention to integrating cultural and psychiatric research methods. This chapter focuses on some of those syndromes from diverse cultural regions, which have received the most intensive research and are associated with psychiatric categories: *Amok, ataques de nervios,* possession syndrome, and *shenjing shuairuo.*

Amok.

Amok is a dissociative episode characterized by a period of depression followed by an outburst of violent, aggressive, or homicidal behavior. Episodes tend to be caused by a perceived insult and are often accompanied by persecutory ideas, automation, amnesia, and exhaustion. Patients return to premorbid states following the episode. *Amok* seems to be prevalent only among males. The term originated in Malaysia, but similar behavior patterns can be found in Laos, Philippines, Polynesia (*cafard* or *cathard*), Papua New Guinea, and Puerto Rico (*mal de pelea*), and among the Navajo (*iich'aa*).

PHENOMENOLOGY. A prototypical episode is composed of the following elements:

1. Exposure to a stressful stimulus or subacute conflict, eliciting in the subject feelings of anger, loss, shame, and lowered self-esteem. The stressor usually appears minor in proportion to the resulting behavior (e.g., an argument with a coworker, verbal insult), but may occasionally be severe (i.e., death of a loved one).
2. A period of social withdrawal and brooding over the precipitating conflict, often involving aimless wandering, and sometimes accompanied by visual perceptual alterations.
3. Transition, usually sudden, to frenzied and extremely violent homicidality, with or without a brief prodromal stage of preparation (e.g., the subject may locate a preferred weapon or reach suddenly for whatever implement is available).
4. Indiscriminate selection of victims who may or may not symbolically represent the original actors in the conflict (e.g., subject attacks only Chinese people who are strangers to him, after a conflict with a Chinese coworker). Occasionally, the subject also attacks animals or objects in his path, or wounds himself, sometimes severely. The subject perseveres at these violent activities despite external attempts to bring him under control.
5. Verbalizations, when present, may be frenzied and guttural, or express internal conflict (e.g., ask forgiveness of a relative before killing him) or split consciousness (e.g., subject admits to a positive relationship with the victim, but denies this for his "spear").
6. Cessation may be spontaneous but usually results from being overpowered or killed. It is typically abrupt and leads to a change in consciousness, usually stupor or sleep.
7. Subsequent partial or total amnesia and report of "unconsciousness" or description of "darkened vision" (*mata gelap*) during the acute episode.
8. Perceptual disturbances or affective decompensations may occur for days or weeks after the acute attack. Psychosis or depression sometimes ensues.

EPIDEMIOLOGY. Epidemiologic rates of *amok* in Malaysia and Indonesia are unknown and may vary regionally and over time. From the available data, *amok* appears to follow an endemic pattern in Malayo-Indonesia with some epidemic increases, the reverse of which has been found for *amok*-like attacks in Laos.

Amok is essentially unknown in women (only one case was found in the literature, and it was considered atypical in that no deaths occurred). It is thought to occur more frequently in men of Malay extraction, Muslim religion, low education, and rural origin, who are between the ages of 20 and 45 years.

PRECIPITANTS. Precipitants of *amok* in Malaysia and Indonesia typically consisted of experiences eliciting in the subject marked feelings of loss, shame, anger, or lowered self-esteem. Although specific triggers were very diverse in nature and presentation, including sudden and gradual stressors, most consisted of interpersonal or social conflicts superficially appearing to generate only mild to moderate stress. These include arguments with coworkers, nonspecific family tensions, feelings of social humiliation, bouts of possessive jealousy, gambling debts, and job loss. Rarely, however, *amok* was precipitated by a severe stressor, such as the simultaneous death of the spouse and child of the subject.

ADDITIONAL CLINICAL FEATURES. It is unclear whether *amok* episodes are associated with indirect suicidal intent on the part of the subject. Anecdotes and cultural views supporting a connection are available, but interviews with surviving subjects have refuted the association.

Rates of relapse are unknown. It is considered very likely in the popular view, leading currently in Malaysia to permanent psychiatric hospitalization of surviving subjects, and, in the past, to banishment or execution.

TREATMENT. Afflicted individuals in 20th-century Malaysia have been exempted from legal or moral responsibility for acts committed while in a state of *amok* using a kind of "insanity defense," which characterizes the attack as "unconscious" and beyond the subject's control. They were subsequently hospitalized, sometimes permanently, and frequently received diagnoses of schizophrenia and were treated with antipsychotic medication. Alternatively, trials have sometimes resulted in criminal verdicts and prolonged imprisonment.

Ataque de Nervios.

Ataque de nervios is an idiom of distress principally reported among Latinos from the Caribbean but recognized among many Latin American and Latin Mediterranean groups. Commonly reported symptoms to include uncontrollable shouting, attacks of crying, trembling, heat in the chest rising into the head, and verbal or physical aggression. Dissociative experiences, seizure-like or fainting episodes, and suicidal gestures are prominent in some attacks but absent in others. A general feature of an *ataque de nervios* is a sense of being out of control. *Ataques de nervios* frequently occur as a direct result of a stressful event relating to the family (e.g., news of a death of a close relative, a separation or divorce from a spouse, conflicts with a spouse or children, or witnessing an accident involving a family member). People may experience amnesia for what occurred during the *ataque de nervios,* but they otherwise return rapidly to their usual level of functioning.

Ataque de nervios (attack of nerves, in Spanish) is a syndrome indigenous to various Latin American cultures, notably those of the Hispanic Caribbean (Puerto Rico, Cuba, and the Dominican Republic). It has received considerable attention in the psychiatric and anthropologic literature since the mid-1950s, mostly in Puerto Rican communities on the island and in populations within the United States.

PHENOMENOLOGY.   An *ataque de nervios* can be described as prototypically composed of the following elements:

1. Exposure to a frequently sudden, stressful stimulus, typically eliciting feelings of fear, grief, or anger, and involving a person close to the subject, such as a spouse, child, family member, or friend. The severity of the trigger ranges from mild–moderate (i.e., marital argument, disclosure of migration plans) to extreme (i.e., physical or sexual abuse, acute bereavement).
2. Initiation of the episode is immediate upon exposure to the stimulus, or after a period of brooding or emotional "shock."
3. Once the acute attack begins, the rapid evolution of an intense affective storm follows, characterized by a primary affect usually congruent with the stimulus (such as anger, fear, grief) and a sense of loss of control (*emotional expressions*).
4. All or some of the following accompany these:
   A. *Bodily sensations:* Trembling, chest tightness, headache, difficulty breathing, heart palpitations, heat in the chest, paresthesias of diverse location, difficulty moving limbs, faintness, blurred vision, or dizziness (*mareos*).
   B. Behaviors (*action dimension*): Shouting, crying, swearing, moaning, breaking objects, striking out at others or self, attempting to harm self with the nearest implement, falling to the ground, shaking with convulsive movements, or lying "as if dead."
5. Cessation may be abrupt or gradual, but it is usually rapid, and often results from the ministration of others, involving expressions of concern, prayers, or use of rubbing alcohol (*alcoholado*). There is a return of ordinary consciousness and reported exhaustion.
6. The attack is frequently followed by partial or total amnesia for the events of the episode, and descriptions such as the following for the acute attack: Loss of consciousness, depersonalization, mind going blank, or general unawareness of surroundings (*alterations in consciousness*). However, some *ataques* appear to exhibit no alterations in consciousness.

EPIDEMIOLOGY.   Risk factors for *ataque de nervios* span a range of social and demographic characteristics. The strongest predictors of *ataque* are female gender, lower formal education, and disrupted marital status (i.e., divorced, widowed, or separated). *Ataque* sufferers also reported less satisfaction in their social interactions, generally and specifically with their spouses. Also, people who experienced an *ataque de nervios* were more likely to describe their health as only fair or poor, to seek help for an emotional problem, and to take medications for this purpose. Persons with *ataque* also reported deriving less satisfaction from leisure time activities and feeling overwhelmed more often.

PRECIPITANTS.   Prototypically, *ataque de nervios* was linked by sufferers to an acute precipitating event or to the summation of many life episodes of suffering brought to a head by a trigger that overwhelmed the person's coping ability. In 92 percent of cases, the *ataque* was directly provoked by a distressing situation, and 73 percent of the time, it began within minutes or hours of the event. A majority of first *ataques* (81 percent) occurred in the presence of others, as opposed to when the sufferer was alone and led to a person receiving help (67 percent). Unlike the typical experience of persons with panic disorder, most patients reported feeling better (71 percent) or feeling relieved (81 percent) after their first *ataque*. The first episodes of *ataque de nervios* are closely tied to the interpersonal world of the sufferer, and they result in an unburdening (*desahogarse*) of one's life problems, at least temporarily.

ADDITIONAL CLINICAL FEATURES.   The association between *ataque de nervios* and a sense of loss of control and of being overwhelmed highlight the importance of the association between the cultural syndrome and other behaviors associated with acute emotional dysregulation. Most concerning among these is the strong relationship between *ataques* and suicidal ideation and attempts. Other related behaviors include loss of aggression control, expressed as attacks on people or property, and dissociative experiences related to the acute *ataque* experience.

SPECIFIC CULTURAL FACTORS.   The complex relationship between *ataque de nervios* and psychiatric diagnosis may be clarified about its broader popular nosology. In the Hispanic Caribbean and other areas of Latin America, *ataque* is part of a popular nosology of *nervios* (nerves), composed of other related categories. Experiences of adversity are linked in this nosology to ensuing "alterations" of the nervous system, which result in its impaired functioning, including the peripheral nerves. This quasi-anatomical damage is evidenced in emotional symptoms, including interpersonal susceptibility, anxiety, and irritability, as well as in physically mediated symptoms, such as trembling, palpitations, and decreased concentration.

TREATMENT.   No treatment studies of *ataque de nervios* have ever been conducted. Typical treatment involves, first, ensuring the safety of the person and those around him or her, given the association between *ataque,* suicidality, and uncontrolled aggressivity. "Talking the person down" is usually helpful, accompanied by expressions of support from relatives and other loved ones; rubbing alcohol (*alcoholado*) to help calm the person is a culturally prescribed way of expressing this support.

"Telling the story" of what led to the *ataque* usually constitutes the principal therapeutic approach in subsequent stages of treatment. Because one of the main functions of the attack is to communicate a feeling of being overwhelmed, indicating receipt of the message and the desire to offer support are usually perceived as therapeutic. The person should be allowed to set the pace of disclosure and to give enough details and circumstances to feel "unburdened" (*desahogado[a]*).

In the case of single or occasional *ataques* in the absence of psychiatric diagnosis, brief follow-up is usually sufficient. This may be discussed with the patient and the family to ensure a full return to the previous healthy state. For recurrent *ataques,* treatment depends on the associated psychopathology, the nature of the precipitants (including traumatic exposure), the degree of family conflict or support, the social context, the previous treatment experiences, and the patient's and family's expectations, among other factors.

Psychotherapy is typically the mainstay of treatment, given the usual source of the overwhelmed behavior in the interpersonal milieu. Pharmacotherapy may also help treat *ataque*-related psychopathology; the primary emphasis should be placed on treating the underlying disorder. Given the slow crescendo of many *ataques,* judicious use of short-acting benzodiazepines also has a role in helping abort an impending episode. However, this should not be the primary form of treatment for recurrent *ataques,* since it only forestalls the principal function of the syndrome as a mode of communication. Instead, psychotherapy and a social activism stance by the therapist that acknowledges the origins of adversity among low-income Latinos in socioeconomic disenfranchisement and ethnic/racial discrimination are usually required to address the interpersonal and sociocultural roots of *ataque de nervios*.

Possession Syndrome.   Involuntary possession trance states are very common presentations of emotional distress around the world.

Cognate experiences have been reported in extremely diverse cultural settings, including India, Sri Lanka, Hong Kong, China, Japan, Malaysia, Niger, Uganda, Southern Africa, Haiti, Puerto Rico, and Brazil. *Possession syndrome* is an umbrella English-language term used to describe South Asian presentations of involuntary possession trance that encompasses multiple names in regional languages and dialects of India and Sri Lanka. These presentations are seen as a form of illness by the person's cultural group because they are involuntary, they cause distress, and they do not occur as a normal part of a collective cultural or religious ritual or performance.

PHENOMENOLOGY. It is important to distinguish at the outset between possession syndrome, as an instance of possession trance, and the broader category of possession. The latter refers to a general ideology describing the full range of direct spirit influences on human affairs, including effects on physical, psychological, spiritual, social, and ecologic realms. By contrast, as a subset of general possession experience, possession trance refers to specific alterations in consciousness, memory, behavior, and identity attributed to direct spirit influence. In addition to pathologic possession, trance states, South Asian cultures authorize multiple examples of normal possession and possession trance. When voluntary and normative, these states are typically seen as instances of religious devotion, mystical ecstasy, social commentary, asceticism, interpersonal relations, existential reflection, and the study of consciousness. This chapter discusses possession syndrome as a pathologic entity with an established phenomenology, that is, as a particular case in the general continuum of etiologic ideas regarding possession illnesses. A prototypical episode is composed of the following elements:

1. Onset occurs typically due to subacute conflict or stress and shows considerable variation. It may be gradual and nonspecific (e.g., diverse somatic complaints, such as dizziness, headaches, abdominal discomfort, hot–cold flashes, listlessness, or difficulty breathing) or sudden and specific, in the form of an abrupt transition to an altered state of consciousness.
2. Behavior during the altered state consists of some or all of the following:
   A. Dramatic, semi-purposeful movements, such as head-bobbing, bodily shaking, thrashing, gyrating, or falling to the ground, accompanied by guttural, incoherent verbalizations, such as mumbling, moaning, or shrieking.
   B. Aggressive or violent actions directed at self or others, including spitting, striking, and impulsive suicidal or homicidal gestures. Verbalizations may be coherent and consist of derogatory comments or threats of violence directed against significant others or the subject (in the third person) and typically considered by observers to be uncharacteristic of the subject's usual behavior.
   C. Specific gestures, comments, or requests denoting the appearance of a known possessing personality by (1) reference to standard attributes of culturally recognizable figures or (2) the name and degree of deceased family members or acquaintances.
3. In all cases, this state is marked by the emergence of one or several secondary personalities distinct from that of the subject. Their specific identities, which may remain undisclosed for some time, adhere to cultural norms regulating permissible agents of possession, which vary by religion, region, and caste. Acceptable agents include spirits of deceased family members, in-law relations, or known village acquaintances who died under specific conditions of distress, and minor supernatural figures of the Hindu pantheon (rarely major deities) and the Islamic spiritual world.

4. Possession by the secondary personality(ies) is episodic, resulting in alternation between the usual personality of the subject and the altered state. The subject in his or her usual identity appears in a daze, exhausted, distressed, or confused about the situation and may report visual or auditory perceptual disturbances regarding the possessing agent and "unconsciousness" and partial or total amnesia for the altered state.
5. Frequently, the specific identities of possessing personalities remain undisclosed for some time, requiring the active ministrations of family members and the intervention of specialized indigenous practitioners. The process of disclosure is conceived as a struggle between the family members and the beneficent agents possessing the healer on the one side, and the troublesome possessing personalities on the other. It is characterized by remarkable reactivity on the part of the subject to environmental cues, including direct questioning, strategic neglect, and aggressive manipulation.
6. The outcome is variable. Total recovery is often reported at the cessation of a single acute episode, which may be of several weeks' duration. Alternatively, prolonged morbidity may result, or even, rarely, death.

Methodologic considerations limit data on the epidemiology, precipitants, and associated psychopathology of subjects with possession syndrome in South Asia. These include a lack of representative community samples and nonsystematic definitions of the syndrome, which shows considerable regional variation.

EPIDEMIOLOGY. Possession syndrome is more common in women than men, with a female-to-male ratio of approximately 3 to 1 in both community and psychiatric cohorts. The age of onset is usually between 15 and 35 years, but many cases reportedly begin in childhood. Attacks may persist well into middle age, and geriatric cases have also been reported.

PRECIPITANTS. Precipitants of possession syndrome are varied but typically consist of marked social or family conflicts, or stressful life transitions, of subacute duration, eliciting strong feelings of vulnerability in persons without firm emotional support. Examples encountered in the literature included marital conflict, abuse, and neglect, at times associated with alcoholism; the arrival of a new bride to the home of her husband's family; delay in arranging a marriage, or in consummating it; forced marriage; widowhood; postpartum status; loss of family social standing; the death of a family member; difficulty finding employment and financial difficulties; alienation from family support; and subordination to other family members and in-laws.

SPECIFIC CULTURAL FACTORS. Possession syndrome constitutes a normative cultural category throughout India and Sri Lanka. It may present initially in a variety of forms, linked by the attribution of spirit etiology. When it presents in a nonspecific fashion, indigenous diagnosis is confirmed by the appearance of the altered state during the therapeutic ritual. It is considered an affliction by its painful, involuntary nature and attributed to the intervention of specific spiritual agencies acting independently or at the behest of a witch. Certain castes and persons in transitional states (e.g., puerperium) are considered most vulnerable to a spirit attack, especially when deprived of emotional and material support.

TREATMENT. Specialized indigenous practitioners and ritual therapies are generally available and widely utilized, but psychiatric treatment is typically avoided. Indigenous treatments include neutralization of the conflict or stress via the communal rituals involved in exorcism, as well as the reformulation of the suffering into beneficent individual and communal practice via initiation into a spirit devotion cult, such as the Siri cult of South India, or education into the roles of oracle (diviner), exorcist, or, rarely, avatar (divine incarnation).

Shenjing Shuairuo.

Shenjing shuairuo ("weakness of the nervous system" in Mandarin Chinese) is a translation and cultural adaptation of the term "neurasthenia," which was transmitted into China from the West and Japan in the 1920s and 1930s. Revived in its modern form by the American neurologist George Beard since 1868, his formulation of neurasthenia (Greek for "lack of nerve strength") originally denoted a heterogeneous syndrome of lassitude, pain, poor concentration, headache, irritability, dizziness, insomnia, and over 50 other symptoms. It was considered at first an "American disease," resulting from the "pressures" of a rapidly modernizing society but was later adopted by European diagnosticians. Its pathophysiology was thought to derive from a lowering of nervous system function on a physical rather than emotional basis, due to excessive demand for its use, especially among the educated and wealthier classes. In Soviet psychiatry, buttressed by Pavlovian research, it was a central component of mental health nosology, which became especially influential in Chinese psychiatry after the communist revolution of 1949.

Although neurasthenia declined in importance in Western classification systems during the 20th century, *Shenjing shuairuo* underwent marked popular and professional development in mainland China, Taiwan, Hong Kong, in Chinese migrant communities, and in Japan, where a similar syndrome is labeled *shinkei suijaku*. From a peak in about 1980, when it may have constituted up to 80 percent of all "neurotic" diagnoses in Chinese societies, *Shenjing shuairuo* has undergone intense psychiatric and anthropologic reexamination. It currently features prominently in the second edition revised *Chinese Classification of Mental Disorders* (CCMD-2-R), under the section on "other neuroses." The CCMD-2-R diagnosis requires three symptoms out of five nonhierarchical symptom clusters, organized as weakness, emotional, excitement, and nervous symptoms, and the fifth category of sleep disturbances. Like other neurotic disorders in the Chinese manual, the condition must last at least 3 months, and should (1) lower the efficiency of work, study, or social function; (2) cause mental distress; or (3) precipitate treatment seeking.

PHENOMENOLOGY. Given the evolution of diagnostic practice regarding *shenjing shuairuo* in Chinese societies over the last decades, which may be labeled the professional approximation of the condition or its "disease" aspect, phenomenologic description in this chapter is based instead on clinical histories of self-identified sufferers, or the "illness" aspect of the syndrome. The following elements are prototypical:

1. Onset is usually gradual, sometimes spanning several years, and typically emerges out of a conflictive, frustrating, or worrying situation that involves work, family, and other social settings, or their combination. A sense of powerlessness in changing the precipitating situation appears central to most illness accounts of the syndrome.

2. Symptoms show substantial individual variation, but usually involve at least some of the following spontaneous complaints: Insomnia, affective dysphoria, headache, bodily pains and distortions (e.g., "swelling" of the head), dizziness, difficulty concentrating, tension and anxiety, worry, fatigue, weakness, gastrointestinal problems, and "troubled vexation" (*fan nao*).

This last emotion has been described as a form of irritability mixed with worry and distress over "conflicting thoughts and unfulfilled desires," that may be partially concealed for the sake of preserving social harmony.

3. The sufferer frequently seeks the sick role, attributing his or her difficulties in meeting work, school, or other social expectations to the syndrome. Sources of treatment vary substantially across Chinese communities, depending on the availability of formal and traditional service sectors.

4. The course is variable and may respond closely to changing interpersonal and social circumstances. Amelioration of the precipitating stressor(s) typically brings about substantial improvement, although residual symptoms appear common.

5. Response to treatment may be strongly mediated by the illness role and its relationship to the intractability of precipitating stressors.

PRECIPITANTS. An empirical assessment of the precipitants of *shenjing shuairuo* has found high rates of work-related stressors, which were made more intractable by the centrally directed nature of mainland Chinese society. These included unwelcome work assignments, job postings that caused family separations, harsh criticism at work, excessive workloads, monotonous tasks, and feelings of inadequacy or incompatibility of skills and responsibilities. Students usually described less severe study-related precipitants, particularly school failure or anxiety over the mismatch between personal or family aspirations and performance. Other interpersonal and family-related stressors included romantic disappointments, marital conflict, and the death of a spouse or other relative. Chinese etiologic understandings of the syndrome commonly invert the Western view of "psychosomatic" presentations, whereby social–interpersonal precipitants cause psychological distress that is displaced onto bodily experience.

ADDITIONAL CLINICAL FEATURES. The clinical course of the syndrome may depend on the associated psychiatric comorbidity and the degree of persistence of the precipitating stressors. One longitudinal study found a complete resolution of *shenjing shuairuo* symptoms and reasonable social adjustment 20 years from the index diagnosis in 83 of 89 cases. Only one case was receiving continued treatment, and no subjects reported the onset of depressive disorder after the *shenjing shuairuo* diagnosis.

Chinese psychiatrists have carried out numerous studies of neurophysiologic and cognitive function in *shenjing shuairuo* patients since the 1950s. Most have reported abnormalities compared to normal controls, including in tests of polysomnography, electroencephalography, psychogalvanic reflexes, gastric function, and memory function. These findings need to be replicated with well-controlled samples using contemporary diagnostic instruments.

SPECIFIC CULTURAL FACTORS. The evolving definitions of *shenjing shuairuo* have emerged from a tradition of syncretism in Chinese medicine between indigenous illness understandings and international contributions. Nineteenth-century Western notions of a weakened nervous system due to overuse (neurasthenia) found an ancient cognate expression in Chinese concepts of bodily meridians or channels (*jing*) binding vital organs in balanced networks along which forces (e.g., *qi*, vital energy, in *yin* and *yang* forms) could be disrupted from their normal, harmonious flow. This gave rise to *shenjing shuairuo*, an illness whereby the *jing* that carry *shen*—spirit or vitality, the capacity of the mind to form ideas and the desire of the personality to live life—have become *shuai* (degenerate) and *ruo* (weak) following undue nervous excitement.

TREATMENT.   When accessing formal sectors of care, most patients used both Western-trained physicians and traditional Chinese doctors. Nonpsychiatric medical settings were preferred, including neurology and general medicine clinics, in concert with cultural understandings of the somatopsychic etiology of *shenjing shuairuo,* emphasizing its physical mediation. The modality of treatment was usually traditional Chinese medicines, which were prescribed by both Western-trained and Chinese-style doctors. This conformed to the balanced status still ascribed to both types of training among Chinese physicians. Polypharmacy was common, combining sedatives, traditional herbs, antianxiety agents, vitamins, and other tonics. Despite the active suppression of religious healing in China, almost a quarter of patients were also engaged in such treatment.

▲ 34.4 Theories of Personality and Psychopathology

SIGMUND FREUD: FOUNDER OF CLASSIC PSYCHOANALYSIS

Psychoanalysis was the child of Sigmund Freud's genius. He put his stamp on it from the very beginning, and it can be fairly stated that, although the science and theory of psychoanalysis have advanced far beyond Freud, his influence is still strong and pervasive. In recounting the progressive stages in the evolution of the origins of Freud's psychoanalytic thinking, it is useful to keep in mind that Freud himself was working against the background of his neurologic training and expertise and in the context of the scientific thinking of his era.

The science of psychoanalysis is the bedrock of psychodynamic understanding. It forms the fundamental theoretical frame of reference for a variety of forms of therapeutic intervention, embracing not only psychoanalysis itself but also various forms of psychoanalytically oriented psychotherapy and related forms of therapy employing psychodynamic concepts. Currently, considerable interest has been generated in efforts to connect psychoanalytic understandings of human behavior and emotional experience with emerging findings of neuroscientific research.

At the same time, psychoanalysis is undergoing a creative ferment in which classical perspectives are continually being challenged and revised, leading to a diversity of emphases and viewpoints, all of which can be regarded as representing aspects of psychoanalytic thinking. This has given rise to the question as to whether psychoanalysis is one theory or more than one. The divergence of multiple theoretical variants raises the question of the degree to which newer perspectives can be reconciled to classical perspectives.

Freud himself inaugurated the spirit of creative modifications in theory. Some of the theoretical modifications of the classic theory after Freud have attempted to reformulate basic analytic propositions while still retaining the spirit and fundamental insights of a Freudian perspective; others have challenged and abandoned fundamental analytic insights in favor of divergent paradigms that seem radically different and even contradictory to basic analytic principles.

Although there is more than one way to approach the diversity of such material, the decision has been made to organize this material along roughly historical lines, tracing the emergence of analytic theory or theories over time, but with a good deal of overlap. However, there is an overall pattern of gradual emergence, progressing from early drive theory to structural theory to ego psychology to object relations, and on to self-psychology, intersubjectivism, and relational approaches.

Psychoanalysis today is recognized as having three crucial aspects: it is a therapeutic technique, a body of scientific and theoretical knowledge, and a method of investigation. This section focuses on psychoanalysis as both a theory and a treatment, but the basic tenets elaborated here have broad applications to nonpsychoanalytic settings in clinical psychiatry.

Life of Freud

Sigmund Freud (1856–1939) (Fig. 34-22) was born in Freiburg, a small town in Moravia, which is now part of the Czech Republic. When Freud was 4 years old, his father, a Jewish wool merchant, moved the family to Vienna, where Freud spent most of his life. Following medical school, he specialized in neurology and studied for a year in Paris with Jean-Martin Charcot. He was also influenced by Ambroise-Auguste Liébeault and Hippolyte-Marie Bernheim, both of whom taught him hypnosis while he was in France. After his education in France, he returned to Vienna and began clinical work with hysterical patients. Between 1887 and 1897, his work with these patients led him to develop psychoanalysis.

Beginnings of Psychoanalysis

In the decade from 1887 to 1897, Freud immersed himself in the serious study of the disturbances in his hysterical patients, resulting in discoveries that contributed to the beginnings of psychoanalysis. These slender beginnings had a threefold aspect: Emergence of psychoanalysis as a method of investigation, as a therapeutic technique, and as a body of scientific knowledge based on an increasing fund of information and fundamental theoretical propositions. These early researches flowed out of Freud's initial collaboration with Joseph Breuer and then, increasingly, from his independent investigations and theoretical developments.

The Case of Anna O

Breuer was an older physician, a distinguished and well-established medical practitioner in the Viennese community (Fig. 34-23). Knowing Freud's interests in hysterical pathology, Breuer told him about the unusual case of a woman he had treated for approximately 1.5 years, from December 1880 to June 1882. This woman became famous under the pseudonym Fräulein Anna O, and the study of her difficulties proved to be one of the essential stimuli in the development of psychoanalysis.

Anna O was, in reality, Bertha Pappenheim, who later became independently famous as a founder of the social work movement in Germany. When she began to see Breuer, she was an intelligent and strong-minded young woman of approximately 21 years of age who had developed several hysterical symptoms connected with the illness and death of her father. These symptoms included paralysis of the limbs, contractures, anesthesias, visual and speech disturbances, anorexia, and distressing nervous cough. Two distinct phases of consciousness also characterized her illness: One relatively standard, but the other reflected a second and more pathologic personality.

Anna was very fond of and close to her father and shared with her mother the duties of nursing him on his deathbed. During her altered states of consciousness, Anna recalled the vivid fantasies and intense

FIGURE 34-22
Sigmund Freud at age 79. (Courtesy of Menninger
Foundation Archives, Topeka, KS.)

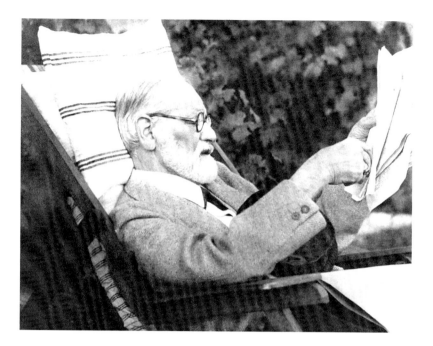

emotions she had experienced while caring for her father. It was with considerable amazement, both to Anna and Breuer, that when she could recall, with the associated expression of affect, the scenes or circumstances under which her symptoms had arisen, the symptoms would disappear. She vividly described this process as the "talking cure" and as "chimney sweeping."

Once the connection between talking through the circumstances of the symptoms and the disappearance of the symptoms themselves had been established, Anna proceeded to deal with each of her many symptoms, one after another. She was able to recall that on one occasion when

her mother had been absent, she had been sitting at her father's bedside and had had a fantasy or daydream in which she imagined that a snake was crawling toward her father and was about to bite him. She struggled forward to try to ward off the snake, but her arm, which had been draped over the back of the chair, had gone to sleep. She was unable to move it. The paralysis persisted, and she was unable to move the arm until, under hypnosis, she could recall this scene. It is easy to see how this kind of material must have made a profound impression on Freud. It provided a convincing demonstration of the power of unconscious memories and suppressed affects in producing hysterical symptoms.

In the course of the somewhat lengthy treatment, Breuer had become increasingly preoccupied with his fascinating and unusual patient and, consequently, spent more and more time with her. Meanwhile, his wife had grown increasingly jealous and resentful. As soon as Breuer began to realize this, the sexual connotations of it frightened him, and he abruptly terminated the treatment. Only a few hours later, however, he was recalled urgently to Anna's bedside. She had never alluded to the forbidden topic of sex during her treatment, but she was now experiencing hysterical childbirth. Freud saw the phantom pregnancy as the logical outcome of the sexual feelings she had developed toward Breuer in response to his therapeutic attention. Breuer himself had been entirely unaware of this development, and the experience was quite unnerving. He was able to calm Anna down by hypnotizing her, but then he left the house in a cold sweat and immediately set out with his wife for Venice on a second honeymoon.

According to a version from Freud through Ernest Jones, the patient was far from cured and later hospitalized after Breuer's departure. It seems ironic that the prototype of a cathartic cure was, in fact, far from successful. Nevertheless, the case of Anna O provided a critical starting point for Freud's thinking and a crucial juncture in the development of psychoanalysis.

The Interpretation of Dreams

In his landmark publication *The Interpretation of Dreams* in 1900, Freud presented a theory of the dreaming process that paralleled his earlier analysis of psychoneurotic symptoms. He viewed the dream experience as a conscious expression of unconscious fantasies or wishes not readily acceptable to conscious waking experience.

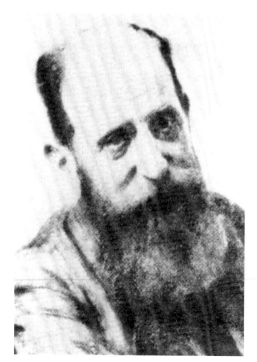

FIGURE 34-23
Joseph Breuer (1842–1925).

Thus, dream activity was considered to be one of the usual manifestations of unconscious processes.

The dream images represented unconscious wishes or thoughts, disguised through a process of a symbolization and other distorting mechanisms. This reworking of unconscious contents constituted the dream work. Freud postulated the existence of a "censor," pictured as guarding the border between the unconscious part of the mind and the preconscious level. The censor functioned to exclude unconscious wishes during conscious states but, during regressive relaxation of sleep, allowed specific unconscious contents to pass the border, only after transforming these unconscious wishes into disguised forms experienced in the manifest dream contents by the sleeping subject. Freud assumed that the censor worked in the service of the ego—that is, as serving the self-preservative objectives of the ego. Although he was aware of the unconscious nature of the processes, he tended to regard the ego at this point in developing his theory more restrictively as the source of conscious processes of reasonable control and volition.

The analysis of dreams elicits material that has been repressed. These unconscious thoughts and wishes include nocturnal sensory stimuli (sensory impressions such as pain, hunger, thirst, urinary urgency), the day residue (thoughts and ideas connected with the activities and preoccupations of the dreamer's current waking life), and repressed unacceptable impulses. Because the sleep state blocks motility, the dream enables partial but limited gratification of the repressed impulse that gives rise to the dream.

Freud distinguished between two layers of dream content. The *manifest* content refers to what is recalled by the dreamer; the *latent* content involves the unconscious thoughts and wishes that threaten to awaken the dreamer. Freud described the unconscious mental operations by which latent dream content is transformed into the manifest dream as the *dream work*. Repressed wishes and impulses must attach themselves to innocent or neutral images to pass the scrutiny of the dream censor. This process involves selecting meaningless or trivial images from the dreamer's current experience, which are dynamically associated with the latent images that they resemble in some respect.

Condensation. *Condensation* is the mechanism by which several unconscious wishes, impulses, or attitudes can be combined into a single image in the manifest dream content. Thus, in a child's nightmare, an attacking monster may come to represent not only the dreamer's father but may also represent some aspects of the mother and even some of the child's primitive hostile impulses as well. The converse of condensation can also occur in the dream work, namely, irradiation or diffusion of a single latent wish or impulse distributed through multiple representations in the manifest dream content. The combination of mechanisms of condensation and diffusion provides the dreamer with a highly flexible and economic device for facilitating, compressing, and diffusing or expanding the manifest dream content, which is derived from latent or unconscious wishes and impulses.

Displacement. The mechanism of *displacement* refers to the transfer of amounts of energy (cathexis) from an original object to a substitute or symbolic representation of the object. Because the substitute object is relatively neutral—that is, less invested with affective energy—it is more acceptable to the dream censor and can pass the borders of repression more easily. Thus, whereas symbolism can be taken to refer to the substitution of one object for another, displacement facilitates distortion of unconscious wishes through the transfer of affective energy from one object to another.

Despite the transfer of cathectic energy, the aim of the unconscious impulse remains unchanged. For example, in a dream, the mother may be represented visually by an unknown female figure (at least one who has less emotional significance for the dreamer), but the naked content of the dream nonetheless continues to derive from the dreamer's unconscious instinctual impulses toward the mother.

Symbolic Representation. Freud noted that the dreamer would often represent highly charged ideas or objects by using innocent images that were in some way connected with the idea or object being represented. In this manner, an abstract concept or a complex set of feelings toward a person could be symbolized by a simple, concrete, or sensory image. Freud noted that symbols have unconscious meanings that can be discerned through the patient's associations to the symbol, but he also believed that certain symbols have universal meanings.

Secondary Revision. The mechanisms of condensation, displacement, and symbolic representation are characteristic of a type of thinking that Freud referred to as *primary process*. This primitive mode of cognitive activity is characterized by illogic, bizarre, and absurd images that seem incoherent. Freud believed that a more mature and reasonable aspect of the ego works during dreams to organize primitive aspects of dreams into a more coherent form. *Secondary revision* is Freud's name for this process, in which dreams become somewhat more rational. The process is related to mature activity characteristic of waking life, which Freud termed *secondary process*.

Affects in Dreams. Secondary emotions may not appear in the dream at all, or they may be experienced in somewhat altered form. For example, repressed rage toward a person's father may take the form of mild annoyance. Feelings may also appear as their opposites.

Anxiety Dreams. Freud's dream theory preceded his development of a comprehensive theory of the ego. Hence, his understanding of dreams stresses the importance of discharging drives or wishes through the hallucinatory contents of the dream. He viewed such mechanisms as condensation, displacement, symbolic representation, projection, and secondary revision primarily as facilitating the discharge of latent impulses, rather than as protecting dreamers from anxiety and pain. Freud understood anxiety dreams as reflecting a failure in the protective function of the dream-work mechanisms. The repressed impulses succeed in working their way into the manifest content in a more or less recognizable manner.

Punishment Dreams. Dreams in which dreamers experience punishment represented a unique challenge for Freud because they appear to represent an exception to his wish-fulfillment theory of dreams. He came to understand such dreams as reflecting a compromise between the repressed wish and the repressing agency or conscience. In a punishment dream, the ego anticipates condemnation on the dreamer's conscience if the latent unacceptable impulses are allowed direct expression in the manifest dream content. Hence, the wish for punishment on the part of the patient's conscience is satisfied by giving expression to punishment fantasies.

Topographical Model of the MIND

The publication of *The Interpretation of Dreams* in 1900 heralded the arrival of Freud's topographical model of the mind, in which he divided the mind into three regions: the conscious system, the preconscious system, and the unconscious system. Each system has its unique characteristics.

The Conscious. The conscious system in Freud's topographical model is the part of the mind in which perceptions coming from the outside world or within the body or mind are brought into awareness. Consciousness is a subjective phenomenon whose content can be communicated only using language or behavior. Freud assumed that consciousness used a form of neutralized psychic energy that he referred to as *attention cathexis,* whereby persons were aware of a particular idea or feeling as a result of investing a discrete amount of psychic energy in the idea or feeling.

The Preconscious. The preconscious system is composed of those mental events, processes, and contents that can be brought into conscious awareness by focusing attention. Although most persons are not consciously aware of the appearance of their first-grade teacher, they ordinarily can bring this image to mind by deliberately focusing attention on the memory. Conceptually, the preconscious interfaces with both unconscious and conscious regions of the mind. To reach conscious awareness, the contents of the unconscious must become linked with words and thus become preconscious. The preconscious system also serves to maintain the repressive barrier and to censor unacceptable wishes and desires.

The Unconscious. The unconscious system is dynamic. Its mental contents and processes are kept from conscious awareness through the force of censorship or repression, and it is closely related to instinctual drives. At this point in Freud's theory of development, instincts were thought to consist of sexual and self-preservative drives, and the unconscious was thought to contain the mental representations and derivatives of the sexual instinct primarily.

The content of the unconscious is limited to wishes seeking fulfillment. These wishes motivate dream and neurotic symptom formation. This view is now considered reductionist.

The unconscious system is characterized by *primary process thinking,* principally aimed at facilitating wish fulfillment and instinctual discharge. It is governed by the pleasure principle and, therefore, disregards logical connections; it has no concept of time, represents wishes as fulfillments, permits contradictions to exist simultaneously, and denies the existence of negatives. The primary process is also characterized by extreme mobility of drive cathexis; the investment of psychic energy can shift from object to object without opposition. Memories in the unconscious have been divorced from their connection with verbal symbols. Hence, when words are reapplied to forgotten memory traits, as in psychoanalytic treatment, the verbal cathexis allows the memories to reach consciousness again.

The contents of the unconscious can become conscious only by passing through the preconscious. When censors are overpowered, the elements can enter consciousness.

Limitations of the Topographical Theory. Freud soon realized that two primary deficiencies in the topographical theory limited its usefulness. First, many patients' defense mechanisms that guard against distressing wishes, feelings, or thoughts were not initially accessible to consciousness. Thus, repression cannot be identical with preconscious, because, by definition, this region of the mind is accessible to consciousness. Second, Freud's patients frequently demonstrated an unconscious need

for punishment. This clinical observation made it unlikely that the moral agency making the demand for punishment could be allied with anti-instinctual forces available to conscious awareness in the preconscious. These difficulties led Freud to discard the topographical theory. However, certain concepts derived from the theory continue to be useful, mainly primary and secondary thought processes, the fundamental importance of wish fulfillment, the existence of a dynamic unconscious, and a tendency toward regression under frustrating conditions.

Instinct or Drive Theory

After the development of the topographical model, Freud turned his attention to the complexities of instinct theory. Freud was determined to anchor his psychological theory in biology. His choice led to terminologic and conceptual difficulties when he used terms derived from biology to denote psychological constructs. *Instinct,* for example, refers to a pattern of species-specific behavior that is genetically derived and, therefore, is more or less independent of learning. Modern research demonstrating that instinctual patterns are modified through experiential learning has made Freud's instinctual theory problematic. Further confusion has stemmed from the ambiguity inherent in a concept on the borderland between the biologic and the psychological: Should the mental representation aspect of the term and the physiologic component be integrated or separated? Although *drive* may have been closer than the instinct to Freud's meaning, in contemporary usage, the two terms are often used interchangeably.

In Freud's view, an instinct has four principal characteristics: source, impetus, aim, and object. The *source* refers to the part of the body from which the instinct arises. The *impetus* is the amount of force or intensity associated with the instinct. The *aim* refers to any action directed toward tension discharge or satisfaction, and the *object* is the target (often a person) for this action.

Instincts

LIBIDO. The ambiguity in the term *instinctual drive* is also reflected in the use of the term *libido.* Briefly, Freud regarded the sexual instinct as a psychophysiological process that had both mental and physiologic manifestations. Essentially, he used the term *libido* to refer to "the force by which the sexual instinct is represented in mind." Thus, in its accepted sense, libido refers specifically to the mental manifestations of the sexual instinct. Freud recognized early that the sexual instinct did not originate in a finished or final form, as represented by genital primacy. Instead, it underwent a complex process of development, at each phase of which the libido had specific aims and objects that diverged in varying degrees from the simple aim of genital union. The libido theory thus came to include all of these manifestations and the complicated paths they followed in the course of psychosexual development.

EGO INSTINCTS. From 1905 on, Freud maintained a dual instinct theory, subsuming sexual instincts and ego instincts connected with self-preservation. Until 1914, with the publication of *On Narcissism,* Freud had paid little attention to ego instincts; in this communication, however, Freud invested ego instinct with libido for the first time by postulating an ego libido and an object libido. Freud thus viewed narcissistic investment as an essentially libidinal instinct and called the remaining nonsexual components the *ego instincts.*

AGGRESSION. When psychoanalysts today discuss the dual instinct theory, they are generally referring to libido and aggression. Freud, however, originally conceptualized aggression as a component of the sexual instincts in the form of sadism. As he became aware that sadism had nonsexual aspects, he made finer gradations, which enabled him to categorize aggression and hate as part of the ego instincts and the libidinal aspects of sadism as components of the sexual instincts. Finally, in 1923, to account for the clinical data he was observing, he was compelled to conceive of aggression as a separate instinct in its own right. The source of this instinct, according to Freud, was mostly in skeletal muscles, and the aim of the aggressive instincts was destruction.

LIFE AND DEATH INSTINCTS.   Before designating aggression as a separate instinct, Freud, in 1920, subsumed the ego instincts under a broader category of life instincts. These were juxtaposed with death instincts and were referred to as *Eros* and *Thanatos* in *Beyond the Pleasure Principle.* Life and death instincts were regarded as forces underlying sexual and aggressive instincts. Although Freud could not provide clinical data that directly verified the death instinct, he thought the instinct could be inferred by observing *repetition compulsion,* a person's tendency to repeat past traumatic behavior. Freud thought that the dominant force in biologic organisms had to be the death instinct. In contrast to the death instinct, eros (the life instinct) refers to the tendency of particles to reunite or bind to one another, as in sexual reproduction. The prevalent view today is that the dual instincts of sexuality and aggression suffice to explain most clinical phenomena without recourse to a death instinct.

Pleasure and Reality Principles.

In 1911, Freud described two basic tenets of mental functioning: the pleasure principle and the reality principle. He essentially recast the primary process and secondary process dichotomy into the pleasure and reality principles and thus took an essential step toward solidifying the notion of the ego. Both principles, in Freud's view, are aspects of ego functioning. The *pleasure principle* is defined as an inborn tendency of the organism to avoid pain and to seek pleasure through the discharge of tension. The *reality principle,* on the other hand, is considered to be a learned function closely related to the maturation of the ego; this principle modifies the pleasure principle and requires delay or postponement of immediate gratification.

Infantile Sexuality.

Freud set forth the three central tenets of psychoanalytic theory when he published *Three Essays on the Theory of Sexuality.* First, he broadened the definition of sexuality to include forms of pleasure that transcend genital sexuality. Second, he established a developmental theory of childhood sexuality that delineated the vicissitudes of erotic activity from birth through puberty. Third, he forged a conceptual linkage between neuroses and perversions.

Freud's notion that sexual drives influence children has made some persons reluctant to accept psychoanalysis. Freud noted that infants are capable of erotic activity from birth, but the earliest manifestations of infantile sexuality are nonsexual and are associated with such bodily functions as feeding and bowel–bladder control. As libidinal energy shifts from the oral zone to the anal zone to the phallic zone, each stage of development is thought to build on and to subsume the accomplishments of the preceding stage. The *oral stage,* which occupies the first 12 to 18 months of life, centers on the mouth and lips and is manifested in chewing, biting, and sucking. The dominant erotic activity of the anal stage, from 18 to 36 months of age, involves bowel function and control. The *phallic stage,* from 3 to 5 years of life, initially focuses on urination as the source of erotic activity. Freud suggested that phallic

erotic activity in boys is a preliminary stage leading to adult genital activity. Whereas the penis remains the principal sexual organ throughout male psychosexual development, Freud postulated that females have two principal erotogenic zones: the vagina and the clitoris. He thought that the clitoris was the chief erotogenic focus during the infantile genital period, but that erotic primacy shifted to the vagina after puberty. Studies of human sexuality have subsequently questioned the validity of this distinction.

Freud discovered that in the psychoneuroses, only a limited number of the sexual impulses that had undergone repression and were responsible for creating and maintaining the neurotic symptoms were normal. For the most part, these were the same impulses that were given overt expression in the perversions. The neuroses, then, were the negative of perversions.

Object Relationships in Instinct Theory.

Freud suggested that the choice of a love object in adult life, the love relationship itself, and the nature of all other object relationships depend primarily on the nature and quality of children's relationships. In describing the libidinal phases of psychosexual development, Freud repeatedly referred to the significance of a child's relationships with parents and other significant persons in the environment.

The awareness of the external world of objects develops gradually in infants. Soon after birth, they are primarily aware of physical sensations, such as hunger, cold, and pain, which give rise to tension, and caregivers are regarded primarily as persons who relieve their tension or remove painful stimuli. Recent infant research, however, suggests that awareness of others begins much sooner than Freud initially thought. Table 34-10 summarizes the stages of psychosexual development and the object relationships associated with each stage. Although the table goes only as far as young adulthood, development is now recognized as continuing throughout adult life.

Concept of Narcissism.

According to Greek myth, Narcissus, a beautiful youth, fell in love with his reflection in the water of a pool and drowned in his attempt to embrace his beloved image. Freud used the term *narcissism* to describe situations in which an individual's libido was invested in the ego itself rather than other persons. This concept of narcissism presented him with vexing problems for his instinct theory and essentially violated his distinction between libidinal instincts and ego or self-preservative instincts. Freud's understanding of narcissism led him to use the term to describe a wide array of psychiatric disorders, very much in contrast to the term's contemporary use to describe a specific personality disorder. Freud grouped several disorders as the narcissistic neuroses, in which a person's libido is withdrawn from objects and turned inward. He believed that this withdrawal of libidinal attachment to objects accounted for the loss of reality testing in psychotic patients; grandiosity and omnipotence in such patients reflected excessive libidinal investment in the ego.

Freud did not limit his use of narcissism to psychoses. In states of physical illness and hypochondriasis, he observed that libidinal investment was frequently withdrawn from external objects and outside activities and interests. Similarly, he suggested that in normal sleep, libido was also withdrawn and reinvested in a sleeper's own body. Freud regarded homosexuality as an instance of a narcissistic form of object choice, in which persons fall in love with an idealized version of themselves projected onto another person. He also found narcissistic manifestations in the beliefs and myths of primitive people, especially those involving the ability to influence external events through the magical omnipotence of thought

Table 34-10
Stages of Psychosexual Development

Oral Stage

Definition	Earliest stage of development in which the infant's needs, perceptions, and modes of expression are primarily centered in mouth, lips, tongue, and other organs related to oral zone and around the sucking reflex.
Description	Oral zone maintains dominance in psychic organization through approximately first 18 mo of life. Oral sensations include thirst, hunger, pleasurable tactile stimulations evoked by the nipple or its substitute, and sensations related to swallowing and satiation. Oral drives consist of two components: libidinal and aggressive. States of oral tension lead to seeking oral gratification, as in quiescence at the end of nursing. Oral triad consists of wishes to eat, sleep, and reach that relaxation that occurs at the end of sucking just before onset of sleep. Libidinal needs (oral erotism) predominate in early oral phase, whereas they are mixed with more aggressive components later (oral sadism). Oral aggression is expressed in biting, chewing, spitting, or crying. Oral aggression is connected with primitive wishes and fantasies of biting, devouring, and destroying.
Objectives	To establish a trusting dependence on nursing and sustaining objects, establish comfortable expression and gratification of oral libidinal needs without excessive conflict or ambivalence from oral sadistic wishes.
Pathologic traits	Excessive oral gratifications or deprivation can result in libidinal fixations contributing to pathologic traits. Such traits can include excessive optimism, narcissism, pessimism (as in depressive states), or demandingness. Envy and jealousy are often associated with oral traits.
Character traits	Successful resolution of the oral phase results in capacities to give to and receive from others without excessive dependence or envy and to rely on others with a sense of trust as well as with a sense of self-reliance and self-trust. Oral characters are often excessively dependent and require others to give to them and look after them and are often extremely dependent on others for maintaining self-esteem. These are readily amalgamated with narcissistic needs.

Anal Stage

Definition	The stage of psychosexual development promoted by maturation of neuromuscular control over sphincters, particularly the anal sphincter, permitting greater voluntary control over retention or expulsion of feces.
Description	This period extends roughly from 1 to 3 yr of age, marked by recognizable intensification of aggressive drives mixed with libidinal components in sadistic impulses. Acquisition of voluntary sphincter control is associated with an increasing shift from passivity to activity. Conflicts over anal control and struggles with parents over retaining or expelling feces in toilet training give rise to increased ambivalence, together with conflicts over separation, individuation, and independence. Anal erotism refers to sexual pleasure in anal functioning, both in retaining precious feces and presenting them as a precious gift to the parent. Anal sadism refers to expression of aggressive wishes connected with discharging feces as powerful and destructive weapons. These wishes are often displayed in fantasies of bombing or explosions.
Objectives	The anal period is marked by greater striving for independence and separation from dependence on and control of parents. Objectives of sphincter control without overcontrol (fecal retention) or loss of control (messing) are matched by attempts to achieve autonomy and independence without excessive shame or self-doubt from loss of control.
Pathologic traits	Maladaptive character traits, often apparently inconsistent, derive from anal erotism and defenses against it. Orderliness, obstinacy, stubbornness, willfulness, frugality, and parsimony are features of anal character. When defenses against anal traits are less effective, anal character reveals traits of heightened ambivalence, lack of tidiness, messiness, defiance, rage, and sadomasochistic tendencies. Anal characteristics and defenses are typically seen in obsessive-compulsive neuroses.
Character traits	Successful resolution of the anal phase provides the basis for development of personal autonomy, a capacity for independence and personal initiative without guilt, a capacity for self-determining behavior without a sense of shame or self-doubt, a lack of ambivalence, and a capacity for willing cooperation without either excessive willfulness or self-diminution or defeat.

Urethral Stage

Definition	This stage was not explicitly treated by Freud but serves as a transitional stage between anal and phallic stages. It shares some characteristics of anal phase and some from subsequent phallic phase.
Description	Characteristics of the urethral phase are often subsumed under phallic phase. Urethral erotism, however, refers to pleasure in urination as well as pleasure in urethral retention analogous to anal retention. Similar issues of performance and control are related to urethral functioning. Urethral functioning may also have sadistic quality, often reflecting persistence of anal sadistic urges. Loss of urethral control, as in enuresis, may frequently have regressive significance that reactivates anal conflicts.
Objectives	At stake are issues of control and urethral performance and loss of control. It is not clear whether or to what extent objectives of urethral functioning differ from those of anal period, except that they are expressed in a later developmental stage.
Pathologic traits	The predominant urethral trait is competitiveness and ambition, probably related to compensation for shame due to loss of urethral control. This may instigate development of penis envy, related to feminine sense of shame and inadequacy in being unable to match male urethral performance. This may also be related to issues of control and shaming.
Character traits	Besides healthy effects analogous to those from the anal period, urethral competence provides a sense of pride and self-competence based on performance. Urethral performance is an area in which the small boy can imitate and try to match his father's more adult performance. Resolution of urethral conflicts sets the stage for budding gender identity and subsequent identifications.

Phallic Stage

Definition	Phallic stage begins sometime during year 3 and continues until approximately the end of year 5.
Description	The phallic phase is characterized by a primary focusing of sexual interests, stimulation, and excitement in the genital area. The penis becomes the organ of principal interest to children of both sexes, with lack of penis in females being considered as evidence of castration. The phallic phase is associated with an increase in genital masturbation accompanied by predominantly unconscious fantasies of sexual involvement with the opposite-sex parent. Threats of castration and the related anxiety are connected with guilt over masturbation and oedipal wishes. During this phase oedipal involvement and conflict are established and consolidated.

Table 34-10
Stages of Psychosexual Development (*Continued*)

Objectives	To focus erotic interest in genital area and genital functions. This lays the foundation for gender identity and serves to integrate residues of previous stages into a predominantly genital–sexual orientation. Establishing the oedipal situation is essential for furtherance of subsequent identifications, serving as a basis for important and perduring dimensions of character organization.
Pathologic traits	Derivation of pathologic traits from phallic–oedipal involvement is sufficiently complex and subject to such a variety of modifications that it encompasses nearly the whole of neurotic development. Issues, however, focus on castration in males and penis envy in females. Patterns of internalization developed from resolution of the Oedipus complex provide another important focus of developmental distortions. The influence of castration anxiety and penis envy, defenses against them, and patterns of identification are primary determinants of the development of human character. They also subsume and integrate residues of previous psychosexual stages, so that fixations or conflicts deriving from preceding stages can contaminate and modify oedipal resolution.
Character traits	The phallic stage provides the foundation for an emerging sense of sexual identity, curiosity without embarrassment, initiative without guilt, as well as mastery not only over objects and persons in the environment but also over internal processes and impulses. Resolution of the oedipal conflict gives rise to internal structural capacities for regulation of drive impulses and their direction to constructive ends. The internal sources of such regulation are the ego and superego, based on introjections and identifications derived primarily from parental figures.

Latency Stage

Definition	This is the stage of relative instinctual quiescence or inactivity of sexual drive during the period from the resolution of the Oedipus complex until pubescence (from about 5–6 yr until about 11–13 yr).
Description	The institution of the superego at the close of the oedipal period and further maturation of ego functions allow for considerably greater degrees of control of instinctual impulses and motives. Sexual interests are generally thought to be quiescent. This is a period of primarily homosexual affiliations for both boys and girls, as well as a sublimation of libidinal and aggressive energies into energetic learning and play activities, exploring the environment, and becoming more proficient in dealing with the world of things and persons around them. It is a period for development of important skills. The relative strength of regulatory elements often gives rise to patterns of behavior that are somewhat obsessive and hypercontrolling.
Objectives	The primary objective is further integration of oedipal identifications and consolidation of gender and sex-role identity. Relative quiescence and control of instinctual impulses allow for development of ego apparatuses and mastery of skills. Further identificatory components may be added to the oedipal ones on the basis of broadening contacts with other significant figures outside the family (e.g., teachers, coaches, and other adult figures).
Pathologic traits	Dangers in the latency period can arise either from the lack of development of inner controls or an excess of them. Lack of control can lead to failure to sufficiently sublimate energies in the interest of learning and the development of skills; an excess of inner control, however, can lead to premature closure of personality development and precocious elaboration of obsessive character traits.
Character traits	The latency period is frequently regarded as a period of relatively unimportant inactivity in the developmental schema. More recently, greater respect has been gained for the developmental processes in this period. Important consolidations and additions are made to basic postoedipal identifications and to processes of integrating and consolidating previous attainments in psychosexual development and establishing decisive patterns of adaptive functioning. The child can develop a sense of industry and capacity for mastery of objects and concepts that allows autonomous functioning and a sense of initiative without risk of failure or defeat or a sense of inferiority. These are all important attainments that need to be further integrated, ultimately as the essential basis for a mature adult life of satisfaction in work and love.

Genital Stage

Definition	The genital or adolescent phase extends from the onset of puberty from approximately ages 11–13 until young adulthood. Current thinking tends to subdivide this stage into preadolescent, early adolescent, middle adolescent, late adolescent, and even postadolescent periods.
Description	Physiologic maturation of systems of genital (sexual) functioning and attendant hormonal systems leads to intensification of instinctual, particularly libidinal, drives. This produces a regression in personality organization, which reopens conflicts of previous stages of psychosexual development and provides opportunity for re-resolution of these conflicts in the context of achieving a mature sexual and adult identity. This period has been described as a "second individuation."
Objectives	Primary objectives are the ultimate separation from dependence on and attachment to parents and establishment of mature, nonincestuous, heterosexual object relations. Related are the achievement of a mature sense of personal identity and acceptance and integration of adult roles and functions that permit new adaptive integrations with social expectations and cultural values.
Pathologic traits	Pathologic deviations due to failure to achieve successful resolution of this stage of development are multiple and complex. Defects can arise from a whole spectrum of psychosexual residues, since the developmental task of adolescence is in a sense a partial reopening, reworking, and reintegration of all of these aspects of development. Previous unsuccessful resolutions and fixations in various phases or aspects of psychosexual development will produce pathologic defects in the emerging adult personality and defects in identity formation.
Character traits	Successful resolution and reintegration of previous psychosexual stages in the adolescent genital phase set the stage normally for a fully mature personality with the capacity for full and satisfying genital potency and a self-integrated and consistent sense of identity. This provides the basis for a capacity for self-realization and meaningful participation in areas of work, love, and in creative and productive application to satisfying and meaningful goals and values.

processes. In the course of normal development, children also exhibit this belief in their omnipotence.

Freud postulated a state of primary narcissism at birth in which the libido is stored in the ego. He viewed the neonate as completely narcissistic, with the entire libidinal investment in physiologic needs and satisfaction. He referred to this self-investment as *ego libido*. The infantile state of self-absorption changes only gradually, according to Freud, with the dawning awareness that a separate person—the mothering figure—is responsible for gratifying an infant's needs. This realization leads to the gradual withdrawal of the libido from the self and its redirection toward the external object. Hence, the development of object relations in infants parallels the shift from primary narcissism to object attachment. The libidinal investment in the object is referred to as *object libido*. If a developing child suffers rebuffs or trauma from the caretaking figure, object libido may be withdrawn and reinvested in the ego. Freud called this regressive posture *secondary narcissism*.

Freud used the term *narcissism* to describe many different dimensions of human experience. At times, he used it to describe a perversion in which persons used their bodies or body parts as objects of sexual arousal. At other times, he used the term to describe a developmental phase, as in primary narcissism. In still other instances, the term referred to a particular object choice. Freud distinguished love objects who are chosen "according to the narcissistic type," in which case the object resembles the subject's idealized or fantasied self-image, from objects chosen according to the "anaclitic," in which the love object resembles a caretaker from early in life. Finally, Freud also used the word *narcissism* interchangeably and synonymously with *self-esteem*.

Ego Psychology

Although Freud had used the construct of the ego throughout the evolution of psychoanalytic theory, ego psychology, as it is known today, really began with the publication in 1923 of *The Ego and the Id*. This landmark publication also represented a transition in Freud's thinking from the topographical model of the mind to the tripartite structural model of ego, id, and superego. He had observed repeatedly that not all unconscious processes could be relegated to a person's instinctual life. Elements of the conscience, as well as functions of the ego, are also unconscious.

Structural Theory of the Mind.
The structural model of the psychic apparatus is the cornerstone of ego psychology. The three provinces—id, ego, and superego—are distinguished by their different functions.

ID. Freud used the term *id* to refer to a reservoir of unorganized instinctual drives. Operating under the domination of the primary process, the id cannot delay or modify the instinctual drives with which an infant is born. The id, however, should not be viewed as synonymous with the unconscious, because both the ego and the superego have unconscious components.

EGO. The ego spans all three topographical dimensions of conscious, preconscious, and unconscious. Logical and abstract thinking and verbal expression are associated with conscious and preconscious functions of the ego. Defense mechanisms reside in the unconscious domain of the ego. The ego, the executive organ of the psyche, controls motility, perception, contact with reality, and, through the defense mechanisms available to it, the delay and modulation of drive expression.

Freud believed that the id is modified due to the impact of the external world on the drives. The pressures of external reality enable the ego to appropriate the energies of the id to do its work. As the ego brings influences from the external world to bear on the id, it simultaneously substitutes the reality principle for the pleasure principle. Freud emphasized the role of conflict within the structural model and observed that conflict occurs initially between the id and the outside world, only to be transformed later to conflict between the id and the ego.

The third component of the tripartite structural model is the superego. The superego establishes and maintains an individual's moral conscience based on a complex system of ideals and values internalized by parents. Freud viewed the superego as the heir to the Oedipus complex. Children internalize parental values and standards at about the age of 5 or 6 years. The superego then serves as an agency that provides ongoing scrutiny of a person's behavior, thoughts, and feelings; it makes comparisons with expected standards of behavior and offers approval or disapproval. These activities occur mostly unconsciously.

The ego-ideal is often regarded as a component of the superego. It is an agency that prescribes what a person should do according to internalized standards and values. The superego, by contrast, is an agency of moral conscience that *proscribes*—that is, dictates what a person should not do. Throughout the latency period and after that, persons continue to build on early identifications through their contact with admired figures who contribute to the formation of moral standards, aspirations, and ideals.

Functions of the Ego.
Modern ego psychologists have identified a set of essential ego functions that characterizes the operations of the ego. These descriptions reflect the ego activities that are generally regarded as fundamental.

CONTROL AND REGULATION OF INSTINCTUAL DRIVES. The development of the capacity to delay or postpone drive discharge, like the capacity to test reality, is closely related to the early childhood progression from the pleasure principle to the reality principle. This capacity is also an essential aspect of the ego's role as a mediator between the id and the outside world. Part of infants' socialization to the external world is acquiring language and secondary process or logical thinking.

JUDGMENT. A closely related ego function is judgment, which involves the ability to anticipate the consequences of actions. As with the control and regulation of instinctual drives, judgment develops in parallel with the growth of *secondary process thinking*. The ability to think logically allows assessment of how contemplated behavior may affect others.

RELATION TO REALITY. The mediation between the internal world and external reality is a crucial function of the ego. Relations with the outside world can be divided into three aspects: the sense of reality, reality testing, and adaptation to reality. The *sense of reality* develops in concert with an infant's dawning awareness of bodily sensations. The ability to distinguish outside the body from the inside is an essential aspect of the sense of reality, and disturbances of body boundaries, such as depersonalization, reflect impairment in this ego function. *Reality testing*, an ego function of paramount importance, refers to the capacity to distinguish internal fantasy from external reality. This function differentiates persons who are psychotic from those who are not. *Adaptation to reality* involves persons' ability to use their resources to develop effective responses to changing circumstances based on previous experience with reality.

Table 34-11
Parallel Lines of Development

Instinctual Phases	Separation–Individuation	Object Relations	Psychosocial Crises
Oral	Autism, symbiosis	Primary narcissism, need-satisfying	Trust or mistrust
Anal	Differentiation, practicing, rapprochement	Need-satisfying, object constancy	Autonomy or shame, self-doubt
Phallic	Object constancy, Oedipal complex	Object constancy, ambivalence	Initiative or guilt
Latency	—	—	Industry or inferiority
Adolescence	Genitality, secondary individuation	Object love	Identity or identity confusion
Adulthood	Mature genitality	—	Intimacy or isolation, generativity or stagnation, integrity or despair

OBJECT RELATIONSHIPS. The capacity to form mutually satisfying relationships is related in part to patterns of internalization stemming from early interactions with parents and other significant figures. This ability is also a fundamental function of the ego, in that satisfying relatedness depends on the ability to integrate positive and negative aspects of others and self and to maintain an internal sense of others even in their absence. Similarly, mastery of drive derivatives is also crucial to the achievement of satisfying relationships. Although Freud did not develop an extensive object relations theory, British psychoanalysts, such as Ronald Fairbairn (1889–1964) and Michael Balint (1896–1970), elaborated extensively on the early stages in infants' relationships with need-satisfying objects and on the gradual development of a sense of separateness from the mother. Another of their British colleagues, Donald W. Winnicott (1896–1971), described the *transitional object* (e.g., a blanket, teddy bear, or pacifier) as the link between developing children and their mothers. A child can separate from the mother because a transitional object provides feelings of security in her absence. The stages of human development and object relations theory are summarized in Table 34-11.

SYNTHETIC FUNCTION OF THE EGO. First described by Herman Nunberg in 1931, the *synthetic function* refers to the ego's capacity to integrate diverse elements into an overall unity. Different aspects of self and others, for example, are synthesized into a consistent representation that endures over time. The function also involves organizing, coordinating, and generalizing or simplifying large amounts of data.

PRIMARY AUTONOMOUS EGO FUNCTIONS. Heinz Hartmann described the so-called primary autonomous functions of the ego as rudimentary apparatuses present at birth that develop independently of intrapsychic conflict between drives and defenses. These functions include perception, learning, intelligence, intuition, language, thinking, comprehension, and motility. In the course of development, some of these conflict-free aspects of the ego may eventually become involved in a conflict. They will develop normally if the infant is raised in what Hartmann referred to as an *average expectable environment.*

SECONDARY AUTONOMOUS EGO FUNCTIONS. Once the sphere where primary autonomous function develops becomes involved with conflict, the so-called *secondary autonomous ego functions* arise in the defense against drives. For example, a child may develop caretaking functions as a reaction formation against murderous wishes during the first few years. Later, the defensive functions may be neutralized or deinstinctualized when the child grows up to be a social worker and cares for homeless persons.

Defense Mechanisms. At each phase of libidinal development, specific drive components evoke characteristic ego defenses. The anal phase, for example, is associated with reaction formation, as manifested by the development of shame and disgust concerning anal impulses and pleasures.

Defenses can be grouped hierarchically according to the relative degree of maturity associated with them. Narcissistic defenses are the most primitive and appear in children and persons who are psychotically disturbed. Immature defenses are seen in adolescents and some nonpsychotic patients. Neurotic defenses are encountered in obsessive-compulsive and hysterical patients as well as in adults under stress. Table 34-12 lists the defense mechanisms, according to George Valliant's classification of the four types.

Theory of Anxiety. Freud initially conceptualized anxiety as "dammed-up libido." Essentially, a physiologic increase in sexual tension leads to a corresponding increase in libido, the mental representation of the physiologic event. This buildup causes the actual neuroses. Later, with the development of the structural model, Freud developed a new theory of a second type of anxiety that he referred to as *signal anxiety.* In this model, anxiety operates at an unconscious level and serves to mobilize the ego's resources to avert danger. Either external or internal sources of danger can produce a signal that leads the ego to marshal specific defense mechanisms to guard against or reduce instinctual excitation.

Freud's later theory of anxiety explains neurotic symptoms as the ego's partial failure to cope with distressing stimuli. The drive derivatives associated with danger may not have been adequately contained by the defense mechanisms used by the ego. In phobias, for example, Freud explained that fear of an external threat (e.g., dogs or snakes) is an externalization of internal danger.

Danger situations can also be linked to developmental stages and can create a developmental hierarchy of anxiety. The earliest dangerous situation is a fear of disintegration or annihilation, often associated with concerns about fusion with an external object. As infants mature and recognize the mothering figure as a separate person, separation anxiety, or fear of the loss of an object, becomes more prominent. During the oedipal psychosexual stage, girls are most concerned about losing the love of the most crucial figure in their lives, their mother. Boys are primarily anxious about bodily injury or castration. After resolving the oedipal conflict, a more mature form of anxiety occurs, often termed *superego anxiety.* This latency-age concern involves the fear that internalized parental representations, contained in the superego, will cease to love, or will angrily punish, the child.

Table 34-12
Classification of Defense Mechanisms

Narcissistic-Psychotic Defenses

These defenses are usually found as part of a psychotic process, but may also occur in young children and adult dreams or fantasies. They share the common note of avoiding, negating, or distorting reality.

Projection	Perceiving and reacting to unacceptable inner impulses and their derivatives as though they were outside the self. On a psychotic level, this takes the form of frank delusions about external reality, usually persecutory, includes both perception of one's own feelings and those of another with subsequent acting on the perception (psychotic paranoid delusions). Impulses may derive from id or superego (hallucinated recriminations).
Denial	Psychotic denial of external reality, unlike repression, affects perception of external reality more than perception of internal reality. Seeing, but refusing to acknowledge what one sees, or hearing and negating what is actually heard are examples of denial and exemplify the close relationship of denial to sensory experience. Not all denial, however, is necessarily psychotic. Like projection, denial may function in the service of more neurotic or even adaptive objectives. Denial avoids becoming aware of some painful aspect of reality. At the psychotic level, the denied reality may be replaced by a fantasy or delusion.
Distortion	Grossly reshaping the experience of external reality to suit inner needs, including unrealistic megalomanic beliefs, hallucinations, wish-fulfilling delusions, and employing sustained feelings of delusional grandiosity, superiority, or entitlement.

Immature Defenses

These mechanisms are fairly common in preadolescent years and in adult character disorders. They are often mobilized by anxieties related to intimacy or its loss. Although they are regarded as socially awkward and undesirable, they often moderate with improvement in interpersonal relationships or with increased personal maturity.

Acting out	The direct expression of an unconscious wish or impulse in action to avoid being conscious of the accompanying affect. The unconscious fantasy, involving objects, is lived out and impulsively enacted in behavior, thus gratifying the impulse more than the prohibition against it. On a chronic level, acting out involves giving in to impulses to avoid the tension that would result from postponement of their expression.
Blocking	An inhibition, usually temporary in nature, of affects especially, but possibly also thinking and impulses. It is close to repression in its effects but has a component of tension arising from the inhibition of the impulse, affect, or thought.
Hypochondriasis	Transformation of reproach toward others arising from bereavement, loneliness, or unacceptable aggressive impulses, into self-reproach in the form of somatic complaints of pain, illness, and so forth. Real illness may also be overemphasized or exaggerated for its evasive and regressive possibilities. Thus, responsibility may be avoided, guilt may be circumvented, and instinctual impulses may be warded off.
Introjection	In addition to the developmental functions of the process of introjection, it also can serve specific defensive functions. The introjection of a loved object involves the internalization of characteristics of the object with the goal of ensuring closeness to and constant presence of the object. Anxiety consequent to separation or tension arising out of ambivalence toward the object is thus diminished. If the object is lost, introjection nullifies or negates the loss by taking on characteristics of the object, thus in a sense internally preserving the object. Even if the object is not lost, the internalization usually involves a shift of cathexis reflecting a significant alteration in the object relationship. Introjection of a feared object serves to avoid anxiety through internalizing the aggressive characteristic of the object, thereby putting the aggression under one's own control. The aggression is no longer felt as coming from outside, but is taken within and utilized defensively, thus turning the subject's weak, passive position into an active, strong one. The classic example is "identification with the aggressor." Introjection can also take place out of a sense of guilt in which the self-punishing introject is attributable to the hostile-destructive component of an ambivalent tie to an object. Thus, the self-punitive qualities of the object are taken over and established within one's self as a symptom or character trait, which effectively represents both the destruction and the preservation of the object. This is also called *identification with the victim.*
Passive-aggressive behavior	Aggression toward an object expressed indirectly and ineffectively through passivity, masochism, and turning against the self.
Projection	On a nonpsychotic level, projection involves attributing one's own unacknowledged feelings to others; it includes severe prejudice, rejection of intimacy through suspiciousness, hypervigilance to external danger, and injustice collecting. Projection operates correlatively to introjection, such that the material of the projection derives from the internalized but usually unconscious configuration of the subject's introjects. At higher levels of function, projection may take the form of misattributing or misinterpreting motives, attitudes, feelings, or intentions of others.
Regression	A return to a previous stage of development or functioning to avoid the anxieties or hostilities involved in later stages. A return to earlier points of fixation embodying modes of behavior previously given up. This is often the result of a disruption of equilibrium at a later phase of development. This reflects a basic tendency to achieve instinctual gratification or to escape instinctual tension by returning to earlier modes and levels of gratification when later and more differentiated modes fail or involve intolerable conflict.
Schizoid fantasy	The tendency to use fantasy and to indulge in autistic retreat for the purpose of conflict resolution and gratification.
Somatization	The defensive conversion of psychic derivatives into bodily symptoms; tendency to react with somatic rather than psychic manifestations. Infantile somatic responses are replaced by thought and affect during development (desomatization); regression to earlier somatic forms or response (resomatization) may result from unresolved conflicts and may play an important role in psychophysiological and psychosomatic reactions.

Table 34-12
Classification of Defense Mechanisms (*Continued*)

Neurotic Defenses

These are common in apparently normal and healthy individuals as well as in neurotic disorders. They function usually in the alleviation of distressing affects and may be expressed in neurotic forms of behavior. Depending on circumstances, they can also have an adaptive or socially acceptable aspect.

Controlling	The excessive attempt to manage or regulate events or objects in the environment in the interest of minimizing anxiety and solving internal conflicts.
Displacement	Involves a purposeful, unconscious shifting of impulses or affective investment from one object to another in the interest of solving a conflict. Although the object is changed, the instinctual nature of the impulse and its aim remain unchanged.
Dissociation	A temporary but drastic modification of character or sense of personal identity to avoid emotional distress; it includes fugue states and hysterical conversion reactions.
Externalization	A general term, correlative to internalization, referring to the tendency to perceive in the external world and in external objects components of one's own personality, including instinctual impulses, conflicts, moods, attitudes, and styles of thinking. It is a more general term than projection, which is defined by its derivation from and correlation with specific introjects.
Inhibition	The unconsciously determined limitation or renunciation of specific ego functions, singly or in combination, to avoid anxiety arising out of conflict with instinctual impulses, superego, or environmental forces or figures.
Intellectualization	The control of affects and impulses by way of thinking about them instead of experiencing them. It is a systematic excess of thinking, deprived of its affect, to defend against anxiety caused by unacceptable impulses.
Isolation	The intrapsychic splitting or separation of affect from content resulting in repression of either idea or affect or the displacement of affect to a different or substitute content.
Rationalization	A justification of attitudes, beliefs, or behavior that might otherwise be unacceptable by an incorrect application of justifying reasons or the invention of a convincing fallacy.
Reaction formation	The management of unacceptable impulses by permitting expression of the impulse in antithetical form. This is equivalently an expression of the impulse in the negative. Where instinctual conflict is persistent, reaction formation can become a character trait on a permanent basis, usually as an aspect of obsessional character.
Repression	Consists of the expelling and withholding from conscious awareness of an idea or feeling. It may operate either by excluding from awareness what was once experienced on a conscious level (secondary repression) or it may curb ideas and feelings before they have reached consciousness (primary repression). The "forgetting" associated with repression is unique in that it is often accompanied by highly symbolic behavior, which suggests that the repressed is not really forgotten. The important discrimination between repression and the more general concept of defense has been discussed.
Sexualization	The endowing of an object or function with sexual significance that it did not previously have, or possesses to a lesser degree, to ward off anxieties connected with prohibited impulses.

Mature Defenses

These mechanisms are healthy and adaptive throughout the life cycle. They are socially adaptive and useful in the integration of personal needs and motives, social demands, and interpersonal relations. They can underlie seemingly admirable and virtuous patterns of behavior.

Altruism	The vicarious but constructive and instinctually gratifying service to others, even to the detriment of the self. This must be distinguished from altruistic surrender, which involves a masochistic surrender of direct gratification or of instinctual needs in favor of fulfilling the needs of others to the detriment of the self, with vicarious satisfaction only being gained through introjection.
Anticipation	The realistic anticipation of or planning for future inner discomfort: Implies overly concerned planning, worrying, and anticipation of dire and dreadful possible outcomes.
Asceticism	The elimination of directly pleasurable affects attributable to an experience. The moral element is implicit in setting values on specific pleasures. Asceticism is directed against all "base" pleasures perceived consciously, and gratification is derived from the renunciation.
Humor	The overt expression of feelings without personal discomfort or immobilization and without unpleasant effect on others. Humor allows one to bear, and yet focus on, what is too terrible to be borne, in contrast to wit, which always involves distraction or displacement away from the affective issue.
Sublimation	The gratification of an impulse whose goal is retained but whose aim or object is changed from a socially objectionable one to a socially valued one. Libidinal sublimation involves a desexualization of drive impulses and the placing of a value judgment that substitutes what is valued by the superego or society. Sublimation of aggressive impulses takes place through pleasurable games and sports. Unlike neurotic defenses, sublimation allows instincts to be channeled rather than dammed up or diverted. Thus, in sublimation, feelings are acknowledged, modified, and directed toward a relatively significant person or goal so that modest instinctual satisfaction results.
Suppression	The conscious or semiconscious decision to postpone attention to a conscious impulse or conflict.

Adapted from Vaillant GE. *Adaptation to Life*. Boston, MA: Little Brown; 1977; Semrad E. The operation of ego defenses in object loss. In: Moriarity DM, ed. *The Loss of Loved Ones*. Springfield, IL: Charles C Thomas; 1967; and Bibring GL, Dwyer TF, Huntington DS, Valenstein AA. A study of the psychological principles in pregnancy and of the earliest mother–child relationship: Methodological considerations. *Psychoanal Stud Child*. 1961;16:25.

Character. In 1913, Freud distinguished between neurotic symptoms and personality or character traits. *Neurotic symptoms* develop due to the failure of repression; *character traits* owe their existence to the success of repression, that is, to the defense system that achieves its aim through a persistent pattern of reaction formation and sublimation. In 1923, Freud also observed that the ego could only give up important objects by identifying with them or introjecting them. This accumulated pattern of identifications and introjections also contributes to character formation. Freud specifically emphasized the importance of superego formation in character construction.

Contemporary psychoanalysts regard character as a person's habitual or typical pattern of adaptation to internal drive forces and external environmental forces. *Character* and *personality* are used interchangeably and are distinguished from the ego in that they mostly refer to styles of defense and directly observable behavior rather than feeling and thinking.

Character is also influenced by constitutional temperament, the interaction of drive forces with early ego defenses and with environmental influences, and various identifications with, and internalizations of, other persons throughout life. The extent to which the ego has developed a capacity to tolerate the delay of impulse discharge and to neutralize instinctual energy determines the degree to which such character traits emerge in later life. Exaggerated development of individual character traits at the expense of others can lead to personality disorders or produce a vulnerability or predisposition to psychosis.

Classic Psychoanalytic Theory of Neuroses

The classic view of the genesis of neuroses regards conflict as essential. The conflict can arise between instinctual drives and external reality or internal agencies, such as the id and the superego or the id and the ego. Moreover, because the conflict has not been worked through to a realistic solution, the drives or wishes that seek discharge have been expelled from consciousness through repression or another defense mechanism. Their expulsion from conscious awareness, however, does not make the drives any less powerful or influential. As a result, the unconscious tendencies (e.g., the disguised neurotic symptoms) fight their way back into consciousness. This theory of the development of neurosis assumes that a rudimentary neurosis based on the same type of conflict existed in early childhood.

Deprivation during the first few months of life because of absent or impaired caretaking figures can adversely affect ego development. This impairment, in turn, can fail to make appropriate identifications. The resulting ego difficulties create problems in mediating between the drives and the environment. Lack of capacity for the constructive expression of drives, especially aggression, can lead some children to turn their aggression on themselves and become overtly self-destructive. Parents who are inconsistent, excessively harsh, or overly indulgent can influence children to develop disordered superego functioning. The severe conflict that cannot be managed through symptom formation can lead to extreme restrictions in ego functioning and fundamentally impair the capacity to learn and develop new skills.

Traumatic events that seem to threaten survival can break through defenses when the ego has been weakened. More libidinal energy is then required to master the excitation that results. The libido thus mobilized, however, is withdrawn from the supply that is usually applied to external objects. This withdrawal further diminishes the strength of the ego and produces a sense of inadequacy. Frustrations or disappointments in adults may revive infantile longings that are then dealt with through symptom formation or further regression.

In his classic studies, Freud described four different types of childhood neuroses, three of which had later neurotic developments in adult life. This well-known series of cases shown in tabulated form in Table 34-13 exemplifies some of Freud's important conclusions: (1) neurotic reactions in the adult are associated frequently with neurotic reactions in childhood; (2) the connection is sometimes continuous but more often is separated by a latent period of nonneurosis; and (3) infantile sexuality, both fantasized and real, occupies a memorable place in the early history of the patient.

Table 34-13
Classic Psychoneurotic Reactions of Childhood

	Conversion Reaction (Dora)	Phobic Reaction (Hans)	Obsessive-Compulsive Reaction (Rat Man)	Mixed Neurotic Reaction (Wolf Man)
Family history	Striking family history of psychiatric and physical illness	Both parents treated for neurotic conflict but not severe	No family history of mental illness	Striking family history of psychiatric and physical illness
Symptoms	Enuresis and masturbation, 6–8 yr; onset of neurosis at 8; migraine, nervous cough, and hoarseness at 12; aphonia at 16; "appendicitis" at 16; convulsions at 16; facial neuralgia at 19; change of personality at 8 from "wild creature" to quiet child	Compulsive questions at 3–3 1/2 yr in regard to sex difference; jealous reaction to sibling birth at 3 1/2; overt castration threat; overt masturbation at 3 1/2; overeating and constipation at 4–5; phobic reaction at 4–5; attack of flu at 5 worsens phobia; tonsillectomy at 5 worsens phobia	Naughty period at 3–4 yr; marked timidity after beating by father at 4; recognizing people by their smells as a child (Renifleur); precocious ego development; onset of obsessive ideas at 6–7	Tractable and quiet up to 3 1/4 yr; "naughty" period at 3 1/4–4 yr; phobias at 4–5 with nightmares; obsessional reaction at 6–7 (pious ceremonials). Disappearance of neuroses at 8
Causes	Seduction by older man; father's illness; father's affair	Seductive care by mother; sibling birth at 3 1/2	Seduction by governess at 4; death of sibling at 4; beating by father at 4	Seduction by older sister at 3 1/4; mother's illness; conflict between maid and governess

Courtesy of E. James Anthony, M.D.

Specific differences are worth noting in the four cases shown in Table 34-13. First, the phobic reactions tend to start at about 4 or 5 years of age, the obsessional reactions between 6 and 7 years, and the conversion reactions at 8 years. The degree of background disturbance is most significant in the conversion reaction and the mixed neurosis, and it seems only slight in the phobic and obsessional reactions. The course of the phobic reaction seems little influenced by severe traumatic factors, whereas traumatic factors, such as sexual seductions, play an essential role in the three other subgroups. It was during this period that Freud elaborated his seduction hypothesis for the cause of the neuroses, in terms of which the obsessive-compulsive and hysterical reactions were alleged to originate in active and passive sexual experiences.

Treatment and Technique

The cornerstone of psychoanalytic technique is free association, in which patients say whatever comes to mind. Free association not only provides analytic content, it helps to induce the regression needed for establishing and working through the transference

neurosis. When this development occurs, all the original wishes, drives, and defenses associated with the infantile neurosis are transferred to the person of the analyst.

As patients attempt to free associate, they soon learn that they have difficulty saying whatever comes to mind without censoring specific thoughts. They develop conflicts about their wishes and feelings toward the analyst that reflect childhood conflicts. The *transference* that develops toward the analyst may also serve as resistance to the process of free association. Freud discovered that *resistance* was not merely a stoppage of a patient's associations, but also an essential revelation of the patient's internal object relations as they were externalized and manifested in the transference relationship with the analyst. The systematic analysis of transference and resistance is the essence of psychoanalysis. Freud was also aware that the analyst might have transferences to the patient, which he called *countertransference*. Countertransference, in Freud's view, was an obstacle that the analyst needed to understand so that it did not interfere with treatment. In this spirit, he recognized the need for all analysts to have been analyzed themselves. Variations in transference and their descriptions are contained in Table 34-14. The basic mechanisms by which transferences are

Table 34-14
Transference Variants

Libidinal Transferences
Follow the classic model and usually in milder forms as positive *transference reactions* but can take the form of more intense and disturbing *erotic transferences*. They are derivatives of phallic-oedipal, libidinal impulses and may be permeated variously by pregenital influences. They can occur with varying degrees of intensity, and in mild forms, may not even require interpretation if they contribute to and support the therapeutic relation. Sigmund Freud recommended that they call for interpretation only when they begin to serve as a resistance.

Aggressive Transferences
Take the form either of negative or more pathologic paranoid transferences. *Negative transferences* are seen at all levels of psychopathology but can predominate in some borderline patients who tend to see the therapeutic relationship in terms of power and victimization, regarding the therapist as omnipotent and powerful, whereas the patient experiences him- or herself as helpless, weak, and vulnerable. Negative transferences are identifiable in varying degrees in all analyses and usually require specific intervention and interpretation.

Transferences of Defense
Opposed to *transferences of impulse;* defense against impulses finds its way into the transference rather than the impulses themselves. In this form of transference, attention shifts from drives to the ego's defensive functioning so that transference is no longer merely repetition of instinctual cathexes but includes aspects of ego functioning as well.

Transference Neurosis
Involves the recreation or more ample expression of the patient's neurosis enacted anew within the analytical relation and at least theoretically mirroring aspects of the infantile neurosis. The transference neurosis usually develops in the middle phase of analysis, when the patient, at first eager for improved mental health, no longer consistently displays such motivation but engages in a continuing battle with the analyst over the desire to attain some kind of emotional satisfaction from the analyst so that this becomes the most compelling reason for continuing analysis. At this point of the treatment, the transference emotions become more important to the patient than alleviation of distress sought initially, and the major, unresolved, unconscious problems of childhood begin to dominate the patient's behavior. They are now reproduced in the transference, with all their pent-up emotion.

The transference neurosis is governed by three outstanding characteristics of instinctual life in early childhood: the pleasure principle (before effective reality testing), ambivalence, and repetition compulsion. Emergence of the transference neurosis is usually a slow and gradual process, although in certain patients with a propensity for *transference regression,* particularly more hysterical patients, elements of transference and transference neurosis may manifest themselves relatively early in the analytical process. One situation after another in the life of the patient is analyzed and progressively interpreted until the original infantile conflict is sufficiently revealed. Only then does the transference neurosis begin to subside. At that point, termination begins to emerge as a more central concern.

Contemporary opinion is divided to its importance and centrality, whether it forms to the extent Freud believed, and whether it is necessary for successful analysis—for some, it remains an essential vehicle for analytical interpretation and therapeutic effectiveness; for others, it may never develop or, to the extent that it does, may play a less central role in the process of cure.

Transference Psychosis
Occurs when failure of reality testing leads to loss of self–object differentiation and diffusion of self and object boundaries. This may reflect an attempt to refuse with an omnipotent object, investing the self with omnipotent powers as defense against underlying fears of vulnerability and powerlessness. Transference psychosis can also include negative transference elements in which fusion carries the threat of engulfment and loss of self that may precipitate a *paranoid transference reaction.*

(continued)

Table 34-14
Transference Variants (*Continued*)

Narcissistic Transferences

Clarified by Heinz Kohut (1971) as variations of patterns of projection of archaic narcissistic configurations onto the therapist. They are based on projections of narcissistic introjective configurations, both superior and inferior—the superior form reflecting narcissistic superiority, grandiosity, and enhanced self-esteem, and the inferior opposite qualities of inferiority, self-depletion, and diminished self-esteem. The therapist comes to represent, in Kohut's terms, either the grandiose self in *mirror transferences* or the idealized parental imago in *idealizing transferences*. In idealizing transferences, all power and strength are attributed to the idealized object, leaving the subject feeling empty and powerless when separated from that object. Union with the idealized object enables the subject to regain narcissistic equilibrium. Idealizing transferences may reflect developmental disturbances in the idealized parent imago, particularly at the time of formation of the ego-ideal by introjection of the idealized object. In some individuals, narcissistic fixation leads to development of the grandiose self. Reactivation in analysis of the grandiose self provides the basis of mirror transferences formation, which occur in three forms: *archaic merger transference,* a less archaic *alter-ego* or *twinship transference,* and *mirror transference in the narrow sense*. In the most primitive merger transference, the analyst is experienced only as an extension of the subject's grandiose self and, thus, becomes the repository of the patient's grandiosity and exhibitionism. In the alter-ego or twinship transference, activation of the grandiose self leads to experience of the narcissistic object as similar to the grandiose self. In the most mature form of mirror transference, the analyst is experienced as a separate person but, nonetheless, one who becomes important to the patient and is accepted by him or her only to the degree that he or she is responsive to the narcissistic needs of the reactivated grandiose self.

Self–Object Transferences

Represent extensions of the self-psychology paradigm beyond merely narcissistic configurations. The self–object involves investment of the self in the object so that the object comes to serve a self-sustaining function that the self cannot perform for itself—either in maintaining fragile self-cohesion or in regulating self-esteem. The other, thus, is not experienced as an autonomous and separate object or agency in its own right but as present only to serve the needs of the self. Transference in this sense reflects a continuing developmental need that seeks satisfaction in the analytical relation.

Self–object transferences reflect the underlying need structure the patient brings to the therapeutic relationship based on the predominant pattern of self–object deprivation or frustration and the corresponding seeking for the appropriate form of self–object involvement. These configurations have been described as the *understimulated self,* the *overstimulated self,* the *overburdened self,* and the *fragmenting self.* Other descriptions of self–object need translate patterns of transference interaction based on narcissistic dynamics into the perspective of the relationship between self and self–object, as in mirror-hungry personalities and ideal-hungry personalities. Variations on the mirroring transference theme include the alter-ego–hungry personality, the merger-hungry personality, and, in contrast, the contact-shunning personality. In transferences derived from such personality configurations, the classic meaning of transference has undergone radical modification. Rather than displacements or projections from earlier object relational contexts, the patient brings to bear a need based in his or her own currently deficient capacity and defective character structure—a need to involve the object in a dependent relationship to complete or stabilize his or her own psychic integration.

Transitional Relatedness

This transference model is based on Donald Winnicott's notion of the transitional object. Transference in more primitive character structures is regarded as a form of *transitional object relation* in which the therapist is perceived as outside the self but is invested with qualities from the patient's own archaic self-image. The transference field in this view is envisioned as a transitional space in which the transference illusion is allowed to play itself out.

Transference as Psychic Reality

Reflects the need of each participant in analysis to draw the other into a stance corresponding to his or her own intrapsychic configuration and needs as a reflection of the individual subject's psychic reality. This regards the classic view of transference, based on displacement or projection from past objects, as inadequate, resulting in further diffusion of meaning of transference as equivalent to the individual's capacity to create a meaningful world or to inform the world with meaning. In this rendition, transference becomes equivalent to the patient's psychic reality so that any distinction between the meanings given to reality and the meanings inherent in transference is lost. Transference in these terms becomes all-encompassing, and whatever distinguishing and dynamic significance it may have had fades into obscurity. In this form of transference, no definable mechanism seems to be at work other than whatever is involved in the subject's psychic reality. The subject's view of his or her environment and impression of objects of his or her experience, including the analytical object, are indistinguishable from ordinary cognitive and affective processes characterizing personal involvement and responsiveness to the world about him or her.

Transference as Relational or Intersubjective

The relational or intersubjective view of transference as emerging from or cocreated by the subjective interaction between analyst and analysand transforms transference into an interactive phenomenon in which individual intrapsychic contributions from either participant are obscured. Transference in this sense is not anything individual to, or intrapsychically derived from, the patient but is based on the present ongoing interaction between analyst and patient coconstructing transference. On these terms, analysis of transference has little to do with past derivatives and everything to do with the ongoing relation with the analyst, primarily in the form of interpersonal enactments. Transference in this sense is no longer a one-person phenomenon but reflects a two-person transference–countertransference interaction. The supposition is that no such thing as transference exists without countertransference and no such thing as countertransference exists without transference. The patient is thus relieved of any burden of a personal dynamic unconscious reflecting developmental vicissitudes and residues of a life history. Transference is created anew in the immediacy of present analytical interaction as the product of mutual influence and communication between analyst and analysand, probably relying on some form of mutual projective identification to sustain the interactive connotation.

Table 34-15
Transference Mechanisms

Displacement

The basic mechanism of classic transference paradigms in which an object representation derived from any level or combination of levels of the subject's developmental experience is displaced to the representation of the new object, namely, the analyst, in the therapeutic relationship. Displacement is the basic mechanism for libidinally based transferences, both positive and erotic, as well as for aggressive and especially negative transferences. By and large, displacement transferences tend to play a more dominant role in neurotic disorders in which phallic–oedipal (and to a lesser degree preoedipal) dynamics tend to play a dominant, although not exclusive, role.

Projection

Process by which qualities or characteristics of the self-as-object, usually involving introjections or self-representations, are attributed to an external object, and the subsequent interaction with the object is determined by the projected characteristics. Thus, the analyst or object may be seen as sadistic—that is, as possessing the sadistic character of the analysand or subject, an aspect of the subject's self that is denied or disowned by the subject. Projection tends to play a more prominent, although again not exclusive, role in formation of transferences in more primitive character disorders but can be found in variously modified forms throughout the spectrum of neuroses. Because projections derive primarily from the configuration of introjects constituting the patient's self-as-object, the effect of projective or externalizing transferences is that the image of the therapist comes to represent part of the patient's own self-organization rather than simply an object representation.

Projections derived from destructive introjects can provide the basis for both negative and paranoid transference reactions. Those based on the victim or introject result in the patient relating to the therapist as his or her victim and him- or herself assuming a hostile or sadistic position as a destructive aggressor or victimizer to the therapist's victim. Then again, projection based on the aggressor or introject results in the patient relating to the therapist as an aggressor and him- or herself assuming a weak, vulnerable, or masochistic position in which he or she becomes a passive and vulnerable victim to the therapist's destructive aggression. Similar patterns can take place around narcissistic issues involving introjective configurations of narcissistic superiority and inferiority.

Projective dynamics in self–object transferences, however, seem to involve more than narcissistic projections because these forms of transference tend to draw the analyst into meeting the pathologic needs of the self. If anything is projected, it is an infantile wished-for imago, one lacking earlier in the patient's experience, as, for example, an empathic and idealized parental figure. On the other hand, transitional transferences, despite their considerable overlap with self–object phenomena, tend to involve a more explicit projective element as the self-related contribution to the transitional experience.

Projective Identification

The concept of projective identification was first proposed by Melanie Klein, arguing that the projection of impulses or feelings into another person brought about an identification with that person based on attribution of one's own qualities to that other. This attribution served as the basis for a sense of empathy and connection with the other. On these terms, projective identification was a fantasy taking place solely in the mind of the one projecting.

Projective identification is often appealed to as a mechanism of transference, or more exactly transference–countertransference interactions, particularly in Kleinian usage. Confusion arises from the failure to clearly distinguish between projection and projective identification. The notion of projective identification added to the basic concept of projection of the notes of diffusion of ego boundaries, a loss or diminishing of self–object differentiation, and inclusion of the object as part of the self.

Later elaborations of the notion of projective identification transformed it from a one-body to a two-body phenomenon, describing interaction between two subjects, one of whom projects something onto or into the other, whereon the other introjects or internalizes what has been projected. Instead of the projection and introjection taking place in the same subject, the projection now takes place in one and the internalization in the other. This latter usage has led to extensive extrapolation of the concept of projective identification to apply to all sorts of object relations, including transference. The emphasis in Kleinian transference is less on the influence of the past on the present but rather the influence of the internal world on the external in the here-and-now interaction with the analyst.

---

effected—displacement, projection, and projective identification—are described in Table 34-15.

Analysts after Freud began to recognize that countertransference was not only an obstacle but also a source of useful information about the patient. In other words, the analyst's feelings in response to the patient reflect how other persons respond to the patient and indicate the patient's own internal object relations. By understanding the intense feelings in the analytic relationship, the analyst can help the patient broaden the understanding of past and current relationships outside the analysis. The development of insight into neurotic conflicts also expands the ego and provides an increased sense of mastery.

ERIK H. ERIKSON

Erik H. Erikson (Fig. 34-24) was one of America's most influential psychoanalysts. Throughout six decades in the United States, he distinguished himself as an illuminator and expositor of Freud's theories and as a brilliant clinician, teacher, and pioneer in psychohistorical investigation. Erikson created an original and highly influential theory of psychological development and crisis occurring in periods that extended across the entire life cycle. His theory grew out of his work first as a teacher, then as a child psychoanalyst, next as an anthropologic field worker, and, finally, as a biographer. Erikson identified dilemmas or polarities in the ego's relations with the family and larger social institutions at nodal points in childhood, adolescence, and early, middle, and late adulthood. Two of his psychosexual historical studies, *Young Man Luther* and *Gandhi's Truth* (published in 1958 and 1969, respectively), were widely hailed as profound explorations of how crucial circumstances can interact with the crises of certain great persons at particular moments in time. The interrelationships of the psychological development of the person and the historical developments of the times were more fully explored in *Life History and the Historical Moment*, written by Erikson in 1975.

Erik Homburger Erikson was born on June 15, 1902, in Frankfurt, Germany, the son of Danish parents. He died in 1994. His father abandoned his mother before he was born, and he was brought up by his mother, a Danish Jew, and her second husband, Theodor Homburger, a German-Jewish pediatrician. Erikson's parents chose to keep his real parentage a secret from him, and for many years he was known as Erik Homburger. Erikson never knew his biologic

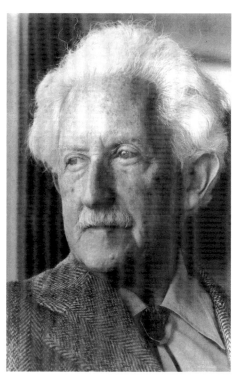

FIGURE 34-24
Erik Erikson (1902–1994).

father; his mother withheld that information from him all her life. Undoubtedly, the man who introduced the term "identity crisis" into the language struggled with his sense of identity. Compounding his parents' deception about his biologic father—their "loving deceit," as he called it—was the fact that, as a blond, blue-eyed, Scandinavian-looking son of a Jewish father, he was taunted as a "goy" among Jews, at the same time being called a Jew by his classmates. His being a Dane living in Germany added to his identity confusion. Erikson was later described as a man of the borders. Much of what he was to study was concerned with how group values are implanted in the very young, how young people grasp onto group identity in the limbo period between childhood and adulthood, and how a few persons, like Gandhi, transcend their local, national. Even temporal identities to form a small band of people with wider sympathies who span the ages.

The concepts of identity, identity crisis, and identity confusion are central to Erikson's thought. In his first book *Childhood and Society* (published in 1950), Erikson observed that "the study of identity…becomes as strategic in our time as the study of sexuality was in Freud's time." By identity, Erikson meant a sense of sameness and continuity "in the inner core of the individual" maintained amid external change. A sense of identity, emerging at the end of adolescence, is a psychosocial phenomenon preceded in one form or another by an identity crisis; that crisis may be conscious or unconscious, with the person being aware of the present state and future directions but also unconscious of the fundamental dynamics and conflicts that underlie those states. The identity crisis can be acute and prolonged in some people.

The young Erikson did not distinguish himself in school, although he did show artistic talent. On graduation, he spent a year traveling through the Black Forest, Italy, and the Alps, pondering life, drawing, and making notes. After that year of roaming, he studied art in his home city of Karlsruhe and later in Munich and Florence.

In 1927 Peter Blos, a high school friend, invited Erikson to join him in Vienna. Blos, not yet a psychoanalyst, had met Dorothy Burlingham, a New Yorker who had come to Vienna to be psychoanalyzed; she had brought her four children with her and hired Blos to tutor them. Blos was looking for a fellow teacher in his new school for the children of English and American parents and students of his new discipline of psychoanalysis. Erikson accepted his offer.

Blos and Erikson informally organized their school—much in the style of the so-called progressive or experimental schools prevalent in the United States. Children were encouraged to participate in curriculum planning and to express themselves freely. Erikson, still very much the artist, taught drawing and painting, but he also exposed his pupils to history and foreign ways of life, including the cultures of the American Indian and Eskimo.

During that period, Erikson became involved with the Freud family, friends of Mrs. Burlingham. He became particularly close to Anna Freud, with whom he began psychoanalysis. Anna Freud, who had been an elementary school teacher, was at that time formulating the new science of child psychiatry, trying to turn attention from the adult's corrective backward look to a neurosis-preventative study of childhood itself. Under Anna Freud's tutelage, Erikson began more and more to turn his attention to childhood, both his own and that of the children whom he saw in the classroom. The analysis was not then the rigidly structured procedure into which it later developed; Erikson met with Miss Freud daily for his analytic hour and frequently saw her socially and as part of the circle of Freud's followers and associates. Still undecided about his future, Erikson continued to teach school while studying psychoanalysis at the Vienna Psychoanalytic Institute. He also studied to become accredited as a Montessori teacher.

In 1929 he married Joan Mowat Serson, an American of Canadian birth. He was hastily made a full member, rather than an associate member of the Vienna Psychoanalytic Society—unorthodoxy that allowed him to leave a Vienna threatened by fascism immediately after his graduation in 1933. Earlier, Erikson had met the Viennese Hanns Sachs, co-founder, along with Otto Rank of the psychoanalytically oriented journal *Imago*. Sachs—who had settled in Boston, where he was associated with the Harvard Medical School—was sure that Erikson would be welcome at Harvard and suggested that he make Boston his home. After a brief stay in Denmark, the Eriksons moved to Boston, where he became the city's only child analyst. He held positions at the Harvard Medical School and Massachusetts General Hospital, served as a consultant at the Judge Baker Guidance Center, and maintained a private practice.

Erikson was much influenced by Cambridge's circle of young social scientists, including anthropologists Margaret Mead and Ruth Benedict. Exposure to the views of those vigorous thinkers helped to shape his theories of child psychology and his cross-cultural approach to human development. Classical psychoanalysis had traditionally concerned itself with pathology and with treating disturbed people. However, Erikson found himself more interested in the normal personality and applying his observations about how young people function and how childhood play affects character formation. Although he remained in the Boston area for only 3 years, he established a solid reputation as a skilled clinician and researcher before moving to Yale University's Institute of Human Relations. There he furthered an interest sparked at Harvard in the work of American anthropologists. In 1938 he traveled to South Dakota to study the children of the Sioux Indians of the Pine Ridge Reservation. His observations about how communal and historical forces powerfully influence child-rearing became a vital contribution to psychology and the study of humans in society.

In 1939 Erikson moved to a post at Berkeley, from which he studied the Yurok Indians, a group of salmon fishers. He left Berkeley in 1950 after refusing to sign what he called a vague, fearful addition to the loyalty oath. He resettled at the Austen Riggs Center in Stockbridge, Massachusetts, working with young people. In 1960 he was appointed to a professorship at Harvard. After he retired from Harvard in 1972, Erickson joined Mount Zion Hospital in San Francisco as a senior consultant in psychiatry. Until his death in 1994, he continued to focus on many of his earlier interests, examining the individual in this historical context and elaborating on concepts of the human life cycle, especially those of old age.

Epigenetic Principle

Erikson's formulations were based on the concept of *epigenesis*, a term borrowed from embryology. His *epigenetic principle* holds that development occurs in sequential, clearly defined stages and that each stage must be satisfactorily resolved for development to proceed smoothly. According to the epigenetic model, if a successful resolution of a particular stage does not occur, all subsequent stages reflect that failure in physical, cognitive, social, or emotional maladjustment.

Relation to Freudian Theory. Erikson accepted Freud's concepts of instinctual development and infantile sexuality. For each of Freud's psychosexual stages (e.g., oral, anal, and phallic), Erikson described a corresponding zone with a specific pattern or mode of behavior. Thus, the oral zone is associated with sucking or

taking-in behavior; the anal zone is associated with holding on and letting go. Erikson emphasized that the development of the ego is more than the result of intrapsychic wants or inner psychic energies. It is also a matter of mutual regulation between growing children and a society's culture and traditions.

Eight Stages of the Life Cycle. Erikson's conception of the eight stages of ego development across the life cycle is the centerpiece of his life's work, and he elaborated on the conception throughout his subsequent writings (Table 34-16). The eight stages represent points along a continuum of development. Physical, cognitive, instinctual, and sexual changes combine to trigger an internal crisis, the resolution of which results in either psychosocial regression or growth and the development of specific virtues. In *Insight and Responsibility*, Erikson defined virtue as "inherent strength," as in the active quality of medicine or liquor. He wrote in *Identity: Youth and Crisis* that "crisis" refers not to a "threat of catastrophe, but a turning point, a crucial period of increased vulnerability and heightened potential, and therefore, the ontogenetic source of generational strength and maladjustment."

STAGE 1: TRUST VERSUS MISTRUST (BIRTH TO ABOUT 18 MONTHS). In *Identity: Youth and Crisis,* Erikson noted that the infant "lives through and loves with" its mouth. Indeed, the mouth forms the basis of its first mode or pattern of behavior, incorporation. The infant is taking the world through the mouth, eyes, ears, and sense of touch. The baby is learning a cultural modality that Erikson termed *to get,* that is, to receive what is offered and elicit what is desired. As the infant's teeth develop, and it discovers the pleasure of biting,

Table 34-16
Erikson's Psychosocial Stages

Psychosocial Stage	Associated Virtue	Related Forms of Psychopathology	Positive and Negative Forerunners of Identity Formation	Enduring Aspects of Identity Formation
Trust vs. mistrust (birth–)	Hope	Psychosis Addictions Depression	Mutual recognition vs. autistic isolation	Temporal perspective vs. time confusion
Autonomy vs. shame and doubt (~18 mo–)	Will	Paranoia Obsessions Compulsions Impulsivity	Will to be oneself vs. self-doubt	Self-certainty vs. self-consciousness
Initiative vs. guilt (~3 yr–)	Purpose	Conversion disorder Phobia Psychosomatic disorder Inhibition	Anticipation of roles vs. role inhibition	Role experimentation vs. role fixation
Industry vs. inferiority (~5 yr–)	Competence	Creative inhibition Inertia	Task identification vs. sense of futility	Apprenticeship vs. work paralysis
Identity vs. role confusion (~13 yr–)	Fidelity	Delinquent behavior Gender-related identity disorders Borderline psychotic episodes		Identity vs. identity confusion
Intimacy vs. isolation (~20s–)	Love	Schizoid personality disorder Distantiation		Sexual polarization vs. bisexual confusion
Generativity vs. stagnation (~40s–)	Care	Mid-life crisis Premature invalidism		Leadership and followership vs. abdication of responsibility
Integrity vs. despair (~60s–)	Wisdom	Extreme alienation Despair		Ideologic commitment vs. confusion of values

Adapted from Erikson E. *Insight and Responsibility.* New York: WW Norton; 1964 and Erikson E. *Identity: Youth and Crisis.* New York: WW Norton; 1968, with permission.

it enters the second oral stage, the active-incorporative mode. The infant is no longer passively receptive to stimuli; it reaches out for sensation and grasps at its surroundings—the social modality shifts to that of *taking and holding* on to things.

The infant's development of essential trust in the world stems from its earliest experiences with its mother or primary caretaker. In *Childhood and Society,* Erikson asserts that trust depends not on "absolute quantities of food or demonstrations of love, but rather on the quality of the maternal relationship." A baby whose mother can anticipate and respond to its needs in a consistent and timely manner despite its oral aggression will learn to tolerate the inevitable moments of frustration and deprivation. The defense mechanisms of introjection and projection provide the infant with the means to internalize pleasure and externalize pain such that "consistency, continuity, and sameness of experience provide a rudimentary sense of ego identity." Trust will predominate over mistrust, and hope will crystallize. For Erikson, the element of society corresponding to this stage of ego identity is religion, as both are founded on "trust born of care."

In keeping with his emphasis on the epigenetic character of psychosocial change, Erikson conceived of many forms of psychopathology as examples of what he termed *aggravated development crisis,* development, which having gone awry at one point, affects subsequent psychosocial change. A person who, as a result of severe disturbances in the earliest dyadic relationships, fails to develop a basic sense of trust or the virtue of hope may be predisposed as an adult to the profound withdrawal and regression characteristic of schizophrenia. Erikson hypothesized that the depressed patient's experience of being empty and being no good is an outgrowth of a developmental derailment that causes oral pessimism to predominate. Addictions may also be traced to the mode of oral incorporation.

STAGE 2: AUTONOMY VERSUS SHAME AND DOUBT (ABOUT 18 MONTHS TO ABOUT 3 YEARS).

In the development of speech and sphincter and muscular control, the toddler practices the social modalities of *holding on and letting go* and experiences the first stirrings of the virtue that Erikson termed *will.* Much depends on the amount and type of control exercised by adults over the child. Control that is exerted too rigidly or too early defeats the toddler's attempts to develop its internal controls, and regression or false progression results. Parental control that fails to protect the toddler from the consequences of their lack of self-control or judgment can be equally disastrous to the child's development of a healthy sense of autonomy. In *Identity: Youth and Crisis,* Erikson asserted: "This stage, therefore, becomes decisive for the ratio between loving goodwill and hateful self-insistence, between cooperation and willfulness, and between self-expression and compulsive self-restraint or meek compliance."

Where that ratio is favorable, the child develops an appropriate sense of autonomy and the capacity to "have and to hold"; where it is unfavorable, doubt and shame will undermine free will. According to Erikson, the principle of law and order has at its roots this early preoccupation with the protection and regulation of will. In *Childhood and Society,* he concluded, "The sense of autonomy fostered in the child and modified as life progresses, serves (and is served by) the preservation in the economic and political life of a sense of justice."

A person who becomes fixated at the transition between the development of hope and autonomous will, with its residue of mistrust and doubt, may develop paranoiac fears of persecution. When psychosocial development is derailed in the second stage, other forms of pathology may emerge. The perfectionism, inflexibility, and stinginess of the person with an obsessive-compulsive personality disorder may stem from conflicting tendencies to hold on and to let go. The ruminative and ritualistic behavior of the person with an obsessive-compulsive disorder may be an outcome of the triumph of doubt over autonomy and the subsequent development of a primitively harsh conscience.

STAGE 3: INITIATIVE VERSUS GUILT (ABOUT 3 YEARS TO ABOUT 5 YEARS).

The child's increasing mastery of locomotor and language skills expands its participation in the outside world and stimulates omnipotent fantasies of broader exploration and conquest. Here the youngster's mode of participation is active and intrusive; its social modality is that of being on the make. The intrusiveness is manifested in the child's fervent curiosity and genital preoccupations, competitiveness, and physical aggression. The Oedipus complex is in ascendance as the child competes with the same-sex parent for the fantasized possession of the other parent. In *Identity: Youth and Crisis,* Erikson wrote that "jealousy and rivalry now come to a climax in a final contest for a favored position with one of the parents: the inevitable and necessary failure leads to guilt and anxiety."

Guilt over the drive for conquest and anxiety over the anticipated punishment are both assuaged in the child through repression of the forbidden wishes and development of a superego to regulate its initiative. This conscience, the faculty of self-observation, self-regulation, and self-punishment, is an internalized version of parental and societal authority. Initially, the conscience is harsh and uncompromising; however, it constitutes the foundation for the subsequent development of morality. Having renounced oedipal ambitions, the child begins to look outside the family for arenas in which it can compete with less conflict and guilt. This is the stage that highlights the child's expanding initiative and forms the basis for the subsequent development of realistic ambition and the virtue of *purpose.* As Erikson noted in *Childhood and Society,* "The 'oedipal' stage sets the direction toward the possible and the tangible which permits the dreams of early childhood to be attached to the goals of active adult life." Toward this end, social institutions provide the child with an economic ethos in adult heroes who begin to replace their storybook counterparts.

When there has been an inadequate resolution of the conflict between initiative and guilt, a person may ultimately develop a conversion disorder, inhibition, or phobia. Those who overcompensate for the conflict by driving themselves too hard may experience sufficient stress to produce psychosomatic symptoms.

STAGE 4: INDUSTRY VERSUS INFERIORITY (ABOUT 5 YEARS TO ABOUT 13 YEARS).

With the onset of latency, the child discovers the pleasures of production. He or she develops industry by learning new skills and takes pride in the things made. Erikson wrote in *Childhood and Society* that the child's "ego boundaries include his tools and skills: the work principle teaches him the pleasure of work completion by steady attention and persevering diligence." Across cultures, this is when the child receives systematic instruction and learns the fundamentals of technology and how to use necessary utensils and tools. As children work, they identify with their teachers and imagine themselves in various occupational roles.

A child unprepared for this stage of psychosocial development, either through an insufficient resolution of previous stages or by current interference, may develop a sense of inferiority and inadequacy. In the form of teachers and other role models, society becomes crucially important in the child's ability to overcome that sense of inferiority and achieve the virtue known as competence.

In *Identity: Youth and Crisis,* Erikson noted: "This is socially a most decisive stage. Since industry involves doing things beside and with others, a first sense of division of labor and of differential opportunity, that is, a sense of the technological ethos of a culture, develops at this time."

The pathologic outcome of a poorly navigated stage of industry versus inferiority is less well defined than in previous stages. However, it may concern the emergence of a conformist immersion into the world of production in which creativity is stifled, and identity is subsumed under the worker's role.

STAGE 5: IDENTITY VERSUS ROLE CONFUSION (ABOUT 13 YEARS TO ABOUT 21 YEARS).
With the onset of puberty and its myriad social and physiologic changes, adolescents become preoccupied with identity. Erikson noted in *Childhood and Society* that youth are now "primarily concerned with what they appear to be in the eyes of others as compared to what they feel they are, and with the question of how to connect the roles and skills cultivated earlier with the occupational prototypes of the day." Childhood roles and fantasies are no longer appropriate, yet the adolescent is far from equipped to become an adult. In *Childhood and Society,* Erikson writes that the integration that occurs in the formation of ego identity encompasses far more than the summation of childhood identifications. "It is the accrued experience of the ego's ability to integrate these identifications with the vicissitudes of the libido, with the aptitudes developed out of endowment, and with the opportunities offered in social roles."

The formation of cliques and an identity crisis occur at the end of adolescence. Erikson calls the crisis normative because it is a typical event. Failure to negotiate this stage leaves adolescents without a stable identity; they suffer from identity diffusion or role confusion, characterized by not having a sense of self and by confusion about their place in the world. Role confusion can manifest in such behavioral abnormalities as running away, criminality, and overt psychosis. Problems in gender identity and sexual role may manifest at this time. Adolescents may defend against role diffusion by joining cliques or cults or by identifying with folk heroes. Intolerance of individual differences is how the young person attempts to ward off a sense of identity loss. Falling in love, a process by which the adolescent may clarify a sense of identity by projecting a diffused self-image onto the partner and gradually seeing it assume a more distinctive shape. An overidentification with idealized figures is how the adolescent seeks self-definition. With the attainment of a more sharply focused identity, the youth develops the virtue of *fidelity*—faithfulness not only to the nascent self-definition but also to an ideology that provides a version of self-in-world. As Erik Erikson, Joan Erikson, and Helen Kivnick wrote in *Vital Involvement in Old Age,* "Fidelity is the ability to sustain loyalties freely pledged in spite of the inevitable contradictions of value systems. It is the cornerstone of identity and receives inspiration from confirming ideologies and affirming companionships." Role confusion ensues when the youth is unable to formulate a sense of identity and belonging. Erikson held that delinquency, gender-related identity disorders, and borderline psychotic episodes can result from such confusion.

STAGE 6: INTIMACY VERSUS ISOLATION (ABOUT 21 YEARS TO ABOUT 40 YEARS).
Freud's famous response to the question of what a normal person should be able to do well, "Lieben und arbeiten" (to love and to work), is one that Erikson often cited in his discussion of this psychosocial stage, and it emphasizes the importance he placed on the virtue of love within a balanced identity. Erikson asserted in *Identity: Youth and Crisis* that Freud's use of the term love referred to "the generosity of intimacy as well as genital love; when he said love and work, he meant a general work productiveness which would not preoccupy the individual to the extent that he might lose his right or capacity to be a sexual and a loving being."

Intimacy in the young adult is closely tied to fidelity; it can make and honor commitments to concrete affiliations and partnerships even when that requires sacrifice and compromise. The person who cannot tolerate the fear of ego loss arising out of self-abandonment (e.g., sexual orgasm, moments of intensity in friendships, aggression, inspiration, and intuition) is apt to become profoundly isolated and self-absorbed. *Distantiation,* an awkward term coined by Erikson to mean "the readiness to repudiate, isolate, and, if necessary, destroy those forces and persons whose essence seems dangerous to one's own," is the pathologic outcome of conflicts surrounding intimacy and, in the absence of an ethical sense where intimate, competitive, and combative relationships are differentiated, forms the basis for various forms of prejudice, persecution, and psychopathology.

Erikson's separation of the psychosocial task of achieving identity from achieving intimacy and his assertion that substantial progress on the former task must precede development on the latter have engendered much criticism and debate. Critics have argued that Erikson's emphasis on separation and occupationally based identity formation fails to consider the importance for women of continued attachment and the formation of an identity based on relationships.

STAGE 7: GENERATIVITY VERSUS STAGNATION (ABOUT 40 YEARS TO ABOUT 60 YEARS).
Erikson asserted in *Identity: Youth and Crisis* that "generativity is primarily the concern for establishing and guiding the next generation." The term *generativity* applies not so much to rearing and teaching one's offspring as it does to a protective concern for all the generations and social institutions. It encompasses productivity and creativity, as well. Having achieved the capacity to form intimate relationships, the person now broadens the investment of ego and libidinal energy to include groups, organizations, and society. *Care* is the virtue that coalesces at this stage. In *Childhood and Society,* Erikson emphasized the importance to the mature person of feeling needed. "Maturity needs guidance as well as encouragement from what has been produced and must be taken care of." Through generative behavior, the individual can pass on knowledge and skills while obtaining a measure of satisfaction in having achieved a role with senior authority and responsibility in the tribe.

When persons cannot develop true generativity, they may settle for pseudoengagement in occupation. Often, such persons restrict their focus to the technical aspects of their roles, at which they may now have become highly skilled, eschewing greater responsibility for the organization or profession. This failure of generativity can lead to profound personal stagnation, masked by various escapisms, such as alcohol and drug abuse, and sexual and other infidelities. Mid-life crisis or premature invalidism (physical and psychological) can occur. In this case, pathology appears not only in middle-aged persons but also in the organizations that depend on them for leadership. Thus, the failure to develop at midlife can lead to sick, withered, or destructive organizations that spread the effects of failed generativity throughout society; examples of such failures have become so common that they constitute a defining feature of modernity.

STAGE 8: INTEGRITY VERSUS DESPAIR (ABOUT 60 YEARS TO DEATH).
In *Identity: Youth and Crisis,* Erikson defined integrity as "the acceptance of one's one and only life cycle and of the persons who have become significant to it as something that had to be and that, by necessity, permitted of no substitutions." From the vantage point of

this stage of psychosocial development, the individual relinquishes the wish that important persons in his life had been different and can love in a more meaningful way—one that reflects accepting responsibility for one's own life. The individual in possession of the virtue of wisdom and a sense of integrity has room to tolerate the proximity of death and to achieve what Erikson termed in *Identity: Youth and Crisis,* a "detached yet active concern with life."

Erikson underlined the social context for this final stage of growth. In *Childhood and Society,* he wrote, "The style of integrity developed by his culture or civilization thus becomes the 'patrimony' of his soul....In such final consolidation, death loses its sting."

When attempting to attain integrity has failed, the individual may become deeply disgusted with the external world and contemptuous of persons and institutions. Erikson wrote in *Childhood and Society* that such disgust masks a fear of death and a sense of despair that "time is now short, too short for the attempt to start another life and to try out alternate roads to integrity." Looking back on the eight ages of man, he noted the relation between adult integrity and infantile trust, "Healthy children will not fear life if their elders have integrity enough not to fear death."

Psychopathology

Each stage of the life cycle has its psychopathological outcome if it is not mastered successfully.

Basic Trust.   An impairment of basic trust leads to basic mistrust. In infants, social trust is characterized by ease of feeding, depth of sleep, smiling, and general physiologic homeostasis. Prolonged separation during infancy can lead to hospitalism or anaclitic depression. In later life, this lack of trust may be manifested by dysthymic disorder, a depressive disorder, or a sense of hopelessness. Persons who develop and rely on the defense of projection—in which, according to Erikson, "we endow significant persons with the evil which actually is in us"—experienced a sense of social mistrust in the first years of life and are likely to develop paranoid or delusional disorders. Basic mistrust is a significant contributor to the development of schizoid personality disorder and, in most severe cases, to the development of schizophrenia. Substance-related disorders can also be traced to social mistrust; substance-dependent personalities have strong oral-dependency needs and use chemical substances to satisfy themselves because of their belief that human beings are unreliable and, at worst, dangerous. If not appropriately nurtured, infants may feel empty, starved not just for food but also sensual and visual stimulation. As adults, they may become seekers after stimulating thrills that do not involve intimacy, which helps ward off feelings of depression.

Autonomy.   The stage in which children attempt to develop into autonomous beings is often called the *terrible twos,* referring to toddlers' willfulness at this period of development. If shame and doubt dominate over autonomy, compulsive doubting can occur. The inflexibility of the obsessive personality also results from an overabundance of doubt. Too rigorous toilet training, commonplace in today's society, requires a clean, punctual, and deodorized body, can produce an overly compulsive personality that is stingy, meticulous, and selfish. Known as anal personalities, such persons are parsimonious, punctual, and perfectionistic (the three P's).

Too much shaming causes children to feel evil or dirty and may pave the way for delinquent behavior. In effect, children say, "If that's what they think of me, that's the way I'll behave." Paranoid

personalities feel that others are trying to control them, a feeling that may have its origin during the stage of autonomy versus shame and doubt. When coupled with mistrust, the seeds are planted for persecutory delusions. Impulsive disorder may be explained as a person's refusal to be inhibited or controlled.

Initiative.   Erikson stated: "In pathology, the conflict over initiative is expressed either in hysterical denial, which causes the repression of the wish or the abrogation of its executive organ by paralysis or impotence; or in overcompensatory showing off, in which the scared individual, so eager to 'duck,' instead 'sticks his neck out.'" In the past, hysteria was the usual form of pathologic regression in this area, but a plunge into a psychosomatic disease is now common.

Excessive guilt can lead to a variety of conditions, such as generalized anxiety disorder and phobias. Patients feel guilty because of normal impulses, and they repress these impulses, with resulting symptom formation. Punishment or severe prohibitions during the stage of initiative versus guilt can produce sexual inhibitions. Conversion disorder or specific phobia can result when the oedipal conflict is not resolved. As sexual fantasies are accepted as unrealizable, children may punish themselves for these fantasies by fearing harm to their genitals. Under the brutal assault of the developing superego, they may repress their wishes and begin to deny them. If this pattern is carried forward, paralysis, inhibition, or impotence can result. Sometimes, in fear of not being able to live up to what others expect, children may develop a psychosomatic disease.

Industry.   Erikson described industry as a "sense of being able to make things and make them well and even perfectly." When children's efforts are thwarted, they are made to feel that personal goals cannot be accomplished or are not worthwhile, and a sense of inferiority develops. In adults, this sense of inferiority can result in severe work inhibitions and a character structure marked by feelings of inadequacy. For some persons, the feelings may result in a compensatory drive for money, power, and prestige. Work can become the main focus of life at the expense of intimacy.

Identity.   Many disorders of adolescence can be traced to identity confusion. The danger is role diffusion. Erikson stated:

Where this is based on a strong previous doubt on one's sexual identity, delinquent and outright psychotic incidents are not uncommon. If diagnosed and treated correctly, those incidents do not have the same fatal significance that they have at other ages. It is primarily the inability to settle on an occupational identity that disturbs young persons. Keeping themselves together, they temporarily overidentify, to the point of apparent complete loss of identity, with the heroes of cliques and crowds.

Other disorders during the stage of identity versus role diffusion include conduct disorder, disruptive behavior disorder, gender identity disorder, schizophreniform disorder, and other psychotic disorders. The ability to leave home and live independently is an essential task during this period. An inability to separate from the parent and prolonged dependence may occur.

Intimacy.   The successful formation of a stable marriage and family depends on the capacity to become intimate. The years of early adulthood are crucial for deciding whether to get married and to whom. Gender identity determines object choice, either straight or gay, but making an intimate connection with another person is a significant task. Persons with schizoid personality disorder remain isolated from others because of fear, suspicion, inability to take risks, or the lack of a capacity to love.

GENERATIVITY.   From about 40 to 65 years, the period of middle adulthood, specific disorders are less clearly defined than in the other stages described by Erikson. Middle-aged persons show a higher incidence of depression than younger adults, which may be related to middle-aged persons' disappointments and failed expectations as they review the past, consider their lives, and contemplate the future. The increased use of alcohol and other psychoactive substances also occurs during this time.

INTEGRITY.   Anxiety disorders often develop in older persons. In Erikson's formulation, this development may be related to persons' looking back on their lives with a sense of panic. Time has run out, and chances are used up. The decline in physical functions can contribute to psychosomatic illness, hypochondriasis, and depression. The suicide rate is highest in persons over the age of 65. Persons facing dying and death may find it intolerable not to have been generative or make significant attachments in life. Integrity, for Erikson, is characterized by an acceptance of life. Without acceptance, persons feel despair and hopelessness that can result in severe depressive disorders.

Treatment

Although no independent Eriksonian psychoanalytic school exists in the same way that Freudian and Jungian schools do, Erikson made many vital contributions to the therapeutic process. Among his most important contributions is his belief that establishing a state of trust between doctor and patient is the essential requirement for successful therapy. When psychopathology stems from basic mistrust (e.g., depression), a patient must reestablish trust with the therapist, whose task, like that of the good mother, is sensitive to the patient's needs. The therapist must have a sense of personal trustworthiness that can be transmitted to the patient.

Techniques.   For Erikson, a psychoanalyst is not a blank slate in the therapeutic process, as the psychoanalyst commonly is in Freudian psychoanalysis. On the contrary, effective therapy requires that therapists actively convey to patients the belief that they are understood. This is done through both empathetic listening and verbal assurances, which enable a positive transference built on mutual trust to develop.

Beginning as an analyst for children, Erikson tried to provide this mutuality and trust while he observed children recreating their worlds by structuring dolls, blocks, vehicles, and miniature furniture into the dramatic situations that were bothering them. Then, Erikson correlated his observations with statements by the children and their family members. He began treatment of a child only after eating an evening meal with the entire family, and his therapy was usually conducted with much cooperation from the family. After each regressive episode in the treatment of a schizophrenic child, for instance, Erikson discussed with every member of the family what had been going on with them before the episode. Only when he was thoroughly satisfied that he had identified the problem did treatment begin. Erikson sometimes provided corrective information to the child—for instance, telling a boy who could not release his feces and had made himself ill from constipation that food is not an unborn infant.

Erikson often turned to play, which, along with specific recommendations to parents, proved fruitful as a treatment modality. Play, for Erikson, is diagnostically revealing and thus helpful for a therapist who seeks to promote a cure, but it is also curative in its own right. Play is a function of the ego and gives children a chance to synchronize social and bodily processes with the self. Children playing with blocks or adults playing out an imagined dramatic situation can manipulate the environment and develop the sense of control that the ego needs. Play therapy is not the same for children and adults, however. Children create models to gain control of reality; they look ahead to new areas of mastery. Adults use play to correct the past and to redeem their failures.

Mutuality, which is essential in Erikson's system of health, is also vital to a cure. Erikson applauded Freud for the moral choice of abandoning hypnosis because hypnosis heightens both the demarcation between the healer and the sick and the inequality that Erikson compares with the inequality of child and adult. Erikson urged that the relationship of the healer to the sick person be one of equals "in which the observer who has learned to observe himself teaches the observed to become self-observant."

Dreams and Free Association.   As with Freud, Erikson worked with the patient's associations to the dream as the "best leads" to understanding the dream's meaning. He valued the first association with the dream, which he believed to be powerful and essential. Ultimately, Erikson listened for "a central theme which, once found, gives added meaning to all the associated material."

Erikson believed that interpretation was the primary therapeutic agent, sought as much by the patient as the therapist. He emphasized free-floating attention as the method that enabled discovery to occur. Erikson once described this attentional stance by commenting that in clinical work, "You need a history and you need a theory, and then you must forget them both and let each hour stand for itself." This frees both parties from counterproductive pressures to advance in the therapy and allows them to notice the gaps in the patient's narrative that signal the unconscious.

Goals.   Erikson discussed four dimensions of the psychoanalyst's job. The patient's desire to be cured and the analyst's desire to cure is the first dimension. Mutuality exists in that patient and therapist are motivated by cure, and labor is divided. The goal is always to help the patient's ego get stronger and cure itself. The second dimension Erikson called objectivity-participation. Therapists must keep their minds open. "Neuroses change," wrote Erikson. New generalizations must be made and arranged in new configurations. The third dimension runs along the axis of knowledge-participation. The therapist "applies selected insights to more strictly experimental approaches." The fourth dimension is tolerance-indignation. Erikson stated: "Identities based on Talmudic argument, on messianic zeal, on punitive orthodoxy, on faddist sensationalism, on professional and social ambition" are harmful and tend to control patients. Control widens the gap of inequality between the doctor and the patient and makes the realization of the recurrent idea in Erikson's thought—mutuality—difficult.

According to Erikson, therapists have the opportunity to work through past unresolved conflicts in the therapeutic relationship. Erikson encouraged therapists not to shy away from guiding patients; he believes therapists must offer patients both prohibitions and permissions. Nor should therapists be so engrossed in patients' past life experiences that current conflicts are overlooked.

The goal of therapy is to recognize how patients have passed through the various stages of the life cycle and how the various crises in each stage have or have not been mastered. Equally important, future stages and crises must be anticipated so that they can be negotiated and mastered appropriately. Unlike Freud, Erikson does not believe that the personality is so inflexible that change cannot occur in middle and late adulthood. For Erikson, psychological growth and development occur throughout the entire span of the life cycle.

The Austen Riggs Center in Stockbridge, Massachusetts, is a repository of Erikson's work, and many of his theories are put into practice there. Erik's wife, Joan, developed an activities program at the Austen Riggs Center as an "interpretation-free zone," where patients could take up work roles or function as students with artists and craftspersons, without the burden of the patient role. This workspace encouraged the play and creativity required for the patients' work development to parallel the process of their therapy.

OTHER PSYCHODYNAMIC SCHOOLS

The men and women discussed in this chapter contributed to psychiatric thought and practice in the early and middle years of the 20th century. Many of these theories of psychopathology evolved as direct offshoots of Freudian psychoanalysis. This, however, is derived from various aspects of psychology, such as learning theory and quantitative methods of personality assessment. The theories selected for the discussion in this section have stood the test of time and are most relevant for psychiatry.

Brief synopses of the theories that exert the most significant influence on current psychiatric thought are listed below in alphabetical order of their proponent. Each of these theories contains insights that merit consideration because they enhance our understanding of the complexities of human behavior. They also illustrate the diversity of theoretical orientation that characterizes psychiatry today.

Karl Abraham (1877–1925)

Karl Abraham, one of Sigmund Freud's earliest disciples, was the first psychoanalyst in Germany. He is best known for his explication of depression from a psychoanalytic perspective and for his elaboration of Freud's stages of psychosexual development. Abraham divided the oral stage into a biting phase and a sucking phase; the anal stage into a destructive-expulsive (anal-sadistic) phase and a mastering-retentive (anal-erotic) phase; and the phallic stage into an early phase of partial genital love (true phallic phase) and a later mature genital phase. Abraham also linked the psychosexual stages to specific syndromes. For example, he postulated that obsessional neurosis resulted from fixation at the anal-sadistic phase and depression from fixation at the oral stage.

Alfred Adler (1870–1937)

Alfred Adler (Fig. 34-25) was born in Vienna, Austria, where he spent most of his life. A general physician, he became one of the original four members of Freud's circle in 1902. Adler never accepted the primacy of the libido theory, the sexual origin of a neurosis, or the importance of infantile wishes. Adler thought that aggression was far more critical, specifically in its manifestation as a striving for power, which he believed to be a masculine trait. He introduced the term *masculine protest* to describe the tendency to move from a passive, feminine role to a masculine, active role. Adler's theories are collectively known as *individual psychology.*

Adler saw individuals as unique, unified biologic entities whose psychological processes fit together into an individual lifestyle. He also postulated a principle of dynamism, in which every individual is future-directed and moves toward a goal. Adler also emphasized

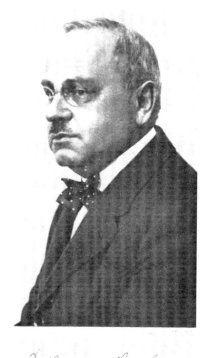

FIGURE 34-25
Alfred Adler (print includes signature). (Courtesy of Alexandra Adler.)

the interface between individuals and their social environment: the primacy of action in the real work over fantasy.

Adler coined the term *inferiority complex* to refer to a sense of inadequacy and weakness that is universal and inborn. A physical defect compromises a developing child's self-esteem, and Adler referred to this phenomenon as *organ inferiority.* He also thought that basic inferiority tied to children's oedipal longings could never be gratified.

Adler was one of the first developmental theorists to recognize the importance of children's birth order in their origin. The first-born child reacts with anger to the birth of siblings and struggles against giving up the powerful position of an only child. They tend not to share and become conservative. The second-born child must continuously strive to compete with the firstborn. Youngest children feel secure because they have *never* been displaced. Adler thought that a child's sibling position results in lifelong influences on character and lifestyle.

The primary therapeutic approach in Adlerian therapy is encouragement, through which Adler believed his patients could overcome feelings of inferiority. Consistent human relatedness, in his view, leads to greater hope, less isolation, and more significant affiliation with society. He believed that patients needed to develop a greater sense of their dignity and worth and a renewed appreciation of their abilities and strengths.

Franz Alexander (1891–1964)

Franz Alexander (Fig. 34-26) emigrated from his native Germany to the United States, where he settled in Chicago and founded the Chicago Institute for Psychoanalysis. He wrote extensively about the association between specific personality traits and certain psychosomatic ailments, a point of view that came to be known as

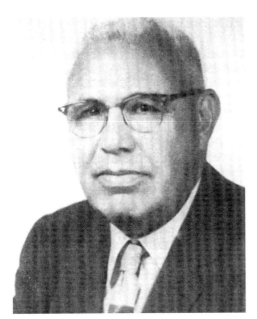

FIGURE 34-26
Franz Alexander. (Courtesy of Franz Alexander.)

the *specificity hypothesis*. Alexander fell out of favor with classic analysts for advocating the *corrective emotional experience* as part of the analytic technique. In this approach, Alexander suggested that an analyst must deliberately adopt a particular mode of relatedness with a patient to counteract noxious childhood influences from the patient's parents. He believed that the trusting, supportive relationship between patient and analyst enabled the patient to master childhood traumas and grow from the experience.

Gordon Allport (1897–1967)

Gordon Allport (Fig. 34-27), a psychologist in the United States, is known as the founder of the humanistic school of psychology, which holds that each person has an inherent potential for autonomous function and growth. At Harvard University, he taught the

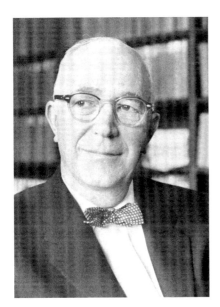

FIGURE 34-27
Gordon Allport. (© Bettmann/Corbis.)

first course in the psychology of personality offered at a college in the United States.

Allport believed that a person's only real guarantee of personal existence is a sense of self. Selfhood develops through a series of stages, from awareness of the body to self-identity. Allport used the term *propriem* to describe strivings related to the maintenance of self-identity and self-esteem. He used the term *traits* to refer to the chief units of personality structure. *Personal dispositions* are individual traits that represent the essence of an individual's unique personality. Maturity is characterized by a capacity to relate to others with warmth and intimacy and an expanded sense of self. In Allport's view, mature persons have security, humor, insight, enthusiasm, and zest. Psychotherapy is geared to helping patients realize these characteristics.

Michael Balint (1896–1970)

Michael Balint was considered a member of the independent or middle group of object relations theorists in the United Kingdom. Balint believed that the urge for the primary love object underlies virtually all psychological phenomena. Infants wish to be loved totally and unconditionally, and when a mother is not forthcoming with appropriate nurturance, a child devotes his or her life to a search for the love missed in childhood. According to Balint, the *basic fault* is the feeling of many patients that something is missing. As with Ronald Fairbairn and Donald W. Winnicott, Balint understood this deficit in internal structure to result from maternal failures. He viewed all psychological motivations stemming from the failure to receive adequate maternal love.

Unlike Fairbairn, however, Balint did not entirely abandon drive theory. He suggested that libido, for example, is both pleasure-seeking and object seeking. He also worked with seriously disturbed patients, and like Winnicott, he thought that certain aspects of psychoanalytic treatment occur at a more profound level than that of the ordinary verbal explanatory interpretations. Although some material involving genital psychosexual stages of development can be interpreted from the perspective of intrapsychic conflict, Balint believed that certain preverbal phenomena are reexperienced in the analysis. The relationship itself is decisive in dealing with this realm of early experience.

Eric Berne (1910–1970)

Eric Berne (Fig. 34-28) began his professional life as a training and supervising analyst in classic psychoanalytic theory and technique, but ultimately developed his school, known as *transactional analysis*. A *transaction* is a stimulus presented by one person that evokes a corresponding response in another. Berne defined psychological games as stereotyped and predictable transactions that persons learn in childhood and continue to play throughout their lives. *Strokes,* the basic motivating factors of human behavior, consist of specific rewards, such as approval and love. All persons have three ego states that exist within them: the *child,* which represents primitive elements that become fixed in early childhood; the *adult,* which is the part of the personality capable of objective appraisals of reality; and the *parent,* which is an introject of the values of a person's actual parents. The therapeutic process is geared toward helping patients understand whether they are functioning in the child, adult, or parent mode in their interactions with others. As patients learn to recognize characteristic games repeatedly played throughout life, they can ultimately function in the adult mode as much as possible in interpersonal relationships.

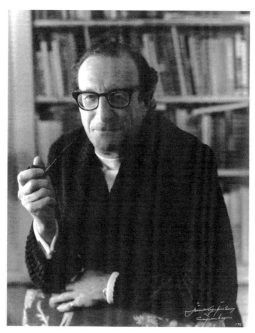

FIGURE 34-28
Eric Berne. (Courtesy of Creative Commons Attribution-Share Alike 4.0 International.)

Wilfred Bion (1897–1979)

Wilfred Bion expanded Melanie Klein's concept of *projective iden-tification* to include an interpersonal process in which a therapist feels coerced by a patient into playing a particular role in the patient's internal world. He also developed the notion that the therapist must contain what the patient has projected so that it is processed and returned to the patient in a modified form. Bion believed that a sim-ilar process occurs between mother and infant. He also observed that "psychotic" and "nonpsychotic" aspects of the mind function simultaneously as sub-organizations. Bion is probably best known for his application of psychoanalytic ideas to groups. Whenever a group gets derailed from its task, it deteriorates into one of three primary states: dependency, pairing, or fight-flight.

John Bowlby (1907–1990)

John Bowlby is generally considered the founder of attachment theory. He formed his ideas about attachment in the 1950s while consulting with the World Health Organization (WHO) on home-lessness in children. He stressed that the essence of attachment is *proximity* (i.e., the tendency of a child to stay close to the mother or caregiver). His theory of the mother–infant bond was firmly rooted in biology and drew extensively from ethology and evolu-tionary theory. A basic sense of security and safety is derived from a continuous and close relationship with a caregiver, according to Bowlby. This readiness for attachment is biologically driven, and Bowlby stressed that attachment is reciprocal. Maternal bonding and caregiving are always intertwined with the child's attachment behavior. Bowlby felt that without this early proximity to the mother or caregiver, the child does not develop a *secure base,* which he considered a launching pad for independence. In the absence of a secure base, the child feels frightened or threatened, and develop-ment is severely compromised. Bowlby and attachment theory are discussed in detail in Section 34.1.

Raymond Cattell (1905–1998)

Raymond Cattell obtained his Ph.D. in England before moving to the United States. He introduced *multivariate analysis* and *factor analysis*—statistical procedures that simultaneously examine the relations among multiple variables and factors—to personality. By examining a person's life record objectively, using personal inter-viewing and questionnaire data, Cattell described various traits representing the building blocks of personality.

Traits are both biologically based and environmentally deter-mined or learned. Biologic traits include sex, gregariousness, aggres-sion, and parental protectiveness. Environmentally learned traits include cultural ideas, such as work, religion, intimacy, romance, and identity. An important concept is the *law of coercion* to the bio-social mean, which holds that society exerts pressure on genetically different persons to conform to social norms. For example, a person with a strong genetic tendency toward dominance is likely to receive social encouragement for restraint, whereas the naturally submissive person will be encouraged toward self-assertion.

Ronald Fairbairn (1889–1964)

Ronald Fairbairn, a Scottish analyst who worked most of his life in relative isolation, was one of the significant psychoanalytic theorists in the British school of object relations. He suggested that infants are not primarily motivated by the drives of libido and aggression but are by an object seeking instinct. Fairbairn replaced the Freudian ideas of energy, ego, and id with the notion of *dynamic structures.* When an infant encounters frustration, a portion of the ego is defensively split off in the course of development and func-tions as an entity to internal objects and other subdivisions of the ego. He also stressed that both an object and an object *relationship* are internalized during development, so that a self is always with an object, and the two are connected with an affect.

Sándor Ferenczi (1873–1933)

Although Sándor Ferenczi, a Hungarian analyst, had been analyzed by Freud and was influenced by him, he later discarded Freud's techniques and introduced his method of analysis. He understood the symptoms of his patients as related to sexual and physical abuse in childhood and proposed that analysts need to love their patients in a way that compensates for the love they did not receive as chil-dren. He developed a procedure known as *active therapy,* in which he encouraged patients to develop an awareness of reality through active confrontation by the therapist. He also experimented with *mutual analysis,* in which he would analyze his patient for a session and then allow the patient to analyze him for a session.

Viktor Frankl (1905–1997)

His experience in Nazi concentration camps profoundly shaped the Austrian neurologist and philosopher Viktor Frankl's distinctive view of human nature and psychopathology. There he concluded that even the most appalling circumstances could be endured if one found a way of making them meaningful. He described his expe-rience in *Man's Search for Meaning,* a book that has been read by millions around the world.

Frankl was both a humanist and an existentialist. He believed that human beings shared with other animals somatic and psy-chological dimensions, but that humans alone also had a spiritual dimension that confers both freedom and responsibility. People find meaning in their lives through creative and productive work, through an appreciation of the world and others, and by freely adopting positive attitudes even in the face of suffering. Those who fail to find meaning face alienation, despair, and existential neuroses. Traditional societies provided a framework of meaning in religion and shared cultural values; in modern society, people must find their sources of meaning, and Frankl attributed many social problems, such as drug abuse and suicide, to their failures to do so.

Because of the spiritual dimension, human beings show self-transcendence and self-distancing. The former refers to the capacity to put other values (e.g., the well-being of a loved one) above self-interest. The latter is the ability to take an external perspective, as seen in a sense of humor. These capacities form the basis for therapeutic interventions in Frankl's version of psychotherapy known as logotherapy. Logotherapy is derived from the Greek word logos, which means thought or reason, and Frankl believed that man instinctively attempts to find universal understanding and harmony in life experiences.

Anna Freud (1895–1982)

Anna Freud (Fig. 34-29), the daughter of Sigmund Freud, ultimately made her own unique contributions to psychoanalysis. Although her father focused primarily on repression as the central defense mechanism, Anna Freud extensively elaborated on individual defense mechanisms, including reaction formation, regression, undoing, introjection, identification, projection, turning against the self, reversal, and sublimation. She was also a key figure in the development of modern ego psychology in that she emphasized that there was "depth in the surface." The defenses marshaled by the ego to avoid unacceptable wishes from the id were in and of themselves complex and worthy of attention. Up to that point, the primary focus had been on uncovering unconscious sexual and aggressive wishes. She also made seminal contributions to child psychoanalysis and studied the function of the ego in personality development. She founded the Hampstead child therapy course and clinic in London in 1947 and served as its director.

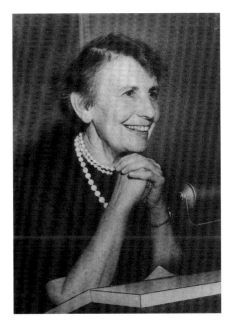

FIGURE 34-29
Anna Freud. (Courtesy of the National Library of Medicine.)

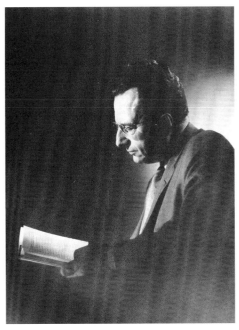

FIGURE 34-30
Erich Fromm. (© Bettmann/Corbis.)

Erich Fromm (1900–1980)

Erich Fromm (Fig. 34-30) came to the United States in 1933 from Germany, where he had received his Ph.D. He was instrumental in founding the William Alanson White Institute for Psychiatry in New York. Fromm identified five character types common to, and determined by, Western culture; each person may possess qualities from one or more types. The types are (1) the *receptive personality* is passive; (2) the *exploitative personality* is manipulative; (3) the *marketing personality* is opportunistic and changeable; (4) the *hoarding personality* saves and stores; and (5) the *productive personality* is mature and enjoys love and work. The therapeutic process involves strengthening the person's sense of ethical behavior toward others and developing productive love, characterized by care, responsibility, and respect for other persons.

Kurt Goldstein (1878–1965)

Kurt Goldstein (Fig. 34-31) was born in Germany and received his M.D. from the University of Breslau. He was influenced by existentialism and Gestalt psychology—every organism has dynamic properties, which are energy supplies that are relatively constant and evenly distributed. When states of tension-disequilibrium occur, an organism automatically attempts to return to its normal state. What happens in one part of the organism affects every other part, a phenomenon known as *holocoenosis.*

Self-actualization was a concept Goldstein used to describe persons' creative powers to fulfill their potentialities. Because each person has a different set of innate potentialities, persons strive for self-actualization along different paths. Sickness severely disrupts self-actualization. Responses to disruption of an organism's integrity may be rigid and compulsive; regression to more primitive modes of behavior is characteristic. One of Goldstein's significant contributions was his identification of the *catastrophic reaction* to brain damage, in which a person becomes fearful and agitated and refuses to perform simple tasks because of the fear of possible failure.

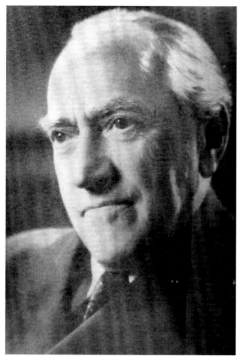

FIGURE 34-31
Kurt Goldstein. (Courtesy of New York Academy of Medicine, New York.)

Karen Horney (1885–1952)

German-born physician-psychoanalyst Karen Horney (Fig. 34-32), who emphasized the preeminence of social and cultural influences on psychosexual development, focused her attention on the differing psychology of men and women and explored the vicissitudes

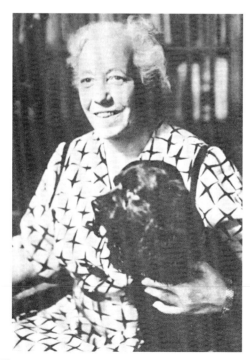

FIGURE 34-32
Karen Horney. (Courtesy of the Association for the Advancement of Psychoanalysis, New York.)

of marital relationships. She taught at the Institute of Psychoanalysis in Berlin before immigrating to the United States. Horney believed that a person's current personality attributes result from the interaction between the person and the environment and are not solely based on infantile libidinal strivings carried over from childhood. Her theory, known as *holistic psychology,* maintains that a person needs to be seen as a unitary whole who influences, and is influenced by, the environment. She thought that the Oedipus complex was overvalued in terms of its contribution to adult psychopathology, but she also believed that rigid parental attitudes about sexuality led to an excessive concern with the genitals.

She proposed three separate concepts of the self: the *actual self,* the total of a person's experience; the *real self,* the harmonious, healthy person; and the *idealized self,* the neurotic expectation, or glorified image that a person feels he or she should be. A person's *pride system* alienates him or her from the real self by overemphasizing prestige, intellect, power, strength, appearance, sexual prowess, and other qualities that can lead to self-effacement or self-hatred. Horney also established the concepts of *basic anxiety* and *basic trust.* The therapeutic process, in her view, aims for *self-realization* by exploring distorting influences that prevent the personality from growing.

Edith Jacobson (1897–1978)

Edith Jacobson, a psychiatrist in the United States, believed that the structural model and an emphasis on object relations are not fundamentally incompatible. She thought that the ego, self-images, and object images exert reciprocal influences on one's development. She also stressed that the infant's disappointment with the maternal object is not necessarily related to the mother's actual failure. In Jacobson's view, disappointment is related to a specific, drive-determined demand, rather than a global striving for contact or engagement. She viewed an infant's experience of pleasure or "unpleasure" as the core of the early mother–infant relationship. Satisfactory experiences lead to the formation of good or gratifying images, whereas unsatisfactory experiences create bad or frustrating images. Normal and pathologic development is based on the evolution of these self-images and object images. Jacobson believed that *fixation* refers to modes of object relatedness rather than modes of gratification.

Carl Gustav Jung (1875–1961)

Carl Gustav Jung (Fig. 34-33), a Swiss psychiatrist, formed a psychoanalytic school known as *analytic psychology,* which includes basic ideas related to but going beyond, Freud's theories. After initially being Freud's disciple, Jung broke with Freud over the latter's emphasis on infantile sexuality. He expanded on Freud's concept of the unconscious by describing the *collective unconscious* as consisting of all humankind's common, shared mythologic and symbolic past. The collective unconscious includes *archetypes*—representational images and configurations with universal symbolic meanings. Archetypal figures exist for the mother, father, child, and hero, among others. Archetypes contribute to *complexes,* feeling-toned ideas that develop from personal experience interacting with archetypal imagery. Thus, a mother complex is determined not only by the mother–child interaction but also by the conflict between archetypal expectation and experience with the real woman who functions in a motherly role.

Jung noted that there are two types of personality organizations: introversion and extroversion. *Introverts* focus on their inner

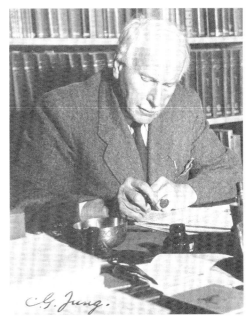

FIGURE 34-33
Carl Gustav Jung (print includes signature). (Courtesy of National Library of Medicine, Bethesda, MD.)

world of thoughts, intuitions, emotions, and sensations; *extroverts* are more oriented toward the outer world, other persons, and material goods. Each person has a mixture of both components. The *persona,* the mask covering the personality, is the face a person presents to the outside world. The persona may become fixed, and the real person hidden from him- or herself. *Anima* and *animus* are unconscious traits possessed by men and women, respectively, and contrast with the persona. *Anima* refers to a man's undeveloped femininity, whereas *animus* refers to a woman's undeveloped masculinity.

Jungian treatment aims to bring about an adequate adaptation to reality, which involves a person fulfilling their creative potentialities. The ultimate goal is to achieve *individuation,* a process continuing throughout life whereby persons develop a unique sense of their own identity. This developmental process may lead them down new paths away from their previous directions in life.

Otto Kernberg (1928–Present)

Otto Kernberg is perhaps the most influential object relations theorist in the United States. Influenced by both Klein and Jacobson, much of his theory is derived from his clinical work with patients who have borderline personality disorder. Kernberg places great emphasis on the splitting of the ego and the elaboration of good and bad self-configurations and object configurations. Although he has continued to use the structural model, he views the id as composed of self-images, object images, and their associated affects. Drives appear to manifest themselves only in the context of internalized interpersonal experience. Good and bad self-representations and object relations become associated, respectively, with libido and aggression. Object relations constitute the building blocks of both structure and drives. Goodness and badness in relational experiences precede drive cathexis. The dual instincts of libido and aggression arise from object-directed affective states of love and hate.

Kernberg proposed the term *borderline personality organization* for a broad spectrum of patients characterized by a lack of an integrated sense of identity, ego weakness, absence of superego integration, reliance on primitive defense mechanisms such as splitting and projective identification, and a tendency to shift into primary process thinking. He suggested a specific type of psychoanalytic psychotherapy for such patients in which transference issues are interpreted early in the process.

Melanie Klein (1882–1960)

Melanie Klein (Fig. 34-34) was born in Vienna, worked with Abraham and Ferenczi, and later moved to London. Klein evolved a theory of internal object relations that was intimately linked to drives. Her unique perspective grew mainly from her psychoanalytic work with children, in which she became impressed with the role of unconscious intrapsychic fantasy. She postulated that the ego undergoes a splitting process to deal with the terror of annihilation. She also thought that Freud's concept of the death instinct was central to understanding aggression, hatred, sadism, and other forms of "badness," all of which she viewed as derivatives of the death instinct.

Klein viewed projection and introjection as the primary defensive operations in the first months of life. Infants project derivatives of the death instinct into the mother and then fear attack from the "bad mother," a phenomenon that Klein referred to as *persecutory anxiety.* This anxiety is intimately associated with the *paranoid-schizoid position,* infants' mode of organizing experience in which all aspects of infant and mother are split into good and bad elements. As the disparate views are integrated, infants become concerned that they may have harmed or destroyed the mother through the hostile and sadistic fantasies directed toward her. At this developmental point, children have arrived at the *depressive position,* in which the mother is viewed ambivalently as having both positive and negative aspects and as the target of a mixture of loving and hateful feelings. Klein was also instrumental in developing child analysis, which evolved from an analytic play technique in which children used toys and played in a symbolic fashion that allowed analysts to interpret the play.

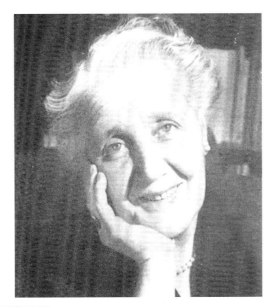

FIGURE 34-34
Melanie Klein. (Courtesy of Melanie Klein and Douglas Glass.)

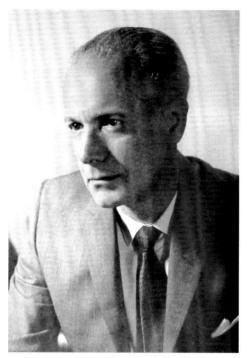

FIGURE 34-35
Heinz Kohut. (Courtesy of New York Academy of Medicine, New York.)

Heinz Kohut (1913–1981)

Heinz Kohut (Fig. 34-35) is best known for his writings on narcissism and the development of self-psychology. He viewed the development and maintenance of self-esteem and self-cohesion as more critical than sexuality or aggression. Kohut described Freud's concept of narcissism as judgmental, in that development was supposed to proceed toward object relatedness and away from narcissism. He conceived of two separate lines of development, one moving in the direction of object relatedness and the other in the direction of greater enhancement of the self.

In infancy, children fear losing the protection of the early mother–infant bliss and resort to one of three pathways to save the lost perfection: the grandiose self, the alter ego or twinship, and the idealized parental image. These three poles of the self manifest themselves in psychoanalytic treatment in terms of characteristic transferences, known as *self-object transferences*. The *grandiose self* leads to a *mirror transference,* in which patients attempt to capture the gleam in the analyst's eye through exhibitionistic self-display. The *alter ego* leads to the *twinship transference,* in which patients perceive the analyst as a twin. The *idealized parental image* leads to an *idealizing transference,* in which patients feel enhanced self-esteem by being in the presence of the exalted figure of the analyst.

Kohut suggested that empathic failures in the mother lead to a developmental arrest at a particular stage when children need to use others to perform self-object functions. Although Kohut originally applied this formulation to narcissistic personality disorder, he later expanded it to apply to all psychopathology.

Jacques Lacan (1901–1981)

Born in Paris and trained as a psychiatrist, Jacques Lacan founded his institute, the Freudian School of Paris. He attempted to integrate the intrapsychic concepts of Freud with concepts related to linguistics and semiotics (the study of language and symbols). Whereas Freud saw the unconscious as a seething cauldron of needs, wishes, and instincts, Lacan saw it as a sort of language that helps to structure the world. His two principal concepts are that the unconscious is structured like a language, and the unconscious is a discourse. Primary process thoughts are uncontrolled free-flowing sequences of meaning. Symptoms are signs or symbols of underlying processes. The role of the therapist is to interpret the semiotic text of the personality structure. Lacan's most basic phase is the mirror stage; it is here that infants learn to recognize themselves by taking the perspective of others. In that sense, the ego is not part of the self but is something outside of, and viewed by, the self. The ego comes to represent parents and society more than it represents the actual self of the person.

Lacan's therapeutic approach involves the need to become less alienated from the self and more involved with others. Relationships are often fantasized, which distorts reality and must be corrected. Among his most controversial beliefs was that the resistance to understanding the real relationship with the therapist can be reduced by shortening the length of the therapy session and that psychoanalytic sessions need to be standardized not to time but, instead, to content and process.

Kurt Lewin (1890–1947)

Kurt Lewin received his Ph.D. in Berlin, came to the United States in the 1930s, and taught at Cornell, Harvard, and the Massachusetts Institute of Technology. He adapted the field approach of physics to a concept called *field theory.* A *field* is the totality of coexisting, mutually interdependent parts. Behavior becomes a function of persons and their environment, which together make up the *life space.* The life space represents a field in constant flux, with *valences* or needs that require satisfaction. A hungry person is more aware of restaurants than someone who has just eaten, and a person who wants to mail a letter is aware of mailboxes.

Lewin applied field theory to groups. *Group dynamics* refers to the interaction among members of a group, each of whom depends on the others. The group can exert pressure on a person to change behavior, but the person also influences the group when change occurs.

Abraham Maslow (1908–1970)

Abraham Maslow (Fig. 34-36) was born in Brooklyn, New York, and completed his undergraduate and graduate work at the University of Wisconsin. Along with Goldstein, Maslow believed in *self-actualization theory*—the need to understand the totality of a person. A leader in humanistic psychology, Maslow described a hierarchical organization of needs present in everyone. As the more primitive needs, such as hunger and thirst, are satisfied, more advanced psychological needs, such as affection and self-esteem, become the primary motivators. Self-actualization is the highest need.

A peak experience, frequently occurring in self-actualizers, is an episodic, brief occurrence in which a person suddenly experiences a powerful transcendental state of consciousness—a sense of heightened understanding, an intense euphoria, an integrated nature, unity with the universe, and an altered perception of time and space. This powerful experience tends to occur most often in the psychologically healthy and can produce long-lasting beneficial effects.

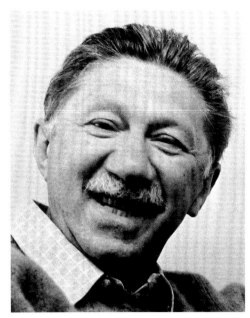

FIGURE 34-36
Abraham H. Maslow. (© Bettmann/Corbis.)

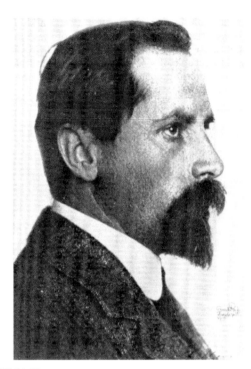

FIGURE 34-37
Adolf Meyer. (From the National Library of Medicine, Bethesda, MD.)

Karl A. Menninger (1893–1990)

Karl A. Menninger was one of the first physicians in the United States to receive psychiatric training. With his brother, Will, he pioneered the concept of a psychiatric hospital based on psychoanalytic principles and founded the Menninger Clinic in Topeka, Kansas. He also was a prolific writer; *The Human Mind,* one of his most famous books, brought psychoanalytic understanding to the lay public. He made a compelling case for the validity of Freud's death instinct in *Man Against Himself.* In *The Vital Balance,* his magnum opus, he formulated a unique theory of psychopathology. Menninger maintained a lifelong interest in the criminal justice system and argued in *The Crime of Punishment* that many convicted criminals needed treatment rather than punishment. Finally, his volume titled *Theory of Psychoanalytic Technique* was one of the few books to examine the theoretical underpinnings of psychoanalysts' interventions.

Adolf Meyer (1866–1950)

Adolf Meyer (Fig. 34-37) came to the United States from Switzerland in 1892 and eventually became director of the psychiatric Henry Phipps Clinic of the Johns Hopkins Medical School. Not interested in metapsychology, he espoused a commonsense psychobiological methodology for the study of mental disorders, emphasizing the interrelationship of symptoms and individual psychological and biologic functioning. His approach to the study of personality was biographical; he attempted to bring psychiatric patients and their treatment out of isolated state hospitals and into communities and was also a strong advocate of social action for mental health. Meyer introduced the concept of *common sense psychiatry* and focused on how a patient's current life situation could be realistically improved. He coined the concept of *ergasia,* the action of the total organism. His goal in therapy was to aid patients' adjustment by helping them modify unhealthy adaptations. One of Meyer's tools was an autobiographical life chart constructed by the patient during therapy.

Gardner Murphy (1895–1979)

Gardner Murphy (Fig. 34-38) was born in Ohio and received his Ph.D. from Columbia University. He was among the first to publish a comprehensive history of psychology and made significant contributions to social, general, and educational psychology. According to Murphy, three essential stages of personality development are the stage of undifferentiated wholeness, the stage of differentiation, and the stage of integration. This development is frequently uneven, with both regression and progression occurring along the way. The four inborn human needs are visceral-, motor-, sensory-, and emergency-related. These needs become increasingly specific in time as a person's experiences mold them in various social and environmental contexts. *Canalization* brings about these changes by establishing a connection between a need and a specific way of satisfying the need.

Murphy was interested in parapsychology. States such as sleep, drowsiness, specific drug, toxic conditions, hypnosis, and delirium tend to be favorable to paranormal experiences. Impediments to paranormal awareness include various intrapsychic barriers, conditions in the general social environment, and heavy investment in ordinary sensory experiences.

Henry Murray (1893–1988)

Henry Murray (Fig. 34-39) was born in New York City, attended medical school at Columbia University, and was a founder of the Boston Psychoanalytic Institute. He proposed the term *personology* to describe the study of human behavior. He focused on *motivation,* a need aroused by internal or external stimulation; once aroused, motivation produces continued activity until the need is reduced or satisfied. He developed the *Thematic Apperception Test* (TAT), a projective technique used to reveal unconscious and conscious mental processes and problem areas.

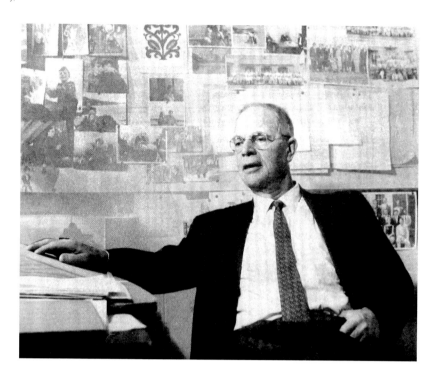

Frederick S. Perls (1893–1970)

Gestalt theory developed in Germany under the influence of several men: Max Wertheimer (1880–1943), Wolfgang Köhler (1887–1967), and Lewin. Frederick "Fritz" Perls (Fig. 34-40) applied Gestalt theory to a therapy that emphasizes the current experiences of the patient in the here and now, as contrasted to the there and then of psychoanalytic schools. In terms of motivation, patients learn to recognize their needs at any given time and how the drive to satisfy these needs may influence their current behavior. According to the Gestalt point of view, behavior represents more than the sum of its parts. A *gestalt,* or a whole, includes and goes beyond the sum of smaller, independent events; it deals with essential characteristics of experience, such as value, meaning, and form.

Sandor Rado (1890–1972)

Sandor Rado (Fig. 34-41) came to the United States from Hungary in 1945 and founded the Columbia Psychoanalytic Institute in New York. His theories of *adaptational dynamics* hold that the organism is a biologic system operating under hedonic control, which is somewhat similar to Freud's pleasure principle. Cultural

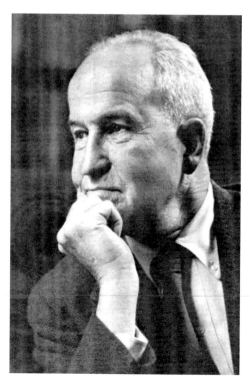

FIGURE 34-39
Henry Murray. (Courtesy of New York Academy of Medicine, New York.)

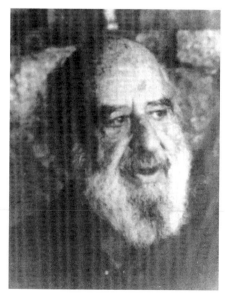

FIGURE 34-40
Fritz Perls. (Courtesy of the National Library of Medicine.)

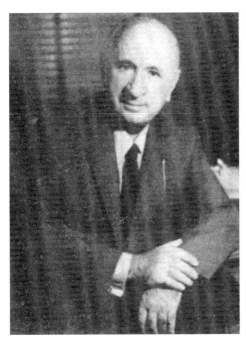

FIGURE 34-41
Sandor Rado. (Courtesy of New York Academy of Medicine.)

factors often cause excessive hedonic control and disordered behavior by interfering with the organism's ability for *self-regulation.* In therapy, the patient needs to relearn how to experience pleasurable feelings.

Otto Rank (1884–1939)

An Austrian psychologist and a protégé of Sigmund Freud, Otto Rank (Fig. 34-42) broke with Freud in his 1924 publication, *The Trauma of the Birth,* and developed a new theory called *birth*

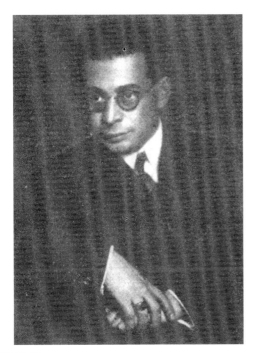

FIGURE 34-42
Otto Rank. (Courtesy of New York Academy of Medicine.)

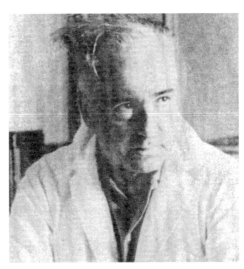

FIGURE 34-43
Wilhelm Reich. (Courtesy of New York Academy of Medicine.)

trauma. Anxiety is correlated with separation from the mother—specifically, with separation from the womb, the source of effortless gratification. This painful experience results in primal anxiety. Sleep and dreams symbolize the return to the womb.

The personality is divided into impulses, emotions, and will. Children's impulses seek immediate discharge and gratification. As impulses are mastered, as in toilet training, children begin the process of will development. If the will is carried too far, pathologic traits (e.g., stubbornness, disobedience, and inhibitions) may develop.

Wilhelm Reich (1897–1957)

Wilhelm Reich (Fig. 34-43), an Austrian psychoanalyst, made significant contributions to psychoanalysis in character formation and character types. The term *character armor* refers to the personality's defenses that serve as resistance to self-understanding and change. The four primary character types are as follows: the *hysterical character* is sexually seductive, anxious, and fixated at the phallic phase of libido development; the *compulsive character* is controlled, distrustful, indecisive, and fixated at the anal phase; the *narcissistic character* is fixated at the phallic stage of development, and if the person is male, he has contempt for women; and the *masochistic character* is long-suffering, complaining, and self-deprecatory, with excessive demand for love.

The therapeutic process, called *will therapy,* emphasizes the relationship between patient and therapist; the goal of treatment is to help patients accept their separateness. A definite termination date for therapy is used to protect against excessive dependence on the therapist.

Carl Rogers (1902–1987)

Carl Rogers (Fig. 34-44) received his Ph.D. in psychology from Columbia University. After attending Union Theological Seminary in New York, Rogers studied for the ministry. His name is most clearly associated with the *person-centered theory* of personality and psychotherapy, in which the central concepts are self-actualization and self-direction. Specifically, persons are born with a capacity to direct themselves in the healthiest way toward a level of completeness called self-actualization. From

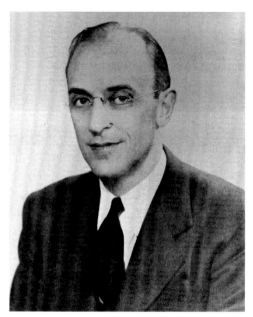

FIGURE 34-44
Carl Rogers. (Courtesy of the National Library of Medicine.)

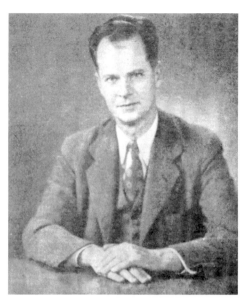

FIGURE 34-45
B. F. Skinner. (Courtesy of New York Academy of Medicine, New York.)

his person-centered approach, Rogers viewed personality not as a static entity composed of traits and patterns but as a dynamic phenomenon involving ever-changing communications, relationships, and self-concepts.

Rogers developed a treatment program called *client-centered psychotherapy.* Therapists attempt to produce an atmosphere in which clients can reconstruct their strivings for self-actualization. Therapists hold clients in unconditional positive regard, which is the total nonjudgmental acceptance of clients. Other therapeutic practices include attention to the present, focus on clients' feelings, emphasis on process, trust in the potential and self-responsibility of clients, and a philosophy grounded in a positive attitude toward them, rather than a preconceived structure of treatment.

Jean-Paul Sartre (1905–1980)

Born in Paris, Jean-Paul Sartre wrote plays and novels before turning to psychology. He was a German prisoner of war from 1940 to 1941 during World War II. Influenced by the ideas of Martin Heidegger, he developed what he called *existential psychoanalysis.* The reflective self was a crucial concept in Sartre's psychology. He recognized that humans alone could reflect on themselves as objects so that the experience of "being" in humans is unique in the natural world. This capacity to reflect leads humans to impose meaning on existence. For Sartre, this meaning allows a human being to create their essence.

Sartre denied the unconscious; he thought that human beings were condemned to be free and to face the fundamental existential dilemma—their aloneness without a god to provide meaning. As a result, each individual creates values and meanings. Neurosis is an escape from freedom, which is the key to maintaining psychological health. Sartre made no distinction between philosophy and psychology. Psychologists, as with philosophers, search for the truth about the world. Part of this truth, in Sartre's view, was the dialectic between consciousness and *being.* Consciousness introduces nothingness and is a negation of being-in-itself. Ideals are revealed in actions, not in professed beliefs.

B. F. Skinner (1904–1990)

Burrhus Frederic Skinner (Fig. 34-45), commonly known as B. F. Skinner, received his Ph.D. in psychology from Harvard University, where he taught for many years. Skinner's seminal work in operant learning laid much of the groundwork for many current methods of behavior modification, programmed instruction, and general education. His global beliefs about the nature of behavior have been applied more widely. It can be argued, than those of any other theorist, except, perhaps, Freud. His impact has been impressive in scope and magnitude.

Skinner's approach to personality was derived more from his fundamental beliefs about behavior than from a specific theory of personality per se. To Skinner, personality did not differ from other behaviors or sets of behaviors; it is acquired, maintained, and strengthened or weakened according to the same rules of reward and punishment that alter any other behavior. *Behaviorism,* as Skinner's basic theory is most commonly known, is concerned only with observable, measurable behavior that can be operationalized. Many abstract and mentalistic hallmarks of other dominant personality theories have little place in Skinner's framework. Concepts such as self, ideas, and ego are considered unnecessary for understanding behavior. Through the process of operant conditioning and the application of basic principles of learning, persons are believed to develop sets of behavior that characterize their responses to the world of stimuli that they face in their lives. Such a set of responses is called *personality.*

Harry Stack Sullivan (1892–1949)

Harry Stack Sullivan (Fig. 34-46) is generally acknowledged as the most original and distinctive American-born theorist in dynamic psychiatry. When psychiatrists use the term *parataxic distortion,* apply the concept of self-esteem, consider the importance of preadolescent peer groups in development, or view a patient's behavior as an interpersonal manipulation, they are applying concepts Sullivan first proposed.

Sullivan described three modes of experiencing and thinking about the world. The *prototaxic mode* is undifferentiated thought

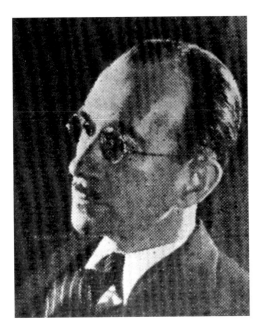

FIGURE 34-46
Harry Stack Sullivan. (Courtesy of the National Library of Medicine.)

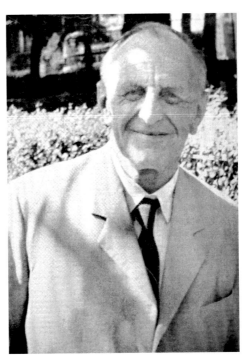

FIGURE 34-47
Donald Winnicott. (Courtesy of New York Academy of Medicine, New York.)

that cannot separate the whole into parts or use symbols. It occurs in infancy and also appears in patients with schizophrenia. In the *parataxic mode,* events are causally related because of temporal or serial connections. Logical relationships, however, are not perceived. The *syntaxic mode* is the logical, rational, and most mature type of cognitive functioning of which a person is capable. These three types of thinking and experiencing occur side by side in all persons; it is the rare person who functions exclusively in the syntaxic mode.

The total configuration of personality traits is known as the *self-system,* which develops in various stages and is the outgrowth of interpersonal experiences, rather than an unfolding of intrapsychic forces. During infancy, anxiety occurs for the first time when infants' primary needs are not satisfied. During childhood, from 2 to 5 years, a child's main tasks are to learn the requirements of the culture and how to deal with influential adults. As a juvenile, from 5 to 8 years, a child needs peers and must learn how to deal with them. In preadolescence, from 8 to 12 years, the capacity for love and collaboration with another person of the same sex develops. This so-called *chum period* is the prototype for a sense of intimacy. In the history of patients with schizophrenia, this experience of chums is often missing. During adolescence, significant tasks include the separation from the family, the development of standards and values, and the transition to heterosexuality.

The therapy process requires the active participation of the therapist, who is known as a *participant-observer.* Modes of experience, particularly the parataxic, need to be clarified, and new patterns of behavior need to be implemented. Ultimately, persons need to see themselves as they are, instead of as they think they are or want others to think they are.

Sullivan is best known for his creative psychotherapeutic work with severely disturbed patients. He believed that even the most psychotic patients with schizophrenia could be reached through the human relationship of psychotherapy.

Donald W. Winnicott (1896–1971)

Donald W. Winnicott (Fig. 34-47) was one of the central figures in the British school of object relations theory. His theory of *multiple*

self-organization included a *true self,* which develops in the context of a responsive *holding environment* provided by a *good-enough mother.* When infants experience a traumatic disruption of their developing sense of self, however, a false self emerges and monitors and adapts to the conscious and unconscious needs of the mother; it thus provides a protected exterior behind which the true self is afforded the privacy that it requires to maintain its integrity.

Winnicott also developed the notion of the *transitional object.* Ordinarily, a pacifier, blanket, or teddy bear, this object serves as a substitute for the mother during infants' efforts to separate and become independent. It provides a soothing sense of security in the absence of the mother.

The case history below illustrates how the different psychodynamic schools discussed in this chapter can be applied to the clinical observations.

Mr. A was a 26-year-old white man who had a history of bipolar I disorder. He was brought in for treatment after not completing the last required course for his advanced degree and being arrested for disturbing the peace. He had consistently lied to his family about where he stood with his coursework and about having skipped an examination that would have qualified him to use his professional degree. He had also not told them that he had been using marijuana almost daily for several years and occasionally used hallucinogens. His arrest for disorderly conduct was for swimming naked in an apartment complex in the middle of the night while taking hallucinogens.

Mr. A's use of marijuana began early in college but became daily during graduate school. He was diagnosed as having bipolar I disorder early in his senior year at college after an apparent episode of mania. His mood disorder was well controlled on lithium (Eskalith). During graduate school, he was episodically compliant with medications, preferring to try to maintain a state of hypomania. He saw a psychiatrist every 3 to 6 months for medication checks. During his 4 years in graduate school, he had two clear episodes of depression and began taking sertraline (Zoloft), 100 mg/day, with questionable benefit. Mr. A believed that he could be a great writer. He spent most of his time reading and trying to write. He dreamed of going to New York and becoming part of a group of avant-garde writers that would parallel the Algonquin Club of the 1930s or the Beat poets of the late 1940s. This aspiration and his marijuana abuse predated his development of bipolar I disorder. He attended class episodically, nonetheless performing adequately. His last class had no final examination but required a paper. He planned to write this paper in the form of a play, involving a dialogue between two thinkers from different times and cultures. His professor was very excited about this idea, but Mr. A kept postponing the task until he was forced to extend his schooling by a year. His other significant interest during this time involved growing and photographing flowers.

Mr. A was born and raised in a large city. His father had been very successful in commercial real estate, and his mother, after raising the children, used the substantial real estate holdings she inherited from her father to set up a business to manage them. Most of the money was placed in trust for the patient and his siblings. His mother had total financial control of the trusts and doled out the proceeds to the children as they needed them. There was no family history of any psychiatric disorders.

The patient described his mother as very loving and caring but intrusive and controlling. For example, the mother arranged the initial treatment but then was angry that the psychiatrist had not called her regularly to report on her adult son's progress. She was also critical of various aspects of the treatment, as reported to her by her son. The patient's two older siblings had attended prestigious colleges and graduate schools but had returned home to work in the mother's real estate management company. The 30-year-old sister was living in the parents' home. The 35-year-old brother had lived at home for a time but then moved out to a location a few blocks away. There was a younger brother, still in college, who also smoked marijuana excessively. He tried to minimize the patient's problems to the family and tried to protect the patient, who desperately had not wanted to return home. Of note is that none of the children were married, although the two older ones had a couple of serious relationships.

The children seemed to regard the mother with affectionate amusement and bemusement. The father was seen as a very caring but undemonstrative man who put much energy into keeping the mother from becoming too upset and encouraged them to do the same. The children often wanted to provoke the mother for her judgmental, detail-oriented intrusiveness. The father discouraged them but occasionally found their provocations amusing.

The family viewed itself as very close, with strong values oriented toward community service and family loyalty. The family belonged to a religious community but expressed their involvement primarily in social service and social action volunteer work, accompanied by generous financial contributions.

The patient had been a very successful debater in high school and recalled his development as very positive but provided few details. He tended to place himself in the role of the outsider, an observer of humanity, which he saw as consonant with the role of a writer. He was proud to have bipolar I disorder and tried to regulate his medications so that he would be hypomanic much of the time, seeing this as enhancing his creativity. He viewed his use of marijuana in the same vein. One of the most distressing aspects of his depressive episodes was that marijuana no longer created a feeling of well-being but made him feel worse. His current depressive episode involved no neurovegetative symptoms. Instead, he presented as flat, numb, apathetic, ashamed, anhedonic, and anergic. He was notably ashamed of being back in his hometown and of living with his parents.

The patient ostensibly understood and accepted his illness well and had read much about it. However, the family had responded to the information "with proper treatment, bipolars can live normal lives," meaning that the information should be kept secret to be treated

normally. Mr. A, on the other hand, was very open with friends at graduate school about his illness and his pride in it and the creativity he associated with it.

The patient had two long-standing recurrent dreams. One involved him flying. The narrative line varied, but the flying theme recurred. Often, he had other magical powers in his dreams, such as the ability to heal, not to be killed by bullets, to save the world or some group of people from mortal danger, and so on. The other recurrent dream was of a hotel lobby. These dreams regularly began with him entering a hotel lobby to meet a group of people, accompanied by a feeling of dread.

POSITIVE PSYCHOLOGY

Positive psychology is an umbrella term describing the scientific study of what makes life most worth living. Research findings from positive psychology are intended to provide a more complete and balanced scientific understanding of the human experience. The new field of positive psychology calls for as much focus on strength as on weakness, as much interest in building the best things in life as in repairing the worst, and as much concern with making the lives of normal people fulfilling as with healing pathology.

Positive psychology does not replace business-as-usual psychology, which often focuses on people's problems and how to remedy them. Instead, positive psychology intends to complement and extend problem-focused psychology. The attention of positive psychologists is increasingly turning to deliberate interventions that promote the well-being of individuals and groups, and again, these should be regarded as supplements to existing therapies.

Positive psychology studies what goes right in life, from birth to death. It is concerned with optimal experience—people being their best and doing their best. Everyone's life has peaks and valleys, and positive psychology does not deny the low points. Its signature premise is nuanced: What is good about life is as genuine as what is bad and deserves equal attention from psychologists. Positive psychology assumes that life entails more than avoiding or undoing problems and that explanations of the good life must do more than reverse accounts of distress and dysfunction.

Empirical Findings

Although still a young field, positive psychology already has a canon of established findings worth considering. Indeed, positive psychology is a bottom-up field, very much defined by its empirical results. Discussed below are some of the things that have been learned about positive experiences, positive traits, positive relationships, and positive institutions.

When psychologists study self-reported happiness and life satisfaction, usually under the rubric of subjective well-being, they administer numerical rating scales. The consistent and perhaps surprising result is that most people in most circumstances, most of the time, score above the scale midpoint, whether they are multimillionaires in the United States or pavement dwellers in Calcutta. This conclusion holds across demographic characteristics like age, sex, ethnicity, and education, each of which has a surprisingly small association with avowed happiness.

The significant correlates of happiness are social. In contrast to the modest demographic correlates of happiness and well-being, consider the following robust correlates:

▶ Number of friends
▶ Being married

▶ Being extroverted
▶ Being grateful
▶ Being religious
▶ Pursuing leisure activities
▶ Employment (not income)

In a study that compared happy people to very happy people, there was one striking difference: good relationships with other people. Of the very happy people in the sample, all had close relationships with others. Psychology research documents very few necessary or sufficient conditions, but these data suggest that good social relationships may be a necessary condition for extreme happiness.

People who are successful in life's venues are, of course, happy, but the less obvious and more interesting finding from experimental and longitudinal research is that happiness foreshadows success in academic, vocational, and interpersonal realms.

Having good relationships with other people is the most critical contributor to a satisfying life and may even be a necessary condition for happiness. Having a "best friend" at work is a strong predictor of satisfaction and even productivity. A good relationship is one in which the amount of positive communication considerably outweighs negative communication.

Positive psychologists have taken a close look at the features of positive communication, describing four ways in which a person can respond to someone else when something happens, including good events such as a raise at work:

▶ Active-constructive responding—an enthusiastic response: "That's great; I bet you'll receive many more raises."
▶ Active-destructive responding—a response that points out the potential downside: "Are they going to expect more of you now?"
▶ Passive-constructive responding—a muted response: "That's nice, dear."
▶ Passive-destructive responding—a response that conveys disinterest: "It rained all day here."

Couples who use active-constructive responding have good marriages. The other responses, if they dominate, are associated with marital dissatisfaction. Although this research has only been done in the context of marriage, it may well generalize to other relationships.

Psychology and psychiatry have a long history of either ignoring religion or regarding it with suspicion. However, research findings have begun to accumulate, showing that religion has particular benefits in various psychological domains. Internalized religious beliefs may help a person to cope with problems and even avoid physical illness in the first place. Religiousness is robustly associated with longevity, happiness, and other indices of a life lived well.

People who are so poor that they cannot meet their basic needs are unhappy, but above extreme poverty, increased income has a surprisingly small relationship with life satisfaction.

Despite the small contribution of income to well-being, whether or not someone is working is much more strongly related to happiness. People who are employed and engaged in what they do are happy, regardless of the status or compensation associated with their job. Happiness and engagement lead people to regard their work as a calling and be more productive at whatever they do, take fewer sick days, and even postpone their retirement.

According to Aristotle's notion of *eudaimonia*—being faithful to one's inner self (demon)—true happiness entails identifying one's virtues, cultivating them, and living by them. Contrast this notion with the equally venerable idea of *hedonism*—pursuing pleasure and avoiding pain—that is the foundation for *utilitarianism,* which in turn provides the underpinning of psychoanalysis and all but the most radical of the behaviorisms. Research shows that eudaimonia consistently trumps pleasure as a predictor of life satisfaction. Those who pursue eudaimonic goals and activities are more satisfied than those who pursue pleasure. This is not to say that hedonism is irrelevant to life satisfaction, just that all things being equal, hedonism contributes less to long-term happiness than does eudaimonia.

Although the study of positive institutions is in its infancy, there is an agreement that institutions that allow people to flourish—whether families, schools, workplaces, or even entire societies—share a core of common characteristics:

▶ Purpose—a shared vision of the moral goals of the institution, one reinforced by remembrances and celebrations
▶ Safety—protection against threat, danger, and exploitation
▶ Fairness—equitable rules governing reward and punishment and the means for consistently enforcing them
▶ Humanity—mutual care and concern
▶ Dignity—the treatment of all people in the institution as individuals regardless of their position

Psychologists, at least in the United States, have long believed that the human condition can be improved by the intelligent application of what they have learned. Positive psychologists are no exception, and many have turned their attention to interventions that make people more happy, hopeful, virtuous, accomplished, and socially involved. In some cases, these applications are running in front of data that would support them, but in other cases, outcome research has been done. Even the most compelling research is not based on follow-up that extends beyond a few years, and the research participants are usually motivated and willing volunteers. How well these interventions will generalize—across diverse people and over time—is a research topic of high priority.

Positive Psychology and Clinical Work

When positive psychology was first described, its stated goal was not to move people from –5 to zero—the goal of conventional psychology and psychiatry—but rather from +2 to +5, within the upper right-hand quadrant of Figure 34-48. This emphasis on *promotion* instead of remediation is an essential feature of a positive psychology perspective, but it does not do justice to this new field and its potential role in clinical work.

Positive Psychology's Vision of Psychological Health.
In its 1948 constitution, the World Health Organization (WHO) defined *health* as "a state of complete physical, mental, and social well-being and not merely the absence of disease or infirmity." In more recent years, this statement has been expanded to include the ability to lead a life that is socially and economically productive. This definition is an essential declaration that health entails more than the absence of illness, but it is circular since "well-being" is a synonym for "health." Work by positive psychologists makes this definition more concrete and useful as a guide for research and intervention.

If one can extrapolate from the sorts of topics that have been studied, positive psychology assumes that people are doing well when they experience more positive feelings than negative feelings, are satisfied with their lives as they have been lived, have identified what they do well, and use these talents and strengths on an

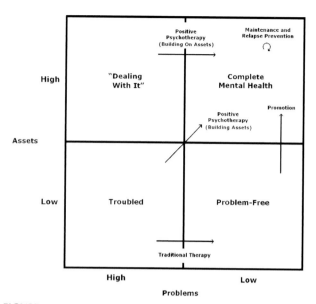

FIGURE 34-48
Mental health and mental illness. These are dimensions. Quadrants are shown for the purpose of illustration only. (From Sadock BJ, Sadock VA, Ruiz P, eds. *Kaplan & Sadock's Comprehensive Textbook of Psychiatry.* 9th ed. Philadelphia, PA: Lippincott Williams & Wilkins; 2009:2942, with permission.)

ongoing basis, are highly engaged in what they do, are contributing members of a social community, and have a sense of meaning and purpose in their lives. Physical health and safety, of course, provide an essential context for psychological well-being. It is difficult to imagine a cultural group in which these components of the good life are not valued. Respect for human diversity need not entail extreme cultural relativism.

Note that this fuller characterization of health reflects the WHO definition and is drawn from research in all of the domains of concern to contemporary positive psychology. The relevant research cautions that health so defined is not unitary. No one can have it all, at least at the same time, given tradeoffs among the psychological states and traits that reflect doing well. Psychological health, therefore, needs to be described with a profile of features and not a single summary score. The fifth edition of the *Diagnostic and Statistical Manual of Mental Disorders* (DSM-5) describes hundreds of psychological problems. However, there may be just as many different manifestations of the good life.

Theory of Psychopathology.   As a perspective on topics that deserve scientific study, positive psychology has no single theory. Like much of contemporary psychology, it instead relies on mid-range theories that draw on various broader perspectives, from evolutionary to behavioral to cognitive to sociocultural models, to make sense of specific phenomena. Different topics are explained with different theories. The eventual integration of psychology may be a worthy goal, but it has not yet been achieved.

At this early point in the development of positive psychology, the lack of a consensual or integrated theory is not a problem. The good psychological life is not yet understood, and positive psychologists are still grappling with the right vocabulary to describe it. Accordingly, championing a single theory at present would be premature, even counterproductive.

It has been argued that positive psychology is a descriptive endeavor, not a prescriptive one. If this means that positive psychology should be an empirical science—informed by replicable

facts—then this claim is reasonable and a defining feature of the entire field. If this means that positive psychology is assumption-free or value-neutral, it becomes much more challenging to defend. After all, positive psychologists make the value judgment that the "good" life is indeed good—that is, desirable, morally and otherwise—and the metatheoretical assumption that the good life can be studied with the conventional methods of psychology. In any event, positive psychology seems no more prescriptive than clinical psychology or psychiatry. It may even be less so, given the theoretical diversity of positive psychology as it now exists.

Positive Psychology Assessment.   The assessment has long been a staple of psychology, and much of it has been tilted—understandably—toward identifying weaknesses, deficiencies, and problems. The positive psychology perspective is that business-as-usual assessment should be expanded (not replaced) by attention to areas of strength and competence. Low life satisfaction can occur in the absence of psychopathology, but it is nonetheless related to psychological and social problems. Conversely, high life satisfaction is linked to good functioning, even in the presence of symptoms.

Positive psychologists have developed an impressive set of measurement instruments that allow someone to break through the zero point of deficiency measures. For example, the healthiest that one can score on a typical measure of depression is zero, but this lumps together people who are blasé with those filled with zest and joy. The distinction seems well worth making, and the self-report surveys and interviews developed by positive psychologists allow it.

Most of the existing positive psychology measures were developed for research purposes, and they are most valid when aggregated to yield conclusions about groups of people. They can also be used ipsatively (i.e., forced to choose between two options), to describe the psychological characteristics of an individual and how they stay the same or change over time, but the cautious use of these descriptions is a point of discussion and a departure in treatment. None is a robust diagnostic test, and none should be treated as if it were. Such prudence is appropriate for all psychological assessments, but it is worth emphasizing in positive psychology measures.

Positive Psychology Techniques.   Positive psychologists have demonstrated that brief interventions in the short term can increase happiness, satisfaction, and fulfillment. In some cases, there is also evidence that they can alleviate depression. For example, patients or clients can be asked to count their blessings:

Every night for 1 week, set aside 10 minutes before you go to bed. Use that time to write down three things that went really well on that day and why they went well. You may use a journal or your computer to write about the events, but you must have a physical record of your writing. It is not enough to do this exercise in your head. The three things you list can be relatively small in importance or relatively large in importance. Next to each positive event in your list, answer the question, "Why did this good thing happen?"

They can also be asked to use their strengths in novel ways. They take the Values in Action Inventory of Strengths (VIA-IS) questionnaire online and identify their most signature strengths of character. Then they are instructed to use these strengths in their daily life:

Every day for the next 7 days, use one of your top five strengths in a way that you have not before. You might use your strength in a new setting or with a new person. It is your choice.

Outcome research shows that various psychotherapies are effective in alleviating problems and usually equally so, despite the different forms they take. One interpretation of the equal effectiveness of different therapies is that nonspecific factors common to all treatments are responsible. Perhaps the types of strategies being studied by positive psychologists reflect these common factors and give names to them. Strategies like instilling hope and building strengths may be the critical factors in the effectiveness of any therapy.

Some qualifications are in order if these techniques are used in the context of treatment. First, the therapist must ascertain a client's readiness to change in the particular ways requested in the exercise and the client's capacity to make the change. Like any psychotherapeutic procedure, these techniques cannot be imposed on the unwilling or unable.

Second, none of these techniques is akin to a crash diet or an antibiotic. The degree to which they have lasting effects is related to how patients or clients integrate them into their regular behavioral routines. Counting blessings for a week will make a person happier for that week, but only if they become habitually grateful will there be a more enduring effect. Research finds—not surprisingly—that the people who showed lasting benefits were those who continued to use the exercise.

Third, these exercises are typically presented as one size fits all, but there is no reason to think that they are equally useful for all patients or clients. Nothing is known about the match of an exercise with a client's particular presenting problems or goals or with a client's age, sex, social class, or ethnicity.

Fourth, little is known about the parameters of these interventions. For example, how many blessings should one count, and how frequently should this be done? With college students, counting blessings three times a week may be more effective in increasing happiness than counting them more frequently. Is this a general phenomenon or one specific to young adults attending college?

Fifth, all interventions run the risk of unintended harm, and although positive psychologists would like to believe that their techniques avoid iatrogenic effects, this assertion cannot be made with thorough confidence. For example, although optimism is related to mental and physical health, it would be simplistic and potentially hazardous to tell patients or clients that positive expectations will solve all their difficulties. Along these lines, if a positive psychology intervention overemphasizes a client's choice and responsibility, considerable damage could be done in cases of abuse and victimization, in which self-blame needs to be undone and certainly not encouraged. Interventions based on positive psychology should not preclude the use of existing therapeutic strategies when these are indicated.

Positive Psychotherapies. *Positive psychotherapies* are beginning to appear: therapeutic interventions based on the theories and findings of positive psychology. What distinguishes these emerging positive psychotherapies from conventional treatments is that their stated goal is not symptom reduction or relief but relatively enhanced happiness, life satisfaction fulfillment, productivity, and the like—one or more components of positive psychology's vision of the good life. These new therapies target people with psychological problems as well as those without them. In the latter case, positive psychotherapies make contact with life coaching.

The possible field of positive psychotherapies is so broad that it needs narrowing, and somewhat arbitrarily, the focus here is on approaches characterized by an explicit *therapeutic alliance* between the positive psychologist and the patient or client. This feature goes by many names and has been variously defined, but its recurring themes include collaboration between therapist and client, an affective bond between them, and an agreement on the goals and tasks of the intervention. Asking people to write about their goals or perform acts of kindness, despite beneficial consequences, may or may not be instances of positive psychotherapy—what matters is the relational context of the request.

TAKING STOCK. The unique and explicit goal of emerging positive psychotherapies is to enhance well-being and to promote the good life among those with obvious psychological problems as well as those without them. They are also similar to more established therapies. Positive psychotherapies are short-term, structured interventions for individuals or small groups. Most can be placed in the cognitive-behavioral realm, although their techniques could be integrated easily into other treatment models. Most positive psychotherapies entail out-of-sessions exercises and homework assignments, the results of which are discussed in sessions. Several positive psychotherapies rely on journal-keeping, and many of these therapies rely on ongoing assessment.

Like other cognitive-behavioral interventions, positive psychotherapies take issue with assumptions of the medical model that people in treatment are ill and that their problems are best described as discrete (present-or-absent) entities as in DSM-5. According to positive psychology, people's weaknesses and strengths exist in degrees.

As emphasized, research support is still accumulating. Enough outcome studies have been conducted to conclude that positive psychotherapies are more than just promising, with effect sizes in the small to moderate range typical of psychological interventions. Not known in most cases is how positive psychotherapies fare in direct comparison with conventional treatments for anxiety or depression. Also, as already mentioned, the boundary conditions of effective positive psychotherapy are unknown.

Many positive psychologists would like to believe that a strengths-based approach to change is superior to one that focuses on the remediation of deficiencies, but this hypothesis has yet to be put to a serious test. The even-handed suspicion is that attention to both strengths and weaknesses is critical and that no useful purpose is served by regarding these as mutually exclusive therapeutic strategies.

References

Contributions from the Psychosocial Sciences

Abramowitz JS, Arch JJ. Strategies for improving long-term outcomes in cognitive behavioral therapy for obsessive-compulsive disorder: insights from learning theory. *Cogn Behav Pract*. 2014;21:20–31.

Akre KL, Ryan MJ. Complexity increases working memory for mating signals. *Curr Biol*. 2010;20(6):502–505.

Bond T. Comparing decalage and development with cognitive developmental tests. *J Appl Meas*. 2010;11(2):158–171.

Boom J. Egocentrism in moral development: Gibbs, Piaget, Kohlberg. *New Ideas Psychol*. 2011;29(3):355.

Bouton ME. *Learning and Behavior: A Contemporary Synthesis*. Sunderland, MA: Sinauer; 2007.

Bouton ME. Learning theory. In: Sadock BJ, Sadock VA, Ruiz P, eds. *Kaplan & Sadock's Comprehensive Textbook of Psychiatry*. 9th ed. Philadelphia, PA: Lippincott Williams & Wilkins; 2009:647.

Byrne JH, ed. *Learning and Memory—A Comprehensive Reference*. New York: Elsevier; 2008.

Crystal JD. Comparative cognition: comparing human and monkey memory. *Curr Biol*. 2011;21(11):R432–R434.

Dickinson D. Zeroing in on early cognitive development in schizophrenia. *Am J Psychiatry*. 2014;171:9–12.

Freud S. *The Standard Edition of the Complete Psychological Works of Sigmund Freud*. Vol. 24. London: Hogarth Press; 1953–1974.

Gerstner JR, Lyons LC, Wright KP Jr, Loh DH, Rawashdeh O, Eckel-Mahan KL, Roman GW. Cycling behavior and memory formation. *J Neurosci*. 2009;29(41): 12824–12830.

Greenberg JR, Mitchell SA. *Object Relations in Psychoanalytic Theory*. Cambridge, MA: Harvard University Press; 1983.

Greenspan S, Curry J. Piaget and cognitive development. In: Sadock BJ, Sadock VA, Ruiz P, eds. *Kaplan & Sadock's Comprehensive Textbook of Psychiatry*. 9th ed. Vol. 1. Philadelphia, PA: Lippincott Williams & Wilkins; 2009:635.

Harris PL. Piaget on causality: the whig interpretation of cognitive development. *Br J Psychol*. 2009;100(S1):229.

Hockenbury D. Learning. In: *Discovering Psychology*. 5th ed. New York: Worth Publishers; 2011:183.

Houdé O, Pineau A, Leroux G, Poirel N, Perchey G, Lanoë C, Lubin A, Turbelin MR, Rossi S, Simon G, Delcroix N, Lamberton F, Vigneau M, Wisniewski G, Vicet JR, Mazoyer B. Functional magnetic resonance imaging study of Piaget's conservation-of-number task in preschool and school-age children: a neo-Piagetian approach. *J Exp Child Psychol*. 2011;110(3):332–346.

Illeris K, ed. *Contemporary Theories of Learning: Learning Theorists... In Their Own Words*. New York: Routledge; 2009.

Kandel ER. The biology of memory: a forty-year perspective. *J Neurosci*. 2009; 29(41):12748–12756.

Kandel ER, Dudai Y, Mayford MR. The molecular and systems biology of memory. *Cell*. 2014;157(1):163–186.

Kosaki Y, Dickinson A. Choice and contingency in the development of behavioral autonomy during instrumental conditioning. *J Exp Psychol Anim Behav Process*. 2010;36(3):334–342.

Laplanche J, Pontalis J-B. *The Language of Psycho-analysis*. New York: Norton; 1973.

Lee SH, Dan Y: Neuromodulation of brain states. *Neuron*. 2012;76(1):209–222.

Lubin FD. Epigenetic gene regulation in the adult mammalian brain: multiple roles in memory formation. *Neurobiol Learn Mem*. 2011;96(1):68–78.

Mahler MS, Pine F, Bergman A. *The Psychological Birth of the Human Infant*. New York: Basic Books; 1975.

Maia TV. Two-factor theory, the actor-critic model, and conditioned avoidance. *Learn Behav*. 2010;38(1):50–67.

Meissner WW. Theories of Personality in Psychotherapy. In: Sadock BJ, Sadock VA, eds. *Kaplan & Sadock's Comprehensive Textbook of Psychiatry*. 9th ed. Vol. 1. Philadelphia, PA: Lippincott Williams & Wilkins; 2009:788.

Mesotten D, Gielen M, Sterken C, Claessens K, Hermans G, Vlasselaers D, Lemiere J, Lagae L, Gewillig M, Eyskens B, Vanhorebeek I, Wouters PJ, Van den Berghe G. Neurocognitive development of children 4 years after critical illness and treatment with tight glucose control: a randomized controlled trial. *JAMA*. 2012;308(16): 1641–1650.

Paller KA, Squire LR. Biology of memory. In: Sadock BJ, Sadock VA, Ruiz P, eds. *Kaplan & Sadock's Comprehensive Textbook of Psychiatry*. 9th ed. Vol. 1. Philadelphia, PA: Lippincott Williams & Wilkins; 2009:658.

Pallini S, Baiocco R, Schneider BH, Madigan S, Atkinson L. Early child-parent attachment and peer relations: A meta-analysis of recent research. *J Fam Psychol*. 2014;28(1):118–123.

Rösler R, Ranganath C, Röder B, Kluwe RH, eds. *Neuroimaging of Human Memory*. New York: Oxford University Press; 2008.

Sigelman CK, Rider EA. *Learning theories. In: Life-Span Human Development*. Belmont, CA: Wadsworth; 2012:42.

Solntseva SV, Nikitin BP. Protein synthesis is required for induction of amnesia elicited by disruption of the reconsolidation of long-term memory. *Neurosci Behavl Physiol*. 2011;41(6):654.

Stern D. *The Interpersonal World of the Infant*. New York: Basic Books; 1985.

Urcelay GP, Miller RR. Two roles of the context in Pavlovian fear conditioning. *J Exp Psychol Anim Behav Process*. 2010;36(2):268–280.

Whitbourne SK, Whitbourne SB. Piaget's cognitive-developmental theory. In: *Adult Development and Aging: Biopsychosocial Perspectives*. 4th ed. Hoboken, NJ: John Wiley & Sons, Inc.; 2011:32.

Normality and Mental Health

Blom RM, Hagestein-de Bruijn C, de Graaf R, ten Have M, Denys DA. Obsessions in normality and psychopathology. *Depress Anxiety*. 2011;28(10):870.

Macaskill A. Differentiating dispositional self-forgiveness from other-forgiveness: Associations with mental health and life satisfaction. *J Soc Clin Psychol*. 2012; 31:28.

Sajobi TT, Lix LM, Clara I, Walker J, Graff LA, Rawsthorne P, Miller N, Rogala L, Carr R, Bernstein CN. Measures of relative importance for health-related quality of life. *Qual Life Res*. 2012;21:1.

Tol WA, Patel V, Tomlinson M, Baingana F, Galappatti A, Silove D, Sondorp E, van Ommeren M, Wessells MG, Panter-Brick C. Relevance or excellence? Setting research priorities for mental health and psychosocial support in humanitarian settings. *Harv Rev Psychiatry*. 2012;20:25.

Vaillant GE. Positive mental health: is there a cross-cultural definition? *World Psychiatry*. 2012;11(2):93.

Vaillant GE. *Spiritual Evolution: A Scientific Defense of Faith*. New York: Doubleday Broadway; 2008.

Vaillant GE, Vaillant CO. Normality and mental health. In: Sadock BJ, Sadock VA, Ruiz P, eds. *Kaplan & Sadock's Comprehensive Textbook of Psychiatry*. 9th ed. Philadelphia: Lippincott Williams & Wilkins; 2009:691.

Wakefield JC. Misdiagnosing normality: Psychiatry's failure to address the problem of false positive diagnoses of mental disorder in a changing professional environment. *J Ment Health*. 2010;19(4):337.

Ward D. 'Recovery': Does it fit for adolescent mental health? *J Child Adolesc Ment Health*. 2014;26:83–90.

Contributions from the Sociocultural Sciences

Aggarwal NK. The psychiatric cultural formulation: translating medical anthropology into clinical practice. *J Psychiatr Pract*. 2012;18(2):73–85.

Bhugra D, Popelyuk D, McMullen I. Paraphilias across cultures: contexts and controversies. *J Sex Res*. 2010;47(2):242–256.

Bhui K, Bhugra D, eds. *Culture and Mental Health*. London: Hodder Arnold; 2007.

Biag BJ. Social and transcultural aspects of psychiatry. In: Johnstone EC, Owens DC, Lawrie SM, Mcintosh AM, Sharpe S, eds. *Companion to Psychiatric Studies*. 8th ed. New York: Elsevier; 2010:109.

Bolton SL, Elias B, Enns MW, Sareen J, Beals J, Novins DK, Swampy Cree Suicide Prevention Team; AI-SUPERPFP Team. A comparison of the prevalence and risk factors of suicidal ideation and suicide attempts in two American Indian population samples and in a general population sample. *Transcult Psychiatry*. 2014;51(1):3–22.

Breslau J, Aguilar-Gaxiola S, Borges G, Kendler KS, Su M, Kessler RC. Risk for psychiatric disorder among immigrants and their US-born descendants: evidence from the National Comorbidity Survey Replication. *J Nerv Ment Dis*. 2007;195(3): 189–195.

Burghardt GM. Darwin's legacy to comparative psychology and ethology. *Am Psychol*. 2009;64(2):102–110.

Burt A, Trivers R. *Genes in Conflict: The Biology of Selfish Genetic Elements*. Cambridge, MA: Belknap Press; 2006.

Chao RC, Green KE. Multiculturally Sensitive Mental Health Scale (MSMHS): Development, factor analysis, reliability, and validity. *Psychol Assess*. 2011;23(4): 876–887.

Confer JC, Easton JA, Fleischman DS, Goetz CD, Lewis DMG, Perilloux C, Buss DM. Evolutionary psychology. Controversies, questions, prospects, and limitations. *Am Psychol*. 2010;65(2):110–126.

Crozier I. Making up koro: multiplicity, psychiatry, culture, and penis-shrinking anxieties. *J Hist Med Allied Sci*. 2012;67(1):36–70.

De Block A, Adriaens PR. *Maladapting Minds: Philosophy, Psychiatry, and Evolutionary Theory*. New York: Oxford University Press; 2011.

De La Rosa M, Babino R, Rosario A, Martinez NV, Aijaz L. Challenges and strategies in recruiting, interviewing, and retaining recent Latino immigrants in substance abuse and HIV epidemiologic studies. *Am J Addict*. 2012;21(1):11–22.

Donlan W, Lee J. Screening for depression among indigenous Mexican migrant farmworkers using the Patient Health Questionnaire-9. *Psychol Rep*. 2010;106(2): 419–432.

Griffith JL. Neuroscience and humanistic psychiatry: a residency curriculum. *Acad Psychiatry*. 2014;1–8.

Guarnaccia PJ, Lewis-Fernandez R, Pincay IM, Shrout P, Guo J, Torres M, Canino G, Alegria M. Ataque de nervios as a marker of social and psychiatric vulnerability: results from the NLAAS. *Int J Soc Psychiatry*. 2010;56(3):298–309.

Haque A. Mental health concepts in Southeast Asia: diagnostic considerations and treatment implications. *Psychol Health Med*. 2010;15(2):127–134.

Jefee-Bahloul H. Teaching psychiatry residents about culture-bound syndromes: implementation of a modified team-based learning program. *Acad Psychiatry*. 2014; 1–2.

Juckett G, Rudolf-Watson L. Recognizing mental illness in culture-bound syndromes. *Am Fam Physician*. 2010;81(2):206.

Kagawa-Singer M. Impact of culture on health outcomes. *J Pediatr Hematol Oncol*. 2011;33(Suppl 2):S90–S95.

Keller MC, Miller G. Resolving the paradox of common, harmful, heritable mental disorders: which evolutionary genetic models work best? *Behav Brain Sci*. 2006; 29(4):385–404; discussion 405–452.

Khalil RB, Dahdah P, Richa S, Kahn DA. Lycanthropy as a culture-bound syndrome: a case report and review of the literature. *J Psychiatr Pract*. 2012;18(1):51–54.

Kohn R, Wintrob RM, Alarcón RD. Transcultural psychiatry. In: Sadock BJ, Sadock VA, Ruiz P, eds. *Kaplan & Sadock's Comprehensive Textbook of Psychiatry*. 9th ed. Philadelphia, PA: Lippincott Williams & Wilkins; 2009:734.

Kortmann F. Transcultural psychiatry: from practice to theory. *Transcult Psychiatry*. 2010:47(2):203–223.

Lewis-Fernández R, Guarnaccia PJ, Ruiz P. Culture-bound syndromes. In: Sadock BJ, Sadock VA, Ruiz P, eds. *Kaplan & Sadock's Comprehensive Textbook of Psychiatry*. 9th ed. Philadelphia, PA: Lippincott Williams & Wilkins; 2009:2519.

Lipton JE, Barash DP. Sociobiology and psychiatry. In: Sadock BJ, Sadock VA, Ruiz P, eds. *Kaplan & Sadock's Comprehensive Textbook of Psychiatry*. 9th ed. Vol. 1. Philadelphia, PA: Lippincott Williams & Wilkins; 2009:716.

Llyod K. The history and relevance of culture-bound syndromes. In: Bhui K, Bhugra D, eds. *Culture and Mental Health*. London: Hodder Arnold; 2007:98.

Millon T. Classifying personality disorders: an evolution-based alternative to an evidence-based approach. *J Pers Disord*. 2011;25(3):279–304.

Ruiz P. A look at cultural psychiatry in the 21st century. *J Nerv Ment Dis*. 2011; 199(8):553–556.

Swartz L. Dissociation and spirit possession in non-Western countries: Notes towards a common research agenda. In: Sinason V, ed. *Attachment, Trauma and Multiplicity: Working With Dissociative Identity Disorder*. 2nd ed. New York: Routledge; 2011:63.

Teo AR, Gaw AC. Hikikomori, a Japanese culture-bound syndrome of social withdrawal? A proposal for DSM-5. *J Nerv Ment Dis*. 2010;198(6):444–449.

Ton H, Lim RF. The assessment of culturally diverse individuals. In: Lim RF, ed. *Clinical Manual of Cultural Psychiatry*. Washington, DC: American Psychiatric Publishing; 2006:3–31.

van der Horst FCP, Kagan J. *John Bowlby – From Psychoanalysis to Ethology: Unravelling the Roots of Attachment Theory*. Hoboken, NJ: John Wiley & Sons, Inc; 2011.

Theories of Personality and Psychopathology

Aviezer H, Trope Y, Todorov A. Body cues, not facial expressions, discriminate between intense positive and negative emotions. *Science.* 2012;338(6111):1225–1229.

Bergmann MS. The Oedipus complex and psychoanalytical technique. *Psychoanal Inq.* 2010;30(6):535.

Breger L. *A Dream of Undying Fame: How Freud Betrayed His Mentor and Invented Psychoanalysis.* New York: Basic Books; 2009.

Britzman DP. *Freud and Education.* New York: Routledge; 2011.

Brown C, Lowis MJ. Psychosocial development in the elderly: an investigation into Erikson's ninth stage. *J Aging Stud.* 2003;17:415–426.

Caldwell L, Joyce A, eds. *Reading Winnicott.* New York: Routledge; 2011.

Capps D. The decades of life: Relocating Erikson's stages. *Pastoral Psychol.* 2004; 53:3–32.

Chodorow NJ. The American independent tradition: Loewald, Erikson, and the (possible) rise of intersubjective ego psychology. *Psychoanal Dialogues.* 2004;14:207–232.

Cotti P. Sexuality and psychoanalytic aggrandisement: Freud's 1908 theory of cultural history. *Hist Psychiatry.* 2011;22(85 Pt 1):58–74.

Cotti P. Travelling the path from fantasy to history: the struggle for original history within Freud's early circle, 1908–1913. *Psychoanal Hist.* 2010;12(2):153–172.

Crawford TN, Cohen P, Johnson JG, Sneed JR, Brook JS. The course and psychosocial correlates of personality disorder symptoms in adolescence: Erikson's developmental theory revisited. *J Youth Adolesc.* 2004;33(5):373–387.

DeRobertis EM. Deriving a third force approach to child development from the works of Alfred Adler. *J Hum Psychol.* 2011;51:492.

DeRobertis EM. Winnicott, Kohut, and the developmental context of well-being. *Hum Psychol.* 2010;38(4):336.

Efklides A, Moraitou D, eds. *A Positive Psychology Perspective on Quality of Life.* New York: Springer Science+Business Media; 2013.

Freud S. *The Standard Edition of the Complete Psychological Works of Sigmund Freud.* Vol. 24. London: Hogarth Press; 1953–1974.

Friedman LJ. Erik Erikson on identity, generativity, and pseudospeciation: a biographer's perspective. *Psychoanal Hist.* 2001;3:179.

Funk R, ed. *The Clinical Erich Fromm: Personal Accounts and Papers on Therapeutic Technique.* New York: Editions Rodopi B.V.; 2009.

Gardner H. Sigmund Freud: Alone in the world. In: *Creating Minds: An Anatomy of Creativity Seen Through the Lives of Freud, Einstein, Picasso, Stravinsky, Eliot, Graham, and Ghandi.* New York: Basic Books; 2011:47.

Giannopoulos VL, Vella-Brodrick DA. Effects of positive interventions and orientations to happiness on subjective well-being. *J Positive Psychol.* 2011;6(2):95.

Guasto G. Welcome, trauma, and introjection: a tribute to Sandor Ferenczi. *J Am Acad Psychoanal Dynam Psych.* 2011;39(2):337.

Hoare CH. Erikson's general and adult developmental revisions of Freudian thought: "Outward, forward, upward." *J Adult Dev.* 2005;12:19–31.

Hoffman L. One hundred years after Sigmund Freud's lectures in America: towards an integration of psychoanalytic theories and techniques within psychiatry. *Hist Psychiat.* 2010;21(84 Pt 4):455–470.

Hollon SD, Wilson GT. Psychoanalysis or cognitive-behavioral therapy for bulimia nervosa: the specificity of psychological treatments. *Am J Psychiatry.* 2014;171(1):13–16.

Huffman JC, DuBois CM, Healy BC, Boehm JK, Kashdan TB, Celano CM, Denninger JW, Lyubomirsky S. Feasibility and utility of positive psychology exercises for suicidal inpatients. *Gen Hosp Psychiatry.* 2014;36(1):88–94.

Kernberg O. Narcissistic personality disorder. In: Clarkin JF, Fonagy P, Gabbard GO, eds. *Psychodynamic Psychotherapy for Personality Disorders: A Clinical Handbook.* Arlington, VA: American Psychiatric Publishing; 2010:257.

Kirshner LA, ed. *Between Winnicott and Lacan: A Clinical Engagement.* New York: Routledge; 2011.

Kiselica AM, Ruscio J. Scientific communication in clinical psychology: examining patterns of citations and references. *Clin Psychol Psychother.* 2014;21(1):13–20.

Kivnick HQ, Wells CK. Untapped richness in Erik H. Erikson's rootstock. *Gerontologist.* 2014;54(1):40–50.

Lachman G. *Jung the Mystic: The Esoteric Dimensions of Carl Jung's Life and Teachings: A New Biography.* New York: Penguin; 2010.

Linley PA, Joseph S, Seligman MEP, eds. *Positive Psychology in Practice.* Hoboken, NJ: Wiley; 2004.

Meissner WW. Classical psychoanalysis. In: Sadock BJ, Sadock VA, Ruiz P, eds. *Kaplan & Sadock's Comprehensive Textbook of Psychiatry.* 9th ed. Vol. 1. Philadelphia, PA: Lippincott Williams & Wilkins; 2009:788.

Meissner WW. The God in psychoanalysis. *Psychoanal Psychol.* 2009;26(2):210.

Mohl PC, Brenner AM. Other psychodynamic schools. In: Sadock BJ, Sadock VA, Ruiz P, eds. *Kaplan & Sadock's Comprehensive Textbook of Psychiatry.* 9th ed. Vol. 1. Philadelphia, PA: Lippincott Williams & Wilkins; 2009:847.

Neukrug ES. Psychoanalysis. In: Neukrug ES, ed. *Counseling Theory and Practice.* Belmont, CA: Brooks/Cole; 2011:31.

Newton DS., Erik H. Erikson. In: Sadock BJ, Sadock VA, eds. *Kaplan & Sadock's Comprehensive Textbook of Psychiatry.* 8th ed. Vol. 1. Philadelphia, PA: Lippincott Williams & Wilkins; 2005:746.[

Palombo J, Bendicsen HK, Koch BJ. *Guide to Psychoanalytic Developmental Theories.* New York: Springer; 2009.

Pattakos A, Covey SR. *Prisoners of Our Thoughts: Viktor Frankl's Principles for Discovering Meaning in Life and Work.* San Francisco: Berrett-Koehler; 2010.

Paul HA. The Karen Horney clinic and the legacy of Horney. *Am J Psychoanal.* 2010;70(1):63–64.

Perlman FT, Brandell JR. Psychoanalytic theory. In: Brandell JR, ed. *Theory & Practice in Clinical Social Work.* 2nd ed. Thousand Oaks, CA: Sage; 2011:41.

Peterson C, Park N. Positive psychology. In: Sadock BJ, Sadock VA, Ruiz P, eds. *Kaplan & Sadock's Comprehensive Textbook of Psychiatry.* 9th ed. Philadelphia, PA: Lippincott Williams & Wilkins; 2009:2939.

Peterson C. *A Primer in Positive Psychology.* New York: Oxford University Press; 2006.

Pietikainen P, Ihanus J. On the origins of psychoanalytic psychohistory. *Hist Psychol.* 2003;6(2):171–194.

Revelle W. Personality structure and measurement: The contributions of Raymond Cattell. *Br J Psychol.* 2009; 100(S1):253.

Reynolds HR. Positive behavior intervention and support: improving school behavior and academic outcomes. *N C Med J.* 2012;73(5):359–360.

Schwartz J. The vicissitudes of Melanie Klein. Or, what is the case? *Attach New Direc Psychother Relation Psychoanal.* 2010;4(2):105.

Shapiro ER, Fromm MG. Eriksonian clinical theory and psychiatric treatment. In: Sadock BJ, Sadock VA, eds. *Comprehensive Textbook of Psychiatry.* 7th ed. New York: Lippincott Williams & Wilkins; 2000.

Sheldon KM, Kashdan TB, Steger MF. *Designing Positive Psychology: Taking Stock and Moving Forward.* New York: Oxford University Press; 2011.

Slater C. Generativity versus stagnation: an elaboration of Erikson's adult stage of human development. *J Adult Dev.* 2003;10:53.

Snyder CR, Lopez SJ. *Oxford Handbook of Positive Psychology.* 2nd ed. New York: Oxford University Press; 2009.

Snyder CR, Lopez SJ, Pedrotti JT. *Positive Psychology: The Scientific and Practical Explorations of Human Strengths.* 2nd ed. Thousand Oaks: Sage; 2010.

Stein M, ed. *Jungian Psychoanalysis: Working in the Spirit of Carl Jung.* Chicago: Open Court; 2010.

Tauber AI. *Freud, The Reluctant Philosopher.* Princeton, NJ: Princeton University Press; 2010.

Thurschwell P. *Sigmund Freud.* 2nd ed. New York: Routledge; 2009.

Van Hiel A, Mervielde I, De Fruyt F. Stagnation and generativity: structure, validity, and differential relationships with adaptive and maladaptive personality. *J Pers.* 2006; 74(2):543–573.

Westermeyer JF. Predictors and characteristics of Erikson's life cycle model among men: a 32-year longitudinal study. *Int J Aging Hum Dev.* 2004;58(1):29–48.

Wulff D. Freud and Freudians on religion: a reader. *Int J Psychol and Rel.* 2003;13:223.

35 ▲

A Brief History of Psychiatry

It is challenging to present a brief history of psychiatry that goes beyond cherry-picking individual moments as it is difficult to decide what advances in science are most relevant to the field. Equally significant are the contributions of related fields, including philosophy, theology, psychology, sociology, and other disciplines that have contributed to our understanding and attitudes about mental health.

Psychiatry was not considered a formal discipline of medicine until relatively recently. However, concern with the causes and treatment of various mental illnesses go back to antiquity. We can often see specific familiar themes and debates from different ages. For example, are mental illnesses truly aberrant, or merely variations of normal behavior. Is there some value in evolutionary fitness or to society, in mental illness? Are mental illnesses diseases of the "mind" or the "body," and what is the difference? Is the pathogen internal, such as a virus, a malfunctioning gene or a dysfunctional immune system, or external, such as a god, demon, industrial life, or a society in general? Who is best suited to treat the diseases—a medical doctor, or some other professional or nonprofessional healer? We see such debates emerge throughout society, and even when some no longer have scientific merit (i.e., mind vs. body debates), they often still linger in the lay understanding of the illnesses and affect how society treats individuals suffering from these disorders.

PSYCHIATRY BEFORE THE MODERN ERA

Many of us think of the roots of medicine beginning in Ancient Greece, and for the western world, that is, in part, true. However, the civilizations of Ancient Asia tended to be more advanced in the medical sciences. For example, psychiatry was practiced as a discipline in Ancient India, and the pre-2nd century CE medical treatise, the Charaka Saṃhitā or Compendium of Charaka, includes sections on psychiatric diseases (Fig. 35-1). Psychiatric hospitals existed in India even before that.

The Greeks tended to see psychiatric illnesses as supernatural disorders, although Hippocrates makes some mention of rudimentary anatomic research into the causes of psychiatric illness. In a broader sense, the Greeks were wrestling with what has become a significant theme in modern psychiatry: whether to view diseases as mere abnormalities or on a continuum with normal. Thus, the ongoing debate between whether we should see such disorders as depression on a continuum with normal sadness and grief, or as a fundamentally different phenomenon has its roots in antiquity. For example, Galen and Plato stressed a categorical approach to disease, whereas Hippocrates took a more dimensional approach, often seeing typical human attributes as being on a continuum with abnormal. This affected treatment approaches: Galen focused on treating the disease process, whereas Hippocrates emphasized treating the individual.

In the Middle Ages, Arab countries included psychiatric wards in their hospitals. The first was built in Baghdad around the early 9th century. Many of the great Islamic medical scholars, including Abu Ali al-Hussain ibn Abdallah ibn Sina (known in the West as Avicenna), wrote on mental disorder treatments.

Psychiatric hospitals appeared in medieval Europe around the 13th century. However, they did not provide treatment and were merely places for custodial care. The best known is probably the Bethlem Royal Hospital, usually shortened to Bethlem, or *Bedlam* (Fig. 35-2). It was founded in 1247 and was not a hospital in the modern sense but rather a place to collect alms for the care of the needy. Although the history is somewhat unclear, it may have taken in and cared for the insane as early as the later 14th century, and there is documentation of mentally ill inmates by the early 15th century. Little is known about the treatments that might have occurred. However, the hospital gradually transitioned from a general hospital to an asylum for the insane by the later 15th century.

PSYCHIATRY IN THE MODERN AGE

Early Modern Age

By the late 17th century, other "lunatic asylums" proliferated, most were privately run. The first building built specifically as an asylum for the insane was the Bethel Hospital Norwich, founded by Mary Chapman. Meanwhile, in France, Louis XIV created what was for Europe the first public mental health system, although again, there was little treatment.

One of the earliest Western treatises on mental illness was the *Anatomy of Melancholy, What it is: With all the Kinds, Causes, Symptomes, Prognostickes, and Several Cures of it. In Three Maine Partitions with their several Sections, Members, and Subsections. Philosophically, Medicinally, Historically, Opened and Cut Up* (usually just called *The Anatomy of Melancholy*) by Robert Burton, a mathematician, astrologer, and scholar at Oxford University (Fig. 35-3). Although going well beyond what we would consider a medical textbook, Burton's book does discuss "melancholy," which includes depressive illnesses, although it takes a much broader view and includes much of the human experience.

Although the medieval focus was theoretically on care, not punishment for the insane, often, the treatments were barbaric. These could include prolonged chained restraint and physical punishments. These practices began to change during the enlightenment, with a call for humanitarian reform. For example, in William Battie's, Treatise on Madness, he criticized the treatments occurring at such hospitals as Bethlem and argued for good hygiene and nutrition as mainstays of treatment. Although many of the somatic treatments he recommended were likely counterproductive (bleeding, purgatives), he did raise psychiatry to the level of a respectable discipline and helped support the humane treatment of mentally ill patients.

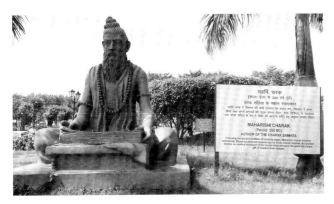

FIGURE 35-1
Charak Monument in Yog Peeth Campus, Father of Medicine & Surgery. (Source: Alokprasad, Balajijagadesh—Own work, CC BY-SA 3.0, https://commons.wikimedia.org/w/index.php?curid=8124213)

Expanding on the concept, the York Retreat in England, founded by William Tuke and the Bicêtre Hospital and then Salpêtrière, in France, under Dr. Philippe Pinel, championed the concept of "moral treatment." These approaches emphasized avoiding restraint—Pinel is famous for removing the patients' chains (Fig. 35-4). His mentor, Jean-Baptiste Pussin, who, with his wife and colleague Marguerite, advocated for moral treatment and began banning chains at the Bicêtre Hospital, which greatly influenced the young Pinel. Pinel extensively elaborated this and took a scientific approach. He was one of the first to present a comprehensive categorization of psychiatric diseases, which reflected a functional view of mental illness emphasizing phenomenology over pathophysiology.

In Edinburgh, Scotland, the pseudoscience of phrenology gained influence in the 18th century under the leadership of William Browne and George and Andrew Combe. Although useless as medical science, it was an important conceptual and philosophical step in that it shifted the concept of mental illness from a moral or philosophical disorder to a material one originating in the physical matter of the brain.

The 19th and Early 20th Century

In the early 19th century, the state began playing a larger role in the Western treatment of mental illness. In 1808, Britain passed the Country Asylums Act, which established public mental asylums.

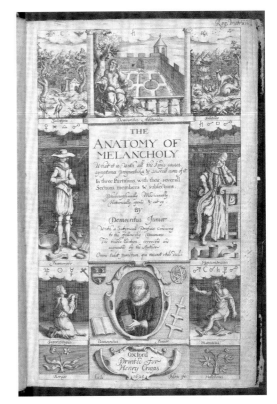

FIGURE 35-3
Robert Burton's The Anatomy of Melancholy, 1628. (Source: The British Library.)

In 1828 the Commissioners in Lunacy were appointed to oversee and license private asylums, partly in response to public concern over the abuses at Bethlem Hospital and similar private asylums. By then, "Bedlam" had become synonymous with "uproar" and "confusion," owing to the mismanagement at the hospital, and scandalous practices, such as continuing to chain patients (Fig. 35-5), and allowing the public to visit the hospital and view patients for their entertainment.

In 1838, France enacted a law regulating asylum services across the country and built the first school for individuals with intellectual disabilities. Similarly, the 1845 Lunacy Act in Britain

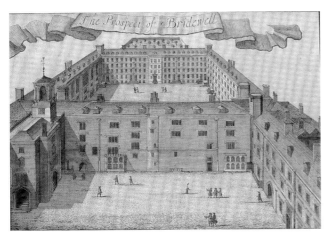

FIGURE 35-2
The Bethlem Royal Hospital. (Source: from John Strype's, An Accurate Edition of Stow's "A Survey of London," 1720. Public Domain.)

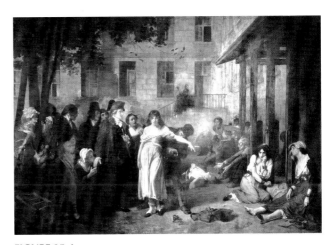

FIGURE 35-4
Pinel, removing the chains from an inmate at the Salpétrière in 1795. (Source: Pinel, médecin en chef de la Salpêtrière en 1795, by Tony Robert Fleury. From the collection at the hôpital de la Pitié-Salpétrière.)

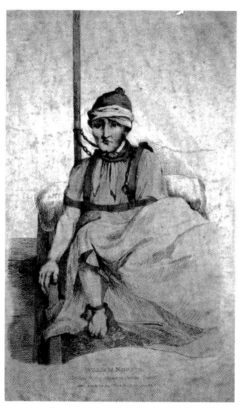

FIGURE 35-5

Etching of James Norris by G. Arnald 1815. (Source: Scan of a public domain image printed in Roy Porter, Madmen: A Social History of Madhouses, Mad-Doctors and Lunatics (Stroud, 2006).)

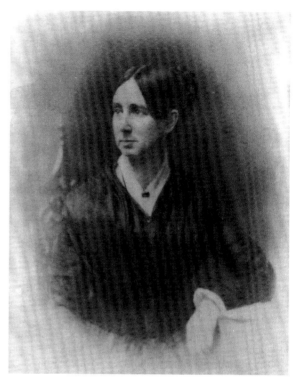

FIGURE 35-6

Dorothea Dix. (Source: United States Library of Congress's Prints and Photographs division (Public domain).)

reclassified mentally ill people as patients requiring treatment. It mandated that asylums be built and required periodic inspections of these facilities.

In the United States, reformers such as Dorothea Dix (Fig. 35-6) helped advocate for the first law to establish a state asylum, which became the Utica State Hospital, founded in about 1850. Dix achieved this after conducting a statewide investigation of the mentally ill poor in Massachusetts, showing that they were treated like prisoners in cages, often naked and physically abused. She later conducted similar investigations in other states, always advocating for moral care for the mentally ill.

The latter half of the 19th century and early 20th century saw the rise of scientific approaches to mental disorders, which advances in the classification of psychiatric disorders and beginning insights into the pathophysiology and etiology of disorders.

The first medical case report formally describing a schizophrenic psychosis was most likely that of Benedict Morel (1809–1873) in 1852, a French psychiatrist, who used the term *démence précoce* to describe deteriorated patients whose illnesses began in adolescence. Subsequent cases describing what was likely schizophrenia include those reported by Greisinger in 1867, Hecker in 1871, and Kahlbaum in 1874. Kalbaum's case was notable as one of the first medical case reports of catatonia.

For much of the 19th and early 20th century in Europe, most psychiatric disorders were thought to derive from either congenital or degenerative diseases. Jules Falret in 1854 described bipolar disorder (*folie circulaire*), and 1882, the German psychiatrist Karl Kahlbaum used the term cyclothymia, describing mania and depression as stages of the same illness.

Emil Kraepelin, building on the work of these predecessors, pioneered the scientific classification of psychiatric disease (Fig. 35-7). Kraepelin declared that all psychiatric disorders were biologic. As etiologic classification was not feasible, he based his

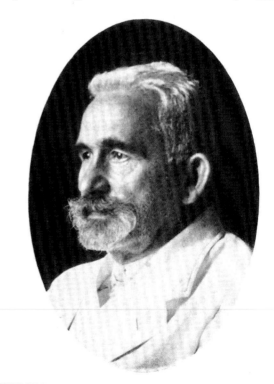

FIGURE 35-7

Emil Kraepelin in 1926. (Source: Wikipedia, original: Münchener Medizinische Wochenschrift], unknown photographer.)

classification on a careful study of disease phenomenology in different patients, in which he noted the similarities and differences in the symptomatology between different diseases.

Kraepelin translated Morel's *démence précoce* into *dementia praecox*, a term that emphasized the change in cognition (dementia) and early onset (praecox) of the disorder. Patients with dementia praecox were described as having a long-term deteriorating course and the clinical symptoms of hallucinations and delusions. Kraepelin distinguished these patients from those who underwent distinct episodes of illness alternating with periods of normal functioning, which he classified as having manic-depressive psychosis. Persistent persecutory delusions characterized another separate condition called paranoia. These patients lacked the deteriorating course of dementia praecox and intermittent symptoms of manic-depressive psychosis.

Eugene Bleuler coined the term schizophrenia, which replaced dementia praecox in the literature. Deriving it from the Ancient Greek words "schizo" ("I split") and "phren" ("mind"), he chose the term to express the presence of schisms among thought, emotion, and behavior in patients with the disorder. This term is often misconstrued, especially by laypeople, to mean split personality, a concept that would be closer to that of the dissociative disorders. Bleuler also stressed that, unlike Kraepelin's concept of dementia praecox, schizophrenia need not have a deteriorating course.

Bleuler identified specific fundamental (or primary) symptoms of schizophrenia to develop his theory about the internal mental schisms of patients. These symptoms included associational disturbances of thought, especially looseness, affective disturbances, autism, and ambivalence, summarized as "the four As": associations, affect, autism, and ambivalence. Bleuler also identified accessory (secondary) symptoms, including the symptoms significant to Kraepelin, such as hallucinations and delusions.

Sigmund Freud (Fig. 35-8) initially also sought a biologic explanation for mental disease. However, realizing that the contemporary scientific tools were not up to the task, he instead developed a psychoanalytic approach based on his experiences with his private patients as he sought to understand the unconscious meanings behind their thoughts, behaviors, and desires. Although Freud was a neurologist and arguably working in psychology, his work was soon adopted by psychiatrists. The psychoanalytic approach became transcendent in the middle of the 20th century, and many psychiatric illnesses were explained in psychoanalytic terms; that is, in terms of conflicts and drives, particularly sexual drives, and stemming from early life experiences. Like many philosophical movements, psychoanalysis may have suffered from its overwhelming popularity, and at times it overreached as it tried to treat illnesses for which it was not suited, or tried to explain many human behaviors and achievements through the lens of psychoanalytic theory. In the latter half of the 20th century, as effective biologic treatments were discovered, many psychiatrists became disenchanted with psychoanalysis's lack of empirical data and seeming resistance to scientific testing. It began to lose influence as a primary approach to understanding and treating psychiatric disease.

The Latter 20th Century

The approach to mental illness, including the specific patients treated, shifted around World War II, as psychiatrists moved out of the asylum to confront very different patients, moving from the treatment of the "insane" to people who were "like us." No longer confined to just the asylum, psychiatrists proved their usefulness in the military arena, treating both patients traumatized by combat and those found unfit to serve in the military for psychological reasons.

Greater importance was attached to the role of the environment on mental illness. This change drew from the work of Adolph Meyer (Fig. 35-9). Meyer, the founder of psychobiology, saw mental disorders as reactions to life stresses. It was a maladaptation that was understandable in terms of the patient's life experiences.

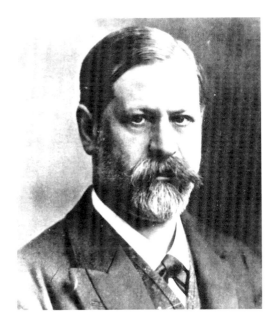

FIGURE 35-8
Sigmund Freud at age 47. (Courtesy of Menninger Foundation Archives, Topeka, KS.)

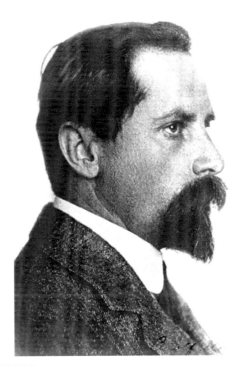

FIGURE 35-9
Adolf Meyer. (Courtesy of National Library of Medicine, Bethesda, M.D.)

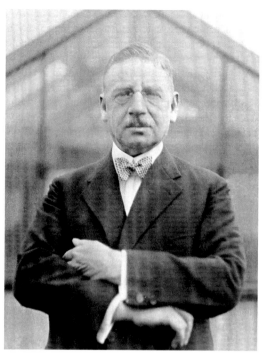

FIGURE 35-10
Otto Loewi. (Source: Creative Commons Attribution 4.0 International.)

Building on Meyer's social perspective and Freud's emphasis on early life experiences, Walter Menninger and others developed the *psychosocial model* of mental illness. Depression was seen not as a neurologic illness but as a failure to adapt. Menninger went as far as to suggest that all psychiatric disorders could be reduced to "one basic psychosocial process: the failure of the suffering individual to adapt to his or her environment."

The second half of the 20th century saw a gradual transition from a psychoanalytic and sociologic understanding of mental illness to a biologic one. Many discoveries helped propel this shift in approach.

Biologic models had existed before. For example, in the 1930s, Papez theorized that emotions were caused by a circuit connecting the limbic lobe, amygdala, septal region, and hippocampus. Electroconvulsive therapy was also developed in the 1930s and used to treat depression as early as the 1940s.

An early influence on biologic explanations for etiology was Otto Loewi's discovery of acetylcholine's role as a neurotransmitter. In proving this, Loewi (Fig. 35-10) employed a now-famous experiment, published in 1921, in which he used the saline solution from one frog heart to stimulate the rate in a second denervated heart, thus proving that a chemical must control the heart rate. He later showed that this chemical was acetylcholine. This was the first experiment that showed that a chemical could cause a response absent of electrical stimulation, thus discovering the critical role of neurotransmitters.

Loewi's experiment is famous, not only for its scientific value but also that the idea for the experiment came in a dream. Although he wrote down the dream when briefly waking from it, he could not make sense of his scribbles the next morning. Fortunately, he went on to have the same dream the next night, and when awakening from that, he rushed to his laboratory to perform what would become Nobel Prize-winning research.

The practical beginning of biologic psychiatry occurred with the serendipitous discovery of several drugs that could treat mental disorders, including chlorpromazine for schizophrenia, imipramine and iproniazid for depression, and lithium carbonate for bipolar disorder. In each case, the initial importance of the drug was not appreciated. For example, chlorpromazine was synthesized from promethazine, an antihistamine, in a search for more stable antihistamine sedatives. It was initially used as an anesthetic adjunct, and its antipsychotic properties were only later recognized after psychiatrists began administering it to manic and psychotic patients, again originally as a sedative.

Imipramine was also first synthesized as an antihistamine, and, following in the footsteps of chlorpromazine, tried as an antipsychotic before some case reports convinced the manufacturers to investigate its role as an antidepressant. Supporting these findings was the discovery that certain drugs, such as reserpine, which irreversibly blocks monoamine transporters, could cause depression through the depletion of monoamines. Not only did it help the development of the first biologic theory for depression, the monoamine theory, but it also lent what was considered the first reproducible example of a chemical causing a mental disorder.

Lithium had been used as a medication since the 19th century, initially for gout. However, the doses needed to, for example, dissolve urate in the body were toxic. It was later used as a salt substitute for hypertensive patients but was largely banned after the toxicity became apparent. Lithium was used for mania in the late 1800s, but this was related to some theories that mood disorders were a type of "brain gout." As that theory waned in popularity, lithium was largely abandoned as a psychotherapeutic. In the late 1940s, John Cade, an Australian physician, rediscovered lithium's value for mania. Because of toxicity concerns, however, it took many decades and much research before it was adopted in the United States and other countries.

Neuroimaging started being used as an investigatory tool in the 1980s, following the discovery by Johnstone and others that patients with schizophrenia had enlarged cerebral ventricles. Pioneers such as Nancy Andreasen conducted the first MRI studies of schizophrenia and developed many of the techniques used by other investigators of the disease.

Genetic explorations also yielded interesting findings, such as the high heritability of certain disorders such as schizophrenia, autism spectrum disorder, and bipolar disorder. Although actual genetic associations have been elusive, the research in genetics lent additional support to the drug research and neuroimaging research which, when combined, created a growing body of research which moved the understanding of the etiology of many mental disorders from childhood parenting and other experiences or social causes to disorders that are, at least in part, inherited.

DEINSTITUTIONALIZATION

The 20th century also saw a shift from the asylum to the office and the community as the center of psychiatric treatment. The influence of the psychoanalytic and psychosocial movements also influenced psychiatry's belief that most psychiatric diseases had at least potential treatments. In 1963, President Kennedy introduced legislation that delegated the NIH to administer community mental health centers, thus beginning the community health movement in the United States (Fig. 35-11). It outlined a plan to discharge patients, including severely mentally ill patients, from institutions and instead treat them in the community. Although a

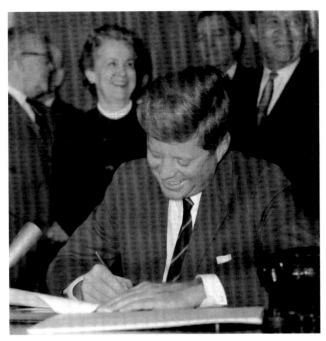

FIGURE 35-11
President John F. Kennedy signs the Mental Retardation Facilities and Community Mental Health Center Construction Act. (Source JFK Library. Public Domain.)

laudable goal, it has been most successful at deinstitutionalization, whereas community centers have been poorly funded and supported. Thus, although most psychiatric patients no longer live in asylums, they may be homeless, living in dangerous environments, or be confined in jails, and in each case, receive little treatment.

THE CLASSIFICATION OF PSYCHIATRIC DISORDERS

Clinical treatment and classification dragged somewhat behind the science. Before the 1960s, many institutions and asylums developed their unique classification systems, and the result was a significant variation in both diagnostic terminology and how those diagnoses were applied. For example, in 1953, the American Psychiatric Association held a conference to develop a research program to evaluate psychiatry therapies. However, the members concluded that such research would be meaningless without a standardized approach diagnosis, which did not then exist.

This problem was further exposed in the United States–United Kingdom study conducted in the 1960s, which showed that many patients diagnosed with schizophrenia would be diagnosed with bipolar disorder in the United Kingdom. This variation results from an overemphasis in the United States on psychotic symptoms as a diagnostic criterion for schizophrenia. Another telling study was the Rosenhan experiment, in which experimenters feigned hallucinations to enter psychiatric hospitals, but usually acted normally once admitted. They were diagnosed with psychiatric disorders and even given antipsychotic drugs (which they flushed down toilets).

The problem was also apparent in such studies as the Baltimore Morbidity Study, which used DSM-I criteria and found inconsistent and unreliable results. The situation was such that in the 1970s, the President's Commission on Mental Health, informally called the Carter Commission, concluded that they could not form meaningful goals for mental health treatment until they understood the disorders better.

This problem led to an attempt to develop more reliable diagnostic systems. In the United States, this coalesced into the Diagnostic and Statistical Manual of Mental Disorders (DSM), developed by the American Psychiatric Association (APA). The first two editions are mostly preliminary works, reflecting the prevalent approaches among psychiatrists. For example, the second edition of the DSM (1968) distinguished between psychotic (defined more broadly than today) and neurotic forms of depression. This division developed into an endogenous/exogenous distinction—virtually depression due to a disease of the brain versus depression that is a reaction to stress, be it current or developmental. Although lacking any empirical validity, the distinction was a convenient way to divide biologic and psychodynamic concepts of depression. This division often drove treatment during much of the 1970s, in which it was thought some forms of depression were better treated with psychotherapy, whereas others should be addressed with medication.

The introduction of the DSM-III in 1980, and its subsequent revisions up to and including DSM-5, represented a significant paradigm change in diagnosis, which was borne of research designed to create more reliable criteria for mental disorders (Fig. 35-12).

Feighner and colleagues at Washington University developed the Feighner, or St. Louis criteria, criteria for 15 major psychiatric categories. This approach represented the first systematic approach that relied entirely on numbers and types of symptoms to diagnose psychiatric disorders. While this was taking place, Robert Spitzer, Jean Endicott, and other researchers at the New York State Psychiatric Institute were developing methods to increase the reliability of psychiatric diagnoses. These groups and other researchers were brought together by the National Institute of Mental Health in the 1970s, where they developed the Research Diagnostic Criteria (RDC), which were essentially an elaboration and expansion of the Feighner criteria.

The RDC prepared the way for the DSM-III, which resulted from the work of the Task Force on Nomenclature and Statistics, headed by Dr. Spitzer, formed by the APA in the early 1970s. The DSM-III eliminated the endogenous/exogenous dichotomy previously inherent in many diagnoses, and eliminated assumptions of cause from the criteria, taking a strictly phenomenal approach. For example, major depression was defined by symptomatic criteria. It also divided the mood disorders, with major depression and bipolar disorder being treated as distinct disorders. Although acknowledging more minor forms of depression, DSM-III's categorical approach created a rigid divide between those with major depressive disorder and those not meeting the criteria for the disorder, a difference that survives to this day. This divide risks neglecting some individuals who do not fit into one of the DSM categories and yet suffer from depression; although DSM includes ways to categorize them, it is likely that in clinical practice, many such patients are treated as if they had no disorder.

However, the benefits of this categorical approach have been that it has created more reliable diagnoses, allowing for research on more homogeneous populations. This strategy bore significant fruit, and there was a pharmaceutical revolution in the 1980s and 1990s, in which researchers developed and introduced new classes of medications, such as the SSRIs and the atypical antipsychotics. Although arguably not more efficacious than the original antidepressants and antipsychotics, the drugs were considered more

Evolution of the DSM System

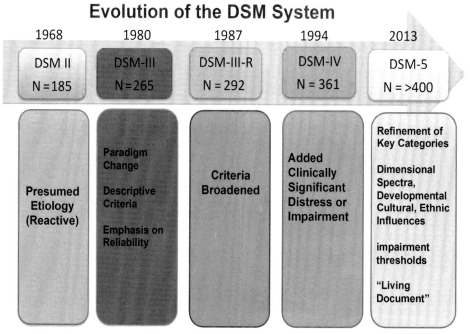

1968	1980	1987	1994	2013
DSM II N = 185	DSM-III N = 265	DSM-III-R N = 292	DSM-IV N = 361	DSM-5 N = >400
Presumed Etiology (Reactive)	Paradigm Change Descriptive Criteria Emphasis on Reliability	Criteria Broadened	Added Clinically Significant Distress or Impairment	Refinement of Key Categories Dimensional Spectra, Developmental Cultural, Ethnic Influences impairment thresholds "Living Document"

FIGURE 35-12

DSM system. Key issues and number of categories.

tolerable, and the result was a considerable increase in the number of patients taking, and benefitting from, psychopharmacological agents. Some have pointed out that this phenomenon also caused abuses and overuse of the drugs for conditions that could be more considered part of the human condition, and there was a predictable backlash in which critics questioned both the safety and efficacy of many psychiatric drugs. Organized psychiatry often found itself on the defensive as it had to make a case for the drugs and contend with critiques that went beyond scientific questions into the effect of the drugs on culture and society.

The DSM-III and its role in contributing to the remedicalization of psychiatry also affected psychological treatments. Although the more reliable criteria made it easier to design studies and enroll suitable populations for treatment studies, it also helped encourage a bias toward psychological treatments that lent themselves to scientific research—ones that were easily manualized and reproducible in a consistent way. Hence, such therapies as cognitive-behavioral therapies, behavioral therapies, and interpersonal therapies gained predominance as treatments for major psychiatric disorders. In contrast, psychoanalytic treatments, whose depth and complexity made them inherently harder to study consistently, became more marginalized and considered "boutique treatments" reserved for those who could pay the sometimes considerable out-of-pocket costs for these therapies.

LOOKING TO THE FUTURE

The combination of new technologies, such as high-resolution functional imagining (Fig. 35-13) and total gene mapping, combined with the ever-increasing ability of computers to manipulate vast amounts of data, has resulted in a remarkable explosion in research on such disorders as schizophrenia, autism, obsessive-compulsive disorder, and major depression during the past decade, and we have made great strides toward understanding the genetics and pathophysiology of these disorders. However, there remains a frustrating gap between basic and clinical research.

In genetics, the limitations of clinical diagnoses for research purposes are clear, and the search for valid biomarkers has been disappointing. It may be that a focus on meaningful endophenotypes may be an essential step. However, the predictive power of many of the proposed endophenotypes remains to be proven.

Pharmacologic research into treating the disorder, after several fruitful decades, has stalled. Clozapine, arguably the most effective antipsychotic, was discovered in the 1960s, the SSRIs became available in the 1980s and 90s, and the subsequent efforts to refine pharmacologic treatment have, so far, fallen short of hopes. Barriers to translational research include the lack of a valid animal

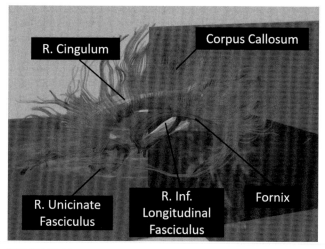

FIGURE 35-13

This image is an example of the high level of detail that neuroimaging technologies can produce to aid investigators. Three-dimensional image reconstructed based on diffusion data acquired on a 3-T General Electric scanner, Brigham and Women's Hospital, Harvard Medical School, Boston, MA, which shows several major white matter fiber bundles (generally differing in colors, converted to grayscale for this book) identified through diffusion tensor imaging.

model for many of the disorders, and efforts are being made in improving how animal testing is performed. In the meantime, new approaches are being attempted that deemphasize the importance of single receptors and emphasize a multi-target approach to psychopharmacology—essentially using "dirty drugs," which had previously been discouraged due to concerns over side effects, as well as moving beyond monoamine targets to include other receptors, including glutamatergic targets and G-protein–coupled receptors.

What is clear, however, is that most psychiatric disorders are very complex disorders that require multifaceted solutions. These solutions include attention to psychosocial treatments as well as pharmacologic. The change from conceptualizing many of the disorders as neurodevelopmental rather than neurodegenerative disorders also highlights the importance of early identification of disorders in the hopes that early interventions can alter the course at a more promising stage.

Table 35-1 presents a summary of some of the significant persons and events in the history of psychiatry.

Table 35-1
A History of Psychiatry Table

Persons and Events in Psychiatry

Person or Event	Country	Publications	Significance
Hippocrates of Cos (ca. 460–370 BCE)		*Hippocratic Writings*. Baltimore, MD: Pelican Classics; 1978	Held that diseases are caused by imbalances in the four humors (blood, phlegm, yellow bile, black bile); melancholia is caused by excess black bile; hysteria is caused by wandering uterus; looked for natural causes of epilepsy, the "sacred disease"; advised dietary treatment of illness; the *Hippocratic Oath* established ideals of ethical conduct for physicians
Plato (427–347 BCE)	Greece	*The Dialogues of Plato*. Jowett B, trans. New York: Random House; 1937	In *Timaeus, Phaedrus,* and *The Republic,* described two kinds of madness: Madness in which the appetitive soul lost the domination of the rational soul and madness inspired by the gods (divine madness)
Aristotle (384–322 BCE)	Greece	Ross WD: *Aristotle*. 6th ed. New York: Routledge; 1995	In *De Anima* and other psychological works, described the affections of desire, anger, fear, courage, envy, joy, hatred, and pity
Galen of Pergamon (130–200)	Asia Minor (Turkey) in the Roman Empire	On the Affected Parts. Siegel R, trans., ed. Basel: Karger; 1976	Consolidated the thoughts of Hippocrates, Plato, and Aristotle; his idea that depression was caused by an excess of black bile was influential until the 19th century
St. Augustine (354–430)	Tageste (Numidia, North Africa)	Confessions. Pusey EB, trans. New York: Modern Library; 1949; Wills G: Saint Augustine. New York: Lipper/Viking; 1999	His *Confessions* was the first book to center on psychological introspection
Avicenna (980–1037)	Persia	A Treatise on the Canon of Medicine of Avicenna. London: Luzac; 1930	His *Canon of Medicine* recognized that certain physical diseases were caused by emotional upsets and was widely read by Christian and Muslim physicians
Constanitus Africanus (ca. 1010–1087)	Carthage, North Africa	Constantino l'Africano. Della melancolia. Rome; 1959	His *Melancholia* made observations on delusional thinking, and, from the first medical school at Salerno, spread Galenic ideas on depression throughout western Europe
Petrarch (1304–1374)	Italy	*De remediis utriusque fortunae*	In his letters and *De remediis,* he developed a rhetoric that aimed to console and comfort the mentally disturbed, so (in the estimation of Stanley Jackson) "he made a significant contribution to the realm of consolatory and therapeutic wisdom"
Henry Kramer and James Sprenger (15th century)	Germany	*Malleus maleficarum (Witches' Hammer)* (1486)	Influential in causing the persecution of persons for witchcraft

(continued)

Table 35-1
A History of Psychiatry Table (*Continued*)

Persons and Events in Psychiatry

Person or Event	Country	Publications	Significance
Paracelsus (ca. 1493–1541)	Einsiedeln (Switzerland), then traveled Europe	Pagel W. "Disease and the stars. 'The animal in man' and lunacy. The psychiatry of Paracelsus." In: *Paracelsus*. 2nd rev. ed. Basel: Karger; 1982:150	Opposed the ideas of Galen; believed that psychiatric illness occurred when an individual's animal instincts were stimulated by the stars and that emotions caused physical illness (hence has been called an early "psychosomaticist"); treatments were mainly psychotherapy, but also included venesection, trephining, and sulfur
Juan Luis Vives (1493–1540)	Born in Spain; from the age of 16 yr lived mainly in Holland and Belgium	*De anima et vita (Of Soul and Life)* (1538); Noreña CG. *Juan Luis Vives and the Emotions*. Carbondale, IL: Southern Illinois University Press; 1989	Described for the first time the importance of psychological associations in forming emotions and in the remembering of past events
Johann Weyer (1515–1588)	Holland	*De Praestigiis Daemonum (The Deception of Demons)* (1563); reprinted in Mora G, ed. *Witches, Devils, and Doctors in the Renaissance*. Binghampton, NY: Center for Medieval and Early Renaissance Studies; 1991	Criticizes the *Malleus* and refutes some of the prevailing beliefs in witchcraft
Juan Huarte de San Juan (ca. 1530–1592)	Spain	*The Examination of Men's Wits* (1575)	An early account of differences in temperaments and dispositions
Giambattista Porta (1535–1615)	Italy	*De humana physiognomia* (1586)	Gave to physiognomy the air of at least a pseudoscience
Felix Plater (1536–1614)	Switzerland	*Practice of Medicine* (1602); *Observations of Diseases Injurious to Body and Mind* (1614)	New classification of diseases based on symptoms, causes, and treatments; careful description of all known psychiatric and organic diseases; the first physician to separate medicine from philosophy and make it a branch of natural science; a pioneer in studying the behavior and neuropathology of the persons with mental handicaps
Robert Burton (1577–1640)	England	*The Anatomy of Melancholy* (1621)	The most famous book on psychiatry in the 17th century; a comprehensive presentation of all previous medical-psychological thought on melancholy, also drawing on the nonmedical literature of Western civilization
Paolo Zacchia (1584–1659)	Italy	*Questiones medico-legales* (1621–1635)	Held that a physician, rather than a priest or lawyer, should evaluate a patient's responsibility for disturbed behavior; the beginning of forensic psychiatry
Thomas Sydenham (1624–1689)	England	Dissertatio epistolaris . . . [1682]. In: The Entire Works of Dr. Thomas Sydenham Newly Made English (1742)	Gave a comprehensive picture of the many symptoms of hysteria, believing that in the form of hypochondriacal complaints, it could exist in men and that it was caused by disturbed animal spirits; his approach to classifying the causes of symptoms resembled the modern psychiatric endeavor of constructing atheoretical classifications of psychiatric illnesses
Thomas Willis (1621–1675)	England	*Two Discourses Concerning the Soul of Brutes* (1683)	Summarized what was known about major psychiatric illnesses; recognized differences in illnesses when there was gross brain disease and when the brain seemed normal, attributing the latter to disturbed animal spirits; attributed hysteria to disturbed animal spirits acting on the brain, not to a wandering uterus

Table 35-1
A History of Psychiatry Table (*Continued*)

Persons and Events in Psychiatry

Person or Event	Country	Publications	Significance
Georg Ernst Stahl (1660–1734)	Germany	*Theoria medica vera* (1707), *De animi morbis* (1708)	Theory of animism; the soul, *anima*, maintains functions of body in health and disease; psychiatric illness is caused either by inhibitions of anima or diseases of the body
William Battie (1703–1776)	England	*A Treatise of Madness* (1758)	First physician who made insanity his full work, raised "the mad business" to a respected specialty, and first used "madness" in the title of his book
Boissier de Sauvages (1706–1767)	France	*Nosologia methodica* (1765)	Nosology divided diseases into classes based on symptoms; although speculative and artificial, it stimulated a rethinking of concepts of disease
John Aiken (1747–1822)	England	*Thoughts on Hospitals* (1771)	First book on hospitals in which "lunatic hospitals" were discussed
Franz Anton Mesmer (1734–1815)	Austria, France	*Memoire sur la découverte du magnetism animal* (1779)	Showed that when a mental therapist used the so-called animal magnetism, it could cure cases of psychiatric illness; led to the discovery of hypnosis
Vincenzo Chiarugi (1759–1820)	Italy	*Regulations of the Hospitals of Santa Maria Nuova and of Bonifazio* (1789)	One of the first attempts to treat the insane inmates of asylums humanely and without restraints
William Cullen (1710–1790)	Scotland	*Nosology, or a Systematic Arrangement of Diseases* (1800)	A great 18th-century nosologist who first used the terms *neurosis* and *neurotic* to describe mental diseases
Philippe Pinel (1745–1826)	France	*A Treatise on Insanity in Which Are Contained the Principles of a New and More Practical Nosology of Mental Disorders* (1801)	Classified mental illness into four main forms and established a new, humane treatment for inmates of insane asylums, which he called "the moral treatment of insanity"
Johann Reil (1759–1813)	Germany	*Rhapsodies about the Application of Psychotherapy to Mental Disturbances* (1803)	The founder of rational psychotherapy, recognizing the therapeutic value of institutional surroundings, music, psychodrama, and occupational therapy; first used the word *psychiatry,* and founded the first psychiatric journal
Benjamin Rush (1745–1813)	United States	*Medical Inquiries and Observations upon the Diseases of the Mind* (1812); Farr C: Benjamin Rush and American psychiatry. *Am J Psychiatry.* 1994;151(Suppl):65	The most famous American physician of his time and the only physician to sign the Declaration of Independence; the first American author of a book on general psychiatry; and the father of American psychiatry
Thomas Sutton (1767–1835)	England	*Tracts on Delirium Tremens* (1813)	First description of alcoholic delirium tremens
William Tuke (1732–1822); Samuel Tuke (1784–1857), grandson of William Tuke; Daniel Hack Tuke (1827–1895), youngest son of Samuel Tuke; John Charles Bucknill (1817–1895)	England	Tuke S. Description of the Retreat, an Institution near York, for Insane Persons of the Society of Friends. York; 1813; Tuke DH, Bucknill JC. *A Manual of Psychological Medicine Containing the History, Nosology, Description, Statistics, Diagnosis, Pathology, and Treatment of Insanity.* London; 1858	W. Tuke founded the York Retreat for the moral treatment of mentally ill Quakers in 1796; S. Tuke's *Description of the Retreat* influenced asylum treatment in England, Europe, and the United States; the *Manual* of D. Tuke and Bucknill was the first comprehensive textbook of psychiatry
Joseph Adams (1756–1818)	England	*A Treatise on the Supposed Hereditary Properties of Diseases…Particularly in Madness and Scrofula* (1814)	First book on the hereditary properties of diseases; argued that it was not a disease that was inherited but a susceptibility to diseases; therefore, prevention and cure were possible

(*continued*)

Table 35-1
A History of Psychiatry Table (*Continued*)

Persons and Events in Psychiatry

Person or Event	Country	Publications	Significance
Franz Joseph Gall (1758–1828), Johann Gaspar Spurzheim (1776–1832)	Austria, Germany	*The Physiognomical System of Drs. Gall and Spurzheim; founded on an anatomical and physiological examination of the nervous system in general and of the brain in particular* (1815)	The beginning of phrenology: Mapping parts of the brain, defining their psychological functions, and making psychological and psychotherapeutic predictions
Johann Christian Heinroth (1773–1843)	Germany	Disturbances of the Mind (1818); Hansen LA. Metaphors of mind and society: The origins of German psychiatry in the revolutionary era. *Isis.* 1998;89:387; Cauwenbergh LS. J Chr A Heinroth (1773–1843) a psychiatrist of the German Romantic era. *Hist Psychiatry.* 1991;2:365	First systematic textbook of psychiatry that attempted to formulate an actual clinical system of psychotherapy; the first to use the word psychosomatic and the first to hold a chair in psychological medicine at the University of Leipzig
Robert Gooch (1784–1830)	England	*An Account of…Diseases Peculiar to Women* (1829)	First account of postpartum psychosis
James Cowles Pritchard (1786–1848)	England	*A Treatise on Insanity and Other Disorders Affecting the Mind* (1835)	Standard textbook of psychiatry covering all of the literature on all known diseases; described moral insanity, later called *psychopathic personality*
Jean Etienne Dominique Esquirol (1782–1840)	France	*Mental Maladies: A Treatise on Insanity* (1838)	Coined the term *hallucination,* described "idiocy," classified insanities into monomania (partial insanity) and general delirium, and recognized both emotional and organic causes of illness; one of the authors of a comprehensive law providing an asylum for every department of France
Isaac Ray (1807–1881)	United States	*Treatise on Medical Jurisprudence of Insanity* (1838)	Founded American forensic psychiatry
James Braid (1795–1860)	England	*Neurypnology; or, the Rationale of Nervous Sleep* (1843)	Entirely separated hypnotism from animal magnetism and began the study of hypnotic phenomena
Daniel M'Naghton (1813–1865)	England	West DJ, Walk A, eds. *Daniel M'Naghton: His Trial and the Aftermath.* London Gaskell Books; 1977	Suffering from persecutory delusions, M'Naghton murdered the secretary of a government official in 1843; at his murder trial, he was ruled not guilty by reason of insanity and was committed to an insane asylum for the rest of his life; the "M'Naghton rule" has influenced English and American legal criteria for acquittal on the basis of insanity
Wilhelm Griesinger (1817–1868)	Germany	*Mental Pathology and Therapeutics* (1845)	Proclaimed that psychiatric diseases are brain diseases and that psychiatry had become a medical specialty
Jacques-Joseph Moreau de Tours (1804–1884)	France	*Du haschich et de l'aliénation mentale* (1845)	Described the effects of his taking hashish, and became the first psychiatrist to experience a drug-induced psychosis
Walter Cooper Dendy (1794–1871)	England	Psychotherapeia, or the remedial influence of mind. *J Psychol Med Ment Pathol.* 1853;6:268	First introduced the term *psychotherapeia* (psychotherapy), which he defined as prevention and remedy of disease by psychical influence and which he predicted would become valuable in psychiatry
Jean-Pierre Falret (1794–1870), Jules Baillarger (1809–1890)	France	Baillarger J. La folie à double forme. *Bull Acad Imp Med.* 1853–1854;19:340; Falret JP. La folie circulaire. *Bull Acad Imp Med.* 1853–1854;19:382; Pichot P. The birth of the bipolar disorder. *Eur Psychiatry.* 1995;10:1	Baillarger and Falret called bipolar disorder "double insanity" and "circular insanity"; in 1899, Kraepelin named this illness *manic-depressive psychosis*

Table 35-1
A History of Psychiatry Table (*Continued*)

Persons and Events in Psychiatry

Person or Event	Country	Publications	Significance
Thomas Kirkbride (1809–1883)	United States	*On the Construction, Organisation, and General Arrangements of Hospitals for the Insane* (1854)	Set a standard for mid–19th century care of the chronically insane that commands respect today
John Conolly (1794–1866)	England	*The Treatment of the Insane without Mechanical Restraints* (1856)	Conolly's work for the nonrestraint system marked the success of a movement that began with Pinel and created a new approach to treating insanity throughout the civilized world
George Robinson (1821–1875)	England	*On the Prevention and Treatment of Mental Disorders* (1859)	Introduced the idea of looking beyond the precincts of the asylum to prevent mental illness
Gustav Theodor Fechner (1801–1887)	Germany	*Elements of Psychophysics* (1860)	Established the relationship between the intensity of stimuli and sensory reactions; called the founder of experimental psychology
Benedict-Augustin Morel (1809–1873)	France	*Traité des maladies mentales* (1860)	Presented cases of insanity and other mental illnesses caused by inherited "mental degeneration" that became worse from one generation to the next
Thomas Laycock (1812–1876)	England	*Mind and Brain* (1860)	Mentioned unconscious functional activity of the brain but did not further develop the idea
Forbes B. Winslow (1810–1874)	England	*On Obscure Diseases of the Brain and Disorders of the Mind* (1860)	First to mention psychical diagnostic tests (psychological tests) and the psychiatric interview
Ewald Hecker (1843–1909)	Germany	Die Hebephrenie. *Arch Pathol Anat Physiol.* 1871:52	First description of "hebephrenia" (later a subgroup of dementia praecox)
Karl Kahlbaum (1828–1899)	Germany	*Die Katatonie oder das Spannungsirresein* (Berlin, 1874)	First description of catatonia (later a subgroup of dementia praecox)
George Miller Beard (1840–1883)	United States	*A Practical Treatise on Nervous Exhaustion (Neurasthenia)* (1880)	Neurasthenia—a disease of mental and physical exhaustion—replaced the diagnosis of hypochondriasis; it became prevalent in the American and European upper classes from approximately 1870 to 1920
Richard von Krafft-Ebing (1840–1902)	Germany	*Psychopathia sexualis* (1886); Oosterhuis H. *Stepchildren of Nature: Kraft-Ebing, Psychiatry, and the Making of Sexual Identity.* Chicago, IL: University of Chicago Press; 2000	Described cases of homosexuality and sexual perversions, claiming that some were caused by degeneration, and coined the terms *sadism, masochism,* and *sexual bondage; Psychopathia* was respected by lawyers and scientists, and it founded the science of sexology
Pierre Janet (1859–1947)	France	*L'automatisme psychologique: Essai de psychologie experimentale sur les formes inferieures de l'active* (Paris, 1889); van der Kolk BA, van der Hart O. Pierre Janet and the breakdown of adaptation in psychological trauma. *Am J Psychiatry.* 1989;146:1530	Showed that severe traumatic experiences caused two types of dissociative symptoms—*hysteria,* with dissociations of feelings or memories related to the experiences, and *psychasthenia,* with obsessions, phobias, and anxieties; the first systematic attempt to show how the mind can dissociate in the face of severe trauma
Herman Emminghaus (1845–1904)	Germany	*Psychic Disturbances of Childhood* (1887)	First textbook of child psychiatry

(*continued*)

Table 35-1
A History of Psychiatry Table (*Continued*)

Persons and Events in Psychiatry

Person or Event	Country	Publications	Significance
Jean-Martin Charcot (1825–1893)	France	Owen ARG. *Hysteria, Hypnosis, and Healing: The Work of JM Charcot.* New York: Garrett Publications; 1971; by Goetz C, Bonduelle M, Gelfand T. *Charcot: Constructing Neurology.* Oxford: Oxford University Press; 1995	In 1882, became the first professor of diseases of the nervous system at the University of Paris, helping to institutionalize neurology as a medical specialty and making Paris an international center for neurologic studies; although he erroneously believed that only hysterics could be hypnotized, he fully delineated and classified the protean manifestations of hysteria, and he was the first to give a psychological account of hysteria and show that some of its symptoms are the result of ideas that dominated the mind of the hysteric
Georges Gilles de la Tourette (1857–1904)	France	Etude sur une affection nerveuse caractérisée par l'incoordination motrice accompagnée d'echolalie et coprolalie. *Arch Neurol (Paris).* 1885;ix:19,158; Yorston G, Hindley N, trans. and intro: Study of a nervous disorder characterized by motor incoordination with echolalia and coprolalia. *Hist Psychiatry.* 1998;9:97; Kushner HI. *A Cursing Brain? The Histories of Tourette Syndrome.* Cambridge, MA: Harvard University Press; 1999	Described a syndrome of involuntary movements and echolalia and coprolalia in nine patients, seven of whom were at the Paris Hôpital de la Salpêtrière, where he was a resident neurologist in training; Jean-Martin Charcot, director of the Salpêtrière and France's leading neurologist, then sanctioned the use of de la Tourette's name for the syndrome
Cesare Lombroso (1835–1909)	Italy	*Genius and Insanity* (1864), *The Delinquent Man* (1876), *The Female Offender* (1893)	Emphasized the study of the individual personality, which gave rise to pathographies—psychopathologically oriented biographies; his books on delinquent men and women stimulated a school of criminal anthropology that engendered the science of criminology
Emil Kraepelin (1856–1926)	Germany	Kraepelin E. *Psychiatrie: Ein Lehrbuch für Studerende und Aerzte.* 6th ed. (1899); *Memoirs.* Berlin: Springer-Verlag; 1987	Divided the major psychoses into two groups: Dementia praecox, which deteriorated to dementia, and manic-depressive psychosis, which did not deteriorate
John Hughlings Jackson (1834–1911)	England	*Selected Writings of John Hughlings Jackson* (London, 1931–1932)	From 1870 to 1900, developed the thesis that psychiatric symptoms are a regression from higher functions that are the products of evolution; the symptoms resulted from activating more primitive functions
Sigmund Freud (1856–1939)	Austria	*The Interpretation of Dreams* (1900), *Three Essays on the Theory of Sexuality* (1905), *Introductory Lectures on Psychoanalysis* (1915–1917)	Discovered the manifestations of the unconscious and how to use them in treating psychiatric patients; described infantile sexuality and how it accounted for adult sexual dysfunctions; founded psychoanalysis
Morton Prince (1854–1929)	United States	*The Dissociation of a Personality* (1905)	Early account of a multiple personality; emphasized techniques of hypnosis and manifestations of the unconscious
Clifford Beers (1876–1943)	United States	*A Mind That Found Itself* (1908)	Account of experiences in psychiatric hospitals that stimulated the mental hygiene movement in the United States
Eugen Bleuler (1857–1939)	Switzerland	*Dementia Praecox or the Group of Schizophrenias* (1911)	Coined the term *schizophrenia* and described its symptoms

Table 35-1
A History of Psychiatry Table (*Continued*)

Persons and Events in Psychiatry

Person or Event	Country	Publications	Significance
Alfred Binet (1857–1911)	France	*A Method of Measuring the Development of the Intelligence of Young Children,* with T. Simon (1911); English translation, 1913	Developed the first practicable intelligence test for children; it has become the prototype for subsequent tests of intellectual ability in children and adults
Hideyo Noguchi (1876–1928)	United States	Noguchi H, Moore JW. A demonstration of the *Treponema pallidum* in the brain in cases of general paralysis. *J Exp Med.* 1913:17	The definitive demonstration, after a century of controversy, that the syphilitic organism causes general paresis; the first time that the cause of a major psychosis became known
Alfred Adler (1870–1937)	Austria	*Study of Organ Inferiority and Its Psychical Compensations* (1917); Stepansky PE. In: *Freud's Shadow: Adler in Context.* Hillsdale, NJ: Analytic Press; 1983	First psychoanalytic defector from Freud; founded the school of individual psychology and coined the terms *life style* and *inferiority complex*
Hermann Rorschach (1884–1922)	Switzerland	*Psychodiagnostik* (1921)	Inkblot test revealed unconscious motivations and ego defenses against them and was used for psychiatric diagnosis; it stimulated the development of other projective diagnostic tests
Julius von Wagner-Jauregg (1857–1940)	Austria	de Rudoli G. *Therapeutic Malaria* (1927); Wagner-Jauregg J. The history of the malaria treatment of general paresis. *Am J Psychiatry.* 1994;151(Suppl):231; Brown EM. Why Wagner-Jauregg won the Nobel Prize for discovering malaria therapy for general paresis of the insane. *Hist Psychiatry.* 2000;11:371	During the decade 1917–1927, showed that general paresis patients underwent remissions when malaria was induced; for the time, it was the most successful organic treatment of a psychosis; for that, he became, in 1927, the first psychiatrist to receive the Nobel Prize; in the 1940s, penicillin became the treatment of choice for paresis
Otto Rank (1884–1939)	Austria, France, United States	*The Myth of the Birth of the Hero* (1909), *The Trauma of Birth* (1924), *Will Therapy* (1936); Lieberman EJ. *Acts of Will: The Life and Work of Otto Rank.* New York: Free Press, Macmillan; 1985	Made important contributions to Freudian psychoanalysis by showing how a person's wishes and fantasies influenced the formation of human myths; breaking with Freud, Rank formed his theory of how the experience of birth influenced a person's mental development and then his technique of will therapy
American Board of Psychiatry and Neurology (ABPN)	United States	Freeman W, Ebaugh F, Boyd D Jr. The founding of the American Board of Psychiatry and Neurology, Inc. *Am J Psychiatry.* 1959;115:769	In 1934, a group of prominent American psychiatrists and neurologists founded the ABPN, comprising equal numbers of psychiatrists and neurologists, with separate qualifications and examinations for psychiatrists and neurologists; the qualifications for psychiatrists included 3 yr of study of psychiatry after an internship, and 2 yr of hospital practice in psychiatry; the original purpose of the ABPN was, in the words of Walter Freeman, "to create standards of ethical practice and professional competence based on adequate fundamental education in the field"; since its founding, it has maintained these standards while keeping abreast of advances in information and technology
Henry A. Murray (1893–1988)	United States	*Thematic Apperception Test.* Cambridge, MA: Harvard University Press; 1943	The Thematic Apperception Test, originated in 1935, is a method used for uncovering conscious and unconscious dominant themes in a person's mental life
Charles Bradley (1902–1979)	United States	Bradley C. The behavior of children receiving Benzedrine. *Am J Psychiatry.* 1937:577; Gross MD. Origin of stimulant use for treatment of attention deficit disorder. *Am J Psychiatry.* 1995;152:298	The first physician to record the successful treatment of what came to be called attention-deficit disorder in children with stimulant medications

(continued)

Table 35-1
A History of Psychiatry Table (*Continued*)

Persons and Events in Psychiatry

Person or Event	Country	Publications	Significance
Cure of pellagra	United States	Roe D. *A Plague of Corn: The Social History of Pellagra*. Ithaca, NY: Cornell University Press; 1973	Pellagra is a niacin-deficiency disease manifested by diarrhea, dermatitis, and dementia; in the South, it was caused by removal of niacin in the milling of corn and was a major cause of dementia; in 1912, Joseph Goldberger (1874–1929), of the U.S. Public Health Service, proved that pellagra was caused by absence of a pellagra-preventive factor in the diet; in 1937, that factor was identified as niacin; since then, with niacin-enriched diets, pellagra has largely vanished; pellagra has also occurred in other countries whose staple grain is maize (American corn)
Genetics of schizophrenia	Germany, United States	Rüdin E. *Studien über Verebung und Entstehung geistiger Störungen. I. Zur Vererbung und Neuetstehung der Dementia Praecox.* [*Studies on the Heredity and Genesis of Mental Diseases. I. On the Heredity and New Formation of Dementia Praecox*]. Berlin: Verlag von Julius Springer; 1916; Kallman FJ. *The Genetics of Schizophrenia*. New York: JJ Augustin; 1938; Rainer JD. The contributions of Franz J. Kallmann to the genetics of schizophrenia. In: Cancro R, Dean SR, eds. *Research in the Schizophrenic Disorders: The Stanley R. Dean Award Lectures*. Vol. 2. Jamaica, New York: Spectrum; 1985	Rüdin (1874–1952) and Kallman (1897–1965) showed that schizophrenia was transmitted by recessive genes (although they differed over how these genes exerted their effects); Kallman first worked under Rüdin in the Max Planck Institute of Psychiatry in Munich, then studied the incidence of schizophrenia among the siblings and descendants of 1,087 hospitalized schizophrenic patients in two Berlin hospitals; when he emigrated to the United States in 1936, he brought the German manuscript of his book on these patients; it was translated into English in 1938 and became a pioneering work; Kallman spent the rest of his life working at the New York Psychiatric Institute, where he established the first full-time medical genetics department in a U.S. psychiatric institution
ECT	Italy	Abrams R. The treatment that will not die. *Psychiatr Clin North Am.* 1994;17:525; Berrios G. The scientific origins of electroconvulsive therapy: A conceptual history. *Hist Psychiatry.* 1997;8:105	Two Italian psychiatrists, Ugo Cerletti (1897–1963) and Lucio Bini (1908–1964), first used ECT in Rome in 1938 to produce convulsions that alleviated symptoms in a schizophrenic patient; it was then found to be more effective in mood disorders than in schizophrenia, and although its use has declined because of psychotropic drugs, modified forms of ECT are used today
Karen Horney (1885–1952)	Germany until 1932, then United States	*The Neurotic Personality of Our Time* (1937), *New Ways in Psychoanalysis* (1939), *Neurosis and Human Growth: The Struggle Toward Self-Realization* (1950); Paris B. *Karen Horney: A Psychoanalyst's Search for Self-Understanding*. New Haven, CT: Yale University Press; 1994	Opposed Freud's theory of the castration complex in women and his emphasis on the oedipal complex and sexuality as influencing neurosis; argued that neurosis was influenced by the culture of the society in which one lived
Adolf Meyer (1866–1950)	Switzerland until 1893, then United States	Meyer A. A short sketch of the problems of psychiatry. *Am J Insanity.* 1896–1897;53:538; Lidz T. Adolf Meyer and the development of American psychiatry. *Am J Psychiatry.* 1996;123:320; Adolf Meyer. In: Havens L, ed. *Approaches to the Mind*. Boston, MA: Little, Brown	From 1912 to 1940, the dominant figure in American psychiatry; his concept of psychobiology viewed the patient as a biologic and psychological unity who became ill because of internal pathology and maladaptations to the environment; he treated patients with medical and nonmedical therapies in community clinics; his work has become part of present-day American psychiatry

Table 35-1
A History of Psychiatry Table (*Continued*)

Persons and Events in Psychiatry

Person or Event	Country	Publications	Significance
Constitution, personality, and mental illness	Germany, United States	Kretschmer E. *Body Build and Character* (1922); Sheldon WH. *Varieties of Human Physique* (1940)	Kretschmer (1888–1964) and Sheldon (1899–1977) postulated that thin, aesthenic individuals were prone to introversion, schizoid tendencies, and schizophrenia, whereas individuals who were short and round were predisposed to be extroverts and had cyclothymic personalities and manic depression; there are many exceptions to these postulates
Führer decree (1939)	Germany	Lifton RJ. The Nazi doctors. In: *"Euthanasia": Direct Medical Killing.* New York: Basic Books; 1986: Chapter 2; Gallagher HG. *By Trust Betrayed: Patients, Physicians, and the License to Kill in the Third Reich.* New York: Henry Holt; 1990; Annas GJ, Grodin MA, eds. *The Nazi Doctors and the Nuremburg Code. Human Rights in Human Experimentation.* Oxford: Oxford University Press; 1992	In October 1939, soon after the outbreak of World War II, a Führer decree ordered doctors to kill patients who had incurable medical illnesses (this grew out of the Nazi doctrine of preserving racial purity by eliminating those who were "biologically unfit"); during the course of the war, approximately 270,000 mental patients were killed by physicians and medical personnel; Henry Friedlander postulated in *The Origins of Nazi Genocide: From Euthanasia to the Final Solution* (1995) that these medical killings, which began in 1940, served as a stimulus and practical model for the Nazi genocide of Jews and Gypsies that began in 1941
MMPI	United States	Buchanan R. The development of the Minnesota Multiphasic Personality Inventory. *J Hist Behav Sci.* 1994;29:148	The MMPI, developed by S. R. Hathaway (1903–1984) and J. C. McKinley (1891–1950) at the University of Minnesota during the early 1940s, became the most widely used and researched psychological personality measurement device; a revised version of the MMPI, MMPI-2, was published in 1989; in 1999, a third edition of MMPI-2 was published, containing the results of new research studies along with a new chapter on forensic applications of MMPI-2
Leo Kanner (1894–1981)	Austria, United States	*Child Psychiatry.* Springfield, IL: CC Thomas; 1935; Autistic disturbances of affective contact. *Nerv Child.* 1943;2:217	The first English-language textbook of child psychiatry and a pioneering description of what Kanner later called "early infantile autism"
Melanie Klein (1882–1960), Anna Freud (1895–1982)	Central Europe, then England	Klein M. *The Psychoanalysis of Children* (1932); Kernberg O. Melanie Klein. In: Kaplan HI, Freedman AM, Sadock BJ, eds. *Comprehensive Textbook of Psychiatry.* 3rd ed. Baltimore, MD: Williams & Wilkins; 1980; Grosskurth P. *Melanie Klein: Her World and Her Work.* New York: Knopf; 1986; Freud A. *The Ego and the Mechanisms of Defence* (1936), *The Psychoanalytic Treatment of Children* (1946), A short history of child analysis. *Psychoanal Study Child.* 1966;21:7; Young-Bruehl E. *Anna Freud: A Biography.* New York: Summit Books; 1988	Klein and A. Freud were pioneers in originating different concepts of child psychoanalysis; Klein's concepts of the "paranoid-schizoid and depressive positions" of very young children has influenced child psychiatry and the treatment of adult borderline and psychotic patients; A. Freud formulated a group of basic concepts of child psychoanalysis and extended the ego psychology work of her father, Sigmund Freud, by delineating the ego defenses, including "identification with the aggressor"
Helene Deutsch (1884–1982)	Europe until 1935, then United States	*The Psychology of Women*, 2 vols. (1945); some forms of emotional disturbance and their relationship to schizophrenia ('As If'). In: Deutsch H, ed. *Neuroses and Character Types.* New York: International Universities Press; 1965: Chapter 20; Roazen P. *Helene Deutsch: A Psychoanalyst's Life.* Garden City, NJ: Anchor Press/Doubleday; 1985	For several decades the most comprehensive Freudian view of the life cycle of women; her most famous clinical concept was the "as if" personality: An apparently normal person who gives a good semblance of adaptation to reality, yet is actually devoid of genuine emotion

(continued)

Table 35-1
A History of Psychiatry Table (*Continued*)

Persons and Events in Psychiatry

Person or Event	Country	Publications	Significance
Ivan Petrovich Pavlov (1849–1936), Andrew Salter (1914–1996)	Russia, United States	Pavlov IP. *Lectures on Conditioned Reflexes.* 2 vols. New York: International Publishers; 1941; Babkin, BP. *Pavlov: A Biography.* Chicago: University of Chicago Press; 1949; Salter A. *Conditioned Reflex Therapy.* New York: Farrar, Straus; 1949	From 1903 to 1936, Pavlov showed how conditioned reflexes influence normal and pathologic thought; Salter then applied conditioned reflex therapy to psychiatric patients by postulating that neuroses result from an excess of cortical inhibition and by emphasizing assertion training; his therapy became one trend in the development of behavioral therapy
NMHA (1946), NIMH (1949)	United States	Grob GN. *From Asylum to Community: Mental Health Policy in Modern America.* Princeton, NJ: Princeton University Press; 1991: Chapters 2–4. Romano J. Reminiscences: 1938 and since. *Am J Psychiatry.* 1990;147:785	Congressional passage in 1946 of the NMHA provided American psychiatry for the first time with generous funds for psychiatric education and research, and led to the creation of the NIMH in 1949, with goals of research in schizophrenia and training of mental health personnel
Erik H. Erikson (1902–1994)	Europe; United States since 1930s	*Childhood and Society* (1950), *Identity and the Life Cycle* (1959); Friedman LJ. *Identity's Architect: A Biography of Erik H. Erikson.* New York: Scribner; 1999; Wallerstein R, Goldberger L, eds. *Ideas and Identities: The Life and Work of Erik Erikson.* Madison, CT: International Universities Press; 1999	Restated Freud's concepts of infantile sexuality, developed concepts of adult identity and identity crisis, and applied psychoanalytic concepts to U.S. cultural life and political history; his *Young Man Luther: A Study in Psychoanalysis and History* (1958) influenced the writing of psychohistory
Carl Rogers (1902–1987)	United States	*Client-Centered Theory* (1951)	Showed that in many patients there existed constructive mental forces that had been previously unrecognized and unemployed and that a therapist, through the use of insight and catharsis, could aid a patient to use these forces to make beneficial changes in his or her life; the approach marked the beginning of a shift of psychotherapy from physicians and psychoanalysts to clinical psychologists and psychiatric social workers
Donald Winnicott (1896–1971)	England	Winnicott D. Transitional objects and transitional phenomena [1951]. In: *Collected Papers: Through Paediatrics to Psychoanalysis.* London: Tavistock, 1958; Kohon H. *The British School of Psychoanalysis: The Independent Tradition.* New Haven, CT: Yale University Press; 1986; Rodman FR. *Winnicott: Life and Work.* New York: Perseus; 2003	Observed the transitional objects to which a young child becomes attached, which provide a bridge between the child's inner and outer worlds and then influence the development of play, creativity, and cultural life in general; a member of the "independent tradition" in British psychoanalysis (i.e., independent from the views of Klein and Anna Freud), which, instead of emphasizing instincts, stressed object relations
Jean Delay (1907–1987), Pierre Deniker (1917–1999)	France	Delay J, Deniker P. Le traitement des psychoses par une méthode neurolytique dérivée de l'hibernothérapie. *C R Congrés Med Alién Neurol France.* 1952;50:497; Thuillier J. *Ten Years That Changed the Face of Mental Illness.* London: Martin Dunitz; 1999; Healy D. *The Creation of Psychopharmacology.* Cambridge, MA: Harvard University Press; 2002	In their first reports on chlorpromazine to French psychiatrists, Delay and Deniker emphasized that patients were quieted like animals in hibernation and called the drug "hibernotherapie"; chlorpromazine and related compounds then came into wide general use for treating patients with psychosis and helped to reduce the number of asylum patients

Table 35-1
A History of Psychiatry Table (*Continued*)

Persons and Events in Psychiatry

Person or Event	Country	Publications	Significance
Harry Stack Sullivan (1892–1949)	United States	Sullivan HS. *The Interpersonal Theory of Psychiatry*. Perry HS, Gawel ML, eds. New York: WW Norton; 1953; Perry HS. *Psychiatrist of America: The Life of Harry Stack Sullivan*. Cambridge, MA: The Belknap Press of Harvard University Press; 1982	The interpersonal theory holds that a person's impulses and strivings cannot be studied in and for themselves, but only as they appear in an interpersonal situation; Sullivan also coined the terms *participant observer* (therapists must be aware of the overt and covert behavior of the patient and their own reactions); *consensual validation* (the awareness of patient and therapist of the terminology they use); and *parataxic distortion* (the patient's distortion of the real person of the therapist necessitated by the patient's personality structure)
Egas Moniz (1874–1955), Walter Freeman (1895–1972)	United States, Europe	Valenstein ES. *Great and Desperate Cures: The Rise and Decline of Psychosurgery and Other Radical Treatments for Mental Illness*. New York: Basic Books; 1986; Pressman JD. *Last Resort: Psychosurgery and the Limits of Medicine*. Cambridge: Cambridge University Press; 1998	During the late 1940s and early 1950s, under the influence of Moniz and Freeman, many patients with severe psychoses and OCD were treated by lobotomy—destruction of the white matter of the frontal lobes of the brain; no adequately controlled studies were ever performed; some patients improved, but others experienced irreversible personality deterioration; with the advent of the psychotropic drugs, the use of lobotomies markedly declined
Advent of the double-blind test	United States	Gold H, Kwit NT, Otto H. The xanthines (theobromine and aminophylline) in the treatment of cardiac pain. *JAMA*. 1937;108:2173; Hampson JL, Rosenthal D, Frank J. A comparative study of the effect of mephenesin and placebo on the symptomatology of a mixed group of psychiatric outpatients. *Bull Johns Hopkins Hosp*. 1954;95:170	In the double-blind test, a drug or a procedure and a placebo are compared in such a way that neither the patient nor the therapists involved in treatment know which preparation is being administered; this type of test was first used in medicine in 1937 to evaluate the efficacy of the xanthines in relieving cardiac pain; it was used in psychiatry in 1954 to evaluate the efficacy of mephenesin, and then lithium, in relieving different psychiatric illnesses; since 1954, the main psychiatric use of double-blind tests has been to evaluate the efficacy of psychotropic drugs and psychiatric procedures
Carl Gustav Jung (1875–1961)	Switzerland	*Psychological Types* (1921), *Two Essays on Analytical Psychology* (1912–1928), *The Structure and Dynamics of the Psyche* (1916–1952), *The Archetypes and the Collective Unconscious* (1934–1955); Kirsch T. *The Jungians: A Comparative and Historical Perspective*. London: Routledge; 2000	After separating from Freud, Jung founded the school of analytical psychology, developing new psychotherapeutic approaches and concepts of the unconscious (especially the collective unconscious) and new personality types, such as introvert and extrovert
Antidepressant drugs	Switzerland, United States	Kuhn R. The treatment of depressive states with an iminodibenzyl derivative (G 22355). Swiss Med J. 1957;87:1135; Loomer HP, Saunders JC, Kline NS. A clinical and pharmacodynamic evaluation of iproniazid as a psychic energizer. Psychiatr Res Rep. 1957;8:129; Healy D. *The Antidepressant Era*. Cambridge, MA: Harvard University Press; 1997; Kuhn R. *Hist Psychiatry*. 2007;17:253	The first reports of the effectiveness of a tricyclic drug, imipramine (G 22355), and an MAOI, iproniazid (Marsilid), in the treatment of depression
B. F. Skinner (1904–1990), Joseph Wolpe (1915–1997)	United States, South Africa	Skinner BF. *Science and Human Behavior*. New York: Free Press; 1953; Wolpe J. *Psychotherapy by Reciprocal Inhibition*. Stanford, CA: Stanford University Press; 1958	Skinner's operant conditioning and Wolpe's reciprocal inhibition were important trends in the development of behavioral therapy

(*continued*)

Table 35-1
A History of Psychiatry Table (*Continued*)

Persons and Events in Psychiatry

Person or Event	Country	Publications	Significance
Development of child psychiatry	United States	Lewis M, ed. *Child and Adolescent Psychiatry: A Comprehensive Textbook.* 2nd ed. Baltimore, MD: Williams & Wilkins; 1996: Chapters 120 (Rafferty F. Effects of health delivery systems on child and adolescent mental health care); 123 (Schowalter J. Recruitment, training, and certification in child and adolescent psychiatry in the United States); 127 (Bernstein D. The discovery of the child: A historical perspective on child and adolescent psychiatry)	After 1945, child psychiatry developed as a psychiatric specialty that separated from adult psychiatry with the formation of the American Academy of Child Psychiatry (1953) and the American Board of Child Psychiatry (1959)
Karl Jaspers (1883–1969)	Germany	*General Psychopathology* (1st ed., 1913; 7th ed., 1959) (English trans., 1963)	Delineated different mental states to show the meaningful connections between different thoughts (without looking for an underlying cause), and to have empathy for both the felt mental state of the patient and the observing mental state of the physician; this view influenced psychotherapy in general and became part of the tenets of existential psychotherapy
Kurt Schneider (1887–1967)	Germany	Schneider K. *Psychopathic Personalities.* London: Cassell; 1958; Schneider K. *Clinical Psychopathology.* New York: Grune Stratton; 1959	In clinical psychiatry, Schneider carried forward—with modifications—the descriptive and phenomenologic approaches of Kraepelin and Jaspers; his work included clinical and phenomenologic descriptions of the experience of delusions and hallucinations and a classification and definition of the primary and secondary symptoms of schizophrenia; *Psychopathic Personalities* described a number of abnormal personality types that he encountered in practice and differentiated from psychotic states
Michel Foucault (1926–1984)	France	*Histoire de la folie* (1961); English trans., *Madness and Civilization: A History of Insanity in the Age of Reason.* New York: Pantheon; 1965	Gave an unconventional history of attitudes toward insanity in Europe from 1500 to 1800; believing that sanity and insanity are largely conditioned by history and the model on which a given society operated, he postulated that creation of the asylum and moral therapy at the end of the 18th century was not progress but an attempt to force insane people to conform to existing social values, and that the authority of the psychiatrist who headed the hospital did not derive from his knowledge of the science of human behavior, but from his association with the power of society; although important historians showed that many of his facts and interpretations contained serious errors, his ideas continue to be debated; *Histoire de la folie* is, in the words of Porter, "easily...the single most influential text of psychiatric historiography in the second half of the century"
Benzodiazepine drugs	United States	Cohen IM. The benzodiazepines. In: Ayd FJ Jr, Blackwell B, eds. *Discoveries in Biological Psychiatry.* Baltimore, MD: Ayd Medical Communications; 1984:130	The benzodiazepines were developed by the pharmaceutical company of Hoffmann-La Roche; chlordiazepoxide (Librium) was first marketed in 1960 and diazepam (Valium) in 1963; the drugs became widely prescribed as anxiolytic drugs in cases of nonpsychotic anxiety

**Table 35-1
A History of Psychiatry Table (*Continued*)**

Persons and Events in Psychiatry

Person or Event	Country	Publications	Significance
Haloperidol in the treatment of Gilles de la Tourette syndrome	France	Seignot JN. Un cas de maladie des tics de Gilles de la Tourette guéri par le R-1625. *Ann Med Psychol.* 1961;cxix:578; The case of Gilles de la Tourette syndrome: A condition of nervous tics cured by R.1625. *Hist Psychiatry.* 1997;8:434	Reported the cure of one case of Tourette syndrome with haloperidol in 1961, when the drug was an experimental compound (R. 1625); However, the patient treated had previously undergone a lobectomy, which easily could have affected his response; Since then, haloperidol has become probably the most commonly prescribed drug for Tourette syndrome
Joint Commission on Mental Illness and Mental Health (1955–1961)	United States	*Action for Mental Health* (1961); Community Mental Health Centers Act of 1963	*Action for Mental Health* recommended psychiatric deinstitutionalization of the care of persons with mental illness by shifting their care from large mental hospitals into community mental health clinics; deinstitutionalization became a reality with the passage of the Community Mental Health Centers Act of 1963
Rene Spitz (1887–1974)	Europe, then United States	*The First Year of Life: A Psychoanalytic Study of Normal and Deviant Development of Object Relations.* New York: International Universities Press; 1965	Showed that, when separated from their mothers during the first year of life, some infants exhibited overt depression, characterized by *marasmus* (a pining away of a physically healthy child), which could result in death; Spitz also observed that indiscriminate smiling at moving faces and masks began between the ages of 2 and 6 mo, and that smiling at familiar faces occurred only after age 6 mo
Classification of mental disorders	United States	DSM-I prepared by the Committee on Nomenclature and Statistics of the APA, G.N. Raines, chair (Mental Hospital Service, Washington, DC, 1952); DSM-II prepared by the Committee on Nomenclature and Statistics of the APA, E. Gruenberg, chair (APA, Washington, DC, 1968); Grob G. Origins of DSM-I: A study in appearance and reality. *Am J Psychiatry.* 1991;148:421	DSM-I replaced several outdated classifications of mental disorders and for the first time provided a glossary of definitions of psychiatric conditions; it was not universally accepted in the United States and most other countries; although DSM-II diagnosed new disease entities, including disorders of childhood and adolescence, its diagnostic methods and criteria were criticized by several leading psychiatrists
Epidemiological evidence for the genetic transmission of schizophrenia	United States, Denmark	Rosenthal D, Kety SS, eds. *The Transmission of Schizophrenia.* London: Pergamon Press; 1968:235 (Wender PH, Rosenthal D, Kety SS. A psychiatric assessment of the adoptive parents of schizophrenics), 345 (Kety SS, Rosenthal D, Wender PH, Schulsinger F. The types and prevalence of mental illness in the biological and adoptive families of adopted schizophrenics), and 377 (Rosenthal D, Wender PH, Kety SS, Schulsinger F, Welner J. Schizophrenics' offspring reared in adoptive homes); Kety SS, Wender PH, Jacobsen B, Ingraham LJ, Jansson L. Mental illness in the biological and adoptive relatives of schizophrenic adoptees: Replication of the Copenhagen study in the rest of Denmark. *Arch Gen Psychiatry.* 1994;51:442	A study of 5,483 Danish adoptees found that 507 had been admitted to a psychiatric hospital, and 33 were classified as having schizophrenic disorders; an equal number of matched adoptees who had no history of psychiatric disorders were identified for comparison; of the 150 biologic relatives of the schizophrenic adoptees, 8.7% had a diagnosis of schizophrenia, compared with 1.9% of the 156 biologic relatives of the nonschizophrenic adoptees; that significant difference indicated that genetic factors were important in the transmission of schizophrenia; these statistics were then replicated by statistics from the rest of Denmark; this method of study was later used to show that other psychiatric disorders (bipolar disorder, suicide, psychopathy, felonious behavior, alcoholism, and hyperactivity in children) were caused by genetic factors; it stimulated molecular geneticists to search for the molecular genetic basis of those disorders

(continued)

Table 35-1
A History of Psychiatry Table (*Continued*)

Persons and Events in Psychiatry

Person or Event	Country	Publications	Significance
Lithium therapy for psychotic excitement	Australia, Denmark, United States	Cade J. Lithium salts in the treatment of psychotic excitement. *Med J Aust.* 1949;36:349; Schou M, Juel-Nielsen N, Stromgren E, Voldby H. The treatment of manic psychoses by the administration of lithium salts. *J Neurol Neurosurg Psychiatry.* 1954;17:250; Schou M. Forty years of lithium treatment. *Arch Gen Psychiatry.* 1997;54:9; J Schioldann: Mogens Abelin Schou (1918–2005)—Half a century with Lithium. *Hist Psychiatry.* 2007;17:247	After the Australian psychiatrist Cade reported that lithium quieted manic patients, the Danish psychiatrist Schou confirmed that finding in a double-blind study; Schou then developed lithium therapy for manic-depressive illness; because of lithium's toxicity and because many psychiatrists questioned its therapeutic effectiveness, it was not approved until 1970 by the U.S. Food and Drug Administration
William H. Masters (1915–2001), Virginia E. Johnson (1925–)	United States	*Human Sexual Response* (1966), *Human Sexual Dysfunction* (1970)	Both books revolutionized knowledge and attitudes about sex; *Response* showed that the female capacity for orgasm greatly exceeds that of most men, that Freud's theories of clitoral and vaginal orgasm needed revision, and that the capacity for meaningful sexual relationships continues into old age; *Dysfunction* stated that most sexual dysfunctions are amenable to some form of counseling; although that statement needed further verification, it gave hope to patients and sex counselors, and it stimulated the discipline of sex therapy
Margaret Mahler (1897–1985)	Central Europe until 1938, then United States	Mahler M, Pine F, Bergman A. *The Psychological Birth of the Human Infant: Symbiosis and Individuation.* New York: Basic Books; 1975; *The Memoirs of Margaret S. Mahler.* Stepansky PE, ed. New York: Free Press; 1988	Delineated the series of stages marking the infant's gradual intrapsychic separation from the mother and its understanding of itself as a distinct individual along with other equally distinct individuals
John Bowlby (1907–1990)	England	*Attachment* (1969), *Separation: Anxiety and Anger* (1973), *Loss: Sadness and Depression* (1980), *A Secure Base: Clinical Applications of Attachment Theory* (1988); Holmes J. *John Bowlby and Attachment Theory.* London: Routledge; 1993	Bowlby's attachment theory is largely based on the belief that a child's social and emotional development depends on the formation, maintenance, and renewal of attachment and affection as bonds between a child and parent (caregiver); deviant emotional and personality development is attributed to the rejection or disruption of ambivalent attachment bonds; loss, or threat of loss, of the attachment figure is viewed as a principal pathogenic agent; Bowlby furthermore believed that when the attachment behaviors of the child are nurtured by the caregiver, the child can develop a sense of security that then allows safe exploration of the world (environment), a positive sense of self, and good relations with others
Jacques Lacan (1901–1981), "the French Freud"	France	*The Language of the Self: The Function of Language in Psychoanalysis* (1968); Turkle S. *Psychoanalytic Politics: Freud's French Revolution.* New York: Basic Books; 1978; Roudinesco E. *Jacques Lacan & Co.: A History of Psychoanalysis in France, 1925–1985.* Chicago: University of Chicago Press; 1990	Emphasized language and the need to make contact with the prelanguage period in the unconscious and rejected the standard 50-min analysis for sessions that were sometimes 10, 5, or even 3 min; founded a school of psychoanalysis, described as a return to Freud; at the time of his death, there were reportedly 5,000 Lacanian analysts in France; the most influential figure in French psychiatry; his ideas influenced literature, language, linguistics, economics, and mathematics; he was an integral part of the political left

Table 35-1
A History of Psychiatry Table (*Continued*)

Persons and Events in Psychiatry

Person or Event	Country	Publications	Significance
Heinz Kohut (1913–1981)	Austria until 1940, then United States	*The Analysis of the Self* (1971); *The Restoration of the Self* (1977); The two analyses of Mr. Z. *Int J Psychoanal.* 1979;60:3; Baker H, Baker M. Heinz Kohut's self psychology: An overview. *Am J Psychiatry.* 1987;144:1; Strozier CS. *Heinz Kohut: The Making of a Psychoanalyst.* New York: Farrar, Straus and Giroux; 2001	Originated the psychoanalytic school of self-psychology, which delineated a new group of developmental needs and three new views of transferences: Mirroring, idealizing, and alter ego
Jean Piaget (1896–1980)	Switzerland	Greenspan S, Curry J. Piaget's approach to intellectual functioning. In: Kaplan HI, Sadock BJ, eds. *Comprehensive Textbook of Psychiatry.* 6th ed. Baltimore, MD: Williams & Wilkins; 1995	Influenced by his observations of his three children, Piaget found four major stages in the formation of thought from infancy through adolescence, with each a necessary prerequisite for the one that follows: (1) *sensorimotor* (up to 2 yr), child learns about space and permanent objects; (2) *preoperational* (2–7 yr), verbal symbols are learned so words come to represent objects; (3) *concrete operations* (7–11 yr), objects become classified according to similarities; (4) *formal operations* (11 yr through end of adolescence), adult logical thinking is used more and more; although there have been criticisms and revisions of these four stages, they will (in the words of Greenspan and Curry) "serve as a basis for understanding social and emotional development and provide a framework for clinical and educational intervention"
NAMI	United States	*NAMI: We Are Family.* Arlington, VA: NAMI; 1979; a 10-page brochure describing the work of NAMI; since then NAMI has published regular annual reports on its work	NAMI, founded in 1979 as an organization of patients with schizophrenia and their family members, has developed new approaches to working with families—counseling, individual family therapy, multifamily therapy groups, and psychoeducational programs—and is probably the most vigorous citizens' group in America that advocates to legislators and the public for the problems of persons with mental illness
Sociobiologic psychiatry	United States, Holland	Van Praag H. Sociobiological psychiatry. *Compr Psychiatry.* 1981;22:441	An approach to the treatment of mental illnesses developed by the Dutch psychiatrist Herman van Praag; it analyzes the possibilities and limitations of pharmacotherapy and psychotherapy and their compatibility when used together in the treatment of psychiatric patients in various diagnostic categories
Roger Sperry (1913–1994)	United States	Some effects of disconnecting the cerebral hemispheres. *Science.* 1982;217:1223; Sperry RW, Levi-Montalcini R. In: Finger S, ed. *Minds Behind the Brain: A History of the Pioneers and Their Discoveries.* New York: Oxford University Press; 2000	In 1981, Sperry shared the Nobel Prize in Physiology or Medicine for his work demonstrating that the left brain hemisphere contains the primary speech capacity, that the right hemisphere is involved with short-term memory, and that the two function independently when the connection between them is cut; this work (funded by grants from the NIMH) suggested that such states as autism and delusions sometimes may be caused by disturbances in the connections between the hemispheres

(continued)

Table 35-1
A History of Psychiatry Table (*Continued*)

Persons and Events in Psychiatry

Person or Event	Country	Publications	Significance
Brief psychotherapy	United States, England	Malan D. *A Study of Brief Psychotherapy*. New York: Plenum Press; 1976; Mann J, Goldman R. *A Casebook in Time-Limited Psychotherapy*. New York: McGraw-Hill; 1982; Davanloo H. *Short-Term Dynamic Psychotherapy*. New York: Jason Aronson; 1980; Sifneos P. *Short-Term Dynamic Psychotherapy Evaluation and Technique*. New York: Plenum Press; 1979; Crits-Cristoph P. The efficacy of brief dynamic psychotherapy: A meta-analysis. *Am J Psychiatry*. 1992;149:151	Aims at producing insight and personality changes in a patient in a short, cost-limited time frame; it includes limiting time devoted to therapy, focusing on a particular problem, actively involving the therapist, engaging in anxiety-provoking confrontations, past–present link interpretations, and problem solving, recapitulating patient's resistances, emphasizing change and progress, and terminating early
Psychology of women	United States	Miller JB. *Towards a New Psychology of Women*. Boston, MA: Beacon Press; 1976; Gilligan C. *In a Different Voice: Psychological Theory and Women's Development*. Cambridge, MA: Harvard University Press; 1982; Levinson D, in collaboration with Levinson J. *The Seasons of a Woman's Life*. New York: Knopf; 1996	Jean Baker Miller, Carol Gilligan, and Daniel Levinson offer different views on women's psychology and the female life cycle
NARSAD	United States	NARSAD activities are reported in *Research* brochures and *Newsletters*	NARSAD was organized in 1986; in 1987, a funding program with 10 grants of $25,000 each was instituted; in 2003, NARSAD reported that in 15 yr, it had awarded $144.4 million to fund 2,153 grants to 1,711 scientists at 312 universities and medical research institutions for research in schizophrenia and depression; in 2007 NARSAD announced that it had awarded 23 Distinguished Investigator grants and 222 Young Investigator grants; it has become the largest nongovernment, publicly funded organization that distributes funds for brain disorder research
Changes in the diagnosis and classification of homosexuality	United States	Bayer R. *Homosexuality and American Psychiatry: The Politics of Diagnosis*. New York: Basic Books; 1981; DSM-III (1980); DSM-III-R (1987)	In 1973, in the light of new clinical information and under political pressure from the National Gay Task Force, the APA changed its diagnosis of homosexuality from a disease to a condition that can be considered a disease only if it is subjectively disturbing to the person; although some APA members protested the decision, it was upheld in a 1974 APA referendum; in the DSM-III, homosexuality was diagnosed as *ego-dystonic homosexuality;* in DSM-III-R, the reference to homosexuality was eliminated; some of the factors that influence a person to have a homosexual orientation are known (biology, family cultural environment, intrapsychic psychodynamics), but others remain unknown
Classification of mental disorders	United States	DSM-III (1980); DSM-III-R (1987); Wilson M. DSM-III and the transformation of American psychiatry: A history. *Am J Psychiatry*. 1993;150:399	The DSM-III reorganized the entire system of classifying diseases, leading to a more detailed, precise, and clear delineation of symptoms and a more medical and less psychoanalytic view of the symptoms; it was widely read and accepted in the United States and became the common language used by workers in psychiatry; the DSM-III-R was published because data from new studies were inconsistent with some of the previous diagnostic criteria and because of the need to review the criteria (along with systematic descriptions of diseases) for clarity and conceptual accuracy

Table 35-1
A History of Psychiatry Table (*Continued*)

Persons and Events in Psychiatry

Person or Event	Country	Publications	Significance
James Masterson (1926–), Otto Kernberg (1928–)	United States	Masterson J. *Psychotherapy of the Borderline Adult: A Developmental Approach.* New York: Brunner/Mazel; 1976; *Narcissistic and Borderline Disorders: An Integrated Developmental.* New York: Brunner/Mazel; 1981; Masterson J, Klein R, eds. *Psychotherapy of the Disorders of the Self: The Masterson Approach.* New York: Brunner/Mazel; 1988; Kernberg O. *Borderline Conditions and Pathological Narcissism.* New York: Jason Aronson; 1975; Kernberg O. *Severe Personality Disorders: Psychotherapeutic Strategies.* New Haven, CT: Yale University Press; 1984	Masterson and Kernberg developed two different psychoanalytic concepts (both emphasizing object relations) for understanding, diagnosing, and treating narcissistic and borderline personality disorders
Psychology and neurophysiology of dreams	United States	Hobson JA, McCarley RW. The brain as a dream state generator: An activation-synthesis hypothesis of one dream process. *Am J Psychiatry.* 1977;134: 1335; McCarley RW. Dreams: Disguise of forbidden wishes or transparent reflections of a distinct brain state? In: Bilder RM, Lefever FF, eds. *Neuroscience of the Mind: On the Centennial of Freud's Project for a Scientific Psychology.* New York: New York Academy of Sciences; 1998:116; Reiser MF. The dream in contemporary psychiatry. *Am J Psychiatry.* 2001;158:351	The Hobson–McCarley activation–synthesis hypothesis of dream formation, based on neurophysiologic research, postulates that dreams are caused by two reciprocally interacting groups of brainstem neurons; although this hypothesis at first tended to view dreams as products of brain physiology that lacked intrinsic psychological importance (and thus refuted Freud's psychoanalytic theory of dreams), this view has lately changed; Reiser suggested that new research has shown that the psychology of dreams is more complex than has been previously thought and postulated "a preliminary psychobiological concept of the dream process" in which "the mind exploits (for memory and cognitive functions) the special physiologic state of the activated dreaming brain"; Reiser emphasized that this concept is not a "final or complete understanding of the dream process," but that it may serve as a stimulus "for further research to both psychoanalysis and cognitive neuroscience"
Theories on the psychology of love	United States	Bergmann MS. *The Anatomy of Loving.* New York: Columbia University Press; 1987; Sternberg RJ. *The Triangle of Love: Intimacy, Passion, Commitment.* New York: Basic Books; 1987; Sternberg RJ, Barnes ML, eds. *The Psychology of Love.* New Haven, CT: Yale University Press; 1988; Gaylin W, Person E, eds. *Passionate Attachments: Thinking about Love.* New York: Free Press; 1988; Person E. *Dreams of Love and Fateful Encounters: The Power of Romantic Passion.* New York: WW Norton; 1988	These books, which appeared within 1 yr of one another, differed in their accounts of the nature of love; no one dominant theory emerged, yet each book offered new information and ideas on the phenomenology of love
Evaluations of psychotherapy	United States	Bruce R, Staples FR, Cristol AH, Yorkston NJ, Whipple KS. *Psychotherapy versus Behavior Therapy.* Cambridge, MA: Harvard University Press; 1975; Elkin I, Shea MT, Watkins JT, Imber SD, Sotsky SM. National Institute of Mental Health Treatment of Depression Collaborative Research Program: General effectiveness of treatments. *Arch Gen Psychiatry.* 1989;48:971	Two methodologically sophisticated studies that concluded that groups of neurotic patients in psychotherapy showed a significant reduction in their symptoms when compared with control groups

(continued)

Table 35-1
A History of Psychiatry Table (*Continued*)

Persons and Events in Psychiatry

Person or Event	Country	Publications	Significance
Eric Kandel (1929–)	Austria, United States after 1939	Kandel E. Psychotherapy and the single synapse: The impact of psychiatric neurobiological research. *N Engl J Med.* 1979;301:1028; From metapsychology to molecular biology: Explorations into the nature of anxiety. *Am J Psychiatry.* 1983;140:1277; Genes, nerve cells, and the remembrance of things past. *J Neuropsychiatry.* 1989;1:103; Biology and the future of psychoanalysis: A new intellectual framework for psychiatry revisited. *Am J Psychiatry.* 1999;156:505; *In Search of Memory: The Emergence of a New Science of Mind.* New York: WW Norton; 2006	Showed connections between psychiatry and neurobiology and research on the CNS of the snail *Aplysia;* developed an experimental system and set of conceptual approaches for studying the biologic basis of simple forms of learning and memory and demonstrated that "learning produces changes in neuronal architecture, changes that result from learned alterations in gene expression"; suggested that normal learning, learning of neurotic behavioral patterns, and unlearning of such detrimental behaviors through psychotherapeutic intervention might involve long-term functional and structural changes in the brain that result from altered gene expression; in his 1999 article, Kandel suggested ways of creating a discipline of neurobiology, cognitive psychology, and psychoanalysis that "would forge a new and deeper understanding of the mind" In 2000, the Nobel Prize for Physiology or Medicine was awarded to three men: Kandel for work in *Aplysia* (the second psychiatrist to receive the prize, after Wagner von Jauregg); Arvid Carlsson, a neuropsychopharmacologist at the University of Gothenburg in Sweden, known for his development of the dopamine hypothesis; and Paul Greengard, a neuroscientist at Rockefeller University in New York City, who studied how such neurotransmitters as dopamine communicate their signals at the cellular level. (Andreasen NC. Three living heroes of contemporary psychiatry. *Am J Psychiatry.* 2000;157:1911)
Aaron Beck (1921–)	United States	Beck A. *Cognitive Therapy and the Emotional Disorders.* New York: International Universities Press; 1976; Beck A, Rush AJ, Shaw BF, Emery G. *Cognitive Therapy of Depression.* New York: Guilford Press; 1979; Beck A, Emery G, Greenberg R. *Anxiety Disorders and Phobias: A Cognitive Perspective.* New York: Basic Books; 1985; Beck A, Freeman A. *Cognitive Therapy of Personality Disorders.* New York: Guilford Press; 1990; Weishaar M. Aaron T. Beck. *Key Figures in Counselling and Psychotherapy.* London: Sage; 1993; Barsky AJ, Ahern DK. Cognitive behavioral therapy for hypochondriasis. A randomized controlled trial. *JAMA.* 2004;291:1464	As formulated by Beck, cognitive therapy is a system of psychotherapy based on a theory of psychopathology and a set of therapeutic principles and techniques that emphasize the reorganization of a person's maladaptive processes of perceiving, thinking, and forming opinions; the study of Barsky and Ahern showed that cognitive-behavioral therapy in six 90-min intervals "appears to have significant beneficial long-term effects on the symptoms of hypochondriasis." On November 16, 2007 Beck was one of five scientists chosen to receive the Lasker Award for his technique of cognitive therapy; the Award is considered the nation's most prestigious medical awards and carries a prize of $100,000. (*The New York Times,* November 17, 2007, Section N, p. 24)

Table 35-1
A History of Psychiatry Table (*Continued*)

Persons and Events in Psychiatry

Person or Event	Country	Publications	Significance
Karl Menninger (1893–1990), William Menninger (1900–1966)	United States	Faulkner H, Pruitt V, eds. *The Selected Correspondence of Karl A. Menninger.* New Haven, CT: Yale University Press; 1988; Friedman LJ. Menninger: *The Family and the Clinic.* New York: Knopf; 1990	The Menninger Clinic (founded in 1920 in Topeka, Kansas) became recognized for its innovative approaches to mental health, scientific excellence, and emphasis on public service; William Menninger introduced new, effective treatments for American psychiatric casualties in World War II; Karl Menninger applied psychoanalytic concepts to American psychiatry and wrote three popular and influential psychiatric-psychoanalytic books: *The Human Mind* (1930), *Man Against Himself* (1938), and *Love Against Hate* (1942); in June 2003, the Clinic moved from Topeka to Houston, Texas, where it became partners with Baylor College of Medicine and the Methodist Hospital
Frederick K. Goodwin (1936–), Kay Redfield Jamison (1946–)	United States	Goodwin FK, Jamison KR. *Manic-Depressive Illness.* New York: Oxford University Press; 1990; 2nd ed., 2007	Offered a new diagnosis and classification of manic-depressive illness as a cluster of related illnesses, including bipolar disease, cyclothymia, and recurrent depressive disease; also offered the most comprehensive review of all information on the disease and all aspects of treatment, including medical (acute and prophylactic) and the role of psychotherapy
A memoir of depression	United States	Styron W. *Darkness Visible: A Memoir of Madness.* New York: Random House; 1990	A national bestseller, described by the *Washington Post* as "a striking addition to the notable personal accounts of mental illness"; has been used by therapists as "an invaluable document" to help patients understand the symptoms of their depression. (*The New York Times,* November 12, 2006, Section 4, p. 11)
SSRIs	United States	"The Story of Prozac," Washington, DC: Pharmaceutical Manufacturers Association; 1993; Grebb J. Serotonin-specific inhibitors. In: Kaplan HI, Sadock BJ, eds. *Comprehensive Textbook of Psychiatry.* 6th ed. Baltimore, MD: Williams & Wilkins; 1995	SSRIs are antidepressants, generally as effective as previous antidepressants but with fewer adverse effects; the first SSRI, fluoxetine (Prozac), developed by Lilly in the 1970s, has become the most widely prescribed antidepressant in the United States; it was followed by sertraline (Zoloft), developed by Roerig in 1992, and paroxetine (Paxil), developed by SmithKline Beecham in 1993
Jerome Frank (1910–2005), E. Fuller Torrey (1937–)	United States	Frank J. *Persuasion and Healing: A Comparative Study of Psychotherapy.* Baltimore, MD: Johns Hopkins University Press; 1961; 2nd rev. ed., 1973; Frank J, Frank JB. *Persuasion and Healing: A Comparative Study of Psychotherapy.* 3rd rev. ed. Baltimore, MD: Johns Hopkins University Press; 1991; Torrey EF. *The Mind Game: Witchdoctors and Psychiatrists.* New York: Emerson Hall; 1972; Torrey EF: *Witchdoctors and Psychiatrists: The Common Roots of Psychotherapy and Its Future.* New York: Harper & Row; 1986 (a revised edition of *The Mind Game*)	These books offered perspectives on the practices of contemporary American psychotherapy and psychotherapists by delineating how psychic changes are effected in a wide range of therapist–patient interactions, including miracle cures, faith healing, Communist thought control, the so-called placebo effect in medicine, special types of individual and group psychotherapies, and the work of traditional healers in third-world countries and among Mexican and Puerto Rican Americans and Navaho

(continued)

Table 35-1
A History of Psychiatry Table (*Continued*)

Persons and Events in Psychiatry

Person or Event	Country	Publications	Significance
Psychiatric epidemiology	United States	Robins LN, Regier DA, eds. *Psychiatric Disorders in America: The Epidemiologic Catchment Area Study*. New York: Free Press; 1991	This NIMH Epidemiologic Catchment Area study, the largest and most sophisticated study of psychiatric epidemiology ever undertaken in the United States, showed that more than 30% of individuals have at least one psychiatric disorder (and many have more than one); that alcoholism and phobic disorder are the most common illnesses, followed by depression; that the uneducated, unmarried, and divorced are more vulnerable; that, more important than race or economic status as a predictor of most illness, the young are more vulnerable than their elders; the study permitted follow-up and evaluation of changes (both overall and in specific areas) to show how particular services are used or not used; it thus continues to provide data for an ongoing discussion of mental health needs and future psychiatric research projects
Forensic psychiatry	United States	Bursztajn H, Scherr A, Brodsky A. The rebirth of forensic psychiatry in light of recent historical trends in criminal responsibility. *Psychiatr Clin North Am*. 1994;1(3):611; Prentice S. A history of subspecialization in forensic psychiatry. *Bull Am Acad Psychiatry Law*. 1995;23(2):195	Changing concepts of criminal responsibility in mid–20th century America, and interactions between the American Academy of Forensic Sciences and the American Academy of Psychiatry and the Law, resulted in forensic psychiatry's becoming officially recognized as a subspecialty by the American Board of Medical Specialties on September 17, 1992, under the designation of "Added Qualification in Forensic Psychiatry"
Epidemic of AIDS and of persons infected with HIV (1981–)	Worldwide	Grmek M. *History of AIDS: Emergence and Origin of a Modern Pandemic*. Princeton, NJ: Princeton University Press; 1990; Berridge V, Strong P, eds. *AIDS and Contemporary History*. Cambridge: Cambridge University Press; 1993; Feldman D, Miller J, eds. *The AIDS Crisis: A Documentary History*. Westport, CT: Greenwood Press; 1998; Bayer R, Oppenheimer G, eds. *AIDS Doctors: Voices from the Epidemic*. Oxford: Oxford University Press; 2000; Treisman G, Angelino F. *The Psychiatry of AIDS: A Guide to Diagnosis and Treatment*. Baltimore, MD: Johns Hopkins University Press; 2004; Mayer K, Pizer H, eds. *The AIDS Pandemic: Impact on Science and Society*. San Diego, CA: Elsevier Academic Press; 2005	Psychiatrists are called on to manage individuals who are at high risk for HIV infection or who are HIV infected and to treat the psychiatric disorders that result from or are comorbid with HIV infection; these disorders include dementia, delirium, anxiety, and disorders of cognition, adjustment, mood, and sleep; because AIDS is largely caused by sexual contact and IV drug use, psychiatrists and mental health professionals need to teach the techniques of safe sex and safe drug use and work with addicts to withdraw from drug; the global incidence of AIDS is steadily increasing

Table 35-1
A History of Psychiatry Table (*Continued*)

Persons and Events in Psychiatry

Person or Event	Country	Publications	Significance
Classification of mental disorders	United States	American Psychiatric Association. *Diagnostic and Statistical Manual of Mental Disorders*. 4th ed. Text rev. Washington, DC: American Psychiatric Association; 2000 (DSM-IV-TR)	The DSM-IV, probably the most ambitious undertaking in the history of American psychiatric nosography, was based on 6 yr of collecting and analyzing relevant information and making field tests of proposed changes in diagnosis; it continued the atheoretical approach to causes, made fewer diagnostic changes than the DSM-III, systematically described each disorder in terms of its associated features, and replaced the DSM-III-R as the diagnostic text used by workers in psychiatry; the DSM-IV-TR contained updated information about the associated features, prevalence, course, and familial pattern of some of the mental disorders that had been described in the DSM-IV; it also gave more comprehensive diagnostic criteria for personality change due to a general medical condition, paraphilias, and tic disorders than those given in the DSM-IV
Clozapine, risperidone, and olanzapine in the treatment of schizophrenia	United States, Canada, Europe, England, South America, South Africa	Kane J, Honigfield G, Singer J, Meltzer H, and the Clozaril Collaborative Study Group: Clozapine for the treatment-resistant schizophrenic. A double-blind comparison with chlorpromazine. *Arch Gen Psychiatry*. 1988;45:789; Kane J, Marder SR. Clozapine benefits and risks. *Schizophren Bull*. 1994;20:23; Ayd FJ Jr. Risperidone (Risperdal): A unique antipsychotic. Int Drug Ther Newslett. 1994;29:5; Marder SR, Meibach RC. Risperidone in the treatment of schizophrenia. *Am J Psychiatry*. 1994;151:825; Kane J. Risperidone. *Am J Psychiatry*. 1994;151:802; Beasley C, Tollefson G, Tran P, Satterlee W, Sanger T. Olanzapine versus placebo and haloperidol acute phase results of the North American double-blind olanzapine trial. *Neuropsychopharmacology*. 1996;14:111; Tollefson G, Kuntz A. Review of recent clinical studies with olanzapine. *Br J Psychiatry*. 1999;37:30; Volavka J, Czobor P, Sheitman B, Lindenmayer JP, Citrome L. Clozapine, olanzapine, risperidone, and haloperidol in the treatment of patients with chronic schizophrenia and schizoaffective disorder. *Am J Psychiatry*. 2002;159:255; Grilly J. The history of clozapine and its emergence in the U.S. market: A review and analysis. *Hist Psychiatry*. 2007;18:39	Clozapine and risperidone have been used successfully since 1989 and 1994 to treat both positive and negative schizophrenic symptoms that have been resistant to other treatments; these drugs each offer the possibility for real and continued improvement of individuals who are persistently psychotic; olanzapine has been in use since September 1996 and is effective in treating positive and negative schizophrenic symptoms; the 2002 study by Volavka et al. on 157 hospital in-patients who had a diagnosis of chronic schizophrenia or schizoaffective disorder showed that clozapine, risperidone, and olanzapine (but not haloperidol) resulted in statistically significant improvements in the positive and negative symptoms of hospital patients: "The overall pattern of results suggests that clozapine and olanzapine have similar general antipsychotic efficacy and that risperidone may be somewhat less effective. Clozapine was the most effective in treatment for negative symptoms. However, the differences were small."

(*continued*)

Table 35-1
A History of Psychiatry Table (*Continued*)

Persons and Events in Psychiatry

Person or Event	Country	Publications	Significance
Publications in psychohistory and psychobiography	United States, England	Lawton H. *The Psychohistorian's Handbook*. New York: Psychohistory Press; 1988; Elovitz P, ed. Clio's Psyche. Understanding the "Why" of Culture, Current Events, History, and Society (1994) (a quarterly periodical published by the Psychohistory Forum, 627 Dakota Trail, Franklin Lakes, NJ 07417); Sabbadini A, ed. *Psychoanalysis and History*. Vol. 1, No. 1. London: Artesian Books; 1998–1999 (since its first issue, this *History* has appeared at regular intervals of twice a year; since 2005 edited by John Forrester, and since 2007 published by Edinburgh University Press); Szaluta J. *Psychohistory: Theory and Practice*. New York: Peter Lang; 1999; Elovitz P. Psychoanalytic scholarship on American Presidents. *Annu Psychoanal*. 2003;31:135; Schultz WT, ed. *Handbook of Psychohistory*. New York: Oxford University Press; 2005	Lawton defined *psychohistory* "as the interdisciplinary study of why man has acted as he has in history, prominently utilizing psychoanalytic principles" (no uniformly accepted definition exists); examined different psychohistorical writings, concepts, and methods of doing interdisciplinary research (most of which date from the appearance of Erikson's *Young Man Luther* in 1958); and called attention to the two best-established journals in the field, started in the 1970s: the *Psychohistory Review* (stopped publication in 1999) and the *Journal of Psychohistory; Clio's Psyche* has short, concise studies by various authors on greatly varied subjects (including the personalities of famous individuals, presidential character, nationalism, ethnic conflicts and the Holocaust, AIDS, movies, psychological issues, psychoeconomics, and the environment); many studies aim to combine primary research with psychological insights; notable interviews with distinguished psychohistorians (in his interview with *Clio,* psychohistorian Peter Loewenberg commented, "I'd like to get away from the idea of applying psychoanalysis to history because I think the integration of psychodynamic perceptions with historical conceptualization should take place at the moment that the historian contacts the data or the archives. Both history and psychoanalysis are fundamentally historical enterprises— they're models of explanation.") *Psychoanalysis and History* has two stated aims: (1) "historiographic studies of the psychoanalytic movement itself, as well as biographical research on aspects of the lives and works of prominent psychoanalysts. Only one century old, psychoanalysis has an already rich and articulated history, having undergone complex external and internal vicissitudes and having developed its identity in most diverse ways in different geographical regions. We intend...to present as yet unpublished documents...which will throw new light on a number of important aspects of our discipline" and (2) "We shall also attempt to apply psychoanalytic ideas—for instance the concept of unconscious processes, of developmental stages, or of relevant defence mechanisms such as repression, splitting, projective identification and 'deferred action' (Nachtraglichkeit)—to the interpretation of historical events"

Table 35-1
A History of Psychiatry Table (*Continued*)

Persons and Events in Psychiatry

Person or Event	Country	Publications	Significance
			Szaluta's book was the first text to present both the theory and practice of psychohistory; the contributions of Freud and post-Freudians were delineated, the pros and cons of psychohistory examined, and major works of psychohistory discussed; Szaluta emphasized how psychohistory differs from traditional history and how it can be insightful in the study of the individual, the family, and the group
			Elovitz discussed how, in almost three decades of research on presidential psychobiography, he was influenced by psychoanalysis to develop a method of "disciplined subjectivity" in which he applied the "nonjudgmental manner of the clinician…to the politician"; he studied his subject's childhood, personality, family background, life crises, defense mechanisms, and patterns of success and failure; throughout the entire process, he carefully monitored countertransference feelings; as a result of following this method, he claimed to understand both the pressures of office and the personalities of presidents and to have insights into "understanding the contradictory desires, the ambivalence, of both the leader and the led"
			A *Handbook of Psychohistory* offers articles on psychohistory and psychobiography that show a variety of different psychological approaches
Paul Wender (1934–)	United States	*Attention-Deficit Hyperactivity Disorder in Adults.* New York: Oxford University Press; 1998	As a result of his 25 yr of studying ADHD in adults, Wender gave new evidence suggesting that ADHD is genetically transmitted and that approximately one-third of children with ADHD reach adulthood with persisting symptoms of the disorder; he also reviewed what was known about ADHD's symptoms, its life course, and the value of treatments with various drugs
Computers and the Internet	United States	The APA has published two books on the use of computers in psychiatry: Lieff J. *Computer Applications in Psychiatry.* Washington, DC: American Psychiatric Publishing; 1987; and Chan CH, Luo JS, Kennedy RS. *Concise Guide to Computers in Clinical Psychiatry.* Washington, DC: American Psychiatric Publishing; 2002; Miller MJ. Computer-based testing of the psychiatric patient. In: Sadock BJ, Sadock VA. *Comprehensive Textbook of Psychiatry.* 7th ed. Philadelphia, PA: Lippincott Williams & Wilkins; 2000	Computers have been applied to practically every area of psychiatry, including recording patient symptoms, facilitating the transfer of records, tracking patients in the community, and establishing databases; they have been used by insurance companies and managed care companies for accounting and monitoring patient care, and, since the 1970s, they have been used with increasing frequency in giving patients psychological tests
		Two articles about the Internet are Alessi NE. The Internet and the future of psychiatry. *Am J Psychiatry.* 1996;153:861 and Rajendran PR. The Internet: Ushering in a new era of medicine. *JAMA.* 2001;285:804	The Internet is a computer communications network that transmits information quickly and easily on a global scale, facilitating contacts between different psychiatrists, and between psychiatrists and patients, and enabling patients to obtain rapid information on the professional qualifications of the psychiatrist who is treating them and the psychiatric medications the psychiatrist has prescribed for them

(*continued*)

Table 35-1
A History of Psychiatry Table (*Continued*)

Persons and Events in Psychiatry

Person or Event	Country	Publications	Significance
			Although the Internet offers unprecedented access to information, including information on psychiatric illnesses, it also can be subject to disinformation, either inadvertent, misleading (e.g., advertising), or malicious (antipsychiatry groups)
Discoveries of genetic variations as causes of mental illnesses	United States, Canada, England, Europe, Australia	Oberlé I, Rousseau F, Heitz D, Kretz G, Davys D. Instability of a 550–base pair DNA segment in fragile X syndrome. *Science*. 1991;252:1097; Yu S, Pritchard M, Kremer E, Lynch M, Nancarrow J. Fragile X genotype characterized by an unstable region of DNA. *Science*. 1991;252:1179; Ying-Hui Fu, Kuhl DPA, Pizzuti A, Pieretti M, Sutcliffe JS. Variation of the CGG repeat at the fragile X site results in genetic instability: Resolution of the Sherman paradox. *Cell*. 1991;67:1047; Schellenberg GD, Bird TD, Wijsman EM, Orr T, Anderson L. Genetic linkage of evidence for a familial Alzheimer's disease locus on chromosome 14. *Science*. 1992;258:668; Mullen M, Houlden H, Windelspecht M, Fidani L, Lombardi C. A locus for familial early-onset of Alzheimer's disease on the long arm of chromosome 14, proximal to the α-1-antichymotrypsin gene. *Nat Genet*. 1992;2:340; The Huntington's Disease Collaborative Research Group: A novel gene containing a trinucleotide repeat that is expanded and unstable on Huntington's disease chromosome. *Cell*. 1993;72:971; Amir RE, Van den Veyver IB, Wan M, Tran CQ, Franke U. Rett syndrome is caused by mutations in X-linked MECP2, encoding methyl-CpG-binding protein 2. *Nat Genet*. 1999;23:185	During 1991–1993, genetic variations were identified as causes for the fragile X syndrome, a common cause of inherited mental retardation; familial early onset of Alzheimer disease; and Huntington disease; in 1999, it was discovered that the MECP2 gene causes Rett syndrome, a pervasive developmental disorder included in the DSM-IV classification
		Hyman S, Moldin S. Genetic science and depression: Implications for research and treatment. In: Weissman MM, ed. *Treatment of Depression: Bridging the 21st Century*. Washington, DC: American Psychiatric Association; 2001:98; Andreasen NC. Schizophrenia. Chapter 8. In: *Brave New Brain: Conquering Mental Illness in the Era of the Genome*. New York, Oxford: Oxford University Press; 2001:199	The 2001 article by Hyman and Moldin stated that, although previous studies had shown that heredity plays a role in the transmission of depression, "a single major gene is an unlikely contributor to etiology; rather, multiple genes of small effect contribute with nongenetic factors in producing vulnerability to the illness"; in the same year, Andreasen observed, "Most experts now think that schizophrenia is clearly multifactorial, involving multiple genes, and possibly even different genes in different individuals, as well as many nongenetic or environmental influences. The fact that multiple genes are probably involved is the main reason why the various reports that 'the schizophrenia gene has been found on chromosome 5' (or 11 or 22 or elsewhere) have not been consistently repeated"

Table 35-1
A History of Psychiatry Table (*Continued*)

Persons and Events in Psychiatry

Person or Event	Country	Publications	Significance
Three books on psychotherapy	United States	Jackson SW. *Care of the Psyche: A History of Psychological Healing*. New Haven, CT: Yale University Press; 1999; Sabo AN, Havens L, eds. *The Real World Guide to Psychotherapy Practice*. Cambridge, MA: Harvard University Press; 2000; Hersen M, Sledge WH, eds. *Encyclopedia of Psychotherapy*. 2 Vols. San Diego, CA: Academic Press; 2002	Jackson's *History* is notable for its delineation of the roles of healer and sufferer throughout history; the essays by Sabo, Havens, and others suggest how, through forming relationships with patients, it is possible to do some effective psychotherapy and to counter the constraints of managed care; the *Encyclopedia* gives concise articles, written by experts, on the major psychotherapies that are now in use, along with studies of the efficacy of each of these therapies
Education of psychiatrists	United States	Luhrmann TM. *Of Two Minds: The Growing Disorder in American Psychiatry*. New York: Knopf; 2000	Depicts contemporary American psychiatry as divided between two views of mental illness: A biomedical model, consisting of symptoms treated by psychopharmacology, and a psychodynamic model, consisting of emotional conflicts, treated by psychotherapy; although Luhrmann states that the use of both models together is necessary in treating patients, she observes that "a combination of socio-economic forces [managed care] and ideology is driving psychotherapy out of psychiatry"; she also observes that this would be bad for psychiatrists and patients and encourages "a way of thinking about mental illness that can strip humanity from its sufferers"
Theory and treatment of depression	United States, England, Switzerland	In a March 1999 New York City meeting of the American Psychopathological Association, leading clinical scientists gave papers on the topic Treatment of Depression, all of which were published as in Weissman MM, ed. *Treatment of Depression: Bridging the 21st Century*. Washington, DC: American Psychiatric Association; 2001	The papers ranged widely in discussing different aspects of depression; Charles Nemeroff and Michael Owens, in "Contribution of modern neuroscience to developing new treatments for psychiatric disorders," reviewed the evidence that CRF is hypersecreted in depressed patients, that "untoward early life experience is associated with a persistent CRF gene expression and CRF neuronal activity, which may underlie the vulnerability of individuals exposed to child abuse or neglect to develop depression in adulthood," and that the recent use of a CRF antagonist for the treatment of major depression has been successful; Steven Hyman and Steven Moldin, in "Genetic science and depression: Implications for research and treatment," delineated the growth in knowledge from the Human Genome Project, the interactions of different genomes with their environments and protein products, *proteomics,* and then suggested that "the greatest benefit from genetic research is likely to come in the development of platforms for drug discovery and for understanding the genetic contributions to drug action"

(continued)

Table 35-1
A History of Psychiatry Table (*Continued*)

Persons and Events in Psychiatry

Person or Event	Country	Publications	Significance
			Other papers gave overviews of various treatments; in the United States, there are 20 FDA-approved antidepressants, which in general are "moderately effective," although none of them cures depression, and "a significant number of people either do not respond or respond only partially"; there are two new physical therapies—transcranial magnetic stimulation and vagus nerve stimulation—that remain to be evaluated; there is evidence that cognitive or behavioral therapy each is effective in the treatment of clinical depression; in an epilogue, Weissman observed, "treatment for depression is more targeted, faster, and with fewer side effects and is aimed at the underlying pathophysiology of depression"
Neuroimaging	United States	Andreasen NC. Mapping the mind. In: *Brave New Brain: Conquering Mental Illness in the Era of the Genome.* Oxford: Oxford University Press; 2001:130; Morihisa JM, ed. *Advances in Brain Imaging.* Washington, DC: American Psychiatric Association, 2001	Beginning in the 1970s and 1980s, techniques of CT and MRI showed how the brain was physically diminished in the dementias and other organic illnesses and how, in some cases of schizophrenia, the ventricles were enlarged; after this discovery, what were known as "functional techniques of neuroimaging"—including functional MRI, single-photon emission computed tomography, and PET—were applied to studying changes in brain activity (blood flow) in mental illness; although Andreasen stated that most of these techniques are still research tools, she also observed that in some illnesses "PET permits us to study the relationship between drug dose and clinical response based on a measurement of the levels and activity in the brain"
The effects of traumatic events on individuals	United States, England, France, Germany, and Italy	Micale MS, Lerner P, eds. *Traumatic Pasts, Psychiatry, and Trauma in the Modern Age, 1870–1930.* Cambridge: Cambridge University Press; 2001	A collection of essays by scholars from different disciplines, describing how individuals in several countries suffered medical and psychological disturbances from the effects of railroad accidents, accidents at work, remembering traumatic events in their lives, and the aftermath of shell shock in World War I; in their essay "Trauma, psychiatry, and history," Lerner and Micale commented that there is no "single, uniform, transhistorically valid concept of psychological trauma," and that although it is "impossible to write a single, unilinear history of trauma," it is possible to write case histories of how individuals experienced trauma and to collate these experiences with the ideas about the nature of trauma that were held by scientists and social groups and that were dominant in the cultures in particular moments in the past

Table 35-1
A History of Psychiatry Table (*Continued*)

Persons and Events in Psychiatry

Person or Event	Country	Publications	Significance
Diagnosis and treatment of borderline personality disorder	United States	Gunderson JG. *Borderline Personality Disorder: A Clinical Guide*. Washington, DC: American Psychiatric Association; 2001; American Psychiatric Association. *Practice Guideline for the Treatment of Patients with Borderline Personality Disorder*. Washington, DC: American Psychiatric Association; 2001; Oldham JM. A 44-year-old woman with borderline personality disorder. *JAMA*. 2002;287:1031	Gunderson' *Guide* and the APA's *Practice Guideline* recommend combinations of long-term psychotherapy (often consisting of cognitive therapy or psychodynamic psychotherapy) and medications that are targeted for specific symptoms, and include low-dose antipsychotics and SSRIs; Oldham observed that, after this treatment, "over time, most patients with borderline personality disorder show substantial improvement"
September 11, 2001, terrorist attacks on the World Trade Center and the Pentagon	United States	Kleinfield NR, Connelly M: 9/11 still strains New York psyche. Poll finds widespread unease and lingering fear of terror. *The New York Times*, September 8, 2003, Section A, pp. A1–A2; Sheehy G: Middletown America. *One Town's Passage from Trauma to Hope*. New York: Random House; 2003; Cancelmo JA, Tylim I, Hoffenberg J, eds. *Terrorism and the Psychoanalytic Space: International Perspectives from Ground Zero*. New York: Pace University Press; 2003	The 9/11 terrorist attacks were notable for their amalgam of violence, loss, and death and for the great variability of the mental and physical reactions that followed from these attacks; whereas some individuals have recovered and formed what Gail Sheehy describes as a "new life," others have suffered from persisting episodes of PTSD, anxiety, depression, physical symptoms, and fears that there will be new terror attacks; 5 yr after the attack two-thirds of New Yorkers said they were still "very concerned" about another attack on their city (*The New York Times*, September 7, 2006)
Overviews of psychoanalysis	United States	Erwin E, ed. *The Freud Encyclopedia: Theory, Therapy, and Culture*. New York: Routledge; 2002; Zaretsky E. *Secrets of the Soul: A Social and Cultural History of Psychoanalysis*. New York: Knopf; 2004	The *Encyclopedia* consists of more than 200 entries by Freud scholars, which include biographical sketches of Freud (with an entry on his family) and of individuals who contributed to the development of psychoanalysis; entries on each of Freud's famous case histories; evaluations of Freud's theories of anxiety and defense, drives, the unconscious and repression, neuroses, and narcissism; the influence of psychoanalysis on such humanistic disciplines as anthropology and cultural studies, history and biography, literary criticism, film studies, and philosophy, as well as on biology and neurobiology; and the history and current state of psychoanalysis in various countries in Europe, the Americas, and Africa, as well as in Great Britain, Australia, Japan, Korea, China, India, and the Philippines *Secrets of the Soul* gives kaleidoscopic overviews of how Freud's ideas were influenced by the social, political, and cultural climates in which these ideas originated; Zaretsky argues that "the idea of a *personal* unconscious was new" and "gave expression to possibilities of individuality, authenticity, and freedom that had only recently emerged" and that then played an important role in "the modernism of the 1920s, the English and American welfare states of the 1940s and 1950s, the radical upheavals of the 1960s, and the feminist and gay-liberation movements of the 1970s"; at the same time, in ways that were complex and paradoxical, psychoanalysis became "a fount of antipolitical, antifeminist, and homophobic prejudice" and led to the creation of other psychotherapies and movements that in many cases replaced it; Zaretsky's book is a pioneering attempt to delineate the historical impact of psychoanalysis

(continued)

Table 35-1
A History of Psychiatry Table (*Continued*)

Persons and Events in Psychiatry

Person or Event	Country	Publications	Significance
Psychosomatic Medicine/ Consultation-Liaison Psychiatry	United States	Blumenfield M, Strain J, eds. *Psychosomatic Medicine*. Philadelphia, PA: Lippincott Williams & Wilkins; 2006	In 2003, the American Board of Psychiatry and Neurology granted a psychiatric subspecialty status to psychosomatic medicine, and in 2005, the first board examination in psychosomatic medicine was held, and in 2017 the name was changed to Consultation-Liaison Psychiatry, the book edited by Blumenfield and Strain consists of a collection of articles giving comprehensive accounts of psychosomatic symptoms in medical, psychiatric, and neurologic illnesses and how these symptoms can be treated
Confinement of the mentally ill in asylums	South Africa, Switzerland, France, Canada, Australia, Germany, United States, Japan, Argentina, Mexico, India, Nigeria, Ireland, and England	Porter R, Wright D, eds. *The Confinement of the Insane. International Perspectives, 1800–1965*. Cambridge: Cambridge University Press; 2003	This volume brings together 14 original research papers by different scholars, each of whom examines the social forces that influenced the confinement of the insane in asylums in different countries during different periods of time in the 19th and 20th centuries; summing up the contents of the papers, Porter concluded that the history of the growth of asylums "proves more complex than it might seem," revealing that "the asylum was neither just a site for care and cure, nor just a convenient place for locking up inconvenient people ('custodialism'). It was many things all at once. And far from being a weapon securely under the control of the [psychiatric] profession, or the state, it was a contested site, subject to continual negotiations among different parties, including families and the patients themselves"
Treatment of schizophrenia	United States	American Psychiatric Association. *Practice Guideline for the Treatment of Patients with Schizophrenia*. 2nd ed. Washington, DC: American Psychiatric Association; 2004	Recommendations that are intended to help psychiatrists in assessing and treating adult patients with schizophrenia in their acute phase, treatment stabilization phase, and stable phase; each recommendation receives one of three categories of endorsement: Recommended with substantial confidence, recommended with moderate confidence, and may be recommended on the basis of individual circumstances; although the *Practice Guideline* is based on synthesis of "current scientific knowledge and rational clinical practice," it is emphasized that it is only a guideline, that it should not be construed to serve as a standard of medical care, and that "the ultimate judgment regarding a particular clinical procedure or treatment plan must be made by the psychiatrist in light of the clinical data presented by the patient and the diagnosis and treatment options available"
College Mental Health	United States	Kadison R, Geronimo I. *College of the Overwhelmed: The Campus Mental Health Crisis and What to Do about It*. San Francisco: Jossey-Bass; 2004	Delineates the mental pressures faced by college students as they confront academic requirements, explore sexuality, and form new interpersonal relationships; as a result of these pressures, "since 1988, the likelihood of a college student suffering depression has doubled, suicidal ideation has tripled and sexual assaults have quadrupled"; on the second half of the book, in a chapter entitled "For students only," Kadison and Geronimo offer proactive ways for students to maintain mental balance and how to seek help if things go wrong

Table 35-1
A History of Psychiatry Table (*Continued*)

Persons and Events in Psychiatry

Person or Event	Country	Publications	Significance
A suppressed psychiatric scandal	United States	Scull A. *Madhouse: A Tragic Tale of Megalomania, and Modern Medicine.* New Haven, CT: Yale University Press; 2005	The madhouse Scull writes about was the Trenton State Hospital in New Jersey from 1907 to 1930, when Henry Cotton was its Superintendent; believing that infections of various body parts were a cause of psychiatric illness, Cotton treated psychiatric patients by surgical extirpation of these parts, which were mainly teeth and tonsils, but which also included stomachs, gallbladders, colons, testicles, and ovaries; when Adolf Meyer had the young psychiatrist Dr. Phyllis Greenacre investigate Cotton's treatments, Greenacre reported that these treatments resulted in deaths, disabilities, and questionable improvement of psychiatric symptoms; however, Meyer suppressed her report; Cotton was demoted from Superintendent to Director of Research; a public scandal was thus averted, and knowledge of Cotton's operations remained unknown for many years until Scull, after doing research based on documents and the recollections of several individuals, uncovered what had been unknown and published his book
Use of amphetamines as antidepressant drugs	United States	Rasmussen N. Making the first antidepressant: Amphetamine in American medicine, 1929–1950. *J Hist Med Allied Sci.* 2006;61:288	Shows how during the 1940s and 1950s amphetamine was a very commonly prescribed remedy for depression and related neurotic conditions, used by both general practitioners and psychiatrists; in the 1960s, although amphetamine was used in a variety of conditions, it largely stopped being used in most psychiatric cases, being replaced by the minor tranquilizers and the MAOI and tricyclic antidepressants
Recollections of treating schizophrenia	United Sates	Seeman M. Forty-five years of schizophrenia: Personal reflections. *Hist Psychiatry.* 2006;17:363	Seeman recollected that, in the 45 yr since she has been treating schizophrenia, "although there have been many advances over this period, understanding of schizophrenia continues to be elusive, and treatments remain imperfect. Therefore, as perspectives shift and the ground moves beneath us, the psychiatric profession need to anchor itself firmly in the stories our [schizophrenic] patients tell us." Whether these stories "be of symptoms, of loss or of survival."
Mental health policy	United States	Frank R, Glide S. *Better But Not Well: Mental Health Policy in the United States Since 1950.* Baltimore, MD: Johns Hopkins University Press; 2006	The mentally ill have improved due to the development of better-tolerated medications (selective serotonin reuptake inhibitors compared with tricyclic antidepressants) and the development of policies such as Medicare, Medicaid, Social Security Disability Insurance, and the expansion of private health insurance; however, the majority of the mentally ill are impoverished, and there has been no increase in their rates of employment; in addition, during the last 50 yr their rates of homelessness have more than doubled, and incarcerations have gone up fivefold
George Mora (1923–2006), and his work in the history of psychiatry	Italy and after 1953 the United States	Works on the history of Italian psychiatry, a wide range of medical and psychiatric topics, a translation of Johann Weyer's *De praestigiis daemonum* (1991) , and with Jeanne Brand, *Psychiatry and Its History: Methodological Problems in Research* (1970)	For a generation Mora was the foremost American authority on the history of psychiatry, as well as the author of the sections of the history of psychiatry for the first four editions of the *Comprehensive Textbook of Psychiatry*

(continued)

Table 35-1
A History of Psychiatry Table (*Continued*)

Persons and Events in Psychiatry

Person or Event	Country	Publications	Significance
Mood disorders	United States	In 2006–2007 two textbooks on mood disorders were published: Stein D, Kupfer D, Schatzberg A, eds. *The American Psychiatric Publishing Textbook of Mood Disorders.* Arlington, VA: American Psychiatric Publishing; 2006; Goodwin FK, Jamison KR. *Manic-Depressive Illness: Bipolar Disorders and Recurrent Depression.* 2nd ed. New York: Oxford University Press; 2007 (1st ed., 1990)	Each of these books gave detailed information on the latest knowledge of the causes, symptoms, and treatments of mood disorders
Albert Ellis (1913–2007)	United States	Ellis published 75 books, including *Overcoming Procrastination, How to Live With a Neurotic, Sex Without Guilt,* and *A Guide to Rational Living*	By late 1953, Ellis had begun developing Rational Emotive Behavior Therapy (REBT), a mode of therapy that aimed at helping individuals make psychological changes by teaching them to challenge their self-defeating thoughts; in 1960, he founded the Albert Ellis Institute to promulgate his work; he continued the shift of psychotherapy from psychoanalysts and from physicians to clinical psychologists and psychiatric social workers, which had been begun by Carl Rogers; in 2003, the American Psychological Association named him the second most influential psychologist of the 20th century, second only to Rogers
Mental Health Policy	United States	Mental Health Parity and Addiction Equity Act of 2008. "Fact Sheet": The Mental Health Parity and Addiction Equity Act of 2008 (MHPAEA). Accessed November 19, 2015. Available at http://www.dol.gov/ebsa/newsroom/fsmhpaea.htm	Enacted in 2008 as part of the Affordable Care Act to address loopholes created by the initial Mental Health Parity Act of 1996. The act (1) includes mental health and substance use disorder benefits in the *Essential Health Benefits;* (2) applies federal parity protections to mental health and substance use disorder benefits in the individual and small group markets; and (3) provides more Americans with access to quality health care that includes coverage for mental health and substance use disorder services
Publication of DSM-5	United States	American Psychiatric Association. *Diagnostic and Statistical Manual of Mental Disorders.* 5th ed. Washington, DC: American Psychiatric Association; 2013	In 2013, this revision to the DSM-IV was published, with several important changes: Aspergers and Autism disorders were subsumed under the term *autism spectrum disorders;* criteria were added to ADHD to facilitate application across the lifespan; symptoms must now be present before age 12 (vs. age 7 in DSM-IV); subtype specifiers of schizophrenia were eliminated due to their limited diagnostic stability, low reliability, and poor validity. In bipolar disorder, a "with mixed features" specifier has been added; Addition of disruptive mood dysregulation disorder and premenstrual dysphoric disorder; Bereavement exclusion now omitted from criterion of MDD; OCD and related disorders are a new diagnostic category and include hoarding disorder excoriation (skin-picking) disorder; Adjustments made to criterion for trauma and stress-related disorders; Creation of gender dysphoria as a new diagnostic class. Substance disorders expanded to include gambling disorder.

Table 35-1
A History of Psychiatry Table (*Continued*)

Persons and Events in Psychiatry

Person or Event	Country	Publications	Significance
Mentally ill and gun violence	United States	Metzl JM, MacLeish KT. Mental illness, mass shootings, and the politics of American firearms. *Am J Public Health.* 2015:240–249	There is increasing focus on mental illness and gun violence in the wake of several mass shootings, which reflects decades-long history of more general debates in psychiatry about guns, violence, and mental competence. Social and political rhetoric following these violent events strengthen implications that mental illness caused these events or earlier detection of these problems might have prevented them. Many states reactively enacted legislation requiring mental health clinicians to report "dangerous patients" to local officials as a way to prevent these people from obtaining firearms. Many argue that the focus should be on prevention efforts that will have a boarder impact on communities such as reexamination of gun laws and improving mental health resources.
Changes in marijuana legislation	United States (23 states)	Wilkinson ST, Yarnell S, Radhakrishnan R, Ball SA, and Cyril D'souza D. Marijuana legalization: Impact on pyschicians and public health." *Annu Rev Med.* 2014	Between 1996 and 2015, 23 states passed laws legalizing marijuana use for medical purposes after numerous studies revealed its therapeutic potential for multiple medical conditions including epilepsy, cachexia, and chronic pain. Several states have legalized small amount of marijuana for recreational use reflecting a growing shift in public opinion regarding the safety or marijuana. Marijuana use and sale remains illegal under federal law and it is still listed as schedule I substance. Many states are calling for federal decriminalization of marijuana but the debate rages on given remaining concerns about legalization and public health effects. Despite efforts to reschedule marijuana, it continues to be classified as a schedule I substance.
United States Drug Enforcement Agency	United States	Wing N. (2015, March 18). DEA Approves Study of Psychedelic Drug MDMA In Treatment of Seriously Ill Patients. Retrieved November 17, 2015, from http://www.huffingtonpost.com/2015/03/18/deadmda-study_n_6888972.htm	MDMA was classified as a schedule I substance in 1985. In the years since, recent studies have shown that the drug can be effective for mental disorders. DEA approved study of MDMA in the treatment of anxiety in people with life-threatening illness. This comes after studies showing that MDMA can be helpful for disorders like PTSD in a supervised treatment setting
Physician-assisted suicide	United States	Dyer O, Caroline W, Garcia Rada A. "Assisted dying: law and practice around the world." *BMJ* (2015); Payne K. Consider Assisted Suicide. Tenn Nurse (2015) Fall;78(3):13; Kopelman LM. *Physician-Assisted Suicide: What Are the Issues?* Dordrecht: Kluwer Academic Publishers; 2001	Medical professional codes have long prohibited physicians involvement in assisting a patient's suicide. However, despite ethical and legal prohibitions, calls for the liberalization of this ban have grown in recent years. Oregon's law permitting physician-assisted dying passed in 1997 is the oldest in the world. Mentally competent and physically able adults who have 6 mo or less to live can get prescription for sedative medications they can take to end their lives. As of 2015, several states have enacted similar legislation, but it still remains illegal in the majority of the country

(*continued*)

Table 35-1
A History of Psychiatry Table (*Continued*)

Persons and Events in Psychiatry

Person or Event	Country	Publications	Significance
The Human Connectome Project	United States	Hagmann P, Kurant M, Gigandet X, Thiran P, Wedeen VJ, Meuli R, Thiran JP (2007). Mapping human whole-brain structural networks with diffusion MRI. *PLoS ONE.* 2, e597; Sporns O, Tononi G, Kotter R. (2005). The human connectome: A structural description of the human brain. *PLos Comput Biol.* 1, e42	The Human Connectome Project aims to map all of the connections in the human brain in an effort to understand how cognitive processes emerge from their morphologic substrates. The project was launched in 2009 as part of broader efforts to increase neuroscience research. The human brain is highly complex and researchers face numerous challenges in data collection, mapping neuronal pathways, and correlating functional connectivity with anatomic connectivity. Data generated from the project could offer significant contributions to research in complex neurologic and psychological disorders

ADHD, attention-deficit/hyperactivity disorder; AIDS, acquired immune deficiency syndrome; APA, American Psychiatric Association; CNS, central nervous system; CRF, corticotropin-releasing factor; CT, computed tomography; DSM, *Diagnostic and Statistical Manual of Mental Disorders;* ECT, electroconvulsive therapy; FDA, U.S. Food and Drug Administration; HIV, human immunodeficiency virus; MAOI, monoamine oxidase inhibitor; MMPI, Minnesota Multiphasic Personality Inventory; MRI, magnetic resonance imaging; NAMI, National Alliance for the Mentally Ill; NARSAD, National Alliance for Research on Schizophrenia and Depression; NIMH, National Institute for Mental Health; NMHA, National Mental Health Association; OCD, obsessive-compulsive disorder; PET, positron emission tomography; PTSD, posttraumatic stress disorder; SSRI, selective serotonin reuptake inhibitor; TR, text revision.
This table was conceived and developed by Ralph Colp Jr, M.D., who contributed to many editions of this book and who died in 2008. It was updated by Dr Benjamin Sadock with the assistance of Kristel Carrington, M.D.

References

Ban TA. Pharmacotherapy of mental illness–a historical analysis. *Prog Neuropsychopharmacol Biol Psychiatry.* 2001;25(4):709–727.

Boland RJ, Keller MB. Diagnostic classification of mood disorders: historical context and implications for neurobiology. In: Charney D, ed. *Neurobiological Foundations of Mental Illness.* 2nd ed. New York: Oxford University Press; 2004.

Cade JF. Lithium salts in the treatment of psychotic excitement. *Med J Aust.* 1949; 2(10):349–352.

Cherry CL. *Quakers and Asylum Reform [Internet].* Oxford University Press; 2013 [cited 2020 Sep 16]. Available at ttp://oxfordhandbooks.com/view/10.1093/oxfordhb/9780199608676.001.0001/oxfordhb-9780199608676-e-026

Digby A. The changing profile of a nineteenth-century asylum: the York Retreat. *Psychol Med.* 1984;14(4):739–748.

Dunea G. The anatomy of melancholy. *BMJ.* 2007;335(7615):351.

Edwards M. Mad world: Robert Burton's the anatomy of melancholy. *Brain.* 2010; 133(11):3480–3482.

Eisdorfer C. The impact of genetics on psychiatry. *Curr Psychiatry Rep.* 2000; 2(3):177–178.

Gerard DL. Chiarugi and pinel considered: soul's brain/person's mind. *J Hist Behav Sci.* 1997;33(4):381–403.

Haider B. The war of the soups and the sparks: the discovery of neurotransmitters and the dispute over how nerves communicate. *Yale J Biol Med.* 2007;80(3): 138–139.

Hassler FA. Charaka Samhita. *Science.* 1893;22(545):17–18.

Healy D. *The Antidepressant Era.* Cambridge, MA: Harvard University Press; 2000. 317 p.

Insel TR, Lehner T. A new era in psychiatric genetics? *Biol Psychiatry.* 2007;61(9): 1017–1018.

Johnstone EC, Crow TJ, Frith CD, Husband J, Kreel L. Cerebral ventricular size and cognitive impairment in chronic schizophrenia. *Lancet.* 1976;2(7992):924–926.

Kendler KS, Muñoz RA, Murphy G. The development of the Feighner criteria: a historical perspective. *Am J Psychiatry.* 2010;167(2):134–142.

Koenig HG, Zaben FA, Khalifa DA. Religion, spirituality and mental health in the West and the Middle East. *Asian J Psychiatr.* 2012;5(2):180–182.

Laffey P. Psychiatric therapy in Georgian Britain. *Psychol Med.* 2003;33(7): 1285–1297.

López-Muñoz F, Alamo C, Cuenca E, Shen WW, Clervoy P, Rubio G. History of the discovery and clinical introduction of chlorpromazine. *Ann Clin Psychiatry.* 2005;17(3):113–135.

Marchant J. The Prozac generation [Internet]. *New Scientist.* [cited 2020 Sep 21]. Available at https://www.newscientist.com/article/mg16822601-000-the-prozac-generation/

Mitchell PB, Hadzi-Pavlovic D. John Cade and the discovery of lithium treatment for manic depressive illness. *Med J Aust.* 1999;171(5):262–264.

Raju TN. The nobel chronicles. 1936: Henry Hallett Dale (1875–1968) and Otto Loewi (1873–1961) *Lancet.* 1999;353(9150):416.

Rosenhan DL. On being sane in insane places. *Science.* 1973;179(4070):250–258.

Shoja MM, Tubbs RS. The disorder of love in the Canon of Avicenna (A.D. 980–1037). *Am J Psychiatry.* 2007;164(2):228–229.

Shorter E. *A History of Psychiatry: From the Era of the Asylum to the Age of Prozac.* New York: Wiley; 1997. 436 p.

Shorter E. History of psychiatry. *Curr Opin Psychiatry.* 2008;21(6):593–597.

Shorter E. History of psychiatry. In: Sadock BJ, Sadock VA, Ruiz PR. *Comprehensive Textbok of Psychiatry.* 10th ed. Wolters Kluwer; 2017.

Shorter E. The history of lithium therapy. *Bipolar Disord.* 2009;11(Suppl 2):4–9.

Shorter E. The history of nosology and the rise of the diagnostic and statistical manual of mental disorders. *Dialogues Clin Neurosci.* 2015;17(1):59–67.

Spitzer RL, Cantwell DP. The DSM-III classification of the psychiatric disorders of infancy, childhood, and adolescence. *J Am Acad Child Psychiatry.* 1980;19(3):356–370.

Staff G. The creation of the Prozac myth. *The Guardian.* 2008. Available at http://www.theguardian.com/society/2008/feb/27/mentalhealth.health1

Turner T. Chlorpromazine: unlocking psychosis. *BMJ.* 2007;334(suppl 1):s7.

Unsworth C. Law and lunacy in psychiatry's 'golden age'. *Oxf J Leg Stud.* 1993; 13(4):479–507.

Webster C, ed. *Health, Medicine, and Mortality in the Sixteenth Century.* Cambridge [Eng.]; New York: Cambridge University Press; 1979. 394 p. (Cambridge monographs on the history of medicine.)

Wikipedia. *History of psychiatry [cited 2020 Sep 16].* Available at https://en.wikipedia.org/w/index.php?title=History_of_psychiatry&oldid=977801655

Wójciak P, Rybakowski J. Clinical picture, pathogenesis and psychometric assessment of negative symptoms of schizophrenia. *Psychiatr Pol.* 2018;52(2):185–197.

Yanni C. *The Architecture of Madness: Insane Asylums in the United States.* Minneapolis: University of Minnesota Press; 2007. 191 p. (Architecture, landscape, and American culture.)

Glossary of Terms Relating to Signs and Symptoms

abreaction: A process by which repressed material, particularly a painful experience or conflict, is brought back to consciousness; in this process, the person not only recalls but also relives the repressed material, which is accompanied by the appropriate affective response.

abstract thinking: Thinking characterized by the ability to grasp the essentials of a whole, to break a whole into its parts, and to discern common properties. To think symbolically.

abulia: Reduced impulse to act and to think, associated with indifference about consequences of action. Occurs as a result of neurologic deficit, depression, and schizophrenia.

acalculia: Loss of ability to do calculations; not caused by anxiety or impairment in concentration. Occurs with neurologic deficit and learning disorder.

acataphasia: Disordered speech in which statements are incorrectly formulated. Patients may express themselves with words that sound like the ones intended but are not appropriate to the thoughts, or they may use totally inappropriate expressions.

acathexis: Lack of feeling associated with an ordinarily emotionally charged subject; in psychoanalysis, it denotes the patient's detaching or transferring of emotion from thoughts and ideas. Also called *decathexis.* Occurs in anxiety, dissociative, schizophrenic, and bipolar disorders.

acenesthesia: Loss of sensation of physical existence.

acrophobia: Dread of high places.

acting out: Behavioral response to an unconscious drive or impulse that brings about temporary partial relief of inner tension; relief is attained by reacting to a present situation as if it were the situation that originally gave rise to the drive or impulse. Common in borderline states.

aculalia: Nonsense speech associated with marked impairment of comprehension. Occurs in mania, schizophrenia, and neurologic deficit.

addiction: Psychological or physical dependence on a drug. Sometimes more broadly used to describe dependence on any potentially pleasurable experience (gambling, sexual activity).

adiadochokinesia: Inability to perform rapid alternating movements. Occurs with neurologic deficit and cerebellar lesions.

adynamia: Weakness and fatigability, characteristic of neurasthenia and depression.

aerophagia: Excessive swallowing of air. Seen in anxiety disorder.

affect: The subjective and immediate experience of emotion attached to ideas or mental representations of objects. Affect has outward manifestations that may be classified as restricted, blunted, flattened, broad, labile, appropriate, or inappropriate. *See also* **mood**.

ageusia: Lack or impairment of the sense of taste. Seen in depression and neurologic deficit.

aggression: Forceful, goal-directed action that may be verbal or physical; the motor counterpart of the affect of rage, anger, or hostility. Seen in neurologic deficit, temporal lobe disorder, impulse-control disorders, mania, and schizophrenia.

agitation: Severe anxiety associated with motor restlessness.

agnosia: Inability to understand the import or significance of sensory stimuli; cannot be explained by a defect in sensory pathways or cerebral lesion; the term has also been used to refer to the selective loss or disuse of knowledge of specific objects because of emotional circumstances, as seen in certain schizophrenic, anxious, and depressed patients. Occurs with neurologic deficit. For types of agnosia, see the specific term.

agoraphobia: Morbid fear of open places or leaving the familiar setting of the home. May be present with or without panic attacks.

agrammatism: Speech in which the patient forms words into a sentence without regard for grammatical rules. Seen in Alzheimer and Pick diseases.

agraphia: Loss or impairment of a previously possessed ability to write.

ailurophobia: Dread of cats.

akataphasia: A form of disordered speech in which thoughts cannot be expressed directly but are expressed indirectly such as by making a similar sound (displacement paralogia) or by being derailed into another thought (derailment paralogia). *See also* **derailment**.

akathisia: Subjective feeling of motor restlessness manifested by a compelling need to be in constant movement; may be seen as an extrapyramidal adverse effect of antipsychotic medication. May be mistaken for psychotic agitation.

akinesia: Lack of physical movement, as in the extreme immobility of catatonic schizophrenia; may also occur as an extrapyramidal effect of antipsychotic medication.

akinetic mutism: Absence of voluntary motor movement or speech in a patient who is apparently alert (as evidenced by eye movements). Seen in psychotic depression and catatonic states.

alexia: Loss of a previously possessed reading facility; not explained by defective visual acuity. *Compare with* **dyslexia**.

alexithymia: Inability or difficulty in describing or being aware of one's emotions or moods.

algophobia: Dread of pain.

alogia: Inability to speak because of a mental deficiency or an episode of dementia.

ambivalence: Coexistence of two opposing impulses toward the same thing in the same person at the same time. Seen in schizophrenia, borderline states, and obsessive-compulsive disorders (OCDs).

amimia: Lack of the ability to make gestures or to comprehend those made by others.

amnesia: Partial or total inability to recall past experiences; may be organic (*amnestic disorder*) or emotional (*dissociative amnesia*) in origin.

amnesic aphasia: Disturbed capacity to name objects, even though they are known to the patient. Also called *anomic aphasia,* dysnomia, nominal aphasia, and amnestic aphasia.

anaclitic: Depending on others, especially as the infant on the mother; analytic depression in children results from an absence of mothering.

analgesia: State in which one feels little or no pain. Can occur under hypnosis and in dissociative disorder.

anancasm: Repetitious or stereotyped behavior or thought usually used as a tension-relieving device; used as a synonym for obsession and seen in obsessive-compulsive (anankastic) personality.

androgyny: Combination of culturally determined female and male characteristics in one person.

anergia: Lack of energy.

anhedonia: Loss of interest in and withdrawal from all regular and pleasurable activities. Often associated with depression.

anomia: Inability to recall the names of objects.

anorexia: Loss or decrease in appetite. In *anorexia nervosa,* appetite may be preserved, but the patient refuses to eat.

anosognosia: Inability to recognize a physical deficit in oneself (e.g., patient denies paralyzed limb).

anterograde amnesia: Loss of memory for events subsequent to the onset of the amnesia; common after trauma. *Compare with* **retrograde amnesia**.

anxiety: Feeling of apprehension caused by anticipation of danger, which may be internal or external.

apathy: Dulled emotional tone associated with detachment or indifference; observed in certain types of schizophrenia and depression.

aphasia: Any disturbance in the comprehension or expression of language caused by a brain lesion. For types of aphasia, see the specific term.

aphonia: Loss of voice. Seen in conversion disorder.

apperception: Awareness of the meaning and significance of a particular sensory stimulus as modified by one's own experiences, knowledge, thoughts, and emotions. *See also* **perception**.

appropriate affect: Emotional tone in harmony with the accompanying idea, thought, or speech.

apraxia: Inability to perform a voluntary purposeful motor activity; cannot be explained by paralysis or other motor or sensory impairment. In *constructional apraxia,* a patient cannot draw two- or three-dimensional forms.

asomatopagnosia: Inability to recognize a part of one's body as one's own (also called *ignorance of the body* and *autotopagnosia*).

astasia abasia: Inability to stand or to walk in a normal manner, even though normal leg movements can be performed in a sitting or lying down position. Seen in conversion disorder.

astereognosis: Inability to identify familiar objects by touch. Seen with neurologic deficit. *See also* **neurologic amnesia**.

asthenia: Weakness or debility.

asyndesis: Disorder of language in which the patient combines unconnected ideas and images. Commonly seen in schizophrenia.

ataxia: Lack of coordination, physical or mental. (1) In neurology, refers to loss of muscular coordination. (2) In psychiatry, the term *intrapsychic ataxia* refers to lack of coordination between feelings and thoughts; seen in schizophrenia and in severe OCD.

atonia: Lack of muscle tone. *See* **waxy flexibility**.

attention: Concentration; the aspect of consciousness that relates to the amount of effort exerted in focusing on certain aspects of an experience, activity, or task. Usually impaired in anxiety and depressive disorders.

auditory hallucination: False perception of sound, usually voices, but also other noises, such as music. Most common hallucination in psychiatric disorders.

audible thoughts: A form of auditory hallucination in which everything the patient thinks or speaks is repeated by the voices. Also known as thought echoing.

aura: (1) Warning sensations, such as automatisms, fullness in the stomach, blushing, and changes in respiration, cognitive sensations, and mood states usually experienced before a seizure. (2) A sensory prodrome that precedes a classic migraine headache.

autistic thinking: Thinking in which the thoughts are largely narcissistic and egocentric, with emphasis on subjectivity rather than objectivity, and without regard for reality; used interchangeably with autism and dereism. Seen in schizophrenia and autistic disorder.

automatic obedience: Strict obedience of command without critical judgment. The person may respond to an inner voice, as in schizophrenia, or to another person's command, as in hypnosis.

automatism: Activity carried out without conscious knowledge.

autoscopy: Seeing oneself or a double as part of a brief hallucinatory experience.

behavior: Sum total of the psyche that includes impulses, motivations, wishes, drives, instincts, and cravings, as expressed by a person's actions or motor activity. Also called *conation*.

bereavement: Feeling of grief or desolation, especially at the death or loss of a loved one.

bizarre delusion: False belief that is patently absurd or fantastic (e.g., invaders from space have implanted electrodes in a person's brain). Common in schizophrenia. In nonbizarre delusion, content is usually within the range of possibility.

blackout: Amnesia experienced by alcoholics about behavior during drinking bouts; usually indicates reversible brain damage.

blocking: Abrupt interruption in train of thinking before a thought or idea is finished; after a brief pause, the person indicates no recall of what was being said or was going to be said (also known as *thought deprivation* or *increased thought latency*). Common in schizophrenia and severe anxiety.

blunted affect: Disturbance of affect manifested by a severe reduction in the intensity of externalized feeling tone; one of the fundamental symptoms of schizophrenia, as outlined by Eugen Bleuler.

bradykinesia: Slowness of motor activity, with a decrease in normal spontaneous movement.

bradylalia: Abnormally slow speech. Common in depression.

bradylexia: Inability to read at normal speed.

bruxism: Grinding or gnashing of the teeth, typically occurring during sleep. Seen in anxiety disorder.

carebaria: Sensation of discomfort or pressure in the head.

catalepsy: Condition in which persons maintain the body position into which they are placed; observed in severe cases of catatonic schizophrenia. Compare with *waxy flexibility* and *cerea flexibilitas*. *See also* **command automatism**.

cataplexy: Temporary sudden loss of muscle tone, causing weakness and immobilization; can be precipitated by a variety of emotional states and is often followed by sleep. Commonly seen in narcolepsy.

catastrophic reaction: Extreme emotional state characterized by restlessness, irritability, crying, anxiety, and uncooperativeness. Seen in patients who have had a stroke.

catatonic excitement: Excited, uncontrolled motor activity seen in catatonic schizophrenia. Patients in catatonic state may suddenly erupt into an excited state and may be violent.

catatonic posturing: Voluntary assumption of an inappropriate or bizarre posture, generally maintained for long periods of time. May switch unexpectedly with catatonic excitement.

catatonic rigidity: Fixed and sustained motoric position that is resistant to change.

catatonic stupor: Stupor in which patients ordinarily are well aware of their surroundings.

cathexis: In psychoanalysis, a conscious or unconscious investment of psychic energy in an idea, concept, object, or person. *Compare with* **acathexis**.

cenesthesia: The general awareness of being alive coming from stimuli arising from the functioning of various bodily organs.

cephalagia: Headache.

cerea flexibilitas: Condition of a person who can be molded into a position that is then maintained; when an examiner moves the person's limb, the limb feels as if it were made of wax. Also called *waxy flexibility*. Seen in schizophrenia.

chorea: Movement disorder characterized by random and involuntary quick, jerky, purposeless movements. Seen in Huntington disease.

circumstantiality: Disturbance in the associative thought and speech processes in which a patient digresses into unnecessary details and inappropriate thoughts before communicating the central idea. Observed in schizophrenia, obsessional disturbances, and certain cases of dementia. *See also* **tangentiality**.

clang association: Association or speech directed by the sound of a word rather than by its meaning; words have no logical connection; punning and rhyming may dominate the verbal behavior. Seen most frequently in schizophrenia or mania.

claustrophobia: Abnormal fear of closed or confining spaces.

clonic convulsion: An involuntary, violent muscular contraction or spasm in which the muscles alternately contract and relax. Characteristic phase in grand mal epileptic seizure.

clouding of consciousness: Any disturbance of consciousness in which the person is not fully awake, alert, and oriented. Occurs in delirium, dementia, and cognitive disorder.

cluttering: Disturbance of fluency involving an abnormally rapid rate and erratic rhythm of speech that impedes intelligibility; the affected individual is usually unaware of communicative impairment.

cognition: Mental process of knowing and becoming aware; function is closely associated with judgment.

coma: State of profound unconsciousness from which a person cannot be roused, with minimal or no detectable responsiveness to stimuli; seen in injury or disease of the brain, in systemic conditions such as diabetic ketoacidosis and uremia, and in intoxications with alcohol and other drugs. Coma may also occur in severe catatonic states and in conversion disorder.

coma vigil: Coma in which a patient appears to be asleep and cannot be aroused. A persistent vegetative state.

command automatism: Condition in which suggestions are followed automatically.

command hallucination: False perception of orders that a person may feel obliged to obey or unable to resist.

complex partial seizure: A seizure characterized by alterations in consciousness that may be accompanied by complex hallucinations (sometimes olfactory) or illusions. During the seizure, a state of impaired consciousness resembling a dreamlike state may occur, and the patient may exhibit repetitive, automatic, or semipurposeful behavior.

compulsion: Pathologic need to act on an impulse that, if resisted, produces anxiety; repetitive behavior in response to an obsession or performed according to certain rules, with no true end in itself other than to prevent something from occurring in the future.

conation: That part of a person's mental life concerned with cravings, strivings, motivations, drives, and wishes as expressed through behavior or motor activity.

concrete thinking: Thinking characterized by actual things, events, and immediate experience rather than by abstractions; seen in young children, in those who have lost or never developed the ability to generalize (as in certain cognitive mental disorders), and in schizophrenic persons. *Compare with* **abstract thinking**.

condensation: Mental process in which one symbol stands for a number of components.

confabulation: Unconscious filling of gaps in memory by imagining experiences or events that have no basis in fact, commonly seen in amnestic syndromes; should be differentiated from lying. *See also* **paramnesia**.

confusion: Disturbances of consciousness manifested by a disordered orientation in relation to time, place, or person.

consciousness: State of awareness, with response to external stimuli.

constricted affect: Reduction in intensity of feeling tone that is less severe than that of blunted affect.

constructional apraxia: Inability to copy a drawing, such as a cube, clock, or pentagon, as a result of a brain lesion.

conversion phenomena: The development of symbolic physical symptoms and distortions involving the voluntary muscles or special sense organs; not under voluntary control and not explained by any physical disorder. Most common in conversion disorder but also seen in a variety of mental disorders.

convulsion: An involuntary, violent muscular contraction or spasm. *See also* **clonic convulsion** and **tonic convulsion**.

coprolalia: Involuntary use of vulgar or obscene language. Observed in some cases of schizophrenia and in Tourette syndrome.

coprophagia: Eating of filth or feces.

cryptographia: A private written language.

cryptolalia: A private spoken language.

cycloplegia: Paralysis of the muscles of accommodation in the eye; observed, at times, as an autonomic adverse effect (anticholinergic effect) of antipsychotic or antidepressant medication.

decompensation: Deterioration of psychic functioning caused by a breakdown of defense mechanisms. Seen in psychotic states.

déjà entendu: Illusion that what one is hearing one has been heard previously. *See also* **paramnesia**.

déjà pensé: Condition in which a thought never entertained before is incorrectly regarded as a repetition of a previous thought. *See also* **paramnesia**.

déjà vu: Illusion of visual recognition in which a new situation is incorrectly regarded as a repetition of a previous experience. *See also* **paramnesia**.

delirium: Acute reversible mental disorder characterized by confusion and some impairment of consciousness; generally associated with emotional lability, hallucinations or illusions, and inappropriate, impulsive, irrational, or violent behavior.

delirium tremens: Acute and sometimes fatal reaction to withdrawal from alcohol, usually occurring 72 to 96 hours after the cessation of heavy drinking; distinctive characteristics are marked autonomic hyperactivity (tachycardia, fever, hyperhidrosis, and dilated pupils), usually accompanied by tremulousness, hallucinations, illusions, and delusions. Called *alcohol withdrawal with perceptual disturbance in DSM-5*. *See also* **formication**.

delusion: False belief, based on incorrect inference about external reality, that is firmly held despite objective and obvious contradictory proof or evidence and despite the fact that other members of the culture do not share the belief.

delusion of control: False belief that a person's will, thoughts, or feelings are being controlled by external forces.

delusion of grandeur: Exaggerated conception of one's importance, power, or identity.

delusion of infidelity: False belief that one's lover is unfaithful. Sometimes called *pathologic jealousy.*

delusion of persecution: False belief of being harassed or persecuted; often found in litigious patients who have a pathologic tendency to take legal action because of imagined mistreatment. Most common delusion.

delusion of poverty: False belief that one is bereft or will be deprived of all material possessions.

delusion of reference: False belief that the behavior of others refers to oneself or that events, objects, or other people have a particular and unusual significance, usually of a negative nature; derived from idea of reference, in which persons falsely feel that others are talking about them (e.g., belief that people on television or radio are talking to or about the person). *See also* **thought broadcasting**.

delusion of self-accusation: False feeling of remorse and guilt. Seen in depression with psychotic features.

dementia: Mental disorder characterized by general impairment in intellectual functioning without clouding of consciousness; characterized by failing memory, difficulty with calculations, distractibility, alterations in mood and affect, impaired judgment and abstraction, reduced facility with language, and disturbance of orientation. Although irreversible because of underlying progressive degenerative brain disease, dementia may be reversible if the cause can be treated. Also known as major neurocognitive disorder in **DSM-5**.

denial: Defense mechanism in which the existence of unpleasant realities is disavowed; refers to keeping out of conscious awareness any aspects of external reality that, if acknowledged, would produce anxiety.

depersonalization: Sensation of unreality concerning oneself. Experiencing one's own behavior, thoughts, or feelings as if they were outside oneself, or as in a dream.

depression: Mental state characterized by feelings of sadness, loneliness, despair, low self-esteem, and self-reproach; accompanying signs include psychomotor retardation or, at times, agitation, withdrawal from interpersonal contact, and vegetative symptoms, such as insomnia and anorexia. The term refers to a mood that is so characterized or a mood disorder.

derailment: Gradual or sudden deviation in train of thought without blocking; sometimes used synonymously with *loosening of association.*

derealization: Sensation of changed reality or feeling detached from one's surroundings.

dereism: Mental activity that follows a totally subjective and idiosyncratic system of logic and fails to take the facts of reality or experience into consideration. Characteristic of schizophrenia. *See also* **autistic thinking**.

detachment: Characterized by distant interpersonal relationships and lack of emotional involvement.

devaluation: Defense mechanism in which a person attributes excessively negative qualities to self or others. Seen in depression and paranoid personality disorder.

diminished libido: Decreased sexual interest and drive. (Increased libido is often associated with mania.)

dipsomania: Compulsion to drink alcoholic beverages.

disinhibition: (1) Removal of an inhibitory effect, as in the reduction of the inhibitory function of the cerebral cortex by alcohol. (2) In psychiatry, a greater freedom to act in accordance with inner drives or feelings and with less regard for restraints dictated by cultural norms or one's superego.

disorientation: Confusion; impairment of awareness of time, place, and person (the position of the self in relation to other persons). Characteristic of cognitive disorders.

displacement: Unconscious defense mechanism by which the emotional component of an unacceptable idea or object is transferred to a more acceptable one. Seen in phobias.

dissociation: Unconscious defense mechanism involving the segregation of any group of mental or behavioral processes from the rest of the person's psychic activity; may entail the separation of an idea from its accompanying emotional tone, as seen in dissociative and conversion disorders.

distractibility: Inability to focus one's attention; the patient does not respond to the task at hand but attends to irrelevant phenomena in the environment.

dread: Massive or pervasive anxiety, usually related to a specific danger.

dreamy state: Altered state of consciousness, the semiconscious state associated with an epileptic attack, particularly from medial temporal epilepsy.

drowsiness: State of impaired awareness associated with a desire or inclination to sleep.

dysarthria: Difficulty in articulation, the motor activity of shaping phonated sounds into speech, not in word finding or in grammar.

dyscalculia: Difficulty in performing calculations.

dysgeusia: Impaired sense of taste.

dysgraphia: Difficulty in writing.

dyskinesia: Uncontrolled, involuntary muscle movement. Seen in extrapyramidal disorders.

dyslalia: Faulty articulation caused by structural abnormalities of the articulatory organs or impaired hearing.

dyslexia: Specific learning disability syndrome involving an impairment of the ability to read; unrelated to the person's intelligence. *Compare with* **alexia**.

dysmegalopsia: A distortion in which the size and shape of objects is misperceived, sometimes called the "Alice in Wonderland" effect. *See also* **illusion**.

dysmetria: Impaired ability to gauge distance relative to movements. Seen in neurologic deficit.

dysmnesia: Impaired memory.

dyspareunia: Physical pain in sexual intercourse, which may be emotionally caused and more commonly experienced by women; may also result from cystitis, urethritis, or other medical conditions.

dysphagia: Difficulty in swallowing.

dysphasia: Difficulty in comprehending oral language (*reception dysphasia*) or in trying to express verbal language (*expressive dysphasia*).

dysphonia: Difficulty in speaking or singing.

dysphoria: Feeling of unpleasantness or discomfort; a mood of general dissatisfaction and restlessness. Occurs in depression and anxiety.

dysprosody: Loss of normal speech melody (*prosody*). Common in depression.

dystonia: Extrapyramidal motor disturbance consisting of slow, sustained contractions of the axial or appendicular musculature; one movement often predominates, leading to relatively sustained postural deviations; acute dystonic reactions (facial grimacing and torticollis) are occasionally seen with the initiation of antipsychotic drug therapy.

echolalia: Psychopathological repeating of words or phrases of one person by another; tends to be repetitive and persistent. Seen in certain kinds of schizophrenia, particularly the catatonic types.

echopraxia: Similar to echolalia, however this represents the repeating or mimicking of the movements of another person.

ego-alien: Denoting aspects of a person's personality that are viewed as repugnant, unacceptable, or inconsistent with the rest of the personality. Also called *ego-dystonia. Compare with* **ego-syntonic.**

egocentric: Self-centered; selfishly preoccupied with one's own needs; lacking interest in others.

ego-dystonic: *See* **ego-alien.**

egomania: Morbid self-preoccupation or self-centeredness. *See also* **narcissism.**

ego-syntonic: Denoting aspects of a personality that are viewed as acceptable and consistent with that person's total personality. Personality traits are usually ego-syntonic. *Compare with* **ego-alien.**

eidetic image: Unusually vivid or exact mental image of objects previously seen or imagined.

elation: Mood consisting of feelings of joy, euphoria, triumph, and intense self-satisfaction or optimism. Occurs in mania when not grounded in reality.

elevated mood: Air of confidence and enjoyment; a mood more cheerful than normal but not necessarily pathologic.

emotion: Complex feeling state with psychic, somatic, and behavioral components; external manifestation of emotion is *affect.*

emotional insight: A level of understanding or awareness that one has emotional problems. It facilitates positive changes in personality and behavior when present.

emotional lability: Excessive emotional responsiveness characterized by unstable and rapidly changing emotions.

encopresis: Involuntary passage of feces, usually occurring at night or during sleep.

enuresis: Incontinence of urine, often during sleep.

erotomania: Delusional belief, more common in women than in men, that someone is deeply in love with them (also known as *de Clérambault syndrome*).

erythrophobia: Abnormal fear of blushing.

euphoria: Exaggerated feeling of well-being that is inappropriate to real events. Can occur with drugs such as opiates, amphetamines, and alcohol.

euthymia: Normal range of mood, implying absence of depressed or elevated mood.

evasion: Act of not facing up to, or strategically eluding, something; consists of suppressing an idea that is next in a thought series and replacing it with another idea closely related to it. Also called *paralogia* and *perverted logic.*

exaltation: Feeling of intense elation and grandeur.

excited: Agitated, purposeless motor activity uninfluenced by external stimuli.

expansive mood: Expression of feelings without restraint, frequently with an overestimation of their significance or importance. Seen in mania and grandiose delusional disorder.

expressive aphasia: Disturbance of speech in which understanding remains, but ability to speak is grossly impaired; halting, laborious, and inaccurate speech (also known as *Broca's, nonfluent,* and *motor aphasias*).

expressive dysphasia: Difficulty in expressing verbal language; the ability to understand language is intact.

externalization: More general term than *projection* that refers to the tendency to perceive in the external world and in external objects elements of one's own personality, including instinctual impulses, conflicts, moods, attitudes, and styles of thinking.

extroversion: State of one's energies being directed outside oneself. *Compare with* **introversion.**

false memory: A person's recollection and belief of an event that did not actually occur. In *false memory syndrome,* persons erroneously believe that they sustained an emotional or physical (e.g., sexual) trauma in early life.

fantasy: Daydream; fabricated mental picture of a situation or chain of events. A normal form of thinking dominated by unconscious material that seeks wish fulfillment and solutions to conflicts; may serve as the matrix for creativity. The content of the fantasy may indicate mental illness.

fatigue: A feeling of weariness, sleepiness, or irritability after a period of mental or bodily activity. Seen in depression, anxiety, neurasthenia, and somatoform disorders.

fausse reconnaissance: False recognition, a feature of paramnesia. Can occur in delusional disorders.

fear: Unpleasurable emotional state consisting of psychophysiological changes in response to a realistic threat or danger. *Compare with* **anxiety.**

flat affect: Absence or near absence of any signs of affective expression.

flight of ideas: Rapid succession of fragmentary thoughts or speech in which content changes abruptly and speech may be incoherent. Seen in mania.

floccillation: Aimless plucking or picking, usually at bedclothes or clothing, commonly seen in dementia and delirium.

fluent aphasia: Aphasia characterized by inability to understand the spoken word; fluent but incoherent speech is present. Also called *Wernicke's, sensory* and *receptive aphasias.*

folie à deux: Mental illness shared by two persons, usually involving a common delusional system; if it involves three persons, it is referred to as *folie à trois,* etc. Also called *shared psychotic disorder.*

formal thought disorder: Disturbance in the form of thought rather than the content of thought; thinking characterized by loosened associations, neologisms, and illogic constructs; thought process is disordered, and the person is defined as psychotic. Characteristic of schizophrenia.

formication: Tactile hallucination involving the sensation that tiny insects are crawling over the skin. Seen in cocaine addiction and delirium tremens.

free-floating anxiety: Severe, pervasive, generalized anxiety that is not attached to any particular idea, object, or event. Observed particularly in anxiety disorders, although it may be seen in some cases of schizophrenia.

fugue: Dissociative disorder characterized by a period of almost complete amnesia, during which a person actually flees from an immediate life situation and begins a different life pattern; apart from the amnesia, mental faculties and skills are usually unimpaired.

galactorrhea: Abnormal discharge of milk from the breast; may result from the endocrine influence (e.g., prolactin) of dopamine receptor antagonists, such as phenothiazines.

generalized tonic–clonic seizure: Generalized onset of tonic–clonic movements of the limbs, tongue biting, and incontinence followed by slow, gradual recovery of consciousness and cognition; also called *grand mal seizure.*

global aphasia: Combination of grossly nonfluent aphasia and severe fluent aphasia.

glossolalia: Unintelligible jargon that has meaning to the speaker but not to the listener. Occurs in schizophrenia.

grandiosity: Exaggerated feelings of one's importance, power, knowledge, or identity. Occurs in delusional disorder and manic states.

grief: Alteration in mood and affect consisting of sadness appropriate to a real loss; normally, it is self-limited. *See also* **depression** and **mourning**.

guilt: Emotional state associated with self-reproach and the need for punishment. In psychoanalysis, refers to a feeling of culpability that stems from a conflict between the ego and the superego (conscience). Guilt has normal psychological and social functions, but special intensity or absence of guilt characterizes many mental disorders, such as depression and antisocial personality disorder, respectively. Psychiatrists distinguish shame as a less internalized form of guilt that relates more to others than to the self. *See also* **shame**.

gustatory hallucination: Hallucination primarily involving taste.

gynecomastia: Female-like development of the male breasts; may occur as an adverse effect of antipsychotic and antidepressant drugs because of increased prolactin levels or anabolic–androgenic steroid abuse.

hallucination: False sensory perception occurring in the absence of any relevant external stimulation of the sensory modality involved. For types of hallucinations, see the specific term.

hallucinosis: State in which a person experiences hallucinations without any impairment of consciousness.

haptic hallucination: Hallucination of touch.

hebephrenia: Complex of symptoms, considered a form of schizophrenia, characterized by wild or silly behavior or mannerisms, inappropriate affect, and delusions and hallucinations that are transient and unsystematized. Hebephrenic schizophrenia is now called *disorganized schizophrenia*.

holophrastic: Using a single word to express a combination of ideas. Seen in schizophrenia.

hyperactivity: Increased muscular activity. The term is commonly used to describe a disturbance found in children that is manifested by constant restlessness, overactivity, distractibility, and difficulties in learning. Seen in *attention-deficit/hyperactivity disorder* (ADHD).

hyperacusis: Extreme sensitivity to sounds.

hyperalgesia: Excessive sensitivity to pain. Seen in somatoform disorder.

hyperesthesia: Increased sensitivity to any sense. It can affect one or more senses.

hypermnesia: Exaggerated degree of retention and recall. It can be elicited by hypnosis and may be seen in certain prodigies; also may be a feature of OCD, some cases of schizophrenia, and manic episodes of bipolar I disorder.

hyperphagia: Increase in appetite and intake of food.

hyperpragia: Excessive thinking and mental activity. Generally associated with manic episodes of bipolar I disorder.

hypersomnia: Excessive time spent asleep. May be associated with underlying medical or psychiatric disorder or narcolepsy, may be part of the Kleine–Levin syndrome, or may be primary.

hyperventilation: Excessive breathing, generally associated with anxiety, which can reduce blood carbon dioxide concentration and can produce lightheadedness, palpitations, numbness, tingling periorally and in the extremities, and, occasionally, syncope.

hypervigilance: Excessive attention to and focus on all internal and external stimuli; usually seen in delusional or paranoid states.

hypesthesia: Diminished sensitivity to tactile stimulation.

hypnagogic hallucination: Hallucination occurring while falling asleep, not ordinarily considered pathologic.

hypnopompic hallucination: Hallucination occurring while awakening from sleep, not ordinarily considered pathologic.

hypnosis: Artificially induced alteration of consciousness characterized by increased suggestibility and receptivity to direction.

hypoactivity: Decreased motor and cognitive activity, as in psychomotor retardation; visible slowing of thought, speech, and movements. Also called *hypokinesis*.

hypochondria: Exaggerated concern about health that is based not on real medical pathology but on unrealistic interpretations of physical signs or sensations as abnormal.

hypomania: Mood abnormality with the qualitative characteristics of mania but somewhat less intense. Seen in cyclothymic disorder.

idea of reference: Misinterpretation of incidents and events in the outside world as having direct personal reference to oneself; occasionally observed in normal persons, but frequently seen in paranoid patients. If present with sufficient frequency or intensity or if organized and systematized, they constitute delusions of reference.

illogic thinking: Thinking containing erroneous conclusions or internal contradictions; psychopathological only when it is marked and not caused by cultural values or intellectual deficit.

illusion: Perceptual misinterpretation of a real external stimulus. *Compare with* **hallucination**.

immediate memory: Reproduction, recognition, or recall of perceived material within seconds after presentation. *Compare with* **long-term memory** and **short-term memory**.

impaired insight: Diminished ability to understand the objective reality of a situation.

impaired judgment: Diminished ability to understand a situation correctly and to act appropriately.

impulse control: Ability to resist an impulse, drive, or temptation to perform some action.

inappropriate affect: Emotional tone out of harmony with the idea, thought, or speech accompanying it. Seen in schizophrenia.

incoherence: Communication that is disconnected, disorganized, or incomprehensible. *See also* **word salad**.

incorporation: Primitive unconscious defense mechanism in which the psychic representation of another person or aspects of another person are assimilated into oneself through a figurative process of symbolic oral ingestion; represents a special form of introjection and is the earliest mechanism of identification.

increased libido: Increase in sexual interest and drive.

ineffability: Ecstatic state in which persons insist that their experience is inexpressible and indescribable and that it is impossible to convey what it is like to one who never experienced it.

initial insomnia: Falling asleep with difficulty; usually seen in anxiety disorder. *Compare with* **middle insomnia** and **terminal insomnia**.

insight: Conscious recognition of one's own condition. In psychiatry, it refers to the conscious awareness and understanding of one's own psychodynamics and symptoms of maladaptive behavior; highly important in effecting changes in the personality and behavior of a person.

insomnia: Difficulty in falling asleep or difficulty in staying asleep. It can be related to a mental disorder, can be related to a physical disorder or an adverse effect of medication, or can be primary (not related to a known medical factor or another mental disorder). *See also* **initial insomnia**, **middle insomnia**, and **terminal insomnia**.

intellectual disability: Limitations in intellectual functioning and adaptive behavior, beginning before age 18 years. Below average intelligence.

intellectual insight: Knowledge of the reality of a situation without the ability to use that knowledge successfully to effect an adaptive change in behavior or to master the situation. *Compare with* **true insight**.

intelligence: Capacity for learning and ability to recall, to integrate constructively, and to apply what one has learned; the capacity to understand and to think rationally.

intoxication: Mental disorder caused by recent ingestion or presence in the body of an exogenous substance producing maladaptive behavior by virtue of its effects on the central nervous system (CNS). The most common psychiatric changes involve disturbances of perception, wakefulness, attention, thinking, judgment, emotional control, and psychomotor behavior; the specific clinical picture depends on the substance ingested.

intropunitive: Turning anger inward toward oneself. Commonly observed in depressed patients.

introspection: Contemplating one's own mental processes to achieve insight.

introversion: State in which a person's energies are directed inward toward the self, with little or no interest in the external world.

irrelevant answer: Answer that is not responsive to the question.

irritability: Abnormal or excessive excitability, with easily triggered anger, annoyance, or impatience.

irritable mood: State in which one is easily annoyed and provoked to anger. *See also* **irritability**.

jamais vu: Paramnestic phenomenon characterized by a false feeling of unfamiliarity with a real situation that one has previously experienced.

jargon aphasia: Aphasia in which the words produced are neologistic; that is, nonsense words created by the patient.

judgment: Mental act of comparing or evaluating choices within the framework of a given set of values for the purpose of electing a course of action. If the course of action chosen is consonant with reality or with mature adult standards of behavior, then judgment is said to be *intact* or *normal*; judgment is said to be *impaired* if the chosen course of action is frankly maladaptive, results from impulsive decisions based on the need for immediate gratification, or is otherwise not consistent with reality as measured by mature adult standards.

kleptomania: Pathologic compulsion to steal.

la belle indifférence: Inappropriate attitude of calm or lack of concern about one's disability. May be seen in patients with conversion disorder.

labile affect: Affective expression characterized by rapid and abrupt changes, unrelated to external stimuli.

labile mood: Oscillations in mood between euphoria and depression or anxiety.

laconic speech: Condition characterized by a reduction in the quantity of spontaneous speech; replies to questions are brief and unelaborated, and little or no unprompted additional information is provided. Occurs in major depression, schizophrenia, and organic mental disorders. Also called *poverty of speech*.

lethologica: Momentary forgetting of a name or proper noun. *See* **blocking**.

lilliputian hallucination: Visual sensation that persons or objects are reduced in size; more properly regarded as an illusion. *See also* **micropsia**.

localized amnesia: Partial loss of memory; amnesia restricted to specific or isolated experiences. Also called *lacunar amnesia* and *patch amnesia*.

logoclonia: Repeated use of the same word. See perseveration.

logorrhea: Copious, pressured, coherent speech; uncontrollable, excessive talking; observed in manic episodes of bipolar disorder. Also called *tachylogia*, *verbomania*, and *volubility*.

long-term memory: Reproduction, recognition, or recall of experiences or information that was experienced in the distant past. Also called *remote memory*. *Compare with* **immediate memory** and **short-term memory**.

loosening of associations: Characteristic schizophrenic thinking or speech disturbance involving a disorder in the logical progression of thoughts, manifested as a failure to communicate verbally adequately; unrelated and unconnected ideas shift from one subject to another. *See also* **tangentiality**.

macropsia: False perception that objects are larger than they really are. *Compare with* **micropsia**.

magical thinking: A form of dereistic thought; thinking similar to that of the preoperational phase in children (Jean Piaget), in which thoughts, words, or actions assume power (e.g., to cause or to prevent events).

malingering: Feigning disease to achieve a specific goal, for example, to avoid an unpleasant responsibility.

mania: Mood state characterized by elation, agitation, hyperactivity, hypersexuality, and accelerated thinking and speaking (flight of ideas). Seen in bipolar I disorder. *See also* **hypomania**.

manipulation: Maneuvering by patients to get their own way, characteristic of antisocial personalities.

mannerism: Ingrained, habitual involuntary movement.

melancholia: Severe depressive state. Used in the term *involutional melancholia* as a descriptive term and also in reference to a distinct diagnostic entity.

memory: Process whereby what is experienced or learned is established as a record in the CNS (registration), where it persists with a variable degree of permanence (retention) and can be recollected or retrieved from storage at will (recall). For types of memory, see **immediate memory**, **long-term memory**, and **short-term memory**.

mental disorder: Psychiatric illness or disease whose manifestations are characterized primarily by behavioral or psychological impairment of function, measured in terms of deviation from some normative concept; associated with distress or disease, not just an expected response to a particular event or limited to relations between a person and society.

mental retardation: Obsolete term, please see **intellectual disability**.

metonymy: Speech disturbance common in schizophrenia in which the affected person uses a word or phrase that is related to the proper one but is not the one ordinarily used; for example, the patient speaks of consuming a *menu* rather than a *meal* or refers to losing the *piece of string* of the conversation rather than the *thread* of the conversation. *See also* **paraphasia** and **word approximation**.

microcephaly: Condition in which the head is unusually small as a result of defective brain development and premature ossification of the skull.

micropsia: False perception that objects are smaller than they really are. Sometimes called *lilliputian hallucination*. *Compare with* **macropsia**.

middle insomnia: Waking up after falling asleep without difficulty and then having difficulty in falling asleep again. *Compare with* **initial insomnia** and **terminal insomnia**.

mimicry: Simple, imitative motion activity of childhood.

monomania: Mental state characterized by preoccupation with one subject.

mood: Pervasive and sustained feeling tone that is experienced internally and that, in the extreme, can markedly influence virtually all aspects of a person's behavior and perception of the world. Distinguished from affect, the external expression of the internal feeling tone. For types of mood, see the specific term.

mood-congruent delusion: Delusion with content that is mood appropriate (e.g., depressed patients who believe that they are responsible for the destruction of the world).

mood-congruent hallucination: Hallucination with content that is consistent with a depressed or manic mood (e.g., depressed patients hearing voices telling them that they are bad persons and manic patients hearing voices telling them that they have inflated worth, power, or knowledge).

mood-incongruent delusion: Delusion based on incorrect reference about external reality, with content that has no association to mood or is mood inappropriate (e.g., depressed patients who believe that they are the new Messiah).

mood-incongruent hallucination: Hallucination not associated with real external stimuli, with content that is not consistent with depressed or manic mood (e.g., in depression, hallucinations not involving such themes as guilt, deserved punishment, or inadequacy; in mania, not involving such themes as inflated worth or power).

mood swings: Oscillation of a person's emotional feeling tone between periods of elation and periods of depression.

motor aphasia: Aphasia in which understanding is intact, but the ability to speak is lost. Also called *Broca's, expressive,* or *nonfluent aphasias.*

mourning: Syndrome following loss of a loved one, consisting of preoccupation with the lost individual, weeping, sadness, and repeated reliving of memories. *See also* **bereavement** and **grief**.

muscle rigidity: State in which the muscles remain immovable; seen in schizophrenia.

mutism: Organic or functional absence of the faculty of speech. *See also* **stupor**.

mydriasis: Dilation of the pupil; sometimes occurs as an autonomic (anticholinergic) or atropine-like adverse effect of some antipsychotic and antidepressant drugs.

narcissism: In psychoanalytic theory, divided into primary and secondary types: primary narcissism, the early infantile phase of object relationship development, when the child has not differentiated the self from the outside world, and all sources of pleasure are unrealistically recognized as coming from within the self, giving the child a false sense of omnipotence; secondary narcissism, when the libido, once attached to external love objects, is redirected back to the self. *See also* **autistic thinking**.

needle phobia: The persistent, intense, pathologic fear of receiving an injection.

negative signs: In schizophrenia: flat affect, alogia, abulia, and apathy.

negativism: Verbal or nonverbal opposition or resistance to outside suggestions and advice; commonly seen in catatonic schizophrenia in which the patient resists any effort to be moved or does the opposite of what is asked.

neologism: New word or phrase whose derivation cannot be understood; often seen in schizophrenia. It has also been used to mean a word that has been incorrectly constructed but whose origins are nonetheless understandable (e.g., *head shoe* to mean *hat*),

but such constructions are more properly referred to as *word approximations.*

neurologic amnesia: (1) Auditory amnesia: loss of ability to comprehend sounds or speech. (2) Tactile amnesia: loss of ability to judge the shape of objects by touch. *See also* **astereognosis**. (3) Verbal amnesia: loss of ability to remember words. (4) Visual amnesia: loss of ability to recall or to recognize familiar objects or printed words.

nihilism: Delusion of the nonexistence of the self or part of the self; also refers to an attitude of total rejection of established values or extreme skepticism regarding moral and value judgments.

nihilistic delusion: Depressive delusion that the world and everything related to it have ceased to exist.

noesis: The functioning of the intellectual or cognitive processes.

nominal aphasia: Aphasia characterized by difficulty in giving the correct name of an object. *See also* **anomia** and **amnesic aphasia**.

nymphomania: Abnormal, excessive, insatiable desire in a woman for sexual intercourse. *Compare with* **satyriasis**.

obsession: Persistent and recurrent idea, thought, or impulse that cannot be eliminated from consciousness by logic or reasoning; obsessions are involuntary and ego-dystonic. *See also* **compulsion**.

olfactory hallucination: Hallucination primarily involving smell or odors; most common in medical disorders, especially in the temporal lobe.

orientation: State of awareness of oneself and one's surroundings in terms of time, place, and person.

overactivity: Abnormality in motor behavior that can manifest itself as psychomotor agitation, hyperactivity (hyperkinesis), tics, sleepwalking, or compulsions.

overvalued idea: False or unreasonable belief or idea that is sustained beyond the bounds of reason. It is held with less intensity or duration than a delusion but is usually associated with mental illness.

panic: Acute, intense attack of anxiety associated with personality disorganization; the anxiety is overwhelming and accompanied by feelings of impending doom.

panphobia: Overwhelming fear of everything.

pantomime: Gesticulation; psychodrama without the use of words.

paramnesia: Disturbance of memory in which reality and fantasy are confused. It is observed in dreams and in certain types of schizophrenia and organic mental disorders; it includes phenomena such as *déjà vu* and *déjà entendu*, which may occur occasionally in normal persons.

paranoia: Unreasonable false beliefs, characterized by delusions of persecution, unwarranted jealousy, or exaggerated self-importance, typically elaborated into an organized system.

paranoid delusions: Includes persecutory delusions and delusions of reference, control, and grandeur.

paranoid ideation: Thinking dominated by suspicious, persecutory, or grandiose content of less than delusional proportions.

paraphasia: Abnormal speech in which one word is substituted for another, the irrelevant word generally resembling the required one in morphology, meaning, or phonetic composition; the inappropriate word may be a legitimate one used incorrectly, such as *clover* instead of *hand*, or a bizarre nonsense expression, such as *treen* instead of *train*. Paraphasic speech may be seen in organic aphasias and in mental disorders such as schizophrenia. *See also* **metonymy** and **word approximation**.

parapraxis: Faulty act, such as a slip of the tongue or the misplacement of an article. Freud ascribed parapraxes to unconscious motives.

paresis: Weakness or partial paralysis of organic origin.

paresthesia: Abnormal spontaneous tactile sensation, such as a burning, tingling, or pins-and-needles sensation.

perception: Conscious awareness of elements in the environment by the mental processing of sensory stimuli; sometimes used in a broader sense to refer to the mental process by which all kinds of data, intellectual, emotional, and sensory, are meaningfully organized. *See also* **apperception**.

perseveration: (1) Pathologic repetition of the same response to different stimuli, as in a repetition of the same verbal response to different questions. (2) Persistent repetition of specific words or concepts in the process of speaking. Seen in cognitive disorders, schizophrenia, and other mental illness. *See also* **verbigeration**.

phantom limb: False sensation that an extremity that has been lost is, in fact, present.

phobia: Persistent, pathologic, unrealistic, intense fear of an object or situation; the phobic person may realize that the fear is irrational but, nonetheless, cannot dispel it. For types of phobias, see the specific term.

pica: Craving and eating of nonfood substances, such as paint and clay.

polyphagia: Pathologic overeating.

positive signs: In schizophrenia: hallucinations, delusions, and thought disorder.

posturing: Strange, fixed, and bizarre bodily positions held by a patient for an extended time. *See also* **catatonic posturing**.

poverty of content of speech: Speech that is adequate in amount but conveys little information because of vagueness, emptiness, or stereotyped phrases.

poverty of speech: Restriction in the amount of speech used; replies may be monosyllabic. *See also* **laconic speech**.

preoccupation of thought: Centering of thought content on a particular idea, associated with a strong affective tone, such as a paranoid trend or a suicidal or homicidal preoccupation.

pressured speech: Increase in the amount of spontaneous speech; rapid, loud, accelerated speech, as occurs in mania, schizophrenia, and cognitive disorders.

primary process thinking: In psychoanalysis, the mental activity related directly to the functions of the id and characteristic of unconscious mental processes; marked by primitive, prelogical thinking and by the tendency to seek immediate discharge and gratification of instinctual demands. Includes thinking that is dereistic, illogic, magical; normally found in dreams, abnormally in psychosis. *Compare with* **secondary process thinking**.

projection: Unconscious defense mechanism in which persons attribute to another those generally unconscious ideas, thoughts, feelings, and impulses that are in themselves undesirable or unacceptable as a form of protection from anxiety arising from an inner conflict; by externalizing whatever is unacceptable, they deal with it as a situation apart from themselves.

prosopagnosia: Inability to recognize familiar faces that is not due to impaired visual acuity or level of consciousness.

pseudocyesis: Rare condition in which a nonpregnant patient has the signs and symptoms of pregnancy, such as abdominal distention, breast enlargement, pigmentation, cessation of menses, and morning sickness.

pseudodementia: (1) Dementia-like disorder that can be reversed by appropriate treatment and is not caused by organic brain disease. (2) Condition in which patients show exaggerated indifference to their surroundings in the absence of a mental disorder; also occurs in depression and factitious disorders.

pseudologia fantastica: Disorder characterized by uncontrollable lying in which patients elaborate extensive fantasies that they freely communicate and act on.

psychomotor agitation: Physical and mental overactivity that is usually nonproductive and is associated with a feeling of inner turmoil, as seen in agitated depression.

psychosis: Mental disorder in which the thoughts, affective response, ability to recognize reality, and ability to communicate and relate to others are sufficiently impaired to interfere grossly with the capacity to deal with reality; the classical characteristics of psychosis are impaired reality testing, hallucinations, delusions, and illusions.

psychotic: (1) Person experiencing psychosis. (2) Denoting or characteristic of psychosis.

rationalization: An unconscious defense mechanism in which irrational or unacceptable behavior, motives, or feelings are logically justified or made consciously tolerable by plausible means.

reaction formation: Unconscious defense mechanism in which a person develops a socialized attitude or interest that is the direct antithesis of some infantile wish or impulse that is harbored consciously or unconsciously. One of the earliest and most unstable defense mechanisms, closely related to repression; both are defenses against impulses or urges that are unacceptable to the ego.

reality testing: Fundamental ego function that consists of tentative actions that test and objectively evaluate the nature and limits of the environment; includes the ability to differentiate between the external world and the internal world and to accurately judge the relation between the self and the environment.

recall: Process of bringing stored memories into consciousness. *See also* **memory**.

recent memory: Recall of events over the past few days.

recent past memory: Recall of events over the past few months.

receptive aphasia: Organic loss of ability to comprehend the meaning of words; fluid and spontaneous, but incoherent and nonsensical, speech. *See also* **fluent aphasia** and **sensory aphasia**.

receptive dysphasia: Difficulty in comprehending oral language; the impairment involves comprehension and production of language.

regression: Unconscious defense mechanism in which a person undergoes a partial or total return to earlier patterns of adaptation; observed in many psychiatric conditions, particularly schizophrenia.

remote memory: Recall of events in the distant past.

repression: Freud's term for an unconscious defense mechanism in which unacceptable mental contents are banished or kept out of consciousness; important in normal psychological development and in neurotic and psychotic symptom formation. Freud recognized two kinds of repression: (1) repression proper, in which the repressed material was once in the conscious domain, and (2) primal repression, in which the repressed material was never in the conscious realm. *Compare with* **suppression**.

restricted affect: Reduction in intensity of feeling tone that is less severe than in blunted affect but clearly reduced. *See also* **constricted affect**.

retrograde amnesia: Loss of memory for events preceding the onset of the amnesia. *Compare with* **anterograde amnesia**.

retrospective falsification: Memory becomes unintentionally (unconsciously) distorted by being filtered through a person's present emotional, cognitive, and experiential state.

rigidity: In psychiatry, a person's resistance to change, a personality trait.

ritual: (1) Formalized activity practiced by a person to reduce anxiety, as in OCD. (2) Ceremonial activity of cultural origin.

rumination: Constant preoccupation with thinking about a single idea or theme, as in OCD.

satyriasis: Morbid, insatiable sexual need or desire in a man. *Compare with* **nymphomania**.

scotoma: (1) In psychiatry, a figurative blind spot in a person's psychological awareness. (2) In neurology, a localized visual field defect.

secondary process thinking: In psychoanalysis, the form of thinking that is logical, organized, reality oriented, and influenced by the demands of the environment; characterizes the mental activity of the ego. *Compare with* **primary process thinking**.

seizure: An attack or sudden onset of certain symptoms, such as convulsions, loss of consciousness, and psychic or sensory disturbances; seen in epilepsy and can be substance induced. For types of seizures, see the specific term.

sensorium: Perceptual awareness or the sensory apparatus considered as a whole. Sometimes used interchangeably with *consciousness.*

sensory aphasia: Organic loss of ability to comprehend the meaning of words; fluid and spontaneous, but incoherent and nonsensical, speech. *See also* **fluent aphasia** and **receptive aphasia**.

sensory extinction: Neurologic sign operationally defined as failure to report one of two simultaneously presented sensory stimuli, despite the fact that either stimulus alone is correctly reported. Also called *sensory inattention.*

shame: Failure to live up to self-expectations; often associated with fantasy of how person will be seen by others. *See also* **guilt**.

short-term memory: Reproduction, recognition, or recall of perceived material within minutes after the initial presentation. *Compare with* **immediate memory** *and* **long-term memory**.

simultanagnosia: Impairment in the perception or integration of visual stimuli appearing simultaneously.

somatic delusion: Delusion pertaining to the functioning of one's body.

somatic hallucination: Hallucination involving the perception of a physical experience localized within the body.

somnolence: Pathologic sleepiness or drowsiness from which one can be aroused to a normal state of consciousness.

spatial agnosia: Inability to recognize spatial relations.

speaking in tongues: Expression of a revelatory message through unintelligible words; not considered a disorder of thought if associated with practices of specific Pentecostal religions. *See also* **glossolalia**.

stereotypy: Continuous mechanical repetition of speech or physical activities; observed in catatonic schizophrenia.

stupor: (1) State of decreased reactivity to stimuli and less than full awareness of one's surroundings; as a disturbance of consciousness, it indicates a condition of partial coma or semicoma. (2) In psychiatry, used synonymously with *mutism* and does not necessarily imply a disturbance of consciousness; in *catatonic stupor*, patients are ordinarily aware of their surroundings.

stuttering: Frequent repetition or prolongation of a sound or syllable, leading to markedly impaired speech fluency.

sublimation: Unconscious defense mechanism in which the energy associated with unacceptable impulses or drives is diverted into personally and socially acceptable channels; unlike other defense mechanisms, it offers some minimal gratification of the instinctual drive or impulse.

substitution: Unconscious defense mechanism in which a person replaces an unacceptable wish, drive, emotion, or goal with one that is more acceptable.

suggestibility: State of uncritical compliance with influence or of uncritical acceptance of an idea, belief, or attitude; commonly observed among persons with hysterical traits.

suicidal ideation: Thoughts or act of taking one's own life.

suppression: Conscious act of controlling and inhibiting an unacceptable impulse, emotion, or idea; differentiated from repression in that repression is an unconscious process.

symbolization: Unconscious defense mechanism in which one idea or object comes to stand for another because of some common aspect or quality in both; based on similarity and association; the symbols formed protect the person from the anxiety that may be attached to the original idea or object.

synesthesia: Condition in which the stimulation of one sensory modality is perceived as sensation in a different modality, as when a sound produces a sensation of color.

syntactical aphasia: Aphasia characterized by the fluent production of words, however the inability to form normal grammatical constructions.

systematized delusion: Group of elaborate delusions related to a single event or theme.

tactile hallucination: Hallucination primarily involving the sense of touch. Also called *haptic hallucination.*

tangentiality: Oblique, digressive, or even irrelevant manner of speech in which the central idea is not communicated.

tension: Physiologic or psychic arousal, uneasiness, or pressure toward action; an unpleasurable alteration in mental or physical state that seeks relief through action.

terminal insomnia: Early morning awakening or waking up at least 2 hours before planning to wake up. *Compare with* **initial insomnia** and **middle insomnia**.

thought broadcasting: Feeling that one's thoughts are being broadcast or projected into the environment. *See also* **thought withdrawal**.

thought disorder: Any disturbance of thinking that affects language, communication, or thought content; the hallmark feature of schizophrenia. Manifestations range from simple blocking and mild circumstantiality to profound loosening of associations, incoherence, and delusions; characterized by a failure to follow semantic and syntactic rules that is inconsistent with the person's education, intelligence, or cultural background.

thought insertion: Delusion that thoughts are being implanted in one's mind by other people or forces.

thought latency: The period of time between a thought and its verbal expression. Increased in schizophrenia (*see* **blocking**) and decreased in mania (*see* **pressured speech**).

thought withdrawal: Delusion that one's thoughts are being removed from one's mind by other people or forces. *See also* **thought broadcasting**.

tic disorders: Predominantly psychogenic disorders characterized by involuntary, spasmodic, stereotyped movement of small groups of muscles; seen most predominantly in moments of stress or anxiety, rarely as a result of organic disease.

tinnitus: Noises in one or both ears, such as ringing, buzzing, or clicking; an adverse effect of some psychotropic drugs.

tonic convulsion: Convulsion in which the muscle contraction is sustained.

trailing phenomenon: Perceptual abnormality associated with hallucinogenic drugs in which moving objects are seen as a series of discrete and discontinuous images.

trance: Sleeplike state of reduced consciousness and activity.

tremor: Rhythmical alteration in movement, which is usually faster than one beat a second; typically, tremors decrease during periods of relaxation and sleep and increase during periods of anger and increased tension.

true insight: Understanding of the objective reality of a situation coupled with the motivational and emotional impetus to master the situation or change behavior.

twilight state: Disturbed consciousness with hallucinations.

twirling: Sign present in autistic children who continually rotate in the direction in which their head is turned.

unconscious: (1) One of three divisions of Freud's topographic theory of the mind (the others being the conscious and the preconscious) in which the psychic material is not readily accessible to conscious awareness by ordinary means; its existence may be manifest in symptom formation, in dreams, or under the influence of drugs. (2) In popular (but more ambiguous) usage, any mental material not in the immediate field of awareness. (3) Denoting a state of unawareness, with lack of response to external stimuli, as in a coma.

undoing: Unconscious primitive defense mechanism, repetitive in nature, by which a person symbolically acts out in reverse something unacceptable that has already been done or against which the ego must defend itself; a form of magical expiatory action, commonly observed in OCD.

unio mystica: Feeling of mystic unity with an infinite power. Although this can be a religious phenomenon, it can also be a type of delusion.

vegetative signs: In depression, denoting characteristic symptoms such as sleep disturbance (especially early morning awakening), decreased appetite, constipation, weight loss, and loss of sexual response.

verbigeration: Meaningless and stereotyped repetition of words or phrases, as seen in schizophrenia. Also called *cataphasia.* *See also* **perseveration**.

vertigo: Sensation that one or the world around one is spinning or revolving; a hallmark of vestibular dysfunction, not to be confused with dizziness.

visual agnosia: Inability to recognize objects or persons.

visual amnesia: Inability to remember the appearance of objects or to recognize familiar words

visual hallucination: Hallucination primarily involving the sense of sight.

waxy flexibility: Condition in which a person maintains the body position into which they are placed with slight resistance to movement giving it a waxy feel. See also **cerea flexibilitas**.

word approximation: Use of conventional words in an unconventional or inappropriate way (metonymy or of new words that are developed by conventional rules of word formation) (e.g., *hand shoes* for *gloves* and *time measure* for *clock*); distinguished from a *neologism,* which is a new word whose derivation cannot be understood. *See also* **paraphasia**.

word salad: Incoherent, essentially incomprehensible, mixture of words and phrases commonly seen in far-advanced cases of schizophrenia. *See also* **incoherence**.

xenophobia: Abnormal fear of strangers.

zoophobia: Abnormal fear of animals.

Index

Page numbers followed by *f* indicate figures, page numbers followed by *t* indicated tables, and page numbers in **boldface** indicate main discussions.